Vascular Surgery

Vascular Surgery

A COMPREHENSIVE REVIEW

SIXTH EDITION

Wesley S. Moore, M.D.
Professor of Vascular Surgery
University of California Los Angeles
Division of General Surgery
University of California Los Angeles School of Medicine
Los Angeles, California

W.B. SAUNDERS COMPANY
Philadelphia London New York St. Louis Sydney Toronto

W.B. SAUNDERS COMPANY
A Harcourt Health Sciences Company

The Curtis Center
Independence Square West
Philadelphia, Pennsylvania 19106

Library of Congress Cataloging-in-Publication Data

Vascular surgery: a comprehensive review/Wesley S. Moore [editor].—6th ed.

p.   cm.

ISBN 0–7216–9313–X

1. Blood-vessels—Surgery.   I. Moore, Wesley S.

RD598.5 .V374   2002   617.4′13—dc21   2001020591

Manuscript Editor: Mary Reinwald
Production Manager: Mary B. Stermel
Illustration Specialist: Rita Martello
Book Designer: Marie Gardocky Clifton
Cover Designer: Catherine Bradish

VASCULAR SURGERY: A Comprehensive Review   ISBN 0–7216–9313–X

Printed in the United States of America.

Last digit is the print number: 9   8   7   6   5   4   3   2   1

This textbook of vascular surgery is dedicated to Leslie and Susan Gonda in grateful recognition of their foresight and generosity in funding the vascular centers at UCLA and the Mayo Clinic. Because of their philanthropic efforts, the quality of care will be improved for thousands of patients with vascular disorders, and educational opportunities will be expanded for many generations of healthcare professionals.

WESLEY S. MOORE, M.D.

Contributors

William M. Abbott, M.D.

Chief, Vascular Surgery, Massachusetts General Hospital, Boston, Massachusetts

Vascular Grafts: Characteristics and Rational Selection of Prostheses

Ahmed M. Abou-Zamzam, Jr., M.D.

Assistant Professor of Surgery, Division of Vascular Surgery, University of California-Loma Linda School of Medicine, Loma Linda, California

Nonatherosclerotic Vascular Disease

Samuel S. Ahn, M.D.

Professor of Surgery, Division of Vascular Surgery, University of California, Los Angeles, UCLA School of Medicine; Attending Surgeon and Director of Endovascular Surgery, UCLA Medical Center, Los Angeles, California

Endovascular Surgery

Niren Angle, M.D.

Assistant Professor of Surgery, Division of Vascular Surgery, University of California, Los Angeles, Los Angeles, California

Thrombolytic Therapy for Vascular Disease; Acute Arterial and Graft Occlusion; Prosthetic Graft Infections; Varicose Veins: Chronic Venous Insufficiency

J. Dennis Baker, M.D.

Professor of Surgery, Division of Vascular Surgery, University of California, Los Angeles, UCLA School of Medicine; Chief, Vascular Surgery Section, West Los Angeles Veterans Administration Medical Center, Los Angeles, California

The Vascular Laboratory

Jeffrey L. Ballard, M.D.

Professor of Surgery, Loma Linda University School of Medicine; Program Director, Vascular Surgery Residency, Loma Linda University Medical Center, Loma Linda, California

Anatomy and Surgical Exposure of the Vascular System

Wiley F. Barker, M.D.

Professor Emeritus, Surgery, University of California, Los Angeles, School of Medicine, Los Angeles, California

History of Vascular Disease

Michael Belkin, M.D.

Associate Professor of Surgery, Harvard Medical School; Staff, Brigham and Women's Hospital, Boston, Massachusetts

Evaluation of Cardiac Risk in Patients with Vascular Disease; Aortoiliac Occlusive Disease

Robert S. Bennion, M.D.

Associate Professor of Surgery, University of California, Los Angeles, UCLA School of Medicine, Los Angeles, California

Hemodialysis and Vascular Access

John J. Bergan, M.D.

Professor of Surgery, University of California, San Diego, San Diego; Staff Surgeon, Scripps Memorial Hospital, La Jolla, California

Varicose Veins: Chronic Venous Insufficiency

Ramon Berguer, M.D., Ph.D.

Professor of Surgery, Division of Vascular Surgery, Wayne State University School of Medicine; Chief, Section of Vascular Surgery, Harper Hospital, Detroit, Michigan

Reconstruction of the Supraaortic Trunks and Vertebrobasilar System

Frederic S. Bongard, M.D.

Professor of Surgery, University of California, Los Angeles, UCLA School of Medicine, Los Angeles; Chief, Division of Trauma and Critical Care, Harbor-UCLA Medical Center, Torrance, California

Vascular Trauma

Alexander W. Clowes, M.D.

Professor, Department of Surgery, University of Washington School of Medicine; Chief, Vascular Surgery, University of Washington Medical Center, Seattle, Washington

Anatomy, Physiology, and Pharmacology of the Vascular Wall

Richard H. Dean, M.D.

Professor of Surgery, Wake Forest University School of Medicine; Senior Vice President for Health Affairs, Wake Forest University, Winston-Salem, North Carolina

Renovascular Disease

Ralph G. DePalma, M.D.

Professor of Surgery, Uniformed Services University of the Health Sciences; National Director of Surgery, Department of Veterans Affairs, Acute Care Group, Washington, District of Columbia

Atherosclerosis: Pathology, Pathogenesis, and Medical Management; Vasculogenic Erectile Dysfunction

Magruder C. Donaldson, M.D.

Associate Professor of Surgery, Harvard Medical School; Staff, Brigham and Women's Hospital, Boston, Massachusetts
> Evaluation of Cardiac Risk in the Patient with Vascular Disease; Aortoiliac Occlusive Disease

Janette D. Durham, M.D.

Associate Professor of Radiology, University of Colorado, School of Medicine; Staff, University of Colorado Health Sciences Center, Denver, Colorado
> Congenital Vascular Malformations of the Extremities

James M. Edwards, M.D.

Associate Professor of Surgery, Division of Vascular Surgery, Oregon Health Sciences University, Portland, Oregon
> Nonatherosclerotic Vascular Disease

Michael M. Farooq, M.D.

Assistant Professor of Surgery, University of California, Los Angeles, UCLA School of Medicine; Vascular Surgeon, UCLA Medical Center, Los Angeles, California
> Myointimal Hyperplasia

D. Preston Flanigan, M.D.

Clinical Professor of Surgery, University of California, Irvine; Director, Vascular Laboratory and Wound Care Center, St. Joseph Hospital, Orange, California
> Aneurysms of the Peripheral Arteries

Julie Ann Freischlag, M.D.

Professor of Surgery, University of California, Los Angeles, UCLA School of Medicine; Director, University of California Gonda (Goldschmied) Vascular Center, Los Angeles, California
> Prosthetic Graft Infections

Hugh A. Gelabert, M.D.

Associate Professor of Surgery, Division of Vascular Surgery, University of California, Los Angeles, UCLA School of Medicine, Los Angeles, California
> Primary Arterial Infections and Antibiotic Prophylaxis; Portal Hypertension

Bruce L. Gewertz, M.D.

Dallas B. Phemister Professor and Chairman, Department of Surgery, University of Chicago, Chicago, Illinois
> Visceral Ischemic Syndromes

Jerry Goldstone, M.D.

Professor of Surgery and Chief, Division of Vascular Surgery, Case Western Reserve University School of Medicine; Chief, Vascular Services, University Hospitals of Cleveland, Cleveland, Ohio
> Aneurysms of the Aorta and Iliac Arteries

Antoinette S. Gomes, M.D.

Professor of Radiology and Medicine, University of California, Los Angeles, UCLA School of Medicine, Los Angeles, California
> Principles of Vascular Imaging and Interventional Radiology

Lazar J. Greenfield, M.D.

Frederick A. Coller Distinguished Professor of Surgery and Chairman, Department of Surgery, University of Michigan School of Medicine; Surgeon-in-Chief, University of Michigan Hospitals, Ann Arbor, Michigan
> Venous Thromboembolic Disease

Ian N. Hamilton, Jr., M.D.

Assistant Professor, Department of Surgery, Chattanooga Unit, University of Tennessee College of Medicine, Chattanooga, Tennessee
> Thoracoabdominal Aortic Aneurysms

Kimberley J. Hansen, M.D.

Professor of Surgery, Wake Forest University School of Medicine, Winston-Salem, North Carolina
> Renovascular Disease

Larry H. Hollier, M.D.

Professor, Mount Sinai School of Medicine; Chairman, Department of Surgery, and Surgeon-in-Chief, Mount Sinai Hospital, New York, New York
> Thoracoabdominal Aortic Aneurysms

Glenn C. Hunter, M.D.

Professor of Surgery, Department of Surgery, Section of Vascular Surgery, University of Arizona College of Medicine; Attending Surgeon, University Medical Center, Veterans Administration Medical Center, Tucson, Arizona
> Noninfectious Complications in Vascular Surgery

Fernando E. Kafie, M.D.

Division of Vascular Surgery, University of California, Los Angeles, UCLA School of Medicine, Los Angeles, California
> Thrombolytic Therapy for Vascular Disease

Ted R. Kohler, M.D.

Professor of Surgery, University of Washington School of Medicine; Chief, Vascular Surgery, Veterans Administration Puget Sound Health Care System, Seattle, Washington
> Anatomy, Physiology, and Pharmacology of the Vascular Wall

Michael E. Landis, M.D.

Clinical Fellow in Surgery, Harvard Medical School; Staff, Massachusetts General Hospital, Boston, Massachusetts
> Vascular Grafts: Characteristics and Rational Selection of Prostheses

Gregory J. Landry, M.D.

Assistant Professor of Surgery, Division of Vascular Surgery, Oregon Health Sciences University, Portland, Oregon
> Nonatherosclerotic Vascular Disease

Timothy K. Liem, M.D.

Clinical Assistant Professor of Surgery, Oregon Health Sciences University; Attending Surgeon, Providence St. Vincent Medical Center and Legacy Emanuel and Good Samaritan Hospitals, Portland, Oregon
> Hemostasis and Thrombosis

Evan C. Lipsitz, M.D.

Assistant Professor of Surgery, Department of Surgery, Albert Einstein College of Medicine; Attending Vascular Surgeon, Monte Fiore Medical Center, New York, New York

Femoral-Popliteal-Tibial Occlusive Disease

Herbert I. Machleder, M.D.

Emeritus Professor of Surgery, University of California, Los Angeles, UCLA School of Medicine, Los Angeles, California

Vascular Disease of the Upper Extremity and the Thoracic Outlet Syndromes

James M. Malone, M.D.

Clinical Professor of Surgery, University of Arizona College of Medicine, Tucson, Arizona; Professor of Surgery, Mayo Graduate School of Medicine, Rochester, Minnesota

Lower Extremity Amputation

John A. Mannick, M.D.

Professor of Surgery, Harvard Medical School; Staff, Brigham and Women's Hospital, Boston, Massachusetts

Evaluation of Cardiac Disease in the Patient with Vascular Disease; Aortoiliac Occlusive Disease

Michael L. Marin, M.D.

Professor of Surgery and Henry Kaufmann Professor of Vascular Surgery, Mount Sinai School of Medicine; Chief, Division of Vascular Surgery, Mount Sinai Medical Center, New York, New York

Endovascular Grafting

David S. Maxwell, M.D. (deceased)

Formerly Professor of Anatomy and Cell Biology, University of California, Los Angeles, UCLA School of Medicine; Professor of Surgery and Anatomy, Charles Drew Medical School, Los Angeles, California

Embryology of the Vascular System

James F. McKinsey, M.D.

Associate Professor of Clinical Surgery and Director of Medical Student Education for Surgery, University of Chicago, Chicago, Illinois

Visceral Ischemic Syndromes

Louis M. Messina, M.D.

Professor of Surgery, and Edwin J. Wylie Chair and Chief, Division of Vascular Surgery, University of California, San Francisco, School of Medicine, San Francisco, California

Splanchnic and Renal Artery Aneurysms

Timothy A. Miller, M.D., F.A.C.S.

Professor of Surgery, Division of Plastic and Reconstructive Surgery, University of California, Los Angeles, UCLA School of Medicine; Chief of Plastic Surgery Section, Veterans Affairs Greater Los Angeles Healthcare System, Los Angeles, California

Lymphedema and Tumors of the Lymphatics

Gregory L. Moneta, M.D.

Professor, Oregon Health Sciences University, Portland, Oregon

Natural History and Nonoperative Treatment in Chronic Lower Extremity Ischemia

Wesley S. Moore, M.D.

Professor of Surgery, University of California, Los Angeles, UCLA School of Medicine; Director of Vascular Surgery, UCLA Center for the Health Sciences, Los Angeles, California

Endovascular Grafting; Extracranial Cerebrovascular Disease: The Carotid Artery; Myointimal Hyperplasia

Nicholas J. Morrissey, M.D.

Fellow, Division of Vascular Surgery, Mount Sinai School of Medicine; Fellow in Vascular Surgery, Mount Sinai Hospital, New York, New York

Thoracoabdominal Aortic Aneurysms

Mark R. Nehler, M.D.

Assistant Professor and Associate Program Director, University of Colorado Health Sciences, Denver, Colorado

Natural History and Nonoperative Treatment in Chronic Lower Extremity Ischemia

Malcolm O. Perry, M.D.

Professor Emeritus, Vascular Surgery, University of Texas Southwestern Medical School; Chairman, Department of Surgery, St. Paul Medical Center, Dallas, Texas

Vascular Trauma

Charles M. Peterson, M.D.

Program Director, Blood Diseases Program, National Heart, Lung, and Blood Institute, National Institutes of Health, Bethesda, Maryland

Influence of Diabetes Mellitus on Vascular Disease and Its Complications

John M. Porter, M.D.

Professor of Surgery, Oregon Health Sciences University, Portland, Oregon

Nonatherosclerotic Vascular Disease; Natural History and Nonoperative Treatment in Chronic Lower Extremity Ischemia

William J. Quiñones-Baldrich, M.D.

Professor of Surgery, Section of Vascular Surgery, University of California, Los Angeles, UCLA School of Medicine, Los Angeles, California

Thrombolytic Therapy for Vascular Disease; Acute Arterial and Graft Occlusion

Kyung M. Ro, M.D.

Student, University of California, Davis, School of Medicine, Davis, California

Endovascular Surgery

Robert B. Rutherford, M.D.

Emeritus Professor of Surgery, University of Colorado School of Medicine, Denver, Colorado

> Congenital Vascular Malformations of the Extremities; Role of Sympathectomy in the Management of Vascular Disease and Related Disorders

Lewis B. Schwartz, M.D.

Assistant Professor of Surgery, University of Chicago, Chicago, Illinois

> Visceral Ischemic Syndromes

Donald Silver, M.D.

Professor Emeritus of Surgery, University of Missouri School of Medicine; Staff Surgeon, University of Missouri Health Sciences Center, Columbia, Missouri

> Hemostasis and Thrombosis

James C. Stanley, M.D.

Professor of Surgery, University of Michigan; Head, Section of Vascular Surgery, University of Michigan Hospital, Ann Arbor, Michigan

> Splanchnic and Renal Artery Aneurysms

D. Eugene Strandness, Jr., M.D.

Professor of Surgery, University of Washington School of Medicine; Attending Physician, University of Washington Medical Center, Seattle, Washington

> Hemodynamics for the Vascular Surgeon

Charles A. Taylor, Ph.D.

Assistant Professor of Surgery, Stanford University School of Medicine, and Professor of Mechanical Engineering, Stanford University, Stanford, California

> Hemodynamic Factors in Atherosclerosis

Lloyd M. Taylor, Jr., M.D.

Professor, Oregon Health Sciences University, Portland, Oregon

> Natural History and Nonoperative Treatment in Chronic Lower Extremity Ischemia

Frank J. Veith, M.D.

Professor and Vice-Chairman, Department of Surgery, Albert Einstein College of Medicine; The William J. won Liebig Chair in Vascular Surgery, Montefeore Medical Center, New York, New York

> Femoral-Popliteal-Tibial Occlusive Disease

Alex Westerband, M.D.

Vascular Surgery, Department of Surgery, University of Arizona College of Medicine, Tucson, Arizona

> Noninfectious Complications in Vascular Surgery

Anthony D. Whittemore, M.D.

Professor of Surgery, Harvard Medical School; Chief of Vascular Surgery, Brigham and Women's Hospital, Boston, Massachusetts

> Evaluation of Cardiac Risk in the Patient with Vascular Disease; Aortoiliac Occlusive Disease

Samuel E. Wilson, M.D.

Professor of Surgery, University of California, Irvine, School of Medicine, Orange, California

> Hemodialysis and Vascular Access

Charles L. Witte, M.D.

Professor of Surgery, University of Arizona College of Medicine, Tucson, Arizona

> Physiology and Imaging of the Peripheral Lymphatic System

Marlys H. Witte, M.D.

Professor of Surgery, University of Arizona College of Medicine, Tucson, Arizona

> Physiology and Imaging of the Peripheral Lymphatic System

Lance E. Wyatt, M.D.

Clinical Fellow in Surgery, Harvard Medical School; Resident in Plastic Surgery, Harvard Plastic Surgery Residency Training Program, Boston, Massachusetts

> Lymphedema and Tumors of the Lymphatics

Christopher K. Zarins, M.D.

Chidester Professor of Surgery, Stanford University School of Medicine; Chief of Vascular Surgery, Stanford University Medical Center, Stanford, California

> Hemodynamic Factors in Atherosclerosis

Gerald B. Zelenock, M.D.

Chairman, Department of Surgery, William Beaumont Hospital, Royal Oak, Michigan

> Splanchnic and Renal Artery Aneurysms

R. Eugene Zierler, M.D.

Professor of Surgery, University of Washington School of Medicine; Attending Physician, University of Washington Medical Center, Seattle, Washington

> Hemodynamics for the Vascular Surgeon

Preface to the Sixth Edition

The sixth edition of this book continues the tradition of presenting the topics related to the practice of vascular surgery in a complete and comprehensive manner, but, at the same time, keeping the book to a manageable size. This permits the reading of complete chapters as opposed to simply looking for individual items in a large reference textbook. Vascular surgery continues to be a rapidly evolving and changing field with respect to new technology and outcome data. Frequency of new editions is crucial in keeping this textbook and its readers up to date. For this reason, we have settled on a three-year revision cycle. In this edition, all of the original chapters have been either thoroughly revised or replaced to reflect the most current information.

Finally, we continue to believe in the importance of offering challenging questions at the end of the chapters to give the readers an opportunity for self-assessment.

WESLEY S. MOORE

Preface to the First Edition

During the past 20 years of rapid growth and development in vascular surgery, many graduates of general surgery programs found that their training in vascular surgery represented a valuable new resource for their hospital and practice communities. That training in vascular surgery often provided an important edge in establishing a new practice led to the widespread use of the term *general and vascular surgery* on the community announcements and business cards of new surgeons.

Yet in 1969, a survey conducted by a committee composed of James A. DeWeese, F. William Blaisdell, and John H. Foster discovered that among the 83 residents graduating from the 22 general surgery training programs surveyed, only 19 had performed more than 40 arterial reconstructive procedures during the course of their training, and more than half of the graduating residents had performed fewer than 20 arterial reconstructive procedures. The DeWeese committee, which had been established in 1969 to develop a document on optimal resources in vascular surgery, thus concluded that there was considerable suboptimal vascular surgery being performed in the United States, owing to a combination of both inadequate training and continued deficiencies in vascular surgery experience following training. A survey of the frequency of vascular operations in 1143 hospitals across the United States had revealed that in over 75% of these hospitals, fewer than 10 aneurysm resections and 10 femoropopliteal arterial reconstructions were conducted annually. This discovery led to the unfortunate conclusion that many surgeons were performing only occasional vascular operations, often leading to poor results.

The substance of the DeWeese report was reviewed by the two national vascular societies and their responsible leadership. This paved the way for, among other things, the definition of adequate training in vascular surgery and the recommendation that physicians who wish to practice vascular surgery spend an additional year of training to guarantee adequate experience in the specialty. To ensure prospective candidates that a given fellowship program in vascular surgery would provide a broad and responsible experience, the vascular societies established a committee for program evaluation and endorsement from which program directors could request review. Programs reviewed and found to meet the criteria of appropriate education as established by the committee would be announced annually.

Program evaluation by the joint council of the two national vascular societies was taken on as a temporary responsibility because the role would ultimately become the purview of the Residency Review Committee and the Liaison Committee for Graduate Medical Education. It was recognized that once adequate training programs were developed, the certification of candidates successfully completing training rested with the American Board of Surgery.

After approximately 10 years of experience, debate, and review, the American Board of Medical Specialties approved an application by the American Board of Surgery to grant "Certification of Special Competence in General Vascular Surgery." The first examination for certification was given to qualified members of the American Board of Surgery and Thoracic Surgery in June 1982. The second written examination was held in November 1983 in several centers across the United States.

The intent of this textbook is to provide a comprehensive review of vascular surgery, together with the related medical and basic science disciplines. This edition of the text has been developed to accompany a postgraduate course designed to help candidates prepare for the examination leading to certification in general vascular surgery. Accordingly, a list of questions designed to aid the reader in self-examination completes each chapter. All question sets simply represent the authors' opinion, a fair and adequate survey of the material covered, as none of the chapter authors is a member of the American Board of Surgery (this would be a conflict of interest).

Although chapter outlines were suggested by an editorial committee, the final chapter test represents, in the opinion of its authors, core material in each subject. Particular effort to identify and separate generally accepted concepts from new or controversial material was made. Although this book was designed as a comprehensive review to prepare for an examination, it is also in view of its organization and content, a comprehensive text of vascular surgery.

WESLEY S. MOORE

Contents

History of Vascular Disease

Wiley F. Barker

History is not unchanging, for it is only that which has been remembered or written down. Its value depends upon those who write it and preserve it. Much personal interpretation of such material is necessarily involved, and this is especially true the closer the observer is to the scene and time of the action. A historical view needs some distance in time for proper perspective. In the last few years, there have been immense developments in molecular biology and in techniques of minimally invasive surgery and interventional endovascular manipulations. We may stand so close to the dramatic changes brought into being, that although these changes must be recognized, the acutely contemporaneous developments are still difficult to interpret. Despite their incalculable promise for the future, as Mao-Tse Tung is said to have replied when asked about the effect of the French Revolution on the revolution in China, "It's much to soon to tell."

This history is presented as a series of scenes and acts; as with many modern stage plays, different actors appear in different scenes in different roles. It must be recognized that many scenes are concurrent and yet they must be observed from different points of view, depending on the immediate subject at hand. Finally, the whole ultimately fits together, as one scene prepares the reader to understand either the scene just past or the one to come.

PROLOGUE

Although some may argue that Guy de Chauliac or Ambroise Paré should properly be called the sire of surgery, John Hunter may be a better choice for the favorite candidate, and certainly for the prototype of the vascular surgeon. He was an unbelievably productive and tireless worker, shaped in the same Scottish mold as his brother William, who was 10 years older. John, however, was largely unlettered, whereas William had become sophisticated thanks to an elegant education at Glasgow. Yet they shared a frenetic capacity for work and an incurable curiosity.

To place the Hunters in a clear perspective with regard to nonmedical history, one should remember that they were contemporaries of George Washington and Benjamin Franklin. William was born in Scotland in 1718, his brother

John was born in 1728; William died in 1783 and John in 1793.[1, 2]

William Hunter had preceded John to London, where he soon established a busy practice and interested himself in many medical subjects, including aneurysms. In fact, he proposed the theory that a carelessly used lancet during bloodletting might enter both artery and vein, and that healing might occur in such a way that the two channels might be connected. He thus imagined an arteriovenous fistula; however, because imagination was not enough, he soon found an actual patient[3] and described the clinical manifestations with great accuracy. William's primary activity, however, was focused on obstetrics and on the teaching of anatomy. In this latter project, John started out as his assistant.

Mr. John Hunter is remembered for many things, but most especially for his studies of the dynamics and efficiency of collateral arterial circulation. This he described on the basis of his observations of the vessels feeding the antlers of a stag after he had interrupted the major arteries in the neck. Most of his renown came for his ligation of the femoral artery at a distance from a popliteal aneurysm—in "Hunter's canal."[1, 2]

To be sure, others earlier practiced proximal ligation of arteries. In the third century, a Roman surgeon, Antyllus, described proximal and distal ligation of the artery followed by incision of the aneurysm and removal of its contents, a formidable operation without either anesthesia or asepsis.[4] In 1680, Mathaeus Purmann,[5] faced with a large aneurysm in the antecubital space, carried out ligation of the vessels and excision of the aneurysmal mass. Shortly thereafter, Anel,[6] in 1714, described an operation in which he placed *one* ligature on the artery just at the proximal extent of the aneurysm. The reason for the apparent differences between these several surgical approaches and Hunter's is not hard to understand. Most of Anel's patients suffered from a false aneurysm caused by bloodletting in an otherwise healthy artery, whereas the femoropopliteal aneurysms treated by Hunter were caused by degenerative processes, probably a mixture of lues and trauma.[1, 6, 7] Hunter had seen that the ligature would at times cut through the artery when placed too close to the popliteal aneurysm, and so he chose a more remote site easily reached by the surgeon, which would preserve collaterals through the deep femoral system.

Many other surgeons were ligating aneurysms in various anatomic sites at this time—Sir Astley Cooper, one of John Hunter's students, soon established himself as one of the early vascular surgeons when he ligated the carotid for aneurysm in 1805[8] as well as the aorta for iliac artery aneurysm[9]—but only these few important names from the early part of the 19th century have remained with us.

Ligation was substantially the only procedure in arterial surgery that could be used at this time. To be sure, Hallowell, in Newcastle-on-Tyne, had carried out an arterial repair of an artery torn during bloodletting.[10] The laceration was a short one, and at the suggestion of Richard Lambert, he placed a short (1/4-inch) steel pin through the edges of the wound, thus everting them. He then looped a ligature around the area, approximating the edges of the wound, intima to intima, with apparent success. Hallowell wrote to Dr. William Hunter concerning this in 1761, foreseeing that if this were a successful technique, " . . . we might be able to cure wounds of some arteries that would otherwise require amputation, or be altogether incurable." That Hallowell wrote to William rather than John is probably owing to William's work on arteriovenous fistulae caused by inept bloodletting. Twelve years later (1773), Conradus Asman[11] reviewed the work and attempted some disastrous experiments himself. He soon concluded that such a procedure could not possibly work and that Lambert and Hallowell's efforts had probably failed. After Asman's criticism, the matter of arterial repair rested quietly for nearly another hundred years.

John Hunter's less well-known contributions are scattered throughout the immense museum he left to the Royal College of Surgeons of England, and they hint at a greater understanding of arterial pathology than would be generally achieved until a half century had passed. His accomplishments included dissections of several atherosclerotic aortic bifurcations (specimens P.1177 and P.1178) showing the lesion that Leriche would describe 150 years later, a carotid bifurcation with an ulcerated atheroma from a patient who died of a ruptured luetic thoracic aneurysm (specimen P.1171), and an extracranial internal carotid aneurysm (specimen P.282) in a patient whose neatly described symptoms appear as almost a classical paradigm of transient ischemic episodes.[12] To cap it all, in a postmortem specimen, Hunter had dissected the atheromatous layers (although the term "atheroma" had not yet come into use) from the remaining healthy wall of an atherosclerotic terminal aorta (specimen P.1176), foreshadowing the endarterectomy of dos Santos by more than 150 years. Regrettably, most of Hunter's notes have not survived to give us more than this fragmentary view of his understanding of vascular disease.

Hunter and his student, later known as Sir Astley Cooper, seemed to hold with the teleological belief of the times, that in the "senile" or "spontaneous gangrene" of older persons, thrombosis of the major vessels supervened so that the patient would not bleed to death when the gangrenous part separated.[13] It was Cruveilhier[14] who first clearly recognized the true sequence of events and stated that the term "gangrene due to obstruction of the arteries" by thickening and by thrombosis should replace the terms "spontaneous" and "senile" gangrene, but he attributed the concept to Dupuytren. Thus, gangrene due to occlusion of the arteries was recognized in the early 19th century. The understanding that there were symptoms of a functional nature less dramatic than the terminal morphologic changes of gangrene was not expressed clearly until Barth[15] described in 1835 a patient who manifested classical claudication complicated by heart failure due to mitral valvular disease, which caused her demise. Barth's report included a description of thrombosis of the terminal aorta, with a sketch that suggests that the lesion was a thrombosed hypoplastic terminal aorta, a long-standing contracted atherosclerotic lesion, or a combination of both. Barth reiterated Hunter's observation that the obstructing material could easily be separated from the residual arterial wall.

Although Charcot has most commonly been credited with the description of "intermittent claudication in the horse and in man,"[16] his 1858 report cited Barth as having observed and described claudication very precisely in humans 20 years earlier. Charcot, however, details the vanishing pulses, the cold extremity, and what we now recognize as the loss of sympathetic tone in a horse in the throes of a spasm of severe claudication. This phenomenon was well recognized in the veterinary world by Bouley.[17] Regarding his human patient, Charcot related the functional symptoms to an occlusion of the common iliac artery distal to a traumatic aneurysm, itself secondary to a bullet wound suffered 20 years before. In this patient, he described symptoms similar to those seen in the horse, but in addition he delineated the "herald" hemorrhage of an aortoenteric fistula.

Such information was of little use to the surgeon, however, until arterial repair became a reality. Consistent with the observations of Asman,[11] several German masters pronounced ex cathedra that arterial repair (as opposed to ligation) was impossible. Langenbeck[18] stated in 1825 that because the primary requirement for healing is perfect rest, so long as the movements (pulsations) of the arterial wall would continue, the wound could never heal. Heinecke[19] was certain that the subject would bleed to death through the suture holes and the apposed edges of the arterial wall. Repair of venous injuries, however, was becoming an established procedure: the lateral ligature, in which a clamp is placed on the defect in the venous wall and a ligature tied around the puckered wall, had been performed in 1816 (Travers, cited by Jassinowsky[20]). The first lateral suture of a venous defect (an erosion of the common jugular vein from an infected neck wound) was undertaken by Czerny[21] in 1881, but the patient died of sepsis and hemorrhage. Schede[22] is credited by Jassinowsky[20] with the first successful repair of a large venous injury (one to the common femoral vein). Furthermore, Eck[23] had reported the experimental creation of a portocaval fistula. The original description suggests he had little to confirm his success. Among a series of eight dogs, one survived less than 24 hours, six lived 2 to 6 days, and the one survivor " . . . tired of life in the laboratory and ran away after 2 months."[23] The doctoral dissertation of Jassinowsky,[20] written in 1889 as purely library research work, reviews the published information on arterial suture and concludes that it could not be successful at that moment, but that there might be hope in the future. Only 2 years later, however, it was Jassinowsky himself who did succeed, and in 1891 he reported his successful animal experiments on arterial suture.[24] The fine floss silk suture he described was passed carefully two thirds of the way through the media; he tried to avoid penetrating the intima except in very thin-walled vessels. Dorfler[25] modified Jassinowsky's method and passed the suture through all thicknesses of the arterial wall, recognizing that the arterial suture in the lumen of the vessel did no harm if uninfected; he said that it soon became covered with a glistening membrane. Shortly thereafter, in 1896, Jaboulay and Briau[26] described successful end-to-end carotid arterial anastomoses using an everting "U"-shaped suture.

Jaboulay was one of the surgeons at Lyon under whose influence Alexis Carrel studied. When Sadi Carnot, the President of the Republic of France, was assassinated and died in 1894 because no one dared to try to repair his wounded portal vein, Carrel was highly critical, for he believed the blood vessels could be sutured as well as any other tissue.[27] He soon began to undertake experimental arterial anastomoses. Some of the earliest of these were arteriovenous communications in which the high-flow system ensured patency. Carrel's contributions to technical arterial surgery included methods that vascular surgeons use routinely today.[28, 29] He devised the triangulation suture to facilitate end-to-end anastomosis; he described the patch technique to anastomose a small vessel to the side of a larger one (as in replantation of an inferior mesenteric artery); and he pioneered the use of vessel grafts and organ transplantation. His work, however, was not fully accepted in the United States for many years. Part of the rationale for this lack of acceptance stemmed from disputations that arose between Carrel and his coworker for a year, E. A. Guthrie.[30]

Nonetheless, European surgeons not only accepted but also began to follow Carrel's lead. In 1906, Goyanes[31] of Madrid resected a popliteal aneurysm and then restored arterial continuity with an in situ venous graft using the popliteal vein, probably the first successful clinical vascular replacement.

Surgeons in America were at this time beginning vascular surgery in their own way. In New Orleans, in 1888, Rudolph Matas[32] described a landmark operation. He had stumbled into the surgical procedure for which he is commonly remembered—endoaneurysmorrhaphy—when the aneurysm for which he had ligated the proximal brachial artery with apparent success began to pulsate again 10 days later. He chose to reoperate and to ligate the brachial artery distally. Even after this distal ligation, the pulsation remained, and he was forced to open the aneurysm, clean out the sac (the ancient Antyllian operation), and oversew the other arteries feeding the aneurysm from inside the sac. Matas' operation differed from that of Antyllus in that he used a suture to obliterate the feeding vessels from within the sac instead of ligating them after extensive dissection outside the sac, thus avoiding the risk of interfering with the nerves and collateral vessels and other adherent anatomic structures. It was many years before he again performed an endoaneurysmorrhaphy, for he continued to treat most of his patients successfully by simple proximal ligation.[33] Matas ultimately expanded his technique to include "restorative" and "reconstructive" modifications and

to report an approach to the arteriovenous fistula through the venous component,[34] as had been proposed by Bickham.[35]

J. B. Murphy[36] of Chicago performed a series of experiments on animals in which he successfully restored flow by invagination of the proximal into the distal vessel; then, in 1897, he presented a successful human case. Sterling Edwards revived this anastomotic technique of invagination briefly in his recommendations for the use of the first braided nylon grafts.[37]

Murphy's invagination techniques were reflected in other nonsuture methods of anastomosis: Nitze[38] and Payr[39] used small metal or ivory rings through which the vessel was drawn, everted, and tied in place; this unit was then inserted into the mouth of the distal vessel, and another ligature secured it there. This should be recognized as substantially the Blakemore tube,[40] which was used, albeit without signal success, in World War II.[41]

During the same period, William Stewart Halsted was beginning his tenure at Johns Hopkins Hospital, where an abundance of vascular trauma and of luetic aneurysms commanded his attention. In the early 1900s, Carrel visited Halsted and described his work, including his early arteriovenous anastomoses. As a result, Halsted *almost* made history in 1907[42] when, faced with the dilemma of a patient whose popliteal artery and vein had been sacrificed during an en bloc dissection of a sarcoma of the popliteal space, he went to the other leg, took the saphenous vein, reversed it, and anastomosed the distal saphenous vein to the proximal femoral artery. For his distal anastomosis, however, he chose the popliteal *vein*. Although the graft pulsated for 40 minutes, it soon thrombosed. One can only imagine what a dramatic leap forward vascular surgery would have made then if Halsted, with his superb surrounding cast of talented surgeons, had chosen the popliteal artery for the distal anastomosis and achieved in 1907 a truly successful arterial reconstruction!

Meanwhile, German surgeons such as Höpfner,[43] Lexer,[44, 45] and Jeger[46] became familiar with the use of vein grafts. Höpfner described the bypass procedure, which was illustrated in an encyclopedic book by Jeger. This book, as republished posthumously in 1937, included a foreword that described Jeger's replantation of the completely severed arm of a German soldier, an operation that Jeger had performed in 1914. A year later, while on the Russian front, Jeger came to an untimely death when he was stricken with typhus.

Lexer[45] collected and reported on 65 vein transplants, of which some 13 were his personal cases. In 8 of these 13 cases, Lexer had obtained a distal pulse. This report prompted a Polish surgeon, Weglowski,[47] to present his own personal series of 51 cases, mostly traumatic in origin, operated on between 1914 and 1921. In 40 patients, he was able to document good distal pulses and normal arterial tracings. Yet all this seemed forgotten over the next 25 years, as Germany suffered its agonies in the interbellum years, and as the forceful and charismatic personality of René Leriche appeared on the scene. His role is described in a later section.

ARTERIAL SUBSTITUTES

Up until this point in the narrative history, the surgeon, in the few instances in which he was bold enough to make attempts, used the material most obvious to him for arterial substitution, namely, the saphenous vein. These replacements were usually short—less than 10 cm. A later section deals with the use of longer segments as the primary mode of replacement, but the use of other materials was one of the major steps in the history of vascular surgery.

Following the experience in the laboratory reported by Abbe,[48] Tuffier[49] used rigid tubes of metal and of paraffined glass in World War I, but without much success. Similar tubes were tried in World War II, but the results were no better than with immediate ligation of the artery.[41]

The replacement of the aorta required more than a vein. Hufnagel chose a more inert surface than the glass tubes of Tuffier—methylmethacrylate[50]—and designed a tube with better hemodynamic characteristics. Tubes of this type functioned remarkably well in animal experiments except for the difficulties in securing them within a major artery such as the aorta without the risk of ultimate erosion. The arterial homograft and the use of pliable plastic fabrics substantially eliminated the use of the rigid tube.

The arterial homograft seemed at first to be a quite successful substitute when sutured into the thoracic or the abdominal aorta. Initially, fresh grafts were used, but later they were preserved in Tyrode's solution.[51, 52] The techniques of freezing[53] and then lyophilization[54] allowed the development of artery banks. Early successes were soon erased by late failures of the homografts, and a truly satisfactory aortic substitute remained a desperate need.

In 1952, Voorhees, Jaretzki, and Blakemore[55] observed that fabric threads in the heart soon became covered with endothelium. Dörfler[25] had made a similar gross observation 60 years earlier but had not carried the observation to its conclusion. Voorhees and his associates at Columbia[55] experimented not only with Vinyon-N, but also with parachute silk and other materials. Braided and crimped nylon tubes were introduced by Edwards and Tapp[37] but nylon was soon found to lose strength rapidly and proved unsatisfactory. Many other fabrics were tried, but most were quickly discarded. In 1955, Deterling and Bhonslay[56] summarized the current status of graft materials. Orlon[57] and Teflon[58] were both tried. Szilagyi and colleagues[59] and Julian and associates[60] introduced variations of Dacron. The transcripts of the vascular surgery meetings of the late 1950s might be mistaken for a textile journal, as various weaves, deniers, calendarizing, and the advantages of braid versus knit versus taffeta weaves were discussed. The summation of the principles of vascular grafting by Wesolowski and Dennis[61] and Wesolowski and coworkers[62] enunciated the importance of the principle of porosity, but the substantially nonporous Teflon was to undercut that thesis.

It was the knitted Dacron introduced by DeBakey and associates,[63] however, that placed a potentially successful graft in the hands of every surgeon. Subsequent modifications by the addition of velour to the surface by Sauvage and colleagues[64] and Cooley and associates[65] were refinements to this outstanding contribution. The concept that the fabric tube could become "encapsulated" and might develop a firm new endothelial surface has been pursued as a goal but has not been achieved.

The immediate porosity of the grafts has at times been troublesome, especially in patients whose situations require heparinization, or in whom even minor blood loss from a weeping graft might be intolerable. Impregnation with either collagen[66] or albumin[67] has been a dramatic step forward. The use of Teflon in the form of an extruded, expanded, and flexible tube, as introduced by Soyer and colleagues[68] (Goretex), rather than a woven or knitted fabric as a venous substitute, has come nearly full circle from the impermeable tubes of Hufnagel.[57] It is now substantially the only fully artificial replacement commonly used in infrainguinal arterial reconstructions.[69]

Modified biological substitutes other than the arterial homograft have also been used, however. Rosenberg and associates[70] used bovine carotid arteries that had been subjected to enzymatic treatment to remove all of the tissue-specific protein except the basic structural collagen of the bovine artery. Sawyer's group[71] attempted to modify the bovine heterograft by inducing a negatively charged lining in an effort to inhibit thrombosis. Dardik and co-workers[72] used treated umbilical vein grafts supported with a mesh of Dacron as a peripheral arterial substitute.

ABDOMINAL AORTIC ANEURYSM

Beyond the management of trauma to the arteries, the aneurysm is one of the great themes that has bound vascular surgeons together for many years, and the management of the abdominal aneurysm is certainly one of vascular surgery's major accomplishments. Vesalius is said to have been the first to describe an abdominal aneurysm.[73] The technical maneuvers that have been described previously concerning the ligation of aneurysms in various anatomic sites usually involved aneurysms of the peripheral vessels; aneurysms of the trunk were sacrosanct, because proximal control was not feasible.

Sir Astley Cooper (1768–1849), a student of John Hunter, continued many of Hunter's studies, including evaluation of collateral arterial supplies. In 1805, he ligated the common carotid for aneurysm,[8] but he opened the door for even wider surgical applications when, in 1818, he ligated the abdominal aorta to control external hemorrhage from an aneurysm of the external iliac artery that had eroded to the surface of the skin of the flank, bleeding openly at that site.[9]

Various other methods for accomplishing obstruction of an aneurysm were attempted. Colt, at the end of the 19th century, in an attempt to initiate thrombosis in the aneurysm, used wire to pack the aneurysm.[74] Blakemore and King[75] revived interest in this procedure in 1938, and many other surgeons undertook modifications of the wiring technique but largely without success.

The major actors in the next scene are again Rudolph Matas of New Orleans and William Stewart Halsted of Baltimore. Their interest in the management of trauma to the vessels and in the management of the late sequelae of trauma provided material for the fertile imaginations of the many surgeons who were emboldened to follow in their footsteps. Reid,[76] in 1926, reported the experience of the Johns Hopkins Hospital with aneurysms, which is properly that of its chief, Halsted. Although these aneurysms included many varieties, both anatomic and etiologic, this treatment of the abdominal aneurysm was substantially a failure. These operations were only a preparation for the last gasp of treatment of aneurysms of the abdominal aorta by ligation. Matas finally accomplished a successful aortic ligation (just below the renal arteries). He reported it first in 1923[77] and again later in the *Annals of Surgery* in 1940.[78] In that same issue of the *Annals of Surgery* was a similar paper by Elkin,[79] as well as the hint of a coming era of vascular reconstruction in the report by I. A. Bigger[80] of Virginia. He had ligated the neck of an abdominal aneurysm using fascia that he expected to loosen gradually to allow restoration of flow. With the protection of this temporary control, he performed a plication of the aneurysm, restoring the aorta to its proper caliber. The patient had a protracted survival not only without recurrence of the aneurysm but also with restoration of femoral pulses.

Other experiences with the aorta prepared the way for present-day management of the abdominal aneurysm. Alexander and Byron[81] resected a thoracic aneurysm associated with coarctation of the aorta and successfully oversewed the ends of the vessel. Regrettably, that patient ultimately died of renovascular hypertension.[82] Various attempts were made to use either reactive cellophane[83] or the irritating plasticizer in it, dicetyl phosphate,[84] as a means of inducing sclerosis that might restrain the dilatation of the aneurysm. Again, results were unsatisfactory.

About this time, however, cardiac surgery began to emerge. During the first decade of the 20th century, Jeger[46] proposed valved venous bypasses from the left pulmonary veins to the left ventricle to bypass mitral stenosis, and a valved venous graft from the left ventricle to the innominate artery to bypass aortic stenosis, but no clinical experiments are known. In the mid-1920s, Cutler, Levine, and Beck[85] attempted to treat mitral stenosis surgically but with minimal success. A valvulotome was used, inserted through a ventricular approach. Nonetheless, the influence of these attempts led Gross to the successful ligation[86] and then division[87] of the patent ductus arteriosus. In Baltimore, Blalock and Taussig,[88] began their series of pioneering surgical procedures on various cardiac anomalies, of which the first and most dramatic was the "blue baby" operation, the creation of a systemic shunt from the subclavian artery to the pulmonary artery for congenital pulmonic stenosis. Crafoord and Nylin[89] reported the successful end-to-end anastomosis of the aorta after resection of an aortic coarctation. Gross and Hufnagel[90] carried out their first case after Crafoord's case but before it appeared in print. Successful repair of the coarctation demonstrated that lesions of the thoracic and abdominal segments of the aorta were amenable to a surgical approach.

In 1947, Hufnagel[51] reported on the use of rapid freezing for the preservation of arterial homografts for interposition in the repair of long aortic coarctations. Gross and associates,[52] who at first seemed to fear that frozen vessels could not survive, published a laboratory and clinical report on their experiences with homografts preserved in electrolyte solutions for use in various cardiac operations, but particularly for the management of coarctation of the aorta. Swan and coworkers[91] soon used a homograft for a thoracic aneurysm associated with a coarctation. The report of Estes[92] that defined the grave risk to life for the patient who had an abdominal aneurysm provided the surgeon with justification to consider *elective* resection of the aneurysm instead of attempting treatment only after it was too late in

the game, when the odds were hopeless. In 1951, Oudot[93] reported the use of an aortic homograft to treat an aortic obstruction (Leriche syndrome) after resecting the bifurcation. He set the stage for the successful resection of an abdominal aortic aneurysm and replacement with a homograft by Charles Dubost and colleagues[94] on the 19th of March, 1951. Schaffer and Hardin[95] had actually preceded Dubost by 4 weeks, but the publication of their operation appeared considerably later. Dubost's operation was then followed by those of Julian and coworkers,[96] Brock,[97] DeBakey and Cooley,[98] and Bahnson.[99] It is a curious twist of fate to find that Dubost had left the practice of colorectal surgery to become a cardiac surgeon after he had seen Blalock and Bahnson perform cardiac operations while they were visiting France in the late 1940s. Resection and replacement were to be the primary components of routinely successful treatment of the aortic aneurysm, but Freeman and Leeds,[100] Wylie and colleagues,[101] and Barker[102] had included successful aneurysm repairs of abdominal aneurysms in their series of lesions treated by endarterectomy in 1951, but endarterectomy with arterioplasty for this lesion was poor second to replacement.

Szilagyi and associates'[103] classical study of the benefits of the operation provided confirmation and justification of the procedure that thoroughly confirmed the surgical treatment of the material that Estes had proposed.

The complicated abdominal aneurysm still posed a major problem. Ellis and colleagues[104] were among the first to implant the renal arteries into the graft when the aneurysm was found to include their orifices. Etheredge and coworkers[105] extended this operation to resect a major thoracoabdominal aortic aneurysm. They used a heparinized plastic shunt of the type described in Schaffer's resection and replacement of an abdominal aneurysm with a homograft in March of 1951. Etheredge established the shunt, divided the aorta, and performed the proximal anastomosis. He then moved the clamp down the graft after each successive visceral anastomosis was completed, and finished with the lower aortic anastomosis to the graft. Shumacker[106] modified Etheredge's operation slightly, placing the graft as a permanent bypass, dividing the aorta just below the anastomosis, continuing with attachment of the individual visceral branches, and, finally, performing an obliterative endoaneurysmorrhaphy.

DeBakey and associates[107] reported in 1956 a series of complicated thoracoabdominal aneurysms that were resected by a technique similar to that of Shumacker. In 1973, Stoney and Wylie[108] popularized the long thoracoabdominal incision for the approach to this lesion. The great advance in the management of these complicated lesions was made by Stanley Crawford,[109] who introduced a direct approach to the aneurysm. In this procedure, the aorta is clamped above and below and then opened longitudinally throughout the length of the aneurysm. A fabric graft is sewn into the lumen of the proximal aorta and both anastomoses are completed. The major groups of arteries, including the lower intercostals, are then sewn into the wall of the fabric tube using the expeditious Carrel patch method of anastomosis. This direct method has greatly simplified the approach to lesions that might otherwise have been resected and replaced with great difficulty.

The placement of a graft within the lumen of an aneurysm, whether abdominal, thoracic, or peripheral, was logically extended by a technique that allows one to place the graft through a short arteriotomy from a distance, through either the femoral or the external iliac artery. The evolution of this method stems circuitously from Dotter and coworkers.[110] In 1983, they attempted to improve the results of simple arterial dilatation or maintain patency of a graft with small endarterial spiral coils. After several generations of devices that did not acquire wide acceptance, Palmaz and his associates[111] introduced a metal mesh stent. This device can be expanded by balloon dilatation that secures the stent in place. Introduced originally to maintain patency of a segment of artery that has undergone percutaneous dilatation, this method was at first used in occlusive disease, but Parodi and coworkers[112] modified the technique to secure a fabric graft that had been placed within an aneurysm. First used as a tube graft, modifications soon allowed placement of bifurcation grafts.[113–115] The dramatic decrease in morbidity and mortality owing to the use of this method has led to widespread use, although not all aneurysms are amenable to it.

Unquestionably, the development of the endovascular manipulations so briefly described in the previous paragraph is one of the major historical steps in vascular surgery, as is the introduction of other endarterial procedures for the treatment of arterial obstructions. Regrettably, the relatively benign nature of these operations has opened the door to a series of misunderstandings with other medical specialties whose practitioners, although not surgeons, have nonetheless undertaken these procedures. The lack of standardized methods of reporting of experience in the nonvascular literature and the overly enthusiastic promotion of the method clouds the value of these methods. Comparison of methods and results should be made possible by accurate and standardized methods of analysis. It is hoped that a rational, cooperative approach will be followed in the future. This argument becomes one of important clinical and ethical relevance that is not yet clearly in the purview of history.

PERIPHERAL ARTERIAL ANEURYSMS

The peripheral arterial aneurysm was one of the first arterial lesions treated by the surgeon, but its importance paled beside the advances made in the management of the aortic aneurysm described in the previous paragraphs. The history of treatment by ligation in earlier centuries has been detailed in the first sections of this chapter.

In 1949, Linton[116] used Leriche's principle of arteriectomy and sympathectomy for the management of a series of 14 patients who had popliteal aneurysm, an ingenious approach that in his series resulted in no amputations. The patient received a preliminary sympathectomy, then shortly—although sometimes at the same séance—underwent resection of the aneurysm with ligation of the proximal and distal vessel but with no effort made to restore continuity of the main arterial channel.

The ability to replace vessels of the size of the popliteal artery promptly brought to the fore the concept that the popliteal aneurysm had a risk-benefit pattern similar to that of the abdominal aneurysm. If operations were done

electively, the results were excellent, but once thrombosis occurred, the risk to the limb was grave, as Whychulis and associates[117] and Gifford and colleagues[118] previously reported. Wylie,[119] in a discussion of the methods of Whychulis and associates[117] and Edwards,[120] introduced the procedure of exclusion of the aneurysm and restoration of flow through a bypass technique.

OCCLUSIVE ARTERIAL DISEASE

As mentioned earlier, it was not until the middle of the 19th century that the relationship between arterial occlusions and either clinical symptoms or gangrene became clearly established. Repair of acute injuries had been accomplished, but the management of more chronic arterial obstructions had not yet become a surgical target. The effective arterial suture anastomosis was developed at Lyon through the ideas of Jaboulay and Carrel. After World War I, another surgeon from Lyon assumed a major role in vascular surgery.

René Leriche, born in 1879, was educated and trained at Lyon, where his seniors were Jaboulay and Carrel. After completing his training, Leriche stayed in the service of Professor Poncet until the latter died. Shortly thereafter, Jaboulay was killed. "Surgery in Lyon was decimated," said Leriche.[121] Then came World War I, with its forced dislocations and peregrinations. After he was demobilized, Leriche worked in a trauma hospital in Lyon for several years. There, he saw many patients with post-traumatic neuralgias. These confirmed his theory of the role of the sympathetic nervous system in this problem and the possible treatment by periarterial sympathectomy, about which he had first published in 1916.[122] Then, seeing patients with arterial thrombosis due to "artérite," a loose and nonspecific term used to describe arterial occlusion in general, Leriche came to the conclusion that if the patient were seen before the occluding thrombosis was too widespread, a local resection of the thrombosed artery would provide relief. Because many patients did well after this simple procedure and soon developed relatively warm feet, he concluded that the collateral circulation in these patients must usually have been satisfactory and that the coldness of the extremity must have been due to vasospasm instead of insufficient arterial flow. He therefore applied the principle of sympathectomy, first as a periarterial operation, then as an arteriectomy (excising the obstructed segment), and then as a division of the sympathetic rami.

Diez,[123] dissatisfied with the results of periarterial sympathectomy, modified that operation into the lumbar ganglionectomy. At nearly the same time, Royle[124] and Hunter[125] introduced the same procedure for the fruitless management of spasm in striated muscle in patients with poliomyelitis. The use of this operation for the management of pain syndromes and for the management of ischemic extremities remains, although it is controversial.

It seems likely that the force of Leriche's personality led European surgical thought along lines that diverged from accepting already known techniques of vascular grafting. This is not to say that Leriche actively spoke against the use of grafts. In fact, it is said that he often stated it would have been ideal to connect the two ends of a severed artery by a graft, but the distance always seemed too great. Instead, he chose to offer arterial excision and sympathectomy, an approach that had less benefit but also less risk.

One of Leriche's most important early observations included the definition of the syndrome to which his name is attached, the atherosclerotic obliteration of the terminal aorta and the iliac arteries. He described this in 1923,[126] during the period in which he was beginning to evaluate arteriectomy. It was 17 years, however, before he found a case suitable for performance of resection of the aortic bifurcation and lumbar sympathectomy.[127]

Leriche's surgical clinic became famous, and he collected around him great surgeons who came to learn: DeBakey, Learmonth, dos Santos, and Kunlin to name only a few.

Here, it is necessary to flash back briefly to 1909, for in that year Murphy[128] removed an embolus from the common iliac artery and restored flow into the femoral system. Although locally successful, distal thrombosis required a distal amputation. Two years later, Labey, as cited by Mosney and Dumont,[129] performed the fully successful removal of an embolus from the artery of a patient. Embolectomy was thereafter performed with occasional success worldwide, but it did not become a fully satisfactory procedure because of the need for great haste in operating before extensive distal thrombosis supervened. After the clinical introduction of heparin by Murray,[130] it became possible to extend the indications and limiting time restrictions for embolectomy and to improve the results.

Surgeons such as João Cid dos Santos[131] and his father Reynaldo undertook the use of heparin to prevent thrombosis after reviving the old Matas endoaneurysmorrhaphy. The younger dos Santos believed that with the protection of heparin, he might be able to remove chronically adherent arterial emboli and their associated thrombus and have healing occur without rethrombosis. Finding a patient with advanced renal disease and a seriously ischemic extremity, dos Santos removed the clot and reestablished flow. His immediate glow of success was dimmed when he was upbraided by the pathologist for having removed the intima as well. This episode he later described as "the moment of the fall of the myth of the need for an intact endothelium." After another successful case, in which he removed a chronic thrombosis of the subclavian, axillary, and brachial arteries secondary to the arterial distortion by scalenus anticus syndrome, he sent his report to René Leriche. Leriche presented the work in the name of dos Santos to the French Academy of Surgery,[132] and endarterectomy as well as modern vascular reconstructions had begun. It is interesting to note that in neither of dos Santos' first two patients was the lesion primarily that of atherosclerotic thrombosis.

Subsequently, Freeman and Leeds,[100] Wylie and associates,[101] and others[102] in this country adopted the operation, using the open technique that was primarily claimed by Bazy, Hugier, and Reboul.[133] In the report of Wylie's work of September 1951, he described endoaneurysmectomy and endarterectomy of the aorta. Cannon and I had undertaken six procedures without success, but in the summer of 1951 Wylie visited our institution, and in October 1951, I performed the first successful endarterectomy in our series.[102] As seen from a historical point of view, that opera-

tion consisted of a combination of the Matas endoaneurysmorrhaphy and the dos Santos endarterectomy (or, rather, the technique as revised by Reboul). An abdominal aneurysm was endarterectomized, tailored to a proper size, and wrapped with fascia lata. The endarterectomy in continuity was performed throughout the length of the left iliofemoralpopliteal system. In fact, these operations were only extensions of the repair of an aneurysm performed by Bigger in 1940.[80]

Cannon and Barker[134] later introduced the long closed endarterectomy using intraluminal strippers, which was a modification of the original method of dos Santos. Several varieties of endarterectomy loops were devised by Butcher[135] and by Vollmar and coworkers[136] among others. A period of early success was followed by disenchantment with the difficulty of the operation in comparison with the increasingly popular grafting procedures.

Leriche and his close associate, Kunlin, had not had great technical success with the operation of endarterectomy, especially in the femoral artery system. Kunlin[137] revived the vein graft in the form of a long venous bypass graft. Kunlin had published initial accounts of his first series before the above report, but this report provides the greatest detail. Veins had been used in earlier years, but only for very short (4 to 8 cm) replacements on rare occasions during the prior 40 years. This is the technique that has persisted as the basic method of arterial reconstruction ever since.

Saphenous vein grafting, however, was useful only in the femoral and iliofemoral system, and it remained for Jacques Oudot to perform a comparable operation on the aorta[93] using an aortic homograft, which thoracic and cardiac surgeons were already using as a graft in segments of the thoracic aorta for coarctation and for other thoracic aortic lesions. Oudot was presented with a 51-year-old patient who had claudication as a result of a proximal left iliac and distal aortic occlusion. The anatomic lesion is commonly pictured in descriptions of Oudot's operation as a simple bifurcation graft, common iliac to common iliac, but, in fact, the operation was a much more complicated procedure. He approached the aorta through a left flank incision and resected the bifurcation. The patient's internal iliacs were found to be thrombosed and were ligated. The external iliac arteries of the graft were very small, but the graft's internal iliacs were large. Oudot therefore anastomosed the graft's internal iliacs to the patient's external iliacs. He did the left-sided anastomosis first, however, and then found that his restoration obstructed his view and hindered manipulations of the right-sided anastomosis. This difficult anastomosis thrombosed promptly. Oudot made the best of a bad situation and pointed out that he had done a perfect experiment; there was still some argument from the camp of Leriche as to whether grafting at this level would be worthwhile. On the right side, Oudot had performed substantially nothing more than an arteriectomy; on the left, he had reconstituted the lumen. The right side was warm but pulseless and fatigued easily, whereas the left side had a pulse and did not tire.

Six months later, Oudot[138] reoperated on the patient, who was still complaining of right-sided claudication; he performed an iliac-to-iliac "extra-anatomic" bypass, as had been suggested by Kunlin earlier.

A few months later, Oudot climbed the Himalayan massif, Annapurna, with the French team, and shortly after his return to France he was killed in an automobile accident at the age of 40.

The saga of the treatment of arterial disease continues with the development and then the failure of artery banks and then with the introduction of the plastic prosthesis, but by 1952, the stage was set for nearly everything that is done today. Robert Linton's espousal[139] of the reversed saphenous vein in 1952 confirmed the approach of Kunlin and established the procedure of choice for peripheral reconstruction for many years.

Endarterectomy did not die: It persists in carotid operations and in local tailoring of the femoral vessels to prepare them for attachment of a graft, but only rarely is it used in the aorta. Edwards[140] made one important attempt to revive femoral endarterectomy by the use of a long venous patch throughout the length of the endarterectomy. This procedure worked well except when the patch was so wide it created a stagnant column of blood in the femoral artery. Because its use was limited to procedures that ended proximal to the distal portion of the popliteal artery and because the operation was exceedingly tedious, the procedure fell out of favor.

However, closed endarterial procedures have become commonplace. Dotter and Judkins[141] proposed the use of a stiff dilator, a procedure that was not widely accepted. Gruntzig and Hopff[142] modified this method by using a balloon that could distend and fracture the stenotic plaque. Others, injecting drugs or small emboli of biologic and nonbiologic materials, have been able to control arterial or venous hemorrhage, thrombose small aneurysms, and control the multiple arteriovenous connections of vascular malformations.

Endarterial manipulations have been extended to include not only dilatations and placement of emboli of several kinds in bleeding arteries but also, by development of newer methods, attempts at removal of the atherosclerotic lesion by endarterial manipulations through a percutaneous route. A major requirement for endarterial procedures was believed to be endarterial visualization, beyond that given by contrast radiography. Endarterial visualization began effectively with the work of Greenstone and others.[143]

Bom[144] introduced a different mode—endoluminal ultrasonography—to visualize the interior of the artery. Actual removal of the plaque by several mechanical means followed this technique. Simpson and associates[145] used a side-biting forceps in a catheter, whereas Kensey and colleagues[146] employed a catheter through which a rapidly rotating, auger-like tip is passed, and Ahn and coworkers[147] advocated a high-speed rotary burr. Others have used various forms of laser energy to destroy the plaque,[148] one that recognizes the difference between plaque and normal arterial wall,[149] or a laser-heated probe that "melts" the atheroma.[150] Further mechanical dilatation often accompanies these initial coring methods. These procedures appear to offer only limited removal of the atheromatous material and much less satisfactory results than the classical techniques of endarterectomy. Appraisal of these methods belongs in the clinical rather than the historical section of this volume.

Dotter and others[110] proposed the addition of intraluminal stents to maintain patency of grafts as well as vessels that had been dilated. The use of intraluminal stents was referred to in an earlier section.

Two other major breakthroughs in the use of the saphenous vein must receive comment.

First, a major advance in care of the ischemic extremity came about by the extension of the vein graft to much more distal sites. It is likely that early unfavorable experience with endarterectomy in vessels smaller than the popliteal artery may have held back common use of the tibial arteries as the distal site of attachment of the graft. Palma[151] published, in 1960, descriptions of vein graft insertions into the tibial arteries. Later information from Palma (personal communication, September 16, 1988) indicates that these were performed as early as 1956. McCaughan described the exposure of the distal popliteal artery in 1958,[152] but his terminology included a description of the artery more commonly known as the tibioperoneal trunk as the "distal popliteal artery." In that paper of July 1957, McCaughan described a successful graft into the tibial vessels using an exposure in the upper third of the calf. In 1960, he presented six additional patients with grafts into the tibial segment.[153] In 1966, McCaughan[154] went one step further when he reported four grafts in which the distal site of the graft was the posterior tibial artery at the ankle. George Morris and others,[155] in 1959, and Tyson and DeLaurentis,[156] in 1966, were other pioneers in the use of infrapopliteal procedures.

The other extension of distal femoral reconstruction was the application of the in situ vein graft with destruction of valvular competence within the vein by Karl Victor Hall.[157] This was the procedure used by Goyanes[31] in his replacement of a popliteal aneurysm, but Goyanes fortunately did not find any valves in the popliteal segment he used. The procedure did not receive much attention until revitalized by Leather and associates[158] in 1981. Many variations on the theme of the distal bypass have been introduced, combining free grafts and in situ methods. Dardik and associates[159] introduced not only the use of the tanned human umbilical vein but also a distal arteriovenous fistula. This was not so much a revival of Carrel's earlier attempts to revascularize an extremity through the veins, but rather an attempt to provide a sufficient outflow for a long graft to assure its patency, with some of the graft flow still directed through the distal arterial tree. DeLaurentis and Friedman[160] introduced a method of sequential multiple bypasses in the extremity, and Veith and associates[161] carried this method to its ultimate extent, with bypasses from one tibial artery to another, even with bypasses beginning and ending below the malleolus. Nehler[162] and associates applied this small vessel bypass technique to management of small vessel disease in the hand.

A different approach to the ischemic limb was early advocated by Peter Martin and coworkers,[163] who introduced an extended form of profundaplasty. This work was preceded by earlier contributions by the French surgeons Oudot and Cormier,[164] but since that time, Miller and colleagues,[165] Cohn and others,[166] and Towne and associates[167] have added useful concepts to the management of ischemia with the help of the profunda femoris artery.

None of these great advances of reconstructive surgery,

however, have been helpful in the management of the frustrating syndrome of thromboangiitis obliterans. It is likely that von Winiwarter[168] did describe the pathologic process of this disease, but his description is ambiguous. Certainly, Leo Buerger[169] gave a description of most of the clinical picture. Neither von Winiwarter nor Buerger noted the association with tobacco or the involvement of the upper extremities.

One major contribution rounds out this section. In 1963, Thomas Fogarty and associates[170] devised one of the most useful technical methods in the management of occlusive arterial disease when they introduced the balloon embolectomy catheter for the extraction of clot in the treatment of embolization. This technique has been modified for use in many other arterial and venous operations and has even been adapted to many general surgical uses.

ARTERIAL TRAUMA

Arterial injuries have always been a challenge to the surgeon. Trauma was the source of Hallowell's first arterial repair. During the years that followed the Civil War, Weir Mitchell and colleagues[171] described the syndrome of burning pain ("causalgia") that followed many arterial injuries, and it was this lesion that intrigued Leriche[122] and led him to his interest in the sympathetic nervous system. Halsted remarked on the fascination that arterial injuries held for the surgeon. During World War I, Makins[172] surveyed the injuries to blood vessels incurred by the British forces. DeBakey and Simeone[173] provided a similar service for the United States forces after World War II, noting that almost no benefit derived from the vascular surgical techniques then available because of the incidental and associated surgical problems and the matters of delay.

So it was that few arterial injuries were treated definitively—except for ligation—until the Korean War. Before that time, the main interest in arterial injuries seemed to lie in the estimation of the prognosis for survival of the limb and in the selection of the appropriate level for ligation of the artery.

During the Korean War, however, Jahnke and Howard,[174] Hughes,[175] and Spencer and Grewe[176] participated in a program in which acute vascular injuries were treated by the use of fresh vein grafts. Whelan and others[177] and Rich and Hughes[178] continued this use of the techniques of arterial repair in Vietnam. The Registry of Vascular Injuries from Vietnam as maintained at the Walter Reed Army Medical Center under the direction of Rich has continued to yield a monumental body of information concerning acute vascular repair. Civilian medical centers have carried over the applications of these techniques to the everyday pattern of injuries to the vessels.

The arteriovenous fistula is one of the sequelae of trauma to the major vessels that poses a special challenge to surgeons. Its acute effects on the distal circulation, its systemic effects as a major left-to-right shunt, and its local changes, which result in increased blood flow through the feeding arterial supply, have all been intriguing examples of the body's adaptability—or lack of it.

The arteriovenous fistula was first described by William Hunter.[3] The lesion did not become common until the end of the 19th century, as weapons and the injuries they caused changed. Volumes have been written in interpretation of the diverse physiologic parameters involved in this lesion, but, as early as 1913, Soubbotitich[179] noted that simple ligation of the proximal artery should never be done. Not long after, Lexer[44] introduced the "ideal" operation, consisting of resection of the aneurysmal sac and restoration of flow through the artery with a short venous graft if the ends of the artery could not be brought back together. Reconstruction of the vein was desirable but not mandatory. Bickham[35] had suggested approaching the repair of the artery through the venous component of the sac, with repair of the vein if possible, a modification of the Matas endoaneurysmorraphy. For the most part, however, until the era of the Korean War, in the 1950s and even later, the commonest form of surgical management was quadruple ligation and excision of the sac and fistula. Such an operation depends on the development of sufficient collateral circulation to the distal limb to allow the limb to survive after arterial interruption, but the surgery must occur before the extra load placed on the heart by the left-to-right shunt causes serious cardiac disability. The timing of the operation became a matter of most delicate clinical judgment. Emile Holman,[180] who had developed during his training at Johns Hopkins a lifelong interest in the arteriovenous fistula, was the most eminent contributor to the understanding of the physiology of the arteriovenous fistula. With the advent of prompt exploration and repair of acute arterial injuries, it was anticipated that the number of late arteriovenous fistulas would be greatly reduced, but this has not been the case.

OCCLUSIVE DISEASE OF THE EXTRACRANIAL CEREBROVASCULAR ARTERIES

The critical nature of the blood flow to the brain through the great arteries of the neck was recognized by the ancient Greeks, who named the carotid artery after the symptoms that followed its occlusion—asphyxia, or stupor. The clinical importance of carotid artery obstruction has been only slowly accepted by the neurologic community in general, however, despite the fact that eminent neurologists such as Savory,[181] Hunt,[182] and Fisher[183, 184] had made the critical clinical observations relating arterial lesions and atheroembolic phenomena many years before surgical treatment became accepted.

The first elective attempt to restore flow to the ischemic brain was made by Carrea and associates[185] in 1951, but this operation was not reported until 1955. The proximal portion of the diseased internal carotid artery was excised, and flow was restored by an anastomosis of the unusually large distal external carotid artery to the cut end of the internal carotid. A slightly different reconstruction of a carotid bifurcation that was injured by a gunshot wound was accomplished by Lefèvre[186] in 1918. The carotid bulb was resected, the common carotid ligated, and the external carotid anastomosed to the internal carotid to provide to the brain the arterial supply from the rich anastomoses of the external carotid.

The most widely acclaimed carotid early reconstruction—

and the one that truly began the era of modern carotid surgery—was the resection of the carotid bifurcation and the restoration of carotid flow by anastomosis of the common carotid to the internal carotid artery by Eastcott, Pickering, and Rob[187] in 1954, but this was not the classical carotid endarterectomy. Denton Cooley and colleagues,[188] William Roe,[189] and Michael DeBakey[190] were among the first to successfully perform true carotid endarterectomies.

As was the case with Estes and his paper justifying the approach to the abdominal aneurysm, so the report to the National Research Council of Great Britain by Yates and Hutchinson[191] indicated the importance of occlusive disease of the carotid and vertebral arteries. In Rochester (Minnesota), Whisnant and associates[192] identified the risk of stroke in the presence of transient ischemic attacks and provided the solid basis for operation on the carotid artery. Hollenhorst[193] called attention to the bright cholesterol emboli that are pathognomonic of atherosclerotic embolization, but Julian and associates[194] and Moore and Hall[195] further identified the role of embolization as the major cause of transient cerebral ischemic symptoms. Additional landmark studies of the morphology of the carotid plaque and its evolution were presented by Imparato and coworkers[196] and by Lusby and associates.[197] Moore and Hall[198] and other of Wylie's colleagues called attention to the role of carotid back-pressure in identifying patients whose brains need protection during the period of operative occlusion.

Operation for the symptomatic patient was soon relatively well accepted, but prophylactic operation for the prevention of stroke remains controversial in asymptomatic patients whose carotid lesions are identified by a bruit or by a measurable change in retinal artery pressure or by some other noninvasive laboratory test. Work by Thompson and colleagues[199] is the predominant authoritative basis for the prophylactic operation, despite criticism concerning lack of perfect controls. Subsequently, Dixon and associates[200] brought forth more evidence concerning the role of large and asymptomatic ulcerations of the carotid bifurcation. Berguer and coworkers[201] have shown that many "asymptomatic" patients with carotid lesions actually demonstrate multiple small cerebral infarcts that have not been clearly reflected in the patient's symptoms. An immense body of controversial literature has been published concerning the use of anticoagulant or antiplatelet agents to prevent thrombosis or thromboembolization, but these modalities remain an adjunct to the highly effective operation of carotid endarterectomy when performed by trained surgeons.

Moore[202] has summarized the several early multicenter randomized trials of carotid endarterectomy that have been performed for comparison of carotid endarterectomy with nonsurgical methods. These have shown such an excellence of effectiveness that many criticisms of the operation have been quieted. Confirmatory reports have stemmed from the many subsequent multicenter trials.

The inability of the surgeon to clear the totally occluded bifurcation safely and effectively has been addressed by the use of microsurgical techniques. Yasargil, Krayenbuhl, and Jacobson[203] first brought this technique to the attention of the American vascular world, and since then, many neurosurgeons have become skillful in the performance of extracranial-to-intracranial bypass. Subsequently, however, a randomized study indicated serious doubts about the value of this technique in preventing strokes.[204]

VISCERAL VASCULAR OCCLUSIONS

One of the most important lesions in relatively small arteries has been the occlusive lesion in the coronary arteries. Longmire, Cannon, and Kattus[205] carried out a few successful coronary endarterectomies in 1958. The difficulties associated with endarterectomy in small vessels led others to the use of the vein graft, first used as a replacement by Favoloro[206] and then as a bypass by Johnson and associates[207] in 1969.

Renal arterial insufficiency has been treated successfully for many years. Goldblatt and others[208] recognized the importance of renal ischemia and others came to explain the details of the deranged physiology. Freeman and associates[209] were among the first to treat this lesion successfully, and they opened the vast area of renovascular hypertension to successful surgical management. Decamp and colleagues,[210] Poutasse,[211] and Foster and associates[212] have been leaders in the perfection of these techniques.

The recognition of the several forms of fibromuscular hyperplasia in the renal artery was followed by its identification in the internal carotid artery by Connett and Lansche.[213] Ehrenfeld and associates[214] put the surgical management of this lesion on a firm footing.

Occlusive disease occurs much less frequently in the mesenteric vessels than in most other visceral beds but is nonetheless a frequently lethal lesion. It is commonly recognized only when it has reached an advanced stage and has occasioned extensive intestinal necrosis. Dunphy,[215] however, in 1936, related the progression of symptoms of mesenteric ischemia to the status of frank intestinal infarction. Fifteen years later, Klass[216] removed an embolus from the superior mesenteric artery successfully, although the patient died of his primary cardiovascular disease. The first series of endarterectomized patients treated by Barker and Cannon[102] included one patient with a successful mesenteric endarterectomy, although the patient died of acute renal failure. Five years later, Shaw and Rutledge[217] carried out an embolectomy of the superior mesenteric artery without concomitant bowel resection. The following year, Shaw and Maynard[218] identified two patients who had both malabsorption and mesenteric ischemia and treated them successfully with endarterectomy. In the meantime, Mikkelsen and Zaro[219] reported similar experiences from California, and they clarified the term *intestinal angina*.

The meandering mesenteric collaterals so well described by Kountz, Laub, and Connolly[220] provided a radiographic sign of the presence of serious insufficiency of the celiac axis and superior mesenteric vessels, which should be cause for careful evaluation of these vessels, whether found at operation or in the radiologic suite.

One of the important nonsurgical lesions that mimics obstructive mesenteric vascular disease is the nonocclusive form of mesenteric vascular insufficiency identified by Heer and associates,[221] which occurs in forms of cardiogenic shock wherein the cardiac output is low and mesenteric vascular resistance is high.

The extrinsic compression syndrome of the celiac axis is

a subject capable of generating considerable discussion. Marable and associates[222] first described this as compression by the arcuate ligament of the diaphragm. Some authors have believed that other anatomic structures, such as the neural components of the celiac ganglion, may also be involved. Many support the existence of this lesion as a cause of serious symptoms, but others forcefully deny its existence.[223]

VASCULAR MISCELLANY

There are many technical and mechanical advances that cannot properly be placed in any one of the previously described compartments of the history of vascular surgery. One of these is the concept of the *extra-anatomic bypass.* The term itself is controversial: It has been suggested that this implies a bypass outside of the body instead of outside of the classical anatomic routes, but its usage is so well established that it is retained here. It was proposed by Kunlin[137] and actually carried out as an ilioiliac bypass by Oudot in 1951.[138] Although rerouting of flow through short shunts for one reason or another had been done by many surgeons, the first dramatic step was taken by Blaisdell, DeMattei, and Gauder,[224] who led a graft from the thoracic aorta extraperitoneally to the femoral artery. Shortly thereafter, this anatomic arrangement was modified as the axillofemoral and then as the axillobifemoral graft in 1963.[225]

The axillofemoral bypass was first advised as a means of establishing flow to the extremity in the presence of an infected aortic reconstruction that had to be removed. Similarly, in 1969, Guida and Moore[226] described the bypass through the obturator foramen to avoid infection in the groin. Shaw and Baue[227] expanded this concept 2 years later. Vetto[228] reported the femorofemoral bypass in 1962, 11 years after Oudot's ilioiliac operation. Today the pattern of unusual anatomic configurations seems limited only by the patient's needs and the surgeon's ingenuity.

One of the important indications for replacement of the classical aortic prosthesis is the development of an aortoenteric fistula. These lesions have plagued surgeons since the first aortic grafts were performed. Elliott, Smith, and Szilagyi[229] contributed one of the first important papers to the understanding of this problem. Later, Busuttil and associates[230] defined the common primary role of a false aneurysm at the aortic suture line and clarified the management.

One of the great advances in nephrology was the introduction of hemodialysis in the mid 1950s as described by Kolff,[231] but hemodialysis by the nephrologist demands access to the vascular system. Vascular access surgery lacks the glamor of much of the rest of vascular surgery, but it is a significant portion of vascular surgical practice. The construction and maintenance of an access that functions well is eminently demanding of surgical skill and judgment. The first approaches involved external silicone tubing that connected the arterial and venous systems in the arm.[232] The natural progression was to the use of a direct arteriovenous fistula that resulted in dilated veins suitable for recurrent punctures by Brescia and his team.[233] The introduction of an autologous vein graft to allow a better fistula and

better access to the vein[234] was soon followed by the use of other shunts, both biological[235] and plastic.

In a similar pattern are the problems of the varied thoracic outlet syndromes whose care is shared with orthopedists, neurosurgeons, and physiotherapists. Although first recognized and treated surgically in 1861,[236] clear anatomic understanding came about through the works of J. B. Murphy[237]; of Adson and Coffey[238]; and of Ochsner, Gage, and DeBakey.[239] It appeared to early authors that a cervical rib was the offending anatomic structure, but Adson and Coffey introduced solidly the concept of entrapment of the brachial plexus and accompanying artery by the anterior scalene muscle. Naffziger[240] confirmed the mechanical origins of the syndrome and demonstrated the anterior approach. Falconer and Li[241] proposed the resection of the first rib for relief of the costoclavicular compression of the vessels. Edward Edwards[242] offered a thesis consolidating evolutionary causation of these syndromes, pointing out that the human is one of the few animals in whom there is a descent of the shoulder girdle and the heart that leads to the draping of the great vessels over the highest rib, whatever that might be.

The surgical approaches to this area have been varied—paraspinal and anterior supraclavicular—but Roos[243] introduced the transaxillary approach.

The commonest form involves the nerves and arteries, but a slightly different anatomic arrangement is responsible for the Paget-Schroetter syndrome, involving obstruction of the venous system. McLeery and associates[244] early defined the anatomic problem of intermittent venous obstruction from the subclavius and anterior scalene muscles.

VENOUS SURGERY

The history of venous surgery is in one sense older and in another sense newer than that of arterial surgery. Venous repairs were undertaken before arterial repairs were generally successful. Most of the first generation of arterial surgeons learned about the vagaries of the venous system as their first experiences in vascular surgery. Varicose veins, venous thrombosis, pulmonary embolism, and the postphlebitic extremity have been the four major topics.

Varicose veins were treated surgically in Da Costa's era by extensive local resection, through incisions at times nearly the entire length of the leg. Homans[245] is given credit for the introduction of the concept of interruption of the saphenous vein in the groin to control regurgitant flow down the saphenous system, but Trendelenberg[246] had performed a similar operation in 1890. Babcock[247] devised techniques to strip or avulse veins by means of extraluminal strippers; the Mayo external stripper has been for many years a useful instrument to facilitate dissection of the vein.[248]

Pulmonary embolism has long been a major problem for physicians in all areas of medical practice. In 1908, Trendelenburg[249] introduced the operation of pulmonary embolectomy. This operation has been infrequently undertaken and usually unsuccessful, but its rare successes have continued to challenge surgeons to improve it. It is an operation that can be applied more frequently today because of the ability to support the patient's cardiovascular system until the operation can be performed. Its role may be displaced by the ability of the radiologist to place catheters in the pulmonary artery and dissolve the clot with thrombolytic agents.

In 1934, the true relationship between deep, bland venous thrombosis of the leg veins and pulmonary embolism was clarified by John Homans of Boston,[250] who matched the ends of a thrombus taken from the pulmonary artery at autopsy with residual clot in the popliteal vein and thus indicated that this must have been the source of the embolus. Homans recognized that the great venous sinuses in the soleal veins are capable of returning large quantities of blood during exercise, but that at other times blood may indeed be stagnant there. Thus, given the other factors of Virchow's triad (stagnant flow, endothelial injury, increased coagulability), one might anticipate spontaneous thrombosis at this site. In fact, subsequent studies with radioiodinated fibrinogen have shown an alarming rate of thrombosis in this area; fortunately, only a very small proportion of these thromboses yield thrombi that propagate into the mainline channels and produce serious clinical problems.

The next step in the management of the patient with venous thrombosis was also made by Homans,[251, 252] who introduced the ligation of the femoral (superficial) vein where it joins the deep femoral system in the groin. This procedure must be viewed in the context of the times; there was no practical anticoagulant commonly in use. Allen,[253] Veal,[254] and others quickly took up this operation.

Disappointment came to Homans when a patient, whose superficial femoral vein he and I had ligated, propagated a clot through the deep femoral system and into the common femoral vein and suffered a fatal embolism, despite superficial femoral interruption.

The level of venous ligation was moved upward[252] because of similar failures of superficial femoral vein interruption. First the common femoral and then the external iliac veins were ligated bilaterally. These operations could be performed under local anesthesia through groin incisions, but because it was soon recognized that bilateral ligation of the iliac veins was indicated, the level was shortly raised to the vena cava. It is hard to identify who first did ligate the vena cava for pulmonary embolism, but Northway and Buxton,[255] O'Neill,[256] and Collins and coworkers[257] are all credited with early reports.

It seems unfortunate that as anticoagulants became commonly available—first Coumadin (Endo Labs) and then heparin—their use was not commonly combined with ligation; ligation and anticoagulation were on an "either one or the other" basis. Simple ligation without anticoagulant therapy was associated with a serious frequency of increased thrombosis in the stagnant systems below the ligature, which often led to severe postphlebitic symptoms. Anlyan and colleagues,[258] Bowers and Leh,[259] and others seriously criticized interruption and, in fact, gave rise to a school that treated venous thrombosis with increasingly large doses of heparin.[260] The extent of the postphlebitic syndrome, however, seems to be more clearly related to the extent of the inflammatory thrombophlebitic process and its destruction of the valves than it does to ligation or to the level of ligation.[261] The successful use of large doses

of heparin has greatly diminished the need for venous interruption.

Another approach to venous interruption, however, was to maintain some flow through the cava and still prevent the passage of emboli to the lungs by plication of the cava with sutures.[262] Some extravascular occlusive devices were suggested by Moretz and associates,[263] by Miles and colleagues,[264] and by Adams and DeWeese.[265] Mobin-Uddin's invention of a transvenous umbrella[266] and Greenfield and associates' transvenous wire trap[267] and its successors have reduced even further the need for major venous interruption by open surgical methods.

The problems of the postphlebitic extremity remain. This syndrome was well described by Homans,[268] but his contributions to its therapy were not particularly fruitful, except that his regimen included some of the best forms of nonoperative therapy. Trout,[269] Linton,[270] and Dodd and Cockett[271] separately advocated methods that accomplish subfascial interruption of the communicating veins in the lower leg; this procedure remains a surgical standard.

The re-creation of a venous drainage channel that is protected from regurgitant flow has offered a new approach to this old problem. Kistner[272] demonstrated the technique of making an incompetent valve into a competent one. Venous transposition is another approach chosen by Dale[273] and by Palma.[274] Taheri and coworkers[275] have described the results of a free graft of a valved segment of the axillary vein into the diseased femoral system. Taheri and others[276] have gone in further with the attempts to develop prosthetic venous valves.

HIGHLIGHTS IN DIAGNOSTIC MODALITIES

The diagnosis of both arterial and venous diseases has long depended on the use of contrast radiography. One of the first to use this successfully was Brooks,[277] who injected sodium iodide to demonstrate the lesions of Buerger's disease in digital vessels. Moniz[278] described "arterial encephalography" for neurologic lesions in the living patient in 1927. His presentation was not only a seminal paper; it recognized the needs of the radiographer in terms that are pertinent more than 70 years later.

In the audience at Moniz' presentation were Reynaldo dos Santos and his son, João Cid dos Santos. The father[279] soon published the basic technical approach to the arteriography of the vessels of the abdomen and their branches. Each of these authors foresaw the great advances in the development of rapid cassette changers and contrast media with less toxicity, but the techniques of image enhancement and subtraction by electronic means are more recent contributions.[280]

One of the major technical advances was Seldinger's technique,[281] which, instead of using a single needle for the injection of the contrast material, used a catheter passed over a wire that in turn is introduced through the primary arterial puncture. The wire is advanced to the desired site, and then the appropriate catheter is advanced over the wire. Wire and catheter can be alternated so that injections can be made at different sites and at different rates. This method allows the radiologist to place a catheter at almost any site in the body. The culmination of these technical advances is intravenous injection, digitalization of the signal from the fluoroscopic screen, and enhancement of the output and its clarification by subtraction.

A totally different aspect of radiology was signaled by such work as that of Dotter and Judkins,[141] who used a rigid dilator passed through a large catheter-sheath under fluoroscopic guidance to dilate narrowed arteries; this has led to the burgeoning field of *interventional* rather than purely diagnostic radiology.

The growth of vascular surgery has lately been almost synonymous with the development of methods of noninvasive diagnosis of peripheral vascular disease. This is an outgrowth of those methods commonly taken for granted, which had their humble beginnings in the stethoscope, the sphygmomanometer,[282] and the ophthalmoscope.

The measurement of many physiologic parameters in the laboratory was brought to bear on the patient by such physicians as Winsor,[283] whose evaluation of pressure gradients remains a critical basis for the clinical estimation of the severity of arterial obstruction. Other parameters commonly measured in the early vascular diagnostic laboratories included digital and segmental plethysmography and skin temperature and resistance, both before and after sympathetic blockade.

Pachon[284] introduced a modification of the sphygmomanometer and the segmental plethysmograph as the oscillometer, which provided a very rough measure of the volume of the distensile arterial pulse wave. The figures obtained bear no physiologic definition, but comparisons at different levels in one extremity, of comparable levels in different extremities, and of one site on successive occasions did provide the surgeon with some objective evidence of change. Although the stethoscope is used by all physicians, its role in the evaluation of murmurs over the peripheral arteries was clarified and codified by Edwards and Levine[285] and then by Wylie and McGuiness.[286] It is intriguing to remember that Barth[15] listened to the carotid arteries in his patient with aortic obstruction in 1835.

One of the interesting early techniques was that of Baillart,[287] who used the ophthalmoscope and ophthalmodynamometry to evaluate lesions of the eye. Operator sensitivity and reproducibility—critical aspects of many similar techniques— were such that the utility of the technique was not great. Kartchner and coworkers,[288] however, introduced a recording device to reproduce relative pressure curves within the ocular globe and to compare the peak time of the retinal artery pulse wave, which is reflected in the globe's pressure on each side, as well as with the arrival of the pulse wave in the ear lobe, which enabled estimation of the severity of obstruction in the carotid system. Gee and associates[289] developed a method to evaluate backpressure in the totally occluded carotid to predict the necessity for the use of shunt during operative carotid occlusion. Their method has, however, come to be of greater value in the evaluation of forward-pressure beyond the stenotic carotid, because it provides more precise measurement of the pressures, but it does not provide the accurate time relationships of Kartchner's system. Each of these was a useful step but was only a step to superior diagnostic methods.

Ultrasonography is one of the most popular modalities

in its many ramifications. Leopold and associates[290] used classical ultrasonic imaging (B mode) techniques to outline the aorta as well as other abdominal viscera. Ultrasonography in another form (i.e., in either the continuous or the gated Doppler mode that allows measurement of the shift in frequency of the ultrasonic signal reflected from moving red blood cells) was introduced by Strandness and colleagues[291] and by Sumner and Strandness.[292] Combined with a sphygmomanometer, this method has become one of the most useful and standard means of evaluating peripheral arterial disease and of identifying segmental pressure differences, just as Winsor had done with less satisfactory equipment. The use of the ultrasonic flow detector was soon modified by Brockenbrough[293] to determine the direction of flow through the supraorbital artery, which is reversed in the presence of high-grade obstruction of the ipsilateral carotid artery. Machleder and Barker[294] dramatized the technique, but the extreme operator sensitivity limits its use considerably. Technical improvements have made it possible to use this method to evaluate intracranial flow at the base of the brain[295, 296] and even visceral branches in the abdomen.[297]

Imaging of the crude Doppler signal was introduced by Thomas and others,[298] who simply mounted a Doppler probe on a scanning device. Sophistication of these scanning methods with a combination of the regular ultrasonic B-mode scanning to display the anatomy and to obtain a reference point from which pulsed Doppler reflections can be read allows exact identification of blood flow patterns, especially by color coding velocities at the site within the lumen in arteries that can be "reached" by the Doppler signal.[299] This method was at first used in the carotid bifurcation, but it has been extended to common use in peripheral arterial sites, in the mesenteric vessels,[297] and as a monitoring device at the operating table.[300]

As carotid angiography has been shown in the many recent randomized trials to contribute a major proportion of the morbidity and mortality to carotid surgery, the duplex color-coded scan imaging has rapidly replaced the more expensive and dangerous method of carotid contrast angiography as the primary diagnostic tool. It provides highly accurate anatomic data as well as physiologic information, although there are still needs for arteriography in some patients.

A new twist on computerized tomography was introduced radiologically by Kalender and associates.[301] Among the first presentations to the vascular surgeons was a paper by Rubin and others.[302] This form of spiral computerized tomography has also come into more common use, and although its images may lose some of the detail obtained by other methods, it does provide a superb overall picture of the course and collaterals of an arterial segment, and its software allows manipulation so that the image can be visualized from many different angles appearing in three dimensions.

Evaluation of the venous side of the circulation has not provided such exact information. Cranley and coworkers[303] introduced phleborrheography, which evaluates the changes in venous pulse, outflow, and respiratory excursions in the diagnosis of deep venous disease of the legs. Less sophisticated, easier to handle, but perhaps less informative is Wheeler's impedance plethysmography.[304]

The Doppler velocity probe, despite some drawbacks of operator sensitivity, remains a useful method for identifying obstruction in the available superficial major veins, such as in the groin, the popliteal space, and the axilla. It can also be used in the postphlebitic extremity to identify both regurgitant flow in superficial channels and flow from communicating veins and can be used even in the presence of brawny edema that otherwise obscures much of the venous system from sight and palpation.

Just as the duplex scan in carotid surgery has become popular, so has color-assisted duplex imaging come to be an important part of the evaluation of the venous system.[305]

References

1. Dobson J: John Hunter. Edinburgh, E & S Livingstone, 1969.
2. Gray EA: Portrait of a Surgeon. A Biography of John Hunter. London, Robert Hale, 1952.
3. Hunter WA: History of aneurism of the aorta with some remarks on aneurisms in general. Med Obs Inquiries 1:323, 1757.
4. Cames C: Wörtliche Uebersetzung des Werkes des römischen Artzes Antyllus: Düsseldorf, Michael Trilitsch Verlag, 1941, p 107.
5. Purmann MG: Chirurgia Curiosa, Edition of 1716, p 612.
6. Erichsen Sir JE: Observation on Aneurism (Anel). London, Sydenham Society, 1844, p 216.
7. Erichsen Sir JE: Observation on Aneurism (Hunter). London, Sydenham Society, 1844, p 404.
8. Brock RC: Astley Cooper and carotid artery ligation. Guy's Hospital Reports (Special Number) 117:219, 1968.
9. Tyrell FG: The lectures of Sir Astley Cooper, Bart, FRCS, on the principles and practice of surgery (4th American edition from the last London edition). Philadelphia, Carey EL, Hart A, 1835, pp 212–214.
10. Lambert R: Letter from Mr Lambert to Dr Hunter: Giving an account of a new method of treating an aneurism. Med Obs Inquiries, June 15, 1761.
11. Asman C: Inaugural dissertation. Groningen, The Netherlands, University of Groningen, 1773.
12. Blane G: (Communication without title). Transactions Soc Improvement Med Chir Knowledge 2:1, 1800.
13. Cooper Sir A: The lectures of Sir Astley Cooper, Bart, FRCS, On the Principles and Practice of Surgery, 2nd ed. London, FC Westley, 1830, p 98.
14. Cruveilhier J: Senile Gangrene. Anatomie Pathologique du Corps Humain, Section 27 (Malades des Arteres, 1–8, Plate v. 27), Paris, 1835–1842.
15. Barth (No initial): Observation d'une obliteration complet de l'aorte abdominale, recuillie dans le service de M. Louis, suivie de reflections. Arch Gen Med, Second Series, 8:26–53, 1835.
16. Charcot JM: Obstruction artérielle et claudication intermittente dans le cheval et dans l'homme. Mem Soc Biol 1:225–238, 1858.
17. Bouley J: Claudication intermittente des membres postérieures par l'oblitération des artères fémorales. Recueil de Médecin Vétérinaire 8:517, 1831.
18. Langenbeck CJM: Pathology and Therapy of Surgical Illnesses, vol 3. Göttingen, Heimatsverlag, 1825, p 414.
19. Heinecke W: Bluting, Blutstillung, Transfusion nebst Luftentritt und Infusion. In Billroth T, Luecke H (eds): Deutsche Chirurgie. Stuttgart, Verlag von Ferdinand Enke, 1885.
20. Jassinowsky A: Die Arteriennaht: Eine experimentelle Studie. Inaugural dissertation for the Degree of Doctor of Medicine, Dorpat (now Tartu), Estonia, University of Tartu, 1889.
21. Czerny V: On lateral closure of vein wounds. Langenbeck's Arch Chir 28:671, 1881.
22. Schede M: Einege Bemerkungen über die Naht von Venenwunden. Arch Klin Chir 43:548, 1883.
23. Eck NV K: voprosu o perevyazkie vorotnois veni. Prevaritelnoye soobshtshjenye. Woen Med J (St Petersburg) 130:1–2, 1877 (as cited by Child CG III: Eck's fistula. Surg Gynecol Obstet 96:375–376, 1953).
24. Jassinowsky A: Ein Beitrag zur Lehre von der Gefässnaht. Arch Klin Chir 40:816–841, 1891.
25. Dörfler J: Ueber Arteriennaht. Beitr Klin Chir 22:781–825, 1899.
26. Jaboulay M, Briau E: Recherches expérimentales sur la suture et la greffe artérielles. Bull Lyon Med 81:97–99, 1896.
27. Edwards P, Edwards WS: Alexis Carrel, Visionary Surgeon. Springfield, IL, Charles C Thomas, 1974.
28. Carrel A: Les anastomoses vasculaires et leur technique opératoire. Union Med Can 1904, 33:521–527.
29. Carrel A: The surgery of blood vessels, etc. Johns Hopkins Hosp Bull 190:18–28, 1907.
30. Harbison SP: The origins of vascular surgery: The Carrel-Guthrie letters. Surgery 52:406–418, 1962.
31. Goyanes J: Nuevos trabajos de chirurgia vascular, substitucion plastica de los arterios por las venas o arterioplatica venosa, applicada como nuevo metodo al tratamiento de los aneurismas. El Siglo Med 53:546–549, 561–568, 1906.
32. Matas R: Traumatic aneurism of the left brachial artery. Med News 53:462–466, 1888.
33. Cohn I Sr: Rudolph Matas. New York, Doubleday and Company, 1960.
34. Matas R: Some experiences and observations in the treatment of arteriovenous aneurisms by the intrasaccular method of suture (endoaneurismorrhaphy) with special reference to the transvenous route. Ann Surg 71:403–427, 1920.
35. Bickham WS: Arteriovenous aneurisms. A case of traumatic arteriovenous aneurism of the common femoral artery and vein unsuccessfully treated by a new method of compression—and finally cured by the proximal ligation of the external iliac artery extraperitoneally—with the suggestion that the application to these aneurisms of the Matas method of operation used for ordinary aneurisms—and the mention of some other recent methods of operating. Ann Surg 39:767–775, 1904.
36. Murphy JB: Resection of arteries and veins injured in continuity . . . end-to-end suture . . . experimental and clinical research. Med Rec 51:73–88, 1897.
37. Edwards WS, Tapp JS: Chemically treated nylon tubes as arterial grafts. Surgery 38:61–76, 1955.
38. Nitze F: Kleinere Mittheilungen Kongres im Moskau. Zentralbl Chir 39:1042, 1897.
39. Payr E: Beiträge zur Technik der Blutgefässe und der Nervennaht nebst Mittheilungen die Verwundung eines resorbibaren Metalles in der Chirurgie. Arch Klin Chir 62:67–93, 1900.
40. Blakemore AH, Lord JW Jr, Stefko PL: The severed primary artery in war wounded: A nonsuture method of bridging arterial defects. Surgery 12:488–508, 1942.
41. Elkin ED, DeBakey ME: Vascular Surgery (Surgery in World War II, vol 4). Washington, DC, Office of the Surgeon General, 1955.
42. Halsted WS: (in discussion of a paper by Matas R) Some of the problems related to the surgery of the vascular system: Testing the efficiency of the collateral circulation as a preliminary to the occlusion of the great surgical arteries. Trans Am Surg Assoc 28:49–51, 1910.
43. Höpfner E: Ueber Gefässnaht, Gefässtransplantionen und Replantationen von amputieren Extremitäten. Arch Klin Chir 70:417–471, 1903.
44. Lexer E: Die ideale Operation des arteriellen und des arteriellvenösen Aneurysma. Arch Klin Chir 83:459–477, 1907.
45. Lexer E: 20 Jahre Transplantionsforschung in der Chirurgie. Arch Klin Chir 138:251–302, 1925.
46. Jeger E: Die Chirurgie der Blutgefässe und des Herzens (replication of 1913 edition). Berlin, Springer-Verlag, 1973.
47. Weglowski R: Ueber de Gefässtransplantation. Zentralbl Chir 40:2241–2243, 1925.
48. Abbe R: The surgery of the hand. N Y Med J 1894, 59:33–40, 1894.
49. Tuffier M: De l'intubation dans les plaies des grosses artères. Bull Acad Med 74:455–460, 1915.
50. Hufnagel CA: Permanent intubation of the thoracic aorta. Arch Surg 54:382–389, 1947.

51. Hufnagel CA: Preserved homologous arterial transplants. Bull Am Coll Surg 32:231, 1947.
52. Gross RE, Hurwitt ES, Bill AH Jr, Peirce EC II: Preliminary observations on the use of human arterial grafts in the treatment of certain cardiovascular defects. N Engl J Med 239:578–579, 1948.
53. Deterling RA Jr, Coleman CC, Parshley MS: Experimental studies on the frozen homologous aortic graft. Surgery 29:419–440, 1951.
54. Marangoni AG, Cecchini LP: Homotransplantation of arterial segments by the freeze-drying method. Ann Surg 134:977–983, 1951.
55. Voorhees AB Jr, Jaretzki A III, Blakemore AH: Use of tubes constructed of Vinyon-"N" cloth in bridging arterial defects. Ann Surg 135:332–336, 1952.
56. Deterling RA, Bhonslay SB: An evaluation of synthetic materials and fabrics suitable for blood vessel replacement. Surgery 38:7189, 1955.
57. Hufnagel CA: The use of rigid and flexible plastic prosthesis for arterial replacement. Surgery 37:165–174, 1955.
58. Girvin GW, Wilhelm MC, Merendino KA: The use of Teflon fabric as arterial grafts. An experimental study in dogs. Am J Surg 92:240–247, 1956.
59. Szilagyi DE, France LC, Smith RF, et al: Clinical use of an elastic Dacron prosthesis. Arch Surg 77:538–551, 1958.
60. Julian OC, Deterling RA, Dye WS, et al: Dacron tube and bifurcation prosthesis produced to specification. Surgery 41:50–61, 1957.
61. Wesolowski SA, Dennis CA (eds): Fundamentals of Vascular Grafting. New York, The Blakiston Division, McGraw-Hill Book Company, 1963.
62. Wesolowski SA, Fries CC, Karlson KE, et al: Porosity: Primary determinant of ultimate fate of synthetic vascular grafts. Surgery 50:91–96, 1961.
63. DeBakey ME, Cooley DA, Crawford ES, Morris GC Jr: Clinical application of a new flexible knitted Dacron arterial substitute. Arch Surg 77:713–724, 1958.
64. Sauvage G, Berger KE, Wood SJ, et al: An external velour surface for porous arterial prosthesis. Surgery 70:940–953, 1971.
65. Cooley DA, Wukasch DC, Bennet JC, et al: Double velour knitted grafts for aorto-iliac replacement. In Sawyer PN, Kaplitt MJ (eds): Vascular Grafts. New York, Appleton-Century-Crofts, 1978.
66. Quiñones-Baldrich WJ, Moore WS, Ziomek S, Chvapil M: Development of a "leak-proof" knitted Dacron vascular prosthesis. J Vasc Surg 3:895–903, 1986.
67. Guidion R, Snyder R, Martin L, et al: Albumin coating of a knitted polyester arterial prosthesis: An alternative to preclotting. Ann Thorac Surg 37:457–465, 1984.
68. Soyer T, Lempinen M, Cooper P, et al: A new venous prosthesis. Surgery 72:864–872, 1972.
69. Veith FJ, Gupta SK, Ascer E, et al: Six-year prospective multicenter randomized comparison of autologous saphenous vein and expanded polytetrafluoroethylene grafts in infrainguinal arterial reconstructions. J Vasc Surg 3:104–114, 1986.
70. Rosenberg NL, Henderson J, Lord GW, et al: Use of enzyme treated heterografts as arterial substitutes. Arch Surg 85:192–197, 1969.
71. Sawyer PN, Stancezewski B, Lucas TR, et al: Experimental and clinical evaluation of a new negatively charged bovine heterograft for use in peripheral and coronary revascularization. In Sawyer PN, Kaplitt MJ (eds): Vascular Grafts. New York, Appleton-Century Crofts, 1978.
72. Dardik H, Ibrahim IM, Sprayregan S, et al: Clinical experiences with modified human umbilical cord vein for arterial bypass. Surgery 79:618–624, 1976.
73. Leonardo RA: History of Surgery. New York, Froben Press, 1943, p 139.
74. Power DA: The palliative treatment of aneurysms by "wiring" with Colt's apparatus. Br J Surg 9:27–36, 1921.
75. Blakemore AH, King BG: Electrothermic coagulation of aortic aneurysms. JAMA 111:1821–1827, 1938.
76. Reid M: Aneurysms in the Johns Hopkins Hospital. All cases treated in the surgical service from the opening of the hospital to January 1922. Arch Surg 12:1–73, 1926.
77. Matas R: Ligation of the abdominal aorta: Report of the ultimate result, one year, five months and nine days after the ligation of the abdominal aorta for aneurysm of the bifurcation. Ann Surg 81:457–464, 1925.
78. Matas R: Aneurysm of the abdominal aorta at its bifurcation into the common iliac arteries. Ann Surg 112:909–922, 1940.
79. Elkin DC: Aneurysm of the abdominal aorta: Treatment by ligation. Ann Surg 112:895–905, 1940.
80. Bigger IA: Surgical treatment of aneurysm of the aorta: Review of literature and report of two cases, one apparently successful. Ann Surg 112:879–894, 1940.
81. Alexander J, Byron FX: Aortectomy for thoracic aneurysm. JAMA 126:1139–1145, 1944.
82. Alexander JT, Byron FX: Aortectomy for thoracic aneurysm: A supplemental report. JAMA 132:22, 1946.
83. Pearse HE: Experimental studies on the gradual occlusion of large arteries. Ann Surg 122:923–937, 1940.
84. Yeager G, Cowley RA: Studies on the use of polythene as a fibrous tissue stimulant. Ann Surg 128:509–520, 1948.
85. Cutler EC, Levine SA, Beck CC: The surgical treatment of mitral stenosis. Arch Surg 9:689–821, 1924.
86. Gross RE: A surgical approach for ligation of a patent ductus arteriosus. N Engl J Med 220:510–514, 1939.
87. Gross RE: Complete surgical division of the patent ductus arteriosus. Surg Gynecol Obstet 78:36–43, 1944.
88. Blalock A, Taussig HB: The surgical treatment of malformations of the heart in which there is pulmonary stenosis or pulmonary atresia. JAMA 128:189–202, 1945.
89. Crafoord C, Nylin G: Congenital coarctation of the aorta and its surgical treatment. J Thorac Surg 14:347–361, 1945.
90. Gross RE, Hugfnagel CA: Coarctation of the aorta. Experimental studies regarding its correction. N Engl J Med 233: 287–293, 1945.
91. Swan H, Maaske C, Johnson M, et al: Arterial homografts: II. Resection of thoracic aneurysm using a stored human arterial transplant. Arch Surg 61:732–737, 1950.
92. Estes JE Jr: Abdominal aortic aneurysm: A study of 102 cases. Circulation 2:258–264, 1950.
93. Oudot J: La greffe vasculaire dans les thromboses du carrefour aortique. Presse Med 59:234–236, 1951.
94. Dubost C, Allary M, Oeconomos N: Resection of an aneurysm of the abdominal aorta: Reestablishment of the continuity by a preserved human arterial graft, with result after five months. Arch Surg 64:405–408, 1952.
95. Schaffer PW, Hardin CW: The use of temporary and polythene shunts to permit occlusion, resection and frozen homologous artery graft replacement of vital vessel segments. Surgery 31:186–199, 1952.
96. Julian OC, Grove LVJ, Dye WS, et al: Direct surgery of arteriosclerosis. Resection of abdominal aorta with homologous aortic graft replacement. Ann Surg 138:387–403, 1953.
97. Brock RC: Reconstructive arterial surgery. Proc Soc Med 46:115–130, 1953.
98. DeBakey ME, Cooley DA: Surgical treatment of aneurysm of abdominal aorta by resection and restoration of continuity with homograft. Surg Gynecol Obstet 97:257–266, 1953.
99. Bahnson HT: Considerations in the excision of aortic aneurysms. Ann Surg 138:377–386, 1953.
100. Freeman NE, Leeds FH: Vein inlay graft in treatment of aneurysm and thrombosis of abdominal aorta: Preliminary communication with report of 3 cases. Angiology 2:579–587, 1951.
101. Wylie EJ Jr, Kerr E, Davies O: Experimental and clinical experiences with use of fascia lata applied as a graft about major arteries after thromboendarterectomy and aneurysmorrhaphy. Surg Gynecol Obstet 93:257–272, 1951.
102. Barker WF, Cannon JA: An evaluation of endarterectomy. Arch Surg 66:488–495, 1953.
103. Szilagyi DE, Smith RE, DeRusso FJ, et al: Contribution of abdominal aortic aneurysmectomy to prolongation of life. Ann Surg 164:678–699, 1966.
104. Ellis FH, Helden RA, Hines EA Jr: Aneurysm of the abdominal aorta involving the right renal artery: Report of a case with preservation of renal function after resection and grafting. Ann Surg 142:992–995, 1955.
105. Etheredge SN, Yee JY, Smith JV, et al: Successful resection of a large aneurysm of the upper abdominal aorta and replacement with homograft. Surgery 38:1071–1081, 1955.
106. Shumacker HB Jr: Innovation in the operative management of the thoracoabdominal aneurysm. Surg Gynecol Obstet 136:793–794, 1973.
107. DeBakey ME, Creech O, Morris GC: Aneurysm of the thoracoabdominal aorta involving the celiac, mesenteric and renal arteries. Report of four cases treated by resection and homograft replacement. Ann Surg 144:549–573, 1956.

108. Stoney RJ, Wylie EJ: Surgical management of arterial lesions of the thoracoabdominal aorta. Am J Surg 126:157–164, 1973.
109. Crawford ES: Thoraco-abdominal aortic aneurysms involving renal, superior mesenteric and celiac arteries. Ann Surg 179:763–772, 1974.
110. Dotter CT, Buschman RW, McKinney MK, Rösch J: Transluminal expandable Nitinol coil stent grafting: Preliminary report. Radiology 147:251–260, 1983.
111. Palmaz JC, Sibbitt RR, Reuter SR, et al: Expandable intraluminal graft: Preliminary study. Radiology 156: 73–77, 1985.
112. Parodi J, Palmaz JC, Barone HD: Transfemoral intraluminal graft implantation for abdominal aortic aneurysms. Ann Vasc Surg 5:491–499, 1991.
113. White GH, Yu W, May J, et al: A new nonstented balloon expandable graft for straight or bifurcated endoluminal bypass. J Endovasc Surg 1:16–24, 1994.
114. Moore WS: The role of endovascular grafting technique in the treatment of abdominal aortic aneurysm. Cardiovasc Surg 3:109–114, 1995.
115. Moore WS, Vescera CL: Repair of abdominal aortic aneurysm by transfemoral endovascular graft placement. Ann Surg 220:331–341, 1994.
116. Linton RR: The arteriosclerotic popliteal aneurysm. A report of 14 patients treated by preliminary lumbar sympathectomy and aneurysmectomy. Surgery 2:41–58, 1949.
117. Whychullis AR, Spittel JS Jr, Wallace RB: Popliteal aneurysms. Surgery 68:942–952, 1970.
118. Gifford RW Jr, Hines EA Jr, Janes JM: An analysis and follow-up study of one hundred popliteal aneurysms. Surgery 33:284–293, 1953.
119. Wylie EJ (in discussion of Whycullis[117] above).
120. Edwards WS: Exclusion and saphenous bypass of popliteal aneurysm. Surg Gynecol Obstet 128:829–830, 1969.
121. Leriche R: Souvenirs de ma Vie Mort. Paris, Editions du Seuil, 1956.
122. Leriche R: De la causalgie envisagée comme une névrite du sympathetique et de son traitement par la dénudation et l'excision des plexus nerveux périartèriels. Presse Med 23:178–180, 1916.
123. Diez J: Le traitement des affections trophiques et gangréneuses des membres inférieurs par la resection du sympathique lombosacre. Rev Neurol 33:184–192, 1926.
124. Royle N: A new operative procedure in the treatment of spastic paralysis and its experimental basis. Med J Aust 1:77–86, 1924.
125. Hunter JI: The influence of the sympathetic nervous system in the genesis of rigidity in striated muscle in spastic paralysis. Surg Gynecol Obstet 39:721–743, 1924.
126. Leriche R: Des obliterations artérielles hautes (obliteration de la terminacion de l'aorte) comme causes des insuffisances circulatoires des membres inférieurs. Bull Mem Soc Chir (Paris) 49:1404–1406, 1923.
127. Leriche R: De la résection du carrefour aortico-iliaque avec double sympathectomie lombaire pour thrombose artéritique de l'aorte. Le syndrome de l'oblitération terminoaortique par artérite. Presse Med 48:601–604, 1940.
128. Murphy JB: Removal of an embolus from the common iliac artery, with re-establishment of circulation in the femoral. JAMA 52:1661–1663, 1909.
129. Mosny N, Dumont MJ: Embolie fémorale au cours d'un rétrécissement mitral pur. Artèriotomie. Guérison. Bull Acad Natl Med (Paris) 66:358–361, 1908.
130. Murray GDW: Heparin in thrombosis and embolism. Br J Surg 27:567–598, 1939.
131. dos Santos JC: From embolectomy to endarterectomy or the fall of a myth. J Cardiovasc Surg 17:113–128, 1976.
132. dos Santos JC: Sur la désobstruction des thromboses artérielles anciennes. Mem Acad Chir 73:409–111, 1947.
133. Bazy L, Hugier J, Reboul H, et al: Technique des "endartérectomies" pour artérites oblitérantes chroniques des membres inférieures, des iliaques, et de l'aorte abdominale inferiéur. J Chir 65:196–210, 1949.
134. Cannon JA, Barker WF: Successful management of obstructive femoral arteriosclerosis by endarterectomy. Surgery 38:48–60, 1955.
135. Butcher HR Jr: A simple technique for endarterectomy. Surgery 44:984–989, 1958.
136. Vollmar J, Laubach K: Chirurgische Behandlung der arterielle Embolie. Ring-desobliteration der Stombahn. Munchen Med Wochanschr 107:756–763, 1965.
137. Kunlin J: Le traitement de l'ischémie artéritique par la greffe veineuse longue. Revue de Chirurgie. Rev Chir 70:206–235, 1951.
138. Oudot J: Un deuxième cas de greffe de la bifurcation aortique pour thrombose de la fourche aortique. Mem Acad Chir 77:644–645, 1951.
139. Linton RR: Some practical considerations in surgery of blood vessel grafts. Surgery 38:817–834, 1955.
140. Edwards WS: Composite reconstruction of the femoral artery with saphenous vein after endarterectomy. Surg Gynecol Obstet 111:651–653, 1960.
141. Dotter CT, Judkins MP: Percutaneous transluminal treatment of arteriosclerotic obstruction. Radiology 84:631–643, 1956.
142. Gruntzig A, Hopff H: Perkutane Recanalisation chronischer arterieller Arterienverschlusse mit einem neuen Dilatations-katheter: Modification der Dotter-Technik. Dtsch Med Wochenschr 99:2502–2505, 1974.
143. Greenstone SM, Shore JM, Heringman EC, Massell TB: Arterial endoscopy (arterioscopy). Arch Surg 93:811–812, 1966.
144. Bom N: Intra-arterial ultrasonic imaging for recanalization by spark erosion. SPIE 904:107–109, 1988.
145. Simpson JB, Johnson DE, Thapliyal HV, et al: Transluminal atherectomy: A new approach to the treatment of atherosclerotic vascular disease. Circulation 72(Suppl 2): III–146, 1985.
146. Kensey KR, Nash JE, Abrahams C, Zarins CK: Recanalization of obstructed arteries with a flexible, rotating tip catheter. Radiology 165:387–389, 1987.
147. Ahn SS, Auth DC, Marcus DR, Moore WS: Removal of focal atheromatous lesions by angioscopically guided high-speed rotary atherectomy: Preliminary experimental observations. J Vasc Surg 7:292–300, 1988.
148. Grundfest WS, Litvack F, Forrester JS, et al: Laser ablation of human atherosclerotic plaque without adjacent tissue injury. J Am Coll Cardiol 5:929–933, 1985.
149. Murphy-Chetorian D, Kosek J, Mok W, et al: Selective absorption of ultraviolet laser energy by human atherosclerotic plaque treated with tetracycline. Am J Cardiol 55:1293–1297, 1985.
150. Abela GS, Fenech A, Crea F, Conti CR: "Hot-tip": Another method of laser vascular recanalization. Lasers Surg Med 5:327–335, 1985.
151. Palma EC: Treatment of arteritis of the lower limbs by autogenous vein grafts. Minerva Cardioangiol Eur 8:36–49, 1960.
152. McCaughan JJ Jr: Surgical exposure of the distal popliteal artery. Surgery 44:536–539, 1958.
153. McCaughan JJ Jr: Study of 100 consecutive bypass grafts of the femoral artery. Memphis Med J 35:227–237, 1960.
154. McCaughan JJ Jr: Bypass graft to the posterior tibial artery at the ankle: Case reports. Am Surg 32:126–130, 1966.
155. Morris GC Jr, DeBakey ME, Cooley DA, Crawford ES: Arterial bypass below the knee. Surg Gynecol Obstet 108:321–332, 1959.
156. Tyson RR, DeLaurentis DA: Femorotibial bypass. Circulation 33/34(Suppl I 1):183–188, 1966.
157. Hall KV: The great saphenous vein used in situ as in arterial shunt after extirpation of the vein valves. Surgery 51:492–495, 1962.
158. Leather RP, Shah DM, Karmody AM: Infrapopliteal bypass for limb salvage: Increased patency and utilization of the saphenous vein "in situ." Surgery 90:1000–1008, 1981.
159. Dardik H, Sussman B, Ibrahim IM, et al: Distal arteriovenous fistula as an adjunct to maintaining arterial graft patency for limb salvage. Surgery 94:478–486, 1983.
160. DeLaurentis DA, Friedman P: Segmental femorotibial bypass: Another approach to the inadequate saphenous vein problem. Surgery 71:400–404, 1972.
161. Veith FJ, Ascer E, Gupta SJ, et al: Tibiotibial vein bypass grafts: A new operation for limb salvage. J Vasc Surg 2:552–557, 1985.
162. Nehler MR, Dalman RL, Harris EJ: Upper extremity arterial bypass distal to the wrist. J Vasc Surg 16:633–642, 1992.
163. Martin P, Renwick S, Stephenson C: On the surgery of the profunda femoris artery. Br J Surg 55:539–542, 1968.
164. Oudot J, Cormier JM: La localization la plus fréquente de l'artérite segmentaire celle de l'artère fémorale superficielle. Presse Med 61:1361–1364, 1953.
165. Miller T, Niazmand R, Barker WF: Femoral artery reconstruction under local anesthesia: Maximal results from minimal risks. Am J Surg 122:513–516, 1971.
166. Cohn LH, Trueblood W, Crowley LG: Profunda femoris reconstruction in the treatment of femoropopliteal occlusive disease. Arch Surg 103:475–479, 1971.

167. Towne JB, Bernhard VM, Rollins DL, et al: Profundaplasty in perspective: Limitations in the long-term management of limb ischemia. Surgery 90:1037–1046, 1981.

168. Von Winiwarter F: Ueber eine eigentümliche Form von Endarteritis und Endophlebitis mit Gangrän des Fusses. Arch Klin Chir 23:202–225, 1879.

169. Buerger L: Thrombo-angiitis obliterans: A study of the vascular lesions leading to presenile spontaneous gangrene. Am J Med Sci 136:567–580, 1908.

170. Fogarty TJ, Cranley JJ, Krause RJ, et al: A method of extraction of arterial emboli and thrombi. Surg Gynecol Obstet 116:241–244, 1963.

171. Mitchell SW, Morehouse GR, Keen WW: Gunshot Wounds and Other Injuries of Nerves. Philadelphia, Miller, 1864, pp 100–118.

172. Rich NL, Hughes CW: Vietnam: Vascular Registry: A preliminary report. Surgery 65:218–226, 1969.

173. Makins GH: On Gunshot Wounds to the Blood-Vessels. Bristol, John Wright and Sons, 1919.

174. DeBakey ME, Simeone FA: Battle injuries of the arteries in World War II. Ann Surg 123:534–579, 1946.

175. Jahnke EJ Jr, Howard JM: Primary repair of major arterial injuries. Arch Surg 66:646–649, 1953.

176. Hughes CW: Acute vascular trauma in Korean War casualties. An analysis of 180 cases. Surg Gynecol Obstet 99:91–100, 1954.

177. Spencer FC, Grewe RV: The management of arterial injuries in battle casualties. Ann Surg 141:304–313, 1955.

178. Whelan TJ, Burkhalter WE, Gomez CA: Management of war wounds. Adv Surg 3:227–350, 1968.

179. Soubbotitich V: Military experience of traumatic aneurysms. Lancet 2:720–721, 1913.

180. Holman E: Arteriovenous Aneurysms: Abnormal Communication between the Arterial and Venous Circulation. New York, Macmillan, 1937.

181. Savory WS: Case of a young woman in whom the main arteries of both upper extremities and of the left side of the neck were throughout completely obliterated. Med Chir Trans London 39:205–235, 1856.

182. Hunt JR: The role of the carotid arteries in the causation of vascular lesions of the brain with remarks on certain special features of the symptomatology. Am J Med Sci 147:704–713, 1914.

183. Fisher M: Occlusion of the internal carotid artery. Arch Neurol Psychiatr 65:346–377, 1951.

184. Fisher M: Occlusion of the carotid arteries: Further experiences. Arch Neurol Psychiatr 72:187–204, 1954.

185. Carrea R, Mollins M, Murphy G: Surgical treatment of spontaneous thrombosis of the internal carotid artery in the neck. Carotidcarotideal anastomosis. Report of a case. Acta Neurol Latinoam 1:71–78, 1955.

186. Lefèvre MH: Sur un cas de plaie du bulbe carotidien per balle, traitée par ligature de la carotid primitive et l'anastomose bout à bout de la carotid externe avec la carotid interne. Bull Mem Soc Chir 44:923–928, 1918.

187. Eastcott HHG, Pickering GW, Rob C: Reconstruction of internal carotid artery in a patient with intermittent attacks of hemiplegia. Lancet 2:994–996, 1954.

188. Cooley DA, Al-Naaman YD, Carton CA: Surgical treatment of arteriosclerotic occlusion of common carotid artery. J Neurosurg 13:500–506, 1956.

189. Roe WA: An early successful carotid endarterectomy, not previously reported. Presented at Southern California Vascular Surgery Society, Coronado, CA, September 11–12, 1992.

190. DeBakey ME: Successful carotid endarterectomy for cerebrovascular insufficiency: Nineteen year followup. JAMA 233:1083–1085, 1975.

191. Yates PO, Hutchinson EC: Cerebral infarction: The role of stenosis of the extracranial arteries. Med Res Council Spec Report (London) 300:1–95, 1961.

192. Whisnant JP, Matsumoto N, Eleback LR: Transient cerebral ischemic attacks in a community: Rochester, Minnesota, 1955 through 1969. Mayo Clin Proc 48:194–198, 1973.

193. Hollenhorst RW: Significance of bright plaques in the retinal arterioles. JAMA 178:23–29, 1961.

194. Julian OC, Dye WS, Javid H, Hunter JA: Ulcerative lesions of the carotid artery bifurcation. Arch Surg 86:803–809, 1963.

195. Moore WS, Hall AD: Ulcerated atheroma of the carotid artery: A cause of transient cerebral ischemia. Am J Surg 116:237–242, 1968.

196. Imparato AM, Riles TJ, Gorstein F: The carotid bifurcation plaque: Pathologic findings associated with cerebral ischemia. Stroke 10:238–245, 1979.

197. Lusby RJ, Ferrell LD, Ehrenfeld WA, et al: Carotid plaque hemorrhage: Its role in production of cerebral ischemia. Arch Surg 1982, 117: 147–148, 1982.

198. Moore WS, Hall AD: Carotid artery back pressure: A test of cerebral tolerance to temporary carotid artery occlusion. Arch Surg 99:702–710, 1969.

199. Thompson JE, Patman RD, Talkington CM: Asymptomatic carotid bruit. Ann Surg 188:308–316, 1978.

200. Dixon S, Pais SO, Raviola C, et al: Natural history of nonstenotic, asymptomatic ulcerations of the carotid artery: A further analysis. Arch Surg 117:1493–1498, 1982.

201. Berguer R, Sieggreen MY, Lazo VA, Hodakowski GT: The silent brain infarct in carotid surgery. J Vasc Surg 3:442–447, 1986.

202. Moore WS: Indications for carotid endarterectomy. Results of randomized trials. Paper presented at the 29th Annual "Controversial Areas in General Surgery," UCLA Extension Program, Palm Springs, California, Apr 2, 1992 .

203. Yasargil MG, Krayenbuhl KA, Jacobson JH II: Microneurosurgical arterial reconstruction. Surgery 67:221–223, 1970.

204. EC/IC Bypass Group: Failure of extracranial-intracranial bypass to reduce the risk of ischemic stroke: Results of an international randomized trial. N Engl J Med 313:1191–1200, 1985.

205. Longmire WP Jr, Cannon JA, Kattus HA: Direct-vision coronary endarterectomy for angina pectoris. N Engl J Med 259:993–999, 1958.

206. Favoloro RG: Saphenous vein autograft replacement of severe segmental coronary artery occlusion. Ann Thorac Surg 5:334–339, 1968.

207. Johnson WD, Flemman RJ, Lepley D Jr, et al: Extended treatment of severe coronary artery disease: A total surgical approach. Ann Surg 170:460–470, 1969.

208. Goldblatt H, Lynch J, Hanzal RF, et al: Studies on experimental hypertension. J Exp Med 59:347–379, 1934.

209. Freeman NE, Leeds FH, Elliott WG, Roland SI: Thromboendarterectomy for hypertension due to renal artery occlusion. JAMA 156:1077–1079, 1954.

210. DeCamp P, Snyder CH, Bost RB: Severe hypertension due to congenital stenosis of artery to solitary kidney: Correction by splenorenal anastomosis. Arch Surg 75: 1023–1026, 1957.

211. Poutasse EF: Surgical treatment of renal hypertension: Results in patients with occlusive lesions of renal arteries. J Urol 82:403–411, 1959.

212. Foster JH, Dean RH, Pinkerton JA, et al: Ten years' experience with renovascular hypertension. Ann Surg 177:755–766, 1973.

213. Connett MC, Lansche JM: Fibromuscular hyperplasia of the internal carotid artery. Report of a case. Ann Surg 162:59–62, 1965.

214. Ehrenfeld WK, Stoney RJ, Wylie EJ: Fibromuscular hyperplasia of the internal carotid artery. Arch Surg 95:284–287, 1967.

215. Dunphy JE: Abdominal pain of vascular origin. Am J Med Sci 92:109–113, 1936.

216. Klass J: Embolectomy in acute mesenteric occlusion. Ann Surg 34:913–917, 1951.

217. Shaw RS, Rutledge RH: Superior-mesenteric-artery embolectomy in treatment of massive mesenteric infarction. N Engl J Med 257:595–598, 1957.

218. Shaw RS, Maynard EP: Acute and chronic thrombosis of the mesenteric arteries associated with malabsorption. Report of two cases successfully treated by thromboendarterectomy. N Engl J Med 258:874–878, 1958.

219. Mikkelsen WP, Zaro JA: Intestinal angina: Report of a case with preoperative diagnosis and surgical relief. N Engl J Med 260:912–914, 1959.

220. Kountz SL, Laub DR, Connolly JE: "Aortoiliac steal" syndrome. Arch Surg 92:490–497, 1966.

221. Heer FW, Silen W, French WS: Intestinal gangrene without apparent vascular occlusion. Am J Surg 110:231–238, 1965.

222. Marable SA, Molnar E, Beman FJ: Abdominal pains secondary to celiac axis compression. Am J Surg 111:493–495, 1966.

223. Szilagyi DE, Rion RL, Elliott JP, et al: The celiac artery compression syndrome: Does it exist? Surgery 178:232–246, 1973.

224. Blaisdell FW, DeMattei GA, Gauder PJ: Extraperitoneal thoracic aorta to femoral bypass graft as replacement for an infected aortic bifurcation prosthesis. Am J Surg 102:583–585, 1961.

225. Blaisdell FW, Hall AD: Axillary-femoral artery bypass for lower extremity ischemia. Surgery 54:563–568, 1963.

226. Guida PM, Moore SW: Obturator bypass technique. Surg Gynecol Obstet 128:1307–1316, 1969.

227. Shaw RS, Baue AE: Management of sepsis complicating arterial reconstructive surgery. Surgery 53:75–86, 1963.

228. Vetto RM: The treatment of unilateral iliac artery obstruction with a transabdominal subcutaneous femorofemoral graft. Surgery 52:342–345, 1962.

229. Elliott JP, Smith RF, Szilagyi DE: Aorto-enteric and paraprosthetic-enteric fistulas: Problems of diagnosis and management. Arch Surg 108:479–490, 1974.

230. Busuttil RW, Rees W, Baker JD, et al: Pathogenesis of aortoduodenal fistula. Surgery 85:1–13, 1979.

231. Kolff WJ: The first clinical experience with the artificial kidney. Ann Intern Med 62:609–619, 1965.

232. Quinton WE, Dillard DH, Scribner BH: Am Soc Artificial Int Org 6:104–113, 1960.

233. Brescia MJ, Cimino JE, Appel K, Hurwich BL: Chronic hemodialysis using venipuncture and surgically created arteriovenous fistula. N Engl J Med 275: 1089–1092, 1966.

234. May J, Tiller D, Johnson J, Sheil AGR: Saphenous-vein arteriovenous fistula in regular dialysis treatment, N Engl J Med. 280:770, 1969.

235. Haimov M, Burrows L, Baez A, et al: Alternatives for vascular access for hemodialysis. Experience with autogenous vein autografts and bovine heterografts. Surgery 75:447–452, 1974.

236. Coote H: Exostosis of the left transverse process of the seventh cervical vertebra, surrounded by blood vessels and nerves; successful removal. Lancet 1:360–361, 1861.

237. Murphy JB: The clinical significance of cervical ribs. Surg Gynecol Obstet 3:514–520, 1906.

238. Adson AW, Coffey JR: Cervical rib: A method of anterior approach for relief of symptoms by division of the scalenus anticus. Ann Surg 85:839–857, 1927.

239. Ochsner A, Gage M, DeBakey ME: Scalenus anticus (Naffziger) syndrome. Am J Surg 28:669–693, 1935.

240. Naffziger HC, Grant WT: Neuritis of the brachial plexus mechanical in origin. Surgery Gynecol Obstet, 1938, 67:722–730, 1938.

241. Falconer MA, Li FWP: Resection of the first rib in costoclavicular compression of the brachial plexus. Lancet 1:59–63, 1962.

242. Edwards E: Anatomic and clinical comments on shoulder girdle syndromes. In Barker WF: Surgical Treatment of Peripheral Vascular Disease. New York, McGraw-Hill, 1962.

243. Roos DB: Transaxillary approach for the first rib resection to relieve thoracic outlet syndrome. Ann Surg 163:354–358, 1966.

244. McLeery RS, Kesterson JE, Kirtley JA, Love, RB: Subclavius and anterior scalene muscle compression as a cause of intermittent obstruction of the subclavian vein. Ann Surg 133:588–601, 1951.

245. Homans J: The etiology and treatment of varicose ulcer of the leg. Surg Gynecol Obstet 24:300–311, 1917.

246. Trendelenberg F: Ueber die Unterbindung der Vena saphena magna bei Unterschenkelvaricen. Beitr Klin Chir 7:195–210, 1890.

247. Babcock WW: A new operation for the extirpation of varicose veins. N Y Med J 86:153–156, 1907.

248. Mayo CH: The surgical treatment of varicose veins. St Paul Med J 6:695–699, 1904.

249. Trendelenburg F: Ueber die operative Behandlung der Embolie der Lungenarterie. Arch Klin Chir 86:686–700, 1908.

250. Homans J: Thrombosis of the deep veins of the lower leg causing pulmonary embolism. N Engl J Med 211:933–997, 1934.

251. Homans J: Venous thrombosis in the lower extremity: Its relation to pulmonary embolism. Am J Surg 38:316–326, 1937.

252. Homans J: Deep quiet thrombosis in the lower limbs: Preferred levels for interruption of the veins: Iliac section or ligation. Surg Gynecol Obstet 79:70–82, 1944.

253. Allen AW Management of thromboembolic disease in surgical patients. Surg Gynecol Obstet 96:107–114, 1953.

254. Veal JR: Prevention of pulmonary complications by high ligation of the femoral vein. JAMA 121:240–244, 1943.

255. Northway O, Buxton RW: Ligation of the inferior vena cava. Surgery 18:85–94, 1945.

256. O'Neill EE: Ligation of the inferior vena cava in the prevention and treatment of pulmonary embolism. N Engl J Med 232:641–646, 1945.

257. Collins CG, Jones JR, Nelson WE: Surgical treatment of pelvic thrombophlebitis. New Orleans Med Surg J 1943, 95:324–329, 1943.

258. Anlyan WG, Campbell FH, Shingleton WW, et al: Pulmonary embolism following venous ligation. Arch Surg 64:200–207, 1952.

259. Bowers RF, Leh SM: Late results of inferior vena cava ligation. Surgery 37:622–628, 1955.

260. Conti S, Daschbach M, Blaisdell FW: A comparison of high-dose versus conventional-dose heparin therapy for deep vein thrombosis. Surgery 92:972–980, 1982.

261. Barker WF, Mandiola S: Postphlebitic syndrome after vena caval interruption. In Foley WT (ed): Advances in the Management of Cardiovascular Disease. Chicago, Year Book, 1980, pp 31–42.

262. Spencer FC: Plication of the inferior vena cava for pulmonary embolism. Surgery 62:388–392, 1968.

263. Moretz WH, Rhode CM, Shepherd MH, et al: Prevention of pulmonary emboli by partial occlusion of the inferior vena cava. Am Surg 25:617–626, 1959.

264. Miles RM, Richardson RR, Wayne L, et al: Long-term results with the serrated Teflon vena cava clip in the prevention of pulmonary embolism. Ann Surg 169:881–891, 1969.

265. Adams JT, DeWeese JA: Partial interruption of the inferior vena cava with a new plastic clip. Surg Gynecol Obstet 123:1087–1088, 1966.

266. Mobin-Uddin K, Smith PE, Martinez LD, et al: A vena cava filter for the prevention of pulmonary embolus. Surg Forum 18:209–211, 1967.

267. Greenfield LJ, Peyton MD, Brown PP, et al: Transvenous management of pulmonary embolic disease. Ann Surg 180:461–468, 1974.

268. Homans J: The late results of femoral thrombophlebitis and their treatment. N Engl J Med 235:249–253, 1934.

269. Trout H: Ulcers due to varicose veins and lymphatic blockage. W V Med J 34:54–60, 1938.

270. Linton RR: The communicating veins of the lower leg and the technique for their ligation. Ann Surg 107:582–593, 1938.

271. Dodd K, Cockett FB: The Pathology and Surgery of the Veins of the Lower Limb. Edinburgh, E & S Livingstone, 1956.

272. Kistner RL: Surgical repair of the incompetent vein valve. Arch Surg 110:1336–1342, 1975.

273. Dale WA: Venous crossover grafts for the relief of iliofemoral venous block. Surgery 57:608–612, 1976.

274. Palma EC, Esperoti R: Vein transplants and grafts in the surgical treatment of the postphlebitic syndrome. J Cardiovasc Surg 1:94–107, 1960.

275. Taheri SA, Lazar L, Elias S, et al: Surgical treatment of postphlebitic syndrome with vein valve transplant. Am J Surg 144:221–224, 1982.

276. Taheri SA, Rigan D, West P, et al: Experimental prosthetic vein valve. Am J Surg 156:111–114, 1988.

277. Brooks B: Intra-arterial injection of sodium iodide. JAMA 82:1016–1019, 1924.

278. Moniz E: L'encéphalographie artérielle, son importance dans la localization des tumeurs cérébrales. Rev Neurol (Paris) 2:72–90, 1927.

279. dos Santos R, Lamas A, Caldas P: L'arteriographie des membres, de l'aorte et des ses branches abdominales. Bull Mem Soc Natl Chir 55:587–601, 1929.

280. Kruger RA, Mistretta CA, Crummy AB, et al: Digital K-edge subtraction radiography. Radiology 125:243–245, 1951.

281. Seldinger SI: Catheter replacement of the needle in percutaneous angiography. Acta Radiol 39:368–376, 1953.

282. Erlanger J: Blood pressure estimations by indirect methods: I. The mechanisms of the oscillatory criteria. Am J Physiol 39:401–446, 1915–1916.

283. Winsor T: Pressure gradients. Influence of arterial disease on the systolic blood pressure gradients of the extremity. Am J Med Sci 220:117–126, 1950.

284. Pachon V: Sur la méthode des oscillations et les conditions correctes de son emploi en sphygmomanométrie clinique. C R Soc Biol (Paris) 66:733–735, 1909.

285. Edwards EA, Levine HD: Peripheral vascular murmurs. Mechanisms of production and diagnostic significance. Arch Intern Med 90:284–300, 1952.

286. Wylie EJ, McGuiness JS: The recognition and treatment of arteriosclerotic stenosis of major arteries. Surg Gynecol Obstet 97:425–433, 1953.

287. Baillart P: La pression artérielle dans les branches de l'artère centrale de la retine: Nouvelle technique pour la determiner. Ann d'Occul 154:648–666, 1917.

288. Kartchner MM, McRaw LP, Crain V, et al: Oculoplethysmography:

An adjunct to arteriography in the diagnosis of extracranial occlusive disease. Arch Surg 106:528–535, 1973.

289. Gee WG, Mehigan JI, Wylie EJ: Measurement of collateral hemispheric blood pressure by ocular pneumoplethysmography. Am J Surg 130:121–127, 1975.

290. Leopold GR, Goldberger LE, Bernstein EF: Ultrasonic detection and evaluation of abdominal aortic aneurysm. Surgery 72:939–945, 1972.

291. Strandness DE, Schultz RD, Sumner DS, et al: Ultrasonic flow detection: A useful technique in the evaluation of peripheral vascular disease. Am J Surg 113:311–320, 1967.

292. Sumner DS, Strandness DE Jr: The relationship between calf blood flow and ankle blood pressure in patients with intermittent claudication. Surgery 65:763–771, 1969.

293. Brockenbrough EC: Screening for Prevention of Stroke: Use of a Doppler FlowMeter. Washington/Alaska Regional Medical Program, Information and Education Resource Unit, 1969.

294. Machleder HI, Barker WF: The stroke on the wrong side: Use of the Doppler ophthalmic test in cerebrovascular screening. Arch Surg 105:943–947, 1972.

295. Bendick PJ, Jackson VP: Evaluation of vertebral arteries by duplex sonography. J Vasc Surg 1986, 3:523–530, 1986.

296. Lindegaard KF, Bakke SJ, Grolimund P, et al: Assessment of intracranial hemodynamics in carotid artery by transcranial Doppler ultrasound. J Neurosurg 63:890–898, 1985.

297. Jager K, Bollinger A, Valli C, Amman R: Measurement of mesenteric blood flow by duplex scanning. J Vasc Surg 3:462–469, 1986.

298. Thomas GI, Spencer MD, Jones TW, et al: Non-invasive carotid bifurcation mapping: Its relation to carotid surgery. Am J Surg 128:168–174, 1974.

299. Barber FE, Baker DW, Arthur CW, et al: Ultrasonic duplex echo-Doppler scanner. IEEE Trans Biomed Eng 21:109–113, 1974.

300. Flanigan DP, Douglas DJ, Mach I, et al: Intraoperative ultrasonic imaging of the carotid artery during carotid endarterectomy. Surgery 100:893–899, 1986.

301. Kalender WA, Seissler W, Klotz E, Vock P: Spiral volumetric CT with single-breath-hold technique, continuous transport and continuous scanner rotation. Radiology 176:181–190, 1990.

302. Rubin GD, Walker PJ, Dake MD, et al: Three dimensional spiral computed tomographic angiography: An alternative imaging modality for the abdominal aorta and its branches. J Vasc Surg 18:656–665, 1993.

303. Cranley JJ, Canos JJ, Sull WF, et al: Phleborheographic technique for diagnosing deep venous thrombosis of the lower extremities. Surg Gynecol Obstet 141:331–339, 1975.

304. Wheeler HB, Pearson D, O'Connell D: Impedance plethysmography: Technique, interpretation and results. Arch Surg 104:164–169, 1972.

305. Comerota AJ, Katz ML, Greenwald L, et al: Should venous duplex imaging replace hemodynamic tests? J Vasc Surg 11:53–61, 1990.

2

Embryology of the Vascular System

David S. Maxwell

It is quite evident that the vascular apparatus does not independently and by itself "unfold" into the adult pattern. On the contrary, it reacts continuously in a most sensitive way to the factors of its environment, the pattern in the adult being the result of the sum of the environmental influences that have played upon it throughout the embryonic period. We thus find that this apparatus is continuously adequate and complete for the structures as they exist at any particular stage as the environmental structures progressively change; the vascular apparatus also changes and thereby is always adapted to the newer conditions. Furthermore, there are no apparent ulterior preparations at any time for the supply and drainage of other structures which have not yet made their appearance. For each stage it is an efficient and complete going-mechanism, apparently uninfluenced by the nature of its subsequent morphology.

GEORGE L. STREETER (1918)

In this quotation from George Streeter, an observation made more than 80 years ago, we see exemplified the finest tradition of the working scientist: years of attention to the most minute details of his subject, which eventuate in the broadest and most comprehensive view of the fundamental issues. In this statement, Streeter says in summary all that needs to be said and virtually all that can be said about the development of the vascular system, save for some specific details that serve only to embellish the theme he has laid out.

The story of the development of the vascular system encompasses the life span of the organism. This system retains the ability to grow, change, regenerate, and add on in response to changing needs on the part of tissues, from the earliest stages of embryonic life to the final breath. Thus, it supports normal growth, wound healing, and revascularization of tissues endangered by restricted flow in existing vessels, just as it supports the new growth of tumors, and transiently develops a highly efficient transport and exchange system through the uteroplacental circulation of pregnancy. All this is accomplished by the opening of—and enlargement of preexisting—vessels and the bud-

ding of new vascular growth from preexisting stem vessels. That it may fail eventually to respond in some instances to adequately supply myocardium or the central nervous system is not as remarkable as that it does respond so well for so long. It must seem that in the embryonic and fetal history of the vascular system there would be clues to the mysteries that surround this responsiveness throughout life. Furthermore, in the prenatal unfolding of the vascular system lie the origins of the various cardiovascular malformations to which the human organism is subject. We do not yet know whether the mechanisms of growth and the stimuli to vascularization of the embryo and fetus are the same as those that encourage and sustain the responsiveness of the vasculature in the postnatal organism.

In this summary chapter, I do not attempt to review the enormous literature on the subject, and I sacrifice many exciting details in the interest of a simple narrative exposition of the high points. The organizational scheme takes us first to a short history of the heart, which is simply a greatly modified blood vessel, followed by descriptions of the development of the large arteries and veins. I conclude with some comments on the growth of small vessels, which, like acorns, must appear and flourish first to produce the mighty trunk and branches of the vascular tree.

EARLY HISTORY

An organism of a cubic millimeter or so in volume (depending on the surface area and other factors related to the effectiveness of diffusion) may thrive without a vascular system. The human embryo enjoys the elaboration of a vascular system from its earliest stages, almost as if it anticipated that its bulk would soon require a highly sophisticated transport system. As the embryonic disk becomes recognizable, blood islands rapidly accumulate around the periphery of the disk. These isolated "puddles" begin to coalesce and communicate with one another until the embryo resembles a bloody sponge. Most prominent is the precephalic region in which the seemingly random coalescence of blood islands forms a network in the region soon to be identified as the *cardiogenic plate* (Fig. 2–1A).

In these earliest stages of development, the vascular system manifests one of its greatest mysteries: to what extent is the developmental pattern dictated by tissue needs and demands (possibly through the release of angiogenic factors, or through stimulus provided by metabolic products) and to what extent by factors such as extravascular pressures restricting flow in one set of possible blood channels and forcing enlargement of adjacent alternate routes of blood flow? And to what extent is the overall pattern dictated genetically? The *similarity* of the vascular tree from one individual to another urges the speculative favoring of a detailed genetic code. The *variability* from

one to the other, each pattern seemingly equally efficient in supporting tissues and organs, argues for development according to need and use and to mechanical and other adventitious factors.

In the case of the heart, a detailed genetic code is surely the guiding factor. Here, curiously, we begin with a parallel pair of cardiac tubes that fuse into one large tube; the latter then divides internally into the right and left hearts. At first glance, this seems inefficient; why not simply have each original tube of the pair form a right or left heart? The reason is clear when we examine the details of internal division of the heart, in which the single outflow tract is divided in such a way as to connect the right heart to the primitive vessels supplying the pulmonary circuit and connecting the remaining members of the branchial arch arteries to the left heart.

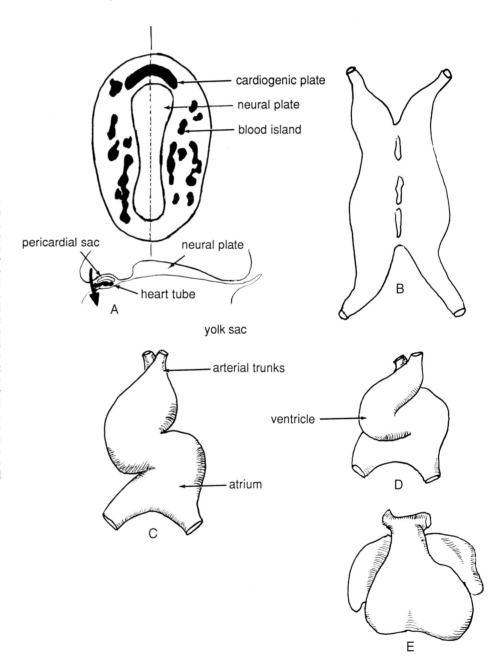

Figure 2–1. *A,* Embryonic disk from above, head of embryo up. Dotted line indicates plane of longitudinal section below, cranial end to the left. In the section, the pericardial sac is above the heart tube, but as the head folds under the forebrain (direction of the *large arrow*), the positions of the heart and sac will be reversed, with the heart invaginating from above the pericardial sac. *B,* The two parallel primitive heart tubes (from dorsal view) fusing in the midline to form a single heart tube and a single-chambered heart. *C–E,* Successive stages of the folding of the heart tube, viewed from the front. The venous end of the tube swings posteriorly to form the atria, whereas the arterial end (ventricles) remains anterior. *C–E,* represent the "loop stage" (see Delacruz et al[1]). (Adapted from Moore KL: The Developing Human, 3rd ed. Philadelphia, WB Saunders, 1982; and Rushmer RF: Cardiovascular Dynamics, 2nd ed. Philadelphia, WB Saunders, 1961.)

HEART

Our interest in the heart in this chapter is restricted to its development as that bears on the origins of the great vessels. The heart is simply a highly modified artery from both the histologic and the embryologic viewpoints. Histologically, it resembles a muscular artery because it has three layers to its walls: *adventitia* (epicardium), *tunica media* (myocardium), and *tunica intima* (endocardium). At the beginning, the heart tubes are simply a parallel pair of vessels, seemingly little different from the other components of the random network of primitive blood vessels. Nonetheless, the fusion of these two tubes and the development of a feeble myocardial investment around the endothelium lead quickly to irregular contractions of the musculature with feeble and inefficient ejection of blood. Subsequent events display the development of septa, dividing the single-chambered heart into right and left halves, and the appearance of valves that dictate unidirectional flow. The heart is beating with increasing regularity and with an efficiency-improving peristalsis and force as the myocardial element thickens and cytodifferentiates, and presumably from these first feeble sporadic beats, there is a stirring of the blood contents of the primitive vessels, perhaps with some benefit to the growing tissues around them and perhaps beginning to stimulate the enlargement of those channels that will survive into later embryonic stages. Beginning to channel blood through preferred pathways leads to closure and disappearance of less satisfactory routes and enlargement of the more successful channels into definitive blood vessels soon worthy of names recognizable in terms of the adult circulatory pattern. Channel formation from blood islands might be influenced simply by the choice of the lowest resistance of the available pathways.

The now-fused heart tube (see Fig. 2–1B) begins to invaginate the presumptive pericardial cavity, acquiring its visceral and parietal layers of pericardium while still a single-chambered heart configured as a simple, relatively straight tube. As the somites begin to appear in the neck and trunk region, the heart tube begins to fold on itself, first bulging ventrally, further invaginating the pericardial sac. The heart that is now swinging ventrocaudally comes to lie in front of the head and will continue its descent down the front of the neck and into the anterior chest. The ventrally directed bulge created by the U-shaped fold of the heart characterizes the "loop stage."[1] The ventral limb of the U is the arterial outflow path, and the dorsal limb of the U will become the venous inflow tract (see Fig. 2–1C through E). By the 10-somite stage, approximately 3 weeks' ovulation age, the heart has begun to fold in a coronal plane as well, directing the ventricular region to the left and forming a recognizable outflow tract, now termed the bulbus cordis, whose distal part is called the truncus arteriosus (see Fig. 2–1C). At this stage, the heart is still a single-chambered structure innocent of valves but rather completely enclosed in a pericardial sac and demonstrably beating, albeit irregularly. There is no single primordium, no segment of the primitive heart tube, that can be identified as leading to a specific cardiac cavity in the early postloop stage. Instead, there are microscopically and experimentally identifiable zones, each of which gives origin to a specific anatomic region of a definitive "cardiac cavity." These primordia are most accurately termed "primitive cardiac regions"; thus, referring to segments of the heart tube as forerunners of the chambers of the fully formed heart is misleading.[1] The folds in the heart tube and the peristaltic nature of myocardial contraction lead to a predetermined direction of flow out through the bulbus cordis, the folds acting as inefficient "valves" to so direct the flow. Such early vitality is not surprising because the cardiovascular system is the earliest formed and functional of the organ systems of the body. The heart is disproportionately large for the size of the embryo at this stage, and this disproportion remains until birth, with only a modest decline in heart-body ratio toward birth. This obviously is due to the fact that the heart must support not only the growing tissue of the organism but also the embryo's share of the enormous placental circulation.

It is worth digressing for a moment at this time to emphasize the functional problems faced by the developing heart. It is required to form and to function in such a way as to support the growth of and to maintain the developing organism in an intrauterine (aquatic) environment; that is, to support an organism incapable of independent gas exchange itself and dependent on the placenta for oxygen and nutriment and for other metabolic exchange. Its lungs are developed rather late and require only to be supplied with enough blood to support their growth. To perfuse the embryonic lungs with a rate of blood flow commensurate with an air-breathing existence would be energetically inefficient and perhaps an impediment to their growth and development, but during the early stages of development of the cardiovascular system, the lungs are simply not sufficiently developed to be called anything other than buds, volumetrically incapable of containing any significant quantity of blood. So the heart must develop a mechanism whereby it can support the organism in an aquatic environment with extensive exchange across a placenta and provide adequate distribution of blood throughout the growing body of the embryo, yet it must simultaneously develop a configuration that will enable it to shift its mode of function instantly at birth to the support of the organism by way of pulmonary gas exchange. Simply put, in fetal and embryonic life the two sides of the heart may function as two pumps operating "in parallel," with the output of both ventricles distributed to the placenta and to the growing tissues of the body, and with no interdependence of the output. Yet the two hearts must have the means to shift from functioning "in parallel" to "in tandem" at birth, wherein the outflow of one heart becomes the inflow of the other, and blood is obligated to first perfuse the pulmonary circuit, to return to the heart, and then to perfuse the systemic circuit, and so on. One emphasis of this survey is to focus on the development of this organ's features that render it capable of these sequential and different modes of function.

ARTERIES

During the early folding of the heart and with identification of a bulbus cordis and truncus arteriosus as an outflow tract, the aortic arches are beginning to form. The truncus arteriosus is continuous with a ventral aorta. This large, single-channeled artery is connected to a pair of dorsal aortae through a series of branchial (pharyngeal) arch arteries. The developing pharynx passes through a period in its development in which it is said to mimic the development of the gill apparatus of fish. Outpouchings of the pharyngeal wall grow as pockets toward the surface, where they are met or at least approached by corresponding infoldings of the ectodermal surface. Normally, these outpouchings and infoldings neither meet nor coalesce to form gill slits or fistulae. The supporting tissue on either side of the pouches is endowed with a cartilaginous supporting bar, a nerve, and a blood vessel, respectively known as the branchial arch (pharyngeal) cartilage, branchial arch nerve, and branchial arch artery. The first such cartilaginous bar is Meckel's cartilage, in front of the first pharyngeal pouch; the second, Reichert's cartilage, lies between the first and second pouches, and so on. The pharynx is supported by six arch complexes, surrounding and intervening between the pharyngeal pouches. The arteries of these arches are the connectives from the ventral aorta to the dorsal aortae, and they appear in sequence from cranial to caudal. Rarely are more than three such arch arteries identifiable at one time; in this case as elsewhere in the embryo the cranial development leads or precedes that occurring more caudally. As the fourth arch artery appears, the first is being transformed into its successor structures and ceases to be identifiable as an arch artery. In humans, it seems that there are five such arch arteries, numbered 1, 2, 3, 4, and 6, in recognition of the dropping out in phylogeny of the fifth arch artery, which plays no significant role in human development (the fifth pharyngeal pouch becomes fused with the fourth at its opening into the pharynx; its rudimentary arch between the fourth and fifth pouches contributes to the formation of the larynx). In contrast to the constancy of innervation of the derivatives of the pharyngeal arches, the vascular supply to the arches is subject to later, often extensive modification. The motor nerve to an arch persists throughout phylogeny and throughout ontogenetic development in supplying the derivatives of that arch (first arch, mandibular nerve; second arch, facial nerve; third arch, glossopharyngeal nerve; fourth through sixth arches, recurrent and superior laryngeal nerves and vagal pharyngeal nerve). The geometric representation of the arch artery pattern and the fate of those arteries is summarized in Figure 2–2. The paired dorsal aortae sweep posteriorly and fuse in the midline to form a single dorsal aorta (see Fig. 2–2 inset) posterior to entry points of the arch arteries.

The lungs begin their development as a ventrally directed outgrowth from the pharynx, and the single tube that will become the trachea descends into the presumptive chest cavity, where it branches into a pair of lung buds. These buds from the beginning receive a small blood supply from branches of the sixth aortic arch arteries (see Fig. 2–2A). Clearly, the sixth arch arteries will play a role in the development of the pulmonary arterial tree. The developmental problem posed here is that the sixth arch arteries are initially part of the systemic circulation, simply representing the caudalmost of the branchial arch arteries springing from the truncus arteriosus and uniting with the dorsal aortae. In the division of the heart tube into right and left hearts, some provision must be made for joining

the right ventricular outflow tract to the sixth arch arteries and joining the remainder of the great branchial arch system and aortae with the left ventricle. The rationale for fusion of primitive heart tubes into a single channel and subsequent division is now clear in this need to divide the bulbus cordis and truncus arteriosus into a pulmonary and an aortic artery. In the manner of that division, we can see the solution to the problem of connecting the right ventricle and the developing pulmonary artery to the lungs and connecting the remainder of the arch arteries to the systemic circulation and to the left ventricle. The interested reader is encouraged to examine the beautifully illustrated paper of Congdon[2] for further clarification of this point.

We turn now to the division of the heart into four chambers that make up two separate hearts, with provision for a parallel mode of function before birth and a tandem mode after birth. The umbilical veins (after the sixth week, a single left umbilical vein) return blood to the fetal heart by their union with the inferior vena cava. This return route sees the umbilical vein enter the liver, where a shunt, the *ductus venosus*, bypasses the complex hepatic circulation and shunts the blood directly into the inferior vena cava. Thus, the right atrium receives a supply of freshly oxygenated blood, in contrast to the adult condition. Before separation of the right and left atrium that placental return is into the single atrial chamber, which is diagrammatically depicted in Figure 2–3A. The single chamber undergoes a constriction in the plane of the atrioventricular orifices (and the *atrioventricular sulcus* on the exterior of the heart). From the margins of this constriction, endocardial cushions grow inward to begin the formation of the tricuspid and mitral valves. The single atrium begins its separation into two halves by the downgrowth from the dorsocranial wall of a filmy crescentic curtain, the *septum primum* (see Fig. 2–3B). The leading invaginated edge of the crescent grows down toward the floor of the single atrium, that floor now forming by virtue of the growth of the atrioventricular valve primordia. Figure 2–3B shows the septum primum from the right side as it progresses toward complete closure of the single atrial chamber in its midline, and we see that just before the *foramen primum* closes, a group of perforations in the dorsocranial part of the partition form (see Fig. 2–3B) and then coalesce into a *foramen secundum* (see Fig. 2–3C). This is necessary, inasmuch as throughout this developmental sequence, the heart is pumping blood to and returning it from the placenta, and the returning blood must be shunted from the right side of the heart into the left atrium in large volume to sustain the systemic circulation. *Thus, at no point in fetal life may the right and left atria be functionally separate.* During the time when the placental circulation is intact, the pressure in the right atrium exceeds that in the left atrium, and a right-to-left shunt will be operative. Thus, the foramen secundum opens just in time to continue that shunt as the foramen primum closes. Now, on the right side of the septum primum, a much more robust and rigid septum secundum begins its downgrowth following the same pattern as that of the septum primum (see Fig. 2–3C), a crescent-shaped leading edge growing down from above toward the endocardial cushions that will finally separate the atria from the ventricles. This downgrowth of the septum secundum comes to overlie the orifice of the

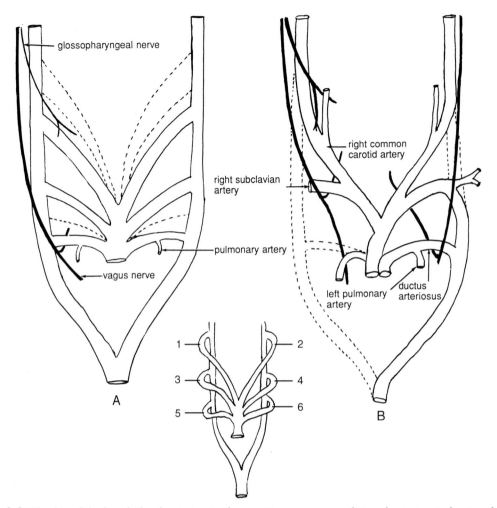

Figure 2–2. The fate of the branchial arch arteries. *A,* The primitive arrangement of six arch arteries. Arches 1 and 2 have formed and been accommodated into the vessels of the head (*dotted lines* indicate arteries that are no longer "arches," i.e., 1, 2, and 5; see text). Arches 3, 4, and 6 connect the ventral aorta (aortic sac and truncus arteriosus) with the paired dorsal aortae. These latter fuse posteriorly to form a single dorsal aorta. *B,* The subsequent disposition of these vessels. The dotted lines indicate vessels that normally disappear, and include the right sixth arch beyond the right pulmonary artery. The glossopharyngeal nerve (motor to the third arch) and the recurrent laryngeal nerve (motor to the sixth arch derivatives) are shown. The recurrent is a branch of the vagus "recurring" around the sixth arch in *A,* and in *B,* these nerves recur around the ductus arteriosus and around the right subclavian. *Inset,* The first three aortic arch arteries from the front (*ventral*) view, during the branchial period (schematic: at no time are all arch arteries evident at the same time). The paired dorsal aortae unite into a single dorsal aorta posterior to the entry of the arch arteries. The postbranchial period, during which time the heart descends from the branchial region into the chest, is characterized by the modification of the arch system into the adult disposition of the derived arteries.

foramen secundum. Fortunately, the septum secundum is sturdy and relatively unyielding, whereas the septum primum is thin and curtainlike. As long as the free lower edge of the septum secundum fails to reach the floor of the atrium, thus forming the *foramen ovale,* the elevated pressure in the right atrium pushes blood through the ovale, deflecting the septum primum and allowing blood to pass through the foramen secundum into the left atrium and permitting continuation of the obligatory right-to-left shunt. Inasmuch as the downgrowth of the septum secundum is arrested, leaving a fixed foramen ovale, such a shunt operates throughout the intrauterine life of the organism. The orifice of the foramen ovale is just above and medial to the orifice of the inferior vena cava (see Fig. 2–3D), so inferior caval (i.e., placental) blood is preferentially directed into that foramen, and thence into the left atrium, with remarkably little mixing of this oxygenated blood with the oxygen-poor blood returning via the superior vena cava.

The division of the ventricles and the single aortic outflow path is, at the same time, simpler to understand but more critically complex. The ventricle begins to divide by the upward growth of a muscular partition of myocardium from the cardiac apex toward the truncus arteriosus (Fig. 2–4A). This will form the muscular part of the interventricular septum. At the same time, a pair of ridges, the spiral ridges, grow toward each other as outgrowths of the walls of the truncus arteriosus. These will fuse together to form a *spiral septum,* dividing the septum from above down. The lower ends of the spiral ridges contribute to the formation of the final septal closure (see Fig. 2–4B). This is an extraordinarily complex phenomenon involving early histologic changes and probably initiated by hemodynamic influences and subsequently controlled by genetic factors (see the careful analysis by Fanapazir and Kaufman[3]). Where the three cushions meet, the membranous interventricular septum is formed. Figures 2–4C and 2–4D sche-

Figure 2–3. The single early atrium is represented as a hollow sphere, from an anterolateral view. The atrioventricular canals are the lower part of the cutaway sphere. *A,* The dotted line indicates the plane of division into right and left atria. The entry of the superior and inferior venae cavae (right atrial segment of the sphere) and the pulmonary arteries (left segment of the sphere) are indicated by entering tubes. *B–D,* Successive stages in development of interatrial septum. *B,* The septum primum grows down, leaving a free margin as the ostium primum. As this ostium prepares to close, holes appear in the upper posterior part of the septum, which in *C* have coalesced into an ostium secundum. *C,* The septum secundum begins to grow down to the right of the septum primum, covering over the ostium secundum on that side. The free margin of the septum secundum does not close over *D,* leaving the foramen ovale open. The right atrial contents flow into the left atrium via the foramen ovale and ostium secundum. (Adapted from Tuchmann-Duplessis H, David HG, Haegel P: Illustrated Human Embryology. New York, Springer-Verlag, 1972.)

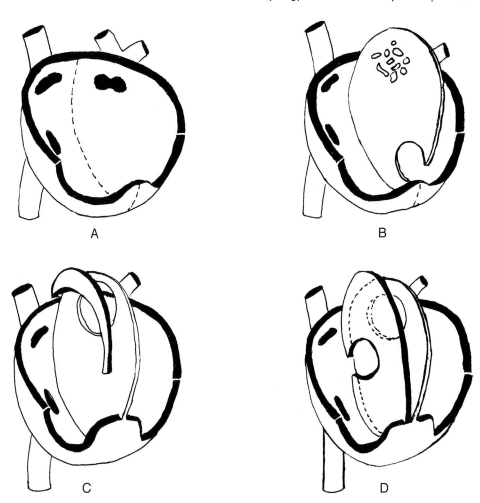

matically depict the spiral arrangement of the division of the truncus arteriosus whereby the single outflow tract is divided into pulmonary and aortic tubes, each connected to its corresponding ventricular cavity. The complexity of the closure lies in the precise pitch of the spiral septum, which must occur to align its lower end with the upthrusting muscular cushion to meet accurately in a single plane, or other interference in the fusion of those cushions into a complete membranous septum will lead to a membranous interventricular septal defect. Misalignment of the spiral ridges may result in failure of the great arteries to form and to function independently through the accident of a pulmonary-aortic fistula. Misalignment of the lower end of the dividing arteries and asymmetry in the positioning of the spiral ridges could lead to such errors as overriding aorta with right ventricular contents partially ejected into the aorta. The features of the tetralogy of Fallot can be readily interpreted as a result of such misalignment in the truncus division: The tetralogy consists of *overriding aorta, pulmonary stenosis,* and *membranous septal defect* (due presumably to asymmetric division of the proximal truncus arteriosus), and *right ventricular hypertrophy* (secondary to the right-to-left shunt through the overriding aorta and to the stenotic pulmonary artery).

A superbly illustrated and truly classical account of early experimental findings and an excellent historical review of the anatomy and physiology of fetal circulation is to be found in the book by Barclay and associates,[4] and more recent summaries may be obtained in standard works (Arey,[5] Clemente,[6] Hamilton and Mossman,[7] Moore,[8] Sabin,[9] and Tuchmann-Duplessis and associates[10]).

The original plan of five pairs of aortic arch arteries (see Fig. 2–2) becomes modified by incorporation of the first two arch arteries into the internal carotid system, dropping out of the paired dorsal aortae between the third and fourth arches, and participation in the formation of the common carotid arteries by the third arches. Caudal to the lost segments of dorsal aortae, the fourth arches become the roots of the subclavian arteries, the right sixth is lost distal to its pulmonary branch, and the left sixth becomes the left pulmonary, with the segment distal to the pulmonary "branch" serving as the *ductus arteriosus* (see Fig. 2–2B). This arterial shunt vessel develops specialized muscle in its tunica media, which is stimulated to contract and shut down the shunt vessel after birth. It is believed that abnormal migration of some of this specialized smooth muscle into the aortic wall accounts for aortic stenosis, the stricture having developed in the aorta at the site of this ectopic "ductus" muscle after birth.

The closure of this right-to-left shunt on the arterial side at birth results in a great increase in pulmonary blood flow (the resistance of pulmonary vessels drops dramatically with inflation of the lungs and elongation of *helicine* arteries). On the venous side, the rise in left atrial pressure and

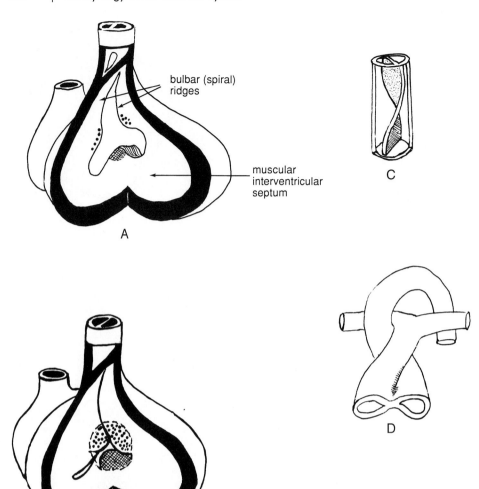

bulbar (spiral) ridges

muscular interventricular septum

A

B

C

D

Figure 2–4. Stages in the division of the ventricle and the formation of the great arteries from the truncus arteriosus and bulbus cordis. *A,* The ventricle has begun to divide by formation of the muscular part of the interventricular septum by growth of the musculature of the ventricular wall. The bulbus cordis is dividing into two vessels, beginning with the growing together of two spiral ridges. *B,* The two spiral ridges meet and fuse to divide the bulbus cordis into two outflow tracts: the pulmonary artery and the ascending aorta. The ridges at their lower extremities (stippled cushions) meet a muscular cushion derived from the muscular interventricular septum (hatched), to form the membranous part of the interventricular septum (outlined in *dotted lines*). The spiral character of the arterial division connects the sixth arch arteries to the right ventricle, and the left ventricle to the other arch arteries and their derivatives. *C,* Spiral septum shown diagrammatically, in a cutaway cylinder representing the single bulbus cordis. The hatched surface of the septum may be taken as the aortic side of the division, and the stippled side, as the pulmonary surface of the septum. The two resulting arteries must spiral around one another as in *D;* derived from a single tube, they are constrained to remain wrapped in a single pericardial sleeve. (Adapted from Tuchmann-Duplessis H, David HG, Haegel P: Illustrated Human Embryology. New York, Springer-Verlag, 1972; and Moore KL: The Developing Human. Philadelphia, WB Saunders, 1982.)

loss of umbilical venous return arrest the interatrial right-to-left shunt. Elevated left atrial pressure results in the two interatrial septa operating as a flap valve, closing the foramen ovale by applying the curtain-like septum primum against the left (see Fig. 2–3D).

Certainty in the derivation of the arteries of the head is not easy to achieve. The vessels form from a loose network of interconnected vessels, in which it is often not possible even to distinguish between arteries and veins.[11] The artery of the first arch becomes a part of the internal carotid artery, which also forms in part from persistence of the rostral parts of the dorsal aortae. The second arch artery appears in the form of the *stapedial artery.* This artery of the tympanic cavity passes through the annulus (obturator foramen) in the stapes, and in some mammals it persists in this form. In humans, this form of stapedial artery may remain into adulthood as a surgically troublesome vascular anomaly. This artery of the second arch for a time supplies three branches (supraorbital, infraorbital, and mandibular), distributed with the divisions of the trigeminal nerve. An anastomosis between the infraorbital and mandibular branches of the stapedial artery and the external carotid is said to give rise to the maxillary artery and its middle meningeal branch. It is further argued that the orbital

anastomotic branch of the middle meningeal artery is the remnant of the original supraorbital branch of the stapedial artery. Some information is indicated in the phylogenetic history of the artery. In most mammals, the originally small external carotid artery, as it grows forward, taps the origin of the stapedial artery and appropriates its branches, which at one stroke reduces the size and causes the disappearance of the original stapedial artery, and extends the distribution of the external carotid. As Romer[12] colorfully put it, "the process is analogous to 'stream piracy,' whereby one river taps the headwaters of another." Padget[13] offers a detailed discussion and critical appraisal of the literature of the general mammalian stapedial artery and of the human artery, and her discussion is recommended to the interested reader.

The third arch artery forms the common carotid arteries and the first segments of the internal carotid arteries. Thus, it is probable that portions of the first three arches all contribute to the external carotid arteries. The left fourth arch forms the arch of the aorta, and the left dorsal aorta distal to the point of union of this arch forms the descending aorta along with the single dorsal aorta more caudally (see Fig. 2–2B). The entirety of the right dorsal aorta is lost. The right horn of the aortic sac forms the brachiocephalic artery, from which the right common carotid and subclavian arteries spring.

The sixth arches are associated with the pulmonary blood supply, first as the source of the small twigs to the lung buds. Those twigs and their parent stems from the truncus arteriosus become the definitive pulmonary arteries. Now, it should be clear why the complex twist of the spiral septum dividing the truncus arteriosus is necessary. In dividing the truncus, it is essential to connect the right ventricle to the origins of the sixth arches from the truncus, leaving the more rostral arch arteries connected to the part of the truncus connected to the left ventricle. The arch arteries spring from a single vessel, the truncus, and must end as arteries arising from separate arteries: the sixth arising from the pulmonary artery and the first through fourth from the aortic component of the truncus. The twisting division of the truncus accounts also for the intertwined course of the pulmonary artery and the ascending aorta, and their derivation from a single vessel, the truncus, accounts for these great arteries being wrapped in a single pericardial sleeve (see Fig. 2–4D).

The branchial arches develop nerve supplies along with their vascular supplies, and it is an axiom of anatomy that once nerve supply is established, it is never lost. The motor nerves of the branchial arches supply the structures derived from those arches henceforth, no matter what developmental events ensue. In Figure 2–2, the position of the glossopharyngeal nerve as the motor nerve of the third arch can be seen, and the recurrent laryngeal branch of the vagus as the motor nerve of the sixth arch, as these nerves are drawn caudally by the descent of the heart and growth of the branchial arch system. The "recurrent" branch of the vagus is in fact the motor nerve derived from the *nucleus ambiguus* of the brainstem, which happens to distribute by way of the vagus, having emerged from the brainstem as the cranial root of the spinal accessory nerve (XI). The recurring course of the nerve is accounted for by its inherited requirement of lying caudal to the sixth arch artery. The distal part of the left sixth arch artery becomes the ductus arteriosus (the *ligamentum arteriosum* after birth). Thus arises the asymmetry in the courses of the two recurrent laryngeal nerves. The left nerve is constrained to occupy its original relationship to its arch artery as that artery is drawn down into the chest by the descent of the heart. The right nerve loses that constraint as the sixth arch drops out distal to the origin of the pulmonary artery. The only persisting arch to prevent the nerve's remaining in the neck as the heart descends is the fourth arch on the right side (the right subclavian artery), around which we find the nerve "recurring" in the adult human (see Fig. 2–2B). The surgeon who finds in thyroid surgery that the right recurrent nerve does not come up around the subclavian artery should take that as a warning that a developmental abnormality in the formation of the right subclavian artery might be expected (e.g., a retroesophageal right subclavian). In that event, the right subclavian forms from the right seventh intersegmental artery and part of the right dorsal aorta, the right fourth arch artery and right dorsal aorta having involuted cranial to the origin of the seventh intersegmental artery (see Moore[8] and other embryology texts).

The developing embryo in its earliest stages is supported by a yolk sac of nutriment, sustaining growth until the placenta is sufficiently developed to assume those duties. The embryo lies on the surface of the yolk sac, with the interior of the latter in continuity with the developing gastrointestinal tract. The digestive tract cranial to the yolk sac is termed the "foregut," that caudal to the yolk sac is termed the "hindgut," and that directly connected to the yolk sac is termed the "midgut." Three aortic branches, midline and unpaired, arise to supply each of these segments of the digestive tract, and these arteries remain the source of arterial blood for those portions of the tract and their derivatives. Thus, the celiac artery is the artery of the foregut and the derivatives of the foregut, including the liver and spleen. The artery of the midgut is the superior mesenteric artery; the artery of the hindgut is the inferior mesenteric artery. During development, the digestive tract outgrows the room available for it in the abdominal cavity and temporarily "herniates" out into the umbilical cord. Its return from this extraabdominal sojourn is accompanied by a rotation that accounts for the disposition of the stomach, the duodenum, and the bowel in the adult. The axis of rotation around which this reentry into the abdomen occurs is the superior mesenteric artery (see the exquisitely illustrated account of Dott[14]).

The kidneys begin their development in the pelvis and migrate cranially to their final position on the posterior abdominal wall. The pelvic kidneys derive their arterial blood supply from the iliac system, and as they ascend, the previous arterial supply drops out and new vessels from the aorta are established. The ascent and the history of the previous blood supply are to be read in the sources of small vessels supplying the ureter, the origins of these indicating the stems of vessels formerly supplying the kidney. Should the "ascent" of the kidney be arrested, the blood supply at the time, of course, remains the supply into adulthood. So the ascent of the horseshoe kidney is arrested by the overhanging inferior mesenteric artery, and the horseshoe kidney has arterial blood supplied from common iliac vessels or the aorta at a level lower than the origin of the normal renal arteries. So, too, accessory renal arteries usually arise below the renal arteries and enter the inferior pole of the kidney, attesting to a previous source of blood that did not entirely disappear with ascent to the final renal destination.

The limbs seem to be organized, around a central arterial stem, so from the beginning, an axial artery is identifiable. Figure 2–5 depicts the changes in circulatory pattern for the two limbs. Generally, the axial artery in large part disappears and certainly ceases to be the principal source of limb blood.

In the upper limb, the axial artery passes down the core of the limb to the hand plexus. It is a continuation of the subclavian and axially system, already established in the 5-mm embryo, and is the forerunner of the brachial artery and, more distally, the interosseous artery. The upper limb axial artery sprouts a median branch and an ulnar arterial branch on the medial side of the stem artery. The median temporarily joins with the ulnar in the volar arch. A radial sprout follows on the preaxial side of the limb, and this new branch usurps the median's connection with the volar arch. The distal axial artery persists as the anterior interosseous. This pattern is completed before the end of the

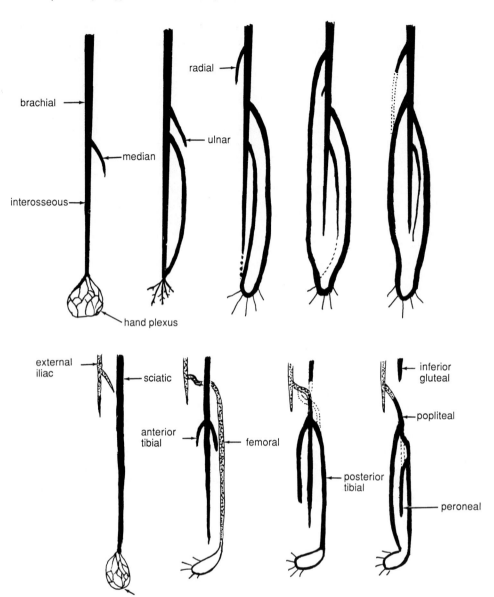

Figure 2–5. The development of the arterial pattern of the limbs; top row (left to right), upper limb; lower row, lower limb. *Upper limb,* Initially the limb is organized around a single axial artery, the brachial and its interosseous continuation, terminating in a hand plexus. The hand plexus will develop into the palmar arches. The stem artery gives rise in succession to the median, ulnar, and radial arteries. The median normally has an evanescent existence as a major vessel, losing its connection with the hand plexus, which it usurped from the axial vessel. See text for details. *Lower limb,* The axial vessel for the lower limb is the sciatic, which remains in the adult as the inferior gluteal, and portions of the popliteal and peroneal arteries. The femoral arises from the external iliac, and appropriates the distal part of the sciatic to dominate the vascular distribution of the limb. The anterior tibial arises as a branch of the popliteal; the posterior tibial is developed from the union of the femoral with the popliteal. Notice in the third figure from the left an upper segment of the femoral is lost, allowing the popliteal to become interposed. See text for details. (Adapted from Arey LB: Developmental Anatomy, 7th ed. Philadelphia, WB Saunders, 1965.)

second month, and the early dominance of the axial and the median arteries is permanently lost. The median artery persists as a branch of the anterior interosseous artery, serving as the nutrient artery of the median nerve. It may persist in a much enlarged form as an anomaly, accompanying the median nerve into the palm, and retaining its connection with—and contribution to—the palmar arterial arches.

Figure 2–5 shows the steps by which the adult pattern of arterial supply to the lower limb is derived from the axial artery of the limb bud. The axial vessel is the sciatic artery, a direct branch of the umbilical. It is the primary source of the blood for the limb bud in the 9-mm embryo. The major stem artery for the limb becomes the femoral, as the latter continues the course of the external iliac. The femoral annexes the foot plexus of the sciatic and the origin of this axial vessel. The remaining proximal "stump" of the once-dominant sciatic artery persists as the inferior gluteal artery. A branch of the latter, the artery of the sciatic nerve, is all that remains of the former glory of the sciatic artery.

The distal parts of the sciatic stem, appropriated by the femoral near its origin from the external iliac, give rise to the anterior tibial artery, which connects with the plantar arch distally. The newer, more distal femoral establishes a new connection to the distal sciatic so that it and the plantar arch come to branch from the sciatic. The most distal segment of the sciatic shifts its origin to the posterior tibial as the peroneal, and the adult pattern is established. The remnants of the sciatic persist (from above down) as the inferior gluteal with its small artery of the sciatic nerve, the popliteal artery, and the peroneal artery. In the adult arterial plan, these persisting segments of the original sciatic artery no longer have any continuity with each other in any significant way.

The umbilical arteries, carrying blood to the placenta for gas and metabolite exchange, appear as large branches of the internal iliac arteries and persist unmodified throughout gestation. These arteries develop robust branches to the upper surface of the urinary bladder. At birth, the segments of the umbilical arteries distal to the origin of the arteries to the bladder are obliterated and remain as fibrous cords, the medial umbilical ligaments. The stem of these arteries and the branches to the bladder are henceforth known as the *superior vesicle arteries*.

VEINS

As the arterial distribution system develops, appropriate return pathways arise simultaneously. The venous system is extensively interconnected, with great capacity for collateral routes of venous return, and arteries generally are accompanied by corresponding veins. The short review of the venous system here focuses only on the great systems of veins that arise early in embryonic life and that give rise to the major collecting pathways recognizable in the normal adult. Thus, even such important but developmentally simple systems as the pulmonary venous system are not subjects of discussion here.

A passing comment on venous valves is appropriate here, however, to draw attention to a provocative analysis and comparative study of superficial veins in the limbs of primates.[15] The number and spacing of venous valves is dictated genetically and is relevant to the need to maintain optimum pressures within capillary beds to ensure a balance in fluid exchange in tissues. The distance between venous valves in the limbs is just that needed to provide the transcapillary pressure gradients required for an equilibrium in fluid efflux and return to the vascular bed and is not, as previously supposed, an adaptation to counter the effects of gravity in the bipedal posture.

The veins of the embryo fall into three major groups: vitelline (omphalomesenteric) veins, umbilical veins, and the cardinal system of veins. The coalesced blood islands that give rise to undifferentiated blood networks develop a venous side, as they do an arterial side, as directions of blood flow become established through them. Preferential pathways emerge on the venous side, giving rise to larger and more dominant veins that undergo modification as regional or organ-specific changes occur. Many of the venous channels developed in support of fetal life disappear as the need for them vanishes through subsequent development.

The vitelline veins are the veins of the yolk sac. They pass through the intestinal portal of the umbilical cord, alongside the (at first) wide channel of communication between the sac and the midgut region of the alimentary canal. A vitelline plexus is formed of communicating venous channels between the vitelline veins in the *septum transversum,* and as the liver develops in the septum, it infringes on the vitelline plexus, breaking it up into hepatic sinusoids. The vitelline pathway from the septum transversum into the heart persists, in spite of this encroachment, as hepaticocardiac channels. The right channel of this return persists as the terminal segment of the inferior vena cava (Fig. 2–6). The vitelline plexus also surrounds the duodenum during the stage of hepatic growth, and the plexus is further distorted when the herniated midgut returns in a spiraling motion into the abdominal cavity. It is this rotation during the return that brings the duodenum into its transverse position and fixes this position of the duodenum by peritonealization. This position forces the

blood in the surrounding plexus to shunt from the right to the left vitelline vein, which is the segment of the vitelline system lying just caudal to the transversely oriented duodenum. The left vitelline vein then sends its blood directly across to the liver by way of its dorsal anastomosis with the persistent cranial end of the right vitelline vein.

The portal vein thus formed does not spiral around the duodenum as so commonly described and illustrated but instead is short and straight with the duodenum spiralling around it. The ease with which these changes take place may be readily understood if the two following basic facts are appreciated: (1) the essentially plexiform nature of the embryonic vascular system and (2) the natural tendency for blood to seek the most direct route of flow because of hydrodynamic factors. (Refer to the clear sequence of illustrations of this development in Figs. 225 through 230 of the fourth edition of *Hamilton, Boyd and Mossman's Human Embryology,*[7] p 274.)

The umbilical veins, entering the abdominal cavity by way of the umbilicus, must also traverse the septum transversum to arrive at the heart, and their septal segments within the septum also become enmeshed with the vitelline veins in the hepatic plexus of sinusoids. In the 5-mm embryo, the umbilical veins communicate extensively with the vitelline plexus in the liver. Two days later, the right umbilical vein undergoes atrophy, and all placental blood returns to the fetal heart via the left vein. The left vein's channel through the liver enlarges to accommodate this enhanced flow and forms the *ductus venosus,* a direct channel through the liver between the left umbilical vein and the inferior vena cava. This channel, of course, obliterates at birth with cessation of flow through the umbilical system, and the intrahepatic shunt is replaced by the *ligamentum venosum.* Thus, there is said to be a sphincter in this shunt that regulates umbilical flow, a particularly important feature to prevent overloading the fetal heart during uterine contractions. This sphincter's closure at birth contributes to the prompt obliteration of the shunt. The course of the left umbilical vein caudal to the liver is in the free margin of the ventral mesentery. The obliterated umbilical vein between umbilicus and liver is the *ligamentum teres hepatis* of the adult, lying in the free margin of the falciform ligament; the latter is the adult counterpart of the ventral mesentery between the liver and the anterior abdominal wall.

The cardinal veins are the body wall veins of the embryo and fetus. There are several sets designated by distinguishing names—a source of considerable confusion for the student of human anatomy. The *anterior cardinal veins* (also termed "precardinal" veins) drain the cranial region of the early embryo. The *posterior cardinal veins* drain the caudal portion and arise slightly later than the anterior cardinals. The *subcardinal veins* appear shortly after the posterior cardinal veins and are derived in conjunction with the rapidly growing progenitor of the kidney, the *mesonephros.* The term "*supracardinal*" veins is sometimes employed to designate lateral sympathetic, or thoracolumbar line veins, or paraureteric veins. To limit the number of "cardinal veins" one must attend to, I avoid use of "supracardinal veins" here in discussing the veins of the posterior body wall anterior to the segmental vessels, using instead "*lateral sympathetic.*"

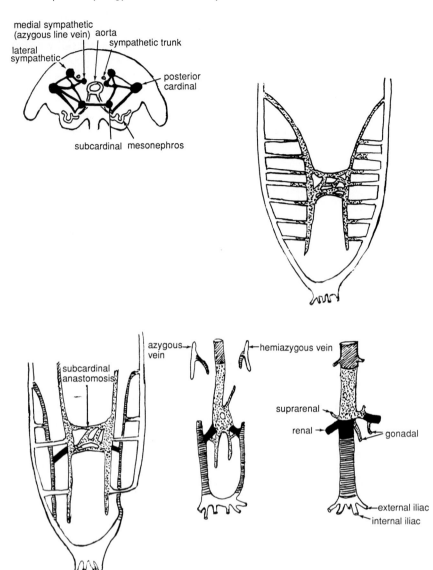

Figure 2–6. The development of the large veins. *Upper left,* A schematic cross-section of the embryo to show the relative positions and extensive interconnections of the major body wall veins. *Upper right* and *lower row* (left to right), succession of stages in the development of the inferior vena cava and the related body wall veins. See key in lower row for identification of the component veins, making up the inferior vena cava *(lower right)*. For simplicity, the azygous and hemiazygous veins are depicted as if they arose from the lateral sympathetic veins, but, in fact, they arise as derivatives from the parallel medial sympathetic (azygous line) veins. See text for details. (Adapted from Williams PL, Wendell-Smith CP, Treadgold S: Basic Human Embryology, 2nd ed. Philadelphia, JB Lippincott, 1969; and Hollinshead WH, Rosse L: Textbook of Anatomy, 4th ed. Philadelphia, Harper & Row, 1985.)

The primary head vein of the embryo evolves into the complex system of dural sinuses and venous pathways of the head, and the reader is referred to the classical accounts of Streeter[16] and Padget,[11, 13] whose illustrations make amply clear the changes leading to the adult pattern. The anterior and posterior cardinal veins unite behind the heart to form the common cardinal veins, or ducts of Cuvier (right and left). The union of the ducts of Cuvier is the ductus venosus at the venous end of the heart. Part of the ductus venosus becomes incorporated into the walls of the atria, most notably the right atrium.

The posterior cardinal veins are the first of a series of caudal longitudinal body wall veins, which form an interconnected system (see Fig. 2–6) giving rise to the caudal body wall venous drainage and to the inferior vena cava and azygous system of veins.

The subcardinal veins appear soon after the posterior cardinal veins as a pair of veins along the medial side of the urogenital folds. They are associated with the mesonephros and probably arise as a series of longitudinal anastomoses for the plexuses of the mesonephroi. They drain the mesonephroi and the germinal epithelium and terminate cranially and caudally by connecting with the posterior cardinal veins (see Fig. 2–6). The subcardinal veins unite with each other and along their lengths with the posterior cardinal veins through anastomoses; the multiple transverse anastomoses of these veins are probably their most distinctive feature. One of these anastomoses is the intersubcardinal anastomosis between the two veins ventral to the aorta. The right subcardinal vein establishes a communication with the liver sinusoids and that segment becomes the hepatic segment of the inferior vena cava (see Fig. 2–6). The preaortic anastomosis comes into play in the establishment of the vena cava inferior to that segment.

The lateral sympathetic ("supracardinal") veins appear soon after the hepatic segment of the inferior vena cava, anterior to the segmental vessels. They appear first as a plexus but quickly become a longitudinal trunk, ending cranially in the posterior cardinal vein, and posteriorly anastomosing with the subcardinal vein, especially strongly on the right side. The part caudal to that latter anastomosis persists, and most of the remainder of the lateral sympathetic veins regress, the persisting right caudal segment surviving as the infrarenal part of the inferior vena cava (see Fig. 2–6). As the lateral sympathetic veins appear, a medial pair (medial sympathetic or azygous line veins) also arise but medial to the sympathetic trunk in the abdominal wall. These link across the midline, and by the dropping out of an intermediate segment on the left side, form the azygous system of veins.

The adult pattern is completed by the emerging dominance of the right common cardinal vein. The left upper intercostal spaces drain into the remainder of the left common cardinal vein, which connects with the left brachiocephalic vein after the lateral part of the left common cardinal is lost. The left superior intercostal vein is formed in part by the left posterior and anterior cardinal veins. The potential communication between the two may persist as a left superior vena cava; and the latter's position may be identified in the normal adult as the oblique cardiac vein (of Marshall), which in the adult may be traced at times to the left superior intercostal vein as a reminder of that origin.

The inferior vena cava has a complex origin. The hepatic segment, as noted previously, is derived from the cranial segment of the right vitelline vein and the hepatic sinusoids. A prerenal segment forms distal to this as an anastomosis between the hepatic segment and the right subcardinal vein. This latter vein forms the prerenal segment (down to the junction of the renal veins). A renal segment is formed from a renal collar (note the preaortic anastomosis between the subcardinals described previously). The renal collar is an anastomosis involving this preaortic anastomosis and anastomoses between the right subcardinal and lateral sympathetic veins. A postrenal segment forms from the lumbar part of the right lateral sympathetic vein down to the level of the common iliac veins. The common iliacs join with the lower part of the inferior vena cava as the postcardinal veins degenerate, forcing the iliacs to find this secondary route of venous return to the heart. The definitive renal veins, as the kidneys come to rest in the adult position, are formed as connections to the inferior vena cava through the anastomoses between subcardinals and lateral lumbar veins. On the left side, the longer path to the inferior vena cava is accomplished through recruitment of this anastomosis between the subcardinal veins. On the right, this anastomosis is incorporated into the formation of the renal segment of the inferior vena cava, and the situation is less complex.

The multiple sources incorporated into the inferior vena cava, including anastomoses across the midline, may lead to some bizarre malformations. Most dramatic of these may be the retrocaval ureter, which is clearly not a malformation of the ureter or a misguided path of ascent of the kidney but must be interpreted as incorporation of unusual components of the renal collar into the inferior vena cava. Fortunately, this is a very rare occurrence, but accounts in the literature agree on this interpretation as a caval rather than a ureteric malformation.[17–19]

GROWTH OF NEW VESSELS

It would be helpful to know whether the development of new blood vessels in the fetus and during postnatal growth of the organism is a model for vascular proliferation under other circumstances. It is very likely that this is so, although the factors that might serve to stimulate and direct such growth might be quite different. The central nervous system (CNS) provides a model that has been much studied by a variety of means. The relative maturity of the brain at birth provides an existing and fully functional vascular tree that might be taken as a model of a relatively mature vascular system. The further growth and development of the CNS dictates the need for postnatal neovascularization to support the further maturation of the tissue.

Examination of the vascularization of the CNS, in addition to the interest derived in relation to vascular proliferation, addresses a fundamental issue in vascular growth during development: To what extent is development of a vascular bed a permissive condition for the subsequent onset of function; that is, to what extent is it anticipatory of and necessary for function? Or, conversely, to what extent is the development of a vasculature the response to the greater metabolic demands of a tissue that is increasing in or beginning to achieve the functional levels expected of it at full maturation?

Study of CNS regions at the time of onset of measurable function (e.g., auditory system) reveals that vascular sprouting parallels such events in their time courses (Skolnik and Maxwell, unpublished). Such observations cannot distinguish cause and effect, and perhaps they must go hand in hand, functional and vascular maturation identically timed or responsive to some common signal from yet another source. Greater temporal resolution would have to be applied than we have been able to bring to bear on this question to date.

It is possible to describe the manner of new vessel growth in the CNS and to derive some quantitative information therefrom. Rowan and Maxwell[20] studied the postnatal rat cerebral cortex, which is structurally and cytologically quite immature at birth and undergoes a remarkable degree of postnatal maturation in the first 3 weeks after birth. CNS blood vessels display alkaline phosphatase activity alone among CNS tissue elements. Using a simple histochemical procedure, it is possible to visualize small vessels in the light and electron microscopes, relying on the enzyme reaction to label vessels, and those cells that are in the process of becoming vessels through cytodifferentiation, with no ambiguity whatsoever.[21] It has been a matter of widely accepted dogma that new vessels in the CNS and perhaps elsewhere begin as a proliferation of solid cords of cells that later "canalize" (develop lumens). Such a mechanism seems improbable on purely mechanistic grounds, and this does not seem to be the case in the CNS. In this tissue, postnatal growth of new vessels seems to occur by budding from preexisting vessels, the buds recognizable by their enzyme content, and by the presence of lumens, although collapsed and empty. The lumens are not identifiable by light microscopy, so the interpretation of solid cords of cells is quite understandable. The buds or sprouts have characteristic cytoplasmic protuberances, or fingers, which "explore" in advance of the growth of the sprout, seeming to seek the most appropriate path or perhaps sensing the direction where vessel growth will best satisfy the perceived need. Figures 2–7, 2–8, 2–9, and 2–10 show a series of such sprouts from the rat cerebral cortex.

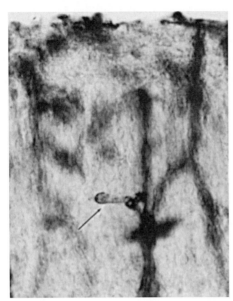

Figure 2–7. Light micrograph of rat cerebral cortex, reacted for alkaline phosphatase. A vascular sprout *(arrow)* is seen in the superficial cortex 2 days postnatal; cortical surface at the top. (×1548.) (Reproduced courtesy of Dr. R. Rowan.)

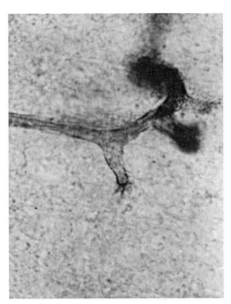

Figure 2–8. Light micrograph of rat cerebral cortex, reacted for alkaline phosphatase. A vascular sprout in middle third of the rat cortex, 7 days postnatal. Delicate exploratory fingers, or pseudopodia, are seen at the tip of the sprout. (×3148.) (Reproduced courtesy of Dr. R. Rowan.)

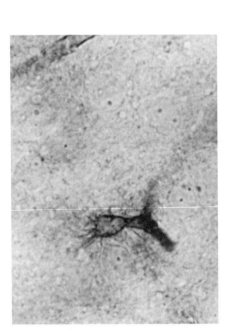

Figure 2–9. Light micrograph of rat cerebral cortex, reacted for alkaline phosphatase. Vascular sprout, middle third of the cortex, 8 days postnatal. Pseudopodia are evident at the tip. (×3148.) (Reproduced courtesy of Dr. R. Rowan.)

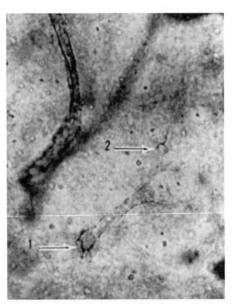

Figure 2–10. Light micrograph of rat cerebral cortex, reacted for alkaline phosphatase. A branched sprout with two tips *(arrows)*. A larger tip (1) extends down and to the left of the stem vessel; a smaller tip extends upward (2). The parent sprout and the two sprout tips are much less intensely stained than the mature vessels dominating the upper and left parts of the photograph. (×3148.) (Reproduced courtesy of Dr. R. Rowan.)

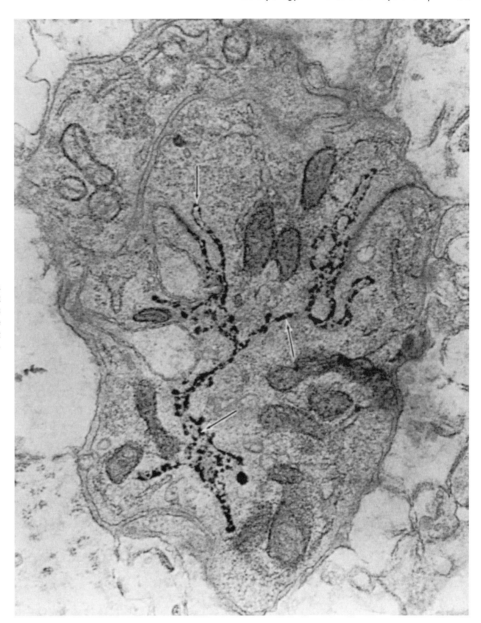

Figure 2–11. Electron micrograph of a sprout in the middle third of the cortex 8 days postnatal. The unopened lumen is delicately outlined by deposition of enzyme (alkaline phosphatase) reaction product and is indicated by arrows. (×42,200.) (Reproduced courtesy of Dr. R. Rowan.)

These sprouts presumably link up with a venous channel, and hemodynamics, which should serve to open the lumen as a capillary link, is thus established. Figure 2–11 is an electron micrograph of such a sprout, in which the unopened state of the lumen is evident. Inasmuch as it is CNS arteries that prominently display alkaline phosphatase activity, and the sprouts at the earliest detectable stages also display this enzyme, we presume that postnatal vascularization proceeds by arteriolar sprouting, with subsequent linkage with the venous bed. An excellent historical review of the study of growth and differentiation of blood vessels and statement of the current status of the field are to be found in Eriksson and Zarem's chapter[22] in *Microcirculation.*

The factors that may induce an arteriole to sprout may be multiple, possibly legion. An enormous literature on angiogenic factors is available for the CNS and for other tissues, including tumors. Attention must be drawn here, however, to a series of papers announcing a major achievement by Vallee's group at Harvard.[23–25] These investigators isolated and analyzed an angiogenic factor from human carcinoma cells, and for the first time, an angiogenic factor was isolated, its amino acid sequence determined, and its genetic code identified. Curiously, this factor, "angiogenin," is remarkably similar in its amino acid sequence to a ribonuclease, and the unraveling of the biologic meaning of this similarity and possible relationship will be fascinating to watch in the literature. This is not to say that only one angiogenic protein is the cause of neovascularization. There may be many, perhaps different ones operating in the embryo and fetus, compared with those in the adult in wound healing, and perhaps again even another set operating in neoplasms. There is abundant evidence that tissue metabolites are capable of stimulating vascular development (e.g., high carbon dioxide and low oxygen content in tissue fluids). A complex list of possibilities will have to be sorted out to determine which of such factors act to stimulate production and/or release of specific angiogenic factors from cells (and which cells) and which are sufficient factors in their own right, acting directly on preexisting vessels.

It may not be satisfying to conclude a survey such as this with a dismaying array of presently unanswered questions. It is compelling evidence, however, that the questions are there and that the vigorous activity in laboratories around the world will yield some answers. The control of neovascularization, of which the embryo is such a master, may allow us to apply the lessons the embryo has to teach us to a wide spectrum of problems afflicting the adults in our clinics and hospitals.

References

1. Delacruz M, Sanchez-Gomez C, Palomino MA: The primitive cardiac regions in the straight tube heart (stage 9) and their anatomical expression in the mature heart: An experimental study in the chick embryo. J Anat 165:121–131, 1989.
2. Congdon ED: Transformation of the aortic-arch system during the development of the human embryo. Carnegie Contr Embryol 14(68):47–110, 1922.
3. Fanapazir K, Kaufman MH: Observations on the development of the aorticopulmonary spiral septum in the mouse. J Anat 158:157–172, 1988.
4. Barclay AE, Franklin KJ, Prichard MML: The Foetal Circulation. Oxford, Blackwell Scientific, 1946.
5. Arey LB: Developmental Anatomy, 7th ed. Philadelphia, WB Saunders, 1965.
6. Clemente CD: Gray's Anatomy, 30th American ed. Philadelphia, Lea & Febiger, 1985.
7. Hamilton WJ, Mossman HW: Hamilton, Boyd and Mossman's Human Embryology, 4th ed. Baltimore, Williams & Wilkins, 1972.
8. Moore KL: The Developing Human, 3rd ed. Philadelphia, WB Saunders, 1982.
9. Sabin FR: Origin and development of the primitive vessels of the chick and pig. Carnegie Contr Embryol 6:63–124, 1917.
10. Tuchmann-Duplessis H, David HG, Haegel P: Illustrated Human Embryology. New York, Springer-Verlag, 1972.
11. Padget DH: Development of the cranial venous system in man, from the viewpoint of comparative anatomy. Carnegie Contr Embryol 36(247):79–140, 1957.
12. Romer AS: The Vertebrate Body, 4th ed. Philadelphia, WB Saunders, 1970.
13. Padget DH: The development of the cranial arteries in the human embryo. Carnegie Contr Embryol 32:205–261, 1948.
14. Dott NM: Anomalies of intestinal rotation: Their embryology and surgical aspects: With report of five cases. Br J Surg 11:252–286, 1923.
15. Thiranagama R, Chamberlain AT, Wood BA: Valves in superficial limb veins of humans and nonhuman primates. Clin Anat 2:135–145, 1989.
16. Streeter GL: The developmental alterations in the vascular system of the brain of the human embryo. Carnegie Contr Embryol 9:5–38, 1918.
17. Derbes VJ, Dial WA: Postcaval ureter. J Urol 36:226–233, 1936.
18. Gruenwald P, Surks SN: Pre-ureteric vena cava and its embryological explanation. J Urol 49:195–261, 1943.
19. Randall A, Campbell EW: Anomalous relationship of the right ureter to the vena cava. J Urol 34:565–583, 1935.
20. Rowan RA, Maxwell DS: Patterns of vascular sprouting in the postnatal development of the cerebral cortex of the rat. Am J Anat 160:246–255, 1981.
21. Rowan RA, Maxwell DS: An ultrastructural study of vascular proliferation and vascular alkaline phosphatase activity in the developing cerebral cortex of the rat. Am J Anat 160:257–265, 1981.
22. Eriksson E, Zarem HA: Growth and differentiation of blood vessels. In Kaley G, Altura BM (eds): Microcirculation, vol I. Baltimore, University Park Press, 1977, pp 393–419.
23. Fett JW, Strydom DJ, Lobb RR, et al: Isolation and characterization of angiogenin, an angiogenic protein from human carcinoma cells. Biochemistry 24:5480–5486, 1985.
24. Kurachi K, Davie CW, Strydom DJ, et al: Sequence of the cDNA and gene for angiogenin, a human angiogenesis factor. Biochemistry 24:5494–5499, 1985.
25. Strydom DJ, Fett JW, Lobb RR, et al: Amino acid sequence of human derived angiogenin. Biochemistry 24:5486–5494, 1985.

Anatomy, Physiology, and Pharmacology of the Vascular Wall

Alexander W. Clowes and Ted R. Kohler

NORMAL ANATOMY

Although the vasculature is a series of tubes whose primary function is to act as nonthrombogenic conduits for blood, in fact it is quite diverse in structure and function. Not only do the vessels act as conduits, they also act as capacitors, and they regulate the molecular and cellular traffic between the vascular and extravascular spaces. This latter function is largely a property of small vessels (particularly postcapillary venules). Because the cellular elements (endothelium and smooth muscle cells) in the microvasculature are the same as in the large vessels, we might expect the cells located in arteries and veins to have some of the same regulatory properties as when they are located in the arterioles and venules. As is discussed later in this chapter, the similar properties of the endothelium and smooth muscle cells in large and small vessels may account for some of the abnormal properties of vessels undergoing atherosclerotic change or thickening after transplantation (transplant atherosclerosis).

The vasculature has distinct anatomic and physiologic features. Arteries are divided into three categories: large elastic arteries, medium-sized muscular arteries, and small arteries. All arteries possess three layers, or tunics, called the intima, media, and adventitia. The intima, the innermost layer of the wall lying inside the internal elastic lamina and directly adjacent to the flowing blood, is composed of endothelium at the luminal surface and subendothelial extracellular matrix. In some vessels, one or more layers of smooth muscle cells are present; this so-called intimal cushion of smooth muscle cells may in some circumstances be the progenitor of the fibrous intimal plaque. The media,

bounded by the internal and external elastic laminae, contains smooth muscle cells embedded in a matrix of collagen, elastin, and proteoglycans. The adventitia lies outside the external elastic lamina and is composed of loose connective tissue, fibroblasts, capillaries, occasional leukocytes (particularly mast cells), and small nerve fibers.

The large elastic arteries of the body include the aorta and its major branches, while the medium-sized muscular arteries include most of the distributing vessels to the organs. These two classes of arteries, like all vessels, have all three layers represented in the wall. They differ principally in the amount of elastic tissue present in the media. The aortic wall is composed of well-defined lamellar units consisting of commonly oriented and elongated smooth muscle cells with their surrounding matrix, including a meshwork of collagen, and a layer of elastin.[1,2] The number of lamellar units in the aortas of various mammalian species, encompassing a wide range of body sizes, is proportional to the radius, regardless of variations in wall thickness.[1] As a result, the average tension per lamellar unit is remarkably constant. This lamellar unit represents the structural and functional unit of the aortic wall. Wall stress, which is pressure times radius divided by thickness, is fairly constant as a result of the linear relationship between wall thickness and radius and the fact that blood pressure is independent of species and size. This results in a good match between the strength of the wall and the tangential distending force within it. Increases in pressure, as occur in hypertension or in the wall of thin vein grafts placed in the arterial circulation, or increases in vessel diameter that occur when vessels dilate in response to increased flow, result in increased stress and compensatory increases in wall thickness.

In the elastic arteries, the media is composed of layers of smooth muscle cells interspersed with clearly defined lamellae of elastin. The media of muscular arteries is also

From Clowes AW: Series of atherosclerosis. In White RA (ed): Atherosclerosis: Human Pathology and Experimental Animal Methods and Models. Boca Raton, Fla, CRC Press, 1989, pp 3–15.

composed of smooth muscle cells but lacks discrete elastic lamellae, except for the internal and external elastic layers (Fig. 3–1). The elastin is present only as thin fibers. In the largest elastic arteries with more than 28 elastic layers, a microvasculature (vasa vasorum) penetrates the media from the adventitial side and provides a nutrient supply to the deep layers of the wall.[3] The inner layers receive nutrients directly from the lumen.

As arteries become smaller, there is a progressive loss of elastic tissue to the point that the internal and external elastic lamellae become discontinuous and fragmented, and the clear distinction between the various layers is lost. At the arteriolar level, the wall is composed of an endothelium, a layer of smooth muscle, and a filamentous collagenous adventitia. Compared with other arteries in the body, the small arteries have a relatively thick media and a large ratio of media to lumen, in keeping with their function as resistance vessels.

As has been pointed out by others,[4] the differentiation of these three types of arteries is of great pathologic significance, because each class of vessels is subject to particular types of disease. Atherosclerosis is confined to elastic and muscular arteries, and medial calcific sclerosis to muscular arteries. Small arteries develop diffuse fibromuscular thickening and hyalinization.

Veins tend to be much larger and more thin walled than arteries. The intima contains only an endothelial layer. The internal elastic layer is clearly evident only in the larger veins, and the media contains relatively few smooth muscle cells, collagen, and little elastin. In the veins of the extremities, there are thin bicuspid valves containing mainly endothelium and connective tissue.

REGULATION OF LUMINAL AREA

Although a description of the structures of the normal vasculature underscores the point that endothelial and smooth muscle cells are the principal cellular elements, such a description does not provide any insight into the mechanisms that regulate wall structure and function under normal circumstances or during the development of pathologic lesions. Furthermore, such a description does not give a clue to how a vessel adjusts its mass and dimensions in response to external stimuli (hypertension, increased blood flow, vascular injury) or to how it maintains a nonthrombogenic state. To understand these physiologic responses, we must consider the functions of the individual cellular elements and the activities of these cells when they exist together as an organ in the fully formed vessel.

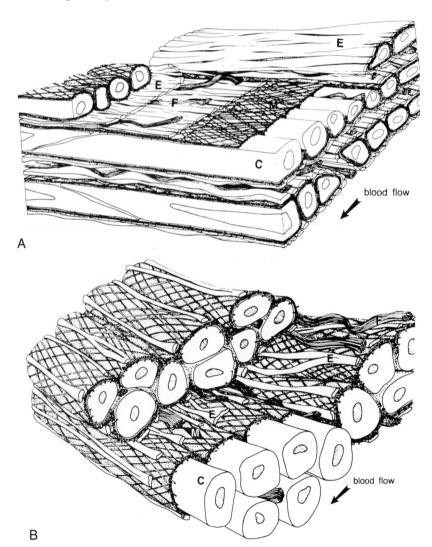

blood flow

A

blood flow

B

Figure 3–1. Schematic representation of the lamellar organization of elastic (A) and muscular (B) arteries. Each unit is composed of a group of commonly oriented smooth muscle cells (C) surrounded by matrix (M) consisting of basal lamina and a fine meshwork of collagen and surrounded by elastic fibers (E) oriented in the same direction as the long axes of the cells. Wavy collagen bundles (F) lie between the elastic fibers. The elastic lamellae are much better defined in the elastic arteries (A) than in the muscular arteries (B). (From Clark JM, Glagov S: Transmural organization of the arterial media: The lamellar unit revisited. Arteriosclerosis 5:19–34, 1985.)

Both developing and mature vessels respond to changes in blood flow by adjusting their diameter in a manner that maintains constant shear. A striking example of this change is found in an artery proximal to an arteriovenous fistula.[5] The vessel enlarges and can, over the course of a lifetime, become aneurysmal. Conversely, diameter is reduced when outflow is diminished. This has been observed in mature and developing arteries and in vessels where flow is reduced by a proximal obstruction.[6–8] Diseased arterial segments also respond to changes in flow. A coronary artery with an enlarging atherosclerotic intima will presumably develop luminal stenosis, and, therefore, the blood velocity in that stenosis increases. This increase in blood velocity in turn causes vasodilatation. In fact, a diseased coronary artery can dilate and maintain normal luminal dimensions despite changes in wall structure so long as the intimal lesion does not exceed 40% of the area inside the internal elastic lamina.[9] At this point, pathologic narrowing begins. The endothelium senses changes in blood velocity and shear and translates this biomechanical information into biochemical signals that regulate vessel diameter. Vessels denuded of endothelium do not respond to changes in flow.[10] Acute diameter changes occur by altering vasomotor tone.[6] If the change in flow is chronic, arterial wall structure remodels to the new caliber, and vasomotor tone returns to normal. This is demonstrated in the work of Langille and O'Donnell,[6] who showed that the reduction in lumen that accompanies partial ligation of carotid outflow in rabbits initially is reversible by application of topical vasodilators, but later becomes fixed.

Pharmacologic agents regulating vascular wall contraction can be classified as endothelial and nonendothelial dependent.[11] Furchgott and Zawadzki[12] reported in 1980 that the relaxation of isolated rabbit aorta and other arteries induced by acetylcholine and other agonists for muscarinic receptors depended on the presence of endothelial cells. After removal of the endothelial cells, acetylcholine no longer induced relaxation; instead, it caused contraction. A large number of agents, including acetylcholine, arachidonic acid, adenosine triphosphate (ATP) and adenosine diphosphate (ADP), bradykinin, histamine, norepinephrine, serotonin, thrombin, and vasopressin, have been shown to produce an endothelium-dependent relaxation of arteries. Other substances, such as adenosine and adenosine monophosphate (AMP), papaverine, isoproterenol, nitrovasodilators (such as sodium nitroprusside), and prostacyclin, do not require the presence of endothelial cells to elicit relaxation. The endothelial-dependent relaxation results from release of nitric oxide, which stimulates guanylate cyclase of the underlying smooth muscle cells and causes an increase in cyclic guanosine monophosphate (cGMP). Nitric oxide is derived from L-arginine,[13] and is present in higher concentrations in small resistance vessels than in larger conduit arteries.

In addition to expressing a relaxing factor, endothelium can express contracting factors.[11, 12] The contracting factors appear to be responsible for contractions in some systemic vessels induced by arachidonic acid and hypoxia and in isolated cerebral vessels by stretch. One of these factors is a peptide, endothelin, which has been isolated from cultured endothelial cells and is a potent vasoconstrictor. Increase in shear stress suppresses the expression of the gene for endothelin and increases the production of nitric oxide synthase (NOS) by endothelial cells. It is likely that these endothelial-derived relaxing and constricting factors contribute to long-term vascular adaptation in response to increased blood flow. As is discussed later in the chapter, regulation of wall structure and vessel diameter is closely linked. Nitric oxide inhibits smooth muscle cell growth, whereas endothelin promotes it. Certain pathologic conditions in which endothelium is either missing or abnormal are associated with acute and chronic vasospasm; it is quite possible that the acute problems of atypical angina (coronary vasospasm) and cerebrovasospasm after cerebral hemorrhage are in part manifestations of abnormal endothelial function and abnormal secretion of these factors.[14]

REGULATION OF MEDIAL AND INTIMAL THICKENING

Arterial wall thickening is a prominent feature of most pathologic processes. In hypertensive animals and humans, arteries exhibit medial thickening, whereas after endothelial denudation or in the presence of hypercholesterolemia, they develop a thick intima.[15–17] Exactly how these responses are regulated is not clear, although it is certain that in each instance, proliferation of smooth muscle cells and accumulation of extracellular matrix are important components. In addition, in hypercholesterolemic subjects, the accumulation of lipid and lipid-filled macrophages contributes to the intimal lesion.

Because smooth muscle accumulation is a central feature of most forms of vascular thickening, it is worth discussing the mechanisms of growth control as we currently understand them.[18] During growth and development, smooth muscle cells proliferate; they revert spontaneously to a quiescent state in adult vessels. In the adult rat, smooth muscle cells turn over at the rate of 0.06% per day, a number barely detectable with available methods.[19] How the early rapid growth and late quiescence are regulated is not known, but this must be of importance to the problem of primary hypertension and local susceptibility to atherosclerotic change.

Of the models of smooth muscle growth in vivo, perhaps the best characterized is the balloon injury model.[20] In this model, smooth muscle proliferation is stimulated by the passage of an inflated balloon catheter along an artery. The artery is at once stretched and denuded of its endothelium. Immediately thereafter, platelets begin to adhere to the wall wherever endothelium is missing; they then spread and degranulate.

In most situations, endothelial denudation and platelet adherence are followed 1 to 2 days later by the onset of medial smooth muscle proliferation and migration of these cells across the internal elastic lamina to form a neointima.[19] In the ballooned rat carotid, this can be a most dramatic response, with a marked increase in the thymidine labeling index (a measure of proliferation) (Fig. 3–2). Intimal cells commit to proliferation early after injury. If entry into the cell cycle is blocked by giving the animals heparin during the first few days after injury, the number of dividing cells and the mass of neointima are significantly reduced.[21] Not all smooth muscle cells in the intima respond

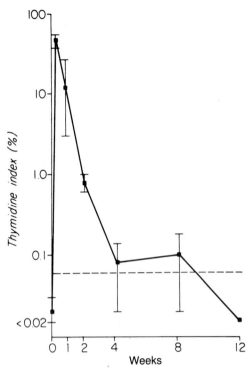

Figure 3–2. Smooth muscle cell proliferation rates following balloon catheter injury of the rat carotid artery, as measured by the percentage of cells that incorporate thymidine. Proliferation is greatest at 48 hours and falls rapidly thereafter. (Adapted from Clowes AW, Reidy MA, Clowes MM: Kinetics of cellular proliferation after arterial injury: I. Smooth muscle growth in the absence of endothelium. Lab Invest 49:327–333, 1983.)

equally to mitogenic stimuli, probably because there is a mixture of cells derived from either the mesoderm or the ectoderm.[22]

A link between smooth muscle proliferation and earlier platelet granule release has been proposed based on studies characterizing the proteins within the granules.[16] Among them are several growth factors, including platelet-derived growth factor (PDGF), transforming growth factor β (TGFβ), and an epidermal growth factor–like protein.[23] Where these granule proteins go after being released from the platelets is not known. One hypothesis suggests that these factors accumulate in the artery wall and stimulate subsequent smooth muscle growth.

The reaction-to-injury hypothesis was first proposed many decades ago as a general mechanism for atherogenesis and has been refined in view of more recent information.[16] Although attractive in theory, it is based on rather slim evidence mainly derived from experiments in thrombocytopenic animals. Injured arteries in these animals showed very little intimal thickening.[24] Later work using thrombocytopenic rats suggests that platelets may be more important in stimulating migration than in cell proliferation.[25] These animals had reduced intimal thickening even though smooth muscle cell proliferation was not measurably altered. Additional work using anti-PDGF antibodies or infusion of PDGF after balloon injury supports this concept.[26, 27]

This early proliferation in the media of the injured artery does not lead to an increase in wall thickness; the wall thickens only after smooth muscle cells migrate from the media and proliferate in the intima. This process persists for a period of time and subsides spontaneously whether or not endothelium reappears at the luminal surface. The intimal mass is further increased by the accumulation of extracellular matrix synthesized by the smooth muscle cells[28] (Fig. 3–3).

Although little is known of what starts or stops the intimal thickening process, there are several observations that are interesting and perhaps important. The first is that the surface of the injured artery accumulates a single layer of platelets. Fibrin and microthrombi are only seen at the luminal surface when the artery is reinjured after an intimal thickening has formed or in small craters in association with adherent macrophages in hypercholesterolemic animals. Thus, active fulminant thrombosis is not a usual feature of injured vessels; when it occurs, it must represent a major aberration of vessel function.[29] Second, in models demonstrating early re-endothelialization or partial de-endothelialization without medial injury, intimal thickening does not develop, although one or two rounds of medial smooth muscle proliferation can occur. This result suggests that endothelium may play a role in suppressing smooth muscle growth and migration from the media to the intima. We know that smooth muscle growth inhibitors can be extracted from the vessel wall, that endothelium can synthesize a heparin-like molecule that inhibits smooth muscle cell growth in vitro, and that heparin itself can suppress both proliferation and migration of smooth muscle cells in vitro and in vivo.[30] Endothelium also releases nitric oxide, a growth inhibitor whose production is flow dependent (see later). Taken together, these findings suggest that endothelium can inhibit smooth muscle proliferation and that the quiescent state of smooth muscle cells in the normal arteries of adult animals may be an actively maintained one rather than one attributable to the lack of growth factors. Finally, there is the more general concept emerging that the cells of the vascular wall "speak" to each other and regulate the function of one another.

The possibility of cell-cell communication has now been considered briefly twice: in regard to chronic vasodilatation in response to increased blood velocity and in regard to control of smooth muscle cell proliferation and migration. Let us examine the kinds of messages and the participants in more detail, particularly with regard to growth control and the maintenance of the antithrombotic state. At the outset, we can state that at least in vitro there is evidence for direct cell-cell communication by means of intercellular junctions; there is also evidence for communication by means of molecules secreted into the extracellular space and acting at a distance.

Direct cell-cell junctional communication has been demonstrated in monolayers of endothelium[31] and in mixed cell populations between endothelium and smooth muscle cells.[32] Gap junctions have been demonstrated morphologically between endothelial cells and between endothelium and smooth muscle cells in vivo and in vitro. The significance of these direct links has in general not been defined, although in culture pericytes and smooth muscle cells can inhibit endothelial growth when the cells are in contact with one another.[32] Plasma membrane preparations from confluent large vessel endothelium also actively inhibit

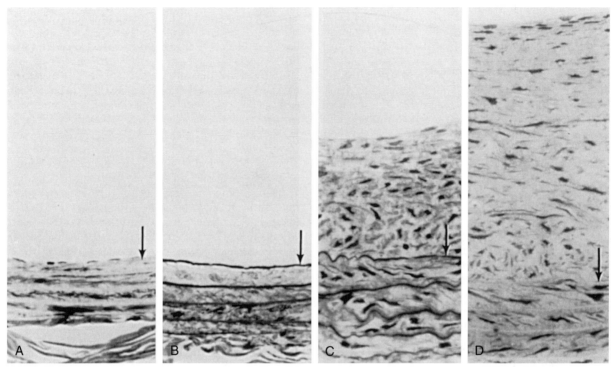

Figure 3–3. Histologic cross-sections of the region lacking endothelium of injured left carotid arteries. *A*, Normal vessel. Note single layer of endothelium in intima. *B*, Denuded vessel at 2 days. Note loss of endothelium. *C*, Denuded vessel at 2 weeks. Intima is now markedly thickened because of smooth muscle proliferation. *D*, Denuded vessel at 12 weeks. Further intimal thickening has occurred. Internal elastic lamina is indicated by the arrow. Lumen is at the top. (From Clowes AW, Reidy MA, Clowes MM: Kinetics of cellular proliferation after arterial injury: I. Smooth muscle growth in the absence of endothelium. Lab Invest 49:327–333, 1983.)

growing endothelial cells.[33] In vivo capillary endothelial growth is associated with absence of pericytes, and cessation of growth is associated with their reappearance. In addition, the intercellular links might help to regulate endothelial proliferation and endothelial-mediated vascular relaxation in collateral vessels by propagating signals from one cell to the next upstream from a large vessel occlusion. They would also provide a mechanism for a local response in a vessel without the need for the release and wide dissemination of potent vasoactive or growth-regulatory substances.

Cell-cell communication at a distance is likely to be mediated by secreted soluble factors. As mentioned previously, the blood platelet, which in reality is a fragment of a megakaryocyte, carries within it an array of potent mitogens. The notion that platelets are involved in wound-healing processes came from morphologic studies of injured vessels and the observation that whole blood serum contains much more growth-promoting activity than serum prepared from blood depleted of all cellular elements, including platelets (plasma-derived serum). These findings led to the discovery of PDGF, a basic dimeric protein[34] with a molecular weight of approximately 30,000. It is transported in the blood in the alpha granule of the platelet and is released along with other alpha granule proteins. PDGF is by itself extremely potent and is active as a smooth muscle mitogen in trace amounts (nanograms per milliliter). It also exhibits a range of other activities (stimulates smooth muscle migration, contraction, and matrix synthesis) on smooth muscle and other types of cells, although it is not a mitogen for endothelium. When placed in a wound chamber in vivo, it induces a granulation tissue response.[35]

The structure of the gene for PDGF is nearly identical to that of the oncogene v-*sis*, a gene associated with cellular transformation by the simian sarcoma virus.[36, 37] This discovery, coupled with the finding that a variety of cells (including normal cells) synthesize and secrete active PDGF, raises the possibility that normal wound healing and malignant, unscheduled growth of tumor cells might have striking similarities with subtle differences in gene regulation. It also led to a search for growth factors in vascular wall cells. We now have solid evidence that endothelium, smooth muscle cells, and leukocytes, including macrophages, can express the PDGF gene (c-*sis*) in vitro and in vivo.[34] What role the gene product, the PDGF protein, plays in wall function remains to be resolved. The work mentioned here using anti-PDGF antibodies or infusion of PDGF in animals undergoing carotid injury by balloon catheter suggests that the primary role of PDGF is to stimulate smooth muscle cell migration rather than proliferation.[26, 27]

Recent work suggests that intracellular mitogens released from injured medial smooth muscle cells are primarily responsible for stimulating cell proliferation. First, smooth muscle cell proliferation occurs when arteries are injured by hydrostatic distention that does not cause significant endothelial injury.[38] In this case, there is very little smooth muscle cell migration, probably because of the lack of platelet factor release.[38] Second, very little smooth muscle cell proliferation is observed when the endothelium is injured by using a fine nylon loop that does not damage the media.[39, 40] Basic fibroblast growth factor (bFGF) may be the principle mitogen responsible for smooth muscle cell proliferation after injury. Both bFGF messenger RNA (mRNA) and protein are found in the uninjured vessel wall.[41] Infusion or local administration of bFGF after arterial injury causes a marked increase in smooth muscle cell replication and intimal thickening.[41, 42] Conversely, infusion of antibodies to bFGF causes a significant reduction in smooth muscle cell proliferation.[43] bFGF does not appear to be mitogenic for cells in uninjured vessels, suggesting that other products of injury are necessary to induce mitogenesis. Cultured smooth muscle cells derived from injured media produce up to five times more PDGF than do cells from uninjured arteries.[44] These injured cells also express mRNA for insulin-like growth factor[45] and TGFβ,[46] both of which are mitogenic for smooth muscle cells in culture. Thus, the smooth muscle cells in the injured media may stimulate cell growth in a paracrine fashion by release of a number of mitogens.

The rate of blood flow, which affects diameter in developing and mature arteries, also influences intimal hyperplasia in injured vessels and vascular grafts. Wall thickening of vein and synthetic grafts is increased in areas of reduced flow[47, 48] and is reduced by high flow[49, 50] (Fig. 3–4). Increased flow causes regression of intima in endothelialized baboon polytetrafluoroethylene grafts.[51] As mentioned earlier, the endothelium responds to changes in shear and releases factors that regulate arterial diameter and wall structure in response to flow. For example, reduced flow causes an increase in PDGF expression in rat carotid arteries.[52] High flow upregulates NOS in synthetic grafts. We have found that the suppressive effect of flow on intimal thickening can be blocked by local infusion of an NOS inhibitor. Flow also appears to affect intimal hyperplasia in balloon-injured rat carotid arteries, even though the endothelium is absent in this model.[53] This implies that surface smooth muscle cells can respond to flow in a manner similar to that of endothelium. Finally, restoration of endothelial cell NOS activity in the denuded wall of injured rat carotid arteries by gene transfer suppresses intimal hyperplasia and increases vessel reactivity.[54]

There are several interesting preliminary observations that permit us now to outline a theory of growth control in the wall. Endothelial cells in vitro can condition the tissue culture medium with growth-promoting factors for smooth muscle cells; a portion of this activity is due to PDGF-like proteins and perhaps to other characterized factors, such as bFGF. Production of PDGF is increased when the cells are exposed to endotoxin or phorbol esters and decreased when the cells are exposed to oxidized low-density lipoprotein.[55] Smooth muscle cells make PDGF in vitro as well; in particular, cells derived from neonatal as opposed to adult aortas and proliferating cells derived from injury-induced intimal thickenings as opposed to quiescent media are prone to do this.[18] Macrophages, when stimulated, increase their production of PDGF. Finally, injured vascular wall cells release intracellular mitogens (e.g., bFGF). These fragmentary results support the concept that "activated" vascular wall cells can amplify the initial stimulus (perhaps an influx of platelet-derived factors) by producing

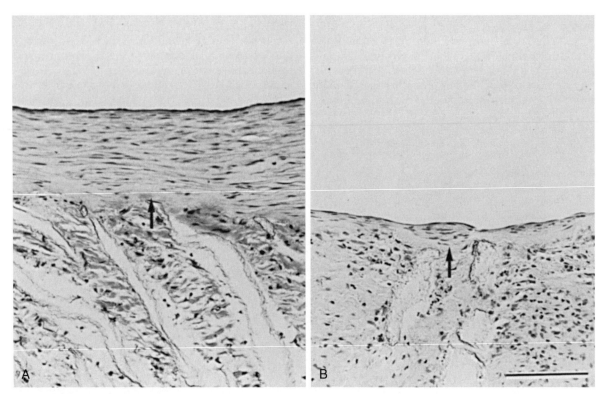

Figure 3–4. Cross-sections of polytetrafluoroethylene grafts 3 months after placement in the aortoiliac circulation in baboons. *A*, Control side with normal flow. *B*, Experimental side with a distal arteriovenous fistula causing increased flow. The arrows indicate the junction of the graft and neointima. (Bar, 100 μm.) (From Kohler TR, Kirkman TR, Kraiss LW, et al: Increased blood flow inhibits neointimal hyperplasia in endothelialized vascular grafts. Circ Res 69:1557–1565, 1991.)

PDGF and other growth-promoting factors that would then act on the cells. Furthermore, these factors might also act to regulate the traffic of leukocytes in and out of the wall; the activated leukocytes could in turn reciprocate by the production of factors affecting the function of the vascular wall cells. What emerges here is the notion that there may be a great deal of cross-talk between the cells of the wall and the blood, with many complex feedback loops[56] (Fig. 3–5).

New possibilities for preventing restenosis are emerging from our increasing understanding of cellular and molecular events. A complete listing of therapeutic strategies is beyond the scope of this chapter, but some recent developments are worth noting. For example, our laboratory has found that blockade of the PDGF β receptor with a chimeric human-murine antibody, in conjunction with heparin, inhibits intimal hyperplasia in a primate arterial injury model.[57] This finding supports the notion that PDGF plays an important role in wall thickening after injury. Platelet glycoprotein-IIb/IIIa blockade with the chimeric antibody abciximab inhibits platelet aggregation and reduces the incidence of repeated procedures, death, or myocardial infarction after coronary angioplasty.[58] A single dose of this drug improved clinical results 3 years after the procedure, suggesting that either platelets have a role in initiating intimal hyperplasia or the drug affects smooth muscle cell proliferation and migration.[59] In this regard, it is interesting to note a clinical trial of ticlopidine showing that 2-year patency rates were improved by the drug in vein grafts of lower extremity arteries.[60]

Many strategies are emerging for local control of smooth muscle cell proliferation following vascular injury. These include antisense oligonucleotides to inhibit cell cycle regulatory proteins and local delivery of radiation.[61–65] Radiation has the potential advantage of affecting adventitial cells. Lumen narrowing after injury results both from the mass of neointima that forms and from remodeling of the vessel to a smaller diameter. Adventitial myofibroblasts contribute to each of these processes by forming a fibrotic scar around the injured vessel and by migrating across the wall into the neointima.[66] It is not yet known if just the right dose of radiation can be delivered to halt the restenosis process.

So far, trials using ^{32}P radioactive β-emitting stents with low activity levels (0.75 to 3.0 μCi) for coronary angioplasty have shown no beneficial effect. Stents with higher activity levels (>3.0 μCi) have reduced intimal hyperplasia within the stent, but the low doses that are delivered to the adjacent artery near the end of the stents may actually encourage edge restenosis, particularly if this segment has been overdilated. This creates a "candy wrapper" appearance with a widely patent stented region flanked on either side by tight stenoses.[67]

REGULATION OF THROMBOSIS BY THE ENDOTHELIUM

Empirical observation demonstrates quite clearly that a normal endothelial-lined artery is resistant to thrombosis. Even with complete cessation of blood flow for a prolonged period of time clotting does not occur, although blood in a damaged vessel clots rather readily. It would seem that endothelium must make one or more antithrombotic or anticoagulant molecules, and this has proved to be true. What is more striking is that the endothelium expresses an extensive array of procoagulant functions as well. Like the growth factors, these procoagulant-anticoagulant functions are regulated by messages coming from the blood or from neighboring cells.[68]

On the anticoagulant side of the balance, the endothelium synthesizes a membrane-associated heparan sulfate that, like heparin, increases the affinity of antithrombin III for thrombin.[69] Because this interaction requires the binding of heparan sulfate to the antithrombin III, the complex must be active at the level of the endothelial surface. Heparan–antithrombin III then rapidly inactivates circulating thrombin and other activated serine proteases in the clotting cascade, including factors VII, IX, and X. Thus, endothelial-derived heparan sulfate can act to impede two aspects of the injury response: the activation of the clotting cascade and the stimulation of smooth muscle proliferation that we referred to earlier.[30] In addition, endothelial cells can inhibit clotting by means of the protein C pathway.[70] Endothelium synthesizes and secretes a protein called

Figure 3–5. Diagram illustrating how injury to the artery might cause endothelial cell (EC) and smooth muscle cell (SMC) disruption and release of intracellular mitogens such as basic fibroblast growth factor (bFGF). bFGF then stimulates medial smooth muscle proliferation. Factors from platelets (PDGF BB) regulate movement of the smooth muscle cells from the media to the intima. Angiotensin II also affects the intimal thickening process. (From Clowes AW, Reidy MA: Prevention of stenosis after vascular reconstruction: Pharmacologic control of intimal hyperplasia—a review. J Vasc Surg 13:885–891, 1991.)

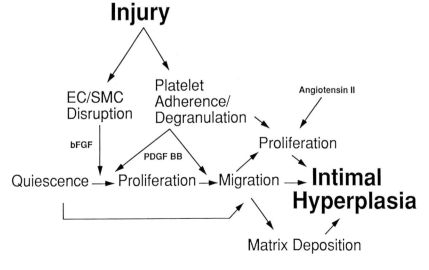

thrombomodulin, which in turn is bound to a surface receptor. The receptor-thrombomodulin complex binds thrombin and in so doing inactivates the proteolytic activity for fibrinogen. The thrombomodulin-thrombin complex activates protein C, and the activated protein C binds to protein S on the endothelial surface. The protein C–protein S complex then can inactivate factor Va, thereby inhibiting the clotting cascade. That this pathway is important is amply demonstrated in homozygous-deficient patients, who develop spontaneous thrombosis. Finally, endothelial cells can inhibit platelet adhesion and aggregation through the synthesis of prostaglandin I₂ and can degrade formed fibrin by activating plasminogen to plasmin.

On the procoagulant side, endothelial cells synthesize and secrete tissue factor, a plasminogen activator inhibitor, and von Willebrand's factor, and they express a number of receptors for factors of the clotting cascade. When the cells are exposed to a variety of inflammatory mediators derived from the blood or from resident macrophages (e.g., endotoxin, interleukin-1 [IL-1], tumor necrosis factor), endothelial cells respond by changing the balance of anticoagulant-procoagulant activities to favor coagulation. Also, the cells synthesize and express IL-1, which potentially could affect the underlying smooth muscle cells.[71] At present, these conclusions are largely based on in vitro experiments; although they have relevance mainly to the microvasculature, they also may prove to be important to large vessels in

view of the recent evidence that not only macrophages but also different populations of lymphocytes are present in the atherosclerotic plaque. Furthermore, the ability of the vascular wall cells to maintain the anticoagulant state at the luminal surface must have a direct bearing on the thrombotic complications associated with end-stage atherosclerosis.

Thrombin generated during thrombosis may play an important role in regulation of smooth muscle cell growth. It is mitogenic for these cells grown in culture. Antithrombin agents block the increase in PDGF gene expression that normally follows injury and can limit smooth muscle cell proliferation following injury.[72] Thrombin may also potentiate cell growth by activating platelets and attracting activated macrophages, which also produce mitogens.

SUMMARY

The normal blood vessel must be viewed not only as a conduit but also as an organ containing endothelial and smooth muscle cells that can respond to physical and chemical stimuli in the blood by adjusting vascular diameter and thickness. Furthermore, vascular wall cells can communicate among themselves and express factors that can regulate cell proliferation and coagulation as well as allow the cells to participate in local inflammatory reactions.

References

1. Wolinsky H, Glagov S: A lamellar unit of aortic medial structure and function in mammals. Circ Res 20:99, 1967.
2. Clark JM, Glagov S: Transmural organization of the arterial media: The lamellar unit revisited. Arteriosclerosis 5:19, 1985.
3. Wolinsky H, Glagov S: Nature of species differences in the medial distribution of aortic vasa vasorum in mammals. Circ Res 20:409, 1967.
4. Cotran RS, Kumar V, Robbins SL: Pathologic Basis of Disease. Philadelphia, WB Saunders, 1989, p 553.
5. Zarins CK, Zatina MA, Giddens DP, et al: Shear stress regulation of artery lumen diameter in experimental atherogenesis. J Vasc Surg 5:413, 1987.
6. Langille BL, O'Donnell F: Reductions in arterial diameter produced by chronic decreases in blood flow are endothelium-dependent. Science 231:405, 1986.
7. Guyton JR, Hartley CJ: Flow restriction of one carotid artery in juvenile rats inhibits growth of arterial diameter. Am J Physiol 248:H540, 1985.
8. Brownlee RD, Langille BL: Arterial adaptations to altered blood flow. Can J Physiol Pharmacol 69:978, 1991.
9. Glagov S, Weisenberg E, Zarins CK, et al: Compensatory enlargement of human atherosclerotic coronary arteries. N Engl J Med 316:1371, 1987.
10. Frangos JA, Eskin SG, McIntire LV, Ives CL: Flow effect on prostacyclin production by cultured human endothelial cells. Science 227:1477, 1985.
11. Furchgott RF, Vanhoutte PM: Endothelium-derived relaxing and contracting factors. FASEB J 3:2007, 1989.
12. Furchgott RF, Zawadzki JV: The obligatory role of endothelial cells in the relaxation of arterial smooth muscle by acetylcholine. Nature 288:373–376, 1980.
13. Moncada S, Higgs EA, Hodson HF, et al: EDRF and EDRF-related substances. The L-arginine:nitric oxide pathway. J Cardiovasc Pharmacol 17(Suppl 3):S1–S9, 1991.
14. Freiman PC, Mitchell GG, Heistad DD, et al: Atherosclerosis impairs endothelium-dependent vascular relaxation to acetylcholine and thrombin in primates. Circ Res 58:783, 1986.

15. Wolinsky H: Long-term effects of hypertension on the rat aortic wall and their relation to concurrent aging changes: Morphological and chemical studies. Circ Res 30:301, 1972.
16. Ross R: Pathogenesis of atherosclerosis—an update. N Engl J Med 314:488, 1986.
17. Steinberg D: Lipoproteins and the pathogenesis of atherosclerosis. Circulation 76:508, 1987.
18. Schwartz SM, Campbell GR, Campbell JH: Replication of smooth muscle cells in vascular disease. Circ Res 58:427, 1986.
19. Clowes AW, Reidy MA, Clowes MM: Kinetics of cellular proliferation after arterial injury: 1. Smooth muscle growth in the absence of endothelium. Lab Invest 49:327, 1983.
20. Baumgartner HR, Studer A: Consequences of vessel catheterization in normal and hypercholesterolemic rabbits [in German]. Pathol Microbiol 29:393, 1966.
21. Clowes AW, Clowes MM: Kinetics of cellular proliferation after arterial injury. IV Heparin inhibits rat smooth muscle mitogenesis and migration. Circ Res 58:839–845, 1986.
22. Topouzis S, Majesky MW: Smooth muscle lineage diversity in the chick embryo. Two types of aortic smooth muscle cell differ in growth and receptor-mediated transcriptional responses to transforming growth factor-beta. Dev Biol 178:430–445, 1996.
23. Bowen-Pope DF, Ross R, Seifert RA: Locally acting growth factors for vascular smooth muscle cells: Endogenous synthesis and release from platelets. Circulation 72:735, 1985.
24. Friedman RJ, Stemerman MB, Wenz B, et al: The effect of thrombocytopenia on experimental arteriosclerotic lesion formation in rabbits, smooth muscle cell proliferation and re-endothelialization. J Clin Invest 60:1191, 1977.
25. Fingerle J, Johnson R, Clowes AW, et al: Role of platelets in smooth muscle cell proliferation and migration after vascular injury in rat carotid artery. Proc Natl Acad Sci U S A 86:8412, 1989.
26. Ferns GAA, Raines EW, Sprugel KH, et al: Inhibition of neointimal smooth muscle accumulation after angioplasty by an antibody to PDGF. Science 253:1129, 1991.
27. Jawien A, Bowen-Pope DF, Lindner V, et al: Platelet-derived growth

factor promotes smooth muscle migration and intimal thickening in a rat model of balloon angioplasty. J Clin Invest 89:507, 1992.

28. Clowes AW, Reidy MA, Clowes MM: Mechanisms of stenosis after arterial injury. Lab Invest 49:208, 1983.

29. Reidy MA: A reassessment of endothelial injury and arterial lesion formation. Lab Invest 53:513, 1985.

30. Clowes AW, Clowes MM: Regulation of smooth muscle proliferation by heparin in vitro and in vivo. Int Angiol 6:45, 1987.

31. Larson DM, Carson MP, Haudenschild CC: Junctional transfer of small molecules in cultured bovine brain microvascular endothelial cells and pericytes. Microvasc Res 34:184–199, 1987.

32. Orlidge A, D'Amore PA: Inhibition of capillary endothelial cell growth by pericytes and smooth muscle cells. J Cell Biol 105:1455, 1987.

33. Heimark RL, Schwartz SM: The role of membrane-membrane inter-actions in the regulation of endothelial cell growth. J Cell Biol 100:1934, 1985.

34. Ross R, Raines EW, Bowen-Pope DF: The biology of PDGF. Cell 46:155, 1986.

35. Sprugel KH, McPherson JM, Clowes AW, Ross R: Effects of growth factors in vivo. I. Cell ingrowth into porous subcutaneous chambers. Am J Pathol 129:601, 1987.

36. Doolittle RF, Hunkapillar MW, Hood LE, et al: Simian sarcoma virus oncogene, v-*sis*, is derived from the gene (or genes) encoding a platelet-derived growth factor. Science 221:275, 1983.

37. Waterfield MD, Scrace GT, Whittle N, et al: Platelet-derived growth factor is structurally related to the putative transforming protein p28-*sis* of simian sarcoma virus. Nature 304:35, 1983.

38. Clowes AW, Clowes MM, Fingerle J, Reidy MA: Kinetics of cellular proliferation after arterial injury. V. Role of acute distention in the induction of smooth muscle proliferation. Lab Invest 60:360–364, 1989.

39. Tada T, Reidy MA: Endothelial regeneration. IX. Arterial injury fol-lowed by rapid endothelial repair induces smooth-muscle-cell prolif-eration but not intimal thickening. Am J Pathol 129:429, 1987.

40. Fingerle J, Au YPT, Clowes AW, Reidy MA: Intimal lesion formation in rat carotid arteries after endothelial denudation in absence of medial injury. Arteriosclerosis 10:1082, 1990.

41. Lindner V, Lappi DA, Baird A, et al: Role of basic fibroblast growth factor in vascular lesion formation. Circ Res 68:106, 1991.

42. Edelman ER, Nugent MA, Smith LT, Karnovsky MJ: Basic fibroblast growth factor enhances the coupling of intimal hyperplasia and prolif-eration of vasa vasorum in injured rat arteries. J Clin Invest 89:465, 1992.

43. Lindner V, Reidy MA: Proliferation of smooth muscle cells after vascular injury is inhibited by an antibody against basic fibroblast growth factor. Proc Natl Acad Sci U S A 88:3739, 1991.

44. Walker LN, Bowen-Pope DF, Reidy MA: Production of platelet-derived growth factor-like molecules by cultured arterial smooth muscle cells accompanies proliferation after arterial injury. Proc Natl Acad Sci U S A 83:7311, 1986.

45. Cercek B, Fishbein MC, Forrester JS, et al: Induction of insulin-like growth factor I messenger RNA in rat aorta after balloon denudation. Circ Res 66:1755, 1990.

46. Majesky MW, Lindner V, Twardzik DR, et al: Production of trans-forming growth factor b_1 during repair of arterial injury. J Clin Invest 88:904–910, 1991.

47. Berguer R, Higgins RF, Reddy DJ: Intimal hyperplasia. Arch Surg 115:332, 1980.

48. Rittgers SE, Karayannacos PE, Guy JF: Velocity distribution and intimal proliferation in autologous vein grafts in dogs. Circ Res 42:792, 1978.

49. Kohler TR, Kirkman TR, Kraiss LW, et al: Increased blood flow inhibits neointimal hyperplasia in endothelialized vascular grafts. Circ Res 69:1557, 1991.

50. Kraiss LW, Kirkman TR, Kohler TR, et al: Shear stress regulates smooth muscle proliferation and neointimal thickening in porous polytetrafluoroethylene grafts. Arterioscler Thromb Vasc Biol 11:1844, 1991.

51. Mattsson EJ, Kohler TR, Vergel SM, Clowes AW: Increased blood flow induces regression of intimal hyperplasia. Arterioscler Thromb Vasc Biol 17:2245–2249, 1997.

52. Mondy JS, Lindner V, Miyashiro JK, et al: Platelet-derived growth factor ligand and receptor expression in response to altered blood flow in vivo. Circ Res, 81:320–327, 1997.

53. Kohler TR, Jawien A: Flow affects development of intimal hyperplasia following arterial injury in rats. Arterioscler Thromb Vasc Biol 12:963, 1992.

54. von der Leyen HE, Gibbons GH, Morishita R, et al: Gene therapy inhibiting neointimal vascular lesion: In vivo transfer of endothelial cell nitric oxide synthase gene. Proc Natl Acad Sci U S A 92:1137–1141, 1995.

55. DiCorleto PE, Bowen-Pope DF: Cultured endothelial cells produce a platelet-derived growth factor–like protein. Proc Natl Acad Sci U S A 80:1919, 1983.

56. Libby P, Salomon RN, Payne DO, et al: Functions of vascular wall cells related to development of transplantation-associated coronary arteriosclerosis. Transplant Proc 21:1, 1989.

57. Hart CE, Kraiss LW, Vergel S, et al: PDGFbeta receptor blockade inhibits intimal hyperplasia in the baboon. Circulation 99:564–569, 1999.

58. The EPISTENT Investigators: Randomised placebo-controlled and balloon-angioplasty–controlled trial to assess safety of coronary stent-ing with use of platelet glycoprotein-IIb/IIIa blockade. Evaluation of platelet IIb/IIIa inhibitor for stenting [see comments]. Lancet 352:87–92, 1998.

59. Topol EJ, Ferguson JJ, Weisman HF, et al: Long-term protection from myocardial ischemic events in a randomized trial of brief inte-grin beta3 blockade with percutaneous coronary intervention. EPIC Investigator Group. Evaluation of platelet IIb/IIIa inhibition for pre-vention of ischemic complication [see comments]. JAMA 278:479–484, 1997.

60. Schomig A, Neumann FJ, Kastrati A, et al: A randomized comparison of antiplatelet and anticoagulant therapy after the placement of coro-nary-artery stents [see comments]. N Engl J Med 334:1084–1089, 1996.

61. Mann MJ, Gibbons GH, Kernoff RS, et al: Genetic engineering of vein grafts resistant to atherosclerosis. Proc Natl Acad Sci U S A 92:4502–4506, 1995.

62. Wilcox JN, Waksman R, King SB, Scott NA: The role of the adventitia in the arterial response to angioplasty: The effect of intravascular radiation. Int J Radiat Oncol Biol Phys 36:789–796, 1996.

63. Meerkin D, Bonan R, Crocker IR, et al: Efficacy of beta radiation in prevention of post-angioplasty restenosis. An interim report from the beta energy restenosis trial. Herz 23:356–361, 1998.

64. Waksman R, Robinson KA, Crocker IR, et al: Endovascular low-dose irradiation inhibits neointima formation after coronary artery balloon injury in swine. A possible role for radiation therapy in restenosis prevention. Circulation 91:1533–1539, 1995.

65. Teirstein PS, Massullo V, Jani S, et al: Three-year clinical and angio-graphic follow-up after intracoronary radiation: Results of a random-ized clinical trial. Circulation 101:360–365, 2000.

66. Wilcox JN, Waksman R, King SB, Scott NA: The role of the adventitia in the arterial response to angioplasty: The effect of intravascular radiation [review]. Int J Radiat Oncol Biol Phys 36:789–796, 1996.

67. Albiero R, Adamian M, Kobayashi N, et al: Short- and intermediate-term results of ^{32}P radioactive beta-emitting stent implantation in patients with coronary artery disease: The Milan dose-response study. Circulation 101:18–26, 2000.

68. Hawiger JJ: Hemostasis, bleeding, and thromboembolic complications of trauma and infection. In Clowes GHA Jr (ed): Trauma, Sepsis and Shock. The Physiological Basis of Therapy. New York, Marcel Dekker, 1988, p 123.

69. Marcum J, McKenney J, Rosenberg R: The acceleration of thrombin-antithrombin III complex formation in rat hind quarters via heparin-like molecules bound to endothelium. J Clin Invest 74:341, 1984.

70. Esmon CT: Protein C. Prog Hemost Thromb 7:1984, pp 25–54.

71. Libby P, Ordovas JM, Auger KH, et al: Endotoxin and tumor necrosis factor induce interleukin-1 beta gene expression in adult human vascular endothelial cells. Am J Pathol 124:179, 1986.

72. Harker LA, Hanson SR, Runge MS: Thrombin hypothesis of throm-bus generation and vascular lesion formation. Am J Cardiol 75:12B–17B, 1995.

Questions

1. In normal arteries, most of the smooth muscle cells are found in
   (a) the intima
   (b) the media
   (c) the adventitia
   (d) none of the above

2. Arteries respond to an increase in blood flow by
   (a) contracting
   (b) dilating
   (c) intermittently contracting
   (d) intermittently dilating

3. Endothelial cells synthesize and secrete substances that cause
   (a) vasodilatation
   (b) vasoconstriction
   (c) both vasodilatation and vasoconstriction
   (d) none of the above

4. Injured arteries thicken due to
   (a) medial smooth muscle hyperplasia
   (b) intimal smooth muscle hyperplasia
   (c) intimal endothelial hyperplasia
   (d) none of the above

5. The reaction-to-injury hypothesis was proposed to explain the initial stages of atherosclerosis. Which element of this hypothesis has not been proved?
   (a) smooth muscle cells are important components of the plaque
   (b) thrombus can accumulate on atherosclerotic lesions
   (c) platelets contain potent growth factors

   (d) growth factors released from platelets stimulate smooth muscle growth in vivo

6. Platelet-derived growth factor (PDGF) is found in
   (a) platelets
   (b) smooth muscle cells
   (c) endothelium
   (d) all of the above

7. Smooth muscle cells respond to PDGF by
   (a) proliferating
   (b) synthesizing matrix
   (c) migrating
   (d) all of the above

8. Based on in vitro studies, endothelial cells appear to express molecules that regulate the behavior of the blood at the luminal surface. Which of the following endothelial-derived molecules act to sustain the anticoagulant state?
   (a) heparan sulfate
   (b) von Willebrand's factor
   (c) plasminogen activator inhibitor
   (d) thrombomodulin
   (e) prostacyclin

9. Which of the molecules listed in question #8 are procoagulants?

10. In general, inflammatory mediators (e.g., interleukin-1) cause endothelial cells to express
   (a) increased procoagulant activities
   (b) increased anticoagulant activities
   (c) increased endothelial-derived relaxing factor
   (d) none of the above

Answers

1. b   2. b   3. c   4. b   5. d   6. d   7. d   8. a,d,e   9. b,c   10. a

4

Anatomy and Surgical Exposure of the Vascular System

Jeffrey L. Ballard

A well-planned surgical exposure facilitates even the most difficult operative procedure. Awareness of the relationship of surface anatomy to underlying vascular structure allows precise incision placement. This minimizes tissue trauma and reduces the likelihood of wound infection. Detailed knowledge of vascular anatomy helps to prevent injury to vital structures in the operative field. In this chapter, anatomic relationships and variations that may be encountered during common vascular exposures are highlighted. Several alternate surgical approaches are also described. Sources given in the reference list supply the reader with additional detailed information.

Exposure of the carotid bifurcation is discussed first. This is followed by a systematic discussion of anatomy and surgical exposure of the peripheral vascular system ending with commonly used approaches for the arterial circulation in the leg and foot.

EXPOSURE OF THE CAROTID BIFURCATION

The common carotid artery bifurcates approximately 2.5 cm below the angle of the mandible. Normally, the sternocleidomastoid muscle, the posterior belly of the digastric muscle, and the omohyoid muscle bound the carotid bifurcation. Thus, a skin incision placed along the anterior border of the sternocleidomastoid muscle facilitates exposure of the carotid sheath.

The surgeon must be aware of the location of important cranial and somatic nerves during carotid endarterectomy. The mandibular ramus of the facial nerve is vulnerable to injury during this operation. Nerve damage by retraction or surgical dissection can cause temporary or permanent dysfunction. Turning the head toward the opposite side draws the mandibular ramus well below the mandible and increases the possibility of facial nerve injury.

The great auricular nerve (C-2 and C-3 dermatomes) should be protected in its location on the sternocleidomas-toid muscle just anterior to and below the ear. Damage to this nerve results in numbness of the posterior aspect of the auricle and may cause distressing ipsilateral postoperative occipital headaches.

The common facial vein comes into view as the incision is deepened. This vessel courses superficial to the carotid bifurcation to join the internal jugular vein. It serves as an important landmark during the dissection. Several small vessels coursing toward the sternocleidomastoid muscle are nutrient branches from the superior thyroid artery and vein. These vessels should be ligated and divided to avoid troublesome postoperative bleeding. In the typical carotid dissection, the common carotid artery should be exposed above the level of the omohyoid muscle. Once this vessel is isolated, further distal dissection along its medial aspect facilitates exposure of the superior thyroid and external carotid arteries. Dissection in the "V" of the carotid bifurcation should be avoided because this area is extremely vascular. It is wise to encircle the internal carotid artery well above the level of gross atherosclerotic disease. This dissection is usually 1 to 2 cm above the bifurcation and thereby avoids the highly vascular carotid sinus tissue.

The descending branch of the hypoglossal nerve (ansa cervicalis) is located anterior and parallel to the sternocleidomastoid muscle. If this branch is followed upward, the main hypoglossal nerve trunk can be located. Division of the descending branch of the hypoglossal nerve near its origin allows the main nerve trunk to be displaced upward and forward, thus providing higher exposure of the internal carotid artery. A nutrient vein and artery to the sternocleidomastoid muscle course in immediate relation to this nerve at this level. Care should be taken to avoid injury to the underlying hypoglossal nerve when these vessels are ligated and divided. This maneuver allows the nerve to retract superomedially and out of harm's way. Division of this artery/vein "sling" about the hypoglossal nerve facilitates exposure of the internal carotid artery under the posterior belly of the digastric muscle.

The surgeon must also be constantly aware of the location of the vagus nerve and its branches. It lies within the carotid sheath between the common carotid artery and the internal jugular vein. Normally, it is directly behind the internal carotid artery at its origin. Care must be taken to prevent injury to the nerve at this vulnerable location. Additional care is required to prevent vagus nerve injury during redo carotid exposure. This is owing to the fact that in these cases the nerve, which can be encased in scar tissue, frequently courses anterior to the carotid bifurcation. The superior laryngeal nerve arises from the vagus nerve above the carotid bifurcation, passes behind the internal carotid artery, and descends medial to the superior thyroid artery. Care must be taken during mobilization of this vessel not to injure the superior laryngeal nerve or its external branch (Fig. 4–1). The external branch of the superior laryngeal nerve may sometimes pass between branches of the superior thyroid artery or be adherent to it. Table 4–1 lists the locations and tests for function of the important nerves encountered during carotid endarterectomy and includes special remarks about each.

An arteriotomy should be created just proximal to the carotid bulb and lateral to the carotid flow divider. This incision is then lengthened distally through the diseased internal carotid artery (ICA) under direct vision to a point at which there is normal-appearing intima. It is critical not to make this arteriotomy on the anterior aspect of the ICA near the carotid sinus because this is a relatively fixed area that is hard to reapproximate without creating a focal narrowing that is at risk for restenosis. It is wise to find the correct endarterectomy plane at the level of the carotid bulb. Thereafter, endarterectomy first proceeds proximally, and the specimen is excised sharply with Potts scissors at the level of the common carotid artery. Everting the external carotid artery into the carotid bulb facilitates endarterectomy at this level. Then, one must carefully find the plaque transition point between the atherosclerotic plaque

to be removed and the remaining nondiseased ICA. This is the critical step in the performance of a technically sound carotid endarterectomy and, if done correctly, tacking sutures are rarely required. Meticulous care is then taken to ensure that no loose areas of media remain through the endarterectomized surface. In our practice, Dacron patch angioplasty reapproximates the arteriotomy, and intraoperative duplex ultrasound scanning completes the procedure. The reader is referred to *Wylie's Atlas of Vascular Surgery*[1] for color illustrations of the steps in performing carotid endarterectomy.

The value of cranial nerve protection during carotid surgery is emphasized by the reports of Evans and coworkers[2] and Hertzer and colleagues.[3] The vagus nerve is the cranial nerve most commonly injured during carotid endarterectomy. Evans and associates prospectively studied the incidence of cranial nerve injury during carotid surgery. Observations were made by surgeons and by a speech pathologist before and after carotid endarterectomy. There was a 4% incidence of preoperative vagus nerve dysfunction when a surgeon made the evaluation. However, a 30% incidence of preoperative dysfunction of cranial nerve X was noted when the evaluation was made by a speech pathologist. Two days after the endarterectomy, the surgeon's evaluation demonstrated a 14.6% incidence of vagal nerve deficit, whereas the speech pathologist's evaluation reported a 35% incidence of superior laryngeal or recurrent nerve dysfunction!

These data support the wisdom of a thorough vocal cord evaluation before performing carotid endarterectomy because of the high incidence of unrecognized vagal nerve dysfunction. Examination of vocal cord function is of particular importance when reoperation is planned or when operating on the contralateral side soon after the first, at which time paresis of cord function may still persist.

EXPOSURE OF THE HIGH INTERNAL CAROTID ARTERY

One of the most difficult vascular surgical exposures is that of the high internal carotid artery. The surgeon must contend with many vital nerve structures within a confined space. This is frequently made more difficult by a space-occupying vascular lesion or the presence of vascular injury with hemorrhagic staining and displacement of the tissues. Structures that overlie the high internal carotid artery in the neck include the facial nerve, the parotid gland, the ramus of the mandible, and the mastoid and styloid processes. The hypoglossal nerve, glossopharyngeal nerve, digastric and stylohyoid muscles, and occipital and posterior auricular arteries cross it. The distal cervical internal carotid artery courses progressively deeper to enter the petrous canal of the temporal bone.

Exposure routinely begins at the level of the common carotid artery proximal to the carotid bifurcation. The omohyoid muscle serves as a landmark for the proximal extent of this exposure. The dissection continues distally, protecting the vagus nerve, which lies immediately behind the internal carotid artery. The hypoglossal nerve is exposed, and the descending branch is divided to displace the hypoglossal nerve forward. The digastric and stylohyoid muscles

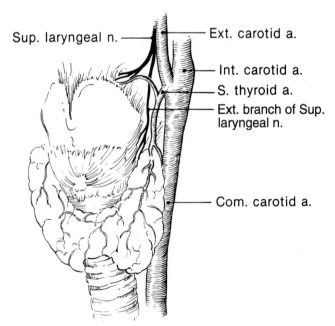

Sup. laryngeal n. —

Ext. carotid a.

Int. carotid a.

S. thyroid a.

Ext. branch of Sup. laryngeal n.

Com. carotid a.

Figure 4–1. Note the vulnerable location of the external branch of the superior laryngeal nerve to the superior thyroid artery.

TABLE 4-1

Regional Nerves Encountered During Carotid Endarterectomy

NERVE BRANCH	LOCATION ENCOUNTERED	TEST FOR FUNCTION	REMARKS
Mandibular ramus of facial nerve (cranial nerve VII)	Deep to platysma muscle Can be 5–10 mm below inferior margin of mandible	Ask patient to show teeth—check for paralysis of lower lip	Gentle use of retractors on mandible; nerve is pulled down when head is rotated to opposite side for operative exposure
Great auricular nerve (C-2 and C-3)	Anteromedial surface of SCM muscle anterior to and below ear	Anesthesia of ear and adjacent scalp	Causes disturbing occipital headache when damaged
Cutaneous cervical nerve (C-2 and C-3)	Subcutaneous on deep fascia	Anesthesia of skin below mandible	Should warn patient preoperatively regarding possible sensory loss
Glossopharyngeal nerve branch (cranial nerve IX)	Between external and internal carotid arteries (carotid sinus nerve, also known as "nerve of Herring")	None	Manipulation of nerve may cause bradycardia and/or hypotension; atropine IV or local infiltration of nerve with lidocaine relieves circulatory changes
Vagus nerve (cranial nerve X)	Within carotid sheath; between internal jugular vein and common carotid artery; directly behind internal carotid artery	Indirect laryngoscopy for vocal cord function	Dissect "right on" distal common and internal carotid arteries and avoid "past pointing" with vascular occluding clamps
External branch of superior laryngeal nerve (branch of cranial nerve X)	Adjacent and medial to superior thyroid artery	Loss of function of cricothyroid muscle	Inability to reproduce high tones
Hypoglossal nerve (cranial nerve XII)	Main nerve trunk crosses the internal and external carotid arteries 1–2 cm above carotid bifurcation; SCM artery and vein branches sling around nerve	Extended tongue deviates to side of injured nerve	Visualize descending branch first and follow it to main nerve trunk; careful ligation of SCM muscular arterial and venous branches to preserve dry operative field

IV, intravenous; SCM, sternocleidomastoid.

are divided to facilitate this exposure. In addition, the styloid process and the stylohyoid ligament are excised. The glossopharyngeal and the superior laryngeal nerves must be identified and preserved. It becomes evident that one is now working in a progressively narrowing triangle with inadequate space for performing any major vascular reconstructive procedure.

Anatomic dissection in human cadaver specimens demonstrates that division of the posterior belly of the digastric muscle facilitates exposure of the internal carotid artery to the middle of the first cervical vertebra. Anterior subluxation of the mandible improves exposure to the superior border of the first cervical vertebra. The addition of styloidectomy to the maneuvers described here extends the exposure cephalad approximately 0.5 cm.[4]

Fisher and associates[5] described a unique technique of wire fixation of the mandible to hold its subluxed position during the operative procedure. The 12 to 15 mm of space obtained converts the triangle described earlier into a narrow rectangle (Fig. 4–2). It is important to avoid dislocation of the mandible, because serious injury can occur to the temporomandibular joint and even to the contralateral internal carotid artery. In the discussion of Fisher and associates' paper, Stanley suggested that a towel clip placed on the angle of the mandible through two small stab incisions would allow the subluxation to be fixed by minimal retraction. Dossa and associates[6] also suggested that temporary mandibular subluxation can be accomplished in a safe and expeditious manner using diagonal interdental/Steinmann pin wiring. Figure 4–3 shows a diagram of the relationship of the mandibular condyle to the auricular eminence and infratemporal fossa.

In situations requiring more room for vascular reconstruction, transection of the mandibular ramus with either translocation or temporary removal of the condyle and ramus fragment affords wider exposure. Wylie and associates[7] described this approach with detailed color illustrations of the involved anatomy.

Following induction of anesthesia, arch bars and wires immobilize the mandible. The usual carotid endarterectomy incision is extended posteriorly to a point behind the ear. The carotid bifurcation and internal carotid artery are exposed as described previously. The mandibular ramus of the facial nerve is protected. The angle of the mandible is exposed and the periosteum elevated toward the mandibular notch anteriorly and posteriorly. The mandibular ramus is divided vertically using a power saw posterior to the foramen of the inferior alveolar artery and nerve. The posterior bone fragment is gently rotated out and upward as the pterygoid muscles are divided, thus allowing its removal. The bone fragment is preserved in chilled lactated Ringer's solution until it is replaced after arterial reconstruction.

Once the mandibular ramus is removed, the digastric and stylohyoid muscles are divided and the dissection is continued to the skull base. Care should be taken to protect the hypoglossal, glossopharyngeal, and vagus nerves, which are in immediate relation to the high internal carotid artery.

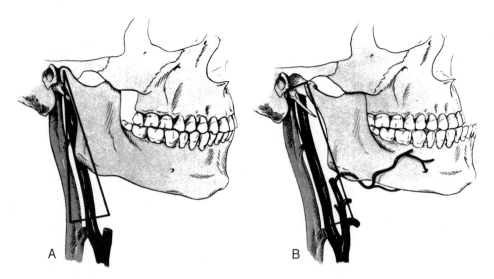

Figure 4–2. These diagrams show how the narrow triangle of exposure (*A*) for the high internal carotid artery is expanded to a narrow rectangle (*B*) by anterior subluxation of the condyle of the mandible. (From Fisher DF Jr, Clagett GP, Parker JI, et al: Mandibular subluxation for high carotid exposure. J Vasc Surg 1:727, 1984.)

The mandibular fragment is returned to its anatomic location after completion of internal carotid artery reconstruction and interrupted nonabsorbable sutures close the temporomandibular joint capsule. A thin titanium plate is used to fix the mandibular fragment in place. The cervical fascia and platysma muscle are closed in layers, followed by routine skin closure.

EXPOSURE OF AORTIC ARCH BRANCHES AND ASSOCIATED VEINS

The most widely accepted direct route employed for surgical exposure of the innominate and proximal left common carotid arteries, as well as the superior vena cava and its confluent brachiocephalic veins, is through a full median sternotomy. However, we have recently described a less invasive surgical exposure for the direct treatment of these aortic arch branch vessels and associated major veins.[8] Similar to a median sternotomy, this surgical approach provides excellent exposure of the aortic arch branch vessels with the exception of the left subclavian artery. This is owing to the fact that the aortic arch passes obliquely posterior and to the left after its origin from the base of

the heart, thus making the first portion of the left subclavian artery inaccessible from this anterior approach.

Mini-sternotomy is effected by first making a limited skin incision measuring 7 to 8 cm in the midline. This should extend from the sternal notch to just past the angle of Louis. The manubrium and upper sternum are divided in the midline down to the third intercostal space with a narrow blade mounted on a redo sternotomy oscillating saw (Stryker, Kalamazoo, MI). The sternum is then transected transversely at the third intercostal space, creating an upside down "T" incision (Fig. 4–4). Care is taken to not injure the internal mammary vessels, which are adjacent to the sternum. After accurate hemostasis along the periosteal edges, a Rienhoff or other similar pediatric sternal retractor is placed to open the upper sternum. The skin incision can be extended upward along the anterior border of either sternocleidomastoid muscle, with division of the strap muscles to expose the proximal right common carotid artery or the more distal left common carotid artery. This extension can also be used to expose the carotid bifurcation.

The two lobes of the thymus gland are separated in the midline, and if the surgeon carefully observes the pleural bulge during positive pressure inspiration, entry into either pleural space can be avoided. Nutrient vessels to the thy-

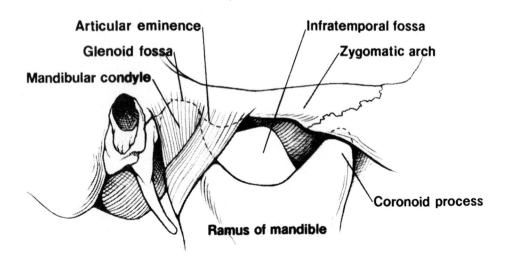

Articular eminence
Glenoid fossa
Mandibular condyle
Infratemporal fossa
Zygomatic arch
Coronoid process
Ramus of mandible

Figure 4–3. Anterior subluxation moves the condyle of the mandible to the articular eminence but not to the infratemporal fossa as would occur with dislocation of the mandible. (From Fisher DF Jr, Clagett GP, Parker JI, et al: Mandibular subluxation for high carotid exposure. J Vasc Surg 1:727, 1984.)

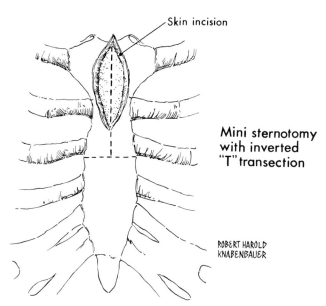

Skin incision

Mini sternotomy
with inverted
"T" transection

ROBERT HAROLD
KNABENBAUER

Figure 4–4. Skin incision and "mini-sternotomy" sternal division. (From Sakopoulos AG, Ballard JL, Gundry SR: Minimally invasive approach for aortic branch vessel reconstruction. J Vasc Surg 31(1P + 1):200, 2000.)

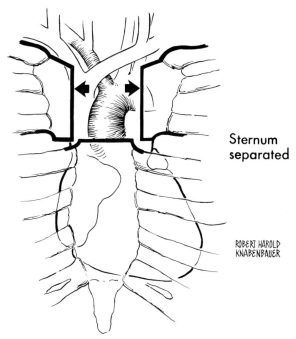

Sternum
separated

ROBERT HAROLD
KNABENBAUER

Figure 4–5. Upper sternum is divided and separated, exposing the ascending aorta and arch vessels. (From Sakopoulos AG, Ballard JL, Gundry SR: Minimally invasive approach for aortic branch vessel reconstruction. J Vasc Surg 31(1P + 1):200, 2000.)

mus gland are carefully ligated and divided, keeping a dry field for visibility. These vessels arise from the internal thoracic artery and drain into the internal thoracic or brachiocephalic veins. The upper pericardium is then opened vertically and the edges are sewn to the skin with silk suture.

The left brachiocephalic vein can be visualized in the upper portion of the wound. A thymic vein may join this vessel inferiorly, and an inferior thyroid vein may require ligation and division as it joins the brachiocephalic vein superiorly. After complete mobilization of the left brachiocephalic vein, the anterior surface of the aortic arch can be visualized, as well as the origin of the innominate artery. The base of the heart and the innominate and left common

carotid arteries are thus exposed (Fig. 4–5). The recurrent laryngeal nerve must be protected during exposure of the innominate artery bifurcation. It courses from the vagus nerve anteriorly around the origin of the subclavian artery to return in the tracheoesophageal groove to its termination in the larynx.

Innominate and/or left common carotid artery endarterectomy, patch angioplasty, or bypass can then be performed in the usual fashion (Fig. 4–6). After the procedure, a 19 French Blake drain (Johnson & Johnson, Cincinnati, Oh)

Figure 4–6. Artist's rendering of surgical exposure of the innominate artery with visible atherosclerotic stenosis: *A*, Repair by proximal exclusion and ascending aorta to innominate artery bypass. *B*, Repair by endarterectomy and patch angioplasty. (From Sakopoulos AG, Ballard JL, Gundry SR: Minimally invasive approach for aortic branch vessel reconstruction. J Vasc Surg 31(1P + 1): 200, 2000.)

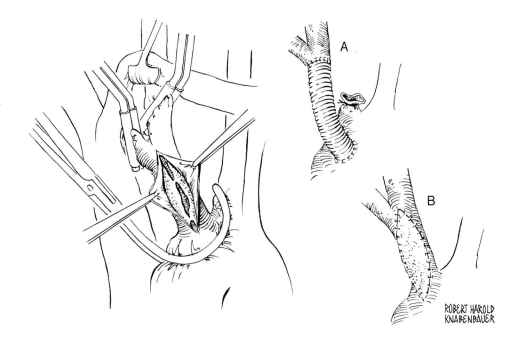

ROBERT HAROLD
KNABENBAUER

is placed in the mediastinum and brought out laterally through one of the intercostal spaces. This is connected to a Heimlich valve grenade suction device. Chest tubes are not used. Two wires are used to bring the upper and lower sternal edges of the "T" together and two more are placed in the manubrium. If needed, another wire placed as a "figure-of-eight" at the level of the second intercostal space completely rejoins the divided upper sternum. After approximating the muscular and subcutaneous planes in two layers, the skin is closed in a subcuticular fashion.

Origin of the Right Subclavian Artery and Vein

The origin of the right subclavian artery is exposed through a sternotomy incision with extension above and parallel to the clavicle. The right sternohyoid and sternothyroid muscles are divided, followed by exposure of the scalene fat pad. Branches of the thyrocervical trunk are divided and the dissection is deepened to expose the anterior scalene muscle. The phrenic nerve should be identified and protected as it courses from lateral to medial across the surface of the anterior scalene muscle to pass into the superior mediastinum. The proximal right subclavian artery comes into view with division of the anterior scalene muscle just above its insertion on the first rib.

Traumatic vascular injury at the confluence of the subclavian artery and internal jugular and subclavian veins is difficult to manage solely through a supraclavicular approach. Ideally, sternotomy for proximal vascular control should be followed by supraclavicular extension of the

incision. However, in the event that the injury is exposed without proximal control, the incision should be promptly extended via a sternotomy while an assistant maintains compression of the vessels against the undersurface of the sternum to temporarily control hemorrhage (Fig. 4–7). Alternatively, temporary percutaneous balloon occlusion of the distal innominate artery from a femoral artery approach can be life saving and greatly facilitate this exposure.

Origin of the Left Subclavian Artery

The left subclavian artery arises from the aortic arch posteriorly and from the left side of the mediastinum. Therefore, it cannot be adequately exposed for vascular reconstruction through a sternotomy incision. Traumatic injuries and aneurysms of the proximal left subclavian artery should be approached through the left side of the chest. The preferred exposure is an anterolateral thoracotomy through the fourth intercostal space or the bed of the resected fourth rib.

If the vascular injury or aneurysm is extensive, it is wise to prepare the left upper extremity for inclusion in the operative field so that it can be positioned for a second supraclavicular incision. This allows ready access to the second portion of the subclavian artery to gain distal vascular control. Anterolateral exposure of the left side of the chest also facilitates partial occlusion of the aortic arch for lesions involving the origin of the subclavian artery. The phrenic and vagus nerves must be identified and preserved after the pleura is opened and before the dissection of the first portion of the subclavian artery.

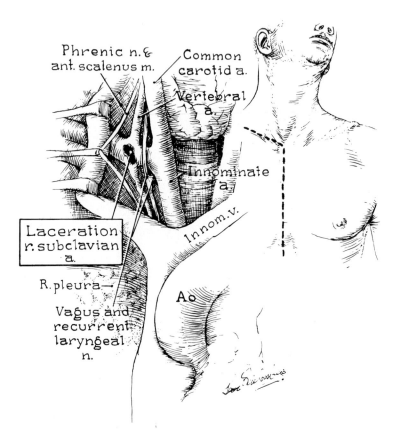

Figure 4–7. Exposure of the anterior aortic arch branches through a median sternotomy incision. Note the location of the phrenic, vagus, and recurrent laryngeal nerves, which must be identified and protected. Ao, Aorta. (From Ernst C: Exposure of the subclavian arteries. Semin Vasc Surg 2:202, 1989.)

In situations in which there is exigent bleeding into the pleural space from a traumatic injury of the proximal left subclavian artery, prompt vascular control can be obtained by an anterior thoracotomy in the third or fourth intercostal space. This exposure facilitates placement of a vascular clamp across the origin of the bleeding subclavian artery (Fig. 4–8). An inframammary incision is preferred in females, with the breast mobilized superiorly for the exposure just described.

Subclavian and Vertebral Arteries

Exposure of the second portion of the subclavian artery is accomplished through a supraclavicular incision beginning over the tendon of the sternocleidomastoid muscle and extending laterally for 8 to 10 cm. The platysma muscle is divided and the scalene fat pad mobilized superolaterally. Thyrocervical vessels are ligated and divided as encountered, with exposure of the anterior surface of the anterior scalene muscle. The phrenic nerve can be seen coursing in a lateral to medial direction over this muscle and should be gently mobilized and preserved. The thoracic duct must also be protected at its termination with the confluence of the internal jugular, brachiocephalic, and subclavian veins. Unrecognized injury may result in a lymphocele or lymphocutaneous fistula.

The anterior scalene muscle is divided just above its point of insertion on the first rib to facilitate exposure of the subclavian artery. Division of this muscle should be done under direct vision and without cautery as the brachial plexus is immediately adjacent to the lateral aspect of the anterior scalene muscle. The origin of the left vertebral artery arises from the medial surface of the subclavian artery medial to the anterior scalene muscle and behind the sternoclavicular joint. The internal thoracic artery, which originates from the inferior surface of the subclavian artery

opposite the thyrocervical trunk, should be protected as the subclavian artery is dissected free of surrounding tissue. Figure 4–9 depicts the essential anatomy of this exposure.

Resection of subclavian artery aneurysms and emergency exposure for vascular injury involving the second and third portions of this vessel require wide exposure. This can be accomplished by resecting the clavicle, including the periosteum. The latter structure, when preserved, results in reossification of a deformed clavicle.

The surgical exposure of the vertebral artery is described in detail in Chapter 32 of this text and in the surgical literature.[9] Injuries to the intraosseous portion of the vertebral artery with associated hemorrhage are best managed by embolic occlusion proximal and, if possible, distal to the area of injury.

AXILLARY ARTERY EXPOSURE

The proximal axillary artery is exposed by a short incision made between the clavicular and sternal portions of the pectoralis major muscle. Branches of the thoracoacromial vessels are divided to expose the axillary vein first and then the axillary artery above and posterior to the vein. Dissection medial to the pectoralis minor muscle provides appropriate exposure of the axillary artery for axillofemoral bypass graft origin. If additional exposure is required laterally, a portion of the pectoralis minor muscle can be divided near its insertion into the coracoid process of the scapula.

The second portion of the axillary artery is more difficult to expose because it lies directly behind the pectoralis major muscle. Extension of the previously mentioned incision continues across the distal portion of the pectoralis major muscle at the anterior axillary fold and out onto the midline of the proximal medial surface of the arm (Fig. 4–10). The tendinous portion of the muscle is divided near its insertion to expose the axillary contents. The pectoralis

Figure 4–8. Anterior thoracotomy with placement of an occluding vascular clamp for control of exigent bleeding from the proximal left subclavian artery. (From Trunkey D: Great vessel injury. In Blaisdell F, Trunkey D [eds]: Trauma Management, vol 3. Cervicothoracic Trauma. New York, Thieme, 1986, p 255.)

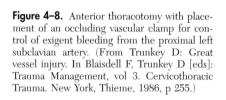
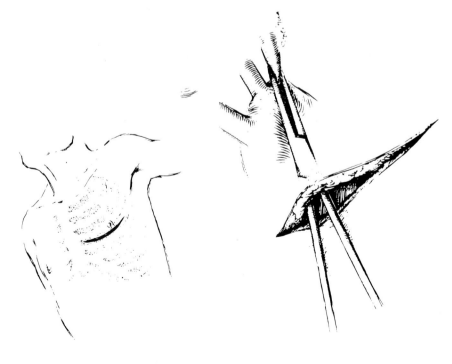

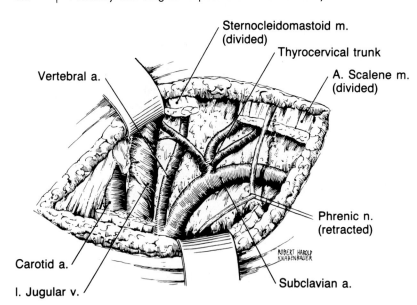

Vertebral a.

Sternocleidomastoid m. (divided)

Thyrocervical trunk

A. Scalene m. (divided)

Phrenic n. (retracted)

Carotid a.

I. Jugular v.

Subclavian a.

Figure 4–9. Exposure of the second portion of the left subclavian artery via a supraclavicular incision. Note that both the sternocleidomastoid and the anterior scalene muscles are divided for this exposure.

minor muscle can also be divided if more medial exposure is desired.

THORACIC OUTLET EXPOSURE

Either a supraclavicular or a transaxillary approach facilitates decompression of the thoracic outlet. Roos has described the transaxillary approach for first rib resection in the management of thoracic outlet syndrome.[10] However, evolution of thought regarding thoracic outlet syndrome has led us to favor supraclavicular exposure of the superior thoracic aperture. Essential anatomic elements of this approach have been detailed in *Wylie's Atlas of Vascular Surgery*.[11]

A transverse supraclavicular incision based 1.5 cm above the medial half of the clavicle is deepened to develop subplatysmal flaps and to expose the scalene fat pad. Reflection of the fat pad superolaterally facilitates exposure of the anterior scalene muscle. This exposure also requires

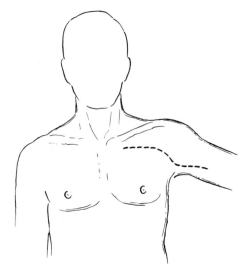

Figure 4–10. Incision employed for the exposure of the axillary artery.

ligation and division of the transverse cervical artery and vein and resection of the omohyoid muscle.

Identification and careful manipulation of the phrenic nerve are essential to avoid excessive traction or injury. Complete removal of the anterior scalene muscle begins at the level of the first rib and ends at the transverse processes of the cervical vertebrae. Subtotal removal of the scalenus medius muscle in a plane parallel and just inferior to the long thoracic nerve exposes all five roots and three trunks of the brachial plexus.

This unencumbered exposure of the brachial plexus facilitates neurolysis and complete mobilization of the nerve roots. Additional myofibrous bands or bony anomalies are removed at this time. If the course of the lower trunk and C-8 to T-1 nerve roots are deviated by the first rib, the rib should be partially or totally removed to free the path.

Incision of Sibson's fascia and displacement of the dome of the pleura inferiorly help to fully expose the inner aspect of the first rib. Gentle anteromedial retraction of the plexus ensures adequate posterior division of the first rib. Anteriorly, the rib is transected distal to the scalene tubercle. A counterincision just below the clavicle can be used to facilitate anterior transection of the first rib. This approach is useful for rib resection in association with axillosubclavian vein thrombosis. Final removal of the first rib requires division of intercostal muscle attachments to the second rib and division of any other soft tissue.

The scalene fat pad can be wrapped around the plexus if split in a sagittal plane. Repositioning of the fat pad decreases dead spaces and may help to prevent incorporation of the brachial plexus into the healing scar tissue. The wound is closed in layers after secure hemostasis and reapproximation of the sternocleidomastoid muscle.

EXPOSURE OF THE DESCENDING THORACIC AND PROXIMAL ABDOMINAL AORTA

No single approach lends itself so well to extensive exposure of the thoracic and abdominal aorta as a properly positioned thoracoabdominal incision. After pulmonary artery and radial arterial line placement and dual-lumen tracheal intubation, the patient is placed in a modified right lateral decubitus position, with the hips rotated 45 degrees from horizontal. This allows exposure of both groins. A beanbag device is helpful to support the patient's position on the operating table. The free left upper extremity should be passed across the upper chest and supported on a cushioned Mayo stand. In this way, thoracoabdominal aortic exposure is gained by unwinding the torso as described by Stoney and Wylie.[12]

The rib interspace to enter depends primarily on the extent of thoracic aorta to be exposed. The fourth or fifth intercostal space is used when the entire thoracoabdominal aorta from subclavian artery origin through abdominal aorta is to be exposed, whereas the seventh or eighth intercostal space allows mid- to terminal thoracic aortic exposure plus wide abdominal aortic visualization. Dividing the respective lower rib posteriorly facilitates this exposure. On occasion, two interspaces (for instance, fourth and ninth) may be entered under one thoracoabdominal incision to facilitate proximal descending thoracic and abdominal aortic exposure. The thoracic incision is continued across the costal margin in a paramedian plane to the level of the umbilicus (Fig. 4–11). If the terminal aorta and iliac vessels are to be exposed, the incision is extended to the left lower quadrant.

With the left lung deflated, the origin of the left subclavian artery and proximal descending thoracic aorta can be gently dissected free of surrounding tissue to facilitate cross-clamping. The vagus and recurrent laryngeal nerves are densely adherent to the aorta just proximal to the subclavian artery. Meticulous care should be taken not to

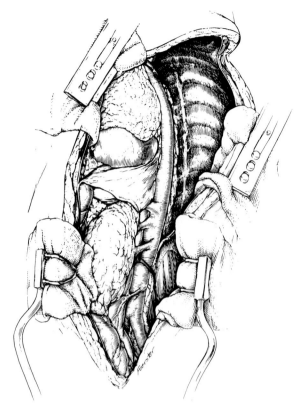

Figure 4–12. Thoracoabdominal aortic exposure from the origin of the left subclavian artery to the common iliac arteries. (From Rutherford RB: Thoracoabdominal aortic exposures. In Rutherford RB [ed]: Atlas of Vascular Surgery: Basic Techniques and Exposures. Philadelphia, WB Saunders, 1993, p 233.)

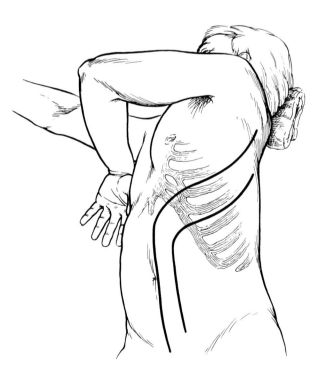

Figure 4–11. Incision options for thoracoabdominal aortic procedures are based on extent of thoracic aorta to be exposed and desire to stay in an extraperitoneal plane. (From Rutherford RB: Thoracoabdominal aortic exposures. In Rutherford RB [ed]: Atlas of Vascular Surgery: Basic Techniques and Exposures. Philadelphia, WB Saunders, 1993, p 223.)

injure these structures. Division of the inferior pulmonary ligament exposes the middle and distal descending thoracic aorta. The diaphragm is radially incised toward the aortic hiatus, and the left diaphragmatic crus is divided to expose the terminal descending thoracic aorta. Alternatively, just the central tendinous portion of the diaphragm can be divided, or it can be incised circumferentially at a distance of approximately 2.5 cm from the chest wall.

The left retroperitoneal space is developed in a retronephric extraperitoneal plane because surgical exposure of the thoracoabdominal aorta is greatly facilitated by forward mobilization of the left kidney. Division of the median arcuate ligament and lumbar tributary to the left renal vein allows further medial rotation of abdominal viscera and left kidney. Clearing the posterolateral surface of the thoracoabdominal aorta facilitates aortotomy. With this exposure, the origins of the left renal, celiac, and superior mesenteric arteries can then be visualized and dissected free as indicated by the disease process present (Fig. 4–12).

Preservation of the blood supply to the spinal cord is critical in this extensive operation. Brockstein and associates[13] have stressed the importance of the arteria radicularis magna (artery of Adamkiewicz) in providing circulation to the anterior spinal artery (Fig. 4–13). This vessel is a branch of either a distal intercostal or a proximal lumbar artery. It has been identified as proximal as T-5 and as distal as L-4.[13] However, the artery generally arises at the T-8 to L-1 level. Therefore, it is unwise to ligate any large

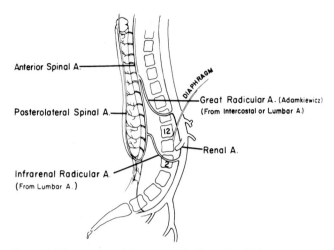

Figure 4–13. Diagram of the great and infrarenal radicular arteries supplying the anterior spinal artery. (From Szilagy DG, Hageman JH, Smith RF, et al: Spinal damage in surgery of the abdominal aorta. Surgery 83: 38, 1979.)

intercostal or proximal lumbar artery until the aorta has been opened so that an assessment of arterial back-bleeding can be made under direct vision.

Closure of this extensive aortic exposure begins by re-approximating the diaphragm with 2-0 Prolene suture. A posterior (No. 28 French or No. 32 French) chest tube is placed under direct vision, and the ribs are then reapproximated with interrupted No. 1 Vicryl suture. Occasionally, a segment of the cartilaginous costal arch is excised to provide stable rib approximation. Thoracic musculature is reapproximated in layers with 1-0 Vicryl suture. In the abdomen, the posterior rectus sheath is reapproximated and then the anterior rectus sheath is closed with a running No. 1 PDS suture. Finally, skin is reapproximated with a running 3-0 subcuticular suture.

RETROPERITONEAL EXPOSURE OF THE ABDOMINAL AORTA AND ITS BRANCHES

Transperitoneal aortic exposure is generally regarded as the standard operative approach to the abdominal aorta. However, retroperitoneal aortic exposure has gained wider acceptance among vascular surgeons because it affords a more direct route to the aorta and facilitates complex aortic reconstruction above the level of the renal arteries. We and others have demonstrated that in comparison to trans-peritoneal aortic exposure, the retroperitoneal approach is associated with decreased perioperative morbidity, earlier return of bowel function, fewer respiratory complications, decreased intensive care and hospital stay, and lower overall cost.[14–16]

For this aortic exposure, the patient is positioned on the operating table with the kidney rest at waist level. After pulmonary artery and radial arterial line placement and tracheal intubation, the patient is turned to the right lateral decubitus position, with the pelvis rotated posteriorly to allow exposure of both groins. The kidney rest is elevated and the operating table gently flexed to open the space

between the left anterior superior iliac spine and the costal margin (Fig. 4–14). The free left upper extremity is positioned as described earlier.

The incision begins over the lateral border of the rectus muscle approximately 2 cm below the level of the umbilicus and is carried laterally over the tip of the 12th rib. This decreases the chance of injury to the main trunk of the intercostal nerve within the 11th intercostal space. In males, resection of a significant portion of this rib facilitates retroperitoneal aortic exposure. However, in females, 12th rib resection is not always required. The anterior rectus sheath is opened to allow transection of the left rectus abdominis muscle. Inferior epigastric vessels are divided between silk ligatures to avoid troublesome postoperative bleeding. The incision is carried laterally through the external and internal oblique muscle fibers. Careful incision of the most lateral aspect of the posterior rectus sheath facilitates development of an extraperitoneal plane. The remaining posterior sheath is divided toward the midline, and, laterally, transversus abdominis muscle fibers are split toward the 12th rib.

The peritoneum is gently swept off the posterior rectus sheath, the transversus abdominis fibers, and the diaphragm to allow safe entry into the left retroperitoneal space. This space is best entered laterally. The peritoneum and its contents are swept medially off the psoas muscle toward the diaphragm along with Gerota's fascia with the contained left kidney. With careful manual control of the left kidney/peritoneal contents and countertraction upward

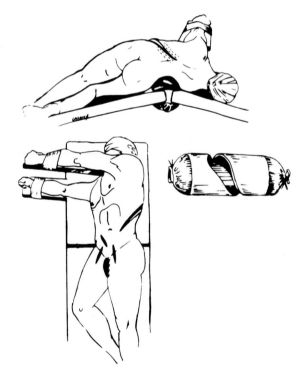

Figure 4–14. Positioning for exposure of the retroperitoneal aorta. *Top,* Flexion of table increases exposure. *Bottom left,* The hips are positioned at a 45-degree angle with the table, and the left arm is passed across the chest. *Bottom right,* The position unwinds the torso for greater exposure. Incisions for exposure of the right iliac and common femoral arteries are shown in the bottom left. (From Shepard A, Scott G, Mackey W, et al: Retroperitoneal approach to high-risk abdominal aortic aneurysms. Arch Surg 126:157, 1973.)

on the diaphragm, further medial rotation of the left kidney and viscera allows exposure of the aorta from the left diaphragmatic crus to its bifurcation. The Omni-Tract retraction system (Omni-Tract Surgical, Minneapolis, Minn) is critical for maintaining this exposure.

The left renal artery is readily identified and serves as the main landmark for suprarenal as well as infrarenal aortic exposure (Fig. 4–15). Just above this level, division of the median arcuate ligament and left diaphragmatic crus facilitates exposure of the supraceliac aorta (Fig. 4–16). The celiac and superior mesenteric arteries can be dissected free for a significant length after careful incision of the enveloping neural tissue that surrounds both vessels. The distal thoracic aorta is readily accessible if the dissection is carried proximally between the crura and in an extrapleural plane. This extended exposure facilitates repair of suprarenal aortic disease and transaortic renal or mesenteric endarterectomy as well as antegrade bypass to these vessels.

Visceral and Renal Artery Exposure

This left flank approach is ideal for visceral and renal artery exposure. The celiac artery and proximal aspects of its major branches are readily accessible. In addition, the splenic artery can easily be mobilized off the posterior aspect of the pancreas to facilitate extra-anatomic splenorenal bypass. Hepatorenal bypass requires a right retroperito-

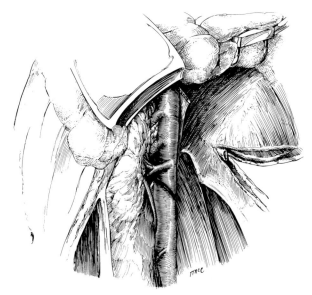

Figure 4–16. Division of the median arcuate ligament and left diaphragmatic crus facilitates suprarenal and supraceliac exposure. (From Rutherford RB: Thoracoabdominal aortic exposures. In Rutherford RB [ed]: Atlas of Vascular Surgery: Basic Techniques and Exposures. Philadelphia, WB Saunders, 1993, p 207.)

neal approach. There are no major branches that emanate from the superior mesenteric artery for a distance of up to 5 cm distal to its origin. Therefore, bypass or endarterectomy of the superior mesenteric artery well beyond its orifice is possible without ever entering the peritoneal space. The first major branch is usually the middle colic artery, which arises from the anterior and right lateral surface of the superior mesenteric artery as it emerges from the pancreas. This branch is the usual site for an embolus to lodge. It is important to remember that in addition to a possible replaced right hepatic artery, the common hepatic artery occasionally arises from the superior mesenteric artery.[17] In both circumstances, the replaced artery arises from the proximal aspect of the superior mesenteric artery just past its origin and courses back toward the right upper quadrant.

Dissection at the origin of the left renal artery and along the posterolateral aspect of the infrarenal aorta exposes the large communicating vein connecting the renal to the hemiazygous vein. Once this venous tributary (often two tributaries are encountered) is divided, the left renal vein can be elevated off the infrarenal aorta to facilitate cross-clamping. This maneuver facilitates right renal artery exposure as the origin of this vessel comes into view with superolateral retraction of the left renal vein. This retroperitoneal surgical exposure also allows dissection of either renal artery to its branch vessels in preparation for endarterectomy or bypass.

In order to carry out transaortic renal endarterectomy with direct visualization of a clean end point, it is necessary to dissect the renal arteries well beyond their respective origins. In addition, the segment of aorta to be isolated must be completely mobilized with control of any adjacent lumbar arteries. This eliminates troublesome back-bleeding that can obscure vision after creation of an aortotomy. Proximal exposure of the suprarenal aorta should include

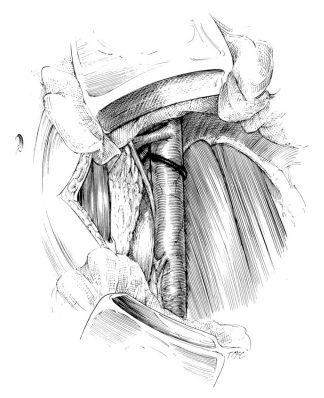

Figure 4–15. Left renal artery serves as landmark for this dissection. Note iliolumbar venous tributary just distal to the left renal artery. (From Rutherford RB: Thoracoabdominal aortic exposures. In Rutherford RB [ed]: Atlas of Vascular Surgery: Basic Techniques and Exposures. Philadelphia, WB Saunders, 1993, p 201.)

at least the origin of the superior mesenteric artery so that an aortic clamp can be placed above this level. This is necessary if there is little distance between the origins of the renal arteries and mesenteric vessels. Transaortic endarterectomy is accomplished either by transecting the aorta below the level of the renal arteries or by making a longitudinal aortotomy posterolateral to the left renal artery and/or superior mesenteric artery. Aortotomy can also be carried to the supraceliac aorta to facilitate visceral endarterectomy. Any of these visceral vessels can also be transected well beyond the disease process to facilitate direct end-to-end bypass. The ability to extensively mobilize the renal and mesenteric arteries is a major advantage of this retroperitoneal surgical exposure.

The inferior mesenteric artery is the primary blood supply to the left colon and is located by carrying the infrarenal dissection inferiorly along the posterolateral aspect of the aorta. In some large aneurysms, the thickened wall of the aorta obscures the actual origin of the inferior mesenteric artery. Division of this mesenteric vessel flush with the aorta is generally well tolerated. However, its inadvertent division distal to the left colic branch may result in sigmoid colon infarction. This complication is much more likely to occur when there is arteriosclerotic occlusion of the marginal artery of Drummond.[18] In patients with visceral artery occlusive disease, the left colic artery communicates with the left branch of the middle colic artery to become the meandering mesenteric artery (also known as the central anastomotic artery). This artery provides collateral circulation between the superior and inferior mesenteric arteries and vice versa (Fig. 4–17).[17]

Beyond the pelvic brim, the left common and external iliac arteries are readily accessible for vascular control.

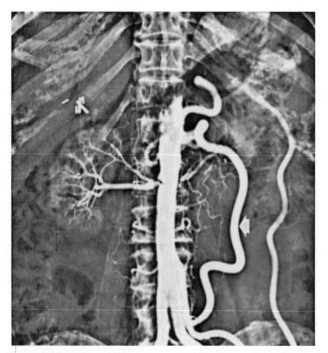

Figure 4–17. Angiogram from a patient with occlusion of the celiac and superior mesenteric arteries. Note the large inferior mesenteric artery with a central anastomotic artery (*arrow*) and a large marginal artery (*lateral position*) providing collateral circulation.

Ligating and dividing the inferior mesenteric artery flush with the aorta facilitates exposure of the distal anterolateral surface of the infrarenal aorta and the right common and external iliac arteries. It is wise to remember that the common iliac veins and vena cava are densely adherent to the posteromedial aspect of the left common iliac artery and the posterolateral aspect of the right common iliac artery. Vascular control of these vessels is safest after gently elevating them off their respective underlying major vein. This maneuver also facilitates transection of the distal common iliac artery under direct vision so that end-to-end aortoiliac reconstruction can be accomplished. If the iliac anastomosis cannot be performed at this level, it is wise to graft end to end to the internal iliac artery and then jump a separate graft to the external iliac artery. With this graft configuration, even an aneurysmal internal iliac artery may be simultaneously excluded (by opening it) and bypassed to the level of its first branch vessel. This helps to maintain vital pelvic perfusion.

Wound closure is accomplished in layers using No. 1 Vicryl suture for the posterior rectus sheath, transversalis fascia, transversus abdominis, and internal oblique muscle layers. The anterior rectus sheath and external oblique aponeurosis are closed with No. 1 PDS suture. Subcuticular skin closure with 3-0 Vicryl suture completes this multilayer wound closure.

ALTERNATE RENAL ARTERY EXPOSURE

The distal right renal artery can be exposed through a right-sided flank incision, which is a "mirror image" of the incision described in the section on retroperitoneal exposure of the aorta. With the patient on the operating table in a modified left lateral decubitus position, the retroperitoneal space is entered laterally after division of the abdominal wall muscles. The peritoneum and contents are gently mobilized anteriorly and medially, including the right kidney enclosed in Gerota's fascia. The renal artery is palpated distally and carefully dissected free of surrounding tissue. The inferior vena cava is also identified and mobilized after ligation of two or three paired lumbar veins. The vena cava can be gently elevated to expose the right posterolateral aspect of the aorta. Partial aortic occlusion with a side-biting vascular clamp is employed for anastomosis of the proximal bypass graft. Thereafter, a distal end-to-end anastomosis completes renal artery revascularization.

An extra-anatomic revascularization procedure for the right kidney is described by Moncure and associates.[19] This exposure employs a right subcostal incision extending into the right flank. The hepatic flexure of the colon is mobilized and rotated to the left. The duodenum is kocherized toward the midline to expose the right kidney. The renal artery is located behind and just above the right renal vein. Next, the hepatic artery is palpated in the hepatoduodenal ligament and the gastroduodenal artery identified. The common hepatic artery proximal to the gastroduodenal artery is dissected free. An end-to-side anastomosis of the bypass graft to the hepatic artery is constructed first. The bypass graft is then routed over the hepatoduodenal ligament and anastomosed to the transected end of the renal artery to revascularize the kidney. Figure 4–18 demon-

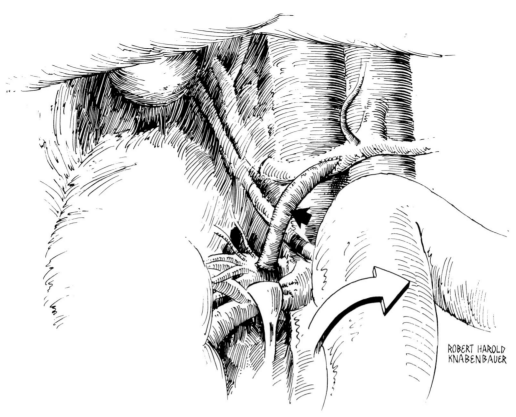

Figure 4–18. Illustration of hepatic-to-right renal artery bypass. The duodenum is kocherized *(open arrow)* for exposure. The reverse saphenous vein bypass is identified *(solid arrow)*. Note the retraction of the right renal vein for exposure.

strates the essential anatomy and a side-to-side distal anastomosis. However, end-to-end reconstruction is easier to accomplish.

The left renal artery can be exposed peripherally for extra-anatomic bypass by using the same incision described earlier in this section for retroperitoneal exposure of the abdominal aorta. Once the pararenal aorta is exposed, the tail of the pancreas is separated from the left adrenal gland to expose the splenic artery for bypass to the left renal artery (Fig. 4–19).[19] Inflow can also be obtained from the

aorta proximal or distal to the renal artery. This bypass can originate from the side of the aorta with destination to the transected left renal artery.

ALTERNATE EXPOSURE OF THE ABDOMINAL AORTA AND ITS BRANCHES

A helpful modification of the standard midline abdominal incision that can be used to expose the proximal abdominal

Figure 4–19. Flank exposure of the left renal artery. See text for details.

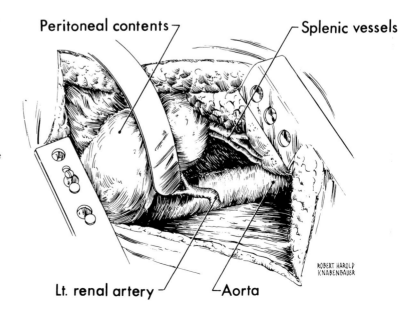

Peritoneal contents — Splenic vessels

Lt. renal artery — Aorta

aorta without entering the chest is illustrated in Figure 4–20. An inverted hockey-stick incision is employed beginning at the left midcostal margin. The left rectus muscle is transected and the oblique and transversus muscles are divided in the direction of the skin incision. The incision is continued down the linea alba to the symphysis pubis. The left side of the colon is mobilized by incising the peritoneum along the white line of Toldt from the pelvis to the lateral peritoneal attachments of the spleen. The spleen is gently mobilized and brought forward toward the midline by incising the splenorenal and splenophrenic ligaments.

Dissection is continued by forward mobilization of the spleen, pancreatic tail, and splenic flexure of the colon between the mesocolon and Gerota's fascia, with care not to damage the adrenal gland medially or the adrenal vein at its junction with the left renal vein. This left-to-right transperitoneal medial visceral rotation affords excellent exposure of the supraceliac and visceral aorta, including the renal arteries (Fig. 4–21). This exposure is facilitated by forward displacement of the left kidney along with the rest of the mobilized viscera. Division of the median arcuate ligament and diaphragmatic crura exposes the distal thoracic aorta without entering the left chest.

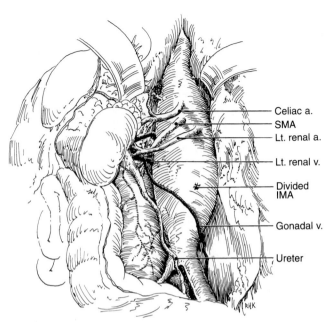

Figure 4–21. Transperitoneal medial visceral rotation with the left kidney rotated forward for repair of a supraceliac aortic aneurysm. IMA, Inferior mesenteric artery. (From Ballard JL: Management of renal artery stenosis in conjunction with aortic aneurysm. Semin Vasc Surg 9:221, 1996.)

TRANSPERITONEAL EXPOSURE OF THE ABDOMINAL AORTA AT THE DIAPHRAGMATIC HIATUS

Exposure of the supraceliac aorta at the diaphragmatic hiatus is life saving for early control of exigent hemorrhage in the case of a ruptured abdominal aortic aneurysm. It is also useful for temporary control of the aorta during repair of aortocaval or aortoenteric fistulas and infected aortic grafts. Less frequently, this exposure is suitable for revascularization of the celiac trunk and its proximal branches or the superior mesenteric artery.

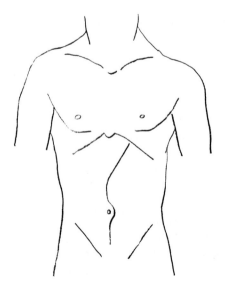

Figure 4–20. Modified abdominal incision for greater left upper quadrant exposure during transperitoneal medial visceral rotation. (From Deiparine MK, Ballard JL: Correspondence re: "Transperitoneal medial visceral rotation." Ann Vasc Surg 9:607, 1995.)

This exposure through the lesser sac is facilitated by downward retraction of the stomach and lateral retraction of the esophagus. The aortic pulse is palpated, and the arching fibers of the diaphragm at the aortic hiatus are divided directly over the aorta. The periaortic fascia is opened and the index and middle fingers are passed medially and laterally to the aorta. Gentle blunt finger dissection between the diaphragmatic fibers and the aorta creates space on either side of the aorta. This maneuver is critical, because any overlying muscle fibers would allow a vascular occluding clamp to slide up and off the aorta. No effort is made to completely encircle the aorta because an intercostal or proximal lumbar artery or vein can be avulsed with troublesome bleeding. At this point, a partially opened aortic clamp is advanced over the dorsal hand and fingers that have been appropriately positioned to cross-clamp the aorta and interrupt blood flow. This exposure is illustrated in Figure 4–22.

Celiac artery reconstruction requires more exposure. A generous incision is made in the posterior parietal peritoneum, and the diaphragmatic crura are completely divided. The inferior phrenic arteries should be isolated, ligated, and divided. The aortic branch to the left adrenal gland is also usually visualized and sacrificed. Dissection is continued distally to expose the celiac artery, which can be palpated at its origin from the anterior surface of the aorta. Dense fibers of the median arcuate ligament are divided along with the neural elements forming the celiac plexus. This tissue is quite vascular; thus, stick ties and cautery are useful for hemostasis. Once the celiac trunk has been exposed, the common hepatic artery is dissected free of surrounding tissue as it courses toward the liver hilum. Sympathetic nerve fibers can be seen to entwine on the surface of this vessel. There is usually a 3- to 4-cm segment of the hepatic artery that is free of branches and therefore useful as a site for vascular anastomosis. The splenic artery is palpable at the superior border of the pancreas and courses to the left toward the splenic hilum. Here, again, there is a 4- to 5-cm segment free of branches that can be used for placement of a vascular anastomosis. The left gastric artery is the smallest of the three main branches of the celiac artery. It courses anteriorly to follow the lesser curvature of the stomach and should be protected during this exposure.

The supraceliac aorta can also be used as the bypass origin for superior mesenteric artery reconstruction. The proximal anastomosis is made on the anterior surface of the aorta after the aortic hiatus is opened as described earlier. Using careful finger dissection, a tunnel must then be created behind the pancreas. The bypass graft is passed through the tunnel and anastomosed to the distal patent superior mesenteric artery. Kinking of the bypass, such as can occur with retrograde aortic-to-superior mesenteric artery bypass grafts during replacement of bowel, is unlikely in this tunneled position.

Anterior exposure of the superior mesenteric artery inferior to the transverse mesocolon requires opening the posterior parietal peritoneum lateral to the third and fourth portions of the duodenum (Fig. 4–23). The left renal vein is identified and mobilized as described previously for exposure of the renal arteries. The left renal vein is retracted downward and the dissection carried upward on the aorta until the superior mesenteric artery origin can be palpated. It usually arises from the left side of the anterior surface of the aorta. The artery is immediately encased by the superior mesenteric sympathetic nerve plexus, which must be incised for exposure. Bleeding from the vascular plexus tissue is controlled by cautery and suture ligatures. The

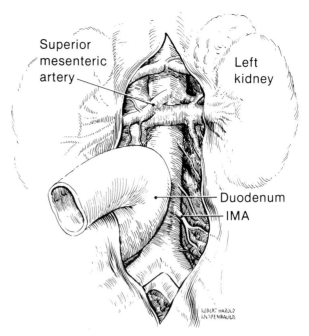

Figure 4–23. Infracolic exposure of the superior mesenteric artery. The pancreas and transverse colon are not shown but are retracted upward and forward. See text for details. IMA, inferior mesenteric artery.

overlying transverse mesocolon and pancreas significantly limit this exposure.

TRANSPERITONEAL EXPOSURE OF THE INFRARENAL ABDOMINAL AORTA

A midline abdominal incision from the xiphoid to the symphysis pubis is commonly used for anterior exposure of the infrarenal abdominal aorta. One major disadvantage of this approach is incomplete visualization of the proximal abdominal aorta and/or renal artery origins. This potential lack of exposure is improved by proximally extending the midline incision around the xiphoid process and completely mobilizing the third and fourth portions of the duodenum. The dissection continues through the posterior peritoneum just lateral to the duodenum and medial to the inferior mesenteric vein to avoid damaging the circulation to the left—or sigmoid—colon. This is particularly important in dealing with ruptured abdominal aortic aneurysms, where landmarks are frequently obscured by an extensive retroperitoneal hematoma. The duodenum can nearly always be visualized and used as a landmark during this exposure.

It is wise to palpate the aortic bifurcation and expose the common iliac arteries from the midline, thereby avoiding injury to the ureters. Fibers of the sympathetic nerves arch over the left common iliac artery in males, and damage to these sympathetic fibers can result in erectile dysfunction and retrograde ejaculation. Figure 4–24 shows the relationship of the infrarenal sympathetic nerve fibers to the terminal aorta and iliac arteries. Incising along the white line of Toldt and mobilizing the sigmoid or proximal ascending colon toward the midline can readily identify the external iliac arteries. Graft limbs coursing out to this

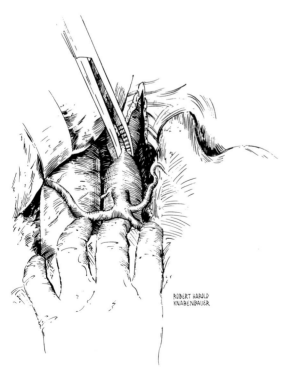

Figure 4–22. Exposure of the abdominal aorta at the diaphragm. See text for details.

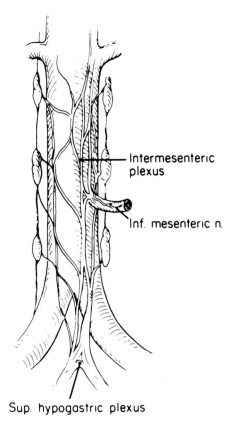

Figure 4–24. Relationship of the infrarenal sympathetic nerves to the aorta and iliac arteries. Note the condensation of nerve elements coursing over the left common iliac artery origin. (From Weinstein MH, Machleder HI: Sexual function after aortoiliac surgery. Ann Surg 181:787, 1975.)

level should be passed under both the colon mesentery and ureter.

TRANSPERITONEAL EXPOSURE OF THE RENAL ARTERIES

The left main renal artery originates from the posterolateral surface of the aorta. Usually, this location is at the level of the upper border of the left renal vein where it crosses over the abdominal aorta. The right renal artery often arises at a slightly lower level. Anterior exposure of either renal artery origin involves incision of the posterior parietal peritoneum just lateral to the fourth portion of the duodenum. Additional exposure is obtained by continuing this incision along the distal third portion of the duodenum.

The left renal vein is identified and carefully mobilized. Frequently, there is a small parietal vein that terminates in the inferior margin of the left renal vein over the aorta. Otherwise, there are two major venous tributaries to be identified, ligated, and divided. The first is located by following the inferior margin of the left renal vein laterally to the termination of the left gonadal vein. Next, the dissection is carried laterally along the superior surface of the left renal vein until the confluence of the left adrenal vein is identified. It should be ligated flush with the renal vein and divided. The entire left renal vein can then be mobilized on a silastic vascular loop.

Cautious dissection is advisable in this area, as there is an important large communicating vein arising from the posterior surface of the proximal left renal vein. This vein communicates with the adjacent lumbar vein and thence to the hemiazygous system and superior vena cava. The presence of this venous collateral allows acute ligation of the left renal vein without impairment of renal function. This lumbar venous communication should be preserved if at all possible during this anterior transperitoneal approach.

Once the left renal vein is mobilized, attention should be directed to exposing the left lateral surface of the aorta above and below the level of the left renal vein. The left renal artery arising from the posterolateral surface of the aorta is thus exposed. Autonomic nerve elements are encountered on the renal artery but can be divided without concern. Gentle placement of a vein retractor under the left renal vein with upward retraction by an assistant greatly facilitates this exposure. A silastic loop placed about the renal artery origin aids in the mobilization and dissection of this vessel.

The right renal artery is more difficult to expose, because it passes directly behind the inferior vena cava on its course to the renal hilum. The origin of this artery is palpated as it emerges from the right posterolateral aspect of the aorta. Care should be taken not to injure the right adrenal branch, which arises 5 to 10 mm from the origin of the right renal artery. The size of this vessel may be 2 to 3 mm when renal artery stenosis is present because it becomes a very important collateral to the distal right renal artery via capsular branches. In the event that the entire right renal artery and its branches must be exposed, the surgeon must completely mobilize the vena cava above and below the artery by carefully ligating and dividing all adjacent lumbar veins.

The subhepatic space is entered and the duodenum kocherized to allow exposure of the right renal vein as it joins the inferior vena cava. The renal vein is mobilized on a silastic loop to aid in identification of the main renal artery lying beneath the vein. Exposure of the renal artery is complete when this distal dissection joins the medial exposure already described.

EMERGENCY EXPOSURE OF THE ABDOMINAL AORTA AND VENA CAVA

Vascular exposure of injured vessels within the abdomen is best carried out through a generous midline abdominal incision. Location of the hematoma determines the exposure to be employed. Because the abdominal circulation arises in a retroperitoneal location, the overlying viscera need to be rotated medially or elevated superiorly in order to expose the aorta and its major branches and the caval and portal venous circulation.

Kudsk and Sheldon[20] have classified the retroperitoneal space into three zones (Fig. 4–25). The presence of a central hematoma (zone 1) indicates injury to the aorta, the proximal renal/visceral arteries, the inferior vena cava, or the portal vein. An expanding, zone 1 retroperitoneal hematoma with extension to the left indicates a proximal aortic or adjacent major branch vessel injury. Transperito-

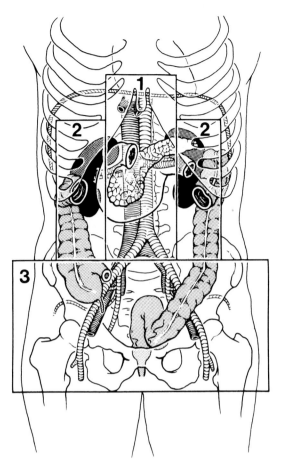

Figure 4–25. Anatomic zones for exploration of retroperitoneal hematomas. See text for details. (From Kudsk KA, Sheldon GF: Retroperitoneal hematoma. In Blaisdell FW, Trunkey DD [eds]: Trauma Management, vol 1. Abdominal Trauma, 2nd ed. New York, Thieme Medical Publishers, 1993, p 400.)

neal left-to-right medial visceral rotation swiftly and widely exposes the aorta from the diaphragm to its bifurcation. Exposure can be facilitated by division of the left rectus muscle transversely in the left upper quadrant or by the modified abdominal incision described earlier in the chapter. The splenic flexure is mobilized, including the spleen and the left kidney, with rotation of these viscera to the right. The origins of the celiac, superior mesenteric, and renal arteries are likewise exposed (Fig. 4–26).

The presence of a zone 1 retroperitoneal hematoma with extension into the right flank is indicative of major caval, portal venous, or proximal injury to a major arterial branch in the right upper quadrant. Exposure is gained by incising the peritoneum lateral to the ascending colon and reflecting this structure medially followed by duodenal kocherization. This right-to-left medial visceral rotation exposes the entire vena cava from the iliac confluence to the liver (Fig. 4–27).

Incising the hepatoduodenal ligament above the duodenum exposes the portal vein. The common bile duct is retracted laterally, and the hepatic artery is palpated and isolated for inspection. Thereafter, retracting the hepatic artery toward the midline facilitates examination of the portal vein. The right side of the aorta can be inspected as well as the proximal right renal artery if rotation and

mobilization of the overlying bowel are continued to the midline.

Lateral hematomas (zone 2) indicate injury to distal visceral and renal vessels. Despite their lateral location, it is wise not to enter a large hematoma to control exigent hemorrhage until central aortic exposure has been secured for possible cross-clamping. Retroperitoneal pelvic hematomas (zone 3) usually indicate torn branches of the iliac vessels associated with pelvic fractures. These may not require exploration unless the hematoma is expanding or there is evidence of large vessel injury demonstrated by angiography.

EXTRAPERITONEAL EXPOSURE OF THE ILIAC ARTERIES

This exposure begins with an oblique incision in the lower quadrant of the abdomen on the side of involved iliac artery occlusive disease. It is good practice to start the incision near the pubic tubercle with extension obliquely lateral, staying medial to the anterior superior iliac spine of the pelvis. The external oblique aponeurosis is opened in the direction of its fibers, and the incision is continued into the fleshy portion of this muscle. The internal oblique and transversus abdominis muscles are divided in the direction of the incision to enter the preperitoneal space. The peritoneum is gently rotated medially to expose the external iliac artery. The ureter, which is adherent to the peritoneum and usually retracts with the peritoneal contents, is vulnerable to injury as it courses across the iliac bifurcation. Exposure of the common iliac artery requires extension of the incision proximally and laterally into the flank region.

Care should be taken not to injure the ilioinguinal or genitofemoral nerves during exposure or retraction. Their location on the anterior surface of the psoas muscle is vulnerable. Combination of this incision with a curvilinear incision over the common femoral artery permits exposure from the terminal common iliac artery to the proximal superficial or deep femoral arteries (Fig. 4–28). The iliac artery exposed in this extraperitoneal fashion is particularly appealing as an inflow source in cases in which there is extensive scarring at the groin from previous peripheral vascular procedures.

EXPOSURE OF THE COMMON FEMORAL ARTERY

A curvilinear incision placed directly over the palpable pulse, with extension above as well as below the groin crease, provides excellent exposure of the common femoral artery and its branches. An incision made just medial to the midpoint of the inguinal ligament suffices in the absence of a palpable pulse. Frequently, the diseased artery can be rolled beneath the index finger, and this guides the plane of deeper dissection. It is important to remember to check for posterior branches, because an aberrant medial femoral circumflex artery can arise anywhere along the posterior surface of the common femoral artery. Failure to control this vessel can result in troublesome bleeding when the common femoral artery is opened.

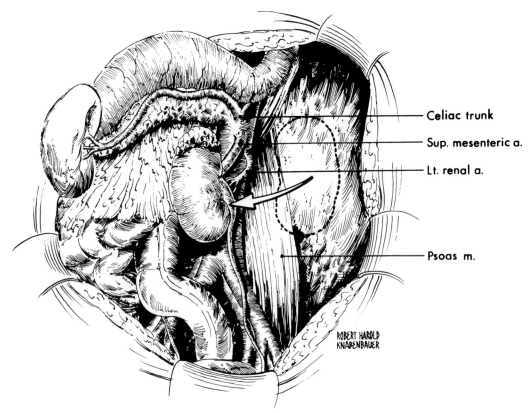

Celiac trunk

Sup. mesenteric a.

Lt. renal a.

Psoas m.

ROBERT HAROLD
KNABENBAUER

Figure 4–26. Rotation right of intraabdominal contents including the left kidney for complete visualization of the abdominal aorta. Rotation of the kidney forward and to the right *(arrow)* from the renal fossa *(dotted outline)*. (From Smith LL, Catalano RD: Exposure of vascular injuries. In Bongard FS, Wilson SE, Perry MO [eds]: Vascular Injuries in Surgical Practice. Norwalk, Conn, Appleton & Lange, 1991, p 18.)

Gentle dissection about the origin of the profunda femoris artery is important. The lateral femoral circumflex artery arises from the lateral side of the deep femoral artery, and this vessel can be easily injured. Care should also be taken to identify the lateral femoral circumflex vein, which courses from a lateral to a medial direction across the origin of the profunda femoris artery. Division of this vein facilitates arterial mobilization and distal dissection. This maneuver is paramount if the proximal profunda femoris artery is to be used as an inflow source, and it provides excellent exposure for eversion endarterectomy.

EXPOSURE OF THE DEEP FEMORAL ARTERY

The profunda femoris artery is located 1.5 cm medial to the femur and lies on the pectineus and adductor brevis muscles. In cases in which the deep femoral artery is being exposed as an initial procedure, the dissection is aided by flexion and external rotation of the thigh to relax the involved muscles. Colborn and associates[21] have described the surgical anatomy of the deep femoral artery. The reader is well advised to consult this excellent and well-illustrated article.

The deep femoral artery can be a useful inflow or outflow source in a patient with a hostile groin after previous surgical exposures. Nuñez and associates[22] have described a practical approach to the middle and distal thirds

of this artery that avoids a scarred femoral bifurcation. This surgical dissection begins lateral to the sartorius muscle. Figure 4–29 demonstrates the incision over the lateral aspect of the sartorius muscle and branches of the lateral femoral circumflex artery. These branches are followed medially to the profunda femoris artery after the incision is deepened between the vastus medialis and adductor longus muscles. Complete mobilization of the artery at this level requires division of overlying venous tributaries to the deep femoral vein. This dissection can then safely be extended distally or, if needed, proximally to the femoral bifurcation.

Alternatively, the distal third of the profunda femoris artery can be exposed by a surgical plane of dissection that is posterior to the adductor longus muscle in the medial thigh.[23] This exposure is deepened between the gracilis and adductor longus muscles to the medial aspect of the profunda femoris artery. Knee flexion relaxes the involved muscles and aids in this exposure.

EXPOSURE OF THE POPLITEAL ARTERY

The popliteal artery is exposed from a medial approach with few exceptions. The proximal and distal portions of this vessel are readily exposed. However, the medial head of the gastrocnemius muscle and the tendinous insertions of the long adductor muscles obscure the midportion of the artery at the joint space of the knee. A posterior

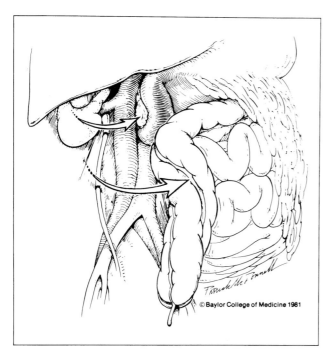

Figure 4–27. Rotation left of intraabdominal viscera by mobilization of the right colon and by kocherization of the duodenum. The right kidney can also be mobilized to inspect the posterior surface of the vena cava if necessary. (Reproduced with the permission of Dohrmann M, original illustrator.)

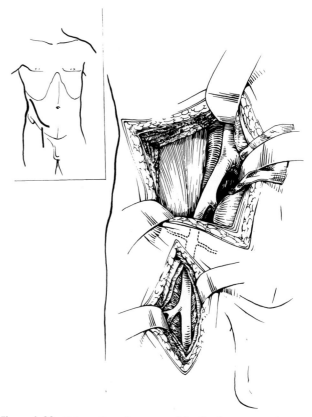

Figure 4–28. Extraperitoneal exposure of the distal common and external iliac arteries. Counterincision at groin facilitates iliofemoral reconstruction.

approach to the midpopliteal artery is useful for isolated disorders such as popliteal entrapment or cystic adventitial disease.

The proximal popliteal artery is exposed through an incision placed in the groove between the vastus medialis and sartorius muscles. The greater saphenous vein lies just posterior to this incision and care must be taken to preserve it during the dissection. The sartorius muscle is retracted

posteriorly and investing fascia incised longitudinally, preserving the saphenous nerve, which is usually seen lying on the deep fascial surface. Once the fascia is opened, the popliteal artery can be palpated in its location under the adductor magnus tendon.

Figure 4–29. Lateral approach to the deep femoral artery. *Upper right,* The incision is lateral to the sartorius muscle. *Lower left,* The exposure of the profunda femoris vessel. See text for details.

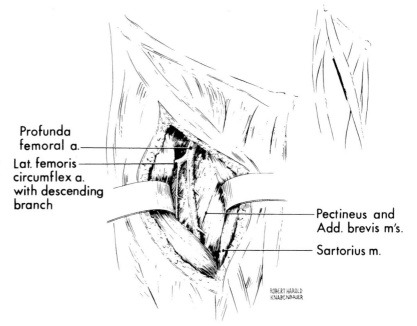

Profunda femoral a.

Lat. femoris circumflex a. with descending branch

Pectineus and Add. brevis m's.

Sartorius m.

Although not usually necessary, additional exposure can be obtained distally by dividing the tendon of the medial head of the gastrocnemius muscle. Gentle insertion of the left index finger behind its tendinous origin aids in isolating this structure and protecting the underlying neurovascular bundle. Should additional distal exposure be necessary, the tendinous insertions of the sartorius, semimembranosis, semitendinosis, and gracilis muscles may be divided. It is well to mark these tendons with identifying sutures to aid in their subsequent repair.

The terminal popliteal artery and tibioperoneal trunk are exposed through an incision placed approximately 1.5 cm posterior to the medial margin of the tibia. Once again, the surgeon must be aware of the greater saphenous vein and protect it in its subcutaneous location. The thick muscular fascia overlying the gastrocnemius muscle is incised to enter the popliteal space. The popliteal vein is usually encountered first within the neurovascular sheath. Gentle downward retraction of the vein facilitates dissection of the popliteal artery, which lies superolateral to the vein. The origin of the anterior tibial artery arises anteriorly and laterally from the terminal popliteal artery. Further exposure of the tibioperoneal trunk and proximal peroneal and posterior tibial arteries requires the division of the soleus muscle fibers arising from the medial margin of the tibia. Division of overlying venous tributaries between the often-paired popliteal veins facilitates this exposure.

Lateral Exposure of the Popliteal Artery

A lateral approach to the popliteal artery can be employed when previous medial exposure has resulted in dense tissue scarring, making repeat procedures extremely difficult. The incision for the above-knee popliteal artery is placed between the iliotibial tract and the biceps femoris muscle as described by Veith and associates.[24] The dissection is deepened through the fascia lata posterior to the junction of the lateral intramuscular septum and the iliotibial tract to enter the popliteal space. The popliteal vein is encountered first within the vascular sheath. It can be mobilized and retracted posteriorly to allow exposure of the popliteal artery. The tibial and peroneal nerves are also posterior and loosely adherent to the hamstrings. They naturally fall out of harm's way with retraction of the biceps femoris, semimembranosus, and semitendinosus muscles.

The lateral approach to the below-knee popliteal artery begins with an incision over the head and proximal one fourth of the fibula. As the incision is deepened, care must be taken to preserve the common peroneal nerve as it courses around the neck of the fibula (Fig. 4–30). The biceps femoris tendon is divided. The ligamentous attachments to the head of the fibula are also divided, and the proximal fibula is removed. The entire below-knee popliteal artery, anterior tibial artery origin, and tibioperoneal trunk are accessible after removal of the bone fragment (Fig. 4–31). The proximal posterior tibial and peroneal arteries can be exposed if more of the distal fibula is resected.

EXPOSURE OF THE TIBIAL AND PERONEAL ARTERIES

Management of lower extremity ischemic vascular disease requires accurate knowledge of the arterial and venous

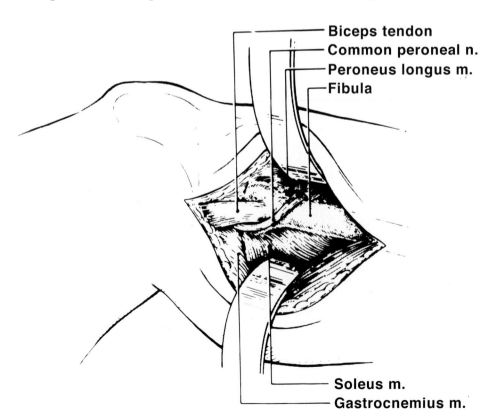

- Biceps tendon
- Common peroneal n.
- Peroneus longus m.
- Fibula

- Soleus m.
- Gastrocnemius m.

Figure 4–30. Lateral approach to the distal popliteal artery. Note the common peroneal nerve coursing around the neck of the fibula. (From Veith F, Ascer E, Gupta S: Lateral approach to the popliteal artery. J Vasc Surg 6:119, 1987.)

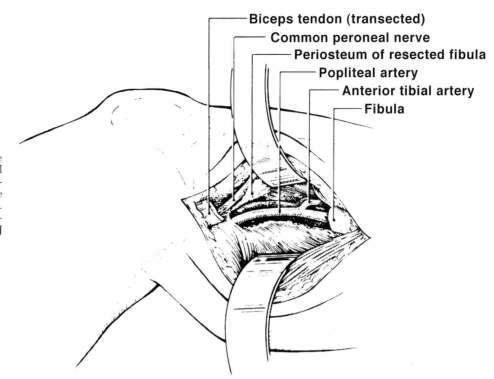

- **Biceps tendon (transected)**
- **Common peroneal nerve**
- **Periosteum of resected fibula**
- **Popliteal artery**
- **Anterior tibial artery**
- **Fibula**

Figure 4–31. Lateral approach to the distal popliteal artery after the removal of the proximal fibula. Note the transected tendon of the biceps muscle and the intact common peroneal nerve. (From Veith F, Ascer E, Gupta S: Lateral approach to the popliteal artery. J Vasc Surg 6:119, 1987.)

circulation of the leg. It is important to keep in mind the relationship of the three major leg arteries to the tibia and fibula as well as the compartments of the leg. Figure 4–32 demonstrates these important relationships. Note the anterior tibial vessels lying on the interosseous membrane in the anterior compartment. The peroneal artery, which is adjacent to the medial margin of the fibula in the deep posterior compartment, lies in close proximity to the trans-

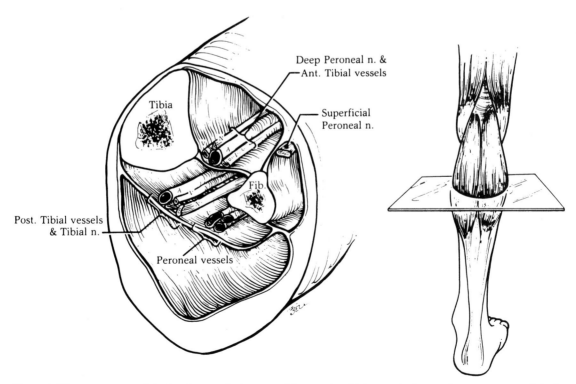

- Tibia
- Deep Peroneal n. & Ant. Tibial vessels
- Superficial Peroneal n.
- Post. Tibial vessels & Tibial n.
- Fib.
- Peroneal vessels

Figure 4–32. Cross-section of the leg showing the location of the anterior tibial artery in the anterior compartment of the leg and the posterior tibial and peroneal arteries in the deep posterior compartment. (From Briggs S, Seligson D: Management of extremity trauma. In Richardson D, Polk H, Flint M [eds]: Trauma: Clinical Care and Pathophysiology. Chicago, Year Book Medical, 1987, p 544.)

verse crural intermuscular septum. The posterior tibial vessels are medial to the peroneal artery and veins, but also above the intermuscular septum and in the deep posterior compartment of the leg.

Surgical exposure of the crural vessels requires patience and great care. There are numerous small muscular branches, and each artery has two accompanying veins with their respective tributaries to protect. Careless dissection leads to bleeding that obscures the operative field and increases the likelihood of injury to these delicate vascular structures.

Anterior Tibial Artery

This vessel travels between the tibialis anterior and the extensor digitorum longus muscles in the proximal portion of the anterior compartment of the leg. The extensor hallucis longus muscle crosses over the artery from lateral to medial in the distal leg above the level of the flexor retinaculum. Surgical exposure of the anterior tibial artery is best afforded either in the proximal leg or just above the flexor retinaculum proximal to the ankle.

A skin incision made approximately 2.5 cm lateral to the anterior border of the tibia facilitates proximal exposure of the anterior tibial artery. Deepening the dissection between the two muscle bellies assists this surgical exposure. Dorsiflexion and internal rotation of the foot aid in identification of the groove between these two muscles. The muscles are gently separated down to the anterior tibial artery, which lies between its two accompanying veins and anterior to the deep peroneal nerve on the interosseous membrane.

Alternatively, a dissection course that passes between the extensor hallucis longus and extensor digitorum longus laterally and the tibialis anterior muscle medially exposes the artery just above the flexor retinaculum.[23] The upper portion of the flexor retinaculum can be divided to improve distal exposure. However, complete division of this retinaculum is not recommended. If the anterior tibial artery is unsuitable for vascular reconstruction at this level, the dissection should skip down to the dorsalis pedis artery below the inferior portion of the retinaculum.

Posterior Tibial Artery

Extending the incision described earlier for medial exposure of the tibioperoneal trunk facilitates proximal exposure of the posterior tibial artery. This requires incising the origin of the soleus muscle from the medial border of the tibia. Tributary veins traveling through this muscle origin may cause troublesome bleeding. These should be ligated to keep the operative field dry. Immediately deep to the soleus fibers, the posterior tibial vessels can be observed coursing between the tibialis posterior and the flexor digitorum longus muscles. The tibial nerve, which crosses the artery posteriorly from medial to lateral, must be protected. This exposure can be challenging, as there is a dense network of venous tributaries overlying the origin of the posterior tibial artery.

Exposure of the middle aspect of the posterior tibial artery is best achieved distal to the lower edge of the soleus muscle fibers in the medial calf.[23] This dissection into the deep posterior compartment of the leg continues above the intermuscular septum to expose the neurovascular bundle. The artery must be carefully dissected free from its accompanying paired veins and tibial nerve.

Peroneal Artery

The proximal and middle aspects of the peroneal artery can be exposed using the same medial leg incisions that were described for exposure of the posterior tibial artery. Once this latter artery is exposed, the dissection continues on the intermuscular septum to a deeper level. The peroneal artery is located adjacent to the medial border of the fibula. This exposure is quite deep and therefore more difficult in a large leg.

Resecting a short segment of the fibula through a lateral incision over this bone can also expose the peroneal artery. This incision should be placed below the entrance of the peroneal nerve into the anterior compartment of the leg. The peroneal vessels lie just deep to the medial border of the fibula. Once this short segment of bone is removed, the vessels are exposed. Careful division and removal of the fibula are essential, as the accompanying venous plexus that surrounds the peroneal artery is easy to disturb and may cause significant bleeding. Surprisingly little postoperative morbidity is associated with this exposure.

EXPOSURE OF PEDAL ARTERIES

A detailed understanding of the pedal arterial circulation is important because distal bypass sites in the foot are frequently used for limb-threatening ischemic vascular disease. Ascer and associates have described various surgical approaches as well as results of these distal lower extremity bypass procedures.[25] Figure 4–33 shows the branches and distribution of the distal anterior and posterior tibial arteries in the foot.

Distal Posterior Tibial Artery and Plantar Branches

Exposure of the terminal posterior tibial artery with its concomitant veins and tibial nerve is accomplished by a retromalleolar incision. The dissection is continued distally by division of the flexor retinaculum. The neurovascular bundle is surrounded by fatty tissue and the artery is usually superior to the nerve. Further dissection may require sequential incisions to accurately follow the course of the terminal posterior tibial artery into the plantar surface of the foot. Small self-expanding retractors facilitate this exposure, as the plantar tissues are thick and rigid. The plantar aponeurosis and the flexor digitorum brevis muscle can be incised to expose the medial and lateral

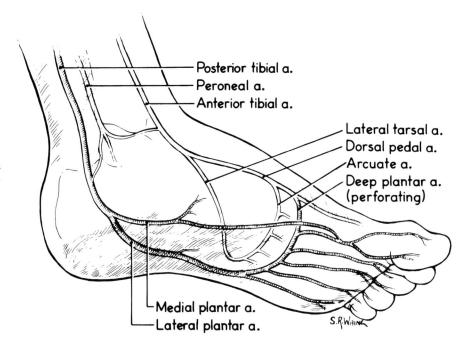

Figure 4–33. Anatomy of the arterial circulation of the foot. (From Ascer E, Veith F, Gupta S: Bypasses to plantar arteries and other tibial branches: An extended approach to limb salvage. J Vasc Surg 8:434, 1988.)

plantar arteries (Fig. 4–34). This latter vessel continues distally into the foot to form the deep plantar arch.

Dorsal Pedal Artery and Lateral Tarsal Branch

These vessels are approached through a longitudinal incision lateral to the extensor hallucis longus tendon. The inferior extensor retinaculum is partially incised just distal to the ankle joint to expose the proximal dorsalis pedis artery and lateral tarsal branch. The lateral tarsal artery

usually arises at the level of the navicular bone and beneath the extensor digitorum brevis muscle. This artery communicates with the arcuate artery in the midfoot. Therefore, it is an important collateral blood supply to the dorsum of the foot. Division of the inferior extensor retinaculum is not required for more distal exposure of the dorsal pedal artery. It is necessary to protect the distal deep peroneal nerve coursing medial to this artery.

Deep Plantar Artery

This vessel is the main continuation of the dorsal pedal artery at the level of the metatarsal bones. It is best ap-

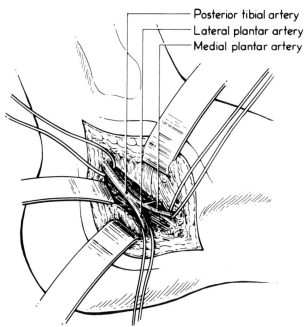

Figure 4–34. Exposure of the terminal left posterior tibial artery using a retromalleolar incision. The terminal branches of this vessel are shown, the larger being the lateral plantar branch. See text for details. (From Ascer E, Veith F, Gupta S: Bypasses to plantar arteries and other tibial branches: An extended approach to limb salvage. J Vasc Surg 8:436, 1988.)

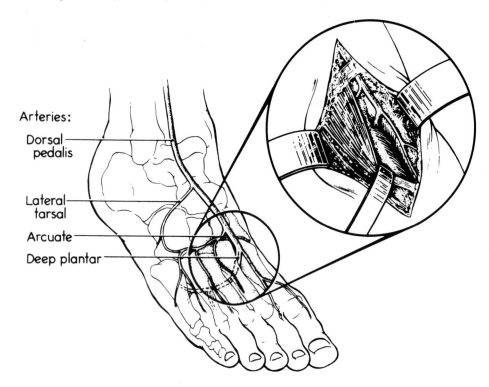

Arteries:

Dorsal pedalis

Lateral tarsal

Arcuate

Deep plantar

Figure 4–35. Diagram of the arterial circulation on the dorsum of the foot. The insert shows the origin of the deep plantar branch as it courses between the two heads of the first dorsal interosseous vessel. See text for details. (From Ascer E, Veith F, Gupta S: Bypasses to plantar arteries and other tibial branches: An extended approach to limb salvage. J Vasc Surg 8:437, 1988.)

proached through a curvilinear incision over the dorsum of the foot lateral to the extensor hallucis longus tendon. The artery is followed distally until it divides into the first dorsal metatarsal and deep plantar branches. The latter vessel descends between the two heads of the first dorsal interosseous muscle to anastomose with the lateral plantar branch. This forms the deep plantar arch of the foot (Fig. 4–35). Adequate exposure of the deep plantar branch requires retraction of the extensor hallucis brevis muscle. The periosteum of the second metatarsal bone is then carefully elevated and a portion of the bone is removed by a rongeur to provide adequate exposure for distal arterial anastomosis (Fig. 4–36). This exposure requires delicate dissection otherwise because injury to adjacent arterial branches and venous tributaries may obscure the operative field or create ischemia to marginally viable tissues.

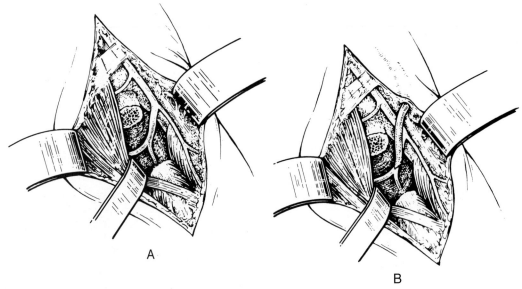

A

B

Figure 4–36. *A,* Shows the deep plantar arch branch following resection of a portion of the second metatarsal bone. *B,* Shows the distal anastomosis of a bypass to this vessel. (From Ascer E, Veith F, Gupta S: Bypasses to plantar arteries and other tibial branches: An extended approach to limb salvage. J Vasc Surg 8:437, 1988.)

References

1. Effeney DJ, Stoney RJ: Extracranial cerebrovascular disease. In Effeney DJ, Stoney RJ (eds): Wylie's Atlas of Vascular Surgery. Philadelphia, JB Lippincott, 1992, pp 18–57.
2. Evans W, Mendelowitz D, Liapis C, et al: Motor speech deficit following carotid endarterectomy. Ann Surg 196:461, 1982.
3. Hertzer N, Feldman B, Beven E, et al: A prospective study of the incidence of injury to the cranial nerves during carotid endarterectomy. Surg Gynecol Obstet 151:781, 1980.
4. Mock CN, Lilly MP, McRae RG, Carney WI Jr: Selection of the approach to the distal internal carotid artery from the second cervical vertebra to the base of the skull. J Vasc Surg 13:846, 1991.
5. Fisher D, Clagett G, Parker J, et al: Mandibular subluxation for high carotid exposure. J Vasc Surg 1:727, 1984.
6. Dossa C, Shepard AD, Wolford DG, et al: Distal internal carotid exposure: A simplified technique for temporary mandibular subluxation. J Vasc Surg 12:319, 1990.
7. Wylie E, Stoney R, Ehrenfeld W, Effeney D: Nonatherosclerotic disease of the extracranial carotid arteries, vol 2. In Egdahl R (ed): Manual of Vascular Surgery. New York, Springer-Verlag, 1986.
8. Sakopoulos AG, Ballard JL, Gundry SR: Minimally invasive approach for aortic branch vessel reconstruction. J Vasc Surg 31(1 Pt 1):200, 2000.
9. Berguer R: Distal vertebral artery bypass: Technique, the "occipital connection," and potential uses. J Vasc Surg 2:621, 1985.
10. Roos D: Surgical treatment of the thoracic outlet syndromes. In Jamison CW (ed): Current Operative Surgery: Vascular Surgery. London, Bailliere & Tindall, 1985.
11. Effeney DJ, Stoney RJ: Extracranial cerebrovascular disease. In Effeney DJ, Stoney RJ (eds): Wylie's Atlas of Vascular Surgery. Philadelphia, JB Lippincott, 1992, p 210.
12. Stoney R, Wylie E: Surgical management of arterial lesions of the thoracolumbar aorta. Am J Surg 126:157, 1973.
13. Brockstein B, Johns L, Gewertz BL: Blood supply to the spinal cord: Anatomic and physiologic correlations. Ann Vasc Surg 8:394, 1994.
14. Ballard JL, Yonemoto H, Killeen JD: Cost effective aortic exposure: A retroperitoneal experience. Ann Vasc Surg 14:1, 2000.
15. Sicard GA, Reilly JM, Rubin BG, et al: Transabdominal versus retroperitoneal incision for abdominal aortic surgery: Report of a prospective randomized trial. J Vasc Surg 21:174, 1995.
16. Darling RC III, Shah DM, McClellan WR, et al: Decreased morbidity associated with retroperitoneal exclusion treatment for abdominal aortic aneurysm. J Cardiovasc Surg 33:65, 1992.
17. Uflacker R: Abdominal aorta and branches. In Uflacker R (ed): Atlas of Vascular Anatomy—An Angiographic Approach. Baltimore, Williams & Wilkens, 1997, p 405.
18. Tollefson DFJ, Ernst CB: Gastrointestinal and visceral ischemic complications of aortic reconstruction. In Bernhard VM, Towne JB (eds): Complications in Vascular Surgery. St. Louis, Quality Medical Publishing, 1991, p 135.
19. Moncure A, Brewster D, Darling R, et al: Use of the splenic and hepatic arteries for renal revascularization. J Vasc Surg 3:196, 1986.
20. Kudsk KA, Sheldon GF: Retroperitoneal hematoma, vol 1. In Blaisdell FW, Trunkey DD (eds): Trauma Management: Abdominal Trauma. New York, Thieme-Stratton, 1982, p 281.
21. Colborn GL, Mattar SG, Taylor B, et al: The surgical anatomy of the deep femoral artery. Am Surg 61:336, 1995.
22. Nunez A, Veith F, Gupta S, et al: Direct approaches to the distal portions of the deep femoral artery for limb salvage bypasses. J Vasc Surg 8:576, 1988.
23. Rutherford RB: Exposure of lower extremity vessels. In Rutherford RB (ed): Atlas of Vascular Surgery: Basic Techniques and Exposures. Philadelphia, WB Saunders, 1993, p 112.
24. Veith F, Ascer E, Gupta S: Lateral approach to the popliteal artery. J Vasc Surg 6:119, 1987.
25. Ascer E, Veith F, Gupta S: Bypasses to plantar arteries and other tibial branches: An extended approach to limb salvage. J Vasc Surg 8:434, 1985.

Review Questions

1. Of the following nerves, the one most likely to be injured during carotid endarterectomy is
   (a) recurrent laryngeal nerve
   (b) vagus nerve (X)
   (c) hypoglossal nerve (XII)
   (d) superior laryngeal nerve
   (e) glossopharyngeal nerve (IX)

2. Structures contributing to thoracic outlet compression syndrome may include (true or false)
   (a) subclavius muscle
   (b) first rib
   (c) scalenus anticus
   (d) congenital cervical rib
   (e) sternocleidomastoid muscle

3. Concerning lower extremity circulation (true or false)
   (a) the deep femoral artery is accessible only by an approach that is lateral to the sartorius muscle
   (b) it is possible to expose the popliteal artery above and below the knee by lateral or medial approaches
   (c) the lateral tarsal artery is the largest distal branch of the posterior tibial artery
   (d) the deep plantar arch is formed by the deep plantar artery and the lateral plantar artery

4. During repair of an infrarenal abdominal aortic aneurysm (true or false)
   (a) autonomic nerve fibers crossing the left common iliac artery should be protected to preserve erectile function
   (b) a large anastomotic artery appearing on arteriography between the superior and inferior mesenteric arteries indicates satisfactory perfusion of the left colon with little risk of ischemia if the inferior mesenteric artery is ligated
   (c) a large lumbar artery near the renal arteries should be preserved because this may represent a significant contribution to the anterior spinal artery
   (d) the left renal vein may be safely ligated and divided to facilitate aortic exposure if the lumbar and adrenal tributaries are maintained for collateral circulation
   (e) initial aortic control at the diaphragm safely facilitates infrarenal vascular control in a patient with injured aortic branch vessels or ruptured aortic aneurysm

5. Patients with celiac and superior mesenteric artery occlusive disease would be expected to have (true or false)
   (a) a large central anastomotic artery
   (b) retrograde filling of the superior mesenteric artery
   (c) a large marginal artery of Drummond
   (d) a low incidence of left colon ischemia following inferior mesenteric artery ligation

6. Renal artery reconstruction
   (a) may be performed via a left or right retroperitoneal approach
   (b) may be difficult in the obese or previously operated patient if an anterior transabdominal approach is used
   (c) is facilitated in the high-risk patient using splenic artery-to-left renal artery bypass or hepatic artery-to-right renal artery bypass
   (d) is more difficult with regard to exposure and revascularization of the right renal artery due to its retro-vena cava position
   (e) all of the above

7. Regarding carotid artery exposure (true or false)
   (a) the distal internal carotid artery is crossed posteriorly by the hypoglossal nerve (XII)
   (b) the vagus nerve (X) passes posterolateral to the carotid bifurcation
   (c) distal exposure is safely facilitated by anterior dislocation of the mandible
   (d) distal exposure may be facilitated by division of the posterior belly of the digastric muscle and the stylohyoid muscle
   (e) anteriorly the distal internal carotid artery is covered by the parotid gland

8. Regarding trauma to the great vessels (true or false)
   (a) exposure of the proximal left subclavian artery is best accomplished via sternotomy
   (b) temporary right third interspace thoracotomy may be used to control exigent hemorrhage from the innominate artery
   (c) right subclavian exposure via a simple supraclavicular incision is adequate for most traumatic injuries in this area
   (d) exposure of either common carotid artery origin is best accomplished via a sternal splitting incision extended along the anterior border of the appropriate sternocleidomastoid muscle

9. Exposure of the infrapopliteal arteries involves the following anatomic relationships (true or false)
   (a) the anterior tibial artery passes posterior to the interosseous membrane
   (b) lateral exposure of the peroneal artery requires segmental fibular resection
   (c) the tibial nerve crosses the posterior tibial artery anteriorly
   (d) the posterior tibial artery lies deep to the transverse crural intermuscular septum

10. The arteria radicularis magna (artery of Adamkiewicz)
    (a) is important in providing circulation to the anterior spinal artery
    (b) may supply up to two thirds of the spinal cord
    (c) appears as a branch of either a distal intercostal or proximal lumbar artery
    (d) is rarely identified via standard arteriography preoperatively
    (e) all of the above

Answers

1. b	2. (a) T	3. (a) F	4. (a) T	5. (a) T	6. e	7. (a) F	8. (a) F	9. (a) F	10. e
	(b) T	(b) T	(b) F	(b) T		(b) T	(b) F	(b) T	
	(c) T	(c) F	(c) T	(c) T		(c) F	(c) F	(c) F	
	(d) T	(d) T	(d) T	(d) F		(d) T	(d) T	(d) F	
	(e) F		(e) T			(e) T			

5

Hemostasis and Thrombosis

Timothy K. Liem and Donald Silver

Most of the bleeding that occurs during surgery or in association with trauma is mechanical and usually can be controlled. Occasionally, bleeding is caused or accelerated by congenital or acquired defects of the hemostatic mechanisms. The vascular surgeon must understand the hemostatic system sufficiently to either arrest bleeding or restore hemostasis or both, according to the patient's needs.

There is increasing evidence that a significant number of acute arterial and venous thrombotic disorders are associated with congenital and acquired hypercoagulable states. The vascular surgeon also should be able to recognize and manage the common thrombophilic states and should be able to restore arterial and venous blood flow not only by mechanical means but also by pharmacologic means.

HEMOSTASIS

Hemostasis is the process by which bleeding from injured tissue is controlled. Although hemostasis is a dynamic process, it can be divided into four components: vessel response to injury, platelet activation and aggregation, activation of coagulation with clot stabilization, and mobilization of the fibrinolytic pathway. Each component has numerous modulatory mechanisms that are also described.

Components of Hemostasis

Vessel Response

When a vessel is injured, the interaction of humoral, neurogenic, and myogenic events leads to temporary vasoconstriction in the muscular arteries and arterioles. Mechanisms for vasoconstriction remain poorly understood, but they may include the release of thromboxane A_2 (TXA_2) by activated platelets, endothelin by endothelial cells, bradykinin, and fibrinopeptide B. Vasoconstriction has less of a role in obtaining hemostasis in veins and venules.

In normal vessels, endothelial cells cover the luminal surface, forming a monolayer with tight cell-cell interaction. The endothelium weighs approximately 1.5 to 2.0 kg and has a volume equal to that of the liver.[1] Once regarded as a passive barrier between the blood and the underlying thrombogenic subendothelium, the endothelium is now recognized as a biologically active organ that participates in and modulates various physiologic processes, including hemostasis and thrombosis.

In their quiescent state, endothelial cells are actively antithrombotic (Table 5–1). They synthesize and secrete *prostacyclin* (PGI_2) and *nitric oxide* (NO), potent vasodilators and inhibitors of platelet aggregation. *Heparan sulfates* are heparin-like mucopolysaccharides that are synthesized and expressed by macrovascular and microvascular endothelial cells. They accelerate the activity of antithrombin III (AT III), thereby inactivating thrombin and several other serine protease coagulation factors. *Thrombomodulin* (TM), a glycoprotein expressed on the endothelial surface of all organs with the exception of the brain, also inactivates thrombin.[2] The thrombomodulin-thrombin complex in turn is a potent activator of protein C.[3] *Protein S* is a cofactor

TABLE 5–1

The Endothelial Cell as Modulator of Hemostasis

THROMBOGENIC FUNCTION	EFFECT
Loss of NO° and PGI_2 after injury	Loss of vasodilating stimulus
von Willebrand factor synthesis	↑ Platelet adhesion
Factor V synthesis	↑ Thrombin
Expression of tissue factor	↑ Thrombin
Binds factors VIIa and IXa	↑ Thrombin
Surface membrane site for prothrombinase complex	↑ Thrombin
Plasminogen activator inhibitor synthesis	↑ Thrombin
ANTITHROMBOTIC FUNCTION	
NO and PGI_2 synthesis	Vasodilating stimulus
PGI_2 synthesis and granule release	↓ Platelet aggregation
Thrombomodulin synthesis	↓ Factors Va and VIIIa
Protein S synthesis	↓ Factors Va and VIIIa
Heparin sulfates synthesis	↓ Thrombin
Tissue-type plasminogen activator (t-PA) and urokinase synthesis	↓ Plasmin
Tissue factor pathway inhibitor	↓ Factors IXa and Xa

°NO, nitric oxide; PGI_2, prostacyclin.

for activated protein C and is synthesized by both endothelial cells and the liver.[4, 5] *Activated protein C* inactivates factor Va and factor VIIIa. These factors greatly accelerate the conversions of prothrombin (II) to thrombin (IIa) and factor X to Xa. *Tissue factor pathway inhibitor* (TFPI) is a potent inhibitor of the external coagulation pathway. TFPI is expressed by megakaryocytes and capillary endothelium, and the majority is bound to the endothelial surface.[6, 7] It is released in response to heparin administration and binds to the factor VIIa/tissue factor/Xa complex, inhibiting the further conversion of factor X to Xa and factor IX to IXa. The endothelium also synthesizes *tissue-type plasminogen activator* (t-PA) and *urokinase*. Both are serine proteases that bind to fibrinogen and remain bound to fibrin. These proteases convert plasminogen to plasmin, the enzyme responsible for fibrinolysis.

The endothelium possesses substantial procoagulant activity and acts as a template for hemostasis when stimulated after vessel injury (see Table 5–1). *Tissue factor* (thromboplastin, factor III) is a low molecular weight lipoprotein that is constitutively expressed by most cells, including vascular adventitia, central nervous tissue, lung, and placental tissue. It is also expressed in the epithelium of the skin, mucosa, bronchus, and glomeruli. Endothelial cells and blood cells do not express tissue factor on their surfaces unless stimulated by agonists such as interleukin 1 (IL-1), thrombin, or endotoxin. Vessel injury causes endothelial denudation and activation, which result in exposure of blood to tissue factor. Low circulating levels of activated factor VII (VIIa) bind to tissue factor via a calcium ion-dependent interaction that is enhanced by the presence of factor X. This complex catalyzes the conversion of factor IX to IXa and factor X to Xa, leading to thrombin formation.

Endothelial cells and megakaryocytes synthesize and secrete *von Willebrand factor* (vWf), which is necessary for platelet adhesion to the vessel wall. vWf has binding sites for collagen, platelet glycoproteins Ib and IIb–IIIa, and factor VIII. vWf and factor VIII circulate together as a complex, although they are the products of two distinct genes. Endothelial cells, in addition to the liver, synthesize *factor V*. Factors V and VIII are cleaved by thrombin into their activated states (Va and VIIIa), and then become integral components of the membrane-bound prothrombinase and tenase complexes, respectively (mostly on the platelet surface but also on the endothelium).[8, 9] The prothrombinase and tenase complexes accelerate the formation of thrombin (IIa) and factor Xa (Fig. 5–1). Endothelial cells also synthesize a *plasminogen activator inhibitor* (PAI-1), which rapidly inactivates circulating t-PA. When the plasminogen activator becomes incorporated within a thrombus or hemostatic plug, it is more slowly inactivated by PAI-1.

Platelet Activities

Platelets are small, discoid-shaped, anuclear cells with an average circulatory life span of 8 to 12 days. There are

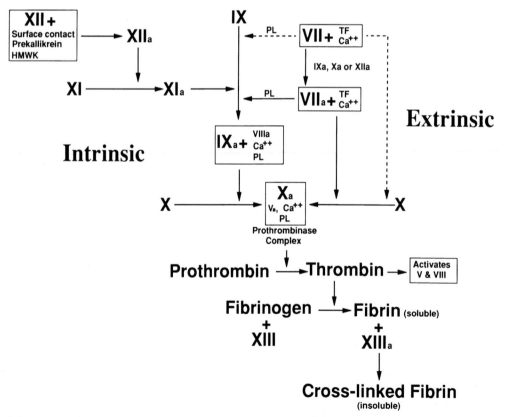

Figure 5–1. The intrinsic and extrinsic pathways of coagulation. The intrinsic pathway is initiated by surface contact, the extrinsic pathway is initiated by the release of tissue factor (TF) from tissues injured during surgery or trauma. Factor VIIa possesses an activity 100 times greater than that of factor VII. The pathways are interrelated and operate in tandem to achieve hemostasis. *PL,* phospholipid from activated platelet or endothelial membranes.

usually 200,000 to 400,000 platelets/mm³ in human blood. Platelets are released as cytoplasmic fragments of mega-karyocytes within bone marrow.

The platelet surface membrane is composed of a phospholipid bilayer, glycoproteins, and proteins. Carbohydrate moieties of the glycoproteins make up the outer layer, known as the glycocalyx, with which circulating proteins interact. Surface receptors are known to exist for thrombin, adenosine diphosphate (ADP), epinephrine, TXA₂, fibrinogen, collagen, platelet activating factor, serotonin, vasopressin, vitronectin, fibronectin, laminin, vWf, and the Fc receptor, FcγRIIA.[10] The intercellular adhesion receptors P-selectin, platelet endothelial cell adhesion molecule-1 (PECAM-1), and intercellular adhesion molecule-2 (ICAM-2) most likely mediate the recognition and attachment to monocytes, neutrophils, and leukocytes.[11, 12]

Platelets contain three types of storage granules: (1) amine storage or *dense* granules, which contain serotonin, ADP, adenosine triphosphate (ATP), and calcium; (2) protein storage or *alpha* granules, which contain coagulation proteins (high-molecular-weight kininogen [HMWK], fibrinogen, fibronectin, factor V, vWf, platelet factor 4), growth factors (PDGF, TGF-α, TGF-β), and adhesion proteins (fibronectin, thrombospondin, P-selectin); and (3) *lysosomes*, which contain numerous proteases, glycosidases, and acid hydrolases.

The initial stage of hemostasis, consisting of vasoconstriction and platelet plug formation, is termed "primary hemostasis." After vascular injury, platelets adhere within seconds to the subendothelial matrix (via binding to exposed collagen fibrils, vWf, thrombospondin, fibronectin, and laminin). Collagen binds to the platelet via the glycoprotein (GP) Ia–IIa complex and GP IV, whereas, vWf binds primarily to the platelet GP Ib-IX-V complex and to a lesser degree, the GP IIb–IIIa complex. Collagen-induced platelet activation results in loss of the discoid shape and release of prothrombotic alpha and dense granule contents. Shape change occurs when attachments between actin filaments and the cell membrane are severed. Subsequent actin elongation results in the formation of filopods and lamellipodia that allow more efficient platelet-platelet interaction. The granule release reaction further amplifies platelet activation and aggregation via vWf, fibronectin, ADP, serotonin, and the release of fibrinogen, factor V, and platelet factor 4.

Platelet activation is associated with numerous downstream signals that include protein kinase C activation, generation of inositol trisphosphate (IP₃), intracellular calcium mobilization (via phospholipase-C), and generation of arachidonic acid (via phospholipase-A₂). Arachidonic acid (AA) is converted by cyclooxygenase-1 (prostaglandin H synthase-1) to the prostaglandin endoperoxides PGG₂ and PGH₂. PGG₂ is then converted to TXA₂ by thromboxane synthetase. TXA₂, PGG₂, and PGH₂ stimulate further aggregation and platelet granule release.[13]

The concomitant generation of thrombin via the coagulation cascade and the release of ADP from platelet-dense granules further amplify platelet activation and aggregation. Regardless of the agonist, the final common pathway for platelet aggregation involves a conformational change in the GP IIb–IIIa complex, with the reversible exposure of binding sites for fibrinogen. Circulating fibrinogen and

fibrinogen released from alpha granules form bridges between adjacent platelets.[14]

Numerous medications inhibit platelet function at several steps in the activation and aggregation pathway. Aspirin irreversibly inhibits platelet cyclooxygenase-1, inhibiting thromboxane-mediated platelet aggregation for the life of the platelet. Ticlopidine and clopidogrel inhibit ADP-mediated platelet activation and aggregation.[15, 16] Novel GP IIb–IIIa inhibitors prevent platelet aggregation by blocking the binding of fibrinogen.[17]

Platelets are dynamically involved in the coagulation cascade. Procoagulant phospholipids (platelet factor 3) are exposed on the platelet membrane after stimulation by thrombin and collagen. These phospholipids provide a binding site for the prothrombinase complex. Platelets also release factor V from alpha granules. Factor V becomes activated and membrane bound, acting as a receptor for the binding of activated factor X. Additionally, platelets have surface receptors for factors XI, activated XI, and HMWK.

Coagulation Activation

The platelet plug, required for normal hemostasis, deaggregates as its fibrinogen bridges dissociate unless thrombin is generated and fibrin stabilization of the plug occurs (secondary hemostasis). The formation of fibrin requires the interaction of platelet aggregates, endothelial cells, and plasma coagulation proteins.

Thirteen plasma coagulation proteins have been designated by the Roman numerals I through XIII (an "a" follows the Roman numeral when the factor has been activated). Most of these factors are synthesized in the liver. Although factor VIII and vWf circulate together via a tight non-covalent bond, they are the products of two unrelated genes. Recently, the nomenclature regarding factor VIII and vWf was clarified by the International Committee on Thrombosis and Haemostasis. Currently, the factor VIII protein, antigenic level, and functional activities are referred to as VIII, VIII:Ag, and VIII:C, respectively. vWf protein and antigenic levels are referred to as vWf and vWf:Ag.[18] The hepatic synthesis of factors II, VII, IX, and X is vitamin K-dependent. When vitamin K is not available, these factors are synthesized and released, but they are not biologically active.

The sequence of enzymatic events leading to thrombin formation has been termed the "coagulation cascade" (see Fig. 5–1). The intrinsic pathway is activated when plasma is exposed to a negatively charged surface such as subendothelium, collagen, or endotoxin. Factor XII is activated to XIIa by the interaction of HMWK, prekallikrein, and the negatively charged surface. However, the physiologic significance of factor XII activation is unclear because deficiencies in factor XII, HMWK, and prekallikrein are not associated with any clinical bleeding diatheses.

The extrinsic pathway to thrombin production probably is the more physiologic route for the generation of thrombin and fibrin. It is initiated by the exposure of tissue factor (TF), which is constitutively expressed in the vascular adventitia and subendothelium. TF binds to low levels of circulating factor VIIa in the presence of calcium (TF-

VIIa).[19, 20] This complex activates factor X to Xa, and factor IX to IXa.[21] Factor Xa by itself does not generate thrombin efficiently. However, factors Xa and thrombin can activate factor VII to VIIa, factor V to Va, and factor VIII to VIIIa. The latter two active cofactors are critical components of the phospholipid membrane-associated prothrombinase and tenase complexes, respectively (see Fig. 5–1). The prothrombinase (Xa-Va-Ca^{2+}-phospholipid) and tenase (IXa-VIIIa-Ca^{2+}-phospholipid) complexes are 10^5 to 10^6 times more active than their serine protease factors acting independently.[20] The tenase complex is also about 50 times more efficient in activating factor X than TF-VIIa. The vital role for these complexes is clinically evident. Unlike factor XII deficiency, deficiencies of tissue factor and factors V (parahemophilia), VII, VIII (hemophilia A), IX (hemophilia B), X, and XI may be associated with significant bleeding diatheses. The clinical significance of factor XI deficiency indicates that physiologic amplification of the thrombotic process probably requires an additional intrinsic pathway positive feedback that involves activation of factor XI to XIa by thrombin.

Thrombin proteolytically cleaves fibrinopeptides A and B from the fibrinogen molecule. The resulting fibrin monomers polymerize and propagate to form a gel. Thrombin also activates factor XIII to XIIIa in a reaction that is greatly accelerated (greater than 80-fold) by the presence of fibrin.[22] Factor XIIIa covalently cross-links adjacent fibrin monomers, forming a stable clot that is more resistant to lysis by plasmin.

Coagulation Inhibition

Several mechanisms have evolved to control the rate of thrombin and fibrin formation. *Antithrombin III* (AT III) is a serine protease inhibitor that is synthesized in the liver and endothelial cells. AT III inhibits numerous coagulation factors including thrombin (IIa), TF-VIIa, and factors IXa, Xa, XIa, and XIIa, but its most important targets are factors IIa and Xa. AT III activity is enhanced at least 1000-fold whenever it binds to circulating heparin or endothelial-bound heparin-like molecules. After the AT III-heparin complex binds to an activated coagulation factor, the heparin dissociates and continues to act as a catalyst for the formation of other AT III-serine enzyme complexes.

Tissue Factor Pathway Inhibitor

TFPI is a Kunitz-type enzyme inhibitor that is synthesized by the endothelium and megakaryocytes.[23, 24] It binds to the TF-VIIa-Xa complex and inhibits the further conversion of factors X to Xa and IX to IXa.[25] TFPI is constitutively expressed on the endothelium, and it circulates bound to plasma lipoproteins (hence the former name lipoprotein-associated coagulation inhibitor). TFPI activity and antigen levels increase several-fold after the administration of heparin.

Thrombomodulin

TM is a proteoglycan expressed on the surface of most endothelial cells, except within the central nervous system.[2]

TM readily binds to thrombin, causing a conformational change in the substrate binding site. The thrombin molecule is rendered incapable of binding active coagulation factors but is able to bind and activate circulating protein C. TM also accelerates the inactivation of thrombin by AT III.[26, 27] A procoagulant function for TM also has been found: TM accelerates the activation of thrombin-activatable fibrinolysis inhibitor (TAFI) compared with free thrombin alone.[28]

Protein C and Protein S

Protein C and protein S are both synthesized by the liver, but protein S also has been found in endothelium and platelets.[29, 30] Both proteins undergo several post-translational modifications including the γ-carboxylation of glutamine residues via a vitamin K-dependent reaction. Protein S (a nonenzymatic cofactor for protein C) circulates either free or bound to the C4b binding protein. Activated protein C (APC) binds to protein S on the endothelial or platelet surface and cleaves several peptide bonds in factors Va and VIIIa, resulting in the decreased formation of the prothrombinase and tenase complexes.

Heparin Cofactor II

Heparin cofactor II is another specific thrombin inhibitor, which forms a stable 1:1 complex with thrombin. Heparin, heparan-like molecules, and dermatan sulfate accelerate the activity of heparin cofactor II. Unlike AT III, heparin cofactor II cannot inhibit other coagulation factors. The plasma concentration of heparin cofactor II (70 µg/L) is much lower than that of AT III (150 mg/L), and it is unlikely that heparin cofactor II plays a major role in the regulation of hemostasis.

Fibrinolysis

Plasminogen, an inactive precursor that is synthesized in the liver, can be converted to plasmin by several plasminogen activators (PAs). Circulating t-PA (synthesized in the endothelium) does not activate plasminogen efficiently. However, t-PA and plasminogen both have high affinity for fibrin, which acts as a template for accelerated plasminogen activation (greater than 1000-fold).[31, 32] Thus, the primary role for t-PA–activated plasmin is the degradation of fibrin into fibrin degradation products. However, exogenously administered t-PA also may activate plasminogen, which is bound to one of the fibrin degradation byproducts (the DD[E] complex), resulting in the release of free plasmin.[33, 34] This may lead to the limited breakdown of fibrinogen, factor V, and factor VIII, and to a systemic fibrinolytic state.

Three types of urokinase plasminogen activators (u-PA) have been studied. The precursor, *pro-urokinase* (single-chain urokinase plasminogen activator [scu-PA]), has a low level of enzymatic activity and no affinity for fibrin, but it does demonstrate specificity against fibrin-bound plasminogen. This may be caused by a conformational change in the plasminogen, exposing the critical peptide bond and making it more susceptible to activation by scu-PA.[35] scu-PA is readily converted by plasmin or kallikrein to the more active *two-chain urokinase plasminogen activator* (tcu-PA), which has a high-molecular weight and a low-molecular weight form. Commercially produced urokinase is composed primarily of the low-molecular weight variant. tcu-PA activates circulating plasminogen and fibrin-bound plasminogen equally well, resulting in a more pronounced systemic fibrinolysis.[36] u-PA-activated plasmin also performs numerous other functions related to cell migration and remodeling, including the activation of matrix metalloproteinases.[37] Monocytes and endothelial cells express the u-PA receptor, which binds to u-PA and localizes plasmin to the cell surface.

Each step within the plasminogen activation system has a known inhibitor. *Plasminogen activator inhibitor* (PAI)-1 is released by endothelial cells, platelets, and hepatocytes. This inhibitor efficiently inactivates t-PA and tcu-PA, and performs other functions including the inhibition of thrombin and smooth muscle cell migration. PAI-2 is a less potent inhibitor of t-PA and tcu-PA, but its role in physiologic hemostasis remains uncertain. PAI-2 is released into the circulation during pregnancy, indicating a greater role for hemostasis during pregnancy and delivery. Neither PAI-1 nor PAI-2 inhibits prourokinase (scu-PA). α_2-*Antiplasmin* inactivates circulating plasmin more readily than it does fibrin-bound plasmin, thus decreasing overall systemic fibrinolysis. Other less specific proteases that inhibit fibrinolysis are α_1-protease inhibitor and α_2-macroglobulin.

Preoperative Evaluation

A good history and thorough physical examination detect the majority of bleeding disorders preoperatively. Laboratory testing is warranted if a bleeding disorder is present or suspected. Careful questioning should distinguish a congenital bleeding disorder from an acquired one. Determining the pattern of inheritance may further aid in identifying a congenital deficiency. A history of bleeding problems beginning in childhood or at the beginning of menses implies an inherited bleeding disorder. A history of postoperative or spontaneous bleeding in a family member is important because many patients with inherited disorders do not experience serious bleeding until challenged by an operative procedure or trauma. All patients should be asked about bleeding after tooth extraction, minor trauma, circumcision, and other surgical procedures.

An acquired hemostatic disorder should be suspected in adults who bleed during or following surgery or trauma but who have no previous history of bleeding disorders. However, some patients with congenital disorders, such as von Willebrand disease (vWd), may not demonstrate their bleeding diatheses until challenged. Patients with liver disease are at increased risk for developing a coagulopathy during surgery, after trauma, and after massive transfusion. Patients resuscitated with greater than 20 mL/kg of hetastarch in 24 hours are at risk for bleeding from decreased platelet adhesiveness and deficiencies in coagulation proteins. Patients receiving more than 1.5 mg/kg of dextran in 24 hours are also at increased risk for bleeding as a result

of impaired platelet function and reduced plasma concentration of vWf. A detailed history of drug use is also important because many drugs alter platelet function and predispose patients to bleeding complications.

Physical examination should include a thorough inspection for ecchymoses, petechiae, purpura, hemangiomas, jaundice, hematomas, and hemarthroses. Petechiae, ecchymoses, and mucocutaneous bleeding (epistaxis, gastrointestinal or genitourinary bleeding, menorrhagia) are more commonly associated with defects in primary hemostasis. Bleeding into deep tissues (hemarthroses, muscle, and retroperitoneal hematomas) tends to occur with defects in coagulation. Splenomegaly may be associated with thrombocytopenia. Signs of hepatic insufficiency should be noted because these patients may have decreased production of coagulation proteins. Patients suffering from myeloproliferative disorders, some malignant neoplasms, collagen disorders, or renal insufficiency are at increased risk for bleeding complications.

The "screening" laboratory tests include platelet count and examination of peripheral blood smear; bleeding time; and prothrombin time (PT), activated partial thromboplastin time (aPTT), and thrombin time. The bleeding time, a very sensitive test for hemostasis, is prolonged with qualitative platelet deficiencies as well as with decreased levels of fibrinogen and factors V and vWF. The PT assesses the extrinsic pathway and is prolonged by deficiencies of prothrombin, fibrinogen, and factors V, VII, and X. The aPTT is prolonged by deficiencies of factors in the intrinsic pathway, including VIII, IX, XI, and XII. To a lesser extent, aPTT detects factor deficiencies in the common pathway: V, X, prothrombin, and fibrinogen. The aPTT is also prolonged by heparin. The lupus anticoagulant prolongs phospholipid-dependent coagulation reactions in vitro: PT, aPTT, and dilute Russell's viper venom time. However, it does not cause clinical bleeding. The thrombin time is prolonged by hypofibrinogenemia, fibrin abnormalities, and heparin.

Platelet Disorders

Hemorrhagic complications may occur because of quantitative or qualitative platelet disorders that are acquired or congenital in origin. Thrombocytopenia and qualitative platelet defects are among the most common causes of bleeding in surgical patients. Spontaneous bleeding may occur when platelet counts fall below 20,000/mm³. Platelet counts between 30,000 and 50,000/mm³ are adequate to assure hemostasis provided that there are no associated functional platelet or coagulation disorders. Platelet counts of 50,000 to 100,000/mm³ are required to restore hemostasis during bleeding.

Thrombocytopenia

Thrombocytopenia may occur from increased platelet destruction, abnormal production, dilution, or temporary sequestration (usually in the spleen). Increased destruction may occur via nonimmune versus immune mechanisms. Nonimmune-mediated thrombocytopenia occurs in hemolytic-uremic syndrome (HUS), thrombotic thrombocytopenic purpura (TTP), disseminated intravascular coagulation (DIC), and some vasculitides. In these syndromes, platelets are stimulated to aggregate within the microcirculation, often affecting the brain, kidneys, heart, lungs, and adrenal glands.[38] Early plasmapheresis and plasma transfusion (platelet-poor fresh frozen plasma [FFP], cryoprecipitate-poor plasma), along with high-dose glucocorticoid administration, can reverse most cases of TTP.[39, 40] Platelet transfusions should be used only for intracerebral or other life-threatening hemorrhagic complications. The treatment for HUS varies considerably, but may include hemodialysis, heparin therapy, and plasma exchange, depending on the duration and severity of the illness. GP IIb–IIIa inhibitors may become a useful adjunct in HUS.[41]

Immune-mediated platelet destruction may occur with certain collagen vascular diseases (lupus erythematosus), immune thrombocytopenic purpura (ITP), and lymphoproliferative disorders (chronic lymphocytic leukemia, non-Hodgkin's lymphoma), or it may be drug induced. Acute ITP is a postinfectious thrombocytopenia, which occurs predominantly in children, and is usually self-limited. Chronic ITP is idiopathic and results when autoimmune antibodies are generated against the platelet membrane. Initial therapy for chronic ITP consists of corticosteroids (prednisone, methylprednisolone) followed by splenectomy in nonresponders. Severely thrombocytopenic patients with major hemorrhagic complications and patients requiring urgent surgery can be treated with platelet transfusions, intravenous gamma globulin (IV IgG), and plasmapheresis.

Some drugs may induce thrombocytopenia via the formation of antigen-antibody complexes on the platelet surface, increasing platelet destruction (quinidine, quinine, sulfonamides, penicillins, valproic acid, heparin). In general, discontinuation of the drug reverses the thrombocytopenia within 2 to 5 days. Adjuvant therapy for active bleeding may include corticosteroids, platelet transfusions, and, in some cases, IV IgG. Heparin-induced thrombocytopenia is a prothrombotic condition that is discussed further under Thrombosis.

Impaired platelet production may be caused by aplastic anemia, megakaryocytic aplasia, radiation, myelosuppressive drugs, viral infections, vitamin B_{12} and folate deficiencies, and several other drugs (ethanol, estrogens, interferon, thiazides). Thrombocytopenia also has been described in association with numerous congenital disorders (Fanconi's aplastic anemia, sex-linked recessive thrombocytopenia, Alport's syndrome).

Thrombocytopenia commonly occurs after massive transfusions of banked blood. Only 10% of platelets remain viable in blood held in cold storage for longer than 24 hours. In general, the replacement of one blood volume decreases the platelet count by one third to one half.[42] Despite this, abnormal bleeding is uncommon, and the routine administration of platelets following massive transfusion is not warranted unless hemorrhage is ongoing.[43] Hypothermia (temperature lower than 32°C) also may cause thrombocytopenia, the mechanism of which remains unclear. However, sequestration of platelets during hypothermia is well documented. Platelets appear to activate, release alpha granule products, aggregate, and sequester in the portal circulation. Rewarming may cause a significant portion to return to the circulation. Cold-induced coagulopathy is best prevented by transfusing warmed blood products and maintaining the core body temperature above 32°C.

The centrifugation of one unit of whole blood yields 8 to 10×10^{10} platelets. Approximately 4 to 8 units of whole blood are required to yield enough platelets for administration in the average adult. Current apheresis techniques can yield between 2.5 to 10×10^{11} platelets from a single donor (over 1–2 hours). One unit of single donor platelets usually increases the platelet count by 10,000/mm^3/m^2 body surface area.

Qualitative Disorders of Platelet Function

Qualitative platelet disorders should be suspected when bleeding occurs in patients with normal coagulation studies and platelet counts. Qualitative disorders may be congenital or acquired; acquired disorders are much more common. Disturbances of platelet adherence and aggregation rarely cause bleeding spontaneously but certainly exacerbate bleeding secondary to surgery and trauma. Congenital qualitative disorders of platelet function include vWd, Bernard-Soulier syndrome, Glanzmann's thrombasthenia, storage pool diseases, and diseases of platelet activation.

von Willebrand disease (vWd) is the most common inherited bleeding disorder, characterized by a deficiency or defect in vWf. vWd has been classified into 6 subtypes (1, 2A, 2B, 2M, 2N, 3), with type 1 being the most common (70%).[44] Type 1 vWd is usually transmitted as an autosomal dominant trait with incomplete penetrance. In general, patients manifest epistaxis, ecchymoses, menorrhagia, and post-traumatic/postsurgical bleeding. Decreased platelet adherence causes prolongation of the bleeding time. The aPTT also may be elevated because most patients with vWd have concomitant decreases in their factor VIII coagulation activity (VIII:C). Ristocetin agglutination of platelets is impaired but can be corrected with the addition of vWf-rich cryoprecipitate.

Treatment of vWd may consist of replacement (cryoprecipitate, purified factor VIII concentrates, platelet transfusions) versus nonreplacement therapy (vasopressin, antifibrinolytic agents). Approximately 80% of patients with type 1 vWd respond to deamino (-D-arginine) vasopressin (DDAVP) with increased vWf:Ag and VIII:C (within 60 minutes), which may last for 4 to 6 hours. Unfortunately, response to therapy cannot be predicted without trial administration. Repeated administration of DDAVP (every 12 hours) may be required in patients with type 1 vWd who undergo surgical procedures. Most type 2 and type 3 patients do not respond to DDAVP. Antifibrinolytic agents (ϵ-aminocaproic acid, tranexamic acid) have been used for the treatment of mucocutaneous bleeding and for prophylaxis during oral surgical procedures.[45] Patients who are unresponsive to DDAVP may require replacement therapy during the perioperative period. Until recently, cryoprecipitate (rich in vWf, factors VIII and XIII, and fibronectin) was the treatment of choice. More recently, some purified factor VIII concentrates (which contain large quantities of multimeric vWf) and a newly formulated vWf concentrate have been used successfully.[46] There are no clear guidelines regarding the amount and frequency of administration; replacement therapy is largely empiric. The bleeding time and factor VIII levels are used to monitor response to replacement therapy.

Bernard-Soulier syndrome is transmitted as an autosomal recessive trait and is characterized by a deficiency in the GP Ib-IX-V complex (primary binding site for vWf). These patients have prolonged bleeding times (>20 min), mild to moderate thrombocytopenia, and absent ristocetin-induced platelet agglutination. Heterozygous patients have one half the normal amount of GP Ib-IX-V, but demonstrate normal platelet responses. Platelet transfusions are the mainstay of therapy, but they are limited by the development of antibodies to human leukocyte antigens (HLAs) (alloimmunization) and to the GP Ib-IX-V complex. The use of HLA cross-matched and leukocyte-depleted platelets should minimize alloimmunization. Other unproved therapies may include DDAVP and corticosteroids.

Glanzmann's thrombasthenia is a rare autosomal recessive trait in which platelet membranes lack GP IIb–IIIa receptors, leading to failure of platelet aggregation regardless of the initial stimulus. These patients have normal platelet counts, markedly prolonged bleeding times, deficient clot retraction, and normal ristocetin-induced agglutination. Patients who are heterozygous exhibit normal platelet aggregation responses. As with Bernard-Soulier syndrome, platelet transfusions are the primary form of therapy. Again, the use of HLA cross-matched and leukocyte-depleted platelets is optimal.

Storage pool diseases are a group of rare hereditary disorders characterized by deficiencies in platelet granules or their contents or both. These include deficiencies in α-granule contents (Gray platelet syndrome), δ-granule storage diseases (Wiskott-Aldrich syndrome, Hermansky-Pudlak syndrome, Chediak-Higashi syndrome), and αδ-granule storage disease.[47] Cryoprecipitate and platelet transfusions may be used in the perioperative period. DDAVP also has been used to decrease the requirement for transfusions.

Acquired qualitative platelet abnormalities may be caused by certain drugs, uremia, cirrhosis, myeloproliferative disorders, and dysproteinemias. Aspirin irreversibly acetylates platelet cyclooxygenase-1, inhibiting thromboxane- and endoperoxide-mediated platelet activation for the life of the platelet. The effect of aspirin on the bleeding time is variable and may depend largely on the technique used to perform the test.[48, 49] Nonsteroidal anti-inflammatory drugs (indomethacin, phenylbutazone, ibuprofen) reversibly inhibit cyclooxygenase. Numerous antibiotics including some β-lactams, cephalosporins, and nitrofurantoin impair platelet aggregation and prolong the bleeding time. Mechanisms may include inhibition of agonist binding to the membrane receptor and inhibition of intracellular signal transduction. Platelet GP IIb–IIIa inhibitors (abciximab, eptifibatide, tirofiban) block the binding of fibrinogen to the GP IIb–IIIa receptor and effectively prevent platelet aggregation in a dose-dependent fashion. Correction of bleeding may be accomplished with platelet transfusions.

Uremia causes defective platelet adherence and aggregation, resulting in a prolonged bleeding time. Clinical manifestations may include petechiae, ecchymoses, and mucocutaneous bleeding. The pathophysiology remains unclear but may involve impaired thromboxane and calcium metabolism and/or defective platelet-subendothelial adhesion (via vWf). DDAVP has been shown to shorten bleeding times preoperatively in uremic patients.[50] DDAVP, 0.3 to 0.4 μg/kg IV over 15 to 30 minutes, improves the bleeding time in most patients within 1 hour. Hemodialysis, peritoneal dialysis, and infusions of cryoprecipitate and conjugated estrogens also have been used with some success.[51]

Coagulation factor deficiencies, DIC, dysfibrinogenemias, impaired thrombopoiesis, platelet sequestration, and impaired platelet aggregation all contribute to the hemostatic defects that are associated with liver failure. Therapy is nonspecific but may include DDAVP and platelet transfusions for severe thrombocytopenia.

Coagulation Disorders

Congenital Disorders

Congenital disorders of coagulation usually involve a single factor. Preoperative transfusion of the appropriate factor is necessary and may be required during surgery and postoperatively. Deficiencies of factor XII, HMWK, and prekallikrein cause prolongation of the aPTT but do not cause significant bleeding diatheses. Deficiencies of the remaining factors may result in serious bleeding after surgery or trauma.

Hemophilia A (factor VIII deficiency) is the most common of the inherited coagulation defects, with a prevalence of 1:10,000 males. *Hemophilia B* (Christmas disease, factor IX deficiency) has a prevalence of approximately 1:50,000 males. Both are X-linked recessive disorders that are clinically indistinguishable. The severity of these disorders depends on the levels of factor VIII or IX that are present. Severely affected individuals (factor levels <1%) during infancy or early childhood manifest spontaneous hemarthroses and deep tissue hematomas. Patients with mild to moderate hemophilia (factor levels >5%) may develop hemorrhagic complications only after surgery or trauma.

Patients with hemophilia A who require major surgery should receive factor VIII replacement to achieve 100% of normal activity just before the procedure. Each unit infused per kilogram of body weight increases the factor VIII level by approximately 0.02 U/mL (normal activity is 1 U/mL).[52] Levels should be monitored postoperatively and replacement therapy should be repeated every 12 hours to maintain at least 50% of normal activity until all wounds are healed.[53] Factor VIII levels may be restored using donor-directed cryoprecipitate, virus-inactivated factor VIII concentrate, or recombinant factor VIII. DDAVP (increases factor VIII levels) and ε-aminocaproic acid may be used as adjunctive therapies in patients with mild hemophilia to reduce or avoid the need for replacement therapy during oral or minor surgical procedures.

Patients with hemophilia B should have at least 50% of normal activity before major surgery, and for the first 7 to 10 days postoperatively. Factor IX may be replaced with prothrombin complex concentrates (containing factors II, VII, IX, and X), purified factor IX, or recombinant factor IX. Replacement therapy may be limited by several factors. Prothrombin complexes are associated with the development of arterial or venous thromboses in some patients. In addition, therapy with recombinant factor IX may not achieve as much activity when compared with purified factor IX. This may be due to the need for post-translational modifications (γ-carboxylation) that are not present in recombinant factor IX. In addition, replacement therapy for hemophilia A and B is complicated by the development of inhibitors to factors VIII and IX in approximately 15% of patients. Alternative strategies include the use of high-dose factor VIII, recombinant factor VIIa, and attempts to induce immune tolerance.

Rare coagulation factor deficiencies of factors II, V, VII, and X occur with a prevalence of 1:500,000 to 1:1,000,000. They are usually transmitted with an autosomal recessive pattern. The most severe complications occur with deficiencies of factors II and X.[54] In general, only low levels of factor activity are required for normal hemostasis (10% to 20% of normal). Replacement therapy for factors II and X may be accomplished with FFP or factor concentrates. Factor IX concentrates contain significant amounts of factors II and X and may be used for their replacement. The short half-life of factor VII requires a more frequent replacement schedule using factor VII concentrates. Recombinant factor VIIa also may be used for factor VII deficiencies. Factor V deficiencies may be treated with FFP because factor V concentrates are not yet commercially available.

Abnormalities of fibrinogen and fibrinolysis are also heritable abnormalities. Afibrinogenemia is a very rare disorder that is transmitted as an autosomal recessive trait; hypofibrinogenemia may occur in heterozygous individuals. Clinical manifestations include gastrointestinal and mucous membrane bleeding, hemarthroses, intracranial hemorrhage, and recurrent fetal loss. The PT and aPTT, which are markedly prolonged, usually correct when mixed with normal plasma. Replacement therapy with cryoprecipitate is usually reserved for active bleeding, for the perioperative period, and for prophylaxis during pregnancy. The level of fibrinogen necessary for hemostasis ranges between 50 and 100 mg/dL. Each unit of cryoprecipitate usually increases the fibrinogen level by approximately 10 mg/dL.[55]

Dysfibrinogenemias are a heterogenous group of disorders that may cause defective fibrin formation, polymerization, cross-linkage, or impaired fibrinolysis. Patients may manifest mild to moderate bleeding diatheses (30%) or recurrent thromboses (20%).[56] The PT and aPTT usually are prolonged. Functional assays for fibrinogen are abnormal, whereas antigenic assays are normal. Cryoprecipitate is indicated for hemorrhage but contraindicated for acute thrombotic episodes.

Congenital hyperfibrinolytic states may result in delayed bleeding. The congenital hyperfibrinolytic states include heterozygous and homozygous α$_2$-antiplasmin deficiencies and functionally abnormal or deficient PAI-1.[57] The whole blood clot lysis time and the euglobulin clot lysis time are characteristically shortened. Antifibrinolytic agents (ε-aminocaproic acid or tranexamic acid) are recommended for the management of active bleeding.[58]

Acquired Disorders

Patients develop acquired coagulation disorders because of deficiencies of coagulation proteins, synthesis of nonfunctioning factors, and consumption or inadequate replacement of coagulation proteins.

Hepatic insufficiency may cause decreased plasma levels of several coagulation factors (including factors II, V, VII, IX, X, XIII, and fibrinogen) because of a decreased synthetic capacity, defective post-translational modification (γ-carboxylation), and increased breakdown of activated factors (because of subclinical DIC). Thrombocytopenia also may occur because of increased splenic sequestration. However, levels of factor VIII and vWf may be elevated because they are synthesized in extrahepatic locations. Correction of the coagulation factor deficits and the thrombocytopenia is accomplished with FFP and platelet transfusions, respectively. Vitamin K administration alone does not completely reverse the coagulopathy.

Vitamin K deficiency may cause a bleeding diathesis as a result of the synthesis of nonfunctional forms of the vitamin K-dependent coagulation factors II, VII, IX, and X. Normal sources of vitamin K include dietary intake (green leafy vegetables, soybean oil) and vitamin K synthesis by normal intestinal flora. Vitamin K deficiency may be caused by poor dietary intake, decreased intestinal absorption of vitamin K, decreased production by the gut flora, and liver failure. This situation more commonly arises in patients receiving antibiotic bowel preparations or long-term parenteral nutrition (without vitamin K supplementation). Vitamin K deficiency also occurs in patients who have a prolonged recovery after intestinal surgery and in those with intrinsic bowel diseases (Crohn's disease, celiac sprue, ulcerative colitis) as well as in patients with obstructive jaundice. Vitamin K should be administered preoperatively to patients with hepatic insufficiency, obstructive jaundice, malabsorption states, or malnutrition. Patients with an intact enterohepatic circulation can receive vitamin K orally (2.5 to 5 mg), with normalization of the PT within 24 to 48 hours. Slow IV administration should be used in patients with biliary obstruction or malabsorption. Patients who require urgent correction of the PT should receive slow IV vitamin K and replacement therapy (FFP or prothrombin concentrates).

DIC is characterized by the systemic generation of fibrin, often resulting in the thrombosis of small and medium-sized blood vessels. The consumption of clotting factors and platelets also results in impaired coagulation and hemorrhagic complications. DIC is mediated by several cytokines (including tumor necrosis factor-alpha [TNF-α] and IL-6), which result in the systemic generation of TF, thrombin, and fibrin.[59] Fibrinolytic activity, which is initially increased via the release of t-PA, becomes depressed in response to elevated PAI-1.[59, 60] DIC may develop in association with bacterial infections (gram-positive and gram-negative infections), trauma, malignancy, obstetrical complications, hemolytic transfusion reactions, giant hemangiomas (Kasabach-Merritt syndrome), and aortic aneurysms. A compensated DIC (present in more than 80% of patients who undergo major surgery), in which coagulation factors and platelets are replaced as they are consumed, may be asymptomatic or may appear with ecchymoses and petechiae. Surgery, trauma, hypotension, or transfusion reactions may exacerbate the coagulopathy and hypofibrinolysis, leading to excessive bleeding and intravascular thrombosis.

A combination of laboratory tests may help to confirm the clinical diagnosis of DIC. These include detection of thrombocytopenia or a rapidly decreasing platelet count, prolongation of the PT and aPTT, and the presence of fibrin degradation products (D-dimer assay, latex agglutination for FDP). Extrinsic pathway coagulation proteins (factors II, V, VII, and X) and physiologic coagulation inhibitors (AT III, protein C) usually are depressed, whereas vWf and factor VIII levels may be increased.[61] The fibrinogen level is variably affected by DIC.

The first goal of management is the elimination of the cause of the DIC. When this is possible, the intravascular coagulation ceases with the return of normal hemostasis. In severe DIC, with ongoing blood loss, patients are best managed by replacement of deficient blood elements using FFP(up to 6 units per 24 hours) and platelets while the precipitating cause of the DIC is eliminated.[59] Administration of AT III and protein C concentrates may retard the consumption of coagulation factors, although this remains to be proved. Some trials have demonstrated a benefit with the administration of heparin or low molecular weight heparin (LMWH).[62, 63] Given that patients with DIC already have a coagulopathy, heparin should be used cautiously (lower dosages of 300 to 500 units/hour IV) with careful clinical observation and laboratory monitoring. Direct thrombin inhibitors (hirudin, recombinant thrombomodulin), activated protein C, and extrinsic pathway inhibitors (recombinant TFPI) are under investigation as well.

THROMBOSIS

In 1856, Virchow suggested that thrombus formation was the result of an interaction between an injured surface, stasis, and the hypercoagulability of blood. One or more components of Virchow's triad can be invoked when determining the etiology of an in vivo thrombosis. Hypofibrinolysis is the only major process not recognized by Virchow that contributes to intravascular thrombosis.

Most of the inherited thrombophilic conditions, with the exception of congenital hyperhomocysteinemia, are more closely associated with venous than with arterial thromboembolism. Acquired conditions such as the presence of antiphospholipid antibodies and heparin-associated antibodies have a well-recognized association with both arterial and venous thromboses. The more common inherited and acquired hypercoagulable states are discussed later, as are the indications for testing and the optimal timing for the performance of these assays. The more commonly used antithrombotic agents as well as alternative agents are discussed with regard to the management of established thromboses and prophylaxis against thromboembolism.

Prothrombotic Conditions

Inherited Prothrombotic Conditions

Activated protein C (APC) resistance is most commonly caused by a mutation in the factor V gene, during which Arg506 is replaced with Gln (factor V Leiden), making activated factor V resistant to degradation by APC.[64] It is the most common inherited hypercoagulable condition, occurring in approximately 12% to 33% of patients with venous thromboembolism.[65-68] This is compared with a prevalence of 3% to 6% in control populations.[66-68] The white population is affected more commonly than black, Asian, or Native American populations. Individuals who are heterozygous for the factor V mutation have a 2.7-fold to 7-fold increased risk for venous thromboembolism, whereas homozygous patients may have an 80-fold increased risk.[67, 68] A small percentage of patients with APC resistance do not have the Leiden mutation. Other factor V mutations (factor V Cambridge, factor V HR2 haplotype) also may cause APC resistance.[69, 70]

Functional APC resistance can be detected by performing the aPTT in the presence and absence of purified APC. In general, an aPTT ratio (aPTT with APC/aPTT without APC) of less than 2.0 is considered a positive study (normal 2.4–4.0). Numerous factors may affect the accuracy of the aPTT ratio, including protein C deficiency, the presence of anticoagulants, and antiphospholipid antibodies. Modifications to this functional assay have improved its sensitivity and specificity.[71] DNA testing using the polymerase chain reaction to amplify the factor V Leiden mutation has already become standardized. The optimal management of patients with APC resistance remains to be defined. APC-resistant individuals in high-risk situations (e.g., pregnancy, surgery) should receive thrombosis prophylaxis. Those patients with prior thrombotic episodes may benefit from long-term warfarin therapy. This is especially true for patients with multiple prior episodes, thromboses in unusual locations, and multiple inherited thrombophilic mutations.

Prothrombin 20210A is a mutation (G to A substitution) in the prothrombin gene at nucleotide 20210, resulting in increased levels of plasma prothrombin.[72] The prothrombin 20210A mutation is present in 18% of selected patients with strong family histories of venous thromboembolism, 6.2% of unselected patients with a first episode of thrombosis, and 2.3% of healthy controls. The prevalence is even higher in southern European whites.[73] A significant number of patients have more than one congenital thrombophilic condition, further increasing their risk for venous thromboembolism.[72, 74]

AT III deficiency was the first reported congenital thrombophilic condition.[75] It is transmitted with an autosomal dominant pattern and has a prevalence of 1:5000 in the population.[76] AT III deficiency has been detected in approximately 1% of patients with venous thromboses, conferring a risk which may be as high as 50-fold.[77, 78] The lifetime risk for developing a thrombotic episode ranges between 17% and 50%.[79] Although thromboembolism may occur spontaneously, usually it is associated with a precipitating event such as surgery, trauma, or pregnancy. Arterial thromboses, although less common than venous thromboses, also occur. AT III levels may be reduced to less than 80% of normal in other conditions, including hepatic insufficiency, DIC, acute venous thrombosis, sepsis, nephrotic syndrome, and in patients receiving heparin or estrogen supplementation.

The mainstay of therapy in AT III-deficient patients with venous thromboembolism is still heparin anticoagulation, although supranormal dosages may be required.[80] AT III concentrates may be appropriate in patients who do not achieve adequate anticoagulation with heparin alone. The minimum level of AT III necessary to prevent thrombosis is unknown; however, it is suggested that levels be adjusted to greater than 80% of normal activity. Antithrombin may be replaced with AT III concentrate (1 U/kg increases the AT III activity by 1% to 2%), or alternatively, FFP. Asymptomatic patients should receive thrombosis prophylaxis during high-risk situations such as prolonged immobilization, surgery, or pregnancy. However, long-term warfarin therapy is usually reserved for AT III-deficient patients who have experienced thrombotic events.

Protein C and protein S deficiencies include a number of disorders. Congenital protein C deficiency may be transmitted as an autosomal dominant or recessive trait and has a prevalence of 1:200 to 1:500.[81, 82] The incidence of thrombosis varies, depending on the population in question. Studies identifying protein C deficiency in healthy blood donors demonstrate a low prevalence of venous thrombosis, whereas studies that screen patients with venous thromboembolism find a higher prevalence of protein C deficiency compared with controls.[77, 81–83] Overall, inherited protein C deficiency is associated with approximately a 7-fold increased risk for developing a first venous thromboembolic event.[83] Common sites for venous thromboses include the lower extremities, mesenteric veins, and cerebral venous sinuses. Functional and immunologic assays are available to establish the diagnosis of protein C deficiency. Normal adults have protein C antigen levels ranging from 70% to 140% of normal. Patients with antigen levels less than 55% are likely to have heterozygous protein C deficiency.

Approximately 60% of the total protein S circulates bound to C4b complement-binding protein.[84] Deficiency states may occur with decreased total protein S, decreased free protein S, and decreased functional protein S activity (with total and free protein S concentrations in the normal range). Histories of patients with congenital protein S deficiencies are very similar to those of patients with protein C deficiency, although arterial thromboses also have been described in patients with protein S deficiency. Protein S may be measured with functional assays, assessing the ability to catalyze the inhibition of factor Va by APC, or immunologic assays.

Both protein C and protein S are vitamin K-dependent proteins synthesized in the liver. Consequently, plasma levels may be decreased in patients with hepatic insufficiency. Acquired protein C and protein S deficiencies also may occur with warfarin administration, vitamin K deficiency (malabsorption, biliary obstruction), sepsis, DIC, acute thromboses, and in patients receiving some chemotherapeutic medications. Because C4b also is an acute-phase reactant, inflammatory conditions may increase C4b levels, causing a decrease in free protein S and an increased tendency toward thrombosis.[85]

Heparin is the first line of therapy in the management of acute thromboembolic episodes in patients with known protein C and S deficiencies. Because warfarin-induced skin necrosis is more likely to occur in patients with protein C deficiency, heparin therapy should overlap with the first 4 or 5 days of warfarin therapy, and large loading dosages of warfarin should be avoided. Longer term treatment with warfarin is effective in the prevention of recurrent venous thromboembolic episodes in patients with protein C and protein S deficiencies. FFP occasionally may be required to restore functional levels of protein C and protein S.

Abnormalities of fibrinogen and fibrinolysis include dysfibrinogenemias, which may impair any of the steps involved in the generation and cross-linkage of fibrin. They have been reported in association with bleeding diatheses (30%) as well as with venous thromboembolism (20%). Therapeutic alternatives have been described earlier.

Elevated factor XI is a mild risk factor for the development of venous thrombosis.[86] Factor XI levels in the 90th percentile or greater confer a 2.2-fold relative risk for the development of venous thrombosis. Even lower factor XI levels demonstrate a linear dose-response relationship with thrombotic risk. The underlying cause for elevated factor XI levels remains to be determined.

Acquired Prothrombotic Conditions

Many clinical disorders predispose to thrombosis by activating the coagulation system or causing platelet aggregation. Soft tissue trauma, thermal injuries, and operative dissection all predispose to thrombosis through release of tissue factor and activation of the extrinsic coagulation pathway.

Sepsis predisposes to thrombosis via multiple mechanisms. Gram-positive bacteria may directly cause platelet aggregation and subsequent thrombosis. Gram-negative bacterial endotoxin may stimulate platelet aggregation but may also, through interaction with leukocytes and endothelial cells, cause tissue factor-like activation of the coagulation system. Endotoxin is known to be a major stimulus for the development of DIC.

As many as 11% of patients with malignancies have venous thromboembolic complications.[87] Pancreatic, prostate, gastrointestinal, and lung cancers have a particularly strong association with thrombosis. Conversely, patients with idiopathic venous thromboembolism also are more likely to be diagnosed with cancer (up to 7.6%).[88] Aggressive screening for occult malignancies in patients with venous thromboembolism has not yet been shown to be cost-effective or to result in improved long-term survival.

Pregnancy and oral contraceptive usage are associated with a fourfold increased risk for venous thromboembolism.[78, 89, 90] The risk may be three to five times greater in the immediate postpartum period. Even very low dosages of estrogen (as used in hormonal replacement) are associated with a twofold to fourfold increased risk for thrombosis.[91, 92] Although the exact mechanism is unclear, these women demonstrate increased levels of thrombin and fibrinogen, with decreased levels of protein S and plasminogen activators.

Antiphospholipid antibodies (APA), including lupus anticoagulants (LA) and anticardiolipin antibodies (ACA), are IgG, IgM, or IgA immunoglobulins, which are directed against phospholipid-binding proteins (prothrombin and β_2-GP I). These antibodies interfere with in vitro phospholipid-dependent clotting assays, such as aPTT, kaolin clotting time (KCT), and the dilute Russell viper venom time tests. In vivo, antiphospholipid antibodies may promote thrombosis by interfering with the activation of protein C.[93]

The presence of APA is associated with a 9-fold increased risk for venous thrombosis. Clinical manifestations of the antiphospholipid syndrome may include venous and arterial thromboses (coronary, cerebral) and recurrent fetal loss. LA also is associated with arterial thrombosis. As many as 50% of LA-positive patients who undergo vascular surgical procedures develop a thrombotic complication.[94] Patients with thrombotic episodes should receive heparin and warfarin anticoagulation. Long-term warfarin therapy (at higher intensity, International Normalized Ratio [INR] >3) has been shown to reduce the recurrence of thrombosis.[95] Warfarin may be discontinued when the IgM and/or IgG immunoglobulins are no longer detectable.

Heparin-associated antibodies (HAAbs) and heparin-induced thrombocytopenia (HIT) are important considerations for patients receiving anticoagulation therapy. Heparin-associated antibodies (HAAb), IgG and IgM, target the heparin-platelet factor 4 complex. These immune complexes bind to the Fcγ-RII platelet receptor, causing pathophysiologic platelet activation, aggregation, and thrombocytopenia. The incidence of HAAb formation varies widely, depending on the indications for heparin, the type of heparin that is used, and the tests used to detect HAAbs. LMWHs are associated with a significantly decreased incidence of HAAb formation and HIT.[96] Up to 20% of patients who undergo vascular surgical procedures develop HAAbs, which are associated with a greater than twofold increased risk for thrombotic complications.[97] The incidence of HIT ranges between 2% and 9%, depending on the type of heparin that is used, the route of administration, and the definition of thrombocytopenia that is used.[98, 99] Most authors use a platelet count of less than 100,000/mm³ to define HIT-associated thrombocytopenia. However, thrombocytopenia is not a prerequisite for the development of thrombotic complications.

The diagnosis of HIT may be made according to the following criteria:

1. The development of thrombocytopenia or a significantly decreased platelet count while receiving heparin
2. Resolution of thrombocytopenia after cessation of heparin
3. Exclusion of other causes for thrombocytopenia
4. A positive HAAb assay (2-point platelet aggregation assay, serotonin release assay, enzyme-linked immunosorbent assay)

Patients who develop HIT or thrombosis in the setting of a positive HAAb assay should discontinue heparin immediately. Most patients require continued anticoagulation with alternative agents such as recombinant hirudin and danaparoid. Long-term antithrombotic therapy with warfarin remains effective.

Hyperhomocysteinemia may be caused by inborn errors of metabolism (cystathionine β-synthase deficiency, methylene tetrahydrofolate reductase variant), or, more commonly, by acquired deficiencies in vitamins B$_6$, B$_{12}$, and folic acid. Elevated homocysteine is an independent risk factor for myocardial infarction, stroke, and peripheral arterial atherothrombosis.[100] It is also an independent risk factor for venous thrombosis, with an odds ratio of approximately 2 to 2.5.[101–103] The risk may be much higher in patients with combined hyperhomocysteinemia and other thrombophilic conditions.[104, 105] Homocysteinemia may be detected using fasting plasma levels or after methionine loading (100 mg/kg). Elevated homocysteine levels may be effectively reduced with folate, vitamin B$_6$, and B$_{12}$ supplementation.[106] Whether vitamin supplementation and correction of hyperhomocysteinemia are protective against venous thromboses remains to be determined.

Surgery and trauma are very strong risk factors for the development of venous thrombosis. Venous thromboembolism occurs in up to 25% of patients undergoing general surgical procedures without thrombosis prophylaxis. Orthopedic procedures (hip and knee replacement, hip fracture repair) are associated with an even greater risk for venous thromboembolism (45% to 61%). The incidence of venous thromboembolism in trauma patients depends on the severity of injury. Multisystem trauma is associated with a greater than 50% incidence.[107]

Myeloproliferative diseases (polycythemia vera, chronic myelogenous leukemia, myeloid metaplasia, essential thrombocytosis), hypergammaglobulinemia, and hyperfibrinogenemia may predispose to thrombosis by causing a hyperviscous state. At clinical presentation, patients manifest cerebral (arterial and venous), coronary, pulmonary, and peripheral arterial and venous thromboemboli. HUS and TTP cause microvascular thromboses and thrombocytopenia.

Indications and Timing for Thrombophilia Screening

Before 1993, inherited prothrombotic conditions were detected in less than 10% to 15% of patients with venous thromboembolism. Since the discovery of factor V Leiden and the prothrombin 20210A mutation, the number of patients with detectable thrombophilia has increased significantly. Patients who develop venous thromboembolism at a young age, patients with recurrent thrombosis, and those with a positive family history or thromboses in unusual locations are candidates for screening. Patients who develop warfarin-induced skin necrosis also have a significant chance of having protein C deficiency. Patients with suspected thrombophilia should be screened for APC resistance, prothrombin 20210A mutation, APA, hyperhomocysteinemia, HAAbs, and deficiencies of AT III, protein C, and protein S. Patients with arterial thrombosis who require screening for thrombophilia should be tested for APA (including LA and ACA), HAAbs, and hyperhomocysteinemia.

Because acute thrombosis may be associated with transient depletion of AT III, protein C, and protein S, screening should not be performed during this period. Heparin and warfarin therapy also interfere with screening tests for APC resistance, whereas warfarin decreases functional and antigenic levels of protein C and protein S. Accurate screening is most easily accomplished approximately 2 to 3 weeks after the patient has discontinued warfarin therapy. If the risk of recurrent thromboembolism is deemed too great to discontinue warfarin, the patient may be converted to subcutaneous heparin or LMWH during this 2- to 3-week period. Protein C and S levels should not be affected by heparin administration. Testing for the presence of

HAAbs should be performed after heparin has been discontinued, because false-negative results may be obtained for up to 72 hours.

Management of Established Thrombosis

Unfractionated heparin, warfarin, and aspirin are the most commonly used antithrombotic agents. Several newer drugs recently have been made available by the Food and Drug Administration for limited indications. These include danaparoid, recombinant hirudin, ticlopidine, clopidogrel, and several GP IIb–IIIa receptor antagonists. Although numerous other agents are in development or in clinical trials (recombinant TFPI, GP Ib inhibitors, other factor IIA and Xa inhibitors), they are not discussed in this chapter.

Unfractionated and Low Molecular Weight Heparins

Unfractionated bovine lung and porcine intestinal heparin have been the mainstay of therapy for episodes of acute arterial (coronary, cerebral, peripheral arterial) and venous (deep venous) thromboses for the past several decades. Unfractionated heparins (UH) are glycosaminoglycans composed of repetitive disaccharide units (uronic acid and glucosamine) with molecular weights ranging from 4000 to 40,000 daltons. LMWHs are derived from the enzymatic or alkaline degradation of UH purified from porcine intestinal mucosa. The average molecular weight of the various preparations ranges from 3000 to 6000 Da.[108]

UH and LMWH bind to AT III via a specific pentasaccharide sequence that is present in only 30% of molecules. This exposes an active site for the neutralization of numerous activated coagulation factors. Factor Xa is inactivated via this mechanism. In contrast, factor IIa (thrombin) inactivation requires the formation of a ternary complex in which thrombin and AT III bind to heparin molecules with at least 18 to 20 saccharide units. Only 25% to 50% of LMWH molecules contain this critical length, thus reducing their anti-IIa activity while maintaining anti-Xa activity. UH and LMWH also cause a twofold to 6-fold increase in TFPI, via release from the endothelial surface. TFPI forms a complex with factors VIIa, Xa, and TF, inhibiting the conversion of factor IX to IXa and factor X to Xa.

UH binds to numerous plasma proteins (platelet factor 4, vitronectin, and fibronectin), platelet glycoprotein receptors, and vascular endothelium. This may be responsible for the variable bioavailability and anticoagulant response. Heparin is cleared via the reticuloendothelial cells (saturable) and kidneys (nonsaturable), resulting in a dose-dependent half-life that ranges from 45 to 150 minutes. LMWHs demonstrate less binding to plasma proteins and endothelium, resulting in a greater bioavailability and a more predictable therapeutic response. As a result, weight-adjusted dosages may be administered without therapeutic monitoring. LMWHs are cleared primarily via the kidneys, with plasma half lives that are twofold to fourfold longer than that of UH.

UH may be administered as an IV bolus of 80 to 100 U/kg, followed by an infusion of 15 to 18 U/kg/hour. The aPTT is monitored every 6 hours until the dosage and therapeutic response have stabilized. The therapeutic range of 1.5 to 2.5 times control varies from one laboratory to another and should be standardized by protamine titration. Platelet counts should be monitored on a regular basis to allow the early detection of HIT. LMWHs are rapidly absorbed after subcutaneous (SC) injection. The dosage varies according to the commercial preparation used. Some preparations with longer half lives require only once-a-day dosing.

Heparinoids

Danaparoid (Organon Inc., West Orange, New Jersey) is the most widely tested heparinoid. It is composed of heparan sulfate (83%), dermatan sulfate (12%), and chondroitin sulfate (5%). Like LMWH, danaparoid is derived from animal intestinal mucosa. It has a mean molecular weight of 6000 Da. The heparan sulfate component of danaparoid binds to AT III via the specific pentasaccharide sequence, with preferential inactivation of factor Xa. The dermatan sulfate component of danaparoid also has slight anti-IXa activity through a mechanism involving heparin cofactor II. Rapid anticoagulation may be achieved with an IV bolus of 2250 to 2500 U (adjustment for weight may be required) followed by a continuous infusion with a stepwise decreasing rate (400 U/hr for 2–4 hr, then 300 U/hr for 2–4 hr, then 150–200 U/hr).[109]

Danaparoid has been used successfully as an alternative antithrombotic agent in patients with HIT. However, danaparoid carries a 10% to 20% rate of cross-reactivity with antiheparin antibodies.[109, 110] Before using danaparoid in HIT-positive patients, cross-reactivity testing should be performed. Centers that do not routinely test for cross-reactions against danaparoid may use alternative antithrombotic agents such as recombinant hirudin.

Hirudin and Direct Thrombin Inhibitors

Hirudin is a 65 amino acid polypeptide derived from the salivary gland of the medicinal leech (*Hirudo medicinalis*). Recombinant hirudin (lepirudin, Hoechst Marion Roussel Inc., Kansas City, Missouri) is more widely available and has similar pharmacologic properties. Hirudin forms a stoichiometric complex with thrombin blocking the catalytic site, substrate groove, and anion binding site, preventing the formation of fibrin, and factors Va, VIIIa, and XIIIa.[111] Hirudin also inhibits thrombin-induced platelet activation and aggregation. Lepirudin is initiated with an IV bolus of 0.4 mg/kg, followed by a continuous infusion of 0.15 mg/kg/hr. Therapy may be monitored using the aPTT (therapeutic range 1.5–2.5 times reference) or a more recently developed assay, the ecarin clotting time.[112] After an initial distribution phase, hirudin follows first-order elimination kinetics. It is excreted via the kidneys and has a half-life ranging from 1 to 2 hours. Patients with renal insufficiency or failure and patients weighing more than 110 kg require significant dosage adjustments.

Lepirudin has been used successfully as an alternative anticoagulant in patients with HIT.[113] However, the rate of adverse events still remains significant (up to 30%), probably reflecting the severity of illness in HIT patients. Numerous clinical trials also have compared hirudin with heparin in the treatment of patients undergoing coronary angioplasty and coronary thrombolysis, and patients with unstable angina. Hirudin was associated with a decreased risk for ischemic events compared with heparin therapy. Some trials also demonstrated an increased incidence of major hemorrhage, although this complication usually occurred when hirudin was given in conjunction with thrombolytic agents. As with heparin, hirudin has the potential to cause an immunologic reaction. Approximately 40% of patients develop detectable antihirudin antibodies. Unlike heparin antibodies, however, these are not associated with the development of any resistance to therapy nor with thromboembolic or bleeding complications.[114]

Warfarin

Coumarin derivatives, including warfarin, block the vitamin K-dependent γ-carboxylation of glutamine residues on factors II, VII, IX, and X, and proteins C and S. This results in the production of vitamin K-dependent proteins, which have a decreased number of Gla residues and decreased enzymatic activity. A reduction in the number of Gla residues from the usual 10 to 13 to 6 decreases the coagulation factor biologic activity by more than 95%. An antithrombotic state depends on the replacement of functional coagulation factors present in the circulation with the altered coagulation proteins. Factor VII and protein C have the shortest half lives—approximately 6 hours each. Factor II and factor X have longer half lives of approximately 72 and 36 hours, respectively. Although warfarin may prolong the prothrombin time within 24 hours owing to factor VII depletion, an antithrombotic state is not usually attained for 2 to 4 days.

Warfarin is rapidly absorbed and reaches a maximum plasma concentration within 2 to 12 hours. Ninety-seven percent of warfarin circulates bound to albumin, with the unbound portion responsible for the anticoagulant effect. The amount of warfarin required to cause a prolongation of the prothrombin time depends on the amount of dietary vitamin K, the age of the patient, and comorbid conditions (liver failure, obstructive jaundice, starvation). Numerous medications also have been found to potentiate or interfere with the activity of warfarin (Table 5–2). Patients on long-term oral anticoagulation who begin or stop a medication that may interfere with or potentiate warfarin activity should be monitored with more frequent prothrombin time measurements.

Warfarin therapy is initiated by the oral intake of 5 to 7.5 mg once a day. Reduced dosages should be given to elderly patients and patients with liver disease or those with vitamin K deficiency as a result of malnutrition or long-term parenteral feeding. Because factor II and factor X depletion may not be effective for 2 to 4 days, heparin or an alternative agent should be administered during the first few days of warfarin therapy for patients in whom immediate anticoagulation is necessary. The PT assay is

TABLE 5 – 2

Common Drug Interactions with Oral Anticoagulants*†

POTENTIATE	ANTAGONIZE
acetaminophen	barbiturates
anabolic steroids	carbamazepine
cephalosporins	chlordiazepoxide
chloral hydrate	cholestyramine
cimetidine	dicloxacillin
ciprofloxacin	griseofulvin
clofibrate	nafcillin
cotrimoxazole	rifampin
disulfiram	sucralfate
erythromycin	vitamin K
fluconazole	
isoniazid	
itraconazole	
metronidazole	
omeprazole	
phenylbutazone	
phenytoin	
piroxicam	
propafenone	
propoxyphene	
propranolol	
quinidine	
sulfinpyrazone	
tamoxifen	
tetracycline	

*Hirsh J, Dalen JE, Anderson DR, et al: Oral anticoagulants: Mechanism of action, clinical effectiveness, and optimal therapeutic range. Chest 114(Suppl): 445S–469S, 1998.

†Wells PS, Holbrook AM, Crowther NR, et al: The interaction of warfarin with drugs and food: A critical review of the literature. Ann Intern Med 121:676–683, 1994.

most commonly used to monitor warfarin therapy. This test is sensitive to changes in activity of factors II, VII, IX, and X. The PT assay is performed by adding thromboplastin and calcium to citrated plasma. Thromboplastins vary according to their ability to activate the external coagulation cascade and are graded by the International Sensitivity Index (ISI). The INR attempts to standardize PT assays, which use different thromboplastins, according to the following equation:

$$INR = [\text{patient prothrombin time (sec)}/\text{population prothrombin time (sec)}]^{ISI}$$

PT should be monitored on a daily basis for the first 4 to 5 days of warfarin therapy. The INR usually achieves the desired range during this period. A longer period of daily monitoring is required in patients resistant to warfarin. Once the therapeutic range is attained, the PT can be monitored 2 to 3 times per week and, when stable, every 4 to 6 weeks. Many patients are receiving heparin at the time that warfarin is initiated. Concomitant administration of heparin prolongs the PT. This is due to the inactivation of factors IIa, IXa, and Xa by AT III. It should be expected that the PT will decrease when heparin is discontinued. The effect of heparin on the PT can be reduced by removing the heparin from the test plasma or by stopping the heparin infusion 4 to 6 hours before obtaining blood for the PT.

The primary complication of warfarin therapy is hemorrhage, which occurs in 3% to 12% of patients.[115] Less common complications include alopecia, urticaria, dermatitis, fever, nausea, diarrhea, abdominal cramping, and hypersensitivity reactions. Dermal gangrene is a rare complication (0.01% to 0.1% of patients receiving warfarin) caused by the rapid depletion of protein C before depletion of factors II, IX, and X.[116] This risk increases to approximately 3% in patients with protein C deficiency.[117] Concomitant UH or LMWH administration should decrease the risk of this complication.

Thromboembolism Prophylaxis

Venous Thromboembolism Prophylaxis

The incidence of venous thrombosis and pulmonary embolism may be reduced by either limiting venous stasis or administering drugs to inhibit coagulation, or a combination of both of these approaches. Stasis is reduced by ambulation and pneumatic compression of the lower extremities.

Intermittent pneumatic compression (IPC) devices reduce lower extremity venous stasis, enhance fibrinolytic activity, and increase plasma levels of TFPI.[118] *Elastic stockings* also decrease stasis and increase venous flow velocities. Both devices appear to decrease the incidence of deep venous thrombosis (DVT) in patients who undergo general, urologic, and gynecologic surgical procedures. The incidence of DVT in control patients ranges from 20% to 27%, whereas the use of IPC is associated with DVT incidence of 10% to 18%.[119, 120] IPC devices also decrease the incidence of DVT in patients undergoing hip or knee replacement. However, mechanical prophylaxis alone is probably not sufficient in patients undergoing total hip replacement and should be supplemented with either LMWH or adjusted-dose UH or warfarin.[107] IPC provides effective thrombosis prophylaxis in patients who undergo neurosurgical procedures (6% with IPC, 23% in controls).[121]

The effectiveness of IPC devices is limited by a lack of compliance among patients and nursing staff. Intermittent pneumatic foot compression devices may improve patient acceptance. However, these newer devices are less effective than other forms of DVT prophylaxis, especially in patients undergoing orthopedic procedures.[122]

Subcutaneous heparin is used to decrease incidence of venous thromboembolism, which develops in 19% to 25% of general surgical patients.[107] The incidence is even greater in patients with numerous risk factors (older age, malignancy, inherited thrombophilia, prior venous thromboembolism). Subcutaneous UH (5000 U SC 2 hours preoperatively, followed by 5000 U every 8 to 12 hours postoperatively) decreases the overall incidence of venous thrombosis to approximately 8%.[107] The incidence of pulmonary embolism is reduced as well. This regimen is probably adequate in moderate- and high-risk general surgical patients. Two large meta-analyses have demonstrated that LMWH confers no additional protection in this population and may be associated with an increased risk of hemorrhagic complications.[123, 124]

However, fixed low-dose UH prophylaxis is not as effective in patients with hip fractures or in those undergoing total hip or knee replacement. Orthopedic and very high-risk general surgical patients (those with additional risk factors) should receive more effective DVT prophylaxis (LMWH, adjusted-dose warfarin, adjusted-dose UH, or combination prophylaxis with intermittent pneumatic compression). The aPTT does not require monitoring in patients receiving fixed-dose UH or LMWH prophylaxis. Platelet counts should be monitored for the detection of HIT.

LMWH produces fewer thromboembolic complications than UH. Patients who undergo major orthopedic procedures without DVT prophylaxis are at very high risk for thromboembolic complications (45% to 61%). Depending on the preparation, LMWH decreases the incidence significantly (15% to 31%) compared with fixed-dose UH (27% to 42%).[107, 125] Preoperative initiation of LMWH (vs. beginning in the postoperative period) may decrease the overall incidence of DVT in patients undergoing hip replacement (10% preoperative vs. 15.3% postoperative), without increasing the incidence of hemorrhage.[126] There is also evidence that longer durations of prophylaxis are more effective. Several randomized trials have found a significantly lower rate of thrombosis with 21 to 35 days of LMWH administration.[127–129] The additional use of IPC devices may decrease the incidence even further.

Numerous randomized trials have compared various LMWH preparations (enoxaparin, certoparin, dalteparin, nadroparin, parnaparin, reviparin, tinzaparin) against UH as DVT prophylaxis in general surgical patients. Only 4 out of 29 trials identified a significant improvement with LMWH.[130] Although the dosage regimens varied widely between trials, there was a tendency toward superior prophylaxis with LMWH when higher dosages were used. Very high-risk patients who undergo general surgical procedures (multiple risk factors, malignancy, thrombophilia) may benefit most from LMWH prophylaxis. The optimal timing for the first prophylactic dose of LMWH remains in question. General surgical patients who receive the first dose before surgery do not appear to experience any additional hemorrhagic complications.[131]

Warfarin has been established in several studies as efficacious prophylaxis against venous thromboembolism. Sevitt and Gallagher found that the incidence of clinical venous thrombosis in patients with hip fractures decreased from 28.7% in the control group to 2.7% in the group treated with oral anticoagulation. At autopsy, the incidence of thrombosis in the two groups was 83% and 14%, respectively.[132] In other studies, oral anticoagulants, with an INR range of 2.0 to 3.0, were effective in preventing venous thrombosis in patients undergoing orthopedic and gynecologic surgery.[133, 134] Very high-risk patients, such as those undergoing major orthopedic procedures, should receive either LMWH or adjusted-dose warfarin. LMWH may be more effective than warfarin, but the difference is probably small. If warfarin is selected, it should be started preoperatively or immediately after surgery. The dosage should be adjusted to achieve a target INR between 2.0 and 3.0.[107] With warfarin, the duration of prophylaxis easily may be extended in patients who continue to have risk factors for venous thromboembolism (immobility, malignancy, a history of previous venous thrombosis).

Arterial Thromboembolism Prophylaxis

Arterial thrombosis occurs in regions with disturbed flow or disrupted endothelial coverage (as with plaque rupture or endarterectomy). Subendothelial collagen and vWf initiate platelet adhesion and activation, whereas TF activates the coagulation cascade, leading to the generation of thrombin and fibrin. Arterial thrombi contain relatively higher concentrations of platelets. As a result, most long-term arterial antithrombotic regimens focus on the inhibition of platelet function.

Aspirin acetylates platelet cyclooxygenase-1 (prostaglandin H synthase-1), blocking the conversion of arachidonic acid to the prostaglandin endoperoxides PGH_2 and PGG_2. This effectively inhibits the synthesis of TXA_2 for the lifespan of the platelet. Aspirin also inhibits PGI_2 synthesis by endothelial cells. However, endothelial cells have nuclei and can synthesize new prostacyclin synthetase, reversing the effects of aspirin. Noncoated aspirin is rapidly disintegrated and absorbed in the stomach. Enteric-coated aspirin dissolves in the more neutral to alkaline pH within the duodenum. Enteric coating does not significantly delay the bioavailability compared with noncoated aspirin.

The Antiplatelet Trialists' Collaboration reviewed 145 randomized trials involving approximately 70,000 "high-risk" patients and 28,000 "low-risk" patients.[135] Subsequent vascular events were significantly reduced in patients with (1) acute myocardial infarction, (2) a past history of myocardial infarction, (3) a past history of stroke or transient ischemic attack, and (4) a history of other vascular events including unstable angina, stable angina, vascular surgery, angioplasty, atrial fibrillation, valvular disease, and peripheral vascular disease. High-risk patients who were treated with antiplatelet therapy had a one-third reduction in the rate of nonfatal myocardial infarction, a one-third reduction in nonfatal strokes, and a one-sixth reduction in vascular death. The most widely tested antiplatelet agent was aspirin (75–325 mg/day). This study and others have demonstrated that lower dosages of aspirin (75 mg/day) also are effective in reducing the risks of myocardial infarction and stroke in high-risk patients.[135–138] The total rate of vascular events (including nonfatal myocardial infarction, nonfatal stroke, and vascular death) in low-risk patients was not significantly altered by long-term antiplatelet therapy.[135] Patients who underwent saphenous or prosthetic infrainguinal bypass procedures also were reviewed. Those who received antiplatelet therapy (mostly using aspirin with or without dipyridamole) had a 43% reduction in lower extremity vascular graft or native arterial occlusion.[139]

Ticlopidine and clopidogrel are thienopyridine derivatives that irreversibly inhibit ADP-mediated platelet activation. Intact ticlopidine and clopidogrel have no effect on platelets in vitro, suggesting that their metabolites may be the more potent platelet inhibitors. They are both rapidly absorbed after oral administration and are highly bound to plasma proteins (albumin and lipoproteins). Ticlopidine may alter platelet function within 24 to 48 hours, but maximum inhibition is not achieved for 8 to 11 days. Clopidogrel induces a dose-dependent inhibition of platelet aggregation that is more rapid (within 2 hr).

Ticlopidine significantly improves the patency of femoropopliteal and femorotibial saphenous vein grafts (66% vs.

51% at 2 yr) compared with placebo.[140] Compared with aspirin, ticlopidine also is associated with a decreased risk of stroke (10% versus 13%).[141] Other studies have demonstrated a decreased risk of myocardial infarction in patients with unstable angina and improved walking distance in patients with claudication.[142, 143] However, no studies have demonstrated that ticlopidine is superior to aspirin in improving lower extremity vascular graft patency. In addition, widespread use of ticlopidine is limited by the potentially severe side effects of pancytopenia and neutropenia.

Clopidogrel has been advocated as an antiplatelet agent with an efficacy superior to that of aspirin. The CAPRIE (Clopidogrel versus Aspirin in Patients at Risk of Ischaemic Events) study evaluated more than 19,000 patients with a history of (1) recent ischemic stroke, (2) recent myocardial infarction, or (3) symptomatic atherosclerotic peripheral vascular disease.[144] Clopidogrel was associated with a relative risk reduction of 8.7% for future ischemic events, representing an absolute reduction of only 0.5% (5.32% with clopidogrel, 5.83% with aspirin). Clopidogrel may be more beneficial as a combination therapy agent because aspirin and clopidogrel inhibit platelet function via different signal transduction pathways (TXA_2 and ADP inhibition). Clopidogrel is not associated with neutropenia.

Glycoprotein IIb–IIIa inhibitors have been evaluated for stroke prevention in clinical trials. Fibrinogen binds to the platelet GP IIb–IIIa receptor via the amino acid sequence Arg-Gly-Asp (RGD), representing the final common pathway for platelet aggregation regardless of the platelet agonist. The first GP IIb–IIIa inhibitor to be developed was c7E3 (abciximab), the antigen-binding fragment (Fab) of a monoclonal anti-GP IIb–IIIa antibody. Subsequently, naturally occurring RGD peptides (trigramin, bitistatin) have been isolated from the venom of several species of vipers. Synthetic RGD peptides (eptifibatide, tirofiban, lamifiban) as well as more potent KGD analogues recently have been manufactured and have undergone clinical trials.[17] Most trials have involved patients after coronary angioplasty and patients with unstable angina or myocardial infarctions.[145–147] Thus far, GP IIb–IIIa inhibitors have not played any significant role in the long-term prevention of stroke or complications related to peripheral vascular disease.

The major risk of using GP IIb–IIIa receptor antagonists is bleeding. Abciximab has a very short half-life (range 10–30 min) caused by rapid binding to the platelet GP IIb–IIIa receptor. Significant platelet function inhibition continues for up to 48 hours after infusions are discontinued.[146] Synthetic RGD peptides (eptifibatide, tirofiban) demonstrate more reversible platelet inhibition. The half lives of these agents range from 2 to 2.5 hours, with most of the elimination occurring via the kidneys. Platelet function generally returns to near normal within 4 to 8 hours.

Warfarin has an established role in the prevention of thromboembolism in selected patients with atrial fibrillation and prosthetic heart valves. Other possible indications for long-term warfarin include the prevention of myocardial ischemia and the prevention of systemic embolism after acute myocardial infarction.[148]

Several studies also indicate that warfarin may improve the patency of lower extremity bypass grafts. In a randomized trial involving 130 patients who underwent femoropopliteal vein bypass surgery, Kretschmer and coworkers[149, 150] found an improved patency, limb salvage, and overall survival in patients receiving phenprocoumon (a coumarin derivative). Flinn and colleagues[151] also found that warfarin improved patency in patients with infrageniculate prosthetic grafts. More recent studies involving patients at high risk for failure (suboptimal vein, poor outflow, redo procedures) have confirmed an improved patency

with warfarin plus aspirin compared with aspirin alone.[152] Long-term warfarin therapy is a reasonable option for most patients with prosthetic infrainguinal or axillofemoral bypass grafts, suboptimal venous conduit, or poor outflow tracts (e.g., isolated popliteal arteries). Patients who are treated with warfarin should receive overlapping UH, LMWH, or IV heparin, until the therapeutic INR is achieved (target INR range 2.0–3.0).

References

1. Engelberg H: Endothelium in health and disease. Semin Thromb Hemost 14:1–11, 1988.
2. Ishii H, Salem HH, Bell CE, et al: Thrombomodulin: An endothelial anticoagulant protein is absent from human brain. Blood 67:362–365, 1986.
3. Esmon CT, Owen WG: Identification of an endothelial cell cofactor for thrombin-catalyzed activation of protein C. Proc Natl Acad Sci U S A 78:2249–2252, 1981.
4. Naworth PP, Brett J, Steinberg S, et al: Endothelium and protein S: Synthesis, release and regulation of anticoagulant activity (abstract). Thromb Haemost 58:49, 1987.
5. Stern D, Brett J, Hams K, et al: Participation of endothelial cells in the protein C-protein S anticoagulant pathway: The synthesis and release of protein S. J Cell Biol 102:1971–1978, 1986.
6. Werling RW, Zaccharski LR, Kisiel W, et al: Distribution of tissue factor pathway inhibitor in normal and malignant human tissues. Thromb Haemost 69:366–369, 1993.
7. Osterud B, Bajaj MS, Bajaj SP: Sites of tissue factor pathway inhibitor (TFPI) and tissue factor expression under physiologic and pathologic conditions. Thromb Haemost 73:873–875, 1995.
8. Rodgers GM, Shuman MA: Enhancement of prothrombin activation on platelets by endothelial cells and mechanism of activation of factor V. Thromb Res 45:145–152, 1987.
9. Tracy PB, Eide LL, Mann KG: Human prothrombinase complex assembly and function on isolated peripheral blood and cell populations. J Biol Chem 260:2119–2124, 1985.
10. Bennett JS: The molecular biology of platelet membrane proteins. Semin Hematol 27:186–204, 1990.
11. Kansas GS: Selectins and their ligands: Current concepts and controversies. Blood 88:3259–3287, 1996.
12. Diavco TG, deFougerolles AR, Bainton DF, et al: A functional integrin ligand on the surface of platelets: Intercellular adhesion molecule-2. J Clin Invest 94:1242–1251, 1994.
13. Silver MJ, Smith JB, Ingerman CM, et al: Arachidonic acid-induced human platelet aggregation and prostaglandin formation. Prostaglandins 4:863–875, 1973.
14. Nachman RL, Leung LLK: Complex formation of platelet membrane glycoproteins IIb and IIIa with fibrinogen. J Clin Invest 69:263–269, 1982.
15. Ito MK, Smith AR, Lee ML: Ticlopidine: A new platelet aggregation inhibitor. Clin Pharm 11:603–617, 1992.
16. Herbert JM, Frehel D, Vallee E, et al: Clopidogrel, a novel antiplatelet and antithrombotic agent. Cardiovasc Drug Rev 11:180–198, 1993.
17. Lefkovits J, Plow EF, Topol EJ: Platelet glycoprotein IIb/IIIa receptors in cardiovascular medicine. N Engl J Med 332:1553–1559, 1995.
18. Marder VJ, Mannucci PM, Firkin BG, et al: Standard nomenclature for factor VIII and von Willebrand's factor: A recommendation by the International Committee on Thrombosis and Haemostasis. Thromb Haemost 54:871–872, 1985.
19. Morrissey JH, Macik BG, Neuenschwander PF, Comp PC: Quantitation of activated factor VII levels in plasma using a tissue factor mutant selectively deficient in promoting factor VII activation. Blood 81:734–744, 1993.
20. Mann KG: Biochemistry and physiology of blood coagulation. Thromb Haemost 82:165–174, 1999.
21. Osterud B, Rapaport SI: Activation of factor IX by the reaction product of tissue factor and factor VII: Additional pathway for initiating blood coagulation. Proc Natl Acad Sci U S A 74:5260–5264, 1977.
22. Janus TJ, Lewis SD, Lorand L, et al: Promotion of thrombin-catalyzed activation of factor XIII by fibrinogen. Biochemistry 22:6269–6272, 1983.
23. Bajaj MS, Kuppuswamy MN, Saito H, et al: Cultured normal human hepatocytes do not synthesize lipoprotein-associated coagulation inhibitor: Evidence that endothelium is the principal site of its synthesis. Proc Natl Acad Sci U S A 87:8869–8873, 1990.
24. Novotny WF, Girard TJ, Miletich JP, Broze GJ Jr: Platelets secrete a coagulation inhibitor functionally and antigenically similar to the lipoprotein associated coagulation inhibitor. Blood 72:2020–2025, 1988.
25. Rapaport SI: The extrinsic pathway inhibitor: A regulator of tissue factor-dependent blood coagulation. Thromb Haemost 66: 6–15, 1991.
26. Esmon CT: The regulation of natural anticoagulant mechanisms. Science 235:1348–1352, 1987.
27. Esmon CT: The roles of protein C and thrombomodulin in the regulation of blood coagulation. J Biol Chem 264:4743–4746, 1989.
28. Nesheim M, Wang W, Boffa M, et al: Thrombin, thrombomodulin, and TAFI in the molecular link between coagulation and fibrinolysis. Thromb Haemost 78:386–391, 1997.
29. Fair DS, Marlar RA, Levin EG: Human endothelial cells synthesize protein S. Blood 67:1168–1171, 1986.
30. Schwarz HP, Heeb MJ, Wencel-Drake JD, et al: Identification and quantitation of protein S in human platelets. Blood 66: 1452–1455, 1985.
31. Hoylaerts M, Rijken DC, Lijnen HR, et al: Kinetics of the activation of plasminogen by human tissue plasminogen activator. Role of fibrin. J Biol Chem 257:2912–2919, 1982.
32. Horrevoets AH, Pannekoek H, Nesheim ME: A steady-state template model that describes the kinetics of fibrin-stimulated [Glu1]- and [Lys78]-plasminogen activation by native tissue-type plasminogen activator and variants that lack either the finger or kringle-2 domain. J Biol Chem 272: 2183–2191, 1997.
33. Stewart RJ, Fredenburgh JC, Weitz JI: Characterization of the interactions of plasminogen and tissue and vampire bat plasminogen activators with fibrinogen, fibrin, and the complex D-dimer noncovalently linked to fragment E. J Biol Chem 273:18292–18299, 1998.
34. Olexa SA, Budzynski AZ: Binding phenomena of isolated unique plasmic degradation products of human cross-linked fibrin. J Biol Chem 254:4925–4932, 1979.
35. Gurewich V, Pannell R, Louie S, et al: Effective and fibrin-specific clot lysis by a zymogen precursor form of urokinase (pro-urokinase). A study in vitro and in two animal species. J Clin Invest 73:1731–1739, 1984.
36. Weitz JI, Stewart RJ, Fredenburgh JC: Mechanism of action of plasminogen activators. Thromb Haemost 82:974–982, 1999.
37. Collen D: The plasminogen (fibrinolytic) system. Thromb Haemost 82:259–270, 1999.
38. Moake JL: Studies on the pathophysiology of thrombotic thrombocytopenic purpura. Semin Hematol 34:83–89, 1997.
39. Bell WR, Braine HG, Ness PM, et al: Improved survival in thrombotic thrombocytopenic purpura-hemolytic uremic syndrome. Clinical experience in 108 individuals. N Engl J Med 325:398–403, 1991.
40. Kwaan HC, Soff GA: Management of thrombotic thrombocytopenic purpura and hemolytic uremic syndrome. Semin Hematol 34:159–166, 1997.
41. Taylor FB, Coller BS, Chang AC, et al: 7E3 F(ab')2, a monoclonal antibody to the platelet GP IIb/IIIa receptor, protects against microangiopathic hemolytic anemia and microvascular thrombotic renal

failure in baboons treated with C4b binding protein and a sublethal infusion of *Escherichia coli*. Blood 89:4078–4084, 1997.

42. Murphy S: Platelet transfusion therapy. In Loscalzo J, Shafer AI (eds): Thrombosis and Hemorrhage, 2nd ed. Baltimore, Williams & Wilkins, 1998, pp 1119–1134.

43. Reed RL II, Ciavarella D, Heimbach DM, et al: Prophylactic platelet administration during massive transfusion. A prospective, randomized, double-blind clinical study. Ann Surg 203:40–48, 1986.

44. Sadler JE: A revised classification of von Willebrand disease. For the Sub-committee on von Willebrand Factor of the Scientific and Standardization Committee of the International Society on Thrombosis and Haemostasis. Thromb Haemost 71:520–525, 1994.

45. Logan LJ: Treatment of von Willebrand's disease. Hematol Oncol Clin North Am 6:1079–1094, 1992.

46. Foster PA: A perspective on the use of FVIII concentrates and cryoprecipitate prophylactically in surgery or therapeutically in severe bleeds in individuals with von Willebrand disease unresponsive to DDAVP: Results of an international survey. Thromb Haemost 74:1370–1379, 1995.

47. Nurden AT: Inherited abnormalities of platelets. Thromb Haemost 82:468–480, 1999.

48. Rodgers RP, Levin J: A critical reappraisal of the bleeding time. Semin Thromb Hemost 16:1–20, 1990.

49. Mielke CH Jr: Influence of aspirin and platelets on the bleeding time. Am J Med 74:72–78, 1983.

50. Mannucci PM: Desmopressin (DDAVP) for treatment of disorders of hemostasis. Prog Hemost Thromb 8:19–45, 1986.

51. Shafer AI: Acquired disorders of platelet function. In Loscalzo J, Shafer AI (eds): Thrombosis and Hemorrhage, 2nd ed. Baltimore, Williams & Wilkins, 1998, pp 707–725.

52. Forbes CD: Clinical aspects of the genetic disorders of coagulation. In Ratnoff OD, Forbes CD (eds): Disorders of Hemostasis, 3rd ed. Philadelphia, WB Saunders, 1996, pp 138–185.

53. DiMichele DM, Green D: Hemophilia-factor VIII deficiency. In Loscalzo J, Shafer AI (eds): Thrombosis and Hemorrhage, 2nd ed. Baltimore, Williams & Wilkins, 1998, pp 757–772.

54. Peyvandi F, Mannucci PM: Rare coagulation disorders. Thromb Haemost 82:1207–1214, 1999.

55. Roberts HR, Bingham MD: Other coagulation factor deficiencies. In Loscalzo J, Shafer AI (eds): Thrombosis and Hemorrhage, 2nd ed. Baltimore, Williams & Wilkins, 1998, pp 773–802.

56. Ebert RF: Dysfibrinogenemia: An overview of the field. Thromb Haemost 65:1317, 1991.

57. Schleef RR, Higgins DL, Kellemer E, et al: Bleeding diathesis due to decreased functional activity of type I plasminogen activator inhibitor. J Clin Invest 83:1747–1752, 1989.

58. Stump DS, Fletcher BT, Nesheim ME, et al: Pathologic fibrinolysis as a cause of clinical bleeding. Semin Thromb Hemost 16:260–273, 1990.

59. Levi M, ten Cate H: Disseminated intravascular coagulation. New Engl J Med 341:586–592, 1999.

60. Biemond BJ, Levi M, ten Cate H, et al: Plasminogen activator and plasminogen activator inhibitor I release during experimental endotoxaemia in chimpanzees: Effect of interventions in the cytokine and coagulation cascades. Clin Sci 88:587–594, 1995.

61. Spero JA, Lewis JH, Hasiba U: Disseminated intravascular coagulation. Findings in 346 patients. Thromb Haemost 43:28–33, 1980.

62. Feinstein DI: Treatment of disseminated intravascular coagulation. Semin Thromb Hemost 14:351–362, 1988.

63. Sakuragawa N, Hasegawa H, Maki M, et al: Clinical evaluation of low-molecular-weight heparin (FR-860) on disseminated intravascular coagulation (DIC)—a multicenter co-operative double-blind trial in comparison with heparin. Thromb Res 72: 475–500, 1993.

64. Bertina RM, Loelemann BPC, Koster T, et al: Mutation in blood coagulation factor V associated with resistance to activated protein C. Nature 369:64–67, 1994.

65. Svensson PJ, Dahlbäck B: Resistance to activated protein C as a basis for venous thrombosis. N Engl J Med 330:517–522, 1995.

66. Koster T, Rosendaal FR, de Ronde H, et al: Venous thrombosis due to poor anticoagulant response to activated protein C: Leiden thrombophilia study. Lancet 342:1503–1506, 1993.

67. Rosendaal FR, Koster T, Vandenbroucke JP, Reitsma PH: High risk of thrombosis in patients homozygous for factor V leiden (activated protein C resistance). Blood 85:1504–1508, 1995.

68. Ridker PM, Hennekens CH, Lindpaintner K, et al: Mutation in the gene coding for coagulation factor V and the risk of myocardial infarction, stroke, and venous thrombosis in apparently healthy men. N Engl J Med 332:912–917, 1995.

69. Williamson D, Brown K, Luddington R, et al: Factor V Cambridge: A mutation (Arg306→Thr) associated with resistance to activated protein C. Blood 91:1140–1144, 1998.

70. Bernardi F, Faioni EM, Castoldi E, et al: A factor V genetic component differing from factor V R506Q contributes to activated protein C resistance phenotype. Blood 90:1552–1557, 1997.

71. Le DT, Griffin JH, Greengard HS, et al: Use of a generally applicable tissue factor-dependent factor V assay to detect activated protein C-resistant factor Va in individuals receiving warfarin and in individuals with a lupus anticoagulant. Blood 85:1704–1711, 1995.

72. Poort SR, Rosendaal FR, Reitsma PH, et al: A common genetic variation in the 3′-untranslated region of the prothrombin gene is associated with elevated prothrombin levels and an increase in venous thrombosis. Blood 88:3698–3703, 1996.

73. Rosendaal FR, Doggen CJM, Zivelin A, et al: Geographic distribution of the 20210 G to A prothrombin variant. Thromb Haemost 79:706–708, 1998.

74. De Stefano V, Martinelli I, Mannucci PM, et al: The risk of recurrent deep venous thrombosis among heterozygous carriers of both factor V Leiden and the G20210A prothrombin mutation. New Engl J Med 341:801–806, 1999.

75. Egeberg O: Inherited antithrombin deficiency causing thrombophilia. Thromb Diath Haemorrh 13:516–530, 1965.

76. Tait RC, Walker ID, Perry DJ: Prevalence of antithrombin deficiency in the healthy population. Br J Haematol 87:106–112, 1994.

77. Heijboer H, Brandjes DPM, Büller HR, et al: Deficiencies of coagulation-inhibiting and fibrinolytic proteins in outpatients with deep-vein thrombosis. N Engl J Med 323: 1512–1516, 1990.

78. Rosendaal FR: Risk factors for venous thrombotic disease. Thromb Haemost 82:610–619, 1999.

79. Demers C, Ginsberg JS, Hirsh J, et al: Thrombosis in antithrombin III-deficient persons: Report of a large kindred and literature review. Ann Intern Med 116:754–761, 1992.

80. Schulman S, Tengborn L: Treatment of venous thromboembolism in individuals with congenital deficiency of antithrombin III. Thromb Haemost 68:634–636, 1992.

81. Miletich J, Sherman L, Broze G Jr: Absence of thrombosis in subjects with heterozygous protein C deficiency. N Engl J Med 317:991–996, 1987.

82. Tait RC, Walker ID, Reitsma PH, et al: Prevalence of protein C deficiency in the healthy population. Thromb Haemost 73: 87–93, 1995.

83. Koster T, Rosendaal FR, Briët E, et al: Protein C deficiency in a controlled series of unselected outpatients: An infrequent but clear risk factor for venous thrombosis (Leiden Thrombophilia Study). Blood 85:2756–2761, 1995.

84. Dahlbäck B, Stenflo J: High molecular weight complex in human plasma between vitamin K-dependent protein S and complement component C4b-binding protein. Proc Natl Acad Sci U S A 78:2512–2516, 1981.

85. D'Angelo A, Vigano-D'Angelo S, Esmon CT, Comp PC: Acquired deficiencies of protein S. J Clin Invest 81:1445–1454, 1988.

86. Meijers JCM, Tekelenburg WLH, Bouma BN, et al: High levels of coagulation factor XI as a risk factor for venous thrombosis. N Engl J Med 342:696–701, 2000.

87. Sack GH, Levin J, Bell WR: Trousseau's syndrome and other manifestations of chronic disseminated coagulopathy in individuals with neoplasms: Clinical, pathophysiologic, and therapeutic features. Medicine 56:1–37, 1977.

88. Prandoni P, Lensing AW, Buller HR, et al: Deep-vein thrombosis and the incidence of subsequent cancer. N Engl J Med 327:1128–1133, 1992.

89. World Health Organization: Venous thromboembolic disease and combined oral contraceptives: Results of international multicentre case-control study. World Health Organization Collaborative Study of Cardiovascular Disease and Steroid Hormone Contraception. Lancet 346:1575–1582, 1995.

90. Vandenbroucke JP, Koster T, Briët E, et al: Increased risk of venous thrombosis in oral-contraceptive users who are carriers of factor V Leiden mutation. Lancet 344:1453–1457, 1994.

91. Grodstein F, Stampfer MJ, Goldhaber SZ, et al: Prospective study of exogenous hormones and risk of pulmonary embolism in women. Lancet 348:983–987, 1996.

92. Hulley S, Grady D, Bush T, et al: Randomized trial of estrogen plus progestin for secondary prevention of coronary heart disease in postmenopausal women. Heart and estrogen/progestin replacement study (HERS) research group. JAMA 280:605–613, 1998.

93. Freyssinet JM, Wiesel ML, Gauchy J, et al: An IgM lupus anticoagulant that neutralizes the enhancing effect of phospholipid on purified endothelial thrombomodulin activity—a mechanism for thrombosis. Thromb Haemost 55:309–313, 1986.

94. Ahn SA, Kalunian K, Rosove M, Moore WS: Postoperative thrombotic complications in patients with the lupus anticoagulant: Increased risk after vascular procedures. J Vasc Surg 7:749–756, 1988.

95. Kamashta MA, Cuadrado MJ, Mujic F, et al: The management of thrombosis in the antiphospholipid-antibody syndrome. N Engl J Med 332:993–997, 1995.

96. Warkentin TE, Levine MN, Hirsh J, et al: Heparin-induced thrombocytopenia in patients treated with low-molecular-weight heparin or unfractionated heparin. N Engl J Med 332:1330–1335, 1995.

97. Calaitges JG, Liem TK, Spadone D, et al: The role of heparin-associated antiplatelet antibodies in the outcome of arterial reconstruction. J Vasc Surg 29:779–786, 1999.

98. Schmitt BP, Adelman B: Heparin-associated thrombocytopenia: A critical review and pooled analysis. Am J Med Sci 305:208–221, 1993.

99. Warkentin TE, Kelton JG: Heparin-induced thrombocytopenia. Prog Hemost Thromb 10:1–34, 1991.

100. Guba SC, Fonseca V, Fink LM: Hyperhomocysteinemia and thrombosis. Semin Thromb Hemost 25:291–309, 1999.

101. den Heijer M, Koster T, Blom HJ, et al: Hyperhomocysteinemia as a risk factor for deep-vein thrombosis. N Engl J Med 334:759–762, 1996.

102. Simioni P, Prandoni P, Burlina A, et al: Hyperhomocysteinemia and deep-vein thrombosis: A case-control study. Thromb Haemost 76:883–886, 1996.

103. den Heijer M, Rosendaal FR, Blom HJ, et al: Hyperhomocysteinemia and venous thrombosis: A meta-analysis. Thromb Haemost 80:874–877, 1998.

104. Ridker PM, Hennekens CH, Selhub J, et al: Interrelation of hyperhomocyst(e)inemia, factor V Leiden, and the risk of future venous thromboembolism. Circulation 95:1777–1782, 1997.

105. Mandel H, Brenner B, Berant M, et al: Coexistence of hereditary homocystinuria and factor V Leiden-effect on thrombosis. N Engl J Med 334:763–768, 1996.

106. den Heijer M, Brouwer IA, Bos GMJ, et al: Vitamin supplementation reduces blood homocysteine levels. A controlled trial in patients with venous thrombosis and healthy volunteers. Arterioscler Thromb Vasc Biol 18:356–361, 1998.

107. Clagett GP, Anderson FA, Geerts W, et al: Prevention of venous thromboembolism. Chest 114(Suppl):531S–560S, 1998.

108. Nader HB, Walenga JM, Berkowitz SD, et al: Preclinical differentiation of low molecular weight heparins. Semin Thromb Hemost 25(Suppl 3):63–72, 1999.

109. Magnani HN: Heparin-induced thrombocytopenia (HIT): An overview of 230 patients treated with Orgaran (Org 10172). Thromb Haemost 70:554–561, 1993.

110. Kikta MJ, Keller MP, Humphrey PW, et al: Can low molecular weight heparins and heparinoids be safely given to patients with heparin-induced thrombocytopenia syndrome? Surgery 114: 705–710, 1993.

111. Markwardt F: Hirudin and derivatives as anticoagulant agents. Thromb Haemost 66:141–152, 1991.

112. Pötzsch B, Madlener K, Seelig C, et al: Monitoring of r-hirudin anticoagulation during cardiopulmonary bypass—assessment of the whole blood ecarin clotting time. Thromb Haemost 77:920–925, 1997.

113. Greinacher A, Völper H, Janssens U, et al: Recombinant hirudin (lepirudin) provides safe and effective anticoagulation in patients with the immunologic type of heparin-induced thrombocytopenia: A prospective study. Circulation 99:73–80, 1999.

114. Eichler P, Olbrich K, Pötzsch B, et al: Anti-hirudin antibodies in patients treated with recombinant hirudin for more than five days, a prospective study. Thromb Haemost (Suppl):PS2014, 1997.

115. Liem TK, Silver D: Coumadin: Principles of use. Semin Vasc Surg 9:354–361, 1996.

116. Cole MS, Minifee PK, Wolma FJ: Coumarin necrosis: A review of the literature. Surgery 103:271–277, 1988.

117. Pescatore P, Horellou HM, Conard J, et al: Problems of oral anticoagulation in an adult with homozygous protein C deficiency and late onset of thrombosis. Thromb Haemost 69: 311–315, 1993.

118. Chouhan VD, Comerota AJ, Sun L, et al: Inhibition of tissue factor pathway during intermittent pneumatic compression: A possible mechanism for antithrombotic effect. Arterioscler Thromb Vasc Biol 19:2812–2817, 1999.

119. Colditz GA, Tuden RL, Oster G: Rates of venous thrombosis after general surgery: Combined results of randomized clinical trials. Lancet 2:143–146, 1986.

120. Clagett GP, Reisch JS: Prevention of venous thromboembolism in general surgical patients. Ann Surg 208:227–240, 1988.

121. Agnelli G: Prevention of venous thromboembolism after neurosurgery. Thromb Haemost 82:925–930, 1999.

122. Bounameaux H: Integrating pharmacologic and mechanical prophylaxis of venous thromboembolism. Thromb Haemost 82: 931–937, 1999.

123. Nurmohamed MT, Rosendaal FR, Buller HR, et al: Low-molecular-weight heparin versus standard heparin in general and orthopaedic surgery: A meta-analysis. Lancet 340: 152–155, 1992.

124. Koch A, Bouges S, Ziegler S, et al: Low molecular weight heparin and unfractionated heparin in thrombo-prophylaxis after major surgical intervention: An update of previous meta-analyses. Br J Surg 84:750–759, 1997.

125. Nicolaides AN, Bergqvist D, Hull R, et al: Prevention of venous thromboembolism. International consensus statement. Int Angiol 16:3–38, 1997.

126. Hull RD, Brant RF, Pineo GF, et al: Preoperative vs postoperative initiation of low-molecular-weight heparin prophylaxis against venous thromboembolism in patients undergoing elective hip replacement. Arch Intern Med 159: 137–141, 1999.

127. Bergqvist D, Benoni G, Björgell O, et al: Low-molecular-weight heparin (enoxaparin) as prophylaxis against venous thromboembolism after total hip replacement. N Engl J Med 335:696–700, 1996.

128. Dahl OE, Andreassen G, Aspelin T, et al: Prolonged thromboprophylaxis following hip replacement surgery—results of a double-blind prospective, randomized, placebo-controlled study with dalteparin (Fragmin). Thromb Haemost 77:26–31, 1997.

129. Lassen MR, Borris LC, Anderson BS, et al: Efficacy and safety of prolonged thromboprophylaxis with a low molecular weight heparin (dalteparin) after total hip arthroplasty—the Danish Prolonged Prophylaxis (DaPP) Study. Thromb Res 89: 281–287, 1998.

130. Breddin HK: Low molecular weight heparins in the prevention of deep-vein thrombosis in general surgery. Semin Thromb Hemost 25(Suppl 3):83–89, 1999.

131. Bjerkeset O, Larsen S, Reiertsen O: Evaluation of enoxaparin given before and after operation to prevent venous thromboembolism during digestive surgery: Play-the-winner designed study. World J Surg 27:584–589, 1997.

132. Sevitt S, Gallagher NG: Prevention of venous thrombosis and pulmonary embolism in injured patients. Lancet 2:981–989, 1959.

133. Powers PH, Gent M, Jay RM, et al: A randomized trial of less intense postoperative warfarin or aspirin therapy in the prevention of venous thromboembolism after surgery for fractured hip. Arch Intern Med 149:771–774, 1989.

134. Poller L, McKernan A, Thomson JM, et al: Fixed minidose warfarin: A new approach to prophylaxis against venous thrombosis after major surgery. BMJ 295:1309–1312, 1987.

135. Antiplatelet Trialists' Collaboration: Collaborative overview of randomised trials of antiplatelet therapy-I: Prevention of death, myocardial infarction, and stroke by prolonged antiplatelet therapy in various categories of patients. BMJ 308:81–106, 1994.

136. Lindblad B, Persson NH, Takolander R, et al: Does low-dose acetylsalicylic acid prevent stroke after carotid surgery? A double-blind, placebo-controlled randomized trial. Stroke 24: 1125–1128, 1993.

137. Juul-Moller S, Edvardsson N, Jahnmatz B, et al: Double-blind trial of aspirin in primary prevention of myocardial infarction in patients with stable chronic angina pectoris. Lancet 340:1421–1425, 1992.

138. The SALT Collaborative Group: Swedish Aspirin Low-Dose Trial (SALT) of 75 mg aspirin as secondary prophylaxis after cerebrovascular ischaemic events. Lancet 338:1345–1349, 1991.

139. Antiplatelet Trialists' Collaboration: Collaborative overview of randomised trials of antiplatelet therapy—II: Maintenance of vascular graft or arterial patency by antiplatelet therapy. BMJ 308:159–168, 1994.

140. Becquemin JP: Effect of ticlopidine on the long-term patency of saphenous-vein bypass grafts in the legs. N Engl J Med 337:1726–1731, 1997.

141. Hass WK, Easton JD, Adams HP, et al: A randomized trial comparing ticlopidine hydrochloride with aspirin for the prevention of stroke in high-risk patients. N Engl J Med 321: 501–507, 1989.

142. Balsano F, Rizzon P, Violi F, et al: Antiplatelet treatment with ticlopidine in unstable angina: A controlled multicenter clinical trial. Circulation 82:17–26, 1990.

143. Arcan JC, Blanchard J, Boissel JP, et al: Multicenter double-blind study of ticlopidine in the treatment of intermittent claudication and the prevention of its complications. Angiology 38:802–811, 1988.

144. Caprie Streering Committee: A randomised, blinded, trial of clopidogrel versus aspirin in patients at risk of ischaemic events (CAPRIE). Lancet 348:1329–1339, 1996.

145. Califf RM, and the EPIC Investigators: Use of a monoclonal antibody directed against the platelet glycoprotein IIb/IIIa receptor in high-risk coronary angioplasty. N Engl J Med 330: 956–961, 1994.

146. Simoons ML, de Boer MJ, van den Brand MJ, et al: Randomized trial of a GPIIb/IIIa platelet receptor blocker in refractory unstable angina. Circulation 89:596–603, 1994.

147. Kleiman NS, Ohman EM, Califf RM, et al: Profound inhibition of platelet aggregation with monoclonal antibody 7E3 Fab after thrombolytic therapy. J Am Coll Cardiol 22:381–389, 1993.

148. Hirsh J, Dalen JE, Anderson DR, et al: Oral anticoagulants: Mechanism of action, clinical effectiveness, and optimal therapeutic range. Chest 114(Suppl):445S–469S, 1998.

149. Kretschmer G, Wenzl E, Piza F, et al: The influence of anticoagulation treatment on the probability of function in femoropopliteal vein bypass surgery: Analysis of a clinical series (1970 to 1985) and interim evaluation of a controlled clinical trial. Surgery 102:453–459, 1987.

150. Kretschmer G, Herbst F, Prager M, et al: A decade of oral anticoagulant treatment to maintain autologous vein grafts for femoropopliteal atherosclerosis. Arch Surg 127:1112–1115, 1992.

151. Flinn WR, Rohrer MJ, Yao JST, et al: Improved long-term patency of infragenicular polytetrafluoroethylene grafts. J Vasc Surg 7:685–690, 1988.

152. Sarac TP, Huber TS, Back MR, et al: Warfarin improves the outcome of infrainguinal vein bypass grafting at high risk for failure. J Vasc Surg 28:446–457, 1998.

Questions

1. The following are examples of the procoagulant nature of endothelial cells except:
   (a) expression of tissue factor (thromboplastin)
   (b) expression of thrombomodulin
   (c) synthesis of factor V
   (d) synthesis of von Willebrand factor (vWf)
   (e) synthesis of plasminogen activator inhibitor

2. Which of the following is not true regarding platelet aggregation?
   (a) adenosine diphosphate (ADP) released from dense granules initiates platelet-platelet interaction leading to loose aggregation
   (b) thromboxane A_2 stimulates platelet aggregation and granule release
   (c) von Willebrand factor is essential for normal platelet aggregation
   (d) thrombin can induce platelet aggregation via activation of phospholipase and protein kinase C
   (e) regardless of the stimulant, aggregation involves the reversible expression of fibrinogen receptors on the platelet surface

3. Which of the following is not a vitamin K-dependent coagulation factor?
   (a) factor II
   (b) factor V
   (c) factor VII
   (d) factor IX
   (e) factor X

4. Major regulators of the coagulation cascade include all of the following except:
   (a) antithrombin III
   (b) protein C
   (c) protein S
   (d) tissue factor pathway inhibitor
   (e) heparin cofactor II

5. The extrinsic pathway to thrombin formation is initiated by:
   (a) platelet aggregation and release of dense granule contents
   (b) exposed subendothelial collagen
   (c) tissue factor, a lipoprotein released by injured tissues
   (d) the activation of factor XII
   (e) the combined interaction of HMWK, prekallikrein, and a negatively charged surface

6. All of the following statements regarding von Willebrand disease are true except:
   (a) defects of primary hemostasis commonly cause petechiae and ecchymoses
   (b) hemophilic disorders commonly cause hemarthroses and deep tissue hematomas
   (c) von Willebrand disease is the most common inherited bleeding disorder
   (d) type 1 von Willebrand disease is usually unresponsive to DDAVP
   (e) cryoprecipitate and some factor VIII concentrates are rich in vWf

7. One unit of single donor apheresis platelets will usually raise the platelet count by:
   (a) 1,000 /mm³/m²
   (b) 5,000 /mm³/m²
   (c) 10,000 /mm³/m²
   (d) 20,000 /mm³/m²
   (e) 40,000 /mm³/m²

8. Which of the following statements regarding thrombophilic conditions are true?
   (a) Elevated homocysteine levels are associated with arterial and venous thromboses
   (b) The prothrombin 20210A mutation results in resistance to antithrombin III
   (c) Warfarin is ineffective in patients with antiphospholipid syndrome
   (d) Testing for hypercoagulable conditions should not be performed during warfarin therapy
   (e) Antithrombin concentrates are the mainstay of therapy for antithrombin-deficient patients with venous thromboembolism

9. Following major surgical procedures in patients with hemophilia A, factor VIII:C plasma activity should be at least:
   (a) 5 per cent of normal
   (b) 25 per cent of normal
   (c) 50 per cent of normal
   (d) 75 per cent of normal
   (e) 100 per cent of normal

10. All of the following statements regarding low molecular weight heparin are true except:
    (a) LMWHs demonstrate less binding to plasma proteins and endothelium
    (b) LMWHs preferentially inactivate factor Xa over factor IIa

(c) LMWH thrombosis prophylaxis is superior to unfractionated heparin prophylaxis in orthopedic surgery patients
(d) LMWH is clearly superior to unfractionated heparin for routine general surgical procedures

11. Which of the following statements regarding danaparoid and hirudin are true?
    (a) there is no significant cross-reactivity between danaparoid and heparin in patients with heparin-associated antibodies
    (b) hirudin is a direct thrombin inhibitor, preventing the formation of fibrin
    (c) hirudin therapy does not have to be adjusted in patients with renal failure
    (d) approximately 40% of patients receiving hirudin will develop antibodies, resulting in resistance to further therapy
    (e) danaparoid may be used successfully in most patients with heparin-associated antibodies

Answers

1. b   2. c   3. b   4. e   5. c   6. d   7. c   8. a, d   9. c   10. d
11. b, e

6

Atherosclerosis: Pathology, Pathogenesis, and Medical Management

Ralph G. DePalma

Vascular surgeons continue to encounter complications of atherosclerosis as their most common clinical challenge. Atherosclerosis cannot be considered in this overview as comprehensively as one might wish. However, progress in lesion classification, a better understanding of the disease's pathogenesis, and progress in medical treatment offer important opportunities for a more comprehensive approach to surgical as well as medical therapy.

In developing an understanding of this disease process, one must distinguish prevention from secondary treatment. When active interventions are considered, vascular surgeons understand, perhaps better than many practitioners, the need for a precise approach geared toward particular vascular lesions in specific sites. For example, a stenotic lesion composed of smooth muscle and well-organized collagen, although producing a consistent degree of distal ischemia, is a much "safer" lesion than a plaque containing an unstable core of atheromatous debris beneath a tenuous cap. The location and natural history of individual lesions are familiar to vascular surgeons. The smooth stenosis of an adductor hiatus plaque in the femoral artery is clearly not as threatening as a carotid or coronary plaque with a soft core and friable cap.

Additionally, variations in the patterns and rates of progression of atherosclerosis have been appreciated;[1, 2] these have important clinical implications for treatment. Considering the atherosclerotic process as a single disease leads to serious oversimplification.

Some view atherosclerosis as a polypathogenic process comprising a group of closely related vascular disorders rather than as a single disease.[3, 4] Were multiple risk factors (including dyslipidemias, smoking, diabetes, hypertension and hyperhomocysteinemia) to be considerd as "etiologic" factors, a single disease view would not be logically valid. Nevertheless, this chapter describes the lesions of atherosclerosis as a single entity. Theories of pathogenesis are addressed relative to their usefulness for prediction and control of this disease. Although direct interventions for certain lesions in specific sites are the safest approach in well-defined instances, for example, carotid atheromas, medical therapy is clearly preferable in other situations, for example, stable claudication due to infrainguinal atherosclerosis.

PATHOLOGY

General Concepts

Atheroma is derived from the Greek *athere* meaning porridge or gruel. Sclerosis means induration or hardening. A gruel-like color and consistency and induration or hardening exist to various degrees in different plaques, different disease stages, and different individuals. In 1755, von Haller, as noted by Haimovici and DePalma,[5] first applied the term *atheroma* to a common type of plaque that, on sectioning, exuded a yellow, pultaceous content from its core. Figure 6–1 illustrates a typical fibrous plaque containing a central atheromatous core with a fibrous or fibromuscular cap, macrophage accumulation, and round cell adventitial infiltration. Although a classic definition of atherosclerotic plaque describes the lesion as "a variable combination of changes in the *intima* of arteries consisting of focal accumulation of lipids, complex carbohydrates, blood and blood products, fibrous tissue and calcium deposits,"[6] this description does not encompass adequately the spectrum of atherosclerotic lesions. Advanced plaques invade the media; atheromas at certain stages produce bulging or even enlarged arteries; and round cell infiltration, medial changes, and neovascularization characterize many advanced atherosclerotic lesions. The process involves the entire arterial wall. The descriptions that follow

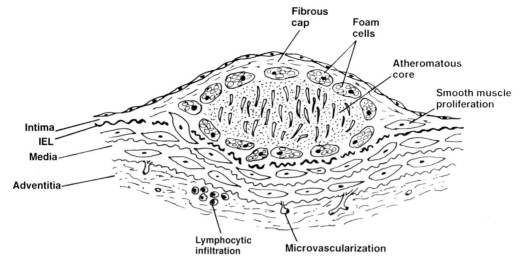

Figure 6–1. Schema of typical atheroma on type IV lesion. Note central lipid core, fibrous cap, macrophage accumulation, and zone of synthetically active smooth muscle at the "shoulders" of the core. Note tendency of the lesion to bulge outward, neovascularization, and adventitial lymphocyte infiltration. *IEL*, internal elastic lamina. (Modified from DePalma RG: Pathology of atheromas. In Bell PRF, Jamieson CW, Ruckley CV [eds]: Surgical Management of Vascular Disease. London, WB Saunders, 1992, pp 21–34.)

consider progressively severe types of plaque, accepted under the rubric of atheromas. Certain lesions, however, might not evolve in the same way.

The development and role of the lipid atherosclerotic core and its relationship to the cap have been recognized as causing plaque complications. An important insight[7] is the finding that the "core" develops early in atherosclerosis, accumulating in the deep aspects of early lesions before actual fibrous plaque formation begins.

Fatty Streaks

Fatty streaks are gross, minimally raised, yellow lesions found frequently in the aorta of infants and children. These lesions contain lipids deposited intracellularly in macrophages and in smooth muscle cells. A recent special report provided by Stary and colleagues[8] defined initial, fatty streaks and intermediate lesions of atherosclerosis as follows: Type I lesions in children are the earliest microscopic lesions, consisting of an increase in intimal macrophages with the appearance of foam cells. Type II lesions are grossly visible; in contrast to type I lesions, type II lesions stain with Sudan III or IV. Fatty streaks are characterized by foam cells and lipid droplets, also in intimal smooth muscle cells, and heterogeneous droplets of extracellular lipids. Type III lesions are considered intermediate lesions; they are usually the bridge between the fatty streak (Fig. 6–2) and the prototypical atheromatous fibrous plaque, the type IV plaque,[9] illustrated in Figure 6–1. Type III lesions occur in plaque expression–prone localities in the arterial tree,[10] that is, sites exposed to forces that cause increased low-density lipoprotein (LDL) influx, particularly low shear stress.[11]

The fatty streak type II lipids are chemically similar to those of the plasma,[12] although the plasma lipids might enter the arterial wall in several ways. The plasma threshold level for LDL entry into the arterial wall is unknown.

As described in a review of pathogenesis,[13] LDL accumulation may occur because of (1) alterations in the permeability of the intima, (2) increases in the interstitial space in the intima, (3) poor metabolism of LDL by vascular cells, (4) impeded transport of LDL from the intima to the media, (5) increased plasma LDL concentrations, or (6) specific binding of LDL to connective tissue components, particularly proteoglycans in the arterial intima. Experimental studies show that LDL cholesterol accumulates in the intima even before lesions develop and in the presence of intact endothelium. These observations are quite similar to those of early lesion formation described by Aschoff[14] early in the 20th century and Virchow[15] in the 19th century.

A second event in early atherogenesis, as shown in animal experiments, is binding of monocytes to the endothelial lining, with their subsequent diapedesis into the subintimal layer to become tissue macrophages.[16–18] Experimentally, fatty streaks are populated mainly by monocyte-derived macrophages. These lipid-engorged scavenger cells mainly become the foam cells that characterize fatty streaks and other lesions. An important observation is that LDL must be altered in some manner,[19] such as by oxidation or acetylation, to be taken up by the macrophages to form foam cells. Oxidized LDL (OxLDL) is a powerful chemoattractant for monocytes. Another aspect of this theory suggests that the endothelium modifies LDL to promote foam cell formation.

The interactions of plasma LDL levels with the arterial wall are the subject of intense interest. LDLs traverse the endothelium mostly through receptor-independent transport, but also through cell breaks.[20] Endothelial cells,[21] smooth cells,[22] and macrophages[23] are all capable of promoting oxidation of LDL. The OxLDL, in turn, further attracts monocytes into the intima and promotes their transformation into macrophages. Macrophages produce cytokines, including platelet-derived growth factor (PDGF), transforming growth factor beta (TGFβ), and interleukin-1 (IL-1). The OxLDL also induces gene prod-

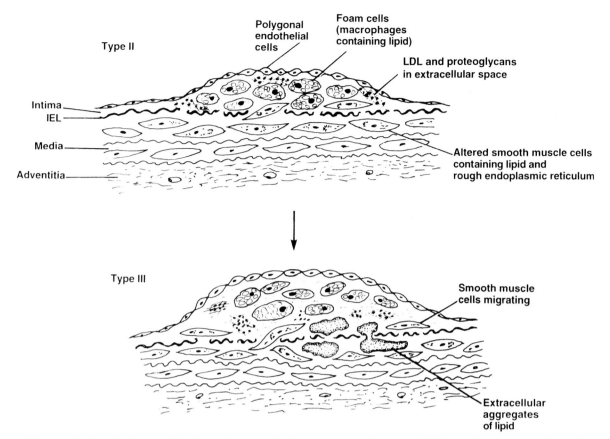

Figure 6–2. Type IIa fatty streak lesions with foam cells. Note low-density lipoprotein (LDL) particles in matrix and altered smooth muscle cells with developed rough endoplasmic reticulum also containing lipid particles. Note evolution to intermediate, more advanced lesion (type III) now containing extracellular aggregates or pools of lipid deep in the intima and extending into media. (From DePalma RG: Atherosclerosis: Theories of etiology and pathogenesis. In Sidawy AN, Sumpio BE, DePalma RG [eds]: Basic Science of Vascular Disease. Armonk, NY, Futura Publishing, 1997.)

ucts ordinarily unexpressed in normal vascular tissue. A notable example is tissue factor (TF), the cellular initiator of the coagulation cascade that is expressed by atheroma monocytes and foam cells.[24] Expression of TF requires the presence of bacterial lipopolysaccharide, suggesting that hypercoagulability in atherosclerosis could be enhanced by endotoxemia.

The large numbers of macrophages and T lymphocytes in the lesion suggest a cellular immune response; oxidized lipoproteins, heat shock proteins, and microorganisms are possible antigens. Recent work analyzing endarterectomy specimens by immunohistochemistry and reverse transcription–polymerase chain reaction (PCR)[25] showed proinflammatory T cell cytokines, IL-2, and interferon-7 in a large proportion of plaques. A helper T cell 1 (Th1)–type cellular immune response probably takes place in the atherosclerotic plaque.

Endothelium

Animal studies reveal that endothelial cells tend to be oriented away from the direction of flow; these cells show increased stigmata or stomata, increased proliferation, and a decrease in microfilament bundles. In humans and animals, endothelial cells become polyhedral or rounded; in humans, increased formation of multinucleated cells and

cilia occurs. Animal studies reveal increased proliferation and cell death, with retraction and exposure of subendothelial foam cells. The endothelium becomes more permeable to macromolecules in experimental models; in humans, it exhibits increased mural thrombus formation and TF expression. Leukocyte adherence increases with expression of a monocyte adhesion molecule (VCAM1). Endothelium-derived relaxing factor and prostacyclin release are decreased with enhanced vasoconstriction.

Media

Experimentally, the smooth muscle shows increased proliferation with increased rough endoplasmic reticulum, phenotypic change, and increased production of altered intracellular and extracellular matrices. These, in humans, include increased expression of type I and type III collagen, dermatan sulfate, proteoglycan, and stromolysins. The smooth muscle cells produce cytokines, including macrophage colony-stimulating factor (M-CSF), tumor necrosis factor (TNF), and monocyte chemoattractant protein-1 (MCP-1). The myocytes accumulate native and modified lipoproteins both by native receptor pathways and by nonspecific phagocytosis; these cells also express increased lipoprotein lipase activity and experimentally display a scavenger receptor similar to that of foam cells.

Macrophages

Macrophages proliferate and express MCP-1, M-CSF, TNF, IL-1, and PDGF, as well as CD immune antigens and TF,[25] as previously mentioned. Macrophages contain increased free and esterified cholesterol and increased acetyl coenzyme A (CoA), cholesterol acyltransferase, and acid cholesterol ester hydrolase. Neutral cholesterol ester hydrolase is decreased. The altered cells also express the scavenger receptor 15-lipoxygenase and exhibit increased lipoprotein oxidation products in humans and in animal models.

The extensive changes outlined indicate the complexity of the morphologic, functional, biochemical, and genetic expressions of the arterial wall in early atherosclerosis. The reader is referred to the original report[8] for comprehensive details, with references for the cellular alterations given.[21]

Gelatinous Plaques

Another type of early atheroma precursor is the intimal gelatinous lesion. These were also first described, in 1856, by Virchow,[15] and noted later by Haust,[26] as important progenitors of advanced atherosclerosis. The methodical study of these lesions has been relatively neglected, but their identification and composition was described by Smith.[27]

Virtually all the plasma proteins, particularly the hemostatic components, are capable of entering the arterial intima; these are thought to be mainly responsible for the lesions. Gelatinous lesions are translucent and neutral in color, with central areas that are grayish or opaque. Certain lesions are characterized by finely dispersed, perifibrous lipid along with collagen strands around the lesions. Grossly, gelatinous lesions feel soft. With gentle lateral pressure, the plaque "wobbles." Gelatinous plaques are often observed during arterial surgery; I am struck by the frequency with which these appear in heavy smokers. The gelatinous material separates easily from the underlying arterial wall without entering the usual endarterectomy plane. Gelatinous plaques are commonly seen in the aorta and occur as extensive areas of flat, translucent thickenings, particularly in the lower abdominal segment. These lesions are characterized by low lipid content and high fluid content. Protein content is variable, but in some plaques, numerous smooth muscle cells are present and the lesions contain substantial amounts of cross-linked fibrin.

Fibrous Plaques

Figure 6–1 typifies the more advanced atherosclerotic lesion, the fibrous or type IV plaque. These are composed of large numbers of smooth muscle cells and connective tissue, which form a fibrous cap over an inner yellow (atheromatous) core. This soft core contains cholesterol esters, mainly cholesteryl oleate, believed to be derived from disrupted foam cells. A second type of particle contains both free cholesterol and cholesterol linoleates. The early core is associated with vesicular lipids rich in free cholesterol.[7] The particles are thought to be derived directly from LDL, possibly by modification of LDL by specific lipolytic enzymes capable of hydrolyzing LDL cholesterol esters.[13] Lipoprotein aggregation and fusion are thought to be the chief pathway of cholesterol ester accumulation. Fibrous plaques are also composed of large numbers of smooth muscle cells, connective tissue cells, and macrophages. Emphasis has been placed on the composition and integrity of the cap, because this structure stabilizes the atheroma, preventing intraluminal rupture of the soft core.[28]

Fibrous plaques appear later than, and often in similar locations as, fatty streaks. Some but not all fibrous plaques are believed to be derived from fatty streaks; other precursors such as the gelatinous plaques or injured arterial areas may also lead to fibrous plaque formation. A mural thrombus can be converted into an atheroma, as demonstrated by chronic intraarterial catheter implantation.[29]

Fibrous plaques protrude into the arterial lumen in fixed cut sections; however, when arteries are fixed at arterial pressure, they produce an abluminal or external bulge. For example, coronary plaques in vivo must occupy at least 40% of the arterial wall before angiographic detection is possible,[30] and atheroma growth can be compensated for by arterial enlargement within certain limits.[31] Remodeling of coronary arteries in subhuman primates and humans has been recently stressed.[32] However, with lesion growth ulceration, rupture, or overlying thrombosis, the arterial lumen is ultimately compromised. When this occurs, distal ischemia develops. A unique adaptive response involving dilatation, with atheromatous involvement of the entire arterial wall and participation of inflammatory cells and immunologically active T lymphocytes, may predispose to aneurysm formation.

During evolution from fatty streak to fibrous plaque in early stages, cholesterol esters appear in the form of ordered arrays of intracellular lipid crystals. In intermediate type III and fibrous plaques, the lipids assume isotropic forms and occur extracellularly.[33] These cholesterol esters and oxysterols are quite irritating and cause severe inflammatory reactions in the connective tissue;[34] they probably behave similarly within the arterial wall. Thus, periarterial inflammation, fibrosis, and lymphocytic infiltration occur. Advancing neovascularization from the adventitia characterizes intermediate fibrofatty and fibrous plaque lesions. Atherosclerotic lesions contain immunoglobulin G (IgG) in large quantities, as well as other immunoglobulins and complement components. The contained IgG recognizes epitopes characteristic of oxidized LDL, indicating that immunologic processes characterize more advanced atherosclerotic plaques.[35] This process can exhibit systemic effects; patients with carotid atherosclerosis have higher antibody ratios of anti-OxLDL and IgM than comparable nonatherosclerotic controls.[36]

Recent experiments[37] suggest that atherogenesis is related to chronic inflammation, driven, in the main, by activation of the complement and monocyte-macrophage systems. In this view, enzymatic degradation, *not oxidation*, becomes a central event.

Complicated Plaques

Fibrous plaques become complicated by calcification, ulceration, intraplaque hemorrhage, or extensive necrosis.

These are late developments in atherosclerosis; such changes relate to the clinical complications of stroke, gangrene, and myocardial infarction. Aneurysm formation may represent a unique genetic or immune interaction with atherosclerosis. Alternatively, aneurysms have been viewed as nonspecific or inflammatory, degenerative, or purely mechanical arterial responses. We have reported a high prevalence of risk factors for atherosclerosis in patients with abdominal aortic aneurysms along with concurrent atherosclerotic involvement of other arteries.[38]

As have the early lesions,[8] the advanced lesions of atherosclerosis have been described and classified.[9] The type IV lesion, or atheroma, is potentially symptom producing. Extracellular lipid is thought to be the precursor of the core that characterizes type IV lesions. Lesions that contain a thick layer of fibrous connective tissue are characterized as type V lesions, whereas those with fissures, hematoma, or thrombus are characterized as type VI lesions. Type V lesions have been further described as largely calcified (type Vc) or consisting mainly of connective tissue with little or no lipid or calcium (type Vb). Atherosclerotic aneurysms are included in this definition of advanced atherosclerosis.

THEORIES OF ATHEROGENESIS

Lipid Hypothesis

Virchow's[15] original concept was that the cellular changes characterizing atherosclerosis were reactive responses to lipid infiltration. Later, Aschoff[14] remarked: "From plasma of low cholesterin content no deposition of lipids will occur even though mechanical conditions are favorable." As can be seen from fatty streak and fibrous plaque evolution, lipids, particularly LDL cholesterol, play a pivotal role in lesion morphology, composition, and evolution. Early experiments by Anitschkow,[39] in which cholesterol was fed to rabbits to produce atherosclerosis, appeared to validate a simple "lipid filtration hypothesis." However, the situation is pathogenically more complex. Atherosclerosis develops in various species in proportion to the ease with which an experimental regimen displaces the normal lipid pattern toward hypercholesterolemia, particularly hyperbetalipoproteinemia. At the same time, arterial susceptibility varies among location, species, and individuals.

Canine and subhuman primate (rhesus and cynomolgus monkey) models of atherosclerosis revealed plaque progression in response to dietary manipulation[40-48] and plaque regression in response to serum cholesterol lowering. However, lesion production in susceptible species is not the result of simple dietary cholesterol overload. Any diet that causes hypercholesterolemia induces experimental atherosclerosis. The presence of excess, or even any, cholesterol is not necessary in atherogenic diets. In developmental subhuman primate feeding experiments, reduction of cholesterol content to 0.5% combined with sugar and eggs produced rapidly progressive plaques when high cholesterol addition (up to 7% by weight) did not.[41, 42] In rabbits, a variety of semipure, purified cholesterol-free diets with various interactions of amino acids induced hypercholesterolemia and atherosclerosis.[49]

Epidemiologic observations provide important circumstantial evidence linking hyperlipidemia to atherosclerosis.[50] Compelling evidence for the view that elevated LDL cholesterol is also an etiologic factor in atherosclerosis is demonstrated by genetic hyperlipidemias, in spite of objections[51] that highly cellular lipid-laden atheromas may be different lesions in these patients. These metabolic disorders are most often due to a lack or abnormality of LDL receptors on hepatocytes, which causes an ability to internalize and metabolize LDL.[52] The resulting serum cholesterol levels are markedly elevated early in life; individuals with the homozygous condition die prematurely from atherosclerosis, rarely living beyond the age of 26 years.

Unfortunately, the heterozygous condition is not uncommon, with total cholesterol levels ranging up to 350 mg/dL. These individuals account for 1 in 500 live births[53] and will suffer from premature atherosclerosis, generally in middle age. The atheromas of these patients, to this observer, are similar in morphology to those seen in individuals with the acquired hyperlipidemias or premature atherosclerosis associated with heavy smoking.

This unfortunate natural experiment is powerful evidence that elevated LDL cholesterol is a relentless factor in plaque inception and the rapid progression of atherosclerosis to lethal consequences. Recent experience with liver transplantation has been successful[54] in retarding the progress of this type of atherosclerosis. Familial hypercholesterolemias are characterized by autosomal dominant disorders produced by at least 12 different molecular defects of the LDL receptors. Familial abnormalities of high-density lipoprotein (HDL), a negative risk factor for atherosclerosis, also exist. Not only is the status of LDL and HDL metabolism important in pathogenesis but surface proteins of the lipoprotein complex or apoproteins are also relevant.

Thrombogenic Hypothesis

In the mid-19th century, Rokitansky[55] postulated that fibrinous substances deposited on the arterial intimal surface as a result of abnormal hemostatic elements in the blood could undergo metamorphosis into atheromatous masses containing cholesterol crystals and globules. The Rokitansky theory held that typical atheromatous lesions resulted mainly from degeneration of blood proteins (i.e., fibrin essentially deposited in the arterial intima). Duguid[56] repopularized this theory in 1946. In particular experimental models, usually rabbits, indwelling arterial catheters or arterial injury[57] results in cholesterol accumulation in lesions without the necessity of added dietary cholesterol. The gelatinous plaques[26, 27] may, under certain circumstances, evolve in a manner such that accumulation of blood proteins dominates lesion development.

Mesenchymal Hypothesis— Hemodynamic Effects

The proliferation of smooth cells in the intima and subsequent production by these cells of connective tissue elements are considered by some to be the primary and crucial steps in atherogenesis.[58, 59] Proteoglycan, an important arterial wall element, may be responsible for trapping infiltrated LDL, even if LDL is not elevated in the blood. Collagen is the other space-filling component of advanced atherosclerotic lesions. Hauss and colleagues[60] proposed that the migration of smooth muscle cells from the media to the intima, with proliferation and production of connective tissue, is a nonspecific reaction of the artery to any injury and that atherosclerosis simply reflects a generic arterial response. Chisolm and colleagues[13] termed this the "nonspecific" mesenchymal hypothesis. These scenarios are similar to wound-healing sequences in response to any injury. In part, this theory attempts to explain why physical factors such as shear stress, vasoactive agents, and different types of injuries induce similar sequences of events in the vessel wall.

Stehbens,[51] highly skeptical of the lipid hypothesis, stated that "atherosclerosis constituted the degenerative and reparative process consequent upon the hemodynamically induced engineering fatigue of the blood vessel wall." He postulated that "the vibrations consisting of the pulsations associated with cardiac contractions and the vortex shedding generated in the blood vessels at branchings, unions, curvatures, and fusiform dilatations (carotid sinus) over a lifetime are responsible for fatigue failure after a certain, but individually variable, number of vibrations." In this view, atherosclerosis, a process of wear and tear, becomes an inexorable process associated with aging. Hypertension[61] and tachycardia induced in experimental animals through atherogenic feeding caused accelerated plaque development, whereas bradycardia induced by sinoatrial node ablation in monkeys reduced coronary and carotid atherosclerosis.[62, 63]

Monoclonal Hypothesis—Smooth Muscle Proliferation

The morphologic similarity of smooth muscle proliferation in some atherosclerotic lesions to uterine smooth muscle myomas led Benditt and Benditt[58] to suggest that atherosclerotic lesions are derived from a singular or, at most, a few mutated smooth muscle cells that, like tumor cells, proliferate in an unregulated fashion. This theory is based on the finding of only one allele for glucose-6-phosphate dehydrogenase in lesions from heterozygotes. A homology exists between the β chain of human PDGF and the protein product of the v-*sis* oncogene, which is a tumor-causing gene derived from simian sarcoma virus. Tumor-forming cells in culture express the genes for one or both of the PDGF chains and secrete PDGF into the medium.[13] This hypothesis considers events causing smooth muscle cell proliferation as critical in atherogenesis. Actions of other growth factors, which might either stimulate or inhibit cell proliferation, depend on circumstances as well as on macrophage-derived cytokine activity. For example, the finding of TGFβ receptors in human atherosclerosis[64] provides evidence for an acquired resistance to apoptosis. Resistance to apoptosis may lead to proliferation of resistant cell subsets associated with progression of lesions. A multiplicity of factors influence smooth muscle proliferation, transformation, and collagen secretion. It must be remembered that *all* arterial cells (endothelium, macrophages, and smooth muscle) elaborate chemotactic and growth factors.

Response-to-Injury Hypothesis

As a result of experimental data and deductive reasoning, Ross and Glomset[65] initially postulated two pathways for the promotion of atheroma formation. In the first (as, e.g., in hypercholesterolemia), monocyte and macrophage migration occurred without endothelial denudation. In some instances, endothelial loss might occur with platelet carpeting of bare areas. In this event, platelets would stimulate proliferation of smooth muscle by releasing PDGF.

In a second pathway, the endothelium itself is postulated to release growth factors stimulating smooth muscle proliferation. Experimental rabbit arterial balloon injury shows that regrowing endothelium induces myointimal proliferation beneath its advancing edges, stimulating accumulation of collagen[66] and glycosaminoglycans.[67] As mentioned previously, stimulated smooth muscle itself releases growth factors, leading to a continued autocrine proliferative response. In the initial iteration of this theory, the second pathway was postulated to be relevant to atheroma stimulated by diabetes, possibly in relation to insulin-derived growth factors, cigarette smoking, or hypertension. Although hypertension causes endothelial injury, striking differences occur between the behavior of smooth muscle cells in atherosclerosis and in hypertension. Atherosclerosis stimulates an overt smooth muscle proliferative response. In most instances, pure hypertension causes thickening of the arterial wall by virtue of increased protein synthesis without an increase in cell number.[68]

The reasons for examining atherosclerosis and arterial wall injury are evident, particularly to vascular surgeons. Arterial trauma, such as clamping or balloon injury, can produce stenoses and vascular injuries (ranging from minor to severe) and initiate myointimal hyperplasia or atheroma. This theory of atherogenesis implies that the process is simply a response to injury. In this scenario, physical or chemical agents cause endothelial denudation. This leads to platelet adherence and subsequent release of PDGF,[69] which then triggers smooth muscle migration from the media to the intima, smooth muscle cell proliferation, and lipid accumulation. Such a sequence clearly applies in specific situations of injury to the arterial wall in which the internal elastic lamina is disrupted.

However, the injury hypothesis as a global theory of atherogenesis has not been supported by subsequent investigations. Arterial denudation is a *rare event* in early atherogenesis in humans and animals, although endothelial cells can be injured or dysfunctional and remain in place.[70] It is now recognized that there probably exists a systemic endothelial dysfunction in atherosclerosis[71] that has profound effects on systemic vasodilatation, as well as all entry through intact endothelium.

Because all the arterial wall cells can secrete growth factors that, if not identical to PDGF and its derivatives, are very similar, it is not necessary to postulate endothelial physical disruption.

The responses of the arterial wall after injury remain of

considerable practical interest in both atherogenesis and intimal hyperplasia. With injury, early medial smooth muscle proliferation is the first step, influenced primarily by basic fibroblast growth factor (bFGF).[72] Migration and production of extracellular matrix are the second and third stages of injury. These mechanisms are relevant to trauma-provoked atheromas, which occur as a result of clamping or balloon injuries even with modestly elevated levels of LDL cholesterol.[73] Other mitogens include angiotensin II, which causes smooth muscle to proliferate and induces expression of other growth factors.[74, 75] One of these growth factors is TGFβ, which exhibits either stimulatory or inhibitory effects in different circumstances. Injury also induces medial angiotensinogen gene expression along with angiotensin receptor expression.[76] Other smooth muscle antigens include thrombin, catecholamine, and possibly endothelin. Thus, atheromas developing in a setting of injury (mechanical, immunologic, or infectious) are probably influenced by these trauma-induced growth factors in varying degrees and sequences. In turn, plasma LDL elevation accentuates neointimal hyperplasia[77, 78] without actual atheroma formation in the classic sense.

Lesion Arrest/Regression

In considering pathogenesis and, more importantly, therapy, the phenomenon of regression must also be considered. Regression of atherosclerosis in response to lowered serum cholesterol has been demonstrated in autopsy studies of starved humans,[14] in animal models,[79] and in pioneering clinical angiographic trials.[80] In humans, trials of vascular end points have shown some impressive examples of regression in coronary arteries, but more commonly, only slight regression with slowing of progression and drastic reductions in coronary events.[81]

As atherosclerotic plaques in experimental animals regress, plaque bulk is reduced mainly by lipid egress. This has been shown convincingly in experiments using hypercholesterolemic dogs[40, 41] and monkeys.[44, 45] The exact mechanisms of atherogenesis and lesion regression or atheroexodus are incompletely understood. However, we demonstrated regression using serial observations of lessened bulk of individual plaques, lessened luminal encroachment as shown by edge defects on sequential angiography, and lessened plaque lipid and altered fibrous protein content measured histologically and chemically.[45] An important technical aspect of this research was the confirmation of regressive changes via immediate autopsy or surgical observation and biopsy. The changes observed grossly or histopathologically closely followed observed regressive angiographic changes.[52, 53]

Such correlative observations are not readily obtained in humans. Lessening of luminal intrusion on sequential angiography does, experimentally, coincide with decreased plaque size and lessened lipid content. In some instances of regression, fibrous protein increases; in other circumstances it decreases. Potentially, fibrosis limits regression, but this process also converts a soft atheromatous plaque into a more stable, fibrotic plaque. Active lesions, particularly in the coronary arteries, are not necessarily the most occlusive ones, and although angiographic edge changes

may be minimal, a reduction in coronary events has been associated with plaque stabilization. To produce regression consistently, serum cholesterol must be reduced, generally to below 200 mg/dL. Experimentally, serum cholesterol levels also exist above which lesions inevitably progress.[45, 48] This threshold in humans might approximate a total serum cholesterol of 150 to 170 mg/dL or an LDL level of 100 mg/dL, the levels Roberts[82] cited in populations in which atherosclerosis is virtually absent.

MEDICAL MANAGEMENT

General Considerations

The fact that, in certain areas of the world, populations free of coronary disease show total cholesterol levels below 150 mg/dL and LDL cholesterol levels below 100 mg/dL led Roberts[82] to question the primacy of other "atherosclerotic risk factors" that are not uncommon in these populations. In considering the usefulness of the lipid hypothesis in treatment rather than prevention, considerable positive evidence has accumulated to support this hypothesis, though with certain caveats.

The complications and deleterious clinical events associated with atherosclerosis are not singular and univariate but multiple and interactive. In the late pathogenesis of atheromas, the resulting instability of the fibrous plaques probably involves more than simple continued lipid accumulation. Considering possible etiologic concepts, Holman and colleagues[83] in 1960 indicated that "a sharp line of distinction exists between atherogenesis and the subsequent evolution of lesions that may or may not precipitate the disease, for the factors involved in the evolution of lesions beyond the stage of fatty streaks may be entirely different from the factors that initiate fatty streaks." Among these factors are altered fibrous proteins, the accumulation of blood elements, cap rupture, and inflammatory and immune mechanisms. Hypotheses of pathogenesis and etiology are constantly tested by manipulating risk factors associated with atherosclerosis. Among all the interventions intended to produce plaque stabilization or regression, only lipid manipulation (i.e., decreasing LDL cholesterol or increasing HDL cholesterol) has promoted favorable changes in the atheroma itself. *In humans, these lipid reductions also generally require cessation of smoking.*

In regression trials overall, the most favorable plaque changes in terms of arrest or regression occur with the most lipid reduction. Blankenhorn and Hodis[80] reviewed these data, noting that regression and stabilization are 1.5 to 2 times more common in treated subjects than in those receiving placebos. Although the angiographic studies do show plaque regression trends, these changes are usually small compared with lesion stabilization. Ornish and colleagues[54] reported favorable clinical results using serial coronary angiography among patients randomly assigned to an experimental group consuming a 10% fat, 12 mg cholesterol diet and undergoing smoking cessation, stress management training, and exercise. After 1 year, 82% of the treated group showed regressive changes in coronary artery plaques that depended, somewhat, on the amount of initial lesion encroachment.

A rational treatment goal would stabilize the plaque itself. Increased fibrous protein synthesis would produce a stable, fibrotic plaque as opposed to a soft, friable plaque containing an unstable, atheromatous core covered by a tenuous cap. In evaluating these hypotheses with a view toward better prediction and control of this process, treating or ameliorating the atheroma itself and providing quantifiable evidence of favorable change have been obtained with effective lipid reduction. Desirable changes include more fibrotic, smaller plaques, which permit enhanced blood flow and are more stable than soft, bulky, friable lesions.

Atherosclerosis is often segmental; the deleterious effects of atheromas can be effectively treated by bypassing or removing arterial lesions. These observations were, over four decades ago, uniquely surgical insights.[4] Such interventions, now including endovascular approaches, are the most important means of treatment for advanced atheromas, including particular patterns of coronary involvement, high-grade carotid lesions, and aortic disease. Strictly surgical approaches to treatment do not prevent disease progression; with certain disease patterns, life expectancy remains shortened. Continued smoking after reconstruction often makes matters worse after an ill-advised intrainguinal reconstruction for stable claudication. Prevention of superimposed embolic phenomena and clotting can be influenced by aspirin, urokinase, and anticoagulants. Modification of inflammatory responses by manipulation of cytokine-derived or immunologic modulating factors could be fruitful. This requires the ability to monitor and influence interactions occurring in lesions and to detect systemic inflammatory responses.

Another productive approach might be to decrease arterial spasm, which is provoked by relatively minor plaques, particularly in coronary or cerebral arteries. Atherosclerotic plaques impair the normal effect of endothelium-derived relaxing factor[85, 86] and cause failure of vasodilator responses in coronary and cerebral arteries.[87] Dietary treatment of experimental atherosclerosis restores endothelium-dependent relaxation responses within certain limits,[88] whereas long-term inhibition of nitric oxide synthesis by feeding promotes experimental atherosclerosis.[89]

Clinical Management

I believe it advisable to screen for total serum cholesterol levels in outpatients, particularly when vascular disease is present or suspected. When total serum cholesterol is greater than 200 mg/dL, fasting blood samples are obtained to measure HDL cholesterol levels. The LDL cholesterol level is calculated by the formula LDL cholesterol = total cholesterol − HDL cholesterol − triglycerides/5. This formula holds for fasting patients when triglycerides are below 400 mg/dL. Serum cholesterol levels must be obtained with patients on a regular diet outside the hospital. With acute illness, sudden inexplicable decrements in total serum cholesterol occur.

I have long supplied patients who have hyperlipidemia with information on diet and recommended exercise in the form of walking. The National Cholesterol Education Program recommends dietary approaches as a first step,

with more aggressive treatment for patients with atherosclerotic vascular diseases. The recommendations include consideration of age and sex in choosing therapy and routine determination of HDL cholesterol level initially, with greater emphasis on physical activity and weight loss as the first lines of therapy. Drug treatment is delayed in patients with a low risk of coronary heart disease (e.g., no smoking, diabetes, or hypertension) or an age of less than 45 years (men) or 55 years (women). More emphasis is now placed on a high level of HDL cholesterol, because this is a powerful negative risk factor.

Drug Therapy for Hyperlipidemia

Currently available drugs include cholestyramine and colestipol (bile acid sequestrants), nicotinic acid (a B complex vitamin), 3-hydroxy-3-methylglutaryl CoA–reducing agents (such as lovastatin and pravastatin, which inhibit cholesterol biosynthesis), and gemfibrozil (a fibric acid derivative that has an unknown mechanism of action). The drug probucol and the natural vitamins E and C are antioxidants. One coronary disease trial examining use of vitamin E supplements suggested an associated 40% lower risk of coronary disease.[90, 91] The reader is referred to a review by LaRosa[81] for detailed information regarding drug therapy. Combining therapies that both lower LDL cholesterol and raise HDL cholesterol is considered highly desirable. In this context, the statin drugs, possibly combined with niacin in nondiabetics, have exhibited dramatic reductions in coronary events that may involve nonlipid actions that affect endothelial function, inflammatory responses, plaque stability, and thrombus formation.[92]

Control of Associated Risk Factors

Cigarette smoking is the most powerful risk factor for atherosclerotic disease and for its clinical complications among patients seen by vascular surgeons. This addiction is directly related to limb amputation, high mortality due to ischemic heart disease, and failure of aortic and femoropopliteal grafts.[93-95] The manner in which cigarette smoking promotes atherosclerosis and graft thrombosis is incompletely understood. Carbon monoxidemia possibly predisposes to arterial wall injury, producing increased plasma flux and entry of LDL and other proteins as well as increased platelet reactivity, peripheral vasoconstriction, and lowered HDL levels.[96]

Clinical practice guidelines[97] should include, at a minimum:

1. All smokers should be offered smoking cessation treatment at every office visit.
2. Clinicians should ask about and record the tobacco use status of every patient.
3. Cessation treatment even as brief as 3 minutes may be effective.
4. The more intense the treatment, the more effective it is in achieving long-term abstinence.
5. Nicotine replacement therapy (short-term), clinician-delivered support, and life skills training are effective components of treatment.

6. Routinely, on an institutional basis, *identify* or *intervene* with all tobacco users at every visit.

To these guidelines, I would add another: Do not perform *elective* interventions for continued smokers for claudication alone. This often makes matters worse.

Hypertension

The control of hypertension prolongs life and reduces coronary mortality.[97] In experimental animals, atherosclerosis associated with hyperlipidemia is accelerated by chronic hypertension.[98] However, as with the risk factor of cigarette smoking, Asian and Caribbean populations show hypertension with low incidence of atherosclerotic disease and an absence of hyperlipidemia. Treatment of hypertension with thiazide diuretics was disadvantageous in terms of coronary outcome in a subgroup of men in the multiple risk factor intervention trial.

Lifestyle alterations in hypertension include weight reduction, reduced dietary sodium intake, reduced alcohol intake, increased physical activity, and—quite probably—increased calcium intake.[99]

Exercise

Regular exercise decreases total serum cholesterol, LDL, and fasting triglycerides and has variable effects on HDL.[100] The preventive effects of exercise are well documented, and a sedentary lifestyle is an important risk factor for coronary disease.[101] No study, however, has shown a direct effect of exercise on atherosclerotic plaques; experimental and clinical data have, in contrast, demonstrated arrest or regression of plaques with lipid reduction. Strenuous unsupervised exercise can be dangerous in the presence of preexisting atherosclerotic disease[102] and does not compensate for persistent uncorrected hyperlipidemia or continued cigarette smoking. This is an important message for patients with vascular disease.

Beneficial effects of exercise in peripheral vascular disease (i.e., increased walking distance) relate to improved skeletal muscle oxidative metabolism.[103] Exercise is also important secondary therapy. Often, exercise programs may be more effective for claudication over the long term than surgical or endovascular intervention, particularly in infrainguinal atherosclerosis. In patients with known coronary atherosclerosis, exercise prescriptions must be carefully structured. Before prescribing strenuous exercise, stress testing or monitoring to detect silent ischemic heart disease is recommended.

Diabetes

One of the most important risk or actual pathogenetic factors promoting atherosclerosis is diabetes. In its singular form, diabetes is associated with severe infracrural and coronary atherosclerosis. A current diabetes control trial[104] reveals favorable reduction in microvascular complications with "tight control" using insulin; unfortunately, this trial was not designed to study end points of macrovascular atherosclerotic complications. Diabetes, as it affects atherogenesis, has not been studied extensively in animal models of atherosclerosis.

Causes of enhanced atherogenesis in diabetes include abnormalities in apoprotein and lipoprotein particle distributions, particularly elevated levels of lipoprotein (a),[105] an independent thromboatherosclerotic risk factor. In poorly controlled diabetes, a procoagulant state exists. Not only do glyco-oxidation and oxidation contribute to LDL entry into macrophages but glycation of proteins and plasma in the arterial wall could contribute further to accelerated atherosclerosis in diabetics. Hormones, growth factors, cytokine-enhanced smooth muscle cell proliferation, and increased foam cell formation are also postulated to be unique aspects of atherogenesis in diabetes mellitus.[106]

Both hyperinsulinemia and insulin resistance are associated with atherosclerosis,[107] and both are associated with type 2 diabetes. Both insulin and glucose stimulate the growth of diabetic infragenicular smooth muscle cells.[108] One possible mechanism to account for atherogenesis is impaired vasoactivity; a study[109] showed that troglitazone, an insulin-action enhancer, corrects impaired brachial artery vasoactivity in patients with occult diabetes (impaired glucose tolerance). This suggests that agents that enhance insulin action may be advantageous. In view of the utility of tight control on preventing microvascular and infectious complications, control of blood glucose on a consistent basis appears advisable. With any given level of LDL, coronary heart disease risk is tripled in patients with diabetes relative to those without,[110] an important consideration in medical management. In the diabetic, elevated triglyceride levels most commonly accompany severely elevated cholesterol levels; this particular combination greatly increases the risk of adverse coronary events.

Antioxidants (Vitamins E and C; Probucol)

The thesis that oxidized LDL accelerates atherosclerosis is based on observations that incubation of macrophage with native LDL does not lead to foam cell formation, whereas incubation with oxidized or acetylated LDL promotes macrophage-to-foam cell formation. In addition, oxidized LDL formation may release proinflammatory products affecting the arterial wall, including cytokines and other cytotoxic products. It has been reported that IL-10, an anti-inflammatory cytokine, blocks atherosclerotic events in vitro and in vivo.[111]

Theoretically, antioxidants may inhibit the proinflammatory response. Yet it has been recently stated that dietary supplementation with antioxidant vitamins is far from proven.[112] Trials with vitamin E supplementation in preventing coronary events have yielded conflicting results, however. Further trials are needed to prove this thesis. Probucol has not proved effective in initial trials.

Inflammatory Components in Plaque Formation

Recent experiments suggest an alternative hypothesis, that atherogenesis is related to chronic inflammation driven by activation of the complement and monocyte systems.[37] Thus enzymatic degradation, not oxidation, may be the central event.

Possibly related to inflammatory and oxidative changes are data suggesting that elevated total body iron stores, particularly in men, relate to atherosclerotic events. Epidemiologic evidence for this thesis is supported by longitudinal data; for example, a study of total body iron stores and stroke risk.[113] A falling ferritin level, for example, due to blood donation or bleeding, was associated with improvement in atherosclerotic disease, whereas a rising ferritin level was associated with disease progression. In addition, changes in the ferritin level over time predicted fatal and nonfatal vascular events. A Veterans Administration cooperative, prospective, randomized single-blind clinical trial (FeAST, Leo R. Zarcharski, Principal Proponent) is now testing the hypothesis that reducing total body iron stores by phlebotomy to ferritin equivalence of 25 μg/mL (the level in healthy menstruating women) may reduce mortality by 30% in a patient population with advanced peripheral vascular disease. It should be noted that iron in the ferrous form is a powerful inflammatory and oxidizing agent. With this hypothesis, both iron intake and excess vitamin C intake might be considered undesirable, because vitamin C enhances iron absorption.

Homocysteine and Folic Acid Supplementation

Elevated levels of homocysteine have emerged as a risk factor for thromboatherosclerotic disease.[114] These could be lowered by increasing folic acid intake. However, data from a group in Salt Lake City[115] suggest that individuals developing the high homocysteine levels associated with coronary risk generally require higher genetic and environmental risk exposure. These include a particular heat-labile protein genetic mutation and a low folic intake. Elevated plasma homocysteine levels in subjects with peripheral vascular disease are associated significantly with death caused by coronary heart disease, likely thrombotic in nature.[116] It is not known whether therapy with folate or vitamins B_{12} or B_6 will control this process. Mandatory folic acid supplementation as a public health initiative remains controversial.

Antiplatelet and Anticoagulant Therapy

Platelet therapy has not produced regressive effects on established lesions, although anti-inflammatory effects probably occur; these favorable effects also relate to anti-thrombotic effect. Currently smaller, rather than larger doses of aspirin are considered advantageous. In prevention, 325 mg of aspirin on alternate days was effective in the Physicians' Health Study.[117] Data concerning intraplaque hemorrhage in carotid lesions in patients receiving aspirin are conflicting.

Results of a long-term study of the effects of clopidogrel indicate a small but statistical advantage in the long-term effects of this therapy over aspirin therapy alone. This population included patients with recent myocardial infarctions, recent stroke, or established peripheral arterial disease.[118] The largest relative risk reduction for clopidogrel, compared with aspirin, was in fatal and nonfatal myocardial infarction—19.2%.[119] Further observations on the efficacy of antiplatelet therapy are needed.

It has been reported that antiplatelet therapy and oral anticoagulants reduce the risk of graft occlusion and ischemic events after infrainguinal bypass surgery.[120] Oral anticoagulant therapy appears to be the more effective treatment in the high-risk patient. The evidence for the beneficial effects of antiplatelet and oral anticoagulant therapy was based on a small number of trials; no proof exists as to which modality is the more effective in the prevention of graft occlusion and ischemic events. A randomized comparison of aspirin with oral anticoagulants has been suggested. Some clinicians use both agents.

Vasoactive Drugs

Other nonlipid strategies, beyond cholesterol reduction, include the use of β-adrenergic receptor blocking agents to reduce catecholamine release, calcium channel blockers to reduce wall stress and inhibit lipid intake, nitrates to relax vascular smooth muscle by nitric oxide release, and angiotensin-converting enzyme inhibitors, which block atherogenic effects on angiotensin II. Nonlipid vasoactive strategies also require further human studies and comparative trials.

Atherosclerosis and Infection

Recent connections between infection and atherosclerosis have been cited. The strongest appear to exist between cytomegalovirus (CMV) and *Chlamydia pneumoniae*. A comprehensive review[121] summarizes the status of evidence to support these possible relationships. These data are based on case control studies and histologic and culture evidence from plaques. In terms of causation, when microorganisms are suggested as risk factors for a chronic disease, Koch's postulates may not be fulfilled, as pointed out by High.[121] CMV is a ubiquitous virus. The first suggestion that a similar virus could induce atherosclerosis in chickens with cholesterol acting as a cofactor was made in the late 1970s.[122] Evidence for a role of CMV in atherosclerosis also comes from the finding of a high incidence of restenosis after coronary atherectomy in patients who are seropositive.[123] To date, no interventional studies using anti-CMV therapy have been performed in patients with atherosclerosis.

In the case of *C. pneumoniae*, a twofold higher risk of IgG and IgA antibodies to *C. pneumoniae* was found in patients with coronary syndromes compared with controls.[124] Since then, many studies confirm the association, with odds ratios ranging from 1.5 to 10 and an average of about 2.5. The association of this organism with atherosclerotic tissue is much more specific than for CMV. *C. pneumoniae* has actually been isolated from atheromatous material. A lack of an animal model inhibits research, however. One experiment, using rabbits nasally inoculated with the organism and fed a cholesterol-enhanced diet, showed accelerated atherosclerosis which was prevented by azithromycin.[125] Oral therapy trials using roxithromycin and azithromycin have been done in humans with suggestive reductions in coronary events. These trials now encourage larger randomized trials of antibiotic therapy for secondary prevention and, possibly, for primary prevention. It has been suggested that the effects of macrolides may relate to an anti-inflammatory action rather than an antibiotic effect. These promising observations are of great interest.

SUMMARY

A general concept has arisen in the notion that medical therapy will induce plaque stabilization thus reducing adverse clinical events. These effects may be correlated with observations that monocyte-derived macrophages and foam cell accumulation cause instability and cap rupture. Therapies that minimize these responses potentially reduce clinical complications of unstable or vulnerable plaques. In addition to conventional treatments, mainly lipid reduction, additional approaches will likely be tested to minimize inflammatory responses associated with atherosclerosis.

References

1. DeBakey ME, Lawrie GM, Glaeser DH: Patterns of atherosclerosis and their surgical significance. Ann Surg 201:115, 1985.
2. DePalma RG: Patterns of peripheral atherosclerosis: Implications for treatment. In Shepard J (ed): Atherosclerosis—Developments, Complications and Treatment. New York, Elsevier, 1987, pp 161–174.
3. McMillan GC: Development of atherosclerosis. Am J Cardiol 31:542, 1973.
4. DeBakey ME: Atherosclerosis: Patterns and rates of progression. In Gotto AM Jr, South LL, Allen B (eds): Atherosclerosis Five: Proceedings of the Fifth International Symposium. New York, Springer-Verlag, 1980, p 3.
5. Haimovici H, DePalma RG: Atherosclerosis: Biologic and surgical considerations. In Haimovici H, Ascer E, Hollier LH, et al (eds): Vascular Surgery: Principles and Techniques, 4th ed. Cambridge, Mass, Blackwell Science, 1996, pp 127–157.
6. Report of Study Group, Classification of Atherosclerotic Lesions. WHO Tech Rep Ser 143:1958.
7. Guyton JR, Kemp KF: Development of the lipid-rich core in human atherosclerosis. Arterioscler Thromb Vasc Biol 16:4–11, 1996.
8. American Heart Association (Stary HC [Chair], Chandler AB, Glagov S, et al): A definition of initial fatty streak and intermediate lesions of atherosclerosis: A report from the committee on vascular lesions of the council on atherosclerosis. Arterioscler Thromb Vasc Biol 14:840, 1994.
9. American Heart Association (Stary HC [Chair], Chandler AB, Glagov S, et al): A definition of advanced types of atherosclerotic lesions and a histological classification of atherosclerosis. Arterioscler Thromb Vasc Biol 15:1512, 1995.
10. Cornhill JF, Hederick EE, Stary HC: Topography of human aortic sudanophilic lesions. Monogr Atherosclerosis 15:13, 1990.
11. Glagov S, Zarins C, Giddens DP, et al: Hemodynamics and atherosclerosis: Insights and perspectives gained from studies of human arteries. Arch Pathol Lab Med 112:1018, 1988.
12. Insull W Jr, Bartch GE: Cholesterol, triglyceride and phospholipid content of intima, media and atherosclerotic fatty steak in human thoracic aorta. J Clin Invest 45:513, 1966.
13. Chisolm GM, DiCarleto PE, Erhart LA, et al: Pathogenesis of atherosclerosis. In Young JR, Graor RA, Olin JW, Bartholomew JR (eds): Peripheral Vascular Diseases. St Louis, Mosby–Year Book, 1991, pp 137–160.
14. Aschoff L: Atherosclerosis. In Lectures on Pathology. New York, Hoeber, 1924, pp 131–153.
15. Virchow R: Gesammelte Abhandlungen zur Wissenschaftlichen Medicin. Frankfurt, Meidinger John, 1856, p 496.
16. Fagiotto A, Ross R, Harker L: Studies of hypercholesterolemia in the nonhuman primate, I: Changes that lead to fatty streak formation. Arterioscler Thromb Vasc Biol 4:323, 1984.
17. Fagiotto A, Ross R: Studies of hypercholesterolemia in the nonhuman primate, II: Fatty streak conversion to fibrous plaque. Arteriscler Thromb Vasc Biol 4:341, 1984.
18. Gerrity RG: The role of monocyte in atherogenesis, I: Transition of blood borne monocytes into foam cells in fatty lesions. Am J Pathol 103:181, 1981.
19. Steinberg D, Parthasarathy S, Carew TE, et al: Beyond cholesterol:
20. Wiklund O, Carew TF, Steinberg D: Role of the low density lipoprotein receptor in the penetration of low density lipoprotein into the rabbit aortic wall. Arterioscler Thromb Vasc Biol 5:135, 1985.
21. Steinbrecher UP: Role of superoxide in endothelial-cell modification of low density lipoprotein. Biochim Biophys Acta 959:20, 1988.
22. Heinecke JW, Baker L, Rosen L, Chait A: Superoxide mediates modification of low density lipoprotein by arterial smooth muscle cells. J Clin Invest 77:757, 1986.
23. Parthasarathy S, Printz DJ, Boyd D, et al: Macrophage oxidation of low density lipoproteins generates a form recognized by the scavenger receptor. Arterioscler Thromb Vasc Biol 6:505, 1986.
24. Brand K, Banka CL, Mackman N, et al: Oxidized LDL enhances lipopolysaccharide induced tissue factor expression in human adherent monocytes. Arterioscler Thromb Vasc Biol 14:790, 1994.
25. Frostegard J, Ulgren AK, Nyberg P, et al: Cytokine expression in advanced human atherosclerotic plaques: Dominance of inflammatory (Th1) and macrophage stimulating cytokines. Atherosclerosis 145:33, 1999.
26. Haust MD: The morphogenesis and fate of potential and early atherosclerotic lesions in man. Hum Pathol 2:1, 1971.
27. Smith EB: Fibrin in the arterial wall. Atherosclerosis 70:186, 1988.
28. Davies MJ, Thomas A: Thrombosis and acute coronary artery lesions in sudden cardiac ischemic death. N Engl J Med 310:1137, 1984.
29. Moore S: Thromboatherosclerosis in normolipemic rabbits: A result of continued endothelial damage. Lab Invest 29:478, 1973.
30. Stiel GN, Stiel LSG, Schofer J, et al: Impact of compensatory enlargement of atherosclerotic arteries on angiographic assessment. Circulation 80:1603, 1989.
31. Glagov S, Weisenberg E, Zarins C, et al: Compensatory enlargement of human atherosclerotic coronary arteries. N Engl J Med 316:1371, 1987.
32. Clarkson TB, Prichard RW, Morgan TM, et al: Remodeling of coronary arteries in human and nonhuman primates. JAMA 271:289, 1994.
33. Hata Y, Hower J, Insull W Jr: Cholesterol ester–rich inclusions from human aortic fatty streak and fibrous plaque lesions of atherosclerosis. Am J Pathol 75:423, 1974.
34. Baranowski A, Adams CWM, Bayliss-High OB, et al: Connective tissue responses to oxysterols. Atherosclerosis 41:255, 1982.
35. Yla-Herttuala S, Palinski W, Butler S, et al: Rabbit and human atherosclerotic lesions contain IgG that recognizes epitopes of oxidized LDL. Atheroscler Thromb Vasc Biol 13:32, 1993.
36. Maggi E, Chiesa R, Milissano G, et al: LDL oxidation in patients with severe carotid atherosclerosis: A study of in vitro and in vivo oxidation markers. Atheroscler Thromb Vasc Biol 14:1892, 1994.
37. Schmiedt W, Kinscherf R, Deigner HP, et al: Complement CG deficiency protects against diet-induced atherosclerosis in rabbits. Arteriosclerosis Thromb Vasc Biol 18:1790, 1998.
38. DePalma RG, Sidawy AN, Giordano JM: Associated etiological and atherosclerotic risk factors in abdominal aneurysms. In Greenhalgh RM, Mannick JA (eds): The Cause and Management of Aneurysm. London, WB Saunders, 1990, pp 37–46.
39. Anitschkow R: Experimental atherosclerosis in animals. In Cowdry

Modifications of low density lipoprotein that increase its atherogenicity. N Engl J Med 320:915, 1989.

V (ed): Arteriosclerosis: Review of Problem. New York, Macmillan, 1933.

40. DePalma RG, Hubay CA, Insull W Jr, et al: Progression and regression of experimental atherosclerosis. Surg Gynecol Obstet 131:633, 1970.

41. DePalma RG, Insull W Jr, Bellon EM, et al: Animal models for study of progression and regression of atherosclerosis. Surgery 72:268, 1972.

42. DePalma RG, Bellon EM, Insull W Jr, et al: Studies on progression and regression of experimental atherosclerosis: Techniques and application to the rhesus monkey. Med Primatol 3:313, 1972.

43. DePalma RG, Bellon EM, Klein L, et al: Approaches to evaluating regression of experimental atherosclerosis. In Manning GM, Haust MD (eds): Atherosclerosis: Metabolic, Morphologic and Clinical Aspects. New York, Plenum Press, 1977, p 459.

44. DePalma RG, Bellon EM, Koletsky S, et al: Atherosclerotic plaque regression in a rhesus monkey induced by bile acid sequestrant. Exp Mol Pathol 31:423, 1979.

45. DePalma RG, Klein L, Bellon EM, et al: Regression of atherosclerotic plaques in rhesus monkeys. Arch Surg 115:1268, 1980.

46. DePalma RG: Angiography in experimental atherosclerosis: Advantages and limitations. In Bond JG, Insull W Jr, Glagov S, et al (eds): Clinical Diagnosis of Atherosclerotic Lesions: Quantitative Methods of Evaluation. New York, Springer-Verlag, 1983, p 99.

47. DePalma RG, Koletsky S, Bellon EM, et al: Failure of regression of atherosclerosis in dogs with moderate cholesterolemia. Atherosclerosis 27:297, 1977.

48. DePalma RG, Bellon EM, Manalo PM, Bomberger RA: Failure of antiplatelet treatment in dietary atherosclerosis: A serial intervention study. In Gallo LL, Vahouny GV (eds): Cardiovascular Disease: Molecular and Cellular Mechanisms, Prevention, Treatment. New York, Plenum Press, 1987, p 407.

49. Kritchevsky D: Atherosclerosis and nutrition. Nutrition 2:290, 1986.

50. LaRosa JC: Cholesterol lowering, low cholesterol and mortality. Am J Cardiol 72:776, 1993.

51. Stehbens WE: The Lipid Hypothesis of Atherosclerosis. Austin, Tex, RG Landes, 1993.

52. Brown MS, Goldstein JL: Lipoprotein receptors in the liver: Control signals for plasma cholesterol traffic. J Clin Invest 72:743, 1983.

53. Schonfeld G: Inherited disorders of lipid transport. Endocrinol Metab Clin North Am 19:211, 1990.

54. Hoeg JM: Familial hypercholesterolemia: What the zebra can teach us about the horse. JAMA 271:543, 1994.

55. Rokitansky C von: A Manual of Pathological Anatomy. Translated by Dan GE. London, Sydenham Society, 1852.

56. Duguid JB: Thrombosis as a factor in the pathogenesis of coronary atherosclerosis. J Pathol 58:207, 1946.

57. Bjorkerud JS, Bondjers G: Arterial repair and atherosclerosis after mechanical injury: 2 tissue response after induction of a total necrosis (deep longitudinal injury). Atherosclerosis 14:259, 1971.

58. Benditt EP, Benditt JM: Evidence for a monoclonal origin of human atherosclerotic plaques. Proc Natl Acad Sci U S A 70:1753, 1973.

59. Schwartz SM: Cellular proliferation in atherosclerosis and hypertension. Proc Soc Exp Biol Med 173:1, 1983.

60. Hauss WH, Junge-Hulsing G, Hollanden HJ: Changes in metabolism of connective tissue associated with aging and arterio- or atherosclerosis. J Atherosclerosis Res 6:50, 1962.

61. Koletsky S, Roland C, Rivera-Velez JM: Rapid acceleration of atherosclerosis in hypertensive rats on a high fat diet. Exp Mol Pathol 9:322, 1968.

62. Beere PA, Glagov S, Zarins CK: Retarding effects of a lowered heart rate on coronary atherosclerosis. Science 226:180, 1989.

63. Beere PA, Glagov S, Zarins CK: Experimental atherosclerosis at the carotid bifurcation of the cynomolgus monkey: Localization, compensatory enlargement and sparing effect of lowered heart rate. Arterioscler Thromb Vasc Biol 12:1245, 1992.

64. McCaffrey TA, Du B, Fu C, et al: The expressions of TGF-beta receptors in human atherosclerosis: Evidence for acquired resistance to apoptosis due to receptor imbalance J Mol Cell Cardiol 31:1627, 1999.

65. Ross R, Glomset JA: The pathogenesis of atherosclerosis. N Engl J Med 295:369, 1976.

66. Chidi CC, DePalma RG: Collagen formation by transformed smooth muscle after arterial injury. Surg Gynecol Obstet 152:8, 1981.

67. Wight TV, Curwen KD, Litrenta MM, et al: Effect of endothelium on glycosaminoglycan accumulation in the injured rabbit aorta. Am J Pathol 113:156, 1983.

68. Schwartz SM, Ross R: Cellular proliferation in atherosclerosis and hypertension. Prog Cardiovasc Dis 26:355, 1984.

69. Ross R, Glomset F, Kariya B, et al: A platelet dependent factor that stimulates the proliferation of arterial smooth muscle cells in vitro. Proc Natl Acad Sci U S A 71:1207, 1974.

70. Ross R: The pathogenesis of atherosclerosis: A perspective for the 1990s. Nature 362:801, 1993.

71. Anderson TJ, Gerhard MD, Meridith IT, et al: Systemic nature of endothelial dysfunction in atherosclerosis. Am J Cardiol 75:7113, 1995.

72. Lindner V, Lappi DA, Baird A, et al: Role of basic fibroblast growth factor in vascular lesion formation. Circ Res 68:106, 1991.

73. DePalma RG, Chidi CC, Sternfeld WC, Koletsky S: Pathogenesis and prevention of trauma provoked atheromas. Surgery 82:429, 1977.

74. Campbell-Bodwell M; Robertson AL Jr: Effects of angiotensin II and vasopressin on human smooth muscle cells in vitro. Exp Med Pathol 35:265, 1981.

75. Itoh H, Mukuyawa M, Pratt RE, et al: Multiple autocrine growth factors modulate vascular smooth muscle in response to angiotensin II. J Clin Invest 91:2268, 1993.

76. Viswanathan M, Stromberg C, Seltzer A, et al: Balloon angioplasty enhances expression of angiotensin II; ATI receptors in neointima of rat aorta. J Clin Invest 90:1707, 1992.

77. Stevens SL, Hilgarth K, Ryan US, et al: The synergistic effect of hypercholesterolemia and mechanical injury on intimal hyperplasia. Ann Vasc Surg 6:55, 1992.

78. Baumann DS, Doblas M, Dougherty A, et al: The role of cholesterol accumulation in prosthetic vascular graft anastomotic intimal hyperplasia. J Vasc Surg 19:435, 1994.

79. St Clair RSW: Atherosclerosis regression in animal models: Current concepts of cellular and biochemical mechanisms. Prog Cardiovasc Dis 26:109, 1983.

80. Blankenhorn DH, Hodis HN: Arterial imaging and atherosclerosis reversal. Arterioscler Thromb Vasc Biol 14:177, 1994.

81. LaRosa JC: Lipid Lowering. In LaRosa JC (ed): Medical Management of Atherosclerosis. New York, Marcel Dekker, 1998, pp 1–30.

82. Roberts WC: Atherosclerotic risk factors: Are there ten or is there only one? Am J Cardiol 64:552, 1989.

83. Holman RLH, McGill HC Jr, Strong JP, Geer JC: Atherosclerosis—the lesion. Am J Clin Nutr 8:84, 1960.

84. Ornish D, Brown SE, Shewritz LW, et al: Can lifestyle changes reverse coronary heart disease? The Lifestyle Heart Trial. Lancet 336:129, 1990.

85. Chester AH, O'Neill GS, Moncada S, et al: Low basal and stimulated release of nitric oxide in atherosclerotic epicardial coronary arteries. Lancet 336:897, 1990.

86. Forstermann U, Mugge A, Alheid U, et al: Selective attenuation of endothelium-mediated vasodilation in atherosclerotic human coronary arteries. Circ Res 62:185, 1988.

87. Heistad DD, Breese K, Armstrong ML: Cerebral vasoconstrictor response to serotonin after dietary treatment of atherosclerosis: Implications for transient ischemic attacks. Stroke 18:1068, 1987.

88. Harrison DG, Armstrong ML, Freiman DC, Heistad DD: Restoration of endothelium dependent relaxation by dietary treatment of atherosclerosis. J Clin Invest 80:1808, 1987.

89. Naruse K, Shimizu K, Muramatsu M, et al: Long term inhibition of NO synthesis promotes atherosclerosis in the hypercholesterolemic rabbit thoracic aorta. Atheroscler Thromb Vasc Biol 14:746, 1994.

90. Rimm EB, Stampfer MJ, Aschenio A, et al: Vitamin E consumption and risk of coronary heart disease in men. N Engl J Med 328:1450, 1993.

91. Stampfer MJ, Hennekers CH, Manson JE: Vitamin E consumption and risk of coronary heart disease in women. N Engl J Med 328:1444, 1993.

92. Rosenson RS, Tangney CC: Antiatherothrombotic properties of statins: Implications for cardiovascular event reduction. JAMA 279:1643, 1998.

93. Wray R, DePalma RG, Hubay CA: Late occlusion of aortofemoral bypass grafts: Influence of cigarette smoking. Surgery 70:696, 1971.

94. Robiesek F, Daugherty HK, Mullen DC: The effect of continued cigarette smoking on the patency of synthetic vascular grafts in Leriche syndrome. J Thorac Cardiovasc Surg 70:107, 1975.

95. Ameli FM, Stein M, Prosser RJ, et al: Effects of cigarette smoking on outcome of femoropopliteal bypass for limb salvage. J Cardiovasc Surg (Torino) 30:591, 1989.

96. Garrison RJ, Kannel WB, Feinleib M, et al: Cigarette smoking and HDL cholesterol. Atherosclerosis 30:17, 1978.

97. Borhani NO, Blaufox MD, Folk BF: Incidence of coronary heart disease and left ventricular hypertrophy in hypertension detection and follow-up programs. Prog Cardiovasc Dis 29(Suppl):55–62, 1989.

98. Kolestsky S, Roland C, Rivera-Velez JM: Rapid acceleration of atherosclerosis in hypertensive rats on a high fat diet. Exp Mol Pathol 9:322, 1968.

99. Stone NJ: Lifestyle interventions in atherosclerosis. In LaRosa JC (ed): Medical Management of Atherosclerosis. New York, Marcel Dekkor, 1998 pp 91–113.

100. Beard CM, Barnard RJ, Robbins DC: Effects of diet and exercise on qualitative and quantitative measures of LDL and its susceptibility to oxidation. Arterioscler Thromb Vasc Biol 16:201, 1996.

101. Powell KE, Thompson PD, Caspersen CJ, Kendrick JS: Physical activity and the incidence of coronary heart disease. Annu Rev Public Health 8:253, 1987.

102. Williams LR, Ekers MA, Collins PS, Lee JF: Vascular rehabilitation: Benefits of a structured exercise/risk modification programs. J Vasc Surg 14:320, 1991.

103. Hiatt WR, Regensteiner JG, Hargarten ME: Benefit of exercise conditioning for patients with peripheral arterial disease. Circulation 81:2, 1990.

104. The Diabetes Control and Complication Trial Research Group: The effect of intensive treatment of diabetes on the development and progression of long-term complications in insulin-dependent diabetes mellitus. N Engl J Med 329:977, 1993.

105. Loscalzo J: Lipoprotein (a): A unique risk factor for atherothrombotic disease. Arteriosclerosis 10:672, 1990.

106. Bierman EI: Atherogenesis in diabetes. Arterioscler Thromb Vasc Biol 12:647, 1992.

107. Goldberg RB: Insulin resistance and atherosclerosis. In LaRosa JC (ed): Medical Management of Atherosclerosis. New York Marcel Dekkor, 1998 pp 283–316.

108. Avena R, Mitchell ME, Neville RF, Sidawy AN: The additive effects of glucose and insulin on the proliferation of vascular smooth muscle cells. J Vasc Surg 28:10339, 1998.

109. Avena R, Mitchell ME, Nylen ES, et al: Insulin action enhancement normalizes brachial artery vasoactivity in patients with peripheral vascular disease and occult diabetes. J Vasc Surg 28:1024, 1998.

110. Stamler J, Vaccaro O, Nealon JD, Westworth D: Diabetes and other risk factors and 12 year cardiovascular mortality for men screened for MRFIT. Diabetes Care 16:434, 1993.

111. Pindersky Oslund LJ, Hedrick CC, Olvera T, et al: Interleukin-10 blocks atherosclerotic events in vitro and vivo. Arterioscler Thromb Vasc Biol 19:2847, 1999.

112. Witzum JL: Role of antioxidants in prevention of coronary artery disease. In LaRosa JC (ed): Medical Management of Atherosclerosis, New York, Marcel Dekker, 1998, pp 41–42.

113. Kiechl S, Willeit J, Landis M, et al: Body iron stores and the risk of carotid atherosclerosis. Circulation 96:3300, 1997.

114. Taylor LM Jr, Porter JM: Elevated plasma homocysteine as a risk factor for atherosclerosis. Semin Vasc Surg 6:36, 1993.

115. Williams RR, Hopkins PN, Wu L, Hunt SC: Applied genetics now and gene therapy in the future. In LaRosa JC (ed): Medical Management of Atherosclerosis. New York, Marcel Dekker, 1998, pp 247–268.

116. Taylor LM, Moneta GL, Sexton GJ, et al: Prospective blinded study of the relationship between plasma homocysteine and the progression of symptomatic peripheral arterial disease. J Vasc Surg 29:8, 1999.

117. Goldhaber SZ, Manson JE, Stumpfer MJ, et al: Low-dose aspirin and subsequent peripheral arterial surgery in the Physicians' Health Study. Lancet 340:143, 1992.

118. CAPRIE Steering Committee: A randomized blinded trial of clopidogrel in patients at risk for ischemic events. Lancet 348:1329, 1996.

119. Gent M: Benefit of clopidogrel in patients with coronary disease. Circulation 96 (Suppl):I–476, 1997.

120. Tangelker MJO, Lawson JA, Algre A, Eikelboom BC: Systematic review of randomized controlled trials of aspirin and oral anticoagulants in the prevention of graft occlusion and ischemic events after infrainguinal bypass surgery. J Vasc Surg 30:701, 1999.

121. High KP: Atherosclerosis and infection due to *Chlamydia pneumoniae* or cytomegalovirus: Weighing the evidence. Clin Infect Dis 28:746, 1999.

122. Fabricant DG, Fabricant J, Litrenta MM, Minick CR: Virus-induced atherosclerosis. J Exp Med 148:335, 1978.

123. Zhou YF, Leon MB, Waclawiw MA, et al: Association between prior cytomegalovirus infection and re-stenosis after coronary atherectomy. N Engl J Med 335:625, 1996.

124. Saikku P, Matilla K, Nieminen MS, et al: Serological evidence of an association of a novel *Chlamydia* with chronic coronary disease and acute myocardial infarction. Lancet 2:983, 1988.

125. Muhlestein JB, Anderson JL, Hammond EG, et al: Infection with *Chlamydia pneumoniae* accelerates the development of atherosclerosis and treatment with azithromycin prevents it in a rabbit model. Circulation 97:633, 1998.

126. Gurfinkle E, Bozovich G, Darsca A, et al: Randomized trial of roxithromycin in non-Q wave coronary syndromes. ROXIS pilot study. Lancet 350:404, 1997.

127. Gupta S, Leatham EW, Carrington D, et al: Elevated *Chlamydia pneumoniae* antibodies, cardiovascular events, and azithromycin in male survivors of myocardial infarction. Circulation 96:404, 1997.

Questions

1. The fibrous plaque
   (a) is an early lesion of atherosclerosis
   (b) is a complicated lesion
   (c) contains mainly fibrous tissue
   (d) is localized in the intima
   (e) contains a yellow "core"

2. The earliest lesions of atherosclerosis are
   (a) denuded areas of endothelium
   (b) increased intimal macrophages containing lipid
   (c) minor breaks in the internal elastic lamina
   (d) focal adventitial lymphocytic infiltration
   (e) small areas of fibrin deposition

3. In atherosclerosis, smooth muscle cells of early lesions produce all these except
   (a) lipoproteins
   (b) type I collagen
   (c) type III collagen
   (d) cytokines
   (e) stromolysins

4. The "core" of a typical fibrous plaque consists mainly of
   (a) inflammatory cells
   (b) fibrin and fibrinogen
   (c) cholesteryl oleate and free cholesterol
   (d) lysosomal enzymes
   (e) proteoglycans

5. Complicated atherosclerotic plaques can be derived from
   (a) mechanical injury
   (b) thrombogenesis at sites of catheter insertion
   (c) immunologic injury
   (d) none of the above
   (e) all of the above

6. Consistent experimental production of atherosclerotic plaques requires
   (a) feeding of a high cholesterol diet
   (b) hyperbetalipoproteinemia
   (c) hormonal manipulation
   (d) balloon injury
   (e) genetically bred animals

7. Metabolic disorders promoting high low-density lipoprotein cholesterol and atherosclerosis
   (a) are exceedingly rare
   (b) are associated with type 1 diabetes
   (c) occur in about 1 in 500 live births
   (d) are related to surface defects in high-density lipoprotein protein moiety
   (e) can be treated with diet in most cases

8. Regression/arrest of atherosclerotic lesions occurs
   (a) only in experimental animals
   (b) by loss of fibrous plaque proteins
   (c) by maintaining cholesterol levels between 200 and 250 mg/dL
   (d) by lipid egress from plaques
   (e) by stress reduction using meditation

9. "Undesirable" changes in plaques include all of the following except
   (a) fibrous tissue transformation
   (b) macrophage infiltration of the cap
   (c) cytokine production by monocytes
   (d) leakage of blood products into the core
   (e) adventitial lymphocyte infiltration

10. Currently accepted clinical management includes all of the following except
    (a) lipid reduction
    (b) smoking cessation
    (c) programmed exercise
    (d) macrolide antibiotics
    (e) control of diabetes

Answers

| 1. e | 2. b | 3. a | 4. c | 5. e | 6. b | 7. c | 8. d | 9. a | 10. d |

7

Hemodynamic Factors in Atherosclerosis

Christopher K. Zarins and Charles A. Taylor

Atherosclerosis is a degenerative process of the artery wall with well-recognized systemic risk factors such as hyperlipidemia, hypertension, and cigarette smoking. However, many individuals at high risk for atherosclerosis are free of significant plaque formation, whereas others with no recognized risk factors develop extensive lesions. Furthermore, morbidity and mortality usually result from localized plaque deposition rather than diffuse disease. Certain vessels, such as the abdominal aorta, carotid arteries, coronary arteries, and peripheral arteries, are particularly susceptible to plaque formation, whereas others, such as upper extremity vessels, are rarely involved. Even in susceptible arteries, plaque deposition is focal. The distal internal carotid is almost always free of disease despite marked atherosclerosis in the adjacent carotid bifurcation.

Several hypotheses have been proposed to account for the unique and focal pattern of atherosclerotic plaque formation. The knowledge that blood flow exerts stresses on vessel walls and affects mass transport to arterial tissue has led to the hypothesis that fluid dynamic forces are localizing factors in atherogenesis. Differences in local susceptibility and reactivity of the artery wall may also play a significant role. The purpose of this chapter is to examine both hemodynamic and artery wall factors that may determine the focal nature of plaque deposition and to consider the specific conditions that promote atherosclerosis in several highly vulnerable sites in the arterial tree.

HEMODYNAMIC FACTORS IN PLAQUE LOCALIZATION

Blood does not flow uniformly in the arterial tree because of variations in geometric configuration and resistance to flow. Differing lumen diameters, curvatures, branchings, and angles produce local disturbances in the primary flow field, resulting in regions of altered shear stress and boundary conditions with areas of separation, secondary flow patterns, and turbulence. Characterization of these conditions at specific sites becomes much more complex when the pulsatile nature of blood flow is taken into consideration. Branch points are known to be particularly vulnerable to plaque formation and are subject to wide variation in hemodynamic conditions. Thus, it is not surprising that a wide variety of hemodynamic factors have been implicated in plaque pathogenesis, including high and low wall shear stress, flow separation and stasis, oscillation of flow, turbulence, and hypertension.[1]

Wall Shear Stress

Wall shear stress (π_w) in arteries is the tangential drag force produced by blood moving across the endothelial surface. It can be approximated by the Hagen-Poiseuille formula:

$$\pi_w = \frac{4\,\mu Q}{\pi r^3}$$

where μ = viscosity of blood, Q = blood flow, and r = radius. Wall shear stress is a function of the velocity gradient of blood near the endothelial surface and is directly proportional to blood flow and blood viscosity and inversely proportional to the cube of the vessel radius. Thus, for a given flow rate, a small change in vessel radius has a large effect on wall shear stress.

High Shear Stress

High shear stress has been thought to potentiate plaque formation by producing endothelial injury and disruption, thereby exposing the underlying artery wall to circulating platelets and lipids.[2, 3] Areas of high shear stress can be produced in the aorta of experimental animals by constricting the lumen. This reduces radius and increases flow velocity and results in marked elevations in wall shear. In 1968, Fry[4] constricted the canine aorta with a mechanical intraluminal device and increased wall shear stress to ap-

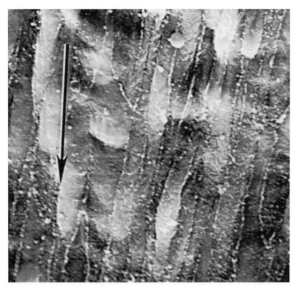

Figure 7–1. Scanning electron micrograph of endothelial surface of a coarctate monkey aorta. Six months after coarctation, there was a 70% lumen stenosis, a 15 mm Hg pressure gradient, and high-flow velocity and shear stress within the coarctation channel. The endothelial surface in the center of the coarctation channel, as well as elsewhere in the aorta, was intact, with no evidence of endothelial disruption or damage. Direction of blood flow is indicated (arrow). (From Zarins CK, Bomberger RA, Glagov S: Local effects of stenosis: Increased flow velocity inhibits atherogenesis. Circulation 64[Suppl II]:II–221, 1981.)

proximately 400 dynes/cm². This represented a 20-fold increase above the normal level of 15 to 20 dynes/cm²,[5] and resulted in endothelial damage and an increase in endothelial permeability. Other studies reported the in vivo finding of damaged and disrupted endothelial cells in high shear stress areas such as aortic ostial flow dividers.[6] To-

gether, these findings were taken as evidence that high shear stress was an initiating factor in atherogenesis.

It is now recognized that the reported in vivo endothelial abnormalities were due to experimental artifacts and that under normal circumstances there is no morphologic evidence of endothelial denudation or disruption either in high or low shear areas in the arterial tree.[7] Furthermore, when shear stress was elevated by aortic coarctation and studied after 10 days to 9 months rather than acutely, there was no evidence of endothelial damage or denudation in the high shear coarctation channel[8] (Fig. 7–1). Thus, if endothelial damage occurred acutely as a result of very high shear, it healed rapidly with no scarring or residual intimal thickening. Specific injury to the endothelium and aortic wall by clamping and suturing to produce a constriction also healed without evidence of endothelial abnormality or intimal thickening in the high shear stress area (Fig. 7–2).

The relationship between high shear stress and plaque formation has been studied in monkeys with aortic coarctation that were fed an atherogenic diet. Extensive intimal plaques formed in the aorta proximal to the coarctation, but within the high shear stress coarctation channel, plaque formation was inhibited[8] (Fig. 7–3). Thus, there is no evidence that high shear stress results in endothelial damage, and rather than promoting plaque formation, high shear appears to inhibit plaque deposition.[9] Such a feedback inhibition may serve to limit the rate of plaque deposition in developing stenoses, which produce local elevations in wall shear stress.

Low Shear Stress

The earliest atherosclerotic lesions in experimental atherosclerosis develop at the upstream rims of aortic ostia, which

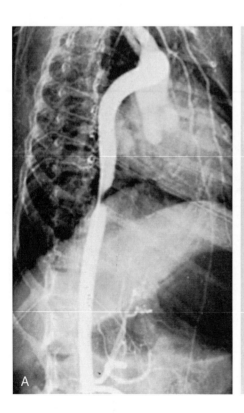

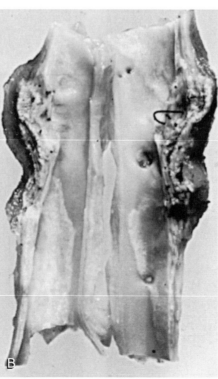

Figure 7–2. Coarctation of aorta in a monkey fed an atherogenic diet for 6 months. The coarctation was produced by suture and is demonstrated by angiography (A). The excised coarcted aortic segment (B) reveals that the prior arterial wall injury has healed fully, and there is no evidence of endothelial disruption or plaque formation within the stenosis. Intimal plaque formed proximal and distal to the stenosis, suggesting that plaque formation was inhibited in the narrowed high shear stress area. (From Zarins CK, Bomberger RA, Glagov S: Local effects of stenosis: Increased flow velocity inhibits atherogenesis. Circulation 64[Suppl II]:II–221, 1981.)

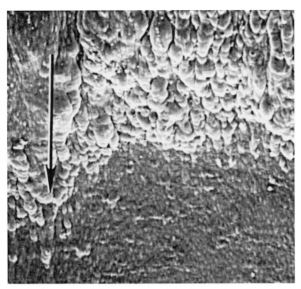

Figure 7–3. Scanning electron micrograph of intimal surface of coarctation channel of a monkey fed an atherogenic diet. Note the abrupt cessation of intimal plaque at the entry into the stenotic area *(arrow)*. The inhibition of plaque formation coincides with the area of increased shear stress. (From Zarins CK, Bomberger RA, Glagov S: Local effects of stenosis: Increased flow velocity inhibits atherogenesis. Circulation 64[Suppl II]:II–221, 1981.)

sinus (Fig. 7–5). Flow visualization and computational fluid dynamics studies demonstrate that as flow from the common carotid artery enters the bifurcation, flow streamlines are compressed toward the flow divider and inner wall of the internal carotid artery, where flow is rapid and laminar and shear stress is high (Fig. 7–6). Plaques do not form in this area. Along the outer wall of the sinus, a large area of flow separation develops in which flow velocity and shear stress are low. The earliest intimal plaques develop in this region, as do late, complicated, and clinically significant lesions.[13] In the region of flow separation, there is a reversal of axial flow and slow fluid movement upstream. However, the region of separation is not simply a zone of stasis and recirculation but is a zone of complex secondary flow patterns, including counterrotating helical trajectories (Fig. 7–7). Flow reattaches distally in the sinus, and the distal internal carotid, which is almost always free of plaque, has relatively rapid axial flow throughout its cross-section.

Particles of dye are carried rapidly along the inner wall but are cleared very slowly from the outer region of flow separation and low flow velocity. Particles in the region of flow separation have an *increased residence time* and would have greater opportunity to interact with the vessel wall. Time-dependent lipid particle–vessel wall interactions

are regions of low shear stress. Similar plaque localization has been noted in humans (Fig. 7–4), and Caro and associates[10] have suggested that low wall shear rates may retard the mass transport of atherogenic substances away from the wall, resulting in increased intimal accumulation of lipids. In addition, low shear stress may interfere with turnover at the endothelial surface of substances essential both to artery wall nutrition and to the maintenance of optimal endothelial metabolic function.[11]

Correlative studies of plaque localization in the human carotid bifurcation with quantitative model flow studies have shown that intimal plaques form in the low shear stress region of the carotid sinus opposite the flow divider and not in the high shear stress region along the inner wall of the internal carotid artery.[12, 13] Shear stress values of zero and below were recorded in the region most likely to develop plaque,[13] and it has been suggested that a threshold value below which plaque deposition occurs may exist.[12] Similar quantitative correlative studies of the human aortic bifurcation have also shown that plaques localize in regions of low shear stress rather than high shear stress.[14]

Flow Field Changes

A number of flow field alterations other than shear stress changes occur at branch points and have been implicated in plaque localization.[5] These changes are particularly prominent in the carotid bifurcation because of the presence of the carotid sinus and may account for the marked vulnerability of this site to atherosclerosis. The carotid sinus has twice the cross-sectional area of the distal internal carotid artery and this, together with the effects of branching and angulation, results in a large area of *flow separation and stasis* along the outer wall of the carotid

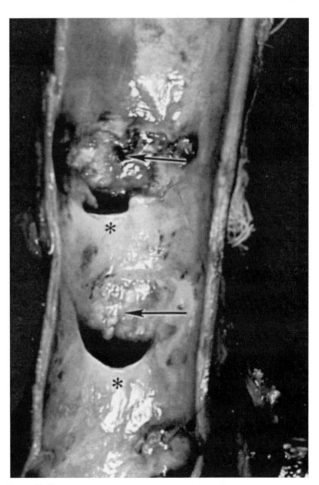

Figure 7–4. Human aorta demonstrating plaque deposition at upstream rim of celiac and superior mesenteric ostia *(arrows)*. These are areas of low shear stress. The flow divider *(asterisks)* is exposed to high shear stress and is free of plaque.

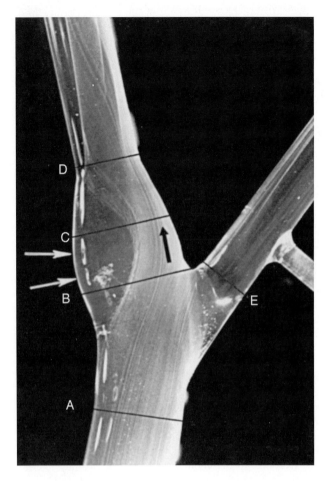

Figure 7–5. Hydrogen bubble flow visualization studies in a glass model human carotid bifurcation under steady flow conditions. Flow is rapid, laminar, and longitudinal along the inner wall of the carotid sinus *(black arrow)*. Along the outer wall, there is a large area of flow separation *(white arrows)*. A–E, Refer to tissue sections taken in a corresponding human carotid bifurcation that demonstrated that early intimal plaques formed in the area of flow separation. (From Zarins CK, Giddens DP, Bharadvaj BK, et al: Carotid bifurcation atherosclerosis: Quantitative correlation of plaque localization with flow velocity profiles and wall shear stress. Circ Res 53:502, 1983.)

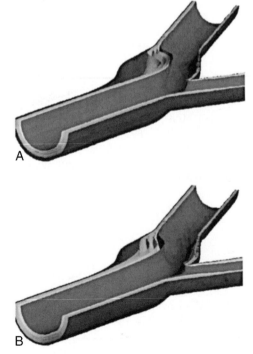

Figure 7–6. Surfaces of constant velocity magnitude for pulsatile flow in a carotid artery model calculated using Computational Fluid Dynamics at *A*, peak systole and *B*, mid-diastole. Surfaces depict range from 0 cm/sec along the vessel wall to 20 cm/sec in the vessel interior in increments of 5 cm/sec. Half of the model is removed for visualization purposes. The maximum value of velocity magnitude is approximately 60 cm/sec in the carotid artery, so a surface of 5 cm/sec represents relatively slow blood flow. Note that along the outer wall of the carotid sinus region, there is a large separation between the zero velocity surface, representing the vessel wall, and the 5 cm/sec surface. This separation corresponds to a low-velocity region and is observed at all times during the cardiac cycle. Also note that the flow surfaces are close together along the inner wall of the bifurcation near the flow divider, as well as in the proximal common carotid and distal internal carotid arteries, corresponding to steep gradients of velocity and high shear stress. (From Taylor CA, Hughes TJR, Zarins CK: Computational investigations in vascular disease. Comp Phys 10:224, 1996.)

During early systole, the region of flow separation disappears with forward flow throughout the cross-sectional area of the sinus. During late systole, however, the region of separation and flow reversal becomes prominent along the outer wall, and there is a reversal in the shear stress directional vector.[18] During diastole, conditions are similar to those seen under steady flow conditions. The magnitudes of velocity and shear are low in this region and correlate strongly with plaque localization. Alternating positive and negative shear stress vectors (oscillations) along the outer wall of the carotid sinus have also been shown to correlate strongly with early plaque deposition.[12]

Particle tracking studies reveal *increased residence time* along the outer wall, which is caused by oscillation of fluid velocity about a mean value close to zero. This delays the convection of fluid and traps fluid elements near the outer wall for several cycles despite the absence of a clear region of stasis or of an area of permanent boundary layer separation (Fig. 7–9). Increased residence time increases the duration of exposure of the lumen surface to circulating atherogenic agents and favors time-dependent transendothelial diffusion as well as intimal entrapment of atherogenic particles.[1]

Thus, variations in shear stress direction associated with pulsatile flow may lead to increased endothelial permeability, whereas even relatively high shear stresses that remain unidirectional may not be injurious.[19] The oscillating shear stress pattern may cause an increased ingress of plasma constituents through the endothelial monolayer by effects on the stability of intercellular junctions. Endothelial cells normally align in the direction of flow[20, 21] in an overlapping arrangement. Changing shear stress may cause cyclic shifts in the relationship between shear stress direction and the orientation of intercellular overlapping borders. This hypothesis agrees well with reports of increased permeability of cultured, confluent endothelial cells subjected to changes in shear stress[22] and increased Evans blue dye

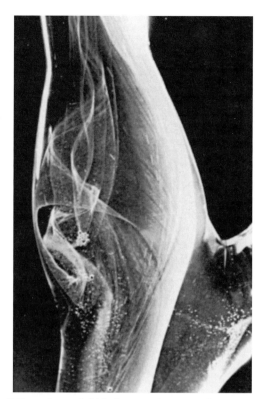

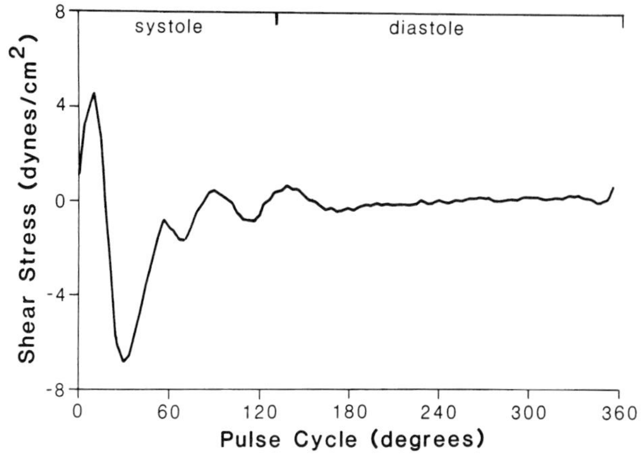

Figure 7–7. Hydrogen bubble flow visualization study in a glass model human carotid bifurcation demonstrating complex helical flow patterns within the area of flow separation. There is a reversal of axial flow, slow fluid movement upstream, and increased fluid residence time. (From Zarins CK, Giddens DP, Bharadvaj BK, et al: Carotid bifurcation atherosclerosis: Quantitative correlation of plaque localization with flow velocity profiles and wall shear stress. Circ Res 53:502, 1983.)

would thus be facilitated in the slow flow region, making it more likely for plaque formation to occur. In addition, blood-borne cellular elements that may play a role in atherogenesis are likely to have an increased probability of deposition or adhesion to the vessel wall in regions of increased residence time.[15] Flow separation has been shown to favor deposition of platelets in vitro,[16] which may stimulate cell proliferation and induce intimal thickening and plaque formation. Radiographic and ultrasound studies have confirmed the presence of flow separation and stasis in patients in this outer wall region of the carotid bifurcation.[17] Not only do early plaques localize in this region but extensive, complicated, stenotic, and ulcerated lesions have the same pattern of distribution along the outer wall of the carotid sinus.

Oscillation of Flow

Under conditions of *pulsatile flow*, the flow field considerations are more complex. Conditions along the inner wall of the carotid sinus are similar to those seen under steady flow conditions.[18] Flow velocity and shear stress are high, and flow remains laminar. There are fluctuations in magnitude of velocity and shear but no change in velocity or shear stress direction.

Along the outer wall, where plaque forms, pulsatile flow produces an *oscillating shear stress* pattern (Fig. 7–8).

Figure 7–8. Wall shear stress along the outer wall of the carotid sinus measured in a glass model human carotid bifurcation under conditions of pulsatile flow. Wall shear stress oscillates from positive to negative values during systole but has very little oscillation during diastole. Shear stress oscillation occurs in areas of the carotid sinus in which there is intimal plaque deposition. (From Ku DN, Giddens DP, Zarins CK, et al: Pulsatile flow and atherosclerosis in the human carotid bifurcation: Positive correlation between plaque location and low and oscillating shear stress. Arterioscler Thromb Vasc Biol 5:293, 1985.)

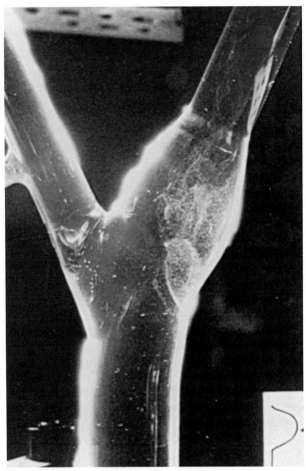

Figure 7–9. Hydrogen bubble flow visualization study under conditions of pulsatile flow demonstrating persistence of bubbles in the region of flow separation. The bubbles have remained for two pulse cycles after clearance of the mainstream bubbles, indicating increased residence time of fluid elements in the region of the outer sinus wall where plaques form. (From Ku DN, Giddens DP: Pulsatile flow in a model carotid bifurcation. Arteriosclerosis 3:31, 1983.)

staining in relation to differences in endothelial organization[23] that may be attributable to changing flow patterns.

Since oscillation of shear stress direction is a systolic event, the number of such oscillations is directly related to the number of systoles, or heart rate. *Heart rate* has been implicated as an independent risk factor in coronary atherosclerosis and is discussed further in the section dealing with the coronary arteries.

Turbulence

Turbulence implies random movement of elements in a flow field. Blood flow turbulence depends on blood flow velocity, artery diameter, and blood viscosity. Extreme or abrupt changes in geometry due to intraluminal projections, severe stenoses, or other obstacles in the flow stream can cause focal turbulence.[24] Although turbulent flow has often been implicated as a factor in plaque pathogenesis,[25, 26] both experimental atherosclerosis studies and in vitro observations in the model carotid bifurcation fail to support this suggestion.

Flow field disturbances such as flow separation, recirculation, and vortex formation may occur in various regions of the arterial tree under normal and abnormal conditions. However, turbulence does not develop in the absence of abnormal geometry such as stenoses or shunts. Experimentally induced arteriovenous anastomoses,[27] stenoses,[28, 29] or aneurysms[30] can produce intimal thickenings with some features of atherosclerosis. However, regions immediately distal to severe stenoses, where significant turbulence has been demonstrated,[31, 32] are free of atherosclerotic lesions.[33–35]

In the human carotid bifurcation, in the region where plaques form, although there is a zone of complex secondary and tertiary flow patterns (including counterrotating helical trajectories [see Fig. 7–7]), there is no turbulence.[36] This is true under a wide range of Reynolds numbers and flow conditions, including both steady and pulsatile flow. Furthermore, in vivo noninvasive pulsed Doppler ultrasound studies of carotid arteries in normal human subjects do not exhibit turbulence.[37] Thus, although it is clear that strong secondary flow patterns exist in the normal carotid bifurcation in areas of early plaque formation, turbulence does not. Turbulence may develop late, however, as a result of severe carotid stenosis and thus would be a result, rather than a cause, of atherosclerotic plaques.

Hypertension

Postmortem studies have revealed that hypertension is associated with an increase in both the extent and severity of atherosclerosis.[38] Numerous epidemiologic studies have identified hypertension as an important risk factor for the development of clinical complications of atherosclerosis, such as myocardial infarction and stroke.[39–41] Yet, clinical data comparing the development of myocardial infarction or stroke in persons with and without control of mild to moderate hypertension revealed no significant difference, suggesting that other factors, possibly interacting with hypertension, may be important.[42]

Thus, the effects of hypertension may be different in different portions of the arterial tree as a result of other local hemodynamic variables. It is well known, for example, that hypertension is a more important factor in cerebrovascular disease and stroke than in coronary artery or peripheral occlusive disease.[40] The occurrence of severe atherosclerosis in clinically normotensive individuals and the sparing of vessels distal to stenoses, even in the presence of elevated blood pressure, indicate that although hypertension may potentiate or enhance atherogenesis, it may not be in itself a necessary atherogenic factor.

Experimentally, hypertension has been implicated as an important etiologic factor in plaque pathogenesis.[43] When hypertension was induced by midthoracic aortic coarctation in atherosclerotic primates, there was increased plaque deposition in the aorta proximal to the coarctation.[44, 45] However, other hemodynamic conditions also existed in the region proximal to the coarctation, including decreased flow velocity, decreased shear stress, increased pulse pressure and wall motion, and increased wall tension. In the aorta distal to the coarctation, mean blood pressure was also elevated because of the presence of renovascular hy-

TABLE 7–1

Effect of Coarctation on Atherosclerosis in Cynomolgus Monkeys

STENOSIS	PROXIMAL AORTA		DISTAL AORTA	
	No Stenosis	70% Stenosis	No Stenosis	70% Stenosis
Surface atherosclerosis (%)	56.0 ± 7.0	74.0 ± 8.0	54.0 ± 9.0	12.0 ± 4.0°
Mural cholesterol (mg/mm²)	9.1 ± 4.1	9.7 ± 1.7	4.6 ± 0.8	2.1 ± 0.6°
DNA content (mg/mm²)	0.77 ± 0.07	0.75 ± 0.10	0.50 ± 0.07	0.23 ± 0.03°
Collagen content (mg/mm²)	23.0 ± 3.0	27.0 ± 1.0	22.0 ± 2.0	15.0 ± 2.0°
Elastin content (mg/mm²)	42.0 ± 2.0	56.0 ± 5.0°	29.0 ± 1.0	29.0 ± 6.0°

° Statistically significantly different.
Adapted from Bomberger RA, Zarins CK, Taylor KE, et al: Effect of hypotension on atherogenesis and aortic wall composition. J Surg Res 28:402–409, 1980.

pertension, but plaque deposition in the distal aorta was almost entirely absent[35] (Table 7–1). Inhibition of plaque deposition, despite the presence of hypertension and marked hyperlipidemia, was associated with decreased pulse pressure,[8, 35] decreased wall motion,[46] and decreased arterial wall metabolism.[47] Hypertension enhanced experimental plaque formation but inhibited plaque regression[48] and enhanced plaque progression,[49] despite reduction of hypercholesterolemia. These observations suggest that factors other than blood pressure per se may be of primary importance in atherogenesis. Thus, although hypertension is important in the clinical complication of atherosclerosis, the nature of its role in plaque pathogenesis remains unclear.

ARTERY WALL SUSCEPTIBILITY

In addition to the interaction of intraluminal hemodynamic conditions with the systemic and lipid environment, local susceptibility and responses of the artery wall are important in the development of atherosclerotic lesions. The artery wall is composed of the intima, which is covered on the luminal surface by a monolayer of endothelial cells; the media, which contains smooth muscle cells, collagen, and elastin; and the adventitia, which contains a network of vasa vasorum.

Endothelial Injury

Endothelial injury and the response to endothelial injury have been implicated in plaque pathogenesis. According to this hypothesis[50] the endothelial lining of arteries is damaged by one of several factors, including mechanical forces such as shear stress and hypertension, chemical agents such as hyperlipidemia or homocysteine, immunologic reactions, or hormonal dysfunction. The injury hypothesis also encompasses the response to such injury, including platelet deposition, release of platelet-derived growth factor, leukocyte adhesion and diapedesis, cellular proliferation, and lipid deposition.[51–53] Focal, repeated endothelial injury would account for the localized nature of plaque deposition.

Although widely quoted, direct evidence for this hypoth-

esis is lacking. There is no in vivo evidence of spontaneous endothelial injury or disruption, with or without platelet adherence, in areas at risk for future lesion development.[54, 55] In addition, there is no direct evidence that experimentally induced endothelial damage or removal results in eventual sustained lesion formation.[7] On the contrary, evidence has been advanced that the formation of experimental intimal plaques may require the presence of a continuous endothelial covering.[7, 54] Moreover, the role of platelets in atherogenesis remains unclear, and platelet-derived growth factor has now been isolated from tissue other than platelets.[56] Previous studies have been aimed at the examination of functional alterations in intact endothelium.[57–59] Activated endothelial cells become permeable to low-density lipoprotein (LDL), have higher replication rates, and develop prothrombotic properties. They express surface glycoproteins that promote the adhesion of neutrophils, monocytes, and platelets. Activated endothelium also promotes the transition of smooth muscle cells from the contractile to the synthetic phenotype, which promotes smooth muscle cell proliferation and cholesterol accumulation.[59] Thus, although mechanical endothelial injury is unlikely to be a significant contributing factor to plaque initiation, endothelial cell function plays an important role in the responses and functions of the artery wall.

Medial Functional State and Metabolism

The functional state of the media appears to be important in plaque pathogenesis. Under conditions in which there is increased pulse pressure, increased wall motion, and increased wall tension, such as exist proximal to aortic coarctation, there is smooth muscle cell proliferation, increased biosynthetic activity, and plaque formation.[35] Similar increases in metabolic activity of medial smooth muscle cells can be demonstrated in vitro.[60] Cyclic stretching of elastin membranes on which were grown smooth muscle cells resulted in increased biosynthesis of collagen, hyaluronate, and chondroitin 6-sulfate.[61] Thus, plaques form readily in areas where medial smooth muscle cells are metabolically active.

Conversely, distal to severe aortic coarctations, despite an increase in mean pressure, pulse pressure is decreased and aortic wall motion is diminished.[46] This is accompanied by atrophy of the media with loss of smooth muscle cells and a significant reduction in DNA content[35] (see Table 7–1). Metabolic function is diminished, with decreased glycolysis[47] and decreased collagen synthesis. Under these conditions, intimal plaque does not form despite a high mean blood pressure and marked hypercholesterolemia, with total serum cholesterol levels of 700 to 900 mg/dL.

Further evidence for the importance of the media in plaque formation can be found in the healing of arterial injuries in the presence of marked hypercholesterolemia. Standard, focal, transmural necrotizing injuries were produced in hypercholesterolemic rabbits. Despite endothelial sloughing at the time of injury, the endothelium was completely regenerated after 4 days. After 30 days, however, in many instances the media had not healed. Those injury sites with a healed, intact media developed intimal thickening at the site of injury. However, those in which the media failed to heal and became atrophic had no intimal thickening but rather became aneurysmal.[62] These observations suggest that an intact, metabolically active media is necessary for intimal plaque formation.

ARTERY WALL ADAPTATION

Artery walls can adapt to enlarging intimal plaques by dilating to maintain a normal lumen diameter. Hemodynamic forces appear to be important in this adaptation.[63] Vessels in high-flow positions, such as arteries feeding an arteriovenous fistula,[64] autogenous aortorenal bypass grafts,[65] and collateral arteries carrying increased flow around an obstruction, tend to enlarge. Conversely, lumen diameter is reduced in arteries with low flow, distal to arteriovenous fistulas, in arteries supplying atrophic or amputated extremities, or in vascular bypass grafts that are too large in relationship to the runoff bed.

Arteries proximal to a chronic arteriovenous fistula have markedly increased blood flow and flow velocity. However, there is no increase in wall shear stress due to artery dilatation and increase in lumen radius.[66, 67] Kamiya and Togawa[68] have suggested that shear stress acts to regulate lumen diameter through an alteration in protein flux in the artery wall. Guyton and Hartley[69] have suggested that arteries dilate as a result of an increase in flow pulsatility and peak velocity, which are sensed by endothelial cells and signaled to medial smooth muscle cells. The response appears to be dependent on the presence of an intact endothelial surface[70] and may be mediated through endothelial-derived vasoactive agents.

Atherosclerotic Artery Enlargement

In experimental diet-induced atherosclerosis in monkeys, coronary arteries[71] and carotid arteries[72] have been noted to enlarge as intimal plaques increase in size. Atherosclerotic artery enlargement has also been demonstrated in human coronary,[73, 74] carotid, and superficial femoral arteries,[75] as well as in the abdominal aorta. Artery enlargement can compensate for the enlarging intimal plaque and prevent lumen encroachment or stenosis[73] (Fig. 7–10). However, this compensatory mechanism appears to be effective in preventing stenosis for relatively small plaques that occupy less than 40% of internal elastic lamina cross-sectional area.[73] Larger plaques result in lumen encroachment and stenosis. Compensatory enlargement in response to intimal plaques can be excessive in certain arterial segments, resulting in a larger than normal caliber.[74] This may predispose to aneurysmal enlargement. Thus, the development of stenosis may be a balance between plaque deposition on the one hand (which tends to narrow the lumen) and artery enlargement on the other (which can maintain a normal lumen caliber or predispose to aneurysm formation). Hemodynamic forces may play a role in the size regulation of atherosclerotic arteries through normal endothelial-dependent artery wall responses or through direct effects of the plaque on the underlying artery wall.

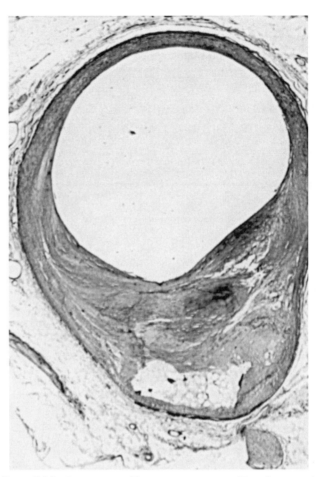

Figure 7–10. Cross-section of human coronary artery. Note the eccentric plaque deposition, oval contour of the external surface of the artery, and relatively rounded contour of the lumen. Arteries with enlarging intimal plaques tend to enlarge to maintain lumen diameter. This adaptive response of the artery wall is important in maintaining lumen patency.

PLAQUE LOCALIZATION

Carotid Bifurcation

Carotid bifurcation atherosclerosis occurs primarily along the outer wall of the internal carotid artery in the area of the carotid sinus. This has been noted on postmortem specimens,[76, 77] on angiograms of patients with severe carotid stenosis,[78] in carotid bifurcation plaques removed during carotid endarterectomy,[76, 79] and in experimental carotid plaques.[72] Angiographic studies in patients have demonstrated static zones and boundary layer separation at the outer wall of the carotid sinus in the region where plaques form,[17] and Doppler spectrum analyses have confirmed flow separation and stasis in this area of the carotid bifurcation in patients.[40] Quantitative correlative studies demonstrate that the earliest carotid plaques form in the area subjected to low shear stress, oscillating shear stress, flow separation, and flow stasis.[12, 13] Late, complex lesions and ulcerations also occur in this region, and it is possible that the hemodynamic conditions may promote not only plaque formation but also plaque complication, ulceration, and thrombosis (Fig. 7–11).

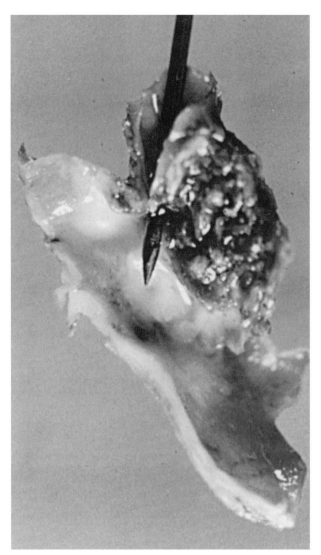

Figure 7–11. Sagittal section of plaque removed during carotid endarterectomy. Probe is in the lumen of the internal carotid artery. Note prominent complex plaque along the outer wall of the carotid sinus. This is the same region in which flow separation, low shear stress, and oscillation of shear stress occurred in model flow studies (see Figs. 7–5 through 7–9).

Coronary Arteries

The pattern of plaque localization in human coronary arteries is similar to that seen at the carotid bifurcation, because plaques tend to localize preferentially in the left anterior descending coronary artery just distal to the major proximal branch point.[80] This is a region of low flow velocity and low and oscillating wall shear stress opposite the flow divider.[81] If oscillation of shear stress direction, which occurs mainly during systole, is a major factor in plaque localization, coronary arteries may be at greater risk than other systemic arteries, because the coronary arteries are subjected to two systolic episodes and one diastolic episode of flow acceleration and deceleration during each cardiac cycle. Coronary arterial flow decreases initially in systole during the isovolumetric contraction and rapid ejection phases, increases briefly when peak systolic aortic pressure exceeds intracoronary pressure, and decreases again during

the remainder of systole as intramyocardial pressure increases the resistance to flow.[82] Flow reversal during systole has been demonstrated with tachycardia and in concentric left ventricular hypertrophy. During isovolumetric relaxation, as intramyocardial and intraventricular pressures decline, coronary flow accelerates rapidly, then decreases slowly as aortic pressure falls and intraventricular pressure builds again late in diastole.

If other determinants of coronary flow are held constant, net coronary flow is directly proportional to heart rate.[83] Conversely, the diastolic time interval is inversely related to heart rate.[84] As heart rate increases, the time spent in diastole when flow is greatest decreases markedly. Because phasic fluctuation in coronary flow is predominantly a systolic occurrence, both the frequency and magnitude of oscillations in shear stress direction should be directly dependent on heart rate. Thus, the frequent preferential localization of plaques in the coronary arteries compared with the renal or other peripheral arteries may be related to the fact that the coronary arteries experience at least twice as many oscillations of flow velocity over time as other major arteries. Thus, during a 1-year period, a resting heart rate of 80 results in 10.5 million more systoles than a resting heart rate of 60, emphasizing the remarkable cumulative effect of a modest change in heart rate on flow conditions in the coronary arteries.

To test the hypothesis that heart rate is an important risk factor in coronary atherosclerosis, we produced sinoatrial node ablation in cynomolgus monkeys. This resulted in a 20% reduction in mean heart rate and a reduction in the magnitude of heart rate fluctuation. After 6 months on an atherogenic diet, animals with a low heart rate had a 50% reduction in intimal plaque area, a 50% reduction in maximum lesion size, and a 50% reduction in percentage stenosis.[85] Similarly, there was a significant reduction in carotid bifurcation atherosclerosis.[72] Thus, heart rate reduction had a protective effect on both coronary and carotid atherosclerosis in monkeys.

Heart rate has also been directly implicated as an independent risk factor in human coronary atherosclerosis. A number of major prospective clinical studies have found high heart rates in men at rest to be predictive of future manifestations of coronary heart disease.[86, 87] Conversely, low heart rates are thought to protect against the development of coronary atherosclerosis.[88] Although increased resting heart rate seems to correlate significantly with an atherogenic lipid profile in sedentary men, suggesting a possible metabolic pathway for the effect of heart rate on coronary artery disease,[89] both theoretical and experimental evidence suggests that hemodynamic factors associated with cyclic myocardial contraction predispose the coronary arteries selectively to atherosclerosis. Hemodynamic factors such as hypertension, altered shear stress, and flow disturbances have also been implicated in plaque localization and progression in several locations in the coronary arteries,[19] but a selective effect in the coronary tree has not been emphasized.

Abdominal Aorta

Human and experimental atherosclerotic lesions are prone to localize in regions of the arterial tree exposed to relatively low flow rates. The human abdominal aorta may be particularly vulnerable to early and rapid development of atherosclerosis because of relatively low flow velocities compared with the remainder of the aorta. One fourth of the cardiac output is delivered to the renal arteries at rest.[90] Renal artery flow, together with celiac and superior mesenteric artery flow, thus ensures a relatively constant high-volume flow through the proximal aorta. In contrast, the volume of flow in the aorta below the renal arteries is greatly dependent on the muscular activity of lower extremities. The infrarenal abdominal aorta may be the appropriate size for a physically active bipedal existence, but with an increasingly sedentary lifestyle, the infrarenal human abdominal aorta may be subjected to relatively slower flow velocities than the suprarenal aorta during a major portion of the day. This effect may be further accentuated by the tendency of the aorta to dilate with age. Thus, a slower flow pattern in the abdominal aorta may tend to favor intimal proliferation and the ingress of lipids, with the formation of atherosclerotic plaques. It is hypothesized that the beneficial effect of exercise in retarding the progression of cardiovascular disease is due, at least in part, to the elimination of adverse hemodynamic conditions, including high particle residence time and low wall shear stress.

Model flow[91] and computational fluid dynamics[92, 93] studies of the aorta have provided qualitative information on abdominal aorta hemodynamics and confirm that under resting and postprandial conditions, the infrarenal aorta experiences velocity direction oscillation, vortex formation, and increased fluid residence time, whereas the suprarenal aorta has laminar flow. Recent computational fluid dynamics investigations to quantify hemodynamic conditions in the abdominal aorta demonstrate that under resting conditions the infrarenal aorta experiences low wall shear stress and flow reversal during most of the cardiac cycle, with the effects being most pronounced during diastole. However, the complex, recirculating flow patterns present at rest disappeared under simulated moderate levels of lower limb exercise (Fig. 7–12). Mean shear stress below the level of the renal arteries was less than 1 dyne/cm² under simulated resting conditions but increased by over 400% under simulated moderate exercise conditions to values above those in the lesion-resistant suprarenal aorta. Particle residence time, defined by the time it took 90% of instantaneously released particles to clear the infrarenal aorta, was reduced by a factor of 3 under moderate exercise conditions.[92] These investigations support the body of evidence that moderate levels of exercise have a beneficial effect on limiting atherosclerosis. Further studies are needed to examine the duration of exposure to exercise conditions needed to achieve benefit.

Aneurysm Formation

Hemodynamic factors are important in both plaque localization and adaptive enlargement of atherosclerotic arteries. These processes may also play a role in aneurysm formation. The association between atherosclerosis and abdominal aortic aneurysms has long been recognized, and it is well-known that patients undergoing operation for aortic

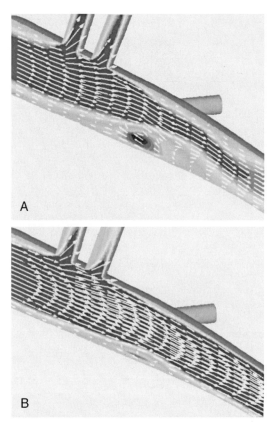

Figure 7–12. Midplane slice of an abdominal aorta computational model displaying contours of axial velocity and the velocity vector field at mid-diastole for simulated (A) resting conditions and (B) moderate exercise conditions. Note that under resting conditions, a large vortex develops along the posterior wall of the aorta. This region of flow stasis and high particle residence time disappears with moderate levels of simulated lower limb exercise, such as might be obtained with a brisk walk. (From Taylor CA, Hughes TJR, Zarins CK: Computational investigations in vascular disease. Comp Phys 10:224, 1996.)

aneurysmal disease are generally 8 to 10 years older than patients undergoing operation for aortoiliac occlusive disease. This suggests that aortic aneurysm formation may be a later stage of atherosclerotic aortic degeneration.[93] Intimal plaque formation in the aorta stimulates adaptive enlargement of the aorta and is usually associated with atrophy and degeneration of the aortic wall underlying the plaque. If plaque degeneration, ulceration, or atrophy were to subsequently develop, this would leave an enlarged thin-walled aorta prone to progressive aneurysmal enlargement. Experimental studies from our laboratory have demonstrated that aneurysms form in diet-induced atherosclerosis with prolonged atherogenic regimens associated with plaque and artery wall atrophy.[94] A controlled trial of lesion regression by lowering of serum cholesterol in experimental animals resulted in aneurysmal enlargement of the abdominal aorta.[95] These findings suggest that the interaction between the plaque and artery wall and evolution of the plaque over time may be important in the pathogenesis of aneurysms.

Alterations in blood flow in the aorta may also influence aneurysm pathogenesis by local alterations in wall shear. An increased incidence of abdominal aortic aneurysms as a very late finding in World War II amputees supports this hypothesis.[96]

POTENTIAL ROLE OF HEMODYNAMICS IN SURGICAL PLANNING

Investigations into hemodynamic factors in atherosclerosis generally use idealized models representing the average anatomy of a group of individuals. These idealized models can be modified in a systematic fashion to investigate the effect of variations in anatomy on flow conditions and are useful for quantifying hemodynamic factors in blood vessels prone to vascular disease. However, to determine the exact flow conditions in a given individual's vascular system for clinical diagnosis or surgical planning, models that more faithfully represent individual anatomic features and flow conditions are necessary.[97] Patient-specific computer models have been created by extracting anatomic information from imaging sources, including computed tomography (CT) and magnetic resonance imaging (MRI). These models are then discretized into a finite element mesh to obtain a finite number of points where the hemodynamic variables of velocity and pressure are computed from appropriate input conditions (Fig. 7–13). Adverse hemodynamic conditions, including recirculating flow, low shear stress, and high particle residence times, can be identified, and alter-

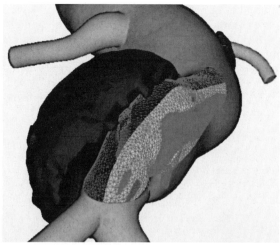

Figure 7–14. Axial component of velocity along a plane through the aortic bifurcation. A slice plane was used to remove the top of the aneurysm for visualization of the flow. The top part of the model is then redisplayed in wireframe. Also shown is the large mural thrombus along the side wall of the aneurysm. The flow decelerates as it enters the aneurysmal cavity, and a vortex develops in the anterior to posterior direction immediately proximal to the bifurcation. Reverse and stagnant flow is observed close to the wall of the aneurysm along the anterior and posterior walls of the aorta. (From Taylor CA, Hughes TJR, Zarins CK: Computational investigations in vascular disease. Comp Phys 10:224, 1996.)

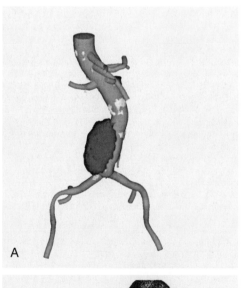

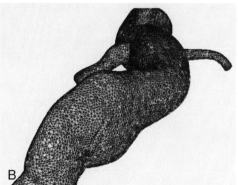

Figure 7–13. Three-dimensional reconstruction of an abdominal aorta from spiral computed tomography. *A,* Geometric model showing skin, blood flow domain, mural thrombus, and calcifications and *B,* close-up of finite element mesh in aneurysmal region used for computer simulation. (From Taylor CA, Hughes TJR, Zarins CK: Computational investigations in vascular disease. Comp Phys 10:224, 1996.)

native surgical procedures to minimize these adverse conditions can be evaluated (Fig. 7–14).

As our knowledge of the importance of hemodynamic factors in atherosclerosis increases, the possibility of using this information to improve patient care will emerge. New, predictive methods using hemodynamic computer modeling hold the potential to enable the evaluation of the long-term efficacy of surgical procedures and vascular prostheses. These new computational methods can provide a means to augment the information that can be obtained from medical imaging studies. In the coming years, surgeons could decide which procedure to perform based on not only *diagnostic* information provided by medical imaging data sources but also *predictive* physiologically based computer models using knowledge of the role of hemodynamic factors in atherosclerosis.

CLINICAL IMPLICATIONS

Clinical efforts to control systemic risk factors such as hyperlipidemia, smoking, and hypertension have been shown to be effective in limiting morbidity and mortality due to atherosclerotic plaques. Control of localizing hemodynamic factors is also possible and may be important in inhibiting plaque formation, enhancing artery wall adaptation, and, perhaps, promoting regression of established plaques. Increased cardiac output and blood flow brought on by increased flow velocity and increased wall shear stress would tend to limit plaque formation and promote artery lumen dilatation. Experimental[98] as well as clinical[88] evidence supports the beneficial effects of exercise on coronary atherosclerosis. Increased flow with exercise serves to limit flow stasis and particle residence time, thus limiting time-dependent lipid–vessel wall interaction. Significant benefit in coronary atherosclerosis can also be anticipated by reduction in heart rate by exercise,[98] modification of psychosocial stress,[99] and drug therapy. Indeed, exercise programs that improve fitness levels can result in a 44% lower risk of all causes of mortality and a 52% lower risk of cardiovascular-related mortality in men.[100] Thus, a comprehensive approach to controlling clinical complications of atherosclerosis should address not only systemic but also local factors in plaque pathogenesis.

References

1. Glagov S, Zarins CK, Giddens DP, Ku DN: Hemodynamics and atherosclerosis. Arch Pathol Lab Med 112:1018–1031, 1988.
2. Ross R, Harker L: Hyperlipidemia and atherosclerosis. Science 193:1094–1100, 1976.
3. Ross R: The pathogenesis of atherosclerosis: An update. N Engl J Med 314:488–500, 1986.
4. Fry DL: Acute vascular endothelial changes associated with increased blood velocity gradients. Circ Res 22:165–197, 1968.
5. Giddens DP, Zarins CK, Glagov S: Response of arteries to nearwall fluid dynamic behavior. Appl Mech Rev 43:S96–S102, 1990.
6. Reidy MA, Bowyer DE: Scanning electron microscopy of arteries. The morphology of aortic endothelium in haemodynamically stressed areas associated with branches. Atherosclerosis 26:181–194, 1977.
7. Reidy MA: Biology of disease: A reassessment of endothelial injury and arterial lesion formation. Lab Invest 53:513–520, 1985.
8. Zarins CK, Bomberger RA, Glagov S: Local effects of stenosis: Increased flow velocity inhibits atherogenesis. Circulation 64(Suppl 2):II-221–II-227, 1981.
9. Bassiouny HS, Lieber BB, Giddens DP, et al: Quantitative inverse correlation of wall shear stress with experimental intimal thickening. Surg Forum 39:328–330, 1988.
10. Caro CG, Fitz-Gerald JM, Schroter RC: Atheroma and arterial wall shear: Observation, correlation and proposal of a shear dependent mass transfer mechanism for atherogenesis. Proc R Soc Lond B Biol Sci 117:109–159, 1971.
11. Robertson AJ Jr: Oxygen requirements of the human arterial intima in atherogenesis. Prog Biochem Pharmacol 4:305–316, 1968.
12. Ku DN, Giddens DP, Zarins CK, et al: Pulsatile flow and atherosclerosis in the human carotid bifurcation: Positive correlation between plaque location and low and oscillating shear stress. Arterioscler Thromb Vasc Biol 5:293–302, 1985.
13. Zarins CK, Giddens DP, Bharadvaj BK, et al: Carotid bifurcation atherosclerosis: Quantitative correlation of plaque localization with flow velocity profiles and wall shear stress. Circ Res 53:502–514, 1983.
14. Friedman MH, Hutchins GM, Bargeron CB, et al: Correlation between intimal thickness and fluid shear in human arteries. Atherosclerosis 39:425–436, 1981.
15. Gerrity RG, Goss JA, Soby L: Control of monocyte recruitment by chemotactic factor(s) in lesion-prone areas of swine aorta. Arterioscler Thromb Vasc Biol 5:55–66, 1985.
16. Parmentier EM, Morton WA, Petschek HE: Platelet aggregate formation in a region of separated blood flow. Phys Fluids 20:2012–2021, 1981.
17. Fox JA, Hugh AE: Static zones in the internal carotid artery: Correlation with boundary layer separation and stasis in model flows. Br J Radiol 43:370–376, 1976.
18. Ku DN, Giddens DP: Pulsatile flow in a model carotid bifurcation. Arterioscler Thromb Vasc Biol 3:31–39, 1983.
19. Fry DL: Hemodynamic forces in atherogenesis. In Scheinberg P (ed): Cerebrovascular Disease. New York, Raven Press, 1976, pp 77–95.
20. Nerem RM, Levesque MJ, Cornhill JF: Vascular endothelial morphology as an indicator of the pattern of blood flow. J Biomech Eng 103:171–176, 1981.
21. Clark JM, Glagov S: Luminal surface of distended arteries by scanning electron microscopy. Eliminating configurational artefacts. Br J Exp Pathol 57:129–135, 1976.
22. Dewey CF, Bussolari SR, Gimbrone MA, et al: The dynamic response of vascular endothelial cells to fluid shear stress. J Biomech Eng 103:177–185, 1981.
23. Fry DL: Responses of the arterial wall to certain physical factors. Ciba Found Symp 12:93–125, 1973.
24. Giddens DP, Khalifa AMA: Turbulence measurements with pulsed Doppler ultrasound employing a frequency tracking method. Ultrasound Med Biol 8:427–437, 1982.
25. Davies PF, Remuzzi A, Gordon EJ, et al: Turbulent fluid shear stress induces vascular endothelial cell turnover in vitro. Proc Natl Acad Sci U S A 83:2114–2117, 1986.
26. Gutstein WH, Farrell GA, Armellini C: Blood flow disturbance and endothelial cell injury in pre-atherosclerotic swine. Lab Invest 29:134–149, 1973.
27. Davis PF, Stehbens WE: The biochemical composition of haemodynamically stressed vascular tissue: I. The lipid, calcium, and DNA concentration in experimental arteriovenous fistulae. Atherosclerosis 56:27–37, 1985.
28. Schneiderman G, Ellis CG, Goldstick TK: Mass transport to walls of stenosed arteries: Variation with Reynolds number and blood flow separation. J Biomech 12:869–877, 1979.
29. Subbiah MT, Kottke IA, Kottke BA, et al: Regional differences in cholesterol content of aorta in response to experimental coarctation in spontaneously atherosclerosis susceptible pigeons. Basic Res Cardiol 75:583–589, 1980.
30. Stehbens WE: Predilection of experimental arterial aneurysms for dietary-induced lipid deposition. Pathology 13:735–747, 1981.
31. Lieber BB: Ordered and random structures in Pulsatile Flow through Constricted Tubes [thesis]. Atlanta, Georgia Institute of Technology, 1985.
32. Khalifa AMA, Giddens DP: Characterization and evolution of post-stenotic flow disturbances. J Biomech 14:279–296, 1981.
33. Ku DN, Zarins CK, Giddens DP, et al: Reduced atherogenesis distal to stenosis despite turbulence and hypertension [abstract]. Circulation 74(Suppl 2):II-334, 1986.
34. Coutard M, Osborne-Pellegrin MJ: Decreased dietary lipid deposition in spontaneous lesions distal to a stenosis in the rat caudal artery. Artery 12:82–98, 1983.
35. Bomberger RA, Zarins CK, Taylor KE, Glagov S: Effect of hypotension on atherogenesis and aortic wall composition. J Surg Res 28:402–409, 1980.
36. Bharadvaj BK, Mabon RF, Giddens DP: Steady flow in a model of the human carotid bifurcation: Part II. Laser Doppler anemometer measurements. J Biomech Eng 15:363–378, 1982.
37. Ku DN, Giddens DP, Phillips DJ, et al: Hemodynamics of the normal human carotid bifurcation: In vitro and in vivo studies. Ultrasound Med Biol 11:13–26, 1985.
38. Glagov S, Rowley DA, Kohut R: Atherosclerosis of human aorta and its coronary and renal arteries. Arch Pathol Lab Med 72:558–571, 1961.
39. Chabanian AV: The influence of hypertension and other hemodynamic factors in atherogenesis. Cardiovasc Dis 26:177–196, 1983.
40. Kannel WB, Schwartz MJ, McNamara PM: Blood pressure and risk of coronary heart disease: The Framingham Study. Dis Chest 56:43–52, 1969.
41. Robertson WB, Strong JP: Atherosclerosis in persons with hypertension and diabetes mellitus. Lab Invest 18:538, 1969.
42. Medical Research Council Working Party: MCR trial of treatment of mild hypertension: Principal results. BMJ 291:97–104, 1985.
43. Breterton KN, Day AJ, Skinner SL: Hypertension-accelerated atherogenesis in cholesterol-fed rabbits. Atherosclerosis 27:79–87, 1977.
44. Bomberger RA, Zarins CK, Glagov S: Subcritical arterial stenosis enhances distal atherosclerosis. Resident Research Award. J Surg Res 30:205–212, 1981.
45. Hollander W, Madoff I, Paddock J, Kirkpatrick B: Aggravation of atherosclerosis by hypertension in a subhuman primate model with coarctation of the aorta. Circ Res 38(Suppl 2):63–72, 1976.
46. Lyon RT, Runyon-Hass A, Davis HR, et al: Protection from atherosclerotic lesion formation by reduction of artery wall motion. J Vasc Surg 5:413–420, 1987.

47. Cozzi PJ, Lyon RT, Davis HR, et al: Aortic wall metabolism in relation to susceptibility and resistance to experimental atherosclerosis. J Vasc Surg 7:706–714, 1988.

48. Zarins CK, Bomberger RA, Taylor KE, et al: Artery stenosis inhibits regression of diet-induced atherosclerosis. Surgery 88:86–92, 1980.

49. Xu C-P, Glagov S, Zatina MA, Zarins CK: Hypertension sustains plaque progression despite reduction of hypercholesterolemia. Hypertension 18:123–129, 1991.

50. Ross R, Glomset J: The pathogenesis of atherosclerosis. N Engl J Med 295:369–377, 1976.

51. Ross R: George Lyman Duff Memorial Lecture. Atherosclerosis: A problem of the biology of arterial wall cells and their interactions with blood components. Arteriosclerosis 1:293–311, 1981.

52. Ip JH, Fuster V, Badimon L, et al: Syndromes of accelerated atherosclerosis: Role of vascular injury and smooth muscle proliferation. J Am Coll Cardiol 15:1667–1687, 1990.

53. Schwartz S, Heimark R, Majesky M: Developmental mechanisms underlying pathology of arteries. Physiol Rev 70:1177–1209, 1990.

54. Zarins CK, Taylor KE, Bomberger RA, et al: Endothelial integrity at aortic ostial flow dividers. Scanning Electron Microsc 3:249–254, 1980.

55. Taylor KE, Glagov S, Zarins CK: Preservation and structural adaptation of endothelium over experimental foam cell lesions. Arterioscler Thromb Vasc Biol 9:881–894, 1989.

56. DiCorleto PE, Bowen-Pope DF: Cultured endothelial cells produce a platelet-derived growth factor-like protein. Proc Natl Acad Sci U S A 80:1919, 1983.

57. Bevilacqua MP, Pober JS, Majeau GR, et al: Interleukin 1 (IL-1) induces biosynthesis and cell surface expression of procoagulant activity in human vascular endothelial cells. J Exp Med 160:618–623, 1984.

58. Einhorn S, Eldor A, Vladavsky I, et al: Production and characterization of interferon from endothelial cells. J Cell Physiol 122:200–204, 1985.

59. Whatley R, Zimmerman G, McIntyre T, Prescott S: Lipid metabolism and signal transduction in endothelial cells. Prog Lipid Res 29:45–63, 1990.

60. Glagov S, Grande JP, Xu C-P, et al: Limited effects of hyperlipidemia on the arterial smooth muscle response to mechanical stress. J Cardiovasc Pharmacol 14(Suppl 6):S90–S97, 1989.

61. Leung DYM, Glagov S, Mathews MU: Cyclic stretching stimulates synthesis of matrix components by arterial smooth muscle cells in vitro. Science 191:475–477, 1976.

62. Bomberger RA, Zarins CK, Glagov S: Medial injury and hyperlipidemia in development of aneurysms or atherosclerotic plaques. Surg Forum 31:338–340, 1980.

63. Zarins CK: Adaptive responses of arteries. J Vasc Surg 9:382, 1989.

64. Schumacker HB Jr: Aneurysm development and degenerative changes in dilated artery proximal to arteriovenous fistula. Surg Gynecol Obstet 130:636, 1970.

65. Szilagyi DE, Elliott JP, Hagerman JH, et al: Biologic fate of autogenous vein implants as arterial substitutes. Surgery 178:232–246, 1973.

66. Zarins CK, Zatina MA, Giddens DP, et al: Shear stress regulation of artery lumen diameter in experimental atherogenesis. J Vasc Surg 5:413–420, 1987.

67. Masuda H, Bassiouny HS, Glagov S, Zarins CK: Artery wall restructuring in response to increased flow. Surg Forum 40:285–286, 1989.

68. Kamiya A, Togawa T: Adaptive regulation of wall shear stress to flow change in the canine carotid artery. Am J Physiol 239:H14–H21, 1980.

69. Guyton JH, Hartley CJ: Flow restriction of one carotid artery in juvenile rats inhibits growth of arterial diameter. Am J Physiol 248:H540–H546, 1985.

70. Langille BL, O'Donnell F: Reductions in arterial diameter produced by chronic diseases in blood flow are endothelial-dependent. Science 231:405–407, 1986.

71. Bond MD, Adams MR, Bullock BC: Complicating factor in evaluating coronary artery atherosclerosis. Artery 9:21, 1981.

72. Beere PA, Glagov S, Zarins CK: Experimental atherosclerosis at the carotid bifurcation of the cynomolgus monkey: Localization, compensatory enlargement and the sparing effect of lowered heart rate. Atheroscler Thromb Vasc Biol 12:1245–1253, 1992.

73. Glagov S, Weisenberg E, Kolettis G, et al: Compensatory enlargement of human atherosclerotic coronary arteries. N Engl J Med 316:1371–1375, 1987.

74. Zarins CK, Weisenberg E, Kolettis G, et al: Differential enlargement of artery segments in response to enlarging atherosclerotic plaques. J Vasc Surg 7:386–394, 1988.

75. Blair JM, Glagov S, Zarins CK: Mechanism of superficial femoral artery adductor canal stenosis. Surg Forum 41:359–360, 1990.

76. Imparato AM, Riles TS, Gorstein F: The carotid bifurcation plaques: Pathologic findings associated with cerebral ischemia. Stroke 10:238–245, 1979.

77. Solbert LA, Eggen DA: Localization and sequence of development of atherosclerotic lesions in the carotid and vertebral arteries. Circulation 43:711–724, 1971.

78. Bauer RB, Sheehan S, Weehsler N, et al: Arteriographic study of sites, incidence and treatment of arteriosclerotic cerebrovascular lesions. Neurology 12:698–711, 1962.

79. Bassiouny HS, Davis H, Masawa N, et al: Critical carotid stenoses: Morphologic and biochemical similarity of symptomatic and asymptomatic plaques. J Vasc Surg 9:202–212, 1989.

80. Montenegro MR, Eggen DA: Topography of atherosclerosis in the coronary arteries. Lab Invest 18:586–593, 1968.

81. Tang TD, Giddens DP, Zarins CK, Glagov S: Velocity profile and wall shear measurements in a model human coronary artery. Adv Bio Eng Am Soc Mech Eng 17:261–263, 1990.

82. Granata L, Olsson RA, Huvos A, et al: Coronary inflow and oxygen usage following cardiac sympathetic nerve stimulator in unanesthetized dogs. Circ Res 16:114, 1965.

83. Laurent D, Bolenc-Williams C, Williams FL, et al: Effects of heart rate on coronary flow and cardiac oxygen consumption. Am J Physiol 185:355–364, 1956.

84. Boudoulas H, Rittgers SE, Lewis RP, et al: Changes in diastolic time with various pharmacologic agents. Circulation 60:164–169, 1979.

85. Beere PA, Glagov S, Zarins CK: Retarding effect of lowered heart rate on coronary atherosclerosis. Science 226:180–182, 1984.

86. Schroll M, Hagerup LM: Risk factors of myocardial infarction and death in men aged 50 at entry. Dan Med Bull 24:252–255, 1977.

87. Dyer AR, Persky V, Stamler J, et al: Heart rate as a prognostic factor for coronary heart disease and mortality: Findings in three Chicago epidemiologic studies. Am J Epidemiol 112:736–749, 1980.

88. Williams PT, Wood PD, Haskell WL, Vranizan KM: The effects of running mileage and duration on plasma lipoprotein levels. JAMA 24:2674–2679, 1982.

89. Williams PT, Haskell WL, Vranizan KM, et al: Associations of resting heart rate with concentrations of lipoprotein subfractions in sedentary men. Circulation 71:441–449, 1985.

90. Guyton AC: Textbook of Medical Physiology, 2nd ed. Philadelphia, WB Saunders, 1961, p 356.

91. Ku DN, Glagov S, Moore JE Jr, Zarins CK: Flow patterns in the abdominal aorta under simulated post prandial and exercise conditions: An experimental study. J Vasc Surg 9:309–316, 1989.

92. Taylor CA, Tropea BI, Hughes TJR, Zarins CK: Effect of graded exercise on aortic wall shear stress. Surg Forum 46:331–334, 1995.

93. Zarins CK, Glagov S: Aneurysms and obstructive plaques: Differing local responses to atherosclerosis. In Bergan JV, Yoo JST (eds): Aneurysms: Diagnosis and Treatment. New York, Grune & Stratton, 1982, pp 61–82.

94. Zarins CK, Glagov S, Wissler RW, Vesselinovitch D: Aneurysm formation in experimental atherosclerosis: Relationship to plaque evolution. J Vasc Surg 12:246–256, 1990.

95. Zarins CK, Xu C-P, Glagov S: Aneurysmal enlargement of the aorta during regression of experimental atherosclerosis. J Vasc Surg 15:90–101, 1992.

96. Vollmar JF, Pauschinger P, Paes E, et al: Aortic aneurysms as late sequelae of above-knee amputation. Lancet 2:834–835, 1989.

97. Taylor CA, Hughes TJR, Zarins CK: Computational investigations in vascular disease. Comp Phys 10:224–232, 1996.

98. Kramsch D, Aspen AJ, Abramowitz BM, et al: Reduction of coronary atherosclerosis by moderate conditioning exercise in monkeys on an atherogenic diet. N Engl J Med 305:1483–1489, 1981.

99. Kaplan JR, Manuck SB, Clarkson TB, et al: Social stress and atherosclerosis in normocholesterolemic monkeys. Science 220:733–735, 1983.

100. Blair SN, Kohl HW, Barlow CE, et al: Changes in physical fitness and all-cause mortality. JAMA 273:1093–1098, 1995.

Questions

1. Wall shear stress is affected most by a change in the
   (a) viscosity of blood
   (b) flow rate
   (c) vessel radius
   (d) blood pressure
   (e) cardiac output

2. The earliest atherosclerotic lesions in experimental atherosclerosis develop
   (a) at the upstream rims of aortic ostia
   (b) in regions of high shear stress
   (c) in regions of turbulent flow
   (d) in the common carotid artery
   (e) in the renal arteries

3. Low wall shear rates
   (a) may retard the mass transport of atherogenic substances away from the wall
   (b) may result in increased intimal accumulation of lipids
   (c) may interfere with turnover at the endothelial surface of substances essential to artery wall nutrition
   (d) are observed in the carotid sinus opposite the flow divider
   (e) all of the above

4. Which of the following is false?
   (a) the carotid sinus has twice the cross-sectional area of the distal internal carotid artery
   (b) the outer wall of the carotid sinus is an area of flow separation and stasis
   (c) flow visualization studies demonstrate that flow in the carotid artery is turbulent
   (d) shear stress is low along the flow divider of the carotid artery bifurcation
   (e) all of the above

5. Pulsatile flow results in
   (a) less complex flow fields
   (b) turbulent flow along the inner wall of the carotid sinus
   (c) high shear stress along the outer wall of the carotid sinus
   (d) alternating positive and negative shear stress vectors along the outer wall of the carotid sinus
   (e) all of the above

6. Hypertension is
   (a) associated with a decrease in the severity of atherosclerosis
   (b) the primary risk factor for the development of clinical complications of atherosclerosis

   (c) the result of elevated shear stress
   (d) a more important factor in coronary artery disease than in cerebrovascular disease
   (e) an important etiologic factor in plaque pathogenesis

7. Which of the following is true?
   (a) endothelial injury is the primary factor in plaque pathogenesis
   (b) the endothelial lining of arteries is observed to be damaged in vivo by shear stress
   (c) focal, repeated endothelial injury accounts for the localized nature of plaque deposition
   (d) there is no direct evidence that experimentally induced endothelial damage or removal results in eventual sustained lesion formation
   (e) there is no evidence that the formation of experimental intimal plaques requires the presence of a continuous endothelial covering

8. The functional state of the media
   (a) appears to be important in plaque pathogenesis
   (b) is unaffected by increased pulse pressure
   (c) is unrelated to wall tension
   (d) is unimportant for plaque formation
   (e) none of the above

9. Artery walls can adapt in response to
   (a) enlarging intimal plaques
   (b) increased flow
   (c) decreased flow
   (d) hypertension
   (e) all of the above

10. The human abdominal aorta
    (a) experiences high shear stress along the posterior wall below the renal arteries
    (b) may be particularly vulnerable to early and rapid development of atherosclerosis because of relatively low flow velocities compared with the remainder of the aorta
    (c) experiences relatively minor changes in flow with lower limb exercise
    (d) flow patterns are observed to be undisturbed under resting conditions in model flow and computational fluid dynamics studies
    (e) is observed to have velocity direction oscillation, vortex formation, and increased fluid residence time in the infrarenal portion relative to the suprarenal portion

Answers

1. c   2. a   3. e   4. c   5. d   6. e   7. e   8. a   9. e   10. e

8

Nonatherosclerotic Vascular Disease

Gregory J. Landry, Ahmed M. Abou-Zamzam, Jr.,
James M. Edwards, and John M. Porter

Although the majority of arterial abnormalities occupying the interest of vascular surgeons are caused by atherosclerosis, a significant minority result from a variety of inflammatory, acquired, congenital, and developmental abnormalities. Those in the medical specialties who may be expected to be familiar with the diagnosis and treatment of these conditions generally rely on vascular surgeons for this function. The newly emerging field of vascular medicine has yet to make a significant impact on the practicing vascular surgeon. Clearly, the complete vascular surgeon must be familiar with the entire spectrum of vascular disease, not just that resulting from atherosclerosis.

This chapter briefly describes the pathogenesis, symptoms, diagnosis, and treatment of a variety of nonatherosclerotic vascular diseases. Covered topics include vasospastic disorders, the vasculitides, heritable arteriopathies, anatomic anomalies, homocysteinemia, and a variety of other uncommon disease processes that may be presented to the vascular surgeon.

VASOSPASTIC DISORDERS

Raynaud's syndrome (RS), variant angina, and migraine headache are the most frequent vasospastic disorders seen in clinical practice. RS is by far the most common vasospastic condition referred to the vascular surgeon and is considered in detail herein.

Raynaud's Syndrome

Since the initial description by Maurice Raynaud in 1862, episodic digital ischemia (RS) has remained an enigmatic clinical entity. The digital ischemia in patients with this condition is traditionally manifest as tricolor changes: white, blue, and red, although one or more of these color changes are frequently absent. The affected digits return to normal 15 to 20 minutes after removal of the precipitating stimulus (usually environmental cold or emotional stress), and, importantly, the fingers remain normal between attacks.

The prevalence of RS in the general population varies with climate and, probably, ethnic origin. In cool, damp climates such as the Pacific Northwest, Scandinavia, and Great Britain, the prevalence approaches 20% to 25%.[1] It is not known whether the lower prevalence in warm, dry climates is due to a decreased occurrence of the syndrome or merely lack of patient complaints. RS occurs in all age groups but is most frequent in young women.[2]

The mechanism of vasoconstriction in RS has been a subject of intense debate for over a century. Raynaud speculated that sympathetic nervous system hyperactivity was responsible, a position disproved by Sir Thomas Lewis, who in the 1920s demonstrated that blockade of digital nerve conduction did not prevent vasospasm.[3] Lewis then proposed the attractive theory of a "local vascular fault," the nature of which remains undefined.

In recent years, the focus in RS pathophysiology has been on alterations in peripheral adrenoceptor activity. Increased finger blood flow was noted in patients following α-adrenergic blockade with drugs such as reserpine. Oral and intraarterial reserpine was the cornerstone of medical management of RS for several years but is unfortunately no longer available.[4] Angiograms of an RS patient before and after cold exposure and before and after intraarterial reserpine are shown in Figure 8–1. Research in canine models demonstrated increased α_2-receptor sensitivity to cold exposure, an observation confirmed in our laboratory using human vessels.[5, 6]

α_2-Adrenoceptors appear to play a major role in the production of the symptoms of RS. α_2-Receptors are present in a pure population on human platelets. Receptor levels in circulating cells appear to mirror tissue levels. Owing to the difficulty of obtaining digital arteries from human subjects, we and others have measured levels of

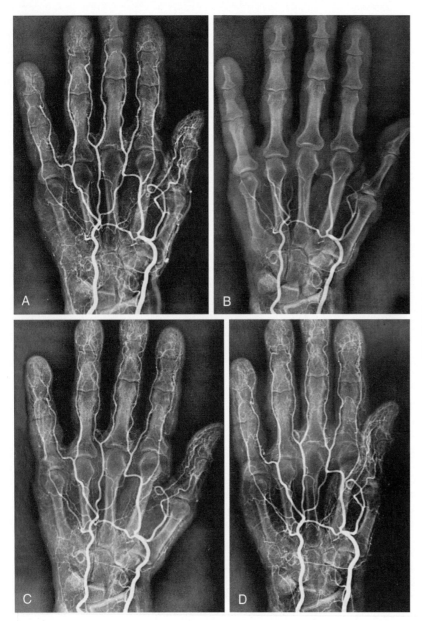

Figure 8–1. Hand angiograms of a Raynaud's syndrome patient before and after cold exposure both before and after administration of intraarterial reserpine. A marked vasospastic response to cold exposure, which is blocked by reserpine administration, is demonstrated. *A,* Before cold, before reserpine; *B,* after cold, before reserpine; *C,* before cold, after reserpine; *D,* after cold, after reserpine.

platelet α adrenoceptors. An increased level of platelet α_2 adrenoceptors in patients with RS has been demonstrated.[7–9] Increased finger blood flow during body cooling was noted in human controls treated with the α_2-adrenergic antagonist yohimbine,[10] but this finding has not been confirmed by others.[11] Possible mechanisms of α_2-adrenergic–induced RS include an elevation in the number of α_2 receptor sites, receptor hypersensitivity, and alterations in the number of receptors exposed at any one time.

The response of subcutaneous resistance vessels to acetylcholine has been shown to be diminished in patients with RS compared with controls, indicating a possible endothelium-dependent mechanism.[12] The possible roles of the vasoactive peptides endothelin, a potent vasoconstrictor, and calcitonin gene-related peptide (CGRP), a vasodilator, have also been investigated. Serum endothelin levels have been noted to significantly increase with cold exposure in patients with RS compared with controls.[13, 14] Depletion of endogenous CGRP may also contribute, as

increased skin blood flow in response to CGRP infusion has been demonstrated in patients with RS compared with that in controls.[15]

Based on observations primarily at the Mayo Clinic 70 years ago by Allen and Brown,[16] patients with Raynaud's symptoms have been traditionally classified as having "Raynaud's disease," or "Raynaud's phenomenon," depending on the presence or absence of an associated systemic disease process. However, Raynaud's phenomenon may precede the development of an associated disease by years. In addition, this system does not address the underlying palmar and digital artery disease that may be present. We have chosen to refer to patients with cold- or stress-induced digital ischemia as having RS, thus avoiding the semantic conflict of "disease" versus "phenomenon."

We have found it useful to subdivide patients with RS into two distinct pathophysiologic groups, obstructive and vasospastic, based on the presence or absence of arterial occlusive disease. Patients with vasospastic RS have patent digital arteries and normal digital artery pressures at room temperature. These patients have an abnormally forceful vasoconstrictive response to cold exposure or emotional stress, leading to digital arterial closure and episodic digital ischemic symptoms. Patients with obstructive RS have significant obstruction of either the palmar and digital arteries or the proximal arm arteries, with a concomitant reduction in resting digital arterial pressure. In these patients, a normal vasoconstrictive response to cold appears sufficient to cause digital arterial closure with resultant episodic digital ischemia.

In patients with obstructive RS, the mechanism of the obstructive process is variable. Patients with connective tissue disease typically have an autoimmune vasculitis, which is probably the mechanism underlying the widespread digital and palmar artery occlusions frequently present. Patients who work with vibrating tools have a similar process and frequently develop a peculiar fibrotic form of palmar and digital artery obstruction presumably associated with injury from repeated shear stress.[17] Hypercoagulable states may appear with digital artery occlusions, as can emboli from various sources, including valvular heart disease and subclavian, axillary, and ulnar aneurysms. Atherosclerosis involving the upper extremities is rarely seen in the younger age group but is frequently observed in older patients, especially men.

A number of diseases have been recognized in association with RS, among which the connective tissue diseases are the most frequent, with scleroderma being the most common. Associated diseases recognized in our patients with RS are shown in Table 8–1. The prevalence of RS in patients with diagnosed connective tissue disorders has been reported to be 70% to 90%.[18] Estimates of the percentage of patients with RS with an associated disease range from 40% to 80%.[1, 19–23] It is important to note that the data from most series come from tertiary care referral centers; therefore, they may not reflect the actual incidence in the general population and may overestimate the actual prevalence of associated diseases. Clearly, most individuals with RS view the condition as a nuisance and do not seek medical advice.

The diagnosis of RS is made by history and physical examination. Noninvasive vascular laboratory testing is used to differentiate obstructive from vasospastic RS. Symptoms are typically described as coldness, numbness, or mild discomfort. Significant pain during attacks is conspicuously absent. Classically, both hands are involved, with frequent sparing of the thumbs. The lower extremities are infrequently involved. Most episodes are induced by cold; however, the cold threshold varies from patient to patient. Emotional stimuli induce attacks in occasional patients. Episodes typically commence with blanching of one or several fingers extending as far as the metacarpophalangeal joint, rarely involving the palm or extending proximally to the wrist. This phase corresponds to vasoconstriction with the absence of blood in digital arteries. After rewarming, the first blood to reach the skin is desaturated, leading to finger cyanosis. Finally, reactive hyperemia leads to digital rubor. Episodes usually last as long as the cold stimulus is present and resolve within 10 to 15 minutes of rewarming. The hands and fingers are normal between attacks.

A history suggestive of an associated connective tissue

TABLE 8–1

Associated Diseases in the Oregon Health Sciences University (OHSU) Series of 1089 Raynaud's Syndrome Patients

DISORDER	PATIENTS (n)
Autoimmune Disease	*290*
Scleroderma	95
Undifferentiated connective tissue disease	24
Mixed connective tissue disease	23
Systemic lupus erythematosus	17
Sjögren's syndrome	16
Rheumatoid arthritis	9
Positive serology	106
Other Diseases	*301*
Atherosclerosis	46
Trauma	44
Hematologic abnormalities	42
Carpal tunnel syndrome	35
Frostbite	32
Buerger's disease	28
Vibration	21
Hypersensitivity angiitis	18
Hypothyroidism	13
Cancer	13
Erythromelalgia	8
No Associated Disease	*498*
Total	*1089*

From Landry G, Edwards JM, McLafferty RM, et al: Long-term outcome of Raynaud's syndrome in a prospective analyzed cohort. J Vasc Surg 23:76–86, 1996.

disease, including arthralgias, dysphagia, sclerodactyly, xerophthalmia, or xerostomia, as well as any prior history of large vessel occlusive disease, malignancy, hypothyroidism, frostbite, trauma, use of vibrating tools, and drug use, should be carefully sought. Carpal tunnel syndrome occurs in approximately 15% of patients with RS.[24] The examiner should carefully evaluate the pulses and assess the digits for evidence of active or healed ulceration, sclerodactyly, telangiectasias, and calcinosis. The optimal serologic evaluation has not been defined. We routinely obtain a complete blood cell count, erythrocyte sedimentation rate, antinuclear antibody titer, and rheumatoid factor. Patients who present with sudden-onset digital ischemia should be evaluated for hypercoagulable states. Tests for specific connective tissue diseases are obtained based on clinical suspicion. Importantly, the physical examination in patients with RS is frequently normal, and the diagnosis relies on history and noninvasive tests.

Routine vascular laboratory testing consists of digital photoplethysmography and digital blood pressures. The digital photoplethysmographic recording provides qualitative information on the character of the arterial waveform.[25] Normal digital blood pressure is within 30 mm Hg of brachial pressure. Patients with obstructive RS have blunted waveforms, whereas patients with vasospastic RS have either normal waveforms or a "peaked pulse." The peaked pulse pattern, first described by Sumner and Strandness,[26] appears to reflect increased vasospastic arterial resistance.

A cold challenge test is performed to verify cold sensitivity.[27] This test is performed with a liquid-perfused cuff placed on the proximal phalanx of the target finger. The cuff is inflated to suprasystolic pressure for 5 minutes while it is perfused with cold water. The pressure at which blood flow is detected on deflation of the cuff is recorded. A control finger on the same hand is tested at room temperature. The test is repeated at several temperatures, and the result is expressed as the percentage drop in finger systolic pressure with cooling. In our experience, this test has an overall sensitivity and accuracy of approximately 90%.[28]

Duplex scanning does not appear to have a major role in the diagnosis of RS, although it can be used to search for proximal arterial obstructive or aneurysmal disease. Laser Doppler imaging is a promising new modality that quantifies digital microvascular blood flow and may have future diagnostic applications in RS.[29] Angiography was used extensively in the past, particularly in the evaluation of patients with obstructive RS. Vasospastic or obstructive RS can be diagnosed on the basis of history, physical examination, serologic tests, and noninvasive studies alone. Patients with an underlying systemic disease process and bilateral palmar and digital arterial obstructive disease documented by vascular laboratory testing do not require angiography to confirm digital artery occlusive disease. Patients with unilateral disease, particularly patients who have only one or two digits of one arm involved, should be considered for angiography to determine both the presence of bilateral disease and the presence of any proximal arterial disease. These patients should also undergo transthoracic or transesophageal echocardiography to rule out a cardiac source of emboli.

We advise all patients with RS to avoid tobacco use, although a recent multicenter epidemiologic study suggested that RS is not strongly influenced by tobacco consumption.[30] Cold avoidance is a hallmark of conservative treatment. Medications that have been associated with the causation of RS symptoms, such as ergot alkaloids and β-blockers, should be avoided if any appropriate alternative therapies exist. More than 90% of patients with RS respond adequately to these simple conservative measures and require no additional treatment. The small number of patients who develop digital ulcers in association with obstructive RS can also be managed conservatively. A healing rate of 85% has been achieved with simple treatment consisting of soap and water scrubs, antibiotics as selected by culture, and conservative débridement.[31] Those patients with severe symptoms and all who develop ulcers are offered pharmacologic therapy.

Our current medication of choice for the treatment of RS is extended-release nifedipine (30 mg every night). Approximately two thirds of patients placed on nifedipine experience subjective benefit. Ten to 20 percent of patients are unable to continue the medication because of unacceptable side effects, including headache, ankle swelling, pruritus, and, rarely, severe fatigue.[32, 33] The newer, second-generation calcium channel blockers such as amlodipine, isradipine, nicardipine, and felodipine also appear to be effective in patients with RS and may be associated with fewer adverse effects.[34] Our second-line drug is Dibenzyline (phenoxybenzamine hydrochloride), an α-adrenergic blocking agent. A number of our patients take medication only during the cold portion of the year or in anticipation of cold exposure. Low-dose sublingual nifedipine (5 mg)

taken 15 to 30 minutes prior to cold exposure has been shown to act as an effective prophylaxis to cold-induced peripheral vasospasm.[35] Angiotensin II receptor blockade with losartan has been shown in a study to be clinically beneficial in improving vasospastic symptoms.[36] Other studies have implicated *Helicobacter pylori* as a possible etiologic agent for RS with improvement of symptoms with *H. pylori* eradication.[37] Pentoxifylline is added on an empirical basis to the nifedipine regimen if ulcerations are present. As a rule, patients with vasospastic RS respond more favorably to medical therapy than do those with occlusive RS.

Active research continues in the treatment of RS with the prostaglandins PGE_1, PGE_2, and PGI_2. Intravenous iloprost, a stable analog of PGI_2, has been shown to be effective in the treatment of RS associated with systemic sclerosis.[38, 39] In recent placebo-controlled double-blind studies, intravenous iloprost was associated with both decreased frequency of Raynaud's episodes and increased frequency of ulcer healing.[39, 40] Several multicenter clinical trials have examined the efficacy of oral forms of iloprost. Although some groups have detected modest improvements in patients with RS, particularly if associated with systemic sclerosis,[41] others have found no benefit when compared with placebo.[42, 43] Clinical trials with other prostaglandins such as oral and intravenous PGE_1 have resulted in less promising results.[44, 45]

Temperature biofeedback in which patients are taught hand warming through behavioral techniques has been demonstrated to reduce symptom frequency in 66% to 92% of patients with vasospastic RS.[46] Transcutaneous electrical nerve stimulation (TENS), which has been described as causing vasodilatation, demonstrated only mild increases in skin temperature, with no improvements in digital plethysmography or transcutaneous partial pressure of oxygen (Po_2) in test hands and a negligible effect on symptoms.[47] Acupuncture has also been suggested in a study as a possible treatment alternative with a significant reduction in frequency and severity of attacks.[48]

Cervicothoracic sympathectomy has been suggested by some as an effective treatment for RS.[49, 50] In our experience, it has never been of lasting benefit, and we do not recommend it for any patient with RS, including those with ischemic ulcerations. In contrast to upper extremity sympathectomy, excellent results have been achieved with lower extremity sympathectomy, with long-term symptomatic relief noted in more than 90% of patients undergoing this procedure.[51] Lumbar sympathectomy remains a viable option in the very rare patient with severely symptomatic lower extremity vasospasm.

Periarterial neurectomy is performed by removing the adventitia of the common digital artery. Several modifications of this technique have been published, generally characterized by increasing lengths of adventitial stripping to facilitate more distal sympathectomy.[52, 53] However, digital periarterial sympathectomy has not been proved any more effective than cervicothoracic sympathectomy, and its use is discouraged.

A minority of patients with RS have an identifiable proximal cause of upper extremity arterial insufficiency demonstrated on angiogram. Patients with subclavian, axillary, or brachial artery obstruction from atherosclerosis, emboli, proximal arterial aneurysms, or other causes are

TABLE 8-2

Long-Term Outcome of Oregon Health Sciences University (OHSU) Raynaud's Syndrome Patients as Classified by Initial Presentation

INITIAL CLASSIFICATION	INITIAL PRESENCE OF CONNECTIVE TISSUE DISEASE (%)	FINAL PRESENCE OF CONNECTIVE TISSUE DISEASE (%)	PRESENCE OF DIGITAL ULCERATION (%)	REQUIREMENT FOR DIGITAL OR PHALANGEAL AMPUTATION (%)
Spastic, negative serology	0	2.0	5.2	1.6
Spastic, positive serology	48.6	57.0	15.5	1.4
Obstructive, negative serology	0	8.5	48.2	19.0
Obstructive, positive serology	72.9	81.2	55.6	11.6

From Landry G, Edwards JM, McLafferty RM, et al: Long-term outcome of Raynaud's syndrome in a prospective analyzed cohort. J Vasc Surg 23:76–86, 1996.

appropriate surgical candidates and can expect excellent results from operative intervention. Restoration of normal hand circulation usually eliminates obstructive RS symptoms. Reconstruction of the palmar arch and direct microvascular bypass of occluded segments of palmar and digital arteries have been successfully employed in a small number of patients.[54, 55] Arteriovenous reversal at the wrist has recently been advocated as a method of providing retrograde arterial perfusion to ischemic hands for limb salvage.[56] These procedures, however, are applicable to only a few carefully selected patients.

The long-term outcome of patients with RS is not known with certainty. We recently reviewed our experience with over 1000 RS patients followed for up to 23 years and found RS to be a relatively benign condition in the majority of patients.[23] We divided patients into four groups at presentation (vasospastic RS with negative serologies, vasospastic RS with positive serologies, obstructive RS with negative serologies, and obstructive RS with positive serologies) to determine whether this classification scheme provided prognostic information. Patients with no evidence of an associated disease or arterial obstruction did extremely well with minimal risk of severe finger ischemia or development of an associated disease, whereas those with obstruction and positive serologies were most likely to develop worsening finger ischemia and ulceration. A summary is presented in Table 8–2. Patients without a diagnosable connective tissue disorder but with one or more clinical signs or laboratory tests suggesting such a disease have a much higher incidence of later being diagnosed with a connective tissue disorder. Current estimates of progression range from 2% to 6% in patients with initially negative serologic tests, to 30% to 75% in patients with positive serologic tests at presentation.[1, 22, 23, 57] Although fingertip débridements and occasional distal phalanx amputations are required to aid ulcer healing, we have performed major interphalangeal finger amputations in only 2 of more than 1000 patients with RS whom we have evaluated and treated.

SYSTEMIC VASCULITIS

Vasculitis has a deceptively simple definition—inflammation, often with necrosis and occlusive changes of the blood vessels—but its clinical manifestations are diverse and complex.[58] The term *arteritis* has been used to describe many of these syndromes, yet *vasculitis* is a more precise term, as many of the entities involve veins as well as arteries. Vasculitis may be generalized or localized. Our knowledge of this condition is incomplete, and the currently used classification systems are chaotic and filled with exceptions and overlapping syndromes. Some classification systems have focused on the etiology of the vasculitis, with groupings of "idiopathic" and "secondary." Although this is a useful system when considering disease processes, reclassification may be necessary as further knowledge is gained regarding etiology. In our opinion, the most useful classification system is based on the size of the vessels involved by the vasculitic process[59] (Table 8–3).

The etiology and pathogenesis of most vasculitides are quite complex and are presently either unknown or incompletely understood. Earlier attempts to associate vasculitis with a single mechanism of immune complex–induced injury have not been substantiated in the majority of vasculitides.[60] The basic pathologic mechanism of vasculitis currently implicates immune-mediated injury, which may include recognition of a vascular structure as antigen, deposition of immune complexes in a vessel wall with complement activation and injury, direct deposition of antigen in a vessel wall, or a delayed hypersensitivity reaction. The inciting antigen has been detected infrequently.

TABLE 8-3

Vasculitides of Potential Vascular Surgical Importance

Large Vessel Vasculitis
Giant cell (temporal) arteritis
Takayasu's disease
Radiation-induced arterial damage

Medium-Sized Vessel Vasculitis
Polyarteritis nodosa (classic PAN)
Kawasaki disease
Drug abuse arteritis
Behçet's disease
Cogan's syndrome
Vasculitis associated with malignancy

Small Vessel Vasculitis
Hypersensitivity vasculitis
Henoch-Schönlein purpura
Essential cryoglobulinemic vasculitis
Vasculitis of connective tissue diseases

The majority of vasculitides are associated with a cellular immunoreaction involving the production of soluble mediators including cytokines, arachidonic acid metabolites, and fibrinolytic and coagulation byproducts. The production of cytokines results in neutrophilic, eosinophilic, monocytic, and lymphocytic interactions at the inflammatory site. Endothelial cells express cell membrane receptors specific for many of these inflammatory cells. Binding of inflammatory cells to the endothelial cell triggers intracellular production of additional endothelial cytokines that affect the local inflammatory environment. Complement binding is thought to aid the attachment of leukocytes to endothelial cells. Platelet interactions with both intact and injured endothelium may contribute to the inflammatory process through activation of coagulation pathways and release of cytokines capable of stimulating and modifying immune responses. For a complete description of these cellular, immune, and inflammatory interactions, the interested reader is directed to available excellent summaries.[60, 61]

The vascular surgeon attends to the sequelae of vasculitic injury in these diseases. Thrombosis, aneurysm formation, hemorrhage, or arterial occlusion may all follow or accompany transmural damage created by the inflammatory reactions on the vascular wall. An abbreviated list of the vasculitides that have potential vascular surgical significance is presented in Table 8–3 and is considered in this section.

LARGE VESSEL VASCULITIS

Giant Cell Arteritis Group

The two conditions included in the giant cell arteritis group are systemic giant cell, or temporal, arteritis and Takayasu's arteritis. Although these have fairly distinctive clinical patterns, as noted in Table 8–4, the two entities likely represent different manifestations of the same disease process.[62] The microscopic pathologic findings of the conditions are similar, and individual tissue sections are frequently impossible to categorize as clearly one or the other. Both conditions consist of localized periarteritis with inflammatory mononuclear infiltrates and giant cells, along with disruption and fragmentation of the elastic fibers of the arterial wall. The arterial inflammation begins and is most pronounced in the media. In both conditions, the intensity of the cellular infiltrate and number of giant cells are variable. Interestingly, giant cells are not necessary to make the diagnosis of giant cell arteritis.[63]

Giant cell arteritis and Takayasu's disease both have a propensity for the insidious development of aneurysms of the thoracic and abdominal aorta, each of which may be accompanied by dissection.[64] Both may be associated with slowly progressive occlusive lesions of the upper extremity, carotid, visceral, and renal arteries. The main differences between these two disease entities are the age and sex of the afflicted individuals.[65]

Systemic Giant Cell Arteritis (Temporal Arteritis)

Systemic giant cell arteritis (GCA) is essentially limited to patients older than 55 years of age, occurs three times as frequently in women as men, and is more prominent in whites. The annual incidence in white females older than 50 years of age is about 16 cases per 100,000.[66] A viral etiology has been suspected but not confirmed.[67] Polymyalgia rheumatica, a clinical syndrome of 4 or more weeks of aching and stiffness of the hip and shoulder girdle muscles associated with an elevated erythrocyte sedimentation rate, is present in 50% to 75% of patients with temporal arteritis.[68]

GCA is a disease process that may involve any large artery of the body, although it has a propensity to involve branches of the carotid artery. The clinical history usually begins with a febrile myalgic process involving primarily the back, shoulder, and pelvic regions. Headache, malaise, anorexia, and weight loss are common. The most characteristic complaint is severe pain along the course of the temporal artery accompanied by tenderness and nodularity of the artery together with overlying skin erythema. The involvement is frequently bilateral. Visual disturbances occur in more than 50% of patients. The mechanism of the visual alterations may be ischemic optic neuritis, retrobulbar neuritis, or occlusion of the central retinal artery. Unilateral blindness occurs in as many as 17% of patients with GCA, followed by contralateral blindness in one third of these patients within 1 week.[69]

GCA is of concern to cardiac and vascular surgeons because it may cause aneurysms or stenoses of the aorta or its main branches. Both true thoracic aortic aneurysms and dissecting aneurysms may occur. Patients with GCA have a 17-fold increased risk of thoracic aortic aneurysms and a 2.4-fold increased risk of abdominal aortic aneurysms compared with age-matched controls.[70] Some have speculated that early, adequate steroid therapy will minimize the likelihood of these serious complications, although convincing evidence is lacking.[62] Successful cardiovascular surgery

TABLE 8–4

Clinical Patterns in Giant Cell Arteritis

	TEMPORAL ARTERITIS	TAKAYASU'S ARTERITIS
Age, sex	Elderly white females	Young females
Pathology	Inflammatory cellular infiltrates; giant cells	Same
Area of involvement	Branches of carotid usually; may involve any artery	Aortic arch and branches; pulmonary artery
Complications	Blindness	Hypertension, stroke
Response to steroids	Excellent	Unpredictable—unproved

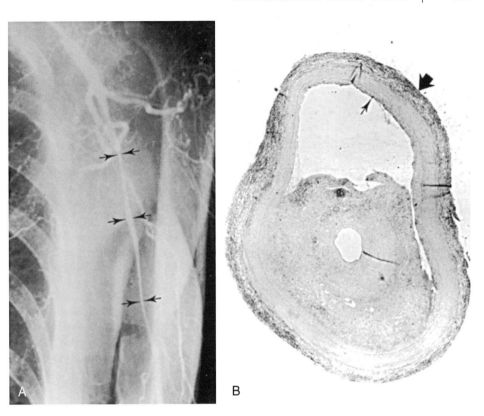

Figure 8–2. *A*, Typical giant cell arteritis showing smooth tapering of axillary artery *(arrows)*. *B*, Photomicrograph of axillary artery involved with giant cell arteritis showing transmural inflammation *(large arrow)* and inner zone of fibrosis *(small arrow)*. (From Rivers SP, Baur GM, Inahara T, Porter JM: Arm ischemia secondary to giant cell arteritis. Am J Surg 143:554–558, 1982.)

has occasionally been performed for the thoracic aortic complications.[71]

Klein and associates[72] found that 14% of patients with GCA had evidence of symptomatic large artery involvement. Symptomatic subclavian-axillary occlusion is a frequent presenting symptom of GCA.[73] Outside of the head and neck, the areas most commonly involved, in decreasing order, are the upper extremities, the upper and lower extremities, and the lower extremities. Coronary and mesenteric involvement have been described.[74] The angiographic features most suggestive of GCA include long segments of smooth stenosis interspersed with normal segments, smoothly tapered occlusions, absence of irregular plaques and ulcerations, and distribution of these abnormalities among the subclavian, axillary, and brachial arteries[72] (Fig. 8–2).

The diagnosis of GCA is suspected clinically and confirmed by the finding of an elevated erythrocyte sedimentation rate and a temporal artery biopsy showing the typical pathologic changes.[63] Bilateral sequential temporal artery biopsies are frequently performed if the results of unilateral biopsy are inconclusive, but, in 97% of cases, the two specimens show the same findings.[75] Characteristic findings on color flow duplex scans have been described, and duplex scanning may supplant temporal artery biopsy as the diagnostic procedure of choice.[76] The importance of a precise and early diagnosis lies in the early initiation of steroid therapy. Prompt steroid therapy will frequently result in restoration of pulses and prevention of lasting visual disturbances. Most important, vascular reconstructive surgery during the acute phase of GCA is relatively contraindicated. Surgical procedures fail in a high percentage of patients unless accompanied by high-dose steroid administration.[63, 73] Patients may present without myalgias,

fever, headaches, or other suggestions of systemic disease, making a high index of suspicion key to diagnosis. The life expectancy of patients with GCA is the same as that of the general population.[77]

Takayasu's Disease

Takayasu's disease frequently affects the aorta and its major branches and, in contrast to GCA, the pulmonary artery. The majority of the patients are Asian, about 85% are female, and the age at onset occurs between 3 and 35 years. The disease has two recognized stages. The first stage is characterized by fever, myalgia, and anorexia in about two thirds of patients. These symptoms may be followed by multiple arterial occlusive symptoms, with manifestations dependent on disease location.

The cardiovascular areas of involvement have been characterized as types I, II, III, and IV and are shown diagrammatically in Figure 8–3. Type I is limited to involvement of the arch and arch vessels and occurs in 8.4% of patients. Type II involves the descending thoracic and abdominal aorta and accounts for 11.2% of cases. Type III has involvement of the arch vessels and the abdominal aorta and its branches and accounts for 65.4% of cases. Type IV has primarily pulmonary artery involvement with or without other vessels and accounts for 15% of patients.[78] Most of the lesions are stenotic, although localized aneurysms have been reported. Arteriography has traditionally been the imaging modality of choice. However, both color flow duplex scanning[79, 80] and computed tomography (CT)–angiography have emerged as important alternatives.[81] Both of these studies give both luminal and mural information about the involved vessels. Interestingly, predilection for

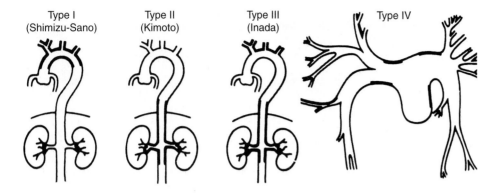

Type I (Shimizu-Sano) Type II (Kimoto) Type III (Inada) Type IV

Figure 8–3. Diagrammatic representation of the recognized types of Takayasu's arteritis. The areas of arterial involvement are shown in heavy lines. (From Lupi-Herrera E, Sanchez-Torres G, Marcustiamer J, et al: Takayasu's arteritis: Clinical study of 107 cases. Am Heart J 93:94–103, 1977.)

the thoracic aorta predominates in Japan, whereas predilection for the abdominal aorta predominates in India.[82]

Cardiovascular findings include diminished peripheral arterial pulsations and hypertension. The hypertension may be due to aortic coarctation or renal artery stenosis. The possible relationship of this disease to the middle aortic, or abdominal coarctation, syndrome is described in a subsequent section. Neurologic symptoms may result from hypertension or central nervous system ischemia associated with large artery occlusion or stenosis. Coronary artery involvement in Takayasu's disease is rare. The cardiac pathologic feature most frequently found is nonspecific and appears to result from heart failure associated with systemic and pulmonary hypertension.

The role of surgery in lesions of the arch vessels, visceral arteries, and renal arteries is uncertain. Successful surgical management of aneurysmal and stenotic lesions requires bypass graft implantation into disease-free arterial segments and continuation of corticosteroid therapy.[83, 84] Interventional techniques have been employed using percutaneous transluminal angioplasty with mixed success.[85–88] Endarterectomy has resulted in early failure and generally is not recommended.

Available information suggests a conservative surgical approach to these patients. A poor long-term outcome is predicted by the presence of major complications (retinopathy, hypertension, aortic insufficiency, aneurysm formation) and a progressive disease course.[89] Overall survival at 15 years is approximately 83%. Aneurysms of the aorta or branch arteries should be treated on their own merits just as atherosclerotic aneurysms in the same locations are. Visceral and arch vessel lesions appear best managed with bypass grafts. It is clear that optimal treatment of these difficult patients requires judicious adherence to vascular surgical principles, as well as close cooperation between the vascular surgeon and the internist.

Radiation-Induced Arterial Damage

Radiation given for treatment of regional malignancy causes well-recognized changes in arteries within the irradiated field. The primary changes consist of intimal thickening and proliferation, medial hyalinization, and cellular infiltration of the adventitia. Normal endothelium has a very slow rate of turnover, and following irradiation endothelial cells do not proliferate. Pleiomorphic endothelial cells may develop as a result of irradiation, with exposure

of the basement membrane leading to thrombosis of small vessels.[90] The effects of radiation on the smooth muscle cell are less well understood. Impairment of nitric oxide–mediated endothelium-dependent relaxation has been suggested.[91] Irradiation also leads to severe inflammation and destruction of the elastic lamellae of small vessels, which can cause aneurysmal dilatation; however, small arteries are most likely to occlude.[92] Postirradiation changes in large arteries often resemble atherosclerosis[93, 94] (Fig. 8–4).

Of considerable importance is the reported tendency of arteries in an irradiated area to show stenosis years later. An unusually large incidence of carotid artery stenosis in patients years after neck irradiation, along with an increased likelihood of stroke, has been described.[94] The lesions found vary between diffuse scarring and areas of typical atheromatous narrowing, with a preponderance of the latter. Radiation may stimulate the development of atherosclerosis, although experimental evidence is inconclusive. Whatever the mechanism of arterial injury, patients who have had regional irradiation, especially of the cervical region, should have careful vascular follow-up, including noninvasive vascular laboratory examinations.

Vascular surgery on irradiated arteries may be performed using standard techniques. Prosthetic and autogenous bypass grafts, as well as endarterectomy, have all been performed satisfactorily.[95] Prudence suggests avoidance of a prosthetic graft in a field in which infection may be expected, such as a radical neck dissection after irradiation, and we preferentially use autologous vein reconstruction. Late graft infections occurring 2 to 5 years after surgery have been described.[96] Currently, there is no defined role for endovascular treatment of radiation-induced arterial disease.[97]

MEDIUM-SIZED VESSEL VASCULITIS

Polyarteritis Nodosa

Polyarteritis nodosa (PAN) is a disseminated disease characterized by focal necrotizing lesions involving primarily medium-sized muscular arteries. This disease has a male-to-female preponderance of 2:1, with a peak incidence in the forties. The clinical manifestations of PAN are varied. PAN may involve only one organ or may involve multiple organs simultaneously or sequentially over time. The most frequent manifestations of PAN include a characteristic crescent-forming glomerulonephritis, polyarteritis, poly-

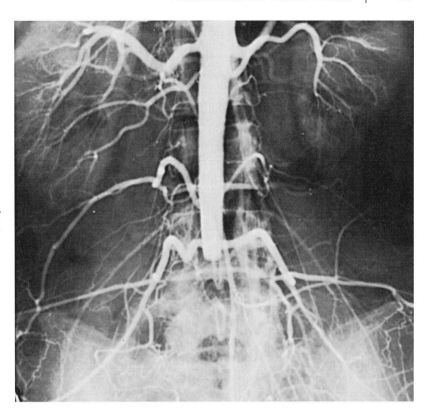

Figure 8–4. Radiation arteritis. Arteriograms in a 40-year-old woman who had received extensive internal and external irradiation for treatment of carcinoma of the cervix. There is a typical absence of atherosclerotic disease of the infrarenal aorta.

myositis, and abdominal pain, first described by Arkin in 1930.[98]

The essential pathologic feature of PAN is focal transmural arterial inflammatory necrosis. The process begins with medial destruction, followed by a sequential acute inflammatory response, fibroblastic proliferation, and endothelial damage. Immune complexes do not appear to be involved in the endothelial degeneration. The vascular injury is resolved as intimal proliferation, thrombosis, or aneurysm formation, all of which may culminate in luminal occlusion with consequent organ ischemia and infarction.[99]

The erythrocyte sedimentation rate, C-reactive protein, and factor XIII–related protein, all nonspecific serologic markers of inflammation, are elevated in PAN.[99] Mild anemia and leukocytosis are frequent. Antineutrophil cytoplasmic antibodies (ANCAs) have been detected in patients with systemic vasculitis, including PAN, Wegener's granulomatosis, Churg-Strauss syndrome, temporal arteritis, and Kawasaki disease.[100] Cytoplasmic (cANCA), perinuclear (pANCA), and "snow-drift" (xANCA) staining patterns have been recognized. These patterns, however, do not presently permit stratification of the systemic vasculitides by ANCA patterns, nor do they correlate with disease activity.

The hallmark of PAN is the formation of aneurysms associated with inflammatory destruction of the media, with the most frequently involved organs including the kidney, heart, liver, and gastrointestinal tract. A detailed arteriographic study of 17 patients with PAN reported that 10 of the patients had multiple arterial aneurysms involving the hepatic, renal, and mesenteric circulations.[101] Another study detected multiple visceral aneurysms in 15 of 26 patients with PAN and made the observation that visceral aneurysms are markers for a more severe clinical course of PAN.[102]

Rupture of intraabdominal PAN aneurysms has been well described and may represent a surgical emergency.[103] Curiously, these aneurysms have been documented to regress on occasion after vigorous steroid and cyclophosphamide therapy, which should be recommended for all asymptomatic visceral aneurysms.[104] An arteriogram of a patient with PAN showing the typical visceral and renal artery aneurysms is shown in Figure 8–5. Visceral PAN lesions may also lead to visceral artery narrowing incident to the inflammatory process, which may progress to occlusion. The visceral ischemia may manifest as cholecystitis, appendicitis, enteric perforation, gastrointestinal hemorrhage, or ischemic stricture formation with bowel obstruction.[103, 105]

Steroid therapy has improved 5-year survival from 15% before the routine use of steroids to the current 50% to 80% 5-year survival.[106] Cyclophosphamide may be added to the steroid regimen in acute severe cases.[104, 107] It has been suggested that prognosis can be predicted at the time of presentation based on the absence or presence of creatinemia, proteinuria, cardiomyopathy, and gastrointestinal or central nervous system involvement. Five-year mortality with zero, one, or two or more of these signs was 12%, 26%, and 46%, respectively.[108] During the acute phase of PAN, renal and gastrointestinal lesions account for the majority of the mortality, whereas cardiovascular and cerebral events account for the mortality in chronic cases.[106]

To date, little vascular surgical experience with PAN has been reported. The multiplicity of diseased areas renders elective vascular repair of all lesions impossible, and there is no accurate way to recognize the dangerous ones. The role of vascular surgery in intestinal revascularization in PAN is presently undefined.

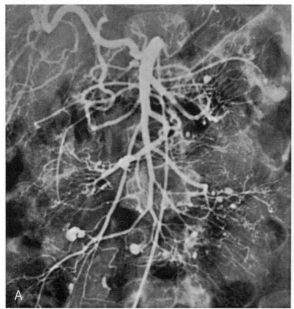
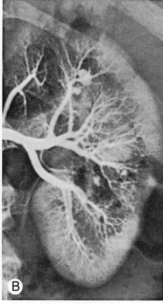

Figure 8–5. *A*, Arteriogram showing multiple visceral aneurysms in a patient with polyarteritis nodosa. *B*, Same patient showing multiple renal artery aneurysms.

Kawasaki Disease

In the 1960s an unusual febrile exanthematous illness swept Japan. Tomisaku Kawasaki observed 50 cases in the department of pediatrics at the Japan Red Cross Medical Center and termed the disease the mucocutaneous lymph node syndrome (MCLS).[109, 110] Over the next decade, the spread of the disease was noted worldwide, and it came to be known as Kawasaki disease.[111] During a recent 2-year period in Japan, over 11,000 cases were reported.[112] The disease is not limited to those of Asian descent and occurs in all ethnic groups, although children of Japanese or mixed Japanese ancestry appear to be most susceptible.

As the disease has become better known, strict clinical criteria have evolved for diagnosis: (1) high fever present for 5 or more days; (2) bilateral congestion of ocular conjunctiva; (3) changes of the mucous membranes of the oral cavity, including erythema, dryness, and fissuring of the lips or diffuse reddening of the oropharyngeal mucosa; (4) changes of the peripheral portions of the extremities, including reddening and induration of the hands and feet and periungual desquamation; (5) polymorphous exanthem; and (6) acute nonsuppurative swelling of the cervical lymph nodes. The presence of a prolonged high fever and any four of the five remaining criteria, in the absence of concurrent evidence of bacterial or viral infection, establishes the diagnosis.[113]

Kawasaki disease has a unimodal peak incidence at 1 year of age; it has not been described in neonates and is rarely observed for the first time in those over the age of 5 years.[112] The acute symptoms may persist for 7 to 14 days before improvement as the fever subsides. Notable laboratory features include elevation of the erythrocyte sedimentation rate and C-reactive protein, and thrombocythemia.[114] Recently, von Willebrand's factor has been shown to be elevated in Kawasaki disease.[115] A small proportion of patients with acute Kawasaki disease show exacerbation or recrudescence of symptoms and signs during the convalescent phase of the disease within 1 to 3 weeks after initial clinical onset. Some feel that this biphasic pattern

represents a more severe form of Kawasaki disease with a higher incidence of arterial lesions and a worse prognosis.[116]

An infectious etiology has long been assumed given the self-limited nature of the disease, seasonal incidence, and geographic outbreaks.[114] However, no single infectious agent has been demonstrated. An immunologic defect has also been postulated, as there appears to be an altered immunoregulatory state in these patients, with decreased numbers of T cells and an increased proportion of activated helper T4 cells. The significance of these changes is not known. The most serious disease manifestation is coronary arteritis, which is likely present in all children with this disease. The spectrum of documented coronary artery pathologic changes consists of active arteritis, thrombosis, calcification, and stenosis, although the distinguishing feature of Kawasaki disease is the formation of diffuse fusiform and saccular coronary artery aneurysms.

Reports employing routine echocardiography in patients with Kawasaki disease have demonstrated coronary artery aneurysms in 25%, with the aneurysms typically appearing in the second week of illness and reaching maximum size from the third to eighth week after the onset of fever.[117] Echocardiography may show dilatation of the right, left, or anterior descending coronary arteries, while the circumflex coronary artery is rarely involved.[118]

Serial arteriographic studies have shown a considerable capacity for all types of coronary arterial lesions to evolve. The aneurysms may regress, leaving a patent arterial lumen, or the arterial segment may become stenotic. Most stenotic lesions regress with maintenance of a patent lumen, but a few do progress to occlusion. Stenotic lesions demonstrated by coronary angiography are most frequently seen in the left anterior descending artery.[119] Patients older than 2 years of age with fever lasting longer than 14 days and pericardial effusion and those not treated with anticoagulant agents appear to have a higher incidence of aneurysm formation.[117] Patients treated with immune globulin have shown a decreased incidence of aneurysm formation.[119] New coronary arterial lesions infrequently occur after 2 weeks. Regression of the coronary arterial lesions occurs over a 2-month period, although some lesions have remained unchanged for more than a year before regression.[120]

Systemic arteritis also occurs in Kawasaki disease, with iliac arteritis as prevalent as coronary arteritis. Aneurysm formation is far less frequent in the systemic arteries than in the coronary arteries, with one report identifying systemic arterial aneurysms (axillary and iliac) in 3.3% of 662 patients with Kawasaki disease with coronary artery aneurysms.[121] The healing process in the systemic arterial lesions may lead to focal arterial stenosis or aneurysm formation, just as in the coronary arteries. Peripheral arterial involvement of the subclavian and axillary artery coexisting with coronary artery aneurysms is seen in Figure 8–6.

Thrombosis of coronary artery aneurysms is the over-whelming cause of death in the early stages of Kawasaki disease, causing acute myocardial infarction or arrhythmia. Coronary aneurysm rupture has also been described. With the initiation of antithrombotic therapy with aspirin and, more recently, immunoglobulin therapy, the mortality from Kawasaki disease has decreased from 2.0% to 0.3% over the past two decades.[119] Currently, there is a consensus that aspirin and immunoglobulin therapy should be initiated in the acute phase of the disease, at least for all children younger than 12 months of age. Immune globulin is given intravenously for 4 days at a dose of 400 mg/kg/day. Aspirin is given orally for 14 days at a dose of 100 mg/kg/day, then continued in low-dose form (3 to 5 mg/kg/day) for an additional 8 weeks.[122, 123]

Coronary artery bypass grafting was first used in Kawasaki disease in 1976.[124] The first procedure used saphenous

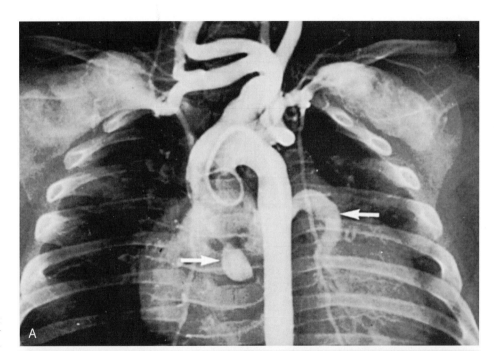

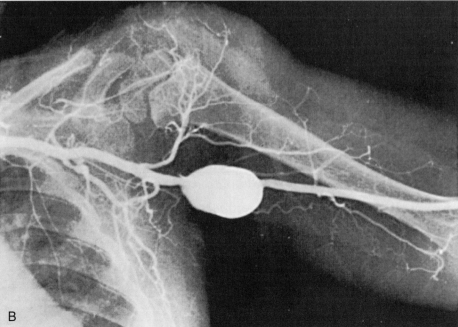

Figure 8–6. *A*, Arteriogram of an infant with Kawasaki disease showing coronary artery aneurysms *(white arrows)* and massive subclavian artery aneurysms. *B*, Arteriogram of a 2-year-old child showing a large axillary artery aneurysm resulting from Kawasaki disease.

vein as conduit, and several more reports followed. Concerns over the use of saphenous vein and its potential for growth with the child have been raised. Few long-term follow-up studies exist, yet the evidence suggests inferior 5-year patency for saphenous vein grafts with Kawasaki disease. These results led to the use of the internal mammary artery (unilateral or bilateral)[125] and the right gastroepiploic artery[126] for coronary revascularization in patients with Kawasaki disease. Internal mammary arterial grafts have been demonstrated to have improved patency (77% vs. 46%) and reduced late cardiac death (1% vs. 3%) at 7 years compared with saphenous vein grafts in a recent multicenter study.[127] Cardiac transplantation for severe ischemic heart disease as a sequela of Kawasaki disease is considered in patients who are not considered candidates for revascularization because of distal coronary stenosis or aneurysms and those with severe irreversible myocardial dysfunction.[128]

Aneurysms of the abdominal aorta and iliac, axillary, brachial, mesenteric, and renal arteries have been observed as late sequelae of the systemic vasculitis. When these lesions become symptomatic from occlusion, expansion, or embolization, most surgeons proceed with standard repair techniques with interposition grafting. Although experience is limited, surgical repair of the aneurysms has been accomplished safely.[129]

Drug Abuse Arteritis

In 1970, Citron and associates[130] published an important report describing the occurrence of necrotizing arteritis indistinguishable from PAN in a group of intravenous drug abusers. Methamphetamine was the drug most frequently abused. These patients developed multiple arterial aneurysms and areas of arterial stenosis resulting from fibrosis occurring in areas of previous arterial necrosis. Four of these 14 patients died of acute disease, with combinations of renal failure, central nervous system dysfunction, and localized intestinal necrosis and perforation. Isolated cerebral angiitis has also been reported in the setting of methamphetamine as well as cocaine abuse.[131, 132] No medical therapy is of proven effectiveness for this condition.

A second type of arterial obstruction has been reported in drug abuse patients that represents arterial damage following the accidental intraarterial injection of drugs during attempted intravenous injections. The most frequently reported drugs have been parenteral barbiturates intended for intravenous injection, in which case arterial injury and thrombosis appear to result from chemical damage, perhaps related to the low pH of the injectate.[133] Another pattern of arterial damage results from the accidental injection of drug preparations intended for oral use. The practice of dissolving tablets in water for intravenous injection is enormously harmful because of the large number of substances (such as silica and tragacanth) in tablets. When this material is accidentally injected intraarterially, significant distal ischemia may result from obstruction of the small arteries by the inert materials[134] (Fig. 8–7).

No convincing evidence has demonstrated the value of any specific treatment in these patients. A variety of therapeutic efforts have been tried, including anticoagulation, regional sympathetic block, and the administration of vasodilators, without proof of efficacy. The outcome ap-

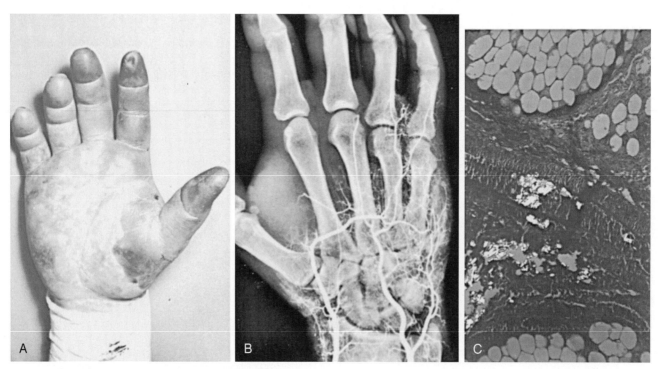

Figure 8–7. *A,* Hand photograph of a 22-year-old man who injected a pentazocine tablet dissolved in tap water into his radial artery. The hand was severely ischemic, with gangrenous changes of the radial side. *B,* Arteriogram showing massive arterial obstruction of the common and proper digital arteries to the thumb, index, and long fingers. *C,* Slide from amputation specimen under polarized light showing bright refractile silica particles in the hand arteries.

pears determined at the time of injection by the quantity and concentration of injectate reaching the distal arterial bed. Nonetheless, heparin anticoagulation is favored if the patient is seen acutely and has no contraindications to this treatment. Compartment syndrome requiring fasciotomy is an infrequent but reported sequela.[135]

Behçet's Disease

In 1937, Behçet[136] described three patients with iritis and associated oral and genital mucocutaneous ulcerations, an association subsequently termed "Behçet's disease." Over one half of these patients have joint involvement. The underlying pathologic lesion is a vasculitis, which results in both venous thromboses and specific arterial lesions. Venous thrombosis is the most frequent vascular disorder in Behçet's disease, affecting up to 30% of patients.[137] Arterial lesions are distinctly less frequent and include occlusive and aneurysmal disease, which when present have a high mortality rate (up to 20%).[138] This systemic disease largely affects individuals from the Mediterranean area and East Asia.

The pathogenesis of vascular damage in Behçet's disease appears to be an immune-mediated destructive process. A humoral-mediated etiology has been suggested by the identification of enhanced neutrophil activity and circulating immune complexes in affected patients.[139] Specific T-cell subsets have also been identified in high concentrations at the sites of vascular involvement, indicating a cellular-mediated process.[140] Activation of complement within the vessel wall may lead to destruction of the media and subsequent aneurysm formation. Vasa vasorum occlusion may in turn lead to transmural necrosis of the large muscular arterial walls, with perforation and pseudoaneurysm formation and injury to adjacent tissues.[141]

Behçet's disease may have a genetic component, as there is an increased incidence of the HLA-B51 allele among patients with Behçet's disease.[142] Both viral and bacterial etiologies have been proposed, although definitive evidence is lacking.[143]

Large artery involvement is an uncommon but serious complication of Behçet's disease. Arterial aneurysms, while distinctly less common than the mucocutaneous, ophthalmic, or arthritic lesions, are the most frequent cause of death in patients with Behçet's disease.[138] Aneurysms have been described in numerous arteries, including the carotid, popliteal, femoral, iliac, and subclavian, but the aorta is the most frequent site of aneurysm formation in this disease.[144, 145] Curiously, the aneurysms frequently appear phlegmonous, suggesting acute bacterial infection, although cultures are invariably negative. The arterial aneurysms are frequently multiple and may be metachronous. Unfortunately, interposition bypass grafts have a high incidence of thrombosis in addition to the propensity to develop anastomotic pseudoaneurysms, with long-term graft patencies being the exception rather than the norm. The use of an aortic endograft in a patient with Behçet's disease was recently described.[146]

Venous involvement is prominent, and lower extremity superficial or deep vein thrombosis occurs in 12% to 27% of patients.[137] Thrombosis of the superior or inferior vena cava occurs less frequently but may be fatal. Lifelong anticoagulation is recommended in patients with Behçet's disease who develop venous thrombosis, but the role of prophylactic anticoagulation is uncertain.

Immunosuppressive agents, including azathioprine and corticosteroids, have been used with some success for nonarterial symptoms.[141] Although corticosteroids may prevent blindness and limit discomfort associated with the mucocutaneous disease, they unfortunately do not appear to alter the progression or course of the underlying vascular disease. Currently, no uniformly satisfactory therapy exists for Behçet's disease; however, early diagnosis and meticulous reconstructive management of identified arterial aneurysms have provided long-term limb salvage in some patients despite the well-recognized propensity for arterial graft complications.[141] Vigilant follow-up is required once large artery disease is recognized. Because this population is at high risk for arteriographic complications, periodic noninvasive imaging and hemodynamic assessment of the arterial system appear prudent.[147]

Cogan's Syndrome

Cogan's syndrome is a rare condition consisting of interstitial keratitis and vestibuloauditory symptoms. It is a disease primarily of young adults, with the mean age of onset in the third decade. It is occasionally associated with a systemic vasculitis similar to PAN.[148] Aortitis with subsequent development of clinically significant aortic insufficiency occurs in 10% of patients with Cogan's syndrome. Mesenteric vasculitis and thoracoabdominal aneurysms have also been described in association with Cogan's syndrome.[149, 150]

Daily administration of high-dose corticosteroids has been successful in reversing both the visual and auditory components of Cogan's syndrome, although deafness may be irreversible. The response of the aortitic component to steroids used singly or in combination with cyclosporine is less well established.[151] Surgical therapy, including aortic valve replacement, mesenteric revascularization, and thoracoabdominal aortic aneurysm repair, is occasionally indicated and can be performed safely.

Vasculitis Associated with Malignancy

Vasculitis associated with malignancy is infrequent. A strong association has been made between a systemic necrotizing vasculitis resembling PAN and hairy cell leukemia.[152] The vasculitis in this situation presents after the diagnosis of the leukemia and is indistinguishable from classic PAN. An immune-mediated mechanism is postulated. More frequently, vasculitides involving small vessels have been described in association with lymphoproliferative disorders.[153] These have primarily cutaneous manifestations and minimal visceral involvement and often are referred to as "paraneoplastic vasculitides."[154]

Vasculitis associated with solid tumors is rare, but resolution with tumor excision has been reported.[155] RS has been reported in association with carcinoma and lymphoproliferative malignancies.[156] These cases were characterized by cold-induced ischemia, which frequently leads to digital artery occlusion and ischemic ulcerations. The symptoms of finger ischemia preceded the diagnosis of malignancy, and several of these patients experienced marked improvement of their hand lesions after removal of the tumor.

SMALL VESSEL VASCULITIS

Hypersensitivity Vasculitis Group

The entities in the hypersensitivity vasculitis group include classic hypersensitivity vasculitis, mixed cryoglobulinemic vasculitis, and Henoch-Schönlein purpura. These conditions appear to result from antigen exposure followed by antigen-antibody immune complex deposition in small arteries and arterial damage. Hypersensitivity vasculitis usually has prominent skin involvement. In some conditions a drug, environmental chemical, or the hepatitis B virus may be implicated as the inciting antigen, but in over half, no causative agent is identified. Henoch-Schönlein purpura is a self-limited disease that occurs primarily in children and affects the skin, gastrointestinal tract, and kidneys. The disease course and findings are similar in cryoglobulinemic vasculitis, which may be associated with a hematologic malignancy or hepatitis B infection.[157]

The clinical syndromes typically associated with this group of diseases include skin rash, fever, and evidence of organ dysfunction, none of which specifically concern vascular surgeons. It is clear, however, that some of these syndromes may present with arteritic involvement substantially limited to the hands and fingers. In these patients, the clinical picture is typically that of severe and widespread palmar and digital arterial occlusions and digital ischemia. The vasculitis may be treated with steroids, with the occasional use of immunosuppressive agents or plasmapheresis. The treatment of hand lesions can otherwise follow the approach outlined later in this chapter for Buerger's disease.[158]

Vasculitis of Connective Tissue Diseases

The connective tissue diseases often are complicated by vasculitis.[62] These diseases have associated immunologic abnormalities, and the occurrence of vasculitis in these patients likely results from immune-mediated damage, as described for other vasculitides.[159] Vasculitis frequently accompanies scleroderma, rheumatoid arthritis, and systemic lupus erythematosus.

Scleroderma is a generalized disorder of connective tissue, the microvasculature, and small arteries. It is characterized by progressive scarring and small vessel occlusion in the skin, gastrointestinal tract, kidneys, lungs, and heart. CREST syndrome (*c*alcinosis, *R*aynaud's syndrome, *e*sophageal dysmotility, *s*clerodactyly, *t*elangiectasias) describes a variant of scleroderma with limited cutaneous involvement. The vasculitis associated with scleroderma results in fibrinoid necrosis and concentric thickening of the intima with deposition of layers of mucopolysaccharide.

Scleroderma is the most frequent connective tissue dis-

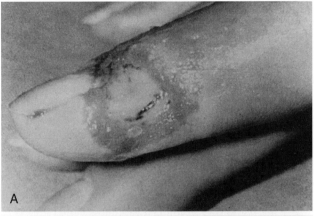
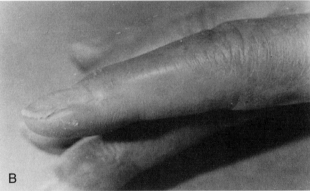

Figure 8–8. Photographs of a patient with scleroderma and a digital ulcer. *A,* Digital ulcer; *B,* healed ulcer following conservative management.

ease recognized in our patients with RS as well as those with digital ulceration[23] (Fig. 8–8). Approximately 80% to 97% of patients with scleroderma have symptoms of RS. In our experience, the RS usually begins as vasopastic and progresses to obstructive RS in a number of patients.

The vasculitis associated with rheumatoid arthritis involves primarily small arteries with a predilection for vasa nervorum and the digital arteries. Intimal proliferation with medial necrosis and progression to fibrosis with vessel occlusion occur. Symptoms of mononeuritis multiplex are common following involvement of small arteries. Cutaneous lesions are often present and include digital ulcers, nail fold infarcts, and palpable purpura.[160] Rarely, there is coronary, mesenteric, or cerebral artery involvement. Patients with rheumatoid arthritis who have positive ANCAs or higher titers of rheumatoid factor have a more aggressive disease course with a more frequent incidence of rheumatoid vasculitis.[161, 162] The presence of vasculitis portends a poor prognosis for patients with rheumatoid arthritis.

The vasculitis of systemic lupus erythematosus is believed to be due to deposition of immune complexes.[163] The most frequent clinical vascular problem in lupus is RS, which may affect 80% of patients. Other vasculitic manifestations include palpable purpura and mononeuritis multiplex. Thrombotic disorders of the arterial and venous system occur in patients with lupus and appear related to the "lupus anticoagulant," not vasculitis. IgA anti–double-stranded DNA (dsDNA) antibodies and anti–endothelial cell antibodies (AECAs) are markers of more virulent vasculitic involvement.[164, 165]

The management of the vasculitides associated with the connective tissue diseases is primarily steroid therapy.[163] Steroids appear to have little or no role in the treatment of the occlusive vascular lesions of scleroderma. Immunosuppressive therapy with cyclophosphamide has also been shown to have modest benefit in selected patients.[166] The treatment of RS associated with lupus or scleroderma is as described earlier.

BUERGER'S DISEASE

Buerger's disease, also known as thromboangiitis obliterans, is a clinical syndrome characterized by the occurrence of segmental thrombotic occlusions of small and medium-sized arteries in the lower, and frequently the upper, extremities, accompanied by a prominent arterial wall inflammatory cell infiltration.[167] Buerger's disease is a discrete entity pathologically and is clinically distinct from either atherosclerosis or immune arteritis.[168] Affected patients are predominantly young male smokers (mean age, 34 years), who usually present with distal limb ischemia, frequently accompanied by localized digital gangrene.

Buerger's disease appears to be on the decline in North America, although there has been an increase in the incidence in women. Women currently constitute up to 20% of patients in certain series.[169] Whether there is a true decline in incidence or simply more uniform application of strict diagnostic criteria is unclear. The increasing proportion of women has been attributed to the increase in the prevalence of smoking in women.[170] A large volume of patients continue to be reported from East and Southwest Asia. In patients with peripheral vascular disease, the reported incidence of Buerger's disease is 0.75% in North America, 3.3% in Eastern Europe, and 16.6% in Japan.[171]

Approximately 40% to 50% of patients with Buerger's disease have a history of superficial migratory thrombophlebitis, RS, or both.[169] The arterial lesions of Buerger's disease usually occur in the distal portions of both upper and lower extremities and may be accompanied by digital gangrene, especially of the toes. Although there have been rare, well-documented reports, both arteriographically and pathologically, of iliac and visceral artery involvement,[172, 173] the overwhelming majority of patients with thromboangiitis obliterans have disease limited to the arteries distal to the elbow and knee. In North America, about 50% of patients with Buerger's disease have isolated lower extremity involvement, 30% to 40% have upper and lower extremity involvement, and about 10% have isolated upper extremity involvement.[169]

The acute lesion of Buerger's disease is a non-necrotizing inflammation of the vascular wall with a prominent component of intraluminal thrombosis. In contrast to both atherosclerosis and immune arteritis, the internal elastic lamina remains intact in Buerger's disease. Therefore, while often considered a vasculitis, Buerger's disease is not a true vasculitis, as it lacks vascular wall necrosis. Both T- and B-cell–mediated activation of macrophages or dendritic cells in the intima have been implicated in the pathogenesis of Buerger's disease.[172] The chronic phase of Buerger's disease includes a decline in hypercellularity with the production of perivascular fibrosis and frequent recanalization of the luminal thrombus. Adjacent veins and nerves are frequently involved in the perivascular inflammatory process.

From an examination of our patients, as well as a review of published experience, we propose the diagnostic criteria for Buerger's disease listed in Table 8–5.[169] The major criteria are essential for diagnosis, whereas the minor criteria are supportive. Central to the diagnosis is the onset of symptoms before age 45 years, a uniform exposure to tobacco, and absence of arterial lesions proximal to the knee or elbow. It is essential to exclude other frequent causes of limb ischemia in young adults. In North America, atherosclerosis is much more prevalent than Buerger's disease, and major atherosclerotic risk factors such as hyperlipidemia, diabetes, and hypertension must be absent. Proximal sources of emboli (cardiac, proximal arterial occlusive, or aneurysmal disease), underlying autoimmune disease, hypercoagulable states, trauma, and local lesions (popliteal entrapment, adventitial cystic disease) must also be excluded. We recognize that these criteria are so restrictive that some patients with Buerger's disease will be excluded, but we believe these strict criteria are essential to eliminate the diagnostic uncertainty obvious in many publications of purported Buerger's disease.

After the clinical criteria have been met, objective confirmation of distal occlusive disease limited to small and medium-sized vessels is required. This may be satisfied by four-limb digital plethysmography, distinct histopathologic findings when available, or arteriography. The arteriographic findings reveal that the extremity arteries proximal to the popliteal and distal brachial levels are normal, proximal atherosclerosis and vascular calcification are absent, and there is an abrupt transition from a normal, smooth proximal vessel to an area of occlusion.[168] Involvement

TABLE 8–5

Criteria for Diagnosis of Buerger's Disease

Major Criteria

Onset of distal extremity ischemic symptoms before age 45 yr
Tobacco use
Exclusion of
    Proximal embolic source (cardiac, TOS, ASO, aneurysms)
    Trauma and local lesions (entrapment, adventitial cyst)
    Autoimmune disease
    Hypercoagulable states
    Atherosclerosis
    Atherosclerotic risk factors (diabetes, hypertension, hyperlipidemia)
No evidence of arterial disease proximal to popliteal or distal brachial
    arteries
Objective documentation of distal occlusive disease by either
    Plethysmography
    Histopathology
    Arteriography

Minor Criteria

Migratory superficial phlebitis
RS
Upper extremity involvement
Instep claudication

ASO, arteriosclerosis obliterans; RS, Raynaud's syndrome; TOS, thoracic outlet syndrome.
From Mills JL, Porter JM: Buerger's disease: A review and update. Semin Vasc Surg 6:14–23, 1993.

tends to be segmental rather than diffuse and is commonly symmetrical. In the upper extremity, the ulnar or radial artery is frequently occluded, and extensive digital and palmar arterial occlusion is uniformly present. In the lower extremity, the infrageniculate vessels are extensively diseased with diffuse plantar arterial occlusion. Tortuous "corkscrew" collaterals frequently reconstitute patent distal arterial segments and, although not pathognomonic, are suggestive of Buerger's disease (Fig. 8–9).

Arteriography, while desirable, is not essential for the diagnosis of every case of Buerger's disease.[169] Arteriography may be omitted when a patient's history is typical of Buerger's disease, there are no associated atherogenic risk factors, the serologic tests for autoimmune disease and hypercoagulable states are negative, and vascular laboratory examination reveals diffusely abnormal digital plethysmographic tracings in all four extremities accompanied by a conspicuous absence of proximal large artery occlusive disease.

Digital plethysmography frequently provides especially important diagnostic information. In the typical Buerger's patient, obstructive arterial waveforms are present in all digits, providing objective evidence of widespread digital arterial occlusion or stenosis. Patients with unilateral digital plethysmographic abnormalities should undergo arteriography to rule out a proximal, potentially correctable arterial lesion causing the digital ischemia. Additionally, patients with symptoms and objective findings localizing their dis-

ease to the distal feet and toes and who have normal hand and finger plethysmography should undergo arteriography to rule out a proximal embolic source for their ischemia.

The etiology of Buerger's disease remains unknown. Although a strong association with tobacco use has been clinically recognized, a causal relationship has not been conclusively demonstrated.[168] Nonetheless, we have never recognized Buerger's disease in a nonsmoker, with the exception of a single patient who used large amounts of snuff. An increased cellular response to tobacco antigen has been noted in patients with Buerger's disease, as well as in healthy smokers compared with nonsmokers. Tobacco is currently considered at least a permissive factor and likely a causative factor.

The major histocompatibility complex, specifically HLA-A9, -B5, -DR4, and -DRw6, has been implicated in Buerger's disease, but its role is unclear.[169, 173] Considerable evidence indicates that an autoimmune process is central to the illness. Several independent investigators have identified elevated levels of anticollagen antibodies in patients with Buerger's disease.[174–176]

The cornerstone of treatment for patients with Buerger's disease is complete tobacco abstinence. The disease typically undergoes remissions and relapses that correlate closely with the cessation and resumption of cigarette smoking. In our clinical series, no patient has sustained further tissue loss following cessation of smoking.[169] Unfortunately, prolonged tobacco abstinence is the exception rather than the norm. Persistent efforts on the part of the physician and family members may ultimately result in smoking cessation. In a report from Japan, an impressive 50% of patients were able to quit smoking.[177]

We use a prolonged conservative local treatment program for areas of finger ulceration and gangrene, with the primary goal being a clean, dry digit.[178] Ischemic ulcer débridement, often including nail removal, is used frequently, accompanied by minimal rongeur removal of exposed phalangeal bone as needed. Any associated infection is treated with antibiotics. Proximal finger amputations are rarely required, and wrist or forearm amputations have never been necessary in our patients with Buerger's disease. Prolonged conservative management is usually rewarded by healing with preservation of maximal digital length, provided smoking has been discontinued. We have found thoracic sympathectomy ineffectual, and we find no convincing evidence that this procedure is of any significant benefit in these patients.

The course of lower extremity Buerger's disease stands in marked contrast to that observed with upper extremity involvement. Ischemic rest pain can be severe, and narcotic analgesics are frequently required. Several large series have reported a 12% to 31% incidence of major leg amputation over a 5- to 10-year period.[179] Our own experience revealed a 31% incidence of major leg amputation.[169] Lumbar sympathectomy for Buerger's disease is not beneficial, and we do not perform or recommend the procedure.

Arteriography should be performed in all patients with threatened limb loss. If arteriography reveals a patent distal vessel and if autogenous vein is available, a distal arterial bypass may be considered.[180] The use of autogenous vein is mandatory. Distal bypass is infrequently feasible because of the diffuse nature of the arterial occlusive disease

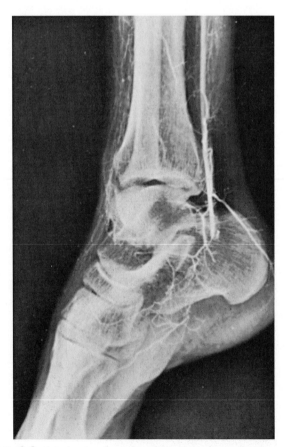

Figure 8–9. Arteriogram of patient with Buerger's disease showing occlusion of the posterior tibial artery at the ankle, total occlusion of the anterior tibial artery, and numerous small collateral vessels.

process. In our experience and that of others, the long-term results of reconstruction are mediocre. However, published Japanese data have suggested that acceptable primary (49%) and secondary (63%) 5-year patency rates can be achieved in lower extremity bypasses, including inframalleolar bypasses, in patients with Buerger's disease.[181]

Many medications have been recommended for the treatment of Buerger's disease, including corticosteroids, PGE$_1$, vasodilators, hemorrheologic agents, antiplatelet agents, and anticoagulants. There is no evidence that any are effective. A randomized European trial comparing the oral prostacyclin analog iloprost with placebo did demonstrate improved pain control with iloprost, but no improvement in wound healing.[182] Preliminary results of gene therapy with intramuscular injection of vascular endothelial growth factor have been promising in promoting ulcer healing.[183]

We have noted anecdotal improvement in pain control with the use of either nifedipine or diltiazem in patients with Buerger's disease accompanied by severe RS. We have also noted benefit from pentoxifylline in patients with rest pain or digital ulceration, especially of the fingers. We often empirically place Buerger's disease patients on antiplatelet therapy because this appears reasonable for the treatment of a disease characterized by widespread, segmental arterial and superficial venous thromboses. Thus, we treat many of our Buerger's disease patients with a combination of nifedipine, pentoxifylline, and aspirin, although we recognize an absence of objective evidence supporting the use of these agents.

Although lower extremity Buerger's disease portends a significantly worse prognosis for limb salvage than atherosclerotic occlusive disease, life expectancy for patients with Buerger's disease approaches that of an age-matched population.[184] This is likely due to a lack of coronary artery involvement in the disease process. Reported survival is 97% at 5 years and 94% at 10 years.[169]

HERITABLE ARTERIOPATHIES

Hereditary disorders of the arterial wall account for a minute fraction of problems encountered by the vascular surgeon. These disorders affect the structure or stability of collagen or elastin, resulting in weakness of the arterial wall. These patients may possess characteristic phenotypic features, but they are often not recognized until the patient presents with a catastrophic vascular complication. The heritable arteriopathies discussed in this chapter include Marfan's syndrome, Ehlers-Danlos syndrome, cystic medial necrosis, and pseudoxanthoma elasticum. Arteriomegaly is also included in this section, although it is not strictly a heritable disease and there are no distinguishing phenotypic features.

Marfan's Syndrome

Marfan's syndrome is an inherited disorder of connective tissue characterized by a panoply of anatomic disorders affecting the skeletal, ocular, and cardiovascular systems with variable phenotypic expression. It is serious largely because of its cardiovascular complications.

The pathologic basis of Marfan's syndrome has been elegantly uncovered. Hollister and colleagues[185] discovered diminished levels of fibrillin in skin biopsies and cultured fibroblasts in patients with Marfan's syndrome. Fibrillin, a large glycoprotein (350 kD), is one of the structural components of the elastin-associated microfibrils. Subsequently, genetic linkage studies identified an abnormal fibrillin gene on chromosome 15 in a group of patients with Marfan's syndrome.[186, 187] Both a reduction in fibrillin formation and abnormalities in the fibrillin molecule have been identified.[188, 189]

The incidence of Marfan's syndrome is estimated to be 1 in 10,000, and there has been no identified race or sex preference.[190] Inheritance is by an autosomal dominant pattern, though nearly 25% of all cases are the result of spontaneous genetic mutations. In its classic form, the syndrome is easily recognizable and consists of abnormalities of the eye (subluxation of the lens), skeleton (arachnodactyly, extreme limb length, pectus excavatum or carinatum, and joint laxity), and cardiovascular system (aortic dilatation and aortic valvular incompetence). The diagnosis is established on the basis of clinical manifestations in most cases. However, some patients have only one or a few of the characteristic features. A recent advance has been the ability to confirm the diagnosis by DNA analysis, whereby quantitative and qualitative defects in fibrillin can be detected.[191] Prenatal diagnosis can be accomplished using chorionic villus sampling.[192]

Patients with Marfan's syndrome develop progressive dilatation of the aortic root with a resultant ascending aortic aneurysm and aortic valve incompetence (Fig. 8–10). A significant number have mitral valve prolapse and mitral insufficiency. Mild aortic isthmus coarctation may be associated with this syndrome, predisposing the patient to ascending aortic dissection. Less frequently, aneurysmal dilatation and dissection involve the pulmonary, coronary, carotid, and splenic arteries and the infrarenal aorta.

If Marfan's syndrome is untreated, the life expectancy of the patient is about 40 years, with 95% of deaths related to cardiovascular causes. Progressive aortic root dilatation leading to aortic dissection or aortic valvular insufficiency accounts for 80% of fatal complications. The remainder of deaths are due to congestive heart failure.

Histopathologic evaluation of aortic segments from patients with Marfan's syndrome has revealed cystic medial necrosis, with disruption of collagen fibers and fibrosis of the media.[193] Immunohistochemical analysis has revealed an upregulation of matrix metalloproteinases (MMPs) and abnormalities in elastin synthesis leading to increased susceptibility to degradation by MMPs.[194] Compared with normal subjects, Marfan's syndrome patients have decreased aortic distensibility and increased aortic stiffness indices in both the ascending and abdominal aortic regions, irrespective of the aortic diameter.[195]

In view of the predictably progressive nature of the aortic dilatation, all patients with Marfan's syndrome should be followed from childhood with annual echocardiograms to detect aortic dilatation.[196] There is some evidence that β-blocker therapy initiated before the development of aortic

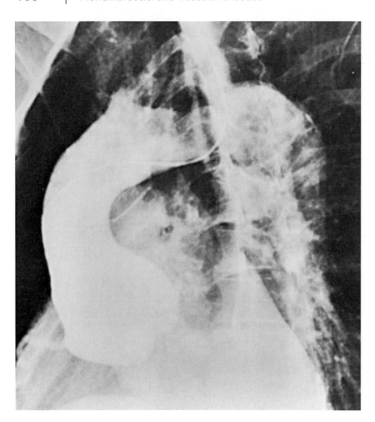

Figure 8–10. Thoracic aortogram of a patient with Marfan's syndrome showing massive aortic dilatation and associated aortic insufficiency.

incompetence may retard the onset of incompetence and perhaps retard aneurysmal degeneration.[197, 198]

Elective repair of the aortic valve and ascending aorta should be accomplished prophylactically before severe aortic insufficiency compromises left ventricular function or the ascending aorta exceeds 6 cm in diameter, at which point the risk of dissection and rupture increases. Surgical intervention typically includes graft replacement of the ascending aorta, with concomitant aortic valve replacement. Occasionally, mitral valve replacement is required. Patients should avoid contact sports, isometric exercises, weightlifting, or physical exertion to the point of exhaustion. With modern surgical techniques, the life expectancy of these patients can be improved considerably, as emphasized by reports with low operative mortality, even in severely symptomatic patients.[199, 200]

Ehlers-Danlos Syndrome

The Ehlers-Danlos syndrome refers to a group of diseases first clearly described by van Meekeren in 1682[201] and later by Ehlers and Danlos, characterized by hyperextensible skin, hypermobile joints, fragile tissues, and a bleeding diathesis primarily related to fragile vessels.[202, 203] Ehlers-Danlos syndrome is the most frequent of the heritable connective tissue disorders and occurs in autosomal dominant, autosomal recessive, and sex-linked patterns. Eleven different types of Ehlers-Danlos syndrome have been described, each with variable clinical signs and symptoms. The specific biochemical defects are known in types IV, VI, VII, and XI and involve defects in collagen

production.[204, 205] For further specific information regarding Ehlers-Danlos syndrome, the reader is referred to standard works.[206]

The extreme fragility of tissues in many patients with Ehlers-Danlos syndrome leads to problems of surgical importance. The skin and soft tissues are easily disrupted, tend to fragment and tear with manipulation, and hold sutures and heal poorly. Wound dehiscence is common when surgery is required.[207] In addition to these significant problems incident to any surgery, a number of patients with Ehlers-Danlos syndrome are prone to arterial disorders that may require surgical intervention.

Ehlers-Danlos syndrome types I, III, and IV frequently have arterial complications. Type IV represents only 4% of all cases of Ehlers-Danlos syndrome but causes the most severe arterial complications. These patients produce little or no type III collagen, which is of major structural importance in vessels, viscera, and skin.[206] Patients are prone to spontaneous rupture of major vessels, aneurysm formation, and acute aortic dissections. Other complications include spontaneous lacerations, false aneurysms, and arteriovenous fistulas. Bleeding or easy bruisability occurs in two thirds of patients with type IV disease. Hemorrhage can be life-threatening despite normal platelet function and coagulation proteins. Defective type III collagen appears to facilitate bleeding by failing to stimulate platelets exposed to subendothelial connective tissue. The media of the arterial wall is thin and disorganized, with fragmented elastic fibers on microscopic examination. There is hyperplasia of the medial cells and increased ground substance in the inner half of the media. Collagen hypoplasia can be seen on skin biopsies with hypertrophy of elastic fibers.[208]

Treatment of spontaneous arterial rupture in patients with Ehlers-Danlos syndrome should be nonoperative, consisting of compression and transfusion whenever possible. If operation for major arterial disruption is required, the therapeutic objective should be ligation to control bleeding if this procedure can be accomplished without tissue loss. Gentle dissection, proximal vessel control with external tourniquets or internal balloon catheters, and the use of carefully applied heavy ligatures reinforced with fine vascular sutures have been emphasized as keys to success. Despite the many pitfalls, major arterial reconstruction can be accomplished in patients with Ehlers-Danlos syndrome, including repair of abdominal aortic aneurysms and aortic dissection.[209] Arteriography carries special risks of vessel laceration and hemorrhage in these patients and should be avoided if possible. Prognosis for patients with type IV Ehlers-Danlos is poor. Forty-four percent of patients with major hemorrhage die before surgical intervention, and there is a 20% mortality with operative intervention.[210]

Cystic Medial Necrosis

Cystic medial necrosis is a condition associated with aortic dissection and manifested pathologically by uniform hyaline degeneration of the media and replacement by a mucoid-appearing basophilic substance. Erdheim[211] believed that the disease was the result of medial replacement by overproduction of mucoid ground substance. Subsequently, numerous studies have shown that the pathologic changes of cystic medial necrosis, with the resultant clinical problems of aortic dissection, spontaneous arterial rupture, and disseminated aneurysm formation, result from a variety of metabolic conditions and syndromes affecting the composition and structure of collagen, elastin, and mucopolysaccharide ground substance. Thus, Marfan's syndrome, Ehlers-Danlos syndrome, any of the mucopolysaccharidoses, and occasionally neurofibromatosis may all present with the typical arterial lesions and pathologic changes identified as cystic medial necrosis. Although the specific biochemical alterations for some of these syndromes have been discovered, for others they remain obscure.

Although most patients with cystic medial necrosis have an identifiable clinical syndrome, the most common of which are Marfan's syndrome and Ehlers-Danlos syndrome, a distinct subpopulation of patients with aortic root disease and histologic findings consistent with cystic medial necrosis fail to show the classic phenotypes of Marfan's syndrome or Ehlers-Danlos syndrome. These patients often seek treatment at an older age and with more advanced vascular disease. Ninety-four percent of the deaths in this patient group are related to cardiovascular disease, with the majority due to aortic dissection, rupture, or sudden death.[212]

The most frequent arterial condition resulting from cystic medial necrosis is aortic dissection, the treatment of which is discussed elsewhere in this text. Aortic dissection from cystic medial necrosis has been reported as a cause of superior vena cava syndrome.[213] Although unusual, cystic medial necrosis has also been reported to involve the pulmonary arteries and the superficial temporal artery.[214] Cystic medial necrosis has also been implicated as a cause of abdominal aortic aneurysms in children.[215] Rarely, patients have a rapidly progressive syndrome of disseminated arterial dissection, spontaneous arterial rupture, and aneurysm formation in which the only discernible lesion has been

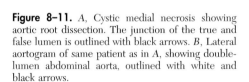
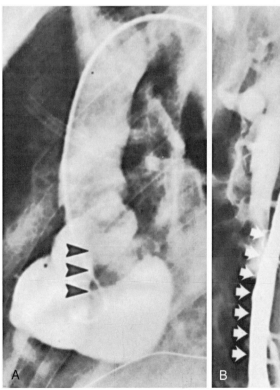
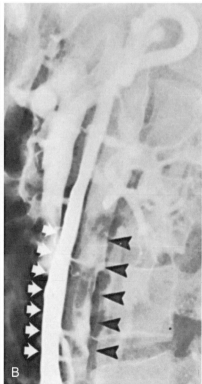

Figure 8–11. *A*, Cystic medial necrosis showing aortic root dissection. The junction of the true and false lumen is outlined with black arrows. *B*, Lateral aortogram of same patient as in *A*, showing double-lumen abdominal aorta, outlined with white and black arrows.

cystic medial necrosis.[216] The angiograms of such a patient are seen in Figure 8–11.

Pseudoxanthoma Elasticum

Pseudoxanthoma elasticum is an inherited disorder of elastic tissue manifested clinically by loose, baggy skin with multiple creases and small yellow-orange cutaneous papules in intertriginous areas. These patients also have changes in the eye (angioid streaks) and distinct vascular abnormalities. The prevalence of pseudoxanthoma elasticum is 1 in 70,000 to 160,000.[217] Studies have demonstrated an autosomal recessive inheritance in the majority, although there is also an autosomally dominant form.[218]

Although the biochemical defect responsible for the syndrome is not known, the basic pathologic change is degeneration of medial elastic fibers, with calcification, fragmentation, and secondary proliferation of the intima leading to luminal narrowing and obstruction. This change results in a markedly abnormal pulse contour due to loss of the elastic recoil and distensibility of vessels and may be demonstrated plethysmographically. Arterial stenoses or occlusions or both are the end results of this pathologic process and may involve the cerebral, coronary, visceral, and peripheral arteries. Radiography frequently reveals extensive arterial calcification in a young patient without obvious risk factors for atherosclerosis. Arterial occlusive disease occurs at an early age, usually presenting in the twenties or thirties. With careful examination, decreased peripheral pulses and evidence of peripheral arterial occlusive disease can be found in 24% to 80% of these patients.[219] Symptoms include intermittent claudication, periodic abdominal pain, and angina. Gastrointestinal hemorrhage is frequent and is believed to originate from the widespread arterial degeneration. Hypertension is common in these patients and is usually ascribed to extensive vascular calcification, although renovascular hypertension has been reported.

Standard techniques of vascular surgery, including autogenous vein bypass and endarterectomy, have been utilized with success in patients with pseudoxanthoma elasticum.[219] Anecdotal benefit from pentoxifylline for the relief of ischemic pain has been reported.[220] The indications for surgery in these patients are the same as for patients with arteriosclerotic occlusive disease.

Arteria Magna Syndrome

Leriche was the first to describe patients with arteria magna syndrome, which is characterized by extreme arterial dilatation, elongation, and tortuosity, which he termed *dolicho et méga-artère*.[221] Since then, many such patients have been recognized, and the terms *arteria magna, arteria dolicho et magna*, and *arteriomegaly* have all been used to describe this condition. Pathologic study reveals that the arterial media of these patients shows a striking loss of elastic tissue.[222]

Angiography in patients with this syndrome reveals characteristic changes. There is arterial widening and tortuosity

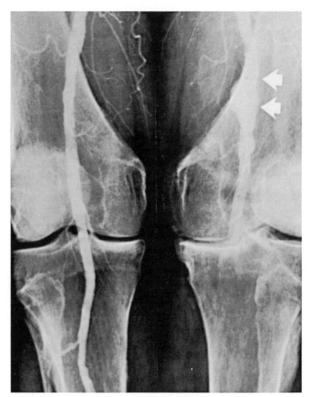

Figure 8–12. Arteriogram of a 68-year-old male showing very dilated popliteal arteries and a left popliteal aneurysm *(arrows)*. This patient's arterial dilatation extended throughout his body, a condition termed "arteria magna syndrome."

(100% of patients), extremely slow arterial flow velocity (100% of patients), and the existence of multiple aneurysms (66% of patients)[223] (Fig. 8–12). The slow arterial flow present in patients with this condition makes arteriography difficult. Large amounts of contrast must be used, and visualization of distal vessels may require multiple injections and special timing sequences with delayed filming.

The propensity for these patients to form arterial aneurysms at multiple sites results in the frequent need for surgical correction. Because of the generalized arterial dilatation in these patients, standard criteria for determining the size of aneurysms to be repaired may not be useful. All patients with arteria magna should have a careful examination of all pertinent sites (aorta, iliac, femoral, popliteal arteries), together with ultrasound imaging of nonpalpable or questionable areas. These examinations should be repeated annually. Any aneurysm that reaches 2 to 2.5 times the size of the parent vessel or becomes symptomatic should be replaced. Arterial occlusions in these patients are almost always thrombotic or embolic complications of aneurysmal disease.

The relationship of arteria magna to typical atherosclerosis is uncertain. The syndrome occurs, albeit rarely, in young people with no evidence of atherosclerosis, and it has been reported in children. Lawrence and colleagues[224] reported a 36% familial incidence among first-degree relative. Clinical experience suggests that most patients in the United States with arteria magna have significant associated atherosclerosis along with the usual risk factors, including tobacco use. In these patients, however, the atherosclerosis is typically nonocclusive, and dilatation predominates.

CONGENITAL CONDITIONS AFFECTING THE ARTERIES

Abdominal Coarctation

Coarctation of the aorta below the diaphragm is a rare but well-recognized condition. Quain[225] described a stricture of the abdominal aorta in 1847 that he believed to be congenital in origin. In 1952, Glenn and coworkers[226] reported the first successful surgical repair, which consisted of bypassing the coarctation with a splenic artery graft. Since that time, the surgical treatment and clinical courses of a large number of patients have been reported.[227] Abdominal coarctation is usually discovered during an evaluation for hypertension. Most patients with abdominal coarctation become symptomatic during their teens, with complaints associated with hypertension, including headache, fatigue, shortness of breath, and palpitations. The hypertension is mediated through the renin-angiotensin system.[228] Severe leg ischemia is distinctly unusual,[229] while moderate claudication is often present. Involvement of the superior mesenteric artery occurs frequently, although symptoms of visceral ischemia have not been reported.

Physical findings in these patients include reduced or absent lower extremity pulses, with a noticeable radial or femoral pulse delay. All patients have prominent abdominal systolic bruits, and many have systolic bruits in the lumbar region or lower posterior thoracic area. The natural history of untreated abdominal coarctation is severe hypertension, with death from either renal or cardiac failure within a few years of the onset of symptoms.[230]

Multiple variants of abdominal coarctation have been described, with the variable factors being the precise location and length of the aortic involvement and the number of visceral branches affected. The origins of the visceral arteries may be involved even when originating from an area of relatively uninvolved aorta. Stenosis or occlusion of the visceral arteries usually does not extend beyond a few millimeters from the origin, implicating a process that is primarily aortic.[227]

Two primary pathogenetic theories have been presented. The first proposes a congenital anomaly representing a failure of normal fusion of the two dorsal aortas of the embryo, resulting in aortic narrowing. The existence of multiple renal arteries in a number of these patients supports this theory, because the formation of a single renal artery is a developmental step that coincides in both location and timing with fusion of the dorsal aortas. The congenital origin of abdominal coarctation in some of these patients may be related to intrauterine injury, as the anomaly has been reported in association with the maternal rubella syndrome.[231] In patients in whom the lesion is congenital, the involved vessels are hypoplastic, without gross or microscopic inflammatory reaction.

The second proposed etiology for abdominal coarctation is inflammation. In this group of patients, microscopic examination of involved arteries reveals pronounced in-

flammatory changes. This lesion is sometimes referred to as the "middle aortic syndrome" to emphasize its acquired rather than congenital etiology.[232] This inflammatory middle aortic narrowing is probably a variant of Takayasu's arteritis and appears to occur with a frequency reflecting the primarily Asian distribution of that disease.[233] Although this arteritis can be successfully treated with corticosteroids during the acute stage, diagnosis is most often made later when the chronic fibrotic and stenotic lesions amenable only to surgical treatment are present.

Arteriography is necessary to define the extent of the lesion and plan treatment (Fig. 8–13). Lateral and oblique views are helpful in detecting the extent of visceral vessel involvement. Renovascular hypertension is assumed, and renin studies or split renal function studies are not necessary unless the potential viability of a poorly visualized kidney (i.e., nephrectomy vs. renal revascularization) is questionable.

Many authors have reported successful surgical treatment of abdominal coarctation by a variety of methods, including aortoaortic bypass, iliac or femoral bypass, prosthetic patch aortoplasty, and splenoaortic anastomosis.[226, 227, 230, 234] In contrast to thoracic coarctation, prosthetic bypass grafting from the descending thoracic aorta to an uninvolved area of the infrarenal aorta, iliac, or femoral arteries has traditionally been the procedure of choice, although some recommend autologous repair with extensive aortic patching.[227, 230] When possible, a single abdominal operative incision is preferable, employing medial visceral rotation to allow optimal exposure of the supraceliac aorta. Alternatively, this operation may also be performed through a thoracoabdominal incision or through separate laparotomy and thoracotomy incisions. Complete revascularization has been reported as a staged procedure.[235] However, single-stage repair is recommended because most of these patients are young and tolerate extensive procedures well.[236] Successful repair of middle aortic coarctation with stent implantation has recently been reported.[237] Restenosis in young patients is a potential problem.[238] In very small children, operation may be delayed to an age (5 to 6 years) at which increased vessel size allows greater chance of successful repair, as long as cardiac and renal function can be preserved by medical management of hypertension.

Results of surgical treatment of abdominal coarctation have been good. Stanley and associates[230] reviewed the results of 73 reported cases and found an 8% operative mortality and 80% excellent or good results. Renal revascularization is most often performed by bypass grafts originating from the thoracoabdominal graft. Autogenous vein and artery, and prosthetic grafts have all been used successfully.[227] Unsuspected proximal stenosis of a visceral artery (splenic) used for renal revascularization has been reported as a cause of failure.[230] Several prophylactic visceral revascularizations have been performed.[239] Speculation that unrecognized preexisting visceral orificial stenosis related to abdominal coarctation may explain the marked female predominance in most atherosclerotic visceral ischemia series remains unproven.

Persistent Sciatic Artery

In the embryo, the axial sciatic artery arises from the umbilical artery and supplies blood to the lower limb,

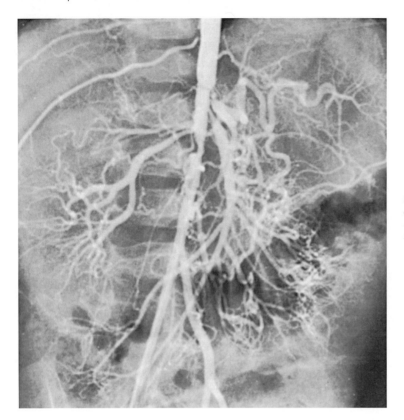

Figure 8–13. Abdominal aortic coarctation in a 2-year-old child showing infrarenal aortic narrowing and high-grade stenoses at the origins of the celiac, superior mesenteric, and right renal arteries with nearly total occlusion of the left renal artery.

following a dorsal course to the popliteal area and then proceeding through the midcalf to the ankle. As development proceeds, this artery is replaced in its upper part by the femoral artery developing from the external iliac artery. By the third month of gestation, the femoral artery predominates, and the vestiges of the sciatic artery remain only as the inferior gluteal artery, the distal popliteal artery, and the peroneal artery.[240]

Rarely, part or all of the sciatic artery may persist into postnatal life as a large artery originating from the internal iliac artery, exiting the pelvis through the sciatic notch in proximity to the sciatic nerve and following a course through the buttock and posterior thigh to join the popliteal artery in the popliteal fossa. The artery may coexist with a normal superficial femoral artery, or the superficial femoral artery may be hypoplastic. In some patients, the entire superficial femoral may be absent, with the sciatic artery being the only vessel in the limb in continuity with the popliteal artery. Persistent sciatic artery is reported to occur with an incidence of 0.03% to 0.06% in large series of femoral arteriograms, with one third of all cases being bilateral.[240, 241]

The anomalous lower extremity blood supply usually remains undetected until later life (mean age of detection, 51 years). Patients eventually present with claudication or more severe lower extremity ischemic symptoms, pulsatile buttock masses, or, rarely, sciatic neuropathy.[242, 243] The anomalous artery has a proclivity for aneurysmal degeneration, with greater than 25% of detected sciatic arteries found to be aneurysmal.[244] The necessity for complete angiographic evaluation of these lesions is obvious. Treatment has usually consisted of aneurysm ligation or excision with femoropopliteal or iliac-popliteal bypass grafting.[241, 244]

Popliteal Entrapment Syndromes

Stuart,[245] in 1879, was the first to describe the anatomic abnormality associated with popliteal entrapment, and Hamming[246] in 1959 reported the first successful treatment of the condition. Love and Whelan[247] coined the term *popliteal artery entrapment syndrome* in 1965. The anatomic basis of this syndrome lies in the anomalous embryonic development of two independent structures, the popliteal artery and the gastrocnemius muscle.[248] Below the knee, the embryonic sciatic artery gives rise to the popliteal and tibial vessels. The femoral artery arises later as the amalgamation of a capillary plexus connecting branches of the external iliac artery proximally and branches of the sciatic artery distally. The femoral and sciatic arteries both contribute to the popliteal artery. The femoral artery becomes dominant as the proximal sciatic artery regresses.

During this period of femoral maturation and sciatic regression, the heads of the gastrocnemius muscles develop. The anlage of the gastrocnemius muscle develops as a single muscle migrating cephalad from its origin on the calcaneus. As the gastrocnemius matures, it divides into larger medial and smaller lateral heads that gain their final attachments on the femoral epicondyles. The medial head of the gastrocnemius migrates from its lateral origin toward the medial epicondyle at the same developmental stage at which the mature popliteal artery is developing from the femoral and sciatic arteries.

The exact etiology of popliteal artery entrapment remains unknown. Anomalies primarily arise from variations in the relationship of the popliteal artery and the medial head of the gastrocnemius muscle itself or from a muscular slip. Less frequently, the popliteus, the plantaris, or the semimembranosus muscle provides the constriction.[249] Insua and associates[250] classified the variants into four groups (Fig. 8–14). In type 1, about 50% of all cases, the popliteal artery deviates medial to the normally placed medial head of the gastrocnemius muscle. Type 2 lesions (25%) involve an abnormal attachment of the medial head of the gastrocnemius, with the popliteal artery passing medially but with less deviation than in type 1. In type 3 (6%), the normally situated popliteal artery is compressed by muscle slips of the medial head of the gastrocnemius. Type 4 lesions have associated fibrous bands on the popliteus muscle compressing the popliteal artery. Compressions of the artery by other structures have been described, but these are rare.[249] Rich and others[251] added type 5 lesions, in which the popliteal vein accompanies the artery in its abnormal course. Additionally, iatrogenic or acquired popliteal artery entrapment syndromes have been described, in which an autogenous vein graft has been improperly tunneled either medial to the medial head of the gastrocnemius or through the medial head of the muscle rather than between the medial and lateral heads.[252]

The true incidence of popliteal artery entrapment syndrome is unknown. The reported incidence is increasing coincidentally with the development of more sophisticated diagnostic tests. A review of 20,000 patients screened with routine vascular laboratory testing identified verifiable popliteal artery entrapment syndrome in less than 1%.[249] However, in an autopsy series, Gibson and colleagues[253] found an incidence of 3.5% in 86 postmortem examinations. Interestingly, all of the patients were older than age 60 years when they died, and the popliteal arteries showed no histologic abnormalities. Clearly, not all entrapped popliteal arteries become symptomatic. About 90% of reported cases have occurred in men; more than half of these patients have become symptomatic when younger than 30 years old. The defect is bilateral in 20% of patients.[254]

Symptoms are due to obstruction of the popliteal artery with gastrocnemius contraction. Premature atherosclerotic changes occur, presumably in relation to repeated microtrauma, and thrombosis, embolism, or aneurysm formation may ensue. Symptomatic patients may manifest acute ischemia due to popliteal artery occlusion (10%) or with progressive intermittent claudication. Calf claudication in patients younger than 40 years of age is sufficiently infrequent that its presence should suggest the possibility of popliteal artery entrapment.

Diagnosis of popliteal artery entrapment syndrome has been difficult, as most patients are asymptomatic at rest. Symptomatic patients may have normal, reduced, or absent pulses of the lower leg. Ankle dorsiflexion or plantar flexion or knee extension may diminish or occlude distal pulses. Continuous wave Doppler, photoplethysmography, and ar-

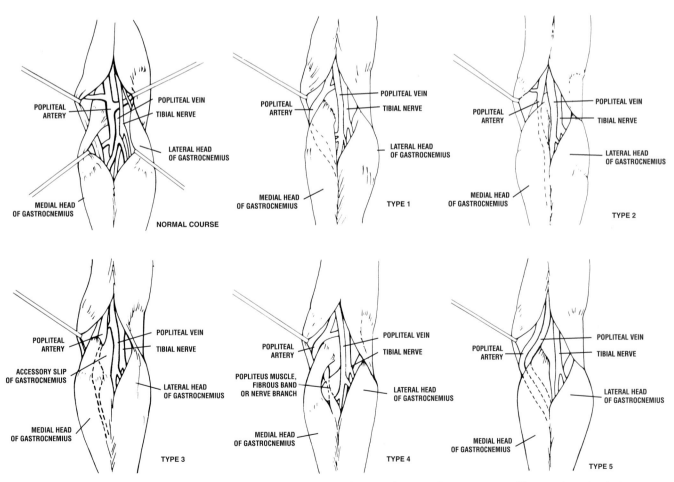

Figure 8–14. Diagram of the types of popliteal artery entrapment. (From Rich NM, Collins G Jr, McDonald PT, et al: Popliteal vascular entrapment: Its increasing interest. Arch Surg 114:1377–1384, 1979.)

terial duplex scanning have been used with these same maneuvers of the leg to provide objective confirmation of popliteal artery entrapment.[255] Others have used progressively more challenging treadmill exercise regimens to elicit symptoms and objective decline in the ankle-brachial index for patients suspected of having popliteal artery entrapment syndrome.[256] However, these noninvasive tests and physical findings are quite nonspecific, as maneuver-induced pulse diminution may occur in normal individuals.

Arteriography demonstrating midpopliteal artery compression or medial deviation with the leg in a position of stress had been the gold standard for the diagnosis of the popliteal artery entrapment syndrome, but it is being replaced by noninvasive techniques. CT and magnetic resonance imaging (MRI) have proved useful in precisely defining anomalous anatomic relationships between the popliteal artery and adjacent muscle groups, as well as assessing the patency of the artery.[257] Furthermore, both examinations provide bilateral detail. Although both CT and MRI may define the entrapment, MRI provides better soft tissue definition and does not require the use of intravenous contrast to localize the vascular structures or define their patency status.[258] Unlike conventional CT scans, MRI can also provide longitudinal views of the popliteal fossa. For these reasons, MRI has assumed the central role in the noninvasive diagnosis of popliteal artery entrapment (Fig. 8–15).

The treatment of this condition is surgical. Identifying the specific type of entrapment preoperatively is both difficult and unnecessary, as the surgical management will only be influenced by the patency of the popliteal artery. If diagnosed early and if minimal arterial changes are present, section of the medial gastrocnemius head may be sufficient. Bypass grafting is required in patients with significant arterial stenosis, occlusion, or aneurysm formation.[259] Autogenous vein is the only acceptable graft across the knee. The original descriptions of the surgical technique for this condition favored a posterior approach to the popliteal fossa.[246] Later, a medial approach was emphasized to expose the entire length of the popliteal artery,

ensure total division of the medial head of the gastrocnemius, and act as a safeguard against iatrogenic popliteal artery entrapment. To date, similar results have been obtained with both techniques. We currently favor the medial approach.

FIBROMUSCULAR DYSPLASIA

Fibromuscular dysplasia (FMD) is a nonatherosclerotic, noninflammatory vascular disease most frequently involving the renal arteries of young white women.[260] Detailed histologic studies have resulted in the recognition of at least four distinct pathologic types: intimal fibroplasia, medial fibroplasia, medial hyperplasia, and perimedial dysplasia.[261]

The first report of FMD by Leadbetter and Burkland in 1938[262] described a patient with renal artery involvement. The majority of cases involve the renal artery, with the carotid and iliac arteries representing distant second and third most likely areas of involvement.[263] Rarely, the external iliac, femoral, popliteal, mesenteric, subclavian, axillary, forearm, vertebral, and coronary arteries may be involved. Ninety percent of adult patients with FMD are female. With renal involvement, 70% of patients display bilateral disease. The more severe disease almost always occurs on the right. Lesions affecting the left renal artery alone occur in fewer than 10% of these patients. The lesions of medial fibroplasia have the classic "string of beads" morphology on angiography (Fig. 8–16).

Medial fibroplasia accounts for 85% of FMD, perimedial dysplasia for 10%, and intimal fibroplasia for 5%. The groups are distinguished from each other by the vessel wall layer primarily affected and by the tissue components that predominate. An increase of fibrous connective tissue, collagen, and ground substance within the media is characteristic of medial fibroplasia. The smooth muscle cell is multipotential and appears to be the source from which the proliferative changes in FMD are derived. The etiology of FMD is unknown. Several theories have been advanced, including (1) arterial stretching, (2) mural ischemia second-

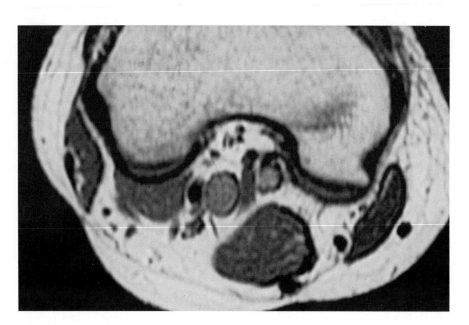

Figure 8–15. A magnetic resonance imaging scan showing the abnormal insertion of the medial head of the gastrocnemius muscle between the popliteal artery and vein. The popliteal artery ends up medial to the medial head of the gastrocnemius muscle.

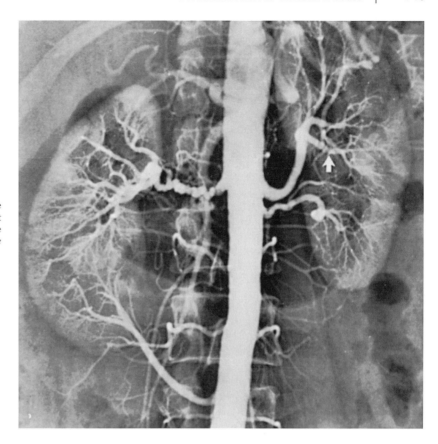

Figure 8–16. Fibromuscular dysplasia (FMD). The superior right renal artery shows typical involvement extending beyond the primary branching. Moderate left kidney segmental artery FMD is present (*white arrow*).

ary to an abnormal distribution of vasa vasorum, (3) estrogenic (or other hormonal) effects on the arterial wall, (4) immunologic insult, and (5) anomalous embryologic development.[264] A familial prevalence of 11% was noted in a recent series.[265]

Symptoms produced by FMD are generally secondary to the associated arterial stenoses and are indistinguishable from those caused by atherosclerosis. The two most frequently seen clinical syndromes are renovascular hypertension and transient cerebral ischemic attacks. Treatment is recommended for arterial stenotic lesions only when they produce significant symptoms. Renovascular hypertension caused by FMD has responded more favorably to surgery than has that caused by atherosclerosis.[265] Results of surgical management of children with renovascular FMD have been encouraging.[266] Percutaneous transluminal angioplasty has been shown to be effective in selected patients.[267] Using logistic regression, factors found to independently predict good response of hypertension to angioplasty included systolic blood pressure before intervention, duration of hypertension, and patient age.[268] Fibromuscular dysplasia of the renal artery may be associated with the formation of renal artery aneurysms and renal artery dissection.

Carotid artery FMD causes symptoms identical to atherosclerotic lesions and, similarly, the disease usually stops before the internal carotid artery enters the base of the skull. Less than 1% of patients undergoing carotid arteriography have FMD.[264] Ten percent to 51% of patients with FMD of the internal carotid artery harbor intracranial aneurysms.[269]

Treatment of symptomatic patients by graduated internal dilatation at the time of surgery is preferred, but patch angioplasty or interposition grafting may be required, depending on the location and extent of involvement.[270] Iliac FMD and femoral artery FMD have been successfully treated by graduated internal dilatation with long-term success,[271] although transluminal angioplasty has been increasingly applied.

ADVENTITIAL CYSTIC DISEASE

Adventitial cystic disease is a rare condition that must always be considered in the differential diagnosis of claudication in a young patient. Arterial stenosis is caused by single or multiple synovial-like cysts in the subadventitial layer of the arterial wall compressing the arterial lumen. The cysts typically contain mucinous degenerative debris or clear, gelatinous material similar to that found in ganglia. Eighty percent of patients with this condition are male, and the median age at presentation is 42 years.[272]

The first case report describing operative management was in 1954.[273] Since then, fewer than 150 cases have been reported. The popliteal artery has been by far the most frequently involved artery, with the femoral and iliac arteries being the next most frequent areas of involvement. Bilateral popliteal involvement has not been reported.

The etiology of adventitial cystic disease is unknown. A direct communication with the adjacent knee joint, similar to a true ganglion, has been demonstrated in selected cases.[274] Others have suggested the presence within the arterial wall of mucin-secreting cell rests derived embryologically from the synovial anlage of the knee joint.[275] The theory that adventitial cystic disease is due to repeated arterial microtrauma has largely been abandoned.

On examination, the finding of a popliteal bruit and the absence of palpable pulses with knee flexion have been noted in a number of patients with adventitial cystic disease involvement of the popliteal artery. Diagnosis is possible using ultrasonography, CT, and MRI.[276] Intravascular ultrasonography has also emerged as a helpful imaging modality.[277] Arteriography may demonstrate segmental popliteal arterial occlusion or may show a "scimitar" sign of luminal encroachment by the cyst in a normally placed vessel that has no other signs of occlusive disease.[278]

Several methods of treatment have been described. Arteries with a small cyst have been successfully treated with CT- or ultrasound-guided needle aspiration[279] or cyst enucleation, although approximately 10% recur following this treatment. In more severely affected patients, segmental arterial replacement may be required. Patients with popliteal occlusion require bypass grafting. Treatment has been successful in more than 90% of reported cases.[272]

COMPARTMENT SYNDROME

Compartment syndrome occurs whenever tissue pressure within a confined space becomes sufficiently elevated to impair perfusion. If untreated, diminished nutritive blood flow results in limb dysfunction secondary to ischemic muscle contracture.[279] The first clinical description of this syndrome was by von Volkmann over a century ago in a report on contracture involving the arm following trauma. He attributed the deformity to a prolonged interruption of the vascular supply to the muscle.[280] In 1926, Jepson[281] reported successful experimental reproduction of the syndrome and demonstrated that early compartment decompression may prevent ischemic muscle paralysis and contracture.

The multiple clinical etiologies for compartment syndrome have been well described by Matsen[282] and are listed in Table 8–6. Any loss of vascular integrity, such as occurs following prolonged ischemia or reperfusion injury, leads to increased edema within a compartment. This edema then compromises venous outflow, increasing venous and capillary pressures, leading to increased compartment and decreased perfusion pressures. Pivotal to the development of the syndrome, whether from external compression or internal tissue swelling, is the production of sufficient intracompartment pressure to impair blood flow to the tissues.

The capillary leak following ischemia and reperfusion is believed to be mediated through inflammatory mediators and oxygen-derived free radicals.[283] The return of oxygenated blood to the microcirculation of ischemic tissue causes activation of inflammatory mediators locally and systemically. Neutrophil adherence to endothelium leads to oxidant release (H_2O_2, O_2, and OH^-) that damages the endothelium. Animal models suggest that treatment with free radical scavengers may mitigate the damage seen in compartment syndrome.[284] Experimentally blocking neutrophil adherence has also been shown to decrease reperfusion injury.[285]

There is no absolute pressure above which compartment

TABLE 8–6

Etiologies of Compartment Syndromes

Decreased compartment volume	Closure of fascial defects
	Application of excessive traction to fractured limbs
Increased compartment content	Bleeding
	Major vascular injury
	Coagulation defect
	Bleeding disorder
	Anticoagulant therapy
	Increased capillary filtration
	Increased capillary permeability
	Reperfusion after arterial revascularization
	Trauma
	Fracture
	Contusion (crush)
	Intensive use of muscles
	Exercise
	Seizures
	Burns
	Intraarterial drug injection
	Cold
	Orthopedic surgery
	Snakebite
	Increased capillary pressure
	Intensive use of muscles
	Venous obstruction
	Diminished serum osmolarity— nephrotic syndrome
Externally applied pressure	Tight casts, dressings, or air splints
	Lying on limb

syndrome will invariably occur, although tissue blood flow diminishes rapidly as intracompartment pressure approaches the level of the diastolic blood pressure. Additionally, conditions such as hypotension or vasoconstriction may lead to the production of the syndrome at lower intracompartment pressures. In addition to the absolute and relative intracompartment pressures, the duration of ischemia is an important factor. Nerve tissue appears to be most susceptible to ischemia, with symptoms occurring within minutes and permanent damage at 2 hours or less. Muscle death begins at approximately 4 hours. Maximal muscle contracture appears to require about 12 hours of ischemia.[282] Skin and subcutaneous tissues are capable of tolerating periods of ischemia that are not tolerated by skeletal muscle or peripheral nerves.[286]

In patients with acute interruption of arterial blood flow, the incidence of compartment syndrome averages 8%.[287] The need for fasciotomy following revascularization is increased if more than 6 hours of ischemia have occurred or if there has been a substantial period of shock in association with the arterial injury. Other circumstances increasing the need for fasciotomy include the occurrence of a tight swelling of the extremity preoperatively or intraoperatively, the combination of arterial and venous injury, and the presence of concomitant soft tissue crush injury. Compartment syndrome may develop in up to 30% of all extremities after combined fracture and arterial injury. Interest in the use of thrombolytic therapy for acute arterial occlusion must be kept in mind as another mode of reperfusion injury. Acute compartment syndrome following thrombolysis has been observed in our own practice and reported in the literature.[288]

In the lower leg, compartment syndrome most frequently occurs in the anterior compartment, followed by the lateral, deep posterior, and superficial posterior compartments. The quadriceps compartment in the thigh and the gluteal compartment in the buttock may be involved. In the upper extremity, the volar forearm compartment is most frequently involved, but involvement of the dorsal forearm, biceps, deltoid, and hand interossei have also been reported.

The accurate diagnosis of compartment syndrome leading to successful treatment is based on the recognition of the early signs and symptoms of increased compartment pressure, as diminished function of the extremity precedes nerve and muscle necrosis by several hours. Clinical signs include fullness and tenderness of the compartment, pain disproportionate to the physical findings, paresthesias of the compartment nerves, and weakness of the involved muscles. The palpable pulse status and Doppler pressures are unreliable reflections of intracompartment pressures. With compression of postcapillary venules and a continued fall in the arteriovenous perfusion gradient, tissue damage may occur despite continued arterial inflow and palpable pulses.[289]

In questionable clinical situations or when the patient is unable to adequately communicate, objective data reflecting either intracompartment pressure or nerve function may be monitored. Continuous or intermittent compartment pressure determinations may be made by the Wick catheter technique, in which a plastic catheter is placed percutaneously into the compartment and is connected to a pressure transducer.[290] A solid-state transducer that fits within a catheter tip in a handheld unit, the "solid-state transducer in catheter" (STIC) monitor, eliminates the artifacts inherent to pressure lines.[291] Surgical decompression is generally recommended for patients who have a compartment pressure of 40 mm Hg or greater or for those who have had a compartment pressure greater than 30 mm Hg for 4 hours. Others have argued that intervention based on fixed pressure is inappropriate and that critical intracompartment pressures occur when within 30 mm Hg of the mean arterial pressure or 20 mm Hg of the diastolic pressure.[292]

Once compartment syndrome occurs, the time delay before treatment becomes the critical factor in determining outcome. Twelve hours appears to be the point beyond which significant residual dysfunction will likely occur despite adequate surgical decompression.[293] All circumferential bandages or casts should be removed on suspicion of increased compartment pressure to allow a complete examination of the extremity. The extremity should be placed at the level of the heart and not elevated, because elevation may further jeopardize ischemic compartment components. If physical examination, pressure measurements, or nerve conduction studies suggest a compartment syndrome, immediate surgical decompression is indicated. Our choice of a decompressive technique is shown in Figure 8–17.

Untreated compartment syndrome results in direct neu-

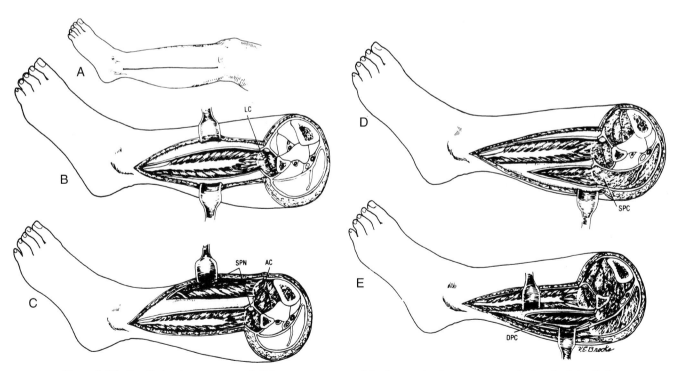

Figure 8–17. Parafibular decompression of all four compartments of the leg. *A,* The skin incision runs the length of the fibula. *B,* The lateral compartment (LC) is opened directly beneath the skin incision. *C,* The anterior compartment (AC) is exposed by retracting the anterior skin flap and is opened over the entire length. Care is taken to preserve the superficial peroneal nerve (SPN). *D,* The superficial posterior compartment (SPC) is exposed by retracting the posterior skin flap and is opened over its entire length. *E,* The lateral compartment is retracted anteriorly, and the superficial posterior compartment is retracted posteriorly after the fibular origin of the soleus muscle is released (not shown). This exposes the deep posterior compartment (DPC), which is opened over its entire length. (From Matsen FA, Winquist RA, Krugmire RB: Diagnosis and management of compartmental syndromes. J Bone Joint Surg 62:286–291, 1980.)

rologic dysfunction or the development of contractures following fibrous replacement of myonecrosis. Symptomatic severity ranges from mild to critical, and amputation may be required. Frequent examination of the blood from patients with compartment syndrome may reveal elevated levels of creatinine phosphokinase as well as hyperkalemia. Subsequently, there may be myoglobinuria and renal failure.[294] In such patients, restoration of normal hemodynamics, the administration of mannitol to enhance urine flow and improve intrarenal blood distribution, and alkalinization of the urine to prevent precipitation of myoglobin within the renal tubules are specific therapeutic measures.[294] Prevention of the reperfusion syndrome has been shown in selective patients after the administration of hypertonic mannitol, presumably as a result of its free radical scavenging.[295] Deep muscle infections are uncommon but potentially life-threatening sequelae.

HOMOCYSTINURIA

Homocystinuria, an inborn error of metabolism in which homocysteine accumulates abnormally in plasma, tissues, and urine, was first described in 1963.[296] Patients with this disorder suffer from multiple abnormalities, including ectopia lentis, mental retardation, thromboembolic disorders, and rapidly progressive arteriosclerotic vascular disease.[296, 297] Three specific enzyme deficiencies, each of which may be responsible for homocystinuria, have been identified: (1) cystathionine β-synthetase (CβS) deficiency,[298] (2) homocysteine methyltransferase (HMT) deficiency,[299] and (3) methylene tetrahydrofolate reductase (MTHFR) deficiency.[300] These enzymes require cofactors, including folate, vitamin B_6 (pyridoxine), and vitamin B_{12} (cobalamin).[301–303] Regardless of the primary cause, all forms of homocystinuria in humans have been associated with premature atherosclerosis, frequently complicated by thrombosis.[297] The occurrence of the same clinical syndrome in patients with different enzyme deficiencies that all result in abnormal accumulation of homocysteine is strong evidence that homocysteine itself is toxic.

Homocysteine is an intermediary, nonstructural amino acid involved in the transulfuration pathway leading to the production of cysteine. In this pathway, a sulfur group is transferred from methionine to serine to produce cysteine. The enzymes CBS, HMT, and MTHFR, as well as the cofactors folate, vitamin B_6, and vitamin B_{12}, are all involved. Any deficiency in these enzymes or cofactors leads to the accumulation of homocysteine. Harker and colleagues[304] have shown that infusion of homocysteine into laboratory animals produces endothelial cell injury and rapid proliferation of atherosclerotic lesions. Treatment of homocysteinemic animals with vitamin B_6 or folate or both improved some of the laboratory and clinical manifestations of homocysteinemia.[305]

Homocysteine exists in human plasma in at least three forms: as the mixed disulfide homocysteinecysteine, as free homocysteine, and as the disulfide homocystine.[306] In nonhomocystinuric conditions, most homocysteine exists in the plasma bound to protein. Men have higher levels of plasma homocysteine than women, and premenopausal women have lower levels than postmenopausal women.[307] Accumu-

lation of homocysteine leads the liver to produce homocysteine thiolactone, which has been implicated as the toxic substance in homocysteinemic atherogenesis. Homocysteine thiolactone alters surface charges and may predispose to cellular aggregation within the vascular lumen.[308] Interestingly, the metabolism of homocysteine thiolactone appears abnormal in patients with arteriosclerosis without homocysteinemia.

The detection of elevated plasma homocysteine has historically required the use of a cumbersome dietary methionine load. Kang and associates[309] simplified these investigations when they demonstrated elevated levels of protein-bound homocysteine in patients with coronary artery disease, without any requirements for dietary methionine loading, through the use of high-performance liquid chromatography. This enables accurate levels to be obtained without the need for fasting or for methionine loading and has become the standard clinical assay.[310]

The arteriosclerotic lesions occurring in homocystinuria, whether resulting from CBS deficiency, HMT deficiency, or MTHFR deficiency, are typical fibrous plaques.[311] Microscopic evaluation reveals medial hypertrophy, elaboration of extracellular matrix and collagen, and degeneration and destruction of the elastic laminae. Lipid deposition in the plaques is characteristically absent.[311]

The prevalence of mild homocysteinemia in the general population is estimated to be 5% to 7%. If a genetic defect is necessary, homozygous thermolabile MTHFR and heterozygous CBS and MTHFR deficiency are the most probable factors.[312] These deficiencies cause an approximately 50% reduction in corresponding enzyme activities and are estimated to occur in 5% to 6% of the population. However, other factors, such as vitamin deficiency and environment, must be involved, as phenotypic expression is not complete.[313] Increasing evidence indicates that mildly elevated levels of plasma homocysteine may be associated with symptomatic atherosclerotic disease.[314]

Evaluation of our patients with peripheral vascular disease has confirmed elevated total plasma homocysteine levels in a significant number of patients compared with age- and sex-matched controls.[315] Stampfer and colleagues,[316] in a retrospective review of prospectively obtained blood samples in the Physicians' Health Study, demonstrated an association between elevated plasma homocysteine levels and myocardial infarction. Arnesen and coauthors[317] showed that elevated homocysteine levels predicted myocardial infarction in a general population in Norway. Perry and coauthors[318] and Verhoef and associates[319] both found that elevated homocysteine levels were related to ischemic strokes.

Our data have established elevated homocysteine levels as an independent risk factor for death from cardiovascular disease in patients with lower extremity disease and cerebrovascular disease.[320] Norwegian investigators have also prospectively demonstrated a strong relationship between homocysteine levels and early mortality rates in patients with established coronary artery disease.[321]

Investigations have focused on lowering these supranormal plasma homocysteine levels through alteration of the homocysteine-methionine pathways using pharmacologic doses of the cofactors for these enzymatic pathways, specifically folic acid, vitamin B_6, and vitamin B_{12}.[322] Elevated levels of plasma homocysteine can be reliably reduced to normal by the administration of folate in most patients. Patients who are resistent to folate therapy often respond to vitamin B_6, vitamin B_{12}, choline, or betaine. These substances appear to be able to reduce homocysteine levels regardless of the underlying cause of elevated homocysteine.

Treatment of homocysteinemia with various vitamins has the potential for being essentially nontoxic. At present, there are no convincing data that lowering the homocysteine level in patients with vascular disease will yield any true benefit. Although intuitively one would expect clinical

improvement once the toxic homocysteine levels have declined, serial evaluation of the progression of peripheral vascular disease in groups randomized to treatment and nontreatment is necessary to determine clinical benefit.

We are currently involved in a prospective, randomized study to determine the role of homocysteine in vascular disease. This study involves a treatment period to determine whether folic acid therapy slows disease progression in individuals with elevated homocysteine levels. We are hopeful that this and other prospective studies currently under way will help to further elucidate the role of homocysteinemia in vascular disease.

References

1. Edwards JM: Raynaud's syndrome: Basic data. Ann Vasc Surg 8:509–513, 1994.
2. Fraenkel L, Zhang Y, Chaisson CE, et al: Different factors influencing the expression of Raynaud's phenomenon in men and women. Arthritis Rheum 42:306–310, 1999.
3. Lewis T: Experiments relating to the peripheral mechanism involved in spasmodic arrest of the circulation in the fingers, a variety of Raynaud's disease. Heart 15:7, 1929.
4. Kontos HA, Wasserman AJ: Effect of reserpine in Raynaud's phenomenon. Circulation 39:259–266, 1969.
5. Harker CT, Ousley PJ, Bowman CJ, Porter JM: Cooling augments alpha-2-adrenoceptor–mediated contractions in the rat tail artery. Am J Physiol 260:H1166–H1171, 1991.
6. Janssens WJ, Vanhoutte PM: Instantaneous changes in alpha-adrenoceptor affinity caused by moderate cooling in canine cutaneous veins. Am J Physiol 234:330–337, 1978.
7. Graafsma SJ, Wollersheim H, Droste HT, et al: Adrenoceptors on blood cells from patients with primary Raynaud's phenomenon. Clin Sci 80:325, 1991.
8. Keenan EJ, Porter JM: Alpha₂-adrenergic receptors in platelets from patients with Raynaud's syndrome. Surgery 94:204, 1983.
9. Edwards JM, Phinney ES, Taylor LM, et al: Alpha₂-adrenergic receptor levels in obstructive and spastic Raynaud's syndrome. J Vasc Surg 5:38, 1987.
10. Coffman JD, Cohen RA: Alpha₂-adrenergic and 5-HT₂ receptor hypersensitivity in Raynaud's phenomenon. J Vasc Med Biol 2:101–106, 1990.
11. Cooke JP, Creager SJ, Scales KM, et al: Role of digital artery adrenoceptors. Vasc Med 2:1–7, 1997.
12. Smith PJ, Ferro CJ, McQueen DS, Webb DJ: Impaired cholinergic dilator response of resistance arteries isolated from patients with Raynaud's disease. Br J Clin Pharmacol 47:507–513, 1999.
13. Zamora MR, O'Brien RF, Rutherford RB, et al: Serum endothelin-1 concentrations and cold provocation in primary Raynaud's phenomenon. Lancet 336:1144, 1990.
14. Leppert J, Ringquist A, Karlberg BE, Ringquist I: Whole-body cooling increases plasma endothelin-1 levels in women with primary Raynaud's phenomenon. Clin Physiol 18:420–425, 1998.
15. Shawket S, Dickerson C, Hazelman B, et al: Selective suprasensitivity to calcitonin gene-related peptide in the hands in Raynaud's phenomenon. Lancet 2:1354–1357, 1989.
16. Allen EV, Brown GE: Raynaud's disease: A critical review of minimal requisites for diagnosis. Am J Med Sci 83:187–200, 1932.
17. McLafferty RB, Edwards JM, Ferris BL, et al: Raynaud's syndrome in workers who use vibrating pneumatic air knives. J Vasc Surg 30:1–7, 1999.
18. Medsger TA: Progressive systemic sclerosis and related disorders. In Panush RF (ed): Principles of Rheumatology. New York, John Wiley & Sons, 1981, pp 331–350.
19. Priollet P, Vayssairat M, Housset E: How to classify Raynaud's phenomenon: Long-term follow-up study of 73 cases. Am J Med 83:494–498, 1987.
20. Harper FE, Maricq HR, Turner RE, et al: A prospective study of Raynaud's phenomenon and early connective tissue disease: A five-year report. Am J Med 72:883–888, 1982.
21. Kallenberg CCGM, Wouda AA: Systemic involvement and immunologic findings in patients presenting with Raynaud's phenomenon. Am J Med 69:675–680, 1980.
22. Edwards JM, Porter JM: Associated diseases with Raynaud's syndrome. Vasc Med Rev 1:51–58, 1990.
23. Landry G, Edwards JM, McLafferty RM, et al: Long-term outcome of Raynaud's syndrome in a prospective analyzed cohort. J Vasc Surg 23:76–86, 1996.
24. Porter JM, Snider RL, Bardana EJ, et al: The diagnosis and treatment of Raynaud's phenomenon. Surgery 77:11, 1975.
25. Holmgren K, Baur GM, Porter JM: The role of digital photoplethysmography in the evaluation of Raynaud's syndrome. Bruit 5:5–9, 1981.
26. Sumner D, Strandness DE: An abnormal finger pulse associated with cold sensitivity. Ann Surg 175:294–298, 1972.
27. Nielson SL, Lassen NA: Measurement of digital blood pressure after local cooling. J Appl Physiol 43:907–910, 1977.
28. Gates KH, Tyburczy JA, Zupan T, et al: The noninvasive quantification of digital vasospasm. Bruit 8:34–37, 1984.
29. Clark S, Campbell F, Moore T, et al: Laser doppler imaging—a new technique for quantifying microcirculatory flow in patients with primary Raynaud's phenomenon and systemic sclerosis. Microvasc Res 57:284–291, 1999.
30. Palesch YY, Valter I, Carpentier PH, Maricq HR: Association between cigarette and alcohol consumption and Raynaud's phenomenon. J Clin Epidemiol 52:321–328, 1999.
31. Mills JL, Friedman EI, Taylor LM Jr, et al: Upper extremity ischemia caused by small artery disease. Ann Surg 206:521, 1987.
32. Rodeheffer RJ, Rommer JA, Wigley F, et al: Controlled double-blind trial of nifedipine in the treatment of Raynaud's phenomenon. N Engl J Med 308:880–883, 1983.
33. Fisher M, Grotta J: New uses for calcium channel blockers. Drugs 46:961–975, 1993.
34. Sturgill MG, Seibold JR: Rational use of calcium-channel antagonists in Raynaud's phenomenon. Curr Opin Rheumatol 10:584–588, 1998.
35. Weber A, Bounameaux H: Effects of low-dose nifedipine on a cold provocation test in patients with Raynaud's disease. J Cardiovasc Pharmacol 15:853–855, 1990.
36. Pancera P, Sansone S, Secchi S, et al: The effects of thromboxane A₂ inhibition (picotamide) and angiotensin II receptor blockade (losartan) in primary Raynaud's phenomenon. J Intern Med 242:373–376, 1997.
37. Gasbarrini A, Massari I, Serricchio M, et al: *Helicobacter pylori* eradicates and ameliorates primary Raynaud's phenomenon. Dig Dis Sci 43:1641–1645, 1998.
38. Wigley FM, Wise RA, Seibold JR, et al: Intravenous iloprost infusion in patients with Raynaud phenomenon secondary to systemic sclerosis. Ann Intern Med 120:199–206, 1994.
39. Wigley FM, Seibold JR, Wise RA, et al: Intravenous iloprost treatment of Raynaud's phenomenon and ischemic ulcers secondary to systemic sclerosis. J Rheumatol 19:1407–1414, 1992.
40. Kyle MV, Belcher G, Hazleman BL: Placebo-controlled study showing therapeutic benefit of iloprost in the treatment of Raynaud's phenomenon. J Rheumatol 19:1403–1406, 1992.
41. Black CM, Halkier-Sorensen L, Belch JJ, et al: Oral iloprost in Raynaud's phenomenon secondary to systemic sclerosis: A multicen-

tre, placebo-controlled, dose-comparison study. Br J Rheumatol 37:952–960, 1998.

42. Vayssairat M: Controlled multicenter double blind trial of an oral analog of prostacyclin in the treatment of primary Raynaud's phenomenon. J Rheumatol 23:1917–1920, 1996.

43. Wigley FM, Korn JH, Csuka ME, et al: Oral iloprost treatment in patients with Raynaud's phenomenon secondary to systemic sclerosis: A multicenter, placebo-controlled, double-blind study. Arthritis Rheum 41:670–677, 1998.

44. Wise RA, Wigley F: Acute effects of misoprostol on digital circulation in patients with Raynaud's phenomenon. J Rheumatol 21:80–83, 1994.

45. Katoh K, Kawai T, Narita M: Use of prostaglandin E$_1$ (lipo-PGE$_1$) to treat Raynaud's phenomenon associated with connective tissue disease: Thermographic and subjective assessment. J Pharm Pharmacol 44:442–444, 1992.

46. Freedman RR: Physiological mechanisms of temperature biofeedback. Biofeedback Self Regul 16:95–115, 1991.

47. Mulder P, Dompeling EC, van Slochteren-van der Boor JC, et al: Transcutaneous electrical nerve stimulation (TENS) in Raynaud's phenomenon. Angiology 42:414–417, 1991.

48. Appiah R, Hiller S, Caspary L, et al: Treatment of primary Raynaud's syndrome with traditional Chinese acupuncture. J Intern Med 241:119–124, 1997.

49. Lowell RC, Gloviczki P, Cherry KJ, et al: Cervicothoracic sympathectomy for Raynaud's syndrome. Int Angiol 12:168, 1993.

50. Nicholson ML, Hopkinson BR, Dennis MJS: Endoscopic transthoracic sympathectomy: Successful in hyperhidrosis but can the indications be extended? Ann R Coll Surg Engl 76:311–314, 1994.

51. Janoff KA, Phinney ES, Porter JM: Lumbar sympathectomy for lower extremity vasospasm. Am J Surg 150:147–151, 1985.

52. Yee AM, Hotchkiss RN, Paget SA: Adventitial stripping: A digit saving procedure in refractory Raynaud's phenomenon. J Rheumatol 25:269–276, 1998.

53. McCall TE, Petersen DP, Wong LB: The use of digital artery sympathectomy as a salvage procedure for severe ischemia of Raynaud's disease and phenomenon. J Hand Surg [Am] 24:173–177, 1999.

54. Jones NF, Raynor SC, Medsger TA: Microsurgical revascularization of the hand in scleroderma. Br J Plast Surg 40:264–269, 1987.

55. Nehler MR, Dalman RL, Harris EJ, et al: Upper extremity arterial bypass distal to the wrist. J Vasc Surg 16:633–642, 1992.

56. King TA, Marks J, Berrettone BA: Arteriovenous reversal for limb salvage in unreconstructable upper extremity arterial occlusive disease. J Vasc Surg 17:924–933, 1993.

57. Spencer-Green G: Outcomes in primary Raynaud's phenomenon: A meta-analysis of the frequency, rates, and predictors of transition to secondary diseases. Arch Intern Med 158:595–600, 1998.

58. Lie JT: Vasculitis, 1815 to 1991: Classification and diagnostic specificity. J Rheumatol 19:83–89, 1992.

59. Jennette JC, Falk RJ, Andrassy K, et al: Nomenclature of systemic vasculitides: Proposal of an international consensus conference. Arthritis Rheum 37:187–192, 1994.

60. Savage COS: Pathogenesis of systemic vasculitis. In Churg A, Churg J (eds): Systemic Vasculitides. New York, Igaku-Shoin, 1991, pp 7–30.

61. Gauthier VJ, Mannik M: Immune complexes in the pathogenesis of vasculitis. In LeRoy EC (ed): Systemic Vasculitis: The Biological Basis. New York, Marcel Dekker, 1992, pp 401–420.

62. Sheps SG, McDuffie FC: Vasculitis. In Juergens JL, Spittell JA, Gairbaim JF (eds): Peripheral Vascular Disease. Philadelphia, WB Saunders, 1980, pp 493–553.

63. Jacobs MR, Allen NB: Giant cell arteritis. In Churg A, Churg J (eds): Systemic Vasculitides. New York, Igaku-Shoin, 1991, pp 143–158.

64. Joyce JW: Uncommon arteriopathies. In Rutherford RB (ed): Vascular Surgery. Philadelphia, WB Saunders, 1989, pp 276–286.

65. Michel BA, Arend WP, Hunder GG: Clinical differentiation between giant cell (temporal) arteritis and Takayasu's arteritis. J Rheumatol 23:106–111, 1996.

66. Huston KA, Hunder GG, Lie JT, et al: Temporal arteritis: A 25 year epidemiologic, clinical, and pathologic study. Ann Intern Med 88:162–167, 1978.

67. Duhaut P, Bosshard S, Calvet A, et al: Giant cell arteritis, polymyalgia rheumatica, and viral hypotheses: A multicenter, prospective case-control study. J Rheumatol 26:361–369, 1999.

68. Pountain G, Hazleman B: Polymyalgia rheumatica and giant cell arteritis. BMJ 310:1057–1059, 1995.

69. Mehler MF, Rabinowich L: The clinical neuro-ophthalmologic spectrum of temporal arteritis. Am J Med 85:839–844, 1988.

70. Evans JM, O'Fallon M, Hunder GG: Increased incidence of aortic aneurysm and dissection in giant cell (temporal) arteritis. Ann Intern Med 122:502–507, 1995.

71. Healey LA, Wilskie KR: The Systemic Manifestations of Temporal Arteritis. New York, Grune & Stratton, 1978.

72. Klein RG, Hunder GG, Stanson AW, et al: Large artery involvement in giant cell temporal arteritis. Ann Intern Med 83:806–812, 1975.

73. Rivers SP, Baur GM, Inahara T, et al: Arm ischemia secondary to giant cell arteritis. Am J Surg 143:554–558, 1982.

74. Kay RH, Pale R, Herman MV: Unsuspected giant cell arteritis diagnosed at open heart surgery. Arch Intern Med 112:1378–1379, 1982.

75. Boyer LR, Miller NR, Green WR: Efficacy of unilateral versus bilateral temporal artery biopsies for the diagnosis of giant cell arteritis. Am J Ophthamol 128:211–215, 1999.

76. Schmidt WA, Kraft HE, Vorpahl K, et al: Color duplex ultrasonography in the diagnosis of temporal arteritis. N Engl J Med 337:1336–1342, 1997.

77. Matteson EL, Gold KN, Bloch DA, Hunder GG: Long-term survival of patients with giant cell arteritis in the American College of Rheumatology giant cell arteritis classification criteria cohort. Am J Med 100:193–196, 1996.

78. Lupi-Herrera E, Sanchez-Torres G, Marcustiamer J, et al: Takayasu's arteritis. Clinical study of 107 cases. Am Heart J 93:94–103, 1977.

79. Sun Y, Yip PK, Jeng JS, et al: Ultrasonographic study and long-term follow-up of Takayasu's arteritis. Stroke 27:2178–2182, 1996.

80. Taniguchi N, Itoh K, Honda M, et al: Comparative ultrasonographic and angiographic study of carotid arterial lesions in Takayasu's arteritis. Angiology 48:9–20, 1997.

81. Park JH, Chung JW, Lee KW, et al: CT angiography of Takayasu's arteritis: Comparison with conventional angiography. J Vasc Interv Radiol 8:393–400, 1997.

82. Sharma S, Rajani M, Talwar KK: Angiographic morphology in nonspecific aortoarteritis (Takayasu's arteritis): A study of 126 patients from North India. Cardiovasc Intervent Radiol 15:160–165, 1992.

83. Joyce JW: The giant cell arteritides: Diagnosis and the role of surgery. J Vasc Surg 3:827–832, 1986.

84. Robbs JV, Abdool-Carrim ATO, Kadwa AM. Arterial reconstruction for non-specific arteritis (Takayosu's disease): Medium to long term results. Eur J Vasc Surg 8:401–407, 1994.

85. Kerr GS, Hallahan CW, Giordano J, et al: Takayasu arteritis. Ann Intern Med 120:919–929, 1994.

86. Tyagi S, Kaul UA, Nair M, et al: Balloon angioplasty of the aorta in Takayasu's arteritis: Initial and long-term results. Am Heart J 124:876–882, 1992.

87. Rao SA, Mandalam KR, Rao VR, et al: Takayasu arteritis: Initial and long-term follow-up in 16 patients after percutaneous transluminal angioplasty of the descending thoracic and abdominal aorta. Radiology 189:173–179, 1993.

88. Tyagis, Verma PK, Gambhir DS, et al: Early and long-term results of subclavian angioplasty in aortoarteritis (Takayasu's disease): Comparison with atherosclerosis. Cardiovasc Intervent Radiol 21:219–224, 1998.

90. Madrazo AA, Keane WF: Radiation vasculitis. In Churg A, Churg J (eds): Systemic Vasculitides. New York, Igaku-Shoin, 1991, pp 343–349.

91. Sugihara T, Hattori Y, Yamamoto Y, et al: Preferential impairment of nitric oxide–mediated endothelium-dependent relaxation in human cervical arteries after radiation. Circulation 100:635–641, 1999.

92. Fonkalsrud EW, Sanchez M, Zervbavel R, et al: Serial changes in arterial structure following radiation therapy. Surg Gynecol Obstet 145:395–400, 1977.

93. McCready RA, Hyde GL, Bivins BA, et al: Radiation induced arterial injuries. Surgery 93:306–312, 1983.

94. Elerding SC, Fernandez RN, Grotta JC, et al: Carotid artery disease following external cervical irradiation. Ann Surg 194:609–615, 1981.

95. Andros G, Schneider PA, Harris RW, et al: Management of arterial occlusive disease following radiation therapy. Cardiovasc Surg 9:135–142, 1996.

96. Phillips GR 3d, Peer RM, Upson JE, Ricotta JJ: Late complications of revascularization for radiation-induced arterial disease. J Vasc Surg 16:921–924, 1992.

97. Saliou C, Julia P, Feito B, et al: Radiation-induced arterial disease of the lower limb. Ann Vasc Surg 11:173–177, 1997.

98. Arkin A: A clinical and pathological study of periarteritis nodosa. Am J Pathol 6:401–427, 1930.

99. Rosen S, Falk RJ, Jennette JC: Polyarteritis nodosa, including microscopic form and renal vasculitis. In Churg A, Churg J (eds): Systemic Vasculitides. New York, Igaku-Shoin, 1991, pp 57–77.

100. Staud R, Williams RC: Antineutrophilic cytoplasmic antibodies (ANCA) and vasculitis. Compr Ther 20:623–627, 1994.

101. Travers RL, Allison DJ, Brettle RP, et al: Polyarteritis nodosa: A clinical and angiographic analysis of 17 cases. Semin Arthritis Rheum 8:184–199, 1979.

102. Ewald EA, Griffin D, McCune WJ: Correlation of angiographic abnormalities with disease manifestations and disease severity in polyarteritis nodosa. J Rheumatol 14:952–956, 1987.

103. Selke FW, Williams GB, Donovan DL, et al: Management of intra-abdominal aneurysms associated with periarteritis nodosa. J Vasc Surg 4:294–299, 1986.

104. Fauci AS, Katz P, Haynes BF, et al: Cyclophosphamide therapy of severe systemic necrotizing vasculitis. N Engl J Med 301:325–328, 1979.

105. McCauley RL, Johnston MR, Fauci AS: Surgical aspects of systemic necrotizing vasculitis. Surgery 97:104–108, 1985.

106. Cohen RD, Conn DL, Ilstrup DM: Clinical features, prognosis, and response to treatment in polyarteritis. Mayo Clin Proc 55:140–144, 1980.

107. Allen NB, Bressler PB: Diagnosis and treatment of systemic and cutaneous necrotizing vasculitis syndromes. Med Clin North Am 8:243–259, 1997.

108. Guillevin L, Lhote F, Gayraud M, et al: Prognostic factors in polyarteritis nodosa and Churg-Strauss syndrome: A prospective study in 342 patients. Medicine (Baltimore) 75:17–28, 1996.

109. Kawasaki T: MCLS—clinical observations of 50 cases. Jpn J Allergy 16:178–182, 1967.

110. Kawasaki T, Kosaki F, Okawa S, et al: A new infantile acute febrile mucocutaneous lymph node syndrome (MLNS) prevailing in Japan. Pediatrics 54:271–276, 1974.

111. Feigen RD, Schleien CL: Kawasaki disease. Curr Clin Top Infect Dis 4:30, 1983.

112. Yanagawa H, Yashiro M, Nakamura Y, et al: Epidemiologic pictures of Kawasaki disease in Japan: From the nationwide incidence survey in 1991 and 1992. Pediatrics 95:475–479, 1995.

113. Barron KS, Shulman ST, Rowley A, et al: Report of the National Institutes of Health Workshop on Kawasaki disease. J Rheumatol 26:170–190, 1999.

114. Arav-Boger R, Assia A, Jurgenson U, Spirer Z: The immunology of Kawasaki disease. Adv Pediatr 41:359–367, 1994.

115. Nadh MC, Shah V, Dillon MJ: Soluble cell adhesion molecules and von Willebrand factor in children with Kawasaki disease. Clin Exp Immunol 101:13–17, 1995.

116. Landing BH, Larson EJ: Pathological features of Kawasaki disease (mucocutaneous lymph node syndrome). Am J Cardiovasc Pathol 1:215–229, 1987.

117. Laupland KB, Dele Davies H: Epidemiology etiology, and management of Kawasaki disease: State of the art. Pediatr Cardiol 20:177–183, 1999.

118. Capannari TE, Daniels SR, Meyer RA, et al: Sensitivity, specificity, and predictive value of two-dimensional echocardiography in detecting coronary artery aneurysms in patients with Kawasaki disease. J Am Coll Cardiol 7:355–360, 1986.

119. Gribetz D, Landing BH, Larson EJ: Kawasaki disease: Mucocutaneous lymph node syndrome (MCLS). In Churg A, Churg J (eds): Systemic Vasculitides. New York, Igaku-Shoin, 1991, pp 257–272.

120. Kato H, Ichinose E, Yoshioka F, et al: Fate of coronary aneurysms in Kawasaki disease: Serial coronary angiography and long term follow-up study. Am J Cardiol 49:1758–1766, 1982.

121. Inoue O, Akagi T, Ichinose E, et al: Systemic artery involvement in Kawasaki disease. Proceedings of the Third International Kawasaki Disease Symposium, Tokyo, November 29 to December 2, 1988. New York, Allan R Liss, 1988, p 53.

122. Koren G, Rose V, Lavi S, Rowe R: Probable efficacy of high dose salicylates in reducing coronary involvement in Kawasaki disease. JAMA 254:767–769, 1985.

123. Saalouke MG, Venglarcik JS III, Barker DR, et al: Rapid regression of coronary dilatation in Kawasaki disease with intravenous gamma-globulin. Am Heart J 12:905–909, 1991.

124. Kitamura S, Kawashima Y, Fujita T, et al: Aortocoronary bypass grafting in a child with coronary obstruction due to a mucocutaneous lymph node syndrome. Circulation 53:1035–1040, 1976.

125. Myers JL, Gleason MM, Cyren SE, Baylen BG: Surgical management of coronary insufficiency in a child with Kawasaki's disease: Use of bilateral mammary arteries. Ann Thorac Surg 46:459–461, 1988.

126. Takeuchi Y, Gomi A, Okamura Y, et al: Coronary revascularization in a child with Kawasaki disease: Use of a right gastroepiploic artery. Ann Thorac Surg 50:294–296, 1990.

127. Kitamura S, Kameda Y, Seki T, et al: Long-term outcome of myocardial revascularization in patients with Kawasaki coronary artery disease: A multicenter cooperative study. J Thorac Cardiovasc Surg 107:663–673, 1994.

128. Checchia, PA, Pahl E, Shaddy RE, Shulman ST: Cardiac transplantation for Kawasaki disease. Pediatrics 100:695–699, 1997.

129. Sethi S, Ott DA, Nihill M: Surgical management of the cardiovascular complications of Kawasaki's disease. Tex Heart Inst J 10:343–348, 1983.

130. Citron BP, Halpern M, McCarron M, et al: Necrotizing angiitis associated with drug abuse. N Engl J Med 283:1003–1011, 1970.

131. Yu Y, Cooper DR, Wellenstein DE: Cerebral angiitis and intracerebral hemorrhage associated with methamphetamine abuse. J Neurosurg 58:109–111, 1983.

132. Fredericks RK, Lefkowitz DS, Challa VR, Troost BT: Cerebral vasculitis associated with cocaine abuse. Stroke 22:1437–1439, 1991.

133. Ellertson DG, Lazarus AM, Averbach R: Patterns of acute vascular injury after intra-arterial barbiturate injection. Am J Surg 126:813–817, 1973.

134. Lindell TD, Porter JM, Langston C: Intraarterial injection of oral medications. A complication of drug addiction. N Engl J Med 287:1132–1133, 1972.

135. Woodburn KR, Murie JA: Vascular complications of injecting drug misuse. Br J Surg 83:1329–1334, 1996.

136. Behçet H: Über rezidivierende Aphthose durch ein Virus verursachte Geschwur am Mund, am Maule und an den Genitalien. Dermatol Wochenschr 105:1152–1157, 1937.

137. Harris EJ, Nehler MR, Porter JP: Arteritis. Semin Vasc Surg 6:2–13, 1993.

138. Shimutzu T, Ehrlich GE, Inaba G, Hayashi K: Behçet's disease (Behçet's syndrome). Semin Arthritis Rheum 8:223–260, 1979.

139. Ehrlich GE: Vasculitis in Behçet's disease. Int Rev Immunol 14:81–88, 1997.

140. Hamzaoui K, Hamzaoui A, Hentati F, et al: Phenotype and functional profile of T cells expressing gamma-delta receptor from patients with active Behçet's disease. J Rheumatol 21:2301–2306, 1994.

141. Sakane T, Takeno M, Suzuki N, Inaba G: Behçet's disease 341:1284–1291, 1999.

142. Mizuki N, Inoko H, Ohno S: Pathogenic gene responsible for the predisposition to Behçet's disease. Int Rev Immunol 14:33–48, 1997.

143. Lehner T: The role of heat shock protein, microbial and autoimmune agents in the aetiology of Behçet's syndrome. Int Rev Immunol 14:21–32, 1997.

144. Schwartz P, Weisbrott M, Landau M, Antebi E: Peripheral false aneurysms in Behçet's disease. Br J Surg 74:67–68, 1987.

145. Tuzun H, Besirli K, Sayin A, et al: Management of aneurysms in Behçet's syndrome: An analysis of 24 patients. Surgery 121:150–156, 1997.

146. Vasseur MA, Haulon S, Beregi JP, et al: Endovascular treatment of abdominal aneurysmal aortitis in Behçet's disease. J Vasc Surg 27:974–976, 1998.

147. Freyrie A, Paragona O, Cenacchi G, et al: True and false aneurysms in Behçet's disease: Case report with ultrastructural observations. J Vasc Surg 17:762–767, 1993.

148. St. Clair EW, McCallum RW: Cogan's syndrome. Curr Opin Rheumatol 11:47–52, 1999.

149. Ho AC, Roat MI, Venbrux A, Hellmann DB: Cogan's syndrome with refractory abdominal aortitis and mesenteric vasculitis. J Rheumatol 26:1404–1407, 1999.

150. Tseng JF, Cambria RP, Aretz HT, Brewster DC: Thoracoabdominal aortic aneurysm in Cogan's syndrome. J Vasc Surg 30:565–568, 1999.

151. Covelli M, Lapadula G, Pipitone V: Cogan's syndrome: Unsuccessful outcome with early combination therapy. Clin Exp Rheumatol 17:479–483, 1999.

152. Fortin PR, Esdaile JM: Vasculitis and malignancy. In Churg A, Churg J (eds): Systemic Vasculitides. New York, Igaku-Shoin, 1991, pp 327–341.

153. Greer JM, Longley S, Edwards NL, et al: Vasculitis associated with malignancy. Medicine 67:220–230, 1988.
154. Fortin PR: Vasculitides associated with malignancy. Curr Opin Rheumatol 8:30–33, 1996.
155. Kurzrock R, Cohen PR, Markowitz A: Clinical manifestations of vasculitis in patients with solid tumors: A case report and review of the literature. Arch Intern Med 154:334–340, 1994.
156. Andrasch RH, Bardana EJ, Porter JM, et al: Digital ischemia and gangrene preceding renal neoplasm. Arch Intern Med 136:486–488, 1976.
157. Levo Y, Gorevic PD, Kassab HJ, et al: Association between hepatitis B virus and essential mixed cryoglobulinemia. N Engl J Med 296:1501–1504, 1977.
158. Taylor LM, Baur GM, Porter JM: Finger gangrene caused by small artery occlusive disease. Ann Surg 193:453, 1981.
159. Danning CL, Illei GG, Boumpas DT: Vasculitis associated with primary rheumatologic disease. Curr Opin Rheumatol 10:58–65, 1998.
160. Panush RS, Katz P, Longley S, et al: Rheumatoid vasculitis: Diagnostic and therapeutic decisions. Clin Rheumatol 2:321–330, 1983.
161. Braun MG, Csernok E, Schmitt WH, Gross WL: Incidence, target antigens, and clinical implications of antineutrophil cytoplasmic antibodies in rheumatoid arthritis. J Rheumatol 23:826–830, 1996.
162. Voskuyl AE, Zwinderman AH, Westedt ML, et al: Factors associated with the development of vasculitis in rheumatoid arthritis: A case-control study. Ann Rheum Dis 55:190–192, 1996.
163. D'Cruz D: Vasculitis in systemic lupus erythematosus. Lupus 7:270–274, 1998.
164. Witte T, Hartung K, Matthias T, et al: Association of IgA anti-dsDNA antibodies with vasculitis and disease activity in systemic lupus erythematosus. Rheumatol Int 18:63–69, 1998.
165. Navarro M, Cervera R, Font J, et al: Anti-endothelial cell antibodies in systemic autoimmune diseases: Prevalence and clinical significance. Lupus 6:521–526, 1997.
166. Martin-Suarez I, D'Cruz D, Mansoor M, et al: Immunosuppressive treatment in severe connective tissue diseases: Effect of low dose intravenous cyclophosphamide. Am Rheum Dis 56:481–487, 1997.
167. Buerger L: Thromboangiitis obliterans: A study of the vascular lesions leading to presenile spontaneous gangrene. Am J Med Sci 136:567–580, 1908.
168. Mills JL, Porter JM: Thromboangiitis obliterans (Buerger's disease). In Churg A, Churg J (eds): Systemic Vasculitides. New York, Igaku-Shoin, 1991, pp 229–239.
169. Mills JL, Porter JM: Buerger's disease: A review and update. Semin Vasc Surg 6:14–23, 1993.
170. Cutler DA, Runge MS: 86 years of Buerger's disease—what have we learned? Am J Med Sci 309:74–75, 1995.
171. Shionoya S: Buerger's Disease: Pathology, Diagnosis and Treatment. Nagoya, Japan, University of Nagoya Press, 1990.
172. Abu-Dalu J, Giler SH, Urca I: Thromboangiitis obliterans of the iliac artery. Angiology 24:359–364, 1973.
173. Lie JT: Visceral intestinal Buerger's disease. Int J Cardiol 66(Suppl 1):S249–S256, 1998.
173. Papa M, Bass A, Adar R, et al: Autoimmune mechanisms in thromboangiitis obliterans (Buerger's disease): The role of tobacco antigen and the major histocompatibility complex. 111:527–531, 1992.
174. Spittell JA: Thromboangiitis obliterans—an autoimmune disorder. N Engl J Med 308:1157–1158, 1983.
175. Simi'c L, Pirnat L: Immunological aspects of smoking in patients with thromboangiitis obliterans. Vasa 14:349–352, 1985.
176. Adar R, Papa MZ, Halpern Z, et al: Cellular sensitivity to collagen in thromboangiitis obliterans. N Engl J Med 308:1113–1116, 1983.
177. Matsushita M, Shionoya S, Matsumoto T: Urinary cotinine measurement in patients with Buerger's disease: Effects of active and passive smoking on the disease process. J Vasc Surg 14:53–58, 1992.
178. Mills JL, Friedman EI, Taylor LM Jr, Porter JM: Upper extremity ischemia caused by small artery disease. Ann Surg 206:521–528, 1987.
179. Borner C, Heidrich H: Long-term follow-up of thromboangiitis obliterans. Vasa 27:80–86, 1998.
180. Largiader J, Schneider E, Bruner U, Bollinger A: Arterial reconstruction in Buerger's disease (thromboangiitis obliterans). Vasa 15:174–179, 1986.
181. Sasajima T, Kubo Y, Inaba M, et al: Role of infrainguinal bypass in Buerger's disease: An eighteen-year experience. Eur J Vasc Endovasc Surg 13:186–192, 1997.
182. Verstraete M, and the European TAO Study Group: Oral iloprost in the treatment of thromboangiitis obliterans (Buerger's disease): A double-blind, randomized, placebo-controlled trial. Eur J Vasc Endovasc Surg 15:300–307, 1998.
183. Isner JM, Baumgartner I, Rauh G, et al: Treatment of thromboangiitis obliterans (Buerger's disease) by intramuscular gene transfer of vascular endothelial growth factor: Preliminary results. J Vasc Surg 28:964–973, 1998.
184. Callow AD: Thromboangiitis obliterans (Buerger's disease). In Callow AD, Ernst CB (eds): Vascular Surgery: Theory and Practice. East Norwalk, CT, Appleton & Lange, 1995, pp 213–216.
185. Hollister DW, Godfrey MP, Sakai LY, et al: Immunohistologic abnormalities of the microfibrillar-fiber system in the Marfan syndrome. N Engl J Med 323:152–159, 1990.
186. Kainulainen K, Pulkkinen L, Savolainen A, et al: Location on chromosome 15 of the gene defect causing Marfan syndrome. N Engl J Med 323:935–939, 1990.
187. Dietz HC, Cutting GR, Pyeritz RE, et al: Marfan syndrome caused by a recurrent de novo missense mutation in the fibrillin gene. Nature 353:337–339, 1991.
188. Nijbroek G, Sood S, McIntosh I, et al: Fifteen novel FBN1 mutations causing Marfan syndrome detected by heteroduplex analysis of genomic amplicons. Am J Hum Genet 57:8–21, 1995.
189. Auyama T, Francke U, Dietz MC, Furthmayr H: Quantitative differences in biosynthesis and extracellular deposition of fibrillin in cultured fibroblasts distinguish five groups of Marfan syndrome patients and suggest distinct pathogenetic mechanisms. J Clin Invest 94:130–137, 1994.
190. McKusick VA: The defect in Marfan syndrome. Nature 352:279–281, 1991.
191. Schaefer GB, Godfrey M: Quantitation of fibrillin immunofluorescence in fibroblast cultures in the Marfan syndrome. Clin Genet 47:144–149, 1995.
192. Wang M, Mata J, Price CE, et al: Prenatal and presymptomatic diagnosis of the Marfan syndrome using fluorescence PCR and an automated sequencer. Prenat Diagn 15:499–507, 1995.
193. Perejda AJ, Abraham PA, Carnès WH, et al: Marfan syndrome: Structural, biochemical, and mechanical studies of the aortic media. J Lab Clin Med 106:376–383, 1985.
194. Segura AM, Lyna RE, Horiba K, et al: Immunohistochemistry of matrix metallo proteinases and their inhibitors in thoracic aortic aneurysms and aortic valves in patients with Marfan's syndrome. Circulation 98(Suppl)19:II331–II337, 1998.
195. Hirata K, Triposkiadis F, Sparks E, et al: The Marfan syndrome: Abnormal elastic properties. J Am Coll Cardiol 18:57–63, 1991.
196. Kornbluth M, Schnittger I, Eyngorina I, et al: Clinical outcome in the Marfan syndrome with ascending aortic dilatation followed annually by echocardiography. Am J Cardiol 84:752–755, 1999.
197. Rios AS, Silber EN, Bavishi N, et al: Effect of long-term beta blockade on aortic root compliance in patients with Marfan syndrome. Am Heart J 137:1057–1061, 1999.
198. Shores J, Berger KR, Murphy EA, Pyeritz RE: Progression of aortic dilatation and the benefit of long-term β-adrenergic blockade in Marfan's syndrome. N Engl J Med 330:1335–1341, 1994.
199. Finkbohner R, Johnston D, Crawford ES, et al: Marfan syndrome: Long-term survival and complications after aortic aneurysm repair. Circulation 91:728–733, 1995.
200. Gio HVL, Greene PS, Alejo DE, et al: Replacement of the aortic root in patients with Marfan's syndrome. N Engl J Med 340:1307–1313, 1999.
201. Van Meekeren JA: De dilatabilitate extraordinaria cutis. In Observationes Medicochirugicae. Amsterdam, 1682.
202. Ehlers E: Cutis laxa Neigung zu Haemorrhagien in der Haut, Lockerung mehrere Artikulationen. Dermatol Z 8:173–174, 1901.
203. Danlos M: Un cas de cutis laxa avec tumeurs par contusion chronique des condes et des genoux (xanthome juvénile pseudodiabètique de M. M. Hallopeault Mace de Lepinay). Bull Soc F Dermatol Syphilis 19:70, 1908.
204. Tsipouras P, Byers PH, Schwartz RC, et al: Ehlers-Danlos syndrome type IV: Cosegregation of the phenotype to a COL3A1 allele of type III procollagen. Hum Genet 74:41–46, 1986.
205. Prockop DJ, Kivirikko KI: Heritable diseases of collagen. N Engl J Med 34:376, 1984.
206. Steinmann B, Royce PM, Superti-Furga A: The Ehlers-Danlos syndrome. In Royce PM, Steinmann B (eds): Connective Tissue and

Its Heritable Disorders: Molecular, Genetic, and Medical Aspects. New York, Wiley-Liss, 1993, pp 351–407.

207. Freeman RK, Swegle J, Sise MJ: The surgical complications of Ehlers-Danlos Syndrome. Am Surg 62:869–873, 1996.

208. Bellenot F, Boisgard S, Kantelip B, et al: Type IV Ehlers-Danlos syndrome with isolated arterial involvement. Ann Vasc Surg 4:15–19, 1990.

209. Serry C, Agomuoh OS, Goldin MD: Review of Ehlers-Danlos syndrome: Successful repair of rupture and dissection of abdominal aorta. J Cardiovasc Surg 29:530–534, 1988.

210. Mattar SG, Kumar AG, Lumsden AB: Vascular complications in Ehlers-Danlos syndrome. Am Surg 60:827–831, 1994.

211. Erdheim J: Medionecrosis aortae idiopathica cystica. Virchows Arch 276:187–229, 1930.

212. Maraslese DI, Moodie DS, Lytle B, et al: Cystic medial necrosis of the aorta in patients without Marfan's syndrome: Surgical outcome and long-term follow-up. J Am Coll Cardiol 16:68–73, 1990.

213. Roberts AJ, Jaffe RB, Michaels LL, et al: Cystic medial necrosis. A correctable cause of the superior vena cava syndrome. Arch Surg 109:84, 1974.

214. Tredal SM, Carter JB, Edwards JE: Cystic medial necrosis of the pulmonary artery. Arch Pathol 97:183, 1974.

215. Millar AJ, Gilbert RD, Brown RA, et al: Abdominal aortic aneurysms in children. J Pediatr Surg 31:1624–1628, 1996.

216. Read RC, Wolf P: Symptomatic disseminated cystic medial necrosis. N Engl J Med 271:816, 1964.

217. Altman LK, Fialkow PJ, Parker F, Sagbiel RW: Pseudoxanthoma elasticum: An underdiagnosed genetically heterogeneous disorder with protean manifestations. Arch Intern Med 134:1048, 1974.

218. Neldner KH: Pseudoxanthoma elasticum. In Royce PM, Steinmann B (eds): Connective Tissue and Its Heritable Disorders: Molecular, Genetic, and Medical Aspects. New York, Wiley-Liss, 1993, pp 425–436.

219. Carter DJ, Vince FP, Woodword DAK: Arterial surgery in pseudoxanthoma elasticum. Postgrad Med J 52:291, 1976.

220. Takaro TK, Coodley GO: Pentoxifylline for ischemic pain in pseudoxanthoma elasticum. West J Med 159:689–690, 1993.

221. Leriche R: Dolicho et méga-artère: Dolicho et méga-veine. Presse Med 51:554, 1943.

222. Randall PA, Omar MM, Rohner R, et al: Arteria magna revisited. Radiology 132:295, 1979.

223. Thomas ML: Arteriomegaly. Br J Surg 71:690, 1971.

224. Lawrence PF, Wallis C, Dobrin PB, et al: Peripheral aneurysms and arteriomegaly: Is there a familial pattern? J Vasc Surg 28:599–605, 1998.

225. Quain R: Partial contraction of the abdominal aorta. Trans Pathol Soc Lond 1:244, 1847.

226. Glenn F, Keefer EB, Speer DS, et al: Coarctation of the lower thoracic and abdominal aorta immediately proximal to the celiac axis. Surg Gynecol Obstet 94:561, 1952.

227. Hallett JW, Brewster CD, Darling RC, et al: Coarctation of the abdominal aorta: Current options in surgical management. Ann Surg 191:430, 1980.

228. Meacham PW, Dean RH, Lawson JW, et al: Study of the renal pressor system in experimental coarctation of the abdominal aorta. Am Surg 43:771, 1977.

229. Paroni R, Astuni M, Baroni C, et al: Abdominal aortic coarctation inducing aortic occlusion and renovascular hypertension. J Cardiovasc Surg 32:770–773, 1991.

230. Stanley JC, Graham LM, Whitehouse WM: Developmental occlusive disease of the abdominal aorta and the splenic and renal arteries. Am J Surg 142:190, 1981.

231. Siassi B, Glyman G, Emmonouilides GC: Hypoplasia of the abdominal aorta associated with the rubella syndrome. Am J Dis Child 120:426, 1970.

232. Sen PK, Kinore SG, Engineer SD, et al: The middle aortic syndrome. Br Heart J 25:610, 1963.

233. Lande A: Takayasu's arteritis and congenital coarctation of the descending thoracic and abdominal aorta: A critical review. AJR Am J Roentgenol 127:277, 1976.

234. Messina ML, Goldstone J, Ferrell LD, et al: Middle aortic syndrome: Effectiveness and durability of complex arterial revascularization techniques. Ann Surg 204:331–339, 1986.

235. Robicsek F, Daugherty HK, Cook JW, et al: Coarctation of the abdominal aorta with stricture of the major vessels. Surgery 87:545, 1980.

236. Mickley V, Fleiter T: Coarctations of descending and abdominal aorta: Long-term results of surgical therapy. J Vasc Surg 28:206–214, 1998.

237. Brzezinska-Rajsczys G, Qureshi SA, Ksiazyk J, et al: Middle aortic syndrome treated by stent implantation. Heart 81:166–170, 1999.

238. Suarez de Lezo J, Pan M, Romero M, et al: Immediate and follow-up findings after stent treatment for severe coarctation of aorta. Am J Cardiol 83:400–406, 1999.

239. Pierce WS, Vincent WR, Fitzgerald E, et al: Coarctation of the abdominal aorta with multiple aneurysms. Ann Thorac Surg 20:687, 1975.

240. Noblet D, Gasmi T, Mikati A, et al: Persistent sciatic artery: Case report, anatomy, and review of the literature. Ann Vasc Surg 2:390–395, 1988.

241. Greebe J: Congenital anomalies of the iliofemoral artery. J Cardiovasc Surg 18:317, 1977.

242. Steele G, Saunders RJ, Riley J, et al: Pulsatile buttock masses: Gluteal and persistent sciatic artery aneurysms. Surgery 82:201–204, 1977.

243. Gasecki AP, Ebers GC, Vellet AD, Buchan A: Sciatic neuropathy associated with persistent sciatic artery. Arch Neurol 49:967–968, 1992.

244. Wolf YG, Gibbs BF, Guzzetta VJ, Bernstein EF: Surgical treatment of aneurysm of the persistent sciatic artery. J Vasc Surg 17:218–221, 1993.

245. Stuart TP: A note on a variation in the course of the popliteal artery. J Anat Physiol 13:162, 1879.

246. Hamming JJ: Intermittent claudication at an early age, due to an anomalous course of the popliteal artery. Angiology 10:369–371, 1959.

247. Love JW, Whelan TJ: Popliteal artery entrapment syndrome. Am J Surg 109:620–624, 1965.

248. Murray A, Halliday M, Croft RJ: Popliteal artery entrapment syndrome. Br J Surg 78:1414–1419, 1991.

249. Bouhoustos J, Daskalakis E: Muscular abnormalities affecting the popliteal vessels. Br J Surg 68:501–506, 1981.

250. Insua JA, Young JR, Humphries AW: Popliteal artery entrapment syndrome. Arch Surg 101:771, 1970.

251. Rich NM, Collins GJ, McDonald PT, et al: Popliteal vascular entrapment: Its increasing interest. Arch Surg 114:1377–1384, 1979.

252. Brener BJ, Alpert J, Brief DK, et al: Iatrogenic entrapment of femoro-popliteal saphenous vein bypass grafts by the gastrocnemius muscle. Surgery 78:668–674, 1975.

253. Gibson MH, Mills JG, Johnson GE, et al: Popliteal entrapment syndrome. Ann Surg 185:341–348, 1977.

254. Murray A, Halliday M, Croft RJ: Popliteal artery entrapment syndrome. Br J Surg 78:1414–1419, 1991.

255. diMarzo L, Cavallaro A, Sciacca V, et al: Diagnosis of popliteal artery entrapment syndrome: The role of duplex scanning. J Vasc Surg 13:434–438, 1991.

256. Collins PS, McDonald PT, Lim RC: Popliteal artery entrapment. An evolving syndrome. J Vasc Surg 10:484–490, 1989.

257. Rizzo RJ, Flinn WR, Yao JST, et al: Computed tomography for evaluation of arterial disease in the popliteal fossa. J Vasc Surg 11:112–119, 1990.

258. Fermand M, Houlle D, Fiessinger JN, et al: Entrapment of the popliteal artery: MR findings. AJR Am J Roentgenol 154:425–426, 1990.

259. Levien LJ, Veller MG: Popliteal artery entrapment syndrome: More common than previously recognized. J Vasc Surg 30:587–598, 1999.

260. Luscher TF, Lie JT, Stanson AW, et al: Arterial fibromuscular dysplasia. Mayo Clin Proc 62:931–952, 1987.

261. Stanley JC, Gewertz BL, Bove EL, et al: Arterial fibrodysplasia: Histopathologic character and current etiologic concepts. Arch Surg 110:561–566, 1975.

262. Leadbetter WF, Burkland CE: Hypertension in unilateral renal disease. J Urol 39:611–626, 1938.

263. Descotes J, Pelissier PH, Chignier E: Dystrophy of the media with aneurysmal tendency in the abdominal aorta-iliac segments. J Cardiovasc Surg 17:413, 1976.

264. Harrington OB, Crosby VG, Nicholas L: Fibromuscular hyperplasia of the internal carotid artery. Ann Thorac Surg 9:516–524, 1970.

265. Foster JH, Maxwell MH, Franklin SS, et al: Renovascular occlusive disease: Results of operative treatment. JAMA 231:1043–1048, 1975.

265a. Pannier-Moreau I, Grimbert P, Fiquet-Kempf B, et al: Possible familial origin of multifocal renal artery fibromuscular dysplasia. J Hypertens 15(12,Pt2):1797–1801, 1997.

266. O'Neill JA Jr: Long-term outcome with surgical treatment of renovascular hypertension. J Pediatr Surg 33:106–111, 1998.

267. Mahler F, Probst PN, Haertel M, et al: Lasting improvement of renovascular hypertension by trans-luminal dilatation of atherosclerotic and non-atherosclerotic renal artery stenosis. A follow-up study. Circulation 65:611–617, 1982.

268. Davidson RA, Barri Y, Wilcox CS: Predictors of cure of hypertension in fibromuscular renovascular disease. Am J Kidney Dis 28:334–338, 1996.

269. Mettinger KL, Ericson K: Fibromuscular dysplasia and the brain. I. Observations on angiographic, clinical and genetic characteristics. Stroke 13:46, 1982.

270. Chiche L, Bahnini A, Koskas F, Kieffer E: Occlusive fibromuscular disease of arteries supplying the brain: Results of surgical treatment. Am Vasc Surg 11:496–504, 1997.

271. Houston C, Rosenthal D, Lamis PA, et al: Fibromuscular dysplasia of the external iliac arteries: Surgical treatment by graduated interval dilatation technique. Surgery 85:713–715, 1979.

272. Flanigan DP, Burnham SJ, Goodreau JJ, et al: Summary of cases of adventitial cystic disease of the popliteal artery. Ann Surg 189:165–175, 1979.

273. Ejrup B, Hiertonn T: Intermittent claudication. Three cases treated by free vein graft. Acta Chir Scand 108:217, 1954.

274. Galle C, Cavenaile JC, Hoang AD, et al: Adventitial cystic disease of the popliteal artery communicating with the knee joint. J Vasc Surg 28:738–741, 1998.

275. Levien LJ, Benn CA: Adventitial cystic disease: A unifying hypothesis. J Vasc Surg 28:193–205, 1998.

276. Miller A, Salenius JP, Sacks BA, et al: Noninvasive vascular imaging in the diagnosis and treatment of adventitial cystic disease of the popliteal artery. J Vasc Surg 26:715–720, 1997.

277. Do DD, Braunschweig M, Baumgartner I, et al: Adventitial cystic disease of the popliteal artery: Percutaneous US-guided aspiration. Radiology 203:743–746, 1997.

278. Macfarlane R, Livesey SA, Pollard S, Dunn DC: Cystic adventitial arterial disease. Br J Surg 74:89–90, 1987.

279. Koman M, Hardaker WT, Goldner JL: Wick catheter in evaluating and treating compartment syndromes. South Med J 73:303–309, 1981.

280. Eaton RG, Green WT: Volkmann's ischemia: A volar compartment syndrome of the forearm. Clin Orthop 117:58–64, 1975.

281. Jepson PS: Ischemic contracture: Experimental study. Ann Surg 84:785, 1926.

282. Matsen FA: Compartmental Syndrome: A Unified Concept. New York, Grune & Stratton, 1980.

283. DelMaestro RF: An approach to free radicals in medicine and biology. Acta Physiol Scand Suppl 492:153–168, 1980.

284. Perler BA, Tohmeh AG, Bulkley GB: Inhibition of the compartment syndrome by ablation of free radical-mediated reperfusion injury. Surgery 108:40–47, 1990.

285. Mileski WJ, Winn RK, Vetter NB, et al: Inhibition of CD18-dependent neutrophil adherence reduces organ injury after hemorrhagic shock in primates. Surgery 108:206, 1990.

286. Mubarak SJ, Hargens AR: Acute compartment syndromes. Surg Clin North Am 63:539–551, 1983.

287. Mills JL, Porter JM: Basic data related to clinical decision-making in acute limb ischemia. Ann Vasc Surg 5:96–98, 1991.

288. Rudoff J, Ebner S, Canepa C: Limb-compartmental syndrome with thrombolysis. Am Heart J 128(6,pt1):1267–1268, 1994.

289. Whitesides TE, Haney TC, Morimoto K, et al: Tissue pressure measurements as a determinant of the need of fasciotomy. Clin Orthop 113:43–49, 1975.

290. Mubarak SJ, Owen CA, Hargens AR: Acute compartment syndromes: Diagnosis and treatment with the aid of the Wick catheter. J Bone Joint Surg Am 60:1091–1095, 1978.

291. McDermott AGP, Marble AE, Yabsley RH: Monitoring acute compartment pressures with the STIC catheter. Clin Orthop 190:192–197, 1984.

292. Mars M, Hadley GP: Raised intracompartmental pressure and compartment syndromes. Injury 29:403–411, 1998.

293. Mabee JR: Compartment syndrome: A complication of acute extremity trauma. J Emer Med 12:651–656, 1994.

294. Perry MO: Compartment syndromes and reperfusion injury. Surg Clin North Am 68:853–864, 1988.

295. McCord JM: Oxygen-derived free radicals in post-ischemic tissue injury. N Engl J Med 313:154–157, 1985.

296. Carson HAJ, Cusworth DC, Dent CE, et al: Homocystinuria: A new inborn error of metabolism associated with mental deficiency. Arch Dis Child 38:425, 1963.

297. McCully KS: Homocysteine theory of atherosclerosis. Development and current status. Atheroscler Rev 11:157–247, 1983.

298. Mudd SH, Finkelstein JD, Irrevere F, Laster L: Homocystinuria: An enzymatic defect. Science 143:1443–1445, 1964.

299. Mudd SH, Levy HL, Abeles RH: A derangement in the metabolism of vitamin B-12 leading to homocystinuria, cystathionuria, and methyl malonic aciduria. Biochem Biophys Res Commun 35:21–26, 1969.

300. Deloughery TG, Evans A, Sadeghi A, et al: Common mutation in methylenetetrahydrofolate reductase. Correlation with homocysteine metabolism and late-onset vascular disease. Circulation 94:3074–3078, 1996.

301. Smolin LA, Crenshaw TD, Kurtyca D, Benevenga NJ: Homocysteine accumulation in pigs fed diets deficient in vitamin B-6 (pyridoxine). Relationship to atherosclerosis. J Nutr 133:2022–2028, 1983.

302. Kang SS, Wong PWK, Norusis M: Homocysteine due to folate deficiency. Metabolism 36:458–465, 1987.

303. Brattstorm L, Israelsson B, Lindgarde X, et al: Higher total plasma homocysteine in vitamin B-12 deficiency than in heterozygosity for homocystinuria due to cystathionine B–synthetase deficiency. Metabolism 37:175–182, 1988.

304. Harker LA, Ross R, Slichter SJ, Scott CR: Homocystinemia: Vascular injury and arterial thrombosis. N Engl J Med 291:537–543, 1974.

305. Hladovec J: Experimental homocystinemia, endothelial lesions and thrombosis. Blood Vessels 16:202–205, 1979.

306. Refsum H, Helland S, Ueland PM: Radioenzymatic determination of homocysteine in plasma and urine. Clin Chem 31:624–628, 1985.

307. Boers GHK, Smals AGH, Trijbels FJM: Unique efficiency of methionine metabolism in premenopausal women may protect against vascular disease in the reproductive years. J Clin Invest 72:1971–1975, 1983.

308. McCully KS, Carvalho ACA: Homocysteine thiolactone, N-homocysteine thiolactonyl retinamide, and platelet aggregation. Res Commun Chem Pathol Pharmacol 6:349–360, 1987.

309. Kang SS, Wong PWK, Cook HY, et al: Protein bound homocysteine. A possible risk factor for coronary artery disease. J Clin Invest 77:1482–1486, 1986.

310. Fortin LJ, Genest J: Measurement of homocyst(e)ine in the prediction of arteriosclerosis. Clin Biochem 28:155–162, 1995.

311. McCully KS: Vascular pathology of homocysteinemia: Implications for the pathogenesis of atherosclerosis. Am J Pathol 56:111–128, 1969.

312. Kang SS: Critical points for determining moderate hyperhomocyst(e)inemia. Eur J Clin Invest 25:806–808, 1995.

313. Boers GHK, Smals AGH, Trijbels FJM, et al: Heterozygosity for homocystinuria in premature peripheral and cerebral occlusive arterial diseases. N Engl J Med 313:709–714, 1985.

314. Nehler MR, Taylor LM Jr: Homocysteinemia as a risk factor for atherosclerosis: A review. Cardiovasc Surg 5:559–567, 1997.

315. Taylor LM, DeFrang RD, Harris EJ, Porter JM: The association of elevated plasma homocyst(e)ine with progression of symptomatic peripheral arterial disease. J Vasc Surg 13:128–136, 1991.

316. Stampfer MJ, Malinow MR, Willett WC, et al: A prospective study of plasma homocyst(e)ine and risk of myocardial infarction in US physicians. JAMA 268:877–881, 1992.

317. Arnesen E, Refsum H, Bonaa KM, et al: Serum total homocysteine and coronary heart disease. Int J Epidemiol 24:704–709, 1995.

318. Perry IJ, Refsum H, Morris RW, et al: Prospective study of serum homocysteine concentration and risk of stroke in middle aged men. Lancet 346:1395–1398, 1995.

319. Verhoef P, Hennekens CH, Malinow MR, et al: A prospective study of plasma homocyst(e)ine and risk of ischemic stroke. Stroke 25:1924–1930, 1994.

320. Taylor LM Jr, Moneta GL, Sexton GJ, et al: Prospective blinded study of the relationship between plasma homocysteine and progression of symptomatic peripheral arterial disease. J Vasc Surg 29:8–21, 1999.

321. Nygard O, Nordrehaug JE, Refsum H, et al: Plasma homocysteine levels and mortality in patients with coronary heart disease. N Engl J Med 337:230–236, 1997.

322. Brattstrom L. Vitamins as homocysteine-lowering agents. J Nutr 126:S1276–S1280, 1996.

Questions

1. Which group with Raynaud's syndrome has the lowest risk of developing a connective tissue disease?
   (a) vasospastic, negative serologies
   (b) vasospastic, positive serologies
   (c) obstructive, negative serologies
   (d) obstructive, positive serologies
   (e) obstructive, unknown serologies

2. Vasculitis is a central feature in all of the following syndromes except
   (a) Kawasaki disease
   (b) Cogan's syndrome
   (c) Behçet's disease
   (d) Takayasu's disease
   (e) Gilbert's disease

3. The majority of patients with temporal arteritis are encompassed in which of the following groups?
   (a) 50 years, male, white
   (b) 50 years, female, nonwhite
   (c) 50 years, male, nonwhite
   (d) 50 years, male and female, nonwhite
   (e) 50 years, female, white

4. Optimal initial treatment for subacute upper extremity ischemia caused by temporal arteritis is
   (a) steroids
   (b) endarterectomy
   (c) saphenous vein bypass
   (d) thrombolytic therapy
   (e) warfarin anticoagulation

5. Which of the following is of greatest benefit in the treatment of patients with Buerger's disease?
   (a) sympathectomy
   (b) oral vasodilators
   (c) arterial reconstructive surgery
   (d) warfarin anticoagulation
   (e) cessation of tobacco use

6. Extensive vascular calcification in a young patient with normal parathyroid function suggests
   (a) hyperlipidemia
   (b) Hurler's syndrome
   (c) pseudoxanthoma elasticum
   (d) Marfan's syndrome
   (e) Ehlers-Danlos syndrome

7. Abdominal coarctation is most frequently discovered during evaluation for
   (a) claudication
   (b) blue toe syndrome
   (c) weight loss
   (d) hypertension
   (e) abdominal pain

8. Calf claudication in a nonsmoker younger than 30 years of age is most commonly caused by
   (a) popliteal entrapment syndrome
   (b) atherosclerosis
   (c) polyarteritis nodosa
   (d) Takayasu's disease
   (e) homocystinemia

9. The early objective diagnosis of anterior compartment syndrome is best made by
   (a) absent dorsal pedal pulse
   (b) footdrop
   (c) tense swelling
   (d) localized compartment pain
   (e) compartment pressure measurement with Wick or the "solid-state transducer in catheter" monitor

10. All of the following are important in homocysteine metabolism except
    (a) vitamin B_6
    (b) folate
    (c) cobalamin
    (d) ornithine transcarbamoylase
    (e) homocysteine methyltransferase

Answers

1. a   2. e   3. e   4. a   5. e   6. c   7. d   8. a   9. e   10. d

9

Influence of Diabetes Mellitus on Vascular Disease and Its Complications

Charles M. Peterson

THE CLINICAL PROBLEM

Diabetes is described in the *Ebers Papyrus*. Nevertheless, despite being recognized for four millennia, the disease in many ways remains undefined. Diabetes mellitus is a heterogeneous collection of syndromes characterized by hyperglycemia. It is estimated to afflict approximately 14 million inhabitants of the United States.[1] With newer definitions for the diagnosis of the disease,[2] the prevalence of diabetes may be as high as 16 million. Owing to the high prevalence of diabetes mellitus in patients with peripheral arterial disease, screening for this disorder is now recommended on a vascular ward in those who do not already carry the diagnosis.[3]

Insulin-dependent diabetes mellitus (IDDM), or type 1 diabetes, comprises approximately 10% of diabetic patients; the majority have non–insulin-dependent diabetes mellitus (NIDDM), or type 2 diabetes. Other types of diabetes include gestational diabetes mellitus (GDM), which occurs de novo during pregnancy; the type that can occur from toxins or trauma to the insulin-secreting cells (β cells) of the pancreatic islets of Langerhans; or secondary diabetes mellitus due to another disease, which impairs pancreatic function or induces insulin resistance such as occurs in iron overload syndromes, acromegaly, or Cushing's disease.

IDDM, or the type characterized by low or undetectable insulin secretion and a need for administered insulin to sustain life, is generally accepted as primarily autoimmune in etiology.[4] The genetic vulnerabilities and the environmental insults that elicit IDDM are under intense study but remain uncharacterized. The complexity of these interactions is illustrated by the fact that less than 50% of monozygotic twins of a diabetic proband develop IDDM. NIDDM is a highly concordant genetic disease, with nearly 100% of monozygotic twins of a diabetic proband acquiring the disease. The concordance for first- and second-degree relatives increases given the challenge of obesity. NIDDM subjects tend to have insulin levels in the normal to high range yet remain "insulin resistant," with an inadequate ability to secrete insulin in a manner sufficient to lower blood glucose into the normal range.[5]

Clinical practice guidelines are published yearly by the American Diabetes Association (ADA).[6] The new guidelines define a fasting glucose higher than 126 mg/dL as diabetes and impaired fasting glucose between 110 and 126 mg/dL.

Persons with either IDDM or NIDDM tend to be at double jeopardy for the development of vascular disease because they have both glucose toxicity, a result of elevated blood glucose, as the hallmark of the disease, as well as insulin toxicity, derived from elevated insulin levels from peripheral insulin injection (in the case of IDDM and some NIDDM) or elevated endogenous insulin secretion (in the case of most NIDDM). The nature of these toxicities is described in some detail later. This chapter also emphasizes the importance of minimizing these two toxicities through therapeutic approaches that target normal glucose levels without unduly raising insulin levels or promoting hypoglycemia.[7]

The recognition of vascular disease as an obligatory concomitant of diabetes mellitus occurred during this century. Osler noted in 1908 that "The thickening of the arteries in . . . diabetes . . . may be due to the action on the blood vessels of poisons retained within the system."[8] In the 1945 edition of his textbook, 20 years after the use of insulin had become common, Joslin noted that "Arteriosclerosis in the form of gangrene of the lower extremities has decreased while at the same time it has

This chapter was written by Charles M. Peterson in his private capacity. The views expressed in the chapter do not necessarily represent the views of the National Institutes of Health, the Department of Health and Human Services, or the United States.

increased in the heart as coronary disease and in the brain as apoplexy."[9]

It is now generally agreed that diabetes mellitus accelerates the initiation and propagation of vascular disease. At present, 84% of diabetic subjects who live longer than 20 years after diagnosis have some form of vascular disease and 75% of persons with diabetes now die of vascular disease or its complications, primarily myocardial infarction and stroke.[10] Thus, persons with diabetes, regardless of type, have an increased risk for disease of the large and small vessels. In addition, the distribution of large vessel disease is more diffuse.

Diabetes remains problematic for the vascular surgeon for several reasons. The diagnosis of vascular disease in a person with diabetes may be confounded by the presence of sensorimotor polyneuropathy that may mask typical pain patterns of presentation. The outcome of surgical intervention has tended to be less favorable in persons with diabetes because their length of hospital stay tends to be longer, their risk for infection greater, and their probability of an adverse outcome higher than in persons without diabetes. In the 1960s, mortality rates in diabetic patients who had surgery were reported to be 3.6% to 13.2%.[11] In 1983, Hjortrup and colleagues[12] studied morbidity in diabetic and nondiabetic patients who had major vascular surgery and found that there were no deaths in either group and comparable morbidity. Although their theories were unproved, the authors hypothesized that the improvement in statistical outcome in the intervening 20 years was due to improvements in diabetes care.

There appears to be little doubt that diabetes care enhances the outcome of perioperative infection. From 1990 to 1995, Golden and coworkers at Johns Hopkins evaluated 411 adults with diabetes who underwent coronary artery surgery with glucose surveillance six times per day. After simultaneous adjustment for age, sex, race, underlying comorbidity, acute severity of illness, and length of stay in the surgical intensive care unit, patients with higher mean glucose readings were at increased risk of developing infections. Thus, they concluded that in patients with diabetes who undergo coronary artery surgery, postoperative hyperglycemia is an independent predictor of short-term infectious complications.[13]

This chapter reviews the epidemiologic data as well as the mechanisms behind the factors that make the person with diabetes vulnerable to the initiation and propagation of vascular disease, with emphasis placed on the effects on the large vessels. The latter part of the chapter details protocols that have proved useful for the control of glucose in both IDDM and NIDDM patients. In view of the increasing evidence that both acute and chronic risk can be modified by intensive diabetes control protocols, the inclusion of these approaches should be part of the therapeutic armamentarium of the surgeon as well as the specialist in diabetes care. Control of blood pressure and blood lipids is also especially important in the patient with diabetes and is addressed later in this chapter as well.

Cerebrovascular, Cardiovascular, and Peripheral Vascular Disease and Diabetes

There are now several large studies across multiple cultures that attest to the adverse effect of elevated glucose levels on the various forms of large vessel disease. Elevated glucose not only appears to accelerate the appearance of vascular disease but also predicts vascular events and prognosis once a vascular event has occurred. In this section, the major large studies are reviewed because they address the issues of stroke, cardiovascular disease (CVD), and peripheral vascular disease.

A number of studies have documented that the level of glucose at hospital admission is a predictor of outcome and extent of neurologic deficit in persons with acute stroke. For example, Toni and associates[14] attempted to identify predictors and possible pathogenic mechanisms of early neurologic deterioration in patients with acute ischemic strokes and to evaluate their impact on clinical outcome. They studied a continuous series of 152 patients with first-ever ischemic hemispheric strokes who were hospitalized within 5 hours of onset, evaluated according to the Canadian Neurological Scale, and assessed with a computed tomography (CT) scan. The initial subset of 80 patients also underwent angiography. A repeated CT scan or autopsy was performed within 5 to 9 days of a patient's stroke. Progressing neurologic deficit was defined as a decrease of 1 point or more in the global neurologic scale score during hospitalization, compared with the score at entry. Those whose condition deteriorated had been hospitalized earlier and had higher serum glucose levels at admission.

The Oslo Study also found that diabetes and the level of nonfasting glucose predicted the outcome of stroke.[15] The study, started in 1972, included 16,209 men aged 40 to 49 years. Of these, 16,172 had no previous history of stroke and 151 were known to have diabetes. Five diabetic and 80 nondiabetic subjects died of stroke during the 18 years of follow-up, giving a rate ratio of 7.87 (95% confidence interval [CI], 2.48 to 19.14) for diabetic subjects. The rate of mortality for all causes in diabetic subjects was more than five times that of those who were nondiabetic. Nonfasting serum glucose was a predictor of fatal stroke in all participants (diabetic subjects included) without a history of stroke in age-adjusted univariate analysis. The relative risk (RR) was 1.13 (CI, 1.03 to 1.25) by an increase of 1 mmol/L (18 mg/dL) of serum glucose according to results of proportional hazards regression analysis.

Similar observations were made in Scotland, where women were found to be more vulnerable to the effects of glucose than men.[16] Sex-specific CVD, ischemic heart disease (IHD), and stroke mortality rates and relative risks for asymptomatic hyperglycemic subjects (top 5%) were compared with those of normoglycemic individuals (bottom 95%) during a mean follow-up of 11.6 years (range, 10 to 14 years) of 4696 men and 5714 women in the west of Scotland aged 45 to 64 at entry. Univariate analysis showed that asymptomatic hyperglycemia was associated with increased risk of all causes, CVD, IHD, and stroke mortality in both males and females. The degree of this association was greater in women than in men. Using multiple logistic regression analysis to take into account differences in age, systolic and diastolic blood pressure, serum cholesterol, body mass index (BM), and cigarette smoking, high causal blood glucose level was still a significant risk factor for CVD mortality in both males and females.

Within the diabetic population, the level of complications such as retinopathy, preexisting nephropathy, and coronary and peripheral vascular disease, in addition to age, is a predictor of outcome.[17] In a cohort of 2124 diabetic persons identified at multiphasic health checkups during the period from 1979 through 1985, 56 suffered a nonembolic ischemic stroke during the follow-up period, which extended through 1991. For each case subject, one diabetic control subject, matched by sex and year of birth, was selected from the same cohort of diabetic subjects. The estimated relative risk of stroke in diabetic subjects with retinopathy was 2.8 (95% CI, 1.2 to 6.9). After adjustment for age, sex, smoking, use of insulin, average systolic blood pressure, and average random glucose, the estimated relative risk was 4.0 (95% CI, 1.0 to 14.5). The relative risk of stroke in diabetic subjects with retinopathy remained elevated after exclusion of those with complications other than retinopathy.

The Honolulu Heart Program also confirmed the poorer prognosis for vascular disease associated with hyperglycemia.[18] This study examined the association between a variety of baseline lifestyle and biologic factors in a middle-aged cohort of Japanese-American men and the 20-year incidence rates of total atherosclerotic end points and each of the initial clinical manifestations of this disease, including fatal and nonfatal coronary heart disease, angina pectoris, thromboembolic strokes, and aortic aneurysms. Japanese-American men ($n = 2710$) between the ages of 55 and 64 years at the time of the initial clinical examination of the program (1965 through 1968) who had no evidence of coronary heart disease, cerebrovascular disease, cancer, or aortic aneurysms were studied. Among these men, 602 atherosclerotic events developed during the 23-year period of follow-up (1965 through 1988). After adjustment for each of the baseline characteristics examined, significant positive associations between quartile cutoffs of BMI, systolic blood pressure, serum levels of glucose, cholesterol, triglycerides, and uric acid, as well as cigarette smoking, and the occurrence of any atherosclerotic end point were noted.

Within the diabetic population, nonfatal or small infarction, especially with multiple occurrences, is a feature of cerebrovascular disease complicating diabetes mellitus and correlates with elevated blood glucose and blood pressure.[19] Asymptomatic cerebral infarction is not rare in diabetic subjects and can now be pathologically and clinically evaluated accurately with magnetic resonance imaging (MRI).

The Wisconsin Epidemiologic Study also confirmed the finding of elevated risk for vascular disease in the diabetic population.[20] The association of glycemia with cause-specific mortality in a diabetic population was studied in a cohort design based in a primary care setting. Participants all had diabetes, were taking insulin, and were diagnosed when they were younger than 30 years old ($n = 1210$). They were compared with a random sample of diabetic persons diagnosed when they were 30 years old or older ($n = 1780$). Thus, both IDDM and NIDDM were studied, although the National Diabetes Data Group criteria for diagnosis were not used.[21] Glycosylated hemoglobin levels were obtained at baseline examinations. Median follow-up was 10 years in patients with younger onset and 8.3 years in those with older onset. The main outcome measure was cause-specific mortality determined from death certificates. In the younger-onset group, after controlling for other risk

factors in proportional hazards models and considering underlying cause of death, glycosylated hemoglobin level as an index of average glucose control was significantly associated with mortality from diabetes (hazard ratio [HR] for a 1% change in glycosylated hemoglobin, 1.25; 95% CI, 1.13 to 1.38) and IHD (HR, 1.18; 95% CI, 1.00 to 1.40). In the older-onset group, glycosylated hemoglobin was significantly associated with mortality from diabetes (HR, 1.32; 95% CI, 1.21 to 1.43), IHD (HR, 1.10; 95% CI, 1.04 to 1.17), and stroke (HR, 1.17; 95% CI, 1.05 to 1.30), but not cancer (HR, 0.99; 95% CI, 0.88 to 1.10). The authors concluded that "These results suggest . . . benefit to the control of glycemia with respect to death due to vascular disease and diabetes."[21]

The Copenhagen Stroke Study also found that diabetes is a risk factor for stroke and that diabetes influences the nature of stroke.[22] The study evaluated stroke type, stroke severity, the prognosis, and the relation between admission glucose levels and stroke severity and mortality. This community-based study included 1135 acute stroke patients, of whom 233 (20%) had diabetes. All patients were evaluated until the end of rehabilitation by weekly assessment of neurologic deficits (Scandinavian Stroke Scale) and functional disabilities (Barthel Index). A CT scan was performed in 83% of stroke cases. The diabetic stroke patient was 3.2 years younger than the nondiabetic stroke patient ($P < .001$) and had hypertension more frequently (48% vs. 30%, $P < .0001$). Intracerebral hemorrhages were six times less frequent in diabetic patients ($P = .002$). Initial stroke severity, lesion size, and site were comparable between the two groups; mortality was higher in diabetic patients (24% vs. 17%; $P = 0.03$), and diabetes independently increased the relative death risk by 1.8 (95% CI, 1.04 to 3.19). Outcome was comparable in surviving patients with and without diabetes, but patients with diabetes recovered more slowly. Mortality increased with increasing glucose levels on admission in nondiabetic patients independent of stroke severity (odds ratio [OR], 1.2 per 1 mmol/L; CI, 1.01 to 1.42; $P = .04$). Thus, diabetes influences stroke in such aspects as age, subtype, speed of recovery, and mortality. The authors concluded that "the effect of reducing high admission glucose levels in nondiabetic stroke patients should be examined in future trials."[22]

A Finnish study, although of short duration, confirmed the excess risk of elderly diabetic women for acute stroke.[23] The study examined whether NIDDM, its metabolic control and duration, and insulin level predict stroke. Cardiovascular risk factors, including glucose tolerance, plasma insulin, and glycosylated hemoglobin, were determined in a Finnish cohort of 1298 subjects aged 65 to 74 years, and the impact of these risk factors on the incidence of both fatal and nonfatal stroke was investigated during 3.5 years of follow-up. Of 1298 subjects participating in the baseline study, 1069 did not have diabetes and 229 had NIDDM. During the 3.5-year follow-up, 3.4% ($n = 36$) of nondiabetic subjects and 6.1% ($n = 14$) of NIDDM subjects had a nonfatal or fatal stroke. The incidence of stroke was significantly higher in diabetic women compared with nondiabetic women (OR, 2.25; 95% CI, 1.65 to 3.06). In multivariate logistic regression analyses including all study subjects, fasting and 2-hour glucose ($P < .01$ and $P < .05$, respectively), glycosylated hemoglobin A_{1c} (Hb A_{1c}) ($P <$

.01), atrial fibrillation ($P < .05$), hypertension ($P < .05$), and previous stroke ($P < .01$) predicted stroke events. In diabetic subjects, fasting and 2-hour glucose ($P < .01$ and $P < .05$, respectively), glycosylated Hb A_{1c} ($P < .05$), the duration of diabetes ($P < .05$), and atrial fibrillation ($P < .05$) were the baseline variables predicting stroke events. Finally, fasting insulin ($P < .05$), hypertension ($P < .05$), and previous stroke ($P < .01$) were associated with stroke incidence in nondiabetic subjects.

The longer term Honolulu Heart Program confirmed that diabetes confers extra risk for men of thromboembolic stroke but not hemorrhagic stroke.[24] The goal of this study was to determine whether glucose intolerance and diabetes increase the risk of thromboembolic, hemorrhagic, and total stroke, independent of other risk factors. Among the 7549 Japanese-American men aged 45 to 68 years and free of coronary heart disease and stroke during 1965 to 1968, a total of 374 thromboembolic, 128 hemorrhagic, and 36 type-unknown strokes occurred. The incidence of thromboembolic but not hemorrhagic stroke increased with the worsening glucose tolerance category. Compared with the low-normal (glucose less than 151 mg/dL) group, subjects in the high-normal (151 to 224 mg/dL), asymptomatic high ($\geq$225 mg/dL), and known diabetes groups all had significantly elevated age-adjusted relative risks of thromboembolic stroke. After adjustment for other risk factors, relative risks remained significantly elevated for the asymptomatic high and known diabetes groups (RR, 1.43 and 2.45; 95% CI, 1.00 to 2.04 and 1.73 to 3.47, respectively). Associations were the same in hypertensive and nonhypertensive subjects and similar but slightly stronger in younger (aged 45 to 54 years) than in older (aged 55 to 68 years) men.

The Northern Manhattan Stroke Study found that an admission blood glucose level greater than 140 mg/dL was an important predictor of mortality in stroke.[25] Ethanol abuse (RR, 2.5), hypertension requiring discharge medications (RR, 1.6), and elevated blood glucose within 48 hours of index ischemic stroke (RR, 1.2/50 mg/dL) were found to be independent predictors of recurrence.

The aforementioned review emphasizes that the findings of the relationship of glucose and vascular disease appear to hold across various cultures and genetic backgrounds. In a study in Taiwan[26] of 479 NIDDM patients 40 years of age or older from four community primary care health centers, cholesterol, high-density lipoprotein (HDL) cholesterol, plasma glucose, and Hb A_{1c} were studied. The duration of diabetes was associated with the development of stroke, with a relative risk of 1.063 for every 1-year increment ($P = .07$). Significant risk factors were serum cholesterol and Hb A_{1c} levels. For every 1-mg/dL increase in mean total cholesterol level, the relative risk of developing vascular disease increased 1.016-fold ($P = .04$). For every 1% (approximately 35 mg/dL) increase in Hb A_{1c}, the relative risk of developing vascular disease increased 1.170-fold ($P = .01$). Female diabetic subjects had a higher relative risk than men. The risk of CVD is therefore two to three times higher in diabetic than nondiabetic subjects. There is a gender difference; the incidence is two times higher in diabetic men and three times higher in diabetic women.[27–30]

In the nondiabetic group in the Honolulu Heart Program, there was a dose-response relation of glucose intolerance at baseline with coronary heart disease incidence, coronary heart disease mortality, and total mortality. This risk was independent of other risk factors in this cohort of 8006 middle-aged and older Japanese-American men.[31] Therefore, even in the normal range, glucose levels predict risk for vascular disease.

Persons with diabetes have shorter life spans. About 75% of increased mortality in men and 50% in women is caused by CVD. Kleinman and colleagues[27] found that the relative risk of mortality from IHD was 2.8 for men and 2.5 for women after controlling for other confounding variables of hypertension, obesity, age, serum cholesterol, and smoking. In a Utah population, CVD accounted for 48% of all-cause mortality in diabetic subjects.[28] Not only do diabetic subjects have an increased mortality from acute myocardial infarction, they also have an increased rate of congestive heart failure (CHF), cardiogenic shock, and dysrhythmias, not necessarily correlated with the size of the infarct.[30, 32] It is thought that the increased rate of CHF is secondary to hypocontractility, which may be due to microvascular disease, the metabolic effects of diabetes leading to cardiomyopathy, and autonomic dysfunction.[32]

Disease of the large vessels in one area of the vascular tree appears to predict disease in others. Associations of vascular disease are also found with perturbations in coagulation.[33] Heinrich and coworkers[33] investigated the vessel status of coronary and peripheral arteries and those arteries supplying the brain in 929 consecutive male patients admitted to a coronary rehabilitation unit. The severity of coronary atherosclerosis was scored using coronary angiography. Changes in extracranial brain vessels and manifest CVD were determined by B-mode ultrasound and Doppler examination. Peripheral arterial disease was diagnosed using baseline and stress oscillography. There was a significant increase in plasma fibrinogen, plasminogen, D-dimer, and C-reactive protein (CRP) with increasing severity of coronary heart disease. Compared with men who had unaffected arteries, men with three diseased coronary arteries had 58% greater D-dimer concentrations. Patients with cerebrovascular disease and peripheral vascular disease also had significantly higher fibrinogen, D-dimer, and CRP concentrations.

Many of the vascular lesions may also be asymptomatic, emphasizing the potential role of prophylactic screening for vascular lesions in other parts of the vascular tree when an index lesion is identified in a diabetic subject.[34] In a prospective population-based study of Dutch white inhabitants between 50 and 75 years of age, 2484 subjects were screened with respect to glucose tolerance. A group of 173 people with diabetes and a representative age- and sex-stratified sample of 288 nondiabetic subjects were studied in the vascular laboratory. Carotid artery disease was investigated with duplex scanning, arm and leg artery obstructions with real-time frequency analysis of continuous wave Doppler signals, and indirect blood pressure measurements. Comparing diabetic with nondiabetic subjects, the authors found significantly more obstructions of the carotid arteries (8.7% vs. 2.8%), arm arteries (2.3% vs. 0%), and leg arteries (31.8% vs. 18.4%). The same held if only the crural artery obstructions were compared (23.7% vs. 16.0%). More than half of the subjects with a carotid artery obstruction also had leg artery obstructions.[34]

The same group investigated the cross-sectional association between peripheral arterial disease and glycemic level, age, sex, and glucose tolerance.[35] The prevalence rates of ankle-brachial pressure index (ABI) less than 0.90 were 7.0%, 9.5%, 15.1%, and 20.9% in normal glucose-tolerant, impaired glucose-tolerant (IGT), NIDDM, and known diabetic subjects under treatment, respectively (chi-square test for linear trend: $P < .01$). Prevalence rates of any peripheral arterial disease (ABI less than 0.90, at least one monophasic or absent Doppler flow curve, or vascular surgery) were 18.1%, 22.4%, 29.2%, and 41.8% in these categories (chi-square test for linear trend: $P < .0001$). Logistic regression analyses showed that any arterial disease was significantly associated with Hb A_{1c}, fasting, and 2-hour postload plasma glucose after correction for cardiovascular risk factors (ORs and 95% CIs: 1.35; 1.10 to 1.65; 1.20; 1.06 to 1.36; and 1.06; 1.01 to 1.12, respectively). These authors did not find an association with insulin levels and vascular disease.

As recently reviewed, diabetes-related peripheral vascular disease remains a huge public health problem.[36] Although rates of lower extremity amputation and arterial reconstruction declined from 1983 to 1992, by 1996 the rate of major amputation had increased 10.6% since 1979. The earlier 12-year decline was positively correlated with reductions in the prevalence of smoking, hypertension, and heart disease, but not diabetes.[37]

Diabetic subjects with peripheral vascular disease are more likely to have small vessel disease of the foot, as well as large vessel disease elsewhere.[38] These findings may contribute to the higher risk for development of chronic foot ulcers in diabetic patients with peripheral vascular disease. Additional independent predictors of amputation include, besides peripheral vascular disease, sensory neuropathy and foot ulcers.[39]

Doppler studies with the use of the ABI appear as useful in the diabetic as in the nondiabetic population for identifying vascular disease, as documented by the Cardiovascular Health Study of 5084 participants.[40] Risk factors associated with an ABI of less than 1.0 in multivariate analysis included smoking (OR, 2.55), history of diabetes (OR, 3.84), increasing age (OR, 1.54), and nonwhite race (OR, 2.36). In the 3372 participants free of clinical coronary vascular disease, other noninvasive measures of subclinical CVD, including carotid stenosis by duplex scanning, segmental wall motion abnormalities by echocardiogram, and major electrocardiography (ECG) abnormalities, were inversely related to the ABI (all $P < .01$). Therefore, the lower the ABI, the greater the increase in CVD risk; however, even those with modest, asymptomatic reductions in the ABI (0.8 to 1.0) had increased risk of coronary vascular disease.

The risk for amputation in diabetic subjects appears to parallel the risk for vascular disease in general.[41] A case-control study among 10,068 patients from a large health maintenance organization at a multiphasic health checkup between 1964 and 1984 was carried out with an average length of follow-up after baseline of 13.2 years. Case patients were 150 cohort members with a first, nontraumatic lower extremity amputation after baseline. Control subjects were 278 cohort members who did not experience an amputation during follow-up, matched to patients by age, sex, and year of baseline. Level of glucose control ($P < .0001$), duration of diabetes ($P = .04$), and baseline systolic blood pressure ($P = .004$) were independent predictors of amputation, as were microvascular complications (retinopathy, neuropathy, and nephropathy). The observation that type of diabetes (or genetic background) did not predict amputation but that glycemia was predictive lends credence to the "glucose toxicity" hypothesis of vascular risk.

Clinical Studies of Intervention

As noted earlier, there seems to be a consensus that there is a relationship between glucose levels and cardiovascular events that shows a dose response within both the normal and diabetic populations.[42] There also have been several recent intervention studies that test the glucose toxicity hypothesis as well as studies of blood pressure control and lipid control in patients with diabetes mellitus. Table 9-1 summarizes the results of prospective glucose-lowering trials and CVD in people with diabetes mellitus. As can be seen, there is a significant risk reduction associated with seven out of the eight published trials in type 1 and type 2 diabetes.

TABLE 9-1

Glucose-Lowering Trials and Cardiovascular Disease in Diabetes Mellitus (DM)

STUDY	YEARS	Hb A_{1c} INTENSE (%)	Hb A_{1c} CONTROL (%)	TREATMENT	OUTCOME	RELATIVE RISK REDUCTION (%)
UKPDS	10	7.0	7.9	Insulin and sulfonylurea	MI	16
UKPDS	10.7	7.4	8.0	Metformin	MI	39
Kumamoto	6.0	7.1	9.4	Insulin	CV events	46
VACSDM	2.3	7.1	9.3	Insulin and sulfonylurea	CV events	−40
DIGAMI[47]	1.0	7.1	7.9	Insulin	Mortality	29
UGDP	12.5	Fasting glucose 130–146	Fasting glucose 170–186	Insulin	CV deaths	9
Type 1 DM meta-analysis	2–7	7.6	8.7	Insulin	Any event	45
Type 1 DM meta-analysis	2–7	7.6	8.7	Insulin	First event	28

UKPDS, UK Prospective Diabetes Study; VACSDM, Veterans Affairs Cooperative Study on Glycemic Control and Complications in NIDDA; DIGAMI, Diabetes and Insulin Glucose Infusion in Acute Myocardial Infarction; UGDP, University Group Diabetes Program; MI, myocardial infarction; CV, cardiovascular.

TABLE 9–2

Lipid-Lowering Trials and Cardiovascular Disease in Type 2 Diabetes Mellitus

STUDY	n	FOLLOW-UP (YR)	DECREASED LDL (%)	FIRST TREATMENT	OUTCOME	RELATIVE RISK REDUCTION (%)
Helsinki Heart	135	5.0	10	Gemfibrozil	CHD death, nonfatal MI	69
WOSCOPS	76	4.9	26	Pravastatin	CHD death, nonfatal MI	NA
AFCAPS/TexCAPS	155	5.2	25	Lovastatin	CHD death, nonfatal MI, angina	37
Meta-analysis of above primary prevention trials						55
4S	202	5.5	34	Simvastatin	CHD death, nonfatal MI	55
CARE	586	4.9	27	Pravastatin	CHD death, nonfatal MI	13
LIPID[57]	782	6.1	25	Pravastatin	CHD death, nonfatal MI	19
Meta-analysis of secondary prevention studies above						29

WOSCOPS, West of Scotland Primary Prevention Study; AFCAPS/TexCAPS, Air Force/Texas Coronary Atherosclerosis Prevention Study; CARE, Cholesterol and Recurrent Events; 4S, Scandinavian Simvastatin Survival Study; LIPID, Long-Term Intervention with Pravastatin in Ischaemic Disease; F/U, Follow-up; CHD, coronary heart disease; MI, myocardial infarction; NA, not available.

A Stockholm study provided convincing evidence that control of glycemia prevents microvascular complications in IDDM.[43] The Diabetes Control and Complications Trial (DCCT) clearly confirmed that tight control decreased the incidence of microvascular complications in IDDM.[44] The DCCT showed a trend of decreased incidence of CVD, but the result was not statistically significant. The DCCT was not primarily designed to test the hypothesis that blood glucose control would influence the risk for CVD. The patients were too young and it was too early in the course of their diabetes to expect significant cardiovascular event rates. Nevertheless, 17 initial major cardiovascular events were recorded: 14 in the conventional treatment group and 3 in the intensive group.[45] Total major cardiovascular and peripheral vascular events numbered 40 in the conventional group compared with 23 in the intensive group. Thus, with intensive treatment, the risk for cardiac events was reduced by 78%, and the risk for combined cardiac and peripheral vascular events, by 42%. As noted earlier, these risk differences did not achieve the defined limits for statistical significance. On the other hand, a meta-analysis published in 1999 clearly shows that intervention with intensive glucose control has a beneficial effect on both the incidence of the first and any cardiovascular event in type 1 patients[46] (see Table 9–1).

As summarized in Table 9–1, the results in persons with type 2 diabetes are even more convincing. Of particular note is the Diabetes and Insulin Glucose Infusion in Acute Myocardial Infarction (DIGAMI) study, which documented that acute management with intense insulin treatment at the time of myocardial infarct with subsequent insulin therapy has a significant impact on mortality at 1 year.[47] The 1998 publication of the United Kingdom (UK) Prospective Diabetes Study has reinforced the clinical goal of obtaining Hb A_{1c} values at or below 7% in these patients.[48, 49]

My own studies of peripheral vascular risk in IDDM documented that an intensive program of glucose control documented by glycosylated hemoglobin and multiple, daily blood glucose self-monitoring measures could reverse lesions of the red blood cell, polymorphonuclear leukocyte, platelet, and fluid phase of coagulation associated with diabetes.[50–54] In addition, basement membrane thickening,

nerve conduction, and the ABI were found to improve after a 9-month program of intensive glucose control and exercise. In view of the association of the ABI and risk in diabetic subjects noted earlier, these studies still provide some of the most compelling evidence for programs of glucose control and exercise in persons with diabetes to avoid or even facilitate the reversal of large vessel disease. In view of these findings, the goal of treatment of diabetes is to aggressively treat elevated blood glucose and blood pressure and abnormal lipid profiles.

Table 9–2 summarizes the major lipid-lowering trials in patients with type 2 diabetes. There are three primary randomized trials for primary prevention and an equal number for secondary prevention of CVD. Meta-analysis of these trials shows an overall RR reduction of 55% for primary prevention and 29% for secondary prevention. The 4S study also documented the cost-effectiveness of lipid lowering.[55] In persons with coronary heart disease with normal fasting glucose, simvastatin reduced the average cost of CVD-related hospitalizations by $3585, which offset 60% of the cost of drug. For those with impaired fasting glucose, average CVD-related hospitalization costs were reduced by $4478, which offset 74% of the drug cost. For diabetic subjects, there was a net cost savings of $1801 per subject. Current American Diabetes Association guidelines recommend low-density lipoprotein (LDL) cholesterol targets of less than 2.59 mmol/L (100 mg/dL) for diabetic subjects with one additional cardiovascular risk factor and an intervention level of 3.36 mmol/L (130 mg/dL) with a target of 2.59 mmol/L for all other subjects with diabetes.[56] As shown by the Long-Term Intervention with Pravastatin in Ischaemic Disease (LIPID) study, patients appear to benefit from statin therapy over a wide range of initial lipid levels.[57]

Table 9–3 summarizes the trials of blood pressure lowering in persons with type 2 diabetes. As emphasized in a recent Cochrane Library review,[58] primary intervention trials indicate a treatment benefit for coronary vascular disease but not for total mortality in people with diabetes. For both short- and long-term secondary prevention, there is a benefit for total mortality in persons with diabetes. Most of the published data of randomized control trials of antihypertensive therapy in diabetes for all-cause mortality

TABLE 9-3

Blood Pressure (BP)–Lowering Trials and Cardiovascular Disease in Type 2 Diabetes Mellitus

STUDY	YEARS	BP INTERVENTION (mm Hg)	BP CONTROL (mm Hg)	FIRST TREATMENT	OUTCOME		RELATIVE RISK REDUCTION (%)
UKPDS	9.0	144/82	154/87	Captopril/atenolol	CVD		29
					Stroke		20
					MI		42
SHEP	4.5	145/70	155/70	Chlorthalidone	CVD		45
					Stroke		26
Syst-Eur[60]	2.0	153/78	162/82	Nitrendipine	CV		62
					Stroke		69
HOT	3.8	140/81	144/85	Felodipine	CV + stroke		51
ABCD	5.6	130/80	135/85	Nisoldipine/enalapril	MI		−12
Overall primary prevention							38
Cochrane primary prevention	5.0			Various	CVD mortality and morbidity		30
Cochrane secondary prevention	>1			Various	CVD mortality and morbidity		11

UKPDS, UK Perspective Diabetes Study; SHEP, Systolic Hypertension in the Elderly; Syst-Eur, Systolic Hypertension in Europe Trial; HOT, Hypertension Optimal Treatment; ABCD, Appropriate Blood Pressure Control in Diabetes; CVD, cardiovascular disease; MI, myocardial infarction.

and CVD outcomes are taken from the hypertension trials not specific to diabetes.

It has been suggested that it is cost-effective to treat all patients with type 2 diabetes with angiotensin-converting enzyme (ACE) inhibitors.[59] This approach is reinforced by the publication of the Heart Outcomes Prevention Evaluation (HOPE), a placebo-controlled study of over 9000 subjects that indicated that ramipril substantially lowers the risk of death, heart attack, stroke, coronary revascularization, heart failure, and complications related to diabetes mellitus in a high-risk group of patients with preexisting vascular disease. The results are remarkable both for the magnitude of the treatment effect (an overall reduction of 22% in the primary outcome of myocardial infarction, stroke, or death from cardiovascular causes) and the rather small reduction (3.2 mm Hg) in blood pressure. The authors also noted a marked reduction in the incidence of complications related to diabetes and new cases of diabetes in those taking ramipril.[59]

There has been less enthusiasm for calcium channel blockers in persons with diabetes.[60] Nevertheless, there is evidence that they can be effective as well, as shown in Table 9–3.

EVIDENCE FOR THE INFLUENCE OF GLUCOSE ON THE PATHOPHYSIOLOGY OF VASCULAR DISEASE

Hyperglycemia is associated with vascular disease, as documented earlier. The reasons for this association remain speculative. Table 9–4 documents some of the hypothesized means by which glucose might influence pathologic vascular changes. These factors are now discussed in some detail.

Glycation and Advanced Glycation End Products, or Early and Late Maillard Reactions

In 1976, it became clear that a minor hemoglobin component, Hb A_{1c}, resulted from a post-translational modification of hemoglobin A by glucose and that there was a clinical relationship between Hb A_{1c} and fasting plasma glucose, the peak on the glucose tolerance test, the area under the curve on the glucose tolerance test, and mean glucose levels over the preceding weeks.[61-64] It soon became apparent that an improvement in ambient blood glucose levels resulted in correction (inter alia) of Hb A_{1c} levels[50-54] and that these nonenzymatic glycosylation reactions might provide a hypothesis that could explain a number of the pathologic sequelae of diabetes mellitus via

TABLE 9-4

Glucose Toxicity Hypothesis: Hyperglycemia Initiates or Propagates Vascular Disease by Multiple Mechanisms

I. Glycation of proteins and genetic material leading to dysfunctional or toxic products
II. Interference with the fluid, vascular, and platelet phases of coagulation
III. Perturbations in oxidation-reduction pathways
IV. Production of abnormal lipid metabolism
V. Vascular: volume shifts associated with changes in glycemia or intracellular osmotic shifts associated with alternative metabolic pathways invoked when glucose is elevated are toxic to the vascular tree
VI. Abnormal insulin/proinsulin levels in response to hyperglycemia contribute to vascular disease
VII. Perturbations in the immune system, including lymphokine production and polymorphonuclear leukocyte function, contribute to vascular disease

toxicity arising from glucose adduct formation with proteins or nucleic acids.[64]

As early as 1912, Louis-Camille Maillard[65] suggested that the chemical reactions that now bear his name might play a role in the pathologic changes associated with diabetes mellitus. The ability of reducing sugars to react with the amino groups of proteins is now widely recognized, as is the natural occurrence of many nonenzymatically glycosylated proteins. Important details as to the nature of such reactions are, however, still unclear.

The initial step (or early Maillard reaction) involves the condensation of an amino moiety with the aldehyde form of a particular sugar. Only a very small fraction of most common sugars is normally present in the aldehyde form.[66, 67] A number of transformations are possible following the addition of an amine to a sugar carbonyl group. Considerable evidence now exists that supports the involvement of an Amadori-type rearrangement for the adduct of glucose with the N-terminal of the β chain of hemoglobin. The labile Schiff base aldimine adduct is transformed into a relatively stable ketoamine adduct via the Amadori rearrangement.

Because hemoglobin circulates in its red blood cell for approximately 120 days, there is little opportunity in this cell for late Maillard reactions, or nonenzymatic browning, to occur. In these late Maillard reactions, the Amadori product is degraded into deoxyglucosones that react again with free amino groups to form chromophores, fluorophores, and protein cross-links.[68, 69] In tissues that are longer lived, these reactions may be important mediators of diabetic changes as well as the aging process. Although the structure of a large number of nonenzymatic browning products has been elucidated, few have been obtained under physiologic conditions, thus making detection in vivo difficult and their pathologic role uncertain.[70] Table 9–5 summarizes some of the observations and hypotheses whereby glycation might promote pathologic changes in persons with elevated blood glucose.

The Maillard reaction is ubiquitous in nature. The accumulation of advanced glycation end products (AGEs) in tissues in the human body has been implicated in the complications of diabetes, aging, and renal failure.[71] The links between these reactions and the pathogenesis of nephropathy, macro- and microangiopathy, and cataracts in diabetic subjects is increasingly strong.[72] AGEs accumulate in vivo on long-lived proteins in the vascular wall collagen and basement membranes as a function of age and levels of glycemia.[73] They are capable of producing cross-linking of proteins and have been shown to display diverse biologic activities, including increased endothelial cell permeability,[74] binding to receptors on macrophages and endothelial mesangial cells,[75–77] activation of macrophages with secretion of cytokines after AGE ligand-receptor interaction,[78] quenching of nitric oxide with the consequent inhibition of vascular dilatation,[79] enhancing oxidative stress,[80] and oxidation of LDL.[81] Thus, there is a growing body of evidence supporting a connection between circulating and tissue-accumulated AGEs and diabetic complications.

Coagulation Factors

The coagulation cascade has been implicated in diabetes-related complications through disorders of the platelet,

TABLE 9–5

Hypotheses Regarding the Potential Role of Nonenzymatic Glycation and Browning in the Pathologic Changes Associated with Diabetes Mellitus

I. Structural proteins
  A. *Collagen:* decreased turnover, flexibility, solubility, strength; increased aggregating potential for platelets; binding of immunoglobulins; cross-linking; and immunogenicity
  B. *Lens crystallins and membrane:* opacification, increased vulnerability to oxidative stress
  C. *Basement membrane:* increased permeability, decreased turnover, increased thickness
  D. *Extracellular matrix:* changes in binding to other proteins
  E. *Hemoglobin:* change in oxygen binding
  F. *Fibrin:* decreased enzymatic degradation
  G. *Red blood cell membrane:* increased rigidity
  H. *Tubulin:* cell structure and transport
  I. *Myelin:* altered structure and immunologic recognition
II. Carrier proteins
  A. *Lipoproteins:* alternative degradative pathways and metabolism by macrophages and endothelial cells, increased immunogenicity
  B. *Albumin:* alteration in binding properties for drugs and in handling by the kidney
  C. *IgG:* altered binding
III. Enzyme systems
  A. Cu-Zn superoxide dismutase
  B. *Fibrinogen:* altered coagulation
  C. *Antithrombin III:* hypercoagulable state
  D. *Purine nucleoside phosphorylase:* aging of erythrocytes
  E. *Alcohol dehydrogenase:* substrate metabolism
  F. *Ribonuclease A:* loss of activity
  G. *Cathepsin B:* loss of activity
  H. N-acetyl-D-glucosaminidase: loss of activity
  I. *Calmodulin:* decreased calcium binding
IV. Nucleic acids
  A. Age-related changes, congenital malformations
V. Potentiation of other diseases of postsynthetic protein modification
  A. Carbamylation-associated disorders in uremia
  B. Steroid cataract formation
  C. Acetaldehyde-induced changes in alcoholism

fluid phase, and vascular components of clotting. The following section briefly reviews the association of abnormalities in glucose metabolism and their relationship to these factors.

The Platelet

The platelet, when obtained from patients with diabetes mellitus, has long been recognized as showing abnormal behavior in in vitro[50] and in vivo studies.[54] In general, the correction of hyperglycemia is associated with an improvement in platelet behavior and release. A discussion of the potential role of the platelet in vascular disease in general is discussed elsewhere in this book. The lesion of the platelet associated with hyperglycemia appears to be in a hypersensitivity to stimuli. Thus, platelet aggregation in vitro may occur spontaneously with stirring in plasma obtained from persons with Hb A_{1c} greater than 10%, with concomitant release of vasoactive substances, including serotonin, adenosine diphosphate (ADP), prostaglandins, and so on. The increased functional properties of diabetic platelets result in part from the primary release of larger platelets with enhanced thromboxane formation capacity and increased numbers of the functional glycoprotein receptors GPIB and GPIIB/IIIA, which are synthesized in megakaryocytes.[82] Insulin exerts an antiaggregating effect, but the effect is diminished in the obese and in subjects with NIDDM.[83] Increased platelet aggregation to arachidonic acid has also been linked to reduced antioxidant properties seen in persons with diabetes.[84]

Platelet-rich or fibrin clots are less amenable to lysis in patients with diabetes than in controls.[85] Furthermore, the release of platelet plasminogen activator inhibitor 1 (PAI-1) in whole blood has been found to be increased in NIDDM subjects.[86] PAI-1 levels have been noted to decrease with lowering of blood glucose in NIDDM.[87] Therefore the platelet not only contributes to a prethrombotic state in persons with diabetes but also to problems of clot lysis in hyperglycemic subjects.

The publication of the EPISTENT (Evaluation of Platelet IIb/IIIa Inhibitor for Stenting Trial)[88] substudy provides the most extensive evaluation of stenting and platelet IIb/IIIa blockade in persons with diabetes and provides additional evidence for a role of the platelet in the morbidity and mortality of heart disease and the associated processes in diabetes. The trial involved 491 diabetic patients who were divided into three groups. One group received both a stent and abciximab. A second group underwent balloon angioplasty and also received the drug. The third group had a stent implanted but received only placebo. The reblockage rate was cut in half in the patients who received both the stent and the drug. Those patients had an 8.1% reblockage rate in the 6 months after the procedure, which was about half that of the other two groups. Ongoing trials of eptifibatide and tirofiban should help define the role of whether platelet IIb/IIIa receptor blockers should be used routinely to reduce restenosis after stenting in diabetic subjects as well as the role of activated platelets and endothelium in pathologic conditions.[88] These agents will become more attractive, in part due to the report of thrombotic thrombocytopenic purpura associated with ticlodipine in the setting of coronary artery stents.[89]

The Fluid Phase of Coagulation

Fibrinogen is increasingly recognized as a potential cardiovascular risk factor.[90–92] Fibrinogen levels generally have been found to be elevated in diabetes. Fibrinogen synthesis is increased in part because of increased turnover and feedback to the liver with fragment D and because insulin has been found to increase fibrinogen synthesis.[93]

Early studies of fibrinogen kinetics in diabetic subjects documented a reversible disorder of fibrinogen kinetics associated with hyperglycemia that was corrected with normal glucose levels or heparin administration, consistent with a lesion of antithrombin III activity in hyperglycemic subjects.[94, 95] These findings were recently confirmed by the PLAT Group study.[96]

Oxidative stress, accentuated in diabetic subjects, has been linked to thrombin activation, and a correlation between markers of oxidative stress and fibrinogen has been reported in diabetic subjects. Thus, oxidative stress, which is mediated by hyperglycemia and compounded by glycation, may represent an additional link between diabetes

and hyperfibrinogenemia.[97–99] Glycated fibrin is also less susceptible to plasmin degradation.[100]

The Endothelial Phase of Coagulation

Studies now indicate that elevated glucose levels can be toxic to vascular endothelial cells through multiple mechanisms.[101] Having observed that glucose levels mimicking diabetic hyperglycemia induce in vitro endothelial cell overexpression of extracellular matrix molecules, decreased replication, and increased levels of transforming growth factor β (TGFβ) messenger RNA (mRNA), Cagliero and colleagues[101] examined whether the effects of high glucose are mediated by autocrine TGFβ. Whereas the inhibitory effect of high glucose levels on endothelial cell replication was reversible, that of TGFβ was not. Both perturbations induced upregulation of fibronectin expression, but the effects were additive. Thus there are growth-inhibitory effects of high glucose levels that are independent of TGFβ, and high glucose levels and TGFβ exert their effects through distinct pathways and at different loci.

Pieper and coworkers[102] attempted to evaluate the relative roles of hyperglycemia and insulin lack on endothelial cell dysfunction in diabetes. Rats were continuously infused with glucose or saline for 72 hours to achieve peak plasma glucose concentrations of approximately 25 mM. Plasma insulin rose by 12-fold in glucose-infused rats. Blood pressure was not altered by this intervention. Aortic rings taken from control rats relaxed to administration of the endothelium-dependent vasodilators acetylcholine and A-23187, and to the endothelium-independent vasodilator nitroglycerin. Relaxation to acetylcholine but not to A-23187 or nitroglycerin was impaired in glucose-infused rat aortic rings. Incubation in vitro with either indomethacin or superoxide dismutase did not restore the impaired relaxation to acetylcholine in rings taken from glucose-infused rats. Thus, hyperglycemia with hyperinsulinemia selectively impairs receptor-dependent, endothelium-dependent relaxation. These studies are consistent with the idea that elevated glucose may be a common pathway leading to endothelial dysfunction in IDDM and NIDDM.

Baumgartner-Parzer and associates[103] have recently shown that adhesion molecule gene expression can be modulated by ambient glucose levels as well. These authors found an increase in intercellular adhesion molecule 1 (ICAM-1) but not platelet endothelial cell adhesion molecule expression in response to a high glucose level in human umbilical vein endothelial cells. These findings are also consistent with specific abnormalities in endothelial dysfunction occurring in diabetes.

In vivo–generated NO circulates in plasma mainly as an adduct of serum albumin. Compared to free NO, this NO adduct is relatively long-lived, and exhibits vasodilating and platelet inhibitory properties. Farkas and Menzel[104] have documented that proteins lose their NO-stabilizing function after advanced glycosylation, thus providing another mechanism by which AGE-modified proteins can promote vascular disease.

Lipids

Hyperlipidemia is a normal concomitant of hyperglycemia. Both triglycerides and cholesterol levels tend to improve with normalization of blood glucose levels as documented by ambient glucose levels and glycated hemoglobin levels.[51] Furthermore, glycation of LDL and modification by AGEs leads to a more atherogenic pattern of lipid metabolism.[105] The presence of renal failure accelerates the pathologic changes associated with the presence of AGEs.[106, 107] Thus, improvement in glycemia corrects at least some of the perturbations of lipid metabolism unique to the individual with diabetes.

Oxidation-Reduction Pathways

Both metabolism of excess glucose and the Amadori rearrangement product resulting from excess glycation can promote pro-oxidant activity.[108, 109] Lipid peroxides are thought to be formed by free radicals and may play an important role in the development of atheromatous vascular disease. Velazquez and colleagues[110] investigated the relationship between lipids, lipoproteins, coagulation factors, and lipid peroxides (measured as thiobarbituric acid reacting species (TBARS) in NIDDM patients with macrovascular disease. Eighteen diabetic and 20 nondiabetic subjects with clinical evidence of IHD or peripheral vascular disease were investigated, together with 28 healthy subjects without evidence of vascular disease. TBARS concentrations, as a measure of oxidation status, did not differ significantly in nondiabetic (mean, 5.0 [95% CI, 4.5 to 5.7] mmol/L) and diabetic groups (5.6 [range, 5.1 to 6.0] mmol/L) with macrovascular disease, although values were higher in both groups of patients with vascular disease by comparison with control subjects (2.7 [range, 2.4 to 3.1] mmol/L; $P < .001$). Significant univariate correlations between TBARS concentrations and measures of blood glucose control (fructosamine, blood glucose, and Hb A_{1c}) were found for all 66 subjects ($P < .01$ to 0.001). Thus, diabetes confers a pro-oxidant internal environment consistent with the promotion of vascular disease.

Vascular Volume Shifts

In our studies of fibrinogen turnover, it became apparent that it was important to correct for vascular volume shifts induced by changes in glucose. When blood glucose was elevated from 100 mg/dL to 300 mg/dL, a rise in vascular volume of 8% was documented by double-labeling techniques.[95] The implications for these types of recurrent volume shifts and the resultant stresses on the vascular tree have not been studied.

Insulin Levels

In NIDDM there is thought to be an increased atherogenic potential related to the presence of insulin resistance, hyperinsulinemia, central obesity, and dyslipidemia. This syndrome, now known as syndrome X,[111] was called previously CHAOS (CAD, hypertension, NIDDM, obesity, cerebrovascular accident) or the "deadly quartet" of upper body obesity, glucose intolerance, hypertriglyceridemia, and hypertension. All were associated with early development of coronary artery disease (CAD). Because of these syndromes, insulin resistance with hyperinsulinemia has been studied as a risk factor in itself for CVD. There have been several epidemiologic studies showing a correlation of hyperinsulinemia with CVD.[111–113] Angiographically documented CAD has been linked with impaired glucose and insulin metabolism.[111]

The proposed pathophysiology of hyperinsulinemia and atherosclerotic disease is complicated. Hyperinsulinemia is associated with increased triglycerides, increased very low–density lipoproteins (VLDLs) and decreased HDL, central obesity, vascular intimal hyperplasia, and possibly hypertension, each of which may accelerate the development of atheroma. However, some studies implicate proinsulin as the culprit, rather than insulin itself, and suggest that exogenous insulin does not increase the risk of CVD.[114, 115] Intervention studies of the effect of glucose control on the initiation and progression of large vessel disease in persons with diabetes mellitus are sorely needed. These interactions have been modified to include a role for insulin and glucose in regulating central sympathetic activity.[116] Thus, the links between obesity, diet, insulin resistance, hyperinsulinemia, sympathetic activity, and lipid disorders are becoming more completely defined.

Immunologic Mechanisms

There are multiple potential interactions of the immune system in the genesis of vascular disease. A number of the cytokine-lymphokine perturbations induced by glycation have been discussed earlier. Immune perturbations specific to diabetes and the development of vascular disease have not yet been identified. Because diabetes is heterogeneous and exhibits similar vascular changes despite the etiology of the phenotype, it is unlikely that a particular genetic lesion of the immune system will be linked to the accelerated vascular disease seen in diabetes.

The one lesion in the immune system of importance to the surgeon is that of the polymorphonuclear leukocyte. The polymorphonuclear leukocyte functions abnormally in the person with hyperglycemia, with decreased adherence, migration, chemotaxis, and killing.[50, 117] The lesion of the polymorphonuclear leukocyte reverses within a marrow transit time of 14 days.[50] Therefore, the optimal surgical candidate is one who has had normoglycemia for 2 weeks prior to surgery.

Inflammatory Processes

The Atherosclerosis Risk in Communities study found a role for inflammation and endothelial dysfunction in the pathogenesis of type 2 diabetes.[118] It also appears that circulating inflammatory factors such as tumor necrosis factor α (TNF-α) and interleukin 6 (IL-6) may cause insulin resistance and obesity.[119, 120]

Smoking

The Speedwell study emphasized the critical role of smoking in the genesis of vascular disease, especially in persons with diabetes.[121] Systolic blood pressure, fasting plasma glucose, triglycerides, and white blood cell count were all independently associated with the development of intermittent claudication, angina, and death, but the most striking association was with smoking.

OTHERS AT RISK FOR DIABETES- OR HYPERGLYCEMIA-ASSOCIATED VASCULAR DISEASE

Impaired Glucose Tolerance

Approximately 16% of American adults aged 40 to 74 years have IGT and approximately 6.6% have diabetes.[122] Because 1% to 5% of those with IGT and 5% to 10% of those at high risk for NIDDM become diabetic each year, IGT is an important risk factor for diabetes.[123–127] In addition, macrovascular disease is present, and mortality rates are higher in individuals with IGT.[124, 128, 131] It appears that individuals with IGT have diabetic risk factor values (as defined later) that fall between the values for normoglycemic individuals and those for diabetic individuals. Harris[129] has suggested "that IGT and NIDDM may have similar natural histories and may reflect a continuum of declining glucose tolerance from IGT to overt diabetes."

Physical Inactivity and Obesity as Risk Factors for NIDDM

Over the last few decades, the importance of physical activity for disease prevention and health maintenance has been increasingly recognized. The benefits of exercise and increased physical activity include enhanced insulin sensitivity and glucose effectiveness, decreased risk for hypertension, reduced blood pressure, improved plasma lipids and lipoproteins, decreased obesity and improved body fat distribution, enhanced immunologic function, decreased anxiety and depression, improved sleep, improved psychological characteristics in both normal and psychiatric patients, and disease prevention.[132]

Obesity and an unfavorable body fat distribution, with increased abdominal fat, are well-established risk factors for diabetes, confounded by ethnicity and family history.[133–135] For obese individuals, the rates of diabetes are higher in Hispanics than in African Americans, and the rates in African Americans in turn are higher than in whites. Up to 50% of obese Native Americans develop diabetes.[123] Data from the second National Health and Nutrition Examination Survey[136] revealed that 24.2% of men and 27.1% of women aged 20 to 74 years were overweight (BMI = 27.8 kg/m² and BMI = 27.3 kg/m² for men and women, respectively). It is estimated that in the United States there are 34 million overweight adults, 12.5 million of whom were judged to be "severely overweight."[137]

In a study of 8715 men (mean age, 42 years) followed for an average of 8.2 years, the age-adjusted death rate increased with higher levels of fasting glucose, and fit men had a lower age-adjusted all-cause death rate compared with unfit men regardless of glycemic status.[138] Fit men with a fasting blood glucose (FBG) less than 6.4 mM had the lowest age-adjusted death rate (21.4 per 10,000 person-years). Within each class of glycemic status (FBG < 6.4 mM, FBG 6.4 to 7.8 mM, or FBG = 7.8 mM or diagnosed NIDDM), those who were fit had lower mortality rates compared with those who were unfit. Men who were fit but in the highest glycemic status group had an age-adjusted all-cause mortality rate (45.9 per 10,000 person-years) similar to that of men who were unfit but in the lowest glycemic status group. The data suggest that fit men with an FBG of 7.8 mM or with NIDDM are at risk of death similar to that of men who are unfit with a normal FBG. The authors suggested that because cardiorespiratory fitness can be improved by regular physical activity, using exercise to improve fitness could be a "cornerstone to the effective management of patients with abnormal blood glucose profiles or NIDDM."[138]

No primary prevention projects for NIDDM have used increased physical activity or exercise as the sole intervention for the prevention or deferment of disease.[138–140] Nevertheless, there is evidence for an association between exercise and diabetes from societies that have abandoned a traditional, active lifestyle for a more sedentary "modern" lifestyle. There is a dramatic increase in NIDDM in people who become more sedentary.[141, 142] Conversely, physically active societies have lower rates of NIDDM than more sedentary societies.[143–148]

Ethnicity as a Risk Factor for NIDDM

Ethnic minority populations in the United States have high rates of IGT and are at higher risk for NIDDM.[148] Minorities are especially afflicted with obesity, especially minority women. Age-adjusted percentages of overweight and severely overweight are 24.6% and 9.6%, respectively, for white women, 45.1% and 19.7% for African American women, and 41.5% and 16.7% for Mexican American women. Although it is acknowledged that some races tend to be "heavier" without adverse health effects, and perhaps the norms and standards need to be adjusted for different races, maintaining a normal weight according to the overall population norm was associated with a 23% lower risk of mortality than being persistently overweight.

Results from the National Health and Nutrition Examination Survey Epidemiologic Follow-up Study[149] suggest that the higher rate of lower extremity amputations in black compared with white Americans with diabetes is not attributable to biologic causes but rather to a combination of social and environmental factors, including obesity. The findings included an analysis of more than 14,000 people who participated, 2240 of whom had diabetes at baseline or in whom it developed during the study. The authors found during 20 years of follow-up that the age-adjusted rate of all lower extremity amputations was 2.8 times higher in black than in white subjects. Diabetes and its duration were strong predictors of risk, as were hypertension, smoking, low educational level, and low socioeconomic status.[149]

Positive Family History

Mitchell and colleagues[150] compared the prevalence of NIDDM and IGT in 4914 subjects of white, African American, and Hispanic origin. Men with a parental history of diabetes (in one or both parents, regardless of which parent) had a higher prevalence of diabetes and IGT than men without a parental history. In women, only a maternal history (or maternal and paternal but not paternal alone) was associated with a higher prevalence of NIDDM and IGT.

Gestational Diabetes

A history of GDM, defined as glucose intolerance of variable severity with onset or first recognition during pregnancy,[151] represents an independent risk factor for the development of subsequent diabetes.[152–164] (GDM also is generally viewed by obstetricians as a potential risk factor for adverse pregnancy outcome.) The original criteria put forth by O'Sullivan and Mahan[165] for the diagnosis of GDM were developed and validated for their predictive value for subsequent diabetes.

Because of the different means used to diagnose diabetes during pregnancy and to define diabetes outside of pregnancy, the prevalence of subsequent diabetes after GDM has been reported to be 19% to 87% for combined glucose intolerance and diabetes and 6% to 62% for diabetes alone. When only the O'Sullivan and Mahan[165] criteria were used for the diagnosis of GDM, the prevalence of subsequent diabetes using the National Diabetes Data Group criteria[21] varied from 2.7% to 20.9%, depending on the length of follow-up.

PROTOCOLS TO IMPROVE GLUCOSE CONTROL BEFORE, DURING, AND AFTER SURGERY

The rationale for near-normal glucose levels has been established earlier. Other considerations for the patient with diabetes who faces surgery with less than optimal control of metabolism in an acute situation include hemodynamic instability during anesthesia due to dehydration and osmotic shifts. As noted earlier and in a 1999 review,[166] the patient is more prone to infection,[13, 167] will have decreased wound healing,[168] and may have increased free fatty acids, the metabolism of which places a higher requirement for myocardial oxygen consumption.[169] This section is intended to provide guidelines in various situations encountered in preparation for surgery, perioperatively, and postoperatively.

Preparation for Elective Surgery

Ideally, all patients with the diagnosis of diabetes should be in good glucose control before elective surgery. *Good glucose control* is defined as the glycemic level that provides the optimal setting for elective surgery, minimizes the risk of infection, facilitates healing, and prevents thrombogenesis. From the earlier discussions in this chapter, the ideal targets for glucose control are 80 to 100 mg/dL before meals and no higher than 180 mg/dL 1 hour after meals. Maintenance of these glucose targets achieves a HbA_{1c} level reported to be associated with the lowest risk of diabetic complications (<7%).

Standing Insulin Orders: A Way to Improve Glucose Control in the Hospital

When a patient with diabetes is admitted to the hospital, the usual outpatient dose of insulin is not appropriate.

First, the patient is generally put to bed, with a resultant increase in insulin requirement of 10% to 20%, depending upon his or her usual daily activity level. Second, there is an increased insulin requirement associated with the psychological and physical stress (infection, trauma, inflammation, surgery) of the hospitalization. Therefore, the patient's usual doses of insulin generally need to be adjusted. The only way to achieve a "perfect" dose of insulin is to measure the blood glucose frequently and visit the patient frequently. Alternatively, the admitting orders could be written to start with a prescription that is near the estimated needs, and allow the staff to automatically adjust each insulin dose based on the blood glucose response to that dose. To this end, we developed the standing orders described later. In the following discussion NPH (neutral protamine Hagedorn) insulin and regular insulin use are emphasized because of their long-term familiarity to clinicians. Those interested in newer insulins may wish to consult a 1999 review.[170] The use of short-acting insulins such as insulin lispro may be substituted for regular insulin in the doses given and may have advantages owing to the rapid onset of action and peak effect with less delayed hyperinsulinemia and hypoglycemia.

Calculating the 24-Hour Insulin Requirement

The increasing insulin requirements for increasingly stressful states are listed in Table 9–6. Standing orders (Fig. 9–1) start with a default calculation of 0.6 units/kg/24 hours in persons who are not NPO (nothing by mouth). This dose is safe and generally an undercalculation. If, however, it is clear to the admitting physician that 0.6 unit per day may be too low, the standing orders state that all handwritten orders on the sheet will be followed. Thus, one may override the standing orders by writing in a higher constant when calculating the 24-hour insulin requirement.

TABLE 9 – 6

Increased Insulin Requirements for Stress

The 24-hour insulin requirement (BIG I) is calculated based on the degree of stress of the patient:

I = 0.6 unit times the patient's weight in kilograms for a person who is healthy and physically active

I = 0.7 unit times the patient's weight in kilograms for a person who is premenstrual or is put to bed rest or who is mildly stressed, be it infectious, physical trauma, or psychological stress

I = 0.8–2.0 units times the patient's weight in kilograms for a person who is moderately to severely stressed. Note stess doses of steroids may require 1.0–2.0 units/kg

    Patient's weight: _____ kg

    Constant chosen for BIG I: _____

    Thus, I = _____ units/24 hr

BIG I is then fractioned into

    4/9 I = prebreakfast NPH = _____ units of NPH

    2/9 I = prebreakfast reg = _____ units of reg

    1/6 I = predinner reg = _____ units of reg

    1/6 I = 11 PM NPH = _____ units of NPH

NPH, neutral protamine Hagedorn (insulin); reg, regular insulin.

☐ 1. Routine: NPH plus Regular schedule.

Nursing will calculate and administer the starting dose of insulin as outlined below:

I = 0.6 x weight Kg/24 hours divided so that 4/9 of dose is NPH given before breakfast and 1/6 of dose is NPH given before bedtime.

Regular insulin is given before breakfast as 2/9 of dose and before dinner as 1/6 of dose. The regular insulin is titrated on the blood glucose.

0730: NPH = 4/9 dose = _____.

Check last pre Dinner BS:

If the pre Dinner BS is < 70, then decrease the AM NPH by 2 units.
If the pre Dinner BS is 71 - 120, then no change in the AM NPH.
If the pre Dinner BS is > 120, then increase the AM NPH by 2 units.

Regular = 2/9 dose = _____ to be adjusted according to the following scale:

BS < 70 = _____ = (2/9 I dose) - 3% of the total insulin requirement.
71 - 100 = _____ = 2/9 I dose.
101 - 140 = _____ = (2/9 I dose) + 3% of I.
> 141 = _____ = (2/9 I dose) + 6% of I.

If the BS 1 hour after the meal is < 110, then decrease the corresponding next day mealtime regular insulin by 2 units.
If the BS 1 hour after the meal is 111 - 150, no change in the corresponding next day mealtime regular insulin.
If the BS 1 hour after the meal is > 151, then increase the corresponding next day mealtime regular insulin by 2 units.

1130 Pre lunch: Regular insulin is given based on the following scale:

BS < 120 = 0 insulin.
121 - 140 = 1/18 I = _____.
141 - 180 = 1/18 I + 2 units = _____.
> 181 = 1/18 I + 4 units = _____.

1700 Pre dinner: Regular is 1/6 dose = _____ and based on the following scale.

BS < 70 = _____ = (1/6 I dose) - 3% of I.
71 - 100 = _____ = 1/6 I dose.
101 - 140 = _____ = (1/6 I dose) + 3% of I.
> 141 = _____ = (1/6 I dose) + 6% of I.

If the BS 1 hour after the meal is < 110, then decrease the corresponding next day mealtime regular insulin by 2 units.
If the BS 1 hour after the meal is 111 - 150, no change in the corresponding next day mealtime regular insulin.
If the BS 1 hour after the meal is > 151, then increase the corresponding next day mealtime regular insulin by 2 units.

2330 Bedtime NPH: Give 1/6 of dose = _____

If the pre Breakfast BS is < 70, then decrease the Bedtime NPH by 2 units.
If the pre Breakfast BS is 71 - 120, then no change in the Bedtime NPH.

If the pre Breakfast BS is > 121, then check the last HS and 3AM BS:
If the HS, 3AM, and pre Breakfast BS are > 121, then increase the Bedtime NPH by 2 units.
If the 3AM BS is < 70 (regardless of the HS or pre Breakfast BS), decrease the Bedtime NPH by 2 units.
If the HS, and the 3AM BS are 70 - 120, but the pre Breakfast is > 121, then increase the Bedtime NPH by 2 units.

NOTE: ALL ORDERS CHECKED OR HAND WRITTEN WILL BE FOLLOWED

_____   _____   _____
Physician's Signature   Date   Time

Figure 9–1. Standing orders for insulin for hospitalized diabetic patients.

Frequency of Monitoring and Charting Glucose

To ensure monitoring of the peak response to the insulins and peak postprandial response to the foods, eight blood glucose tests are required each day: before and 1 hour after each meal, before bed, and at 3 AM. These blood glucose levels are charted on the insulin worksheet illustrated in Figure 9–2. The initial calculations of such insulin requirements are written on the worksheet, as are all subsequent insulin changes.

The standing orders allow the nurses to adjust each of the injections daily. The percentage change for the sliding scales is 3% of the total insulin requirement. The sliding scale is adjusted as a percentage of the total dose because these orders apply to small children as well as obese adults. A 2-unit change to correct for the following day is included to make orders slightly easier to follow, but if a patient is very small or very large, one may override the orders and rewrite them, making smaller or larger changes for the subsequent dose.

Automatic Adjustments by Standing Orders

Each dose of insulin will be changed as outlined in the established orders (see Fig. 9–1) by the nursing staff. The AM dose of NPH insulin is adjusted according to the predinner blood sugar. For example, if the predinner blood sugar is too low, then the AM NPH insulin for the following morning will be decreased by 2 units.

The NPH insulin dose at bedtime requires three blood glucose checks before it can be safely adjusted. The NPH insulin dose before bed is designed to "fix the fasting" or conquer the wake-up blood glucose for the following morning. Other forces come into play, however, which may make the interpretation of a high fasting blood glucose difficult. There are six ways to end up with a high fasting blood glucose level:

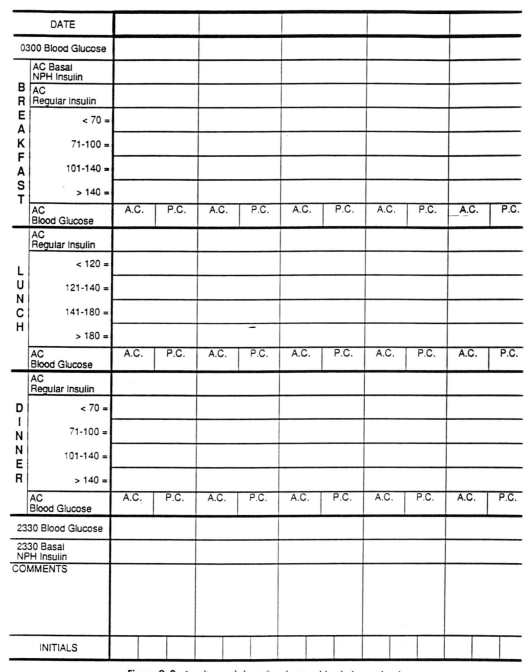

Figure 9–2. Insulin worksheet for charting blood glucose levels.

1. One can go to bed with a high glucose level because of a persisting high dinner level and stay elevated all night long. The cause is either not enough regular insulin at dinner or too much dinner.
2. One can go to bed with a normal blood glucose level, but have a bedtime snack, which then produces the high wake-up glucose level. This can be avoided by having a smaller bedtime snack.
3. One can go to bed with a normal blood glucose level, but "drift up" throughout the night because the NPH insulin dose at bedtime was inadequate.
4. One can go to bed with a normal blood glucose level, become hypoglycemic in the middle of the night, and wake up with a high level because of the counterregula-

tory hormonal response to the low blood glucose. The cause is too much bedtime NPH insulin or an inadequate bedtime snack.
5. One can go to bed with a high glucose level, yet still have a hypoglycemic reaction in the middle of the night, mount a counterregulatory response, and wake up with a high glucose level. In this case, the cause is not enough regular insulin at dinner (or too much dinner) and too much bedtime NPH insulin.
6. One can have a normal bedtime glucose level that stays normal until after 3 AM, when the blood glucose level rises with increasing insulin needs (the dawn phenomenon). More bedtime insulin is needed.

Thus, the adjustment of the bedtime dose of NPH requires

all three readings: bedtime, 3 AM, and wake-up blood glucose levels.

If the wake-up blood glucose level is low (less than 70 mg/dL), decrease the bedtime NPH insulin dose by 2 units. If the wake-up level is high and if the previous night's bedtime and 3 AM levels were also high, then the 11 PM NPH insulin dose should be increased by 2 units. If the 3 AM glucose reading is low, no matter what the bedtime or the wake-up blood glucose was, cut back on the bedtime dose of NPH insulin. Here, the physician would need to write separate orders to indicate if the quantity of food at dinner or at the bedtime snack should be adjusted. The established orders (see Fig. 9–1) would also increase the NPH insulin dose before bedtime if the wake-up blood glucose level is high but the bedtime and 3 AM blood glucose levels are normal, because there is room for a little more bedtime NPH insulin to conquer the fasting.

The 3 AM "Touch-up" Insulin Dose

One additional order that can speed the normalization process is to prescribe regular insulin at 3 AM. If the blood glucose level is high at 3 AM, it definitely will be high at 7:30 AM due to the dawn-associated rise in counterregulatory hormones. Therefore, a convenient and worthwhile addition to these orders is a sliding scale for regular insulin at 3 AM, which is generally the same as the lunchtime "touch-up":

$$BS < 120 = 0$$

$$BS\ 121\ to\ 140 = 1/18\ I$$

$$BS\ 141\ to\ 180 = 1/18\ I + 2\ units$$

$$BS > 181 = 1/18\ I + 4\ units$$

where BS = blood sugar and I = total insulin dose per 24 hours.

It is worth noting that bedtime regular insulin is dangerous. Between the hours of 11 PM and 3 AM, patients are more sensitive to regular insulin because of low levels of counterregulatory hormones. It is generally preferable to leave a high bedtime glucose level untreated but wake the patient at 3 AM and give regular insulin at that time if the blood glucose is still elevated.

The protocol for standing insulin orders was designed to go hand in hand with a 40% carbohydrate diet consisting of three meals and three snacks. The diet is generally calculated based on body weight. A general guideline is 30 kcal/kg for malnourished adults, 25 kcal/kg for persons of ideal body weight, and 18 kcal/kg for the obese patient.

Hypoglycemia Prevention

Although the standing orders for insulin begin with 0.6 units/kg/24 hours, which is most likely an undercalculation, it is always best to pair this protocol with a protocol for hypoglycemia. Suggested hypoglycemia orders are given in Table 9–7.

TABLE 9 – 7

Standing Orders for Hypoglycemia

Routine: nursing staff will carry out protocol outlined below:
A. For asymptomatic blood glucose (BS) < 60 mg/dL:
    Give 8 oz milk and recheck BS in 15 min.
B. For symptomatic blood glucose < 60 mg/dL:
    Give 8 oz milk and recheck BS in 15 min.
    If BS < 60 mg/dL, give another 8 oz milk and recheck BS in 15 min.
    If BS still < 60 mg/dL, give 8 oz orange juice, and a slice of bread.
C. When the patient is either unable to take fluids, lethargic, or argumentative:
    Give 0.15 mg glucagon SC and repeat BS in 10 min.
    If BS < 60 mg/dL, give another 0.15 mg glucagon SC and repeat BS in 10 min.
    Once BS > 60 mg/dL but < 120 mg/dL and patient is able to hear, give 8 oz milk.
D. When patient is unresponsive:
    Give 1.0 mg glucagon IM and then call the physician.
    Check BS in 10 min.
    If patient still unresponsive, start IV line of 1000 mL D_{10} to run wide open.
    Recheck BS in 10 min, turn down IV line to 100 mL/hr when BS > 80 mg/dL.

BS, blood sugar; D_{10}, 10% dextrose in water; SC, subcutaneously.

Deriving the "Personal Lag Time" for Insulin Action

At times, the health care professional may actually create brittle diabetes. All that may be needed is an injection of regular insulin at the moment the meal is ingested. The simple sugars in foods peak as sugar in the blood stream in 15 to 20 minutes. Complex carbohydrates peak as sugar in the blood stream in 60 minutes.

Regular insulin injected under the skin requires about 45 minutes before an effect can be documented in terms of a decrement in blood glucose. The hypoglycemic action of the injected insulin does not peak for 2 to 3 hours. The result is that after an injection of insulin given at the same time as a meal with a fairly large percentage of calories as carbohydrate, blood glucose peaks at about 1 hour after the start of the meal, and the patient is hypoglycemic at 3 hours, concomitant with the peak in insulin action. Such an occurrence might be referred to as iatrogenic reactive hypoglycemia. Counterregulatory hormones secreted (and extra food ingested) in response to the hypoglycemia lead to a marked rise in glucose (usually 250 to 350 mg/dL) approximately 3 hours later, which in turn prompts the need for additional insulin.

To convert this type of brittle diabetes into smoother glycemic profiles, one needs to change the timing of the injection of regular insulin in relationship to the meal. Increasing the lag time between the insulin injection and the ingestion of food can dampen glycemic excursions despite no change in meal plan or dose of insulin. The usual optimal lag time for abdominal injections is 30 to 40 minutes. The usual lag time for leg injections is 40 to 50 minutes.

Several approaches can shorten the lag time between insulin injection and action. First, insulin lispro has a rapid peak and rapid disposal compared with regular insulin. Thus, it can be given when food arrives or even after ingestion of a meal after calculation of the ingested carbohydrate. Second, the warmer the skin temperature, the faster the insulin is absorbed. A hot washcloth placed immediately over the injection site accelerates absorption. Third, muscle activity at the site of injection shortens lag time. Thus, exercise can speed insulin absorption.

Suggested Sliding Scale for Insulin

A simple way to think about insulin action is to assume that hypoglycemia increases insulin sensitivity and hyperglycemia increases insulin resistance. Therefore, a premeal sliding scale for regular insulin might not only include a scale of graded doses of insulin but also a scale of lag times for beginning the meal after the injection. In practice, it is often prudent on a busy inpatient ward to await the arrival of food before the injection of insulin in order to avoid hypoglycemia. As noted earlier, the use of insulin lispro obviates the problem.

Nothing by Mouth (NPO) Orders

Compliance with NPO orders might be simpler if all patients used an insulin infusion pump; then the patient merely skips the breakfast bolus and maintains the basal infusion of insulin. However, this advice presupposes that the patient is on a perfectly calculated basal infusion of insulin (that dose of insulin that keeps the patient normoglycemic during fasting). Unfortunately, many patients are on a basal infusion rate that is adjusted higher than the basal need to provide extra insulin to cover extra calories or foods that slowly convert to glucose (such as protein and high fiber carbohydrates). Thus, even "well-controlled" patients using a pump may need to be instructed to decrease the basal infusion rate by 20% for as long as they are NPO or to adjust the calculated basal infusion to 0.25 units/kg/24 hours, whichever is lower. A good starting point is 0.3 units/kg/24 hours as a basal constant infusion. The blood glucose is measured before bed, at 3 AM, at 7 AM, and every 2 hours thereafter. These frequent checks allow for increasing or decreasing the basal rate or "touching up" with insulin, intravenous (IV) glucose, or glucagon, as needed.

If a patient is on an NPH insulin system, the doses during the fasting period are calculated (0.1 × weight [kg]) to be given every 8 hours that the patient is NPO. The blood glucose should be measured at midnight, 3 AM, 8 AM, and then every 2 hours until the operation. If the blood glucose is elevated, then touch-up doses of regular insulin, similar to the Ultralente insulin protocol, may be given.

If the patient is hospitalized and an IV line is started, hypoglycemia and hyperglycemia can be avoided with IV infusions at 2 mL/kg/hour based on blood glucose checks every hour (during the procedure and recovery) or every other hour. The guidelines for maintaining normoglycemia on IV infusion are outlined in Table 9–8.

These algorithms for maintenance of normoglycemia

Guidelines for Intravenous Infusion Based on Blood Glucose Values

BLOOD GLUCOSE (mg/dL)	INFUSION AT 2 mL/kg/hr
<70	D_{10}
70–120	D_5
>120	Normal saline at 2 mL/kg/hr
>150	Use touch-up insulin IV (0.02 unit) while normal saline is continued at 2 mL/kg/hr and adjust rate based on hourly readings

D_{10}, 10% dextrose in water; D_5, 5% dextrose in water.

during periods of fasting are essentially the same as those used to prescribe a true basal insulin dose or the dose of insulin that maintains normal blood glucose levels in a person with IDDM when he or she does not eat. During periods of increasing stress, such as surgery, extra insulin may be needed. Nevertheless, these guidelines and the surveillance system provide a relatively simple and safe approach to fasting for the patient with IDDM or NIDDM.

Enteral and Parenteral Nutrition in the Diabetic Patient

Given a severely stressful situation, or after the administration of high-dose corticosteroids, the population estimated to become frankly hyperglycemic rises to over 25% (referred to as "stress-induced" diabetes). Furthermore, when highly concentrated glucose solutions are given intravenously to a stressed person, the percentage of hyperglycemic individuals rises to over 50%.[171] It can be seen that a significant number of surgical patients require additional attention to enteral and parenteral nutrition because of elevated blood glucose values if optimal glucose levels are to be maintained.

Enteral Route

There are multiple formulas for tube-feeding patients. They differ by protein concentration and composition, density, fat, and carbohydrate percentage. These basic formulas contain 45% to 60% carbohydrate. The elemental formulas contain low residue and thus are completely absorbed from the jejunum. These elemental diets have more than 70% carbohydrates and sugars. Corn syrup usually is the carbohydrate used. There are two formulas with a low percentage of carbohydrate: one is for pulmonary patients to help lower the respiratory quotient (28% carbohydrate) and the other is designed for diabetic patients with 38% high-fiber carbohydrate. The carbohydrate content of the formula directly affects the resultant blood glucose level achieved and the lower the carbohydrate content of a formula, the lower the resultant blood glucose level maintained. If hyperglycemia is documented by blood glucose determinations every 4 hours, insulin may be given as a constant infusion IV or subcutaneously (SC). One unit of regular

T A B L E   9 – 9

Enteral Nutrition: Normal Fasting for the Patient with Normal Glucose Tolerance and for the Non–Insulin-Dependent Diabetes Mellitus Patient Who Has Normal Fasting Glucose without Insulin

1. Monitor fingerstick blood glucose q6h for 2 days. If all glucose levels remain <180 mg/dL, then frequency of monitoring may be decreased to once a day.
2. If hyperglycemia occurs, continue to monitor blood glucose q6h and
3. Begin insulin to be given as a continuous infusion when the enteral nutrition is being infused to be 1 (one) unit of regular insulin for every 10 g of carbohydrate (CHO) in the feeding.
4. Based on the blood glucose every q6h, change the insulin dose for tomorrow to be:
   <80 = decrease ratio (0.5 unit/10 g CHO)
   81–180 = no change in ratio (1.0 unit/10 g CHO)
   >81 = increase ratio (1.5 units/10 g CHO)

CHO, carbohydrate.

insulin per 10 g of carbohydrate is given over 24 hours in the formula. Table 9–9 summarizes the protocol for blood glucose monitoring and initiating insulin in the nondiabetic patient.

If a patient with known NIDDM has a normal fasting blood glucose before the enteral infusion is started, this patient may have insulin started with the enteral infusion to be 1.0 unit of regular insulin for every 10 g of carbohydrate given over the 24 hours in the formula (Fig. 9–3). Most severely stressed NIDDM patients have fasting hyperglycemia even if their interim fasting glucose level is normal. In the majority of cases, NIDDM patients require both a basal insulin infusion, calculated as 0.3 unit of regular insulin times the weight in kilograms, plus the "meal requirement," which is 1.0 unit of regular insulin for every 10 g of carbohydrate in the formula (Table 9–10).

IDDM patients who require enteral nutrition may also be given insulin for their basal and formula-related needs as in Table 9–10. If the patient is severely ill or is also taking glucocorticoids, the basal insulin dose may be calculated as 1.0 unit/kg body weight and the formula-related insulin dose may start at 1 unit/10 g carbohydrate. The blood glucose may be checked every 4 to 6 hours, and if elevated, additional insulin as SC regular insulin may be given by the floor nursing staff using the following scale:

BS < 180 = no extra regular insulin

BS 181 to 240 = 6 units regular insulin

BS 241 to 300 = 8 units regular insulin

BS > 301 = 10 units regular insulin

If these blood glucose checks are between 80 and 180 mg/dL, no change in the carbohydrate ratio is necessary. If the blood glucose level is less than 80 mg/dL, then the ratio may be decreased to 0.5 unit regular insulin per 10 g carbohydrate. If the blood glucose is greater than 180 mg/

T A B L E   9 – 1 0

Enteral Nutrition for Person with Known Non–Insulin-Dependent Diabetes and Elevated Fasting Glucose

1. Monitor blood glucose q6h.
2. Begin enteral nutrition and insulin infusion at the same time.
3. Insulin infusion is calculated as the sum of the basal and carbohydrate (CHO)-related need.

Basal need is dependent on stress level and weight

Stress Level	Units of Regular Insulin
Mild	0.3 × weight (kg)
Moderate	0.5 × weight (kg)
Severe	1.0 × weight (kg)
Steroid therapy (maximum doses) regardless of degree of illness	1.0 × weight (kg)

CHO-related need: 1 unit regular insulin for every 10 g CHO in enteral nutrition

4. Adjustment for tomorrow's dose is made such that the insulin-CHO ratio is changed based on today's blood glucose levels:
   <80 = decrease ratio (0.5 unit/10 g CHO)
   81–180 = no change in ratio (1.0 unit/10 g CHO)
   >81 = increase ratio (1.5 units/10 CHO)

CHO, carbohydrate.

dL, increase the insulin-to-carbohydrate ratio to 1.5 units/10 g carbohydrate (Table 9–11).

Intravenous Parenteral Nutrition

Most normal, healthy persons become hyperglycemic if they are given intravenous solutions with a concentration of 20% dextrose or more. For the person with normal glucose tolerance, only the dextrose load needs to be covered with insulin at a dose of 1.0 unit regular insulin per 10 g dextrose. For example, if 500 g of dextrose is infused

T A B L E   9 – 1 1

Intravenous Nutrition for the Patient with Normal Glucose Tolerance and the Non–Insulin-Dependent Diabetes Mellitus Patient with Normal Fasting Blood Glucose

1. Monitor blood glucose q6h for 2 d and then bid as long as blood glucose remains normal
2. If hyperglycemia occurs, continue to monitor q6h.
3. Regular insulin may be given SC q6h for the immediate treatment of hyperglycemia:
   <180 = 0 units
   181–240 = 6 units
   241–300 = 8 units
   >301 = 10 units
4. Begin with an IV solution that has insulin in the bag calculated to 1.0 unit of regular insulin for every 10 g of dextrose in the bag.
5. Adjust tomorror's insulin dose based on today's blood glucose levels such that the ratio of insulin to grams of dextrose is changed:
   <80 = decrease ratio (0.5 unit/10 g CHO)
   81–180 = no change in ratio (1.0 unit/10 g CHO)
   >181 = increase ratio (1.5 units/10 g CHO)

CHO, carbohydrate; SC, subcutaneously.

ENTERAL NUTRITION ORDER

DATE & TIME	
	1. FEEDING TUBE:
	☐ Nasogastric ☐ Nasoduodenal ☐ Gastrostomy ☐ Jejunostomy
	Feeding Tube: Type _____ French Size _____
	☐ Abdominal X-ray to confirm tube placement and termination point prior to
	feeding initiation.

	2. FORMULA	**DESCRIPTION**	**INDICATIONS**
	ISOTONIC (1KCAL/cc)		
	☐ Jevity	Contains fiber	Normal bowel function
	☐ Glucerna	Low carbohydrate	Abnormal glucose tolerance
	☐ Osmolite HN	High nitrogen	Low intestinal residue
	HYPERTONIC (1.5KCAL/cc)		
	☐ Ensure Plus	High calorie	Increased caloric needs, volume restriction
	☐ Pulmocare	High fat/Low carbohydrate	Respiratory failure
	ELEMENTAL (1KCAL/cc)		
	☐ Vital HN	Hydrolyzed	Impaired GI function
	OTHER:		

	3. DELIVERY
	METHOD: ☐ Continuous Other:
	STRENGTH: ☐ Full ☐ 3/4 ☐ 1/2 Other:
	RATE/FEEDING SCHEDULE: ☐ 25cc/hr ☐ 50cc/hr Other: _____ cc/hr
	Increase rate to _____ cc/hr after _____ hrs.
	Other feeding schedule:
	ADDITIONAL WATER: Total additional water volume, including
	flushes/medications, to be _____ cc/24hrs.
	Briskly irrigate tubing with 30cc water BEFORE and AFTER
	medication administration or if feeding is interrupted for more
	than 5 minutes.

	4. MONITORING:
	GASTRIC RESIDUALS: Check residuals every _____ hrs. If greater than _____ cc,
	hold feeding for _____ hr(s). Recheck residual. Restart
	feeding at _____ cc/hr, when residual less than _____ cc.
	EXAMPLE: For 50cc/hr, check residual q 4 hrs & hold if 200cc.
	WEIGHT: ☐ Weigh patient on initiation of feeding and M/W/F.

	5. LABORATORY: ☐ CHEM 20 AND TRANSFERRIN NOW AND WEEKLY
	OTHER LABORATORY:

	DATE	**TIME**	**SIGNATURE**
	NOTE: ALL ORDERS CHECKED OR HANDWRITTEN WILL BE FOLLOWED		

Figure 9–3. Enteral nutrition order form for diabetic patients.

over 24 hours (usually 2.5 L of a D_{20} solution), 50 units of regular insulin may be placed in the dextrose solution to be infused over 24 hours. The blood glucose may be checked every 4 to 6 hours and extra regular insulin given as detailed above. The dose of insulin for the solution for the following day may be adjusted such that if the blood glucose level is 80 to 180 mg/dL, no change in the ratio of 1.0 unit regular insulin per 10 g dextrose need be made. If the blood glucose is less than 80 mg/dL, then the ratio may be decreased to 0.5 unit/10 g dextrose. If the blood glucose level is greater than 180 mg/dL, then the ratio may be increased to 1.5 units/10 g dextrose. If a patient remains hyperglycemic while receiving 500 g of dextrose over 24 hours despite 50 units of insulin, the insulin dose may be increased to 75 units of regular insulin for 500 g dextrose (1.5 units/10 g dextrose) (Fig. 9–4 and Table 9–12).

For the patient with fasting hyperglycemia before parenteral nutrition is started, a basal insulin need must be added to the dextrose-insulin–related need. The basal dose depends on body weight, severity of illness, and the administration of steroids. Tables 9–11 and 9–12 list the incremental increase in insulin response with increasing need in NIDDM. The dextrose-related need must be added to the basal need for all diabetic patients.

TOTAL PARENTERAL NUTRITION ORDER FORM

ADMINISTER OVER 24 HOURS; ALL TPN SOLUTIONS WILL BEGIN AT 1800 HOURS DAILY.
ALL CHANGES, ADDITIONS OR DELETIONS <u>MUST</u> BE RECEIVED BY 1400 HOURS.

1. Select One Only:

☐ **Custom** FORMULA AND RATE   **or**   ☐ **Standard** FORMULA (SET RATES DO NOT CHANGE)

CUSTOM:	**PER DAY**
Usual requirements:	
Total daily KCals:	25-35 KCal/kg/day
Protein: 1 - 2 gm/kg or	10-15 % of total KCal
Dextrose:	45-55% of total KCal
Lipids:	25-35% of total KCal
PROTEIN: (4 KCal/gm)	_____ gm/day
DEXTROSE: (3.4 KCal/gm)	_____ KCal/day
LIPIDS: (10 KCal/gm)	_____ KCal/day
RATE: (for custom only)	_____ ml/hr

Start at _____ ml/hr for 4 hours, then increase to rate above.

NOTE: TPN typically requires 2-3 liters.
Call Pharmacy at ext. 2863 for LEAST POSSIBLE VOLUME, or assistance.

STANDARD:		**PER DAY**
☐ PERIPHERAL	2.4 Liters	1652 KCal
Protein 3.5%	84gm	336 KCal
Dextrose 10%	240gm	816 KCal
Lipids 20% 250 ml	50gm	500 KCal
Total Volume = 2400 ml		**Rate: 100 ml/hr**
☐ CENTRAL	2 Liters	1564 KCal
Protein 3.5%	70gm	280 KCal
Dextrose 13%	260gm	884 KCal
Lipids 20% 200 ml	40gm	400 KCal
Total Volume = 2000 ml		**Rate: 83 ml/hr**
*** for 50 kg patient (30 KCal/kg)		
☐ CENTRAL	2.4 Liters	2214 KCal
Protein 4.25%	102gm	408 KCal
Dextrose 16%	384gm	1306 KCal
Lipids 20% 250 ml	50gm	500 KCal
Total Volume = 2400 ml		**Rate: 100 ml/hr**
*** for 70 kg patient (30 KCal/kg)		

☐ Delete lipids
☐ Start at 50ml/hr for 4hr

2. Select Additives FOR All TPN
(BOTH CUSTOM AND STANDARD)

ADDITIVES:		mark this box for standard additives ⌐	**PER DAY** Custom and/or additional orders
Item	Range		
NaCl	60-150	20	meq/day
Na Acetate		50	meq/day
Na Phosphate	10-25mM	12	mM/day
K Phosphate			mM/day
K Acetate			meq/day
KCl	40-80	40	meq/day
MgSO4	15-30	10	meq/day
Ca Gluconate	9-18	9	meq/day
Vitamins [MVI-12]	10 ml	10	ml/day
Trace elements	3 ml	3	ml/day
Reg Insulin 1U/10gm or 3U/100 KCal Dextrose (plus if diabetic add .3U/kg)			U/day
Heparin 1000 U/L	2-3000 U		U/day
Folic acid	1 mg		mg/day
Vit. K 10mg Monday to MWF	1-3x wk		mg/day every Monday
OTHER: _____			

3. MONITORING:

☐ Glucose monitoring Q6H x 5D, then BID.
☐ Renal panel, Phosphorus & Magnesium ordered daily x 3, then MWF.
☐ Serum transferrin, CHEM 20 ordered now & 1 week after start of TPN.
☐ Triglycerides now & 48 hrs after start of TPN.
☐ Daily Weights.
☐ Other:_____

NOTE HOSPITAL POLICY:

- Dextrose 10% will replace TPN during interruptions at same rate.
- Nutrition Support Team (NST) will provide basic assessment and monitoring.
- For new orders received by Pharmacy after 1800, Standard Peripheral TPN formula will be used until 1800 the following day per physician approval. Rate and additives will remain as ordered.

_____ _____
Physician Signature   Date

Figure 9–4. Intravenous parenteral nutrition order form for diabetic patients.

The parenteral solutions may have both the basal insulin need and the dextrose need placed in the bottles to be infused over 24 hours. The three-in-one bags contain an entire day's nutritional needs in one bag. In addition, the day's insulin requirement (basal plus dextrose-related needs) may all be put in one bag.

There is a new product available for peripheral nutrition that substitutes dextrose with glycerol. Because glycerol does not require insulin for metabolism, this product (ProcalAmine), does not raise the blood glucose level of diabetic patients.

In summary, prevention and treatment of hyperglycemia in up to 50% of all patients given parenteral or enteral nutrition is necessary to optimize care in the severely ill patient. The protocols outlined here are designed to monitor and avoid potentially dangerous iatrogenic hyperglycemia.

Matching Insulin to Food

The correlation of postprandial glucose to percentage carbohydrate in a fixed caloric meal is excellent for the dinner meal and quite good for breakfast and lunch. The amount of insulin required to cover carbohydrate in the evening meal is generally about 1.0 unit/10 g carbohydrate and for breakfast, about 1.5 units/10 g carbohydrate. The amount of insulin required to cover lunch usually falls between that required to cover breakfast and dinner. Nevertheless, the above ratios are approximations. An insulin-carbohydrate ratio for each meal is ideally established for each patient. The advantage in developing the skill of matching insulin and carbohydrate lies in the freedom to vary meal composition. It is not only useful for persons on an insulin pump but also for patients on a fixed meal plan if they choose to eat out or vary the meal plan. If an individual

TABLE 9–12

Intravenous Nutrition for Insulin-Dependent Diabetes Mellitus Patients and Non–Insulin-Dependent Diabetes Mellitus Patients with Fasting Hyperglycemia

1. Monitor blood glucose q6h.
2. Begin IV solution and insulin together in the same bag.
3. Insulin dosage is calculated as the sum of the basal and the dextrose-related insulin needs.

Basal need is dependent on stress level and weight

Stress Level	Units of Regular Insulin
Mild	$0.3 \times$ weight (kg)
Moderate	$0.5 \times$ weight (kg)
Severe	$1.0 \times$ weight (kg)
Steroid therapy (maximum doses) regardless of degree of illness)	$1.0 \times$ weight (kg)

Dextrose-related need: 1 unit regular insulin for every 10 g dextrose in the infusion solution.

4. Adjustment for tomorrow's dose is made such that the insulin-CHO ratio is changed based on today's blood glucose levels.

   <80 = decrease ratio (0.5 unit/10 g CHO)
   81–180 = no change in ratio (1.0 unit/10 g CHO)
   >181 = increase ratio (1.5 units/10 g CHO)

CHO, carbohydrate.

knows that an ingested meal is going to exceed the normal carbohydrate quota for a meal, an upward adjustment in the insulin dose may be made by calculating the extra insulin needed from the number of grams of carbohydrate to be ingested above the established quota of the prescribed diet. The approach is equally useful when calories and carbohydrate are eliminated from a meal or diet as might occur in a weight-loss program.

Oral Hypoglycemic Agents and Suggested Protocols for NIDDM Patients to Achieve a Target Glycosylated Hemoglobin of Less Than 7% Outside the Hospital

If a given treatment protocol is not achieving fasting blood glucose levels of 80 to mg/dL and 1-hour postprandial glucose levels less than 180 mg/dL, the present medications may be discontinued and the following scheme followed:

1. Glipizide 10 mg three times a day (30 minutes before each meal with an additional 10 mg added if there is a particular meal which is problematic).[172]
2. If fasting blood glucose and the postprandial glucose levels are not in the target ranges after 2 weeks of this scheme, glipizide may be discontinued and a trial of glyburide 10 mg twice a day prescribed.[173]
3. If the fasting blood glucose and the postprandial glucose levels are not in the target ranges after 2 weeks, metformin may be added starting at a dose of 500 mg twice a day and titrated upward until target blood glucose levels are achieved or a maximum of 2500 mg per day is reached.[174–177] Contraindications to metformin include renal or hepatic disease or cardiac compromise.

If the target fasting blood glucose is not achieved despite the maximum doses of metformin and sulfonylurea agents, NPH insulin may be started at bedtime beginning at a dose of 0.1 unit/kg and increasing the dose by 2.0-unit increments per day until the fasting blood glucose is in the target ranges.[177–180]

Acarbose at a dosage up to 100 mg three times a day may be considered as adjunctive therapy. This agent is a disaccharidase inhibitor and therefore prevents the postprandial rise in glucose after complex carbohydrate ingestion. Also on the horizon are several new classes of drugs, including "insulin sensitizers" and drugs that increase the first phase of insulin secretion from the beta cells. These new agents may minimize the need for insulin therapy when sulfonylurea agents and metformin fail to improve glucose control.

Insulin-sensitizing drugs are also available as adjunctive therapy. The main class of these drugs includes the thiazolidinediones. Troglitazone, the first agent on the market, has been associated with poorly understood hepatic toxicity and hence should be avoided in patients with hepatic disease. Whether the newer approved agents, rosiglitazone and pioglitazone, have such toxicities remains to be seen.

Meglitinides stimulate insulin secretion and have been found to be useful in type 2 diabetes. These agents are taken 15 to 30 minutes before a meal. Repaglinide is the first of this class of agent to be available. It appears to be effective, and the behavioral modification associated with premeal drug delivery may be an advantage.

Table 9–13 outlines an ongoing care protocol for persons with diabetes who are at risk for or have vascular disease. For the reasons detailed throughout the chapter, the emphasis is on control of blood glucose, lipids, and blood pressure. In addition, the issues of aspirin or platelet therapy, vaccination against influenza and pneumonia, smoking

TABLE 9–13

Maintenance Therapy for Diabetes Vascular Disease Prevention

I. Blood glucose control
  A. Target Hb_{1c} of $\leq 7\%$
  B. Monitor blood glucose and target premeal values of 80–120 mg/dL and bedtime values of 100–140 mg/dL
II. Blood pressure control
  A. ACE inhibitor for all adult subjects with diabetes or if microalbuminuria present
  B. Target level of $<130/85$ mm Hg
III. Blood lipid control
  A. Target LDL of <100 mg/dL
  B. Target triglyceride level < 200 mg/dL
IV. Antiplatelet therapy
  A. Aspirin if >30 yr old
  B. Clopidogrel
  C. Ticlopidine (associated with TTP)
  D. Platelet IIb/IIIa inhibitor
IV. Miscellaneous treatment
  A. Vaccination for influenza and pneumococcus
  B. Smoking cessation
  C. Foot care program
  D. Exercise plan
  E. Nutrition plan

Hb A_{1c}, hemoglobin A_{1c}; ACE, angiotensin-converting enzyme; LDL, low-density lipoprotein; TTP, thrombotic thrombocytopenic purpura.

cessation, foot care, exercise, and nutrition should all be considered as part of the management plan. Although these issues, with the exception of blood glucose control, do not differ qualitatively from those associated with vascular disease in the nondiabetic population, a few points are noteworthy. Every patient with diabetes needs to be considered for angiotensin-converting enzyme inhibitor therapy. The findings of the HOPE study reinforce previously noted findings that ramipril substantially lowers the risk of death, heart attack, stroke, coronary revascularization, heart failure, and complications related to diabetes mellitus in a high-risk group of patients with preexisting vascular disease. The study was stopped early by the data and safety monitoring board because of the obvious benefit of ramipril.[181]

Another treatment that warrants some comment is aspirin. It is generally agreed that aspirin is underutilized by persons with diabetes for a number of reasons.[182] Aspirin has been found to have greater benefit in diabetic patients than in those without diabetes in improving survival in the presence of CAD.[183] Also of note is that in the Wisconsin Epidemiologic Study of Diabetic Retinopathy, daily aspirin use by persons with diabetes was inversely associated (OR, 0.11) with lower extremity amputation.[184] Thus, the American Diabetes Association recommends aspirin for all diabetic patients older than 30 years.[167]

References

1. Garber AJ: Clinical perspectives on type 2 diabetes in North America. Diabetes Metab Rev 11(Suppl 1):S81–86, 1995.
2. Schwartz LM, Woloshin S: Changing disease definitions: Implications for disease prevalence. Analysis of the Third National Health and Nutrition Examination Survey, 1988–1994. Effective Clin Pract 2:96–99, 1999.
3. Stuart WP, Wolf B, Macaulay EM, Cross KS: Screening for diabetes on a vascular ward: Lessons from an audit. J R Coll Surg Edinb 43:11–12, 1998.
4. Lernmark A: Insulin-dependent diabetes mellitus. In Davidson JK (ed): Clinical Diabetes Mellitus. New York, Georg Thieme, 1991, p 35.
5. Reaven GM, Laws A: Insulin resistance, compensatory hyperinsulinaemia, and coronary heart disease. Diabetologia 37:948–952, 1994.
6. American Diabetes Association: Clinical Practice Recommendations 2000. Diabetes Care 23 (Suppl 1):S1–S116, 2000.
7. Clark CM, Adlin V (eds): Risks and benefits of intensive management in non–insulin dependent diabetes mellitus. Ann Intern Med 124(Suppl):1–186, 1996.
8. Osler W, McCrae T: Diseases of the arteries. In Modern Medicine, Its Theory and Practice, 4th ed. Philadelphia, Lea & Febiger, 1908, pp 426–427.
9. Joslin EP: A Diabetic Manual. Philadelphia, Lea & Febiger, 1945, p 141.
10. Wellman KF, Volk BW: Historical review. In Volk BW, Wellman KF (eds): The Diabetic Pancreas. New York, Plenum Press, 1977, pp 1–14.
11. Galloway JA, Shuman CR: Diabetes and surgery. A study of 667 cases. Am J Med 34:177–192, 1963.
12. Hjortrup A, Rasmussen B, Kehlet H: Morbidity in diabetic and nondiabetic patients after major vascular surgery. BMJ 257:1107–1108, 1983.
13. Golden SH, Peart-Vigilance C, Kao WHL, Brancati FL: Perioperative glycemic control and the risk of infectious complications in a cohort of adults with diabetes. Diabetes Care 22:1408–1414, 1999.
14. Toni D, Fiorelli M, Gentile M, et al: Progressing neurological deficit secondary to acute ischemic stroke. A study on predictability, pathogenesis, and prognosis. Arch Neurol 52:670–675, 1995.
15. Haheim LL, Holme I, Hjermann I, Leren P: Nonfasting serum glucose and the risk of fatal stroke in diabetic and nondiabetic subjects. 18-year follow-up of the Oslo Study. Stroke 26:774–777, 1995.
16. Janghorbani M, Jones RB, Gilmour WH, et al: A prospective population based study of gender differential in mortality from cardiovascular disease and "all causes" in asymptomatic hyperglycaemics. J Clin Epidemiol 47:397–405, 1994.
17. Petitt DB, Bhatt H: Retinopathy as a risk factor for nonembolic stroke in diabetic subjects. Stroke 26:593–596, 1995.
18. Goldberg RJ, Burchfiel CM, Benfante R, et al: Lifestyle and biologic factors associated with atherosclerotic disease in middle-aged men. 20-year findings from the Honolulu Heart Program. Arch Intern Med 155:686–694, 1995.
19. Kameyama M, Fushimi H, Udaka F: Diabetes mellitus and cerebral vascular disease. Diabetes Res Clin Pract 24(Suppl):S205–208, 1994.
20. Moss SE, Klein R, Klein BE, Meuer SM: The association of glycemia and cause-specific mortality in a diabetic population. Arch Intern Med 154:2473–2479, 1994.
21. National Diabetes Data Group: Classification and diagnosis of diabetes mellitus and other categories of glucose intolerance. Diabetes 28:1039–1057, 1979.
22. Jorgensen H, Nakayama H, Raaschou HO, Olsen TS: Stroke in patients with diabetes. The Copenhagen Stroke Study. Stroke 25:1977–1984, 1994.
23. Kuusisto J, Mykkanen L, Pyorala K, Laakso M: Non–insulin-dependent diabetes and its metabolic control are important predictors of stroke in elderly subjects. Stroke 125:1157–1164, 1994.
24. Burchfiel CM, Curb JD, Rodriguez BL, et al: Glucose intolerance and 22-year stroke incidence. The Honolulu Heart Program. Stroke 25:951–957, 1994.
25. Sacco RL, Shi T, Zamanillo MC, Kargman DE: Predictors of mortality and recurrence after hospitalized cerebral infarction in an urban community: The Northern Manhattan Stroke Study. Neurology 44:626–634, 1994.
26. Fu CC, Chang CJ, Tseng CH, et al: Development of macrovascular diseases in NIDDM patients in northern Taiwan. A 4-yr follow-up study. Diabetes Care 16:137–143, 1993.
27. Kleinman JC, Donahue RP, Harris MI, et al: Mortality among diabetics in a national sample. Am J Epidemiol 128:389–401, 1988.
28. Cardiovascular disease risk factors and related preventive health practices among adults with and without diabetes—Utah, 1988–1993. MMWR Morb Mortal Wkly Rep 44:804–809, 1995.
29. Nathan DM: The pathophysiology of diabetic complications: How much does the glucose hypothesis explain? Ann Intern Med 124:86–89, 1996.
30. Kannel WB, McGee DL: Diabetes and glucose tolerance as risk factors for cardiovascular disease: The Framingham Study. Diabetes Care 2:120–126, 1979.
31. Rodriquez BL, Lau N, Burchfiel CM, et al: Glucose intolerance and 23-year risk of coronary heart disease and total mortality: The Honolulu Heart Program. Diabetes Care 22:1262–1265, 1999.
32. Fava S, Azzopardi J, Muscat HA, Fenech FF: Factors that influence outcome in diabetic subjects with myocardial infarction. Diabetes Care 16:1615–1618, 1993.
33. Heinrich J, Schulte H, Schonfeld R, et al: Association of variables of coagulation, fibrinolysis and acute-phase with atherosclerosis in coronary and peripheral arteries and those arteries supplying the brain. Thromb Haemost 73:374–379, 1995.
34. Mackay AJ, Beks PJ, Dur AH, et al: The distribution of peripheral vascular disease in a Dutch Caucasian population: Comparison of type II diabetic and non-diabetic subjects. Eur J Vasc Endovasc Surg 9:170–175, 1995.
35. Beks PJ, Mackaay AJ, de Neeling JN, et al: Peripheral arterial disease in relation to glycaemic level in an elderly Caucasian population: The Hoorn study. Diabetologia 38:86–96, 1995.
36. Akbari CM, LoGerfo FW: Diabetes and peripheral vascular disease. J Vasc Surg 30:373–384, 1999.
37. Feinglass J, Brown JL, LoSasso A, et al: Rates of lower-extremity amputation and arterial reconstruction in the United States, 1979–1996. Am J Public Health 89:1222–1227, 1999.

38. Adler AI, Boyko EJ, Ahroni JH, Smith DG: Lower-extremity amputation in diabetes. The independent effects of peripheral vascular disease, sensory neuropathy, and foot ulcers. Diabetes Care 22:1029–1035, 1999.

39. Jorneskog G, Brismar K, Fagrell B: Skin capillary circulation is more impaired in the toes of diabetic than non-diabetic patients with peripheral vascular disease. Diabet Med 12:36–41, 1995.

40. Newman AB, Siscovick DS, Manolio TA, et al: Ankle-arm index as a marker of atherosclerosis in the Cardiovascular Health Study. Cardiovascular Heart Study (CHS) Collaborative Research Group. Circulation 88:837–845, 1993.

41. Selby JV, Zhang D: Risk factors for lower extremity amputation in persons with diabetes. Diabetes Care 18:509–516, 1995.

42. Coutinho M, Gerstein HC, Wang Y, Yusuf S: The relationship between glucose and incident cardiovascular events: A metaregression analysis of published data from 20 studies of 95,783 individuals followed for 12.4 years. Diabetes Care 22:233–240, 1999.

43. Reichard P, Nilsson BY, Rosenqvist U: The effect of long term intensified insulin treatment on the development of microvascular complications of diabetes mellitus. N Engl J Med 329:304–309, 1993.

44. The Diabetes Control and Complications Trial Research Group: The effect of intensive treatment of diabetes on the development and progression of long-term complications in insulin-dependent diabetes mellitus. N Engl J Med 329:977–986, 1993.

45. The DCCT Research Group: The effect of intensive diabetes management on macrovascular events and risk factors in the Diabetes Control and Complications Trial. Am J Cardiol 75:894–903, 1995.

46. Lawson M, Gerstein HC, Tsui E, Zinman B: Effect of intensive therapy on early macrovascular disease in young individuals with type 1 diabetes. A systematic review and meta-analysis. Diabetes Care 22 (Suppl 2):B35–B39, 1999.

47. Malmberg K, Ryden L, Efendic S, et al: Randomized trial of insulin-glucose infusion followed by subcutaneous insulin treatment in diabetic patients with acute myocardial infarction (DIGAMI study): Effects on mortality at 1 year. J Am Coll Cardiol 26:57–65, 1995.

48. UK Prospective Diabetes Study (UKPDS) Group: Intensive blood glucose control with sulphonylureas or insulin compared with the conventional treatment and risk of complications in patients with type 2 diabetes (UKPDS 33). Lancet 352:837–853, 1998.

49. UK Prospective Diabetes Study (UKPDS) Group: Effect of intensive blood glucose control with metformin on complications in overweight patients with type 2 diabetes (UKPDS 34). Lancet 352:954–965, 1998.

50. Peterson CM, Jones RL, Koenig RJ, et al: Reversible hematologic sequelae of diabetes mellitus. Ann Intern Med 86:425–429, 1977.

51. Peterson CM, Koenig RJ, Jones RL, et al: Correlation of serum triglyceride levels and hemoglobin A_{1c} concentrations in diabetes mellitus. Diabetes 26:507–509, 1977.

52. Peterson CM, Jones RL, Dupuis A, et al: Feasibility of improved glucose control in patients with insulin dependent diabetes mellitus. Diabetes Care 2:329–335, 1979.

53. Peterson CM, Jones RL, Esterly JA, et al: Changes in basement membrane thickening and pulse volume concomitant with improved glucose control and exercise in patients with insulin dependent diabetes mellitus. Diabetes Care 3:586–589, 1980.

54. Jones RL, Paradise C, Peterson CM: Platelet survival in diabetes mellitus. Diabetes 30:486–489, 1981.

55. Herman WH, Alexander CM, Cook JR, et al: Effect of simvastatin treatment on cardiovascular resource utilization in impaired fasting glucose and diabetes. Findings from the Scandinavian Simvastatin Survival Study. Diabetes Care 22:1771–1778, 1999.

56. Goldberg RB: The benefits of lowering cholesterol in subjects with mild hyperglycemia. Arch Intern Med 159:2627–2628, 1999.

57. The Long-Term Intervention with Pravastatin in Ischaemic Disease (LIPID) Study Group: Prevention of cardiovascular events and death with pravastatin in patients with coronary heart disease and a broad range of initial cholesterol levels. N Engl J Med 339:12349–1357, 1998.

58. Fuller J, Stevens LK, Chaturvedi N, Holloway JF: Antihypertensive therapy in diabetes mellitus. In The Cochrane Library, issue 4. Oxford, Update Software, 1998.

59. Golan L, Birkmeyer JD, Welch HG: The cost-effectiveness of treating all patients with type 2 diabetes with angiotensin-converting enzyme inhibitors. Ann Intern Med 131:660–667, 1999.

60. Tuomilehto J, Rastenyte D, Birkenhager WH, et al: Effects of calcium-channel blockade in older patients with diabetes and systolic hypertension. Systolic Hypertension in Europe Trial Investigators. N Engl J Med 340:677–684, 1999.

61. Bunn HF, Haney DN, Kamin S, et al: The biosynthesis of human hemoglobin A_{1c}. J Clin Invest 57:1652–1659, 1976.

62. Koenig RJ, Peterson CM, Kilo C, et al: Hemoglobin A_{1c} as an indicator of the degree of glucose intolerance in diabetes. Diabetes 25:230–232, 1976.

63. Koenig RJ, Peterson CM, Jones RL, et al: Correlation of glucose regulation and hemoglobin A_{1c} in diabetes mellitus. N Engl J Med 295:417–420, 1976.

64. Peterson CM, Jones RL: Minor hemoglobins, diabetic "control" and diseases of postsynthetic protein modification. Ann Intern Med 87:489–491, 1977.

65. Maillard L-C: Réaction générale des acides amines sur les sucres; conséquences biologiques. CR Acad Sci III 154:66–68, 1912.

66. Angyal SJ: The composition of reducing sugars in solution. In Harmon RE (ed): Asymmetry in Carbohydrates. New York, Marcel Dekker, 1979, pp 15–30.

67. Benkovic SJ: Anomeric specificity of carbohydrate utilizing enzymes. Methods Enzymol 63:370–379, 1979.

68. Hayase F, Nagaraj RH, Miyata S, et al: Aging of proteins: Immunological detection of a glucose-derived pyrrole formed during Maillard reaction in vivo. J Biol Chem 263:37858–37864, 1989.

69. Peterson CM (ed): Proceedings of a conference on nonenzymatic glycosylation and browning reactions: Their relevance to diabetes mellitus. Diabetes 31 (Suppl 3):1–82, 1982.

70. Horiuchi S, Shiga M, Araki N, et al: Evidence against in vivo presence of 2-(2-furoyl)-4(5)-(2-furanyl)-1H-imidazole, a major fluorescent advanced end product generated by nonenzymatic glycosylation. J Biol Chem 263:18821–18826, 1988.

71. Vlassara H, Bucala R, Striker L: Pathogenic effects of advanced glycosylation: Biochemical, biological, and clinical implications for diabetes and aging. J Lab Invest 70:138–151, 1994.

72. Brownlee M: Glycation and diabetic complication. Diabetes 43:836–841, 1994.

73. Bucala R, Cerami A: Advanced glycosylation: Chemistry, biology and implications for diabetes and aging. Adv Pharmacol 23:1–19, 1992.

74. Schmidt AM, Mora R, Cao K, et al: The endothelial cell binding site for advanced glycation end products consists of a complex: An integral membrane protein and a lactoferrin-like polypeptide. J Biol Chem 269:9882–9888, 1994.

75. Doi T, Vlassara H, Kirstein M, et al: Receptor specific increase in extracellular matrix production in mouse mesangial cells by advanced glycation end products is mediated via platelet derived growth factor. Proc Natl Acad Sci U S A 89:2873–2877, 1992.

76. Neper M, Schmidt AM, Brett J, et al: Cloning and expression of RAGE: A cell surface receptor for advanced glycation end products of proteins. J Biol Chem 267:14998–15004, 1992.

77. Vlassara H, Moldawer L, Chan B: Macrophage/monocyte receptor for nonenzymatically glycosylated proteins is up-regulated by cachectin/tumor necrosis factor. J Clin Invest 84:1813–1820, 1989.

78. Vlassara H, Brownlee M, Cerami A: Novel macrophage receptor for glucose-modified protein is distinct from previously described scavenger receptors. J Exp Med 164:1301–1309, 1988.

79. Bucala R, Tracey KJ, Cerami A: Advanced glycosylation products quench nitric oxide and mediate defective endothelium-dependent vasodilation in experimental diabetes. J Clin Invest 87:432–438, 1991.

80. Yan DS, Schmidt AM, Anderson GM, et al: Enhanced cellular oxidant stress by the interaction of advanced glycation end products with their receptors/binding proteins. J Biol Chem 269:9889–9897, 1994.

81. Bucala R, Makita Z, Vega G, et al: Modification of low density lipoprotein by advanced glycation end products contributes to the dislipidemia of diabetes and renal insufficiency. Proc Natl Acad Sci U S A 91:7742–7746, 1994.

82. Tschoeppe D: The activated megakaryocyte-platelet-system in vascular disease: Focus on diabetes. Semin Thromb Hemost 21:152–160, 1995.

83. Trovati M, Mularoni EM, Burzacca S, et al: Impaired insulin-induced platelet antiaggregating effect in obesity and in obese NIDDM patients. Diabetes 44:1318–1322, 1995.

84. Di Simpliciao P, de Giorgio LA, Cardaioli E, et al: Glutathione,

glutathione utilizing enzymes and thioltransferase in platelets of insulin-dependent diabetic patients: Relation with platelet aggregation and with microangiopathic complications. Eur J Clin Invest 25:665–669, 1995.

85. Udvardy M, Posan E, Harsfalvi J: Altered lysis resistance of platelet-rich clots in patients with insulin-dependent diabetes mellitus. Thromb Res 79:57–63, 1995.

86. Jokl R, Klein RL, Lopes-Virella MF, Colwell JA: Release of platelet plasminogen activator inhibitor 1 in whole blood is increased in patients with type II diabetes. Diabetes Care 18:1150–1155, 1995.

87. Bahru Y, Kesteven P, Alberti KGMM, Walker M: Decreased plasminogen activator inhibitor-1 activity in newly diagnosed type 2 diabetic patients following dietary modification. Diabet Med 10:802–806, 1993.

88. Marso SP, Lincoff AM, Ellis SG, et al: Optimizing the percutaneous interventional outcomes for patients with diabetes mellitus: Results of the EPISTENT (Evaluation of Platelet IIb/IIIa Inhibitor for Stenting Trial) Diabetic Substudy. Circulation 100:2477–2484, 1999.

89. Bennet CL, Davidson CJ, Raisch DW, et al: Thrombotic thrombocytopenia purpura associated with ticlodipine in the setting of coronary artery stents and stroke prevention. Arch Intern Med 159:2524–2528, 1999.

90. Dormandy J, Ernst E, Matrai A, Flute PT: Hemorrheological changes following acute myocardial infarction. Am Heart J 104:1364–1367, 1982.

91. Handa K, Kono S, Saku K, et al: Plasma fibrinogen levels as an independent indicator of severity of coronary atherosclerosis. Atherosclerosis 77:209–213, 1989.

92. ECAT Angina Pectoris Study Group: ECAT Angina Pectoris Study: Baseline associations of haemostatic factors with extent of coronary arteriosclerosis and other coronary risk factors in 3000 patients with angina pectoris undergoing coronary angiography. Eur Heart J 14:8–17, 1993.

93. Ceriello A, Taboga C, Giacomello R, et al: Fibrinogen plasma levels as a marker of thrombin activation in diabetes. Diabetes 43:430–432, 1994.

94. Jones RL, Peterson CM: Reduced fibrinogen survival in diabetes mellitus: A reversible phenomenon. J Clin Invest 63:485–493, 1979.

95. Jones RL, Jovanovic L, Forman S, Peterson CM: The time course of reversibility of accelerated fibrinogen disappearance in diabetes mellitus: Association with intravascular volume shifts. Blood 63:22–30, 1984.

96. Cortellaro M, Cofrancesco E, Boschetti C, et al: Association of increased fibrin turnover and defective fibrinolytic capacity with leg atherosclerosis. The PLAT Group. Thromb Haemost 72:292–296, 1994.

97. Collier A, Rumley AG, Paterson JR, et al: Free radical activity and hemostatic factors in NIDDM patients with and without microalbuminuria. Diabetes 41:909–913, 1992.

98. Knobl P, Schernthaner G, Schack C, et al: Thrombogenic factors are related to urinary albumin excretion rate in type 1 (insulin-dependent) and type 2 (non–insulin-dependent) diabetic patients. Diabetologia 36:1045–1050, 1993.

99. Ceriello A, Giugliani D, Quatraro A, et al: Metabolic control may influence the increased superoxide anion generation in diabetic serum. Diabet Med 8:540–542, 1991.

100. Brownlee M, Vlassara H, Cerami A: Nonenzymatic glycosylation reduces the susceptibility of fibrin to degradation by plasmin. Diabetes 32:680–684, 1983.

101. Cagliero E, Roth T, Taylor AW, Lorenzi M: The effects of high glucose on human endothelial cell growth and gene expression are not mediated by transforming growth factor-beta. Lab Invest 73:667–673, 1995.

102. Pieper GM, Meier DA, Hager SR: Endothelial dysfunction in a model of hyperglycemia and hyperinsulinemia. Am J Physiol 269:H845–850, 1995.

103. Baumgartner-Parzer SM, Wagner L, Pettermann M, et al: Modulation by high glucose of adhesion molecule expression in cultured endothelial cells. Diabetologia 38:1367–1370, 1996.

104. Farkas J, Menzel EJ: Proteins lose their nitric oxide stabilizing function after advanced glycosylation. Biochim Biophys Acta 1245:305–310, 1995.

105. Bucala R, Makita Z, Vega G, et al: Modification of low density lipoprotein advanced glycation end products contributes to the dislipidemia of diabetes and renal insufficiency. Proc Natl Acad Sci U S A 91:9441–9445, 1994.

106. Gugliucci A, Bendaya M: Renal fate of circulating advanced glycated end products (AGE): Evidence for reabsorption and catabolism of AGE-peptides by renal proximal tubular cells. Diabetologia 39:149–160, 1996.

107. Friedlander MA, Wu YC, Elgawish A, Monnier VM: Early and advanced glycosylation end products. J Clin Invest 97:728–735, 1996.

108. Smith MA, Sayre LM, Vitek MP, et al: Early AGEing and Alzheimer's. Nature 374:316, 1995.

109. Kobayashi K, Watanabe J, Umeda F, et al: Metabolism of oxidized glycated low-density lipoprotein in cultured bovine aortic endothelial cells. Horm Metab Res 27:356–362, 1995.

110. Velazquez E, Winocour PH, Kesteven P, et al: Relation of lipid peroxides to macrovascular disease in type 2 diabetes. Diabet Med 8:752–758, 1991.

111. Reaven GM: Banting Lecture 1998: Role of insulin resistance in human disease. Diabetes 37:1595–1607, 1988.

112. Shinozaki K, Suzuki M, Ikebuchi M, et al: Demonstration of insulin resistance in coronary artery disease documented with angiography. Diabetes Care 19:1–7, 1996.

113. Stout RW: Insulin and atheroma: 20-yr perspective. Diabetes Care 13:631–654, 1990.

114. Wingard DL, Barrett-Connor EL, Ferrara A: Is insulin really a heart disease risk factor? Diabetes Care 18:1299–1304, 1995.

115. Genuth S: Exogenous insulin administration and cardiovascular risk in non–insulin-dependent diabetes mellitus. Ann Intern Med 124:104–109, 1996.

116. Reaven GM, Lithell H, Landsberg L: Hypertension and associated metabolic abnormalities—the role of insulin resistance and the sympathoadrenal system. N Engl J Med 334:374–381, 1995.

117. Bagdade JD: Phagocytic and microbiological function in diabetes mellitus. Acta Endocrinol (Copenh) 83:27–31, 1976.

118. Duncan BB, Schmidt MI, Offenbacher S, et al: Factor VIII and other hemostasis variables are related to incident diabetes in adults. Diabetes Care 22:767–772, 1999.

119. Pickup JC, Mattock MB, Chusney GD, et al: NIDDM as a disease of the innate immune system: Association of acute-phase reactants and interleukin-6 with metabolic syndrome X. Diabetologia 40:1286–1292, 1997.

120. Tracy RP: The relationship between inflammation, coagulation and CVD (Concurrent session: Type 2 diabetes: An inflammatory disease process?) Presented at 59th Annual Scientific Sessions of American Diabetes Association, San Diego, 1999.

121. Bainton D, Sweetnam P, Baker I, Elwood P: Peripheral vascular disease: Consequence for survival and association with risk factors in the Speedwell prospective heart disease study. Br Heart J 72:128–132, 1994.

122. Wahlquist MI, Kayser L, Lassers BW: Fatty acids as a determinant of myocardial substrate and oxygen metabolism in man at rest and during prolonged exercise. Acta Med Scand 193:83–96, 1973.

123. Saad MF, Knowler WC, Pettitt DJ, et al: The natural history of impaired glucose tolerance in Pima Indians. N Engl J Med 319:1500–1506, 1988.

124. Sartor G, Schersten B, Carlstrom S, et al: Ten-year follow-up of subjects with impaired glucose intolerance. Diabetes 29:41–49, 1980.

125. Jarrett RJ, Keen H, McCartney P: The Whitehall study: Ten-year follow-up on men with impaired glucose tolerance with reference to worsening to diabetes and predictors of death. Diabet Med 1:279–283, 1984.

126. Jarrett RJ, Keen H, Fuller JH, McCartney M: Worsening to diabetes in men with impaired glucose tolerance ("borderline diabetes"). Diabetologia 16:25–30, 1979.

127. Kadowaki T, Miyake Y, Hagura R, et al: Risk factors for worsening to diabetes in subjects with impaired glucose tolerance. Diabetologia 26:44–49, 1984.

128. King H, Zimmet P, Raper LR, Balkau B: The natural history of impaired glucose tolerance in the Micronesian population of Nauru: A six-year follow-up study. Diabetologia 26:39–43, 1984.

129. Harris MI: Impaired glucose tolerance in the U.S. population. Diabetes Care 12:464–474, 1989.

130. Keen H, Rose G, Pyke DA, et al: Blood-sugar and arterial disease. Lancet 2:505–508, 1965.

131. Fuller JH, Shipley MJ, Rose G, et al: Coronary heart disease risk and impaired glucose tolerance. Lancet 1:1373–1376, 1980.

132. Blair SN, Kohl HW, Gordon NF, Paffenbarger RS Jr: How much physical activity is good for health? Annu Rev Public Health 13:99–126, 1992.

133. Bjorntorp P: Regional patterns of fat distribution. Ann Intern Med 103:994–995, 1985.
134. Flegel KG, Ezzati TM, Harris MI, et al: Prevalence of diabetes in Mexican American, Cubans, and Puerto Ricans from the Hispanic Health and Nutrition Examination Survey, 1982–84. Diabetes Care 14:628–638, 1991.
135. National Center for Health Statistics: Plan and Operation of the Hispanic Health and Nutrition Examination Survey 1982–1984 (DHHS Publication No. 85–1321). Washington, DC, Government Printing Office, 1985.
136. National Center for Health Statistics: Plan and Operation of the Second National Health and Nutrition Examination Survey, United States—1976–1980. Vital and Health Statistics, Series 1, No. 15 (DHEW Publication No. PHS 81–1317). Washington, DC, Government Printing Office, 1981.
137. Kuczmarski RJ: Prevalence of overweight and weight gain in the United States. Am J Clin Nutr 55:495S–502S, 1992.
138. Kohl HW, Gordon NF, Villegas JA, Blair SN: Cardiorespiratory fitness, glycemic status, and mortality risk in men. Diabetes Care 15:184–192, 1992.
139. Stern MP: Kelly West lecture: Primary prevention of type II diabetes mellitus. Diabetes Care 14:399–410, 1991.
140. King H, Kriska AM: Prevention of type II diabetes by physical training. Diabetes Care 15(Suppl 4):1794–1799, 1992.
141. Kriska AM, LaPorte RE, Pettitt DJ, et al: The association of physical activity with obesity, fat distribution and glucose intolerance in Pima Indians. Diabetologia 36:863–869, 1993.
142. Kawate R, Yamakido M, Nishimoto Y, et al: Diabetes and its vascular complications in Japanese migrants on the island of Hawaii. Diabetes Care 2:161–170, 1979.
143. West KM: Epidemiology of Diabetes and Its Vascular Lesions. New York, Elsevier. 1978.
144. Eaton SB, Konner M, Shostak M: Stone agers in the fast lane: Chronic degenerative disease in evolutionary perspective. Am J Med 84:739–749, 1988.
145. Lindgarde F, Saltin B: Daily physical activity, work capacity and glucose tolerance in lean and obese normoglycemic middle-aged men. Diabetologia 20:134–138, 1981.
146. Cederholm J, Wibell L: Glucose tolerance and physical activity in a health survey of middle-aged subjects. Acta Med Scand 217:373–378, 1985.
147. Eriksson K-F, Lindgarde F: Impaired glucose tolerance in a middle-aged male urban population: A new approach for identifying high-risk cases. Diabetologia 33:526–531, 1990.
148. Harris MI: Epidemiological correlates of NIDDM in Hispanics, whites, and blacks in the U.S. population. Diabetes Care 14(Suppl 3):639–648, 1991.
149. Resnick HE, Vlsania P, Phillips CL: Diabetes mellitus and nontraumatic lower extremity amputation in black and white Americans. The National Health and Nutrition Examination Survey Epidemiologic Follow-up Study, 1971–1992. Arch Intern Med 159:2470–2475, 1999.
150. Mitchell BD, Valdez R, Hazuda HP, et al: Differences in the prevalence of diabetes and impaired glucose tolerance according to maternal or paternal history of diabetes. Diabetes Care 16:1262–1267, 1993.
151. Summary and recommendations of the Third International Diabetes Workshop-Conference on Gestational Diabetes. Diabetes 40(Suppl 2):197–201, 1991.
152. Kjos SL, Buchanan TA, Greenspoon JS, et al: Gestational diabetes mellitus: The prevalence of glucose intolerance and diabetes mellitus in the first two months post partum. Am J Obstet Gynecol 163:93–98, 1990.
153. O'Sullivan JB: Diabetes mellitus after GDM. Diabetes 40(Suppl 2):131–135, 1991.
154. Lam KSL, Li DF, Lauder IJ, et al: Prediction of persistent carbohydrate intolerance in patients with gestational diabetes. Diabetes Res Clin Pract 12:181–186, 1991.
155. Catalano PM, Vargo KM, Bernstein IM, Amini SB: Incidence and risk factors associated with abnormal post partum glucose tolerance in women with gestational diabetes. Am J Obstet Gynecol 165:914–919, 1991.
156. Damm P, Kuhl C, Bertelsen A, Molsted-Pedersen L: Predictive factors for the development of diabetes in women with previous gestational diabetes mellitus. Am J Obstet Gynecol 167:607–661, 1992.
157. Stangenberg M, Agarwal N, Rahman F, et al: Frequency of HLA genes and islet cell antibodies and result of post partum oral glucose tolerance tests (OGTT) in Saudi Arabian women with abnormal OGTT during pregnancy. Diabetes Res Clin Pract 14:9–13, 1990.
158. Larsson G, Spjuth J, Ranstam J, et al: Prognostic significance of birth of large infant for subsequent development of maternal non-insulin dependent diabetes. A prospective study over 20–27 years. Diabetes Care 9:359–364, 1986.
159. O'Sullivan JB: Gestational diabetes: Factors influencing the rates of subsequent diabetes. In Sutherland HW, Stowers JM (eds): Carbohydrate Metabolism in Pregnancy and the Newborn. New York, Springer-Verlag, 1978, pp 425–435.
160. Coustan DR, Carpenter MW, O'Sullivan PS, Carr SR: Gestational diabetes: Predictors of subsequent disordered glucose metabolism. Am J Obstet Gynecol 168:1139–1145, 1993.
161. Dornhorst A, Bailey PC, Anyaoku V, et al: Abnormalities of glucose intolerance following gestational diabetes. Q J Med 77:1219–1228, 1990.
162. Mestman JH, Anderson GV, Guadelupe V: Follow-up study of 360 subjects with abnormal glucose metabolism during pregnancy. Obstet Gynecol 39:421–425, 1972.
163. Persson B, Hanson U, Hartling SG, Binder C: Follow-up of women with previous gestational diabetes: Insulin, C-peptide, and proinsulin response to oral glucose load. Diabetes 40(Suppl 2):136–141, 1991.
164. Benjamin E, Winters D, Mayfield J, Gohdes D: Diabetes in pregnancy in Zuni Indian women. Diabetes Care 16:1231–1235, 1993.
165. O'Sullivan JB, Mahan CM: Criteria for the oral glucose tolerance test in pregnancy. Diabetes 13:278–285, 1964.
166. Jacober SJ, Soweres JR: An update on perioperative management of diabetes. Arch Intern Med 159:2405–2411, 1999.
167. Cruse PJ, Foord R: A 5-year prospective study of 23,649 surgical wounds. Arch Surg 107:206–210, 1973.
168. Goodson WH, Hunt TK: Studies of wound healing in experimental diabetes mellitus. J Surg Res 22:221–227, 1977.
169. Wahlquist MI, Kayser L, Lassers BW: Fatty acids as a determinant of myocardial substrate and oxygen metabolism in man at rest and during prolonged exercise. Acta Med Scand 193:83–96, 1973.
170. Bolli GB, Di Marchi RD, Park GD, et al: Insulin analogues and their potential in the management of diabetes mellitus. Diabetologia 42:1151–1167, 1999.
171. Harris M: Diabetes In America. Alexandria, Va, American Diabetes Association, 1995.
172. Peterson CM, Sims RV, Jones RL, Rieders F: Bioavailability of glipizide and its effect on blood glucose and insulin levels in patients with non–insulin dependent diabetes. Diabetes Care 5:497–450, 1982.
173. United Kingdom Prospective Diabetes Study Group: Relative efficacy of randomly allocated diet, sulphonylurea, insulin or metformin in patients with newly diagnosed non–insulin dependent diabetes followed for three years. BMJ 310:83–88, 1995.
174. Jackson RA, Hawa MI, Jaspan JB, et al: Mechanism of metformin action in non–insulin-dependent diabetes. Diabetes 36:632–640, 1987.
175. Hermann LS, Schersten B, Bizen PO, et al: Therapeutic comparison of metformin and sulfonylurea, alone and in various combinations. A double-blind controlled study. Diabetes Care 17:1100–1109, 1994.
176. Defronzo RA, Goodman AM, and the Multicenter Metformin Study Group: Efficacy of metformin in patients with non–insulin dependent diabetes mellitus. N Engl J Med 333:541–549, 1995.
177. UK Prospective Diabetes Study Group: Study design, progress, and performance. Diabetologia 34:877–890, 1991.
178. Stolar MW, and the Endocrine Fellows Foundation Study Group: Clinical management of the NIDDM patient. Impact of the American Diabetes Association practice guidelines, 1985–1993. Diabetes Care 18:701–707, 1995.
179. Bloomgarden ZT: The American Diabetes Association Annual Meeting, 1994: Treatment issues for NIDDM. Diabetes Care 17:1078–1084, 1994.
180. American Diabetes Association: Standards of medical care for patients with diabetes. Diabetes Care 17:616–622, 1994.
181. Yusuf S, Sleight P, Pogue J, et al: Effects of an angiotensin-converting-enzyme inhibitor, ramipril, on cardiovascular events in high-risk patients. The Heart Outcomes Prevention Evaluation Study Investigators. N Engl J Med 342:145–153, 2000.
182. Wood DM, Plehwe WE, Colman PB: Aspirin usage in a large teaching hospital diabetes clinic setting. Diabet Med 16:605–608, 1999.

183. Hepaz D, Gottlieb S, Graff E, et al: Effects of aspirin treatment on survival in non–insulin-dependent diabetic patients with coronary artery disease. Israeli Bezafibrate Infarction Prevention Study Group. Am J Med 105:494–499, 1998.

184. Moss SE, Klein R, Klein BE: The 14 year incidence of lower extremity amputations in a diabetic population. The Wisconsin Epidemiologic Study of Diabetic Retinopathy. Diabetes Care 22:951–959, 1999.

Questions

1. Which of the following statements most accurately reflects the course of the diabetic patient following the discovery of insulin?
   (a) The diabetic patient lives longer
   (b) Mortality from coma and sepsis has decreased
   (c) Mortality from vascular disease has increased
   (d) Control of glucose prevents microvascular disease of the eye and kidney as well as neuropathy
   (e) All of the above

2. Abnormal glucose tolerance or diabetes is found more frequently in which of the following?
   (a) Relatives of a person with diabetes
   (b) Hispanic and black minorities
   (c) Women with a history of gestational diabetes
   (d) The obese and unfit
   (e) All of the above

3. Which statement is most accurate?
   (a) Diabetes is a single known genetic disease
   (b) Diabetes is characterized by low insulin levels
   (c) The person with diabetes may be at excess risk for vascular disease because of both increased insulin levels and increased glucose levels
   (d) Diabetes in pregnancy does not increase the risk of eye disease

4. Which of the following statements is not true?
   (a) Diabetic patients tend to have a higher prevalence of stroke, myocardial infarction, and peripheral vascular disease
   (b) Diabetic patients tend to have more diffuse large vessel disease
   (c) The most likely cause of death in a person with diabetes is vascular disease
   (d) Most cardiovascular deaths in persons with diabetes are the result of microvascular disease

5. Which of the following statements are not true regarding stroke?
   (a) Nonfasting serum glucose predicts outcome, including speed of recovery and mortality
   (b) Women are less vulnerable to the increased vascular risk associated with hyperglycemia than men
   (c) Systolic and diastolic blood pressures predict risk in diabetic patients
   (d) Cholesterol and body mass index are risk factors for stroke
   (e) Glycosylated hemoglobin predicts risk
   (f) Persons with diabetes are at increased risk for thrombotic but not hemorrhagic stroke

6. Which statement is not true?
   (a) The risk of cardiovascular disease is two to three times higher in persons with diabetes than nondiabetic subjects
   (b) The risk of vascular disease associated with diabetes is secondary to obesity, lipid disorders, and increased blood pressure, but not diabetes per se
   (c) The increased prevalence of congestive heart failure in diabetic patients with coronary artery disease has been attributed to microvascular disease and autonomic dysfunction
   (d) Large vessel disease in one area of the vascular tree predicts disease in other areas as well
   (e) Many vascular lesions in persons with diabetes are asymptomatic

7. Which of the following statements are not true?
   (a) The ABI is not a good screening tool for persons with diabetes
   (b) Intervention studies in persons with diabetes have shown improvement in the ABI after 9 months of normoglycemia and exercise
   (c) The prevalence of foot ulcers in diabetic patients with peripheral vascular disease is increased in part due to problems with the microcirculation and neuropathy
   (d) Glucose control, blood pressure, and duration of diabetes are all independent predictors of amputation

8. Which of the following probably contribute to vascular disease in hyperglycemic subjects?
   (a) Glycation and advanced glycation end products
   (b) Perturbations in the fluid phase of coagulation
   (c) Increased reactivity of the platelet
   (d) Endothelial cell dysfunction
   (e) Increased oxidative stress
   (f) Vascular volume shifts
   (g) All of the above

9. Which of the following statements is most accurate regarding the indications for vascular reconstruction in the diabetic patient?
   (a) It should be performed primarily for limb salvage rather than claudication
   (b) It should be avoided in subjects with severe neuropathy
   (c) It should be performed less frequently because of poorer outcome statistics
   (d) It should be performed for the same indications in diabetic and nondiabetic patients

10. Physiologic blood glucose control with careful glucose monitoring before, during, and after surgery is important for which of the following reasons?
    (a) Minimizes the risk of infection
    (b) Increases wound healing and strength
    (c) Avoids hypoglycemia
    (d) Minimizes the risk of a prothrombotic state
    (e) All of the above

Answers

1. e   2. e   3. c   4. d   5. b   6. b   7. a   8. g   9. d   10. e

10

Primary Arterial Infections and Antibiotic Prophylaxis

Hugh A. Gelabert

PRIMARY ARTERIAL INFECTIONS

Primary arterial infections are unusual problems that, by their very nature, are poorly understood and difficult to manage. The essential feature of such conditions is the destruction of a major artery by an infectious process. The secondary manifestations are aneurysm formation, embolization, and hemorrhage in the face of systemic septic illness. The presentations vary from indolent to cataclysmic. Successful management requires familiarity with the processes involved and the ability to make prompt decisions at the time of surgery. The goal of this chapter is to review primary arterial infections in terms of their pathophysiology, diagnosis, and treatment.

Working Definition

In general terms, a primary arterial infection is a condition in which infectious agents invade and destroy the wall of an artery, resulting in disruption and pseudoaneurysm formation. These events, occurring in the absence of prosthetic grafts or endovascular stents, would constitute a primary arterial infection.

Historical Perspective

One of the earliest reports of arterial infections was that offered by Ambroise Paré in the 16th century. He described suture ligation and excision of vessels that had become infected after battle injuries. This early treatment subsequently became a mainstay of therapy, and in combination with the modern techniques of vessel substitution, remains such today. Rokitansky[1] and others[2] recognized, early in the 19th century, an association between arterial infection and aneurysm formation. Osler, in 1885,[3] presented the first comprehensive description of this relationship. In addressing the Royal College of Physicians, he

described a 30-year-old man who had succumbed to fever, chills, and pneumonia. At autopsy, the patient was found to have endocarditis involving the aortic valve, as well as multiple aneurysms of the thoracic aorta. Based on carefully described pathologic findings, Osler[3] proposed a causal relationship between infection of the aortic wall and subsequent aneurysm formation. Because of a similarity between the beaded appearance of these aneurysms and fungal vegetations, he introduced the term "mycotic aneurysm," and thus the concept of primary arterial infection.

Historical Definitions

There is no universally accepted definition of primary arterial infection. Moreover, there continues to be confusion regarding the general classification of native arterial infections. The term mycotic aneurysm was initially introduced by Osler to signify those infected aneurysms found in association with bacterial endocarditis. Currently, the term has come to denote an infected aneurysm of any type. Additionally, the majority of the published literature has focused on specific subtypes of arterial infections, namely aneurysmal dilatation associated with arterial infection and illnesses resulting from infection of a traumatic pseudoaneurysm. Another problem is that there exists considerable disparity among the several definitions that have been proposed. Finally, it should be recognized that with the exception of a secondarily infected arterial aneurysm, most of these lesions are, in fact, infected pseudoaneurysms. Most arise by the local destruction of the arterial wall and the fibrous encapsulation of an expanding hematoma, and thus these lesions do not have the histologic components of an arterial wall. Thus, the very term mycotic aneurysm is frequently a misnomer. In this chapter, we use the following definition to describe a primary arterial infection: the direct invasion or extension of a specific pathogen into the intima, media, or adventitia of a native artery, irrespective of the preexisting state of the underlying artery or source of the pathogen. The term mycotic aneurysm is used to denote both true aneurysms and false aneurysms.

Pathogenesis

Five basic mechanisms have been implicated in the development of primary arterial infections. They may broadly be grouped as (1) mycotic aneurysm, (2) microbial arteritis with aneurysm formation, (3) infected aneurysm, (4) mechanical injury with contamination, and (5) arteritis from contiguous spread.

Mycotic Aneurysm

Osler, in coining the term mycotic aneurysm, both named the condition and described what was to be the most prevalent etiology in the preantibiotic era. As he described it, the true mycotic aneurysm is limited to the unique clinical condition characterized by bacterial endocarditis with septic embolization from valvular vegetations. These septic emboli lodge within the arterial wall, where a suppurative infection develops. The arterial wall is destroyed by the infection and the resultant pseudoaneurysm is recognized as a mycotic aneurysm. In subsequent years, the term has acquired a broader significance and has become synonymous with the broad syndrome—primary arterial infection.

Considerable confusion has arisen because the term mycotic aneurysm has been applied to various types of infected aneurysms. Crane[4] attempted to classify mycotic aneurysms into primary and secondary types. He introduced the term "primary mycotic aneurysm" to refer to infected aortic aneurysms not associated with endocarditis or an infectious focus. In contrast, "secondary" types were those that formed as a result of preceding endocarditis. Ponfick[5] and Eppinger[6] were among the first to characterize the anatomic features of these aneurysms pathologically. Ponfick proposed that the initial insult to the arterial wall was a mechanical injury inflicted by the embolization of septic material.[5] Eppinger, in 1887, provided further support for the theory of septic emboli by culturing the same strain of bacteria from both vegetative lesions and the wall of an aneurysm in a patient with endocarditis. He applied the term "embolomycotic" to describe the combination of infectious and embolic components that lead to the formation of mycotic aneurysms.[6]

Microbial Arteritis with Aneurysm Formation

The second mechanism of arterial infection involves the microbial "seeding" of arteries during an episode of bacteremia. "Microbial arteritis with aneurysm formation" occurs when a normal or atherosclerotic artery becomes infected and the weakened artery subsequently becomes aneurysmal.

In 1906, the German pathologist Weisel described distinctive pathologic changes in arterial walls that occurred during the course of an infectious disease but were not of embolic origin.[7] Lewis and Schrager[8] and Cathcart[9] presented case reports of infected peripheral aneurysms that developed in normal arteries of patients with osteomyelitis and typhoid fever, respectively. Despite these reports, nearly 30 years passed before consideration was given to the mechanism by which bacteremia led to arterial infection. Crane, in 1937, described an infected aneurysm that occurred in a patient with hypoplasia of the aorta but with no associated bacterial endocarditis or other identifiable source of infection.[4] He proposed that the combination of the "force of the blood stream" and abnormal development of the aorta allowed bacteria to invade that portion of the aorta. This resulted in an arterial infection, disruption of the aortic wall, and, subsequently, an infected pseudoaneurysm. Revell[10] extended the concept of aortic bacterial seeding one step further and proposed that the route of infection was through the aortic vasa vasorum. Hawkins and Yeager,[11] acknowledging the resistance of arterial intima to infection, suggested that an intimal defect such as that produced by arteriosclerosis would allow bacterial localization and infection.

Infected Aneurysm

Infected aneurysm refers to the infection of a preexisting aneurysm, most often by hematogenous microbiologic seeding of the aneurysm. The original aneurysms are most commonly atherosclerotic; however, they may also be the result of trauma or arteritis. The mechanism of infection is hematogenous spread of the bacteria to the aneurysm. The diseased artery becomes host to the bacterial pathogens when these lodge within the intramural thrombus and arteriosclerotic intima. Although some of these infected aneurysms may proceed to rapid expansion and rupture, many appear to remain quiescent. These are often discovered in the course of incidental microbiologic investigation of aneurysm contents.

Mechanical Injury with Contamination

A third means by which arterial infections occur is that of mechanical arterial injury by contaminated instruments. The instrument serves to inoculate the artery. This type of infection can occur as an inadvertent arterial puncture with a contaminated needle in drug abuse, as an accidental contamination during radiologic procedures, during placement of hemodynamic monitoring catheters, or as a result of traumatic injury. The combination of mechanical disruption of the intima, along with the seeding of the arterial lesion with pathogenic bacteria, leads to the formation of suppurative arteritis and destroys a portion of the arterial wall. This subsequently becomes an infected arterial pseudoaneurysm.

Arteritis from Contiguous Spread

The fourth mechanism by which arterial infections develop is spread of the infection from a contiguous focus. Contiguous infections that have been recognized as potential sources of these bacteria include lesions such as osteomyelitis, infected lymph nodes, tuberculous lymph nodes, and abscesses from narcotic injection.[12] Bacteria, and less commonly, mycobacteria or fungi, invade the artery either by direct extension or via lymphatics. They subsequently produce a necrotizing invasive infection of the arterial wall with eventual destruction of the vessel wall. This process, depending on the rate of progression, leads either to pseudoaneurysm formation or free arterial rupture.

Other Forms of Arterial Infection

There are three other, less common, forms of infected aneurysms that are tangentially included in the above classification: syphilitic aortitis, true fungal aneurysms, and primary (spontaneous) aortoenteric fistulas. Because of significant differences in the pathogens and the pathogenesis of these lesions, they merit separate notice.

Syphilitic aneurysms represent a rarely encountered complication of advanced syphilis. These lesions occur in approximately 10% of patients with the tertiary form of the disease.[13] These aneurysms commonly arise in the ascending aorta, frequently involve the aortic valve, and are secondary to treponemal invasion of the vasa vasorum. Reasons for the preference of *Treponema* for this portion of the aorta remain unclear. After spirochete penetration, an infiltrate develops within the vessel wall consisting of plasma cells, epidermal cells, and giant cells. This infiltrate results in destruction of the elastic and muscular components of the tunica media, replacement of the normal wall with fibrous tissue, and dilatation and subsequent formation of saccular aneurysms.

Fungal arterial infections are also extremely rare and most often occur in patients who are immunosuppressed. Common risk factors include diabetes, immunosuppressive medications, or chronic hematologic disorders such as leukemias or lymphomas. The species most often implicated are *Histoplasma capsulatum*, *Aspergillus fumigatus*, *Candida albicans*, and *Penicillium* species. These lesions most commonly result from either colonization of a preexisting aneurysm or infection of a damaged artery.

Spontaneous or "primary" aortoenteric fistulas (AEFs) arise as a consequence of progressive aneurysmal enlargement with gradual erosion into the adjacent gastrointestinal tract. The erosion is thought to be facilitated by the indurated, atherosclerotic artery pressing against a tethered portion of bowel. The most common location for this erosion is the third portion of the duodenum. In reviewing a series of 16,633 autopsies, Hirst and Affeldt[14] reported the incidence of this type of fistula to be 0.05%. Currently, because the majority of patients diagnosed with aortic aneurysms now undergo elective operation, the incidence of these lesions is thought to be considerably lower. Patients with spontaneous AEFs may have an initial or "herald" bleed. This represents the initial hemorrhage of blood into the duodenum. It may stop for a period of time, then resume in a more prolonged and dramatic manner. Clot within the AEF is responsible for the "intermittent" nature of the bleeding episodes. This condition is considerably different from that associated with aortic graft infection, the secondary AEF. The secondary AEF is more common, more dangerous, and more difficult to manage.

Graft excision and remote reconstruction are the standard management of the secondary AEF. In contrast, significant evidence exists that indicates that the primary AEF may be managed by closure of the duodenal rent, débridement of the aorta, and in situ reconstruction with a Dacron prosthesis. The prerequisites of this approach are the absence of purulence at the fistula site, a small defect in the duodenum, and a relatively healthy patient. It should be noted that the management of primary aortic infections (mycotic aneurysms) is similar to that of the primary AEF in that the absence of gross infection along with adequate débridement may allow in situ graft reconstruction of the aorta.[15]

Etiologic Organisms

The organism most commonly associated with microbial aortitis is *Salmonella*. This is followed, in order of frequency, by *Streptococcus*, *Bacteroides*, *Arizona hinshawii*, *Escherichia coli*, and *Staphylococcus aureus*.[15] Studies that focus on subpopulations such as intravenous (IV) drug abusers or femoral mycotic aneurysms will tend to identify a predominance of gram-positive bacteria such as staphylococci and streptococci, along with gram-negative organisms such as *E. coli* and *Pseudomonas*.

The bacteriology of primary arterial infections has undergone considerable transformation since its original description in the mid-1800s (Fig. 10–1). Brown and colleagues[16] and others suggested that the reason for this

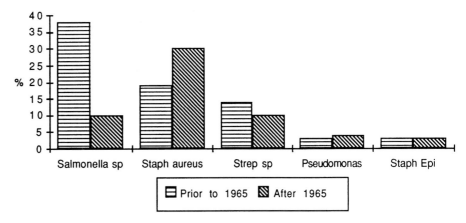

Figure 10–1. Organisms cultured from mycotic aneurysms. *Staph aureus, Staphylococcus aureus; Staph epi, Staphylococcus epidermidis; Strep, Streptococcus.* (From Brown SL, Busuttil RW, Baker JD, et al: Bacteriologic and surgical determinants of survival in patients with mycotic aneurysms. J Vasc Surg 1:541–547, 1984.)

change is antibiotic selective pressure leading to bacterial adaptation. Also, there has been a change in the relative incidence of pathogenic mechanisms with the more common use of invasive diagnostic modalities, as well as the increased illicit use of intravenous (IV) drugs. The majority of arterial infections during the preantibiotic era were true mycotic aneurysms; that is, they were related to bacterial endocarditis. The bacteriology of arterial infections during this period, therefore, was that of endocarditis. Stengal and Wolferth,[17] in 1923, and Revell,[10] in 1945, both reported that the predominant organisms were nonhemolytic streptococci, staphylococci, and pneumococci. Magilligan and Quinn,[18] in a 1986 review, subdivided 91 patients with bacterial endocarditis into two groups: those known to be IV drug abusers (36 patients) and those who were not (55 patients). Of the first group, the most common organisms were *S. aureus* (36%), *Pseudomonas* species (16%), polymicrobial organisms (15%), *Streptococcus faecalis* (13%), and *Streptococcus viridans* (11%). Organisms in the second group (non–IV drug abusers) were *Str. viridans* (22%), *S. aureus* (20%), *Str. faecalis* (14%), and *Staphylococcus epidermidis* (11%). The declining incidence of rheumatic fever and the adoption of early, appropriate antibiotic treatment have resulted in a significant decrease in bacterial endocarditis. This in turn has resulted in a decline in the incidence of Oslerian mycotic aneurysm in recent decades.

Concurrent with the declining incidence of mycotic aneurysms has been an increase in various other types of primary arterial infections. Principal among these are microbial arteritis and infected aneurysms. This may be due, in part, to the increasing age of the population and the simultaneous increase in the prevalence of atherosclerosis. The bacteriology of these arterial infections is different from that of mycotic aneurysms. The microorganisms most commonly associated with microbial arteritis are *Salmonella*, *Staphylococcus*, and *E. coli*. *Salmonella* species, in particular, have a striking propensity for invasion of diseased (atherosclerotic) aortas. In selected series, the involvement of *Salmonella* has been reported to be as high as 50%. The most virulent species, *Salmonella choleraesuis* and *Salmonella typhimurium*, account for over 60% of the reported cases of *Salmonella* arteritis.[19] Less commonly reported organisms associated with microbial arteritis include fungi and anaerobic organisms. Among the latter, *Bacteroides fragilis* has been reported in association with supraceliac aortic aneurysms.

The bacteriology of "infected aneurysms" is similar to that of both mycotic aneurysms and microbial arteritis. Despite this, some variation exists among reported series. Although Bennett and Cherry[20] reported a 66% incidence of *Salmonella* infections, Jarrett and associates[21] described a predominance of gram-positive cocci (59%), with *Staphylococcus aureus* representing 41%. In two prospective studies of patients undergoing aneurysmectomy, cultures obtained from both aneurysm wall and bowel bag revealed a predominance of gram-positive organisms.[21, 22] Both of these series are thought to represent cases of bacterial colonization. Despite the relative infrequency of gram-negative organisms observed in the series of Jarrett and associates, the distinction between gram-negative and gram-positive cultures proved clinically important. Patients with gram-negative bacteria demonstrated a greater likelihood of aortic rupture than those with gram-positive organisms. Specifically, the rupture rate of gram-negative bacterial isolates was 84%, whereas that of gram-positive bacterial cultures was 10%.

According to Brown and associates, the most common infected aneurysms since 1965 are those that occur as a result of mechanical arterial injury with contamination of the vessel wall.[16] The organism most frequently implicated in this type of arterial infection is *S. aureus*. It has been cultured in as many as 30% of their cases. Reddy and associates,[23] in reporting a series of infected femoral false aneurysms, made note of a 65% incidence of *S. aureus*. Cultures also demonstrated a 33% rate of polymicrobial infection.[23] Although arterial infections secondary to contiguous spread are most commonly bacterial, mycobacterial and fungal infections have also been noted to occur in these lesions. As with microbial arteritis, *Salmonella* is the predominant pathogen and *Staphylococcus* is second in frequency (Fig. 10–2).

Anatomic Distribution of Primary Arterial Infections

The anatomic distribution of primary arterial infections varies somewhat, depending on the pathologic type of infection. True mycotic aneurysms, owing to their embolic etiology, may occur in any artery larger than end-digital vessels. They most often involve the larger muscular and elastic arteries. Both Lewis and Schrager[8] and Brown and colleagues,[16] in retrospective reviews, found the most common sites of infection to be abdominal aorta, femoral, and

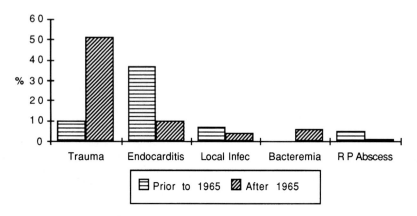

Figure 10–2. Etiology of mycotic aneursyms. Local Infec, local infection; R P Abscess, retroperitoneal abscess. (From Brown SL, Busuttil RW, Baker JD, et al: Bacteriologic and surgical determinants of survival in patients with mycotic aneurysms. J Vasc Surg 1:541–547, 1984.)

superior mesenteric arteries (Fig. 10–3). The predisposition to aortic involvement is thought to be related to the higher incidence of underlying atherosclerotic aneurysms in this location as compared with other anatomic sites.

"Microbial arteritis with aneurysm formation" occurs when a pathogen localizes at the site of an arterial lesion such as an atherosclerotic plaque. As one would anticipate, the arteries most commonly involved are the same ones that demonstrate advanced atherosclerotic changes, namely, the distal aorta, femoral, iliac, and popliteal vessels. "Infected aneurysms" may, in theory, occur at any site within the arterial tree where there is a preexisting aneurysm. It is curious that all series in the literature demonstrate a strong propensity for involvement of the abdominal aorta. Involvement of this artery has been reported to occur in as many as 79% of these cases. Whether this represents a tendency of the bacteria to infect aortic aneurysms or a study bias toward aortic aneurysms is not clear. Certainly, aortic aneurysms have been subjected to closer scrutiny than other peripheral arterial aneurysms. This may account, in part, for this reported predilection.

Arterial infections due to "mechanical injury with contamination" most commonly involve arteries that have minimal soft tissue coverage. There are three main etiologies: accidental drug injection, vascular access, and trauma. Because these etiologies are related to the accessibility of the arteries and their superficial locations, these infections most commonly involve the femoral or brachial arteries. These locations also have an important impact on the presentation of these lesions because femoral and brachial arterial aneurysms are most frequently identified by virtue of the prominence, erythema, and tenderness of the aneurysm rather than by symptoms of arterial sepsis.

Clinical Presentation

The most common clinical presentation in patients with primary arterial infection is fever, leukocytosis, and tenderness over the affected artery. Patients may have a wide range of signs and symptoms depending on the pathophysiology, bacteriology, and location of the infected artery or arteries. Most components of the clinical presentation may be assigned to one of two general groups: signs and symptoms resulting from infection or bacteremia, and signs and symptoms occurring secondary to local arterial involvement or aneurysm formation. Night sweats, general malaise, arthralgias, and increased fatigability in conjunction with fever and leukocytosis occur as a consequence of the recurrent bacteremias associated with primary arterial infections. These are the signs of sepsis caused by the arterial infection. In certain patients, these signs may also be attributed to the primary source of bacteremia. In patients with true mycotic aneurysms, the clinical signs and symptoms of bacterial endocarditis may be difficult to distinguish from those associated with the arterial infection. Similarly, symptoms in patients with arterial lesions that developed by spread from a contiguous suppurative source may derive from either infectious focus.

A second group of signs and symptoms occur as a result of inflammation and aneurysmal dilatation of the infected artery. Localized tenderness is the most readily recognized symptom related to the inflammatory destruction of the arterial wall. Characteristics such as abdominal or peripheral bruits, neurologic defects from nerve compression, or pulsatile masses may be included in this group.

Thrombosis and thromboembolization are common sequelae of such arterial aneurysms. When they appear, they elicit a host of associated symptoms such as ischemic digital or limb pain. Initially, these embolic presentations may be indistinguishable from similar events in uninfected aneurysms. If the embolic material is infected and causes a secondary arterial infection, the mycotic nature of the lesion may be revealed. Other findings of arterial infections include petechial skin lesions and septic arthritis.

Arterial rupture is not an uncommon event in cases of infected arterial aneurysms. This presentation is identical to that of any arterial rupture. If the damaged artery is contained and supported by a capsule of fibrous connective tissue, it may progress to form a pseudoaneurysm, and its principal symptom would be pain. If the rupture is uncontrolled, the presentation is that of hypotensive shock. If the rupture is in a superficial artery that erodes through the skin, the presentation is that of evident life-threatening hemorrhage.

The development of periarterial gas formation signals the presence of a gas-producing organism and should be a clear signal indicating urgency in treating these patients.

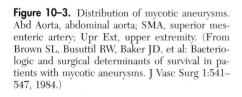

Figure 10–3. Distribution of mycotic aneurysms. Abd Aorta, abdominal aorta; SMA, superior mesenteric artery; Upr Ext, upper extremity. (From Brown SL, Busuttil RW, Baker JD, et al: Bacteriologic and surgical determinants of survival in patients with mycotic aneurysms. J Vasc Surg 1:541–547, 1984.)

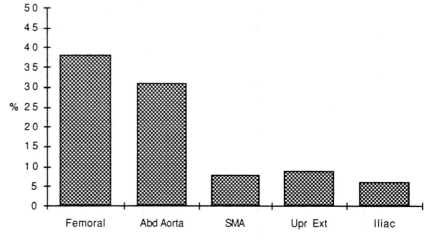

Although this is not a very common presentation, it should be considered in any patient who has unexplained periaortic gas and symptoms suggestive of sepsis.

Diagnostic Testing

The diagnosis of a primary arterial infection is based on the recognition of elements of the clinical presentation along with appropriate use of various testing modalities. The primary factor in making such a diagnosis is a high clinical suspicion and the subsequent search for evidence to support the diagnosis of a primary arterial infection. The choice and use of diagnostic testing are of singular importance in identifying and substantiating the presence of an arterial infection. Because of the potentially fulminant course of these infections, and the fatal outcome of improperly managed cases, both speed and accuracy of diagnosis are crucial. The basic elements of diagnostic testing used in this process include bacteriologic and radiologic techniques.

Blood Cultures

The demonstration of bacterial organisms in association with an arterial lesion is central to the diagnosis of an arterial infection. The bacteria may be detected by either blood cultures or cultures of the arterial wall itself. Blood cultures, by virtue of their availability, are frequently one of the first tests done in patients suspected of having a significant infection. If the patient is floridly bacteremic, the blood culture may detect the circulating bacteria. However, several problems limit the usefulness of blood cultures. The incidence of negative blood cultures testifies to the fact that in only a fraction of symptomatic patients does the blood culture help in the diagnosis. Many patients with arterial infections never have positive blood cultures. In the review of Brown and associates of the University of California, Los Angeles, experience with mycotic aneurysms, only 60% of patients had positive preoperative blood cultures.[16] Finally, many blood cultures may not detect the infectious organism until several days or weeks have elapsed, limiting the test with regard to its ability to have an impact on clinical management.

The presence of bacteria in the blood of the patient may be an important early clue to an arterial infection, but the information from such tests must be evaluated in the proper clinical context. Most bacteremic patients have an evident source of the bacteremia that should be identified and treated. Patients with positive blood cultures and no clinical evidence of a concurrent infection should be considered and examined for possible arterial lesions. The significance of a positive blood culture in an otherwise asymptomatic patient is difficult to determine without considering the patient's underlying problems and risk factors. It should also be noted that patients who are relatively asymptomatic (no systemic manifestations of sepsis) tend to have fewer positive blood cultures. Thus, in the study of Wakefield and coworkers[24] of patients undergoing clean arterial procedures, only 2% of blood cultures were positive, whereas 12% of arteries and 14% of periarterial adi-

pose tissues harbored bacteria. Obvious clues, such as a recently noted aneurysm or history of drug abuse, may serve to promote further investigation.

The type of organism identified in blood cultures may further suggest a source of the infection. Certain pathogens are related to certain types of infections. The association between gram-negative bacteria and urinary tract infections is one example. Similarly, if a blood culture reveals *Salmonella* in a patient with an aneurysm, then an arterial infection should be seriously considered. Although *Staphylococcus* is a common pathogen in arterial infections, its ubiquitous presence on skin often confuses the diagnosis and calls into question the results of the blood culture.

The importance of the preoperative blood culture is difficult to understate. It represents the earliest reliable clue to the presence of an arterial infection. Even in the event of a delayed result, when several days have passed before the blood culture is able to identify the bacteria, the information that the test provides may be invaluable in managing the patient.

Arterial Cultures

Arterial wall cultures may also serve to secure the diagnosis of an arterial infection. The principal drawback to arterial wall cultures is the time they require before revealing information regarding the infection. Patient management must therefore depend on other factors, such as the clinical setting, the index of suspicion, the presence of prior blood culture data, and the results of angiographic studies. The patient's presentation may be important because Wakefield and coworkers discovered that tissue cultures in asymptomatic patients had significantly higher sensitivity than blood cultures.[24] This stands in contrast to symptomatic patients in whom blood cultures tend to have a higher sensitivity than the arterial cultures.

Because clinical decisions cannot always be based on arterial culture results, other techniques are often considered. Intraoperative Gram staining and frozen section of the arterial tissue are among these techniques. Unfortunately, these methods may not provide significant improvement in the detection of bacteria. In the study of Brown and associates, although 60% of patients had positive preoperative blood cultures, only 20% of intraoperative Gram stains were positive.[16] Arterial wall frozen sections have not had widespread use, but they may yet prove helpful. Histologic findings of inflammation and bacterial invasion are strong evidence supporting the diagnosis of arterial infection.

In obtaining both blood and arterial wall cultures, it should be kept in mind that the type of organism may affect the yield of the tests. Brown and associates noted that 60% of available arterial wall cultures were negative.[16] About 25% of their cultures failed to detect any organism at all. Presumably these were difficult organisms to collect and culture. *S. epidermidis* may be difficult to culture without sonicating the specimen. *Treponema pallidum* may require darkfield examination for identification. *Mycobacterium tuberculosis* is a fastidious organism and difficult to grow. These considerations should prompt the special attention of the pathology laboratory, as well as collection of adequate specimens.

Nuclear Imaging: Tagged White Blood Cell Scans

Nuclear imaging has become an important tool in the identification of arterial graft infections but has not served as important a role with regard to the identification of primary arterial infections. The technique is based on the ability of various radioisotope markers to become involved in an inflammatory process. The strength of these tests is their relatively low risk to the patient and the facility of their application. The principal drawback is that the tests may serve to detect many inflammatory lesions, not just those that are the result of an arterial infection. Interpreting the results of a nuclear scan must take into account the clinical condition of the patient in order to improve the diagnostic accuracy. Although the usefulness of these tests has been debated, in the absence of recent trauma or infection, radiolabeled indium or gallium as markers may allow localization of an arterial infection.

Perhaps the most significant problem with the isotopic detection of arterial infections is that these techniques have not been widely applied to this problem. The role of these tests is not well established. As a consequence, in cases wherein the diagnosis of arterial infection is apparent, the tests are forsaken. When the diagnosis of an arterial infection is not established, other testing modalities are frequently used first. Lesions that are not clearly apparent, such as intraabdominal aneurysms, are often better visualized by other forms of imaging (such as angiography, computed tomography [CT] scanning, or magnetic resonance imaging [MRI]. Finally, the specificity and selectivity of the nuclear imaging tests are not well established in these lesions.

Computed Tomography and Magnetic Resonance Imaging

The success of computed imaging techniques such as CT and MRI in identification of a primary arterial infection depends largely on the ability of these scans to resolve the characteristic anatomic features of the lesions. Because of the detailed anatomic data that these scans present, they have become very popular in the evaluation of intraabdominal vascular lesions. There are some significant limitations, however, with regard to their ability to secure the diagnosis of an arterial infection.

The essential diagnostic characteristics of arterial infections include the presence of a focal defect in the wall of the aorta, the saccular shape of the aneurysm, and the edema in the tissues that accompanies the inflammatory reaction. The current reconstruction of CT images does not readily allow recognition of the diagnostic features of mycotic aneurysms. Current scanners detect the presence of an aneurysm in the proximity of the aorta, but they frequently do not have the resolving power to detect small arterial wall defects. Additionally, current CT scanners are

not able to routinely reconstruct images in the same three-dimensional manner as MRI. It is reasonable to expect that the use of more advanced methods of computed reconstruction and higher resolution will improve these abilities.

MRI represents an improvement over CT scanning because current computer analysis of MRI allows more flexible assemblage of the data and facilitates recognition of essential diagnostic characteristics. Additionally, the resolution of MRI may be better than that of CT. MRI does not require intravascular contrast agents, which are frequently needed with CT. Finally, MRI is able to detect tissue differences with regard to certain molecular constituents. An advantage of MRI is its ability to detect the accumulation of water in tissues. This accumulation, tissue edema, is frequently the hallmark of an inflammatory process, and may identify an arterial infection.

Angiography

Angiography is the most widely used technique for the investigation and definition of arterial infections (Fig. 10–4). Its applications include the imaging of both central (abdominal and thoracic) and peripheral arterial lesions. Historically, it was the first method by which the characteristics of primary arterial infections, specifically infectious aortic aneurysms, were identified. Angiography has thus served not only to identify but also to define the characteristics of these lesions. Not surprisingly, angiography is able to surpass computed imaging in identifying the characteristic signs of arterial infections. Additionally, angiography is clearly superior in areas such as the intestinal mesentery and the visceral vessels, where the size of the arterial lesion

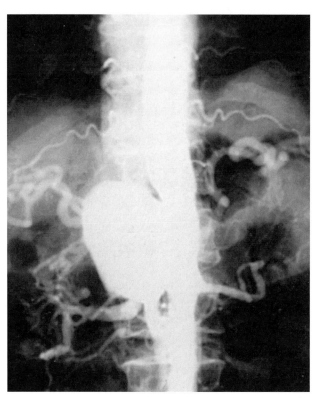

Figure 10–4. Angiogram of aortic mycotic aneurysm.

may be below the resolution of the computed techniques. In the detection of aortic mycotic aneurysms, the angiogram usually provides excellent definition of the defect in the aortic wall, the saccular pseudoaneurysm, as well as the contiguous arterial anatomy. Finally, the arteriogram offers the best definition of the relationship between the visceral vessels and the arterial defect—an essential step in the planning of management. The strength of angiography, then, is the detection of the arterial lesions and the definition of the arterial anatomy. These two elements are essential in planning an arterial reconstruction.

The role of arteriography in the management of a peripheral arterial infection has been questioned. Because some peripheral arterial infections are managed with ligation and débridement without reconstruction, an angiogram may not be necessary. On the other hand, it is important to assess the native circulation before attempting an arterial ligation. Should the limb require urgent revascularization after arterial ligation, an angiogram before the ligation is very helpful in planning the revascularization. It should be noted that an arteriogram obtained after ligation and resection of the vessel is often less than satisfactory. For this reason, an arteriogram of the involved vessels is required in all but emergent cases.

Treatment and Timing of Diagnosis

The diagnosis of a primary arterial infection may be made preoperatively, intraoperatively, or postoperatively. Should the diagnosis be suspected before surgery, preoperative antibiotics may be commenced and the patient may be better informed as to the problems that may be anticipated. Plans may be drawn for contingencies that might require alternative reconstructions.

The diagnosis may be established or confirmed by the findings of surgery. The presence of gross purulence, engorged lymph nodes, and inflamed tissues helps to establish the diagnosis conclusively. Adjunctive tests such as the Gram stain and bacterial cultures may be obtained. The intraoperative findings help to decide the mode of arterial reconstruction; gross infection and pus should be taken as indications for débridement and remote reconstruction. Minimal evidence of infection may suggest reasonably good results from in situ reconstruction.

If the diagnosis is confirmed in the postoperative period by positive bacterial cultures, a prolonged course of antibiotics and graft surveillance would be advised.

Natural History

Given the pathogenesis of a primary arterial infection—bacterial invasion, colonization, and destruction of an artery—the sequence of events that follow this initial insult are predictable and inexorable. Destruction of the arterial wall leads to either the development of an arterial pseudoaneurysm or a life-threatening hemorrhage. Which of these two events occurs is probably related to the rate of progression of the infection, its location, and the subsequent development of an inflammatory response. If the destruction of the arterial wall is gradual and accompanied

by a vigorous inflammatory response, the arterial infection may produce a pseudoaneurysm. If the process of the arterial infection leads rapidly to loss of arterial integrity, the arterial infection will lead to hemorrhage.

Complications of arterial infections include those common to all aneurysms: embolization, thrombosis, and rupture. The incidence of rupture is thought to be increased when the arterial wall is invaded by infectious pathogens. The high rupture rate is reflected in both the virulent course (rapid expansion and progression to rupture), as well as the high mortality of these lesions. For these reasons, mycotic aneurysms are urgent cases that should be repaired as soon as possible. One final complication, which is significantly increased in cases of primary arterial infection, is the rate of infection of the vascular reconstruction. Although the anticipated incidence of graft infection in "clean" cases is less than 1% or 2%, the incidence of graft infection after remote (extra-anatomic) reconstruction in cases of primary arterial infection may be as high as 15%. In older series, when in situ reconstruction was performed in the face of a purulent infection and without concurrent antibiotics, the reinfection rates approached 100%.

Principles of Management

Once the diagnosis has been established, early definitive intervention must be initiated. Two elemental principles form the basis of therapy in primary arterial infections: (1) control of sepsis, and (2) establishment of arterial continuity.

Control of Sepsis

Antibiotic therapy and surgical débridement represent the primary treatment modalities for the control of sepsis in arterial infections. All infected arterial tissue must be débrided. It is important that the arterial resection encompass all inflamed tissues. It should continue to the point where the arterial tissue is normal and healthy. This helps to prevent subsequent recurrence of the infection and disruption of the arterial suture line.

Soft tissues adjacent to the infected artery that appear to be involved in the infection should also be débrided. Major structures such as the vena cava and ureters should be left intact. Retroperitoneal tissues that appear to be involved should be resected. Once all infected tissues have been removed, the wound should be thoroughly irrigated with an antibiotic solution. Ideally, the irrigating solution should contain antibiotic directed toward the suspected pathogens (as detected by preoperative blood cultures). Surgical drains are useful when there is clear evidence of purulence. In the absence of an abscess or fluid collection, drains may not be required. When collateral circulation allows, the excision may be accompanied by proximal and distal ligation and no effort to reconstruct the artery, as first described by Paré.

The use of antibiotics is mandatory in these situations. Broad-spectrum antibiotics should be initiated as soon as a strong clinical suspicion of arterial infection has been established. Blood cultures should be obtained before the initiation of antibiotics. When positive, these cultures should be used in selecting an antibiotic regimen with the highest therapeutic value and fewest side effects. Negative cultures should not preclude the institution of broad-spectrum antibiotics when arterial infection is suspected. The use of high-dose preoperative antibiotics should be directed toward sterilizing the aneurysm and adjacent tissues to minimize bacteremia and local contamination during surgical manipulation of infected tissues. Antibiotics must be continued until the source of the bacteremia has been corrected either surgically or medically. Similarly, the primary source of bacteremia or local bacterial invasion must be controlled as a mainstay of therapy in all types of primary arterial infections. In patients with true mycotic aneurysms, specific consideration must be given to sterilization of cardiac valvular vegetations.

The duration of antibiotic treatment remains somewhat controversial, and several competing regimens have been proposed. Several authors have suggested that IV antibiotics be initiated before surgery and extended for a period of time no less than 6 weeks postoperatively.[25–27] Additionally, these authors recommend that in patients with prosthetic reconstructions, especially those with in situ prosthetic reconstructions, that the patient be placed on a lifelong oral regimen of suppressive antibiotics. Typically, oral trimethoprim-sulfamethoxazole (Bactrim), sulfa drugs, or a first-generation cephalosporin or penicillin is the agent of choice.

Important technical points include the use of monofilament suture material in ligation and oversewing of the arteries. This recommendation is based on the superiority of monofilaments over braided suture in resisting recurrent infection. Additionally, whenever possible, the resected arterial stump should be covered with a pedicle of healthy, viable tissue so as to further reduce the possibility of a recurrent infection, and to accelerate the healing of the arterial segment. In the abdomen, this tissue pedicle is frequently the omentum. A flap of fascia from the prevertebral fascia and ligaments has been used to reinforce the aortic suture line. In the periphery, muscle transposition is the preferred means of obtaining tissue coverage. In the femoral region, this is most readily accomplished by rotating the head of the sartorius.

Nonoperative therapy for arterial infections in specific subsets of patients has been proposed by Kaufman and coworkers.[28] This treatment modality, although effective anecdotally, remains controversial. Further investigation is necessary to evaluate this unique treatment approach.

Reestablishment of Arterial Continuity

Lack of adequate arterial collateralization results in end-organ ischemia when infected arteries are ligated and resected. Accordingly, in these situations, some form of arterial reconstruction must be performed to avoid tissue ischemia. This instance is most common with infections involving the visceral arteries, the aorta, and the femoral artery bifurcation.

Arthur Blakemore, in 1947, was among the first to employ a graft to replace an infected artery when he implanted a Vitallium tube. Since then, a wide range of bypass

materials have been utilized with varying success rates. These include autologous tissues such as saphenous vein and arterial homografts, as well as various synthetic materials such as polytetrafluoroethylene (PTFE), and Dacron. Use of arterial homografts has been disappointing. These conduits were vulnerable to both recurrent infection as well as disruption. The resultant hemorrhage yielded 100% mortality in selected series. Autologous vein grafts are currently considered the optimal material with which to reconstruct most arterial infections. Vein grafts tend to be superior to prosthetic material in resisting recurrent infection. Further, they are durable and familiar to most vascular surgeons. Prosthetic grafts have been used and are the graft of choice in certain instances. These are subject to recurrent infection to a greater extent than autologous vein grafts. They are important in allowing reconstructions that would be difficult or dangerous with autologous tissue. Most prosthetic graft reconstructions of arterial infections are found in extra-anatomic bypasses, and in the rare instances of in situ reconstruction of the paravisceral aorta.

Successful management of arterial infections depends largely on the location and size of the affected artery. General principles indicate that when bypass procedures must be performed, autologous materials such as the patient's own arteries or veins harvested from clean sites should be utilized as the graft of first choice. When prosthetic grafts must be used, every attempt should be made to place them through clean planes, including extra-anatomic bypass when necessary.

Infrarenal Aorta

Primary arterial infections of the infrarenal aorta invariably require excision and graft reconstruction. The standard therapy that has evolved for infections in this location combines excision and débridement of the aneurysm and adjacent tissues with extra-anatomic bypass (e.g., axillofemoral bypass). In a review of spontaneous abdominal aortic infections, Ewart and associates[29] demonstrated a 23% to 63% reoperation rate for graft infection after immediate in situ reconstruction and a 7% recurrent infection rate when patients were initially treated with arterial débridement and remote reconstruction.

Brown and associates, in their review of 51 cases of mycotic aneurysms, noted that the mortality of local graft reconstruction was 32%, whereas extra-anatomic reconstruction patients suffered a 13% mortality rate.[16] Still, the authors advocated in situ reconstruction in selected cases; they proposed that if no gross purulence was encountered intraoperatively, and if the Gram stain was negative, in situ reconstruction utilizing prosthetic (Dacron) material could safely be performed. This approach is predicated on the recommendation that postoperative antibiotics be continued for a minimum of 6 to 8 weeks. Brown and associates demonstrated 63% survival and 19% reinfection rates for aneurysms treated via this approach. In comparison, the rate of infection of extra-anatomic bypasses following repair of mycotic aortic aneurysms has been reported to be as high as 13%.[16]

More recently, experience with in situ reconstruction for primary aortoduodenal fistulas has encouraged some authors to proceed with in situ graft reconstruction of the aorta in instances where there is minimal contamination, no pus, and little extent of the infectious process.[15]

Suprarenal Aneurysms

Because of their unique anatomic characteristics, arterial infections of the paravisceral and suprarenal aorta almost always require immediate in situ arterial reconstruction. It is nearly impossible to bypass the visceral vessels without traversing the bed of the infected paravisceral aorta. Experience gained from these repairs of suprarenal mycotic aneurysms has given credence to the concept of in situ repair with adjunctive lifelong antibiotic therapy.

When combined with débridement of grossly infected tissue and appropriate use of antibiotics, most reported series using this type of reconstruction have demonstrated acceptable morbidity and mortality rates. Chan and associates[25] reported a series of 22 patients with mycotic aneurysms of the thoracic and abdominal aorta. Of these, 13 had involvement of the paravisceral aorta. All 13 required in situ reconstruction. Twelve of the 13 survived surgery and were placed on lifelong suppressive antibiotics. None was reported to have had a clinical recurrence of the infection. In the overall series three patients died; two of the deaths were attributed to multisystem organ failure and aspiration pneumonia. The authors concluded that in situ reconstruction along with surgical débridement and lifelong antibiotics offers the best chance for survival in these difficult patients.[25] It should be noted that although this form of therapy (in situ reconstruction) is inescapable in the reconstruction of infected paravisceral aneurysms, its application to arterial infections at other sites (such as the infrarenal aorta or femoral artery) is less well established and should be approached with caution.

Femoral, Iliac, and Mesenteric Arterial Infections

Other anatomic locations where primary arterial infections are considered relatively common include the femoral, superior mesenteric, and celiac arteries. Attempts at ligation and excision of these vessels for the treatment of primary arterial infections may be associated with a high rate of irreversible ischemia. Currently, the patients who are at greatest risk of developing these infections are IV drug abusers. Because these patients have a tendency to recidivism they are at risk of reinfecting their arterial reconstructions. This has generated debate regarding the best treatment of these patients. The simplest approach is to ligate, resect, and then observe the ligated vascular bed for signs of severe ischemia. Revascularization is performed only if severe ischemia develops. The second choice is to proceed with an autogenous reconstruction at the time of resecting the infected lesion.

The Infected Femoral Pseudoaneurysm

Infections of the vessels of the femoral region are the most common type of arterial infection. In the review by Brown and colleagues, these lesions accounted for 38% of all arterial infections.[16] The most common manifestation is that of an inflamed, tender, pulsatile inguinal mass. The more common complications include erosion through the skin with hemorrhage, embolization, compression of adjacent structures (femoral vein and nerve), and thrombosis. Of these, erosion and hemorrhage are the most feared complications.

The debate regarding reconstruction is of particular interest in the subset of patients with infected pseudoaneurysms of the femoral bifurcation that are the result of IV drug abuse. Because of the addict's tendency to reuse the femoral sites for further drug administration, the arterial reconstruction may be in jeopardy of recurrent infection. If the reconstruction required prosthetic material, then the resultant reinfection would be all the more complicated and dangerous. Finally, the incidence of graft infection after immediate reconstruction is sufficient by itself to warrant hesitation in such reconstructions. Because of these concerns, some authors have advocated simple arterial ligation and resection of the infected tissues. The problem is that simple ligation of the femoral arteries at the level of the arterial bifurcation may have a subsequent amputation rate approaching 33%.[23, 30]

An alternative school holds that the limbs should be reconstructed, and if these are subsequently infected, the infection should be dealt with as necessary. In the course of these reconstructions, the infected arteries and adjacent tissues should be débrided and the reconstruction coursed through uninfected tissues.[31] Finally, the reconstruction should be performed with autogenous tissue if possible.

The third option is to combine both approaches so that the arterial lesion is resected and the adjacent tissues are débrided. The artery is ligated but no reconstructions are performed in the initial setting. The limb is observed for signs of severe ischemia. If the limb appears viable with collateral perfusion alone, no effort is made to reconstruct. If the limb appears severely ischemic, revascularization is attempted. Femoral artery reconstruction should be carried out either with in situ saphenous vein interposition grafting or through an extra-anatomic approach such as a transobturator bypass.

Infection and pseudoaneurysm of the common femoral, superficial femoral, or profunda femoris do not appear to suffer a similar fate. These vessels stand a far better chance of tolerating simple ligation without requiring reconstruction. Wright and Shepard[32] reported a very low incidence of amputation following ligation and resection without amputation in this circumstance. In a series of 39 patients with such infections, they noted an amputation rate of 5%. They further noted that these amputations occurred in two patients who had impaired collateral circulation from prior (contralateral) common femoral artery ligation. In the absence of these two cases, their amputation rate in this group of patients was 0%.[32]

Mesenteric Artery Infections

Mesenteric artery infections tend to appear as pseudoaneurysms within the mesentery of the intestine. These lesions may be asymptomatic, but the more common presentation is that of abdominal pain. These lesions may develop as a consequence of IV drug abuse. Pathophysiologically, they are considered to be the result of mycotic embolization. Because of this, it is necessary to consider the possible source of the emboli as well as the possibility of other embolic targets. In practical terms, this means that these patients should be screened for both cardiac vegetations and other arterial lesions. Preoperative angiography is recommended if possible. Postoperative angiography should be considered if a preoperative study was not obtained.

The mesenteric arterial infections tend to develop rapid expansion and intramesenteric hemorrhage. Alternatively, these aneurysms may result in thrombosis and infarction of the intestine. The management of these vessels is related to the location of the lesion, the available collateral circulation, and the presence and extent of intestinal infarction. Lesions of the proximal mesenteric arteries frequently require reconstruction with autogenous tissues. More distally located pseudoaneurysms may frequently be managed by simple excision. If a small area of intestinal ischemia develops, a limited bowel resection may also be necessary. In instances of extensive intestinal ischemia, a second-look celiotomy may be advisable after restoration of intestinal perfusion.

Arterial Infections of the Upper Extremity

Infection of the arteries of the upper extremities are fairly rare. Collectively, they represented about 10% of arterial infections in the review by Brown and colleagues.[16] Frequently, these lesions are associated with trauma. Like other infections of peripheral vessels, these lesions may appear in a number of ways. The most common presentation is that of an inflamed, tender, pulsatile mass. In the upper extremities, careful inspection should detect evidence of digital embolization: splinter hemorrhages and ischemic lesions.

Because of the extensive collateral blood supply to the upper extremities, infections of the arteries to the upper extremities may often be treated with simple ligation and excision. This is particularly true when the involved segment is between the thyrocervical trunk and the subscapular artery or distal to the profunda brachii. Reconstruction, when required, should be accomplished with a saphenous vein graft or similar autogenous tissues. As with all mycotic aneurysms, pre- and postoperative antibiotics should be given for a prolonged period of time.

Conclusions

Primary arterial infections are relatively rare. These lesions are frequently lethal. They often follow a rapidly progressive course toward expansion and rupture. Only an astute diagnosis along with the correct management allows improved chances of survival. The diagnosis is established by a high index of suspicion along with identification of risk factors and appropriate testing. Once identified, management must be tailored to the organism involved and the site and severity of the infection, as well as the condition of the patient. Surgical excision is almost always necessary

in the course of management. Long-term IV antibiotics (6 weeks) are also almost always required. The subsequent use of lifelong oral antibiotic suppression is strongly recommended for these patients. Optimal care may reduce the mortality of these lesions from nearly 100% to less than 10% to 15%.

PROPHYLACTIC ANTIBIOTIC THERAPY

Although infections of implanted vascular prostheses are relatively uncommon, when they do occur, they are associated with significant morbidity and mortality. Complications of graft infection include pseudoaneurysm, anastomotic disruption, hemorrhage, fistula formation, and sepsis. Infection of a vascular graft almost always requires partial or complete graft removal, which is associated with a high incidence of amputation. Vascular graft infection leads to the patient's death in one fourth to one half of cases in contemporary series. These dire consequences have prompted a continually expanding area of laboratory and clinical investigation into the role of antibiotics in the prevention of vascular graft infection. The widespread use of prophylactic antibiotics in vascular surgery has significantly altered the microbiology and clinical presentation of graft infections. New insights have been gained into the pathogenesis of this process. Alternative methods of antibiotic delivery have been developed in animal models. This section presents the bacteriology and current understanding of the pathogenesis of graft infection, a historical overview of the development of antibiotic prophylaxis in vascular surgery, current recommendations for prophylaxis, and new directions in antibiotic delivery.

Clinical Significance of Graft Infection

The reported incidence of infection after the placement of vascular prostheses ranges from 1% to 6%. This relatively low rate of infection has remained stable over time, despite improvements in technique and the introduction of routine preoperative antibiotic prophylaxis. Two early series, from Hoffert and colleagues[33] in 1965 and Fry and Lindenauer[34] in 1967, reported graft infection rates of 6.0% (12/201) and 1.34% (12/890), respectively. In 1972 Szilagyi and colleagues[35] reported a large series of 3397 cases in which the graft infection rate was 1.9%. Later reports detailed similar findings. The series of Lorentzen and coauthors[36] from 1985 described graft infections in 62 of 2411 patients, a rate of 2.6%. Although the overall incidence of infection has not changed significantly, the use of antibiotic prophylaxis has clearly changed the clinical presentation of most vascular graft infections. Suppurative infections appearing in the first few weeks after graft implantation have given way to more insidious, low-grade, chronic infections.[37, 38]

Infection in prosthetic grafts remains an issue of critical importance in vascular surgery. Reported mortality rates (Table 10–1) from graft infection range from 25% to 75%.[33, 34, 37, 39–42] Mortality has been greatest for proximal grafts, with almost uniform lethality reported in aortic stump sepsis.[34, 35, 39, 43] Despite attempts at reducing mortality in aortic graft infection, it remains relatively high at 24% to

TABLE 10-1

Influence of Graft Site on Incidence and Outcome of Graft Infection

AUTHOR	YEAR	TYPE OF GRAFT	PATIENTS (n)	GRAFT INFECTION RATE (%)*	AMPUTATION RATE (%)†	MORTALITY RATE (%)
Hoffert et al.[33]	1965	Aortoiliac	84	0	NA	NA
		Aortofemoral	30	0	NA	NA
		Iliofemoropopliteal	83	13	75	25
Szilagyi et al.[35]	1972	Aortoiliac	418	0.7	0	66
		Aortofemoral	1244	1.6	21	53
		Iliofemoropopliteal	270	3.0	40	7
Bouhoutsos et al.[59]	1974	Aortoiliac/aortofemoral	412	1.5	0	50
		Iliofemoropopliteal	108	7.4	25	0
Liekweg & Greenfield[40]	1977	Aortoiliac	NR	NR	3	58
		Aortofemoral	NR	NR	11	47
		Iliofemoropopliteal	NR	NR	30	13
Yashar et al.[42]	1978	Aortoiliac	300	1.0	0	33
		Aortofemoral	210	2.9	33	50
		Iliofemoropopliteal	65	4.6	67	0
Casali et al.[105]	1980	Aortoiliac	NR	NR	0	50
		Aortofemoral	NR	NR	25	67
		Iliofemoropopliteal	NR	NR	33	33
Lorentzen et al.[36]	1985	Aortoiliac	515	0.0	NA	NA
		Aortofemoral	1497	3.0	22	29
		Iliofemoropopliteal	489	3.5	53	18
Edwards et al.[53]	1987	Aortic/aortoiliac	769	0.0	NA	NA
		Aortofemoral	1060	0.47	20	40
		Iliofemoropopliteal	583	2.9	12	18

*Primary graft infections only; excludes aortoenteric fistulas.
†Amputation rate among survivors.
NA, not applicable; NR, not reported.

43%.[44–48] Peripheral graft infections are generally associated with lower mortality rates (as low as 6%).[49] Amputation rates are similar for survivors of aortic and peripheral graft infections, ranging from 22.5% to 43%.[35, 40, 50] In more recent series, reported amputation rates range from 24% to 27%.[47–49]

Principles of Antibiotic Prophylaxis

The goal of prophylactic antibiotic therapy is to prevent infection after surgery. The most important indication for antibiotic prophylaxis in vascular reconstructive surgery is the use of prosthetic materials. Synthetic materials provide a protective substrate for bacterial colonization and proliferation. Experimental studies have demonstrated that the presence of a foreign body increases the infectivity of S. aureus 10,000-fold.[51] In light of the potentially catastrophic consequences of vascular graft infection, prophylactic antibiotics are recommended in patients undergoing procedures in which prosthetic materials are employed.

The ideal prophylactic antibiotic should be bactericidal for the most common pathogens causing postoperative infection, adequately concentrated in serum and at the site of surgery. It should be present in adequate concentrations throughout the surgical procedure, be nontoxic to the patient, and be of a cost reasonable to justify its routine use.

Most vascular graft infections are caused by a few specific bacteria. Therefore, broad-spectrum antibiotic prophylaxis is unnecessary. Selecting an antibiotic with the narrowest spectrum of activity that includes the most common pathogens involved in graft infection will limit the emergence of resistant organisms. Antibiotics that are the principal line of therapy in difficult infections (such as vancomycin in the treatment of S. epidermidis infections) should be reserved for that indication and not used in prophylaxis.

Bacteriology of Graft Infection

Gram-positive cocci, the predominant flora of the skin and dermal appendages, are most often responsible for vascular graft infections. Although the bacteriology of graft infection varies somewhat by anatomic site, when all sites are considered together approximately 60% to 65% of reported cases are currently due to gram-positive organisms. The remaining 35% to 40% are largely due to gram-negative rods, which account for approximately half of all infections in intraabdominal (aortic, aortoiliac) grafts. Although S. aureus has historically been the most frequently cultured pathogen, the introduction of routine antibiotic prophylaxis along with improved culture techniques has led to the emergence of S. epidermidis and other coagulase-negative staphylococci as the most frequent cause of vascular graft infection (Table 10–2). The most commonly cultured gram-negative rod is E. coli, followed by Proteus, Pseudomonas, and Klebsiella.

Changing Bacterial Spectrum of Graft Infection

In early reports from the 1960s and 1970s, S. aureus was identified as the predominant pathogen in vascular graft

TABLE 10-2

Effect of Antibiotic Prophylaxis on the Microbiology of Graft Infection

AUTHOR	YEAR	TYPE OF GRAFT	PROPHYLACTIC ANTIBIOTICS	CULTURED ORGANISMS (%)*				CULTURE NEGATIVE (%)
				S. aureus	*S. epidermidis*	*E. coli*	Other GNRs	
Hoffert et al.[33]	1965	Aortic and distal	No	67	17	8	25	17
Fry & Lindenauer[34]	1966	Aortic	No	67	0	25	8	8
Goldstone & Moore[37]	1974	Aortic and distal	†	41	26	15	11	7
Liekweg & Greenfield[40]	1977	Aortic and distal	No	50	4	13	18	NR
Bandyk et al.[38]	1984	Aortofemoral	Yes	10	60	13	23	10
Yeager et al.[48]	1985	Aortic	Yes	0	50	0	0	33
		Distal	Yes	14	14	0	29	43
Quiñones-Baldrich et al.[54]	1991	Aortic	Yes	13	21	18	45	21

*Expressed as percent of cases from which each organism was cultured.
†Prophylaxis administered in 10 of 27 cases of graft infection.
GNR, gram-negative rod; NR, not reported.

infections. In 1965, Hoffert and colleagues reported that *S. aureus* was cultured in 67% (8/12) of aortal, femoral, and popliteal reconstructions.[33] A series of 890 aortic grafts from Fry and Lindenauer in 1967 also reported that *S. aureus* was cultured in 67% (8/12) of aortic graft cases.[34] In 1967, Smith and colleagues[52] reported on nine cases of femoropopliteal graft infection, eight of which were due to *S. aureus*. In a review of 108 published cases of vascular graft infection reported between 1959 and 1974, Liekweg and Greenfield noted that *S. aureus* was responsible for 50% of cases.[40] This was followed by gram-negative rods (30.5%) and streptococcus (8.5%). Only 3.6% of cases were due to *S. epidermidis*.

Goldstone and Moore were among the first to note the impact of antibiotic prophylaxis on the presentation and bacteriology of graft infection.[37] They retrospectively reviewed the incidence of graft infection before and after the initiation of routine antibiotic prophylaxis. During the preantibiotic prophylaxis period (1959–1966), the vascular graft infection rate was 4.1% (9/222). From 1966 to 1973, when prophylactic antibiotic use became routine, the graft infection rate dropped to 1.5% (5/344). Of all staphylococcal infections treated at our institution between 1959 and 1973, 14 of 18 (78%) occurred before the routine use of prophylactic antibiotics.

Reviews of graft infection since the advent of routine antibiotic prophylaxis demonstrate an increasing incidence of late infections due to fastidious organisms such as *S. epidermidis* and other coagulase-negative staphylococci. Bandyk and colleagues presented a report of 30 patients treated for aortofemoral graft infections from 1972 to 1982, 60% of which were due to *S. epidermidis*.[38] The time of presentation influenced the microbiology of graft infection. Four of five early (less than 4 months) infections were due to gram-negative rods. Late infections (greater than 4 months) were much more common, totaling 25, and 15 (60%) of these were due to *S. epidermidis*.

In 1985, Yeager and associates[48] reported a 9-year experience in which they managed 14 aortic and 11 peripheral graft infections. Although peripheral graft infections appeared on average 8 months after surgery, aortic grafts appeared on average 5 years postoperatively. Of five primarily infected aortic grafts (not graft-enteric fistulas or erosions) with positive cultures, four were due to *S. epidermidis*. A wide range of organisms were cultured from peripheral grafts, including coagulase-positive and -negative staphylococci, gram-negative rods, anaerobic streptococci, and diphtheroids.

Edwards and associates[53] reported on 24 infections from a series of 2614 aortofemoropopliteal grafts over a 10-year period from 1975 to 1986, of which the majority (29%) were due to *S. aureus*. The authors noted, however, that in only 7 of 24 cases were prophylactic antibiotics administered according to the departmental protocol; thus, this series may be more representative of the preantibiotic era. This observation is supported by the fact that 63% of these infections appeared within 3 months of implantation. Additionally, cultures were negative in 21% of patients, suggesting that the presence of fastidious organisms such as *S. epidermidis* may have been underestimated. In 1991 Quiñones-Baldrich and colleagues[54] reported an 18-year experience (1970 to 1988) with 45 aortic graft infections. Culture results were available for 38 of 45 patients. Gram-negative organisms, most commonly *Pseudomonas* (21%) and *E. coli* (18%), were cultured from 24 (63%) patients. Gram-positive cocci, most frequently *S. epidermidis* (21%), were cultured from 21 (55%) patients. Of note is the fact that cultures grew multiple organisms in 39% of cases, and that there were eight (21%) negative cultures, again suggesting that the incidence of infection due to fastidious organisms may have been underestimated.

Pathogenesis of Graft Infection

Although no certain explanation for graft infections exists, the two principal routes of graft infection are thought to be direct contamination (bacteria present in the surgical wound) and hematogenous or lymphatogenous seeding. It is generally considered that most graft infections are caused by direct intraoperative contamination of the prosthesis. Potential sources of infecting organisms include the patient's skin, breaks in aseptic technique, adjacent active infections, transudation of bowel flora into the peritoneal space, and the diseased arterial tree itself, which may become colonized with pathogenic bacteria.

Skin Flora

The normal skin flora is the most important source of bacteria. Accordingly, preoperative skin preparation influences subsequent infection rates. Kaiser and coworkers[55] have noted a higher rate of infection with a hexachlorophene-ethanol preparation compared with povidone-iodine. Close and colleagues[56] reported that hexachlorophene alone is more effective than when used in combination with ethanol. In a prospective study, Cruse[57] demonstrated that preoperative hexachlorophene showering can be effective in reducing wound infection rates, and that overzealous shaving may actually increase the risk of infection. Wooster and colleagues[58] demonstrated that vascular grafts routinely become contaminated with skin organisms intraoperatively, and suggested that careful attention to aseptic technique can significantly influence the extent to which this happens.

Groin incisions appear to have special significance in the development of vascular graft infections. Grafts involving an inguinal wound have a higher incidence of infection than those that avoid this region.[35, 37, 59] Jamieson and colleagues[39] reported that the presence of a groin incision increased the risk of graft infection 3.5 times, and that the presence of a groin complication such as a seroma or hematoma increased the risk of infection ninefold over patients without groin complications. Up to 33% of groin incisions with hematomas may develop infections.[42] Lorentzen and associates reported that the highest incidence of infection was in patients who underwent aortobifemoral grafting for abdominal aortic aneurysms (5.9%), whereas there were no infections in 425 patients who underwent aortoiliac bypass for aneurysms (213) and occlusive atherosclerosis (212).[36]

Gastrointestinal Flora

The gastrointestinal tract is a potential source of contamination during aortic reconstruction. Cultures of intestinal bag fluid have been reported by some investigators to yield enteric bacteria[40] and skin organisms such as coagulase-negative staphylococci.[22] In a report on 109 bowel bag cultures from abdominal aortic reconstructions, Scobie and colleagues[60] found positive cultures in 14% of patients. *S. epidermidis* was the single most common organism isolated ($n = 11$), whereas enteric flora were cultured in 12.

The impact of concomitant gastrointestinal surgery in the development of vascular graft infection is unclear. In separate series, DeBakey and coauthors,[61] Stoll,[62] and Hardy and coworkers[63] reported a total of 670 patients who underwent aortic graft placement and simultaneous gastrointestinal procedures, with no episodes of graft infection. These authors concluded that such coincident procedures may be safely undertaken. Other investigators, however, have described the development of graft infection in patients undergoing simultaneous appendectomy,[37] cholecystectomy and gastrostomy,[64] and anterior resection.[59]

Arterial Colonization

The native arterial tree may harbor bacteria. The presence of pathogenic bacteria, particularly coagulase-negative staphylococci, in vascular tissues previously not operated on, has been widely documented (Table 10–3). Lalka and colleagues[65] postulated that transient bacteremias resulting from breaks in the skin or mucous membranes may lead to arterial colonization. Bacterial contamination of vascular prostheses may, therefore in some cases, be inevitable. It is not yet clear, however, to what extent the presence of positive arterial wall cultures influences the likelihood of subsequent graft infection.

The 1977 report of Ernst and associates[22] of abdominal aortic aneurysmal wall cultures was one of the first to highlight the presence of pathogenic organisms in the native aorta. The overall incidence of positive cultures was 15%, and cultures were more likely to be positive when atherosclerotic disease was more advanced. Asymptomatic aneurysms were less likely to be culture positive (9%) than symptomatic (13%) or ruptured aneurysms (35%). *S. epidermidis* was the most frequently isolated organism. The late graft sepsis rate was 10% in the culture-positive group versus 2% in the culture-negative group. In a similar report, Buckels and coauthors[66] described an 8% (22/275) incidence of positive cultures from aortic aneurysm contents. The incidence of graft sepsis was 32% (7/22) in patients with positive cultures compared with 2.4% (6/253) in the culture-negative group.

Similar data suggest that lower extremity arteries may also become infected. In 1984, Macbeth and colleagues[67] reported on cultures of arterial wall specimens from 88 clean, elective lower extremity revascularization procedures. Control cultures were taken from adjacent adipose or lymphatic tissue. Although all control cultures were negative, arterial wall cultures were positive in 43% (38/88) of cases. Of these, 71% (27/38) grew *S. epidermidis*. The authors described three graft infections in 335 cases (0.9% infection rate), all of which had positive arterial wall cultures. Also included in this report was a retrospective review of 22 cases of graft infection for which arterial and graft culture data were available. Of patients with positive arterial cultures, 57% (8/14) had suture line disruption, whereas there were no disruptions in the culture-negative group.[67]

Similar information suggests that arteries of the lower extremities may also bear bacteria. Durham and colleagues[68] reported a series of 102 patients undergoing vascular reconstruction with a 44% (75/102) incidence of positive arterial wall cultures. *S. epidermidis* accounted for 56% of the cultured organisms. Six infections (3.5%) occurred over 18 months; all of these patients had prior positive arterial cultures. No patients with negative arterial cultures developed graft infection. The greatest risk for graft infection appeared to be in patients with positive arterial wall cultures undergoing reoperation.

Hematogenous and Lymphatogenous Seeding

Hematogenous seeding of vascular prostheses is yet another potential source of graft infections. Anecdotal reports implicate urinary tract infection,[36, 37] abdominal sepsis,[37, 42, 60] and other infections[35] in the development of vascular graft infections. Laboratory models demonstrate that bacteremia reliably produces prosthetic graft infections.[69–71]

Positive Arterial Wall Cultures: Incidence and Significance

AUTHOR	YEAR	CULTURE SOURCE	POSITIVE CULTURES (%)	ASSOCIATED WITH SUBSEQUENT INFECTION?	FREQUENCY OF *S. epidermidis* AMONG POSITIVE CULTURES
Ernst et al.[22]	1977	Aortic aneurysms	15	Yes	53
Scobie et al.[60]	1979	Aortic aneurysms	23	No	71
Macbeth et al.[67]	1984	Femoropopliteal specimens	43	Yes	71
McAuley et al.[109]	1984	Aortic thrombus	14	No	NR
Buckels et al.[66]	1985	Aortic aneurysms	8	Yes	30
Durham et al.[68]	1987	Aortofemoropopliteal specimens	44	Yes	56
Schwartz et al.[106]	1987	Aortic aneurysms	10	No	54
Ilgenfritz & Jordan[107]	1988	Aortic aneurysms and ASD	20	No	55
Brandimarte et al.[108]	1989	Aortic aneurysms	31	No	NR
Wakefield et al.[24]	1990	Aortofemoropopliteal specimens	12	No	60

ASD, atrial septal defect; NR, not reported.

Other Local and Systemic Factors

Open wounds on the distal lower extremities may be the source of contaminating bacteria. Hoffert and colleagues noted that 75% of patients with graft infections (9/12) had an open, infected lesion on the distal lower extremity at the time of graft implantation.[33] Liekweg and Greenfield reported that 20 of 60 (33%) inguinal infections occurred proximal to open foot infections.[40] Bunt and Mohr[72] described the presence of bacteria cultured from a distally infected extremity in the inguinal lymph nodes of two patients undergoing lower extremity revascularization; both patients developed graft infection.

Prior vascular surgery has been implicated as a risk factor for vascular graft infection. Dense scar tissue, increased bleeding, and lymphatic leak may all contribute to this phenomenon. Goldstone and Moore noted that 45% (12/27) of patients with graft infections had undergone one or more revisions of their original graft before the development of infection in the same region.[37] In 8 of 12 of these patients, the infection was in the groin. In the series of Edwards and coworkers, 9 of 18 (50%) patients had undergone a previous vascular surgery at the site of the graft infection.[53] Similarly, a report from Reilly and colleagues[46] described a history of multiple previous vascular procedures at the site of graft infection in 40% of cases. Johnson and associates[73] found that prior vascular procedures were not a significant risk factor for graft infection; however, only 12 of 135 patients in this series had prior operations at the site of infection.

The immunologic status of patients with vascular disease may also have an impact on the development of graft infection. Systemic disease, malnutrition, and medical debility may suppress the host response to invading microorganisms. Kwaan and colleagues[74] reported on 12 patients with advanced, fulminating graft infections, all of whom had critical deficiencies in immune status as determined by serum albumin, hemoglobin, immunoglobulin, and lymphocyte assays and by response to standard skin test antigens. Eight of 12 patients who received total parenteral nutrition had significant enhancement of immune response and accelerated recovery from the graft infection. Of the four patients who did not receive nutritional support, two had a prolonged convalescence and two subsequently died from complications of graft infection.

Antibiotic Prophylaxis: Experimental Investigations

The suggestion that prophylactic antibiotic therapy may be effective in the prevention of surgical infections was first made 50 years ago.[75–79] In the early 1960s, Alexander and colleagues demonstrated the efficacy of penicillin prophylaxis in experimental wound infections.[80, 81]

Lindenauer and associates reported an experimental demonstration of the importance of antibiotics in preventing graft infection.[41] Three groups of dogs underwent femoral arteriotomy with primary, Teflon patch, or vein patch closure. A fourth group received sham operation alone. Wound were contaminated with 10,000 to 100,000 *S. aureus* organisms. All subjects, except controls, received intramuscular (IM) procaine penicillin. Among control animals, the infection rate was 94% (8 of 9 shams, 3 of 3 arteriotomies, 3 of 3 Teflon patches, 3 of 3 vein patches). In animals treated with penicillin, the infection rate was 0% (15 shams, 5 arteriotomies, 5 Teflon patches, 5 vein patches). Thus, antibiotic therapy may sterilize a contaminated wound even in the presence of a prosthetic arterial patch.

Moore and colleagues[82] tested the utility of antibiotic prophylaxis in a canine model of hematogenous aortic graft contamination. Thirty minutes before laparotomy, dogs were infused IV with 10 million *S. aureus* organisms, and then underwent placement of a Dacron infrarenal aortic graft. The experimental group received an IV dose of cephalothin (25 mg/kg), which was started just prior to the skin incision and continued for 30 minutes after the procedure. Experimental animals then received cephalothin (IM) three times a day for 5 days. Control animals received no antibiotics. Control animals experienced a significantly increased rate of positive cultures (72%), compared with animals that received perioperative cephalothin (24%).

Antibiotic Prophylaxis: Clinical Investigations

Early Experience

Up until the mid-1970s, the use of antibiotics in vascular reconstruction with synthetic materials was largely based on personal preference. It is notable that in the series of Szilagyi and colleagues from 1972, the graft infection rate among 2145 cases in which prophylactic antibiotics were not administered was 1.5%.[35] Fry and Lindenauer had reported an incidence of 1.34% in 890 cases in which no antibiotics were used.[34] These infection rates were comparable with, and often lower than, those reported in series in which prophylactic antibiotics were used.[39] Noting the preponderance of *S. aureus* in vascular graft infections, however, particularly in cases involving an inguinal incision, Szilagyi and colleagues suggested a clinical trial of an antibiotic directed at this organism in reconstructions that required an inguinal anastomosis.[35]

In 1974, Goldstone and Moore published a review of the San Francisco Veterans Administration Hospital experience with vascular prosthetic infection.[37] This series of 566 aortofemoropopliteal reconstructions was divided into two time periods: the years 1959 to 1965, during which time antibiotics were administered postoperatively only; and the years 1966 to 1973, in which prophylaxis included pre-, intra-, and postoperative antibiotics. The incidence of graft infection in the former group was 4.1% (9/222), compared with 1.5% (5/344) in the latter. Although the investigators conceded that greater experience and skill may have contributed to the lower incidence of infection, they maintained that the major factor responsible was the more appropriate use of antibiotics in the second group of patients. The following year, Perdue[83] published a similar retrospective review, which suggested that the institution of routine antibiotic prophylaxis reduced the incidence of wound infections and other nosocomial infections in patients undergoing major arterial reconstructive procedures.

Prospective Trials

The first large prospective, randomized, blinded clinical study of antibiotic prophylaxis in vascular reconstructive surgery was published by Kaiser and colleagues in 1978.[55] In this series, 462 patients undergoing aortofemoropopliteal reconstruction were randomized to receive either 1 g of cefazolin or a saline placebo. There were no graft infections among 225 patients who received cefazolin, compared with 4 (1.7%) of 237 placebo recipients. When superficial skin infections and subcutaneous skin infections were considered in the analysis (Szilagyi class I and II), the overall infection rates were 0.9% in the cefazolin group and 6.8% in the placebo group. Given no adverse drug reactions, and no noted cefazolin resistance, the authors strongly recommended a short course of cefazolin prophylaxis in arterial reconstructive surgery.[55]

In 1980, Pitt and colleagues[84] reported the results of a controlled study of cephradine prophylaxis in vascular procedures involving a groin incision that compared topical, systemic, and topical plus systemic administration. Of 205 patients, 52 had prosthetic grafts placed, whereas the remainder received vein grafts. Infection rates were equivalent in these two groups. Wound infection rates were 0% for topical administration alone and systemic administration alone, 5.9% for patients receiving both, and 24.5% for controls. A differentiation between graft (Szilagyi class III) and isolated wound (Szilagyi class I and II) infections was not made. Minimum follow-up was 4 weeks, but the mean length of follow-up was not indicated. Patients in whom synthetic graft material was used did not experience a higher incidence of wound infection. The authors concluded that topical and systemic prophylaxis were equally efficacious, and that combined prophylaxis was unnecessary.[84] The follow-up interval in this study, however, was not long enough to make conclusive statements.

The benefit of a short course of systemic cephalosporin prophylaxis in vascular reconstructive surgery was subsequently confirmed in a number of other prospective, randomized trials. In 1983, Salzmann[85] reported a trial of cefuroxime (a second-generation agent) and later cefotaxime (a third-generation agent) versus placebo in 300 patients undergoing aortofemoropopliteal reconstruction. The prophylaxis regimen was changed from cefuroxime to cefotaxime midway through the study because the latter was found to be more effective in vitro against the most common graft infection pathogens at the author's institution. Graft infection rates were 2.4% for the placebo group and 0.8% for the prophylaxis group. The incidence of wound infection was 15.1% in the placebo group and 3.0% in the prophylaxis group. No differences in infection rates were noted between the two antibiotics, and the author concluded that either agent could be used effectively in the prophylaxis of postoperative infection.[85]

Addressing the question of duration of treatment for antibiotic prophylaxis, Hasselgren and colleagues[86] compared 1- and 3-day courses of cefuroxime versus placebo in lower extremity arterial reconstruction. There was only one graft infection in this small cohort of 110 patients, and this occurred in the placebo group. The wound infection rate was 16.7% for patients receiving placebo, compared with 3.8% in the 1-day and 4.3% in the 3-day prophylaxis groups. The investigators recommended that prophylactic antibiotic therapy be limited to a short-term course.[86]

Bennion and colleagues[87] examined the utility of antibiotic prophylaxis in patients with chronic renal insufficiency undergoing placement of a prosthetic arteriovenous shunt for hemodialysis. Patients were randomized to receive cefamandole or placebo just before placement of a PTFE graft, followed by two subsequent doses. The wound infection rate for the cefamandole group was 10.5% (2/19), with one graft (Szilagyi class III) infection. The wound infection rate in the placebo group was 42.1% (8/19), with three graft infections.[87] This high rate of infection is not uncommon in renal failure patients, and the study emphasizes the importance of perioperative antibiotic prophylaxis.

Robbs and associates[88] reported a trial of cloxacillin plus gentamicin versus cefotaxime in infrainguinal arterial reconstruction. This group had adopted a 48-hour course of cloxacillin plus gentamycin as their routine prophylaxis due to the predominance of *S. aureus* and gram-negative infections at their institution. Length of follow-up ranged from 6 to 20 months. The wound infection and graft infection rates for patients receiving cloxacillin plus gentamycin were 5.4% (7/129 wounds) and 1.5% (1/63 grafts), respectively. The rates for patients receiving cefotaxime were 6.2% (8/127 wounds) and 3.3% (2/61 grafts). The differences were not statistically significant. The authors concluded that the multiagent 2-day regimen conferred no advantage over the shorter, single-agent regimen.[88]

Comparisons of Antibiotic Regimens

Because it has become evident that a short course of a cephalosporin antibiotic is the ideal prophylaxis for vascular reconstructive procedures, several studies have focused on whether the most widely used cephalosporin, cefazolin, is the most desirable choice. A large number of graft infections, particularly in abdominal grafts, are due to gram-negative rods. A theoretical disadvantage of first-generation cephalosporins such as cefazolin is the fact they are more vulnerable to gram-negative β-lactamase than second- and third-generation agents. Gram-negative activity is thus limited to *E. coli, Proteus,* and *Klebsiella,* and many hospital-acquired strains of these organisms are cefazolin-resistant. It has also been demonstrated that other cephalosporins such as the second-generation agent cefamandole have greater in vitro activities against coagulase-negative staphylococci, which have been found to colonize the native arterial wall in a large number of patients. It is clear from previous studies by Salzmann,[85] and by Hasselgren[86] and Robbs[88] and their coworkers, that second- and third-generation cephalosporins may be used effectively in vascular surgery prophylaxis.

In 1989, Lalka and colleagues examined this issue in a prospective study of arterial wall microbiology and antibiotic penetration.[65] Forty-seven patients undergoing aortofemoropopliteal reconstruction were randomized to receive perioperative cefazolin or cefamandole, 1 g every 6 hours for nine doses. Serial samples of serum, subcutaneous fat, thrombus, atheroma, and arterial wall were obtained for culture and assay of drug levels by high-performance liquid chromatography. Serum and tissue levels of cefazolin were significantly higher than those of cefamandole at almost all time points. Positive arterial wall cultures were obtained in 41.4% of patients, and 68.8% of bacterial isolates were coagulase-negative staphylococci (half of these were slime producers). The arterial wall concentration of both antibiotics at times fell below the geometric mean minimal inhibitory concentration (MIC) for all organisms combined, but this occurred significantly more often with cefamandole. The conclusion was drawn that both antibiotics needed to be administered in larger doses (cefazolin, 1.5 g every 4 hours; cefamandole, 2 g every 3 hours), and that the antibiotics were essentially equal in efficacy if administered appropriately. The investigators corroborated the findings of Mutch and colleagues,[89] that serum antibiotic levels did not correlate well with aortic tissue concentrations of bioactive antibiotic, and suggested that arterial tissue levels rather than serum levels should be a standard for comparison of antibiotic efficacy.[65]

Edwards and colleagues,[90] in 1992, reported a prospective trial of cefazolin versus the more β-lactamase-stable second-generation cephalosporin cefuroxime in patients undergoing aortic and peripheral vascular reconstruction. Prior studies had suggested that some failures of cefazolin prophylaxis were due to the susceptibility of this agent to staphylococcal β-lactamase, and that other cephalosporins may provide better protection than cefazolin in cardiac surgery.[55, 91, 92] Antibiotics were administered just before surgery, redosed intraoperatively, and continued every 6 hours postoperatively for 24 hours. Dosage and administration schedules were based on a prior pharmacokinetic study. The infection rate in the cefazolin group was 1% (3/287) versus 2.6% (7/272) in the cefuroxime group. This difference was not statistically significant. Cefuroxime exhibited lower trough concentrations than cefazolin, and the length of the operative procedure was found to be a risk factor for infection only in the cefuroxime group. The investigators concluded that cefazolin provides better perioperative prophylaxis, despite its lower resistance to β-lactamase, due to its greater antistaphylococcal potency and superior pharmacokinetic profile.[90] Data from this and other studies[55] suggest that intraoperative redosing of cefazolin in prolonged procedures should be more frequent than in routine therapeutic administration, that is, every 4 rather than every 6 hours.

Current Status of Antibiotic Prophylaxis

Antibiotic Selection

Cefazolin is currently the antibiotic of choice for routine vascular surgery prophylaxis. It is relatively inexpensive, has negligible toxicity and a low incidence of severe allergic reactions, and is active against many of the bacteria commonly implicated in graft infection (Tables 10–4 and 10–5). Its pharmacokinetic profile is ideal for this indication, with reliably high peak serum concentrations and a long half-life of elimination compared with other cephalosporins.[90, 93] It penetrates arterial tissue well with drug concentrations exceeding the MIC of common graft infection pathogens in most instances.[65] Cefazolin is active against *S. aureus* (including penicillinase-producing strains), some strains of *S. epidermidis,* and the more commonly encountered gram-negative rods: *E. coli, Proteus,* and *Klebsiella.* Most other gram-negative rods are resistant, including indole-positive *Proteus vulgaris.* Cephalothin, the other first-generation agent in common clinical use, is somewhat more resistant to staphylococcal β-lactamase, yet it is less active against gram-negative organisms. More important, it is cleared from plasma four to five times as rapidly as cefazolin.[93]

Later generation cephalosporins have greater gram-negative activity and the potential benefit of increased resistance to staphylococcal β-lactamase; however, in vitro and in vivo activity against gram-positive cocci is reduced. Many investigators have tailored their choice of antibiotic to the predominant organisms responsible for graft infection at their particular institution. Cefamandole,[65] cefuroxime,[94] and cefotaxime[88] have all been used effectively as prophylactic agents in prospective trials. However, cefamandole has fallen out of favor for routine use due to an association with hypoprothrombinemia and bleeding, particularly in

TABLE 10–4

Wound Infections among Patients Receiving Cefazolin or Placebo Prophylaxis

PROPHYLAXIS	INFECTIONS (n)	PATIENTS (n)	INFECTED (%)	INFECTIONS BY CATEGORY (%)		
				Class I	Class II	Class III
Cefazolin	2	225	0.9°	0	2	0
Placebo	16	237	6.8°	4	8	4
Total	18	462	3.9			

°Difference is significant at $P < .001$. Brachiocephalic procedures are not included.
From Kaiser AB, Clayson KR, Mulherin JL, et al: Antibiotic prophylaxis in vascular surgery. Ann Surg 188:283–289, 1978.

elderly patients and those with renal insufficiency. Cefuroxime has been shown to have antistaphylococcal potency and pharmacokinetic properties inferior to those of cefazolin.[90] The third-generation agents such as cefotaxime have broad anti–gram-negative activity but are generally less active against staphylococci. Moreover, the later generation cephalosporins are, in most instances, significantly more expensive than the first-generation agents. Cefazolin, therefore, remains the antibiotic of choice, except in specific instances where in vitro testing has revealed that another agent more adequately covers the principal pathogens of graft infection.

A potential disadvantage with cefazolin prophylaxis is the inconsistent activity of this agent against the organism that is currently responsible for the greatest number of graft infections, *S. epidermidis*. It has been shown that during hospitalization patients acquire multiply resistant strains of this bacterium.[95, 96] Up to 75% of *S. epidermidis* isolates at some institutions are now cefazolin resistant. Vancomycin is highly active against both *S. epidermidis* and *S. aureus*; resistance in these organisms is rarely encountered. Vancomycin, however, provides no gram-negative coverage. It is the drug of choice for prophylaxis in patients with a history of anaphylaxis to β-lactam antibiotics, often in combination with an aminoglycoside in procedures in which there is significant risk of gram-negative infection, such as aortic reconstruction. Vancomycin is also considered the antibiotic of choice for the prophylaxis of prosthetic hemodialysis access grafts, and for patients known to be colonized with methicillin-resistant *S. aureus*. It is excreted primarily by glomerular filtration and therefore persists in high serum concentrations in patients with end-stage renal disease.

The broad antibacterial spectrum, excellent tissue penetration, and low toxicity of the fluoroquinolones make them potentially ideal agents for the prophylaxis of surgical infections. Limited data are available concerning the use of fluoroquinolones for this indication, but there are reports of efficacy equal or superior to that of cephalosporin antibiotics in the prophylaxis of colorectal,[97, 98] biliary,[97, 99] and urologic surgery.[100–102] Auger and coauthors[103] reported a randomized study of pefloxacin, a nalidixic acid analog, and cefazolin in patients undergoing cardiac surgery. Of 111 patients, 14 receiving pefloxacin developed bacterial colonization at culture sites compared with 11 in the cefazolin group. One patient who received cefazolin developed mediastinitis from a cefazolin-resistant strain of *S. epidermidis*. As yet, there are no published clinical trials of a fluoroquinolone versus a cephalosporin in the prophylaxis of peripheral vascular surgery procedures.

Antibiotic Administration

Prophylactic antibiotics are administered just before surgery and redosed intraoperatively during long procedures.

TABLE 10–5

Antibacterial Spectrum of Selected Antibiotics

ANTIBIOTIC	ANTIBACTERIAL ACTIVITY (MIC-90 in µg/mL)*				
	S. aureus	S. epidermidis	E. coli	Klebsiella spp.	Pseudomonas spp.
Cefazolin	1.0	0.8	5.0	6.0	R
Cephalothin	1.0	0.5	5.0	32.0	R
Cefamandole	1.0	2.0	4.0	8.0	R
Cefuroxime	2.0	1.0	4.0	R	R
Cefotaxime	2.0	8.0	0.25	0.25	>32.0
Vancomycin	1.0	3.0	R	R	R
Penicillin V	ALP (+): >25.0	0.02†	R	R	R
	ALP (−): 0.03				
Oxacillin	0.25	0.2†	R	R	R
Gentamicin	0.6†	2.0†	4.0	1.0	2.0
Ciprofloxacin	0.5	0.25	0.03	0.125	0.5
Rifampin	0.015	0.015	16.0	32.0	64.0

*MIC-90 is the minimal inhibitory concentration for 90% of strains. MIC >64 µg/mL is considered resistant. Values are approximate and may vary among institutions.
†Many strains are resistant.
R, resistant; ALP, alkaline phosphatase.
Data from Mandell, RGD (ed): Principles and Practice of Infectious Diseases, 3rd ed, New York, Churchill Livingstone, 1989.

Pharmacokinetic studies suggest that prophylactic antibiotics should be administered more frequently and in higher doses during surgery than is recommended for routine therapeutic indications (e.g., cefazolin 1.5 g every 4 hours).[55, 90, 104] Prophylaxis is usually continued postoperatively for up to 24 hours, and possibly longer when the theoretical risk exists of postoperative bacteremia from indwelling venous catheters, arterial lines, bladder catheters, endotracheal tubes, and so on. The advantage of continuing coverage beyond the operating room, however, has not been clearly demonstrated. In the absence of these risk factors, there is clearly no advantage in extending antibiotic prophylaxis for longer than 24 hours.

Regimens of prophylaxis should be tailored to the type of vascular reconstruction that is undertaken. Cefazolin prophylaxis is recommended in all procedures involving the placement of prosthetic materials. It is probably not necessary in "clean" vascular procedures of the neck and upper extremities that do not involve the use of synthetic grafts. In contrast, the marked colonization and favorable bacterial environment of the lower abdomen and groin necessitate the use of antibiotic prophylaxis in all aortofemoropopliteal vascular procedures. The risk of gram-negative infection in aortic reconstruction may necessitate the addition of an aminoglycoside, particularly in institutions with a high degree of cefazolin resistance among gram-negative isolates. Alternatively, a second- or third-generation cephalosporin with broader anti–gram-negative activity may be substituted, as this obviates the risk of aminoglycoside-associated nephrotoxicity.

Cephalosporins should be avoided in patients with a history of anaphylaxis to β-lactam antibiotics. Patients with a history of minor allergic reactions to penicillin antibiotics may be given a cephalosporin test dose to determine if cross-reactivity is present. Reduced dosing of cefazolin and most other cephalosporins is recommended in renal insufficiency, based on the calculated creatinine clearance.

There is evidence that remote bacteremia may be implicated in vascular graft infection. Accordingly, oral prophylaxis for procedures that are highly associated with bacteremia, such as tooth extraction, cystoscopy, and colonoscopy, is recommended. Wooster and colleagues[58] demonstrated an incidence of bacteremia in 200 vascular surgery patients undergoing cystoscopy of 64% among inpatients and 8% in outpatients. For procedures such as tooth extraction and colonoscopy, prophylaxis must be tailored to the most common normal flora of the traumatized site. Penicillins are appropriate choices for major dental procedures, whereas broader gram-negative and anaerobic coverage may be warranted in colonoscopy. It should be emphasized, however, that the true risk of graft infection after procedures associated with bacteremia is unclear, and there is currently no consensus on the role of antibiotic prophylaxis in this setting.

References

1. Rokitansky K: Handbuch der pathologischen Anatomie, 2nd ed. 1844, p 55.
2. Koch L: Über Aneurysma der Arteriae mesenterichae superioris [dissertation]. Erlangen, 1851.
3. Osler W: The Gulstonian lectures on malignant endocarditis. BMJ 1:467, 1885.
4. Crane A: Primary multilocular mycotic aneurysm of the aorta. Arch Pathol 24:634, 1937.
5. Ponfick E: Über embolische Aneurysmen, nebst Bemerkungen über das acute Herzaneurysma (Herzgeschwur). Virchows Arch 58:528, 1873.
6. Eppinger H: Pathogenese (Histogeneses und Aetiologie) der Aneurysmen einschliesslich des Aneurysma equiverminosum. Arch Klin Chir 35:404, 1887.
7. Weisel J: Die Erkrankungen arterieller Gefässe im Verlaufe akuter Infektionen. Z Heilkd 27:269, 1916.
8. Lewis D, Schrager V: Embolomycotic aneurysms. JAMA 53:1808, 1909.
9. Cathcart R: False aneurysms of the femoral artery following typhoid fever. South Med J 2:593, 1909.
10. Revell S: Primary mycotic aneurysms. Ann Intern Med 22:431, 1943.
11. Hawkins J, Yeager G: Primary mycotic aneurysm. Surgery 40:747, 1956.
12. Yellin A: Ruptured mycotic aneurysm, a complication of parenteral drug abuse. Arch Surg 112:981, 1977.
13. Lande A, Beckman Y: Aortitis—pathologic, clinical and arteriographic review. Radiol Clin North Am 14:219, 1976.
14. Hirst AJ, Affeldt J: Abdominal aortic aneurysm with rupture into the duodenum: A report of eight cases. Gastroenterology 10:504, 1951.
15. Reddy DJ, Ernst CB: Infected aneurysms: Recognition and management. Semin Vasc Surg 1:541–547, 1984.
16. Brown SL, Busuttil RW, Baker JD, et al: Bacteriologic and surgical determinants of survival in patients with mycotic aneurysms. J Vasc Surg 1:541–547, 1984.
17. Stengal A, Wolferth C: Mycotic (bacterial) aneurysms of intravascular origin. Arch Intern Med 31:527, 1923.
18. Magilligan D, Quinn E: Active infective endocarditis. In Magilligan DJ, Quinn E (eds): Endocarditis: Medical and Surgical Management. New York, Marcel Dekker, 1986, p 207.
19. Wilson S, Van Wagenen P, Passaro EJ: Arterial infection. Curr Probl Surg 15:5–89, 1978.
20. Bennett D, Cherry J: Bacterial infection of aortic aneurysms: A clinicopathological study. Am J Surg 113:321, 1967.
21. Jarrett F, Darling R, Mundth E, et al: Experience with infected aneurysms of the abdominal aorta. Arch Surg 10:1281, 1975.
22. Ernst C, Campbell H, Daugherty M, et al: Incidence and significance of intra-operative bacterial cultures during abdominal aortic aneurysmectomy. Ann Surg 185:626–633, 1977.
23. Reddy D, Smith R, Elliot JJ, et al: Infected femoral artery false aneurysms in drug addicts: Evolution of selective vascular reconstruction. J Vasc Surg 3:718, 1986.
24. Wakefield T, Pierson C, Schoberg D, et al: Artery, periarterial adipose tissue, and blood microbiology during vascular reconstructive surgery: Perioperative and postoperative observations. J Vasc Surg 11:624–628, 1990.
25. Chan F, Crawford E, Coselli J, et al: In situ prosthetic graft replacement for mycotic aneurysm of the aorta. Ann Thorac Surg 47:193–203, 1989.
26. Crawford E, Crawford J: Diseases of the Aorta Including an Atlas of Angiographic Pathology and Surgical Techniques. Baltimore, Williams & Wilkins, 1984.
27. Mundth E, Darling R, Alvarado RH, et al: Surgical management of mycotic aneurysms and the complications of infections in vascular reconstructive surgery. Am J Surg 110:460, 1969.
28. Kaufman J, Smith R, Capel G, et al: Antibiotic therapy for arterial infection: Lessons from the successful treatment of a mycotic femoral artery aneurysm without surgical reconstruction. Ann Vasc Surg 4:592, 1990.
29. Ewart J, Burke M, Bunt T: Spontaneous abdominal aortic infections. Essentials of diagnosis and management. Am Surg 49:37–49, 1983.
30. Johnson J, Ledgerwood A, Lucas C: Mycotic aneurysms: New concepts in therapy. Arch Surg 118:577–582, 1983.
31. Patel K, Semel L, Clauss R: Routine revascularization with resection of infected femoral pseudoaneurysm from substance abuse. J Vasc Surg 8:322–328, 1988.

32. Wright D, Shepard A: Infected femoral artery aneurysm associated with drug abuse. In Stanley J, Ernst C (eds): Current Therapy in Vascular Surgery. Philadelphia, BC Decker, 1990, pp 350–353.

33. Hoffert P, Gensler S, Haimovichi H: Infection complicating arterial grafts. Arch Surg 90:427–435, 1965.

34. Fry WJ, Lindenauer SM: Infection complicating the use of plastic arterial implants. Arch Surg 94:600–609, 1967.

35. Szilagyi DE, Smith RF, Elliott JP, Vrandecic MP: Infection in arterial reconstruction with synthetic grafts. Ann Surg 106:321–323, 1972.

36. Lorentzen JE, Nielsen OM, Arendrup H: Vascular graft infection: An analysis of sixty-two graft infections in 2411 consecutively implanted synthetic vascular grafts. Surgery 98:81–86, 1985.

37. Goldstone J, Moore WS: Infection in vascular prostheses: Clinical manifestations and surgical management. Am J Surg 128:225–233, 1974.

38. Bandyk D, Berni G, Thiele B, Towne J: Aortofemoral graft infection due to *Staphylococcus epidermidis*. Arch Surg 119:102–108, 1984.

39. Jamieson G, DeWeese J, Rob C: Infected arterial grafts. Ann Surg 181:850–852, 1975.

40. Liekweg WG, Greenfield LJ: Vascular prosthetic infections: Collected experience and results of treatment. Surgery 81:335–342, 1977.

41. Lindenauer S, Fry W, Schaub G, Wild D: The use of antibiotics in the prevention of vascular graft infections. Surgery 62:487–492, 1967.

42. Yashar J, Weyman A, Burnard R, Yashar J: Survival and limb salvage in patients with infected arterial prostheses. Am J Surg 135:499–504, 1978.

43. Buchbinder D, Pasch AR, Rollins DL, et al: Results of arterial reconstruction of the foot. Arch Surg 121:673–677, 1986.

44. Edwards MJ, Richardson D, Klamer TW: Management of aortic prosthetic infections. Am J Surg 155:327–330, 1988.

45. O'Hara PJ, Hertzer NR, Beven EG, Krajewski LP: Surgical management of infected abdominal aortic grafts: Review of a 25-year experience. J Vasc Surg 3:725–731, 1986.

46. Reilly L, Stoney R, Goldstone J, Ehrenfeld W: Improved management of aortic graft infection: The influence of operation sequence and staging. J Vasc Surg 5:421–431, 1987.

47. Reilly LM, Altman H, Lusby RJ, et al: Late results following surgical management of vascular graft infection. J Vasc Surg 1:36–44, 1984.

48. Yeager R, McConnell D, Sasaki T, Vetto R: Aortic and peripheral prosthetic graft infection: Differential management and causes of mortality. Am J Surg 150:36–41, 1985.

49. Samson RH, Veith FJ, Janko GS, et al: A modified classification and approach to the management of infections involving peripheral arterial prosthetic grafts. J Vasc Surg 8:147–153, 1988.

50. Conn J, Hardy J, Chavez C, et al: Infected arterial grafts. Ann Surg 101:704–712, 1970.

51. Elek S, Conen P: The virulence of *Staphylococcus pyogenes* for man. A study of the problems of wound infection. Br J Exp Pathol 38:573–586, 1957.

52. Smith R, Lowry K, Perdue G: Management of the infected arterial prosthesis in the lower extremity. Am Surg 33:711–714, 1967.

53. Edwards W, Martin R, Jenkins J, et al: Primary graft infections. J Vasc Surg 6:235–239, 1987.

54. Quiñones-Baldrich WJ, Hernandez JJ, Moore WS: Long-term results following surgical management of aortic graft infection. Arch Surg 126:507–511, 1991.

55. Kaiser A, Clayson K, Mulherin J: Antibiotic prophylaxis in vascular surgery. Ann Surg 188:283–289, 1978.

56. Close A, Stengel B, Love H: Preoperative skin preparation with povidine-iodine. Am J Surg 108:398–401, 1964.

57. Cruse P: A five-year prospective study of 23,649 surgical wounds. Arch Surg 107:206–210, 1973.

58. Wooster D, Louch R, Kradjen S: Intraoperative bacterial contamination of vascular grafts: A prospective study. Can J Surg 28:407–409, 1985.

59. Bouhoutsos J, Chavatsas D, Martin P, Morris T: Infected synthetic arterial grafts. Br J Surg 108–111, 1974.

60. Scobie K, McPhail N, Barber G, Elder R: Bacteriologic monitoring in abdominal aortic surgery. Can J Surg 22:368–371, 1979.

61. DeBakey M, Ochsner J, Cooley D: Associated intraabdominal lesions encountered during resection of aortic aneurysms: surgical considerations. Dis Colon Rectum 3:485–489, 1960.

62. Stoll W: Surgery for intraabdominal lesions associated with resection of aortic aneurysms. WMJ 65:89–90, 1966.

63. Hardy J, Tompkins W, Chavez C, Conn J: Combining intra-abdominal arterial grafting with gastrointestinal or biliary tract procedure. Am J Surg 126:598–600, 1973.

64. Becker R, Blundell P: Infected aortic bifurcation grafts: Experience with 14 patients. Surgery 80:544–549, 1976.

65. Lalka S, Malone J, Fisher D, et al: Efficacy of prophylactic antibiotics in vascular surgery: An arterial wall microbiologic and pharmacokinetic perspective. J Vasc Surg 10:501–510, 1989.

66. Buckels J, Fielding J, Black J, et al: Significance of positive bacterial cultures from aortic aneurysm contents. Br J Surg 72:440–442, 1985.

67. Macbeth G, Rubin J, McIntyre KJG, Malone J: The relevance of arterial wall microbiology to the treatment of prosthetic graft infections: Graft infection vs arterial infection. J Vasc Surg 1:750–756, 1984.

68. Durham J, Malone J, Bernhard V: The impact of multiple operations on the importance of arterial wall cultures. J Vasc Surg 5:160–169, 1987.

69. Moore WS, Chvapil M, Sieffert G, Keown K: Development of an infection resistant vascular prosthesis. Arch Surg 116:1403–1407, 1981.

70. White J, Benvenisty A, Reemtsma K, et al: Simple methods for direct antibiotic protection of synthetic vascular grafts. J Vasc Surg 1:372–380, 1984.

71. Chervu A, Moore WS, Gelabert HA, et al: Prevention of graft infection by use of prostheses bonded with a rifampin/collagen release system. J Vasc Surg 14:521–525, 1991.

72. Bunt TJ, Mohr J: Incidence of positive inguinal lymph node cultures during peripheral revascularization. Am J Surg 50:522–523, 1984.

73. Johnson JA, Cogbill TH, Strutt PJ, Gundersen AL: Wound complications after infrainguinal bypass. Classification, predisposing factors, and management. Arch Surg 123:859–862, 1988.

74. Kwaan J, Dahl R, Connolly J: Immunocompetence in patients with prosthetic graft infection. J Vasc Surg 1:45–49, 1984.

75. Pulaski E, Schaeffer J: The background of antibiotic therapy in surgical infections. Surg Gynecol Obstet 93:1–6, 1951.

76. Pulaski E: Discriminate antibiotic prophylaxis in elective surgery. Surg Gynecol Obstet 108:385–388, 1959.

77. Linton R: The appropriate use of antibiotics in clean surgery. Surg Gynecol Obstet 112:218–220, 1961.

78. Altemeier W, Culbertson W, Vetto M: Prophylactic antibiotic therapy. Arch Surg 71:2–6, 1955.

79. Altemeier W, Culbertson W, Sherman R, et al: Critical re-evaluation of antibiotic therapy in surgery. JAMA 157:305–309, 1955.

80. Alexander J, McGloin J, Altemeier W: Penicillin prophylaxis in experimental wound infections. Surg Forum 11:299–300, 1960.

81. Alexander J, Altemeier W: Penicillin prophylaxis of experimental staphylococcal wound infection. Surg Gynecol Obstet 120:243–254, 1965.

82. Moore W, Rosson C, Hall A: Effect of prophylactic antibiotics in preventing bacteremic infection in vascular prostheses. Surgery 69:825–828, 1971.

83. Perdue G: Antibiotics as an aid in the prevention of infections after peripheral arterial surgery. Am Surg 41:296–300, 1975.

84. Pitt H, Postier R, MacGowan W, et al: Prophylactic antibiotics in vascular surgery. Ann Surg 192:356–364, 1980.

85. Salzmann G: Perioperative infection prophylaxis in vascular surgery: A randomized prospective study. Thorac Cardiovasc Surg 31:239–242, 1983.

86. Hasselgren P, Ivarsson L, Risberg B, Seeman T: Effects of prophylactic antibiotics in vascular surgery. Ann Surg 200:86–92, 1984.

87. Bennion R, Hiatt J, Williams R, et al: A randomized prospective study of perioperative microbial prophylaxis for vascular surgery. J Cardiovasc Surg 26:270–274, 1985.

88. Robbs J, Reddy E, Ray R: Antibiotic prophylaxis in aortic and peripheral arterial surgery in the presence of infected extremity lesions. Drugs 35(Suppl 2):141–150, 1988.

89. Mutch D, Richards G, Brown R, et al: Bioactive antibiotic levels in the human aorta. Surgery 92:1068–1071, 1982.

90. Edwards W, Kaiser A, Kernodle D, et al: Cefuroxime versus cefazolin as prophylaxis in vascular surgery. J Vasc Surg 15:35–42, 1992.

91. Kernodle D, Classen D, Burke J, et al: Failure of cephalosporins to prevent surgical wound infections. JAMA 263:961–966, 1990.

92. Slama T, Sklar S, Misinski J, et al: Randomized comparison of cefamandole, cefazolin, and cefuroxime in open-heart surgery. Antimicrob Agents Chemother 29:744–747, 1986.

93. Mandell G, Sande M: Penicillins, cephalosporins and other beta-lactam antibiotics. In Gilman A, Rall T, Nies A, Taylor P (eds): Goodman and Gilman's The Pharmacologic Basis of Therapeutics, 8th ed. Elmsford, NY, Pergamon Press, 1990, pp 1065–1097.

94. Herbst A, Kamme C, Norgren L, et al: Infections and antibiotic prophylaxis in reconstructive vascular surgery. Br J Vasc Surg 3:303–307, 1989.

95. Levy M, Schmitt D, Edmiston C, et al: Sequential analysis of staphylococcal colonization of body surfaces of patients undergoing vascular surgery. J Clin Microbiol 28:664–669, 1990.

96. Archer G, Tenenbaum M: Antibiotic-resistant *Staphylococcus epidermidis* in patients undergoing cardiac surgery. Antimicrob Agents Chemother 10:269–272, 1980.

97. Cooreman F, Ghyselen J, Penninckx F: Pefloxacin vs. cefuroxime for prophylaxis of infections after elective colorectal surgery. Rev Infect Dis 11(Suppl 5):S1301, 1989.

98. Offer C, Weuta H, Bodner E: Efficacy of perioperative prophylaxis with ciprofloxacin of cefazolin in colorectal surgery. Infection 16(Suppl 1):S46–S47, 1988.

99. Kujath P: Brief report: Antibiotic prophylaxis in biliary tract surgery: Ciprofloxacin vs. ceftriaxone. Am J Med 87(Suppl 5A):255S–257S, 1989.

100. Gombert M, DuBouchet L, Aulicino T, et al: Brief report: Intravenous ciprofloxacin versus cefotaxime prophylaxis during transurethral surgery. Am J Med 87(Suppl 5A):250S–251S, 1989.

101. Cox C: Comparison of intravenous ciprofloxacin and intravenous cefotaxime for antimicrobial prophylaxis in transurethral surgery. Am J Med 87(Suppl 5A):252S–254S, 1989.

102. Christensen M, Nielsen K, Knes J, et al: Brief report: Single-dose preoperative prophylaxis in transurethral surgery: Ciprofloxacin versus cefotaxime. Am J Med 87(Suppl 5A):258S–260S, 1989.

103. Auger P, Leclerc Y, Pelletier L, et al: Efficacy and safety of pefloxacin vs. cefazolin as prophylaxis in elective cardiovascular surgery. Rev Infect Dis 11(Suppl 5):S1302–S1303, 1989.

104. Guglielmo B, Salazar T, Rodondi L, et al: Altered pharmacokinetics of antibiotics during vascular surgery. Am J Surg 157:410–412, 1989.

105. Casali R, Tucker W, Thompson B, Read R: Infected prosthetic grafts. Arch Surg 115:577–580, 1980.

106. Schwartz J, Powell T, Burnham S, Johnson G Jr: Culture of abdominal aortic aneurysm contents, an additional series. Arch Surg 122:777–780, 1987.

107. Ilgenfritz F, Jordan F: Microbiological monitoring of aortic aneurysm wall and contents during aneurysmectomy. Arch Surg 123:506–508, 1988.

108. Brandimarte C, Santini C, Venditti M, et al: Clinical significance of intraoperative cultures of aneurysm walls and contents in elective abdominal aortic aneurysmectomy. Eur J Epidemiol 5:521–525, 1989.

109. McAuley C, Steed D, Webster M: Bacterial presence in aortic thrombus at elective aneurysm resection: Is it clinically significant? Am J Surg 147:322–324, 1984.

Questions

1. Arterial trauma is involved in the pathogenesis of most primary arterial infections. True or false?

2. Prosthetic grafts should be used to replace excised mycotic aneurysms
   (a) if the surgical field is laved with antibiotics
   (b) in the upper extremities
   (c) only if absolutely necessary
   (d) in fungal arterial infections
   (e) never

3. Since 1965, the most common organism associated with microbial aortitis is
   (a) *Salmonella* species
   (b) fungi
   (c) mycobacteria
   (d) *Pseudomonas* species
   (e) *Staphylococcus aureus*

4. In the management of a mycotic mesenteric aneurysm located in the distal arterial arcade (adjacent to the intestine), the recommended management is
   (a) reconstruction with Dacron graft
   (b) reconstruction with PTFE graft
   (c) reconstruction with umbilical vein graft
   (d) reconstruction with vein graft
   (e) ligation and excision without reconstruction

5. The recommended management of an infrarenal mycotic aneurysm involves the use of antibiotics, débridement of infected tissues, and reconstruction through a remote (extra-anatomic), uninfected field. True or false?

6. What is the average reported incidence of prosthetic graft infection?
   (a) 1% to 6%
   (b) 6% to 10%
   (c) 10% to 15%
   (d) greater than 15%
   (e) 0% to 1%

7. The study by Pitt and colleagues revealed that intravenous antibiotics were much more effective than antibiotic irrigation. True or false?

8. Risk factors for prosthetic graft infection include which of the following?
   (a) multiple reoperations
   (b) inguinal incisions
   (c) open, infected wounds on the extremities
   (d) prior graft infections
   (e) positive arterial wall cultures

9. Avenues of infection include which of the following?
   (a) the skin
   (b) the arterial wall
   (c) open wounds on the distal limb
   (d) intestinal transudate accumulated during an aortic bypass
   (e) the Foley catheter

10. What are the most common organisms found in prosthetic graft infections?
    (a) *Proteus* species
    (b) *Escherichia coli*
    (c) *Staphylococcus aureus*
    (d) *Streptococcus viridans*
    (e) *Staphylococcus epidermidis*

Answers

1. true   2. c   3. a   4. e   5. true   6. a   7. false   8. all of them   9. all of them   10. e

11

Congenital Vascular Malformations of the Extremities

Robert B. Rutherford and Janette D. Durham

Congenital vascular malformations (CVMs) comprise a spectrum of developmental abnormalities that may involve all components of the peripheral circulation: arteries, veins, capillaries, and lymphatics. The majority of clinically significant lesions contain primarily arterial and venous elements. Predominantly venous defects are the most common, accounting for almost half of those discovered in children,[1] but because they produce less severe clinical manifestations, they do not predominate in reported series of CVMs that receive interventional treatment (surgery or embolotherapy). Although anomalous lymphatic elements are frequently intermixed with arteriovenous (AV) anomalies, pure lymphatic congenital lesions (e.g., lymphoceles) are infrequently seen. Understandably, therefore, the greatest emphasis in this chapter is on AV malformations (AVMs), which make up just over one third of all CVMs.[1]

Structurally dissimilar CVMs may appear in clinically similar ways. For example, enlarged or swollen legs can result from lymphatic anomalies, pure venous dysplasias, or AVMs, and varicose veins and local signs of venous hypertension can result from either of the latter two. The different etiologies obviously warrant different therapeutic approaches. Therefore, the crux of CVM management lies in the appropriate application of diagnostic tools to arrive at a precise diagnosis. This allows confident and early prognostic projections to be made and guides the selective and properly timed use of appropriate therapeutic interventions. The aims of this chapter are (1) to describe the incidence, etiology, classification, and clinical presentation of CVMs; (2) to propose the appropriate use of a diagnostic approach that has practical advantages over angiography alone; and (3) to discuss the relative merits of current therapeutic options with suggestions for their clinical use.

Arteriovenous malformations are that subset of CVMs that contain both arterial and venous components, but the most common and clinically important AVMs are those containing arteriovenous fistulas (AVFs), which shunt a significant amount of blood directly from artery to vein, bypassing the nutritive capillary bed. Ninety percent of AVMs occur in the extremities, pelvis, body shell of the trunk, and shoulder girdle. The anatomic sites of involvement are shown in Table 11–1. Congenital CVMs with major AV shunting are particularly problematic because they (1) tend to enlarge with time, (2) may steal blood from the distal extremity, (3) cause continual venous hypertension, and (4) may even increase cardiovascular demand. A major focus of this chapter, therefore, is on the diagnostic evaluation of AVMs, emphasizing the identification and quantification of AV shunt flow. This emphasis carries over into the management strategies proposed.

INCIDENCE

CVMs are rare, unless one includes capillary or cavernous hemangiomas of such little consequence that medical attention for diagnosis or intervention is not sought. Thus, they account for only 1 in 10,000 hospital admissions, and with an increasingly conservative approach to therapy, even this may decrease. In the Heim Pal Hospital for Children in Budapest, Hungary, the prevalence was 1.2%, greater than that for congenital heart defects, spina bifida, or cleft lip.[1] However, the literature is weighted by symptomatic or grossly evident cases presented for evaluation for some interventional treatment. Possibly because of this, no American authors have reported experiences exceeding 100 cases. One of the largest personal experiences with congenital AVMs, reported by Szilagyi, and colleagues,[2] was 82 cases and was accumulated over 22 years, between 1952 and 1974 (approximately four new cases a year in a center known for its expertise on this subject). European experiences, often including all CVMs, are significantly larger.[3] Most vascular surgeons see far fewer cases, and the relative rarity of CVMs means that individual surgeons are unlikely to develop a meaningful personal experience with them and may also have difficulty finding reliable therapeutic recommendations in the literature.

TABLE 11-1

Anatomic Sites of Involvement

ARTERY	CASES
Femoral	30
Iliac	20
Popliteal	8
Radial	4
Radial and ulnar	4
Anterior and posterior tibial	4
Anterior tibial	3
Posterior tibial	2
Subclavian	2
Ulnar	2
Axillary	2
Brachial	1
Total	82

From Szilagyi DE, Smith RF, Elliott JP, Hageman JH: Congenital arteriovenous anomalies of the limbs. Arch Surg 111:423–429, 1976.

NOMENCLATURE

The plethora of names applied over time to CVMs reflects their wide spectrum of clinical presentations, which vary from subtle, asymptomatic birthmarks or scattered varicosities to grotesquely deformed extremities and hemodynamic compromise. The long list of designations also reflects a futile attempt by earlier physicians to reduce the protean clinical manifestations into distinct entities. These names include hemangioma simplex, angioma telangiectaticum, hemangioma cavernosum, strawberry birthmark, nevus angiectoides, port-wine mark, angioma arteriole racemosum or plexiform, cirsoid aneurysm, serpentine aneurysm, congenital arteriovenous aneurysm, and congenital arteriovenous fistula. Some categories of lesions have acquired eponyms such as Klippel-Trenaunay syndrome[4] (varicose veins, enlarged limb, and a birthmark) and Parkes Weber syndrome[5] (the same triad *with* AV fistulas). This confusing diversity in nomenclature developed because early authors did not have the modern diagnostic tools by which to demonstrate that these visibly dissimilar lesions shared common vascular components. Reid[6] and Rienhoff[7] in the 1920s were the first to suggest that CVMs result from an arrest or misdirection in development of the primitive vascular system. Pursuit of this concept, soon aided by the frequent use of angiography, eventually allowed this archaic descriptive nomenclature to be replaced by simpler terms that reflect the common congenital etiology of CVMs and the stage and location of the responsible "errors" in embryonic development. Although a universally accepted nomenclature system has not yet been adopted, Szilagyi and coworkers,[2, 8] who originally authored the chapter on CVMs of the extremities in the early editions of this book, recommended one based on the embryologic development of the vascular system (see Classification).

EMBRYOLOGY OF ANGIOGENESIS

The vascular system first appears during the third gestational week as a network of interlacing blood spaces in the primitive mesenchyme.[9] The blood does not yet circulate in any organized fashion, and no separate arterial or venous channel can yet be identified. The vascular system gradually develops by processes of vascular coalescence and cellular differentiation, culminating in the appearance of separate arterial and venous conduits. This process was described by Woollard[10] in 1922 as a sequence that he divided into three stages. During the *undifferentiated* stage (I), primitive blood lakes coalesce into more organized capillary networks. No arterial or venous conduits can yet be recognized. During the *retiform* stage (II), the capillaries formed in stage I themselves coalesce into larger plexiform structures that are the progenitors of arterial and venous channels. During the *maturation* stage (III), histologically mature vascular channels and principal arterial stems appear. The capillary network that persists beyond fetal life into adulthood may be thought of as a remnant from the original blood lakes in stage I.

CLASSIFICATION

A number of classifications have been proposed for CVMs. Malan[11] proposed an elaborate and complete system to accommodate the numerous varieties of clinical lesions. A more workable system, proposed by deTakats[12] in 1931, is based on the concept that abnormal developmental events in utero determine the morphologic characteristics that become apparent ex utero. The classification system proposed by Szilagyi and associates,[2, 8] conceptually similar to that of deTakats, is based on the correlation of clinical and angiographic findings with the stages of angiogenesis and consists of the following categories: (1) cavernous or simple hemangioma; (2) microfistulous AV communications; (3) macrofistulous AV communications; and (4) anomalous development of mature vascular channels (e.g., persistent primitive sciatic artery). Purely venous or lymphatic anomalies (without arterial involvement), although thought also to be of developmental etiology, would be classified as separate categories of vascular malformations in this classification system, as opposed to the Hamburg system, described later. However, the focus of Szilagyi and coauthors on lesions commonly presenting to vascular surgeons has merit in this book, and will be briefly summarized here.

Cavernous or simple (capillary) hemangiomas histologically resemble the unorganized capillary network of stage I and are thought to represent an arrest in development during that stage. The term *hemangioma* means "a tumor of blood vessel origin," which, strictly speaking, is incorrect, because the majority of these vascular "tumors" are non-neoplastic. Hemangiomas in infants may be separated into two categories based on endothelial cell proliferation.[13] The first and more common lesion has a normal rate of endothelial cell turnover and is a vascular malformation with no malignant potential and thus is not literally a "hemangioma." These lesions are typically first seen at birth and grow commensurately with the child. Enlargement results from changes in blood or lymphatic pressure, collateralization, or hormonal modulation. The most common form, superficial capillary or cavernous hemangiomas, are primarily cosmetic concerns. However, some of these so-called birthmarks may be the superficial component of a much more complex CVM, for example, overlie major AV fistulas. The second category of hemangiomatous vascular lesions is characteristically hypercellular with increased cellular turnover and neoplastic proliferative capacity. This lesion is not a vascular malformation but a true hemangioma. Typically, these appear just after birth and show rapid early growth and, usually, slow involution. The latter is almost always the rule with cutaneous or subcutaneous hemangiomas. For this reason, they should be observed, with early intervention reserved primarily for those with rapid growth encroaching upon critical organs or orifices such as the eyes, nose, and mouth. After involution, they may leave an unsightly inelastic scar and require plastic surgery. Some of the more aggressive parenchymal hemangiomas have a poor prognosis if untreated; however, work by White and colleagues[14] with pulmonary hemangiomatosis shows encouraging results using recombinant interferon alfa-2α with clinical arrest of tumor growth.

Microfistulous AV communications are a network of extensive interconnections between arteries and veins that are too small to be seen on angiography. Significant AV shunting can occur in these lesions, as inferred by secondary angiographic findings such as early venous filling, increased vascularity in the area of the mass, and dilatation of the proximal supplying artery, but more commonly the hemodynamic consequences are modest. These lesions represent developmental arrest in angiogenesis during stage II, with the persistence of immature channels resulting from the coalescence of embryonic capillaries.

Macrofistulous AV communications contain multiple, grossly visible interconnections between arteries and veins that are apparent on angiography. The more complex of these lesions usually have hemangiomatous, fistulous, and aneurysmal elements, which have been described as cirsoid ("varicose") or racemose ("cluster-of-grapes–like"). If superficial enough to be palpable, these lesions are characteristically warm and have a bruit or thrill because of very high AV shunt flow. This category of lesions is thought to result from arrest during or just before stage III of angiogenesis, prior to complete vessel maturation.

Anomalous development of mature vascular channels consists of lesions containing mature but aberrant vessels

such as isolated venous angiomas and arterial malformations, such as persistent sciatic artery. This category does not, strictly speaking, include lesions that cause AV shunting, indicating that they have arisen from the end of stage III after vessel maturation and loss of AV connections have occurred.

Any of the types of CVMs described here can, and not infrequently do, coexist in a single mass lesion. In such cases, the lesion is categorized by the dominant or most serious component, the usual order being AV, arterial, venous, lymphatic, and capillary. This is the basis for the Hamburg classification commonly used in Europe[15] (Table 11–2). This is a practical anatomic and pathologic approach to CVM classification, in that it not only identifies the predominant types of defect but also breaks these down into truncular and extratruncular forms. The truncular forms involve the main, axial vessels. Mostly these are further separated into aplasias or hypoplastic (obstructive) lesions and dilatations (e.g., popliteal venous aneurysms) but, in the case of predominantly AV shunting defects, they are simply grouped into superficial or deep lesions. Extratruncular lesions involve the smaller branches or tributaries away from the main vessels and are usually subgrouped as being either diffusely *infiltrating* or more *limited* and localized. This would apply to AV shunting defects (typically small fistulous lesions) or venous defects (typically clusters of venous lakes or angiomas), which may form local mass lesions or diffusely infiltrate throughout subcutaneous tissues and muscle.[16]

CLINICAL FINDINGS

Although patients with CVMs present in myriad ways, certain patterns in presentation have emerged. In general, the age at the time of first clinical presentation for evaluation is inversely related to the severity of the lesion. Younger children have more obvious vascular masses, limb enlargements, or huge "birthmarks." Older children (and adults) more often have subtler signs: for example, developing varicose veins, swelling, limb length discrepancies,

TABLE 11–2

Classification of Congenital Vascular Defects According to Their Type and Anatomic/Pathologic Features (Hamburg Classification)

TYPE	FORMS	
	Truncular	**Extratruncular**
Predominantly arterial defects	Aplasia or obstructive	Infiltrating
	Dilatation	Limited
Predominantly venous defects	Aplasia or obstructive	Infiltrating
	Dilatation	Limited
Predominantly lymphatic defects	Aplasia or obstructive	Infiltrating
	Dilatation	Limited
Predominantly arteriovenous (AV) shunting defects	Deep	Infiltrating
	Superficial	Limited
Combined/mixed vascular defects	Arterial and venous, without AV shunt	Infiltrating hemolymphatic
	Hemolymphatic, with or without AV shunt	Limited hemolymphatic

From Belov S: Anatomopathological classification of congenital vascular defects. Semin Vasc Surg 6(4):219–224, 1993.

or even aching or "heavy" sensations in the affected extremity, in addition to a previously recognized birthmark.

As listed in Table 11–3, birthmarks are the most common finding in patients with congenital AVMs (70%) and should be recognized as potential indicators of more serious underlying defects.[2] Venous varicosities, the second most common finding (60%), can also be associated with venous angiomas (compressible grapelike clusters of large venous spaces) or ambulatory venous hypertension from hypoplastic, aplastic, or dysplastic venous segments or segments with absent valves. The former are the most common extratruncular, and the latter, the most common truncular venous defects. Atypical distribution and early onset distinguish them from the usual varicosities caused by saphenofemoral incompetence.

Asymmetrical limb length can result from significant regional AV shunting, by an incompletely understood mechanism (for they can also occur with predominantly venous defects), or may indicate significant osseous involvement. However, increased girth or, in fact, increased overall dimensions are also seen, sometimes to a striking degree. In the latter instance, osseous and soft tissue changes go hand in hand, but it must be remembered that "giant" hypertrophy of one limb can occur *without* an underlying CVM. In such cases, it is present at birth with little proportional change with time. *Edema,* in contradistinction, may develop with time due to underlying venous or lymphatic abnormalities, assuming the same characteristics as edema of those respective origins.

Ulceration and *bleeding* are late manifestations. A subcutaneously located vascular "tumor" or varix under pressure may bleed readily following minor trauma. Such focal lesions can progress to ulceration just like venous ulcers in patients with other forms of chronic venous insufficiency, but with AVMs the venous hypertension is never totally relieved by elevation, and healing may be further impaired by a degree of superimposed ischemia. Regional or distal "steal" may contribute to the latter and may result in a diminution of distal pulses.

As shown in Table 11–4, *hemangioma* rarely appears alone in those with a congenital AVM. Unless huge or

TABLE 11–3

Incidence of Physical Changes in 82 Affected Extremities

CHANGES	PATIENTS	
	n	*%*
Color changes	57	69.5
Erythema	(33)	
Cyanosis	(24)	
Venous varices	49	59.7
Edema	46	56.0
Increased length	20	24.3
Deformity	9	11.0
Ulceration	8	9.8
Pulse deficit	3	3.6
Bleeding	3	3.6

From Szilagyi DE, Smith RF, Elliott JP, Hageman JH: Congenital arteriovenous anomalies of the limbs. Arch Surg 111:423–429, 1976.

TABLE 11–4

Incidence of Diagnostic Physical Signs in Congenital Arteriovenous Malformations

PHYSICAL SIGN(S)	PATIENTS (N = 82) (n)
Hemangioma, varices, bruit, swelling	17
Varices, swelling	14
Swelling	14
Hemangioma, swelling	10
Varices	9
Hemangioma, varices, bruit, swelling	8
Bruit, swelling	5
Bruit	3
Varices, bruit, swelling	2

From Szilagyi DE, Smith RF, Elliott JP, Hageman JH: Congenital arteriovenous anomalies of the limbs. Arch Surg 111:423–429, 1976.

disfiguring, hemangiomas are usually accepted as a cosmetic problem until additional signs develop. As an isolated finding, *swelling* is more common than varicosities, and *bruit* is rarely the sole indication of an AVM. It is noteworthy that, in the Henry Ford Hospital experience,[2] there were less than one third (32%) with a single physical finding at clinical presentation. On the other hand, the classic triad of "birthmark, varicosities, and limb enlargement," which characterizes the syndromes of Klippel-Trenaunay (without AVFs) and Parkes Weber (with AVFs), was seen in barely 30%, with various other double or triple combinations of signs being seen in the remainder (38%). Nevertheless, significant birthmarks, early-onset varicose veins, and limb asymmetry, either singly or in combination, all warrant further testing and close clinical follow-up over time.

DIAGNOSTIC METHODS FOR PREDOMINANTLY ARTERIOVENOUS SHUNTING DEFECTS

Angiography has been routinely applied in the past as the definitive study or gold standard for evaluating AVMs.[16] However, because of the advent of new noninvasive diagnostic techniques, angiography can now be limited, as in arterial occlusive disease, to those patients who are likely soon to undergo interventional therapy. This is not only because angiography is uncomfortable and invasive and, in children, can be technically difficult, cause arterial injury, and require anesthesia,[17] but also because it does not regularly provide definitive information about anatomic extent (i.e., involvement of muscle, bone, and other surrounding tissues), does not identify microfistulous communications, and does not characterize venous, capillary, or lymphatic abnormalities. This latter information, plus hemodynamic assessment, can better be provided by other, simpler tests, including noninvasive vascular tests, shunt quantification with labeled microspheres, and noninvasive imaging.[18]

Noninvasive Vascular Tests

For over three decades, noninvasive vascular tests have been accepted as the initial, if not primary, means of

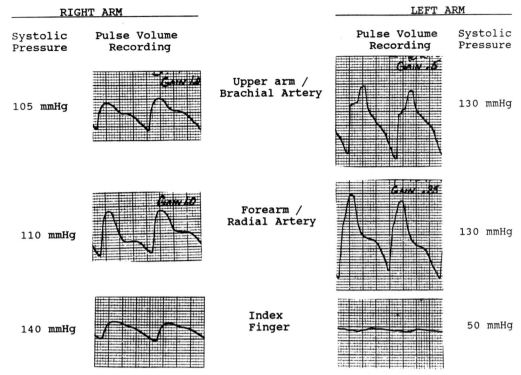

Figure 11–1. Systolic limb pressures (SLP) and pulse volume recording (PVR) in a 13-year-old girl (C.W.) with left palm arteriovenous fistula (AVF) involving distal ulnar and palmar arch arteries. The SLPs illustrate increased systolic pressure and decreased digital pressure distal to the fistula, demonstrating pronounced steal. The PVRs illustrate sharp, high systolic peaks and slightly decreased anacrotic notches proximal to this fistula.

evaluating peripheral vascular diseases. However, it is not generally appreciated that the same noninvasive methods used primarily for evaluating peripheral arterial *occlusion* can also be applied to peripheral AV *shunting*. These tests include segmental limb pressures, segmental plethysmography (or pulse volume recordings), and Doppler analog tracings or velocity waveforms. In addition to these indirect methods, duplex scanning, now that color-flow systems are commonly used, has become an increasingly valuable adjunct.

Segmental limb pressures (SLPs) are systolic arterial pressure determinations at multiple levels along an extremity. The pattern of SLPs can be helpful in localizing peripheral AVFs. Proximal to a fistula, systolic pressure is often *increased*. Distal to a fistula, systolic pressure is usually normal but can be *decreased* secondary to a steal phenomenon.[19] SLPs, then, help locate peripheral AVFs by demonstrating a step-off in systolic pressure from above the fistula to below it when compared with pressures at the same levels in the normal contralateral extremity (Fig. 11–1).

Pulse volume recordings (PVRs) use sensitive, calibrated pneumatic cuffs wrapped around the extremity at multiple levels to monitor the changing limb volume that results from pulsatile arterial flow. This flow is increased proximal to a hemodynamically significant AVF because of lowered vascular resistance. PVR tracings illustrate this increased flow by *sharper, higher systolic peaks*. In addition, because blood flows more readily through the low-resistance fistula than through a normal capillary bed, *the normal anacrotic notch is decreased or absent* (Fig. 11–2). Distal to an AVF, PVRs are often unchanged, although again, if there is a

distal steal, there is a discernible decrease in flow, particularly at the digital level.[19]

Doppler analog tracings or *velocity waveforms* (VWFs) record blood flow velocity. Because of its greater peripheral resistance, the velocity pattern in a resting extremity artery is normally triphasic, with major forward flow in early systole, some flow reversal in later systole, minor forward flow in early diastole, and negligible forward flow in late diastole. As a result of the last, the normal VWF "rests" on (or lies close to) the zero baseline. Significant AVF flow eliminates any end-systolic flow reversal and produces significant flow all through diastole so the VWF tracing proximal to the fistula *never drops near the zero baseline* (Fig. 11–3). In fact, the degree of elevation of the velocity tracing above baseline is directly proportional to fistula flow. The VWF is the most sensitive and least specific noninvasive vascular test for AVFs. Any physiologic or pathophysiologic change causing extremity hyperemia (e.g., exercise, warming, vasodilators, inflammation, relief from ischemia, or recent sympathectomy) can produce a similar pattern to that seen with AVF. Fortunately, in this clinical setting, most of these conditions are easily controlled or clinically ruled out.

There has been a parallel increase in the application of color-flow duplex (CFD) scanning in evaluating peripheral arterial occlusive disease and peripheral AVMs. CFD is no longer limited to superficial lesions. Using appropriate probes, the vascular network of even the larger or deeper AVMs can be fully visualized, and in meaningful color, with turbulent high-flow areas showing up in a network of feeding arteries and veins. AV shunt flow cannot be quanti-

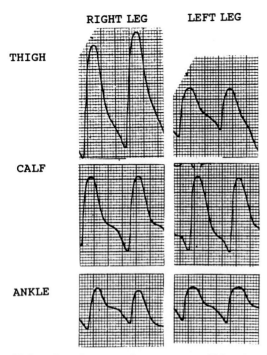

Figure 11-2. Pulse volume recording in a 3-year-old boy (D.W.) with right thigh arteriovenous fistula. This study shows sharpened high systolic peaks and nearly absent anacrotic notches distal to the fibula. Steal is not evident in this study.

fied in AVMs, as it can in angioaccess or some other acquired AVFs, by studying the major inflow artery and comparing it with the normal extremity, but the relative magnitude of fistulous flow can be appreciated. A further advantage over the indirect methods described above is reasonably good anatomic localization. The pulsed Doppler feature of modern CFDs can also be used to perform arterial waveform analysis, and, increasingly, this workhorse of the vascular diagnostic laboratory (VDL) is being applied in this manner to the more obvious, localized cases, with arterial pressures, plethysmography and waveform analysis being reserved for diffuse or equivocal cases. On the other hand, if other imaging techniques (described later) are employed, CFD may be superfluous.

The tests described here have the advantage of being easy, fast, inexpensive, and readily obtainable, being available in any accredited VDL. When used in combination, they detect almost any hemodynamically significant peripheral AVF flow. They are ideal for screening children with birthmarks, unilateral limb enlargement, asymmetry, and early-onset varicosities. However, they are not helpful in detecting AVFs proximal to the upper limb cuff, that is, the groin or axilla, and they miss minor or diffusely distributed microfistulas (constituting together less than 10% to 15% of all extremity AVFs). Obviously, they are not necessary to make the diagnosis in the patient with a discolored, mass lesion associated with local warmth, bruit, and prominent varicosities.

Labeled Microspheres

The labeled microsphere method is a minimally invasive technique that *quantitates* AV shunting in an extremity.[20, 21]

A bolus of technetium (^{99m}Tc)-labeled human albumin microspheres is injected *intraarterially* proximal to an AVF (e.g., in the femoral artery), and the amount of radioactivity subsequently arriving at the lungs is measured with a gamma camera. These microspheres are commonly used today in nuclear medicine departments in lung and other body scans; therefore; this technique is now readily available. Less than 3% of 25- to 35-μm microspheres pass through a normal extremity capillary bed and on to the lungs, where essentially all of them should lodge. To calibrate the amount passing through AVFs and to normalize for differences among patients and microsphere preparations, a second bolus of microspheres is injected *intravenously* in any peripheral vein, because 100% of these microspheres should lodge in the lungs. In this way, the absolute counts measured in the patient's lungs can be converted to a percentage of AV shunting.[20, 21]

The labeled microsphere method is useful both as an

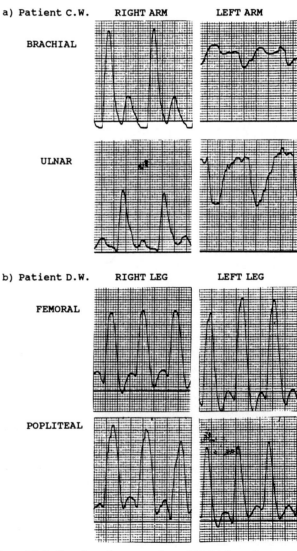

Figure 11-3. Doppler velocity waveforms (VWFs) from the same patients as in Figures 11-1 and 11-2. VWF from C.W. shows extreme elevation in baseline diastolic velocity consistent with large arteriovenous shunting in left arm. VWF from D.W. shows mild elevation in baseline diastolic velocity consistent with lesser arteriovenous shunting in the right leg.

initial diagnostic test and to evaluate therapy. In diagnosis, labeled microspheres distinguish shunting from non-shunting CVMs (e.g., a microfistulous AVM from a pure venous anomaly). The level of shunting has prognostic value. For example, the parents of a child with a 9% AV shunting lesion can be reassured that future symptoms should be mild and easily controlled without intervention, whereas, if the shunt level is 36%, counseling would advise otherwise. In therapy, labeled microspheres measure the decrease in shunting achieved by surgery or embolization. Because AV shunting in congenital AVFs recurs with time after most therapeutic interventions,[2] labeled microspheres may be used after embolization or ablative surgery to quantify recurrence and to time future interventions. The labeled microsphere method cannot be used effectively with the patient under anesthesia because all general and regional anesthesias induce vasodilatation and AV shunting, as does any sympathetic blockade.

Noninvasive Imaging

The resectability of a CVM is determined by its anatomic location, extent, and involvement of important surrounding structures. Computed tomography (CT) and magnetic resonance imaging (MRI) both help to define anatomic involvement of vascular malformations.

CT scanning with contrast enhancement can often demonstrate muscle and bone involvement,[22–24] but highly cellular lesions, having little vascular space, may not enhance, causing an underestimation of a CVM's extent,[25] and diffuse microfistulous AVMs may not be distinguishable from primarily venous anomalies. The optimal technique for contrast infusion (bolus vs. constant infusion) has not yet been determined.[23, 24] and may vary from lesion to lesion. The value of CT scans is also limited by the difficulty in obtaining sections in multiple orientations[26] and the inability to generate information about blood flow.

MRI is superior to CT for evaluating CVMs for several reasons: MRI needs no contrast; it differentiates muscle, bone, fat, and blood vessels,[26] and thus identifies involvement of these tissues by the vascular malformation; it generates axial, coronal, and sagittal sections readily; and it characterizes blood flow through a lesion. High- and low-flow lesions can be distinguished.[25, 27] High-flow lesions increase the risk of developing functional impairment or serious hemodynamic abnormalities in subsequent months or years. Hemorrhage into soft tissues can be observed and aged with MRI, and cellularity can be estimated. Because it accurately assesses both anatomic relationships and flow characteristics with multiplanar views, MRI is more useful than any other single test in the management of CVMs. Its major *current* drawback is a lack of universal availability. The potential clinical value of obtaining an MRI is illustrated in representative longitudinal and axial views (Figs. 11–4 and 11–5, respectively) obtained on a patient referred for operation with a "localized, resectable" AVM based on clinical examination and arteriography (Fig. 11–6).

Magnetic resonance angiography (MRA) has been employed in the evaluation of CVMs.[28] With this technique, vascular contrast is produced noninvasively by the phase response of moving protons. Diastolic and systolic gated

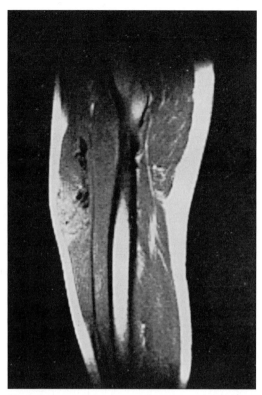

Figure 11–4. Magnetic resonance imaging (MRI), longitudinal view, of right thigh arteriovenous malformation (AVM) in a 19-year-old patient with right thigh congenital vascular malformation (CVM). A high-flow (dark) draining vein and low-flow (light) vascular spaces can be seen to involve the anterior thigh muscles.

images produce, respectively, flow signal and flow void. The difference image is a map of pulsatile flow. These advances have now been developed to the point of clinical applicability, and further improvements will undoubtedly increase the diagnostic accuracy of magnetic resonance technology for CVMs of the extremity in the future.

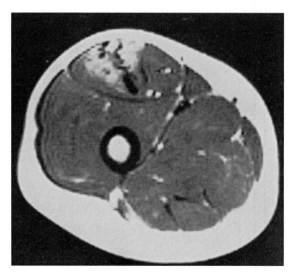

Figure 11–5. Magnetic resonance imaging (MRI), axial view, of right thigh arteriovenous malformation (AVM) in same patient as in Figure 11–4. The vascular mass with high-flow (*dark*) vessels can be observed to involve most of the vastus medialis muscle.

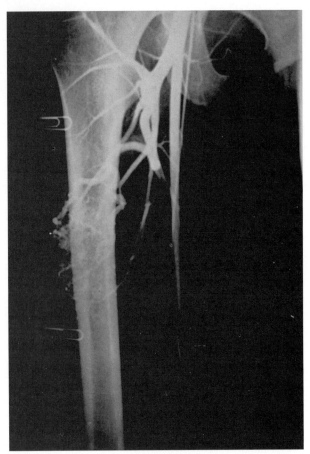

Figure 11–6. Arteriogram of same patient as in Figure 11–4. The arteriogram illustrates an extensive vascular network fed by profunda femoris branches. Early venous filling was seen in later views (not shown).

Advances in CT technology, specifically the 3-dimensional reconstruction of data acquired with the faster helical coil machines, have considerably narrowed the advantages of MRI over standard CT scanning. By subtracting other tissues, the entire CVM can be seen with all its vascular components in appropriate colors. As remarkable as these representations are, the usual vascular software programs show an isolated CVM as if suspended in space, without relationship to surrounding structures, and thus without gauging its anatomic extent. Other tissues, such as bone or muscle, can be included, and this more complex reconstruction, although it might be of great value in selected cases, is not likely to replace MRI in the routine evaluation of CVM mass lesions.

DIAGNOSTIC STUDIES FOR PREDOMINANTLY VENOUS DEFECTS

Although predominantly venous defects constitute the majority of CVMs, until recently they have received relatively little attention. However, depending on the type of venous defect they can demonstrate significant functional or cosmetic problems, and the type of defect also dictates the appropriate diagnostic approach. About 45% of venous defects are truncular (involve axial veins), and these can take the form of avalvulosis or ectasia (with reflux), aneu-

rysm formation (with thromboembolism), or weblike strictures, hypoplastic segments, or agenesis (with obstruction). The latter two, depending on their embryonic onset, may not only be associated with huge varicosities but also persistent embryonal, marginal, lateral, or sciatic veins. Those with Klippel-Trenaunay syndrome often have primarily lateral varicosities and persistent developmental venous pathways. The other 55% of venous defects are extratruncular or peripheral. The commonest of these are venous angiomas, which usually form grapelike clusters of thin-walled venous spaces with only tangential communications with peripheral veins. These may be diffuse throughout the extremity, even involving muscle and bone, or be restricted primarily to the connective tissue spaces above and below the fascia. The localized variety are subcutaneous masses, often large and unsightly.

Truncular defects presenting with venous insufficiency, large atypically distributed varicosities, or even deep venous thrombosis are uncovered by the usual diagnostic approach to these presentations, primarily by duplex scanning, but also with functional tests of venous insufficiency or obstruction used adjunctively (e.g., air plethysmography). Venography may be indicated to define lesions amenable to surgical correction. Patients with the Klippel-Trenaunay triad (birthmark, varicosities, increased limb dimensions) have to be distinguished from the same triad associated with AV fistulas (so-called Parkes Weber syndrome). In this setting, AV fistulas can be ruled in or out by the methods previously described, as a preliminary step. Because the extratruncular lesions cause no venous insufficiency or obstruction, only the large mass lesions are investigated, initially with duplex scanning, but MRI is valuable in estimating their true anatomic extent.

RECOMMENDED DIAGNOSTIC APPROACH

There are three basic diagnostic goals in evaluating patients with CVMs: (1) to establish the diagnosis and categorize the dominant lesion; (2) to define the lesion's anatomic extent and involvement of adjacent structures; and (3) to determine the local, regional, and, if significant, systemic hemodynamic effects. Although the first two goals are directed at defining lesion type and anatomic limits (i.e., potential resectability), the third goal helps to gauge the likely *need* for intervention. Only lesions with significantly increased vascularity and AV shunting are likely to cause significant and progressive functional impairment or affect limb dimensions. The notable exceptions to this are major venous defects and some late maturational defects. In the absence of these flow characteristics, most CVMs may be successfully managed conservatively. Even in the presence of high AV shunt flow, diffuse anatomic involvement may preclude resectability and dictate carefully timed palliative interventions.

With this in mind, diagnostic tests should be employed in a logical sequence that helps to direct management, as indicated in Figure 11–7. Noninvasive vascular tests are obtained, with VWFs for diagnosis of AVFs, and SLPs and PVRs for their localization. With clearly positive noninvasive vascular tests, we recommend an MRI to characterize

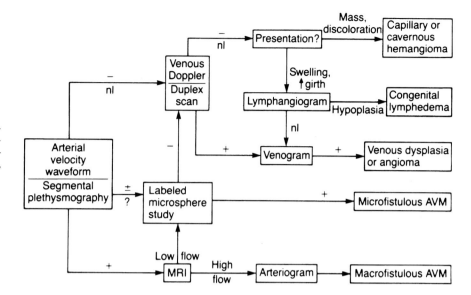

Figure 11–7. Algorithm of diagnostic approach to categorize peripheral congenital vascular malformations. AVM, arteriovenous malformation; +, positive; −, negative; nl, normal.

anatomic extent and confirm flow characteristics. If an extensive, high-flow lesion is seen on MRI, a macrofistulous communication is present, and an arteriogram may be avoided until intervention is necessary. If a low-flow lesion is seen on MRI, a labeled microsphere study would be useful to differentiate microfistulous communications from nonshunting lesions (i.e., venous angiomas, capillary or cavernous hemangiomas).

If *arterial* noninvasive tests are entirely normal at the initial screening, *venous* Doppler studies and duplex scanning may be performed in the same vascular laboratory to identify venous dysplasias or venous angiomas, as detailed above. Normal venous studies then would suggest capillary or cavernous hemangioma in the patient with a birthmark or lymphatic hypoplasia in a patient with diffuse swelling, although minor venous dysplasia or angiomas are not absolutely ruled out without "closed space" venography (performed similar to a Bier block but with contrast instead of an anesthetic agent being injected).[29] Lymphoscintigraphy would confirm lymphedema, if early and not clinically obvious.

Like arteriography, venography and lymphangiography should be reserved for the patient in whom intervention is required because of significant functional or cosmetic problems.[30] With unequal limb length, radiographic documentation of bone age and length is indicated to predict the need for, and timing of, epiphyseal closure.

RECOMMENDED THERAPEUTIC APPROACH

Management of AVMs (outlined in Fig. 11–8) depends on the patient's symptoms as well as the malformation's characteristics. Many lesions are self-limiting, most are incurable, and all invasive treatments have associated complications. Therefore, in those lesions in which surgery and embolotherapy, singly or in combination, can be expected to produce long-term control, interventional therapy should be reserved for specific pressing indications. *Absolute indications* for treatment of symptomatic AVMs include hemorrhage, ischemia from arterial steal, refractory ulceration

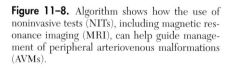

Figure 11–8. Algorithm shows how the use of noninvasive tests (NITs), including magnetic resonance imaging (MRI), can help guide management of peripheral arteriovenous malformations (AVMs).

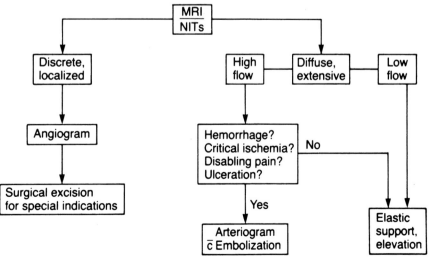

from venous hypertension, and congestive heart failure. *Relative indications* for treatment include disabling pain, limiting claudication and functional impairment of an extremity. Unequal limb length *alone* is not an indication for intervention, because appropriately timed epiphyseal closure in the ipsilateral extremity yields good results.

Therapeutic options include conservative management, surgical resection, and embolotherapy. The most frequently chosen management course is conservative, using support stockings and extremity elevation to control the sequelae of venous hypertension. Although this approach fails to retard the progression of high-flow lesions, it may adequately control symptoms that might otherwise demand aggressive therapy. Primary surgical excision is appropriate only for accessible, localized lesions, and even this is often best performed after embolotherapy to control the local vascularity. If successfully excised, AVMs are cured, although lesions amenable to complete resection are rare (10% or less). Surgical resection is made easier by prior embolization, use of pneumatic tourniquets, autotransfusion, and, occasionally, deep hypothermia. Experience has demonstrated that ligating feeding arteries and performing partial excisions are fruitless. The transient palliation promoted by these techniques does not justify their tendency to complicate or preclude later attempts at embolization.[2]

Embolization may be employed alone or in conjunction with surgery. Preoperative embolization simplifies excision and reduces blood loss during resection of larger lesions (Fig. 11–9). If the anatomic extension of the AVM prevents complete resection, palliative embolization should be undertaken for appropriate indications, as defined previously. Curative embolization has been possible in only a fraction of treated lesions; thus, embolotherapy necessitates a commitment to long-term surveillance and repeated intervention as required.

Currently, embolotherapy is performed in stages. First, an arteriogram is obtained to confirm the diagnosis, characterize the lesion, and identify the primary feeding arteries and draining veins. Selective catheterization of feeding arteries may be necessary to precisely localize AVFs and deliver therapy exactly at the nidus of the lesion. Then embolization is performed, using general anesthesia to obviate pain and improve tolerance for an often lengthy procedure—this is almost always necessary in children. Multiple embolization sessions are generally required for large malformations, to limit contrast volume, anesthesia time, and excessive tissue necrosis. If a combined embolization and surgical approach is elected, the operation should be performed *immediately* after embolization before new vasculature can be recruited. Tissue edema developing 24 to 48 hours after embolization can make surgical resection difficult and tedious.

The goal of embolotherapy for AVMs is to thrombose the so-called nidus of abnormal vasculature that promotes vascular recruitment and AV shunting. Permanent nidus occlusion is desirable because otherwise AVMs typically

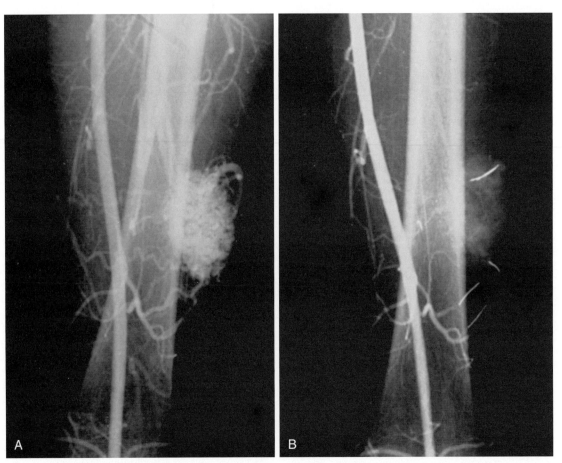

Figure 11–9. Arteriovenous malformation of left thigh (*A*) before and (*B*) after embolotherapy with ethanol.

recur in an almost malignant fashion. Embolization of arterial feeders proximal to the nidus only promotes collateralization and prevents nidus ablation. Therefore, the embolic agents that are most appropriate for embolization include microscopic particles or liquids that can reach the nidus's small-caliber vascular bed. Ivalon (polyvinyl alcohol) particles ranging in size from 100 to 500 μm are useful for precapillary occlusion, allowing embolization of multiple arterial feeders near the nidus. Absolute ethanol and cyanoacrylate adhesives allow obliteration of the nidus itself.

Embolic material is injected only after the feeding arteries are selectively catheterized to avoid the inadvertent embolization of normal vasculature. Improvements in digital imaging, live subtraction fluoroscopy, and road-mapping make this possible. Multiple arteriograms may be required, making digital filming essential. Small, steerable catheter and guidewire systems allow the selective catheterization of lesions that at first glance appear inaccessible. Previous arterial ligation or embolization may prevent a *remote* percutaneous transarterial approach, in which case surgical exposure or *direct* percutaneous puncture and catheterization may be necessary. Blood pressure cuffs, tourniquets, and intraarterial occlusion balloons are often employed to slow blood flow through dynamic lesions and control the deposition of embolic agents.

Leukocytosis, fever, and mild to moderate pain are typically observed following most embolization procedures. Limited tissue necrosis and transient sensory or motor deficits are minor complications that do not require specific treatment. The major complications of embolotherapy include extensive tissue necrosis necessitating skin grafting, inadvertent embolization of normal vasculature, pulmonary embolization, and permanent neurologic loss resulting from embolization of critical vasa nervosum. Although major complications occur infrequently, they emphasize the importance of careful patient selection to ensure that the risk-benefit ratio is in favor of intervention.

Although the best embolic agent remains controversial, the overall approach, therapeutic results, and complication rates are similar among several published patient series. Rosen and colleagues,[31] who advocate the use of cyanoacrylate adhesives, have successfully treated 45 patients with peripheral AVMs, with 79% of patients benefiting from therapy. Thirteen patients appeared cured at 3-year follow-up, 11 patients had residual malformations but were asymptomatic, 12 patients were improved but remained symptomatic, and 9 patients either were unchanged or had worsened. Six percent of patients suffered major complications; for example, two patients had temporary hemiparesis, and one patient had intractable hematuria. Yakes and colleagues[32] used alcohol to treat 10 patients with CMVs—eight AVMs and two venous malformations. Eight of 10 patients benefited from treatment with two apparent cures at 1-year follow-up. The authors reported a 20% major complication rate, including one patient who suffered a fatal pulmonary embolus 4 days post embolization

and one patient who developed an L-3–4 radiculopathy. Widlus and colleagues[33] treated 16 patients with symptomatic AVMs using a combination of tissue adhesive and particles. All patients were improved following treatment. Two patients required skin grafting after a procedure, but no other major complications developed.

These encouraging results support the use of palliative embolization to treat symptomatic AVMs not amenable to complete surgical resection. The combination of better vascular imaging techniques and more limited use of surgery for palliative indications (and its replacement in this setting by embolotherapy, made possible by a decade of technologic refinement) now offers a more optimistic outlook for even the more challenging AVMs.

The treatment of congenital venous defects and anomalies was, in the past, conservative for the most part, being directed at associated venous insufficiency and using traditional methods of compressive therapy and intermittent leg elevation. The primary surgical intervention was directed at resecting the associated varicosities and persistent developmental collateral veins. Depending on the additional involvement of deep and communicating veins and venous insufficiency, symptomatic and cosmetic relief has varied from excellent to unsatisfactory, related, as one would expect, to the relative degree of associated venous insufficiency.[34] European experiences with surgery for venous defects have been more extensive. Loose[35] reported a large experience and recommended a surgical strategy for each defect or combination of defects, with a variety of anticipated results. An update of the Mayo Clinic surgical experience with venous malformations in Klippel-Trenaunay syndrome indicates symptomatic relief in the majority, plus improvement in CEAP (*C*linical, *E*tiologic, *A*natomic, *P*athophysiologic) classification, but recurrent varicosities in the majority.[36]

Clearly, isolated venous defects with significant physiologic effects, such as atretic or hypoplastic deep venous segments with inadequate collateralization,[32] or with potentially serious prognosis, such as popliteal aneurysms,[37] require intervention. For other lesions, such as diffuse ectasia with massive reflux, there is little to be done. Between these two extremes are lesions with little or no venous insufficiency but major cosmetic impact, such as venous angiomatous masses. Surgical excision of these may be indicated if the healed incision produces a better cosmetic result.[38] With venous lesions, sequential sclerosis of abnormal veins in symptomatic areas of these typically diffuse abnormalities is feasible. Direct puncture followed by sclerosis with ethanol or Sotradecol (sodium tetradecyl sulfate) has been described.[38] However, if one considers the potential risk of complications and expense of multiple sessions of ethanol or any other form of sclerotherapy, and the likelihood of persisting discoloration and tender thrombosed masses, it is hard to justify extending this form of therapy from AV fistulas to venous angiomas.

References

1. Tasnadi G: Epidemiology and etiology of congenital vascular malformations. Semin Vasc Surg 6:200–203, 1993.
2. Szilagyi DE, Smith RF, Elliott JP, Hageman JH: Congenital arteriovenous anomalies of the limbs. Arch Surg 111:423–429, 1976.
3. Malan E, Puglionisi A: Congenital angiodysplasias of the extremities. J Cardiovasc Surg 5:87, 1964; 6:255; 1965.
4. Lindenauer SM: The Klippel-Trenaunay syndrome: Varicosity, hypertrophy and hemangioma with no arteriovenous fistula. Ann Surg 162:303–314, 1965.
5. Parkes Weber F: Angioma formation in connection with hypertrophy of limbs or hemihypertrophy. Br J Dermatol 19:231, 1907.
6. Reid MR: Studies on abnormal arteriovenous communications, acquired and congenital: 1. Report of a series of cases. Arch Surg 10:601–638, 1925.
7. Rienhoff WF: Congenital arteriovenous fistula: An embryologic study with the report of a case. Johns Hopkins Hosp Bull 35:271–284, 1924.
8. Szilagyi D, Elliott J, DeRusso F, et al: Peripheral congenital arteriovenous fistulas. Surgery 57:61–68, 1965.
9. Moore KL: The cardiovascular system. In The Developing Human: Clinically Oriented Embryology, 4th ed. Philadelphia, WB Saunders, 1988, pp 286–333.
10. Woollard HH: The development of the principal arterial stems in the forelimb of the pig. Contemp Embryol 14:139–154, 1922.
11. Malan E: Vascular Malformations, Milan, Carlo Erba Foundation, 1974, pp 41–43.
12. deTakats G: Vascular anomalies of the extremities. Surg Gynecol Obstet 55:227–237, 1931.
13. Mulliken J, Glovacki J: Hemangiomas and vascular malformation in infants and children: A classification based on endothelial characteristics. Plast Reconstr Surg 69:412–420, 1982.
14. White CW, Sondheimer HM, Crouch EC, et al: Treatment of pulmonary hemangiomatosis with recombinant interferon α-2a. N Engl J Med 320:1197–1200, 1989.
15. Belov S: Anatomopathological classification of congenital vascular defects. Semin Vasc Surg 6:219–224, 1993.
16. Woolley MM, Stanley P, Wesley JR: Peripherally located congenital arteriovenous fistulae in infancy and childhood. J Pediatr Surg 12:165–176, 1977.
17. Rutherford RB, Pearce WH: Acute problems following diagnostic and interventional radiologic procedures. In Bergan JJ, Yao JST (eds): Vascular Surgery Emergencies. Orlando, Fla, Grune & Stratton, 1986, pp 417–430.
18. Rutherford RB, Anderson BO: Diagnosis of congenital vascular malformations of the extremities: New perspectives. Int Angiol 9:162–167, 1990.
19. Rutherford RB: Noninvasive testing in the diagnosis and assessment of arteriovenous fistula. In Bernstein EF (ed): Noninvasive Diagnostic Techniques in Vascular Disease, 3rd ed. St Louis, Mosby–Year Book, 1985, pp 666–679.
20. Sumner DS, Rutherford RB: Diagnostic evaluation of arteriovenous fistulas: Radionuclide assessment. In Rutherford RB (ed): Vascular Surgery, 3rd ed. Philadelphia, WB Saunders, 1989, pp 1037–1038.
21. Rutherford RB, Fleming RW, McLeod FD: Vascular diagnostic methods for evaluating patients with arteriovenous fistulas. In Diethrich EB (ed): Noninvasive Cardiovascular Diagnosis: Current Concepts. Baltimore, University Park Press, 1978, pp 217–230.
22. Rauch RF, Silverman PM, Korobkin M, et al: Computed tomography of benign angiomatous lesions of the extremities. J Comput Assist Tomogr 8:1143–1146, 1984.
23. Wilson JS, Korobkin M, Genant HK, Bovill EG Jr: Computed tomography of musculoskeletal disorders. AJR 131:55–61, 1978.
24. Bernardino ME, Jing BS, Thomas JL, et al: The extremity soft tissue lesion: A comparative study of ultrasound, computed tomography, and xeroradiography. Radiology 139:53–59, 1981.
25. Pearce WH, Rutherford RB, Whitehill RA, Davis K: Nuclear magnetic resonance imaging: Its diagnostic value in patients with congenital vascular malformations of the limbs. J Vasc Surg 8:64–70, 1988.
26. Cohen JM, Weinreb JC, Redman HC: Arteriovenous malformations of the extremities: MR imaging. Radiology 158:475–479, 1986.
27. Mills CM, Brant-Zawadzki M, Crooks LE: Nuclear magnetic resonance: Principles of blood flow imaging. 142:165–170, AJR, 1984.
28. Meuli RA, Wedeen VJ, Geller SC, et al: MR gated subtraction angiography: Evaluation of lower extremities. Radiology 159:411–418, 1986.
29. Braun SD, Moore AVJ, Mills SR, et al: Closed-system venography in the evaluation of angiodysplastic lesions of the extremities. AJR 141:1307–1310, 1983.
30. O'Donnell TFJ, Edwards JM, Kinmonth JB: Lymphography in congenital mixed vascular deformities of the lower extremities. J Cardiovasc Surg (Torino) 17:535–540, 1976.
31. Rosen RJ, Riles TS, Berenstein A: Congenital vascular malformations. In Rutherford RB (ed): Vascular Surgery, 3rd ed. Philadelphia, WB Saunders, 1989, pp 1049–1061.
32. Yakes WF, Haas DK, Parker SH, et al: Symptomatic vascular malformations: Ethanol embolotherapy. Radiology 170:1059–1066, 1989.
33. Wildus DM, Murray RR, White RI, et al: Congenital arteriovenous malformations: Tailored embolotherapy. Radiology 169:511–516, 1988.
34. Gorenstein A, Katz S, Schiller M: Congenital angiodysplasia of the superficial venous system of the lower extremities in children. Ann Surg 207:213–218, 1988.
35. Loose DA: Surgical treatment of predominantly venous defects. Semin Vasc Surg; 6:252–259, 1993.
36. Noel AA, Gloviczki P, Cherry KJ, et al: Surgical treatment of venous malformations in Klippel-Trenaunay syndrome: An update. J Vasc Surg (in press).
37. Aldridge SC, Comerota AJ, Katz ML, et al: Popliteal venous aneurysm: Report of two cases and review of the world literature. J Vasc Surg 18:708–715, 1993.
38. Yakes WF, Parker SH: Diagnosis and management of vascular anomalies. In Castaneda-Zuniga WR, Tada-Varthy SM (eds): Interventional Radiology, 2nd ed. Baltimore, Williams & Wilkins, 1991, pp 152–189.

Questions

1. Which predominant type of congenital vascular malformation (CVM) is the most common?
   (a) venous
   (b) arterial
   (c) arteriovenous (fistulas)
   (d) lymphatic

2. Which arterial segment is the most common location of a congenital arteriovenous malformation (AVM)?
   (a) femoral
   (b) politeal
   (c) iliac
   (d) popliteal
   (e) infrapopliteal

3. Microfistulous AVMs are due to an inborn error at which stage of limb bud development?
   (a) undifferentiated
   (b) retiform
   (c) syncytial
   (d) maturational

4. Which of the following statements regarding hemangiomas encountered during infancy is/are **NOT** true?
   (a) they have a high endothelial turnover rate
   (b) they may exhibit high flow characteristics
   (c) they are true CVMs
   (d) their growth is commensurate with the child's overall growth

5. Which of the following constitutes the classic triad of AVMs?
   (a) increased limb size
   (b) increased skin warmth
   (c) varicose veins
   (d) a hemangioma-like birthmark
   (e) a bruit

6. Which noninvasive test finding(s) is/are characteristic of lower extremity congenital arteriovenous fistulas?
   (a) increased systolic pressure in a limb segment proximal to the lesion
   (b) end-diastolic velocity close to zero in the proximal artery
   (c) elevated pulse volume recording (plethysmographic tracing) distally in the foot
   (d) velocity waveform in the proximal artery is elevated above baseline

7. Using labeled albumin microspheres to measure the degree of arteriovenous (AV) shunting in the extremity of a child with an apparent CVM is valuable in which of the following?
   (a) for prognostic purposes
   (b) to localize the lesion
   (c) to differentiate microfistulous AVMs from purely venous CVMs
   (d) to estimate AV shunting at the time of arteriography under general anesthesia, thereby saving additional needle punctures

8. MRI holds which of the following advantages over a contrast-enhanced CT scan in evaluating CVMs presenting with mass lesions?
   (a) better flow information
   (b) better definition of anatomic extent
   (c) availability
   (d) multiplanar views
   (e) it is more easily tolerated by children

9. Which of the following is/are true about catheter-directed injections of absolute alcohol into the nidus of AVMs?
   (a) they require multiple sessions
   (b) they must be done under general anesthesia
   (c) they destroy endothelium and cause thrombosis without surrounding tissue necrosis
   (d) they cause permanent nerve injury in close to 10% of cases
   (e) they can permanently control some AVMs

10. Surgery or embolotherapy or both are justified for which of the following indications?
    (a) recurrent hemorrhage from skin lesions
    (b) uneven limb growth
    (c) ischemic ulcer
    (d) symptomatic arterial steal

Answers

1. a   2. c   3. c   4. c, d   5. a, c, d   6. a, d   7. b, c   8. a, b, d   9. a, b, d   10. a, c, d

12

Vasculogenic Erectile Dysfunction

Ralph G. DePalma

The diagnosis and treatment of male erectile dysfunction has progressed remarkably in the past three decades. Erectile dysfunction is defined as: "The persistent or repeated inability to attain, and/or maintain an erection sufficient for satisfactory performance. . . . "[1] Among the reasons for progress in this area are a better understanding of the central role of cavernous sinus in muscle relaxation,[2] and the availability of effective medical therapy for men with primary or new onset erectile dysfunction.[3] Mainly, vascular surgeons require information about prevention of erectile dysfunction during aortoiliac reconstruction; they may also be required to evaluate the contribution of large vessel disease to vasculogenic erectile dysfunction. This chapter emphasizes surgical approaches for prevention of postoperative erectile dysfunction. Current vascular approaches for the primary complaint of erectile dysfunction are also being considered.

PHYSIOLOGY OF ERECTION

Penile erection requires adequate arterial inflow and closure of cavernosal outflow mediated by a complex interplay between neural and local factors.[4, 5] Erection is controlled primarily by relaxation of the smooth muscle of the corporal bodies. These are endothelial-mediated relaxation responses[6] stimulated by neural mechanisms. The role of nitric oxide as the chemical mediator,[7] as well as the importance of adequate oxygenation of the corporal smooth muscle,[8] is key to the development of effective medical therapy. With increased corporal arterial inflow, the emissary veins are compressed against the tunica albuginea, causing venous outflow occlusion. During full erection, cavernosal artery flow virtually ceases. During the flaccid state, there is a constant venous leak, and penile inflow and outflow are balanced. As the corpora do not fill when arterial inflow is insufficient, a venous leak is also present. In the erect state, intercavernous pressure increases from 10 to 15 mm Hg to levels ranging from 80 to 90 mm Hg. Higher pressures that contribute to penile rigidity are generated by perineal muscle contraction.[5]

ETIOLOGY OF ERECTILE DYSFUNCTION

Table 12–1 summarizes general etiologic factors contributing to erectile dysfunction. In modern practice, more cases are now recognized as organic in origin than were appreciated previously; however, in most cases of organic impotence, psychogenic components are also often present. Of 1023 impotent men screened from September 1983 through March 1992, 461 demonstrated some type of arterial inflow problem as judged by noninvasive criteria using penile brachial indices and pulse volume recordings. However, many impotent men exhibit other factors including diabetes, neuropathy (in about 20%), the need to take antihypertensive medications, and other types of cavernous dysfunction, including Peyronie's disease. Older men with multiple factors contributing to impotence are usually not candidates for reconstruction; about 6% to 7%[9] of impotent men ultimately become candidates for vascular intervention. Furthermore, in the author's series, only 15.6% of the men with decreased arterial perfusion exhibited large vessel disease. Thus, when a screening sequence[10] is imposed for surgical case selection, there is a sharp funnel effect in selection of surgical candidates. However, for younger men or older men with large vessel disease, a vascular intervention may be a logical first step for men who fail medical therapy and for those who do not desire prosthetic implantation.[11]

Table 12–2 offers an updated classification of vasculogenic erectile dysfunction. Some type of small vessel, cavernosal, or arteriolar cause appears to be present in 43.3% of men exhibiting abnormal penile perfusion. An additional 41.1% of men with the primary complaint of impotence exhibit a combination of large and small vessel involvement, as can be best ascertained by noninvasive and physical criteria. Most men with the primary complaint of erec-

214

TABLE 12-1

TABLE 12-1

General Etiologic Factors in Erectile Dysfunction

Vasculogenic	Drug-induced
Neurogenic	Psychogenic
Endocrine	

tile dysfunction are very likely to have small vessel rather than large vessel disease.

However, in men with Leriche's syndrome or aortoiliac disease, impotence is an important complaint. Many men younger than 55 years are potent before reconstruction for aneurysm or occlusive disease, and an accurate history of their sexual activity must be obtained. Despite the best surgical techniques to preserve sexual function, impotence can occur after reconstructions for aneurysms and occlusive disease. Importantly, the complaint of impotence has been found to be associated with undiscovered aortoiliac or aneurysmal disease. Therefore, before aortoiliac reconstruction, the surgeon must make careful inquiries into the patient's sexual function and probably carry out selective noninvasive measures of penile artery perfusion.[12] This is particularly important when postoperative sexual function is an expressed concern.

HISTORY AND PHYSICAL EXAMINATION

A history of gradual erectile failure, in the absence of traumatic life events and correlated with symptoms such as claudication, suggests large vessel arteriogenic erectile dysfunction. In these men, both the intensity and duration of atherosclerotic risk factors, mainly cigarette smoking, hypertension, diabetes, and hypercholesterolemia, probably contribute to atherosclerosis. This pattern signals patients with involvement of the aorta or the iliac systems. As reported in 1995,[9] abdominal aneurysms or ulcerative atheromatous disease can cause penile vessel emboli. In these cases, the onset of the dysfunction can be quite sudden. A

TABLE 12-2

Classification of Vasculogenic Erectile Dysfunction

Arterial	
Large vessel	Aorta and branches to internal iliac artery
Small vessel	Anterior division of internal iliac artery and penile arteries
Combined	Atheroembolism from aortoiliac segment
Cavernosal	
Fibrosis	Postpriapic, drug injection, idiopathic with aging
Peyronie's disease	Deformity; venous leakage
Refractory states	Hormonal, diabetic, blood pressure medication
Venous	
Acquired	Various patterns; dorsal vein, crural; spongiosal
Congenital	Cavernous spongiosus leak

history of perineal injuries predisposes to interruption of the cavernosal artery. The immediate onset of erectile failure after urologic, vascular, or rectal operations is an important diagnostic point. Although erectile dysfunction can result from either neural or vascular interruption or both, neural interruption is more commonly associated with ejaculatory disorders. Alcohol and drug abuse contribute to erectile failure, whereas drugs used to treat hypertension and diabetes cause erectile failure because of their neuropathic and metabolic effects. Other hormonal disorders, such as hypogonadism, are less common. The author has detected only two prolactinomas among approximately 1400 men who were screened.[12]

On physical examination, the major findings of aortoiliac disease are decreased femoral pulses or bruits. Sensory testing of the extremities, perineum, or glans may reveal neuropathies associated with diabetic impotence. However, these abnormalities are best quantified by neurovascular testing, using pudendal evoked potentials and measurement of bulbous cavernosal reflex times.[13] Currently, neurologic screening is not routinely employed initially because medical treatment with vasoactive agents is often effective. In cases of postoperative or posttraumatic dysfunction, this testing can be an important factor in decision-making, particularly where prosthetic explantation is an option. A considerable overlap exists between vascular and neurologic dysfunction.[14] The prostate must be examined and nodular abnormalities investigated—prostatic-specific antigen determinations should be routine. Examination is completed by methodical palpation of the corpora cavernosa for Peyronie's plaques and estimation of testicular size. In the majority of men who seek treatment for erectile dysfunction, the physical examination is completely normal.

At this point, the erectile mechanism can be tested in the clinic by intracavernous injection of 10 to 20 μg of Prostin E1.[15] Rigid erection sufficient for intercourse demonstrates adequate arterial inflow and veno-occlusive mechanisms. Provided that aneurysmal disease is ruled out (e.g., by sonography), treatment with oral, injectable, or intraurethral vasoactive agents is indicated as a first step. This may succeed in up to 70% to 80% of cases.

NEUROVASCULAR TESTING

Neurovascular testing[10, 12] can be used primarily to select patients for further studies and as candidates for reconstructive procedures. These tests are also needed in deciding on the dosage of intracavernous injection of vasoactive agents—patients with neurologic deficits are often exquisitely sensitive, and dosage must be reduced.

Penile brachial indices (PBI) are the ratio between systolic pressure detected by a Doppler probe placed distal to the penile cuff and systemic or brachial arm pressure. A cuff of 2.5 cm is used for an average-size penis. The cuff in inflated, then deflated, and reappearance of the Doppler signals in the dorsal artery branch proximal to the corona signals reflow. Normally, this pressure approaches systemic pressure. A PBI above .75 suggests no major obstacle between the aorta and the distal measurement point. Generally, PBIs less than .6 relate to major vascular obstructions in the aortoiliac bed, whereas PBIs between .6 and

.75 are considered abnormal. Flow can be further characterized by use of penile pulse volume recording. Penile pulse volume recording, as I perform it, uses a pneumoplethysmographic cuff (Buffington) with a contained transducer.

This test is performed with the penis in the flaccid state. The variables recorded are the same used for the lower extremity. These include crest time, waveform, and the presence or absence of a dicrotic notch. This technique measures the total pulsation of all penile arteries as the cuff compresses the cavernous tissues. The measurements are taken with the cuff inflated to mean arterial pressure, calculated as diastolic pressure plus one third of systemic pulse pressure. Waveforms on a polygraph with a chart speed of 25 mm per second and sensitivity setting in one will demonstrate in normal patients that the upstroke of the waveform is completed by 0.2 seconds, whereas normal waveform amplitudes vary from 5 or 6 to 30 mm in height. Waveforms can be distinctly abnormal with small vessel disease or cavernosal disorders, whereas PBI is normal.

These noninvasive tests help in the detection of inadequate arterial inflow. However, cases of vasculogenic impotence caused by venous leak or Peyronie's disease or cavernosal fibrosis are not detected. In these instances, color-flow duplex scanning after an intracavernous injection to produce erection can be useful.[12] The noninvasive tests are not completely sensitive and specific. I have found that the combination of penile brachial indices and pulse volume recording predicts an abnormal arteriogram with a sensitivity of 85% and a specificity of 70%. In suspected cases of venogenic impotence (i.e., normal arterial noninvasive tests), we have discovered that 23% of men examined with normal noninvasive studies were found to have associated arterial lesions demonstrated angiographically.[16] Therefore, before small vessel interventions, which are done *only* for those failing medical therapy,[11] both pudendal arteriography and dynamic infusion cavernosography are recommended.

CAVERNOSOMETRY AND CAVERNOSAL ARTERY OCCLUSION PRESSURE

These invasive studies provide quantitative information about arterial inflow and veno-occlusive mechanisms.[12] A calibrated pump provides a flow of warm, heparinized saline via 20-gauge needles inserted into the corpora. During maximum erection, intracavernous pressure at some point equilibrates with arterial inflow pressure. Flow in the deep cavernosal artery stops. This value is called cavernosal artery occlusion pressure (CAOP). CAOP is measured by using Doppler insonation at the point of full erection. It is taken as normal when it is greater than 90 mm Hg. A pressure gradient from brachial levels greater than 30 mm Hg suggests arterial inflow occlusion. Dynamic infusion cavernosography measures the flow required to maintain erection. This value is normally taken to be 40 mL or less after intracavernous injection of a standard papaverine-phentolamine mixture. To visualize venous leaks, diluted nonionic contrast is injected. Spot filming in various obliquities identifies specific abnormal or leaking veins when

cavernosography is positive. As mentioned previously, failure of erection is associated with an excess of venous leakage over inflow. Venous leakage can be due to arterial insufficiency and, as mentioned, before contemplated venous ablation, we recommend routine highly selective pudendal arteriography.

LARGE VESSEL RECONSTRUCTION— PREVENTION OF VASCULOGENIC IMPOTENCE

Given the usual indications for large vessel aortoiliac reconstruction (i.e., aneurysm and occlusive disease), the procedure should provide perfusion of one or both internal iliac arteries wherever possible. Flushing of debris into the internal iliacs should be avoided, and, when possible, endovascular repair should be attempted to maintain internal iliac flow—at least to one internal iliac artery.[17] The dissection must spare the neural fibers about the aorta and the iliac arteries (which are especially rich on the left side) and about the inferior mesenteric artery. In all these cases, a specific history of preoperative sexual activity must be sought. If an elderly couple manifests no interest in this activity, complicated preoperative testing becomes redundant. However, when interest exists, penile brachial indices and pulse volume recordings preoperatively are helpful when compared with postoperative findings. In addition, positive findings of abnormal pudendal and somatosensory evoked potentials are helpful to demonstrate preoperative neuropathy.

OPERATIVE TECHNIQUES

These techniques have been described previously,[18] and illustrations have been reproduced from my 1988 review.[19] Exposure for aortoiliac reconstruction is best accomplished by dissecting the aortoiliac segment from the right side and sparing the nerves and inferior mesenteric artery. In cases of aortoiliac aneurysm, perfusion of the internal iliac is ensured by an inlay technique, illustrated in Figure 12–1. Again, the aneurysmal sac is incised well to the right, avoiding interruption of a dominant left periaortic nerve plexus. The inferior mesenteric artery is sutured from within the aneurysmal sac. Figures 12–2 and 12–3 show techniques for occlusive disease. In men with buttock claudication and impotence related to local disease in the arterial distribution of the internal iliac artery, an extraperitoneal approach with endarterectomy or bypass is a convenient procedure. This approach involves a longitudinal incision along the edge of the rectus muscle with reflection of the peritoneal medially (Fig. 12–4). In renal transplant patients, end-to-side renal artery anastomosis to the external iliac artery avoids division of an internal iliac artery.

Fredberg and Mouritzen described sexual dysfunction in conventional aortoiliac operations.[20] In this series, 55% of men (11/20) with aneurysms were preoperatively impotent, whereas 95% (19/20) were postoperatively impotent. For occlusive disease, 31% (15/48) were preoperatively impotent, and 60% (29/48) were postoperatively impotent.

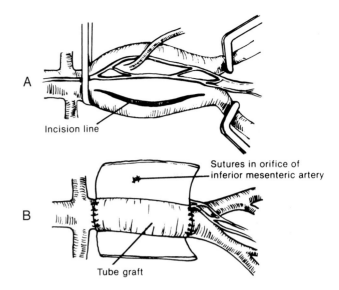

Figure 12–1. Inlay nerve-sparing techniques for aneurysm repair. Note incision on right side of aneurysm. (From DePalma RG: Prevention of sexual dysfunction in aortoiliac surgery. In Jamieson CW [ed]: Current Operative Surgery. Eastborne, East Sussex, Bailliere-Tindall, 1985.)

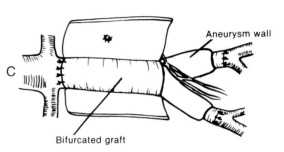

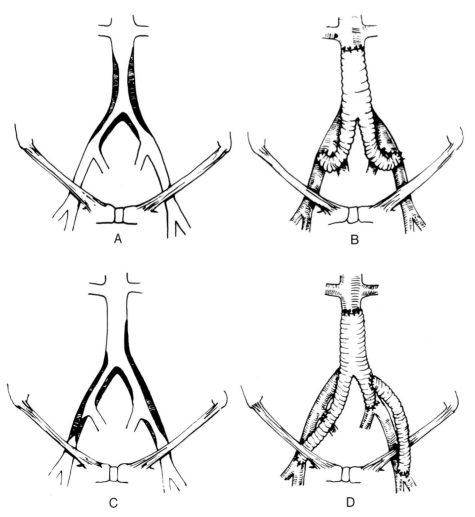

Figure 12–2. Techniques for aortoiliac or aortofemoral bypass: *A* and *B*, End-to-end aortic anastomosis with suprainguinal end-to-side bypass where external iliac and common femoral arteries are spared. *C* and *D*, End-to-end aortic anastomosis with side-to-side reconstruction of right internal iliac and two limbs on left side. (From DePalma RG: Prevention of sexual dysfunction in aortoiliac surgery. In Jamieson CW [ed]: Current Operative Surgery. Eastborne, East Sussex, Bailliere-Tindall, 1985.)

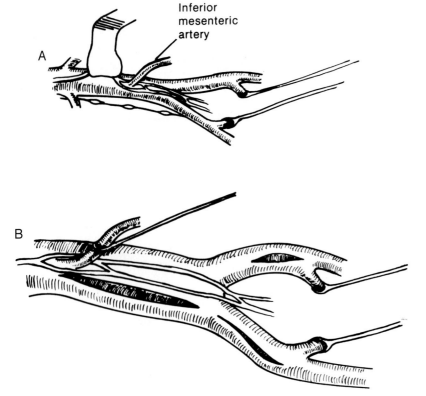

Figure 12–3. Dissection of intrarenal aorta for endarterectomy. *A*, Aorta exposed without mobilization and inferior mesenteric artery spared along with neural fibers. *B*, Internal iliacs controlled and common or external iliacs clamped with minimal mobilization. (From DePalma RG: Prevention of sexual dysfunction in aortoiliac surgery. In Jamieson CW [ed]: Current Operative Surgery. Eastborne, East Sussex, Bailliere-Tindall, 1985.)

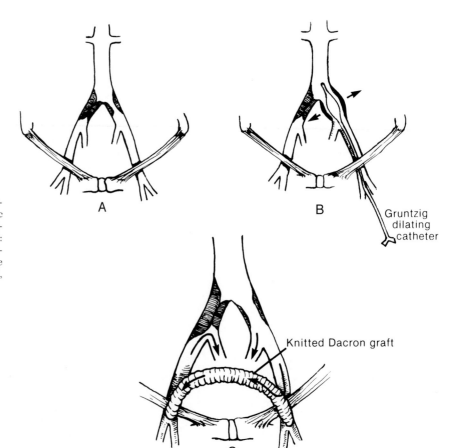

Figure 12–4. Femorofemoral bypass with transluminal angioplasty. *A*, Initial lesion. *B*, Left iliac angioplasty. *C*, Femorofemoral bypass using dilated left iliac donor limb. (From DePalma RG: Prevention of sexual dysfunction in aortoiliac surgery. In Jamieson CW [ed]: Current Operative Surgery. Eastborne, East Sussex, Bailliere-Tindall, 1985.)

In contrast, a series of men whom I operated on using techniques previously described were followed for at least 3 years up to 1990. Of 125 men who underwent an operation for aortoiliac disease, 4 became impotent as a result of emergency operations (rupture) or internal iliac aneurysms. Fifty-three men, average age 64.6, were impotent preoperatively and postoperatively; 30 men, average age 57 years (39–71), were potent preoperatively and postoperatively, whereas 39 men, average age 58.0 years (38–69), impotent preoperatively, regained function postoperatively. Among 125 men undergoing aortoiliac surgery, about 3% were rendered impotent, commonly in emergency settings. Overall, the author was able to restore or maintain function in 54% of men requiring aortoiliac surgery. The average age of men postoperatively potent was 57.5 years (range 38–71), whereas those preoperatively and postoperatively impotent averaged 64.6 years. I have noted in my patients decreasing potency with aging that does not appear to be related to arterial occlusion per se. Schiavi and colleagues[21] have shown age-related decreases in nocturnal penile tumescence in frequency, duration, and degree that correlate with desire, arousal, and coital frequency. Thus, age of patient preoperatively and postoperative aging contribute to diminished sexual function. In my opinion, this decrement in function with age is not linearly related to arterial inflow compromise.

In certain men, femorofemoral bypass combined with intraluminal dilatation of donor external or common iliac arteries is an excellent choice (Fig. 12–5). The procedure completely avoids an aortoiliac dissection, and the results can be quite durable. Objective information with pulse volume recordings before and after femorofemoral bypass correlate with improved patterns of penile plethysmography and pressures after reconstruction.[22]

Common iliac artery transluminal dilatation has been found useful. Transluminal dilatation of the external iliac arteries can improve penile perfusion, relieving steal via the internal iliac and gluteal arteries. Although transluminal dilatation of the common iliac arteries is effective, the internal iliac arteries can be difficult to dilate. However, a report in the Italian literature describes three successful cases among 25 men treated with endovascular interventions for erectile dysfunction.[23] Transluminal dilatation of the pudendal and penile arteries was noted to be plagued by restenosis, and arteriolar dysfunction was suggested.[24]

SMALL VESSEL RECONSTRUCTIONS

Small vessel reconstructions were initially attempted using direct arterialization of the corpus cavernosum. These procedures failed because they induced priapism or thrombosed due to fibrosis at the anastomosis of the artery with the corpus cavernosum. Based on a recent meta-analysis, a guidelines panel stated that the chances of success with venous and arterial surgery do not justify their routine use.[25] These procedures are applicable to the 6% to 7% of men who fail to respond to medical therapy and who do not wish to have a prosthesis.[9, 11] With the availability of effective vasoactive drugs, these procedures are now performed infrequently.

Two types of operations of microvascular bypasses can be used. One involves microvascular bypass into the dorsal artery, and the other involves arterialization of the deep

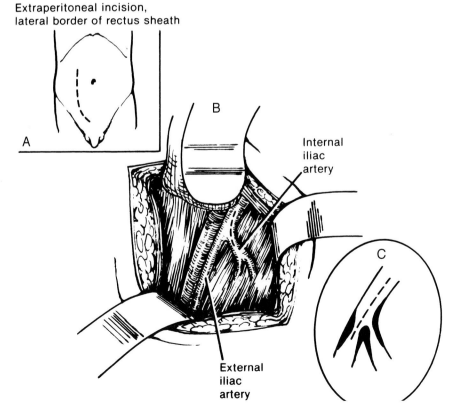

Figure 12–5. Isolated iliac artery endarterectomy. *A,* Incision for retroperitoneal exposure. *B,* Incision for isolated plaque of internal iliac. *C,* Linear incision when external iliac artery also involved. (From DePalma RG: Prevention of sexual dysfunction in aortoiliac surgery. In Jamieson CW [ed]: Current Operative Surgery. Eastborne, East Sussex, Bailliere-Tindall, 1985.)

Extraperitoneal incision, lateral border of rectus sheath

Internal iliac artery

External iliac artery

dorsal vein. The source for inflow is usually the inferior epigastric artery or, in some hands, a vein graft originating from the femoral artery. The author prefers the inferior epigastric artery as inflow source and the direct arterial reconstruction over the deep dorsal vein arterialization.

Patient Selection

The candidate for microvascular correction of erectile dysfunction must be rigorously screened, and have failed to respond to uretic therapy; in addition, the option of prosthetic insertion should be explored with the patient. Ideally, the candidates are young men with a history of trauma or localized disease.[9, 11] Some exhibit diffuse distal penile lesions of unknown origin. The candidate should exhibit absence of neural, hormonal, or medication-induced causes of impotence. I have not accepted diabetic patients for these procedures; the oldest patient selected thus far has been 61.[9] All patients require pudendal arteriography. Appropriate candidates with communication between the dorsal artery and the cavernosal artery are selected using careful visualization of individual penile vessels after intracavernous injection of a vasoactive agent to produce tumescence. As mentioned previously, a full erection masks inflow into the cavernosal artery and is not appropriate for evaluation of the penile microvasculature. The inferior epigastric artery is harvested (ligating side branches) and turned down for microvascular anastomosis to the appropriate dorsal artery.

DEEP DORSAL VEIN ARTERIALIZATION

These candidates are younger individuals with small vessel disease whose dorsal arteries are not suitable for direct bypass. Physiology of this operation was thought to be due to reverse flow via emissary veins into the corpus cavernosum. However, my arteriographic observations and those of others indicate that flow is largely by the circumflex veins into the spongiosum. My follow-up data at 12 to 84 months (average 34.5 months) showed that 33% of these men had spontaneous erections, 47% responded to intracavernous injections (ICI), and 21% remained impotent.[11] Using the inferior epigastric artery, a microvascular anastomosis is done between the inferior epigastric artery and the deep dorsal vein. There is one serious and specific complication of this arterialization—glans hyperperfusion. To prevent this, the anastomosis is performed proximally under the arch of the pubis, and the dorsal vein is ligated proximally and distally, sparing circumflex veins, which provide outflow. When this complication does occur, further distal venous ligation or graft occlusion is urgently required.

VENOUS LIGATION

Success rates for venous ligation have been reported to vary considerably; opinions about this procedure range from advocacy to qualified reservations to condemnations. This variability probably relates to patient selection. At follow-up, ranging 12 to 100 months (average 48 months), 33% functioned spontaneously, 44% used ICI, and the remainder were impotent.[9, 11] Venous ligation implies both direct ligation and excision of the veins in cases selected by dynamic infusion cavernosography. I have confined these procedures to excision of the dorsal vein[26] and have not approached crural veins directly. Other draining veins can be occluded using Gianturco coils inserted by the invasive radiologist. At times, an introducing catheter inserted via the deep dorsal vein is useful. Yu and associates recommended routine dynamic cavernosonography and cavernosometry at 3 months in all cases of venous ligation to rule out sham effect.[27] At this time, additional embolization for new leaks can be done, and with these combined procedures about 70% of men regain erectile function and are able to function with intracorporeal injections.

MEDICAL TREATMENT OF ERECTILE DYSFUNCTION

Medical treatment is almost always used first after an adequate history and physical examination are obtained. The branched logic sequence shown in Figure 12–6 is employed once aneurysms, large vessel disease, and uncontrolled diabetes have been ruled out. Treatment begins with control of risk factors such as cigarette smoking and obesity. It is also possible to alter or minimize antihypertensive treatment by weight control, exercise, or drug change. Some men improve after one or two intracavernosal injections have produced artificial erection, and they then resume spontaneous function.

Specific medical therapy and risk factor modification are done together with initial oral therapy (sildenafil), a selective inhibitor of cGMP–specific phosphodiestrase type 5, which is available in oral form. With dosage titration, this drug was effective in 59% of individuals compared with 20% in the placebo groups.[28] The use of nitrates or terazosin is a specific contraindication to this therapy. Other oral agents (apomorphine) have now also become available.

The majority of men with vasculogenic erectile dysfunction are now treated medically with oral agents or intraurethral or cavernosal injections. Vacuum devices are also available, some without prescription.

From the standpoint of the practicing vascular surgeon, it is important to recognize the requirements for aortoiliac reconstruction that prevent or relieve erectile dysfunction associated with large vessel disease. With conscientious screening and medical treatment, at the most 6% to 7% of men complaining of erectile dysfunction become candidates for vascular surgical intervention. The treatment of men with erectile dysfunction requires a unique sensitivity to the needs and aspirations of the individual, along with careful attention to details of diagnosis and treatment. Outcomes of both medical and surgical interventions are satisfying as effective diagnosis and treatment continue to evolve.

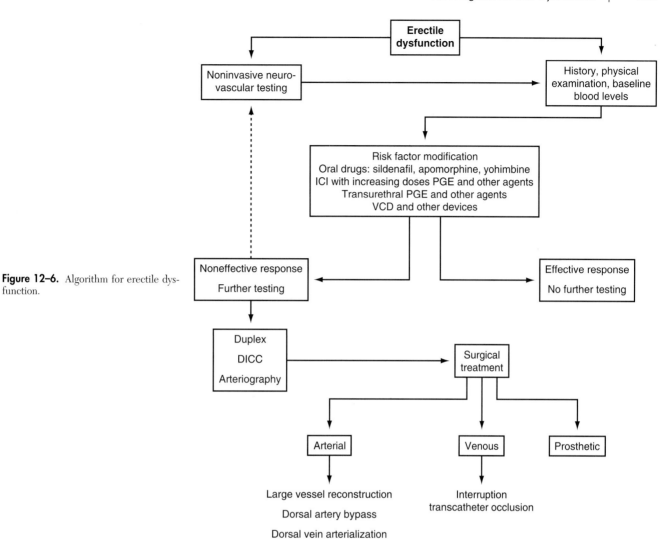

Figure 12–6. Algorithm for erectile dysfunction.

References

1. Process of Care Consensus Panel, Position paper: The process of care model for evaluation and treatment of erectile dysfunction. Int J Impot Res 11:59, 1999.
2. DePalma RG: New developments in the diagnosis and treatment of impotence. West J Med 164:54, 1996.
3. DePalma RG: The best treatment for impotence. Vasc Surg 32:519, 1998.
4. Andersson KE, Wagner G: Physiology of penile erection. Physiol Rev 75:191; 1995.
5. DePalma RG: Anatomy and physiology of normal erections: Pathogenesis of impotence. In Sidawy AN, Sumpio BE, DePalma RG (eds): Basic Science of Vascular Disease, Armonk, NY, Futura 1996, pp 761–774.
6. DeTejada IS, Goldstein I, Azadzoi K, et al: Impaired neurogenic and endothelium-mediated relaxation of penile smooth muscle from diabetic men with impotence. N Engl J Med 32:1025, 1989.
7. Rajfer J, Aronson WJ, Bush PA, et al: Nitric oxide as a mediator of the corpus cavernosum in response to nonadrenergic noncholinergic neurotransmission. N Engl J Med 326:90, 1992.
8. Azadzoi KM, Nehra A, Siroky MB: Effects of cavernosal hypoxia and oxygenation on penile erection [abstract]. Int J Impot Res 6(Suppl I):A26, 1994.
9. DePalma RG, Olding M, Yu GW, et al: Vascular interventions for impotence: Lessons learned. J Vasc Surg 21:576, 1995.
10. DePalma RG, Emsellem HA, Edwards CM, et al: A screening sequence for vasculogenic impotence. J Vasc Surg 5:228, 1987.

11. DePalma RG: Vascular surgery for impotence: A review. Int J Impot Res 9:01, 1997.
12. DePalma RG, Schwab FJ, Emsellem HA, et al: Noninvasive assessment of impotence. Surg Clin North Am 70:119, 1990.
13. Emsellem HA, Bergsrud DW, DePalma RG, et al: Pudendal evoked potentials in the evaluation of impotence [abstract]. J Clin Neurophysiol 359:5, 1988.
14. Fabra M, Porst H: Bulbocavernosus-reflex latencies and pudendal nerve SSEP compared to penile vascular testing in 669 patients with erectile failure and other sexual dysfunction. Int J Impot Res 11:167, 1999.
15. Stackl W, Hasun R, Marberger M: Intracavernous injection of prostaglandin E1 in impotent men. J Urol 140:66, 1988.
16. DePalma RG, Dalton CM, Gomez CA, et al: Predictive value of a screening sequence for venogenic impotence. Int J Impot Res 4:143, 1992.
17. Reis JM, Alves CR, Garro MA, et al: Endovascular surgery for erectile dysfunction. Int J Impot Res 10(Suppl 3):398, 1998.
18. DePalma RG, Edwards CM, Schwab FJ, Steinberg DL: Modern management of impotence associated with aortic surgery. In Bergen JJ, Yao JST (eds): Arterial Surgery: New Diagnostic and Operative Techniques. Orlando, FL, Grune & Stratton, 1988, pp 337–348.
19. DePalma RG: Prevention of sexual dysfunction in aortoiliac surgery. In Jamieson CW (ed): Current Operative Surgery: Vascular Surgery. London, Bailliere-Tindall, 1988, pp 80–96.
20. Fredberg U, Mouritzen C: Sexual dysfunction as a symptom of arte-

riosclerosis and as a complication to reconstruction of the aortoiliac segment. J Cardiovasc Surg 29:149, 1988.

21. Schiavi RC, Schreiner-Engel P, Mandeli J, et al: Healthy aging and male sexual function. Am J Psychiatry 147:766, 1990.

22. Merchant RF Jr, DePalma RG: Effects of femorofemoral grafts on postoperative sexual function: Correlation with penile pulse volume recordings. Surgery 90:962, 1981.

23. Urigo F, Pischedda A, Maiore M, et al: The role of arteriography and percutaneous transluminal angioplasty in the diagnosis and treatment of arterial vasculogenic impotence. Radiol Med 88:86, 1994.

24. Bookstein JJ, Valji K: The arteriolar component in impotence: A possible paradigm shift. AJR 157:932, 1991.

25. Montague DK, Barada JH, Belker AM, et al: Clinical Guidelines Panel on Erectile Dysfunction: Summary Report on the treatment of organic erectile dysfunction. The American Urological Association. J Urol 156:2007, 1996.

26. DePalma RG, Schwab F, Druy EM, et al: Experience in diagnosis and treatment of impotence caused by cavernosal leak syndrome. J Vasc Surg 10:117, 1989.

27. Yu GW, Schwab FJ, Melograna FS, et al: Preoperative and postoperative dynamic cavernosography and cavernosometry: Objective assessment of venous ligation for impotence. J Urol 147:618, 1992.

28. Goldstein I, Lue TF, Padma-Nathan H, et al: Oral sildenafil in the treatment of erectile dysfunction. N Engl J Med 338:1397, 1998.

Questions

1. Penile erection is mediated primarily by
   - (a) dilatation of the internal pudendal artery
   - (b) venous valve closure
   - (c) cavernosal blood O_2 tension
   - (d) relaxation of cavernosal smooth muscle
   - (e) increasing systemic arterial pressure

2. The majority of men with erectile dysfunction exhibit
   - (a) primarily psychogenic dysfunction
   - (b) large vessel atherosclerosis
   - (c) occult aneurysms with embolization
   - (d) neurologic dysfunction
   - (e) small vessel or cavernosal smooth muscle dysfunction

3. Vascular surgery for erectile dysfunction is most often effective with
   - (a) diffuse cavernosal fibrosis
   - (b) occlusion of deep cavernosal arteries
   - (c) venous valvular insufficiency
   - (d) large vessel occlusive disease
   - (e) abnormal neurologic function

4. Penile brachial indices indicate aortoiliac occlusive disease when
   - (a) PBI is between .6 and .75
   - (b) PBI is .6 or less
   - (c) PBI is .8 or less
   - (d) PBI .8 is accompanied by flat pulse volume waves
   - (e) PBI .75 is accompanied by abnormally shaped pulse waves

5. Cavernosal artery occlusion pressure is
   - (a) usually equal to systemic blood pressure
   - (b) measured by pulse volume recording
   - (c) measured by Doppler insonation at full erection during infusion study
   - (d) abnormal when pressure gradients are between 15 and 20 mm Hg below systolic pressure
   - (e) the pressure at which cavernosal flow is enhanced before a rigid erection

6. When a sexually active man expresses concern about possible erectile dysfunction before aneurysm repair, one should
   - (a) reassure the patient and spouse that this is preventable
   - (b) refer the patient to a psychiatrist
   - (c) measure baseline levels of testosterone and prolactin
   - (d) obtain preoperative penile brachial indices and pulse volume recordings
   - (e) obtain preoperative selective pudendal arteriography

7. Useful techniques in preventing postoperative sexual dysfunction in aortic surgery include
   - (a) restoration of flow to internal iliac arteries
   - (b) suture of inferior mesenteric artery within the aortic sac
   - (c) avoidance of the aortic bifurcation
   - (d) retrograde flushing of internal iliacs
   - (e) All of the above

8. Age probably affects potency by
   - (a) decreasing arterial inflow
   - (b) causing nerve deterioration
   - (c) causing smooth muscle dysfunction
   - (d) increasing venous leakage
   - (e) decreasing cardiovascular reserves

9. Artificial erection is most safely obtained by
   - (a) intracavernous papaverine injection
   - (b) intracavernous prostaglandin E_1 injection
   - (c) intracavernous phentolamine injection
   - (d) roller pump cavernosal infusion of 40 mL normal saline/minute
   - (e) all of the above

10. After screening and medical treatment for erectile dysfunction
    - (a) about 6% to 7% of men might become candidates for vascular intervention
    - (b) most will respond to deep dorsal vein arterialization
    - (c) many prefer prosthetic devices
    - (d) most will respond unfavorably and require psychotherapy
    - (e) many need psychological counseling even when therapy is effective

Answers

1. d   2. e   3. d   4. b   5. c   6. d   7. e   8. c   9. b   10. a

13

Hemodynamics for the Vascular Surgeon

R. Eugene Zierler and D. Eugene Strandness, Jr.

Blood flow in human arteries and veins can be described in terms of strict hemodynamic principles. Although the elements of hemodynamics are derived from engineering, mathematics, and physiology, these principles also form the theoretical foundation for the surgical treatment of vascular disease.

The major mechanisms of arterial disease are obstruction of the lumen and disruption of the vessel wall. Arterial obstruction or narrowing may result from atherosclerosis, emboli, thrombi, fibromuscular dysplasia, trauma, or external compression. The clinical significance of an obstructive lesion depends on its location, severity, and duration, as well as the ability of the circulation to compensate by increasing cardiac output and developing collateral pathways. Surgical treatment requires the identification and correction of arterial lesions associated with significant hemodynamic disturbances. Disruption of the arterial wall is caused by ruptured aneurysm or trauma. The tendency of aneurysms to rupture is determined by arterial wall characteristics, intraluminal pressure, and size. In this situation, the role of surgery is to prevent rupture or to reestablish arterial continuity after rupture occurs.

On the venous side of the circulation, the major hemodynamic mechanisms of disease are obstruction and valvular incompetence. These are generally the sequelae of thrombosis in the deep venous system, and they produce venous hypertension in the circulation distal to the involved venous segment. The clinical consequences of venous hypertension are the signs and symptoms of the post-thrombotic syndrome: pain, edema, subcutaneous fibrosis, pigmentation, stasis dermatitis, and ulceration. Treatment of this condition involves elevation, external compression, venous interruption, and, rarely, direct venous reconstruction.

This chapter begins with a discussion of the hemodynamic principles and wall properties that govern arterial flow. The hemodynamic alterations produced by arterial stenoses and their effect on flow patterns in human limbs are considered next. These principles are then related to the treatment of arterial obstruction. Finally, the hemody-

namics of the venous system are briefly reviewed and related to the pathophysiology and treatment of venous disease.

BASIC PRINCIPLES OF ARTERIAL HEMODYNAMICS

Fluid Pressure

The pressure in a fluid system is defined as force per unit area (given in dynes per square centimeter). Intravascular arterial pressure (P) has three components: (1) the dynamic pressure produced by contraction of the heart, (2) the hydrostatic pressure, and (3) the static filling pressure. Hydrostatic pressure is determined by the specific gravity of blood and the height of the point of measurement above a specific reference level. The reference level in the human body is considered to be the right atrium. The hydrostatic pressure is given by:

$$P \text{ (hydrostatic)} = -\rho g h \qquad [1]$$

where ρ is the specific gravity of blood (approximately 1.056 g/cm³), g is the acceleration due to gravity (980 cm/sec²), and h is the distance in centimeters above or below the right atrium. The magnitude of hydrostatic pressure may be quite large. In a man 5 feet 8 inches tall, this pressure at ankle level is approximately 89 mm Hg.[1]

The static filling pressure represents the residual pressure that exists in the absence of arterial flow. This pressure is determined by the volume of blood and the elastic properties of the vessel wall, and it is usually in the range of 5 to 10 mm Hg.

Fluid Energy

Blood flows through the arterial system in response to differences in total fluid energy. Although pressure gradients are the most obvious forces involved, other forms of energy drive the circulation.[2] Total fluid energy (E) can be divided into potential energy (E_p) and kinetic energy (E_k). The components of potential energy are intravascular pressure (P) and gravitational potential energy.

The factors contributing to intravascular pressure have already been discussed. Gravitational potential energy represents the ability of a volume of blood to do work because of its height above a specific reference level. The formula for gravitational potential energy is the same as that for hydrostatic pressure (see Equation 1) but with an opposite sign: $+ \rho gh$. Because the gravitational potential energy and hydrostatic pressure usually cancel each other out and the static filling pressure is relatively low, the predominant component of potential energy is the dynamic pressure produced by cardiac contraction. Potential energy can be expressed as:

$$E_p = P + (\rho gh) \qquad [2]$$

Kinetic energy represents the ability of blood to do work on the basis of its motion. It is proportional to the specific gravity of blood and the square of blood velocity (v), in centimeters per second:

$$E_k = 1/2\rho v^2 \qquad [3]$$

By combining Equations 2 and 3, an expression for the total fluid energy per unit volume of blood (in ergs per cubic centimeter) can be obtained:

$$E + P + (\rho gh) + (1/2\rho v^2) \qquad [4]$$

Fluid Energy Losses

Bernoulli's Principle

When fluid flows from one point to another, its total energy (E) along any given streamline is constant, provided that flow is steady and there are no frictional energy losses. This is in accordance with the law of conservation of energy and constitutes Bernoulli's principle:

$$P_1 + \rho gh_1 + 1/2\rho v_1^2 = P_2 + \rho gh_2 + 1/2\rho v_2^2 \qquad [5]$$

This equation expresses the relationship between pressure, gravitational potential energy, and kinetic energy in an idealized fluid system. In the horizontal diverging tube shown in Figure 13–1, steady flow between point 1 and point 2 is accompanied by an increase in cross-sectional area and a decrease in flow velocity. Although the fluid moves against a pressure gradient of 2.5 mm Hg and therefore gains potential energy, the total fluid energy remains constant because of the lower velocity and a proportional loss of kinetic energy. In other words, the widening of the tube results in the conversion of kinetic energy to potential energy in the form of pressure. In a converging tube, the opposite would occur; a pressure drop and increase in velocity would be noted as potential energy was converted to kinetic energy.

The situation depicted in the preceding example is not observed in human arteries because the ideal flow condi-

A₁=1 cm²　　　**A₂=16 cm²**

V₁=80 cm/sec　　**V₂=5 cm/sec**

P₁=100 mm Hg　　**P₂=102.5 mm Hg**

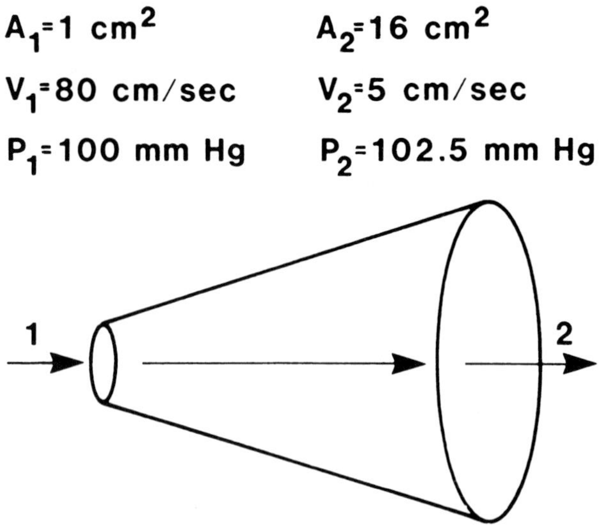

Figure 13–1. Effect of increasing cross-sectional area on pressure in a frictionless fluid system. While pressure increases, total fluid energy remains constant as a result of a decrease in velocity. (Redrawn from Sumner DS: The hemodynamics and pathophysiology of arterial disease. In Rutherford RB [ed]: Vascular Surgery. Philadelphia, WB Saunders, 1977.)

tions specified in the Bernoulli relationship are not present. The fluid energy lost in moving blood through the arterial circulation is dissipated mainly in the form of heat. When this source of energy loss is accounted for, Equation 5 becomes:

$$P_1 + \rho gh_1 + 1/2\rho v_1^2 = P_2 + \rho gh_2 + 1/2\rho v_2^2 + \text{heat} \qquad [6]$$

Viscous Energy Losses and Poiseuille's Law

Energy losses in flowing blood occur either as viscous losses resulting from friction or as inertial losses related to changes in the velocity or direction of flow. The term *viscosity* describes the resistance to flow that arises because of the intermolecular attractions between fluid layers. The coefficient of viscosity (η) is defined as the ratio of shear stress (τ) to shear rate (D):

$$\eta = \frac{\tau}{D} \qquad [7]$$

Shear stress is proportional to the energy loss due to friction between adjacent fluid layers, whereas shear rate refers to the relative velocity of adjacent fluid layers. Fluids with particularly strong intermolecular attractions offer a high resistance to flow and have high coefficients of viscosity. For example, motor oil has a higher coefficient of viscosity than water.[3] The unit of viscosity is the poise, which equals 1 dyne-sec/cm.[2] Because it is difficult to measure viscosity directly, relative viscosity is often used to relate the viscosity of a fluid to that of water. The relative viscosity of plasma is approximately 1.8, whereas for whole blood the relative viscosity is in the range of 3 to 4.

Because viscosity increases exponentially with increases in hematocrit, the concentration of red blood cells is the most important factor affecting the viscosity of whole

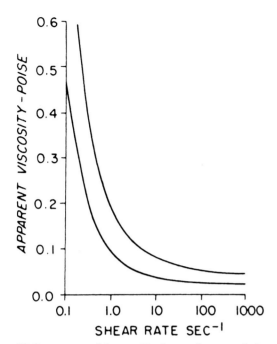

Figure 13–2. Viscosity of human blood as a function of shear rate. Values range between the two lines. (From Strandness DE, Sumner DS: Hemodynamics for Surgeons. New York, Grune & Stratton, 1975.)

blood. The viscosity of plasma is determined largely by the concentration of plasma proteins. These constituents of blood are also responsible for its non-Newtonian character. In a Newtonian fluid, viscosity is independent of shear rate or flow velocity. Because blood is a suspension of cells and large protein molecules, its viscosity can vary greatly with shear rate (Fig. 13–2). Blood viscosity increases rapidly at low shear rates but approaches a constant value at higher shear rates. In most of the arterial circulation, the prevailing shear rates place the blood viscosity on the asymptotic portion of the curve. Thus, for arteries with diameters greater than about 1 mm, human blood resembles a constant-viscosity or Newtonian fluid.

Poiseuille's law describes the viscous energy losses that occur in an idealized flow model. This law states that the pressure gradient along a tube ($P_1 - P_2$ in dynes per square centimeter) is directly proportional to the mean flow velocity ($\bar{V}$, in centimeters per second) or volume flow ($\bar{Q}$, in cubic centimeters per second), the tube length (L, in centimeters), and the fluid viscosity (η, in poises), and is inversely proportional to either the second or fourth power of the radius (r, in centimeters):

$$P_1 - P_2 = \bar{V}\frac{8L\eta}{r^2} = Q\frac{8L\eta}{\pi r^4} \qquad [8]$$

When this equation is simplified to pressure = flow × resistance, it is analogous to Ohm's law of electrical circuits.

The strict application of Poiseuille's law requires the steady, laminar flow of a Newtonian fluid in a straight, rigid, cylindrical tube. Because these conditions seldom exist in the arterial circulation, Poiseuille's law can only estimate the minimum pressure gradient or viscous energy losses that may be expected in arterial flow. Energy losses due to inertial effects often exceed viscous energy losses, particularly in the presence of arterial disease.

Inertial Energy Losses

Energy losses related to inertia (ΔE) are proportional to a constant (K), the specific gravity of blood, and the square of blood velocity:

$$\Delta E = K\ 1/2\rho v^2 \qquad [9]$$

Because velocity is the only independent variable in this equation, inertial energy losses result from the acceleration and deceleration of pulsatile flow, variations in lumen diameter, and changes in the direction of flow at points of curvature and branching.

The combined effects of viscous and inertial energy losses are illustrated in Figure 13–3. When the pressure drop across an arterial segment is measured at varying flow rates, the experimental data fit a line with both linear (viscous) and squared (inertial) terms. The viscous energy losses predicted by Poiseuille's law are considerably less than the total energy loss actually observed.

Vascular Resistance

Hemodynamic resistance (R) can be defined as the ratio of the energy drop between two points along an artery ($E_1 - E_2$) to the mean blood flow (Q):

$$R = \frac{E_1 - E_2}{Q} \cong \frac{P_1 - P_2}{Q} \qquad [10]$$

If the kinetic energy term ($1/2\rho v^2$) is considered to be a small component of the total energy, and the artery is assumed to be horizontal so that the gravitational potential

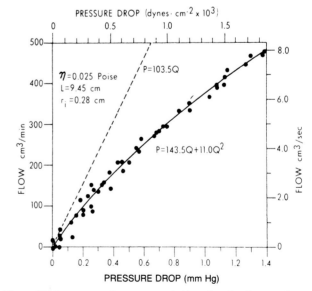

Figure 13–3. Pressure drop across a 9.45-cm length of canine femoral artery at varying flow rates. The experimental data line *(solid)* has both linear and squared terms, corresponding to viscous and inertial energy losses. The pressure-flow curve predicted by Poiseuille's law *(dashed line)* depicts much lower energy losses than those actually observed. (From Sumner DS: The hemodynamics and pathophysiology of arterial disease. In Rutherford RB [ed]: Vascular Surgery. Philadelphia, WB Saunders, 1977.)

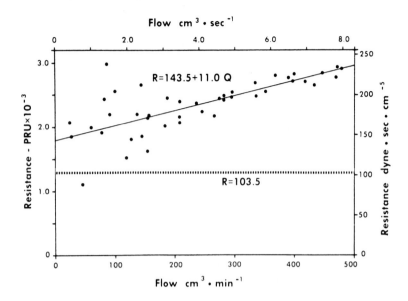

Figure 13–4. Resistance derived from the pressure-flow curve in Figure 13–3. The resistance increases with increasing flow. Constant resistance predicted by Poiseuille's law is shown by the dotted line. (From Sumner DS: The hemodynamics and pathophysiology of arterial disease. In Rutherford RB [ed]: Vascular Surgery. Philadelphia, WB Saunders, 1977.)

energy terms ($\rho g h$) cancel, Equation 4 can be used to express resistance as the simple ratio of pressure drop ($P_1 - P_2$) to flow. Thus, Equation 10 becomes a rearranged version of Poiseuille's law (Equation 8), and the minimum resistance or viscous energy losses are given by the resistance term:

$$R = \frac{8L\eta}{\pi r^4} \qquad [11]$$

The hemodynamic resistance of an arterial segment increases as the flow velocity increases, provided the lumen size remains constant (Fig. 13–4). These additional energy losses are related to inertial effects and are proportional to $1/2P + \rho v^2$.

According to Equation 11, the predominant factor influencing hemodynamic resistance is the fourth power of the radius. The relationship between radius and pressure drop for various flow rates along a 10-cm vessel segment is shown in Figure 13–5. For a wide range of flow rates, the pressure drop is negligible until the radius is reduced to about 0.3 cm; for radii less than 0.2 cm, the pressure drop increases rapidly. These observations may explain the frequent failure of femoropopliteal autogenous vein bypass grafts less than 4 mm in diameter.[4]

The calculation of total resistance (R_t) depends on whether the component resistances ($R_1 \ldots R_n$) are arranged in series or in parallel. This is also analogous to electrical circuits.

$$R_t \text{ (series)} = R_1 + R_2 + \ldots R_n \qquad [12]$$

$$\frac{1}{R_t \text{ (parallel)}} = \frac{1}{R_1} + \frac{1}{R_2} + \ldots \frac{1}{R_n} \qquad [13]$$

The standard physical units of hemodynamic resistance are dyne-seconds per centimeter to the fifth power. A more convenient way of expressing resistance is the peripheral resistance unit (PRU), which has the dimensions of millimeters of mercury per cubic centimeter per minute. One PRU is approximately 8×10^4 dyne-sec/cm[5].

In the human circulation, approximately 90% of the total vascular resistance results from flow through the arteries and capillaries, whereas the remaining 10% results from venous flow. The arterioles and capillaries are responsible for over 60% of the total resistance, whereas the large and medium-sized arteries account for only about 15%.[2] Thus, the arteries that are most commonly affected by atherosclerotic occlusive disease are normally vessels with very low resistance.

Blood Flow Patterns

Laminar Flow

In the steady-state conditions specified by Poiseuille's law, the flow pattern is laminar. All motion is parallel to the

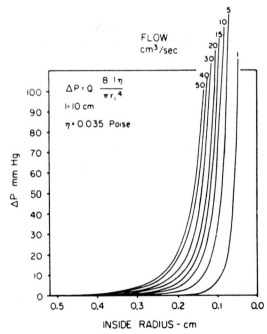

Figure 13–5. Relationship of pressure drop to inside radius of a cylindrical tube 10 cm in length at various rates of steady laminar flow. Flow rates are comparable to those in the human iliac artery. (From Strandness DE, Sumner DS: Hemodynamics for Surgeons. New York, Grune & Stratton, 1975.)

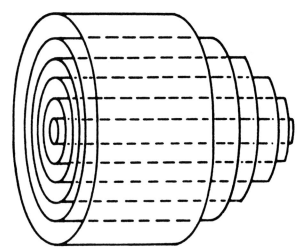

Figure 13–6. Concentric laminae of fluid in a cylindrical tube. Flow is from left to right. The center laminae move more rapidly than those near the periphery, and the flow profile is parabolic. (From Strandness DE, Sumner DS: Hemodynamics for Surgeons. New York, Grune & Stratton, 1975.)

walls of the tube, and the fluid is arranged in a series of concentric layers or laminae like those shown in Figure 13–6. While the velocity within each lamina remains constant, the velocity is lowest adjacent to the tube wall and increases toward the center of the tube. This results in a velocity profile that is parabolic in shape (Fig. 13–7). As previously discussed, the energy expended in moving one lamina of fluid over another is proportional to viscosity.

Turbulent Flow

In contrast to the linear streamlines of laminar flow, turbulence is an irregular flow state in which velocity varies rapidly with respect to space and time. These random velocity changes result in the dissipation of fluid energy as heat. The point of transition between laminar and turbulent flow depends on the tube diameter (d, in centimeters), the mean velocity, the specific gravity of the fluid, and the fluid viscosity. These factors can be expressed as a dimensionless

quantity called the Reynolds number (Re), which is the ratio of inertial forces to viscous forces acting on the fluid:

$$\mathrm{Re} = \frac{d\bar{V}p}{\eta} \qquad [14]$$

In flowing blood at Reynolds numbers greater than 2000, inertial forces may disrupt laminar flow and produce fully developed turbulence. With values less than 2000, localized flow disturbances are damped out by viscous forces. In the normal arterial circulation, Reynolds numbers are usually less than 2000, and true turbulence is unlikely to occur; however, Reynolds numbers greater than 2000 can be found in the ascending aorta, where small areas of turbulence develop.[3] Although turbulent flow is uncommon in normal arteries, the arterial flow pattern is often disturbed.[5] The condition of disturbed flow is an intermediate state between stable laminar flow and fully developed turbulence. It is a transient perturbation in the laminar streamlines that disappears as the flow proceeds downstream. Arterial flow may become disturbed at points of branching and curvature.

When turbulence is the result of a stenotic arterial lesion, it generally occurs immediately downstream from the stenosis and may be present only over the systolic portion of the cardiac cycle when the critical value of the Reynolds number is exceeded. Under conditions of turbulent flow, the velocity profile changes from the parabolic shape of laminar flow to a rectangular or blunt shape (see Fig. 13–7). Because of the random velocity changes, energy losses are greater for a turbulent or disturbed flow state than for a laminar flow state. Consequently, the linear relationship between pressure and flow expressed by Poiseuille's law cannot be applied. This deviation from Poiseuille's law in arterial flow is shown in Figure 13–3.

Boundary Layer Separation

In fluid flowing through a tube, the portion of fluid adjacent to the tube wall is referred to as the boundary layer. This layer is subject to both frictional interactions with the tube wall and viscous forces generated by the more rapidly moving fluid toward the center of the tube. When the tube geometry changes suddenly, such as at points of curvature, branching, or alteration in lumen diameter, small pressure gradients are created that cause the boundary layer to stop or reverse direction. This results in a complex, localized flow pattern known as an area of flow separation or separation zone.[6]

Areas of boundary layer separation have been observed in models of arterial anastomoses and bifurcations.[7, 8] In the carotid artery bifurcation shown in Figure 13–8, the central rapid flow stream of the common carotid artery is compressed along the inner wall of the carotid bulb, producing a region of high shear stress. An area of flow separation has formed along the outer wall of the carotid bulb that includes helical flow patterns and flow reversal. The region of the carotid bulb adjacent to the separation zone is subject to relatively low shear stresses. Distal to the bulb, in the internal carotid artery, flow reattachment occurs and a more laminar flow pattern is present.

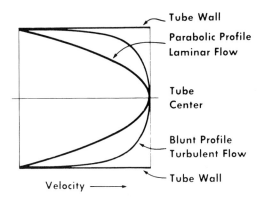

Figure 13–7. Velocity profiles of steady laminar and turbulent flow. Velocity is lowest adjacent to the tube wall and maximal in the center. (From Sumner DS: The hemodynamics and pathophysiology of arterial disease. In Rutherford RB [ed]: Vascular Surgery. Philadelphia, WB Saunders, 1977.)

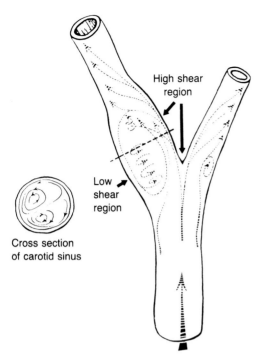

Figure 13–8. Carotid artery bifurcation showing an area of flow separation adjacent to the outer wall of the bulb. Rapid flow is associated with high shear stress, whereas the slower flow of the separation zone produces a region of low shear. (From Zarins CK, Giddens DP, Glagov S: Atherosclerotic plaque distribution and flow velocity profiles in the carotid bifurcation. In Bergan JJ, Yao JST [eds]: Cerebrovascular Insufficiency. New York, Grune & Stratton, 1983.)

The complex flow patterns described in models of the carotid bifurcation have also been documented in human subjects by pulsed Doppler studies.[9, 10] As shown in Figure 13–9, the Doppler spectral waveform obtained near the inner wall of the carotid bulb is typical of the forward, quasi-steady flow pattern found in the internal carotid artery. However, sampling of flow along the outer wall of the bulb demonstrates lower velocities with periods of both forward and reverse flow. These spectral characteristics are consistent with the presence of flow separation and are considered to be a normal finding, particularly in young individuals.[10] Alterations in arterial distensibility with increasing age make flow separation less prominent in older individuals.[11]

The clinical importance of boundary layer separation is that these localized flow disturbances may contribute to the formation of atherosclerotic plaques.[12] Examination of human carotid bifurcations, both at autopsy and during surgery, indicates that intimal thickening and atherosclerosis tend to occur along the outer wall of the carotid bulb, whereas the inner wall is relatively spared.[8] These findings suggest that atherosclerotic lesions form near areas of flow separation and low shear stress. Whether flow separation represents a true causative factor or simply promotes the development of previously existing lesions is not known.

Pulsatile Flow

In a pulsatile system, pressure and flow vary continuously with time, and the velocity profile changes throughout the cardiac cycle. The hemodynamic principles that have been discussed are based on steady flow, and they are not adequate for a precise description of pulsatile flow in the arterial circulation; however, as previously stated, they can be used to determine the minimal energy losses occurring in a specific flow system.

The complex interactions of cardiac contraction, arterial wall characteristics, and blood flow are extremely difficult to define rigorously. For example, estimation of the inertial energy losses in pulsatile flow requires a value for the velocity term (Equation 9); however, in pulsatile flow, velocity varies with both time and position across the flow profile. Furthermore, skewing of the velocity profile may occur as a result of curvature or branching. The resistance term of Poiseuille's law (Equation 11) estimates viscous energy losses in steady flow, but it does not account for the inertial effects, arterial wall elasticity, and wave reflections that influence pulsatile flow. The term *vascular impedance* is used to describe the resistance or opposition offered by a peripheral vascular bed to pulsatile blood flow.[3]

Pulsatile flow appears to be important for optimum organ function. For example, when a kidney is perfused by steady flow instead of pulsatile flow, a reduction in urine volume and sodium excretion occurs.[13] The critical effect of pulsatile flow is probably exerted on the microcirculation. Although the exact mechanism is unknown, transcapillary exchange, arteriolar tone, and lymphatic flow are all influenced by the pulsatile nature of blood flow.

Bifurcations and Branches

The branches of the arterial system produce sudden changes in the flow pattern that are potential sources of energy loss. However, the effect of branching on the total pressure drop in normal arterial flow is relatively small.

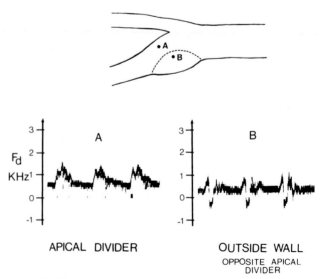

Figure 13–9. Flow separation in the normal carotid bulb shown by pulsed Doppler spectral analysis. The flow pattern near the apical divider (*A*) is forward throughout the cardiac cycle, but near the outside wall (*B*) the spectrum contains both forward (*positive*) and reverse (*negative*) flow components. The latter pattern indicates an area of flow separation. (Reproduced with permission of J. F. Primozich, BS, and D. J. Phillips, PhD.)

Arterial branches commonly take the form of bifurcations. Flow patterns in a bifurcation are determined mainly by the area ratio and the branch angle. The *area ratio* is defined as the combined area of the secondary branches divided by the area of the primary artery.

Bifurcation flow can be analyzed in terms of pressure gradient, velocity, and transmission of pulsatile energy. According to Poiseuille's law, an area ratio of 1.41 would allow the pressure gradient to remain constant along a bifurcation. If the combined area of the branches equals the area of the primary artery, then the area ratio is 1.0 and there is no change in the velocity of flow.[14] For efficient transmission of pulsatile energy across a bifurcation, the vascular impedance of the primary artery should equal that of the branches, a situation that occurs with an area ratio of 1.15 for larger arteries and 1.35 for smaller arteries.[15] Human infants have a favorable area ratio of 1.11 at the aortic bifurcation, but there is a gradual decrease in the ratio with age. In the teenage years, the average area ratio is less than 1.0; in the twenties, it is less than 0.9; and by the forties, it drops below 0.8.[16] This decline in the area ratio of the aortic bifurcation leads to an increase in both the velocity of flow in the secondary branches and the amount of reflected pulsatile energy. For example, with an area ratio of 0.8, approximately 22% of the incident pulsatile energy is reflected in the infrarenal aorta. This mechanism may play a role in the localization of atherosclerosis and aneurysms in this arterial segment.[17]

The curvature and angulation of an arterial bifurcation can also contribute to the development of flow disturbances. As blood flows around a curve, the high-velocity portion of the stream is subjected to the greatest centrifugal force; rapidly moving fluid in the center of the vessel tends to flow outward and be replaced by the slower fluid originally located near the arterial wall. This can result in complex helical flow patterns, such as those observed in the carotid bifurcation.[9] As the angle between the secondary branches of a bifurcation is increased, the tendency to develop turbulent or disturbed flow also rises. The average angle between the human iliac arteries is 54 degrees; however, with diseased or tortuous iliac arteries, this angle can approach 180 degrees.[3] In the latter situation, flow disturbances are particularly likely to develop.

Physical Properties of the Arterial Wall

Composition of the Arterial Wall

Blood vessels are viscoelastic tubes. In this context, viscosity refers to the resistance of a material to shear, and elasticity describes the tendency of a material to return to its original shape after being subjected to a deforming force. As blood proceeds from the large arteries of the thorax and abdomen to the medium-sized arteries of the extremities, the relative amount of elastic tissue in the vessel wall decreases as the amount of collagen and smooth muscle increases. At the level of the arteriole, the wall consists almost entirely of smooth muscle. Thus, the viscoelastic properties of an artery depend primarily on the elastin-collagen ratio. Elastin is the predominant compo-

nent of the thoracic aorta that allows energy to be stored during cardiac systole and returned to the system in diastole. Because collagen is much less extensible than elastin, the more distal arteries, such as the brachial and femoral, do not store much of the pulsatile energy but serve mainly as conduits for blood. The function of the muscular arterioles is to control blood pressure and flow by actively altering the lumen diameter.

As the structure of the arterial wall changes, each successive branching also increases the total cross-sectional area of the arterial tree. The cross-sectional area at the arteriolar level is approximately 125 times that of the aorta; at the capillary level, it has increased approximately 800 times.[3] The reduced elastin-collagen ratio and increased stiffness of the peripheral arteries result in a more rapid pulse wave velocity and a high vascular impedance. Although the impedance of the thoracic aorta must be low to minimize cardiac work, the impedance of peripheral arteries should match the high arteriolar impedance to decrease the reflected components of the pulse wave.

Tangential Stress and Tension

The tangential stress (τ) within the wall of a fluid-filled cylindrical tube can be expressed as

$$\tau = P\frac{r}{\delta} \qquad [15]$$

where P is the pressure exerted by the fluid (in dynes per square centimeter), r is the internal radius (in centimeters), and δ is the thickness of the tube wall (in centimeters). Stress (τ) has the dimensions of force per unit area of tube wall (dynes per square centimeter). Thus, tangential stress is directly proportional to pressure and radius but inversely proportional to wall thickness.

Equation 15 is similar to Laplace's law, which defines tangential tension (T) as the product of pressure and radius:

$$T = Pr \qquad [16]$$

Tension is given in units of force per tube length (dynes per centimeter). The terms *stress* and *tension* have different dimensions and describe the forces acting on the tube wall in different ways. Laplace's law can be used to characterize thin-walled structures such as soap bubbles; however, it is not suitable for describing the stresses in arterial walls.

Arterial Wall Properties in Specific Conditions

AGING AND ATHEROSCLEROSIS. Arterial walls become less distensible with age. This increase in stiffness cannot be explained on the basis of atherosclerosis alone.[3] Alterations in the elastin fibers and elastic lamellae, together with an increase in wall thickness, probably account for this increase in arterial stiffness. Changes associated with aging include fragmentation of elastic lamellae and deposition of collagen between the elastin layers. This tends to maintain the elastin fibers in the extended state. Calcium is also deposited near the elastin fibers and contributes to the increased thickness of the arterial wall.

The effects of atherosclerosis on the mechanical properties of the arterial wall are complex and difficult to distinguish from those due to aging. In the early stages, arterial distensibility may actually increase as elastin fibers are disrupted; however, as the disease progresses, fibrosis and calcification tend to make the arterial wall less distensible.

ENDARTERECTOMY. During an endarterectomy, the atherosclerotic plaque is removed along with the intima and a portion of the media, leaving behind a tube consisting of the outer media and adventitia. This reduces the wall thickness to approximately one third of its original value and should result in an increase in tangential stress, according to Equation 15. As would be expected, endarterectomy decreases the stiffness of an artery to circumferential expansion.[18] Still, the endarterectomized artery remains stiffer and less distensible than a normal artery. This indicates that the components responsible for strength and stiffness are concentrated in the outer layers of the arterial wall. It is because of this anatomic arrangement that endarterectomy is possible.

ANEURYSMS. When the structural components of the arterial wall are weakened, aneurysms may form. Rupture occurs when the tangential stress within the arterial wall becomes greater than the tensile strength. Figure 13–10 shows a tube with an outside diameter of 2.0 cm and a wall thickness of 0.2 cm, dimensions similar to those of atherosclerotic aortas.[1] If the internal pressure is 150 mm Hg, the tangential wall stress is 8.0×10^5 dynes/cm². Expansion of the tube to form an aneurysm with a diameter of 6.0 cm results in a decrease in wall thickness to 0.06 cm. The increased radius and decreased wall thickness increase the wall stress to 98.0×10^5 dynes/cm², assuming that the pressure remains constant. In this example, the diameter has been enlarged by a factor of 3, and the wall stress has increased by a factor of 12.

Although the tensile strength of collagen is extremely high, it constitutes only about 15% of the aneurysm wall.[19] Furthermore, the collagen fibers in an aneurysm are sparsely distributed and subject to fragmentation. The tendency of larger aneurysms to rupture is readily explained by the effect of increased radius on tangential stress (Equation 15) and the degenerative changes in the arterial wall. The relationship between tangential stress and blood pressure accounts for the contribution of hypertension to the risk of rupture.

The diverging and converging geometry of aneurysms can result in complex flow patterns that include areas of boundary layer separation and flow reversal.[20] These patterns explain the frequent accumulation of clot in aneurysms that confines the flow stream to an area not much larger than the native artery. Because this clot increases the effective thickness of the vessel wall, it may reduce tangential stress and provide some protection against rupture. However, the tensile strength of clot and arterial wall is not the same, and the contribution of clot to the integrity of an aneurysm is impossible to predict.[3] Furthermore, the clot within an aneurysm is often not circumferential. In this situation, Equation 15 can be applied to the wall segment without clot, and the tangential stress at that site depends on the maximum internal radius.

Another factor to consider is that in about 55% of ruptured abdominal aortic aneurysms, the site of rupture is in the posterolateral aspect of the aneurysm wall.[21] The posterior wall of the aorta is relatively fixed against the spine, and repeated flexion of the wall in that area could result in structural fatigue. This would produce a localized area of weakness that might predispose to rupture.

HEMODYNAMICS OF ARTERIAL STENOSES

Energy Losses Related to Arterial Stenoses

According to Poiseuille's law (Equation 8), the radius of a stenotic segment has a much greater effect on viscous energy losses than its length. Inertial energy losses, which occur at the entrance (contraction effects) and exit (expansion effects) of a stenosis, are proportional to the square of blood velocity (Equation 9). Energy losses are also influenced by the geometry of a stenosis; a gradual tapering results in less energy loss than an irregular or abrupt change in lumen size. A converging vessel geometry tends to stabilize laminar flow and flatten the velocity profile, whereas a diverging vessel produces an elongated velocity profile and a less stable flow pattern. The energy lost at the exit of a stenosis may be quite significant because of the sudden expansion of the flow stream and dissipation of kinetic energy in a zone of turbulence.

The energy lost in expansion (ΔP) can be expressed in terms of the flow velocity distal to the stenosis (v), and

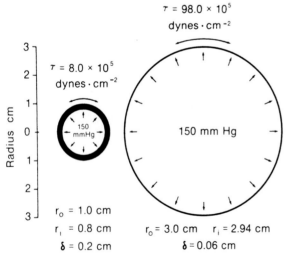

Figure 13–10. End-on view of a cylinder, 2 cm in diameter, that is expanded to 6 cm in diameter, while the wall area remains constant; τ = wall stress, δ = wall thickness, r_1 = inside radius, r_0 = outside radius. (From Sumner DS: The hemodynamics and pathophysiology of arterial disease. In Rutherford RB [ed]: Vascular Surgery. Philadelphia, WB Saunders, 1977.)

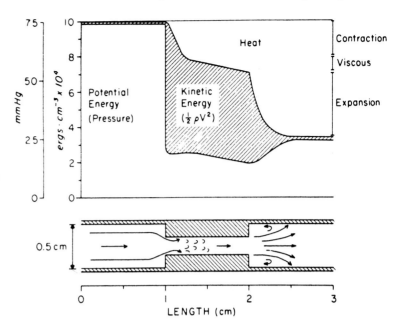

Figure 13–11. Energy losses resulting when blood flows steadily through a 1-cm-long stenosis. Inertial losses *(contraction and expansion)* are more significant than viscous losses. (From Sumner DS: The hemodynamics and pathophysiology of arterial disease. In Rutherford RB [ed]: Vascular Surgery. Philadelphia, WB Saunders, 1977.)

the radii of the stenotic lumen (r_s) and the normal distal lumen (r):

$$\Delta P = k\frac{\rho}{2}v^2\left[\left(\frac{r}{r_s}\right)^2 - 1\right]^2 \qquad [17]$$

Figure 13–11 illustrates the energy losses related to a 1-cm-long stenosis. The viscous losses are relatively small and occur within the stenotic segment. Inertial losses due to contraction and expansion are much greater. Because most of the energy loss in this example results from inertial effects, the length of the stenosis is relatively unimportant.[1]

Bruits and Poststenotic Dilatation

The presence of an audible sound or bruit over an artery is usually regarded as a clinical sign of arterial disease. Stenoses or irregularities of the vessel lumen produce turbulent flow patterns that set up vibrations in the arterial wall. These vibrations generate displacement waves that radiate through the surrounding tissues and can be detected as audible sounds. Such vibrations are probably the main source of sound in the arterial system.[3]

Generally, a soft, midsystolic bruit is associated with a relatively minor lesion that does not significantly reduce flow or pressure. A bruit with a loud diastolic component suggests a stenosis severe enough to reduce flow and produce a pressure drop. Thus, the intensity and duration of a bruit serve as a rough guide to the severity of an arterial stenosis. A bruit may be absent when an artery is nearly occluded or when the flow rate is extremely low.

A dilated area distal to a stenosis is a common clinical finding. Poststenotic dilatation has been observed in the thoracic aorta below coarctations, distal to arterial stenoses at the thoracic outlet, and distal to atherosclerotic lesions. The most likely explanation for this phenomenon is that arterial wall vibrations result in structural fatigue of elastin fibers. In a series of animal model studies, poststenotic

dilatations did not develop unless a bruit was present distal to the stenosis.[22] It appears that vibrations in the audible range may weaken elastin fibers and break down links between collagen fibers. When this occurs, the arterial wall distal to the stenosis becomes more distensible and subject to localized dilatation.

Critical Arterial Stenosis

The degree of arterial narrowing required to produce a significant reduction in blood pressure or flow is called a *critical stenosis*. Because the energy losses associated with a stenosis are inversely proportional to the fourth power of the radius at that site (Equations 8 and 17), there is an exponential relationship between energy loss (pressure drop) and reduction in lumen size. When this relationship is illustrated graphically, the curves have a single sharp bend (Fig. 13–12; also see Fig. 13–5). These observations provide theoretical support for the concept of critical stenosis.[23, 24]

As previously noted, blood flow velocity is a major determinant of fluid energy losses (Equations 8, 9, and 17). Thus, the pressure drop across a stenosis varies with the flow rate. Because flow velocity depends on the distal hemodynamic resistance, the critical stenosis value also varies with the resistance of the runoff bed. In Figure 13–12, a system with a high flow velocity (low resistance) shows a reduction in pressure with less narrowing than a system with low flow velocity (high resistance). The higher flow velocities produce curves that are less sharply bent, making the point of critical stenosis less distinct.

Another observation related to critical stenosis is that the decrease in flow is linearly related to the increase in pressure gradient as long as the peripheral resistance remains constant[24] (Fig. 13–13). In this situation, the curves for pressure drop and flow reduction are mirror images of each other, and the critical stenosis value is the same for both. Many vascular beds are able to maintain a constant

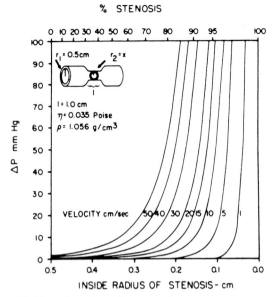

Figure 13–12. Relationship of pressure drop across a stenosis to the radius of the stenotic segment and the flow velocity. (From Strandness DE, Sumner DS: Hemodynamics for Surgeons. New York, Grune & Stratton, 1975.)

level of blood flow over a wide range of perfusion pressures by the mechanism of autoregulation. This is achieved by constriction of resistance vessels in response to an increase in blood pressure and dilatation of resistance vessels when blood pressure decreases. For example, autoregulation permits the brain to maintain normal flow rates down to perfusion pressures in the range of 50 to 60 mm Hg.[25]

Significant changes in pressure and flow begin to occur when the arterial lumen has been reduced by about 50% of its diameter or 75% of its cross-sectional area; however, the concept of critical stenosis is strictly valid only when the flow conditions are specified. Consequently, a stenosis

that is not significant at resting flow rates may become critical when flow rates are increased by reactive hyperemia or exercise. For example, iliac stenoses that do not appear severe by arteriography may be associated with significant pressure gradients during exercise.[26] Because of the complex geometry of atherosclerotic lesions and the wide variation in arterial flow rates, it is often difficult to predict the hemodynamic significance of a lesion based on the apparent reduction in lumen size. Therefore, physiologic testing by blood pressure measurement must be used to document the clinical severity of arterial lesions.[27, 28]

Effect of Stenosis Length and Multiple Stenoses

Poiseuille's law predicts that the radius of a stenosis has a much greater effect on viscous energy losses than its length (Equation 8). If the length of a stenosis is doubled, the viscous energy losses are also doubled; however, reducing the radius by one half increases energy losses by a factor of 16. Furthermore, inertial energy losses are independent of stenosis length and are especially prominent at the exit of a stenosis (see Fig. 13–11 and Equation 17). Because energy losses are primarily due to entrance and exit effects, separate short stenoses tend to be more significant than a single longer stenosis. It has been shown experimentally that when stenoses that are not significant individually are arranged in series, large reductions in pressure and flow can occur.[29] Thus, multiple subcritical stenoses may have the same effect as a single critical stenosis.

Based on the preceding discussion, several points can be made about stenoses in series. When two stenoses are of similar diameter, removal of one provides only a modest increase in blood flow. If the stenoses have different diameters, removal of the least severe has little effect, whereas removal of the most severe improves blood flow significantly.

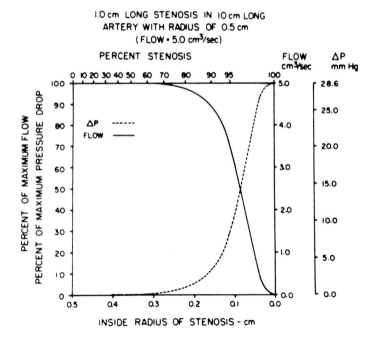

Figure 13–13. Effect of increasing stenosis on blood flow and pressure drop across the stenotic segment. Collateral and peripheral resistances are considered to be fixed. (From Strandness DE, Sumner DS: Hemodynamics for Surgeons. New York, Grune & Stratton, 1975.)

These principles apply only to unbranched arterial segments such as the internal carotid. In the presence of a severe stenosis in the carotid siphon, removal of a less severe lesion at the carotid bifurcation is not likely to result in significant hemodynamic improvement. On the other hand, when the proximal lesion involves an artery that supplies a collateral bed that parallels a distal lesion, removal of the proximal lesion can be beneficial. For example, when there is an iliac stenosis and superficial femoral occlusion, removal of the iliac lesion usually improves perfusion of the lower leg by increasing flow through the profunda-geniculate collateral system.

ARTERIAL FLOW PATTERNS IN HUMAN LIMBS

Collateral Circulation

When arterial obstruction occurs, blood must pass through a network of collateral vessels to bypass the diseased segment. The functional capacity of the collateral circulation varies according to the level and extent of occlusive lesions. As mentioned in the preceding example, the profunda-geniculate system can compensate to a large degree for an isolated superficial femoral artery occlusion; however, the addition of an iliac lesion severely limits collateral flow.

A typical hemodynamic circuit includes the diseased major artery, a parallel system of collateral vessels, and the peripheral runoff bed (Fig. 13–14). The collateral system consists of stem arteries, which are large distributing branches, a midzone of smaller intramuscular channels, and reentry vessels that join the major artery distal to the point of obstruction.[30] These vessels are preexisting pathways that enlarge when flow through the parallel major artery is reduced. The main stimuli for collateral development are an abnormal pressure gradient across the collateral system and increased velocity of flow through the midzone vessels.[31] This mechanism is consistent with the gradual improvement in collateral circulation that results from a regular exercise program in patients with lower extremity arterial occlusive disease.[32]

Collateral vessels are smaller, longer, and more numerous than the major arteries that they replace. Although considerable enlargement may occur in the midzone vessels, collateral resistance is always greater than that of the original unobstructed artery. In addition, the acute changes in collateral resistance during exercise are minimal.[33] Therefore, the resistance of a collateral system is, for practical purposes, fixed.

Distribution of Vascular Resistance and Blood Flow

Unlike collateral resistance, the resistance of a peripheral runoff bed is quite variable. The muscular arterioles are primarily responsible for regulating peripheral resistance and controlling the distribution of blood flow to various capillary beds. Arteriolar tone is mainly determined by the sympathetic nervous system, but it is also subject to the influence of locally produced metabolites.

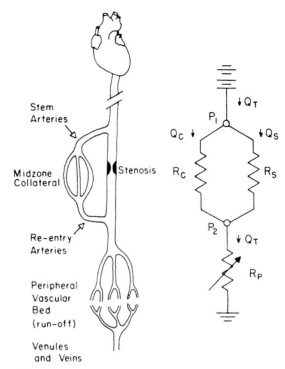

Figure 13–14. Major components of a hemodynamic circuit containing a stenotic artery. The analogous electrical circuit is shown on the right with the heart represented as a battery and the central veins as a ground. Flows are represented by Q_T (total), Q_C (*collateral*), and Q_S (*stenosis*). Resistances are represented by R_C (*collateral*), R_S (*stenosis*), and R_p (*peripheral runoff*); R_C and R_S are fixed. R_p is variable. (From Sumner DS: The hemodynamics and pathophysiology of arterial disease. In Rutherford RB [ed]: Vascular Surgery. Philadelphia, WB Saunders, 1977.)

When discussing blood flow in the lower limb, it is useful to separate vascular resistance into segmental and peripheral components. Segmental resistance consists of the relatively fixed parallel resistances of the major normal or diseased artery and the bypassing collateral vessels, such as the superficial femoral artery and the profunda-geniculate system. Peripheral resistance includes the highly variable resistances of the distal calf muscle arterioles and cutaneous circulation. The total vascular resistance of the limb can be estimated by adding the segmental and peripheral resistances (Equations 12 and 13).

Normally, the resting segmental resistance is very low and the peripheral resistance is relatively high; therefore, the pressure drop across the femoropopliteal segment is minimal. With exercise, the peripheral resistance falls, and flow through the segmental arteries increases by a factor of up to 10, with little or no pressure drop.

With moderate arterial disease, such as an isolated superficial femoral artery occlusion, the segmental resistance is increased as a result of collateral flow, and an abnormal pressure drop is present across the thigh. Because of a compensatory decrease in peripheral resistance, the total resistance of the limb and the resting blood flow often remain in the normal range.[34] During exercise, the segmental resistance remains high and fixed, whereas the peripheral resistance decreases further. However, the capacity of the peripheral circulation to compensate for a high segmental resistance is limited, and exercise flow is less than normal. In this situation, exercise is associated with a still larger pressure drop across the diseased arterial segment. The clinical result is calf muscle ischemia or claudication.

When arterial disease becomes severe, as in combined iliofemoral and tibioperoneal occlusive disease, the compensatory decrease in peripheral resistance may be unable to provide normal blood flow at rest. In this case, there is a marked pressure drop across the involved arterial segments and little or no increase in blood flow with exercise. Claudication is severe, and ischemic rest pain or ulceration may develop.

These changes in the distribution of vascular resistance in the lower limb explain the alterations in blood pressure and flow observed in patients with arterial occlusive disease.

Arterial Pulses and Waveforms

The heart generates a complex pressure pulse that is modified by arterial wall properties and changes in vascular resistance as it progresses distally. Normally, the peak systolic pressure is amplified as it passes down the lower limb.[3] This is due to a progressive decrease in arterial compliance and reflections originating from the relatively high peripheral resistance. Consequently, the systolic pressure at the ankle is higher than that in the upper arm, and the ankle-arm pressure ratio is greater than 1. However, the diastolic and mean pressures gradually decrease as the blood moves distally.

When blood flows through an arterial stenosis or a high-resistance collateral bed, the distal pulse pressure is reduced to a greater extent than the mean pressure.[35] This indicates that the systolic pressure beyond a lesion is a more sensitive indicator of hemodynamic significance than the mean pressure. It is well known that palpable pedal pulses in patients with superficial femoral artery stenosis can disappear after leg exercise. This occurs when increased flow through high-resistance vessels causes a reduction in pulse pressure. The contour of the pressure pulse also reflects the presence of proximal arterial disease. These changes can be demonstrated plethysmographically and include a delayed upslope, rounded peak, and bowing of the downslope away from the baseline.[36]

Changes in the flow pulse are also useful to characterize the state of the arterial system. While the peak pressure increases, the peak of the flow pulse decreases as the periphery is approached.[3] The flow pattern in the major arteries of the leg is normally triphasic (Fig. 13–15). An initial large forward-velocity phase resulting from cardiac systole is followed by a brief phase of flow reversal in early diastole and a third smaller phase of forward flow in late diastole. This triphasic pattern is modified by a variety of factors, including proximal arterial disease and changes in peripheral resistance. For example, body heating, which causes vasodilatation and decreased resistance, abolishes the second phase of flow reversal; on exposure to cold, resistance increases and the reverse-flow phase becomes more prominent. Because a stenotic lesion is accompanied by a compensatory decrease in peripheral resistance, one of the earliest changes noted distal to a stenosis is the disappearance of the reverse-flow phase (see Fig. 13–15).

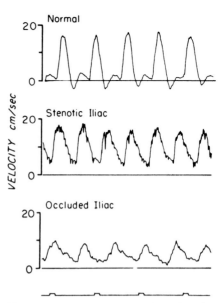

Figure 13–15. Velocity flow waveforms obtained with a directional Doppler velocity detector from the femoral artery of a normal subject, a patient with external iliac stenosis, and a patient with common iliac occlusion. (From Strandness DE, Sumner DS: Hemodynamics for Surgeons. New York, Grune & Stratton, 1975.)

As a stenosis becomes more severe, the distal flow pattern becomes monophasic, with a slow rise, a rounded peak, and a gradual decline toward the baseline in diastole. The character of the flow pulse proximal to an arterial obstruction is variable and depends on the capacity of the collateral circulation. These flow patterns can be studied noninvasively using a Doppler velocity detector and strip-chart recorder.

Pressure and Flow in Normal Limbs

As the pressure pulse moves distally, the systolic pressure rises, the diastolic pressure falls, and the pulse pressure becomes wider. The fall in mean arterial pressure between the heart and ankle is normally less than 10 mm Hg. In normal individuals at rest, the ratio of ankle systolic pressure to brachial systolic pressure (ankle-arm index) has a mean value of 1.11 ± 0.10.[37] Moderate exercise in normal extremities produces little or no drop in ankle systolic pressure. Strenuous effort may be associated with a drop of several millimeters of mercury; however, pressures return rapidly to resting levels after cessation of exercise.

The average blood flow in the normal human leg is in the range of 300 to 500 mL/minute under resting conditions.[3] Blood flow to the muscles of the lower leg is approximately 2.0 mL/100 g/minute. With moderate exercise, total leg blood flow increases by a factor of 5 to 10, and muscle blood flow rises to around 30 mL/100 g/minute. During strenuous exercise, muscle blood flow may reach 70 mL/100 g/minute. After cessation of exercise, blood flow decreases rapidly and returns to resting values within 1 to 5 minutes.

Pressure and Flow in Limbs with Arterial Obstruction

If an arterial lesion is hemodynamically significant at rest, there is a measurable reduction in distal blood pressure. Generally, limbs with a lesion at one anatomic level have ankle-arm indices between 0.9 and 0.5, whereas limbs with occlusions at multiple anatomic levels have indices less than 0.5.[28] The ankle-arm index also correlates with the clinical severity of disease: in limbs with intermittent claudication, the index has a mean value of 0.59 ± 0.15; in limbs with ischemic rest pain, 0.26 ± 0.13; and in limbs with impending gangrene, 0.05 ± 0.08.[37]

Because of the increased segmental vascular resistance in limbs with arterial occlusive disease, the ankle systolic blood pressure falls dramatically during leg exercise. As indicated in Figures 13–16, 13–17, and 13–18, the extent and duration of the pressure drop are proportional to the severity of the arterial lesions. Recovery of pressure to resting levels may require up to 30 minutes.[28]

Resting leg or calf blood flow in patients with intermittent claudication is not significantly different from values obtained in normal individuals. However, the capacity to increase limb blood flow during exercise is quite limited, and pain occurs in the muscles that have been rendered ischemic. The pain of claudication is presumably due to the accumulation of metabolic products that are removed under normal flow conditions. As the occlusive process becomes more severe, the decrease in peripheral vascular resistance can no longer compensate, and resting flow may be less than normal. When this occurs, ischemic rest pain or ulceration may appear. As shown in Figures 13–16, 13–17, and 13–18, the capacity to increase calf blood flow with exercise depends on the severity of arterial disease. With increasing degrees of disease, the hyperemia that follows exercise becomes more prolonged, and the peak

calf blood flow is both decreased and delayed. In some cases, flow may fall below resting levels.[28] The ankle blood pressure returns to normal after peak flows have started to decline.

The changes in blood pressure and flow in lower limbs with arterial occlusive disease provide the basis for noninvasive diagnostic tests. By monitoring the ankle systolic pressure before and after treadmill exercise or reactive hyperemia, two components of the physiologic response can be evaluated: (1) the magnitude of the immediate pressure drop, and (2) the time for recovery to resting pressure. The changes in both of these parameters are proportional to the severity of arterial disease.[38]

Vascular Steal

Hemodynamic arrangements in which one vascular bed draws blood away or "steals" from another can occur in a variety of situations. A vascular steal may arise when two runoff beds with different resistances must be supplied by a limited source of inflow.

Multiple-Level Occlusive Disease

One example of the steal phenomenon involves a limb with lesions in both the iliac and superficial femoral arteries.[1] Between the fixed resistances of these two arterial lesions is the profunda orifice, which supplies the variable resistance of the thigh. The resistance of the distal calf runoff bed is also variable. Under resting conditions, normal leg blood flow can be maintained by a nearly maximal decrease in calf resistance and a moderate decrease in thigh resistance. This is apparent clinically as an abnormally low ankle systolic pressure. With the increased metabolic demands

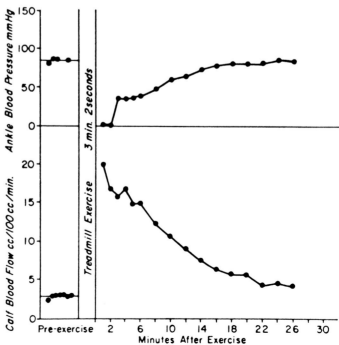

Figure 13–16. Preexercise and postexercise ankle blood pressure and calf blood flow in a patient with severe stenosis of the superficial femoral artery. (From Sumner DS, Strandness DE: The relationship between calf blood flow and ankle blood pressure in patients with intermittent claudication. Surgery 65:763, 1969.)

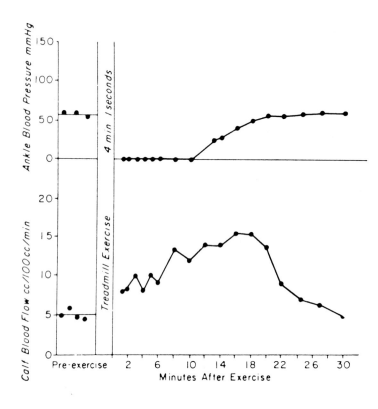

Figure 13–17. Preexercise and postexercise ankle blood pressure and calf blood flow in a patient with iliac stenosis and superficial femoral artery occlusion. (From Sumner DS, Strandness DE: The relationship between calf blood flow and ankle blood pressure in patients with intermittent claudication. Surgery 65:763, 1969.)

Figure 13–18. Preexercise and postexercise ankle blood pressure and calf blood flow in a patient with occlusion of the iliac, common femoral, and superficial femoral arteries. This patient had moderate rest pain and severe claudication. (From Sumner DS, Strandness DE: The relationship between calf blood flow and ankle blood pressure in patients with intermittent claudication. Surgery 65:763, 1969.)

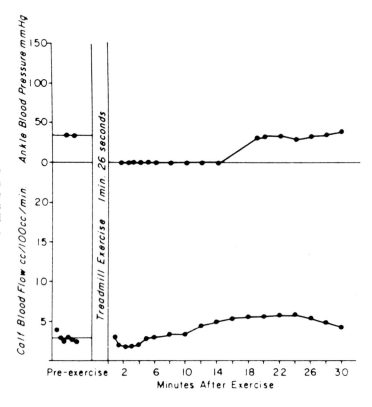

of exercise, the thigh resistance can decrease further, but the calf resistance has already reached its lower limit. This results in a further pressure drop across the proximal iliac lesion, which reduces the pressure perfusing the calf. Blood flow to the calf is decreased until the thigh resistance rises and thigh blood flow begins to fall. In this situation, the effect of exercise is to increase thigh blood flow, decrease calf blood flow, and decrease distal blood pressure. The thigh steals blood from the calf because the proximal iliac lesion restricts inflow to both runoff beds.

Subclavian Steal Syndrome

In the subclavian steal syndrome, reversal of flow in the vertebral artery is associated with subclavian artery occlusion and symptoms of brain stem ischemia.[39] When occlusion is present in the proximal subclavian artery on the left or the innominate artery on the right, the pressure at the origin of the ipsilateral vertebral artery is reduced. This can result in reversal of flow in the vertebral artery, which then serves as a source of collateral circulation to the arm. The increased demands of arm exercise tend to augment the reversed flow, and the patient may experience ischemia of the brain stem. The hemodynamic effect is more severe with innominate artery occlusion than with isolated subclavian occlusion. With innominate occlusion, the origin of the right common carotid is also subject to reduced pressure, and the patterns of collateral circulation to the arm and brain become quite complicated. Blood passing down the vertebral artery on the side of the occlusion may be recovered, in part, by the right common carotid artery; however, during arm exercise, flow in the right common carotid may be reduced.

It is important to distinguish between symptomatic and asymptomatic subclavian steal. The presence of reversed vertebral artery flow, as demonstrated by arteriography, may be a normal variant without clinical significance.[40] In true subclavian steal syndrome, there is often a definite relationship between arm exercise and symptoms of brain stem ischemia. There will also be objective evidence of decreased blood flow to the involved arm, such as a diminished radial pulse and lowered brachial blood pressure relative to the contralateral arm.[41]

Extra-Anatomic Bypass Grafts

When an extra-anatomic bypass is performed, a single donor artery must supply several vascular beds. In the case of a femorofemoral crossover graft, one iliac is the donor artery, the leg ipsilateral to the donor artery is the donor limb, and the contralateral leg is the recipient limb. Studies of crossover grafts in animal models have shown that the immediate effect of the graft is to double the flow in the donor artery.[42, 43] When an arteriovenous fistula is created in the recipient limb, graft flows may increase by a factor of 10 without any evidence of a steal from the donor limb.

These experimental observations are consistent with hemodynamic data from patients with femorofemoral grafts.[44] Improvement in the ankle-arm index on the recipient side can be achieved, even in the presence of significant occlusive disease in both the donor and recipient limbs. Although the ankle-arm index may decrease slightly on the donor side, a symptomatic steal is extremely uncommon. The most important factor contributing to vascular steal with a femorofemoral graft is stenosis of the donor iliac artery. With iliac stenosis, a steal is most likely to occur during exercise, when flow rates are increased. A mildly stenotic iliac can be used as a donor artery when high flow rates are not needed, such as in the treatment of ischemic rest pain. However, when increased flow rates are required to improve the walking distance of a patient with claudication, stenosis of the donor iliac may result in a steal from the donor limb. Occlusive disease in the arteries of the donor limb distal to the origin of the graft does not result in a steal, provided that the donor iliac artery is normal.

These principles also apply to other types of extra-anatomic bypass grafts, including axillary-axillary, carotid-subclavian, and axillofemoral grafts.[42, 45]

HEMODYNAMIC PRINCIPLES AND THE TREATMENT OF ARTERIAL DISEASE

It should be apparent from the preceding discussion that the high fixed segmental resistance of the diseased major arteries and collaterals is responsible for decreased peripheral blood flow. Therefore, to be most effective in improving peripheral blood flow and relieving ischemic symptoms, therapy must be directed toward lowering this abnormally high segmental resistance. Because the peripheral resistance has already been lowered to compensate for the increased segmental resistance, attempts to further reduce the peripheral resistance are seldom beneficial.[46]

Although exercise therapy has been shown to improve collateral function, the degree of clinical improvement is usually modest.[32] In general, exercise therapy is best suited for patients with mild, stable claudication who are not candidates for direct intervention. Another method for improving peripheral blood flow in limbs with arterial disease is medically induced hypertension.[46] The administration of mineralocorticoid and sodium chloride raises systemic blood pressure and increases the head of pressure perfusing the diseased arterial segment. Although this technique has not been widely applied, it has been used successfully in patients with severe distal ischemia and ulceration.

Direct Arterial Intervention

The most satisfactory approach to reducing the fixed segmental resistance is direct intervention by surgical or radiologic techniques. Depending on the nature of the lesions, endarterectomy, embolectomy, replacement grafting, or bypass grafting may be indicated. Percutaneous transluminal angioplasty may also be appropriate in selected cases.[47] In patients with occlusive disease involving a single anatomic level, a successful procedure should return all hemodynamic parameters to normal or near normal. This should be evident as an increase in the ankle-arm index and an improvement in the ankle pressure response to leg exercise.[48] However, because it is seldom possible to perform a perfect arterial reconstruction, it is common to detect a minor degree of residual hemodynamic impairment. When occlusions involve multiple levels, the treatment of one level should result in significant improvement, and the persisting hemodynamic abnormality should then reflect the remaining untreated disease. In such cases, the improvement is usually sufficient to increase claudication distance or relieve ischemic rest pain. The relative severity of lesions at different levels is often difficult to determine clinically; however, the basic principle is to initially treat the most proximal level of hemodynamically significant occlusive disease.

The factors required for optimal function of arterial bypass grafts can be analyzed in terms of basic hemodynamic principles. As previously noted, vessel diameter is the main determinant of hemodynamic resistance, so the diameter of a graft is considerably more important than its length. All prosthetic grafts develop a pseudointimal layer of variable thickness that further reduces the effective diameter.[3] Therefore, whenever the situation permits, a graft with a relatively large diameter should be used. Graft diameter is often limited by arterial size. To minimize energy losses associated with entrance and exit effects, the diameter of a graft should approximate that of the adjacent artery. When arteries of unequal size must be joined, a gradual transition is preferable. Thus, the graft should be slightly smaller than the proximal artery and slightly larger than the distal artery.

Theoretically, end-to-end anastomoses are preferable to those done end to side, because the end-to-end configuration eliminates energy losses due to curvature and angulation. However, these losses appear to be minimal under physiologic conditions, and in most clinical situations the anastomotic angle is determined by technical factors. For example, reversed angulation has been used successfully in the construction of aortorenal and femorofemoral bypass grafts. Nevertheless, as a general rule, the smallest anastomotic angle that is technically feasible should be used. The width of an end-to-side anastomosis should be approximately equal to the diameter of the graft; the length of an anastomosis is less important but does serve as the main determinant of anastomotic angle. A carefully everted suture line also helps to minimize energy losses at anastomoses.

Bifurcation grafts, such as those used for aortofemoral bypass, are subject to the same general hemodynamic considerations as arterial bifurcations and branches. Most commercially available grafts have secondary limbs with diameters that are one half that of the primary tube, resulting in an area ratio of 0.5. In this configuration, each of the secondary limbs has 16 times the resistance of the primary tube, and in parallel they offer 8 times the primary tube resistance. The flow velocity in the secondary limbs is doubled, and almost 50% of the incident pulsatile energy is reflected at the graft bifurcation.[3] As previously discussed, the area ratio determines the hemodynamic characteristics of a bifurcation with respect to pressure gradient, flow velocity, and transmission of pulsatile energy. However, the optimal area ratio for grafts has not been established, and the geometry of bifurcation grafts has received relatively little attention. Instead, the development of prosthetic grafts has emphasized features such as graft material, porosity, and surface characteristics. Despite their theoretical disadvantages, commercially available grafts have functioned extremely well in a variety of clinical applications.

Vasodilators

The rationale for the use of vasodilators is that they lower peripheral vascular resistance and improve limb blood flow. Although this may occur in normal limbs, it is unlikely to be beneficial in limbs in which peripheral resistance is already decreased as a result of arterial disease. There is even a theoretical possibility that dilating vessels in relatively normal areas could divert blood away from the areas of ischemia. Most clinical studies of vasodilator therapy have failed to show a significant effect.[49, 50] There is no conclusive evidence that vasodilators can increase flow in either collateral vessels or severely ischemic tissues. Consequently, there is no theoretical or clinical support for vasodilator therapy.

Sympathectomy

Because the purpose of sympathectomy is to reduce peripheral resistance by release of vasomotor tone, it is subject to the same general criticisms as vasodilator therapy. Because sympathectomy has little, if any, influence on collateral resistance, there is no rational basis for its use in the treatment of intermittent claudication.[51] Furthermore, exercise-induced muscle ischemia alone is a potent stimulus for peripheral vasodilatation.

The use of sympathectomy for cutaneous ischemia has some physiologic basis, because the predominant effect is dilatation of cutaneous arterioles. However, clinical improvement can occur only if the ischemic tissues are capable of further vasodilatation, as demonstrated by reactive hyperemia testing.[36] Beneficial results have been obtained in patients with mild rest pain and superficial ischemic ulcers; patients with severe rest pain and extensive tissue loss are not likely to respond.[51] Although sympathectomy has been recommended as an adjunct to arterial operations, there is little objective evidence that it improves either the early or the late results of arterial reconstructive surgery.[52]

Rheologic Agents

According to Poiseuille's law, hemodynamic resistance is directly proportional to the blood viscosity (Equations 8 and 11). If the pressure remains constant and viscosity is reduced, flow increases in proportion to the fall in viscosity. Procedures for lowering blood viscosity are most often used in the immediate postoperative period to increase flow through a reconstructed arterial segment.

Low-molecular-weight dextran (molecular weight 40,000) is the most commonly used agent for reducing blood viscosity. The increased peripheral blood flow observed after intravenous administration of low-molecular-weight dextran is the result of both peripheral vasodilatation secondary to blood volume expansion and changes in viscosity due to hemodilution.[3] Dextran solutions also influence red blood cell aggregation and platelet function.[53]

An orally administered rheologic agent, pentoxifylline, has been evaluated in a multicenter clinical trial for the treatment of patients with intermittent claudication.[54] Pentoxifylline reduces blood viscosity by improving the membrane flexibility of red blood cells. The drug also has an inhibitory effect on platelet aggregation. During the clinical trial, the distance walked prior to onset of claudication increased in both the pentoxifylline and placebo groups; however, the degree of improvement was significantly greater in those receiving pentoxifylline. It was concluded that pentoxifylline is a safe and effective drug for use in patients with intermittent claudication. Although this agent may provide a modest degree of functional improvement in some patients, its effect on the progression of arterial disease is unknown.

HEMODYNAMICS OF THE VENOUS SYSTEM

The structure of the vein wall is considerably different from that of the companion arteries. Some of these major differences are as follows: (1) the vein wall is much thinner, being anywhere from one third to one tenth as thick as that of the systemic arteries; (2) there is very little elastic tissue in the wall of the vein; (3) the venous media is almost exclusively a muscular layer; (4) venules have no media and no smooth muscle; and (5) a major part of the walls of the larger veins is composed of adventitia. An important characteristic of the veins is the presence of valves, which are essential for proper function. The distribution and number of valves correspond quite well to those regions in which the effects of gravity are greatest. They have a bicuspid structure with a fine connective tissue skeleton covered by endothelium on both surfaces. Their major function is to ensure antegrade flow and prevent reflux from the deep to the superficial veins.

From the clinical standpoint, the area of greatest interest is found below the knee. This is the most common site for the development of venous thrombosis, and it is also the region of the leg where the complications of the post-thrombotic syndrome are evident. The veins of the soleus muscle are often termed the "soleal sinuses" because of their capacious size and lack of venous valves. These sinuses are the most common site for the development of venous thrombosis.

The perforating veins that normally carry blood from the superficial to the deep veins are key elements in venous function. These short channels have the following features: they penetrate the deep fascia; they contain valves; they are found predominantly below the knee; the majority are small and inconstant in location; and they vary in number from 90 to 200.[55] Although not commonly thought of as such, the greater and lesser saphenous veins have all the characteristics of perforating veins. One relatively constant large perforator can be found on the medial aspect of the distal thigh, and this is one of the few that establishes a direct communication between the greater saphenous vein and the deep system of veins. A common misconception is that the perforating veins along the medial aspect of the lower leg communicate directly with the greater saphenous vein. In fact, they communicate most commonly with its major tributary, the posterior arch vein. Normally, there are four relatively constant perforators that join the posterior arch vein, and when these are diseased, they contribute to the pathogenesis of the post-thrombotic syndrome. The region in the vicinity of the lowest two perforating veins is often referred to as the gaiter area.[55]

As discussed later in the chapter, the function of the venous wall and its associated valves becomes evident when the effects of gravity and the calf muscle pump are considered.

Normal Pressure and Flow Relationships

A major factor in venous physiology that explains the capacitance function of these vessels is that they can undergo large changes in volume with very little change in transmural pressure. This is due not to the elastic properties of the walls but rather to the fact that they tend to collapse under the influence of a low transmural pressure. Veins are actually stiffer than arteries when compared at the same distending pressure. This results from the paucity of elastic tissue and the very prominent adventitia, which consists largely of collagen.

One of the remarkable features of the venous system is the wide range of flow rates that can be found. These can vary from high flows to nearly complete stasis. Flow rates depend on a host of complex interactive factors such as body position, level of activity, vascular fluid volume, and ambient temperature. Because it is virtually impossible to measure instantaneous venous flow in either the superficial or the deep veins, it is necessary to look at measurements of venous pressure and relate these to specific conditions or disease states.

Resting Venous Pressure

The pressures that exist in the absence of pulsatile flow are shown in Figure 13–19, which is the hydrostatic model of a 6-foot-tall "dead man." If the case of an open rigid tube is considered, pressure at the top would be zero (atmospheric). In the body, the arteries and veins can be represented as a series of parallel tubes, with the veins being collapsible and the arteries rigid. With the system filled with fluid, but not enough to entirely distend the collapsible tube (venous), the pressure in the collapsed portion of the tube is atmospheric. Pressures in the rigid tube (arterial) must be equal to those in the collapsible tube up to the zero point. Above the zero pressure point, the pressures in the rigid tube are negative, because the collapsed tube representing the veins prevents free communication between the two segments.

When we examine the pressure relationships in a living man, supine and erect, some important facts can be noted[56] (Fig. 13–20). There is a point just below the diaphragm where the pressures in the arteries and veins remain constant regardless of position. This has been termed the "hydrostatic indifferent point" (HIP). This point only

HYDROSTATIC PRESSURE
(mm Hg)

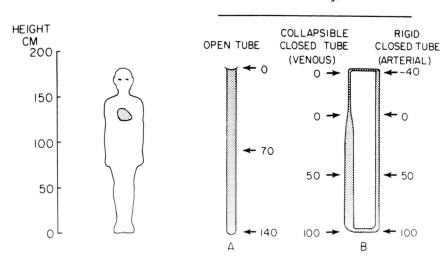

Figure 13–19. Hydrostatic pressures measured in the upright "dead man." *A*, The pressures in the open tube are those expected in a rigid tube of equal height. *B*, The pressures shown are those expected in a system of closed, connected parallel tubes. (From Strandness DE, Sumner DS: Hemodynamics for Surgeons. New York, Grune & Stratton, 1975.)

changes when the subject is placed head down, and then it is located at the level of the right atrium. The zero pressure level is in the region of the right atrium, usually at the level of the fourth intercostal space. The effect of gravity is the same throughout the vascular system in the supine subject. Raising an arm above the head in the erect position does produce some dramatic changes. The arteriovenous pressure gradient in the foot remains the same (83 mm Hg), but in the hand it falls to a level of 31 mm Hg.[57]

Although there is no difference in the pressure gradient across the capillaries in the feet between the supine and the standing position, some important changes do occur. On assuming the standing position, there is a translocation of blood into the veins of the legs that is on the order of 500 mL.[58] There is also a marked increase in the transmural venous pressure at the foot as a result of the effect of gravity. With this increase in pressure, fluid is forced out of the capillaries into the tissues. Although some of this fluid may be picked up by the lymphatics, other factors must come into play if edema is to be prevented. The single most important element in preventing the continued accumulation of interstitial fluid is the calf muscle pump.

This can dramatically lower the pressure in the veins and capillaries, thus promoting the return of interstitial fluid to the circulation.

Pressure Changes During Exercise

Features that distinguish normal subjects from patients with venous disease are best understood by examining the pressure changes that occur with leg exercise. Although patients with chronic arterial disease can usually be distinguished from normal subjects under resting conditions by measurement of distal arterial blood pressure, this is not the case with venous disease. For patients with venous problems, it is only when the muscle pump is activated that the abnormality is apparent. The calf muscle pump produces important changes in venous volume, flow rate, and flow direction. The muscle pump fulfills three useful functions: it lowers the venous pressure in the dependent limb; it reduces venous volume in the exercising limb; and it increases venous return.

With quiet standing, the venous pressure at the level of the foot remains constant, but this is dramatically altered

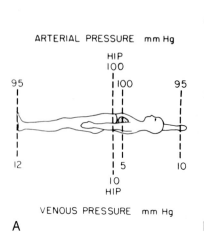

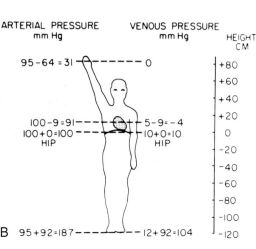

Figure 13–20. The intravascular pressures present in the normal supine (*A*) and erect (*B*) human. The *HIP* (hydrostatic indifferent point) is located just below the diaphragm. (From Strandness DE, Sumner DS: Hemodynamics for Surgeons. New York, Grune & Stratton, 1975.)

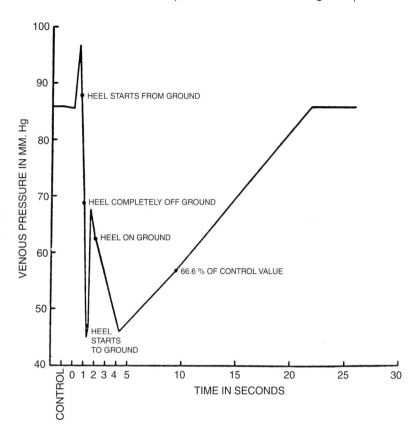

Figure 13–21. Changes in the mean saphenous vein pressure measured at the level of the ankle that occur with a single step. (Redrawn from Pollack AA, Wood EH: Human venous pressure in the saphenous vein at the ankle in during exercise and changes in posture. J Appl Physiol 1:649, 1949.)

with even a single step (Fig. 13–21). As noted in Figure 13–21, at the completion of a single step, the venous pressure is very low and requires several seconds to return to the prestep level.[59] When a normal subject walks, the venous pressure remains at a low and steady level throughout the period of exercise. Calf volume initially falls but gradually increases during exercise as the arterial inflow rises (Fig. 13–22). It is essential to understand that the observed pressure changes at the level of the foot are entirely dependent on intact and functioning venous valves in the distal limb. The calf muscle pump essentially empties the local venous system during contraction. With relaxation, the veins are nearly empty and the venous pressure is very low. These changes are vital to maintaining normal venous return and protecting the limb. As is shown later in the chapter, destruction of the valves dramatically alters these changes.

Venous Flow Patterns

Flow on the venous side of the circulation is influenced by a variety of factors, including respiration, the filling pressure of the right heart, body position, the activity of the calf muscle pump, and the amount of arterial inflow. The patterns of blood flow in the femoral artery and vein are shown in Figure 13–23. Flow velocity in the normal femoral vein is lowest at peak inspiration when the intraabdominal pressure resulting from descent of the diaphragm is at its maximum. In theory, the changes in velocity of venous flow in the subclavian vein should be opposite to those in

the femoral vein; that is, highest at peak inspiration when intrathoracic pressure is at its minimum.

As noted earlier, the presence of competent valves prevents reflux of blood and an increase in venous pressure. This can be shown when the pressure is suddenly increased above a competent iliofemoral valve (Fig. 13–24). A cough and a Valsalva maneuver result in a sharp increase in pressure above the valve but not below it. There is no reflux of blood flow through the valve during either of these maneuvers.

Abnormal Pressure and Flow Relationships

The most common manifestations of abnormal venous function are primary varicose veins and the post-thrombotic syndrome. Current evidence suggests that primary varicose veins are often familial in etiology. The initial abnormality in this condition appears to be incompetence of the terminal valves of the greater and lesser saphenous veins, which permits reflux of blood. With the passage of time, progressive incompetence of the other valves occurs. Dodd and Cockett[60] also include patients with idiopathic perforator vein incompetence in the primary varicose vein group. Although this may be valid, it is likely that many of these incompetent perforators occur secondary to episodes of calf vein thrombosis that result in destruction of the valves.

The flow abnormality produced by loss of valvular competence at any level of the venous system is easily demon-

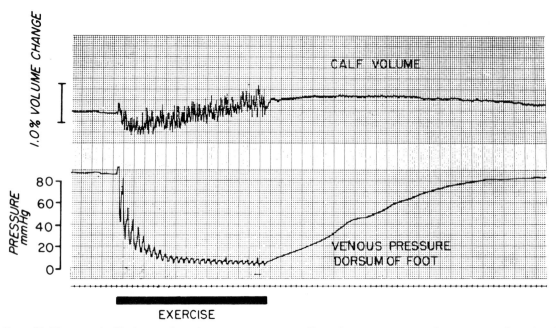

Figure 13–22. Normal calf volume and venous pressure response to calf muscle exercise. Pressure changes measured in a dorsal foot vein. Venous pressure falls rapidly, remains low throughout the period of exercise, and returns slowly to the baseline after calf muscle contraction ceases. (From Strandness DE, Sumner DS: Hemodynamics for Surgeons. New York, Grune & Stratton, 1975.)

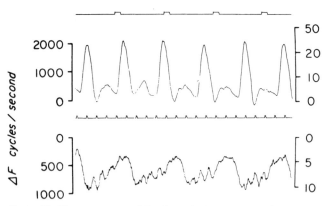

Figure 13–23. Comparison of the flow velocity patterns in the common femoral artery *(top)* and vein *(bottom)* in the supine position with normal respiration. The venous velocity patterns are dominated by the pressure changes that occur with respiration. *F,* Doppler shift frequency, which is proportional to velocity. (From Strandness DE, Sumner DS: Hemodynamics for Surgeons. New York, Grune & Stratton, 1975.)

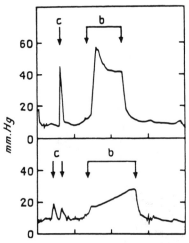

Figure 13–24. Effect of a cough (c) and a Valsalva maneuver (b) on the venous pressure in a patient with a competent valve at the iliofemoral level. *Upper panel,* Pressure changes above the valve; *lower panel,* pressure changes below the valve. (From Ludbrook J, Beale G: Femoral venous valves in relation to varicose veins. Lancet 1:79, 1962.)

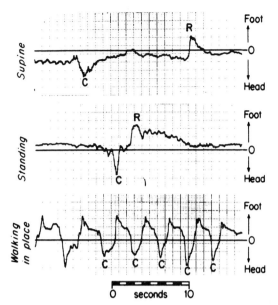

Figure 13–25. Venous velocity changes recorded from an incompetent greater saphenous vein in a patient with primary varicose veins. The effects of muscular contraction (C) and relaxation (R) are indicated for the supine and standing positions. The bidirectional flow that occurs with walking is also shown. (From Strandness DE, Sumner DS: Hemodynamics for Surgeons. New York, Grune & Stratton, 1975.)

strated with a Doppler ultrasonic velocity detector. The flow patterns shown in Figure 13–25 are from the greater saphenous vein of a patient with primary varicose veins. In the supine position, flow with a calf contraction (C) is antegrade with a slight and transient period of reflux during relaxation (R); however, with standing, the opposite is noted, with flow being toward the foot. Walking in place illustrates clearly the rapid changes in direction that occur with each step as a result of loss of valvular competence. When the pressure in the veins on the dorsum of the foot is measured during exercise in a patient with primary varicose veins, the deviations from normal are evident (Fig. 13–26). The pressure does not fall to normally low levels, and it returns to the preexercise level much faster when walking is stopped. If a tourniquet is placed around the upper calf, this pattern is normalized as long as the valves in the deep system are competent.

With the development of acute deep vein thrombosis, two major factors determine the long-term outcome: the location and extent of the residual venous obstruction, and the condition of the valves below the knee in the area of the calf muscle pump.[61–64] Because these vary greatly from one patient to another, it is not surprising that the pressure responses also show a wide variation. Four examples of the types of patterns that can be observed are shown in Figure 13–27. It is clear that even with primary varicose veins, the pressure changes at the level of the foot are abnormal with exercise (see Figs. 13–26 and 13–27). However, patients with this very common condition generally complain of minimal edema and rarely develop ulceration. The factors that appear to be responsible for the development of the post-thrombotic syndrome relate primarily to the status of the deep veins below the knee and the perforating veins.

The most abnormal venous pressures and flows occur in the area where ulceration develops and are due to valvular incompetence in both the distal deep veins and their connections with the superficial venous system. With this combination, the very high pressures that can be generated by activation of the calf muscle pump result in ambulatory venous hypertension in the lower leg.

Browse and Burnand[65] in 1978 offered a reassessment of the factors responsible for the development of the post-thrombotic syndrome. They recognized that the clinical condition could only occur with damage to the deep venous system and postulated that the abnormally high venous pressures would lead to the development of multiple new capillaries in the dermis with large pores in the venular side. As a result, there would be extravasation of large molecules such as fibrinogen and coagulation factors. These, in conjunction with tissue factors, would lead to the conversion of fibrinogen to fibrin. If this were combined with inadequate fibrinolysis, fibrin would accumulate in the tissues and produce a barrier to the diffusion of both oxygen and nutrients. The end result would be tissue anoxia and death of the skin in the affected region.

HEMODYNAMIC PRINCIPLES AND THE TREATMENT OF VENOUS DISEASE

In contrast to the arterial side of the circulation, there are very few direct therapeutic approaches that can correct the underlying hemodynamic abnormalities of venous disease. Although obstruction of inflow to a limb is the most commonly treated arterial abnormality, mechanical interference with venous outflow is a rare cause of chronic venous insufficiency.

One exception to this observation is the patient with venous claudication. This entity is uncommon and may not be recognized. It occurs in the specific clinical setting of

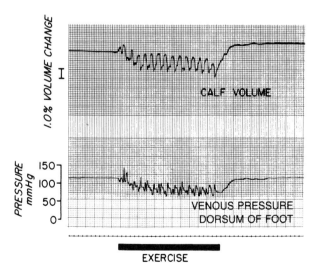

Figure 13–26. Calf volume and venous pressure changes recorded from a dorsal foot vein of a patient with primary varicose veins. The pressure does not fall to the low levels seen in normal subjects, and it returns to the baseline much faster. (From Strandness DE, Sumner DS: Hemodynamics for Surgeons. New York, Grune & Stratton, 1975.)

Hemodynamics for the Vascular Surgeon

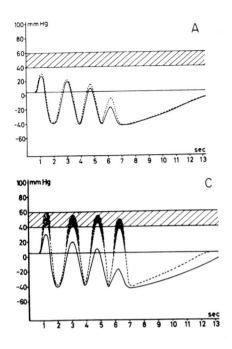
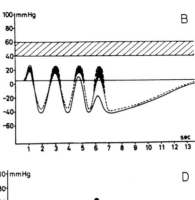
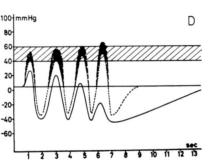

Figure 13–27. The pressure changes in the greater saphenous vein at the ankle during four steps. In each panel, the normal response is noted by the solid line. *A*, Primary varicose veins and no leg ulcers. *B*, Varicose veins, incompetent ankle perforators, normal deep veins, no leg ulcers. *C*, Varicose veins, incompetent ankle perforators, normal deep veins, leg ulcers present. *D*, Varicose veins, incompetent ankle perforators, abnormal deep veins, leg ulcers present. (From Arnoldi CC, Linderholm H: On the pathogenesis of the venous leg ulcer. Acta Chir Scand 134:427, 1968.)

chronic iliofemoral venous occlusion. In most cases, the major deep veins distal to the groin are patent and competent. With vigorous exercise, the patient is unable to adequately decompress the deep venous system, and the thigh becomes tense and very painful. After the patient stops exercising, it often requires 15 to 30 minutes for the pain and tightness to disappear. It is important to recognize that this syndrome rarely occurs with ordinary exercise and thus tends to be seen in relatively young patients who indulge in vigorous activities such as jogging, skiing, or tennis. The underlying mechanism of venous claudication involves the collateral veins that bypass the obstructed segment and have a relatively high, fixed resistance.[66] This high outflow resistance results in a marked increase in venous volume during exercise. In some circumstances it may be feasible to provide therapeutic relief by a crossover saphenous vein graft using the proximal saphenous vein from the opposite limb. This is rarely done because the symptoms in most patients produce only minimal disability.

Other surgical procedures designed to treat chronic venous insufficiency do so by either removing the offending vein or interrupting it at some point in its course. This is done to eliminate sites of reflux and restore the pressure-flow relationship to normal. The value of this particular approach is limited because the most common site of the disease responsible for chronic venous insufficiency is the distal deep veins, an area not amenable to direct surgical intervention.

There has been a good deal of interest in promoting valvular competence in the proximal superficial femoral vein. This has been done by a direct surgical approach through a longitudinal venotomy or by transposition of a competent venous valve.[67, 68] The validity of these techniques can be questioned because there is no evidence to support the concept of the so-called critical valve; the alterations of pressure and flow are nearly always secondary to deep venous abnormalities in the distal limb, and proof of the effectiveness of such an approach is at present lacking.

The most common form of therapy for chronic venous insufficiency is the use of support stockings that provide external compression and thus minimize the amount of edema that occurs during ambulation.[69] The exact mechanism of compression therapy remains poorly understood.[70] In theory, the stocking should reduce the transmural venous pressure gradient in a graduated fashion, with the highest compression pressures in the ankle area and diminishing pressures proximally up the limb. The amount of pressure exerted by a stocking depends on the elastic tension in the garment and the radius of the limb. Compression pressure should be in the range of 80 to 90 mm Hg while standing, 50 to 60 mm Hg while sitting, and 0 mm Hg in the recumbent position. This is obviously not possible with any single stocking, so a compromise must be accepted.

Elevation of the legs above the level of the heart is also a standard method for relieving the symptoms of chronic venous insufficiency. The physiologic basis for the use of elevation depends on three major effects: It reduces venous pressure by decreasing the hydrostatic component related to gravity; it promotes the reabsorption of edema fluid; and it prevents ambulatory venous hypertension. Periodic elevation and external compression therapy are essential for the treatment of chronic venous insufficiency. When strictly adhered to, a regimen of elevation and compression minimizes edema, improves skin nutrition, and avoids ulceration in the majority of patients.

CONCLUSION

The fundamental principles of hemodynamics often seem remote from the everyday clinical problems faced by the vascular surgeon. The purpose of this chapter has been to show how these mathematical and physical concepts provide the basis for a rational approach to the pathophysiology, diagnosis, and treatment of vascular disease. These principles are also important for understanding the noninvasive diagnostic techniques that are discussed elsewhere in this book. The use of objective hemodynamic data is an essential step in the clinical evaluation of patients. This increased reliance on physiologic testing should encourage the vascular surgeon to consider the patient with vascular disease in terms of basic hemodynamic principles.

References

1. Sumner DS: The hemodynamics and pathophysiology of arterial disease. In Rutherford RB (ed): Vascular Surgery. Philadelphia, WB Saunders, 1977, pp 25–46.
2. Burton AC: Physiology and Biophysics of the Circulation, 2nd ed. St Louis, Mosby–Year Book, 1972, pp 86–94.
3. Strandness DE Jr, Sumner DS: Hemodynamics for Surgeons. New York, Grune & Stratton, 1975.
4. Barnes RW: Hemodynamics for the vascular surgeon. Arch Surg 115:216–223, 1980.
5. Attinger EO: Flow patterns in vascular geometry. In Attinger EO (ed): Pulsatile Blood Flow. New York, McGraw-Hill, 1964, pp 179–200.
6. Gutstein WH, Schneck DJ, Marks JO: In vitro studies of local blood flow disturbance in a region of separation. J Atheroscler Res 8:381–388, 1968.
7. Logerfo FW, Soncrant T, Teel T, Dewey F: Boundary layer separation in models of side-to-end arterial anastomoses. Arch Surg 114:1364–1373, 1979.
8. Zarins CK, Giddens DP, Glagov S: Atherosclerotic plaque distribution and flow velocity profiles in the carotid bifurcation. In Bergan JJ, Yao JST (eds): Cerebrovascular Insufficiency. New York, Grune & Stratton, 1983, pp 19–30.
9. Ku DN, Giddens DP, Phillips DJ, et al: Hemodynamics of the normal human carotid bifurcation—in vitro and in vivo studies. Ultrasound Med Biol 1:13–26, 1985.
10. Phillips DJ, Greene FM Jr, Langlois Y, et al: Flow velocity patterns in the carotid bifurcations of young, presumed normal subjects. Ultrasound Med Biol 1:39–49, 1983.
11. Reneman RS, van Merode T, Hick P, et al: Flow velocity patterns in and distensibility of the carotid artery bulb in subjects of various ages. Circulation 71:500–509, 1985.
12. Fox JA, Hugh AE: Localization of atheroma: A theory based on boundary layer separation. Br Heart J 28:388–394, 1966.
13. Milnor WR: Pulsatile blood flow. N Engl J Med 287:27–34, 1972.
14. Malan E, Noseda G, Longo T: Approach to fluid dynamic problems in reconstructive vascular surgery. Surgery 66:994–1003, 1969.
15. McDonald DA: Blood Flow in Arteries, 2nd ed. London, Edward Arnold, 1974.
16. Goaling RG, Newman DL, Bowden NLR, et al: The area ratio of normal aortic junctions—aortic configuration and pulse wave reflection. Br J Radiol 44:850–853, 1971.
17. Lalleman RC, Gosling RG, Newman DL: Role of the bifurcation in atheromatosis of the abdominal aorta. Surg Gynecol Obstet 137:987–990, 1973.
18. Sumner DS, Hokanson DE, Strandness DE Jr: Arterial walls before and after endarterectomy, stress-strain characteristics and collagen-elastin content. Arch Surg 99:606–611, 1969.
19. Sumner DS, Hokanson DE, Strandness DE Jr: Stress-strain characteristics and collagen-elastin content of abdominal aortic aneurysms. Surg Gynecol Obstet 130:459–466, 1970.
20. Scherer PW: Flow in axisymmetrical glass model aneurysms. J Biomech 6:695–700, 1973.
21. Darling RC: Ruptured arteriosclerotic abdominal aortic aneurysms—a pathologic and clinical study. Am J Surg 119:397–401, 1970.
22. Roach MR: Changes in arterial distensibility as a cause of poststenotic dilatation. Am J Cardiol 12:802–815, 1963.
23. Berguer R, Hwang NHC: Critical arterial stenosis—a theoretical and experimental solution. Ann Surg 180:39–50, 1974.
24. May AG, Van de Berg L, DeWeese JA, Rob CG: Critical arterial stenosis. Surgery 54:250–259, 1963.
25. James IM, Millar RA, Purves MY: Observations on the intrinsic neural control of cerebral blood flow in the baboon. Circ Res 25:77–93, 1969.

26. Moore WS, Hall AD: Unrecognized aortoiliac stenosis—a physiologic approach to the diagnosis. Arch Surg 103:633–638, 1971.
27. Carter SA: Response of ankle systolic pressure to leg exercise in mild or questionable arterial disease. N Engl J Med 287:578–582, 1972.
28. Sumner DS, Strandness DE Jr: The relationship between calf blood flow and ankle blood pressure in patients with intermittent claudication. Surgery 65:763–771, 1969.
29. Flanigan DP, Tullis JP, Streeter VL, et al: Multiple subcritical arterial stenosis: Effect on poststenotic pressure and flow. Ann Surg 186:663–668, 1977.
30. Longland CJ: The collateral circulation of the limb. Ann R Coll Surg Engl 13:161–176, 1953.
31. John HT, Warren R: The stimulus to collateral circulation. Surgery 49:14–25, 1961.
32. Skinner JS, Strandness DE Jr: Exercise and intermittent claudication. II. Effect of physical training. Circulation 36:23–29, 1967.
33. Ludbrook J: Collateral artery resistance in the human lower limb. J Surg Res 6:423–434, 1966.
34. Sumner DS, Strandness DE Jr: The effect of exercise on resistance to blood flow in limbs with an occluded superficial femoral artery. Vasc Surg 4:229–237, 1970.
35. Keitzer WF, Fry WT, Kraft RO, et al: Hemodynamic mechanism for pulse changes seen in occlusive vascular disease. Surgery 57:163–174, 1965.
36. Strandness DE Jr, Bell JW: Peripheral vascular disease: Diagnosis and objective evaluation using a mercury strain gauge. Ann Surg 161(Suppl):1–35, 1965.
37. Yao JST: Hemodynamic studies in peripheral arterial disease. Br J Surg 57:761–766, 1970.
38. Zierler RE, Strandness DE Jr: Doppler techniques of lower extremity arterial diagnosis. In Zwiebel WJ (ed): Introduction to Vascular Ultrasonography, 2nd ed. New York, Grune & Stratton, 1986, pp 305–331.
39. Reivich MH, Holling HE, Roberts B, Toole JF: Reversal of blood flow through the vertebral artery and its effect on the cerebral circulation. N Engl J Med 265:878–885, 1961.
40. Gonzales L, Weintraub RA, Wiot JF, Lewis C: Retrograde vertebral artery blood flow: A normal phenomenon. Radiology 82:211–216, 1964.
41. Kelly WA, Strandness DE Jr: The subclavian steal syndrome. In Strandness DE Jr (ed): Collateral Circulation in Clinical Surgery. Philadelphia, WB Saunders, 1969, pp 570–582.
42. Ehrenfeld WK, Harris JD, Wylie EJ: Vascular "steal" phenomenon—an experimental study. Am J Surg 116:192–197, 1968.
43. Shin CS, Chaudhry AG. The hemodynamics of extraanatomic bypass grafts. Surg Gynecol Obstet 148:567–570, 1979.
44. Sumner DS, Strandness DE Jr: The hemodynamics of the femoro-femoral shunt. Surg Gynecol Obstet 134:629–636, 1972.
45. Mozersky DJ, Sumner DS, Barnes RW, et al: The hemodynamics of the axillary-axillary bypass. Surg Gynecol Obstet 135:925–929, 1972.
46. Larsen DA, Lassen NA: Medical treatment of occlusive arterial disease of the legs—walking exercise and medically induced hypertension. Angiologica 6:288–301, 1969.
47. Freiman DB, Ring EJ, Oleaga JA: Transluminal angioplasty of the iliac, femoral, and popliteal arteries. Radiology 132:285–288, 1979.
48. Strandness DE Jr, Bell JW: Ankle pressure responses after reconstructive arterial surgery. Surgery 59:514–516, 1966.
49. Coffman JD, Mannick JA: Failure of vasodilator drugs in arteriosclerosis obliterans. Ann Intern Med 76:35–39, 1972.
50. Strandness DE Jr: Ineffectiveness of isoxuprine on intermittent claudication. JAMA 213:86–88, 1970.
51. Strandness DE Jr: Role of sympathectomy in the treatment of arteriosclerosis obliterans and thromboangiitis obliterans. In Strandness DE

Jr (ed): Collateral Circulation in Clinical Surgery. Philadelphia, WB Saunders, 1969, pp 450–459.

52. Barnes RW, Baker WH, Shanik G: Value of concomitant sympathectomy in aortoiliac reconstruction. Arch Surg 112:1325–1330, 1977.

53. Gruber UF: Dextran and the prevention of postoperative thromboembolic complications. Surg Clin North Am 55:679–696, 1975.

54. Porter JM, Cutler BS, Lee BY, et al: Pentoxifylline efficacy in the treatment of intermittent claudication: Multicenter controlled double-blind trial with objective assessment of chronic occlusive disease patients. Am Heart J 104:66–72, 1982.

55. Strandness DE Jr, Thiele BL: Anatomy of the venous system of the lower limb. In Selected Topics in Venous Disorders. New York, Futura, 1981, pp 1–26.

56. Gauer OH, Thron HL: Postural changes in the circulation. In Hamilton WF, Dow P (eds): Handbook of Physiology. Section 2: Circulation, vol 3. Washington, DC, American Physiological Society, 1965, pp 2409–2439.

57. Holling HE, Verel D: Circulation of the elevated forearm. Clin Sci 16:197–213, 1957.

58. Henry JP, Slaughter OL, Greiner T: A medical massage suit for continuous wear. Angiology 6:482–494, 1955.

59. Pollack AA, Wood EH: Venous pressure in the saphenous vein at the ankle in man during exercise and changes in posture. J Appl Physiol 1:649–662, 1949.

60. Dodd H, Cockett FB: The Pathology and Surgery of the Veins of the Lower Limbs. Edinburgh, Churchill Livingstone, 1976.

61. Strandness DE Jr, Langlois YE, Cramer M, et al: Long-term sequelae of acute venous thrombosis. JAMA 250:1289–1292, 1983.

62. van Bemmelen PS, Bedford G, Beach K, et al: Status of the valves in the superficial and deep venous system in chronic venous disease. Surgery 109:730–734, 1990.

63. Markel A, Manzo RA, Bergelin RO, et al: Valvular reflux after deep vein thrombosis: Incidence and time of occurrence. J Vasc Surg 15:377–384, 1992.

64. Johnson BF, Manzo RA, Bergelin RO, et al: Relationship between changes in the deep venous system and the development of the postthrombotic syndrome after an acute episode of lower limb deep vein thrombosis: A one- to six-year follow-up. J Vasc Surg 21:307–313, 1995.

65. Browse NL, Burnand KG: The postphlebitic syndrome—a new look. In Bergan JJ, Yao JST (eds): Venous Problems. St Louis, Mosby–Year Book, 1978, pp 395–404.

66. Killewich LA, Martin R, Cramer M, et al: Pathophysiology of venous claudication. J Vasc Surg 1:507–511, 1984.

67. Kistner RL: Transvenous repair of the incompetent femoral vein valve. In Bergan JJ, Yao JST (eds): Venous Problems. St Louis, Mosby–Year Book, 1975, pp 493–509.

68. Queral LA, Whitehouse WM, Flinn WR, et al: Surgical correction of chronic deep venous insufficiency by valvular transposition. Surgery 87:688–695, 1980.

69. Husni EA, Ximenes JOC, Goyette EM: Elastic support of the lower limbs in hospital patients—a critical study. JAMA 214:1456–1462, 1970.

70. Mayberry JC, Moneta GL, DeFrang RD, et al: The influence of elastic compression stockings on deep venous hemodynamics. J Vasc Surg 13:91–100, 1991.

Questions

1. Viscous energy losses in flowing blood result from
   (a) changes in the velocity and direction of flow
   (b) friction between adjacent layers of moving blood
   (c) turbulent flow in areas of stenosis
   (d) disturbed flow at points of branching
   (e) areas of boundary layer separation

2. Poiseuille's law states that pressure gradients in an idealized flow model are inversely proportional to
   (a) mean flow velocity
   (b) tube or stenosis length
   (c) blood viscosity
   (d) tube or stenosis radius
   (e) volume flow rate

3. Inertial energy losses in blood flow are related primarily to
   (a) changes in the velocity and direction of flow
   (b) blood viscosity
   (c) the specific gravity of blood
   (d) friction between adjacent layers of moving blood
   (e) the mean blood pressure

4. The critical stenosis value for a particular artery depends on the
   (a) length of the arterial segment
   (b) tangential wall stress
   (c) blood viscosity
   (d) compliance of the arterial wall
   (e) flow rate and peripheral vascular resistance

5. Which of the following statements about the collateral circulation is false?
   (a) collateral vessels are preexisting pathways that enlarge when the parallel major artery is occluded
   (b) the vascular resistance of the collateral bed is relatively fixed
   (c) collateral artery resistance is usually less than that of the original unobstructed parallel artery

   (d) an abnormal pressure gradient across the collateral bed may stimulate further development of collateral pathways
   (e) the midzone of the collateral bed consists of small, intramuscular vessels

6. Which of the following is not related to rupture of arterial aneurysms?
   (a) the volume flow rate through the aneurysm
   (b) the arterial blood pressure
   (c) the internal radius of the aneurysm
   (d) the tensile strength of collagen
   (e) the thickness of the aneurysm wall

7. With an extra-anatomic bypass, such as a femorofemoral crossover graft, a vascular steal from the donor limb is most likely to occur when
   (a) there is occlusive disease in both the donor and recipient limbs
   (b) there is an occlusive lesion in the donor artery
   (c) severe occlusive disease is present in the donor limb
   (d) the recipient limb has only mild occlusive disease
   (e) the donor limb is hemodynamically normal

8. Venous claudication is characterized by all of the following except
   (a) chronic iliofemoral venous occlusion
   (b) thigh pain with vigorous exercise
   (c) high-resistance venous collaterals
   (d) minimal disability with ordinary activities
   (e) valvular incompetence in the tibial veins

9. Which of the following is not a function of the calf muscle pump?
   (a) it lowers venous pressure in the dependent limb
   (b) it reduces the venous volume in the exercising limb
   (c) it improves arterial (nutritive) blood flow to the exercising muscle
   (d) it increases venous return to the right heart

(e) it minimizes the accumulation of interstitial fluid in the distal limb

10. All of the following contribute to the pathogenesis of the post-thrombotic syndrome except
    (a) deep vein thrombosis with obstruction of the deep veins

(b) extravasation of blood components into the subcutaneous tissues
(c) incompetence of the venous valves in the area of the calf muscle pump
(d) the presence of primary varicose veins
(e) ambulatory venous hypertension

Answers

1. b   2. d   3. a   4. e   5. c   6. a   7. b   8. e   9. c   10. d

14

The Vascular Laboratory

J. Dennis Baker

In the early days of vascular surgery, patient assessment was based on a careful history and physical examination. Although a few clinicians used the Collins oscillometer to estimate the pulse pressure in an extremity, there was little available in terms of quantitative assessment of arterial or venous disease. Angiography provided the only objective determination of the patient's pathologic changes. Early experience with arteriography and phlebography demonstrated some of the limitations of these techniques, especially the problem of underestimating the severity of stenotic lesions when single-plane studies were obtained. In addition, the cost, patient discomfort, and risk of complications associated with the contrast studies precluded them from routine use for screening evaluations and for subsequent follow-up.

The growing interest in more accurate differential diagnosis, localization of disease, measurement of its severity, and documentation of progression all stimulated the development of noninvasive techniques. In the 1960s, investigators started working with different plethysmographic techniques for quantitating arterial occlusive disease in the leg. Modification of ultrasonographic equipment to measure blood flow by the Doppler shift principle represented an important step forward in instrumentation and led to rapid development of noninvasive studies. Additional techniques were designed to evaluate carotid artery disease as well as deep venous occlusion and insufficiency. This chapter describes the main diagnostic techniques used in the noninvasive laboratory and discusses their clinical application for patients with vascular disease. Understanding the merits and limitations of each method will help the clinician make the most appropriate use of these tests.

INSTRUMENTATION

Doppler Velocity Measurement Techniques

High-frequency sound waves (2 to 10 MHz) penetrate through soft tissues and are reflected by the different interfaces encountered. Reflection from a moving interface results in the reflected frequency being increased if the motion is toward the point of observation and decreased if away. The magnitude of the shift is determined by:

$$f_s = \frac{2Vf_0 \cos\phi}{C}$$

where f_s is the frequency shift; V, the velocity; f_0, the transmitted frequency; ϕ, the angle between the ultrasound beam and the velocity vector; and C, the speed of sound in tissue (1540 m/sec). For a given velocity, a greater shift f_s is obtained with a higher transmitting frequency. On the other hand, tissue penetration varies inversely with probe frequency, so that the selection of frequency for a given application is a balance between depth and velocity requirements.

Continuous wave (CW) detectors are the simplest systems. The probe has two separate crystals, one transmitting and one receiving continuously. This system detects all velocities within the intersecting paths of the sound beams. If this zone includes more than one vessel (e.g., an artery and a vein), the resulting signal represents both velocities. Pulsed systems use a single crystal, which repeatedly transmits a short burst of sound followed by a waiting period, during which the crystal functions in a receive mode. By selecting the time and duration of the listening phase, one can define a sample volume, the portion of the vessel from which velocity is to be measured.

The shifted frequency obtained from a vessel is within the audible range, so the data can be presented to the examiner as an audio signal. Although qualitative interpretation is helpful in patient examinations, quantitative measurements provide more objective testing. Spectral analyzers can be used to determine the main frequency components obtained from a given vessel. This information is usually displayed on a sonogram, which shows the frequency content in time (Fig. 14–1).

In some applications, it is necessary to have a measure of velocity rather than the raw frequency data. If the probe angle can be measured, the velocity is estimated using the Doppler equation. The accuracy of the estimate depends greatly on the accuracy of the angle measurement. Errors are greatest when the probe is at right angles to flow and

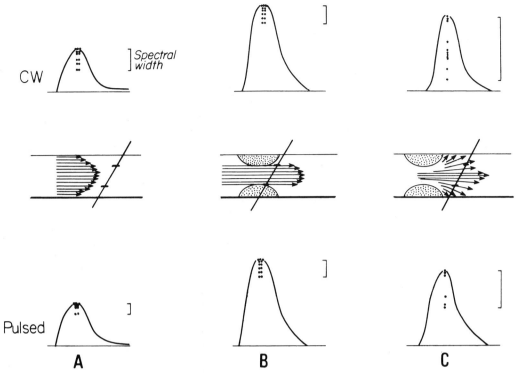

Figure 14–1. Comparison sonograms from continuous-wave (CW) and pulsed Doppler systems. Sonogram displays the different frequency contents detected at each point in time. CW detects all velocities across the vessel, whereas pulsed system detects only those velocity vectors within the sample volume, indicated by the marks on the ultrasound beam. *A*, Normal arterial signals. CW has more low-frequency content, because it detects flow near the walls as well as in center stream. *B*, Within stenosis, there is increased peak frequency, and the frequency distributions of both types of Doppler system are similar, because the sample volume encompasses the entire flow stream. *C*, Beyond stenosis, peak frequency is elevated, with increased frequency distribution resulting from turbulent flow. Spectral width is greater with CW system.

least when at low angles. Whenever possible, velocities should be measured with an angle below 60 degrees.

Duplex Scan

During the 1960s, B mode ultrasound imaging was used for visualization of soft tissue structures. Although early devices had only crude resolution, equipment has improved

to the point that clear, detailed images of vessels can be produced in real time (Fig. 14–2). In general, experience shows that when high-quality imaging is obtained, the diagnostic accuracy is very high; however, in patients with advanced atherosclerosis, it is difficult to obtain optimal studies, and the diagnostic accuracies are lower. A common problem is incomplete imaging of the vessel wall as a result of calcification, which is present in varying degrees in up to half of the patients studied. The interference may be

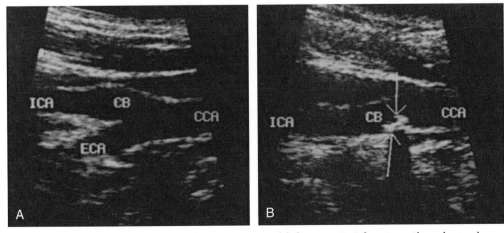

Figure 14–2. B mode images from carotid duplex scan. *A*, Normal bifurcation. *B*, Bifurcation with moderate plaque. Dense appearance with shadowing produced by calcium in the lesion. *CB*, carotid bulb; *CCA*, common carotid artery; *ECA*, external carotid artery; *ICA*, internal carotid artery.

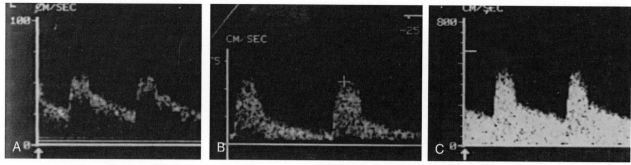

Figure 14–3. Doppler sonograms from carotid duplex scans. *A*, Normal study with normal spectral width. *B*, Moderate stenosis with spectral broadening but no increase in peak frequency. (Note that frequency scales are different in the three records.) *C*, Severe stenosis with high peak velocity and extensive spectral broadening.

limited, but in some vessels there is no visualization of substantial portions of the artery. Although calcified plaques stand out sharply in the ultrasound image, some atheromas are visualized poorly or not at all. A major source of error is that recent thrombus may have the same echo density as flowing blood, so that an occluded vessel may look normal on the ultrasound image.

To overcome the limitations of ultrasound imaging, the research team at the University of Washington developed the duplex scanner, combining a real-time B mode ultrasound image system with a pulsed Doppler detector.[1] The ultrasound image shows not only the vessel under study but also the location of the sample volume of the Doppler beam so that the examiner can position it to study velocity patterns at specific locations in the vessel. The device can study calcified vessels by analyzing the Doppler velocity signal distal to the areas of calcification. The evaluation of the Doppler signal from the common carotid artery and its branches is carried out using spectral analysis (Fig. 14–3). Based on the peak systolic velocity, end-diastolic velocity, and the degree of spectral broadening, a category of stenosis is assigned to the vessel segment.

In the past 20 years, there has been extensive improvement of duplex scanners both in image resolution and Doppler signal processing. The early devices were limited to the study of superficial vessels; however, availability of low-frequency probes (2.0 to 3.5 MHz) permits evaluation of abdominal vessels, including the aorta, the vena cava, and the main visceral branches.

The most recent development is the color-coded Doppler system. A linear array transducer composed of many separate elements is used to produce a grid of sample volumes encompassing the area being covered by the B mode image (Fig. 14–4). A portion of the grid is selected for color coding of velocity information. Each of the sample volumes within the area is examined sequentially. If the returning ultrasound signal has no change in phase or frequency, the amplitude information is used to create the gray-scale image at that point in the matrix. On the other hand, if there is a change in phase or frequency, the information is analyzed in terms of velocity. A color is assigned to represent the mean velocity occurring at that point in the field. Red and blue show flow toward and away from the transducer, respectively. The magnitude of the velocity is represented by the hue of the color: a dark

shade indicates slow flow, and a lighter shade or white shows high flow. The aggregate of the color representation from sample volumes detecting motion produces a real-time representation of the flow patterns within vessels superimposed on the gray-scale image of the stationary tissue. Figure 14–5 (see color insert after p. 250) illustrates examples of the advantages of color duplex scans.

CAROTID ARTERY STUDIES

The internal carotid artery (ICA) poses a unique challenge to physical examination, for it is impossible to palpate a distal pulse. It is not uncommon to find a patient whose carotid pulse in the neck is normal to palpation but who has occlusion of the internal carotid branch. This limitation stimulated development of physiologic tests to assess the status of the ICA. Most of the early tests provided indirect

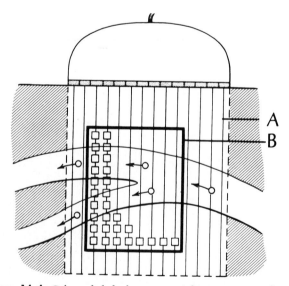

Figure 14–4. Color-coded duplex system. A linear array transducer is used to create a matrix of sample volumes. Gray-scale image is created within area A. Most examinations are carried out with color coding of velocities limited to a portion of the image (area B). Within this portion of the matrix, ultrasound signals from sample volumes with a change in phase or frequency are interpreted as velocity data. Otherwise, the data are coded as part of the gray-scale image.

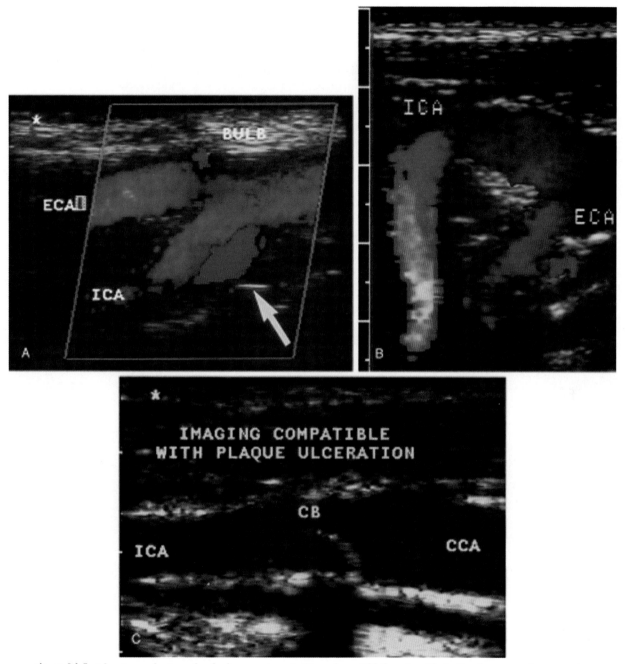

Figure 14-5. Advantages of using color duplex scanning. *A,* Normal carotid bifurcation, illustrating the reverse flow occurring in the bulb during systole *(arrow). B,* Marked tortuosity of internal carotid artery easily demonstrated with color scanner. *C,* Conventional gray-scale image does not provide clear identification of large ulcer.

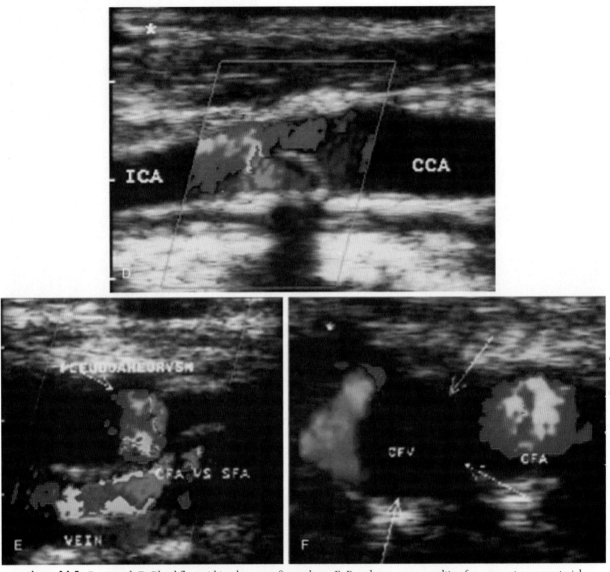

Figure 14-5. *Continued. D,* Blood flow within plaque confirms ulcer. *E,* Pseudoaneurysm resulting from percutaneous arterial catheterization. *F,* Blood flow around partial occluding venous thrombus.

measurement by detecting distal changes in blood flow characteristics produced by advanced stenosis. Common features of the indirect methods are that they detect only lesions that are sufficiently advanced to reduce mean blood flow and they cannot separate a tight stenosis from an occlusion, because the physiologic changes in the distal bed may be indistinguishable.

One of the earliest techniques was the periorbital Doppler examination, using a directional CW detector to study the patterns of collateral flow responses to transient occlusion of branches of the external carotid artery. Although this test used simple instrumentation, diagnosis was based entirely upon qualitative assessment of the changes in the signals detected. A more objective, reproducible test became available with the introduction of the ocular pneumoplethysmograph by Gee and colleagues[2] in 1975. This method used indirect measurement of the ophthalmic artery pressure to detect significant stenosis in the carotid system. Other techniques that were developed include the recording of the Doppler signals in the region of the carotid bifurcation with a handheld CW probe and different systems for analyzing carotid bruits. These methods achieved a variable degree of clinical use in the 1970s and 1980s but were ultimately replaced by duplex scanning.

Duplex Scan

The routine examination covers as much of the common carotid artery (CCA) and its branches as can be visualized with the configuration of the transducer used. In some patients, the origins of the CCAs can be visualized. Figures 14–2A and 14–5A show normal carotid bifurcations. The color image demonstrates the reverse velocity detected in the carotid bulb as the result of the complex flow pattern at the bifurcation. Many older patients have tortuosity such that the CCA, the bulb, and the branches cannot be visualized in a single plane, and careful scanning is required to obtain satisfactory imaging. Figure 14–5B shows an example of tortuosity in an elderly patient. Although such arteries can be studied with a conventional scanner, the color-coded unit simplifies the examination. The scan usually identifies the pathologic regions, but with advanced atherosclerosis it is often difficult to get an adequate image to permit accurate estimation of the degree of stenosis. Much of the classification of stenosis is based on interpretation of the Doppler signal. The two branches are distinguished by the image and the velocity signals. The ICA has a low peripheral resistance at all times, resulting in forward flow throughout diastole, whereas the high resistance in the external carotid results in diastolic flow going to zero. Stenoses produce an increased velocity at the site of the lesion and turbulence beyond (see Fig. 14–1). The turbulence is identified as spectral broadening, seen on the sonogram (see Fig. 14–3). Mild stenoses may not produce a significant increase in peak systolic velocity but are identified by a moderate degree of spectral broadening. Based on the peak systolic velocity and the degree of spectral broadening, the ICA is placed in one of six diagnostic categories, outlined in Table 14–1. Further improvement in accuracy may be obtained using ratios of velocities in the ICA to those in the normal portion of the CCA, especially in the identification of the 80% to 99% category.[3] The diagnosis of ICA occlusion must be based on image as well as Doppler information, because the very low flow found with some "string signs" is below the threshold for velocity detection of many scanners. Newer color duplex devices have improved our ability to find small residual flow channels. The stippled appearance of chronic thrombus and a small diameter of the ICA both point to occlusion. Overall, low-grade stenoses are best assessed with the image, whereas advanced lesions are best evaluated with the Doppler information.

Over the past few years there has been a rapid growth in the use of duplex scanning for carotid diagnosis. Different investigators have demonstrated that the technique can be highly accurate. Studies have shown accuracies in the range of 92% to 96% in the correct identification of severe stenosis.[4-6] When these studies are analyzed in terms of correct category of stenosis, exact agreement is found in 77% to 87%, with poor agreement in only 1% to 2%. Of particular importance is the fact that experienced laboratories make very few errors in separating severe stenosis from occlusion. Mansour and coauthors[7] have reported a 98% positive predictive value and 99% negative predictive value in the correct determination of ICA occlusion.

In addition to estimating the severity of a stenosis, scanners are now being used to study the plaque itself. Most investigators have limited themselves to distinguishing between homogeneous- and heterogeneous-appearing plaques and describing the surface as smooth or irregular. More elaborate approaches to describing morphology are

TABLE 14-1

Categories of Internal Carotid Artery (ICA) Stenosis Determined by Doppler Velocity Criteria

ICA STENOSIS	ICA VELOCITY	SPECTRUM
Normal vessel	Peak systolic velocity < 125 cm/sec	No broadening
1–19%	Peak systolic velocity < 125 cm/sec	Limited broadening in late systole
20–59%	Peak systolic velocity < 125 cm/sec	Broadening throughout systole
60–79%	Peak systolic velocity > 125 cm/sec; end-diastolic velocity < 125 cm/sec	Broadening throughout systole
80–99%	End-diastolic velocity > 125 cm/sec (severe stenoses may have very low velocity)	Broadening throughout systole
Occlusion	No ICA Doppler signal: flow to zero in common carotid artery	

being evaluated, but no single approach has been widely adopted.

Although the majority of attention has been focused on the carotid circulation, laboratories routinely investigate the status of the vertebral arteries. The examination seeks two types of problems: stenosis in the vertebral artery itself and the abnormal flow produced by subclavian steal. In the majority of cases of significant stenosis, the lesion is located at the origin of the vessel. In some cases of severe occlusive disease, there is sufficient asymmetry in the waveforms of the two vertebral arteries to point to the problem side. However, a more complete assessment is obtained by examining the origins. Because of its deeper location, the left vertebral artery is more difficult to study than the right. Ackerstaff and associates[8] found that the status of the ostium could be studied satisfactorily in about 80% of patients. When adequate evaluation of the prevertebral portion was possible, a sensitivity of 80% and a specificity of 97% were achieved in the detection of reductions greater than 50% in diameter. Most clinical cases of subclavian steal are demonstrated by a reverse flow in the vertebral artery on the affected side. Von Reutern and Pourcelot[9] demonstrated that in some cases of subclavian stenosis there is distortion of the waveform rather than complete reversal of flow. The abnormal waveforms may have attenuation of the systolic component or an alternating pattern with reverse flow in systole and forward flow in diastole (Fig. 14–6). Such cases can be more fully assessed by recording the Doppler signal after arm exercise or the induction of reactive hyperemia. In the presence of advanced subclavian stenosis, this stress test produces full reversal of flow.

Applications

Symptomatic Patients

A large portion of transient ischemic attacks and strokes are caused by thromboembolization from arterial plaques in the carotid bifurcation. A duplex scan may be useful for patients who are going to have an angiogram. Identification of the location and severity of lesions in the carotid system may assist in selection of the specific arteriographic technique. Occasionally, the scan may demonstrate a lesion that is underestimated or missed with standard views. Many centers have been using the ultrasound study as the definitive test on which to base the decision to operate. Having a very experienced vascular laboratory with a validated record of high accuracy in carotid scanning is the critical element in using the duplex scan as the definitive test.

Asymptomatic Carotid Stenosis

Increasing numbers of asymptomatic patients are being referred to noninvasive vascular laboratories for evaluation of cervical bruits. Although some of these patients have

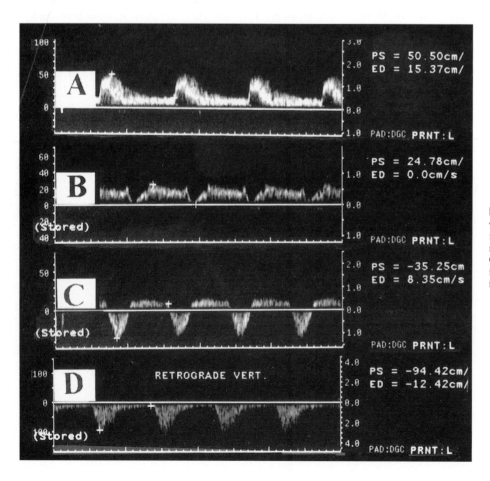

Figure 14–6. Vertebral artery Doppler waveforms. A is normal. B–D are signals recorded on the side of severe subclavian stenosis. B shows attenuated systolic flow. C illustrates reversed flow in systole with forward flow in diastole. D shows complete flow reversal.

bruits radiating from the heart or the great vessels, a considerable proportion of them have bruits originating from the carotid bifurcations. Duplex scanning can provide accurate separation according to category of stenosis (see Table 14–1). Patients with severe stenosis are considered at increased risk of stroke and are evaluated for prophylactic carotid endarterectomy. Lesions that fall in the moderate and advanced categories should have follow-up testing to detect those that progress into the high-risk group. Most people with normal vessels or early disease do not require routine follow-up.

Another indication is screening of patients with advanced atherosclerotic disease in the coronary or peripheral vessels. Owing to the diffuse nature of atherosclerosis, some of these patients have occult carotid bifurcation lesions, with a resulting increased risk of stroke. Screening is carried out most often in patients who are being considered for cardiac or major peripheral arterial operations to detect carotid lesions that may substantially increase the risk of intraoperative and postoperative stroke. Although screening may be appropriate for patients with multiple risk factors or severe occlusive disease in other arteries, routine testing of large populations results in a low yield of stenoses in the 80% to 99% category and is not cost-effective, especially if duplex scanning is used.

Intraoperative Assessment

Over the years, there has been increasing use of completion studies to evaluate the status of the artery operated on before closing. Contrast angiography has been the most common technique used, usually with a single injection into the CCA below the level of the endarterectomy. Another approach has been to examine the repair using a simple CW Doppler unit with subjective evaluation of the signals. This method detects severe residual stenoses but is not sensitive to less severe problems. There has been an increasing use of completion duplex scanning to detect residual defects for correction, and studies have shown satisfactory results.[10–12] Bandyk and colleagues[13] have used a peak systolic velocity greater than 180 cm/second or a velocity ratio greater than 2.4 as criteria to carry out a confirmatory angiogram or to proceed directly to repair.

Postoperative Follow-Up

Recurrent stenosis after carotid endarterectomy remains a clinical problem. Early studies reported as much as 5% symptomatic restenosis and 8% asymptomatic restenosis (as identified by noninvasive testing).[14, 15] More recent studies applying life-table analysis have found 20% to 32% rates for restenosis with greater than 50% diameter reduction.[16, 17] It has been shown that a substantial proportion of the restenoses occur early in the postoperative period. A common practice is to obtain an early postoperative study that can be used as a baseline. Follow-up evaluations are done 6 and 12 months after surgery. If the study results remain normal, noninvasive studies are repeated yearly.

LOWER EXTREMITY ARTERIAL STUDIES

Segmental Extremity Pressure Measurement

Indirect measurement of extremity pressures has been performed since the beginning of the 20th century using a sphygmomanometer and auscultation of the Korotkoff sounds with a stethoscope. Although this technique is universally used for measurement of pressures in the brachial artery, its application in the lower extremity is less practical because of difficulties in listening for Korotkoff sounds in the popliteal space. The technique is certainly not applicable in the distal portions of the extremity because of the small size of the vessels involved. Investigators overcome this limitation by using a variety of plethysmographic devices. In 1959, Winsor[18] first described the clinical measurements of arterial gradients using a plethysmograph. Systolic pressures in the lower extremity were normally higher than those in the upper extremity. He described the blood pressure index (blood pressure of arm/blood pressure of leg), which in normal persons is greater than 1.0. A value greater than 1.0 indicates clinically significant occlusive disease proximal to the point of measurement. Likewise, a gradient between two sampling sites localizes the occlusive disease in the intervening segment. The main limitation of this method is that it detects only occlusive lesions that are sufficiently advanced to reduce the systolic pressure, so that it is not possible to detect early disease. Introduction of the Doppler velocity detector greatly simplified the indirect measurement of extremity pressures. For this application, the Doppler device is simply used to detect the presence or absence of movement of blood in the artery. Measurements made by this method are very reproducible but do not provide diastolic pressure. Plethysmographic techniques are cumbersome and are not used routinely.

In clinical practice, simple screening can be carried out by measuring the pressure at the brachial arteries and at the dorsal pedal and posterior tibial arteries on each side. The ankle index (AI) is determined by dividing the ankle pressure on each side by the higher of the two brachial pressures. The resulting value reflects the severity of the occlusive disease for the entire extremity. Normally, the AI should be greater than 1.0, and values less than 0.95 are abnormal. Figure 14–7 summarizes the general relation between AI values and clinical status. It must be emphasized that this is only a rough correlation and that patients with similar values may have substantial differences in exercise tolerance. Likewise, the index at which rest pain appears varies considerably from patient to patient, ranging from 0.30 to 0.50.

An important limitation of the indirect measurement of extremity pressure occurs in patients with abnormal stiffen-

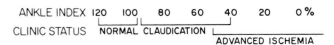

Figure 14–7. Relation of ankle index to patient symptoms.

ing of the vessel wall, most often due to heavy calcification. Such conditions occur in patients with diabetes mellitus but also can be found with other disorders. In these cases, the systolic pressure measured reflects the cuff pressure required to collapse the vessel wall in addition to the pressure required to overcome the intraluminal pressure. In some cases, it is not possible to stop the flow of blood at all. Error due to wall stiffness should be suspected whenever the AI is greater than 1.3 or when its value is out of proportion to the patient's clinical status. In general, a leg with a normal AI should have an easily palpable ankle pulse. In some patients with stiff arteries, it may be possible to obtain an accurate evaluation by measuring the toe pressure. In the normal person, there is a gradient of 20 to 30 mm Hg between the ankle and the toe, so a correction must be made when toe pressures are being used.

Additional information on localization of occlusive disease can be obtained by measuring the pressures at different levels of the leg. The segmental pressure measurements are usually performed by applying cuffs at the thigh, the upper calf, and immediately above the ankle artery. A standard adult-sized cuff (12 cm wide) is satisfactory for calf and ankle determinations, but a thigh cuff (18 cm) should be used above the knee. (Using a narrower cuff above the knee results in artificially high pressure measurements as a result of the size discrepancy between the cuff and the diameter of the thigh. Thigh measurements with an arm cuff usually result in determinations that are 20 to 30 mm Hg higher than those obtained with the wider cuff.) A thigh pressure lower than brachial pressure indicates obstruction proximal to the location of the thigh cuff. Gradients of more than 20 mm Hg between measuring sites are diagnostic of occlusive disease in the intervening segment, and higher gradients are usually associated with more severe lesions.

An important limitation of the use of the wide cuff for thigh measurement is that it is only possible to make a single thigh measurement. As a result, it is not possible to distinguish occlusive disease above the ligament from that in the proximal portion of the superficial femoral artery, because both conditions may result in the same thigh pressure measurement. To overcome this problem, some investigators have recommended using 12-cm–wide cuffs to obtain two separate thigh measurements. When this is done, it is necessary to take into account the 20- to 30-mm Hg artifact that results. In a study comparing the wide-cuff with the two narrow-cuff techniques in the same group of patients, Heintz and coworkers[19] reported an increased accuracy in localization of disease using the two-cuff technique. Both of the methods of thigh pressure measurement are still being used, so it is important to be aware of which method is being reported when reviewing results of patient studies. Although segmental pressures have been used extensively to detect proximal disease, diagnostic errors may occur in 25% of patients. Other techniques should be used when the accurate assessment of the segmental localization is needed.

Stress Testing

Most patients with advanced arterial insufficiency are adequately evaluated by measurements at rest; however, early lesions may not produce sufficient disturbance at resting flow rates to be detected by the usual methods. An example of the problem is the patient with typical symptoms of claudication who has normal or borderline leg pressures. More complete evaluation can be obtained by increasing the flow, thereby accentuating the hemodynamic effect of the stenosis. The simplest and most normal way to increase blood flow is to have the patient walk. The exercise produces a decrease in vascular resistance in the leg, with a resulting increase in flow to the leg. With moderate levels of exercise, there is no change in distal pressures in a normal extremity, but increasing the flow through a moderate stenosis causes an increased resistance at the lesion. The resulting energy loss can be detected by noninvasive tests such as a pressure gradient or the attenuation of the pulse waveform.

The stress test is performed by having the patient walk on a treadmill for 5 minutes or until symptoms force the patient to stop. Most protocols use a low level of exercise (2 mph with a 10% to 12% grade). This level of stress is sufficient to yield an abnormal result in most claudication patients, without undue cardiac stress. Baseline arm and ankle pressures are measured with the Doppler detector. As soon as the patient stops walking, he or she lies down on the examining table for repeat pressure measurements, which are made at 30-second intervals during the first 2 minutes and at 60-second intervals for the remainder of the examination, usually 5 to 10 minutes. The examiner always asks the patient why he or she stopped walking, because in some cases the limiting factor is angina or shortness of breath rather than claudication. Identification of these limitations is an important benefit of the stress test, because it may uncover or emphasize the significance of these other conditions.

One objective measurement of severity of occlusive disease is the exercise tolerance (i.e., the time the patient walks at the standardized rate). Further assessment is based on the changes in extremity pressures. Figure 14–8 shows the time-pressure relations seen in control subjects and in different categories of occlusive disease. Normal people have no significant change in ankle pressures with the modest level of exercise used for the stress test. On the other hand, patients with flow-limiting stenoses have a drop in distal pressures as a result of vasodilatation in the muscles. The amounts of the drop in AI and in the recovery time are both increased by greater severity of occlusive disease. Multiple lesions produce more marked depression of the recovery curve than do single lesions.

There are some situations in which treadmill exercise is not practical or does not offer the best evaluation. In such cases, reactive hyperemia can be used to increase blood flow in the extremities. A thigh cuff inflated above systolic pressure produces local circulatory arrest, resulting in hypoxia and local vasodilatation. When the cuff is released, there is a transient increase in flow, the duration of which is related to the period of ischemia and to the total blood flow to the leg. The magnitude of the pressure drop is comparable to that seen after walking, but the recovery is always more rapid with reactive hyperemia. In contrast to exercise, reactive hyperemia does produce a transient pressure drop (with a rapid recovery) in normal subjects. Criteria for a normal result are (1) lowest AI greater than

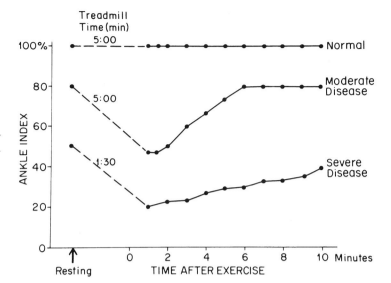

Figure 14–8. Changes in ankle index with exercise. The severity of the arterial stenosis is related to the exercise tolerance and the magnitude of the drop in ankle pressure and recovery time.

0.80 and (2) index returns to 90% of baseline value within 1 minute.[20] The technique provides a useful test method for (1) patients who cannot walk on the treadmill because of disabilities, (2) full evaluation of the less-involved limb in patients with marked asymmetry of their occlusive disease, and (3) patients who are not willing to perform adequately on the treadmill.

Doppler Waveform Analysis

Most commercial Doppler detectors provide an analog signal that is proportional to the velocity of the blood in the vessel studied. This signal can be displayed on a screen or recorded for later analysis. The overall shape of the waveform reflects the status of the vessel proximal to the point studied (Fig. 14–9). In the lower extremity, the normal velocity wave is triphasic, with reverse flow in early diastole. Proximal stenosis first eliminates the reverse flow, and with more severe lesions, there is blunting of the systolic upstroke and increasing flow during diastole. Complete analysis is complicated by the fact that the waveform is also affected by the stenotic lesions below the sampling site. The simplest analysis of Doppler waveforms is the qualitative interpretation of the curves, allowing identification of broad categories of disease. One specific application has been the assessment of the aortoiliac segment. However, the method suffers from a high false-positive rate resulting from the fact that an attenuated wave can be caused by proximal disease, distal disease, or a combination of the two.

A quantitative analysis of the Doppler waveform was described by Gosling and coworkers[21] using a parameter called pulsatility index (PI), obtained by dividing the peak-to-peak frequency shift by the mean frequency shift. The effect of stenosis is defined by the damping factor, the ratio of the distal PI to the proximal PI. Normally, the damping factor is greater than 1.0, and values below this reflect disease between the points of the two measurements. Estimation of severity of disease in the aortoiliac segment by waveform damping is not practical, because it is not normally possible to obtain a Doppler signal from the distal aorta with a CW Doppler.

Segmental Plethysmography

During systole, the blood entering a limb normally causes an increase in the total volume of the extremity, with a return to resting volume during diastole. This phenomenon is responsible for the pulse pressure oscillations seen with the sphygmomanometer while taking blood pressure. The total effect of the volume changes is quite small and can be detected only with the aid of sensitive devices. A variety of plethysmographic recorders have been devised using mercury strain gauge, water displacement, capacitance, and impedance systems, but the majority of these systems have proved to be impractical for routine clinical application. In

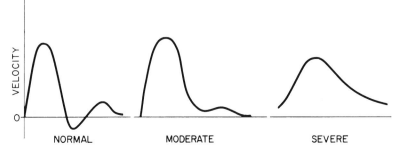

Figure 14–9. Doppler velocity tracings in the leg. Increasing stenosis results in elimination of reverse flow, decrease in systolic peak, and increase in flow during diastole.

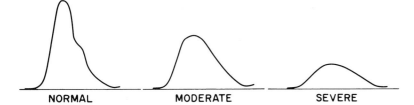

NORMAL   MODERATE   SEVERE

Figure 14–10. Pulse volume recorder tracings in the leg. Increasing stenosis results in loss of the dicrotic notch and flattening of the curve.

the early 1970s, the pulse-volume recorder (PVR) was designed specifically for peripheral arterial diagnosis. The system is based on a calibrated recording air plethysmograph using standard blood pressure cuffs applied at the thigh, calf, and ankle levels. The cuffs are inflated to 65 mm Hg for the recordings to ensure optimal contact of the cuff around the extremity. A sensitive transducer detects the small increase in pressure within the cuff resulting from the volume increase of the extremity during systole. The recorder provides a hard-copy tracing of the pulse wave, which has been demonstrated to be quite similar to arterial pressure waves measured directly.

The primary diagnosis is based on the qualitative evaluation of the PVR waveform.[22] The tracing from each level is categorized as normal, mildly abnormal, moderately abnormal, or severely abnormal. The normal tracing has a brisk, sharp rise to the systolic peak and usually displays a prominent dicrotic notch (Fig. 14–10). Early disease is characterized by the absence of a dicrotic notch and a more gradual, prolonged downslope. Moderate disease is characterized by the rounded systolic peak. Severe occlusive disease produces a flattened wave with a slow upstroke and downstroke. The absolute amplitude measurements are of limited value from patient to patient, because substantial changes result from variations in cardiac output and vasomotor tone. Comparison of amplitudes from one side to the other in the same patient can be of value in assessing unilateral disease. In the presence of bilateral disease, it can be helpful to standardize the amplitude measurements in the lower extremities by comparing them with arm tracings, because most patients do not have major upper extremity occlusive disease. Serial PVR measurements have been shown to be reproducible in patients with stable disease, so that amplitude changes indicate progression of disease.

The PVR has received extensive application in the past 20 years. In most situations, the plethysmographic studies are used in combination with segmental Doppler pressure measurements. Vascular laboratories using the PVR report that it is a useful adjunct to the routine pressure measurements. One particular advantage is the ability to accurately assess the presence or absence of occlusive disease in patients with rigid arteries. In addition, the PVR has improved the detection of aortoiliac stenosis. Kempczinski[23] has reported correct identification of advanced inflow disease in 95% of extremities.

Duplex Scan

In recent years, there has been increasing use of the duplex scan for peripheral arteries. With appropriate scan heads, Doppler signals can be obtained from the aorta down to the tibial branches. Screening for occlusive disease can be done by comparing signals from the distal aorta and more distal sites, looking for attenuation either qualitatively or by measurement of the damping factor (see earlier in this chapter). A more complete assessment is obtained by examining the full length of the segment in question, looking for the increased velocity and spectral broadening produced by a stenosis. The color-coded Doppler scan makes tracking of the vessels and localizing of significant stenoses considerably easier than with conventional scanners. The most common practice is to use the ratio of the peak systolic velocity recorded at the tightest part of the stenosis to the peak systolic velocity recorded in a normal portion of the same artery. A ratio greater than 2.0 defines a greater than 50% diameter reduction of the lumen.[24, 25] Some groups have established additional criteria to distinguish stenosis greater than 75%. Cossman and colleagues[26] consider the stenosis to be greater than 75% if the velocity ratio is greater than 4.0 or the peak velocity in the lesion is greater than 400 cm/second. Gonsalves and Bandyk[27] identify the severe lesion by a velocity ratio greater than 4.0, a peak velocity greater than 300 cm/second, or an end-diastolic velocity greater than 100 cm/second.

Scanning is being used increasingly for visceral vessels and renal arteries of normal and transplanted kidneys. The anterior approach to visceral branches can be made difficult by the presence of bowel gas. Flank approaches and examination of the fasting patient increase the rate of successful studies. Most renal artery stenoses occur at the origins, so that it is necessary to obtain recordings from the proximal part of the vessel. As with peripheral lesions, the focus has been on identifying hemodynamically significant stenoses. A peak systolic velocity greater than 180 cm/second identifies an abnormal vessel, and a ratio of the peak velocity in the stenosis to the peak velocity in the aorta at the level of the renal arteries greater than 3.5 predicts a stenosis with a greater than 60% lumen diameter reduction.[28–30] Another approach has been to use the waveform recorded in the renal hilum.[31] Although recording of hilar signals is usually easier than examination of the main renal arteries, this approach does not seem to be as accurate in the diagnosis of significant stenoses.[30] An important limitation of the duplex scan in the evaluation of renal disease is that accessory branches are rarely found.

Duplex scanning has also been used to study the other visceral branches. The celiac trunk and the proximal superior mesenteric artery can be easily located. On the other hand, the inferior mesenteric artery is often not found unless it provides significant collateral flow because of occlusions in other branches. Unlike the situation with the kidneys, the perfusion to the gut is quite variable, depending upon physiologic responses to feeding. Therefore, it is important to obtain baseline studies of patients in a fasting state. There has not been as much investigation of quantitative criteria to define severe mesenteric disease as in other duplex scan applications. Severe stenosis is identified by significant focal increase in velocity combined with poststenotic turbulence and reduced velocity beyond the stenosis.[32]

Applications

Qualitative Assessment of Specific Vessels

Direct examination with a Doppler detector has been applied in a variety of situations. Preoperative determination of whether there is flow in distal vessels may help plan distal bypass operations in the calf. In the postoperative patient with no distal pulses, it is often possible to detect whether a bypass graft has thrombosed. A more accurate assessment of hand circulation can be achieved by performing a modification of the Allen test, using the Doppler detector to examine flow in the palmar arch during the compression maneuvers. Patency and function of a peritoneovenous shunt (LeVeen or Denver shunt) can be determined.

Severity and Location of Arterial Lesions

The primary use of noninvasive tests in the patient with lower extremity problems is to obtain objective determinations to supplement the physical examination. The measurements permit reproducibility between different examiners as well as from one measurement to the next. In addition, the tests are valuable in measuring progression of arterial disease and assessment of arterial reconstructions. Extremity pressures and pulse plethysmographic recordings are valuable to assess severity of disease; however, duplex scanning must be used for accurate determination of level and extent of lesions. Kohler and associates[24] found a sensitivity of 89% and a specificity of 90% in identification of iliac stenosis greater than 50%. Legemate and coworkers[33] used a velocity increase of 150% and found a sensitivity of 92% and specificity of 98%. It is possible to estimate common femoral artery blood flow with duplex scan measurements, but the high variability in repeat measurements in individual patients limits the clinical usefulness of this approach.[34] Although further refinement of quantitative criteria is required, it is clear that duplex scanning can play an increasing role in evaluation of peripheral arterial insufficiency. A number of groups have had good results using the scan to select patients for transluminal angioplasty.[26, 35, 36] Following the lead of work done with carotid endarterectomy without preoperative angiography, some investigators have reported the feasibility of planning arterial operations with just the ultrasound scan.[37–40] Wain and coauthors[40] reported that duplex mapping is quite accurate down to the popliteal level, but in their experience, the technique was not as good in defining an appropriate target vessel at the crural level.

Intraoperative Assessment

As has been found with carotid surgery, duplex scanning provides an excellent tool for completion assessment after certain other arterial operations. In many operating rooms, scanning can be done more quickly and provide a more complete examination than a conventional contrast angiogram. Often, short, focal defects such as a retained valve are easily seen on scan but may not be well demonstrated, especially with a single film study. Bandyk and associates[13] have promulgated scanning after infrainguinal bypass grafts. The examination involves scanning the full length of the graft, including both anastomoses. A peak systolic velocity greater than 180 cm/second or a velocity ratio greater than 2.4 indicates problem areas for which revision must be considered. Bandyk and associates reported intraoperative revision rates of 14% to 16%. Fifty-two percent of the legs with significant duplex findings not repaired at the time of the original operation underwent subsequent revision.

Intraoperative duplex scanning has also been advocated for renal artery repairs to reduce the risk of early occlusion and possible loss of the kidney. Studies from Bowman Gray and the Mayo Clinic both reported an 11% incidence of detection of defects requiring repair at the time of the original procedure.[42, 43] A focal high-velocity jet with peak systolic velocity greater than 200 cm/second combined with distal turbulence identifies a tight stenosis, whereas lack of flow in the vessel indicates acute thrombosis.[42] Both these findings mandate immediate revision.

Graft Surveillance

Because of the poor secondary patency of vein grafts that thrombose, careful attention has been given to follow-up. As early as 1972, some surgeons advocated noninvasive testing to identify hemodynamic changes. For many years, graft status was monitored with pressure measurements; however, this technique is limited for patients with stiff arteries or with small-caliber distal bypasses. In 1985, Bandyk and associates[44] reported good results with graft surveillance using the duplex scanner to measure the peak systolic velocity. In this study, a peak velocity of less than 40 cm/second was associated with early graft thrombosis. In later years, the surveillance protocol was expanded to include not just a sampling of the graft velocity but a scan of the entire graft.[45, 46] The mapping permits identification of the specific site of the stenosis. A peak systolic velocity of 180 to 200 cm/second indicates a problem. Bandyk and Johnson[46] recommended intervention for any lesion with a peak systolic velocity greater than 300 cm/second or a velocity ratio greater than 3.5. A large proportion are found within the first postoperative year, so that a program of close surveillance is advocated by many authors.[47–49] The fact that significant problems appear later is a reason to continue surveillance beyond the first year, albeit at a reduced frequency.

Amputation Level

There has been much interest in using noninvasive tests to predict the probability of healing major leg amputations. Barnes and colleagues[50] demonstrated that all patients with an AI greater than 70% attained healing at the below-knee level, whereas 25% of patients with lower pressures failed.

From these data, it would be inappropriate to base the decision for above-knee amputation on AI results. The only finding that indicates an above-knee level is the absence of an arterial Doppler signal in the popliteal space.

VENOUS DISEASE

The correct diagnosis of venous disease presented a challenge for many years. In contrast to arterial occlusive disease, venous disease can be difficult to distinguish from other problems on the basis of the physical examination. In the past, diagnosis depended on phlebography, which, in addition to being painful, can precipitate thrombosis in a normal venous system. In the 1960s, Strandness and coworkers[51] and Sigel and colleagues[52] described using the Doppler velocity detector to identify normal and abnormal flow patterns in the veins of the leg. Along with the subsequent development of noninvasive techniques for the arterial system there was a parallel growth of venous diagnosis. In the 1970s and 1980s there was extensive use of physiologic methods such as impedance phlebography (IPG), but these tests have been replaced by duplex scanning.

Doppler Venous Examination

The flow in the veins of an extremity can be evaluated qualitatively with a simple CW Doppler detector. The patient is examined in the supine position with the head slightly elevated. The deep veins are found adjacent to the accompanying arteries. A normal vein has spontaneous flow with a phasic variation with respiration. Breath-holding or a Valsalva maneuver decreases or abolishes flow; with release, there is a transient augmentation of the signal. A quick compression of the extremity distal to the probe produces a brisk augmentation, often followed by a transient decrease on release. Proximal compression decreases or abolishes the flow signal, with augmentation coming on release. Examination of a thrombosed segment of vein shows no flow, and adjacent collateral veins have a high-pitched signal. The patent portion of the vein distal to an obstruction has a continuous flow with no respiratory variation, and the Valsalva maneuver produces no change. Limb compression may produce limited augmentation but clearly less than in the normal vein. The vein segment proximal to an occlusion may have phasic flow similar to normal, but the compression produces little change. The Doppler examination is sensitive to alterations in venous flow patterns, and different forms of extrinsic compression can produce similar changes. Abnormal studies can result from large hematomas, massive edema, or ruptured popliteal cysts. A false-positive test can also occur with advanced pregnancy, ascites, or abdominal masses compressing the inferior vena cava.

Many groups have studied the clinical application of the Doppler venous examination by comparing the results with phlebography. Sumner and Lambeth[53] reviewed a large number of the published studies and found overall diagnostic accuracies ranging from 49% to 96%, with a number showing accuracies more than 90%. Many of the errors were attributed to incomplete examination or lack of examiner experience. The greatest accuracy is obtained in the diagnosis of iliofemoral occlusions, because these produce large and easily detected changes in the venous flow patterns. However, careful testing can produce satisfactory diagnosis of thrombosis below the knee, with accuracies of 84% and 86% reported.[54, 55]

The Doppler venous examination can also detect venous valvular insufficiency. Normally, there should be no flow produced by compression proximal to the probe, because the valves prevent flow toward the probe. With incompetent valves, the proximal compression (or Valsalva maneuver) produces augmentation as a result of the retrograde flow. Demonstration of significant reverse flow is clear evidence of post-thrombotic syndrome.

The Doppler venous examination was an important test for acute deep vein thrombosis (DVT) in the leg, but it has been supplanted by quantitative and imaging techniques. Because of the simplicity of the Doppler examination, it still remains in use, primarily as an extension of the physical examination. An abnormal flow pattern in a patient with borderline physical findings can trigger more complete evaluation by the vascular laboratory. Simple Doppler examination is also helpful in detecting deep venous reflux in the patient with varicose veins.

Duplex Scan

The high resolution available with duplex scanners makes it possible to detect venous thrombosis. In this application, the emphasis is on imaging. Thrombus is seen within the vein lumen with varying degrees of echogenicity (Fig. 14–11). On occasion, fresh thrombus may not appear different from flowing blood; in these instances, additional assessment is obtained by compressing the vein with the probe. Normally, gentle pressure flattens the vein completely (Fig. 14–12). A partial or totally occluding thrombus prevents collapse in response to external pressure. Compression is performed in the transverse mode to ensure accurate evaluation with the maneuver. When examining in the longitudinal orientation, it is possible to move the

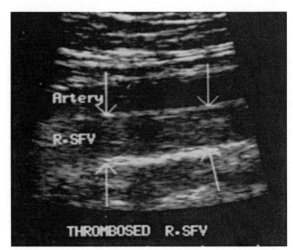

Figure 14–11. B mode scan of venous thrombus. Note the appearance of the vein lumen compared with the normal flow in the adjacent artery. R-SFV, right superficial femoral vein.

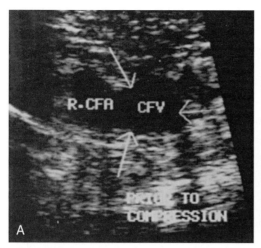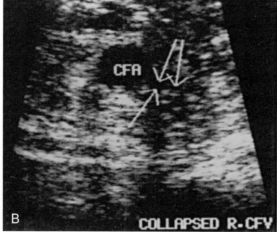

Figure 14–12. Transverse duplex scan. *A*, Normal appearance of vein. *B*, Complete collapse of vein in response to external compression with the probe. R-CFA, right common femoral artery; R-CFV, right common femoral vein.

ultrasound beam off the center of the vein so that the vein appears to collapse when it does not.

Occluded segments can also be identified by the lack of flow on Doppler examination, and examination of flow characteristics should be part of every study. Abnormalities in Doppler velocity signals either at rest or in response to augmentation maneuvers point to lesions that may not be evident with imaging. Color-coded Doppler is especially helpful in detecting partial occluding thrombi (see Fig. 14–5F). The color scanner has also improved the examination of the tibial veins.

Most centers using duplex scanning carry out a detailed examination from the inguinal ligament to the distal end of the popliteal vein. The common and superficial femoral veins are examined in the supine position with moderate leg dependency. (The deep femoral vein is usually not followed beyond its origin.) The popliteal vein is best imaged with the patient in the lateral or prone position. In addition to the deep system, superficial veins can be imaged. The greatest difficulty in many examinations is following the vein through the adductor canal. Many studies do not include tracing all the infrapopliteal branches. The other problem area is the detection of thrombus in the common or external iliac veins. It is difficult to image these; therefore, one often relies on indirect evidence given by the flow signal from the common femoral vein. Proximal occlusion causes a loss of phasic variation with respiration and limited or no change with the Valsalva maneuver. Vogel and coworkers[56] described using the change in common femoral vein diameter during the Valsalva maneuver: an increase of less than 10% indicates iliofemoral thrombosis.

Duplex scan of the deep leg veins for thrombus is technically difficult and requires considerable experience for accurate diagnosis. Experienced investigators have reported sensitivities and specificities on the order of 95% for the diagnosis of thrombus.[56–59] Although most studies have focused on acute thrombosis, Rollins and his associates[58] demonstrated the same high accuracy in the identification of chronic disease as in the acute situation. In addition, they had 89% accuracy in the evaluation of calf veins compared with 93% for the proximal veins.

The duplex scan is also used to evaluate reflux in specific venous segments. Many laboratories perform this evaluation in a casual fashion, examining patients in the recumbent position and using manual compression to cause valve closure. Van Bemmelen and associates[60] emphasized the need to examine the patient in the standing position to re-create the maximum stimulus for reflux. In addition, they recommended using a pneumatic cuff with rapid decompression to provide the necessary reverse flow. A reverse velocity of 30 cm/second is necessary for consistent valvular closure.[61] Manual compression produces a variable amount of reverse flow and often results in incomplete closure. In such a case, slow reverse flow may occur through a normal valve, leading to an interpretation of an abnormal segment.

Venous Reflux Photoplethysmography

The venous reflux resulting from valvular insufficiency has long been recognized as the primary cause of the symptoms and complications of the post-thrombotic syndrome. The first method used to study venous hypertension was the direct measurement by insertion of a needle into a superficial foot vein with pressures determined before, during, and after walking. The response to this test is defined by the magnitude of the pressure drop during walking and the time required for the pressure to return to baseline. The main drawback of ambulatory venous pressure measurement is the need for placing the needle into a foot vein, a procedure that can be difficult or impossible in some patients with advanced post-thrombotic syndrome.

Photoplethysmography (PPG) has been used to study reflux. A light in the probe shines into the superficial layers of the skin, and a photoelectric detector measures the reflected light. The intensity of light reflected varies with the amount of blood in the underlying microcirculation, and the device produces a pulse-wave trace, which is displayed on a strip-chart recorder. The technique is sensitive enough to record the arterial pulsation in the skin. The PPG tracing varies with the venous congestion of the skin, which varies with the venous pressure in the limb. Studies made with simultaneous recording of venous pressure and

PPG signals have demonstrated similar tracing configurations by the two methods.[62, 63]

The test is usually performed with the patient in the sitting position. The sensor is attached with double-sided clear tape over the medial malleolus but should not be directly over a superficial vein. After a short baseline tracing is obtained, the patient is instructed to contract the calf five times in quick succession and then to relax the leg. The recording is continued until the tracing has fully returned to the baseline level. The recovery time is measured from the end of the calf exercise to the point at which the curve returns to baseline (Fig. 14–13). A normal recovery is more than 20 seconds, with many subjects having times of 30 to 60 seconds. Times less than 20 seconds indicate venous reflux, with the severity of the condition being inversely proportional to the recovery time. If an abnormal tracing is obtained, the examination is repeated with a Penrose drain tourniquet (or a narrow cuff inflated to 50 mm Hg) placed above or below the knee to exclude the effect of reflux down the superficial system insufficiency in the face of a normal deep system. Commonly, the tracing improves without being completely normal, indicating combined deep and superficial disease. In some cases of severe reflux combined with persisting iliofemoral occlusion, there may be either no change or a rise in the tracing. These findings indicate very severe disease.

PPG provides a simple, objective method for quantifying venous reflux. The test is easy to perform and interpret. Unlike the Doppler venous examination, which identifies the presence or absence of flow reversal at given levels, the PPG reflects the overall effect of the venous insufficiency in the leg. A limitation of the test is the possibility of having reflux in the deep system with competent valves in the perforating veins. In this situation, the abnormal congestion of the deep system would not be transmitted to the skin and the PPG tracing would be normal.[64]

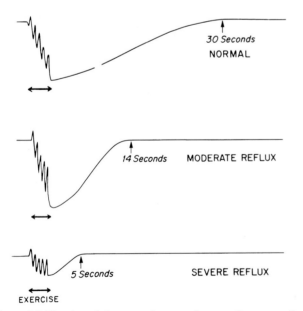

Figure 14–13. Photoplethysmography in evaluation of venous reflux. Incompetent valves result in recovery time less than 20 seconds. Severe insufficiency causes incomplete emptying of the calf during exercise, seen as a limited downward deflection of the tracing.

Applications

Acute Deep Venous Thrombosis

Clinicians have been aware of the fallibility of the physical findings in the diagnosis of acute DVT of the leg, so that most of the effort in the noninvasive diagnosis of venous disease has focused on the acute occlusion.

In the past 10 years, duplex scanning has become the primary modality used to diagnose acute DVT. Many institutions only perform contrast phlebograms in patients with nondiagnostic scans or when the scan cannot be done. This practice has been justified by the high accuracy achieved by different investigators.[56–59] A major advantage of the scan over IPG is the ability to identify the specific location of disease, especially when there is thrombus at multiple levels. Another important advantage is the detection of partial-occluding thrombi, a key limitation of the IPG. In addition to confirming the initial diagnosis, scanning can be used to document change during the therapy.

Recurrent Deep Venous Thrombosis

The diagnosis of recurrent DVT in patients with postthrombotic syndrome presents a great challenge to clinicians. Exacerbation of symptoms may mimic the symptoms of the original thrombosis, and in many cases, patients are readmitted for heparin therapy without objective evidence of recurrence. Although labeled fibrinogen is an excellent method for detecting new thrombus, this test is not available in most nuclear medicine departments. Noninvasive testing may be used to obtain objective diagnosis.

Duplex scanning can identify residual chronic thrombus by its high echogenicity. Other characteristics include thickened vein walls, fibrosed segments of occluded veins, and valvular insufficiency with reverse flow on Doppler examination. These features allow the examiner to use duplex scanning to distinguish recent from chronic clot. This contrasts with the phlebogram, which shows all lesions as filling defects.

Venous Insufficiency

The complications of chronic stasis are usually obvious, but it may be difficult to assess the relative contributions of outflow obstruction and reflux. Although the initial conservative management is similar, further surgical treatment must be directed to the specific etiology. The Doppler examination or the PPG can determine the presence of venous reflux and whether it involves the deep or the superficial system. More recently, duplex scanning has been used to evaluate specific segments, especially in the deep system. Measurement of reverse blood velocities or flows provides a quantitative assessment not available with the simpler tests.[60, 65] This information can help in the selection of procedures such as long saphenous stripping, interruption of communicating veins, and, possibly, the newer methods of venous valve transfer or transposition.

Preoperative Vein Mapping

With the growing use of the greater saphenous vein for in situ bypass grafts, knowledge of the patient's specific anatomy has become more important. Using contrast phlebograms, Shah and associates[66] demonstrated that only 65% of thighs and 45% of calves had a single saphenous trunk. The rest had variants of double systems and cross-connections. Because many surgeons are concerned about the contrast phlebogram inducing acute thrombosis, there has been increasing use of preoperative duplex scanning for mapping superficial veins in both the arms and the legs.[67, 68] The high resolution of the images available on contemporary machines permits satisfactory demonstration of size, course, double segments, and varicosities in most patients. These findings correlate closely with anatomy demonstrated at operation.

Screening Asymptomatic High-Risk Patients

Patients with obesity or previous venous thrombosis and those undergoing major hip, pelvic, or intracranial operations are all at high risk of developing DVT during or shortly after surgery. Some physicians use prophylaxis against thrombosis, whereas others prefer to treat only if thrombosis occurs. For many years, IPG has been used for screening; however, recent reports show that this and other physiologic methods are inadequate. In a study of screening of 537 patients undergoing total hip replacement, Paiement and coworkers[69] found that IPG had a sensitivity of only 24% in detecting thigh thrombosis documented by contrast phlebogram. In a similar study, Comerota and associates[70] found a 20% sensitivity in the detection of asymptomatic thrombi, and the authors attributed the poor accuracy to the high incidence of nonocclusive lesions. These reports show that the physiologic techniques are unsuitable for surveillance of asymptomatic patients and that the duplex scan is the primary test for screening. Studies of asymptomatic, high-risk patients have compared scanning and contrast venography. Although specificity has ranged from 94% to 100%, sensitivity has been between 63% and 79%.[71–73] The results indicate that a negative study may miss asymptomatic thrombi in a significant proportion of patients. The screening role for scanning requires further evaluation.

CONCLUSIONS

The rapid development of noninvasive vascular laboratory techniques in recent years has increased the amount of objective data that can be accumulated about a patient. As is the case with other diagnostic modalities, it is critical to remember that the different tests should always supplement, not replace, the information gained from a careful history and physical examination. It is becoming increasingly common to find medical students or young house staff presenting patients in terms of the results of the vascular laboratory tests rather than describing presenting symptoms and physical findings. Another area of concern is the increasing practice of sending patients to the noninvasive laboratory for "diagnosis of vascular condition" without their having been examined. This practice results in a growing number of inappropriate tests (with the corresponding wasteful cost to the patient).

Optimal use of noninvasive test results requires an understanding of the limitations and errors of the specific examinations. The choice of tests must be based on the questions to be answered. There are some questions that cannot be answered by any of the techniques; for example, these techniques cannot detect small ulcers in the carotid arteries. In addition, it must be remembered that errors, both false-positives and false-negatives, occur with all diagnostic methods, so it is important to be aware of the accuracy of the tests being used. Published studies often represent the best that can be expected, and newly established laboratories often do not achieve results that are as good. Therefore, to apply the noninvasive results appropriately, it is important to find out the accuracy obtained in the laboratory one is using.

References

1. Blackshear WM, Phillips DJ, Thiele BL, et al: Detection of carotid occlusive disease by ultrasonic imaging and pulsed Doppler spectrum analysis. Surgery 86:698–706, 1979.
2. Gee W, Mehigan JT, Wylie EJ: Measurement of collateral cerebral hemispheric blood pressure by ocular pneumoplethysmography. Am J Surg 130:121, 1975.
3. Bluth EI, Stavros AT, Marich KW, et al: Carotid duplex sonography: A multicenter recommendation for standardized imaging and Doppler criteria. Radiographics 8:487–506, 1988.
4. Bendick PJ, Jackson VP, Becker GJ: Comparison of ultrasound scanning/Doppler with digital subtraction angiography in evaluation of carotid arterial disease. Med Instrum 17:220–222, 1983.
5. Langlois Y, Roederer GO, Chan A, et al: Evaluating carotid artery disease—the concordance between pulsed Doppler/spectrum analysis and angiography. Ultrasound Med Biol 9:51–63, 1983.
6. Londrey GL, Spadona DP, Hodgson KJ, et al: Does color-flow imaging improve the accuracy of duplex carotid evaluation? J Vasc Surg 13:659–662, 1991.
7. Mansour MA, Mattos MA, Hood DB, et al: Detection of total occlusion, string sign and preocclusive stenosis in the internal carotid artery by color-flow duplex scanning. Am J Surg 170:154–158, 1995.
8. Ackerstaff RGA, Grosvelt WJHM, Eikelbloom BC, Ludwig JW: Ultrasonic duplex scan of the prevertebral segment of the vertebral artery in patients with cerebral atherosclerosis. Eur J Vasc Surg 2:387–393, 1988.
9. von Reutern GM, Pourcelot L: Cardiac cycle–dependent alternating flow in vertebral arteries with subclavian stenosis. Stroke 9:229–236, 1978.
10. Kinney EV, Seabrook GR, Linney LY, et al: The importance of intraoperative detection of residual flow abnormalities after carotid artery endarterectomy. J Vasc Surg 17:912–923, 1993.
11. Lipski DA, Bergamini TM, Garrison RN, Fulton RL: Intraoperative duplex scanning reduces the incidence of residual stenosis after carotid endarterectomy. J Surg Res 60:3117–3120, 1966.
12. Papanicolaou G, Toms C, Yellin AE, et al: Relationship between intraoperative color-flow duplex findings and early restenosis after carotid endarterectomy: A preliminary report. J Vasc Surg 24:588–596, 1996.
13. Bandyk DF, Mills JL, Gahtan V, Esses G: Intraoperative duplex scanning of arterial reconstructions: Fate of repaired and unrepaired defects. J Vasc Surg 20:426–433, 1994.
14. Kremen JE, Gee W, Kaupp HA, McDonald KM: Restenosis or occlusion after carotid endarterectomy. Arch Surg 114:608–610, 1979.

15. Salvian A, Baker JD, Machleder HI, et al: Etiology and noninvasive detection of restenosis following carotid endarterectomy. Am J Surg 146:29–34, 1983.

16. DeGroote RD, Lynch TG, Jamil Z, Hobson RW: Carotid restenosis: Long-term noninvasive follow-up after carotid endarterectomy. Stroke 18:1031–1036, 1987.

17. Healy DA, Zierler RE, Nichols SC, et al: Long-term follow-up and clinical outcome of carotid restenosis. J Vasc Surg 10:662–669, 1989.

18. Winsor T: Influence of arterial disease on the systolic blood pressure gradients of the extremity. Am J Med Sci 220:117–126, 1959.

19. Heintz SE, Bone GE, Slaymaker EE, et al: Value of arterial pressure measurements in the proximal and distal part of the thigh in arterial occlusive disease. Surg Gynecol Obstet 146:337–343, 1978.

20. Baker JD: Poststress Doppler ankle pressures. Arch Surg 113:1171, 1978.

21. Gosling RG, Dunbar G, King DH, et al: The quantitative analysis of occlusive peripheral arterial disease by nonobtrusive ultrasonic technique. Angiology 22:52–55, 1971.

22. Raines JK: The pulse volume recorder in peripheral arterial disease. In Bernstein EF (ed): Vascular Diagnosis, 4th ed. St Louis, Mosby–Year Book, 1993, pp 534–543.

23. Kempczinski RK: Segmental volume plethysmography in the diagnosis of lower extremity arterial occlusive disease. J Cardiovasc Surg 23:125–129, 1982.

24. Kohler TR, Nance DR, Cramer MM, et al: Duplex scanning for diagnosis of aortoiliac and femoropopliteal disease: A prospective study. Circulation 76:1074–1080, 1987.

25. Leng G, Whyman MR, Donnan PT, et al: Accuracy and reproducibility of duplex ultrasonography in grading femoropopliteal stenoses. J Vasc Surg 17:510–517, 1993.

26. Cossman DV, Ellison JE, Wagner WH, et al: Comparison of contrast angiography to arterial mapping with color-flow duplex imaging in the lower extremities. J Vasc Surg 10:522–529, 1989.

27. Gonsalves A, Bandyk DF: Duplex scanning for lower extremity arterial disease. In AbuRahma A, Bergan J (eds): Noninvasive Vascular Diagnosis. New York, Springer-Verlag, 2000, pp 241–252.

28. Hoffman U, Edwards JM, Carter S, et al: Role of duplex scanning for the detection of atherosclerotic renal artery disease. Kidney Int 39:1232–1239, 1991.

29. Hansen KJ, Tribble RW, Reavis SW, et al: Renal duplex sonography: Evaluation of clinical utilities. J Vasc Surg 12:227–236, 1990.

30. Neumyer MM: Duplex evaluation of the renal arteries. In AbuRahma A, Bergan J (eds): Noninvasive Vascular Diagnosis. New York, Springer-Verlag, 2000, pp 379–390.

31. Stavros TA, Parker SH, Yakes YF, et al: Segmental stenosis of the renal artery: Pattern recognition of the tardus and parvus abnormalities with duplex sonography. Radiology 184:487–492, 1992.

32. Flinn WR, Sandager G: Duplex ultrasonography of the mesenteric circulation. In AbuRahma A, Bergan J (eds): Noninvasive Vascular Diagnosis. New York, Springer-Verlag, 2000, pp 391–399.

33. Legemate DA, Teeuwen C, Hoeneveld H, et al: The potential of duplex scanning to replace aorto-iliac and femoro-popliteal angiography. Eur J Vasc Surg 3:49–54, 1989.

34. Lewis P, Psaila JV, Davies WT, et al: Measurement of volume flow in the human common femoral artery using a duplex ultrasound system. Ultrasound Med Biol 12:777–784, 1986.

35. Edwards JM, Coldwell DM, Goldman ML, Strandness DE: The role of duplex scanning in the selection of patients for transluminal angioplasty. J Vasc Surg 13:69–74, 1991.

36. van der Heijden FHWM, Legemate DA, Leeuwen MS, et al: Value of duplex screening in the selection of patients for percutaneous transluminal angioplasty. Eur J Vasc Surg 7:71–76, 1993.

37. Kohler TR, Andros G, Porter JM, et al: Can duplex scanning replace arteriography for lower extremity arterial disease? Ann Vasc Surg 4:280–287, 1990.

38. Bodily K, Buttorff J, Nordesgaard A, et al: Aorto-iliac reconstruction without arteriography. Am J Surg 171:505–507, 1996.

39. Pemberton M, Nydahl S, Hartshorne T, et al: Can lower extremity reconstruction be based on colour duplex imaging alone? Eur J Vasc Endovasc Surg 12:452–454, 1996.

40. Wain RA, Berdejo GL, Delvalle WN, et al: Can duplex scan arterial mapping replace contrast arteriography as the test of choice before infrainguinal revascularization? J Vasc Surg 29:100–109, 1999.

41. Bandyk DF, Johnson BL, Gupta AK, Esses GE: Nature and management of duplex abnormalities encountered during infrainguinal bypass grafting. J Vasc Surg 24:430–438, 1996.

42. Hansen KJ, O'Niel EA, Reavis SW, et al: Intraoperative duplex sonography during renal artery reconstruction. J Vasc Surg 14:364–374, 1991.

43. Dougherty MJ, Hallett JW, Naessens JM, et al: Optimizing technical success of renal revascularization: The impact of intraoperative color-flow duplex ultrasonography. J Vasc Surg 17:849–857, 1993.

44. Bandyk DF, Cato RF, Towne JB: A low flow velocity predicts failure of femoropopliteal and femorotibial bypass grafts. Surgery 98:799–809, 1985.

45. Bandyk DF, Schmitt DD, Seabrook GR, et al: Monitoring functional patency of in situ saphenous vein bypasses: The impact of a surveillance protocol and elective revision. J Vasc Surg 9:286–296, 1989.

46. Bandyk DF, Johnson BL: Duplex surveillance of infrainguinal bypass grafts. In AbuRahma A, Bergan J (eds): Noninvasive Vascular Diagnosis. New York, Springer-Verlag, 2000, pp 253–267.

47. Bandyk DF, Seabrook GR, Moldenhauer P, et al: Hemodynamics of vein graft stenosis. J Vasc Surg 8:688–695, 1988.

48. Buth J, Disselhoff B, Sommeling C, et al: Color-flow duplex criteria for grading stenoses in infrainguinal vein grafts. J Vasc Surg 14:716–728, 1991.

49. Mattos MA, van Bemmelen PS, Hodgson KJ, et al: Does correction of stenoses identified by color duplex scanning improve infrainguinal graft patency? J Vasc Surg 17:54–66, 1993.

50. Barnes RW, Shanik GD, Slaymaker EE: An index of healing in below knee amputation: Leg blood pressure by Doppler ultrasound. Surgery 79:13–20, 1976.

51. Strandness DE, Schultz RD, Summer DS, Rushmer RF: Ultrasonic flow detection—a useful technique in the evaluation of peripheral vascular disease. Am J Surg 113:311–320, 1967.

52. Sigel B, Popky GL, Wagner DK, et al: A Doppler ultrasound method for diagnosing lower extremity venous disease. Surg Gynecol Obstet 127:339–350, 1968.

53. Sumner DS, Lambeth A: Reliability of Doppler ultrasound in the diagnosis of acute venous thrombosis both above and below the knee. Am J Surg 138:205–210, 1979.

54. Hull RS, Hirsh J, Carter CJ, et al: Diagnostic efficacy of impedance plethysmography for clinically suspected deep-vein thrombosis: A randomized trial. Ann Intern Med 102:21–28, 1985.

55. Barnes RW, Russell HE, Wu KK, Hoak JC: Accuracy of Doppler ultrasound in clinically suspected venous thrombosis of the calf. Surg Gynecol Obstet 143:425–428, 1976.

56. Vogel P, Laing FC, Jeffrey RB, Wing VW: Deep venous thrombosis of the lower extremity: US evaluation. Radiology 163:747–751, 1987.

57. Cronan JJ, Dorfman GS, Scola FH, et al: Deep venous thrombosis: US assessment using venous compression. Radiology 162:191–194, 1987.

58. Rollins DL, Semrow CM, Friedell ML, et al: Progress in the diagnosis of deep venous thrombosis: The efficacy of real-time B-mode ultrasonic imaging. J Vasc Surg 7:638–641, 1988.

59. Sullivan ED, Peter DJ, Cranley JJ: Real-time B-mode venous ultrasound. J Vasc Surg 1:465–471, 1984.

60. van Bemmelen PS, Bedord G, Beach K, Strandness DE: Quantitative segmental evaluation of venous valvular reflux with duplex ultrasound scanning. J Vasc Surg 10:425–431, 1989.

61. van Bemmelen PS, Bedford G, Beach K, Strandness DE: The mechanism of venous valve closure. Arch Surg 125:617–619, 1990.

62. Abramowitz HB, Queral LA, Flinn WR, et al: The use of photoplethysmography in the assessment of venous insufficiency: A comparison to venous pressure measurements. Surgery 86:434–441, 1979.

63. Nicolaides AN, Miles C: Photoplethysmography in the assessment of venous insufficiency. J Vasc Surg 5:405–412, 1987.

64. Barnes RW, Yao JST: Photoplethysmography in chronic venous insufficiency. In Bernstein EF (ed): Noninvasive Diagnostic Techniques in Vascular Disease, 2nd ed. St Louis, Mosby–Year Book, 1982, pp 514–521.

65. Vasdekis SN, Clarke GH, Nicolaides AN: Quantification of venous reflux by means of duplex scanning. J Vasc Surg 10:670–677, 1989.

66. Shah DM, Chang BB, Leopold PW, Corson JD, Leather RP, Karmody AM: The anatomy of the greater saphenous vein system. J Vasc Surg 3:273–283, 1986.

67. Ruoff BA, Cranley JJ, Haannan LA, et al: Real-time duplex ultrasound mapping of the greater saphenous vein before in situ infrainguinal revascularization. J Vasc Surg 6:107–113, 1987.

68. Salles-Cunha SX, Andros G, Harris RW, et al: Preoperative noninvasive assessment of arm veins to be used as bypass grafts in the lower extremities. J Vasc Surg 3:813–816, 1986.

69. Paiement G, Wessinger SJ, Waltman AC, Harris WH: Surveillance of deep vein thrombosis in asymptomatic total hip replacement patients: Impedance phlebography and fibrinogen scanning versus roentgenographic phlebography. Am J Surg 155:400–404, 1988.
70. Comerota AJ, Katz ML, Grossi RJ, et al: The comparative value of noninvasive testing for diagnosis and surveillance of deep vein thrombosis. J Vasc Surg 7:40–49, 1988.
71. Borris LC, Christiansen HM, Lassen MR, et al: Real-time ultrasonography in the diagnosis of deep vein thrombosis in non-symptomatic high-risk patients. Eur J Vasc Surg 4:473–475, 1990.
72. Woolson ST, McCrory DW, Walter JF, et al: B-mode ultrasound scanning in the detection of proximal venous thrombosis after total hip replacement. J Bone Joint Surg Am 72:983–987, 1990.
73. Mattos MA, Londrey GL, Leutz DW, et al: Color-flow duplex scanning for the surveillance and diagnosis of acute deep venous thrombosis. J Vasc Surg 15:366–376, 1992.

Bibliography

AbuRhama A, Bergan J (eds): Noninvasive Vascular Diagnosis. New York, Springer-Verlag, 2000.

Auer AI, Neumyer MM (eds): The Vascular Laboratory: Current Issues and Clinical Developments. Pasadena, Calif, Davies, 2000.

Zwiebel WJ (ed): Introduction to Vascular Ultrasonography, 4th ed. Philadelphia, WB Saunders, 2000.

Questions

1. Measuring thigh pressures with a regular arm blood pressure cuff results in a determination that is
   (a) higher than the actual pressure
   (b) equal to the actual pressure
   (c) lower than the actual pressure

2. An ankle index (ankle pressure/arm pressure) of 160 indicates
   (a) normal arterial system
   (b) significant arterial insufficiency
   (c) pathologic vessel wall stiffness
   (d) arteriovenous fistula in the extremity
   (e) none of the above

3. When evaluating a patient with an exercise stress test, the severity of occlusive disease is evaluated by
   (a) walking time
   (b) magnitude of drop in ankle index
   (c) recovery time
   (d) all of the above
   (e) none of the above

4. Noninvasive cerebrovascular techniques are accurate for all except
   (a) detecting advanced stenosis of the internal carotid artery
   (b) detecting internal carotid occlusion
   (c) detecting arterial ulceration
   (d) detecting abnormal turbulence in the internal carotid artery

5. For a given arterial velocity the magnitude of the Doppler frequency shift is related to
   (a) distance from the probe
   (b) frequency of the probe
   (c) type of system (pulse or continuous wave)
   (d) all of the above
   (e) none of the above

6. Spectral broadening of a Doppler signal is
   (a) greatest proximal to a stenosis
   (b) greatest in the stenosis
   (c) greatest just beyond a stenosis
   (d) the same at all of the above sites

7. Asymptomatic deep venous thrombosis of the leg is best detected by
   (a) impedance plethysmography
   (b) duplex scan
   (c) both
   (d) neither

8. A venous reflux photoplethysmographic examination of a patient with postphlebitic syndrome will show
   (a) increased recovery time
   (b) unchanged recovery time
   (c) decreased recovery time

9. Suitability of a superficial femoral artery for treatment with balloon dilatation can be determined by
   (a) segmental pressures
   (b) volume plethysmography
   (c) duplex scan
   (d) all the above
   (e) none of the above

Answers

| 1. a | 2. c | 3. d | 4. c | 5. b | 6. c | 7. b | 8. c | 9. c |

15

Natural History and Nonoperative Treatment in Chronic Lower Extremity Ischemia

Mark R. Nehler, Lloyd M. Taylor Jr., Gregory L. Moneta, and John M. Porter

Despite the current focus on interventions in vascular surgery, a large percentage of patients who are treated in a busy vascular practice do not require interventional vascular procedures. This is particularly true of patients with chronic lower extremity occlusive disease. Nonoperative therapy, risk factor modification, and education regarding natural history of lower extremity occlusive disease are a large part of treatment at a typical busy vascular surgery clinic. Despite the emergence of vascular medicine as a specialty, there is ample evidence that peripheral vascular disease remains poorly understood among the primary care fields. In addition, with current cost constraints in healthcare resources and education, the situation is not likely to improve noticeably in the near future. Thus, it appears inevitable that the vascular surgeon will continue to play a key role in nonoperative management of multiple vascular conditions.

Owing to the well-recognized fact that the population is aging, management of atherosclerosis plays an important role in adult medical care. Although only 1% to 2% of people younger than 50 years of age suffer from symptoms of intermittent claudication, this figure rises to 5% in those aged 50 to 70 years, and to 10% in those older than age 70.[1-3] New issues in the past 5 years regarding nonoperative management of chronic lower extremity ischemia include pharmacologic data (cilostazol and vascular endothelial growth factor) and more effective smoking cessation (buproprion).

STRATIFYING CHRONIC LOWER EXTREMITY ISCHEMIA

Chronic lower extremity ischemia represents a clinical spectrum. The two important variables are clinical symptoms and measured circulatory impairment. The clinical symptoms may be simple or difficult to stratify regarding severity and natural history. Although, for example, a patient with gangrenous toes on balance represents greater ischemia and potential limb threat than a patient with isolated rest pain, claudication severity is more difficult to stratify. Claudication history has been typically reported as the number of blocks a patient can walk on level ground at a normal speed without having to stop, although clinical trials have shown, curiously, that patients are frequently poor judges of objective walking distance. Claudication pharmaceutical trials have stratified patients based on walking distances (initial or absolute claudication distances) or times during either fixed or graded load treadmill testing. More recently, tools such as the walking impairment questionnaire (WIQ)[4] have been developed to assist in stratifying the claudication history.

Combining the objective measurements of ischemia (ankle/brachial pressure indices, toe pressures, pulse volume recordings) with the clinical situation helps to define the natural history of various patient groups with chronic lower extremity ischemia. Stratifying claudication severity using ankle/brachial index correlates poorly with treadmill walking distances and symptoms.[5, 6] Despite marked improvement in defining vascular populations with chronic lower extremity occlusive disease, there are many unique clinical scenarios in this heterogeneous population that remain less well understood. For example, by no means do all patients with traditional limb-threatening conditions (rest pain, tissue necrosis) suffer near-term amputation without revascularization.

NATURAL HISTORY OF CLAUDICATION

Intermittent claudication describes lower extremity muscular pain (most often calf but may involve thighs and buttocks) induced by exercise and relieved by short periods of rest. It correlates with stage II of the Fontaine classification system. Claudication is caused by arterial obstruction proximal to affected muscle beds, which limits the normal exercise-induced increase in blood flow and produces transient muscle ischemia during exercise. Interestingly, only a fraction of patients with demonstrable peripheral arterial occlusive disease complain of symptoms of intermittent claudication. The presence of asymptomatic lower extremity occlusive disease varies, but the available data indicate that for every patient with intermittent claudication, there are probably three others with similar disease who do not complain of symptoms.[7] It appears that many elderly patients assume that leg pain while walking is a natural part of the aging process. Subjective complaints of intermittent claudication vary in degree and severity based on individual factors, including occupational and recreational habits. Therefore, the number of patients with intermittent claudication who consult their physicians varies markedly from 10% in the inner city[8] to 50% in rural communities.[9]

In addition, physicians frequently are unaware of the existence of peripheral arterial disease in their patient populations. Data from the recent Partners program[10] demonstrated that 13% of a total of 6979 patients older than 50 years of age in the more than 350 primary care practices screened were found to have abnormal ankle/brachial pressure indices, with or without symptoms of intermittent claudication. More importantly, only 24% of those patients found to have chronic lower extremity ischemia had previously been diagnosed with peripheral arterial disease by their physicians.

Once the diagnosis has been made, patients and physicians fear both disease progression and limb loss in addition to the functional limitations due to intermittent claudication. Multiple longitudinal studies of large groups of claudicants with objective criteria for enrollment provide an accurate database.[11–16] Collectively, these studies demonstrated amputation rates of only 1% to 7% at 5 to 10 years of follow-up. However, symptomatic or objective disease progression occurred in 25% of patients over this interval (7%–9% the first year, and 2%–3% annually thereafter). Nearly half of those with disease progression underwent interventions. Continued tobacco use[17] and diabetes mellitus[18] were both correlated with progressive deterioration. However, the most important consistent predictor was the severity of objectively determined arterial occlusive disease at the first patient encounter.[11, 13]

NATURAL HISTORY OF LIMB-THREATENING ISCHEMIA

Limb-threatening ischemia is defined as arterial blood flow that is inadequate to accommodate the metabolic needs of resting tissue. Clinically, limb-threatening ischemia represents either rest pain or tissue necrosis. It corresponds to stage III or IV of the Fontaine classification system. Ischemic rest pain is a burning dysesthesia in the foot, aggravated by limb elevation and improved with dependency, presumably due to the increase in arterial pressure from gravity in a limb with a nonfunctioning venoarteriolar reflex due to ischemia.[19] Necrosis includes ischemic ulcerations or gangrene after minor trauma or surgical incisions involving the foot.

The incidence of critical limb ischemia is not known with certainly. Using multiple different extrapolation methods, it is estimated that between 500,000 and 1 million new cases occur per year.[20, 21] Roughly speaking, this means that one new patient per year develops critical limb ischemia for every 100 patients with intermittent claudication in the population. Most of these patients are elderly.

Major risk factors for advanced limb ischemia include age, smoking, and diabetes. The incidence of major amputation rises markedly with age. A Danish national discharge survey reported that the incidence of major lower extremity amputations increased from 0.3 per 100,000 per year for patients younger than 40 years to 226 per 100,000 per year for those older than 80 years.[22] Smoking is an independent risk factor for the development of peripheral arterial disease, a correlation stronger than that between tobacco use and coronary artery disease. As stated before, continued smoking and heavy smoking are major risk factors for progression of symptoms in patients with intermittent claudication.[17] Diabetes is a major factor. Although diabetes affects only 2% to 5% of Western populations, 40% to 45% of all major amputees have diabetes. Major amputation is more than 10 times more frequent in diabetic patients with peripheral vascular disease than in nondiabetic patients with peripheral vascular disease.[23] The correlation is independent of age and smoking, but diabetic smokers require amputation earlier in life than nondiabetic smokers.[24]

There is a general belief that patients with chronic ischemic rest pain or tissue necrosis inevitably progress to limb loss without prompt revascularization. Clearly, patients with progressive gangrenous changes and constant ischemic pain have an unstable clinical situation requiring prompt therapy.[25] However, abundant clinical experience indicates that patients who have critical limb ischemia with intermittent rest pain may experience noticeable improvement at times when they are presumed to have improved cardiac hemodynamics. During these intervals, small ulcerations may heal with protective dressings alone. Several randomized pharmacologic trials in critical limb ischemia have documented ulcer healing in up to 40% of patients randomized to placebo,[26–28] although in most of these trials, less than half of the control patients were alive without a major amputation after 6 months.[29–31]

Objective circulatory measurement of critical limb ischemia populations provides the best stratification of prognosis. The likelihood of near-term limb loss is related to the severity of ischemia at the time of patient presentation. As a worst-case example, patients with absent ankle arterial Doppler signals have uniformly poor outcomes.[32] In addition, patients with end-stage renal disease have demonstrated poor wound healing and limb salvage despite successful revascularization.[33]

Finally, it is worthwhile to review the natural history of patients undergoing lower extremity amputation. The incidence of major lower extremity amputation appears to have either reached a plateau or decreased in the last decade, possibly owing to improved methods of revascularization and limb salvage.[34–37] It is important to understand that patients who undergo major amputation often do not experience a steady disease progression from claudication to rest pain to tissue necrosis and then to amputation, with or without revascularization attempts. In a review of 713 patients who were undergoing below-knee amputations for ischemia, more than half had experienced no ischemic symptoms as recently as 6 months before the amputation.[38]

Overall, the ratio of below-knee amputations to above-knee amputations is equal and has not significantly changed in several decades.[39–45] However, the introduction of aggressive limb salvage teams has increased the rate of below-knee amputations at single centers.[46] Primary healing of below-knee amputations ranges broadly from 30% to 90%.[38, 46–48] Reamputation to attempt below-knee salvage varies from 4% to 30%.[49–51] It is important to note that half of all below-knee amputees who fail to achieve primary healing ultimately require above-knee amputation.[52–54]

More below-knee amputees achieve ambulation than above-knee amputees,[45, 55, 56] although, overall, the number of major amputees who achieve meaningful independent ambulation is depressingly small. Initial rehabilitation can take up to 9 months or longer. After 2 years, 30% of amputees who had been walking no longer use their prostheses.[45] Advanced age and female gender bode poorly for ambulation.[57] Fifteen percent of amputees require contralateral amputation and another 20% to 30% die within 2 years.[45, 46, 58]

SURVIVAL

Objective testing of both the coronary and carotid circulations in large populations with chronic lower extremity occlusive disease has markedly refined our understanding of the systemic nature of peripheral vascular disease. Hertzer and associates[59] documented coronary anatomy with angiography in 1000 consecutive patients before elective vascular surgery. Coronary atherosclerosis was detected in 90% of all patients. However, symptomatic or electrocardiograph evidence of disease was present in only 47%. More importantly, 14% of asymptomatic patients demonstrated severe, surgically correctable coronary artery disease. Table 15–1 summarizes the data from this important study. Patients in this database were selected because they had advanced peripheral vascular disease that required intervention.

The prevalence of asymptomatic carotid artery disease in patients with chronic lower extremity disease has also been examined. These investigators, like Hertzer and coworkers, screened populations using carotid duplex scans

TABLE 15–1

Incidence of Coronary Artery Disease (CAD) in 1000 Consecutive Peripheral Vascular Disease Patients Screened by Coronary Angiography

	UNSUSPECTED		SUSPECTED	
	Patients	(%)	Patients	(%)
Normal coronary arteries	64	14	21	4
Mild/moderate CAD	218	49	99	18
Advanced compensated CAD	97	22	192	34
Severe correctable CAD	63	14	188	34
Severe incorrectable CAD	4	1	54	10

Data from Hertzer NR, Beven EG, Young JR, et al: Coronary artery disease in peripheral vascular patients: A classification of 1000 coronary angiograms and results of surgical management. Ann Surg 199;223–233, 1984. Table from Taylor LM Jr, Porter JM: Natural history and nonoperative treatment in chronic lower extremity ischemia. In Moore WS (ed): Vascular Surgery: A Comprehensive Review. Philadelphia, WB Saunders, 1993.

before infrainguinal revascularization. The preoperative screening studies showed a 30% incidence of asymptomatic internal carotid artery stenosis greater than 50%.[60–62]

Given the demonstrated prevalence of concomitant coronary and carotid vascular disease, reduced long-term survival in patients with chronic lower extremity ischemia is not surprising. The 5-, 10-, and 15-year mortality rates for patients with intermittent claudication are approximately 30%, 50%, and 70%, respectively—an outlook similar to that of patients who have undergone resection of a Duke's stage B adenocarcinoma of the colon. Multiple risk factors have been defined as important contributors to this increased long-term cardiovascular mortality. These include advanced age at presentation, continued tobacco use,[63] diabetes,[64] and dialysis dependence.[33, 65, 66] Of these, end-stage renal disease is the most pronounced, predicting 2-year survival rates of 50% to 65%, similar to those of patients with metastatic cancer. The most important clinical determinant appears to be the degree of lower extremity circulatory impairment at presentation. Accordingly, 5-year survival rates range from 80% to 90% in claudicant populations managed nonoperatively[67] to 80% in claudicant populations managed operatively[68] and to less than 50% in patients with critical limb ischemia requiring limb salvage surgery[69, 70] (which drops even lower in groups requiring multiple interventions).[71, 72]

Similarly, data exist indicating that survival is inversely related to the degree of objectively determined chronic lower extremity ischemia at presentation.[73] Small series indicate that arterial obstructions below the knee are a particularly ominous sign of abbreviated survival.[74] Therefore, the severity of systemic atherosclerosis is accurately reflected by the severity of the lower extremity disease. The objective data regarding lower extremity ischemia severity accurately predict the long-term prognosis for both life and limb. This knowledge is important in planning individual patient interventions.

More importantly, the diagnosis of chronic lower extremity occlusive disease of any severity identifies patients

TABLE 15-2

Recommendations for Risk Factor Reductions in Patients with Chronic Lower Extremity Ischemia

PARAMETER	TARGET GOAL	THERAPIES
LDL cholesterol	<100 mg/dl	Diet, statins
HDL cholesterol	♂ ≥ 35 mg/dl, ♀ ≥ 45 mg/dl	Diet, exercise, niacin, fibrates
Triglycerides	<150 mg/dl	Diet, exercise, gemfibrizol, niacin
Blood pressure	SBP <130, DBP <85	β-blockers, ACE inhibitors
Antiplatelet	All patients on some form	Aspirin, clopidogrel
Diabetes	Hb A_{1c} < 7%	Insulin, ↑ insulin sensitivity
Tobacco cessation	Complete abstinence	Nicotine replacement, antidepressant

LDL, low density lipoprotein; HDL, high density lipoprotein; SBP, systolic blood pressure; DBP, diastolic blood pressure; Hb A_{1c}, glycosolated hemoglobin.

at risk of early cardiovascular death. This information, particularly in patients with claudication, is likely to be more important than the therapy directed toward the walking disability. Multiple randomized trials in large coronary populations indicate that aggressive risk-factor modification (lipid reduction, antiplatelet therapy, aggressive diabetes management, and blood pressure control) reliably reduce near-term cardiac mortality.[75-84] Table 15-2 describes basic guidelines for risk factor modification based on these trials. Evidence is accumulating that multiple different pharmacologic interventions in these high-risk patients can improve their long-term survival.

CHRONIC LOWER EXTREMITY ISCHEMIA IN YOUNG PATIENTS

Chronic lower extremity ischemia in young patients (<40 years of age) is infrequent. Peripheral vascular disease in young patients has several unique features that the vascular surgeon needs to consider (Table 15-3).[85-91] These patients are almost universally heavy smokers. A prospective study performed detailed evaluation for hypercoagulable states in young patients with chronic lower extremity ischemia and demonstrated that 90% had laboratory abnormalities (deficiencies in natural anticoagulants, defective fibrinolytic

activity, or antiphospholipid antibodies).[89] Another study demonstrated significant abnormalities in low-density lipoprotein (LDL) cholesterol oxidation in young patients with peripheral arterial disease compared with older patients with peripheral arterial disease.[92] Young patients who manifest limb-threatening symptoms frequently progress rapidly to limb loss, despite attempts at revascularization, because of the limited survival of reconstructions and the need for more frequent operative revisions required in these patients.[93, 94] Although survival is reduced in young patients with peripheral vascular disease compared with age-matched controls, on balance, their coronary atherosclerosis does not appear to be as aggressive as that affecting their lower extremities.[95, 96] Initial nonoperative management with aggressive risk factor modification (cessation of tobacco, lipid control) is the therapy of choice in young patients with claudication. This frequently includes a hypercoagulable workup. However, the greater functional expectations and frequent limitations on gainful employment experienced by young patients with claudication complicate their ability to tolerate a prolonged course of nonoperative therapy. Despite this, revascularization attempts should be made very judiciously, with an understanding of the diminished longevity of these procedures in this age group and the higher amputation rates after failures.

NONOPERATIVE TREATMENT OF CHRONIC LOWER EXTREMITY ISCHEMIA

The nonoperative treatment of chronic lower extremity ischemia includes risk factor modification, exercise, and pharmacologic therapy. For the purpose of this discussion, our focus is on smoking cessation, exercise programs, and drug therapy.

Smoking

The paradox of tobacco in Western society is readily evident. Data from several studies[97-99] from the early 1980s regarding the dangers of second-hand smoke has led to legislation restricting tobacco use in public and private facilities. During the past few years, groundbreaking trials have taken place, and tobacco companies have lost several high-profile legal battles. However, despite a very negative public image, the tobacco industry is thriving. The cost of legal expenses has been transferred to the consumer. Young

TABLE 15-3

Chronic Lower Extremity Ischemia Reported in Younger Patients

SOURCE (yr)	PATIENTS	FOLLOW-UP (yr)	STABLE/IMPROVED (%)	WORSE (%)	DEAD (%)	AMPUTATED (%)
McCready et al. (1984)[193]	21	4-6	38	52	10	—
Pairolero et al. (1984)[194]	50	13.5	64	36	10	30
Evans et al. (1987)[195]	153	5.5	—	—	17	16
Valentine et al. (1990)[86]	22	2.2	76	24	4.5	0
Levy et al. (1994)[196]	109	2.3	—	—	—	27

American smokers, particularly women, are actually increasing in number.[100] This continues despite overwhelming evidence regarding the lethal nature of tobacco. The estimated annual excess mortality due to cigarette smoking in the United States exceeds 350,000 deaths, almost as many American lives as were lost in World War II.[101] It is estimated that the annual total direct health care costs from tobacco exceed $16 billion, with indirect costs greater than $37 billion.[102]

Tobacco companies are under fire by state- and individual-sponsored class action lawsuits. The tobacco industry is well defended, however. Their annual legal defense budget is estimated at 900 million dollars. In addition, owing to projected annual payments to be made to individual states from recent settlements, maintaining the tobacco industry will be in the companies' financial interest. The tobacco industry has been able to raise the funds necessary to offset current losses by increasing the price of product. It is projected that a package of cigarettes may cost between $5 and $7 in the near future.[103]

The specific mechanisms through which tobacco exerts adverse effects on arteries remains poorly understood. Multiple toxicities of the innumerable components of tobacco smoke are recognized, including alterations in vascular endothelium, prostaglandin metabolism, platelet function, lipid metabolism, blood viscosity, and coagulation. Several excellent reviews on this subject are available.[104–107] Smoking is associated with acute drops in treadmill walking distances, presumably owing to carbon monoxide.[108] Smokers have an increased risk of peripheral vascular disease progression,[109] myocardial infarction, stroke, and death.[110] Smokers also have an increased risk of major amputation.[111, 112]

Abundant evidence exists regarding the benefit of smoking cessation in the treatment of chronic lower extremity ischemia. Treadmill walking improves after smoking cessa-

tion.[113] In our experience, patients who stop smoking usually experience at least a doubling of previously recorded walking distance. Improved patency of arterial repairs in nonsmokers has been demonstrated for both aortofemoral and femoropopliteal reconstructions[114–117]; degree of tobacco use (measured by carboxyhemoglobin levels) bears directly on the incidence of graft occlusion.[118]

Interestingly, less than half of all persons who experiment with tobacco go on to smoke regularly.[119] Although social environment is a primary determinant of smoking behavior, genetics also plays a role.[120] Nicotine is the active component of tobacco smoke responsible for the positive symptoms of arousal, relaxation, relief of hunger, and enhanced vigilance and task performance that a smoker experiences. Nicotine is also primarily responsible for the tolerance observed in habitual users. Withdrawal symptoms include restlessness, irritability, anxiety, sleep disturbance, delayed reaction times, impaired concentration, and weight gain. The daily smoking cycle (Fig. 15–1) demonstrates that the first few cigarettes of the day produce the greatest positive effect (arousal); by the end of the day, smokers use tobacco to avoid withdrawal symptoms. Overnight abstinence allows considerable resensitization to occur.[121]

Complete cessation of tobacco use is the foundation and the most important part of nonoperative therapy for chronic lower extremity ischemia. Unfortunately, it is also the component of therapy with the poorest rate of success. Each year, approximately 20 to 50 million smokers in the United States try to quit, but only 6% are able to quit long term.[122] The first step is to clearly inform the vascular patient of the harmful effects of tobacco on the vascular system. Although most patients understand the relationship of smoking and lung cancer, less than half understand the relationship between peripheral vascular disease and tobacco.[123] The advice to stop smoking should be repeated at every patient encounter. We prefer stressing the positive

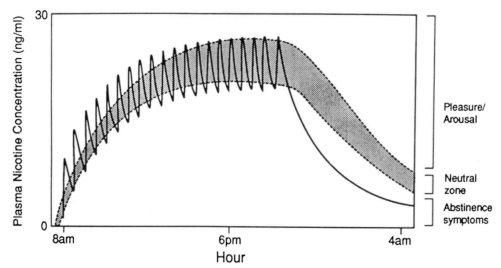

Figure 15–1. Model for the nicotine addiction cycle during daily cigarette smoking. Solid line represents venous plasma nicotine concentrations as individual cigarettes are smoked. The upper dashed line represents the threshold nicotine concentration for producing arousal, and the lower dashed line represents nicotine concentration below which symptoms of withdrawal occur. The shaded area represents nicotine concentrations in which the smoker is comfortable without either arousal or withdrawal stimuli. Note that the threshold levels for both rise progressively during the day because of neuroadaptation, with overnight cessation allowing for drug resensitization. (From Benowitz NL: Cigarette smoking and nicotine addiction. Med Clin North Am 76:415–437, 1992.)

health benefits of cessation, as well as the social and financial freedoms. The latter two issues are becoming more and more pronounced with legislation prohibiting smoking in public places and increasing legal judgments against the tobacco industry, respectively.

Historically, the majority of smokers who quit were able to do so without the help of any formal intervention.[124] However, the development of nicotine replacement therapies has been the cornerstone of smoking cessation for the last decade. Most nicotine replacement agents provide up to 30% of a smoker's regular daily nicotine intake and thus reduce or prevent withdrawal symptoms. Nicotine gum is the oldest form of nicotine replacement, currently available without prescription. The primary drawbacks include the requirement of specific chewing techniques to maximize nicotine release and drug inactivation if beverages are consumed during use due to oral pH changes. Nicotine transdermal patches are easier to use (dose ranging from 7 mg/24 hours to 21 mg/24 hours), the only requirement being skin site rotation. Reported success with this technique has been modest. Reviews of randomized, double-blinded nicotine replacement trials for smoking cessation therapy in young patients (30–40 years old) document biochemically confirmed 6-month abstinence rates varying from 20% to 45% in the treatment groups compared with 5% to 25% in the control groups, depending on the setting (treatment initiation in a smoking cessation clinic being superior to the primary care office).[125–127] No benefit was derived from treatment longer than 8 weeks or from tapering nicotine. Intermediate-dose (14 mg/24 hour) nicotine patches have been used cautiously in patients with symptomatic coronary artery disease.[128] These patients must be warned about the danger of continued smoking while wearing the patch, as myocardial infarction has been reported.[129] In addition, it appears that older patients with cardiovascular disease have only half the abstinence rates compared with controlled trials in a younger population.[130] Finally, nicotine and citrate inhalers have been used in several small, randomized trials with or without nicotine patches.[131, 132] These devices maintain reinforcement of the ritual/sensory phenomena of smoking. Although short-term abstinence with these devices has been effective 20% to 30% of cases, long-term success has been disappointing.

Some therapies for smoking cessation have focused on depression as both an important component of the smoker profile and as a major factor in withdrawal symptoms.[133] The antidepressant agents buproprion and fluoxetine have been used in randomized trials with 12-week biochemically confirmed cessation rates of 30% to 40%.[134, 135] In addition to diminishing withdrawal symptoms (which share many characteristics with chronic depression), these agents appear to attenuate some of the weight gain observed with smoking cessation. These agents have also been used in combination with nicotine replacement (patch or inhaler) with improved results compared with either agent alone.[136]

Finally, research on smoking cessation has centered on the effects of nicotine and neurotransmitters in the brain. Smoking one to two cigarettes increases plasma endorphin levels up to 200% and correlates with nicotine levels.[137] Therefore, trials using opioid antagonists have started. However, a recent 12-week randomized trial of naltrexone in 100 smokers did not demonstrate efficacy.[138]

Exercise

Patients with intermittent claudication typically reduce their walking in response to the discomfort. Severely affected individuals may become nearly housebound. Most patients believe that the pain from claudication indicates injury and avoid further walking to prevent any adverse consequences. Exercise therapy in the management of claudication has been studied for more than 30 years. It is the best documented therapy for claudication, with demonstrated efficacy in exercise performance, quality of life, and functional capacity. Numerous types of exercise programs have been used, with supervised exercise programs clearly superior to those that were not supervised. Initial evaluation includes both functional assessment (we use the walking impairment questionnaire) followed by exercise testing to maximal claudication pain (with either fixed or graded load treadmill testing). Success in the program is defined as improvement in initial and maximal claudication distances on the treadmill, improvement in scores on the questionnaire, or improvement in both.

The typical duration of a supervised exercise program monitored by a skilled nurse or technician is 60 minutes. Patients are encouraged to walk on the treadmill because this activity reproduces walking in the community. The initial workload of the treadmill is set to a speed and grade that produce claudication pain within 3 to 5 minutes. Patients walk at this workload until they experience moderately severe claudication. They rest until the symptoms abate and then resume exercise. This cycle is repeated throughout the supervised exercise session. Patients are reassessed weekly to determine their walking limits and adjust the treadmill settings (increase in speed and/or grade) accordingly as they improve. This scenario induces a training benefit. A typical exercise program lasts from 3 to 6 months. The typical benefits include a 100% to 200% increase in peak exercise performance on the treadmill.[139–146]

The mechanism for this training benefit does not appear to be associated with changes in limb blood flow.[140, 147, 148] Improved extraction of oxygen in substrate has been documented with exercise training.[149, 150] Some studies have demonstrated increases in muscle enzyme activities, but there appears to be poor correspondence with exercise performance.[148, 151] Exercise has been demonstrated to clear intermediates of oxidative metabolism (acylcarnitines) from skeletal muscle, and this has been linked with performance.[140, 152] Therefore, some evidence exists for metabolic improvement after training. In addition, alterations in gait and walking efficiency may contribute to the training response.[153]

Finally, weight reduction may deserve greater emphasis in the management of some patients with chronic lower extremity ischemia. Wyatt and associates measured treadmill walking distances in 20 patients with stable claudication who were carrying progressively greater loads of weight. A linear relationship between excess weight and reduction in treadmill walking distances was observed.[154]

Pharmacologic Therapies

The greater part of drug therapy for patients with chronic lower extremity occlusive disease should focus on therapy for coexisting disease: diabetes or hypertension, risk factor modification (lipid therapy, smoking cessation), and thrombosis prophylaxis (antiplatelet agents). Currently, no pharmacologic therapy has provided significant enough symptomatic relief to gain widespread usage in the therapy of intermittent claudication/critical limb ischemia. To put the data presented in proper perspective, it should be remembered that a supervised exercise program has been reliably shown to increase absolute claudication distance by 100% to 200%.

Pentoxifylline

Hemorrheology is the study of the characteristics of blood flow. Blood viscosity is an important factor affecting flow and is related to hematocrit, plasma protein concentration, platelet aggregation, and erythrocyte deformability. Cellular deformation is important in the microcirculation. Erythrocytes are 8 to 9 μm in diameter, whereas typical capillaries are only 4 to 5 μm in diameter. Therefore, erythrocytes must deform to traverse the capillary bed.

Patients with chronic lower extremity ischemia have abnormal hemorrheology. Blood from patients with claudication demonstrates reduced flow rates through filters with uniform pore size.[155, 156] Multiple studies have demonstrated decreased erythrocyte and leukocyte deformability, increased platelet aggregation, increased leukocyte and platelet adhesion, and increased blood viscosity in patients with chronic lower extremity ischemia.[157–159]

Pentoxifylline improves red cell deformability, lowers fibrinogen levels, decreases platelet aggregation, and increases walking distances in patients with intermittent claudication. Although the improvements have been statistically significant, they have been modest, with less than 10% of patients demonstrating greater than 100% improved walking distances. Subgroups of patients (ankle/brachial index < 0.80 and symptoms lasting >1 year) appear to experience the most benefit. The absolute claudication distance improvement in the larger randomized trials was around 20%. Side effects include gastrointestinal distress. Pentoxifylline has been used in the United States for more than a decade to treat patients with claudication.

Naftidrofuryl

Naftidrofuryl is a serotonin antagonist that has demonstrated improved aerobic metabolism in oxygen-depleted tissues (via stimulation of carbohydrate and fat entry into the tricarboxylic acid cycle); the drug may also reduce both erythrocyte and platelet aggregation.[160] It has been studied exclusively in Europe. Four of five placebo-controlled trials demonstrated efficacy, with a 15% to 40% improvement in absolute claudication distances in patients who used this agent compared with controls.[161–163] This drug is widely used outside of the United States.

Blufomedil

Blufomedil[164, 165] reduces vasoconstriction through both α_1 and α_2 adrenolysis. It has been available in some countries for the treatment of intermittent claudication for more than a decade. Two dated studies with small numbers (total < 150 patients) demonstrated a greater than 40% improvement in absolute claudication distances compared with controls.[166]

Cilostazol

Cilostazol is a phosphodiesterase III inhibitor with vasodilator and antiplatelet actions.[167] Several randomized trials have demonstrated 40% to 50% increase in absolute claudication distance in patients taking cilostazol compared with those taking placebo.[168–170] Effects seem to disappear after discontinuation of the drug.[171] Quality of life assessments using Medical Outcome Study SF-36 questionnaires have also demonstrated efficacy. Side effects include headache, diarrhea, and dizziness. Cilostazol was granted approval for claudication therapy by the United States Food and Drug Agency in 1999.[172]

Antiplatelet Drugs

The use of antiplatelet agents is considered a universal recommendation in patients with chronic lower extremity ischemia. The primary efficacy for these agents in the vascular population is to prevent cardiovascular events. In the Antiplatelet Trialists' Collaboration review of 189 controlled studies in more than 100,000 patients, there was a 25% reduction in myocardial infarction, stroke, and vascular death.[173] There are no compelling data to indicate efficacy in improving walking distances in patients with claudication using antiplatelet therapy.[174, 175]

Clopidogrel blocks the activation of platelets by ADP.[176] The current landmark study randomized clopidogrel or aspirin in the treatment of nearly 20,000 patients with cardiovascular disease (6452 patients had peripheral vascular disease).[177] At 1 to 3 years of follow-up, clopidogrel performed best in the subset of patients with peripheral arterial disease, with an almost 24% relative risk reduction in cardiovascular events. This agent is more expensive than aspirin, and more data are needed to define its clinical role.[178]

Carnitine

Patients with intermittent claudication have metabolic abnormalities in their skeletal muscle. One example is changes observed in carnitine metabolism. Patients with intermittent claudication have an accumulation of acylcarnitines (intermediates of oxidative metabolism) in skeletal muscle, inhibiting transport of free fatty acids into the mitochondria.[179, 180] The amount of acylcarnitine in muscle corresponds to the degree of walking impairment. It has been suggested that supplementation of oral carnitine or propionyl-L-carnitine (acylcarnitine) in patients with intermittent claudication would improve walking distance. The mechanism of action includes promoting pyruvate entry into the citric acid cycle and facilitating transport of free fatty acids into the mitochondria. These actions have been demonstrated in several small phase II trials.[181, 182] Multicenter phase III trials with this agent are in progress.[183] A large phase II–III trial in Europe has confirmed the claudication benefits of propionyl-L-carnitine.[184]

Prostaglandins

Prostaglandin analogs (synthetic prostaglandin E_1 [PGE_1], or prostaglandin E_1 and PGI_2 or prostacyclin) are potent vasodilators that inhibit platelet aggregation.[185] Several randomized trials of prostaglandin infusion therapy for ischemic ulceration have been published.[186–188] No treatment benefits were found, perhaps because of the nearly 40% incidence of improvement in the placebo groups. A single, small intravenous trial in intermittent claudication demonstrated remarkable efficacy (371% increase in absolute claudication distance).[142] The need for intravenous access and frequent vasoactive side effects of flushing and headache make these therapies relatively impractical.

An oral preparation of prostacyclin (Beraprost) has been studied in intermittent claudication. A single phase II study of variable dosages in 164 patients did not demonstrate efficacy over placebo.[183] Again, side effects were reported in more than 50% of patients at the highest dose. Phase III trials of this agent are ongoing.

Vascular Endothelial Growth Factor

Vascular endothelial growth factor is a mitogenic agent designed to develop collateral channels in arterial occlusive disease. Increased collateral vessel development and capillary density have been documented in rabbit skeletal muscle.[189] An anecdotal report described treatment of 10 patients who had critical limb ischemia with two intramuscular injection sessions at 4-week intervals.[190] At 3.7 months, 8 of 10 had clinically improved, with some demonstration of increased flow based on angiography, ankle/brachial index measurement, or both. These data have not been duplicated. Early phase I and phase II trials are ongoing to evaluate this agent in patients with intermittent claudication.

L-Arginine

L-Arginine is an amino acid demonstrated to enhance nitric oxide formation and endothelial-dependent vasodilation in patients with atherosclerosis. Two small trials demonstrated improvements in initial and absolute claudication distances, but larger trials are needed to define L-arginine's role in claudication therapy.[191, 192]

CONCLUSION

Currently, the appropriate management of patients with chronic lower extremity ischemia is a complex clinical issue. Despite the advances in technical issues of revascularization, there remains much that can be done regarding education, risk factor modification, and nonoperative therapy for these patients. These issues make appropriate care of patients with chronic lower extremity ischemia much more than the management of atherosclerotic lesions.

References

1. Criqui MH, Fronek A, Barrett-Connor E, et al: The prevalence of peripheral arterial disease in a defined population. Circulation 71:510–515, 1985.
2. Fowkes FG, Housley E, Cawood EH, et al: Edinburgh Artery Study: Prevalence of asymptomatic and symptomatic peripheral arterial disease in the general population. Int J Epidemiol 20:384–392, 1991.
3. Novo S, Avellone G, Di G, et al: Prevalence of risk factors in patients with peripheral arterial disease. A clinical and epidemiological evaluation. Int Angiol 11:218–229, 1992.
4. Regensteiner JG, Steiner JF, Panzer RJ, Hiatt WR: Evaluation of walking impairment by questionnaire in patients with peripheral arterial disease. J Vasc Med Biol 2:142–152, 1990.
5. Carter SA, Hamel ER, Paterson JM, et al: Walking ability and ankle systolic pressures: Observations in patients with intermittent claudication in a short-term walking exercise program. J Vasc Surg 10:642–649, 1989.
6. Hiatt WR, Regensteiner JG, Hargarten ME, et al: Benefit of exercise conditioning for patients with peripheral arterial disease. Circulation 81:602–609, 1990.
7. Hiatt WR, Hoag S, Hamman RF. Effect of diagnostic criteria on the prevalence of peripheral arterial disease. The San Luis Valley diabetes study. Circulation 91:1472–1479, 1995.
8. Reid DD, Brett GZ, Hamilton PJ, et al: Cardiorespiratory disease and diabetes among middle-aged male civil servants. A study of screening and intervention. Lancet 1:469–473, 1974.
9. Hughson WG, Mann JI, Garrod A: Intermittent claudication: Prevalence and risk factors. Br Med J 1:1379–1381, 1978.
10. Hirsch AT, Criqui MH, Treat-Jacobson D, et al: The Partners Program: A National Survey of Peripheral Arterial Disease Prevalence, Awareness, and Ischemic Risk. Circulation (in press).
11. Dormandy JA, Murray GD: The fate of the claudicant—a prospective study of 1969 claudicants. Eur J Vasc Surg 5:131–133, 1991.
12. Bloor K: Natural history of arteriosclerosis of the lower extremities. Ann R Coll Surg Engl 28:36–51, 1961.
13. Jelnes R, Gaardsting O, Hougaard Jensen K, et al: Fate in intermittent claudication: Outcome and risk factors. Br Med J 293:1137–1140, 1986.
14. O'Riordain DS, O'Donnell JA: Realistic expectations for the patient with intermittent claudication. Br J Surg 78:861–863, 1991.
15. Fowl RJ, Gewirtz RJ, Love MC: Natural history of claudicants with critical hemodynamic indices. Ann Vasc Surg 6:31–33, 1992.
16. Cox GS, Hertzer NR, Young JR, et al: Nonoperative treatment of superficial femoral artery disease: Long-term follow-up. J Vasc Surg 17:172–182, 1993.
17. Cronenwett JL, Warner KG, Zelenock GB, et al: Intermittent claudication: Current results of nonoperative management. Arch Surg 119:430–436, 1984.
18. McDaniel MD, Cronenwett JL: Basic data related to the natural history of intermittent claudication. Ann Vasc Surg 3:273–277, 1989.
19. Anvar MD, Khiabani HZ, Kroese AJ, Stranden E: Alterations in capillary permeability in the lower limb of patients with chronic critical limb ischaemia and oedema Vasa 29:106–111, 2000.
20. Catalano M: Epidemiology of critical limb ischaemia: North Italian data. Eur J Med 2:11–14, 1993.
21. Critical limb ischaemia: Management and outcome. Report of a national survey. The Vascular Surgical Society of Great Britain and Ireland. Eur J Vasc Endovasc Surg 10:108–113, 1995.
22. Eickhoff JH, Hansen HJ, Lorentzen JE: The effect of arterial reconstruction on lower limb amputation rate. An epidemiological survey based on reports from Danish hospitals. Acta Chir Scand (Suppl)502:181–187, 1980.

23. Da Silva A, Widmer LK, Ziegler HW, et al: The Basel longitudinal study: Report on the relation of initial glucose level to baseline ECG abnormalities, peripheral artery disease, and subsequent mortality. J Chronic Dis 32:797–803, 1979.

24. Critical limb ischaemia: management and outcome. Report of a national survey. The Vascular Surgical Society of Great Britain and Ireland. Eur J Vasc Endovasc Surg 10:108–113, 1995.

25. Mahler F: [European consensus concerning chronic critical ischemia of the lower extremities (editorial)]. VASA 19:97–99, 1990.

26. Cronenwett JL, Zelenock GB, Whitehouse Jr WM, et al: Prostacyclin treatment of ischemic ulcers and rest pain in unreconstructible peripheral arterial occlusive disease. Surgery 100:369–375, 1986.

27. Schuler JJ, Flanigan DP, Holcroft JW, et al: Efficacy of prostaglandin E_1 in the treatment of lower extremity ischemic ulcers secondary to peripheral vascular occlusive disease. Results of a prospective randomized, double-blind, multicenter clinical trial. J Vasc Surg 1:160–170, 1984.

28. Eklund AE, Eriksson G, Olsson AG: A controlled study showing significant short term effect of prostaglandin E_1 in healing of ischaemic ulcers of the lower limb in man. Prostaglandins Leukot Med 8:265–271, 1982.

29. Belch JJ, McKay A, McArdle B, et al: Epoprostenol (prostacyclin) and severe arterial disease. A double-blind trial. Lancet 1:315–317, 1983.

30. Norgren L, Alwmark A, Angqvist KA, et al: A stable prostacyclin analogue (iloprost) in the treatment of ischaemic ulcers of the lower limb. A Scandinavian-Polish placebo controlled, randomised multicenter study. Eur J Vasc Surg 4:463–467, 1990.

31. Bliss B, Wilkins D, Campbell WB, et al: Treatment of limb-threatening ischaemia with intravenous Iloprost: A randomised double-blind placebo controlled study. Eur J Vasc Endovasc Surg 5:511–516, 1991.

32. Felix WR, Sigel B, Gunther L: The significance for morbidity and mortality of doppler-absent pedal pulses. J Vasc Surg 5:849–855, 1987.

33. Johnson BL, Glickman MH, Bandyk DF, Esses GE: Failure of foot salvage in patients with end-stage renal disease after surgical revascularization. J Vasc Surg 22:280–285, 1995.

34. Karlstrom L, Bergqvist D: Effects of vascular surgery on amputation rates and mortality. Eur J Vasc Endovasc Surg 14:273–283, 1997.

35. Department of Health and Social Security: Amputation Statistics for England, Wales, and Northern Ireland. (Report). London, 1986.

36. Mattes E, Norman PE, Jamrozik K: Falling incidence of amputations for peripheral occlusive arterial disease in Western Australia between 1980 and 1992. Eur J Vasc Endovasc Surg 13:14–22, 1997.

37. Tunis SR, Bass EB, Steinberg EP: The use of angioplasty, bypass surgery, and amputation in the management of peripheral vascular disease. N Engl J Med 325:556–562, 1991.

38. Dormandy J, Belcher G, Broos P, et al: Prospective study of 713 below-knee amputations for ischaemia and the effect of a prostacyclin analogue on healing. Hawaii Study Group. Br J Surg 81:33–37, 1994.

39. Dowd GS: Predicting stump healing following amputation for peripheral vascular disease using the transcutaneous oxygen monitor. Ann R Coll Surg Engl 69:31–35, 1987.

40. Harrison JD, Southworth S, Callum KG: Experience with the "skew flap" below-knee amputation. Br J Surg 74:930–931, 1987.

41. Valentine RJ, Myers SI, Inman MH, et al: Late outcome of amputees with premature atherosclerosis. Surgery 119:487–493, 1996.

42. Houghton AD, Taylor PR, Thurlow S, et al: Success rates for rehabilitation of vascular amputees: Implications for preoperative assessment and amputation level [see comments]. Br J Surg 79:753–755, 1992.

43. Ratliff DA, Clyne CA, Chant AD, Webster JH: Prediction of amputation wound healing: The role of transcutaneous pO_2 assessment. Br J Surg 71:219–222, 1984.

44. Bunt TJ, Manship LL, Bynoe RP, Haynes JL: Lower extremity amputation for peripheral vascular disease. A low-risk operation. Am Surg 50:581–584, 1984.

45. Kihn RB, Warren R, Beebe GW: The "geriatric" amputee. Ann Surg 176:305–314, 1972.

46. Rush DS, Huston CC, Bivins BA, Hyde GL: Operative and late mortality rates of above-knee and below-knee amputations. Am Surg 47:36–39, 1981.

47. Mooney V, Wagner W Jr, Waddell J, Ackerson T: The below-the-knee amputation for vascular disease. J Bone Joint Surg [Am] 58:365–368, 1976.

48. Jamieson MG, Ruckley CV: Amputation for peripheral vascular disease in a general surgical unit. J R Coll Surg Edinb 28:46–50, 1983.

49. Yamanaka M, Kwong PK: The side-to-side flap technique in below-the-knee amputation with long stump. Clin Orthop 75–79, 1985.

50. Robinson KP: Long posterior flap amputation in geriatric patients with ischaemic disease. Ann R Coll Surg Engl 58:440–451, 1976.

51. Silverman DG, Roberts A, Reilly CA, et al: Fluorometric quantification of low-dose fluorescein delivery to predict amputation site healing. Surgery 101:335–341, 1987.

52. Tripses D, Pollak EW: Risk factors in healing of below-knee amputation. Appraisal of 64 amputations in patients with vascular disease. Am J Surg 141:718–720, 1981.

53. Burgess EM, Matsen FA, III, Wyss CR, Simmons CW: Segmental transcutaneous measurements of PO_2 in patients requiring below-the-knee amputation for peripheral vascular insufficiency. J Bone Joint Surg [Am] 64:378–382, 1982.

54. Finch DR, Macdougal M, Tibbs DJ, Morris PJ: Amputation for vascular disease: The experience of a peripheral vascular unit. Br J Surg 67:233–237, 1980.

55. Pollock SB Jr, Ernst CB: Use of Doppler pressure measurements in predicting success in amputation of the leg. Am J Surg 139:303–306, 1980.

56. Gregg RO: Bypass or amputation? Concomitant review of bypass arterial grafting and major amputations. Am J Surg 149:397–402, 1985.

57. Cameron HC: Amputations in the diabetic: Outcome and survival. Lancet 1964; ii:605–607.

58. Whitehouse FW, Jurgensen C, Block MA: The later life of the diabetic amputee: Another look at the fate of the second leg. Diabetes 17:520–521, 1968.

59. Hertzer NR, Beven EG, Young JR, et al: Coronary artery disease in peripheral vascular patients. A classification of 1000 coronary angiograms and results of surgical management. Ann Surg 199:223–233, 1984.

60. Gentile AT, Taylor LM Jr, Moneta GL, Porter JM: Prevalence of asymptomatic carotid stenosis in patients undergoing infrainguinal bypass Surgery. Arch Surg 130:900–904, 1995.

61. Turnipseed WD, Berkoff HA, Belzer FO: Postoperative stroke in cardiac and peripheral vascular disease. Ann Surg 192:365–368, 1980.

62. Marek J, Mills JL, Harvich J, et al: Utility of routine carotid duplex screening in patients who have claudication. J Vasc Surg 24:572–579, 1996.

63. Violi F, Criqui M, Longoni A, Castiglioni C: Relation between risk factors and cardiovascular complications in patients with peripheral vascular disease. Results from the A.D.E.P. study. Atherosclerosis 120:25–35, 1996.

64. Hertzer NR: Fatal myocardial infarction following lower extremity revascularization. Two hundred seventy-three patients followed six to eleven postoperative years. Ann Surg 193:492–498, 1981.

65. Sanchez LA, Goldsmith J, Rivers SP, et al: Limb salvage surgery in end stage renal disease: Is it worthwhile? J Cardiovasc Surg (Torino) 33:344–348, 1992.

66. Edwards JM, Taylor LM Jr, Porter JM: Limb salvage in end-stage renal disease (ESRD). Comparison of modern results in patients with and without ESRD. Arch Surg 123:1164–1168, 1988.

67. Reunanen A, Takkunen H, Aromaa A: Prevalence of intermittent claudication and its effect on mortality. Acta Med Scand 211:249–256, 1991.

68. Malone JM, Moore WS, Goldstone J: Life expectancy following aortofemoral arterial grafting. Surgery 81:551–555, 1977.

69. Veith FJ, Gupta SK, Samson RH, et al: Progress in limb salvage by reconstructive arterial surgery combined with new or improved adjunctive procedures. Ann Surg 194:386–401, 1981.

70. Taylor LM Jr, Hamre D, Dalman RL, Porter JM: Limb salvage vs. amputation for critical ischemia. The role of vascular surgery. Arch Surg 126:1251–1257, 1991.

71. DeFrang RD, Edwards JM, Moneta GL, et al: Repeat leg bypass after multiple prior bypass failures. J Vasc Surg 19:268–277, 1994.

72. Edwards JM, Taylor LM, Porter JM: Treatment of failed lower extremity bypass grafts with new autogenous vein bypass grafting. J Vasc Surg 11:136–145, 1990.

73. McDermott MM, Feinglass J, Slavensky R, Pearce WH: The ankle-brachial index as a predictor of survival in patients with peripheral vascular disease. J Gen Intern Med 9:445–449, 1994.

74. Kallero KS, Bergqvist D, Cederholm C, et al: Late mortality and morbidity after arterial reconstruction: The influence of arteriosclerosis in popliteal artery. J Vasc Surg 2:541–546, 1985.
75. CAPRIE Steering Committee: A randomised, blinded, trial of clopidogrel versus aspirin in patients at risk of ischaemic events (CAPRIE). Lancet 348:1329–1339, 1996.
76. The Heart Outcomes Prevention Evaluation Study Investigators: Effects of an angiotensin-converting-enzyme inhibitor, ramipril, on cardiovascular events in high-risk patients. N Engl J Med 342:145–153, 2000.
77. Summary of the second report of the National Cholesterol Education Program (NCEP) expert panel on detection, evaluation, and treatment of high blood cholesterol in adults (Adult Treatment Panel II). JAMA 329:3015–3023, 1993.
78. Waters D, Higginson L, Gladstone P, et al: Design features of a controlled clinical trial to assess the effect of an HMG CoA reductase inhibitor on the progression of coronary artery disease. Canadian Coronary Atherosclerosis Intervention Trial Investigators, Montreal, Ottawa, and Toronto, Canada. Control Clin Trials 14:45–74, 1993.
79. Gould AL, Rossouw JE, Santanello NC, et al: Cholesterol reduction yields clinical benefit: Impact of statin trials. Circulation 97:946–952, 1998.
80. Grundy SM: Statin trials and goals of cholesterol-lowering therapy. Circulation 97:1436–1439, 1998.
81. Scandinavian Simvastatin Survival Study Group: Randomised trial of cholesterol lowering in 4444 patients with coronary heart disease: The Scandinavian Simvastatin Survival Study (4S). Lancet 344:1383–1389, 1994.
82. MacGregor AS, Price JF, Hau CM, et al: Role of systolic blood pressure and plasma triglycerides in diabetic peripheral arterial disease. The Edinburgh Artery Study. Diabetes Care 22:453–458, 1999.
83. The HOPE Study Investigators: The HOPE (Heart Outcomes Prevention Evaluation) Study: The design of a large, simple randomized trial of an angiotensin-converting enzyme inhibitor (ramipril) and vitamin E in patients at high risk of cardiovascular events. Can J Cardiol 12:127–137, 1996.
84. Miettinen TA, Pyorala K, Olsson AG, et al: Cholesterol-lowering therapy in women and elderly patients with myocardial infarction or angina pectoris: Findings from the Scandinavian Simvastatin Survival Study (4S) [see comments]. Circulation 96:4211–4218, 1997.
85. Levy PJ, Gonzalez MF, Hornung CA, et al: A prospective evaluation of atherosclerotic risk factors and hypercoagulability in young adults with premature lower extremity. J Vasc Surg 23:36–45, 1996.
86. Valentine RJ, MacGillivray DC, DeNobile JW, et al: Intermittent claudication caused by atherosclerosis in patients aged forty years and younger. Surgery 107:560–565, 1990.
87. Pairolero PC, Joyce JW, Skinner CR, et al: Lower limb ischemia in young adults: Prognostic implications. J Vasc Surg 1:459–464, 1984.
88. Evans WE, Hayes JP, Vermillion BD: Atherosclerosis in the young patient: Results of surgical management. Am J Surg 154:225–229, 1987.
89. Valentine RJ, Kaplan HS, Green R, et al: Lipoprotein (a), homocysteine, and hypercoagulable states in young men with premature peripheral atherosclerosis: A prospective, controlled analysis. J Vasc Surg 23:53–61, 1996.
90. Valentine RJ, Grayburn PA, Vega GL, Grundy SM: Lp(a) lipoprotein is an independent, discriminating risk factor for premature peripheral atherosclerosis among white men. Arch Intern Med 154:801–806, 1994.
91. McCready RA, Vincent AE, Schwartz RW, et al: Atherosclerosis in the young: A virulent disease. Surgery 96:863–869, 1984.
92. Harris LM, Armstrong D, Browne R, et al: Premature peripheral vascular disease: Clinical profile and abnormal lipid peroxidation. Cardiovasc Surg 6:188–193, 1998.
93. Levy PJ, Gonzalez MF, Hornung CA, et al: A prospective evaluation of atherosclerotic risk factors and hypercoagulability in young adults with premature lower extremity. J Vasc Surg 23:36–45, 1996.
94. Harris LM, Peer R, Curl GR, et al: Long-term follow-up of patients with early atherosclerosis. J Vasc Surg 23:576–580, 1996.
95. Valentine RJ, Myers SI, Inman MH, et al: Late outcome of amputees with premature atherosclerosis. Surgery 119:487–493, 1996.
96. Valentine RJ, Myers SI, Hagino RT, Clagett GP: Late outcome of patients with premature carotid atherosclerosis after carotid endarterectomy. Stroke 27:1502–1506, 1996.
97. Lefcoe NM, Ashley MJ, Pederson LL, Keays JJ: The health risks of passive smoking. The growing case for control measures in enclosed environments. Chest 84:90–95, 1983.
98. Weiss ST, Tager IB, Schenker M, Speizer FE: The health effects of involuntary smoking. Am Rev Respir Dis 128:933–942, 1983.
99. Greenberg RA, Haley NJ, Etzel RA, Loda FA: Measuring the exposure of infants to tobacco smoke. Nicotine and continine in urine and saliva. N Engl J Med 310:1075–1078, 1984.
100. Seguire M, Chalmers KI: Late adolescent female smoking. J Adv Nurs 31:1422–1429, 2000.
101. Warner KE: The economics of smoking: Dollars and sense. N Y State J Med 83:1273–1274, 1983.
102. Luce BR, Schweitzer SO: Smoking and alcohol abuse: A comparison of their economic consequences. N Engl J Med 298:569–571, 1978.
103. Geyelin M, Fairclough G: Taking a hit: Yes, $145 billion deals tobacco a huge blow but not a killing one—legal climate may favor appeal of class action; if not, just raise prices—a pack of cigarettes for $7? Wall Street J. 2000.
104. Couch NP: On the arterial consequences of smoking. J Vasc Surg 3:807–812, 1986.
105. Fielding JE: Smoking: Health effects and control. N Engl J Med 313(Pt 1 of 2):491–498, 1985.
106. Fielding JE: Smoking: Health effects and control. N Engl J Med 313(Pt 2 of 2):555–561, 1985.
107. Krupski WC, Rapp JH: Smoking and atherosclerosis. Perspect Vasc Surg 1:103–134, 1988.
108. Aronow WS, Stemmer EA, Isbell MW: Effect of carbon monoxide exposure on intermittent claudication. Circulation 49:415–417, 1974.
109. Cronenwett JL, Warner KG, Zelenock GB, et al: Intermittent claudication: Current results of nonoperative management. Arch Surg 119:430–436, 1984.
110. Violi F, Criqui M, Longoni A, Castiglioni C: Relation between risk factors and cardiovascular complications in patients with peripheral vascular disease. Results from the A.D.E.P. study. Atherosclerosis 120:25–35, 1996.
111. Juergens JL, Barker NW, Hines EA: Arteriosclerosis obliterans: A review of 520 cases with special reference to pathogenic and prognostic factors. Circulation 21:188–195, 1960.
112. McGrath MA, Graham AR, Hill DA, et al: The natural history of chronic leg ischemia. World J Surg 7:314–318, 1983.
113. Quick CR, Cotton LT: The measured effect of stopping smoking on intermittent claudication. Br J Surg (Suppl 69):S24–S26, 1982.
114. Robicsek F, Daugherty HK, Mullen DC, et al: The effect of continued cigarette smoking on the patency of synthetic vascular grafts in Leriche syndrome. J Thorac Cardiovasc Surg 70(1):107–113, 1975.
115. Ameli FM, Stein M, Prosser RJ, et al: Effects of cigarette smoking on outcome of femoral popliteal bypass for limb salvage. J Cardiovasc Surg 30:591–596, 1989.
116. Provan JL, Sojka SG, Murnaghan JJ, Jaunkalns R: The effect of cigarette smoking on the long term success rates of aortofemoral and femoropopliteal reconstructions. Surg Gynecol Obstet 165:49–52, 1987.
117. Myers KA, King RB, Scott DF, et al: The effect of smoking on the late patency of arterial reconstructions in the legs. Br J Surg 65:267–271, 1978.
118. Wiseman S, Kenchington G, Dain R, et al: Influence of smoking and plasma factors on patency of femoropopliteal vein grafts. 299:643–646, 1989.
119. Eissenberg T, Balster RL: Initial tobacco use episodes in children and adolescents: Current knowledge, future directions. Drug Alcohol Depend 59(Suppl 1):S41–S60, 2000.
120. Hughes JR: Genetics of smoking: A brief review. Behav Ther 17:335–345, 1986.
121. Benowitz NL: Cigarette smoking and nicotine addiction. Med Clin North Am 76:415–437, 1992.
122. Smoking cessation during previous year among adults—United States, 1990 and 1991. Morb Mortal Wkly Rep 42:504–507, 1993.
123. Clyne CA, Arch PJ, Carpenter D, et al: Smoking, ignorance, and peripheral vascular disease. Arch Surg 117:1062–1065, 1982.
124. U.S. Department of Health and Human Services: Healthy People: The Surgeon General's Report on Health Promotion and Disease Prevention. U.S. Department of Health and Human Services, Rockville, MD, 1979.
125. Silagy C, Fowler G, Lodge M: Meta-analysis on the efficacy of nicotine replacement therapies in smoking cessation. Lancet 343:139–142, 1994.

126. Fiore MC, Smith SS, Jorenby DE, Baker TB: The effectiveness of the nicotine patch for smoking cessation: A meta-analysis. JAMA 271:1940–1947, 1994.

127. Fiore MC, Jorenby DE, Baker TB, Kenford SL: Tobacco dependence and the nicotine patch: Clinical guidelines for effective use. JAMA 268:2687–2694, 1992.

128. Rennard SI, Daughton DM, Fortman S: Transdermal nictone enhances smoking cessation in coronary artery disease patients. Chest 5S:100, 1991.

129. Shea RW: Press Release. Sturdy Memorial Hospital Medical Alert, 1992.

130. Joseph AM, Norman SM, Ferry LH, et al: The safety of transdermal nicotine as an aid to smoking cessation in patients with cardiac disease. N Engl J Med 335:1792–1798, 1996.

131. Schneider NG, Olmstead R, Nilsson F, et al: Efficacy of a nicotine inhaler in smoking cessation: A double-blind, placebo-controlled trial. Addiction 91:1293–1306, 1996.

132. Westman EC, Behm FM, Rose JE: Airway sensory replacement combined with nicotine replacement for smoking cessation. A randomized, placebo-controlled trial using a citric acid inhaler. Chest 107:1358–1364, 1995.

133. Glassman AH, Helzer JE, Covey LS, Cottler LB, et al: Smoking, smoking cessation, and major depression [see comments]. JAMA 264:1546–1549, 1990.

134. Hurt RD, Sachs DP, Glover ED, et al: A comparison of sustained-release bupropion and placebo for smoking cessation [see comments]. N Engl J Med 337:1195–1202, 1997.

135. Jorenby DE, Leischow SJ, Nides MA, Rennard SI, et al: A controlled trial of sustained-release bupropion a nicotine patch, or both for smoking cessation [see comments]. N Engl J Med 340:685–691, 1999.

136. Blondal T, Gudmundsson LJ, Tomasson K, et al: The effects of fluoxetine combined with nicotine inhalers in smoking cessation—a randomized trial. Addiction 94:1007–1015, 1999.

137. Pomerleau OF, Fertig JB, Seyler LE, Jaffe J: Neuroendocrine reactivity to nicotine in smokers. Psychopharmacology (Berl) 81:61–67, 1983.

138. Wong GY, Wolter TD, Croghan GA, et al: A randomized trial of naltrexone for smoking cessation. Addiction 94:1227–1237, 1999.

139. Creasy TS, McMillan PJ, Fletcher EWL, et al: Is percutaneous transluminal angioplasty better than exercise for claudication? Preliminary results from a prospective randomized trial. Eur J Vasc Surg 4:135–140, 1990.

140. Hiatt WR, Regensteiner JG, Hargarten ME, et al: Benefit of exercise conditioning for patients with peripheral arterial disease. Circulation 81:602–609, 1990.

141. Mannarino E, Pasqualini L, Innocente S, et al: Physical training and antiplatelet treatment in stage II peripheral arterial occlusive disease: Alone or combined? Angiology 42:513–521, 1991.

142. Scheffler P, de la Hamette D, Gross J, et al: Intensive vascular training in stage IIb of peripheral arterial occlusive disease. The additive effects of intravenous prostaglandin E₁ or intravenous pentoxifylline during training. Circulation 90:818–822, 1994.

143. Hiatt WR, Wolfel EE, Meier RH, Regensteiner JG: Superiority of treadmill walking exercise vs. strength training for patients with peripheral arterial disease. Implications for the mechanism of the training response. Circulation 90:1866–1874, 1994.

144. Lievre M, Azoulay S, Lion L, et al: A dose-effect study of beraprost sodium in intermittent claudication. J Cardiovasc Pharmacol 27:788–793, 1996.

145. Regensteiner JG, Meyer TJ, Krupski WC, et al: Hospital vs. home-based exercise rehabilitation for patients with peripheral arterial occlusive disease. Angiology 48:291–300, 1997.

146. Patterson RB, Pinto B, Marcus B, et al: Value of a supervised exercise program for the therapy of arterial claudication. J Vasc Surg 25:312–318, 1997.

147. Mannarino E, Pasqualini L, Menna M, et al: Effects of physical training on peripheral vascular disease: A controlled study. Angiology 40:5–10, 1989.

148. Lundgren F, Dahllof AG, Schersten T, Bylund-Fellenius AC: Muscle enzyme adaptation in patients with peripheral arterial insufficiency: Spontaneous adaptation, effect of different treatments and consequences on walking performance. Clin Sci 77:485–493, 1989.

149. Zetterquist S: The effect of active training on the nutritive blood flow in exercising ischemic legs. Scand J Clin Lab Invest 25:101–111, 1970.

150. Sorlie D, Myhre K: Effects of physical training in intermittent claudication. Scand J Clin Lab Invest 38:217–222, 1978.

151. Holm J, Dahllof A, Bjorntorp P, Schersten T: Enzyme studies in muscles of patients with intermittent claudication. Effect of training. Scand J Clin Lab Invest 31(Suppl 128):201–205, 1973.

152. Hiatt WR, Regensteiner JG, Wolfel EE, et al: Effect of exercise training on skeletal muscle histology and metabolism in peripheral arterial disease. J Appl Physiol 81:780–788, 1996.

153. Scherer SA, Bainbridge JS, Hiatt WR, Regensteiner JG: Gait characteristics of patients with claudication. Arch Phys Med Rehabil 79:529–531, 1998.

154. Wyatt MG, Scott PM, Scott DJ, Poskitt K, et al: Effect of weight on walking distance. Br J Surg 78:1386–1388, 1991.

155. Ehrly AM, Kohler HJ: Altered deformability of erythrocytes from patients with chronic occlusive arterial disease. VASA 5:319–322, 1976.

156. Reid HL, Dormandy JA, Barnes AJ, et al: Impaired red cell deformability in peripheral vascular disease. Lancet 1:666–668, 1976.

157. Ernst EE, Matrai A: Intermittent claudication, exercise, and blood rheology. Circulation 76:1110–1114, 1987.

158. Dormandy JA, Hoare E, Colley J, et al: Clinical, haemodynamic, rheological, and biochemical findings in 126 patients with intermittent claudication. Br Med J 4:576–581, 1973.

159. Johnson G Jr, Keagy BA, Ross DW, et al: Viscous factors in peripheral tissue perfusion. J Vasc Surg 2:530–535, 1985.

160. Waters KJ, Craxford AD, Chamberlain J: The effect of naftidrofuryl (Praxilene) on intermittent claudication. Br J Surg 67:349–351, 1980.

161. Adhoute G, Bacourt F, Barral M, et al: Naftidrofuryl in chronic arterial disease. Results of a six month controlled multicenter study using naftidrofuryl tablets 200 mg. Angiology 37:160–167, 1986.

162. Kriessmann A, Neiss A: Clinical effectiveness of naftidrofuryl in intermittent claudication. Vasa (Suppl):27–32, 1988.

163. Adhoute G, Andreassian B, Boccalon H, et al: Treatment of stage II chronic arterial disease of the lower limbs with the serotonergic antagonist naftidrofuryl: Results after 6 months of a controlled, multicenter study. J Cardiovasc Pharmacol 16(Suppl 3):S75–S80, 1990.

164. Moody AP, al Khaffaf HS, Lehert P, et al: An evaluation of patients with severe intermittent claudication and the effect of treatment with naftidrofuryl. J Cardiovasc Pharmacol 23(Suppl 3):S44–S47, 1994.

165. Trubestein G, Bohme H, Heidrich H, et al: Naftidrofuryl in chronic arterial disease. Results of a controlled multicenter study. Angiology 35:701–708, 1984.

166. Trubestein G, Balzer K, Bisler H, et al: Buflomedil in arterial occlusive disease: Results of a controlled multicenter study. Angiology 35:500–505, 1984.

167. Okuda Y, Kimura Y, Yamashita K: Cilostazol. Cardiovasc Drug Rev 11:451–465, 1993.

168. Money SR, Herd JA, Isaacsohn JL, et al: Effect of cilostazol on walking distances in patients with intermittent claudication caused by peripheral vascular disease. J Vasc Surg 27:267–274, 1998.

169. Beebe HG, Dawson DL, Cutler BS, et al: A new pharmacological treatment for intermittent claudication: Results of a randomized, multicenter trial. Arch Intern Med 159:2041–2050, 1999.

170. Dawson DL, Cutler BS, Meissner MH, Strandness DEJ: Cilostazol has beneficial effects in treatment of intermittent claudication: Results from a multicenter, randomized, prospective, double-blind trial. Circulation 98:678–686, 1998.

171. Dawson DL, DeMaioribus CA, Hagino RT, et al: The effect of withdrawal of drugs treating intermittent claudication. Am J Surg 178:141–146, 1999.

172. Diamantopoulos EJ, Grammoustianos GS, Stavreas NP: Controlled trial of blufemedil in diabetic peripheral occlusive disease. Frankfurt, Zuckschwerdt. International Symposium on Ischemic Diseases and the Microcirculation, 1989, pp 80–84.

173. Antiplatelet Trialists' Collaboration: Secondary prevention of vascular disease by prolonged antiplatelet treatment. Br Med J 296:320–331, 1988.

174. Balsano F, Coccheri S, Libretti A, et al: Ticlopidine in the treatment of intermittent claudication: A 21-month double-blind trial. J Lab Clin Med 114:84–91, 1989.

175. Arcan JC, Blanchard J, Boissel JP, et al: Multicenter double-blind study of ticlopidine in the treatment of intermittent claudication and the prevention of its complications. Angiology 39:802–811, 1988.

176. Herbert JM, Frehel D, Vallee E, et al: Clopidogrel, a novel antiplatelet and antithrombotic agent. Cardiovasc Drug Rev 11:180–198, 1993.
177. CAPRIE Steering Committee: A randomised, blinded, trial of clopidogrel versus aspirin in patients at risk of ischaemic events (CAPRIE). Lancet 348:1329–1339, 1996.
178. Davie AP, Love MP: CAPRIE trial [letter, comment] [see comments]. Lancet 349:355, 1997.
179. Hiatt WR, Nawaz D, Brass EP: Carnitine metabolism during exercise in patients with peripheral vascular disease. J Appl Physiol 62:2383–2387, 1987.
180. Hiatt WR, Wolfel EE, Regensteiner JG, Brass EP: Skeletal muscle carnitine metabolism in patients with unilateral peripheral arterial disease. J Appl Physiol 73:346–353, 1992.
181. Brevetti G, Chiariello M, Ferulano G, Policicchio A, et al: Increases in walking distance in patients with peripheral vascular disease treated with L-carnitine: A double-blind, cross-over study. Circulation 77:767–773, 1988.
182. Brevetti G, Perna S, Sabba C, et al: Superiority of L-propionyl carnitine vs L-carnitine in improving walking capacity in patients with peripheral vascular disease: An acute, intravenous, double-blind, cross-over study. Eur Heart J 13:251–255, 1992.
183. Hiatt WR: Current and future drug therapies for claudication. Vasc Med 2:257–262, 1997.
184. Brevetti G, Diehm C, Lambert D: European multicenter study on propionyl-L-carnitine in intermittent claudication. J Am Coll Cardiol 34:1618–1624, 1999.
185. Weeks JR, Sekhar NC, Ducharme DW: Relative activity of prostaglandins E_1, A_1, E_2 and A_2 on lipolysis, platelet aggregation, smooth muscle and the cardiovascular system. J Pharm Pharmacol 21:103–108, 1969.
186. Cronenwett JL, Zelenock GB, Whitehouse WM Jr, et al: Prostacyclin treatment of ischemic ulcers and rest pain in unreconstructible peripheral arterial occlusive disease. Surgery 100:369–375, 1986.
187. Schuler JJ, Flanigan DP, Holcroft JW, et al: Efficacy of prostaglandin E_1 in the treatment of lower extremity ischemic ulcers secondary to peripheral vascular occlusive disease. Results of a prospective randomized, double-blind, multicenter clinical trial. J Vasc Surg 1:160–170, 1984.
188. Eklund AE, Eriksson G, Olsson AG: A controlled study showing significant short term effect of prostaglandin E_1 in healing of ischaemic ulcers of the lower limb in man. Prostaglandins Leukot Med 8:265–271, 1982.
189. Tsurumi Y, Takeshita S, Chen D, et al: Direct intramuscular gene transfer of naked DNA encoding vascular endothelial growth factor augments collateral development and tissue perfusion. Circulation 94:3281–3290, 1996.
190. Baumgartner I, Pieczek A, Manor O, et al: Constitutive expression of phVEGF165 after intramuscular gene transfer promotes collateral vessel development in patients with critical limb ischemia [see comments]. Circulation 97:1114–1123, 1998.
191. Maxwell AJ, Anderson B: Improvement in walking distance and quality of life in peripheral arterial disease by a nutritional product designed to enhance nitric oxide activity. JACC 33:277a, 1999.
192. Boger RH, Bode-Boger SM, Thiele W, et al: Restoring vascular nitric oxide formation by L-arginine improves the symptoms of intermittent claudication in patients with peripheral arterial occlusive disease. J Am Coll Cardiol 32:1336–1344, 1998.
193. McCready RA, Vincent AE, Schwartz RW, Hyde GL, et al: Atherosclerosis in the young: A virulent disease. Surgery 96:863–869, 1984.
194. Pairolero PC, Joyce JW, Skinner CR, et al: Lower limb ischemia in young adults: Prognostic implications. J Vasc Surg 1:459–464, 1984.
195. Evans WE, Hayes JP, Vermillion BD: Atherosclerosis in the young patient: Results of surgical management. Am J Surg 154:225–229, 1987.
196. Levy PJ, Hornung CA, Haynes JL, Rush DS: Lower extremity ischemia in adults younger than forty years of age: A community-wide survey of premature atherosclerotic arterial disease. J Vasc Surg 18:873–881, 1994.

16

Principles of Vascular Imaging and Interventional Radiology

Antoinette S. Gomes

Angiography is a technique in which radiopaque contrast material is injected into vessels, permitting visualization of the vascular system. The information obtained is used to make a clinical diagnosis, to formulate a preoperative therapeutic plan, and to provide anatomic information that can reduce operative time. Conventional arteriograms can be performed on an inpatient or outpatient basis. In either case, the patient should be closely monitored to avoid the risk of postangiographic complications such as bleeding at the puncture site.

Access to the vascular system is obtained using aseptic technique with percutaneous puncture of the vessel. Patients undergoing routine angiographic procedures should be mildly sedated and well hydrated.

Angiography is performed by several routes. A femoral approach with puncture of the femoral artery below the inguinal ligament is the most widely used. When the femoral vessels are occluded or the catheter cannot be introduced into the femoral artery, an axillary puncture or high brachial artery puncture can be used. This approach is more difficult than the femoral approach owing to the small size and mobility of the vessel. It is associated with a slightly higher risk because of the proximity of the brachial plexus and the increased difficulty of obtaining hemostasis in the soft tissues.[1] Hematoma, direct nerve trauma, and brachial nerve palsy are potential complications with this technique. The incidence of complications in experienced hands is low. When the femoral arteries are not suitable for puncture, a translumbar approach with direct puncture of the abdominal aorta is another alternative. In a small percentage of patients, periaortic bleeding may occur with a possible change in hematocrit. This technique allows good images of the abdomen and legs. It should not be used when there is an aneurysm at the level of catheter entry (T-12) or (L-2–3), a bleeding disorder, an aortic graft at the puncture site, or systemic hypertension.

DIGITAL SUBTRACTION ANGIOGRAPHY

Digital subtraction angiography (DSA) is a form of digital radiography. In digital radiography, x-ray signals are detected electronically, converted to digital form, and processed before being recorded and displayed. Computer subtraction techniques are used to remove uninteresting background information from the image so that the clinically significant details can be displayed with enhanced visibility. In DSA, the aim is to obtain visualization of the vascular system. With digital subtraction techniques and logarithmic amplification of the x-ray signal, one is able to detect and amplify small differences in density.[2–4] This permits detection of very low concentrations of iodinated contrast medium, such as those that occur in the arterial system after the intravenous injection of contrast, or in the venous phase of an arterial injection.

Although the contrast sensitivity is high in DSA, spatial resolution is less than in conventional film-screen arteriograms. As a result, the DSA images are less sharp than those obtained in the conventional arteriogram, but this is acceptable, because it is not always necessary to have high detail to make a diagnosis or plan therapy.

The standard DSA unit consists of an x-ray tube, image intensifier, television camera, and image processor (computer). The subtraction technique most widely used at present is temporal subtraction, in which a mask image obtained before x-ray contrast arrival is stored in the computer memory. Subsequent images obtained during the arrival of the contrast bolus are obtained and then subtracted from the mask. The difference image (the opacified vessels) is displayed and stored. In instances in which motion artifact has occurred between the acquisition of the mask and the subtraction images, postprocessing of the images may then be performed. In postprocessing, a new mask is selected or the mask is shifted to partially compensate and correct the motion artifact. The radiation dose in DSA is similar to, or slightly less than, that in conventional arteriography.[5]

When DSA was first developed, initial interest centered around its use for intravenous angiography. There are, however, serious limitations to the use of intravenous DSA. Motion artifacts interfere with subtraction, and large volumes of contrast may be used with the multiple injections required to evaluate regions of vessel overlap. Intravenous applications are now used infrequently. Currently, the most frequent application of digital techniques is with arterial injections of contrast. Arterial DSA allows arteriography using diluted contrast or reduced volumes of contrast and with reduced film costs. The availability of small French-sized, high-flow catheters makes outpatient digital arteriography feasible. Image quality with arterial DSA is superior to that with intravenous DSA because there is less dilution of the contrast bolus and less of a problem with motion artifact, because the injection site is closer to the structures imaged.

Arterial DSA is now routinely used. Newer imaging systems employ only digital techniques. Using large field of view image intensifiers, arterial DSA routinely supplants conventional film-screen angiography, allowing completion of the study with less contrast and in a shorter time. Arterial DSA facilitates the performance of interventional procedures. The resolution of arterial DSA is less than that with conventional film-screen arteriography, and vessels less than 200 μm are seen better with conventional studies.[6] Arterial DSA, however, has superior contrast detectability when compared with conventional arteriography and offers improved visualization of tumor blushes and venous structures.

TECHNICAL COMPLICATIONS OF ANGIOGRAPHY

The most common angiographic complication is hematoma formation at the catheter site as a result of inadequate compression of the artery or trauma to the vessel after prolonged manipulation of the catheter. This is usually self-limiting and only rarely requires operative evacuation. Loss of pulse may occur because of arterial spasm or thrombus formation.[7] If the pulse is lost during the procedure, vasodilators should be given or a pullout angiogram performed. Surgical treatment of the thrombosed vessel may be necessary. Other complications that may occur at the puncture site include arteriovenous fistulas, false aneurysms, and retroperitoneal hematoma. Subintimal dissection of a catheterized vessel may also occur. These usually heal spontaneously but may result in narrowing or occlusion of the vessel. Distal embolization of blood clot or atheromatous plaque may also occur, with the sequelae determined by the size and location of the dislodged material.

CONTRAST MEDIA

Contrast agents used for angiography can be divided into two major categories: high osmolar agents and low osmolar agents. The older, high-osmolar agents are sodium or methylglucamine salts of triiodo-2,4,6-benzoic acid. Substitutions in the 3,5-acetylamine components distinguish the various agents: iothalamates, diatrizoates, and metrizoates. The sodium salts are less viscous than the methylglucamine salts but more toxic.[8, 9] These contrast agents are available in high, medium, and low concentrations. The osmolarity of these agents is significantly higher than that of blood, which accounts for the sensation of heat, vasodilatation, and pain that patients experience with the injection.

The hyperosmolality of these contrast agents relative to blood is important as it accounts for many of the hemodynamic, cardiac, and unpleasant side effects such as heat vasodilatation and pain associated with contrast agent injections.[10] The newer, lower-osmolar agents have a lower osmolality and a higher ratio between the number of iodine atoms and the number of dissolved particles. The agents include nonionic monomers (metrizamide, iopamidol, ioversol, and iohexol). Also available is a monoacidic dimer (ioxaglate); this has a high ratio of iodine atoms to the number of dissolved particles but still has an ionized anion in solution. These new agents have shown reduced side effects owing to osmolality, reduced organ toxicity, and fewer adverse reactions. They cause less vascular hemodynamic change and less heat and pain after intraarterial and intravenous injections. Less damage to endothelial cells occurs, and less reactivity is induced in the complement and coagulation systems. Also reduced are pulmonary complications, central nervous system (CNS) toxicity, and, probably, nephrotoxicity. The large prospective study by Katayama and colleagues[11] demonstrated a lower overall incidence of adverse reactions in patients who received low-osmolar nonionic contrast media compared with those who received high-osmolar ionic contrast media. In cardiac use, fewer electrocardiographic changes are seen and less ventricular fibrillation is induced.

Because of the higher cost of the newer low-osmolar agents, there has been a tendency to restrict their use to special groups of patients, such as those with renal insufficiency or diabetes, infants, dehydrated patients, patients undergoing high-volume interventional studies, patients undergoing coronary arteriography, and patients with a history of prior adverse reactions to contrast media. In these high-risk patients, the advantages outweigh the increased cost.

These iodinated contrast agents are extracellular agents and are excreted by glomerular filtration. High osmolar agents can produce a transient decrease in renal blood flow and increased vascular resistance.[12] Contrast agents can induce acute renal dysfunction both in patients with and without a history of previous renal disease undergoing angiography.[13] Patients with prior renal failure, proteinuria, diabetes, advanced age, and dehydration are at higher risk for renal dysfunction.[14–16] The changes that occur are usually minimal and transient but can lead to progressive anuria. If managed properly, contrast-induced renal failure usually resolves spontaneously within 7 days.[16] Studies have suggested that renal dysfunction may be dose-related.[17] Hydration of patients prior to angiography is recommended.[18] The administration of mannitol to patients with preexisting renal disease at the time of angiography has also been recommended;[15] however, recent studies have not confirmed its benefit.[19] The use of furosemide (Lasix) with hydration has not been found beneficial. Furosemide administration in combination with dopamine, however, may have a protective effect. The effects on renal function of angiographic contrast media should be considered when extensive angiographic studies are requested and when deciding on the interval between angiography and operation.

Reactions to Contrast Media

In addition to renal dysfunction from a direct nephrotoxic effect, contrast agents may precipitate an allergic reaction.

These reactions may be mild, with hives (urticaria), or they may be severe anaphylactoid reactions characterized by bradycardia, hypotension, wheezing, and shock.[20] In patients with a history of a severe previous reaction, the indications for repeat angiography should be carefully evaluated. The patient should be pretreated with steroids before the study and given antihistamines the day of the examination. A frequently used regimen is prednisone 50 mg orally every 6 hours for three doses leading up to the contrast injection, and diphenhydramine (Benadryl) 50 mg 1 hour before the contrast injection. In addition, intravenous steroids during the examination may be used. An emergency cart should be available.[21, 22] Pretreatment with steroids has been found to block the recurrence of the anaphylactoid symptoms in a high percentage of patients.[21]

ARCH AORTOGRAPHY

The arch aortogram is used to provide visualization of the brachiocephalic vessel origins, carotid bifurcations, and high cervical portions of the carotid arteries. It is usually performed from the femoral approach using a pigtail catheter positioned in the ascending aorta just proximal to the innominate artery. Approximately 50 mL of contrast medium is injected with imaging in both oblique projections. Image acquisition is usually done using a large field-of-view image intensifier with DSA. Conventional film-screen techniques may also be used (Fig. 16–1).

Considerable controversy has existed regarding the merits of the use of arch aortography versus selective arteriography in the evaluation of extracranial carotid disease.

Selective carotid arteriography is easily and safely performed in patients with nonocclusive vascular disease or intracerebral mass lesions. In patients studied for transient ischemic attacks (TIAs), intracranial collateral flow is delicate, and the balance may be upset by hemodynamic changes induced by the placement of catheters in vessels with high-grade stenosis. The slow clearance of contrast from vessels with high-grade stenosis leads to longer cell contact with the contrast agent. The hazards of fibrin deposition on catheters in severely obstructed vessels is increased. Surgical mortality and morbidity are significantly higher in patients operated on for extracranial disease who did not have adequate intracranial visualization. In a series from Duke University,[23] 8% of 350 patients studied for extracranial disease had significant intracranial disease. Johnsrude[23] found that 85% of the patients undergoing evaluation for intracranial disease could be adequately evaluated by multiple-projection aortic arch subtraction studies alone. Other authors have observed similar findings.[24] The complication rate from femoral cerebral angiography with cerebrovascular occlusive disease with this approach has also been reduced.[25] If the arch study does not conform to the results of noninvasive testing, a selective injection can be performed. This offers the advantage of not having to selectively catheterize a tightly stenosed vessel.

ANGIOGRAPHY OF THE EXTREMITIES

Lower Extremities

When visualization of the vessels of the lower extremities is desired, a femoral runoff study is obtained. The standard femoral arteriogram includes a runoff study with filling of

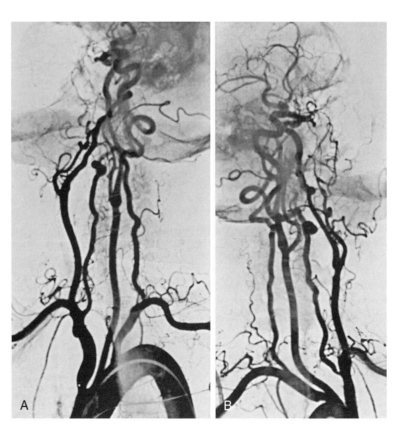

Figure 16–1. Subtraction films of an aortic arch study. *A,* Right posterior oblique position shows mild narrowing at the origin of the innominate artery and normal right carotid and right vertebral arteries. The left common carotid fills well. There is a smooth, nonobstructing plaque in the distal left common carotid artery. The left subclavian and left vertebral arteries are intact. *B,* On the left posterior oblique view, a plaque is seen at the origin of the right subclavian artery. The origin of the left vertebral artery has a 30% to 40% narrowing. Again shown is the plaque in the distal left common carotid artery. The high cervical portions of the right and left internal carotid arteries are well seen.

the vessels of the legs down to the ankles. When a below-knee bypass is planned, filming to the level of the plantar arch may be necessary. A routine study also typically includes an abdominal aortogram with visualization of the aortic bifurcation. In the legs, improved visualization is obtained with reactive hyperemia induced at the time of the study. This can be accomplished using tourniquet constriction with release immediately before injection or with the administration of vasodilators such as papaverine or tolazoline (Priscoline, Ciba-Geigy Pharmaceuticals, Summit, NJ). A standard runoff injection employs 75 to 80 mL of iodinated contrast media for visualization of the pelvis and lower legs. The abdominal injection is made with 40 to 50 mL of contrast medium for visualization of the aortic bifurcation and origins of the renal arteries. With large field-of-view image intensifiers and a stepping table, the entire runoff study is performed using DSA. DSA techniques are particularly helpful for visualization of the arteries in the lower calf and foot and afford improved visualization of delayed, poorly filled vessels distal to sites of obstruction. When visualization of only one leg is needed, the femoral artery on the ipsilateral side may be punctured, or the femoral artery on the opposite side may be punctured and the catheter passed around the aortic bifurcation. It is important that the bifurcation of the superficial femoral and profunda femoral arteries be well visualized. If there is overlap of the vessels at this site, a significant stenosis in either the superficial femoral artery or the profunda femoral artery may be missed. It is often necessary to film the pelvis in the oblique projection with the side of interest elevated to open the bifurcation. In the lower leg, it is also important to avoid overlap of the tibia and fibula during positioning, because overlap of these two structures can result in poor visualization of the underlying runoff vessels. Oblique views may also be required to determine the severity of lesions in the iliac system. Visualization of the vessels in only one projection may result in a severe underestimation of the severity of the lesion. A reduction in vessel cross-sectional area of 75% is considered indicative of a hemodynamically significant lesion. A 50% reduction in diameter is approximately equivalent. When the hemodynamic significance of a stenosis is questioned, a pressure gradient should be measured across the lesion before and after the administration of vasodilators.[26] Gradients that are not hemodynamically significant at rest may be shown to be significant following the administration of the vasodilator. An arterial gradient equal to or greater than 15 mm Hg at rest or following vasodilators is regarded as significant. In interpreting femoral arteriograms, care must be exercised so that vessels are not presumed to be occluded when their failure to opacify is merely the result of an improper filming sequence with filming performed before arrival of the contrast bolus (Figs. 16–2, 16–3, and 16–4).

Upper Extremities

Typical indications for angiography of the upper extremities include evaluation of atherosclerotic vascular disease or trauma, documentation of embolism, or evaluation of arteriovenous fistulas. Angiography of the upper extremities is readily performed via a percutaneous femoral artery approach. Alternatively, if the lesion is distal to the elbow, an antegrade or retrograde brachial artery puncture can be performed. Antegrade axillary punctures are employed rarely. Reactive hyperemia is used to enhance visualization of the vessels of the hand.

Specific Lesions

Atherosclerosis

In the arteries of the lower extremities, atherosclerotic changes occur most frequently in the femoral arteries, iliac arteries, the trifurcation, the popliteal arteries, and the aorta.[27] Lesions in the superficial femoral artery occur most frequently in the region of Hunter's canal. The changes may be evidenced as irregular plaques, ulceration, varying degrees of narrowing and occlusion, or areas of dilatation and elongation. Patients with diabetes usually have diffuse small vessel disease with more frequent involvement below the trifurcation.

In the upper extremities, atherosclerosis involves the subclavian arteries, but rarely extends beyond them.[28] If the occlusion occurs proximal to the vertebral artery origins, a subclavian steal may occur, in which blood flow to the basilar system is decreased as blood preferentially passes retrograde down the vertebral artery into the low-pressure area of the subclavian artery distal to the stenosis. This retrograde filling of the vertebral artery is seen best on delayed films of an aortic arch injection (Fig. 16–5).

Embolism

Emboli to peripheral vessels are seen most commonly at bifurcations.[29, 30] They appear radiographically as filling defects with convex margins. In acute emboli, filling of the arteries distally is usually not seen because of poor collateral formation or propagation of the thrombus. Because a thrombus may form in time in the area of stagnant flow just proximal to an embolus, radiographic differentiation from a thrombus can be difficult. Observations that should differentiate an embolus from a thrombus are absence of atherosclerotic changes in peripheral branches, and small collateral pathways. Thrombus superimposed on an area of stenosis may produce similar changes, but collateral pathways are usually larger and there is usually evidence of atherosclerosis distally. Emboli may be due to clot, foreign bodies, tumor, or subacute bacterial endocarditis (SBE). Emboli most commonly originate in the left atrium. They may arise from aneurysms, atheroma, cardiac tumors, or, paradoxically, from the venous system (Fig. 16–6).

Arteritis

The most commonly seen arteritides are Buerger's disease, Takayasu's disease, and giant cell arteritis.

BUERGER'S DISEASE. Buerger's disease[31–33] involves both upper and lower extremities. It occurs primarily in young

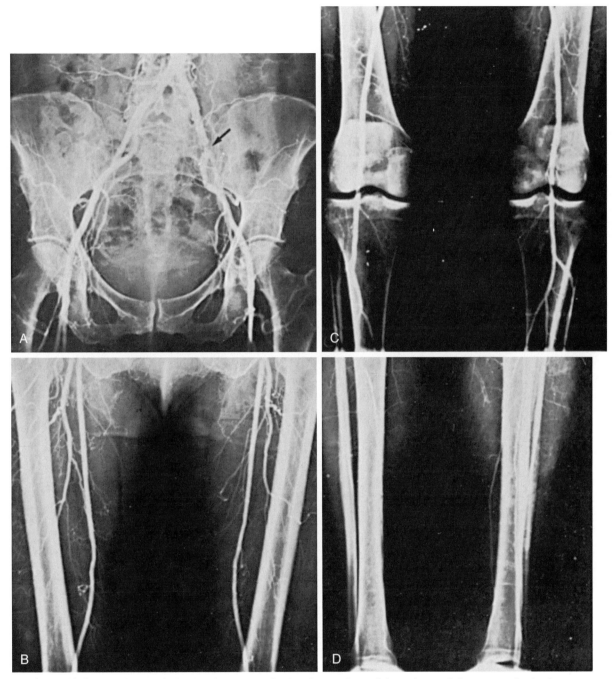

Figure 16–2. Typical femoral runoff study. *A*, View of pelvis showing iliac and femoral artery bifurcations. A localized stenosis is seen in the distal left common iliac artery *(arrow)*. *B*, View of thigh showing patient right and left superficial femoral arteries. *C*, Popliteal artery and trifurcation view showing patent origin of anterior and posterior tibial and peroneal arteries. *D*, Lower leg runoff view showing normal runoff bilaterally.

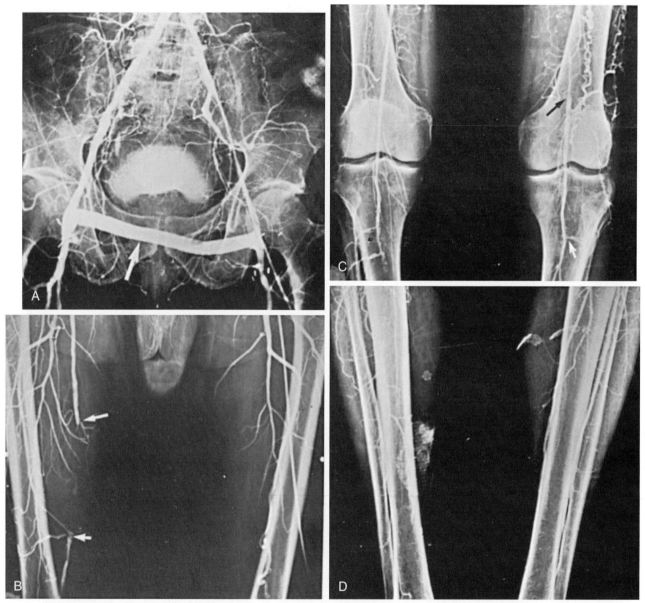

Figure 16–3. Runoff study. *A,* Catheter has passed via a left femoral artery puncture. Injection shows filling of the right common iliac and external iliac arteries with filling of a right femoral-to-left femoral graft *(arrow).* There is subsequent antegrade filling of the left profunda femoral artery. On the right, there is filling of both the profunda femoral and the superficial femoral arteries. *B,* Complete occlusion of the right superficial femoral artery midthigh *(long arrow)* with reconstitution at the level of the adductor hiatus *(short arrow).* To the left is opacification of the left profunda femoral artery with no filling of the left superficial femoral artery. *C,* Filling of the right popliteal artery with occlusion of the distal popliteal artery at the level of the posterior tibial, common peroneal trunk. The right anterior tibial artery is diffusely diseased at its origin. On the left, there is reconstitution of the popliteal artery by myriad collaterals *(black arrow).* The distal popliteal artery gives rise to the anterior and posterior tibial arteries. The left anterior tibial artery has a high-grade stenosis at its origin *(short white arrow).* The peroneal artery is patent. *D,* To the right is reconstitution of the posterior tibial artery just proximal to the ankle; the peroneal artery reconstitutes in the midcalf. The anterior tibial artery is occluded proximally. On the left, the posterior tibial and peroneal arteries fill to ankle level. The left anterior tibial has a high-grade stenosis at its origin but fills distally to the ankle.

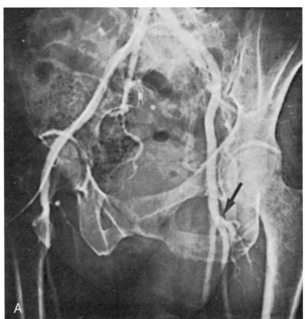

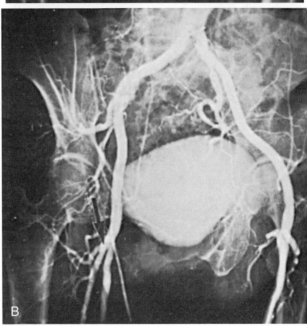

Figure 16–4. Oblique views of the pelvis. When the femoral bifurcations are not well visualized in the posteroanterior view, oblique views with the side of interest elevated should be performed; otherwise, hemodynamically significant bifurcation lesions may be missed. *A*, Right posterior oblique view opens up the left femoral bifurcation *(arrow)*. *B*, Left posterior oblique view opens up right bifurcation *(arrow)*.

male white and Asian smokers. Migratory phlebitis is often associated. Angiographically, mural calcifications are typically absent. The lesions are segmental and symmetrical and involve the distal small and medium-sized vessels with characteristically normal large proximal vessels. The angiogram typically shows absence of significant changes to suggest atheroma in large vessels. Smooth-lined vessels of even caliber are seen down to a point of abrupt occlusion. At the point of occlusion, the collateral pathways have a corkscrew, "spider-leg," or tree-root configuration around the point of focal disease. Corkscrew tortuosity of the superficial femoral and peroneal arteries may be seen. In the upper extremities, an absence of atheroma is again noted. There may be occlusion of the ulnar or radial arteries, or both arteries above the wrist, with typical collateral vessels and recanalization of the radial or ulnar arteries. The palmar arch may be attenuated or interrupted.[30]

TAKAYASU'S DISEASE. This arteritis is seen more frequently in young females and most often involves the arch and brachiocephalic vessels. It can, however, involve the aorta and its branches, as well as the pulmonary arteries. It causes coarctation, occlusion, or aneurysmal dilatation of the affected vessels.[34, 35] The angiograms show narrowing and occlusion of the brachiocephalic vessels, particularly the subclavian arteries. Typically, long coarctations of the thoracic aorta and abdominal aorta occur with concomitant occlusion of renal and mesenteric vessels. Aneurysms of the aorta also occur[34] (Fig. 16–7).

GIANT CELL ARTERITIS. This self-limited arteritis[36-39] usually appears in older patients with the prodrome of polymyalgia rheumatica characterized by fever, malaise, and headache. It has a predilection for medium-sized vessels of the carotid system, especially the temporal arteries, but can involve

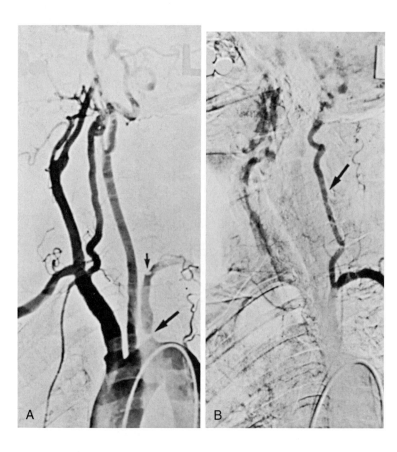

Figure 16–5. Subclavian steal syndrome. *A*, Aortic arch injection in the right posterior oblique position shows a patent innominate, right common carotid, and right vertebral artery. Left common carotid origin is normal. A high-grade stenosis is seen at the origin of the left subclavian artery *(long arrow)*. At the point of expected origin of the left vertebral artery a lucency is identified *(short arrow)*. *B*, Delayed films of the same injection show retrograde filling of the left vertebral artery *(arrow)* with opacification of the proximal left subclavian artery. Findings are typical for a subclavian steal syndrome.

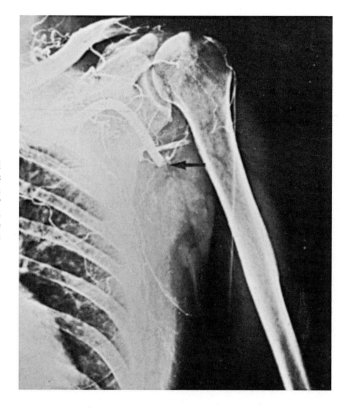

Figure 16–6. Embolic occlusion of proximal brachial, medial, and lateral circumflex humeral arteries. This patient experienced acute pain and loss of pulses in the left arm. Transfemoral selective left subclavian arteriogram shows abrupt termination of the brachial artery with evidence of a lucency indicative of embolus *(arrow)*. In addition, there is a filling defect seen in the anterior humeral circumflex artery and complete occlusion of the posterior humeral circumflex. Note the absence of collateral vessels in this acute embolic occlusion.

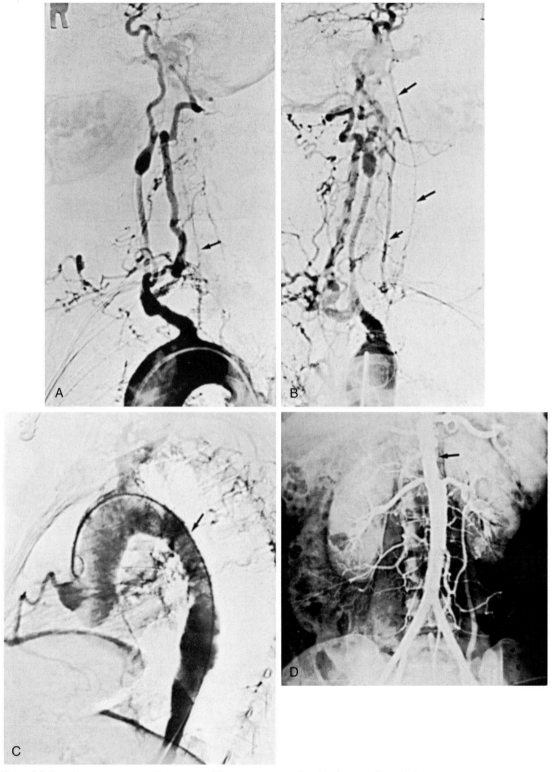

Figure 16–7. Takayasu's arteritis. This 28-year-old woman presented with a history of a right hemiparesis at age 13. *A*, Aortic arch injection in the right posterior oblique projection shows filling of the right innominate artery, the right common carotid, and a hypertrophied left vertebral artery. There is delayed filling of the proximal portion of a narrowed threadlike left common carotid artery *(arrow)*. The left vertebral artery does not opacify on this injection. Extensive collaterals are seen in the neck and supraclavicular region. Both subclavian arteries are occluded proximally. *B*, The left posterior oblique view again shows opacification of the right common carotid artery and right vertebral artery. This film, obtained late in the run, shows better filling of the diffusely narrowed irregular left common carotid artery *(long arrows)*. A segment of this vessel may be recanalized *(lower long arrow)*. There is retrograde filling of the left vertebral artery *(short arrow)*. *C*, Injection into the thoracic aorta shows typical findings of Takayasu's arteritis, with dilation of the ascending aorta, narrowing of the upper thoracic aorta *(arrow)*, followed by an area of dilatation in the descending thoracic aorta. *D*, Abdominal aortogram again shows characteristic findings in Takayasu's arteritis, with narrowing of the abdominal aorta in the segment between celiac axis and origin of the renal arteries *(arrow)*. The infrarenal abdominal aorta is within normal limits. Takayasu's arteritis can extend inferiorly to involve the distal aorta and common iliacs and has been reported to involve the femoral arteries.

the major aortic arch branches, producing upper extremity symptoms. The femoral and popliteal arteries may also be involved. Once the patient's systemic symptoms subside, there are usually residual arterial narrowings. Angiographically, these appear as long segments of smooth arterial stenoses alternating with areas of normal or increased caliber. There is an absence of irregular plaques and ulceration. The radiographic findings may be indistinguishable from those of Takayasu's disease.

Miscellaneous Causes of Occlusive Disease of Medium-Sized and Small Vessels

Medium-sized and small vessel occlusive disease may be the end result of a wide number of diseases, and frequently the diagnosis must be based on laboratory and clinical findings.[40, 41] Chronic recurrent trauma to the hand can produce occlusion of digital vessels. Collagen diseases such as scleroderma can produce spasm and small vessel occlusion. Polyarteritis nodosa can appear with small vessel aneurysms and occlusion. Dysproteinemias, polycythemia vera, and pseudoxanthoma elasticum can manifest with vessel occlusion, as can adverse reaction to drugs such as ergot derivatives and warfarin.[42]

Aneurysms of the Peripheral Vessels

Aneurysms of the peripheral vessels may be fusiform, saccular, mycotic, or false. They are due to a variety of causes, including atherosclerosis, medial degeneration, vasculitis, fibromuscular dysplasia, and trauma. Radiographically, the aneurysm is seen as a collection of contrast media. Laminated thrombus in the wall of the aneurysm may result in failure to diagnose the presence of aneurysms on arteriography. Care should be taken to look for the presence of calcification in the wall of a vessel. In some cases, particularly popliteal artery aneurysms, ultrasonography may be necessary to determine the true size of the aneurysm (Fig. 16–8). Computed tomography (CT) and magnetic resonance imaging (MRI) provide a more accurate assessment of aneurysm size.

Congenital Arteriovenous Malformations

Congenital arteriovenous malformations (AVMs) may be of several types. Macrofistulous malformations are typically hyperdynamic, with increased small or large branching vessels that show early arteriovenous shunting into enlarged draining veins. Malformations may involve small vessels or capillaries only, as in capillary hemangiomas. Angiographically, capillary hemangiomas typically show normal-sized arteries with an intense delayed capillary phase with normal or mildly dilated draining veins. Arteriovenous malformations may also involve only venous structures. These patients typically show normal arteries and capillaries. The dilated veins are seen best on venography.

Angiography of congenital AVMs is necessary to deter-

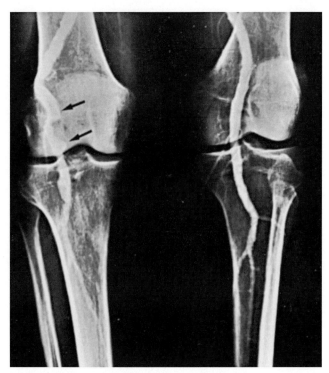

Figure 16–8. Aneurysm of left popliteal artery. Runoff study shows dilatation of the left popliteal artery with intraluminal filling defects consistent with thrombus *(arrows)*. Popliteal artery aneurysms may show as areas of fusiform or saccular dilatation or, in the presence of laminated thrombus, may show only minimal vessel irregularity. Ultrasonography is a useful method for determining the true extent of the aneurysm.

mine the nature and full extent of the malformation and should be performed prior to operative treatment. Angiography invariably reveals these lesions to be larger than appreciated on physical examination. It is of particular importance in the evaluation of hyperdynamic malformations and venous dysplasias. Selective injections with high volumes of contrast medium and rapid filming rates with DSA techniques should be employed (Fig. 16–9). MRI and magnetic resonance angiography (MRA) are also recommended in the evaluation of vascular malformations, as they provide delineation of the extent of the lesion and the relationship of the malformation to other structures.

VASCULAR TRAUMA

Vascular trauma can result from direct injury to the vessel from fracture dislocations, penetrating wounds, blunt trauma, repeated small trauma, or thermal injury. The angiographic findings in arterial trauma vary.[43–45] The most common observation is arterial spasm characterized by tapering and attenuation of the vessel with delayed flow. The vessels are usually draped and stretched in the areas of soft tissue swelling. Abrupt occlusion of the vessel may also be seen. Subintimal tears and dissections may be present. Thrombosis may occur, sometimes with distal emboli. False aneurysms, as well as frank extravasation, may be seen (Fig. 16–10). Arteriovenous fistulas are other sequelae. The arteriovenous fistulas characteristically show

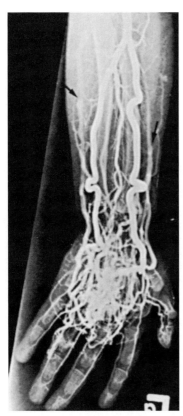

Figure 16–9. Congenital arteriovenous malformation. This 1.5-year-old girl was noted to have a pulsatile mass on the left hand. Transfemoral left subclavian arteriogram reveals markedly dilatated brachial, radial, and ulnar arteries. A dense tangle of vessels is seen projected over the metacarpals. Note the early-draining veins *(arrows)*. This is a hyperdynamic type of arteriovenous malformation that will progressively increase in size.

early filling of venous structures in the area of injury following an arterial injection (Fig. 16–11).

An important point that merits emphasis is that the clinical site of peripheral pulses distal to the site of trauma is not always a reliable indicator of extent of disease. The pulses may be reduced or absent when only spasm is present. Paradoxically, pulses may be good, even when fairly severe trauma to the artery is present.[46, 47] Because of this known disparity between the anatomic and clinical findings, angiography should be used early and often in cases of vascular trauma.

ABDOMINAL AORTOGRAPHY

Abdominal flush aortograms are usually performed via the femoral route. These are performed when evaluation of the abdominal aorta and its major branches is indicated. When specific information regarding organs supplied by major vessels is desired, selective arterial injections are made into the major aortic branches. Newer imaging techniques such as spiral CT angiography and MRA may provide a suitable alternative to conventional aortography when small vessel visualization is not required.

Specific Lesions

Atherosclerotic Disease

Atherosclerotic disease most commonly produces plaques, varying degrees of aortic narrowing, occlusion, and aneurysms of the aorta. Stenosis and occlusion of the aorta and its major branches occur most commonly below the renal arteries. Arteriograms will show localized or diffuse changes and eccentric or concentric narrowing. With high-grade stenoses, collateral vessels occur. When there is complete occlusion, arteriograms demonstrate the level of occlusion and site of reconstitution if the collateral vessels are opacified (Fig. 16–12). It is important to be aware of the major collateral pathways between visceral branches of the aorta. Major collateral pathways occur between the celiac and superior mesenteric artery and inferior mesenteric artery. The arc of Bühler is a fetal remnant connecting between the celiac and superior mesenteric arteries. The middle colic branch of the superior mesenteric artery and the left colic of the inferior mesenteric artery form anastomoses when there is occlusion or stenosis. Another major collateral channel between the superior and inferior mesenteric arteries is via the marginal artery of Drummond.

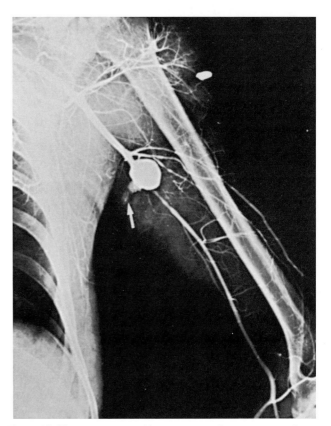

Figure 16–10. Post-traumatic false aneurysm with extravasation. This 34-year-old man was shot in the left shoulder *(the bullet fragment is seen in the upper arm)*. He presented with diminished pulses distally in the left arm and decreased neurologic function in the distribution of the ulnar and median nerves. Selective left axillary artery injection shows a large false aneurysm at the site of vessel disruption. There is evidence of spasm and displacement of the circumflex humeral arteries and muscular branches of the brachial artery in the area of soft tissue swelling. Extravasation of contrast medium is identified *(arrow)*.

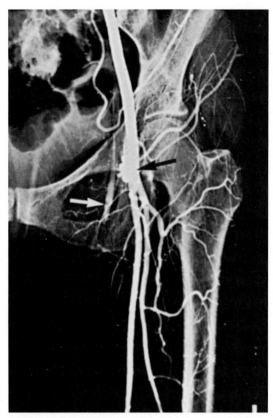

Figure 16–11. Post-traumatic arteriovenous fistula in left groin. This patient had undergone a left transfemoral aortogram for evaluation of hypertension. Two days later, a pulsatile mass appeared in the left side of the groin. A continuous bruit was present. Selective right transfemoral–left external iliac arteriogram reveals a false aneurysm of the common femoral artery at the puncture site *(black arrow)*. Fistulous communication with the femoral vein is present *(white arrow)*.

The arcade of Drummond is an anastomotic marginal colonic artery that runs along the mesenteric surface of the colon and gives off vasa recta to the bowel. This vessel forms an arcade with the marginal artery from the middle colic artery. It is distinct from the arch of Riolan or meandering mesomesenteric anastomosis of Felson, which is a left colic arterial branch that runs cephalad in the mesentery to anastomose with the middle colic artery near the splenic flexure (Figs. 16–13, 16–14, and 16–15).

Abdominal Aneurysms

Abdominal flush aortograms are commonly used to delineate the size and extent of arteriosclerotic aneurysms. The opacified lumen of the aorta does not always indicate the lumen and width of the aneurysm. The plain films obtained before the arrival of contrast must be carefully evaluated for the presence of linear calcifications. These represent calcification in the wall of the aorta. The distance between the linear calcification and the contrast-opacified aorta represents laminated thrombus in the aneurysm. The size of the aneurysm is estimated by measuring the total width of the aorta (Fig. 16–16).

Aneurysms of the hepatic and splenic artery may be identified on a flush injection or may require subselective

catheterization. Splenic aneurysms appear as bulbous, dilated structures and occur more frequently than those in the hepatic artery.

Mycotic aneurysms differ in appearance from atherosclerotic aneurysms in that they characteristically are saccu-

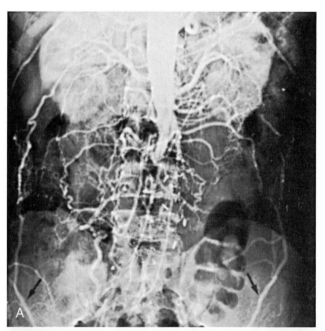

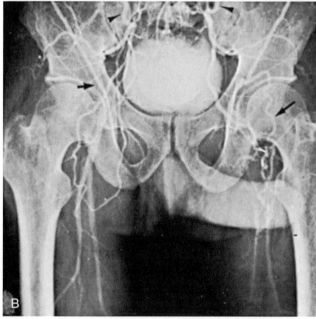

Figure 16–12. Collateral flow to pelvis in occlusion of the infrarenal abdominal aorta. *A,* The aorta is occluded just distal to the inferior mesenteric artery. Large lumbar arteries communicate bilaterally with the deep iliac circumflex arteries *(arrows)*. *B,* The deep iliac circumflex artery on the right *(short arrow)* fills retrograde back to the common femoral artery, which then fills antegrade to give rise to the right superficial and deep femoral arteries. On the left, the deep iliac circumflex communicates with collateral branches of the left femoral circumflex *(long arrow)* and profunda femoral. The iliofemoral arteries *(arrowheads)* also fill from lumbar collaterals retrograde back to the hypogastric arteries. On the left, inferior gluteal branches of the reconstituted hypogastric artery communicate with femoral circumflex branches, which collateralize the superficial and deep femoral arteries.

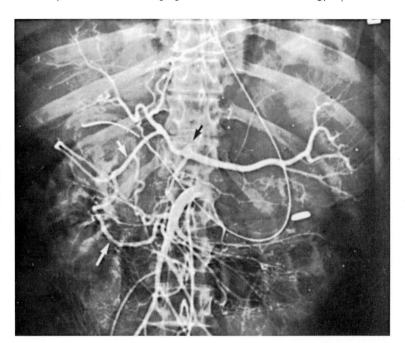

Figure 16–13. Collateral flow in occlusion of celiac axis. On the selective superior mesenteric artery injection there is filling of the inferior pancreatic duodenal artery *(long white arrow)*. This artery fills retrograde to communicate with the gastroduodenal artery *(short white arrow)*, which then fills retrograde back to the celiac trunk *(short black arrow)*. There is filling of the splenic and hepatic arteries. This collateral pathway is important in instances in which there is occlusion of either the celiac axis or the superior mesenteric artery.

lar or rounded in appearance. The lack of associated atherosclerotic changes and calcification aids in the diagnosis. These aneurysms have a propensity for rupture.[48]

Emboli arising from the aneurysms of the left ventricle after myocardial infarction, left atrial tumors, or aneurysms in the midaorta may embolize and produce complete occlusion of the abdominal aorta. Piercing trauma to the abdominal aorta can produce intimal damage, false aneurysms, hemorrhage, and arteriovenous fistulas.

Mesenteric Ischemia

More than 50% of cases of mesenteric ischemia are caused by reduced mesenteric flow from splanchnic vasoconstriction due to reduced cardiac output or shock.[49, 50] The vessels radiographically appear intensely vasoconstricted. Multiple segmental constrictions at the origins of vessels are seen. The finer arterial vessels fill poorly. The changes may be localized or diffuse. Treatment with intraarterial vasodilators such as papaverine and correction of the shock are necessary to prevent irreversible bowel infarction.[51]

In other cases, bowel ischemia is caused by atherosclerotic narrowing with thrombosis or emboli to major visceral branches. Superior mesenteric artery emboli are responsible for 40% to 50% of episodes of acute mesenteric ischemia. These emboli usually originate from a mural or an atrial thrombus.[52, 53]

Occlusions or narrowings involving the origin of the celiac axis, superior mesenteric artery, and inferior mesenteric artery are best seen on an off-lateral view using an abdominal flush injection. Other causes of narrowing include median arcuate ligament compression of the diaphragm, fibromuscular dysplasia, tumors, aneurysms, or arteritis (Fig. 16–17).

Aortic Grafts

Arteriography used to evaluate the status of abdominal and peripheral grafts may reveal a variety of problems. Occlusion of the graft is the most frequently seen problem; others are the development of aneurysms in the host artery near the suture line and stenosis of host arteries at anastomotic sites. Infection or poor healing can result in disruption of the anastomosis, with rupture and retroperitoneal leaking, false aneurysm, fistula, or sinus tract formation (Fig. 16–18). Aortoenteric or aortocaval fistulas may occur. Angiography may be useful if leakage of contrast medium or pseudoaneurysm is seen but is primarily useful for planning the technical aspects of removal of the infected graft and operative repair. Endoscopy is the recommended diagnostic procedure, particularly to rule out other causes of upper gastrointestinal bleeding. It may show erosion of the duodenum. CT may be quite helpful in the stable patient, as often an aneurysm can be visualized, and when there is associated infection, perigraft collections of fluid or gas may be seen.[54]

In aortography of prosthetic grafts, it is preferable to avoid puncture of the graft itself because of the potential disruption of the pseudointima, introduction of infection, or induction of thrombosis. In some instances, however, puncture of a graft is necessary owing to unavailability of other sites of entry. Graft puncture, however, can be performed safely with careful technique,[55] but punctures of infected grafts should be avoided.

GASTROINTESTINAL BLEEDING

Selective arteriography is useful in the detection of bleeding into the peritoneal cavity or bleeding into the gastrointestinal tract. Bleeding sites may be missed angiographically if selective injections are not employed. Bleeding sites are identified angiographically as collections of extravasated radiopaque contrast medium at the site of blood vessel disruption.[56] The bleeding may arise from lesions of the gastrointestinal tract such as ulcers, gastritis, esophageal varices, diverticula, false aneurysms, arteriovenous malformations, hemangiomas, or tumors. Bleeding rates of 0.5

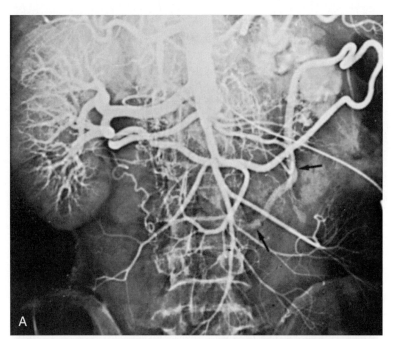

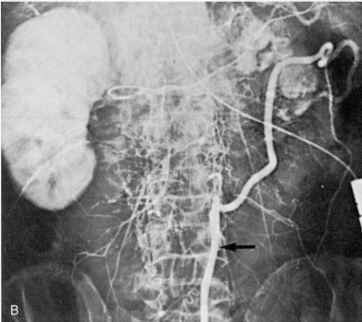

Figure 16–14. Collateral supply to inferior mesenteric artery. *A,* Translumbar aortogram shows complete occlusion of the abdominal aorta just distal to the takeoff of the right renal artery. The left renal artery is occluded. The left kidney is atrophic and calcified secondary to previous tuberculosis. The superior mesenteric artery is visualized. The middle colic branch is markedly hypertrophied. In the region of the splenic flexure, it communicates with a hypertrophied left colic artery, which fills retrograde back to its origin from the inferior mesenteric artery *(arrows). B,* The inferior mesenteric then fills antegrade *(arrow).* This collateral network provides flow to the descending colon and rectum in instances when the inferior mesenteric artery is occluded.

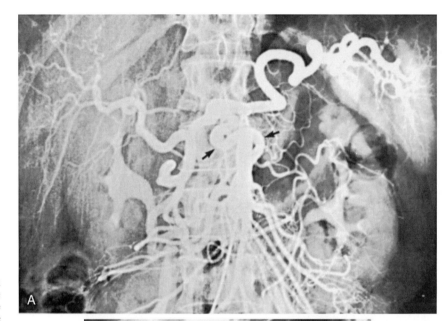

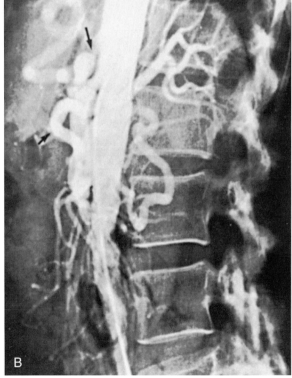

Figure 16–15. Hypertrophied arc of Bühler in celiac axis stenosis. *A,* On this superior mesenteric artery injection there is retrograde filling of the gastroduodenal artery with filling back to the celiac axis and with filling of the splenic artery and hepatic artery. In addition, there is a vessel connecting the superior mesenteric artery with the celiac trunk. This ventral anastomosis represents a remnant of the tenth vitelline artery and is called the arc of Bühler *(short arrows). B,* The lateral view shows a high-grade stenosis at the origin of the celiac axis *(long arrow)* and the ventral position of the arc of Bühler *(short arrow).* The gastroduodenal artery in this patient projects posteriorly.

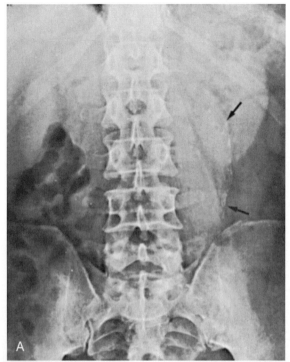

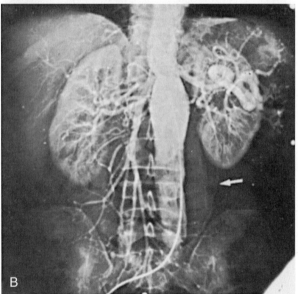

Figure 16–16. Abdominal aortic aneurysm. *A,* Plain films of the abdomen show calcification in the wall of the aneurysm *(arrows). B,* Flush abdominal aortogram shows an infrarenal fusiform abdominal aneurysm extending down to the iliac bifurcation. The origin of the right renal artery was seen on earlier films. The opacified channel does not indicate the true extent of the aneurysm. The calcifications indicate the width of the aneurysm *(arrow).* The soft tissue density between the opacified lumen and the calcified wall of the aorta represents laminated thrombus. In some instances, the calcifications may be very subtle. Abdominal aortic aneurysms can be missed on angiography if this pitfall is not considered.

mL/minute may be detected. Slow-bleeding sites are difficult to localize. Endoscopy should be performed before arteriography for upper gastrointestinal bleeding to help localize the bleeding site and thus minimize the study time and volume of contrast medium required for the arteriogram. With slow bleeding, the success rate is low

unless an anatomic defect is present at the bleeding site. Findings such as the presence of a large early-draining vein may indicate the site of an arteriovenous malformation. Angiodysplasia presents arteriographically as a dense stain with an early-draining vein. Tumor neovascularity or arterial encasement may help localize the site of a slow ooze. A preferable approach to the localization of slowly bleeding sites is the utilization of technetium 99m (^{99m}Tc) sulfur colloid[57] or other ^{99m}Tc-labeled blood pool agents[58] injected intravenously. These blood pool agents collect at the site of hemorrhage as radioactive blood that can be detected using a gamma camera 2 to 40 minutes after injection. These agents can be utilized to detect active sites of bleeding in the gastrointestinal tract and are capable of detecting rates as slow as 0.1 mL/minute. They are particularly useful in the diagnosis of lower gastrointestinal bleeding. The technique can serve as a direct guide to surgery or can aid in delineation of the region to be further studied angiographically.

PORTAL HYPERTENSION

Evaluation of the patient with portal hypertension may be required to demonstrate the site of gastrointestinal bleeding or to provide preoperative vascular evaluation in preparation for a shunt procedure. In the presence of portal hypertension, gastrointestinal bleeding may be from varices or other causes, such as gastritis, Mallory-Weiss tears, or ulcer disease. If selective arterial injections fail to reveal the bleeding site, the bleeding can be assumed to be from varices. Venous bleeding is almost never demonstrated angiographically, and the diagnosis of esophageal bleeding is made on angiography only indirectly by demonstrating portal hypertension and excluding other sites of bleeding.

Portal hypertension may be due to prehepatic obstruction, such as portal vein or splenic vein thrombosis. Intrahepatic obstruction is due to such entities as Laënnec's or biliary cirrhosis. Schistosomiasis causes an intrahepatic presinusoidal obstruction. Suprahepatic obstruction occurs in Budd-Chiari syndrome.

Routine angiographic evaluation of the portal system in patients with portal hypertension can be performed in several ways. Evaluation consists of measurement of the hepatic vein wedge pressure and visualization of the portal system. Hepatic vein wedge pressures are readily obtained by entry into hepatic veins using a catheter that has been passed up the inferior vena cava and into a hepatic vein. In the wedge position, the catheter in the hepatic vein measures the pressure in the communicating sinusoids. The normal sinusoidal pressure is between 3 and 11 mm Hg. This pressure includes not only that within the sinusoids but also the intraabdominal pressure, which can be increased by heart failure or ascites. The true corrected sinusoidal pressure is obtained by subtracting from the wedge pressure the component of pressure transmitted from the inferior vena cava. This can be done by subtracting the wedge pressure from the pressure measured with the catheter lying free within the hepatic vein. The free hepatic vein pressure normally measures between 1 and 6 mm Hg. Therefore, the corrected sinusoidal pressure is normally 1 to 5 mm Hg. The corrected sinusoidal pres-

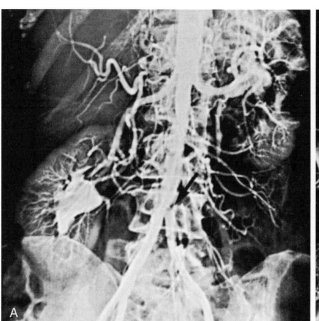

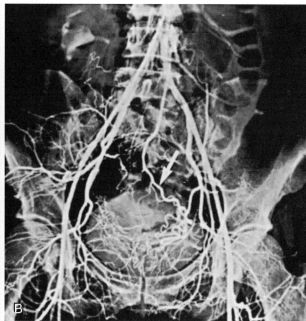

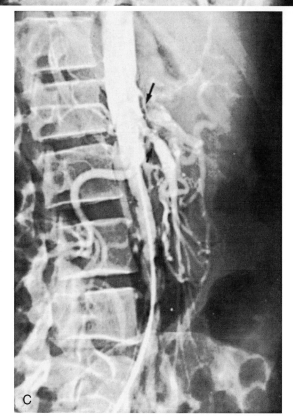

Figure 16–17. Abdominal angina due to superior mesenteric, celiac, and inferior mesenteric artery occlusion. This woman had symptoms of claudication and abdominal angina. *A*, Flush aortogram shows no filling of the celiac axis. The superior mesenteric artery is patent, and there is retrograde filling of the gastroduodenal artery by way of the pancreatic arcade. There is faint opacification of the left splenic artery. There is no filling of the inferior mesenteric artery branches. In addition, a high-grade stenosis is seen at the origin of the left common iliac artery *(arrow)*. *B*, Off-lateral view abdominal aortogram shows a tapered occlusion of the celiac axis at its origin *(long arrow)* and a significant stenosis at the origin of the superior mesenteric artery with poststenotic dilation *(short arrow)*. The inferior mesenteric artery is occluded. *C*, Pelvic arteriogram shows collaterals arising from the left hypogastric artery communicating with the superior hemorrhoidal artery, which fills retrograde back to the main trunk of the inferior mesenteric artery *(arrow)*. This collateral supply to the large bowel is jeopardized by the presence of the high-grade left common iliac stenosis.

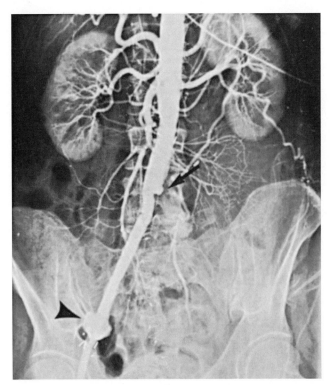

Figure 16–18. Aortobifemoral graft complications. Translumbar aortogram shows the left limb of the aortobifemoral graft to be completely occluded at its origin *(arrow)*. Collaterals are seen along the left lateral aspect of the abdominal wall, which will reconstitute the left superficial and deep femoral arteries distally. The right limb of the graft is patent. A false aneurysm is seen at the distal anastomosis *(arrowhead)*.

sure may be elevated owing to increased resistance at the sinusoidal level, as in cirrhosis or at the postsinusoidal level. With mild portal hypertension, the corrected sinusoidal pressure is 6 to 10 mm Hg. Severe portal hypertension is present when the corrected sinusoidal pressure is 19 mm Hg or higher. In presinusoidal obstruction or portal vein thrombosis, no pressures can be transmitted to the sinusoids, and the hepatic vein wedge pressures are usually normal or subnormal.[59-61]

At present, visualization of the portal vein is most commonly accomplished using arterial portography with injection of the celiac and superior mesenteric arteries and filming carried to the venous phase. Vasodilators such as tolazoline are administered intraarterially to enhance visualization of the venous phase.[62] DSA should be utilized. Adequate volumes of contrast medium are necessary, and filming must be sufficiently delayed. Visualization of the portal vein can be accomplished with the direct injection of contrast into the spleen, but this is rarely done because of the risk of bleeding.[63] A percutaneous transhepatic approach can also be used but is also associated with increased morbidity. Rarely, a transjugular vein approach is used.

Postoperative evaluation of portosystemic shunts can also be accomplished with arterial injections. Delayed films show filling of the inferior vena cava. In many instances, the shunt can be directly cannulated by manipulation of the catheter passed into the inferior vena cava. Pressure gradients may be measured with this technique.

When evaluation of the hepatic veins is desired, direct injection of contrast medium into the hepatic veins is performed. This is indicated in the workup of suspected cases of Budd-Chiari syndrome. In this entity, the hepatic veins appear as a disorganized, spidery network.

SPLENIC ARTERIOGRAPHY

The indications for splenic arteriography have changed with the availability of other noninvasive imaging modalities. Good visualization of the spleen can be accomplished with CT, ultrasonography, or liver scans. CT is capable of detecting both splenic laceration and subcapsular hematomas.[64] Currently, diagnostic angiography is performed infrequently for splenic trauma. A useful algorithm[65] for splenic evaluation is CT or ultrasonography as the primary imaging method. If these studies are normal or diagnostic or show a diffuse infiltrative disease, no further imaging is needed. If the nature of the lesions remains uncertain, angiography is employed as the definitive diagnostic method. The algorithm is short-circuited only if there is a high suspicion of splenic trauma in the precarious patient. Angiography is indicated in the evaluation of splenic artery aneurysms and the diagnosis of splenic arteriovenous fistulas. Other current indications for splenic arteriography include the evaluation of patients with portal hypertension or gastrointestinal bleeding or when differentiation of accessory spleens from vascular pancreatic masses is needed. Splenic arteriography is also performed as part of therapeutic embolization in patients with hypersplenism or trauma or preoperatively to reduce intraoperative blood loss during splenectomy.

Splenic arteriography is performed by selective splenic artery injection.

Typical Angiographic Findings

Extravasation of contrast material is the diagnostic finding in splenic rupture. Mottling of the parenchymal phase is not specific and may be seen with splenic contusion in the absence of rupture. Other characteristic findings are a large avascular area with displacement of the intrasplenic branches, compression of the opacified spleen in the region of the hematoma, and clear fracture in the splenic contour. Simultaneous filling of the splenic artery and vein may be seen.[66, 67]

Splenic artery aneurysms are the most common intraabdominal aneurysms, after those in the aorta and iliac arteries. They are observed most frequently in women of childbearing age and have a high propensity for rupture. Some may be congenital, and others are arteriosclerotic in origin. They may calcify and typically appear as a large, smooth-walled, contrast-filled sac.

RENAL ARTERIOGRAPHY

Although newer imaging techniques have reduced the indications for arteriography of the kidneys, angiography remains the foundation for many diagnostic and interventional procedures involving the kidney. Angiography remains the most accurate method for diagnosing renal vascular hypertension and provides the route by which renal artery stenosis can often be corrected. It is used in the management of vascular injuries to the kidney and pelvis, where it can identify the source of bleeding and provide a route for embolization of the vessel. It is used for vascular mapping in horseshoe kidney and selected cases of renal neoplasm. It also plays an important role in the evaluation of transplanted kidneys.

Evaluation of the renal arteries is performed with a flush aortogram followed by selective arterial injections. Flush injections are utilized to identify accessory renal arteries, which can arise anywhere from the low thoracic aorta down to the iliac artery. These are also necessary for identification of collateral vessels to the kidney when flow in the renal artery is obstructed. The extrarenal collateral vessels arise from the ureteric, gonadal, adrenal, lumbar, and intercostal arteries.[68] The flush injection may provide sufficient information for diagnosis. Selective injections should be performed carefully if there is severe atherosclerotic plaque formation, because elevation of a plaque during injection can result in renal artery occlusion.

Angiographic Findings

Obstruction of the renal arteries may be caused by diseases of the aorta. Atherosclerotic plaques or aneurysms can obstruct renal artery origins. Thrombotic occlusion of the aorta above the renal arteries and aortic dissections that extend into the renal artery can also compromise renal blood flow, as can aortitis, abdominal coarctation, and neurofibromatosis. Atherosclerotic disease of the renal arteries usually involves the proximal third of the artery, producing small plaques or complete occlusion. Atherosclerotic lesions may be eccentric or concentric and may be bilateral. Intrarenal branch stenoses also occur. They may be due to atherosclerotic disease, renal artery dysplasias, thrombosis, embolus, or arteritis. Occasionally, these may be difficult to detect on flush aortography. The parenchymal phase of the arteriogram may show the ischemic area well. When there is a question of branch stenoses, selective arteriography with multiple views is indicated.

Fibromuscular Dysplasia

Fibromuscular dysplasia (FMD), affecting primarily young females, occurs most frequently in the middle and distal third of the main renal arteries.[69, 70] The lesions are usually bilateral. Branch stenoses occur more frequently than in atherosclerotic disease.

Several types of FMDs occur. They include (1) intimal fibroplasia, (2) medial fibroplasia with aneurysms, (3) medial fibromuscular hyperplasia, (4) adventitial hyperplasia, and (5) subadventitial hyperplasia.[71, 72] Angiographically, they may be difficult to distinguish. The commonest type is medial fibroplasia with aneurysms. Angiographically, this typically gives a string-of-beads appearance to the renal artery. The appearance is caused by alternating areas of narrowing due to thickened segments of media partially replaced with collagen, alternating with areas of dilatation where the internal elastic lamina and media are partially disrupted. Focal short stenosis or long segmental stenoses may be due to medial fibromuscular hyperplasia or intimal fibroplasia. In subadventitial perimedial fibroplasia, the segment of the vessel with the string-of-beads appearance is narrower than areas of uninvolved vessel. Tubular lesions characterized by elongated smooth concentric narrowing of the renal arteries may be due to adventitial hyperplasia. Mixed lesions can occur in the same patient. Mural aneurysms may form at the site of medial disruption, and true aneurysms may form in the region of poststenotic dilatation of the renal artery. In a minority of patients, dissection of the renal artery can occur, with the dissection extending into primary or secondary renal branches.

Multiple vessels may be involved, including the carotid arteries, vertebral arteries, and splanchnic and iliac arteries[73] (Fig. 16–19).

Renal Trauma

A clinical radiologic classification has been proposed as an aid to the use of radiographic procedures in the diagnosis of renal trauma.[74] Minor renal injuries are those in which there has been damage to the renal parenchyma but no extension to the renal capsule and no involvement of the pelvocalyceal system. These rarely require arteriography. The intravenous urogram in these patients usually shows a normal urinary tract, with only minimal delay in function on the affected side. Major renal injuries in which both parenchymal and capsular involvement are present usually result in damage to the collecting system. The intravenous urogram in these patients may show extravasation of contrast. Arteriography is indicated in these patients to determine the extent of the injury and the status of the vascular anatomy. When multiple organ involvement is suspected and the patient shows no signs of impending shock, CT may be of value in the detection of early hemorrhage. Critical injuries of the kidney are those in which the renal rupture extends into the pedicle. Exsanguinating hemorrhage may occur in a few minutes. The intravenous urogram is useful in determining the status of the contralateral kidney. The involved kidney is usually nonfunctioning. If the patient is sufficiently stable, arteriography demonstrates the avulsed pedicle or laceration. There is a notable incidence of adjacent organ involvement in pedicle injury. Liver, splenic, or pancreatic damage or damage to the contralateral kidney may be present. Arteriography should encompass an evaluation of these other organs. Thrombosis of the renal artery secondary to trauma is uncommon. It usually involves the left kidney.

Renal Arteriovenous Fistulas

Renal arteriovenous fistulas may be acquired or congenital in origin.[75] Acquired traumatic fistulas are most commonly the result of percutaneous biopsy, occurring in almost 15% of patients undergoing biopsy.[76] Penetrating abdominal trauma is another major cause. Arteriography is indicated and typically shows a dilated renal artery with fistulous

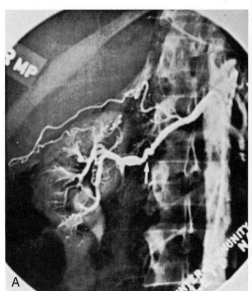

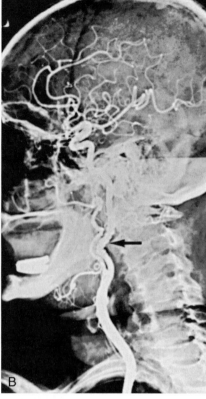

Figure 16–19. Fibromuscular dysplasia. *A,* The middle and distal portion of the right renal artery shows a string-of-beads appearance typical of medial fibroplasia with aneurysm *(arrow). B,* Selective left internal carotid artery injection shows typical string-of-beads appearance of fibromuscular dysplasia (medial fibroplasia with aneurysm) in the proximal portion of the left internal carotid artery *(arrow).*

communication to an early-draining vein. Many of these fistulas can be treated by selected transcatheter arterial occlusion rather than operation.

Renal Artery Aneurysms

Renal artery aneurysms may be congenital, traumatic, degenerative, or inflammatory in origin. They may occur in children but are usually seen in elderly patients, except when they are a sequela of renal artery dysplasia. Hypertension is associated in 72% to 85% of patients.[77] Aneurysms are saccular or fusiform, with the fusiform type seen most frequently in atherosclerotic vascular disease. Approximately 50% of renal artery aneurysms have calcium in their walls. As a rule, calcified aneurysms do not tend to rupture, whereas those without calcium tend to rupture spontaneously.

RENAL DIALYSIS FISTULAS

These surgically constructed arteriovenous fistulas are usually placed in the forearm connecting the radial artery and cephalic vein. The fistulas may be externally created shunts, such as the Scribner shunt,[78] or internal fistulas.[79] The internal fistulas are end-to-side, side-to-side, or end-to-end anastomoses. Dacron prostheses, saphenous veins, or bovine carotid arteries may be interposed between the radial artery and the cephalic vein.[80] Angiography is indicated in the evaluation of these shunts when there is evidence of shunt failure.[81, 82] Problems indicative of faulty shunt function include reduction in the thrill over the

shunt. Increased resistance to return during dialysis suggests stenosis or blockage in the venous limb, whereas decreased flow on withdrawing suggests obstruction in the proximal venous limb or in the artery supplying the fistula. Angiography is used to delineate stenosis or thrombosis. These can occur in either the arterial or the venous limb of the graft. Venous stenoses may arise a considerable distance from the fistula. Pseudoaneurysms develop in the graft at venipuncture sites, and aneurysms may occur in the artery (Figs. 16–20 and 16–21).

Angiographic evaluation of the aforementioned lesions is performed by direct percutaneous puncture and injection into the shunt. Thrombosed shunts are routinely managed with local infusion of a thrombolytic agent followed by balloon angioplasty of any outflow or inflow stenoses (see Ch. 20 for discussion of fibrinolytic therapy and percutaneous transluminal angioplasty). Ischemia of the hand distal to the shunt may also occur. This is best evaluated with a subclavian artery injection performed via the femoral artery approach.

VENOGRAPHY

Extremities

Venography of an extremity is indicated in the evaluation of venous obstruction. The obstruction may be due to thrombosis, tumor invasion, extrinsic compression, or trauma.

Acute venous thrombosis appears radiographically as an intraluminal filling defect outlined by a rim of contrast

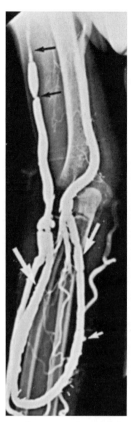

Figure 16–20. Bovine graft arteriovenous fistula. The "U"-shaped limb of the bovine graft is identified *(long white arrows)*. Multiple small false aneurysms are seen at site of previous puncture for dialysis. Note the dilatation of the arterial lumen *(short white arrow)*. Arterialization of vessels is a common finding in long-standing dialysis fistulas. In the venous limb, multiple stenoses are seen in the vein *(black arrows)*.

media. As the thrombus organizes and adheres to the vessel wall, the rim is lost, and complete occlusion of the vessels occurs. Recanalized vessels have a thin, stringy appearance in which the venous valves have been obliterated. Webs may develop, and collateral vessels become prominent. Superficial varices develop.

Lower Extremity Venography

Contrast venography is the most reliable technique for the detection of deep venous thrombosis (DVT).[83–85] Color duplex flow imaging has been found to have high accuracy for detection of DVT above the knee. It is less accurate in the detection of thrombi below the knee. Currently, it is used frequently for screening and may obviate the need for contrast venography.[86] Ascending contrast venography is performed by introducing a 21- or 19-gauge scalp vein needle into a dorsal foot vein and injecting contrast medium. The patient should be on a radiographic tilt table at a 45- to 60-degree tilt with the extremity under study not bearing weight. Nonionic contrast agent is injected and overhead or spot films made as the contrast medium travels up the venous system. Studies are usually done with filming both with and without the application of tourniquets to improve filling of the deep venous system. Complications of the procedure are few but include exacerbation of

thrombophlebitis as a result of endothelial irritation from contact with the contrast medium. Phlebitis may be induced. The incidence of these complications can be reduced if the contrast medium is flushed from the veins with heparinized saline at the end of the study. Extravasation of contrast medium at the injection site may result in a skin slough.

Descending venography is used to assess for incompetence of venous valves in patients with varicose veins and for preoperative evaluation before valve surgery. It is performed by placing a short catheter percutaneously in the femoral vein. With the patient in the upright position (70 to 90 degrees), injection of iodinated contrast is made. Reflux of contrast material inferiorly beyond the midthigh is indicative of incompetent valves.

Upper Extremity Venography

Upper extremity venography is performed with the injection of contrast medium introduced via a scalp vein needle positioned in an arm vein. The technique is useful for the detection of thrombus and in evaluation of patients with venous obstruction due to the thoracic outlet syndrome.

Arteriography is also indicated in the workup of the thoracic outlet syndrome in patients with diminished pulses or asymmetrical cuff blood pressures in the two extremities. It is also indicated when a bruit is present in the affected

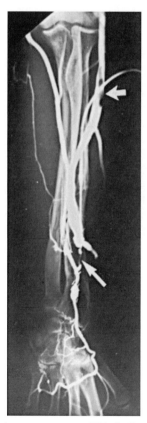

Figure 16–21. Dialysis arteriovenous (AV) fistula. A long, high-grade stenosis is seen in the venous limb of this dialysis AV fistula *(long arrow)*. In addition, an intraluminal filling defect representing thrombus is seen proximally in the venous limb *(short arrow)*. Lesions in the venous limb may arise a considerable distance from the fistula.

extremity or when a source of peripheral emboli is sought. The arteriogram can be performed via a femoral artery approach with the catheter tip positioned in the subclavian artery. As with venography, the arteriogram should be performed with the arm in a neutral position and after maneuvers that elicit symptoms.[87, 88] In positive studies, the site of arterial or venous compression is identified.

Venacavography

Superior venacavography is used primarily for the evaluation of the superior vena cava syndrome, for evaluation of mediastinal masses, and for delineation of superior vena cava anatomy in patients with suspected anomalies of pulmonary or systemic venous return. Scalp vein needles or short intracatheters are placed in each antecubital vein, and contrast medium is injected bilaterally. Radiographic signs of occlusion are intraluminal filling defects and collateral vessels (Fig. 16–22).

Inferior venacavography is indicated in the detection of caval obstruction. It should also be performed before caval umbrella placement. Caval obstruction may be secondary to thrombus, webs, or primary or secondary tumors (Figs. 16–23 and 16–24). The preferred approach is with placement of catheters in both femoral veins and simultaneous injection of contrast medium. Alternatively, a single catheter may be placed just at the origin of the inferior vena cava. In the presence of femoral vein occlusion, the catheter may be introduced via the internal jugular vein or an antecubital vein and passed down the superior vena cava. The cava is easily visualized. If selective renal or adrenal venography is desired, selective catheterization of these vessels can be performed using either a femoral or an antecubital vein approach.

THROMBOLYTIC THERAPY

Thrombolytic therapy plays an important role in the treatment of peripheral vessel occlusion and graft thrombolysis. Streptokinase, urokinase, and recombinant tissue-type plasminogen activator (rt-PA) and reteplase have all been utilized. All are plasminogen activators and produce lysis by stimulating the conversion of plasminogen to its active form, plasmin, a relatively unspecific proteinase that degrades the fibrin matrix of a thrombus. First-generation thrombolytic agents, streptokinase, and urokinase are non–fibrin selective and convert both circulating and fibrin-bound plasminogen to plasmin.[89] Urokinase and streptokinase are not fibrin-specific, and act not only on plasminogen within the clot but also on plasminogen throughout the circulation. Urokinase acts directly on plasminogen to form plasmin; streptokinase must first form an activated complex with plasminogen. The plasmin that is formed subsequently degrades plasma proteins, including fibrin, fibrinogen, plasminogen, and factors V and VIII. A systemic lytic state is achieved that is characterized by depletion of fibrinogen, plasminogen, and α_2-antiplasmin, prolongation of the thrombin time, and accumulation of fibrin split products.

Second-generation thrombolytics such as tissue plasminogen activator (t-PA) are fibrin selective because they preferentially activate fibrin-bound but not fluid-phase plasminogen. The fibrin selectivity of t-PA is due to its high-affinity binding to fibrin. High-fibrin-affinity agents bind directly to fibrin and are avidly taken up by the desirable fibrin plugs that seal vascular defects such as those intracranially or at sites of peptic ulceration or in the retroperitoneum. The third-generation thrombolytic agent, reteplase, is a recombinant plasminogen activator derived from t-PA. Reteplase differs structurally from t-PA and consists of the kringle-2 and protease domains. It is a relatively fibrin-specific thrombolytic agent. The fibrin binding of reteplase at therapeutic concentrations in vitro is about that of urokinase, which is 30% that of t-PA.[90]

Streptokinase was first used in humans in 1959[91] and the clinical use of urokinase soon followed.[92] The first-generation agents, streptokinase and urokinase, were both utilized in the cooperative Urokinase Pulmonary Embolism Trials in the early 1970s.[93, 94] While the benefit of systemic fibrinolytic therapy was noted, it was also noted that systemic therapy was associated with a high incidence of hemorrhagic complications. In an effort to circumvent these complications, Dotter and colleagues[95] proposed a "low-dose regimen" with injection of the streptokinase intraarterially through a catheter with the tip embedded in the clot.[96] Lysis could be achieved with streptokinase doses of 5000 units/hour; however, unpredictable bleeding and a systemic lytic state occurred in a significant number of patients.[97] Similar experience was encountered by other authors.[98, 99] Complete lysis was noted in 44% to 47% of

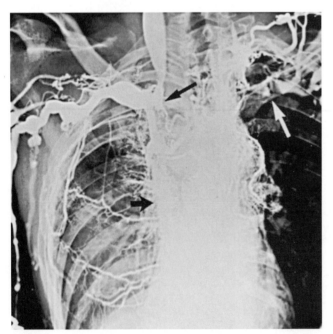

Figure 16–22. Superior vena cava syndrome. This 37-year-old man with carcinoma of the lung developed progressive superior vena cava syndrome. His superior venacavogram, performed by simultaneous injection into right and left antecubital veins, shows complete occlusion of the right subclavian vein (*long black arrow*) with reflux up the right internal jugular vein. Abundant collaterals are present. Mediastinal and intercostal collaterals are identified on the right side communicating with the azygous (*short black arrow*). On the left, there is thrombus with occlusion of the left subclavian vein (*white arrow*) and extensive collaterals to the azygous.

Figure 16–23. Thrombosis of the inferior vena cava. This patient with lymphoma was admitted to the hospital with hemoptysis. During attempted pulmonary angiography, thrombosis of the inferior vena cava was identified. *A,* Shows large intraluminal thrombus in both common iliac veins and in the inferior vena cava *(black arrows).* There is filling of both right and left ascending lumbar veins and extensive paravertebral collaterals. *B,* Oblique view showing extent of thrombus *(white arrow).*

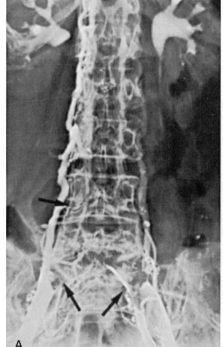
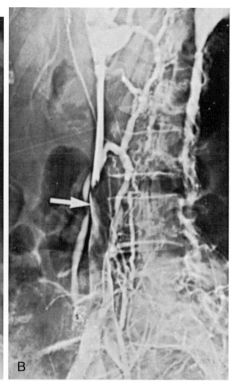

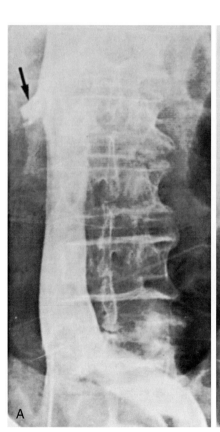
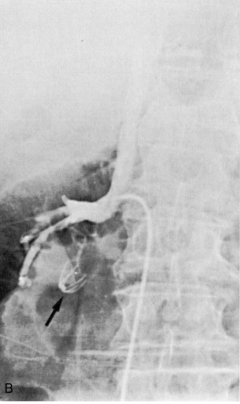

Figure 16–24. Misplaced Mobin-Uddin umbrella. *A,* Inferior venacavogram before umbrella placement shows reflux into right renal vein. Because of poor filling, the wash-in defect in the left renal vein is not identified. *B,* Selective right renal vein injection following placement of the Mobin-Uddin umbrella shows the umbrella *(arrow)* residing outside the inferior vena cava. The umbrella is positioned in an aberrant double right renal vein. The point of entry into the inferior vena cava was not detected. Multiple renal veins occur more frequently on the right side.

patients (Fig. 16–25), but major hemorrhage rates ranged from 8% to 12%.[98, 99]

In spite of the bleeding problems with streptokinase, the technique of delivery of the thrombolytic agent via selectively placed catheters positioned at the site of thrombus is the method by which thrombolytic therapy is currently administered for peripheral vascular occlusions. The

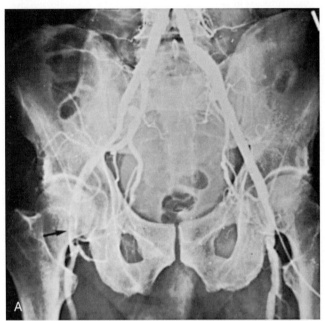

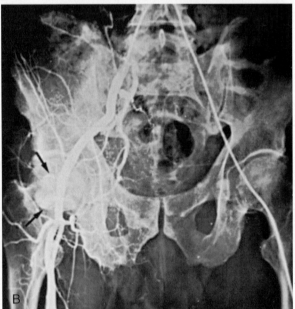

Figure 16–25. Low-dose streptokinase infusion therapy. *A,* Shortly after cardiac catheterization, this patient developed claudication of the right lower extremity. A left transfemoral pelvic arteriogram shows narrowing of the right external iliac artery and intraluminal thrombus in the common femoral artery *(arrow).* The right superficial femoral artery was occluded. He was treated with low-dose intraarterial streptokinase for lysis of the clot for 24 hours. *B,* After treatment with streptokinase, a selective right common iliac artery injection shows normal caliber of the external iliac artery, lysis of the thrombus in the common femoral artery, and filling of the superficial femoral artery. There is, however, also a new false aneurysm *(arrows),* which developed as a result of clot lysis at the previous heart catheterization site.

progression of thrombolysis is monitored by follow-up arteriography and the catheter advanced through the thrombus as needed. The problem of hemorrhage with streptokinase and urokinase is further complicated because there is no one laboratory test that reflects the degree of fibrinolytic therapy or the likelihood of hemorrhage.[100] Bleeding, however, is more likely to occur if the fibrinogen level is less than 100 mg/dL. Additional potential problems that may be encountered with low-dose therapy include sheathing of thrombus around the proximal portion of the catheter, and distal embolization of thrombus fragments during fibrinolytic therapy. Because of the risk of hemorrhage and the lack of specific laboratory monitoring guidelines, contraindications to streptokinase therapy and thrombolytic therapy include recent ischemic CNS events, active bleeding, open wounds, coagulopathy, and recent operation (within 10 days). Bleeding is likely to occur from previous arterial puncture sites, and when lytic infusion is planned, the study should be performed from a single site of catheter entry. Reduction in the dosage of heparin used is also recommended.

Unpredictable bleeding problems and antibody formation to streptokinase interfering with its action resulted in its replacement by urokinase for treatment of peripheral vascular occlusion.

McNamara and Fischer[101] reported complete clot lysis in 70 of 93 (75%) patients using a high-dose urokinase regimen starting with 4000 IU/minute until lysis of a channel through the occlusion with reestablishment of antegrade flow has been accomplished, usually within 2 hours. The dose is then decreased to 1000 to 2000 IU/minute until complete clot lysis has occurred. Intravenous heparin is concomitantly administered. A lower incidence of significant bleeding was observed, 4% versus 13% for streptokinase, and the reported mean infusion time was shorter with urokinase (18 vs. 41 hours).

Cragg and associates[102] compared high-dose and low-dose urokinase regimens in lysis of native arterial and graft occlusions. Their high-dose regimen was 250,000 IU/hour followed by 125,000 IU/hour, and the low dose was 50,000 IU/hour. No significant differences were noted between the high-dose and low-dose groups with respect to mean times to lysis or mean infusion durations. Clinical success was achieved in 65% to 85% of cases. Up until 1998, when it was removed from the market by the Food and Drug Administration (FDA), urokinase was the preferred agent for peripheral arterial, venous, and graft thrombolysis.

t-PA is a serine protease present in most body tissues[103] and similar to the plasminogen activator produced by human vascular endothelial cells.[104] t-PA has a low affinity for circulating plasminogen but a high affinity for fibrin. In the presence of thrombus, both t-PA and plasminogen bind to the fibrin on the surface of the clot. The proteolytic capacity of t-PA increases dramatically in the fibrin domain, and fibrin-bound t-PA activates the conversion of fibrin-bound plasminogen to plasmin, which lyses the thrombus. Because plasmin production is confined primarily to the site of the clot, there should be less derangement of systemic coagulation than that seen with urokinase or streptokinase. The half-life of t-PA in the circulation is 5 minutes. There is evidence that the fibrinolytic activity at the site of a thrombus may continue for several hours after administration is completed.[105] The currently used t-PA is produced by rt-PA. Two-chain and one-chain configurations are available. Currently available rt-PA (manufacturing process G11035) is predominantly single-chain but is likely converted in vivo to the two-chain form by the action of plasmin. The circulating half-life of single-chain rt-PA is on the order of 4 minutes. The contraindications to its use are similar to those of the other thrombolytic agents.

Several different rt-PA dosing regimens have been employed. Risius and colleagues[106] used rt-PA at a dose of 0.1 mg/kg/hour for 1 to 6 hours in 25 patients with lower extremity thromboembolic occlusions (13 thrombosed arteries, 12 thrombosed bypass grafts). The infusion catheter was inserted directly into the thrombus. Thrombolysis occurred in 23 of 25 patients (92%), with time to lysis ranging from 1.0 to 6.5 hours (average lysis time of 3.6 hours). In 15 of 25 patients, fibrinogen levels were maintained above 50% of baseline.

No major complications directly attributable to rt-PA infusions occurred. rt-PA infusions resulted in decreases in plasma fibrinogen, plasminogen, and α_2-antiplasmin levels and in increased plasma levels of fibrin split products. In general, longer infusion times (i.e., higher total dose) resulted in a greater decrease in the aforementioned levels, indicating a systemic lytic state with varying degrees of fibrinolysis.

In the STILE trial rt-PA was administered at a dose of 0.05 μg/kg/hour for a maximum of 12 hours. Systemic heparinization was used and major bleeding complications occurred in 5.6% of patients.[107] Verstraete and associates[108] demonstrated that as rt-PA infusion durations increase, α_2-antiplasmin will be consumed and systemic fibrinogenolysis will occur. In addition, they demonstrated that a large dose infused over a short period of time results in less systemic lytic activity than a small dose infused over a long period of time. Current experience suggests that the fibrin specificity of rt-PA is relative. With longer infusion times, this fibrin specificity can be overcome and fibrinogenolysis can occur.

The role and dose of concomitant heparin therapy during low-dose fibrinolytic therapy is largely undefined. In general, lower doses are recommended, particularly with t-PA.

Reteplase has been recently used for peripheral vascular occlusions (Retavase, Centocor, Malvern, Pa.). It is a nonglycosylated deletion mutein (protein arising from a deletion mutation) of wild-type human t-PA. It consists of the kringle-2 and protease domains but lacks the kringle-1 finger and the growth factor domains of t-PA.[109] It has decreased high-affinity fibrin binding compared to t-PA, and a longer half-life. This reduced high-affinity fibrin binding may result in reduced lysis of old fibrin plugs in the cerebral circulation and hence a lower incidence of intracranial hemorrhage.

Experience with the agent in treatment of peripheral vascular disease is limited. Dosing regimens (unpublished data) have ranged from 0.5 unit/hour, to 0.25 unit/hour. Spontaneous bleeding has been noted after 24 hours with the 0.5-unit/hour regimen. Other than heparin used to maintain patency of vascular sheathes, no added heparin is administered. Further experience with this agent is needed.

Several trials have been undertaken to compare the efficacy of thrombolytic therapy with that of surgery. There have been several randomized trials comparing the efficacy of thrombolytic therapy versus surgery for treatment of peripheral artery ischemia. The Rochester group compared the results of intraarterial urokinase with surgery in patients with limb-threatening ischemia of less than 7 days' duration. Intraarterial thrombolytic therapy was associated with a reduction in the incidence of in-hospital cardiopulmonary complications and a corresponding increase in patient survival rates. Although the cumulative limb salvage rate was similar in the two treatment groups (82% at 12 months), the cumulative survival rate was significantly improved in patients randomized to the thrombolysis group, with the mortality differences primarily attributable to an increased frequency of in-hospital cardiopulmonary complications in the operative group (49% vs. 16%). The decreased mortality from cardiopulmonary complications may reflect the decreased magnitude of required interventions in the thrombolytic group.[110]

The STILE trial randomized patients with native arterial or bypass graft occlusion to optimal surgical procedure or intraarterial catheter–directed thrombolysis with rt-PA or urokinase.[107] Thrombolysis patients required successful catheter placement into the occlusion before lysis.

A composite clinical outcome of death, ongoing recurrent ischemia, and major morbidity was the primary end point. Failure of catheter placement for thrombolysis occurred in 28% of patients. Randomization was terminated early because a significant primary end point occurred on the first interim analysis. Thirty-day outcome demonstrated a significant benefit to surgical therapy, primarily because of a reduction in ongoing ischemia ($P < .001$). Clinical outcome at 30 days, however, was similar, probably because of crossover treatment to surgery.

A significant reduction in planned surgical procedures was observed after thrombolysis. Patients with acute ischemia (0 to 14 days) who were treated with thrombolysis had improved amputation-free survival and shorter hospital stays. However, in patients with chronic ischemia (greater than 14 days' duration), surgical revascularization was found to be more effective and safer than thrombolysis.

Issues to be considered in evaluation of the study design include the following: (1) The high doses of heparin used in the thrombolytic therapy regimen likely contributed to bleeding complications. (2) Thirty percent of patients were randomized within 14 days of worsening ischemia, 44% had symptoms for greater than 1 month before randomization, and 26% had symptoms greater than 2 months. Because the number of patients with chronic ischemia outnumbered patients with acute ischemia by 2.5 to 1, their outcome would have the greatest effect on primary end point analysis. It is not unexpected that surgically treated patients had less ongoing or recurrent ischemia or fewer hemorrhagic complications. Atherosclerotic plaque and organized thrombus are likely the underlying lesions in chronically ischemic patients, and even with partial penetration of the catheter into the thrombus, a lytic agent may not be successful because of proximal thrombus and distal atherosclerotic occlusion.[107] (3) The unusually high number of technical failures due to inability to place a catheter for thrombolysis impacted negatively on the thrombolysis results.

The Thrombolysis or Peripheral Arterial Surgery (TOPAS) study was another multicenter trial to assess thrombolytic therapy and surgery.[111] It compared recombinant urokinase (r-UK) with operation in the treatment of acute peripheral occlusions less than or equal to 14 days in duration. A 12.5% incidence of major bleeding was noted with an increase in risk of hemorrhage when patients received heparin. Because of bleeding complications, the requirement for therapeutic doses of heparin was abolished early in the trial and subtherapeutic doses of heparin subsequently administered. The study determined that intraarterial infusion of urokinase reduced the need for open surgical procedures with no significantly increased risk of amputation or death.

Another recent multicenter trial was the Prourokinase versus Urokinase for Peripheral Occlusions Safety and Efficacy (PURPOSE) trial.[112] Pro-urokinase (r-Pro-UK, a recombinant thrombolytic agent) was compared with urokinase for the treatment of acute lower extremity occlusions. r-Pro-UK is a single-chain zymogen that is assembled into active two-chain urokinase on the surface of the thrombus. It is a relatively fibrin-specific agent, that is, an agent that effects fibrinolysis with degradation of plasma fibrinogen. Only in the milieu of a thrombus in which abundant fibrin fragment E comes in contact with r-Pro-UK, does the zymogen gain intrinsic plasminogenolytic activity.[113] This dose-ranging trial demonstrated that r-Pro-UK has a dose-related safety and efficacy profile. It is, however, not yet clinically available.

TRANSLUMINAL CATHETER RETRIEVAL OF FOREIGN BODIES FROM THE VASCULAR SYSTEM

The majority of foreign bodies removed from the vascular system have been retrieved from the venous system, right heart chambers, or pulmonary arteries. The items most frequently retrieved are catheter fragments, broken-off guidewires, and pacing catheters. From the arterial system, items removed are guidewire fragments and, more recently, Gianturco-Wallace coil occluders.[114]

Foreign body retrieval using catheter technique requires fluoroscopy and is usually accomplished through a percutaneous puncture or cutdown. A sheath may sometimes be employed. Several different types of devices may be used: loop snare catheters (catheters through which a double length of guidewire is passed to make a loop),[115] basket retrievers,[116] hook-tip catheters,[117] or grasping forceps,[118, 119] and, more recently, the Amplatz nitinol gooseneck snare.[120] The nitinol gooseneck snare and wire catch baskets similar to Dormia baskets are the most widely used retrieval instruments. The nitinol gooseneck snare is the easiest to use. Balloon catheters may be used percutaneously to remove items from blood vessels. The removal of foreign bodies utilizing transcatheter techniques is associated with a very low complication rate and presents far less hazard than surgical removal of these items.

PERCUTANEOUS TRANSLUMINAL ANGIOPLASTY

Percutaneous transluminal angioplasty (PTA) is a technique in which specially constructed catheters equipped with a balloon in their distal shaft are passed percutaneously to an area of vessel stenosis. When the catheter has been positioned at the level of stenosis, the catheter is inflated and the stenotic area dilated. The most widely used catheters are those based on the design of Gruntzig.[121, 122] The presently available balloon catheters are made in various sizes. In performing balloon angioplasty, the significance of the stenosis is determined by baseline angiography. In some instances, particularly in large vessels, it is necessary to measure the gradient across the lesion. A guidewire is manipulated across the lesion. A small French-sized catheter is then advanced over the guidewire across the obstruction. The wire is removed and the catheter position verified with injection of contrast. A pullback pressure measurement is made to assess the gradient using vasodilators, if necessary. The guidewire is reintroduced, and the small French-sized catheter is exchanged for a balloon catheter. When the balloon is placed across the lesion, it is inflated. Postdilatation pressures may be recorded to evaluate for residual gradient. Pressure measurements are not usually obtained with small vessels.

Based on experimental studies, Castaneda-Zuniga and coworkers[123] proposed a theory for the mechanism of angioplasty. During balloon dilatation, the atherosclerotic intima is ruptured and partially dehisced. This frees the media from the restraint of the atherosclerotic intima, allowing it to become overstretched with damage to the elastic properties of its elastic collagen and muscle fibers. The increased blood flow through the lesion keeps the media distended as the vessel heals. Vascular angioplasty induces a complex healing process. After initial injury, platelet thrombi and an acute inflammatory response occur, followed by cellular invasion by monocytes-macrophages, proliferation of vascular smooth muscle cells, and extracellular matrix deposition. The injury repair concludes with organization of the matrix and re-endothelialization.[124]

PTA has been used successfully in the dilatation of vessels in multiple sites in the vascular system. In the abdomen and periphery, it has been used in the aorta, mesenteric vessels, and peripheral vessels (Fig. 16–26). It has also been used in cerebral vessels.

PTA has been employed successfully in the treatment of localized aortic stenoses.[125, 126] In a series of 32 patients with mean follow-up of 25 months (range 1 to 96 months) 25 of 28 patients maintained postangioplasty improvement in their ankle-brachial indices (ABIs). Although the technique has been recommended for short stenoses, in this series 41% of stenoses were 2 cm or longer.

In PTA of the iliac arteries, the primary success rate (i.e., ability to cross the lesion and perform dilatation) is approximately 93% to 95%.[127, 128] Iliac PTA is best applied in patients with a short focal stenosis of the iliac arteries. It is generally not recommended for patients with diffuse iliac disease unless they are poor surgical candidates. PTA alone is also not recommended in totally occluded iliac arteries because of the high incidence of complications.[128, 129] Table 16–1 summarizes the results of long-term follow-up with iliac artery PTA.[128-138]

Complication rates with iliac PTA range from 2% to 4%.[132, 134] These rates were compared with surgical results by Malone and colleagues,[139] who reported an immediate patency rate for aortoiliac reconstruction of 99.2% for aor-

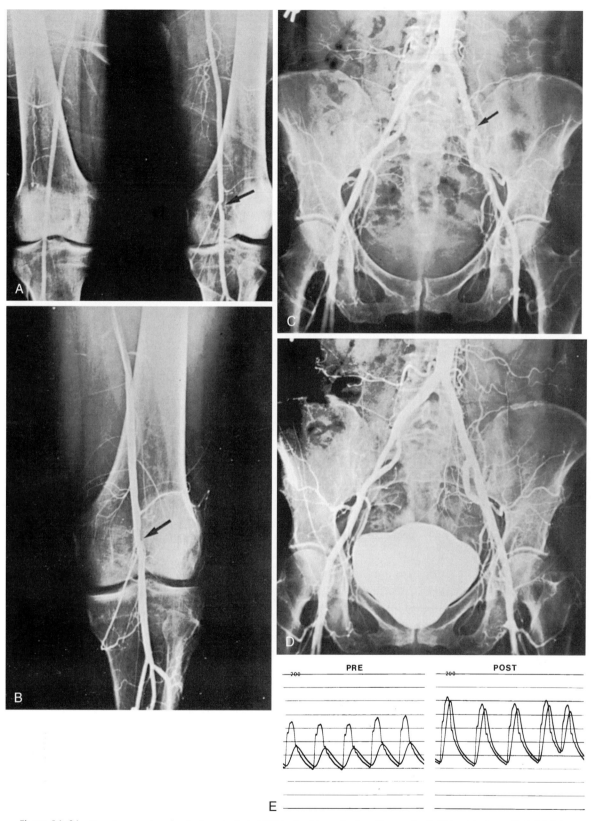

Figure 16–26. Percutaneous transluminal angioplasty (PTA) of pelvic and extremity vessels. *A*, This patient manifested left leg claudication. Femoral runoff study revealed a high-grade localized lesion in the proximal left popliteal artery *(arrow)*. *B*, Gruntzig balloon dilatation was performed. The postdilatation arteriogram shows mild residual deformity at the site of dilatation. Postdilatation, the patient became symptom free. *C*, Pelvic arteriogram in another patient (same patient as in Fig. 16–2) shows a localized left common iliac artery stenosis *(arrow)*. *D*, Post-PTA, the stenosis is relieved. *E*, Pressure tracings measured across the iliac lesion, before and after dilatation, show abolition of the gradient post-PTA.

TABLE 16-1
Iliac Percutaneous Transluminal Angioplasty (PTA)—Long-Term Follow-up

AUTHORS	YEAR	PTAs (No.)	PRIMARY SUCCESS AND RECURRENCE RATES (%)		LONG-TERM FOLLOW-UP (YR) PATENCY RATES (%)					CONTAINS LIFE TABLE	TEST
			Primary	Recurrences	1	2	3	5	7		
Gruntzig[131]	1977	200	93	17	89	86	—	85	—	Yes	b
van Andel et al.[132]	1980	51	96							No	b
Spence et al.[128]	1981	148	93	13[a]	93	82	79	—	—	Yes	c
Kumpe & Jones[135]	1982	65			—	—	82			Yes	b
Johnston et al.[134]	1982	244	90		72	66				Yes	—
Kadir et al.[129]	1983	141	96	8[a]	91	—	89	—	—	Yes	d
Schneider et al.[133]	1982	186			—	—	—	85	—	Yes	b
Schwarten[136]	1984	58		9	—	89				No	e
van Andel et al.[130]	1985	183	96		97	—	—	—	90	Yes	b
Johnston et al.[137]	1987	376	96		78	68	65	60	—	Yes	b
Tegtmeyer et al.[138]	1991	340	93		95	90	89	85	85	Yes	c

[a]Successfully redilatated restenoses were not considered failures.
[b]At least anamnesis, physical examination, and ankle-arm index.
[c]Pulse-volume recordings when indicated.
[d]Ankle-arm index in two thirds of the patients.
[e]Ankle-arm index in combination with digital subtraction angiography.
Adapted from van Andel GJ, van Erp WFM, Krepel VM, Breslau PJ: Percutaneous transluminal dilation of the iliac artery: Long-term results. Radiology 156:321–328, 1985.

tofemoral grafts, with a 4% thrombosis rate each subsequent year. The 5-year patency rate for aortoiliac reconstruction is 91%.[139] Several series have now shown that the long-term results with iliac PTA are comparable to those achieved with reconstructive surgery.[127–129, 132, 140] On the basis of these findings, iliac angioplasty may be considered the sole treatment modality for limb ischemia caused by an isolated iliac lesion or for treatment of an iliac lesion before distal bypass surgery.[128, 133]

PTA of the femoropopliteal arteries has a primary success rate of approximately 84%,[122, 128, 141] which is lower than that of iliac PTA. The incidence of significant complications ranges from 4% to 6%.[122, 141]

The long-term patency rates after femoropopliteal PTA are summarized in Table 16–2.[128, 131, 133, 135, 136, 141–148] Johnston and colleagues[137] noted a lower cumulative patency rate. However, their criteria for success were excessively strict and not always indicative of the status of the dilated segment. Multiple factors affect the outcome of PTA of the femoropopliteal arteries. Experience of the radiologist and catheter configuration have been shown to be important.[141] The success rate with femoropopliteal PTA varies with the site[141] and length of the lesion.[129, 141, 148] Krepel and colleagues[141] obtained a success rate of 97% in superficial femoral artery lesions shorter than 3 cm, compared with 26% in lesions longer than 3 cm. The most significant factor negatively affecting PTA in stenotic femoropopliteal disease is long-segment stenosis. In long lesions of the femoropopliteal vessels, therefore, PTA is not recommended. The long-term results following PTA are better if the lesions are short and concentric and have a regular appearance. Results are also better when the postangioplasty morphology is near normal and the runoff is at least fair.[141]

A meta-analysis by Adar and associates[149] found a 5-year patency of femoropopliteal angioplasty of 60%. Mehta[150] compared PTA with femoropopliteal bypass surgery and reported a 3-year patency rate of 77% in patients who underwent bypass surgery for claudication. In patients undergoing bypass surgery for limb salvage, the 3-year patency rate was 68%.[150] Spence and associates[128] contrasted these results with PTA, in which they observed a 73% patency rate at 3 years in patients undergoing PTA for claudication and a 2-year patency rate of 76.1% in patients undergoing PTA for limb salvage. In the randomized Veterans Administration trial comparing angioplasty with surgery, the 3-year patency rate for femoropopliteal PTA was 59%, not significantly different from that in patients who had undergone surgery.[140] Veith and coworkers[151] obtained in their large series a 66% cumulative life-table limb salvage rate at 6 years for all patients having femoropopliteal-tibial artery reconstructive operations. The subset undergoing a femoropopliteal artery bypass showed a 73% 6-year cumulative life-table analysis limb salvage rate.

Taylor and Porter,[152] in a series of 231 patients undergoing femoropopliteal bypass, reported an operative mortality of 1.4%. Thirty-one percent underwent bypass for claudication, and 64%, for limb-threatening ischemia. The overall primary graft patency for all femoropopliteal grafts was 79% at 5 years. The 5-year patency rate for saphenous vein bypass grafts was 85%, and the 5-year patency for bypass grafts other than saphenous vein was 73%. Patients undergoing a repeat bypass after a prior failed bypass had a patency rate of only 57%.

The mortality and morbidity from PTA are less than the 4% average mortality reported for the femoropopliteal surgery.[150]

Experience with PTA of the infrapopliteal arteries has lagged behind that of PTA of the iliac and femoropopliteal vessels. PTA of these vessels has been considered a high-risk procedure because occlusion of a distal peripheral leg vessel might result in amputation or preclude a bypass operation. The balloon catheters initially available for PTA were not suitable for dilatation of these small distal vessels. The development of small, coaxial, low-profile balloon catheters and small, atraumatic, steerable guidewires, as well

T A B L E   1 6 – 2

Long-Term Results of Femoropopliteal Angioplasty

AUTHORS	YEAR	PTAs (No.)	RECURRENCES	PATENT ARTERIES/FOLLOW-UP PERIOD (YR)[a]					TEST
				2	3	4	5	7	
Gruntzig[131]	1977	184	27	65 (78)[c]	—	—	—	—	d
Greenfield[142]	1980	70	6	84	—	—	—	—	d
Spence et al.[128]	1981	122	20[b]	75	70	—	—	—	e
Freiman et al.[143]	1981	88	—	67	—	—	—	—	d
Kumpe & Jones[135]	1982	50	—	56	—	—	—	—	d
Schneider et al.[133]	1982	682	162	70	—	—	68	—	d
Gallino et al.[147]	1982	200	—	62 (71)[c]	—	69	—	—	d
Colapinto[144]	1983	112	—	58	55	—	—	—	d
Berkowitz et al.[145]	1983	110	30	67	63	—	—	—	d
Mahler et al.[146]	1983	252	—	71	—	—	—	—	d
Krepel et al.[141]	1985	164	38	77	70	70	70	60	d
Johnston et al.[137]	1987	253	—	53	50	44	40	—	d
Capek et al.[148]	1991	217		63	61	61	58		e

[a]All results analyzed by life-table method.
[b]Successfully redilated recurrent stenoses were not considered failures.
[c]Second number is patency rate without "partial" recurrences.
[d]At least anamnesis, physical examination, and ankle-arm index.
[e]Pulse-volume recordings when indicated.
PTAs, percutaneous transluminal angioplasties.
Adapted from Krepel VM, Van Andel GJ, Van Erp WFM, Breslau PJ: Percutaneous transluminal angioplasty of femoropopliteal artery: Initial and long-term results. Radiology 156:325–328, 1985.

as the use of pharmacologic agents such as nifedipine, nitroglycerin, and thrombolytic agents when necessary in addition to heparin, is responsible for the favorable results now achievable with PTA of the infrapopliteal vessels. Also important is the use of digital arteriography, which allows rapid visualization of the runoff vessels.[153] Results of several large series are now available.[154–156] Primary success rates range from 86% to 97%. Schwarten and Cutcliff,[154] in a series of 98 patients with infrapopliteal stenoses or occlusions 5 cm or less in length, reported a 1-year limb salvage rate of 89% and a 2-year (37 limbs) limb salvage rate of 86%. Horvath and coworkers,[156] in a series of 71 patients (103 stenosed crural vessels), used both PTA and laser angioplasty. With life-table analysis for single-vessel runoff, the authors obtained a cumulative patency rate of 92.5% after 6 months (n = 45), 79.8% after 1 year (n = 27), and 64.6% after 3 years (n = 3). Complications have been few. Prompt clinical improvement following infrapopliteal PTA has been noted in patients in whom angioplasty restored straight-line flow to the foot via at least one calf vessel narrowed by no more than 75% of its diameter.[155] The success in these series demonstrates a role for infrapopliteal PTA in appropriately selected patients. These results compare favorably with surgical results at 3 years.

The life-table primary patency rates for isolated popliteal or infrapopliteal runoff vessel surgical bypass grafts range from 59% to 69%,[151, 157–159] with lower rates seen with prosthetic graft material.[155] Cumulative life-table limb salvage rates reported are 51%,[151] 61%,[153] and 82%.[156] These results are obtained in the presence of 5-year patient survival rates ranging from 35% to 44%.[157, 159]

The length of hospitalization, patient costs, and discomfort are significantly less with PTA than with reconstructive surgery. The ease of dilatation and the opportunity for repeat dilatation are additional advantages. The performance of PTA in aortoiliac or femoropopliteal vessels does not preclude later operation. In patients with iliac disease, PTA can be used in conjunction with distal surgery. There is no risk to pelvic autonomic nerves or male sexual functioning. It can be used in obese patients and allows preservation of the saphenous vein for later cardiac or peripheral artery bypass surgery. PTA can also be used to treat inflow or outflow stenoses in patients with failing grafts.[160] Percutaneous balloon angioplasty has also been used in the treatment of venous stenoses in the subclavian veins, the inferior vena cava, and in stenosis in dialysis fistulas.

Presently available data indicate that PTA has an important role in the management of patients with peripheral vascular disease.[161]

RENAL ARTERY PERCUTANEOUS TRANSLUMINAL ANGIOPLASTY

PTA has been demonstrated to be effective in the management of renovascular hypertension due to atherosclerotic disease and to fibromuscular dysplasia (FMD).

Percutaneous Transluminal Angioplasty in Renal Artery Stenosis due to Atherosclerotic Disease

Several studies have now documented that PTA of the renal arteries (PTRA) is an effective method for the long-term management of patients with atherosclerotic renovascular hypertension. In a series of 213 patients reported by Klinge and colleagues,[162] 134 patients had renal artery stenosis caused by atherosclerosis, and 52 had renal artery stenosis from FMD. Initial clinical results could be evaluated in 210 cases, with cure or improvement achieved in

80%. In 23 cases, there was neither clinical nor technical success. The cumulative patency rate at 5 years was 80% in the atherosclerosis group, 89% in the FMD group, and 74% in the indeterminate group. Major complications occurred in 25 patients. Mortality was less than 1%.

Results have been shown to be less favorable in patients with bilateral stenoses; however, in addition to improved blood pressure control, there is evidence that PTRA may in certain cases improve renal function or delay progressive deterioration.[163, 164] In a group of 62 patients with atherosclerotic renal artery disease, Karagiannis and associates[163] observed an overall benefit rate of 70.8% (cured or improved) with PTRA at a mean follow-up of 39 months. Similarly, in a group of 153 patients who underwent PTRA for atherosclerotic stenosis, Losinno and associates[164] observed blood pressure returned to normal in 12%, improved in 51%, and unchanged in 37%. In the entire population of 195 patients, renal function improved in 48% of patients with renal insufficiency due to bilateral stenoses or stenosis in a single functioning kidney. Early studies suggested that PTRA was contraindicated and of little benefit in ostial stenosis.[165] However, later studies have failed to confirm a difference in outcome between ostial and nonostial lesions in patients with renal artery stenosis and have shown that PTRA can play an important role in blood pressure control in this patient population.[166, 167]

Percutaneous Transluminal Angioplasty in Fibromuscular Disease

PTA has been demonstrated to be effective in the management of renovascular hypertension due to FMD. The success rates with PTA for FMD[168, 170] with follow-up to 3 years equal the success rates of bypass surgery for FMD.[171–173] Furthermore, the morbidity, expense, length of hospital stay, and recuperation after PTA are significantly less than those of operation. Recurrence can be treated with repeat PTA, whereas reoperation after failure of bypass surgery usually necessitates nephrectomy.[171] Long-term results with PTA of renal artery stenosis due to FMD have recently been reported by Tegtmeyer and associates.[174] In a series of 66 patients with 85 renal artery stenoses due to FMD followed for as long as 121 months, 26 patients were cured (39%), 39 were improved (59%), and one did not respond to PTA. The cumulative patency rate predicted for 10 years was 87.1%.[174] As a result, PTA is the preferred initial treatment for FMD at many centers (Fig. 16–27).[168–170, 174]

The complications of PTA of renal arteries include renal artery dissection, occlusion, perforation, renal infarction, hematoma, and acute tubular necrosis. In large series, the overall complication rate of PTA varies from 5.7%[168] to 12.5%.[171] Overall surgical results show benefit rates of 74% to 97%,[171, 175] with cure or improvement of hypertension expected in more than 90% of young patients, particularly those with fibromuscular disease or focal atherosclerotic lesions. The similar results of surgery and angioplasty have led to the conclusion that angioplasty is the treatment of choice for uncomplicated fibromuscular disease and nonostial unilateral atheromatous disease of the renal arteries.[169]

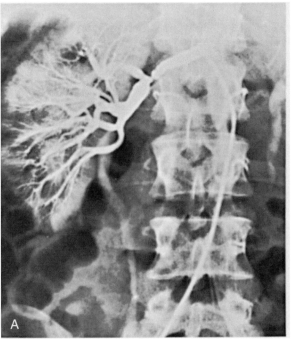

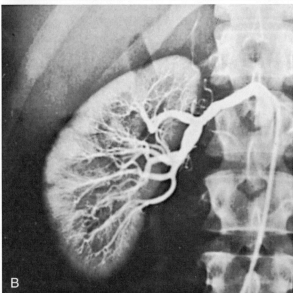

Figure 16–27. Percutaneous transluminal angioplasty (PTA) of renal artery. *A,* Baseline arteriogram in this young hypertensive female patient shows typical string-of-beads appearance of fibromuscular disease. *B,* Post-Gruntzig balloon dilatation arteriogram shows relief of stenosis. This patient is now normotensive.

ANGIOGRAPHIC EMBOLIZATION THERAPY

Transcatheter embolization therapy involves the delivery of occluding agents through catheters selectively positioned in vessels. A wide variety of embolic agents are used. Some are permanent mechanical occluders, such as the Gianturco-Wallace coils,[176] detachable balloons,[177] Ivalon particles,[178] silicone,[179] and bucrylate tissue adhesives.[180] Other agents, such as autologous clot and absorbable gelatin sponge (Gel-foam, Upjohn Co., Kalamazoo, Mich.), are embolic agents that are slowly absorbed by the body over a variable period of time.[181]

A major application of embolization therapy is in the treatment of congenital AVMs. Congenital AVMs are difficult management problems. Surgery is of limited value,[182] being most useful in those situations in which the AVM can be totally excised. Partial removal with ligation of feeders has been shown to be ineffective owing to regrowth of collateral vessels. In those AVMs that cannot be treated by surgical excision or that require amputation, embolization therapy is a useful palliative technique.[183–185] MRI, and in selected cases gadolinium-enhanced MRA, should be obtained in the pretreatment evaluation of these patients. The MRI studies provide information regarding the size and extent of the malformation and the degree of involvement of associated muscle groups or other vital structures. MRI is also useful in the follow-up of these patients. Baseline selective arteriography should be performed in all patients with suspected congenital AVMs before operative or embolization therapy. Arteriography is necessary to delineate the type and extent of the AVM. These lesions are usually more extensive than suspected.

It is important that the interstices of the AVM be occluded and that the embolic agent reach the center of the AVM. Occlusion of the feeding arteries without ablation of the central portion of the AVM is equivalent to ligation of feeding vessels, which has been found to be of little use.

Permanent embolic agents are recommended for occlusion of congenital AVMs. In situations in which the AVM nidus cannot be reached directly owing to previous surgical ligation, direct percutaneous puncture of the AVM is performed, and, using fluoroscopic guidance, the embolic agent is delivered directly into the AVM.

Most patients manifest a systemic response to embolization therapy for several days, characterized by pain, fever, and elevated muscle enzymes. Clinical symptoms respond to supportive therapy. Risks of the procedure include inadvertent distal reflux of particulate or liquid embolic agents or misplacement of the mechanical occluders, with resultant occlusion of inappropriate vessels. These mishaps may necessitate urgent operative embolectomy. Minor complications that have been reported are transient or permanent nerve injury or small areas of skin slough. With proper technique, however, the benefits of the procedure outweigh the risks, and embolization therapy may permit limb salvage. It is an effective palliative therapy, and, should new collateral feeders develop, they can be embolized.[183–185]

Another important application of transcatheter embolization is the treatment of hemorrhage. Embolization therapy has been used successfully in the control of bleeding from bronchial arteries,[186] renal bleeding,[187] splenic bleeding,[62] and gastrointestinal bleeding originating in the stomach. Massive pelvic hemorrhage after trauma or surgery or as a complication of genitourinary tumors can be effectively treated with embolic techniques. Experience has shown that any or all of the branches of the internal iliac artery can be occluded without great risk.[188, 189] Embolization therapy is also used to occlude blood supply to organs such as the spleen before splenectomy and to decrease tumor vascularity before resection. Chemotherapeutic agents may be mixed with a variety of embolic agents to perform chemoembolization of malignant tumors. Embolization therapy is usually performed at the time of diagnostic arteriography.

INFERIOR VENA CAVA FILTERS

The value of inferior vena cava filter placement for prophylaxis against pulmonary embolism has been recognized for many years. Initially, filter placement required a cutdown of the internal jugular vein, but in 1984 percutaneous transjugular and transfemoral placement of the Greenfield filter was described.[190] Currently, a variety of caval filters are available. In addition to improving the functional performance and clot-trapping capability of the filters, an emphasis has been placed by manufacturers on the development of smaller-sized introduction systems more suitable for percutaneous placement. Currently approved filters include the Greenfield stainless steel filter, the Bird's Nest and Modified filter (Cook, Bloomington, Ind.), the Titanium Greenfield filter (Medi-Tech, Watertown, Mass.), the VenaTech filter (L. G. Medical, Chasseneuil, France), the Simon Nitinol filter (Nitinol Medical Technologies, Woburn, Mass.), and the Cordis TrapEase (Cordis Corp., Miami, Fla.)

The Greenfield filter has had the longest availability. It requires a large 24-Fr introducer system with a maximal diameter of 30 mm (recommended for inferior vena cava sizes of 28 mm).[191] It has a reported recurrent embolism rate of 5%[192, 193] and a vena cava occlusion rate of 3% to 5%.[192, 194–196] Optimal filtration of caval blood flow results with angles resulting in less than a 15-degree tilt from the vertical. The large 24-Fr size of the stainless steel Greenfield filter is a disadvantage, and there is an associated 10% to 24% prevalence of sonographically identified femoral vein thrombus.[197] Consequently, it is now rarely used and has been supplanted by filters with a smaller delivery system. The Titanium Greenfield filter is a significantly modified design of the stainless steel Greenfield filter and can be delivered in a 12-French carrier. It has a broader base (38 mm vs. 30 mm) and is recommended for caval diameters up to but not exceeding 28 mm. Initially, its use was associated with a high frequency of vena caval perforation, but this problem has been corrected.[198]

The Bird's Nest and Modified filter, first tested in 1982, has the advantage of a small 12-Fr sheath size. It consists of a series of preshaped wires that assume a mesh configuration resembling a bird's nest.[199, 200] The rate of recurrent pulmonary embolism is reported at 2.7%, and the rate of caval occlusion, 2.9%. Follow-up, however, has been largely clinical. The actual incidence of vena caval occlusion is unknown, but in a subset of 440 patients who underwent radiologic follow-up, caval occlusion was documented in 2.9%. Because of the filter's large size, it can be inserted in venae cavae up to 40 mm in diameter. The VenaTech filter is the FDA-approved version of the LGM filter (L. G. Medical [LGM]). Clinical follow-up shows a recurrent pulmonary embolism rate of 2% and vena caval occlusion rate of 7% in 1-year follow-up.

The Simon Nitinol filter is composed of thermal memory alloy composed of nickel and titanium. The filter wires are in straightened form at cooled temperatures (4°C to

10°C) and re-form to filter configuration at body temperatures.[201] The device is inserted through a 9-French outer sheath and can be delivered via a transfemoral or transjugular route. Multicenter clinical trials show a symptomatic recurrent pulmonary embolism rate of 1.1% and an asymptomatic pulmonary embolism rate of 0.7% diagnosed by ventilation perfusion lung scan or pulmonary angiogram. The vena caval occlusion rate is 7.8% (symptomatic) and 1.9% (asymptomatic).[202] A new 6-Fr nitinol permanent inferior vena cava filter (Cordis TrapEase) is now available. The small French size facilitates delivery.

The major indications for filter placement in venous thromboembolism are (1) contraindication to anticoagulation, (2) failure of adequate anticoagulation, and (3) prophylactic placement in selected high-risk patients.

Controversy surrounds the use of prophylactic filters. Most physicians agree that prophylactic filter placement is reasonable in patients who develop iliofemoral thrombosis while on adequate anticoagulation and in patients who have long free-floating femoral or iliac vein thrombi. Prophylaxis in other high-risk patients, such as those with pulmonary hypertension, is the subject of much dispute. The longevity of these newer filters is not clearly known, and this should be taken into consideration when they are placed in young patients.[202]

VASCULAR STENTS

Vascular stents have been proposed as an endovascular mechanical support to compensate for, or overcome the limitations of, percutaneous angioplasty. They have been employed to manage flow-compromising dissection induced by PTA and to overcome vessel closure during PTA. They have also been proposed as a means of preventing restenosis after PTA.[203] Multiple intraluminal vascular stents are currently in use. The two most frequently used intravascular stents are the Palmaz stent (Johnson & Johnson Interventional Systems, Warren, N.J.) and the Wallstent (Medinvent, Lausanne, Switzerland; Schneider, Minneapolis, Minn.).

The Palmaz stent, a balloon-expandable stent, consists of a slotted, seamless, stainless steel tube of varying diameters mounted on an angioplasty balloon. The Wallstent consists of surgical-grade stainless steel alloy filaments woven to form a tubular braid. It is a self-expanding stent constrained on a special delivery catheter by a membrane that is retracted during delivery. Unlike the Palmaz stent, the catheter is flexible and adapts to vessel curvature. Both stents are currently used intravascularly as an adjunct to percutaneous balloon angioplasty in cases in which relief of stenosis has not been achieved or the stenosis has recurred, or when a spontaneous or postcatheter dissection has occurred. The majority of the vascular experience has been with the deployment of stents in the iliac and renal arteries.

Bosch and Hunink[204] conducted a meta-analysis of aortoiliac stent placement compared with PTA. Published stent studies (n = 8, 816 patients) were compared with PTA studies (n = 6, 1300 patients). After treatment, the mean ABI in the stent studies was significantly higher than in the PTA studies (0.87 vs. 0.76). The immediate technical success rate was 91% in the PTA studies and 96% in the stent studies (P > .05).

The 4-year patency rate after PTA to treat claudication was 65% for stenoses and 54% for occlusions. In the treatment of critical ischemia, the patency rate for PTA was 53% for stenoses and 44% for occlusions. In patients treated with stents for claudication, the 4-year patency rate was 77% for stenoses and 61% for occlusions. For critical ischemia, the patency rate was 67% for stenoses and 53% for occlusions. Analysis showed that 43% fewer long-term failures occurred after stent placement than after PTA.

In the Dutch Iliac Stent Trial,[205] 279 patients with common iliac or external iliac artery disease were randomized to receive direct stent placement (group I, n = 143) or primary angioplasty (group II, n = 136). Angioplasty was followed by stent placement in 59 patients because of a residual pressure gradient across the angioplasty. The complications were 6% for group I and 7% for group II. Cumulative primary patency rates based on duplex scans at 2-year follow-up were similar for both groups: 71.3% in group I vs. 69.9% in group II. Overall comparison of the cumulative patency rates in the two groups showed no difference (P = .2).

A cost-effectiveness analysis was also performed analyzing primary stent placement, PTA, and PTA with selective stent placement.[206] PTA with selective stent placement yielded equivalent complication rates, patency results, and quality-of-life outcomes compared with those of primary stent placement. Because significant differences in the number of complications or rate of reintervention between treatments were not observed, Bosch concluded that primary angioplasty followed by selective stent placement appeared to be the strategy of choice for treating lifestyle-limiting claudication because it was also the most cost-effective procedure.

Palmaz and associates[207] reported their results with 171 iliac artery stent procedures in 154 patients using the Palmaz stent. Of the 261 stents placed, 181 were placed in the iliac arteries, and 80 in the external iliac arteries. Complications occurred in 18 patients (11.7%). At follow-up (average, 6 months; range, 1 to 24 months) 137 patients demonstrated clinical benefit, 113 had become asymptomatic, 11 had no benefit, and 6 improved initially but later developed new symptoms.

Favorable long-term results with iliac artery stenting have been reported by Long and coworkers[208] using the Wallstent and the Strecker stent (Medi-Tech) in a series of 49 patients with 53 iliac artery lesions. Indications for stent deployment included recanalization of total occlusions, 15 lesions (28%); dissection, 22 lesions (42%); post-PTA restenosis, 11 lesions (21%); and immediate post-PTA unsatisfactory results, 5 lesions (9%). Mean follow-up was 15 months (range, 1 to 36 months) with follow-up angiograms in 50 vessels. Complications occurred in 14 patients (26.9%). Primary patency was 85.3% at 12 months and 80.9% at 18 months. Secondary patency was 96.1% at 12 and at 18 months. These results indicate that intravascular stents have a role in the management of iliac artery lesions.

Zollikofer and coworkers[209] reported midterm results with Wallstent placement in 31 patients. Twenty-six iliac and 15 femoropopliteal complex stenoses or occlusions with inadequate response to PTA were treated. In the iliac artery group, 96% of the stents were patent at a mean follow-up of 16 months (range, 6 to 30 months). In the femoropopliteal artery group, of the 11 patients available for follow-up, only 6 had patent stents at 7 to 26 months (mean, 20 months). Four of the six required one to three secondary interventions. Results were clearly superior with the iliac arteries, and the authors recommended that placement in the femoral arteries be performed with caution.

Stent placement has not yet been shown to be efficacious in the femoropopliteal arteries because of stent obstruction by intimal hyperplasia. Zollikofer and coworkers[209] employed Wallstent placement in 15 patients with inadequate response to recanalization and angioplasty for femoropopliteal occlusions. At a mean follow-up of 20 months in 11 patients available for follow-up, only six arteries were patent and four of the six required from one to three secondary interventions.

Martin and colleagues[210] observed a primary patency rate of 61% and a secondary clinical patency rate of 84% at 1 year, with 49% primary and 72% secondary patency rates at 2 years. A 16% major complication rate was noted.

A European single-center prospective study[211] showed conventional femoropopliteal PTA to have a 1-year primary patency rate of 65% compared with a secondary patency rate of 69% after Wallstent placement. Early restenosis occurred in the stent group (38%), as did early thrombosis (19%).

In a recent large multicenter trial[212] comparing PTA with stent implantation, although stenting showed better short-term and mid-term results, primary stenting did not improve long-term clinical and hemodynamic success rates compared with PTA alone.

Renal artery stent placement has been proposed as a means to overcome primary failure of renal angioplasty, to treat restenosis following angioplasty, and to treat the complications of renal angioplasty. Because of the movement of the kidneys, flexible stents such as the Wallstent or Strecker stent have theoretical advantages over the more rigid Palmaz stents. The recurrence rate after renal angioplasty varies from 5% to 33%, with most recurrences developing within a year after PTRA. This has stimulated an increase in the use of stents. Stents have been employed frequently in treatment of ostial lesions, as the immediate technical success rate of PTRA of ostial lesions is in the range of 20% to 24%.[165, 213] Ostial lesions are often caused by bulky plaques along the aortic wall that encroach on and overlap the origin of the renal artery. They may be less responsive to the stretching of the vessel wall and intimal cracking necessary for successful angioplasty. With ostial lesions, exact placement of the stent is important, as those portions of the stent projecting into the aorta tend not to become endothelialized. Although additional results of long-term follow-up from large series are needed, the overall effect on blood pressure seems to be similar to that of balloon angioplasty. Restenosis seems to be a major problem, occurring in 20% to 38% of cases after 1 year.[203, 214] Hennequin and associates[214] reported the results of long-term follow-up in 21 patients who received renal artery stents. At follow-up angiography (range: 12–60 months), 20% of patients had restenosis. Cumulative primary patency was 95%, 85%, and 77% at 7, 9, and 15 months, respectively. Further study is needed to determine whether stent placement may be proposed as a first-line treatment of ostial lesions. Repeat PTRA can usually be performed if restenosis occurs. The use of stents in other vessels, such as the carotid arteries and renal transplant arteries, is under investigation.

Transjugular Intrahepatic Portosystemic Shunts

The transjugular intrahepatic portosystemic shunt (TIPS) procedure is a percutaneous technique used to decompress the portal system. From a percutaneous transjugular approach, a specially designed sheathed puncture needle is passed from the jugular vein down into a hepatic vein radicle. A puncture is then made from the hepatic vein into a branch of the portal vein. The parenchymal tract is dilated, and a metallic stent is placed in the tract. This procedure allows nonoperative decompression of the portal system. It is used in the treatment of variceal bleeding and in the management of intractable ascites. The technique was first performed by Rosch and colleagues,[215] who created an artificial tract between the inferior vena cava and portal vein in swine. Colapinto and coworkers[216] were the first to perform the technique in humans. Their results were limited by early and late shunt occlusion and high mortality. Palmaz and coworkers,[217] using their stent, were able to achieve long-term shunt patency in a canine model of portal hypertension.

The use of the newer vascular stents to maintain patency of the artificial tract between the hepatic vein and portal vein has resulted in improved patency of the shunts.[218] Rossle and associates[219] described results in 100 patients who underwent TIPS with the Palmaz stent for variceal hemorrhage. With mean follow-up of 12 months (±6 months), the authors observed the following: The shunt reduced the portal venous pressure gradient by 57%. At follow-up, stenosis of the shunt was evident in 21 patients, and occlusion in 10 patients. These were all treated successfully by redilatation, thrombolysis, or implantation of a new stent. Hepatic encephalopathy developed in 25% of patients. The major complications of TIPS are hemorrhage (intraabdominal bleeding or capsular bleeding) and, rarely, stent migration. Ninety-two percent of patients remained free of variceal bleeding at 6 months, and 82% at 1 year. The 30-day mortality was 3%, and cumulative 1-year survival, 85%. In a large multicenter trial consisting of patients with variceal bleeding who had failed to respond to sclerotherapy, Coldwell and colleagues[220] noted a 30-day mortality of 0% for patients with Child class A disease, 18% for class B, and 40% for class C. At 6 months, primary patency was 88%, and assisted patency was 94%. Of the major complications due to TIPS, encephalopathy was the most prevalent. The authors concluded that TIPS offers the same safety and efficacy as sclerotherapy and significantly greater short-term survival than surgery until the 6-month anniversary.

The TIPS procedure also may serve as a bridge to liver transplantation and as a preoperative aid to transplantation. It is also used to treat intractable ascites.[221] These and other long-term studies indicate the value of the TIPS procedure and demonstrate that it is a viable therapeutic alternative to surgery and sclerotherapy.

NEW ANGIOGRAPHIC IMAGING TECHNIQUES: MAGNETIC RESONANCE ANGIOGRAPHY AND COMPUTED TOMOGRAPHY ANGIOGRAPHY

Noninvasive imaging of the vascular system can be accomplished using fast CT imaging techniques and MRI.

MRI is a method of imaging based on the behavior of protons when placed in a magnetic field and exposed to radiofrequency waves. Advantages of MRI include a large field of view, which allows imaging of the entire thorax or abdomen on a given scan, the ability to image organs of interest in multiple projections, and the lack of ionizing radiation. Imaging may be done with or without injection of MR contrast media. Flowing blood is well distinguished from soft tissue with MRI. The appearance of flowing blood depends on the particular MRI technique used. With spin echo imaging, flowing blood is seen as signal void (black blood). Spin-echo techniques provide good anatomic definition of large vessels. Smaller vessels, such as the renal or peripheral arteries, are better evaluated using bright blood (gradient echo sequences). A series of images acquired using gradient echo techniques can be processed using the maximum-intensity projection algorithm. This postprocessing algorithm projects the brightest pixels along a user-selected orientation into a projection image. The brightest pixels are assumed to represent flowing blood. The resultant images resemble conventional angiograms, and are called MRA.

Currently, MRA images are acquired using 2-dimensional TOF (time-of-flight), 3-dimensional phase contrast, and 3-dimensional TOF techniques. The 3-dimensional TOF technique with the injection of gadolinium-DTPA (pentetic acid) contrast agent is currently the most widely used technique. MRA has largely replaced contrast angiography for presurgical evaluation of the carotid bifurcation (Fig. 16–28). In many centers, MRA is routinely used to confirm findings of carotid duplex sonography and is used in conjunction with MRI of the brain in patients with suspected cerebrovascular disease. MRI and MRA of the thoracic aorta are used in the diagnosis and follow-up of patients with aortic dissection or aneurysm.[222] MRA is used to evaluate the renal arteries[223, 224] and the peripheral vessels of the extremities.[225, 226] MRI and MRA are often used when there is a contraindication to conventional angiography and are used as an alternative to angiography in patients who are allergic to iodinated contrast material or have renal insufficiency or in whom long-term follow-up would otherwise require repeated arteriography. MRA is also useful for evaluating the central veins, veins of the upper and lower extremities, and veins of the portal system. A limitation of MRA is the inability to accurately assess the degree of stenosis. The extent of a lesion is usually seen;

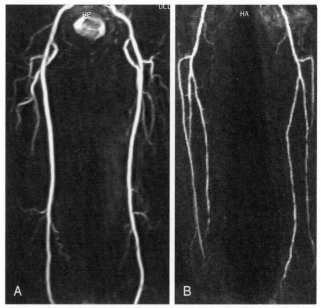

Figure 16–28. Gadolinium-enhanced MRA of the lower extremities. *A,* MRA of the lower pelvis and thighs, down to the level of the popliteal arteries. No abnormalities are noted. *B,* View of the lower legs showing filling of the right and left popliteal arteries. The left anterior tibial artery is occluded proximally. There is evidence of segmental disease in the left peroneal artery and atherosclerotic plaque in the left posterior tibial artery. On the right, there is atherosclerotic plaque in the posterior tibial artery, which terminates just above the ankle. The right anterior tibial and peroneal arteries show no significant disease.

however, stenoses may be overestimated due to slow flow or turbulence, which results in loss of the magnetic resonance signal. These limitations are minimized with the 3-D TOF gadolinium-enhanced MRA techniques.

Spiral CT is a form of fast CT imaging in which continuous rotation of the CT gantry data acquisition system, coupled with continuous movement of the patient through the scanner, allows the rapid acquisition of thin-slice image data. With spiral imaging, continuous volumes of data can be acquired and can be reconstructed to yield an innumerable number of overlapping axial images. Computer algorithms, such as maximum-intensity projections and shaded surface displays, can then reconstruct the data to produce images that resemble conventional angiograms. The ability to track a single bolus injection of contrast medium is improved, and if scanning is done soon after the start of contrast bolus administration, the arterial system can be selectively enhanced. Spiral CT angiography has been used effectively to study aortic dissections, thoracic and abdominal aortic aneurysms, and the renal and carotid arteries.[227] It also has been applied to the diagnosis of pulmonary thromboembolism. Because only a limited volume of tissue can be imaged with the thin-slice technique using iodinated contrast media, spiral CT angiography has limited application in the diagnosis of peripheral vascular disease. Although it affords high-resolution images of larger vessels, it does not currently permit imaging of smaller vessels. Faster CT scans, which will permit imaging of larger volumes, are under development.

References

1. Molnar W, Paul DJ: Complications of axillary arteriotomies: An analysis of 1,762 consecutive studies. Radiology 104:269–276, 1972.
2. Kruger RA, Mistretta CA, Riederer SJ, et al: Computerized fluoroscopy in real time for noninvasive visualization of the cardiovascular system. Radiology 130:49–57, 1979.
3. Mistretta CA, Ort MG, Cameron JR, et al: Multiple images subtraction technique for enhancing low contrast periodic objects. Invest Radiol 8:43–44, 1973.
4. Ort MG, Mistretta CA, Kelcz F: An improved technique for enhancing small period contrast changes in television fluoroscopy. Opt Engl 12:169–175, 1973.
5. Buonocore E, Meany TF, Borkowski GP, et al: Digital subtraction angiography of the abdominal aorta and renal arteries. Radiology 139:281–286, 1981.
6. Brant-Zawadzki M, Gould R, Norman B, et al: Digital subtraction cerebral angiography by intra-arterial injection: Comparison with conventional angiography. AJR 140:347–353, 1983.
7. Jacobsson B, Schlossman D: Thromboembolism of the leg following percutaneous catheterization of the femoral artery for angiography: Predisposing factors. Acta Radiol Diagn 8:109–118, 1969.
8. Fischer HW: Viscosity, solubility and toxicity in the choice of an angiographic contrast medium. Angiology 16:759–763, 1965.
9. Gonzalez L, Stieritz D: Experimental evaluation of sodium methylglucamine iothalamate (MP3064): Cardiovascular responses following proximal aortic injection. Invest Radiol 2:266–271, 1967.
10. Spataro F: Newer contrast agents for urography. Radiol Clin North Am 22:365–380, 1984.
11. Katayama H, Yamaguchi K, Kozuka T, et al: Adverse reactions to ionic and nonionic contrast media: A report from the Japanese Committee on the Safety of Contrast Media. Radiology 175:621–628, 1990.
12. Sherwood T, Lavender J: Does renal flow rise or fall in response to diatrizoate? Invest Radiol 4:327–328, 1969.
13. Older R, Miller J, Jackson D, et al: Angiographically induced renal failure and its radiographic detection. AJR 126:1039–1045, 1976.
14. Pillay V, Robbins P, Schwartz F, et al: Acute renal failure following intravenous urography in patients with long-standing diabetes mellitus and azotemia. Radiology 95:633–636, 1970.
15. Port F, Wagoner R, Fulton R: Acute renal failure after angiography. AJR 121:544–550, 1974.
16. Talner L: Urographic contrast media in uremia. Radiol Clin North Am 10:421–432, 1972.
17. Gomes AS, Baker JD, Martin-Paredero V, et al: Acute renal dysfunction after major arteriography. AJR 145:1249–1253, 1985.
18. Eisenberg RL, Bank WO, Hedgcock MW: Renal failure after major angiography. AJR 136:859–861, 1981.
19. Solomon R, Werner C, Mann D, et al: Effects of saline, mannitol, and furosemide on acute decreases in renal function induced by radiocontrast agents. N Engl J Med 331:1416–1420, 1994.
20. Pendergrass HP, Hodes PJ, Tondreau RL, et al: Further considerations of deaths and unfavorable sequelae following the administration of contrast media in urography in the United States. AJR 74:262–287, 1955.
21. Greenberger P, Patterson R, Kelly J, et al: Administration of radiographic contrast media in high risk patients. Invest Radiol 15:540–549, 1980.
22. Kelly JF, Patterson R, Lieberman P, et al: Radiographic contrast media studies in high risk patients. J Allergy Clin Immunol 62:181–184, 1978.
23. Johnsrude IS: Aortic arch and brachiocephalic angiography. In Johnsrude IS, Jackson DC (eds): A Practical Approach to Angiography. Boston, Little, Brown, 1979, p 296.
24. Hoffman R, Rein B: The routine use of subtraction in aortic arch studies. Radiology 102:575–578, 1972.
25. Haas W, Fields W, North R, et al: Joint study of extracranial arterial occlusion: II. Arteriography, techniques, sites and complications. JAMA 203:159–166, 1968.
26. Castaneda WZ, Knight L, Formanek A, et al: Hemodynamic assessment of obstructive aortoiliac disease. AJR 127:559–561, 1976.
27. Haimovichi H: Patterns of arteriosclerotic lesions of the lower extremities. Arch Surg 95:918–933, 1967.
28. Crawford ES, DeBakey ME, Morris GC: Thrombo-obliterative disease of the great vessels arising from the aortic arch. J Thorac Cardiovasc Surg 43:38–53, 1962.
29. Champion HR, Gill W: Arterial embolus to the upper limb. Br J Surg 60:505–508, 1973.
30. Darling CR, Austen WG, Linton RR: Arterial embolism. Surg Gynecol Obstet 124:106–114, 1967.
31. Lambeth J, Yong N: Arteriographic findings in thromboangiitis obliterans. AJR 109:553–562, 1970.
32. McKusick VA, Harris WS, Otteson OE, et al: Buerger's disease: A distinct clinical and pathologic entity. JAMA 181:5–12, 1962.
33. Wessler S: Thromboangiitis obliterans. Fact or fancy. Circulation 23:165–167, 1961.
34. Lande A, Gross A: Total aortography in the diagnosis of Takayasu's arteritis. AJR 116:165–178, 1972.
35. Lande A, Rossi P: The value of total aortography in the diagnosis of Takayasu's arteritis. Radiology 14:287–297, 1975.
36. Hamrin B, Jonsson N, Landberg T: Involvement of large vessels in polymyalgia rheumatica. Lancet 1:1193–1196, 1965.
37. Harrison C: Giant cell or temporal arteritis: A review. Gen Clin Pathol 1:197–211, 1948.
38. Hauser WA, Ferguson RH, Holley KE, et al: Temporal arteritis in Rochester Minn 1951–1967. Mayo Clin Proc 46:597–602, 1971.
39. Hunder GG, Ward LE, Burbank MK: Giant cell arteritis producing an aortic arch syndrome. Ann Intern Med 66:578–582, 1967.
40. Benedict K, Chang W, McCready F: The hypothenar hammer syndrome. Radiology 111:57–60, 1974.
41. Laws J, Lillie J, Scott J: Arteriographic appearances in rheumatoid arthritis and other disorders. Br J Radiol 36:477–493, 1963.
42. Fagerberg S, Jorulf H, Sandberg C: Ergotism: Arterial spastic disease and recovery studied angiographically. Acta Med Scand 182:769–772, 1967.
43. Love L: Arteriography of peripheral vascular trauma. AJR 102:431–440, 1968.
44. McDonald E, Goodman P, Winestock D: Clinical indications for arteriography in trauma to the extremity: A review of 114 cases. Radiology 116:45–47, 1975.
45. Pochaczevsky R, Mufte M, LaGuerre J, et al: Arteriography of penetrating wounds of the extremities: Help or hindrance? J Can Assoc Radiol 24:354–361, 1973.
46. Lumpkin MB, Logan WD, Couves CM, et al: Arteriography as an aid in the diagnosis and localization of acute arterial injuries. Ann Surg 147:353–358, 1958.
47. Perry MO, Thal ER, Shires GT: Management of arterial injuries. Ann Surg 173:403–408, 1971.
48. Cliff MM, Soulen RL, Finestone AJ: Mycotic aneurysms—a challenge and a clue. Arch Intern Med 126:977–982, 1970.
49. Boley SJ, Sprayregen S, Siegelman SS, Veith FJ: Initial results from an aggressive roentgenological and surgical approach to acute mesenteric ischemia. Surgery 82:848–855, 1977.
50. Ottinger LW, Austen WG: A study of 136 patients with mesenteric infarction. Surg Gynecol Obstet 124:251–261, 1967.
51. Siegelman SS, Sprayregen S, Boley SJ: Angiographic diagnosis of mesenteric arterial vasoconstriction. Radiology 112:533–542, 1974.
52. Boley SJ, Feinstein R, Sammartano RJ: Superior mesenteric embolus. Presented at the American College of Surgeons, Atlanta, October 1980.
53. Ottinger LW: Surgical management of acute occlusion of the superior mesenteric artery. Ann Surg 188:721–731, 1978.
54. Katz PO, Salas L: Less frequent causes of upper gastrointestinal bleeding. Gastroenterol Clin North Am 22:875–889, 1993.
55. Wade GL, Smith DC, Mohr LL: Followup of 50 consecutive angiograms obtained utilizing puncture of prosthetic vascular grafts. Radiology 146:663–664, 1983.
56. Nusbaum M, Baum S: Radiographic demonstration of unknown sites of gastrointestinal bleeding. Surg Forum 14:374–375, 1963.
57. Alavi A, Dann RW, Baum S, et al: Scintigraphic detection of acute gastrointestinal bleeding. Radiology 124:753–756, 1977.
58. Miskowiak J, Nielsen SL, Munck O: Scintigraphic diagnosis of gastrointestinal bleeding with Tc[99m] labeled bloodpool agents. Radiology 141:499–504, 1981.
59. Johnsrude IS: Splanchnic angiography. In Johnsrude IS, Jackson DC (eds): A Practical Approach to Angiography. Boston, Little, Brown, 1979, pp 205–271.

60. Leevy C, Gliedman M: Practical and research value of hepatic vein catheterization. N Engl J Med 258:696–700, 1958.

61. Viamonte M Jr, Warren W, Fomon J: Liver panangiography in the assessment of portal hypertension in liver cirrhosis. Radiol Clin North Am 1:147–167, 1970.

62. Redman H: Mesenteric arterial and venous blood flow changes following selective arterial injection of vasodilators. Invest Radiol 9:193–198, 1974.

63. Leger L: Splenoportography: Diagnostic Phlebography of the Portal Venous System. Springfield, Ill, Charles C Thomas, 1966.

64. Korobkin M, Moss AA, Callen PW, et al: Computed tomography of subcapsular splenic hematoma. Clinical and experimental studies. Radiology 129:441–445, 1978.

65. Shirkhoda A, McCartney WH, Staab EV, et al: Imaging of the spleen: A proposed algorithm. AJR 135:195–198, 1980.

66. Baum S, Roy R, Finkelstein AK, Blakemore AS: Clinical application of selective celiac and superior mesenteric angiography. Radiology 84:279–294, 1965.

67. Haertel M, Ryder D: Radiologic investigation of splenic trauma. Cardiovasc Radiol 2:27–33, 1979.

68. Abrams HL, Comell SH: Patterns of collateral flow in renal ischemia. Radiology 84:1001–1012, 1965.

69. Brewster DC, Darling AC: Optimal methods of aortoiliac reconstruction. Surgery 84:739–748, 1972.

70. Palubinskas AJ, Wylie EJ: Roentgen diagnosis of fibromuscular hyperplasia of the renal arteries. Radiology 76:634–639, 1961.

71. Kincaid OW, Davis GD, Hallerman N, et al: Fibromuscular dysplasia of the renal arteries: Arteriographic features, classification and observations on natural history of the disease. AJR 104:271–282, 1968.

72. McCormack LJ, Dustan HP, Meany TF: Selected pathology of the renal artery. Semin Roentgenol 2:126–138, 1967.

73. Palubinskas AJ, Ripley H: Fibromuscular hyperplasia in extra-renal arteries. Radiology 82:451–454, 1964.

74. Wholey MH, Cooperstone LA: Renal trauma. In Abrams HL (ed): Abrams' Angiography: Vascular and Interventional Radiology, 3rd ed. Boston, Little, Brown, 1983, pp 1231–1237.

75. Love L, Moncada R, Lescher AJ: Renal arteriovenous fistulae. AJR 95:364–371, 1965.

76. Ekelund L, Lindholm T: Arteriovenous fistulae following percutaneous renal biopsy. Acta Radiol 11:38–48, 1971.

77. Hageman JH, Smith RF, Szilagyi E, et al: Aneurysms of the renal artery. Problems of prognosis and surgical management. Surgery 84:563–572, 1978.

78. Quinton W, Dillar D, Scribner BH: Cannulation of blood vessels for prolonged hemodialysis. Trans Am Soc Artif Intern Organs 6:104–113, 1960.

79. Brescia MJ, Cimino JE, Appel K, et al: Chronic hemodialysis using venipuncture and a surgically created arteriovenous fistula. N Engl J Med 275:1089–1092, 1966.

80. Butt KM, Friedman EA, Kountz SL: Angioaccess. Curr Probl Surg 13:36–38, 1976.

81. Gilula LA, Staple TW, Anderson CB, Anderson LS: Venous angiography of hemodialysis fistulas. Radiology 115:555–562, 1975.

82. O'Reilly RJ, Hansen CC, Rosental JJ: Angiography of chronic hemodialysis arteriovenous grafts. AJR 130:1105–1113, 1978.

83. Kirschner LP, Twigg H, Farkas J: Drip infusion venography. Radiology 96:413–415, 1970.

84. Rabinov K, Paulin S: Roentgen diagnosis of venous thrombosis in the leg. Arch Surg 104:134–144, 1972.

85. Thomas ML: Phlebography. Arch Surg 104:145–151, 1972.

86. Rose SC, Zwiebel WJ, Nelson BD, et al: Symptomatic lower extremity deep venous thrombosis: Accuracy, limitations, and role of color duplex flow imaging in diagnosis. Radiology 175:639–644, 1990.

87. Lange EK: Arteriography of thoracic outlet syndrome. In Abrams HI (ed): Abrams' Angiography: Vascular and Interventional Radiology, 3rd ed. Boston, Little, Brown, 1983, pp 1001–1015.

88. Lang EK: Arteriographic diagnosis of the thoracic outlet syndrome. Radiology 84:296–302, 1965.

89. Martin U: Clinical and preclinical profile of the novel recombinant plasminogen activator reteplase. In Sasahara AA, Loscalzo J (eds): New Therapeutic Agents in Thrombosis and Thrombolysis. New York, Marcel Dekker, 1997, pp 495–511.

90. Kohnert U, Rudolph R, Verheijen JH, et al: Biochemical properties of the kringle 2 and protease domains are maintained in the refolded t-PA deletion variant BM 06.022. Protein Eng 5:93–100, 1992.

91. Johnson AJ, McCarty WR: The lysis of artificially induced intravascular clots in man by intravenous infusion of streptokinase. J Clin Invest 38:1627–1643, 1959.

92. Sherry S, Lindemeyer RI, Fletcher AP, et al: Studies on enhanced fibrinolytic activity in man. J Clin Invest 38:810–822, 1959.

93. The Urokinase Pulmonary Embolism Trial. A Cooperative Study. Phase I results. JAMA 214:2163–2172, 1970.

94. The Urokinase Pulmonary Embolism Trial. A National Cooperative Study. Phase II results. JAMA 229:1606–1613, 1974.

95. Dotter CT, Rosch J, Seaman AJ: Selective clot lysis with low dose streptokinase. Radiology 111:31–37, 1974.

96. Rentrop P, Blanke H, Karsch KR, et al: Selective intracoronary thrombolysis in acute myocardial infarction and unstable angina pectoris. Circulation 63:307–317, 1981.

97. Hargrove WC, Barker CF, Berkowitz HD, et al: Treatment of acute peripheral arterial and graft thromboses with low dose streptokinase. Surgery 92:981–993, 1982.

98. Becker GJ, Rabe FE, Richmond BD, et al: Low dose fibrinolytic therapy: Results and new concepts. Radiology 148:663–670, 1983.

99. Mori KW, Bookstein JJ, Heeney DJ, et al: Selective streptokinase infusion: Clinical and laboratory correlates. Radiology 148:677–682, 1983.

100. Martin M: Thrombolytic therapy in arterial thromboembolism. Prog Cardiovasc Dis 21:351–374, 1979.

101. McNamara TO, Fischer JR: Thrombolysis of peripheral arterial and graft occlusions: Improved results using high dose urokinase. AJR 144:769–775, 1985.

102. Cragg AH, Smith TP, Corson JD, et al: Two urokinase dose regimens in native arterial and graft occlusions: Initial results of a prospective, randomized clinical trial. Radiology 178:681–686, 1991.

103. Astrup T, Stage A: Isolation of a soluble fibrinolytic activator from animal tissue. Nature 170:929–930, 1952.

104. Booyse FM, Scheinbuks J, Radek J, et al: Immunological identification and comparison of plasminogen activator forms in cultured normal human endothelial cells and smooth muscle cells. Thromb Res 24:495–504, 1981.

105. Eisenberg PR, Sherman LA, Tiefenbrunn AJ, et al: Sustained fibrinolysis after administration of t-PA despite its short half-life in the circulation. Thromb Haemost 57:35–40, 1987.

106. Risius B, Graor RA, Geisinger MA, et al: Recombinant human tissue-type plasminogen activator for thrombolysis in peripheral arteries and bypass grafts. Radiology 160:183–188, 1986.

107. Results of a prospective randomized trial evaluating surgery versus thrombolysis for ischemia of the lower extremity: The STILE trial. Ann Surg 220:251–266, 1994.

108. Verstraete M, Bounameaux H, DeCock F, et al: Pharmacokinetics and systemic fibrinogenolytic effects of recombinant human tissue-type plasminogen activator (rt-PA) in humans. J Pharmacol Exp Ther 235:506–512, 1985.

109. Martin U, Spooner G, Strein K: Evaluation of thrombolytic and systemic effects of the novel recombinant plasminogen activator BM06.022 compared with alteplase, anistreplase, streptokinase and urokinase in a canine model of coronary artery thrombosis. J Am Coll Cardiol 19:433–440, 1992.

110. Ouriel K, Shortell CK, DeWeese JA, et al: A comparison of thrombolytic therapy with operative revascularization in the initial treatment of acute peripheral arterial ischemia. J Vasc Surg 19:1021–1030, 1994.

111. Ouriel K, Veith FJ, Sasahara AA: A comparison of recombinant urokinase with vascular surgery as initial trial treatment for acute arterial occlusion of the legs. N Engl J Med 338:1105–1111, 1998.

112. Ouriel K, Kandarpa K, Schuerr DM, et al: Prourokinase vs. urokinase for recanalization of peripheral occlusions, safety and efficacy: The PURPOSE Trial. JVIR 10:1083–1091, 1999.

113. Liu JM, Gurewich V: Fragment E-2 from fibrin substantially enhances pro-urokinase-induced Glu-plasminogen activation: A kinetic study using the plasmin resistant mutant pro-urokinase Ala-158-rproUK. Biochemistry 31:6311–6317, 1992.

114. Chuang VP: Non-operative retrieval of Gianturco coils from the abdominal aorta. AJR 132:996–997, 1979.

115. Curry JL: Recovery of detached intravascular catheter or guide wire fragments. A proposed method. AJR 105:894–896, 1969.

116. Lassers BW, Pickering D: Removal of an iatrogenic foreign body from the aorta by means of a ureteric stone catheter. Am Heart J 73:375–378, 1967.

117. Rossi P: "Hook catheter," technique for transfemoral removal of foreign body from right side of the heart. AJR 109:101–106, 1970.
118. King JF, Manley JC, Zeft HJ, et al: Nonsurgical removal of foreign body from right heart. J Thorac Cardiovasc Surg 71:785–786, 1976.
119. Milan VG: Retrieval of intravascular foreign bodies using a modified bronchoscopic forceps. Radiology 129:587–589, 1978.
120. Yedlicka JW Jr, Carlson JE, Hunter DW, et al: Nitinol gooseneck snare for removal of foreign bodies: Experimental study and clinical evaluation. Radiology 178:691, 1991.
121. Gruntzig A, Hopff H: Perkutane Rekanalisation chronischer arterieller Verschlüsse mit einem neuen Dilatationskatheter: Modification der Dotter-Technik. Dtsch Med Wochenschr 99:2502–2505, 1974.
122. Gruntzig A, Kumpe DA: Technique of percutaneous transluminal angioplasty with the Gruntzig balloon catheter. AJR 132:547–552, 1979.
123. Castaneda-Zuniga WR, Formanek A, Tadavarthy M, et al: The mechanism of balloon angioplasty. Radiology 135:565–571, 1980.
124. Faxon DP, Coats W, Currier J: Remodeling of the coronary artery after vascular injury. Prog Cardiovasc Dis 40:129–140, 1997.
125. Tegtmeyer CJ, Kellum CD, Kron IL, Mentzer RM Jr: Percutaneous transluminal angioplasty in the region of the aortic bifurcation: The two balloon technique with results and long-term followup study. Radiology 157:661–665, 1985.
126. Yakes WF, Kumpe DA, Brown SB, et al: Percutaneous transluminal aortic angioplasty: Technique and results. Radiology 172:965–970, 1989.
127. Neiman HL, Bergan JJ, Yao JS: Hemodynamic assessment of transluminal angioplasty for lower extremity ischemia. Radiology 143:639–643, 1982.
128. Spence RK, Frieman DB, Gatenby R, et al: Long-term results of transluminal angioplasty of the iliac and femoral arteries. Arch Surg 116:1377–1386, 1981.
129. Kadir S, White RI, Kaufman SL, et al: Long term results of aortoiliac angioplasty. Surgery 94:10–14, 1983.
130. van Andel GJ, van Erp WFM, Krepel VM, et al: Percutaneous transluminal dilation of the iliac artery: Long term results. Radiology 156:321–323, 1985.
131. Gruntzig A: Die Perkutane Transluminal Re-Kanalisation chronischer Arterienverschlüsse mit einer neuen Dilatationstechnik. Baden-Baden, Germany, Witzstrock, 1977.
132. van Andel GJ: Transluminal iliac angioplasty: Long term results. Radiology 135:607–611, 1980.
133. Schneider E, Gruntzig A, Bollinger A: Langzeitergebnisse nach perkutaner transluminaler Angioplastie (PTA) bei 882 konsekutiven Patienten mit iliakalen und femorpoplitealen Obstruktionen. Vasa 11:322–326, 1982.
134. Johnston KW, Colapinto RF, Baird RJ: Transluminal dilation. An alternative? Arch Surg 117:1604–1610, 1982.
135. Kumpe DA, Jones DN: Percutaneous transluminal angioplasty; radiologic viewpoint. Appl Radiol 11:29–40, 1982.
136. Schwarten DE: Percutaneous transluminal angioplasty of the iliac arteries: Intravenous digital subtraction angiography for followup. Radiology 150:363–367, 1984.
137. Johnston KW, Rae H, Hogg-Johnston B, et al: 5 year results of a prospective study of percutaneous transluminal angioplasty. Ann Surg 206:403–413, 1987.
138. Tegtmeyer CJ, Hartwell GD, Selby JB, et al: Results and complications of angioplasty in aortoiliac disease. Circulation; 83(Suppl 1):I-53–I-60, 1991.
139. Malone JW, Moore WS, Goldstein J: The natural history of bilateral aortofemoral bypass grafts for ischemia of the lower extremities. Arch Surg 110:1300–1306, 1975.
140. Wilson SE, Wolf GL, Cross AP: Percutaneous transluminal angioplasty versus operation for peripheral arteriosclerosis. J Vasc Surg 9:1–9, 1989.
141. Krepel VM, van Andel GJ, van Erp WF, et al: Percutaneous transluminal angioplasty of the femoropopliteal artery: Initial and long term results. Radiology 156:325–328, 1985.
142. Greenfield AJ: Femoral, popliteal and tibial arteries: Percutaneous transluminal angioplasty. AJR 135:927–935, 1980.
143. Freiman DB, Spence RK, Gatenby R: Transluminal angioplasty of the iliac and femoral arteries: Follow up results without anticoagulation. Radiology 141:347–350, 1981.
144. Colapinto RF: Long-term results of iliac and femoropopliteal angioplasty. In Dotter CT, Gruntzig A, Schoop W, Zietler E (eds): Percu-

145. Berkowitz HD, Spence RK, Frieman DB, et al: Long-term results of transluminal angioplasty of the femoral arteries. In Dotter CT, Gruntzig A, Schoop W, Zietler E (eds): Percutaneous Transluminal Angioplasty. Berlin, Springer-Verlag, 1983, pp 207–214.
146. Mahler F, Gallino A, Probst P, et al: Factors influencing early and late follow-up results after percutaneous transluminal angioplasty of the lower limb arteries. In Dotter CT, Gruntzig A, Schoop W, Zietler E (eds): Percutaneous Transluminal Angioplasty. Berlin, Springer-Verlag, 1983, pp 199–201.
147. Gallino A, Mahler F, Probst P, et al: Früh-und Spätergebnisse bei 250 perkutanen transluminalen Dilatationen an den unteren Extremitäten. Vasa 11:319–321, 1982.
148. Capek P, McLean GK, Berkowitz HD: Femoropopiteal angioplasty: Factors influencing long term success Circulation 83(Suppl 1): I-70–I-80, 1991.
149. Adar R, Critchfield GC, Eddie DM: A confidence profile analysis of the results of femoropopliteal percutaneous transluminal angioplasty in the treatment of lower-extremity ischemia. J Vasc Surg 10:57–67, 1989.
150. Mehta S: A Statistical Summary of the Results of Femoropopliteal Bypass Surgery. Newark, Del, WL Gore, 1980, pp 1–32.
151. Veith FJ, Gupta SK, Samson RH, et al: Progress in limb salvage by reconstructive arterial surgery combined with new or improved adjunctive procedures. Ann Surg 194:386–400, 1981.
152. Taylor LM, Porter JM: Clinical and anatomic considerations for surgery in femoropopliteal disease and the results of surgery. Circulation 83(Suppl 1):I-63–I-69, 1991.
153. Casarella WJ: Percutaneous transluminal angioplasty below the knee: New techniques, excellent results. Radiology 169:271–272, 1988.
154. Schwarten DE, Cutcliff WB: Arterial occlusive disease below the knee: Treatment with percutaneous transluminal angioplasty performed with low-profile catheters and steerable guide wires. Radiology 169:71–74, 1988.
155. Bakal CW, Sprayregen S, Scheinbaum K, et al: Percutaneous transluminal angioplasty of the infrapopliteal arteries: Results in 53 patients. AJR 154:171–174, 1990.
156. Horvath W, Oertl M, Haidinger D: Percutaneous transluminal angioplasty of crural arteries. Radiology 177:565–569, 1990.
157. Londry GL, Ramsey DE, Hodgson KJ, et al: Infrapopliteal bypass for severe ischemia: Comparison of autogenous vein, composite, and prosthetic grafts. J Vasc Surg 13:631–636, 1991.
158. Taylor LM, Edwards JM, Porter JM: Present status of reversed vein bypass grafting: Five-year results of a modern series. J Vasc Surg 11:193–206, 1990.
159. Kram HB, Gupta SK, Veith FJ, et al: Late results of two hundred seventeen femoropopliteal artery segments. J Vasc Surg 14:386–390, 1991.
160. Sanchez LA, Gupta SK, Veith FJ, et al: A ten-year experience with one hundred fifty failing or threatened vein and polytetrafluoroethylene arterial bypass grafts. J Vasc Surg 14:729–736, 1991.
161. Pentecost MJ, Criqui MH, Dorros G, et al: Guidelines for peripheral percutaneous transluminal angioplasty of the abdominal aorta and lower extremity vessels. Circulation 89:511–531, 1994.
162. Klinge J, Mali WP, Puylaert C, et al: Percutaneous transluminal angioplasty: Initial and long-term results. Radiology 171:501–506, 1989.
163. Karagiannis A, Douma S, Voyiatzis K, et al: Percutaneous transluminal renal angioplasty in patients with renovascular hypertension; long-term results. Hypertens Res 18:27–31, 1995.
164. Losinno F, Zuccala A, Busato F, Zucchelli P: Renal artery angioplasty for renovascular hypertension and preservation of renal function: Long-term angiographic and clinical follow-up. AJR 162:853–857, 1994.
165. Sos TG, Pickering TG, Sniderman K, et al: Percutaneous transluminal renal angioplasty in patients with renovascular hypertension due to atheroma or fibromuscular dysplasia. N Engl J Med 309:274–279, 1983.
166. Martin LG, Cork RD, Kaufman SL: Long-term results of angioplasty in 110 patients with renal artery stenosis. JVIR 3:619–626, 1992.
167. Eldrup-Jorgenson J, Harvey HR, Sampson LN, et al: Should percutaneous transluminal renal artery angioplasty be applied to ostial renal artery atherosclerosis? J Vasc Surg 21:909–914, 1995.
168. Schwarten DE: Transluminal angioplasty of renal artery stenosis: 70 experiences. AJR 135:969–974, 1980.

169. Sos TA, Sniderman KW, Pickering T, et al: Percutaneous transluminal renal angioplasty: Experience in over 100 arteries. In Kaltenbach M, Rentrop K (eds): Transluminal Coronary Angioplasty and Intracoronary Thrombolysis. Berlin, Springer-Verlag, 1982, pp 412–425.

170. Tegtmeyer CJ, Elson J, Glass TA, et al: Percutaneous transluminal angioplasty: The treatment of choice of renovascular hypertension due to fibromuscular dysplasia. Radiology 143:631–637, 1982.

171. Foster JH, Maxwell MH, Franklin SS, et al: Renovascular occlusive disease: Results of operative treatment. JAMA 231:1043–1048, 1975.

172. Kaufman JJ: Renovascular hypertension: The UCLA experience. J Urol 121:139–144, 1979.

173. Stoney RJ, DeLuccia N, Ehrenfeld WK, et al: Aortorenal arterial autografts: Long range assessment. Arch Surg 116:1416–1422, 1981.

174. Tegtmeyer CJ, Selby JB, Hartwell GD, et al: Results and complications of angioplasty in fibromuscular disease. Circulation 83(Suppl 2):I-155–I-161, 1991.

175. Novick AC, Straffon RA, Steward BH, et al: Diminished operative morbidity and mortality in renal revascularization. JAMA 246:749–753, 1981.

176. Gianturco C, Anderson JH, Wallace S: Mechanical devices for arterial occlusion. AJR 124:428–435, 1975.

177. White RI Jr, Kaufman SL, Barth KH, et al: Embolotherapy with detachable silicone balloons: Technique and clinical results. Radiology 131:619–627, 1979.

178. Tadavarthy SM, Moller JH, Amplatz KA: Polyvinyl alcohol (Ivalon)—a new embolic material. AJR 125:609–616, 1975.

179. Hilal SK, Sane P, Michelson WJ, et al: The embolization of vascular malformations of the spinal cord with low viscosity silicone rubber. Neuroradiology 16:430–433, 1978.

180. Dotter CT, Goldman ML, Rosch J: Instant selective arterial occlusion with isobutyl 2-cyanoacrylate. Radiology 114:227–230, 1975.

181. Barth KH, Strandberg JD, White RI Jr: Long-term followup of transcatheter embolization with autologous clot, oxycel and Gelfoam in domestic swine. Invest Radiol 12:273–280, 1977.

182. Gomes MMR, Bernatz PE: Arteriovenous fistulas: A review and 10 year experience at the Mayo Clinic. Mayo Clin Proc 45:81–102, 1970.

183. Gomes AS, Mali WP, Oppenheim WL: Embolization therapy in the management of congenital arteriovenous malformations. Radiology 144:41–49, 1982.

184. Kaufman SL, Kumar AAJ, Roland JMA, et al: Transcatheter embolization in the management of congenital arteriovenous malformations. Radiology 137:21–29, 1980.

185. Olcott C IV, Newton TH, Stoney RJ, et al: Intra-arterial embolization in the management of arteriovenous malformations. Surgery 79:3–12, 1976.

186. Remy J, Amand A, Fardon H, et al: Treatment of hemoptysis by embolization of bronchial arteries. Radiology 122:33–37, 1977.

187. Wallace S, Chuang VP, Swenson D: Embolization of renal carcinoma. Experience with 100 patients. Radiology 138:563–570, 1981.

188. Higgins CB, Bookstein JJ, Davis GB, et al: Therapeutic embolization for intractable chronic bleeding. Radiology 122:473–478, 1977.

189. Ring EJ, Athanasoulis CA, Wallman AC, et al: Arteriographic management of hemorrhage following pelvic fracture. Radiology 109:65–70, 1973.

190. Tadavarthy SM, Casteneda-Zuniga W, Salomonowitz E, et al: Kimray-Greenfield vena cava filter: Percutaneous introduction. Radiology 151:525–526, 1984.

191. Messmer JM, Greenfield LJ: Greenfield filters: Long-term radiographic follow-up study. Radiology 156:613–618, 1985.

192. Greenfield LJ, Michna BA: Twelve-year clinical experience with the Greenfield vena cava filter. Surgery 104:706–712, 1988.

193. Geisinger MA, Zelch MG, Risius B: Recurrent pulmonary emboli after Greenfield filter placement. Radiology 165:383–384, 1987.

194. Pais S, Tobin K, Austin C, Queral L: Percutaneous insertion of Greenfield inferior vena cava filter: Experience with ninety-six patients. J Vasc Surg 8:460–464, 1988.

195. Pais SO, Tobin KD: Percutaneous insertion of the Greenfield filter. AJR 152:933–938, 1989.

196. Greenfield LJ, Zocco J, Wilk J, et al: Clinical experience with the Kimray-Greenfield vena caval filter. Ann Surg 185:692–698, 1977.

197. Mewissen MW, Erickson SJ, Foley WD, et al: Thrombosis at venous insertion sites after inferior vena caval filter placement. Radiology 173:155–157, 1989.

198. Greenfield LJ, Cho KJ, Pais SO, Van Aman M: Preliminary clinical experience with the titanium Greenfield filter. Arch Surg 124:657–659, 1989.

199. Roehm JOF: The Bird's Nest filter: A new percutaneous transcatheter inferior vena cava filter. J Vasc Surg 1:498–501, 1984.

200. Roehm JOF, Johnsrude IS, Barth MH, Gianturco C: The Bird's Nest inferior vena cava filter: Progress report. Radiology 168:745–749, 1988.

201. Simon M, Kaplow R, Salzman E, Friedman D: A vena cava filter using thermal shape memory alloy: Experimental aspects. Radiology 125:89–94, 1977.

202. Grassi CJ: Inferior vena caval filters: Analysis of five currently available devices. AJR 156:813–821, 1991.

203. Baert AL: Renal artery stent placement. Radiology 191:619–621, 1994.

204. Bosch JL, Hunink MGM: Meta-analysis of the results of percutaneous transluminal angioplasty and stent placement for aortoiliac occlusive disease. Radiology 204:87–96, 1997.

205. Tetteroo E, van der Graaf Y, Bosch JL, et al, for the Dutch Iliac Stent Trial Study Group: Randomized comparison of direct stent placement versus primary angioplasty followed by selective stent placement in patients iliac artery occlusive disease. Lancet 351:153–159, 1998.

206. Bosch JL, for the Dutch Iliac Stent Trial Study Group: Iliac arterial occlusive disease: Cost effectiveness analysis of stent placement versus percutaneous transluminal angioplasty. Radiology 208:641–648, 1998.

207. Palmaz JC, Garcia OJ, Schatz RA, et al: Placement of balloon expandable intraluminal stents in iliac arteries: First 171 procedures. Radiology 174:969–975, 1990.

208. Long AI, Page PE, Raynaud AC, et al: Percutaneous iliac artery stent: Angiographic long-term follow-up. Radiology 180:771–778, 1991.

209. Zollikofer CL, Antonucci F, Pfyffer M, et al: Arterial stent placement with use of the Wallstent: Midterm results of clinical experience. Radiology 179:449–456, 1991.

210. Martin EC, Katzen BT, Benenati JF, et al: Multicenter trial of the Wallstent in the iliac and femoral arteries. JVIR 843–849, 1995.

211. Do DD, Triller J, Walpoth B, et al: A comparison study of self-expandable stents versus balloon angioplasty alone in femoropopliteal artery occlusions. Cardiovasc Intervent Radiol 15:306–312, 1992.

212. Cejna M, Thurnher S, Iliasch H, et al: PTA versus Palmaz stent placement in femoropopliteal artery obstruction: A randomized study. J Vasc Interv Radiol 12:23–31, 2001.

213. Baert AL, Wilms G, Amery A, et al: Percutaneous transluminal renal angioplasty: Initial results and long-term follow-up in 202 patients. Cardiovasc Interv Radiol 13:22–28, 1990.

214. Hennequin LM, Joffre FG, Rousseau HP, et al: Renal artery stent placement: Long-term results with the Wallstent endoprosthesis. Radiology 191:713–719, 1994.

215. Rosch J, Hanafee WN, Snow H: Transjugular portal venography and radiologic portacaval shunt: An experimental study. Radiology 92:1112–1114, 1969.

216. Colapinto RF, Stronell RD, Birch SJ, et al: Creation of an intrahepatic portosystemic shunt with a Gruentzig balloon catheter. Can Med Assoc J 126:267–268, 1982.

217. Palmaz JC, Garcia F, Sibbitt RR, et al: Expandable intrahepatic portacaval shunt in dogs with chronic portal hypertension. AJR 147:1251–1254, 1986.

218. LaBerge JM, Ring EJ, Gordon RL, et al: Creation of transjugular intrahepatic portosystemic shunts with the Wallstent endoprosthesis: Results in 100 patients. Radiology 187:413–420, 1993.

219. Rossle M, Haag K, Ochs A, et al: The transjugular intrahepatic portosystemic stent-shunt procedure for variceal bleeding. N Engl J Med 330:165–171, 1994.

220. Coldwell DM, Ring EJ, Rees CR, et al: Multicenter investigation of the role of transjugular intrahepatic portosystemic shunt in management of portal hypertension. Radiology 196:335–340, 1995.

221. Ochs A, Rossle M, Haag K, et al: The transjugular intrahepatic portosystemic stent-shunt procedure for refractory ascites. N Engl J Med 332:1192–1197, 1995.

222. Yucel EK, Anderson CM, Edelman RR, et al: Magnetic resonance angiography update on applications for extracranial arteries. Circulation 100:2284–2301, 1999.

223. Prince MR: Renal MR angiography: A comprehensive approach. J Magn Reson Imaging 8:511–516, 1998.
224. Hany TF, Leung DA, Pfammatter T, Debatin JF: Contrast-enhanced magnetic resonance angiography of the renal arteries. Invest Radiol 33:653–659, 1998.
225. Baum RA, Sunshine JH, Carpenter JP, et al: Multicenter trial to evaluate vascular magnetic resonance angiography of the lower extremity. JAMA 274:875–881, 1995.
226. Yamashita Y, Mitsuzaki K, Ogata I, et al: Three-dimensional high resolution dynamic contrast-enhanced MR angiography of the pelvis and lower extremities with use of a phased array coil and subtraction: Diagnostic accuracy. J Magn Reson Imaging 8:1066–1072, 1998.
227. Rubin GD, Waller PJ, Dake MD, et al: Three dimensional spiral computed tomographic angiography: An alternative imaging modality for the abdominal aorta and its branches. J Vasc Surg 18:656–665, 1993.

Questions

1. The angiographic approach associated with the highest incidence of complications is
   - (a) the femoral approach
   - (b) the translumbar approach
   - (c) the axillary approach
   - (d) all are associated with equal risk

2. Which of the following statements regarding radiographic contrast media are true?
   - (a) contrast agents can induce renal dysfunction in patients both with and without preexisting renal disease
   - (b) contrast-induced renal failure usually resolves spontaneously within 7 days
   - (c) pretreatment with steroids has been found effective in preventing severe allergic reactions to contrast in patients with a prior history of allergy to x-ray contrast medium
   - (d) the incidence of contrast-induced renal dysfunction is unrelated to the volume of contrast medium administered
   - (e) patients should be dehydrated before arteriography because this results in improved visualization of vessels

3. Takayasu's disease is characterized by which of the following?
   - (a) a corkscrew or tree-root configuration of vessels at the point of vessel occlusion
   - (b) involvement of the aortic arch and branch vessels with coarctation, occlusion, or aneurysmal dilatation of the affected vessels
   - (c) increased incidence in young males
   - (d) coarctation of the abdominal aorta
   - (e) aneurysmal dilatation, irregularity, and occlusion of the small intrarenal branches of the renal artery

4. In the evaluation of patients with arterial trauma, which of the following statements are true?
   - (a) the most common angiographic observation is spasm characterized by tapering and attenuation of vessels with delayed flow or occlusion
   - (b) arteriovenous fistulas and false aneurysm may occur
   - (c) the status of the peripheral pulses is a reliable indicator of the extent of vascular injury
   - (d) active bleeding sites are identified as areas of extravasated contrast
   - (e) arteriography should be avoided because it can result in further vascular injury

5. In the performance of visceral arteriography, which of the following statements are correct?
   - (a) mesenteric ischemia may manifest angiographically as diffuse, intense vasoconstriction of mesenteric vessels in the absence of atherosclerotic changes or embolic occlusion
   - (b) in mesenteric ischemia, one observes atherosclerotic narrowing with thrombosis or emboli to major vessels
   - (c) the best view for visualization of the origins of the celiac, superior mesenteric, and inferior mesenteric arteries is the anteroposterior view
   - (d) major venous bleeding is easier to detect arteriographically than slow arterial bleeding
   - (e) to visualize the portal venous system, direct portal venography with percutaneous splenic puncture or transhepatic portal vein puncture is usually necessary

6. In the radiographic evaluation of the spleen, which of the following statements are correct?
   - (a) arteriography should be performed first in all cases of suspected splenic trauma
   - (b) CT scans, radionuclide studies, and ultrasound scans are of little use in the evaluation of splenic injury
   - (c) splenic artery aneurysms in females are benign and associated with a low incidence of rupture
   - (d) none of the above

7. The single most characteristic finding in fibromuscular dysplasia is
   - (a) complete occlusion of the renal artery
   - (b) renal artery aneurysms
   - (c) areas of narrowing alternating with areas of dilatation in the main renal arteries
   - (d) involvement of the renal arteries
   - (e) none of the above

8. Which of the following statements regarding intraarterial digital subtraction angiography are true?
   - (a) it replaces conventional film-screen arteriography in many cases
   - (b) it provides better resolution than conventional film-screen angiography
   - (c) it is optimally used with large field of view image intensifiers
   - (d) it is of little assistance in the performance of interventional angiographic procedures
   - (e) lower volumes of x-ray contrast medium are used compared with conventional arteriography

9. In which of the following patients is percutaneous transluminal angioplasty most likely to be successful?
   - (a) a 30-year-old woman with fibromuscular disease of the renal arteries
   - (b) an elderly patient with an atherosclerotic ostial stenosis of the renal artery
   - (c) a patient with an 11-cm-long superficial femoral artery occlusion
   - (d) a patient with a high-grade localized stenosis of the common iliac artery
   - (e) a patient with a stenosis at the proximal anastomosis of a femoropopliteal bypass graft

10. Which of the following statements regarding interventional angiography are accurate?
    - (a) transcatheter embolization therapy is useful in the control of bleeding originating in the stomach

(b) in the treatment of post-traumatic pelvic bleeding, embolization of both hypogastric arteries should not be performed

(c) catheter retrieval of broken wires from the venous system is less preferable than operative removal

(d) streptokinase and urokinase therapy is associated with a high incidence of thrombotic complications

(e) in the treatment of congenital arteriovenous malformations, arteriography should be deferred until an attempt at surgical excision has been made

Answers

1. c   2. a, b, c   3. b, d   4. a, b, d   5. a, b   6. d   7. c   8. a, c, e   9. a, d, e   10. a

17

Endovascular Surgery

Samuel S. Ahn and Kyung M. Ro

The development of balloon angioplasty, mechanical atherectomy, stents, and intravascular imaging modalities has created the multidisciplinary field of endovascular surgery. This field can be defined as a diagnostic and therapeutic discipline that utilizes catheter-based systems delivered through a vascular site remote from a lesion, allowing the surgeon to treat the lesion from within the vascular system. This discipline encompasses the subspecialties of vascular surgery, interventional radiology, interventional cardiology, and biomedical engineering and integrates the expertise of these subspecialties for the common purpose of treating peripheral vascular disease. Thus, endovascular surgery provides important, less invasive adjuncts, or alternatives to enhance and replace, in highly selective cases, conventional vascular reconstructive procedures.

Although the concept of endovascular surgery has been known for many years, the field of endovascular surgery is relatively new. Dotter and Jedkins in 1969[1] and Gruntzig and Hopf, in 1974[2] developed and popularized transluminal balloon angioplasty in its modern form. However, the limitations of balloon angioplasty in totally occluded lesions and the high restenosis rates soon became apparent and led to the concepts of mechanically ablating and removing obstructing plaque under direct vision. Mechanical atherectomy emerged, but its results were suboptimal compared to those of balloon angioplasty. Consequently, the disappointing early restenosis rates associated with atherectomy led investigators to focus more on evaluating the long-term results of mechanical and biologic stents, specifically in preventing restenosis. Most recently, endovascular grafting has sparked renewed interest in endovascular surgery. Furthermore, the need for an accurate guidance and assessment tool for these endoluminal procedures to allow direct visualization of arterial lesions led to the development of miniature vascular endoscopes and intravascular ultrasonography.

The purpose of this chapter is to provide the reader with an introduction to the currently available technology and some of the clinical results of some of the various endovascular devices and procedures: balloon angioplasty, atherectomy, stents, and imaging modalities, including angioscopy and intravascular ultrasonography. It is beyond the scope of this chapter to cover endovascular grafting, which is covered separately in Chapter 18.

INTRAOPERATIVE BALLOON ANGIOPLASTY

Percutaneous balloon angioplasty is already covered in detail in another chapter of this textbook and thus is not covered in this chapter. This section deals with the techniques of intraoperative balloon angioplasty.

Balloon Angioplasty: Differences between Intraoperative and Percutaneous Approach

Intraoperative transluminal angioplasty differs from percutaneous balloon angioplasty in several ways.[3] Perhaps the most important difference is that intraoperative balloon angioplasty is used in patients with more severe and advanced peripheral vascular disease. Patients who undergo intraoperative balloon angioplasty often have multilevel and diffuse disease treated by simultaneous conventional vascular procedures in addition to the adjunctive balloon angioplasty. Percutaneous balloon angioplasty, on the other hand, is usually limited to single-level disease in patients with claudication. The second main difference is that intraoperative balloon angioplasty is performed as an adjunctive procedure in the operating room during vascular reconstruction, whereas percutaneous balloon angioplasty is a primary treatment performed in an interventional suite. Perhaps the most useful equipment in the operating room is the more modern, portable, digital "C"-arm fluoroscopy units. Finally, the maintenance of sterility becomes much more important in the operating room because the patient has an open wound. The problem of sterility becomes even more important if a synthetic graft is being implanted, such as an aortobifemoral bypass graft. Otherwise, the balloon angioplasty catheters, guidewires, and introducer sheaths are similar for both intraoperative and percutaneous balloon angioplasty.

Indications

Indications for intraoperative balloon angioplasty continually evolve as various new techniques and devices are developed and new data are reported. As a general rule, balloon angioplasty is most effective in treating short (less than 10 cm) stenotic lesions that are located in relatively large, high-flow vessels. Most adjunctive balloon angioplasty procedures should be performed percutaneously before or after standard surgical revascularization. This applies to inflow as well as outflow lesions. Staged preoperative balloon angioplasty of an inflow lesion allows observation of the treated site to ensure that the balloon angioplasty procedure is successful before embarking on a distal outflow bypass procedure. However, in certain situations, intraoperative balloon angioplasty may serve as an important adjunctive procedure, lessening the extent of surgery required.

Perhaps the most common indication for intraoperative balloon angioplasty is the presence of a clinically suspected but angiographically undocumented iliac artery stenosis or the presence of an unsuspected iliac artery stenosis in conjunction with a totally occluded superficial femoral artery (Fig. 17–1). In this situation, intraoperative measurement of the femoral artery pressure, in the presence of a vasodilator, can unmask an iliac inflow lesion, which can then be treated with intraoperative balloon angioplasty as an adjunct to a femoropopliteal bypass procedure. Similarly, a balloon angioplasty of a donor iliac artery may be performed during a femorofemoral crossover bypass graft (Fig. 17–2). Furthermore, on occasion, retrograde intraoperative balloon angioplasty of a superficial femoral artery stenosis may allow the superficial femoral artery to serve as an important inflow artery to allow a shorter bypass graft distally (Fig. 17–3). This intraoperative dilatation is particularly indicated when an available vein is insufficient to complete a long femoral distal bypass.

Intraoperative balloon angioplasty can also serve to aug-

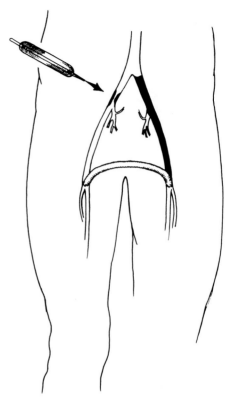

Figure 17–2. Iliac balloon operative transluminal angioplasty (OpTA) provides inflow to a femorofemoral bypass. (From Andros G, Harris RW, Salles-Cunha SX: Technique of intraoperative balloon angioplasty. In Moore WS, Ahn SS [eds]: Endovascular Surgery. Philadelphia, WB Saunders, 1989, pp 209–222.)

ment outflow for a variety of inflow procedures to the common femoral artery, including an aortobifemoral bypass graft (Fig. 17–4), a femorofemoral bypass graft (Fig. 17–5), and a femoral endarterectomy (Fig. 17–6), in the presence of a superficial femoral artery stenosis. Similarly, improved outflow for a femoropopliteal bypass can be achieved by dilating a popliteal artery stenosis (Fig. 17–7) or a tibial artery stenosis (Fig. 17–8). Adjunctive balloon angioplasty of an obstructive popliteal or tibial artery may allow an above-knee femoropopliteal bypass, rather than a below-knee or tibial bypass.

Techniques

Generally, the standard revascularization procedure is performed first but not completed. One of the anastomotic sites is left unfinished to serve as an entry site for the balloon angioplasty catheters. This site is most frequently the common femoral artery. With the femoral anastomosis nearly completed, a standard introducer sheath is inserted proximally or distally, depending on the site of the proposed dilatation. A snare is placed around the introducer sheath to prevent bleeding. The introducer sheath has a self-sealing valve that prevents blood loss during multiple passages of guidewires and catheters. The sheath also has a side arm to allow intraoperative angiography to guide proper positioning of the balloon catheters and to allow completion angiograms. A standard guidewire is passed

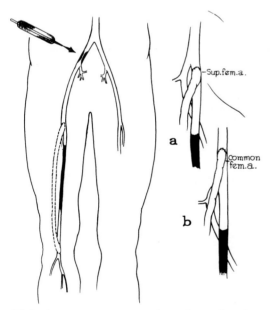

Figure 17–1. Iliac artery operative transluminal angioplasty (OpTA) enhances inflow to a femorodistal bypass. *a*, Graft originating from the superficial femoral artery. *b*, Graft originating from the common femoral artery. (From Andros G, Harris RW, Salles-Cunha SX: Technique of intraoperative balloon angioplasty. In Moore WS, Ahn SS [eds]: Endovascular Surgery. Philadelphia, WB Saunders, 1989, pp 209–222.)

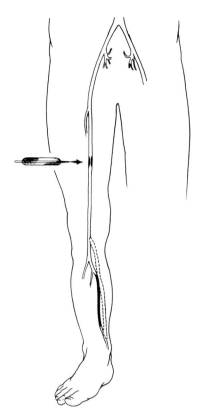

Figure 17–3. Adjunctive *(retrograde)* inflow operative transluminal angioplasty (OpTA) of the superficial femoral artery followed by distal bypass to the paramalleolar posterior tibial artery below the dilated segment. (From Andros G, Harris RW, Salles-Cunha SX: Technique of intraoperative balloon angioplasty. In Moore WS, Ahn SS [eds]: Endovascular Surgery. Philadelphia, WB Saunders, 1989, pp 209–222.)

through the introducer sheath and directed past the stenotic lesion. Then an appropriately sized balloon angioplasty catheter is passed over the guidewire to the site of the obstructive lesion, and balloon dilatation takes place in the standard fashion. Following successful balloon angioplasty, the artery is flushed with heparin irrigation, and the anastomosis is then completed.

Results

The results of intraoperative balloon angioplasty are mostly anecdotal and difficult to evaluate. The simultaneously performed intraoperative balloon angioplasty results are often intermingled with the results of sequential balloon angioplasty and vascular reconstruction. Furthermore, the data are inherently difficult to interpret because of the difficulty in separating the effects of the balloon dilatation procedure from those of the standard revascularization bypass procedure. For instance, in comparing the technical success and short-term outcome of intraoperative versus percutaneous balloon angioplasty, Hsiang and associates[4] reported that their results are similar for both techniques, even though patients who underwent the intraoperative approach had a concomitant surgical procedure performed. Nevertheless, there have been many anecdotal reports of success using this procedure, as summarized by Andros and colleagues.[3]

Limitations and Complications

To quote Andros and coworkers,[3] "The greatest pitfalls of operative balloon angioplasty are not technical, but strategic." First of all, it is important to limit the procedure to carefully selected cases in which the adjunctive balloon angioplasty is indicated and not meddlesome. Failure of an iliac balloon angioplasty site can lead to permanent loss of an otherwise satisfactory femoropopliteal vein bypass. Furthermore, acute occlusion or dissection of a superficial femoral artery stenosis balloon angioplasty site can jeopardize a successful inflow bypass procedure that might otherwise have adequately revascularized the limb by an adequate profundoplasty. Second, it is important to limit the time of arterial occlusion of the balloon-dilated site. The freshly dilated site is often quite thrombogenic, with intimal flaps and dissection that may acutely thrombose in the absence of high blood flow. It is important to perform the standard bypass vascular procedure first, so that the balloon-dilated artery may be exposed to flow immediately following the balloon procedure. These pitfalls reemphasize the preference of attempting preoperative, rather than concomitant intraoperative, balloon dilatation as an adjunct to vascular bypass.

Other complications of intraoperative balloon angioplasty are similar to those of percutaneous balloon angioplasty: acute occlusion, distal emboli, balloon rupture, arterial rupture, and groin hematomas. On the other hand,

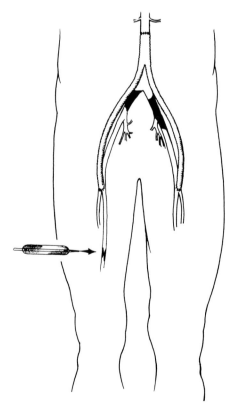

Figure 17–4. Operative transluminal angioplasty (OpTA) of a superficial femoral artery stenosis to increase outflow from an aortobifemoral bypass. (From Andros G, Harris RW, Salles-Cunha SX: Technique of intraoperative balloon angioplasty. In Moore WS, Ahn SS [eds]: Endovascular Surgery. Philadelphia, WB Saunders, 1989, pp 209–222.)

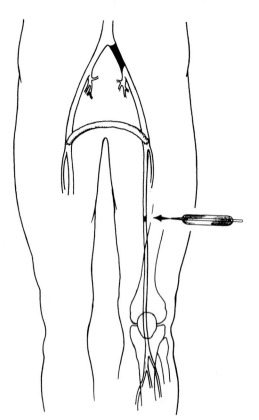

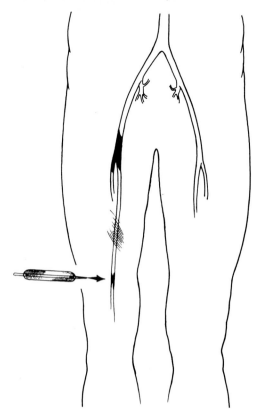

Figure 17–5. Femorofemoral graft with adjunctive outflow balloon angioplasty of the superficial femoral artery on the recipient limb. (From Andros G, Harris RW, Salles-Cunha SX: Technique of intraoperative balloon angioplasty. In Moore WS, Ahn SS [eds]: Endovascular Surgery. Philadelphia, WB Saunders, 1989, pp 209–222.)

Figure 17–6. Common, deep, and proximal superficial femoral artery endarterectomy with complementary intraoperative balloon angioplasty of the midsuperficial femoral artery outflow tract. (From Andros G, Harris RW, Salles-Cunha SX: Technique of intraoperative balloon angioplasty. In Moore WS, Ahn SS [eds]: Endovascular Surgery. Philadelphia, WB Saunders, 1989, pp 209–222.)

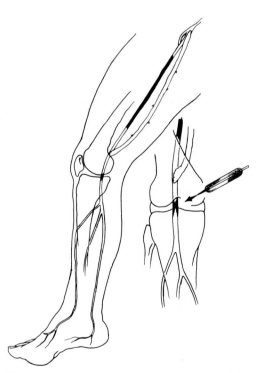

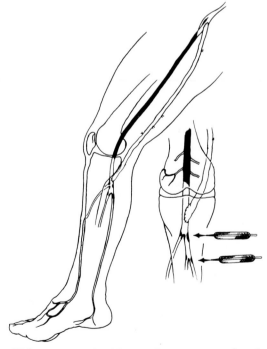

Figure 17–7. Operative transluminal angioplasty (OpTA) of the midpopliteal stenosis allows a femoropopliteal bypass to terminate above the knee. (From Andros G, Harris RW, Salles-Cunha SX: Technique of intraoperative balloon angioplasty. In Moore WS, Ahn SS [eds]: Endovascular Surgery. Philadelphia, WB Saunders, 1989, pp 209–222.)

Figure 17–8. Femoropopliteal bypass obtaining improved outflow with infrapopliteal operative transluminal angioplasty (OpTA). (From Andros G, Harris RW, Salles-Cunha SX: Technique of intraoperative balloon angioplasty. In Moore WS, Ahn SS [eds]: Endovascular Surgery. Philadelphia, WB Saunders, 1989, pp 209–222.)

surgically exposing the artery, using the open technique under controlled situations, may decrease the frequency of these complications.

Comments

Despite its limited indications, intraoperative balloon angioplasty is an important option with which all vascular surgeons should be familiar. Transluminal balloon angioplasty is now a well-established procedure and will likely remain so for some time. Further refinements have been and are currently being made in guidewires and balloon catheters to improve the efficacy of balloon angioplasty in treating various types of lesions.

The technique of transluminal balloon angioplasty requires special skills, expertise, and experience that many surgeons may not have. Optimally, the surgeon should obtain training and supervised clinical experience by working with a qualified vascular surgeon, interventional radiologist, or cardiologist. Such a cooperative effort is needed for optimal results.

PERIPHERAL ATHERECTOMY

Basic Concepts

Atherectomy is the selective removal of atheroma from atherosclerotic diseased arteries performed percutaneously or through a small arteriotomy remote from the diseased site. The concept of debulking plaque is designed to address the limitations of balloon angioplasty, which include its inability to treat complex lesions, acute occlusion, and early restenosis. Such an appealing alternative has led to the development and investigation of at least 12 different atherectomy devices, each with unique features that offer certain advantages and disadvantages over the others. Early clinical results have been promising; however, critical results beyond 6 months have been disappointing. Nevertheless, atherectomy has been shown to enhance immediate results in treating short lesions, with eccentric stenosis or hard, calcified plaque. Atherectomy has been found to be effective in treating recurrent infrainguinal bypass graft stenoses and may be useful in treating failing hemodialysis access grafts.

Of all the atherectomy devices developed in the past 15 years, this section discusses only three that have undergone extensive clinical investigations and are currently available today, and one new promising device. These catheters are characterized by their process of cutting atheroma within the arterial wall and then removing the excised plaque. Extirpative or directional atherectomy shaves or slices atheroma and directly removes the excised plaque from the vessel with a collection chamber. Extirpative catheters include the Simpson Athero Track (Mallinckrodt Medical Inc., St. Louis), the Transluminal Extraction Catheter (TEC) (InterVentional Technologies Inc., San Diego), and the new OmniCath (American BioMed Inc., Georgetown, Tex.). Ablative or rotational atherectomy employs a high-speed rotary device that pulverizes atheroma into microparticles small enough to be aspirated or removed through the reticuloendothelial system. The Auth Rotablator (Boston Scientific Corp., Natick, Mass.) is an ablative catheter.

Simpson AtheroTrack

Device Description

The Simpson AtheroTrack is the improved model of the Simpson AtheroCath. The AtheroTrack offers both over-the-wire and fixed wire shaft design to facilitate introduction to complex or simple stenotic lesions by providing more maneuverability in steering the catheter. The catheter has a housing unit composed of a cutter within a longitudinal opening on one side and a balloon attached on the opposite side (Fig. 17–9). Inflation of the balloon engages the atheroma against a 20-mm cutter window. Then the cutter slices the plaque at 2000 rpm while simultaneously pushing the excised particles into a collection chamber. The catheter also has a tip guard with a hemostasis valve to protect its wire tip. The proximal assembly is composed of a balloon inflation port, a flush port, and an adaptor spline for the drive cable connector. A small lever attached to the cable allows the surgeon to lock the cutter in place before advancing it manually. The AtheroTrack catheter is available in 7-, 8-, 9-, 10-, and 11-French (Fr) sizes.

Technique

Figure 17–10 illustrates the procedure. The AtheroTrack catheter must first advance past the stenotic lesion. Using fluoroscopic guidance, the cutter window is positioned against the stenotic lesion. Then the opposing balloon is inflated to 20 to 40 psi to push the window open, thereby wedging the plaque into it. The motor drive of the cutter is activated, and the plaque is sliced off and pushed into the distal collecting chamber. Multiple passes of the cutter are taken, and the collecting chamber may be rotated to obtain full atherectomy. Once the collecting chamber is full, the catheter needs to be withdrawn to remove the excised particles. Multiple cuts and passages are also required until the final lumen of less than 25% residual stenosis is obtained. A completion angiogram should be performed to assess and document the end result. Repeat atherectomy is performed as needed to obtain complete recanalization.

Indications

The Simpson AtheroTrack is most effective in treating short, discrete, eccentrically placed atheromas. The catheter can be used quite satisfactorily in the iliac, superficial femoral, and popliteal arteries. Like balloon angioplasty, the AtheroTrack can create an arterial lumen larger than that of the catheter used because of its own balloon. Ulcerative plaques are also ideally suited for treatment with Simpson atherectomy. Studies indicate that Simpson atherectomy provides more durable results than balloon angioplasty in treating recurrent infrainguinal bypass graft stenoses.[5, 6] Furthermore, the Simpson atherectomy cathe-

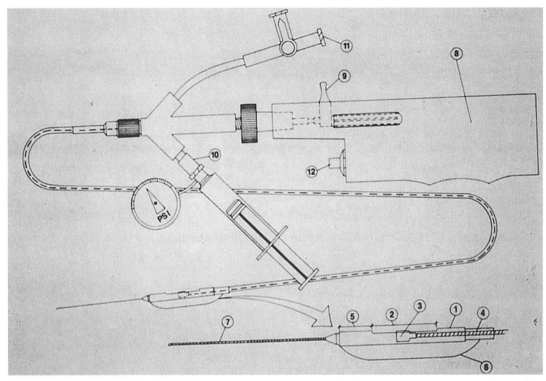

Figure 17–9. Atherectomy catheter system. *1*, Cylindrical housing; *2*, longitudinal opening; *3*, cutter; *4*, cutter drive cable *(to motor)*; *5*, specimen collection area; *6*, balloon support mechanism; *7*, fixed guidewire; *8*, motor; *9*, cutter advance lever; *10*, balloon inflation port; *11*, flush port; *12*, Touhy-Borst opening for cable connector. (From Simpson JB, Selmon MR, Robertson GC, et al: Transluminal atherectomy for peripheral vascular disease. Am J Cardiol 61:96G–101G, 1988.)

ter may be used to treat failing hemodialysis access fistulas.[7, 8] Heavily calcified lesions may create some difficulties for the cutter but do not pose a particular contraindication.

Results

Several clinical studies using the Simpson atherectomy device to treat peripheral arterial occlusive disease re-

ported high initial success rates, varying from 80% to 100%[9–18] (Table 17–1). Graor and Whitlow[12] achieved less than 20% residual stenosis in 100% of lesions 5 cm or smaller and 93% of lesions larger than 5 cm. However, other investigators reported suboptimal intermediate patency results at 6 to 24 months (see Table 17–1). Lugmayr and colleagues[15] and Vroegindewij and associates[16] reported disappointing patencies of 42% and 35%, respectively, at 2 years. These patency results are similar, if not worse, than those previously reported for balloon angioplasty.[19, 20]

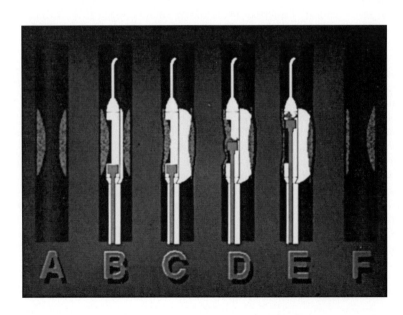

Figure 17–10. The atherectomy procedure. *A*, The lesion before atherectomy. *B*, Atherectomy catheter in position across the lesion. *C*, The balloon support is inflated. *D*, The cutter is advanced. *E*, The specimen is trapped in the housing. *F*, The balloon is deflated and the catheter removed. (From Hinohara T, Robertson GC, Selman MR, Simpson JB: Transluminal atherectomy: The Simpson atherectomy catheter. In Moore WS, Ahn SS [eds]: Endovascular Surgery. Philadelphia, WB Saunders, 1989, pp 310–322.)

T A B L E   1 7 – 1

Results Reported Using the Simpson Atherectomy Device

AUTHORS	PATIENTS (N)	LESIONS (N)	TECHNICAL SUCCESS (%)	PRIMARY PATENCY (%)		
				6 mo	12 mo	24 mo
Simpson et al[9]	61	136	87	69	NA	NA
Polnitz et al[10]	60	94	82	99	72	NA
Hinohara et al[11]	100	195	90	83	NA	NA
Graor & Whitlow[12]	106	106	100 (lesions − 5 cm)	NA	93	88.4
			93 (lesions > 5 cm)	NA	86	73
Dorros et al[13]	126	213	99	45	NA	NA
Kim et al[14]	77	85	92	94	86	86
Lugmayr et al[15]	94	132	95	NA	69	42
Vroegindewij et al[16]	38	38	92	84	42	35
Savader et al[17]	61	136	80	NA	76	58
Wildenhain et al[18]	75	84	92	NA	78	57

NA, not available.

Adjunctive balloon angioplasty is required in some cases to facilitate the passage of the atherectomy catheter or to improve the final lumen further. In such cases, Kim and colleagues[14] tried to compare the results of the Simpson device with those of balloon angioplasty. They compared lesions (n = 68) treated with atherectomy alone with lesions (n = 17) treated with both atherectomy and supplemental balloon angioplasty. Lesions treated with the Simpson device alone achieved patencies of 92%, 84%, and 84% at 1, 2, and 3 years, respectively, and reduced patencies of 78%, 67%, and 57% at 1, 2, and 3 years, respectively, were obtained with the lesions treated by combined atherectomy and balloon angioplasty. In such a study, it is difficult to compare and delineate the effects or influence of each treatment modality. In a more appropriate prospective randomized clinical study, Vroegindewij and coworkers[16] reported 2-year cumulative patency rates of 35% in lesions (n = 38) treated with Simpson atherectomy alone, compared with 56% in lesions (n = 35) treated with balloon angioplasty alone. Although this cumulative patency difference was found to be not statistically significant, the authors did find that atherectomy was associated with a significantly worse patency rate than balloon angioplasty for patients with a lesion length of 2 cm or greater. Furthermore, atherectomy with the Simpson device did not result in an improved clinical and hemodynamic outcome.

The Simpson atherectomy catheter was found to be effective in treating recurrent infrainguinal bypass graft stenoses. Dolmatch and coauthors[5] reported a 92% technical success rate in treating 18 lower extremity bypass grafts (11 polytetrafluoroethylene grafts, 7 autologous saphenous veins) with 23 areas of anastomotic stenosis. The authors were able to sustain this initial success to a high graft patency of 88% at a mean follow-up of 14 months. Additionally, to evaluate the long-term results of Simpson atherectomy, Porter and associates[6] performed 52 procedures (atherectomy alone in 42, atherectomy plus balloon angioplasty in 10) to treat 67 stenoses (28 anastomotic, 39 intragraft) in 44 infrainguinal vein grafts. The authors achieved a remarkable 96% technical success rate by reducing the average diameter stenosis of 81% (range, 50% to 99%) before treatment to 11% (range, 0% to 30%) after treatment. They conducted a long-term follow-up and obtained

primary patency rates of 83%, 80%, and 80% at 1, 2, and 3 years, respectively. Clearly, these initial, intermediate, and long-term results show that the results of Simpson atherectomy are effective and more durable than those previously reported for balloon angioplasty[21, 22] and perhaps similar to those reported for open surgical revision in the treatment of recurrent stenosis in the treatment of recurrent stenosis in infrainguinal bypass grafts.

The Simpson atherectomy catheter has also been used to treat failing hemodialysis access fistulas. In their initial experience, Zemel and colleagues[7] reported a 77% technical success rate using the Simpson device to treat stenotic hemodialysis fistulas in 13 patients. Gray and coworkers[8] reported an 83% technical success and a 50% patency rate at 6 months in treating hemodialysis access with 12 intragraft stenoses. These investigators claimed that the Simpson atherectomy device is safe and effective in the treatment of recurrent stenotic hemodialysis access fistulas. Further clinical trials with a large number of study patients are currently indicated to evaluate the efficacy of this treatment modality with intermediate and long-term follow-up results.

Complications and Limitations

The Simpson atherectomy device is a relatively safe tool. Common complications associated with the device include hematoma caused by bleeding at the atherectomy entry site, pseudoaneurysm, and distal embolization. Graor and Whitlow[12] reported seven cases of hematoma that required major intervention, including one patient who also developed a pseudoaneurysm. Kim and colleagues[14] attributed the 11 cases of hematoma in their study to the bulky 7- to 12-Fr vascular sheaths used and reported three cases of pseudoaneurysm that required surgical repair. Distal embolic problems were also noted, which required surgical intervention in severe cases and urokinase infusion or no treatment if clinically insignificant.

Savader and associates[17] stated that Simpson atherectomy has similar patency compared with that reported for balloon angioplasty[19, 20] in the treatment of femoral and popliteal artery lesions but also a high complication rate of

42.8%: 15 (21.4%) major and 15 (21.4%) minor. The major complications include four puncture-site hematomas, attributed to the use of sheaths 9 Fr or larger, which subsequently underwent vessel repair or required an extended hospital stay; seven embolizations treated with aspiration embolectomy or urokinase therapy or both; two contrast-induced renal failures that required rehydration or dialysis; a pseudoaneurysm that required surgical repair; and a thrombosed arterial lesion within 24 hours treated conservatively. All 15 minor complications were puncture-site hematomas that required no treatment. Apparently, this complication rate is not comparable with those previously reported for balloon angioplasty.[19, 20]

One of the main limitations of the Simpson atherectomy device for general use in the treatment of peripheral arterial occlusive disease is its failure to reduce restenosis. At 6 months, Simpson and coworkers[9] reported a restenosis rate of 36%; Polnitz and associates[10] reported 24% and 11% restenosis rates for concentric and eccentric lesions, respectively; and Dorros and associates[13] reported a significant 55% recurrence rate. In the treatment of recurrent infrainguinal bypass graft stenosis, Dolmatch and colleagues[5] reported a 26% restenosis and reocclusion rate, in contrast to Porter and coworkers'[6] low 12% restenosis rate in treating vein graft stenosis.

The other primary limitation of the Simpson device is its relative ineffectiveness in treating long diffusely diseased segments and long totally occluded lesions. The restenosis rates in these longer lesions are significantly higher. Polnitz and associates[10] observed restenosis at 1 year in 7% of lesions with simple stenosis 5 cm or smaller and 14% of lesions with complex occlusions larger than 5 cm. Furthermore, Vroegindewij and associates[16] found that their treated lesions of 2 cm or greater were associated with a significantly lower patency rate at 1 year (14%) than that of the lesions smaller than 2 cm (50%).

Transluminal Extraction Catheter

Device Description

The TEC is a semiflexible, torque-controlled catheter with a rotating, cone-shaped cutter that tracks over a central guidewire (Fig. 17–11). The cone has openings on the distal tip, and the catheter itself is hollow, so that the particles resulting from atherectomy can be suctioned out of the vessel and collected in a separate collecting chamber (125 mL). The cone-shaped cutter rotates at 700 rpm and leaves relatively large (1 mm) particles. Suction is applied from the proximal port to aspirate the particles into the collecting chamber and thus minimize embolic complications. Furthermore, continuous heparin irrigation is also required via the introducer sheath's side arm to maintain efficiency in the aspiration of excised particles. The catheter is currently available in 5-, 7-, 9-, and 11-Fr sizes.

Technique

Atherectomy with the TEC is performed primarily percutaneously but can be used intraoperatively as well. Because

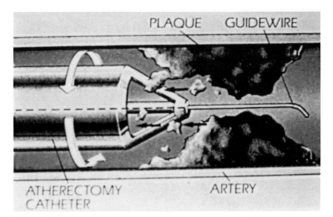

Figure 17–11. The Transluminal extraction catheter (TEC). See text for description.

of the limited size of the TEC, standard balloon angioplasty is often required to achieve a final channel that is adequate in size. Using fluoroscopic guidance, an appropriate-sized introducer sheath is placed into the artery in an antegrade fashion. A guidewire is then passed through the introducer sheath and through the obstructive lesion. Once the guidewire is in place, a 4- or 5-Fr polyethylene exchange catheter is inserted. Then the initial guidewire is replaced with a 0.014-inch TEC guidewire. The exchange catheter is removed, and the TEC is passed over the TEC guidewire until the catheter meets resistance at the obstructive lesion. The atherectomy catheter is then activated, and the motor drive rotates the cutter while suction is applied. The torque tube cutter is passed freely but gently over the guidewire until the obstructive lesion is traversed. Fluoroscopy documents the progress of the atherectomy and the final lumen. Multiple cuts and passages are made if indicated or until a final lumen of less than 25% residual stenosis is achieved. If there is significant residual stenosis, then adjunctive balloon angioplasty is performed to dilate the artery to a final adequate size.

Indications

The TEC device is currently recommended for short stenotic lesions with eccentrically placed atheromas. Previous studies using this atherectomy device indicate suboptimal results in treating total occlusions and long stenotic lesions.[23, 24] Adjunctive balloon angioplasty is usually required in treating such lesions to facilitate or complete the recanalization.

Results

Very few investigators have reported their results using the TEC device in the treatment of peripheral arterial occlusive disease. Wholey and Jarmolowski[23] and Myers and associates[24] reported promising technical success rates of 92% and 86%, and immediate clinical success rates of 90% and 79%, respectively. However, intermediate and long-term follow-up data were not provided in their reports. Wholey and Jarmolowski[23] had a 6-month follow-up on only 50 of the 95 patients, 16 of whom underwent repeat angiography. In treating primarily long stenotic (62%) and occlusive lesions (73%), Myers and associates[24] achieved patency rates of 80% for lesions 5 cm or smaller and 64% for lesions larger than 5 cm at 6 months. Furthermore, adjunctive balloon angioplasty was performed in 76% of all treated lesions.

Complications and Limitations

Complications associated with the TEC device have not been reported in detail. Of the 126 lesions, Wholey and Jarmolowski[23] reported only two (1.6%) thrombotic complications, which were subsequently treated with urokinase infusion. Myers and associates[24] reported only a 6% complication rate in treating primarily long complex lesions: two deaths, catheter fracture requiring removal and replacement in two, thromboembolism in two, and puncture-site bleeding in three patients.

Restenosis and reocclusion are the primary limitations of the TEC device. Of the 16 patients who underwent repeat angiography during follow-up, Wholey and Jarmolowski[23] found restenosis in four patients at 3 months and reocclusion in four whose lesions were longer than 8 cm. Myers and colleagues[24] found restenosis in 26 lesions (18%) and reocclusion in 51 lesions (35%) at 6 months.

OmniCath

Device Description

The OmniCath is a new extirpative atherectomy device currently approved by the Food and Drug Administration (FDA) for investigational use only. It is a radiopaque, torqueable, braided catheter with a hollow cylindrical housing at the distal end. This housing unit contains the cutter within a longitudinal window on one side and a unique unibody tripod composed of extendable wire configuration on the opposite side. The internal beveled cutter spins at 11,000 rpm and is stabilized by an axial guide or track when making a cut (Fig. 17–12). The cutter is activated by hand and rotated by a battery-powered motor via a hollow drive shaft. An idler shaft covers a 2-cm section of the drive shaft at the distal end to minimize or eliminate the potential of tissue wrapping or binding onto the shaft (see Fig. 17–12). The rotating cutter passes back and forth across the lesion, shaving off thin segments of the atheromatous particles with each pass. The atheromatous debris is collected in the housing unit and continuously aspirated through a removal port at the proximal end of the catheter. A radiopaque gold dot just beyond the distal end of the window enhances operative visualization of the device (see Fig. 17–12).

An atraumatic deflector wire pad braces the cutter assembly securely against the obstructive lesion and allows continuous distal perfusion during atherectomy (see Fig. 17–12). This anchoring system can be adjusted and thus regulate the depth of cut by its degree of extension. The extended anchoring wire can withhold a maximum pressure of 27 psi. This mechanism is designed to prevent injury to the vessel wall (i.e., perforation) and thus reduce the likelihood of acute closure and restenosis.

Technique

Atherectomy with the OmniCath is generally performed percutaneously. Using fluoroscopic guidance, the Omni-Cath can be introduced to the obstructive lesion via two techniques: (1) over a 0.014-inch exchange guidewire or (2) placing the catheter onto the exchange guidewire and then inserting this unit into an introducer sheath. The OmniCath is then advanced slowly until the cutting window is positioned against the stenotic lesion. The radiopaque

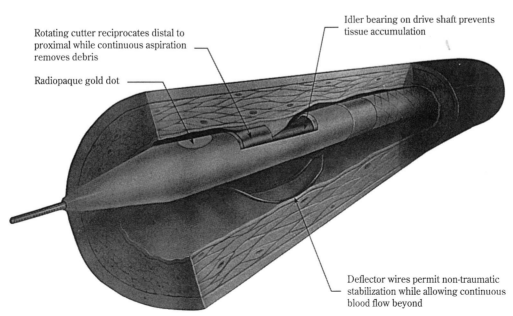

Rotating cutter reciprocates distal to proximal while continuous aspiration removes debris

Idler bearing on drive shaft prevents tissue accumulation

Radiopaque gold dot

Deflector wires permit non-traumatic stabilization while allowing continuous blood flow beyond

Figure 17–12. The new OmniCath atherectomy device with its unique features.

gold dot at the distal end helps confirm the proper positioning of the cutter window. The cutter window is opened by moving the cutter actuation slide to its "advance" position, and then the anchoring deflector wire pad is extended by advancing the wire actuation ring to stabilize the catheter and brace the cutter window against the plaque. Before atherectomy, the guidewire must be withdrawn into the catheter tip, and the aspiration system should be activated for suction. The motor drive of the cutter is then activated, and the cutter is advanced slowly across the obstructive lesion, traversing the full length of the cutter window while aspirating gently. The deflector wire pad may need to be adjusted to maintain a portion of the lesion within the window. Multiple passes across the lesion may be made with the cutter window in the same location. Multiple cuts and passages may be required until a satisfactory angiographic result of less than 25% residual stenosis is obtained. If the catheter is removed before completion of atherectomy, the catheter lumen should be aspirated with heparinized saline to remove all atheromatous debris and blood remaining within the lumen.

Indications

The OmniCath is designed to treat short stenotic lesions with concentrically or eccentrically placed atheromas. It can be used quite satisfactorily in the iliac, superficial femoral, and popliteal arteries. The OmniCath is currently under clinical investigative trial for peripheral atherectomy. Like the Simpson AtheroTrack, the OmniCath appears to be of potential use in the treatment of arteriovenous dialysis grafts.

Results

Preliminary clinical data using the OmniCath device for peripheral atherectomy have not been published, but animal data have been reported by Mazur and coworkers.[25] Concentric and eccentric lesions were induced in the bilateral external iliac arteries of 10 miniature swine which subsequently underwent atherectomy with the OmniCath device. Five swine were sacrificed 3 days after the atherectomy procedure, and the other five at 6 weeks. Histologic sections of the 3-day-old atherectomized lesions showed

that the depth of cuts ranged from partial plaque removal to nearly full luminal thickness of the artery. Histologic sections of the 6-week atherectomized lesions revealed minimal healing response. No evidence of vessel wall injury or significant neointimal proliferation at the anchoring wire deployment sites was found. Angiography revealed 20% luminal narrowing in one lesion at 6 weeks. In evaluating a prototype of the device in microswine, Sapoval and colleagues[26] determined its maneuverability to be satisfactory but its aspiration apparatus to be inefficient. The OmniCath device underwent several modifications before use in humans.

Complications and Limitations

Mazur and associates[25] reported spasm at the atherectomy site in most of the animals, and Sapoval and colleagues[26] reported arterial ruptures in three of four animals. Human clinical trials are currently warranted to determine the safety and efficacy of the OmniCath device in the treatment of peripheral arterial occlusive disease.

Auth Rotablator

Device Description

The Auth Rotablator is a flexible, catheter-deliverable atherectomy device with a variable-sized, football-shaped metal bur on the distal tip (Fig. 17–13). The bur is studded with multiple diamond chips (22 to 45 μm in size) that function as multiple microknives. The bur comes in various sizes, ranging from 1.25 to 6.0 mm in diameter. Progressively larger burs are used incrementally during the recanalization process until a satisfactory lumen is obtained. The bur rotates at 100,000 to 200,000 rpm and tracks along a central guidewire. The guidewire must first traverse the lesion before rotational atherectomy can proceed. The high-speed rotation allows the diamond microchips to preferentially attack a hard calcified atheroma while leaving the surrounding elastic soft tissue of normal arterial wall intact (Fig. 17–14). The device leaves a smooth, polished intraluminal surface and no intimal flaps (Fig. 17–15). Previous canine experiments indicate that the Rotablator pulverizes plaque into particles that are generally smaller than red

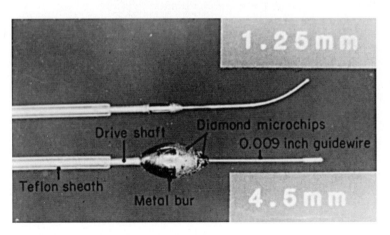

Figure 17–13. Rotablator atherectomy bur and guidewire. Burs 1.25 and 4.5 mm in diameter, respectively, are shown. Note the diamond microchips embedded in the distal half of the bur. Also note the coaxial spring tip *(top)* and semirigid guidewires *(bottom)*. (From Ahn SS: The Rotablator—high-speed rotary atherectomy: Indications, technique, results and complications. In Moore WS, Ahn SS [eds]: Endovascular Surgery. Philadelphia, WB Saunders, 1989, pp 327–335.)

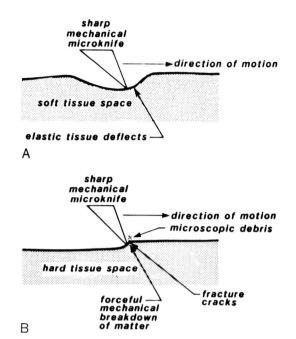

A

B

Figure 17–14. Differential cutting: Its application in soft and hard tissue. *A,* Soft tissue is able to deflect out of the way of the microknife. *B,* Hard tissue is unable to deflect out of the way; the result is fracture and mechanical breakup of atheromatous plaque. (From Ahn SS: The Rotablator—high speed rotary atherectomy: Indications, technique, results and complications. In Moore WS, Ahn SS [eds]: Endovascular Surgery. Philadelphia, WB Saunders, 1989, pp 327–335.)

blood cells and thus pass harmlessly through the reticuloendothelial system.[27]

Technique

Atherectomy with the Auth Rotablator is preferentially performed through an open arteriotomy, although the percutaneous method can be used. The percutaneous technique, however, limits the bur size to 3 mm and ultimately requires subsequent balloon angioplasty. When performing atherectomy alone, an open arteriotomy using a larger-sized bur is preferred. A 9- or 12-Fr introducer sheath is inserted into the artery through the arteriotomy. An angioscope may be inserted to document the lesion and to help with proper placement of the guidewire. Alternatively, conventional fluoroscopy can be used and is more readily available.

First, a small atraumatic guidewire is passed through the lesion, after which an exchange guide catheter is inserted. The initial guidewire is removed, and then a 0.009-inch atherectomy guidewire, which is somewhat stiffer and more rigid to support the rotating bur, is passed through the lesion. The exchange guide catheter is then removed, and the bur is placed over the guidewire to the site of the obstructive lesion. Initially, a bur size half the diameter of the native artery is used; the size of the bur is progressively increased in increments of 0.5 to 1.0 mm. Atherectomy is performed gradually and slowly, recanalizing the artery by advancing the bur over the guidewire. Following atherectomy with the smallest bur, the bur is removed, leaving the guidewire in place. Then the next-sized bur is inserted,

and atherectomy is repeated until an adequate-sized lumen is obtained. The patient is placed on anticoagulation therapy for the first 24 hours postoperatively to prevent early thrombosis. Aspirin is then given long term after the procedure.

Indications

The Auth Rotablator is ideally suited for hard calcified plaque, particularly in diabetic patients who have disabling claudication or limb-threatening ischemia. Recanalization can be achieved expeditiously in short as well as long lesions. Tibial artery lesions, as well as superficial femoral and popliteal artery lesions, can be treated. Stenotic lesions appear better suited for the Rotablator, because a central guidewire must first traverse the lesion. Total occlusions may be treated if the guidewire can be passed initially. Eccentric plaques can be treated quite satisfactorily, because the atherectomy device preferentially attacks calcified plaque.

Results

Clinical studies reported promising technical and immediate clinical success rates with the Auth Rotablator[20–33] (Table 17–2). However, half of these series reported only a short follow-up of 6 months, and patencies obtained at this time interval were suboptimal, ranging from 47% to 82%. Furthermore, patencies obtained at 1 year were worse (31% to 61%).[29, 31, 33]

Ahn and coworkers[29] performed atherectomy with the Auth Rotablator in 20 patients with claudication, ulcer or

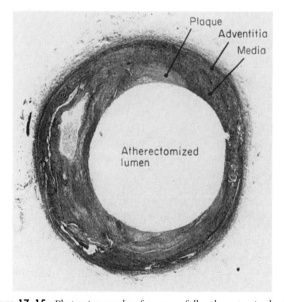

Figure 17–15. Photomicrographs of a successfully atherectomized artery seen in cross-section. Note the smooth, highly polished intraluminal surface denuded of intima and endothelial cells. (Hematoxylin-eosin stain; original magnification ×40.) (From Ahn SS: The Rotablator—high speed rotary atherectomy: Indications, technique, results and complications. In Moore WS, Ahn SS [eds]: Endovascular Surgery. Philadelphia, WB Saunders, 1989, pp 327–335.)

TABLE 17-2

Results Reported Using the Auth Rotablator Device

AUTHORS	PATIENTS (N)	LESIONS (N)	TECHNICAL SUCCESS (%)	IMMEDIATE CLINICAL SUCCESS (%)	PRIMARY PATENCY (%)	
					6 mo	12 mo
Dorros et al[28]	43	82	95	88	NA	NA
Ahn et al[29]	20	42	93	72	66	47
White et al[30]	17	18	94	94	82	NA
CRAG[31]	72	107	89	77	47	31
Henry et al[32]	150	212	97	85	NA	NA
Myers & Denton[33]	34	36	94	92	68	60.7

NA, not available.

gangrene, rest pain, and asymptomatic failing graft. Twenty-five lesions were treated: 20 lesions had 50% to 95% stenosis, and 5 lesions were occluded. Despite the promising technical success rate of 93%, the in-hospital success rate was a disappointing 72% because of complications that developed in 17 of 25 cases (68%). The cumulative patency at 2 years was a dismal 12%.

The Collaborative Rotablator Atherectomy Group[31] (CRAG) reported their experience with the Auth Rotablator from a multicenter trial. Technical angiographic success (less than 25% residual lumen) was achieved in 70 of 79 limbs (89%) and in 82 of 107 arteries (77%). In addition to the nine technical failures, in-hospital thrombosis occurred in nine limbs, resulting in an in-hospital success rate of 77% (61 of 79 limbs). Furthermore, complications occurred in approximately half of the patients, and half of them subsequently underwent an urgent or emergent surgical procedure within 30 days. Six of these patients underwent an amputation, two of which were associated with the device. Late failure was observed in 32 limbs within 15 to 41 months; 4 of the 32 failures also resulted in an amputation. The cumulative patency rate at 2 years was a disappointing 18.6%.

Complications and Limitations

In addition to the poor intermediate and long-term results discussed here, peripheral atherectomy with the Auth Rotablator currently has limited application because of several complications associated with the device. Significant early thromboses were reported by Ahn and colleagues,[29] the CRAG,[31] and Henry and associates.[32] Ahn and coworkers[29] reported five in-hospital cases of thromboses (25%), four of which were associated with hypercoagulable states. The CRAG[31] reported nine cases of early thromboses (11%), two of which subsequently led to amputation. Henry and colleagues[32] correlated the 12 thromboses (8%) in their series with a number of factors, including dissection, elastic recoil, intimal flaps, lengthy lesion, residual stenosis, and vasospasm.

Arterial spasm occurred in 23% of cases reported by Dorros and associates[28] and in 11% of those reported by Henry and colleagues.[32] These spasms occurred mostly in small distal arteries and were attributed to the use of large burs, long rotational sequences, or rotational speed.

Gross hemoglobinuria without any clinical sequelae was found in 63% of cases by Dorros and associates,[28] in 20% by Ahn and associates,[29] and in 13% by the CRAG.[31] These cases were transient and developed in lesions that required larger burs and prolonged rotational sequences.

Contrary to what was reported in previous studies,[27] the atherectomized particles are not always small enough to pass through the reticuloendothelial system safely. Indeed, embolic complications developed in 20% of cases described by Ahn and colleagues,[29] in 10% by the CRAG,[31] and in 1% by Henry and associates.[32] Three of the eight embolic events reported by the CRAG[31] resulted in cutaneous necrosis, and one, in toe amputation.

Like all other atherectomy devices, the Auth Rotablator was also reported to cause dissections, perforations, and puncture-site hematomas.[28–32] Similarly, late restenoses and reocclusions were the significant limiting factors of the Auth Rotablator. Although most of the residual lumina achieved were less than 20%, Ahn and associates[29] reported restenosis in 45% (9 of 20) and reocclusion in 80% (4 of 5) within 18 months. Intimal hyperplasia was believed to be the inciting factor in these cases. The CRAG[31] reported late restenoses and reocclusions in 40% (32 of 79 limbs) during a long-term follow-up of 15 to 41 months. Henry and coworkers[32] reported a 24% restenosis rate, mostly in lesions 7 cm or longer.

Comments

All atherectomy devices that have undergone extensive clinical investigation have failed to improve the restenosis rate of standard balloon angioplasty in the treatment of peripheral arterial occlusive disease. Despite actual removal, debulking, and even polishing of the plaque, the invariable arterial wall trauma still induces intimal hyperplasia. Until the problem of restenosis can be solved, atherectomy will be limited to those instances when balloon angioplasty may be ineffective or contraindicated. Such instances might include the presence of hard, calcified lesions that are difficult to dilate, the presence of intimal flaps or dissections secondary to the balloon angioplasty itself, or ulcerative lesions that have led to thromboembolic complications.

Comments

According to recent reports, the use of atherectomy for the treatment of vein graft stenosis appears promising.[34, 35] Porter and colleagues[34] evaluated their outcomes with the use of atherectomy for the treatment of infrainguinal vein graft stenoses over a 6-year period. With a mean follow-up of 21 months in a group of 42 patients (52 procedures and 67 stenoses), the primary patency rates were 82%, 78%, and 78% at 1, 2, and 3 years, respectively. In a study conducted by Dolmatch and associates[35] for atherectomy of anastomotic bypass graft stenosis, we reported a technical success rate of 92%, with an 88% graft patency rate at 14 months. In 74% of the areas of stenosis, there was less than 50% restenosis at those sites. We also found that the patency rates for those treated with atherectomy alone were the same as for those who were treated with a combined therapy of atherectomy and percutaneous transluminal angioplasty (PTA). The authors concluded that directional atherectomy is an effective treatment method with intermediate patency rates superior to those reported for PTA and comparable with those reported for conventional open revision.

Osborn and colleagues[36] performed a combined therapy of balloon angioplasty and atherectomy in a group of highly selective patients (96 limbs) for the treatment of superficial femoral and popliteal artery stenoses. They reported that at a mean follow-up of 24 months, 71% of limbs maintained their postoperative improvement according to the categorical reporting standards of the Society for Vascular Surgery and the International Society for Cardiovascular Surgery. In addition, in a recent randomized clinical trial comparing the use of balloon angioplasty versus atherectomy (unpublished data), Ahn and associates found that combined therapy of balloon angioplasty and atherectomy yields higher intermediate patency rates than previously reported for either treatment modality alone.

INTRAVASCULAR STENTS

The recognized problem of restenosis after PTA has led to increased interest in intravascular stents. Stents were developed to help address the complications of PTA and are designed to provide a scaffold to maintain the intraluminal structure and patency of the artery. Several different types of stents have been developed and used worldwide, but only a few have undergone critical evaluation. Intravascular stents may be categorized into three basic types: balloon-expandable, self-expanding, and thermal expanding stents. Furthermore, a newly evolved endovascular stent device, the stent graft or covered stent, is briefly described.

Balloon-Expandable Stents

The balloon-expandable stent requires the use of a balloon catheter for its insertion and deployment within the luminal wall of the diseased blood vessel. The stent is mounted onto the balloon and then inflated to properly embed the prosthesis into the wall, creating a stable intraluminal surface that facilitates endothelialization and minimizes stent migration. If necessary, this stent can be expanded further after deployment by repeat balloon dilatation for precise placement.

With the current explosion in stent technology, several balloon-expandable stents have been developed, but only two have undergone clinical investigation: the Palmaz stent (Johnson & Johnson Interventional System Co., Warren, N.J.) and the Strecker stent (Medi-Tech/Boston Scientific Corp., Watertown, Mass.).

Palmaz Stent

Device Description

The Palmaz stent is a stainless steel tube composed of staggered rows of rectangular slots. It is mounted onto an angioplasty balloon catheter used to inflate the malleable steel framework into staggered rows of diamond-shaped slots. This wire mesh structure gives it superior radial compression strength and rigidity. This radial strength prevents elastic recoil after expansion, providing a scaffold to maintain the intraluminal structure and patency of an artery. Its rigidity keeps the stent embedded in the wall of the artery, facilitating rapid endothelialization. Its foreshortening is minimal and thus allows considerable precision in sizing and deployment at the diseased site. Furthermore, the Palmaz stent can be adjusted in diameter if necessary by using a second balloon to reinflate it without subsequent recoil. Conversely, its rigidity carries with it a risk of extrinsic compression in the arterial lumen. Also, it can pose difficulty in deploying the stent in tortuous vessels.

The Palmaz stent is available in different sizes, although only one is currently approved by the Food and Drug Administration (FDA) for use in the iliac artery. The Palmaz P308 stent is 30 mm in its unexpanded length and can be expanded from 8 to 12 mm in diameter. For insertion and deployment, it requires a balloon dilatation catheter 8 to 12 mm in diameter, a 9-Fr introducer, and accessories such as a crimping tool, a crimping tube, and an introducer tube. The crimping tool is used to crimp the stent on the balloon and then deliver it to the lesion site through a 9-Fr vascular access sheath with a hemostatic valve. The introducer tube enables the loaded balloon catheter to advance through the valve. Other, smaller stents and balloons can be inserted through sheaths as small as 7-Fr.

Technique

Using fluoroscopic guidance, a 7- to 10-Fr introducer sheath is inserted over a guidewire and advanced across the obstructed lesion. With this protective sheath in place, the stent-loaded balloon catheter is inserted within the sheath to the lesion site. The protective sheath is withdrawn, unleashing the mounted stent. The final positioning is accomplished by using bony landmarks, external metallic markers (i.e., clamps, scissors), radiopaque rulers, and the contrast imaging with roadmapping capabilities. The balloon is then inflated to expand the stent and the lesion simultaneously, leaving the stent mesh flush within the inner lumen. Repeat balloon inflation is often necessary proximal and distal to the stent to ensure that it is embedded in the arterial wall and not protruding into the lumen. Any residual abnormalities or stenosis cranial or caudal to the stent can then be corrected by dilating the nonstented portion of the vessel using the same balloon. A second stent may be inserted to dilate any residual stenosis proximal or distal to the stent. After stent deployment, the balloon is deflated and withdrawn. Finally, a completion angiogram is performed, and pressure measurements are taken over the angioplasty site.

Indications

In the United States, the Palmaz stent is currently approved by the FDA for the treatment of stenotic or occlusive atherosclerotic lesions and after failed or inadequate balloon angioplasty results in the iliac artery. Failed or inadequate angioplasty results include angiographic residual stenosis of 30% or more, a maximum trans-stenotic mean pressure gradient of 5 mm Hg or more after vasodilatation, or unstable intimal flaps, propagating subintimal or medial dissection. The Palmaz stent confers several advantages, including excellent radial strength, which results in minimal recoil following stent deployment and thus is ideally suited for use in calcified vessels. In other countries, the Palmaz stent has been placed in the superficial femoral and popliteal arteries, as well as in the iliac arteries. Short lesions appear to be most amenable to this stent, and results reported for stent placement in infrainguinal lesions have been suboptimal.

Results

ILIAC STENTING. The Palmaz stent was the first stenting device approved by the FDA for iliac artery applications. Since its introduction, it has been widely used and investigated for lesions in both the iliac and infrainguinal arteries, with several studies reporting impressive high immediate success rates in the iliac arteries (Table 17–3). Indications for use include post–balloon angioplasty restenosis, elastic recoil, dissection induced by endovascular procedures (i.e., balloon angioplasty, atherectomy, or laser recanalization), and stenotic or occlusive atherosclerotic lesions. Intermediate patency rates at 1 and 2 years[37–39] are generally better than those previously reported for balloon angioplasty alone in the iliac artery position.[19, 20]

Palmaz and colleagues[37] coordinated the first and largest multicenter trial using the Palmaz stent in the iliac arteries. Follow-up at 12, 24, and 48 months revealed clinical success rates of 90.9%, 84.1% and 68.6%, respectively (see Table 17–3). These results clearly show the usefulness of stents in improving early results over balloon angioplasty alone.[19, 20] However, as for all reported clinical results, several caveats must be considered before these data can be interpreted further. Because patient entry was relatively infrequent during the early years of the study, the mean follow-up was short (13.3 ± 11.0 months). Furthermore, of the 486 patients, only 16.3% were available for more than 24 months of follow-up evaluation, and 75% had

follow-up of 12 months or less. Most patients in this study had claudication and short (<3 cm) lesions, variables previously determined to be the predictors of successful balloon angioplasty alone.[20] More than 60% of the patients required only one stent, 20% required two stents, and only 15% required three or more stents. Finally, the overall complication rate was 9.9%, with 8% attributed to the stent delivery procedure and 20% attributed to the stent itself. The 30-day mortality rate was 1.9%. Using this same stent, Murphy and coworkers[38] treated 103 limbs with a resultant primary patency rate of 86.2% at 48 months.

Henry and associates[39] reported on Palmaz stent placement in the iliac, femoral, and popliteal arteries of 310 patients, 184 of which were within the iliac system. Immediate clinical improvement was reported in 100% of patients stented in the iliac artery. Primary patency rates were reportedly 94%, 91%, and 86% at 6-month, 1-year, and 2-year follow-up, respectively, and were better than those previously reported for balloon angioplasty.[20, 40] Again, these results are attributed to several variables of the study and must be reviewed. The majority of these patients (89%) were treated for claudication, 52% had good three-vessel runoffs, and 72% of the lesions were shorter than 3 cm, all of which are known predictors for balloon angioplasty success.[20] Additionally, most patients had only one stent placed. Finally, the significant predictors for success in this study were identified lesions 3 cm or shorter and a single stent for one arterial lesion, similar to those previously reported for basic balloon angioplasty.[20] Similarly, Cikrit and colleagues[41] reported 1-, 2-, and 4-year life-table patency rates of 87%, 74%, and 67%, respectively, for single stent placement for occlusive disease. Although limited in the number of treated limbs ($n = 38$), this study noted the need for additional procedures to maintain the long-term patency of the stented limb.

In 1996, Sullivan and colleagues[42] reported a series of 424 limbs with iliac artery stenoses treated with primary stenting. Unlike previously reported studies in which the stents were often placed following a complication or failure of balloon angioplasty, this study involved placement of stents as the primary mode of treatment. Interestingly, the results were similar to those reported for secondary stent placement, with primary patency rates of 89% and 77% at 1- and 2-year follow-up, respectively. Although the majority of stents used were Palmaz stents (86%), a handful of Wallstents were also deployed. In the study conducted by Ballard and colleagues,[43] a combination of the Palmaz stent and Wallstent was also used in 98 limbs to treat disabling claudication or limb-threatening ischemia. A Palmaz stent was chosen for focal lesions in nontortuous vessels or if the puncture site was ipsilateral to the lesion. A Wallstent was preferred for treating longer lesions situated near the inguinal ligament in tortuous vessels and when a contralateral approach was necessitated. The complication rates were high at 19.4%, and the series included six initial treatment failures. Although the cumulative 1-year patency rate was 87.6%, the primary patency rate dropped to 55.3% at 2 years. The authors concluded that major complications were associated with iliac stent placements and patency rates were affected by stent location and progression of distal disease.

TABLE 17-3

Results Reported for Iliac Artery Stenting

AUTHORS	PATIENTS (N)	STENT TYPE	LESIONS (N)	MEAN LESION LENGTH (cm)	IMMEDIATE CLINICAL SUCCESS	COMPLICATION RATE (%)	ACUTE THROMBOSIS RATE (%)	PRIMARY PATENCY (%) 6 mo	12 mo	24 mo	48 mo	RESTENOSIS RATE (%)
Palmaz et al.[37]	486	P	587	3.2	99.2	9.9	1.0	NA	90.9	84.1	68.6	3.3
Murphy et al.[38]	83	P	103	4.0	98.9	9.7	NA	NA	89.3	87.5	86.2	9.0
Henry et al.[39]	184	P	230	3.2	100	NA	0.5	94.0	91.0	86.0	—	0.5°
Cikrit et al.[41]	34	P	38	4.5	18.4	NA	NA	NA	87.0	74.0	67.0	NA
Liermann et al.[46]	52	S	52	4.5	NA	NA	0.0	(98% at mean follow-up = 20 mo)				1.9
Strecker et al.[47]	214	S	214	6.4 (occlusion) 2.8 (stenosis)	100	7.9	3.3	90.0	89.0	87.0	80.0	13.0
Long et al.[48]	61	S	64	6.4	98.0	12.0	1.6	90.0	84.0	69.0	41.0	28.0
Vorwerk et al.[51]	103	W	103	5.1	96.0	11.6	3.9	92.0	87.0	83.0	78.0	17.5
Martin et al.[52]	140	W	171	6.6	95.0	4.3	NA	93.0	81.0	71.0	—	NA
Sapoval et al.[53]	95	W	101	NA	99.0	11.7	NA	NA	79.8	NA	60.8	3.2
Zollikofer et al.[55]	18	W	26	4.6	100	0.0	3.8	(96% at mean follow-up = 16 mo)				16.7
Sullivan et al.[42]	288	W & P	424	NA	87.8	14.1	NA	NA	89.0	76.0	—	18.8
Ballard et al.[43]	72	W & P	145	NA	96.9	19.4	NA	NA	87.6	55.3	—	NA
Murphy et al.[54]	65	W & P	90	5.6	92.0	11.0	NA	NA	68.0	61.0	—	NA

°At 6 months.

P, Palmaz; S, Strecker; W, Wallstent; NA, not available.

INFRAINGUINAL STENTING. Most reports of the use of Palmaz stents in the femoropopliteal arteries have not been as favorable as those reported for its use in the iliac arteries. For lesions treated in the femoral artery, the patency rates reported show improved results over balloon angioplasty, but these cases are plagued by acute thrombosis and high restenosis rates.[39, 44] Furthermore, the results reported for lesions treated in the popliteal artery are worse,[39] demonstrating the inefficacy of the Palmaz stent in arteries with a small diameter.

In the previously described report by Henry and associates,[39] which includes the largest series of infrainguinal stenting, 126 of 310 patients had stent placement in the femoral and popliteal arteries. Immediate clinical success was reported in 97% of femoral and in 80% of popliteal arteries. Although the primary patency rates for femoral stenting were shown to be better than those previously reported for balloon angioplasty, this was not true for stents placed in the popliteal artery—1-, 2-, and 4-year patency rates were all 50% with a restenosis rate of 20% at 6 months. Additional studies conducted by Bergeron and coworkers[44] and Chatelard and Guibourt[45] reported similar primary patency rates in smaller groups of patients.

Complications and Limitations

Serious complications directly related to the Palmaz stent itself include dislodgment of the stent from the catheter delivery system,[37] traumatic crushing of the stent during surgical revascularization at another site,[38] and pseudoaneurysms adjacent to the stented site.[37] The most frequent complications (hematoma,[37–40] distal embolization,[37–40] arterial dissection away from the stent,[37, 38] rupture,[37, 38] and spasms[39]) are related to the puncture site and the relatively large size of the delivery system (9- or 10-Fr). Furthermore, transient contrast-induced renal failures due to contrast volume and postprocedure deaths related to myocardial infarction and stroke have also been reported.[37, 38] The 30-day mortality rates reported by Palmaz and associates[37] and Murphy and coworkers[38] were 1.9% and 1.2%, respectively. Two procedure-related deaths reported by Palmaz and associates were induced by contrast reaction.

The most notable limitation of the Palmaz stent is its rigidity, which precludes its use in tortuous vessels and prevents placement of the device via the contralateral approach. As such, the Palmaz stent should not be placed across articular joints. Like basic balloon angioplasty, the Palmaz stent is also limited by acute thrombosis and restenosis induced by intimal hyperplasia (see Tables 17–3 and 17–4). Murphy and associates[38] and Henry and colleagues[39] correlated thrombosis formation in patients with occlusive lesions or smaller arterial diameter, in whom multiple stents were implanted, and with a hypercoagulable state. Murphy and associates[38] explained further that occluded arteries are already lacking endothelium and denuded of remaining endothelial lining during stent placement. Thus, the remaining endothelium lacks the essential normal tissue templates between stent struts to facilitate re-endothelialization and thrombus prevention. Furthermore, the Palmaz stent does not reduce the restenosis rate. Under- or overdeployment of the stent results in the induction of intimal hyperplasia.[37, 38] Restenosis usually occurs at the native site of the vessel narrowing or occlusion, where flow abnormalities occur and persist proximally and distally to the stent.

Strecker Stent

Device Description

The Strecker stent is a balloon-expandable tubular wire mesh knitted out of a single metallic electropolished tantalum filament with a diameter of 0.1 to 0.15 mm. Its knitting is composed of a series of loosely connected loops to provide flexibility and elasticity. This flexibility allows passage through curved and angulated vessels, making implantation at any site feasible, including arteries near articular joints. Unlike the Palmaz stent, the Strecker stent is compressible in both radial and longitudinal directions. For insertion and deployment, the Strecker stent is premounted onto an angioplasty balloon by specialized sleeves at its ends covered by thin Silastic sheaths. When the balloon is inflated, foreshortening of these sleeves retracts the sheaths and exposes the stent to the arterial lumen. Because of its tantalum metal filament, the stent is highly radiopaque and considered biologically inert.

Because no protective introducer sheath is required, the Strecker stent can be introduced by a delivery system with a relatively small diameter. For peripheral arterial lesions, a stent with a diameter of 4 to 7 mm requires an 8-Fr introducer sheath, whereas a stent with a diameter of 8 to 10 mm requires a 9-Fr sheath. The stent is mounted on a 5- or 6-Fr balloon catheter. The stent is available in expanded diameters of 4 to 12 mm and a maximal length of 8 cm. For renal arterial lesions, stents with a diameter of 4 to 7 mm are available with a length of 1.5 cm and have stronger tantalum filaments of 0.13 mm for increased radial strength.

Technique

The Strecker stent is currently not approved for use in the United States. In Europe and Australia, it has been used primarily to treat insufficient balloon angioplasty results in the iliac artery, as defined previously for Palmaz stents. Limited applications of the Strecker stent in the femoral, popliteal, and renal arteries have been reported but are currently not recommended.

Results

Tables 17–3 and 17–4 summarize the literature on the use of Strecker stent.[46–49] It was difficult to extract such information from the published reports and interpret the data because of inconsistent reporting methods. Thus, more controlled clinical trials with long-term follow-up data are still needed to evaluate the safety and efficacy of the Strecker stent.

Strecker and colleagues[47] conducted the largest study by a single investigative group on use of the Strecker stent in

TABLE 17–4

Results Reported for Iliac Artery Stenting

AUTHORS	PATIENTS (N)	STENT TYPE	LESIONS (N)	MEAN LESION LENGTH (cm)	IMMEDIATE CLINICAL SUCCESS	COMPLICATION RATE (%)	ACUTE THROMBOSIS RATE (%)	PRIMARY PATENCY (%)				RESTENOSIS RATE (%)
								6 mo	12 mo	24 mo	48 mo	
Henry et al.[39]	126	P	126	3.8 SFA	97.0	2.9	3.2		81.0	73.0	65.0	11.0°
				POP	80.0				50.0	50.0	50.0	20.0°
Bergeron et al.[44]	39	P	42	NA	95.0	4.8	4.8	NA	81.0	77.0	—	19.0
Chatelard et al.[45]	35	P	35	NA	100	0.0	6.0	NA	80.4	75.7	—	14.0°
Liermann et al.[46]												
SFA	42	S	42	8.6	NA	NA	2.0	(69% at mean follow-up = 19 mo)				31.0
POP	6	S	6	NA	NA	NA	0.0	(83% at mean follow-up = 19 mo)				16.7
Strecker et al.[47]	131	S	131	6.4 (occlusion) 2.6 (stenosis)	93.0	21.0	6.9	87.0	70.0	54.0	—	21.0
Bray et al.[49]	52	S	57	6.8	100	16.0	10.0	NA	79.0	—	—	43.0
Martin et al.[52]	90	W	109	9.4	95.0	16.7	NA	80.0	61.0	49.0	—	22.0
Zollikofer et al.[55]	13	W	15	13.5	100	NA	28.6	(54% at mean follow-up = 20 mo)				42.9
Gray et al.[56]	55	W & P	57	16.5	NA	24.5	NA	47.0	22.0	—	—	39.0
White et al.[57]	32	W & S	32	4.8 (occlusion) 2.7 (stenosis)	96.9	NA	6.3	93.0	83.0	75.0	—	28.0

°At 6 months.
P, Palmer; S, Strecker; W, Wallstent; SFA, superficial femoral artery; POP, popliteal artery; NA, not available.

333

iliac and femoral artery lesions (see Tables 17–3 and 17–4). Although the reported patency results seem promising, the actual mean follow-up for all patients is relatively short: 16 months for stents in the iliac artery and 13 months for stents in the femoral and popliteal arteries. Accordingly, patency rates reported for lesions in the iliac artery are higher than those previously reported for balloon angioplasty.[19, 20] However, the patency results in the femoropopliteal segments are as disappointing as those of balloon angioplasty, with a high incidence of complications and restenoses even with short follow-up.[20, 40] In treating long arterial lesions (mean length, 6.4 cm), Long and coworkers[48] demonstrated no evidence of improved results over balloon angioplasty. Additionally, the complication and restenosis rates were worse.

Complications and Limitations

The major complications directly attributed to the Strecker stent itself include stent dislocation, displacement,[46–48] and migration.[48] Stent dislocation on the shaft was caused either by the friction with the hemostatic valve of the introducer sheath or with the total occlusive lesions. Stent displacement and migration are attributed to the device's flexibility and lack of radial compression strength. Thus, exact localization and sizing of the diseased lumen must be performed before stent implantation. Stent malfunction reported by Liermann and colleagues[46] included failure of the silicone sleeves to slide back and free the stent after balloon dilation and major shortening of the stent.

The Strecker stent is also limited by acute thrombosis and restenosis (see Tables 17–3 and 17–4). Interestingly, Bray and coworkers[49] reported that 34% of stented lesions in the femoropopliteal arteries progressed from less than 20% residual stenosis at 3 months to more than 50% stenosis at 12 months. Furthermore, the authors observed that the restenosis was in the native artery located proximal or distal to the stent at 3 months and was primarily inside the stent at 12 months.

Self-Expanding Stents

Self-expanding stents are compressed within a small-diameter introducer sheath and then released in the diseased site by withdrawing the sheath while keeping the stent in place. Once the stents are released, they can expand to the predetermined diameter. These stents are further characterized by their high degree of flexibility; thus, they are relatively easy to manage, even in tortuous vessels. However, they lack radial compression strength. One example of such a self-expanding stent is the widely used Wallstent (Schneider, Inc., Minneapolis).

Wallstent

Device Description

The Wallstent is composed of thin stainless steel wires interwoven into braids forming a tube. The crossing points

of the wires are not soldered to each other, resulting in a very flexible stent that can self-expand and move freely in radial and longitudinal directions. It can be introduced into the arterial lumen using a relatively small-diameter introducer catheter (7-Fr). Conversely, its flexibility can cause marked shortening during expansion. Also, because it is made of thin stainless steel, the Wallstent has a low radiopacity and makes precise positioning more challenging.

Technique

The Wallstent is delivered through an introducer catheter with a rolling membrane covering the stent. The stents are available in 50-, 75-, 100-, 125-, and 150-mm lengths compressed within an introducer catheter. The compressed Wallstent within this introducer catheter is inserted over a guidewire and then advanced to the lesion site under fluoroscopic control. After proper positioning for stent deployment is accomplished, the catheter is then slowly withdrawn, which gradually retracts its outer membrane and thus releases the stent. It should be noted that the Wallstent shortens during the release; therefore, proper placement can be somewhat difficult. If the catheter is only partially disengaged, the stent can be pulled back but not advanced forward. Repeated stenting is sometimes necessary to obtain optimal results. If an adequate lumen cannot be obtained, additional dilatation with an angioplasty balloon can be employed.

Indications

The Wallstent has been approved by the FDA for iliac artery applications. These applications include treatment of stenotic or occlusive atherosclerotic lesions and failed or inadequate angioplasty results (as previously defined earlier).

Results

ILIAC STENTING. Unlike most practitioners using stents to salvage failed or inadequate angioplasty results, Vorwerk and Gunther and coworkers[50, 51] used the Wallstent device as the primary treatment for complex iliac artery lesions not amenable to balloon angioplasty. These complex lesions were defined as occlusions, eccentric stenoses, long stenotic segments, ostial lesions, ulcerated plaque, aneurysm formation, and acute complications of balloon angioplasty. The chronic iliac artery occlusions had to be traversed by a guidewire before primary stent placement. Mechanical passage of the occluded segment was attempted in 85 patients and was successful in 63. Accordingly, the stented complex lesions included 63 occlusions and 62 stenoses. The overall patency rates reported were high (see Table 17–3), similar to those reported for the balloon-expandable Palmaz stent.[37–39, 41] Indeed, although the Wallstent is self-expandable, "undersized" balloon dilatation (5 to 7 mm) was used before stent placement in all stenotic lesions and after stent placement in occlusive lesions. Furthermore, in occluded segments, the stents were further dilated with larger balloons (8 to 10 mm) if they did not open to their full diameter. Additionally, 86% of the patients presented with Fontaine stage IIb claudication. Nevertheless, the complication and restenosis rates were surprisingly low, perhaps because of short follow-up duration.

Vorwerk and coworkers[51] further pursued the potential of the Wallstent as the primary treatment for chronic iliac artery occlusions in 103 patients, with 87% of these patients presenting with claudication. Mechanical passage of the occluded segment was attempted in 127 patients. The results reported (see Table 17–3) are similar to those previously reported for balloon angioplasty alone, with slightly higher complication and restenosis rates.

Martin and colleagues,[52] in their multicenter trial of Wallstents placed in the iliac artery, demonstrated a 95% immediate success rate in 140 patients. Furthermore, the 1- and 2-year primary patency rates were 81% and 71%, respectively, which paralleled results reported for the Palmaz stent in the iliac artery. Sapoval and colleagues,[53] in their series of 95 patients (101 lesions), had an immediate success rate of 99% and 1- and 4-year primary patency rates of 79.8% and 60.8%, respectively. Of these 101 lesions, 43 were occlusions.

In a 1998 report by Murphy and associates,[54] 90 iliac lesions in 65 patients were treated with 111 Wallstents and 21 Palmaz stents. There was no specific algorithm used to determine which stent to use and the choice was solely determined by operator preference. The immediate success rate was 92% and the 1- and 2-year primary patency rates were 68% and 61%, respectively. Although there was no observed mortality, the complication rate was 11% and required periprocedural or immediate postprocedural modification of the treatment plan.

INFRAINGUINAL STENTING. As previously indicated for the Palmaz stent,[39, 44, 45] the reports of stent placement in the femoropopliteal area are mediocre and inferior to data reported for the iliac system. Zollikofer and colleagues,[55] in a small series of 13 patients treated predominantly for occlusion, reported a 54% primary patency rate at a mean follow-up of 19 months and a dismal 42.9% restenosis rate. In a larger series of 90 patients (109 lesions) treated exclusively by the Wallstent device, Martin and associates[52] reported 1- and 2-year primary patency rates of 61% and 49%, respectively. However, the relatively favorable outcome compared to the Palmaz and Strecker stent for infrainguinal stenting may be attributed to the fact that a majority of these patients were treated for stenoses and patients with poor runoff were excluded.

Gray and coworkers,[56] in their report of 55 patients treated with Wallstents and Palmaz stents for long-segment superficial femoral artery disease, reported a discouraging 1-year patency rate of 22% and a high restenosis rate of 39%. The poor 1-year patency rate may have been due to the long occlusions and poor runoff. Interestingly, there was little difference in clinical outcome between patients with claudication and those with limb-threatening ischemia.

Complications and Limitations

Aside from its poor radiopacity, the Wallstent has been reported to decrease the patency of the side branches it crosses by as much as 40%.[53] However, the main complication of the Wallstent as the primary stent treatment in iliac artery occlusions is embolization (2.4%[50] and 7.8%[51]), which may subsequently require surgical or percutaneous intervention. Furthermore, a slight tapering of the stent implantation was observed in 25 patients (24.3%[51]). Angiographic follow-up at a mean of 4 months revealed complete resolution of the tapering in 20 of these patients. However, further shortening of the stent and increased diameter were noted in 11 patients (10.7%).

Primary stent treatment in such lesions is also limited by acute thromboses and restenoses (see Tables 17–3 and 17–4). Interestingly, the authors observed that restenosis with the Wallstent occurred in either the proximal, middle, or distal portion of the stented segment, but never in the completely stented lesion.[51]

THERMAL EXPANDING STENTS

Thermal expanding stents are composed of nitinol, a nickel-titanium alloy characterized by its unique property of thermal recovery. The nitinol wire is annealed at 500°C to assume the desired final coil spring configuration. When cooled to 0°C, the coil spring transforms into a straight wire, at which time it may be used for introduction into a Teflon catheter. Once the introducer enters the warm artery (37°C), it recoils back to its annealed shape. Although unique in concept, nitinol stents have not been widely used and are not yet FDA-approved for vascular use.

Stent-Grafts

Recent interest in stents has been focused on this newly evolved type of device. A stent-graft device is composed of an intravascular stent used to maintain the position of an intraluminally placed graft for traumatic arteriovenous fistula and aneurysmal and occlusive disease. Marin and coworkers[58] have successfully treated traumatic arteriovenous fistulas in the brachiocephalic region. Parodi and colleagues[59] have also treated traumatic arteriovenous fistulas in the carotid artery using stent-aided placement of autologous saphenous vein. Several investigators have used the stents to secure polytetrafluoroethylene and Dacron grafts in the iliac and superficial femoral artery position for arterial occlusive disease.[60, 61] These procedures were performed by a balloon dilating the lesion first, placing the graft in position, and then stenting at least the proximal and distal ends of the graft. Occasionally, the entire length of the graft was stented to prevent elastic recoil of the arterial wall. These new techniques are still under investigation and currently are not recommended for general use.

One of the most exciting endovascular therapies being investigated today is the use of stent-grafts to repair aneurysmal disease. Parodi[62] used the Palmaz stent to secure Dacron grafts in the aorta and iliac positions. In 1996, Moore and Rutherford[63] reported the results of transfemoral endovascular repair of abdominal aortic aneurysms using a grafting system developed by EndoVascular Technologies, Inc. (Menlo Park, Calif.) from 13 medical centers in the United States. Details of this new technology are discussed elsewhere in this textbook.

Comments

Stent technology is still rapidly evolving, and long-term follow-up data are sorely needed. Stents have had good success in providing a scaffold to maintain the intraluminal structure and patency of an artery. As such, stents appear to play a role in improving early results after failed or inadequate balloon angioplasty. However, stents induce intimal hyperplasia and thus do not prevent restenosis. The results reported by various clinical investigators are clearly worse in the femoral artery than in the iliac artery position. Currently in the United States, only two stents are approved by the FDA for iliac artery applications. As such, routine use of stents cannot be recommended until additional studies demonstrate that the results with stents are clearly better than those with balloon angioplasty alone.

ANGIOSCOPY

Angioscopy allows direct, visual observation of the intraluminal morphology, thus providing pertinent information of the plaque surface anatomy, degree of ulceration, or differentiation between thrombus and embolus. The following equipment is essential for the angioscopy system to function properly: a flexible fiberoptic scope, a light source, an irrigation system, a camera, a video recorder, and a monitor. Figure 17–16 shows the various components of such a system. The scope itself usually contains three separate components: the light bundle for viewing, the light bundle for illumination, and a transport channel for irrigation or manipulating instruments (Fig. 17–17). Multiple angioscopy systems are now commercially available. A brief description of each of these endoscopes is given in Table 17–5.

Indications

Perhaps the most useful indication for angioscopy is to monitor thromboembolectomy and endarterectomy. White[64] and others[65-68] have clearly shown limitations of blind thromboendarterectomy (Table 17–6). White[64] and Vollmar and Hutschenreiter[68] have shown that angioscopy is superior to conventional angiography for detecting residual intimal flaps following endarterectomy of the iliac artery. Mehigan and Olcott[69] reported the potential benefits

TABLE 17–5

Angioscopy: Overview of Available Instruments

	SCOPE		FIBEROPTIC SYSTEM					
TRADE NAME	Outer Diameter (mm)	Usable Length (cm)	Field of View	Depth (mm)	No. of Bundles (Pixels)	SINGLE VS. SEPARATE UNIT	CHANNELS (IRRIGATION WORKING)	SPECIAL FEATURES
Edwards LIS								
Inoperative	2.3	80	70°	2–5	6000	Disposable separate	1.3 mm integrated	Disposable (potential lower cost)
(2 sizes)	3.0	60	70°	2–15	6000	Disposable separate	1.5 mm integrated	
Percutaneous	1.0	80	70°	2–15	6000	Reusable single	Forward flow irrigating holes	
(2 sizes)	0.85	80	52°	2–15	2000	Reusable single	Forward flow irrigating holes	
Microvasive	6 Fr (2.0)	60	90°	0.2–5.0	2000	Separate Visicath handle with scope; separate scope	Available: 0.6 mm, 0.9 mm	Cost-effective probe; small modular system; interchangeable probes
	8 Fr (2.5)	60	90°	0.2–5.0	2000	Same as 6 Fr	Available 1.1 mm	2 models (8100, 8300); 8300 available with battery pack for light source
	11 Fr (3.5)	60	90°	0.2–5.0	2000	Same as 6 Fr	Available: 0.6 mm, 2.8 mm	Therapeutic accessories (forceps, snares, etc.)
AIS Scopecath	1.5 Fr (0.5)	60	90°	0.2–5.0	2000	Single	Irrigation via coaxial catheter	Smallest diameter available for intraoperative use; coronary artery use; guidewire compatible for positioning; may use fluoroscopy for positioning
Olympus								
PF14	1.4	120	75°	2.1–0.0	32,000*	Single	NA	NA Imaging only
PF22	2.2	120	75°	2.1–0.0	32,000	Single	NA	NA Only scope available with steerability for acute angle vessel visualization (120° in one plane)
PF28	2.8	120	75°	2.1–0.0	32,000	Single	1.0 mm	NA
Karl Storz	2.3	82	65°	1.0–0.0	10 μ†	Single	0.3 mm integrated	Guidewire compatibile for positioning
	3.0	82	60°	1.0–0.0	10 μ†		1.2 mm integrated	In situ valvulotome; grasping and biopsy forceps for working channel
Trimedyne	2.8	105	55°	5.5–14.0	NA	Separate optical lens and catheter	1.15 mm (additional cuff inflation channel)	

*Specification as per manufacturer.
†Pixel number not specified.
NA, not applicable.
From Hernández JJ, Quiñones-Baldrich WJ: Angioplasty: Essential, desirable, and optimal components. In Moore WS, Ahn SS (eds): Endovascular Surgery. Philadelphia, WB Saunders, 1989, pp 39–49.

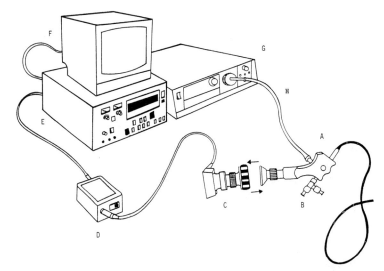

Figure 17–16. Components of an angioscopic system: *A*, angioscope; *B*, irrigation port; *C*, miniature camera; *D*, camera control unit; *E*, videocassette recorder; *F*, monitor; *G*, light source; *H*, light source cable. (From Hernández JJ, Quiñones-Baldrich WJ: Angioplasty: Essential, desirable, and optimal components. In Moore WS, Ahn SS [eds]: Endovascular Surgery. Philadelphia, WB Saunders, 1989, pp 39–49.)

of angioscopically monitoring the completeness of carotid endarterectomy.

Several investigators have also demonstrated the usefulness of angioscopy to monitor the completeness of valvulotomy during in situ saphenous vein bypass grafting.[70, 71] These investigators found retained valves by endoscopic examination following conventional blind valvulotomy. Matsumoto and colleagues[72] also found vascular endoscopy useful for valvulotomy of nonreversed saphenous vein grafts. Chin and Fogarty[73] proposed and developed an integrated angioscopy-valvulotomy system that allows valvulotomy under direct vision.

TABLE 17–6

Limitations of Blind Thromboembolectomy

    Catheter injuries
        Vessel perforation
        Intimal tear or flap
        Subintimal dissection
        Rethrombosis
        Distal embolization
        Myointimal hyperplasia and arterial narrowing
    Inadequate procedure
        Missed thrombus
        Adherent thrombus
        Side branch or small vessel thrombus
        Undetected atherosclerotic lesions
    Absence of information
        No image
        No flow data
        No pressure measurement
    Problems of angiographic control
        Time-consuming
        Postprocedural monitoring only
        Requirement for equipment and technician
        Poor quality of intraoperative angiograms
        Radiation exposure to patient and staff
        Patient exposure to contrast medium
            Anaphylaxis
            Renal failure

From White GF: Angioscopy to monitor arterial thromboembolectomy, In Moore WS, Ahn SS (eds): Endovascular surgery. Philadelphia, WB Saunders, 1989, pp 55–64.

Various investigators have reported on many other indications for vascular endoscopy, including inspection of vascular anastomosis, laser-assisted balloon angioplasty, and mechanical atherectomy.[70, 74, 75] Angioscopy can be useful for grabbing and retrieving organized clot, plaque, or even foreign bodies, using flexible grabbers transported through the working channel of an angioscope[76] (Fig. 17–18). Moreover, flexible biopsy-type cutters can cut residual intimal flaps under direct angioscopic view[76] (Fig. 17–19).

Technique

Angioscopy is usually performed intraoperatively through an open arteriotomy. Proximal control of the inflow is obtained using a vascular clamp or a balloon catheter (Figs. 17–20 and 17–21). Distal back-bleeding can usually be controlled with irrigation injected into the scope. The endoscope may be placed directly into the artery, as shown in Figures 17–19 and 17–20, or may be placed through a standard introducer sheath with a hemostatic valve and a side-arm irrigation channel. Images can be visualized directly or recorded for later viewing. The availability of an irrigation pump or computerized digital angioscopy equipment may enhance one's ability to obtain a satisfactory image and prevent fluid overload by the irrigation.

Results

White[64] has reported residual thrombus after balloon embolectomy in almost all cases. In approximately 80% of 55 cases, the angioscopic findings led to further attempts at clot extraction. In our own experience at the University of California, Los Angeles (UCLA), we found residual thrombus or intimal flaps leading to altered management in 7 of 19 patients undergoing thrombectomy. Grundfest and associates,[70] Mehigan and Olcott,[69] Fleisher and colleagues,[71] and Matsumoto and coworkers[72] have also reported visualization of retained valves that led to reintroduction of the valvulotome in a small but significant number of patients undergoing in situ saphenous vein by-

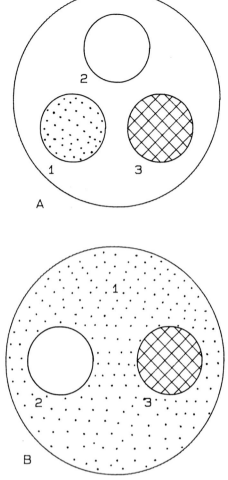

We found that angioscopy allowed safe performance of mechanical atherectomy and aided in monitoring its results.[78] Angioscopy was helpful in the placement of guidewires through the stenotic lesion and in the documentation of residual intimal flaps or thrombus following the procedure. Conventional angiography missed an intimal flap in one patient, and vascular endoscopy allowed placement of a guidewire in another patient in whom conventional angiographic guidance was inadequate.

Complications and Limitations

Angioscopy offers a direct, precise, descriptive color image of endovascular lesions while requiring no contrast dye, radiation, or radiology technician. However, endoscopy is limited by its inability to visualize small runoff vessels and because the overall picture of the vascular tree is too broad. Furthermore, it is difficult to measure the percentage stenosis unless one knows the focal length of the angioscope and the distance from the lesion to the lens. Images of a lumen visualized from a far distance may look quite small, whereas a lumen visualized close up may look quite large. Perhaps the most limiting disadvantage of angioscopy is the requirement for irrigation. Even small amounts of blood can blur or opacify the image; however, overzealous or uncontrolled irrigation can lead to fluid overload or air embolus.

The irrigation pump is now available in many commercial products, and digital angioscopy is being continually refined to overcome the problem of irrigation.

Another potential danger is that one may injure the vascular lumen by passing the scope into the vessel, particularly if the scope is too large for the artery. The late results of vascular endoscopy are not known; therefore, potential injury-induced intimal hyperplasia cannot be completely ruled out at this time.

Finally, angioscopy may allow direct occlusion of the saphenous vein branches during in situ bypass. With further development, such a system could allow in situ saphenous vein bypass with only two incisions: one for the proximal and one for the distal anastomosis.

INTRAVASCULAR ULTRASOUND

Intravascular ultrasound (IVUS) is a promising diagnostic tool that combines ultrasound technology with a catheter-delivered intraluminal system to provide high-resolution,

Figure 17–17. Light bundle patterns. *A*, A single channel (1) contains the light fibers; there are separate working/irrigation (2) and viewing (3) channels. *B*, Light fibers (1) are dispersed around the working and viewing channels (2 and 3). (From Hernández JJ, Quiñones-Baldrich WJ: Angioplasty: Essential, desirable, and optimal components. In Moore WS, Ahn SS [eds]: Endovascular Surgery. Philadelphia, WB Saunders, 1989, pp 39–49.)

pass. Grundfest and associates[70] have also reported anastomotic problems in 23% of patients undergoing bypass procedures. Olcott,[77] however, noted very few intimal flaps or misplaced sutures in anastomotic inspections. Fewer than 5% of patients in Olcott's series required revision of the anastomosis. Our own experience at UCLA has been more consistent with Olcott's data because we have found very few anastomotic problems following bypass surgery.

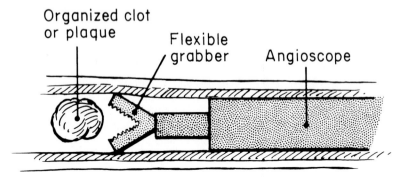

Figure 17–18. A flexible grabbing catheter inserted through a vascular endoscope to retrieve a piece of organized clot or plaque particle. (From Ahn SS: The use of grabbers, cutters, and shavers as an adjunct during endovascular surgery. In Moore WS, Ahn SS [eds]: Endovascular Surgery. Philadelphia, WB Saunders, 1989, pp 514–517.)

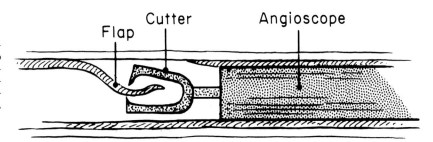

Figure 17–19. A flexible cutter with sharp, piranha-like jaws passed through the vascular endoscope to cut an intimal flap. (From Ahn SS: The use of grabbers, cutters, and shavers as an adjunct during endovascular surgery. In Moore WS, Ahn SS [eds]: Endovascular Surgery. Philadelphia, WB Saunders, 1989, pp 514–517.)

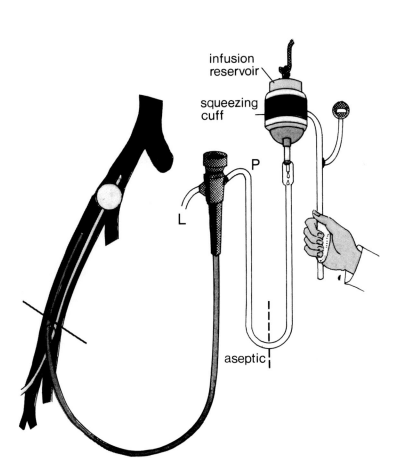

Figure 17–20. Principle of arterial endoscopy at the iliac level using a flexible type B endoscope introduced from a distal arteriotomy at the common femoral artery. Continuous saline perfusion is provided under controlled pressure. *L*, Cold light connection; *P*, perfusion line. (From Vollmar JF, Hutschenreiter JF: Vascular endoscopy for thromboendarterectomy. In Moore WS, Ahn SS [eds]: Endovascular Surgery. Philadelphia, WB Saunders, 1989, pp 87–94.)

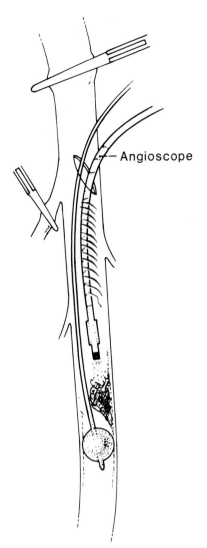

— Angioscope

Figure 17–21. Standard technique of angioscopic thromboembolectomy, with a Fogarty balloon catheter inserted alongside the angioscope, allowing visualization of the thrombectomy process. (From White GH, et al: Angioscopic thromboembolectomy: Preliminary observations with a recent technique. J Vasc Surg 7:495–499, 1988.)

cross-sectional evaluation of the vascular anatomy. Since its inception nearly 50 years ago,[79] technological advances have led to the development of the current high-frequency catheter-tipped transducers that can produce transmural images utilizing small-diameter intraluminal catheters. The increasing role of IVUS in vascular surgery is fueled by the growing implementation of endovascular procedures, in which the utility of IVUS pre-, intra-, or postprocedurally can provide accurate, real-time display of arterial morphology, immediate results of intervention, and extent of dissection, if any.[80] Angiography has historically been used for completion information after endovascular intervention; however, it is limited by its uniplanar view of the vessel and is thus prone to underestimation of residual stenosis. Studies have shown that angiography can misjudge the cross-sectional volume by 40% compared with IVUS.[81–83] Although the innate advantage of angiography is its ability to demonstrate the vascular anatomy in a longitudinal array, the advent of the three-dimensional IVUS format has al-lowed for a similar cross-sectional interpretation of the vessel wall.

Vessel and Plaque Morphology

Numerous investigators have examined the diagnostic potential of IVUS in vitro and in vivo (human and animal models).[84–87] In vitro investigations indicated that measurements of luminal area, diameter, and wall thickness correlated favorably with histopathologic images.[84–87] However, these results should be interpreted with caution, because the elements of the histopathologic specimen examined may not correspond to the exact arterial segment examined by ultrasonography. Quantitative measurement of the vessel dimensions is determined by the relative echogenicity of the internal lamina, external lamina, and adventitia. Elastic arteries have a media that contains a large proportion of elastin and collagen, both elements of which are highly echogenic. There is dampened acoustic impedence between the layers compared to muscular arteries and the distinct layers are not as apparent.[84] On IVUS, elastic arteries are recognized via a media that is as echogenic as the surrounding intima and adventitia. Muscular arteries contain a media composed primarily of smooth muscle cells with minimal collagen and elastin. The media of muscular arteries is poorly echogenic and forms a marked acoustic disparity between the surrounding layers, which results in a three-layered image on IVUS.[88]

Gussenhoven and colleagues[89] proposed four basic echogenic correlations between the plaque component and the atherosclerotic lesion:

1. *Hypoechoic,* representing a significant deposit of lipids and thus often obscured at the sites of total arterial occlusion, severe intimal thickening, or regions of severe calcification
2. *Soft echoes,* representing fibromuscular tissue
3. *Bright echoes,* representing collagen-rich fibrous tissue
4. *Bright echoes with shadowing behind the lesion,* representing calcium

The distinction between fibrous and calcified lesions has been further evaluated by Link and associates[87] and Potkin and coworkers[90] using IVUS. Link and associates[87] examined the use of IVUS within the abdominal aorta and iliac artery and determined sensitivity and specificity of 70% and 53%, respectively, in detecting calcified arteriosclerotic lesions. Potkin and coworkers[90] compared IVUS to histologic sections of excised human coronary arteries, and correctly identified fibrous and calcified plaques in 96% and 100% of cases, respectively.

Clinical Use of Intravascular Ultrasound

In comparison with the gold standard of angiography, IVUS in normal or mildly diseased vessels provides equivalent information; however, in highly diseased or occluded vessels, IVUS provides a more accurate assessment of luminal and vessel diameter.[91] Angiography provides only a planar view of the vessel lumen, whereas IVUS generates a more precise characterization of vessel wall architecture that resembles histologic data of vessel wall thickness and diameter. IVUS, like angiography, is performed via percutaneous access and involves an over-the-wire configuration using an IVUS probe that advances along a 0.014 to 0.038-inch guidewire.[92] Standard angiographic catheters use 5-Fr or 6-Fr sheaths, whereas some 6.2-Fr IVUS catheters require the use of an 8-Fr sheath.[92] The risks associated with the procedure are similar to those of angiography and percutaneous access, and include bleeding or hematoma at the puncture site, pseudoaneurysm formation, and distal embolization.

Several investigators have reported their experiences using IVUS to improve primary patency rates and decrease complication rates after PTA, peripheral atherectomy, and placement of endovascular stent-grafts for peripheral aneurysms.[93] The impetus behind the advancing use of IVUS is to clarify the mechanisms of these endovascular interventions. Long-term clinical outcome of patients after surgery is contingent upon certain characteristics of an atherosclerotic lesion, such as the presence of an ulcerated plaque or thrombus.[94] IVUS can serve as a powerful tool for distinguishing between normal and diseased vessels; furthermore, IVUS can provide information on the eccentricity and histologic type of stenosis prior to intervention to allow for optimal surgical planning. This would afford the surgeon the advantage of being able to strategically target the lesion(s) with a specific therapy based on certain plaque characteristics. In terms of postoperative assessment of intervention, IVUS can provide valuable data on morphologic changes in the arterial wall and the extent of excision following revision.

Evaluation of Percutaneous Transluminal Angioplasty, Stents, and Atherectomy

Recent studies on the role of IVUS in the management of aortoiliac occlusive disease indicated that following stent deployment[95–97] IVUS was able to detect underdeployed stents with greater accuracy than angiography. Several investigators[94, 98, 99] have reported that angiography provides inaccurate information regarding stent deployment in those patients undergoing iliac artery PTA and stent placement. In contrast, IVUS offers a more accurate appraisal of inadequately deployed stents. Arko and colleagues[95] compared the use of angiography with angiography plus IVUS to determine whether the use of IVUS improved the long-term clinical outcome of patients undergoing repair of the iliac artery. They concluded that there was no occurrence of restenoses in the IVUS-assisted group, whereas the non-IVUS group experienced restenoses or occlusion of the stented lesion in 25% of patients at a mean follow-up of 5.5 months. In addition, no patients in the IVUS-assisted group required repeat angiography at follow-up, whereas all failures in the non-IVUS group had to undergo evaluation with angiography.

In such clinical situations, IVUS could potentially curtail the occurrence of restenosis or occlusion of a previously treated lesion and provide the necessary information for choosing the correct angioplasty catheter for proper stent deployment. In addition, the assessment of the outcome after angioplasty or atherectomy may be well suited to IVUS evaluation given its ability to detect dissection or other vessel damage as well as measure postprocedural vessel diameter. Endoluminal stenting of lesions previously treated with balloon angioplasty can improve the patency rate by minimizing the occurrence of technical failures and restenosis.[95] Five-year patency rates of 92% for iliac artery reconstruction have been reported.[100, 101] Sullivan and colleagues,[102] in their evaluation of 288 patients undergoing PTA and stenting of the iliac arteries, concluded that there was a positive correlation between early success rates and the use of multiple stents. IVUS has also been shown to be useful during and immediately after endovascular stent-graft placement for peripheral aneurysms. Van Sambeek and colleagues[96] reported their use of IVUS intraprocedurally in 17 patients undergoing stent-graft placement in the iliac or femoropopliteal arteries and found that in eight cases IVUS showed total exclusion of the aneurysm and no damage to the arterial wall. In the remaining nine patients, IVUS was instrumental in determining the need for additional procedures due to inadequate stent-graft placement.

Muller-Hulsbeck and associates,[97] in their investigation of the use of IVUS for evaluating peripheral arterial stent-grafts placed in 23 patients, performed IVUS investigations immediately after follow-up angiography. At a mean follow-up of 13.9 months, the authors concluded that IVUS detected incompletely expanded stent-grafts in 42% of patients despite postimplantation PTA; moreover, IVUS provided valuable in vivo data on the morphology and distribution of neointimal hyperplasia.

Angiography has provided limited assistance in determining the optimal debulking of plaque required with the use of atherectomy. The restenosis rates and complications of vessel perforation associated with atherectomy reported earlier in this chapter may be due to excessive cutting and resultant incision of the media; the incidence of these complications can potentially be resolved by initial evaluation with IVUS. Incision of the media with atherectomy, whether it is readily apparent on angiography, can impede subsequent healing. Furthermore, calcification poses a notable resistance to atherectomy and IVUS can provide valuable and accurate estimation of the extent of calcification and subsequently guide the clinical course.

Conclusion

The additional quantitative and qualitative data afforded by IVUS at various stages of intervention make it a valuable tool during endovascular procedures and may potentially minimize the risks and complications associated with these procedures. IVUS can influence the management of the intervention at the time of intervention, specify the necessity for any modifications in treatment plans, and help refine the process of selecting patients to undergo these procedures.

CONCLUDING REMARKS

Although endovascular surgery is finally gaining more recognition and acceptance within the medical community, its significance in the treatment of peripheral vascular disease remains questionable. The early results have been somewhat disappointing, and the initial enthusiasm has appropriately turned into more sober, realistic cautiousness. Accordingly, vascular surgeons should practice prudence in the clinical management of their patients (i.e., use FDA-approved devices for FDA-approved applications; conventional vs. endovascular surgery) with optimal care as the primary objective.

The main challenge for the future is controlling restenosis. Apparently, balloon dilatation, debulking or cutting of plaque, or providing a scaffold to maintain the intraluminal structure and patency of an artery reduces the likelihood of restenosis. On the contrary, these endovascular procedures induce intimal hyperplasia, which subsequently results in restenosis. As such, a different approach should be taken to resolve this persistent problem of restenosis. The solution may well lie with pharmacologic manipulation and better understanding the biochemical process of restenosis. If the problem of restenosis is solved, endovascular surgery will have broad applications and will become a dominant treatment modality in peripheral vascular surgery.

References

1. Dotter CT, Jedkins MP: Transluminal treatment of atherosclerotic obstruction: Description of a new technique and preliminary report of this application. Circulation 30:645–670, 1969.
2. Gruntzig A, Hopf H: Perkutane Rekanalisation chronischer arterieller Verschlüsse mit einem neuen Dilationskatheter: Modifikation der Dotter-Technik. Dtsch Med Wochenschr 99:2502–2551, 1974.
3. Andros G, Harris RW, Sales-Cunha SX: Technique of intraoperative balloon angioplasty. In Moore WS, Ahn SS (eds): Endovascular Surgery. Philadelphia, WB Saunders, 1989, pp 209–222.
4. Hsiang YN, Al-Salman M, Doyle DL, Machan LS: Comparison of percutaneous with intraoperative balloon angioplasty for arteriosclerotic occlusive disease. Austr N Z J Surg 63:864–869, 1993.
5. Dolmatch BL, Gray RJ, Horton KM, et al: Treatment of anastomotic bypass graft stenosis with directional atherectomy: Short-term and intermediate results. J Vasc Interv Radiol 6:105–113, 1995.
6. Porter DH, Rosen MP, Skillman JJ, et al: Long term results with directional atherectomy of vein graft stenoses. J Vasc Surg 23:554–567, 1996.
7. Zemel G, Katzen BT, Dake MD, et al: Directional atherectomy in the treatment of stenotic dialysis access fistulas. J Vasc Interv Radiol 1:35–38, 1990.
8. Gray RJ, Dolmatch BL, Buick MK: Directional atherectomy treatment for hemodialysis access: Early results. J Vasc Interv Radiol 3:497–503, 1992.
9. Simpson JB, Selmon MR, Robertson GC, et al: Transluminal atherectomy for occlusive peripheral vascular disease. Am J Cardiol 61:96–101, 1988.
10. Polnitz A, Nerlich A, Berger H, Hofling B: Percutaneous peripheral atherectomy. J Am Coll Cardiol 15:628–688, 1990.
11. Hinohara T, Selmon MR, Robertson GC, et al: Directional atherectomy: New approaches for treatment of obstructive coronary and peripheral vascular disease. Circulation 81(Suppl 4):IV-79–IV-91, 1990.
12. Graor R, Whitlow P: Transluminal atherectomy for occlusive peripheral vascular disease. J Am Coll Cardiol 15:1551–1558, 1990.
13. Dorros G, Iyer S, Lewin R, et al: Angiographic follow-up and clinical outcome of 126 patients after percutaneous directional atherectomy (Simpson AtheroCath) for occlusive peripheral vascular disease. Cathet Cardiovasc Diagn 22:79–84, 1991.
14. Kim D, Gianturco LE, Porter DH, et al: Peripheral directional atherectomy: 4-year experience. Radiology 183:773–778, 1992.
15. Lugmayr H, Pachinger O, Deutsch M: Long term results of percutaneous atherectomy in peripheral arterial occlusive disease. Rofo Fortschr Geb Rontgenstr Neuen Bildgeb Verfahr 158:532–535, 1993.
16. Vroegindewij D, Tielbeek AV, Buth J, et al: Directional atherectomy vs. balloon angioplasty in segmental femoropopliteal artery disease: 2-year follow-up with color flow duplex scanning. J Vasc Surg 21:255–269, 1995.
17. Savader SJ, Venbrux AC, Mitchell SE, et al: Percutaneous transluminal atherectomy of the superficial femoral and popliteal arteries: Long term results in 48 patients. Cardiovasc Interv Radiol 17:312–318, 1994.
18. Wildenhain PM, Wholey MH, Jarmolowski CR, Hill KL: Infrainguinal directional atherectomy: Long-term follow-up and comparison with percutaneous transluminal angioplasty. Cardiovasc Interv Radiol 17:305–311, 1994.
19. Becker GJ, Katzen BT, Dake MD: Noncoronary angioplasty. Radiology 170:921–940, 1989.
20. Johnston KW, Rae M, Hogg-Johnston SA, et al: Five-year results of a prospective study of percutaneous transluminal angioplasty. Ann Surg 206:403–413, 1987.
21. Perler BA, Osterman FA, Mitchell SE, et al: Balloon dilatation versus surgical revision of infra-inguinal autogenous vein graft stenoses: Long-term follow-up. J Cardiovasc Surg 31:656–661, 1990.
22. Whittemore AD, Donaldson MC, Polak JF, Mannick JA: Limitations of balloon angioplasty for vein graft stenosis. J Vasc Surg 14:340–345, 1991.
23. Wholey MH, Jarmolowski CR: New reperfusion devices: The Kensey catheter, the atherolytic reperfusion wire device, and the transluminal extraction catheter. Radiology 172:947–952, 1989.
24. Myers KA, Denton MJ, Devine TJ: Infrainguinal atherectomy using the transluminal endarterectomy catheter: Patency rates and clinical success for 144 procedures. J Endovasc Surg 1:61–70, 1994.
25. Mazur W, Ali NM, Rodgers GP, et al: Directional atherectomy with the OmniCath: A unique new catheter system. Cathet Cardiovasc Diagn 31:79, 1994.
26. Sapoval MR, Gaux JC, Bruneval P, Peronneau P: Animal evaluation of the prototype OmniCath atherectomy catheter. Cardiovasc Interv Radiol 17:226, 1994.
27. Ahn SS, Arca M, Brauel G, et al: Histologic and morphologic effects of rotary atherectomy on human cadaver arteries. Ann Vasc Surg 4:563–569, 1990.
28. Dorros G, Iyer S, Zaitoun R, et al: Acute angiographic and clinical outcome of high speed percutaneous rotational atherectomy (Rotablator). Cathet Cardiovasc Diagn 22:157–166, 1991.
29. Ahn SS, Eton D, Yeatman LR, et al: Intraoperative peripheral rotary atherectomy: Early and late clinical results. Ann Vasc Surg 6:272–280, 1992.
30. White CJ, Ramee SR, Escobar A, et al: High speed rotational ablation (Rotablator) for unfavorable lesions in peripheral arteries. Cathet Cardiovasc Diagn 30:115–119, 1993.
31. The Collaborative Rotablator Atherectomy Group [CRAG]: Peripheral atherectomy with the Rotablator: A multicenter report. J Vasc Surg 19:509–515, 1994.
32. Henry M, Amor M, Ethevenot G, Henry I, Allaoui M: Percutaneous peripheral atherectomy using the Rotablator: A single center experience. J Endovasc Surg 2:51–66, 1995.
33. Myers KA, Denton MJ: Infrainguinal atherectomy using the Auth Rotablator: Patency rates and clinical success for 36 procedures. J Endovasc Surg 2:67–73, 1995.
34. Porter DH, Rosen MP, Skillman RG, et al: Mid-term and long-term results with directional atherectomy of vein graft stenoses. J Vasc Surg 23:554–567, 1996.
35. Dolmatch BL, Gray RJ, Horton KM, et al. Treatment of anastomotic bypass graft stenosis with directional atherectomy: Short-term and intermediate-term results. J Vasc Interven Radiol 6:105–113, 1995.
36. Osborn JJ, Pfeiffer RB, String ST: Directional atherectomy and balloon angioplasty for lower extremity arterial disease. Ann Vasc Surg 11:278–283, 1997.
37. Palmaz JC, Laborde JC, Rivera FJ, et al: Stenting of the iliac arteries with the Palmaz stent: Experience from a multicenter trial. Cardiovasc Intervent Radiol 15:291–297, 1992.
38. Murphy KD, Encarnacion CE, Le VA, Palmaz JC: Iliac artery stent

placement with the Palmaz stent: Follow-up study. J Vasc Interv Radiol 6:321–329, 1995.

39. Henry M, Amor M, Ethevenot G, et al: Palmaz stent placement in iliac and femoropopliteal arteries: Primary and secondary patency in 310 patients with 2–4 year follow-up. Radiol 197:167–174, 1995.
40. Stanley B, Teague B, Raptis S, et al: Efficacy of balloon angioplasty of the superficial femoral artery and popliteal artery in the relief of leg ischemia. J Vasc Surg 23:679–685, 1996.
41. Cikrit DF, Gustafson DA, Dalsing MC, et al: Long-term follow-up of the Palmaz stent for iliac occlusive disease. Surgery 118:608–614, 1995.
42. Sullivan T, Teague B, Raptis G, et al: Efficacy of balloon angioplasty of the superficial femoral artery and popliteal artery in the relief of leg ischemia. J Vasc Surg 23:679–685, 1996.
43. Ballard JL, Sparks SR, Taylor FC, et al: Complications of iliac artery stent deployment. J Vasc Surg 24:545–553, 1996.
44. Bergeron B, Pinot JJ, Poyen V, et al: Long term results with the Palmaz stent in the superficial femoral artery. J Endovasc Surg 2:161–167, 1995.
45. Chatelard PH, Guibourt CH: Long-term results with a Palmaz stent in the femoropopliteal arteries. J Cardiovasc Surg 37(Suppl 1):67–72, 1996.
46. Liermann D, Strecker EP, Peters J: The Strecker stent: Indications and results in iliac and femoropopliteal arteries. Cardiovasc Interv Radiol 15:298–305, 1992.
47. Strecker EP, Hagen B, Liermann D, et al: Current status of the Strecker stent. Cardiol Clin 12:673–687, 1994.
48. Long AL, Sapoval MR, Beyssen BM, et al: Strecker stent implantation in iliac arteries: Patency and predictive factors for long term success. Radiology 194:739–744, 1995.
49. Bray AE, Liu WG, Lewis WA, et al: Strecker stents in the femoropopliteal arteries: Value of duplex ultrasonography in restenosis assessment. J Endovasc Surg 2:150–160, 1995.
50. Vorwerk D, Gunther RW: Stent placement in iliac arterial lesions: Three years of clinical experience with the Wallstent. Cardiovasc Interv Radiol 15:285–290, 1992.
51. Vorwerk D, Gunther RW, Schurmann K, et al: Primary stent placement for chronic iliac artery occlusions: Follow-up results in 103 patients. Radiology 194:745–749, 1995.
52. Martin CC, Katzen BT, Benenati JF, et al: Multicenter trial of the Wallstent in the iliac and femoral arteries. JVIR 6:843–849, 1995.
53. Sapoval MR, Chatellier G, Long AL, et al: Self-expandable stents for the treatment of iliac artery obstructive lesions: Long-term success and prognostic factors. AJR 166:1173–1179, 1996.
54. Murphy TP, Khwaja AA, Webb EE: Aortoiliac stent placement in patients treated for intermittent claudication. JVIR 9:421–428, 1998.
55. Zollikofer CL, Antonucci F, Pfyffer M, et al: Arterial stent placement with use of Wallstent: Midterm results of clinical experience. Radiology 179:449–456, 1991.
56. Gray BH, Sullivan TM, Childs MB, et al: High incidence of restenosis/reocclusion of stents in the percutaneous treatment of long-segment superficial femoral artery disease after suboptimal angioplasty. J Vasc Surg 25:74–83, 1997.
57. White G, Liew S, Waugh R, et al: Early outcome and intermediate follow-up of vascular stent in femoral and popliteal arteries without long-term anticoagulation. J Vasc Surg 21:270–281, 1995.
58. Marin ML, Veith FJ, Cynamon J, et al: Initial experience with transluminally placed endovascular grafts for the treatment of complex vascular lesions. Ann Surg 222:449–469, 1995.
59. Parodi JC, Barone HD, Schonholz C: Transfemoral endovascular treatment of aortoiliac aneurysms and arteriovenous fistulas with stented Dacron grafts. In Veith FJ (ed): Current Critical Problems in Vascular Surgery, vol 5. St Louis, Quality Medical Publishing, 1993, pp 264–268.
60. Raillat C, Rousseau H, Joffre F, Roux D: Treatment of iliac artery stenoses with the Wallstent endoprosthesis. AJR 154:613–616, 1990.
61. Rees CR, Palmaz JC, Garcia O, et al: Angioplasty and stenting of completely occluded iliac arteries. Radiology 172:953–959, 1989.
62. Parodi JC: Endovascular repair of abdominal aortic aneurysms and other arterial lesions. J Vasc Surg 21:549–557, 1995.
63. Moore WS, Rutherford RB: Transfemoral endovascular repair of abdominal aortic aneurysm: Results of the North American EVT phase 1 trial. J Vasc Surg 23:543–553, 1996.
64. White GF: Angioscopy to monitor arterial thromboembolectomy. In Moore WS, Ahn SS (eds): Endovascular Surgery. Philadelphia, WB Saunders, 1989, pp 55–64.

65. Byrnes G, MacGowen WA: The injury potential of the Fogarty balloon catheter. J Cardiovasc Surg 75:590–593, 1975.
66. Stoney RJ, Ehrenfeld WK, Wylie EJ: Arterial rupture after insertion of a Fogarty catheter. Am J Surg 115:830–831, 1968.
67. Holm J, Schersten T: Subintimal dissection secondary to the use of the Fogarty catheter. J Cardiovasc Surg 74:684–686, 1974.
68. Vollmar JF, Hutschenreiter S: Vascular endoscopy for venous thrombectomy. In Moore WS, Ahn SS (eds): Endovascular Surgery. Philadelphia, WB Saunders, 1989, pp 87–94.
69. Mehigan JT, Olcott C: Video angioscopy as an alternative to intraoperative arteriography. Am J Surg 152:139–145, 1986.
70. Grundfest WS, Litvack F, Sherman T, et al: Delineation of peripheral and coronary detail by intraoperative angioscopy. Ann Surg 202:394–400, 1985.
71. Fleisher HL III, Thompson BW, McCowan TC, et al: Angioscopically monitored saphenous vein valvulotomy. J Vasc Surg 4:360–364, 1986.
72. Matsumoto H, Yang Y, Hashizume M: Direct vision valvulotomy for non-reversed vein graft. Surg Gynecol Obstet 165:181–183, 1987.
73. Chin AK, Fogarty TJ: Angioscopic preparation for saphenous vein in situ bypass grafting. In Moore WS, Ahn SS (eds): Endovascular Surgery. Philadelphia, WB Saunders, 1989, pp 74–81.
74. Abele GS, Seeger JM, Barbieri E, et al: Laser angioplasty with angioscopic guidance in humans. J Am Coll Cardiol 8:184–192, 1986.
75. Ahn SS, Auth D, Marcus DR, Moore WS: Removal of focal atheromatous lesions by angioscopically guided high-speed rotary atherectomy: Preliminary experimental observations. J Vasc Surg 7:292–300, 1988.
76. Ahn SS: The use of grabbers, cutters, and shavers as an adjunct during endovascular surgery. In Moore WS, Ahn SS (eds): Endovascular Surgery. Philadelphia, WB Saunders, 1989, pp 514–517.
77. Olcott C: Angioscopic inspection of an anastomosis: Indications and techniques. In Moore WS, Ahn SS (eds): Endovascular Surgery. Philadelphia, WB Saunders, 1989, pp 50–55.
78. Ahn SS, Curtis BV, Marcus DR, et al: Intraoperative vascular endoscopy: Early and late results. Ann Vasc Surg 10:443–451, 1996.
79. Bom N, Ten Hoff H, Lance CT, et al: Early and recent intraluminal ultrasound devices. Int J Card Imaging 4:79, 1989.
80. Issner JM, Rosenfield K, Losordo DW, et al: Percutaneous ultrasound examination as an adjunct to catheter-based interventions: Preliminary experience in patients with peripheral vascular disease. Radiology 175:61–70, 1990.
81. Katzen BT, Benenati JF, Becker GJ, et al: Role of intravascular ultrasound in peripheral atherectomy and stent deployment [abstract]. Circulation 84(Suppl 2):2152, 1991.
82. Arko F, McCollough R, Manning LG, et al: Use of intravascular ultrasound in the endovascular management of atherosclerotic aortoiliac occlusive disease. Am J Surg 172:546–550, 1996.
83. Pandian NA, Kreis A, Brockway B, et al: Ultrasound angioscopy: Real-time, two-dimensional, intraluminal ultrasound imaging of blood vessels. Am J Cardiol 62:493–494, 1988.
84. Nishimura RA, Edwards WD, Warnes CA, et al: Intravascular ultrasound imaging: In vitro validation and pathological correlation. J Am Coll Cardiol 16:145–154, 1990.
85. Tobis JM, Mallery J, Mahon D: Intravascular ultrasound imaging of human coronary arteries in vivo: Analysis of tissue characterizations with comparison of in vitro histological specimens. Circulation 83:913–926, 1991.
86. Gussenhoven WJ, Essed CE, Frietman P, et al: Intravascular echogenic assessment of vessel wall characteristics: A correlation with histology. Int J Card Imaging 4:105–116, 1989.
87. Link TM, Kerber S, Poppelman M, et al: In vitro correlation of intravascular ultrasound and direct magnification radiography for calcified arterial lesions. Invest Radiol 29:420–426, 1994.
88. Fitzgerald PJ, St Goar FG, Connolly AJ, et al: Intravascular ultrasound imaging of coronary arteries: Is three layers the norm? Circulation 86:154–158, 1992.
89. Gussenhoven EJ, Essed CE, Frietman P: Intravascular ultrasonic imaging: Histological and echogenic correlation. Eur J Vasc Surg 3:571–576, 1989.
90. Potkin BW, Bartorelli AL, Gessert JM, et al: Coronary artery imaging with intravascular high-frequency ultrasound. Circulation 81:1575–1585, 1990.
91. Fitzgerald PJ, Yock PG: Mechanisms and outcomes of angioplasty and atherectomy assessed by intravascular ultrasound imaging. J Clin Ultrasound 21:579–588, 1993.

92. Wilson EP, White RA: Intravascular ultrasound. Surg Clin North Am 78:561–574, 1998.
93. Evan JL, Ng KH, Wiet SG, et al: Accurate three-dimensional reconstruction of intravascular ultrasound data: Spatially correct three-dimensional reconstruction. Circulation 53:567–576, 1996.
94. Korogi Y, Hirai T, Takahashi M: Intravascular ultrasound imaging of peripheral arteries as an adjunct to balloon angioplasty and atherectomy. Cardiovasc Interv Radiol 19:1–9, 1996.
95. Arko F, Mettauer M, McCollough R, et al: Use of intravascular ultrasound improves long-term clinical outcome in the endovascular management of atherosclerotic aortoiliac occlusive disease. J Vasc Surg 27:614–623, 1998.
96. Van Sambeek M, Gussenhoven EJ, van Overhagan H, et al: Intravascular ultrasound in endovascular stent-grafts for peripheral aneurysms: A clinical study. J Endovasc Surg 5:106–112, 1998.
97. Muller-Hulsbeck S, Schwartzenberg H, Hutzelmann A: Intravascular ultrasound evaluation of peripheral arterial stent-grafts. Invest Radiol 35:97–104, 2000.
98. Tobis JM, Mahon DJ, Goldberg SL, et al: Lessons from intravascular ultrasonography: Observations during interventional angioplasty procedures. J Clin Ultrasound 21:589–607, 1993.
99. Hartlooper A, van Essen JA, van der Lugt A, et al: Validation of automated contour analysis of intravascular ultrasound images after vascular intervention. J Vasc Surg 27:486–491, 1998.
100. Gunther RW, Vorwerk D, Antonucci F, et al: Iliac artery stenosis or obstruction after unsuccessful balloon angioplasty: Treatment with a self-expandable stent. AJR 156:389–393, 1991.
101. Williams JB, Watts PW, Nguyen PA, Petersen CL: Balloon angioplasty with intraluminal stenting as the initial treatment modality in aorto-iliac occlusive disease. Am J Surg 168:202–204, 1994.
102. Sullivan TM, Childs MB, Bacharach JM, et al: Percutaneous transluminal angioplasty and primary stenting of the iliac arteries in 288 patients. J Vasc Surg 25:829–838, 1997.

Questions

1. Intraoperative balloon angioplasty is different from percutaneous transluminal balloon angioplasty in the following manner
   (a) it generally is used when the patient has more severe symptoms
   (b) it generally is used in multilevel or diffuse occlusive disease
   (c) intraoperative balloon angioplasty is usually performed as an adjunct to conventional open vascular procedures
   (d) all of the above

2. Factors associated with worse results in patients undergoing balloon angioplasty include
   (a) short lesions
   (b) high-flow vessels
   (c) small vessels
   (d) all of the above

3. Indications for peripheral atherectomy include
   (a) short, stenotic calcified lesions that do not respond to dilatation
   (b) ulcerated lesions with embolic symptoms
   (c) restenosis of vein graft
   (d) all of the above

4. Intravascular stents prevent
   (a) restenosis
   (b) arterial recoil
   (c) thrombosis
   (d) all of the above

5. Stents are currently FDA-approved for general use in
   (a) iliac arteries
   (b) superficial femoral and popliteal arteries
   (c) carotid arteries
   (d) all of the above

6. Stents are currently hampered by
   (a) acute thrombosis
   (b) intima hyperplasia
   (c) increased puncture site hematoma
   (d) all of the above

7. Angioscopy provides accurate information regarding
   (a) intravascular thrombus
   (b) runoff vessels
   (c) percent stenosis
   (d) all of the above

8. Intravascular ultrasonography provides accurate information regarding
   (a) lesions distal to the probe
   (b) runoff vessels
   (c) cross-sectional percent stenosis
   (d) all of the above

9. Restenosis secondary to intima hyperplasia is the Achilles' heel of
   (a) balloon angioplasty
   (b) atherectomy
   (c) stents
   (d) all of the above

10. Endovascular grafting
    (a) is currently experimental
    (b) is currently more efficient and effective than traditional vascular bypass
    (c) will eventually eliminate the role of vascular surgeons in the management of vascular disease
    (d) all of the above

Answers

1. d   2. c   3. d   4. b   5. a   6. d   7. a   8. c   9. d   10. a

18

Endovascular Grafting

Wesley S. Moore and Michael L. Marin

Conventional vascular grafting is a well-established, highly successful, and durable treatment for aneurysm and occlusive and traumatic arterial disease. However, developing less invasive approaches that achieve the same end result is clearly more desirable. For example, transabdominal repair of abdominal aortic aneurysm can be performed with mortality rates well under 5% in centers of excellence. Nevertheless, community-based reports document mortality rates in excess of 10%, and this figure probably applies to the majority of patients being considered for conventional repair.[1] The development of an endovascular approach to placement of vascular grafts in sites remote from the point of introduction has opened the possibility of achieving repair of a variety of complex lesions with minimal morbidity and mortality. The objectives of this chapter are to review the experimental background, describe the surgical techniques, and update the results of endovascular grafting for repair of abdominal aortic aneurysm, peripheral aneurysm, arterial occlusive disease, and trauma.

HISTORICAL BACKGROUND

The first attempt to cutaneously place a prosthesis within the lumen of an artery was reported by Dotter in 1969.[2] This innovative investigator described his experience with placing a coiled spring, which served as an endarterial tube graft, in the popliteal artery of a dog. This field of experimentation lay dormant until 1983, when Cragg and colleagues[3] described their experience with "nonsurgical" placement of an arterial endoprosthesis made from nitinol wire. Further development of a nonsuture approach for repair of aortic defects was described by LeMolle and colleagues[4] when they reported the insertion of a prosthetic graft using a rigid attachment system at each end. This technique was originally used for thoracic aortic dissection and subsequently was employed in the abdominal aorta. The approach was either by a transthoracic or transabdominal incision. The aorta was opened, the prosthesis was inserted, and the prosthesis was held stationary by placing a tie around the outside of the aorta and securing the prosthesis within the aorta by tying the ligature, thus effectively sandwiching the aortic tissue between the tie and the prosthesis. In 1986, Balko and colleagues[5] devised a method of placing a polyurethane prosthesis into the abdominal aorta through a transfemoral approach. This was the first report in which this device was used in humans. Patients scheduled for conventional repair of abdominal aortic aneurysm initially had exposure of the femoral artery with transfemoral placement of the endovascular prosthesis. The authors did not intend this to be the definitive repair but used the technique only to determine feasibility. They then proceeded with conventional open operation and removed the endovascular graft. Nonetheless, they demonstrated the feasibility of placing the graft into the abdominal aortic aneurysm and effectively bridging the defect.

The first definitive repair of abdominal aortic aneurysms using transfemoral insertion of a prosthetic graft was reported in 1991.[6] World attention was initially focused on the publication by Parodi and colleagues[6] from Buenos Aires. However, that same year, in a more obscure publication, Volodos and colleagues[7] described their clinical experience with the use of a self-fixing synthetic prosthesis for repair of aneurysms in the thoracic and abdominal aorta as well as the iliac arteries. Parodi's technique utilized a conventional Dacron prosthesis to which a balloon-expandable Palmaz stent was sewn on the proximal end of the graft. A delivery system was fabricated that permitted the device to be passed into position over a guidewire using an open femoral arteriotomy. Parodi initially used this technique in patients who were at increased risk of death with conventional aneurysm repair. He clearly demonstrated the feasibility as well as the success of his approach and demonstrated the surgical technique in major surgical centers all over the world.

A review of the records of the United States Patent Office clearly documents that a number of inventors anticipated the possibility of using this approach clinically, and patents appeared as early as 1988.[8]

Chuter and colleagues[9] reviewed aortic anatomy in a large series of patients with abdominal aortic aneurysm and came to the conclusion that it would be necessary to have a bifurcated graft for endovascular repair if utilization of the endovascular approach was to become clinically competitive with open operation. In 1993, he and his colleagues described a bifurcated graft and demonstrated the technique of experimental implantation in dogs.[10]

During this same time frame, Endovascular Technologies, Inc. (EVT, Menlo Park, Calif.) developed a system for repair of aortic aneurysm. They demonstrated the feasibility of tube graft implantation experimentally and subsequently made application to the U.S. Food and Drug Administration (FDA) for permission to begin clinical investigation of this device. The first clinical implantation of the EGS system from EVT took place at the University of California, Los Angeles (UCLA) Medical Center on February 10, 1993.[11, 12]

As clinical experience with endovascular repair of abdominal aortic aneurysm was beginning to accumulate, Marin and colleagues[13] began to explore the feasibility of applying endovascular techniques to the repair of arterial occlusive lesions as well as to traumatic arterial defects and peripheral aneurysms.

ENDOVASCULAR GRAFT REPAIR OF ABDOMINAL AORTIC ANEURYSM

The Parodi Technique

Parodi's technique is applied in an operating room setting. The patient's femoral artery is exposed under local or epidural anesthesia. The patient is prepared and draped for a standard aneurysm resection, should that become necessary. The artery is punctured, and a guidewire is advanced up the aorta to the level of the diaphragm. An aortogram is then performed and compared with previously obtained imaging studies. The areas of stent deployment are defined, as well as the measurement of the proposed graft for utilization. Graft fixation is achieved by the initial placement of a modified balloon-expandable Palmaz stent (Johnson & Johnson International Systems, Warren, N.J.), which is partially inserted into the lumen of the graft and sutured at two points 180 degrees apart. The stent is attached to a balloon catheter, and the graft is then rotated or wrapped tightly around the balloon catheter and inserted into a delivery sheath. The graft within the delivery sheath is then loaded over the guidewire and advanced, under fluoroscopy, into an appropriate position. The sheath is then retracted, and the balloon is inflated to expand the stent and secure the graft in its proximal subrenal location. The sheath is then withdrawn, which allows the entire graft length to expand. A second stent is then placed in the distal portion of the graft at the level of the bifurcation of the iliac arteries. Parodi also described a technique that enables grafting to take place in the absence of a distal neck. This uses a tapered graft that goes from the aorta to one iliac artery. The contralateral common iliac artery is then occluded by insertion of a series of inflatable balloons. The operation is completed with placement of a crossover femorofemoral bypass graft, thus effectively restoring blood flow to both lower extremities and leaving antegrade flow to one hypogastric artery and providing retrograde flow to the contralateral hypogastric artery.

Parodi updated his series in a presentation to the Eighth Annual Meeting of the Eastern Vascular Society in May 1994.[14] Between September 1990 and April 1994, he treated 50 patients with abdominal aortic aneurysm, with or without iliac aneurysms or with an isolated iliac aneurysm. The anatomic distribution included eight patients with an aortoaortic graft with proximal stent, 28 patients with an aortoaortic graft and two stents, 15 patients with an aortoiliac graft combined with femorofemoral bypass, and 2 patients with an ilioiliac graft for iliac aneurysm alone. The aneurysms ranged in size from 3.8 to 12.0 cm. Half the patients were categorized as being "high risk." Parodi classified 40 of the 50 procedures (80%) as successful. He defined success as the complete exclusion of the aneurysm with restoration of normal blood flow. Four patients (8%) died in the perioperative interval. Two of the four deaths occurred secondary to massive peripheral embolization; the patients succumbed to multiorgan system failure. Three patients were noted to have proximal perigraft leaks into the aneurysm sac. One was of no consequence. However, the second patient, with a large proximal leak, died of aneurysm rupture 2 months after graft placement. Two patients experienced distal leaks. One leak sealed spontaneously, and the second was still patent when the patient subsequently died of pulmonary and cardiac complications 8 months later. During a mean follow-up of 17 months, one late procedure-related death and four unrelated deaths occurred. Of the remaining 41 patients, 6 required secondary operations, 2 open and 4 endovascular. The remaining patients were doing well at the time of the report.[14]

CURRENTLY APPROVED ENDOVASCULAR DEVICES

Two devices have completed Food and Drug Administration (FDA)–approved protocol evaluations. Both were reviewed by an FDA panel in June 1999, and both received conditional approval by the FDA in September 1999. They are currently being implanted under strict guidelines for indications as well as training of the implant teams. These devices are the Ancure system by Guidant (formerly Endovascular Technologies, EVT, Menlo Park, CA) and the AneuRx system by Medtronics (Santa Rosa, CA). Multiple other devices are currently in various stages of investigation in the United States, as well as in use in Europe and Australia.

The Ancure System

The first prototype of this device, termed the EGS system, was a unit body tube graft. As mentioned, the first implant of this device took place at UCLA Medical Center on February 10, 1993. This was the first clinical case of a device specifically constructed for implantation in aneurysm repair, under FDA-approved investigational protocol, to be implanted in the United States.[11, 12] The implant was successful, and the patient lived for another 5 years free of his aneurysm burden until his ultimate death from a malignancy. With this implant, phase I of a three-phase trial was begun at three West Coast centers. In September 1994, the first bifurcated graft was introduced with successful implantation in two patients at UCLA. This opened phase II of the trial, with participation expanded to 21 centers across the country.[15–17] The design of the trial was a prospective, nonrandomized concurrent comparison of endovascular repair with conventional open repair. A third graft configuration, consisting of an aorto-uni-iliac system in combination with a crossover femororfemoral bypass and contralateral iliac occluder, was later introduced as a separate study of patients with combined aortic and iliac aneurysm. The results of these three devices in comparison with open repair were recently updated. The data from the tube and bifurcated graft studies in comparison with open repair were the basis for FDA submission and approval. The aorto-uni-iliac configuration is currently in submission to the FDA for inclusion in the clinical armamentarium.[18]

Patient Evaluation

Patients are usually referred with a diagnosis of abdominal aortic aneurysm made either by ultrasound or computed tomography (CT) scanning. However, the careful measurement required for preparing an Ancure graft mandates a very tight protocol of imaging. The first study that is performed is a CT scan using 3-mm cuts, which is optimally performed with spiral reconstruction. For a patient to be considered for a tube graft repair there must be a neck between the renal arteries and the aneurysm, as well as a distal neck between the aneurysm and the bifurcation of the aorta into the iliac arteries. The proximal neck must be at least 15 mm in length and have a diameter that does not exceed 26 mm. The distal neck diameter should not exceed 26 mm and should be at least 1 cm in length. If a satisfactory proximal neck is present but there is no distal neck, the patient may be a candidate for a bifurcated graft provided the iliac arteries are satisfactory for both access as well as achieving a good seal with the limbs of the graft. Specifically, the iliac arteries may neither be aneurysmal nor have occlusive disease that would preclude passage of the device. Currently available ratios between graft body and limb are 2:1. If there is an iliac artery aneurysm present, then the aortic aneurysm and the iliac artery aneurysm can be repaired using the aorto-uni-iliac system, with a limb extending through the iliac aneurysm to a point either in the distal iliac artery or the external iliac artery, excluding the hypogastric artery. The same can be accomplished using a long-limb bifurcated graft, provided the operator is willing to sacrifice both hypogastric arteries.

If the CT scan reveals acceptable anatomy, the final step of imaging is a contrast aortogram performed with a marker catheter. The marker catheter has radiopaque marks placed at 1-cm intervals. This provides the opportunity to measure the length of the graft required as well as to reconfirm the diameter measurements achieved on the CT scan. The aortogram also provides additional information concerning the number and location of the renal arteries and information concerning the mesenteric circulation. Specifically, if the inferior mesenteric artery is patent and provides collateral blood flow in the distribution of an unsuspected occlusive lesion in the celiac or superior mesenteric artery, this would represent a relative contraindication to endovascular repair. Likewise, if aberrant renal arteries are coming off in the proximity of the aneurysm or distally, this is also a relative contraindication to endovascular repair. Occlusive lesions in the distribution of the celiac, superior mesenteric, or renal arteries may be treated in advance with balloon angioplasty to convert an otherwise unacceptable candidate to one who has the option of endovascular grafting. Additional information that can be obtained on angiography concerns angulation of the proximal neck, as well as tortuosity of the iliac arteries. If the angulation or tortuosity is severe, endovascular grafting may be difficult if not impossible.

Technique

It is our recommendation that all implants be performed in an operating room setting, under either general or regional anesthesia, and that the patient be suitably prepared for both endovascular grafting and open repair should conversion be required. In the series performed at UCLA Medical Center, we have not used a specialized operating room for implantation. We use a standard operating table, specifically the Skytron 3100. This has a sliding table top, which enables us to place the operating table pedestal in an extreme eccentric position and permits full-length body fluoroscopic imaging. In addition, we use a portable digital fluoroscopy unit during implantation with an angiography software pack that provides road-mapping, digital subtraction angiography, and replay capability. Before placing the patient on the operating table, a marker board is placed on the table. This board has movable horizontal cursors that are radiopaque. Once the patient is on the table, preparatory imaging is carried out to make sure that the cursors span an excursion from the 11th rib to the pelvis. These will ultimately be positioned at the level of the renal arteries and aortic bifurcation for specific marking prior to graft implantation. After induction of anesthesia, the abdomen and both groins are surgically prepared and draped with sterile linen in the usual manner.

One femoral artery is selected for placement of the large sheath and is designated as ipsilateral. Several factors are taken into consideration in this designation, including the size of the iliac and femoral arteries, the presence or absence of tortuosity in the iliac system, and any association with mild arterial occlusive disease in the access vessels. With all other factors being equal, the right femoral artery is usually selected as ipsilateral because that is more convenient for a right-handed surgeon. However, when appropriate, the left side is equally appropriate. A vertical incision is used to expose the proximal femoral artery at the level of the inguinal ligament. If there is tortuosity of the external iliac artery, the circumflex branches of the common femoral artery can be divided. This will allow additional mobilization of the external iliac artery beneath the inguinal ligament, with a pull down of the external iliac artery to remove tortuosity. If a tube graft is being used, only one femoral artery requires exposure. If a bifurcated graft or an aorto-uni-iliac system is contemplated, both femoral arteries require exposure. Once femoral artery exposure is complete, the next step is to obtain an angiogram with road map imaging. The femoral artery is punctured with an angiogram needle through which a 0.035-inch guidewire is advanced under fluoroscopic control. The

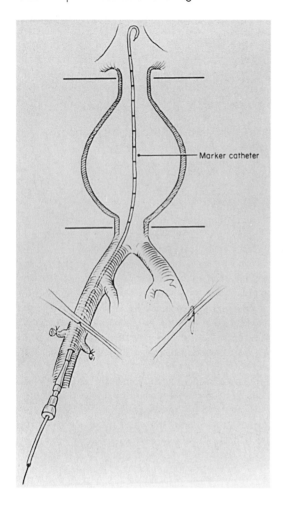

Figure 18–1. An angiogram sheath in place with a pigtail catheter placed in the suprarenal position. The catheter has transverse radiopaque marks that are spaced 1.0 cm apart and permit the exact measurement of the distance between the points of proximal and distal deployment for proper graft length measurement. Also noted are horizontal marks, which are a part of the marker board and have been positioned to show the optimum points of deployment for the proximal and distal attachment systems. (From Moore WS, Rutherford RB, for the EVT Investigators: Transfemoral endovascular repair of abdominal aortic aneurysm: Results of the North American EVT phase 1 trial. J Vasc Surg 23:543–553, 1996.)

needle is removed and replaced with a 7.0-French sheath. The guidewire is then advanced well into the suprarenal aorta. A pigtail marker angiogram catheter is then loaded over the guidewire and inserted, under fluoroscopic control, into the suprarenal aorta (Fig. 18–1).

An angiogram using a pressure injector is then carried out. The optimal image is selected and road-mapped. This will identify the level of the renal arteries as well as the aortic bifurcation. The cursors on the marker board are then adjusted to carefully delineate these two points. For the tube graft, they will be the extremities of the tube graft. For the bifurcated graft system, this then permits final intravascular measurement to ensure that the proper length of graft has been selected.

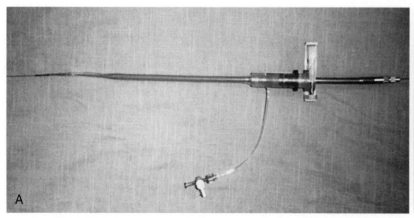
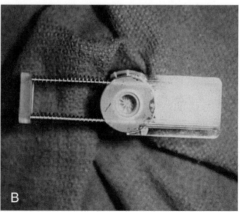

Figure 18–2. *A,* A photograph of the Endovascular Technologies (EVT) sheath with obturator in position. The sheath is loaded over a guidewire and advanced under fluoroscopic control. *B,* Close-up of the valve system of the EVT sheath. The valve is in a closed position. It is actuated by compressing the gated lever, which opens this diaphragm. There is also a more proximal backup valve, which is opened and closed with a wheel. (From Moore WS, Rutherford RB, for the EVT Investigators: Transfemoral endovascular repair of abdominal aortic aneurysm: Results of the North American EVT phase 1 trial. J Vasc Surg 23:543–553, 1996.)

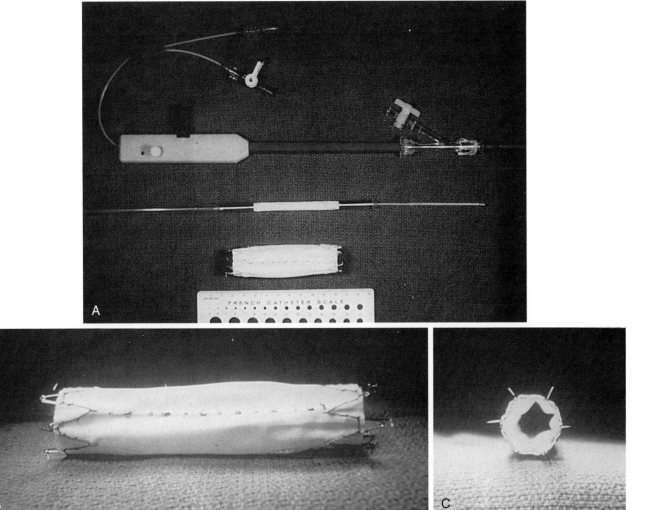

Figure 18–3. *A,* This photograph demonstrates the components of the Endovascular Technologies (EVT) graft delivery system. The *upper portion* shows the handle with irrigating ports and the actuating knob for proximal deployment. The *middle panel* shows a close-up of the graft within the capsule and covered with a transparent jacket. The *lower portion* shows the graft expanded. *B,* A close-up of the expanded prosthetic graft. This is a lightweight woven polyester prosthesis to which self-expanding attachment systems have been sewn at each end. *C,* An end-on view of the graft demonstrating six hooks that are used to engage the aorta and that are driven into place with the expansion of the intrinsic balloon catheter. (From Moore WS, Rutherford RB, for the EVT Investigators: Transfemoral endovascular repair of abdominal aortic aneurysm: Results of the North American EVT phase 1 trial. J Vasc Surg 23:543–553, 1996.)

Once the horizontal cursors are set, the patient is given 5000 units of heparin intravenously. A superstiff guidewire is then passed up the angiogram catheter well into the thoracic aorta, and the angiogram catheter and sheath are removed. The femoral artery is clamped proximally and distally. A transverse oblique arteriotomy is then made through the puncture site. A large 23-French sheath that is a part of the Guidant system is loaded over the guidewire and extended up the femoral artery as the proximal clamp is removed. This is done, under fluoroscopic control, up the iliac system and finally into the aorta (Fig. 18–2).

The obturator within the sheath is then advanced to dilate the distal portion of the sheath. While this is in position, the Ancure tube system can be prepared. The obturator is then removed, and a double-valve system is used for hemostatic control. The Ancure tube graft system of appropriate diameter and length is then loaded over the guidewire and inserted over the sheath. Under fluoroscopic

control, it is positioned according to the location of the horizontal cursors (Fig. 18–3). The jacket that covers the graft is then retracted, and proximal attachment system deployment is achieved by releasing the proximal attachment ring. Once the attachment system has been deployed, the balloon that is intrinsic to the catheter is then advanced so that it is positioned across the attachment system. Three separate inflations are carried out. The balloon is inflated to achieve an appropriate profile, and the pressure within the balloon should not exceed 2 atm. Balloon inflation sets the pins of the attachment system into the aorta for fixation. The distal attachment system is then deployed in a similar fashion. A completion angiogram is then obtained to assure all flow through the graft, with no evidence of any endoleak.

The preliminary steps for deployment of a bifurcation graft are identical up to the point of placement of the large working sheath in the ipsilateral artery. Once this sheath is in place, then the contralateral femoral artery is punctured with an angiogram needle through which a 0.035-inch guidewire is advanced under fluoroscopic control into the aorta. The needle is removed and replaced with a 12-Fr sheath. An Amplatz sheath is then advanced over the guidewire to place its radiopaque-tipped marker at the aortic bifurcation. The guidewire is removed and replaced with an Amplatz snare. The snare is then opened at the bifurcation.

The bifurcated graft catheter delivery system is then suitably prepared. The graft catheter delivery system is loaded over the guidewire on the ipsilateral side and advanced up to the sheath valve. The pullwire assembly from the bifurcated graft delivery system is then inserted into the ipsilateral sheath and advanced fluoroscopically. The pullwire is passed through the open Amplatz snare, and the snare is tightened to capture the pullwire. While advancing the pullwire on the ipsilateral side, it is then brought down on the contralateral side to exit the sheath.

At this point, the graft catheter delivery system is advanced into the sheath and passed up the sheath into the aorta while pulling the pullwire on the contralateral side. As the leading edge of the graft catheter delivery system enters the distal aorta, a careful check is made to be certain that the pullwire is separated from the ipsilateral guidewire. If there has been a circumferential wrap, then rotational maneuvers of the graft catheter delivery system will need to be performed until there is clear separation between the pullwire and the guidewire. Once this is done, then the graft catheter delivery system is advanced well up above the suprarenal aorta so that the distal portion of the graft limbs is above the aortic bifurcation.

The jacket on the catheter delivery system is then retracted, which will allow the contralateral limb to unfold. The pullwire is attached to the contralateral limb, and this is drawn down to achieve separation. The whole system is then brought down toward the aortic bifurcation until the proximal attachment system is positioned immediately below the renal arteries and each graft limb is well within the respective iliac artery.

Once the proximal attachment system is appropriately positioned below the lowest renal artery, the proximal attachment system is deployed and seated with three separate inflations of the intrinsic balloon catheter. A torque catheter is then loaded over the pullwire and advanced under fluoroscopic control until it locks in position at the site of the contralateral distal attachment capsule. The torque catheter allows the operator to rotate either clockwise or counterclockwise the contralateral graft limb to adjust the rotation to an optimal position to avoid twist. This is achieved by looking at radiopaque markers along the graft limb and making certain that they are all lined up on the same side of the guidewire. The graft limb is extended to its full length to avoid redundancy. At this point, the contralateral distal attachment system is deployed, and the intrinsic fine nitinol wire is advanced up the contralateral limb into the body of the graft. A balloon angioplasty catheter is then loaded over the guidewire into the contralateral limb, and the balloon is gently inflated at the distal attachment site to complete its seating. Finally, the ipsilateral distal attachment system is deployed, and the principal intrinsic balloon and the graft catheter are drawn distally to position the balloon across the attachment site, and this is inflated to seat the ipsilateral attachment site. The used graft catheter delivery system is then withdrawn, leaving the guidewire in place. A balloon angioplasty catheter is then loaded over the ipsilateral guidewire, and a series of simultaneous balloon inflations between the ipsilateral and contralateral sites is carried out along the entire length of each graft limb into the graft bifurcation. This ensures that the graft limbs are fully expanded, and if there is any extrinsic compression on a graft limb from disease within the iliac artery, the balloon inflation will dilate and remove the extrinsic compression. A completion angiogram is then obtained to confirm the technical result and to be certain that there is no evidence of endoleak. The catheters and sheaths are then removed, the arteriotomy is repaired, and the groin incisions are closed.

The patient is returned to the recovery room for observation. If everything is stable, the patient is returned to a regular hospital room for overnight observation. Discharge usually takes place the following morning.

Our follow-up protocol is to see the patient within the week for a wound check and pulse examination. If all is well, our next visit will be in 6 months, at which time a contrast-enhanced CT scan is obtained to determine whether an endoleak is present and to document the size of the aneurysmal sac. If an endoleak is present, then we have the patient return in 6 months and repeat the examination. If no endoleak is present, the patient is seen once a year thereafter.

Results

The results of the multi-institutional phase I trial of the tube graft implantation have been reported.[16]

Between February 10, 1993 and December 6, 1994, 46 patients in 13 centers underwent repair of abdominal aortic aneurysm by transfemoral endovascular repair using a tube graft implantation. Individual center experience varied with the use of from 1 to 13 implants. Patient ages ranged from 54 to 84 years, with a mean age of 71.6 years. There were 41 men and 5 women.

A review of the 30-day complication rates revealed no postoperative deaths, one mild myocardial infarction, six episodes of superficial cellulitis that responded to antibiotics, and nine instances of postoperative fever that responded without specific treatment. Seven patients required conversion to open repair at the time of implantation for a variety of reasons. There was no instance of major thromboembolism or mesenteric ischemia. Two patients were noted to have small petechiae on their extremities suggestive of minor episodes of thromboembolism. These resolved without tissue loss. On late follow-up, one patient died 8 months after implantation because of respiratory failure due to underlying chronic obstructive pulmonary disease. There was no instance of late aneurysm rupture. Two late complications were identified. These included a perigraft leak into the aneurysmal sac and metallic fracture of the attachment systems. Initially, 17 implants were noted to have perigraft leaks into the aneurysmal sac. The source was the proximal fixation site in 5 and the distal fixation site in 10 (type I). Type II endoleaks were identified in two patients. These came from either the lumbar branches or back flow from the inferior mesenteric artery. Of the 17 initial leaks, 5 resolved spontaneously, either by the time of hospital discharge or on 6-month follow-up. Eight persisted and continued to undergo careful follow-up but to date have shown no adverse effect. During late follow-up, careful review of plain abdominal films revealed evidence of fractures of components of the attachment systems. These usually occurred in the form of a pin fracture. This was seen in a total of nine patients, and the implant program at that time was placed on hold until the cause could be identified and remedied. The attachment systems underwent reengineering, and the implant program was reimplemented in late 1995. Since that time, there have been no further problems with attachment system fracture.

Early results from the combined European and Australian experience have also been published.[17] The results of all three devices were presented at the endovascular issues section during the 54th Annual Meeting of the Society for Vascular Surgery in combination with the 48th Annual Meeting of the International Society for Cardiovascular Surgery in June 2000. The results of this presentation have just been published. This report summarized the results of 153 patients undergoing tube graft repair, 268 patients undergoing bifurcated graft repair, and 121 patients undergoing aorto-uni-iliac endograft repair for complex aortoiliac aneurysms. These were compared with 111 patients who underwent open aneurysm repair and served as a control group. Successful implantation was achieved in 94.2% of the aortoiliac group, in 90.3% of the bifurcation group, and in 92% of the tube group. There was no significant difference in 30-day operative mortality. It was 4.2% in the aortoiliac group, 2.6% in the bifurcation group, 0% in the tube group, and 2.7% in the control group. Cardiac complications were similar for the aortoiliac and control groups at 22% and 20.7%, respectively. However, they were significantly less for the bifurcation and tube groups at 13.4% and 10.5%, respectively. Pulmonary problems were significantly reduced in all endograft groups compared with controls. Transient renal dysfunction occurred in more of the endograft groups compared with controls, presumably due to the use of intraoperative contrast material. Median blood loss, intensive care unit use, and hospital stays were significantly reduced in all endograft groups compared with controls. The incidence of type I endoleak at the end of 1 year was 2.4% in the aortoiliac group, 2.3% in the bifurcation group, and 3.8% in the tube group. It is noteworthy that no late ruptures have occurred in any group.[18]

The Medtronic AneuRx System

Patient workup for the AneuRx system is similar to that described for the Ancure system. The AneuRx system is a component system that can be assembled within the patient. This provides greater versatility concerning issues of size discrepancy than does the unit body system of Ancure. The AneuRx graft is a fully stented graft as opposed to the Ancure system, which is only stented at its extremities. There are both advantages and disadvantages of these differences.

The insertion of the AneuRx system involves surgical exposure of both common femoral arteries. Following systemic heparinization, introducer sheaths are inserted into the common femoral arteries bilaterally. Guidewire access and an angiogram catheter are passed up one sheath, and an aortogram with road-mapping is obtained to document anatomy and outline points for deployment. The smaller sheath is then removed from the ipsilateral femoral artery, and an arteriotomy is performed to permit the passage of a 21-Fr sheath. The AneuRx primary bifurcated endograft delivery system is then inserted under fluoroscopic control and positioned initially by the renal arteries. The graft cover is then retracted 2 to 3 cm. The graft is slowly pulled down to a position immediately below the lowest renal artery. The graft cover can then be fully retracted, allowing the endograft to expand to full deployment. The contralateral limb is then accessed with guidewires. The 8.0-Fr sheath is removed and replaced with a 16-Fr sheath under fluoroscopic guidance. A delivery catheter is then inserted into the 16-Fr sheath and advanced up to the gate area. Radiopaque markers on the contralateral graft limb are used to obtain proper alignment in the gate area. The 16-Fr sheath is pulled back to the end of the graft cover, and the iliac limb is deployed in a manner similar to that of the main graft. A completion angiogram is then performed from the renal arteries to the iliac bifurcations to check for proper graft placement and endoleak. If endoleak is documented, additional components can be added to treat type I endoleak at both the proximal and distal extremities of the bifurcated graft. The guidewires and sheath are then removed and the femoral arteries repaired. The follow-up of the patient is similar to that described for the Ancure system.

The AneuRx trial, which is under FDA protocol, was a prospective randomized multicenter clinical trial that compared endovascular repair with open surgical repair. One hundred ninety patients underwent endovascular repair, and 60 underwent open surgical repair and served as a control group. The results indicate that there was no difference in perioperative mortality rates between the two groups. However, patients who had endovascular repair of abdominal aortic aneurysm demonstrated significant reductions in blood loss, days in the intensive care unit, and total hospital stay. Major morbidity was reduced from 23% in the open group to 12% in the endovascular group. Stent-graft migration occurred in three patients on late follow-up and resulted in late endoleaks, which could be corrected by endovascular means. In the initial trial, there were no late aneurysm ruptures. However, during the course of follow-up, nine ruptures have been reported.[19, 20]

Endoleak

As experience with endovascular repair of abdominal aortic aneurysm grew, a complication specific to this approach has emerged as the principal weakness of endovascular repair. This is the concept of endoleak. *Endoleak* is defined as a failure to exclude the aneurysmal sac fully from arterial blood flow, and the concern is that pressurization of the aneurysmal sac may persist and ultimately lead to rupture. White and colleagues[21] developed the classification of en-

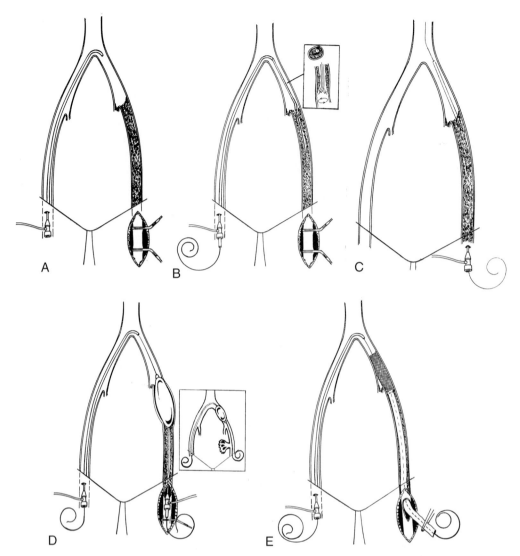

Figure 18–4. Two techniques for arterial recanalization can be used to create a wide tract within the diseased iliac arteries. *A, B,* When the contralateral iliac artery is patent, recanalization is carried out by means of a contralateral, percutaneously inserted guidewire "up and over" the aortic bifurcation, developing a prograde arterial wall dissection plane. This technique allows maximal control of arterial inflow and ensures that the recanalization process begins within the true arterial lumen. *C,* When the "up-and-over" approach is not technically feasible, retrograde recanalization can be used. *D,* After successful wire recanalization is performed, the iliac artery is dilatated to 8 mm along the entire length of the diseased vessel. *E,* An endovascular stented graft is then inserted within a delivery catheter to "reline" the vessel tract. A proximal stent fixes the graft proximally within the inflow vessel lumen.

doleak that has been universally accepted. They described four types of endoleak. Type I endoleak occurs when there is an incomplete seal of either the proximal or distal attachment system in the aorta or iliac arteries. Type II endoleak is essentially back flow from persistently patent lumbar or inferior mesenteric arteries. Type III endoleaks are specific to component endografts. A type III endoleak occurs when one component disconnects from another, allowing blood flow directly into the aneurysmal sac. In addition, a disadvantage of the fully stented graft has been the development of an erosion of the graft fabric by a portion of the stent, leading to direct flow into the aneurysmal sac. This is also in the category of a type III endoleak. Finally, type IV endoleak has to do with porosity of the graft material. Type IV endoleaks are usually self-limiting once the porous graft seals with fibrin.[21]

ENDOVASCULAR GRAFTING OF OCCLUSIVE DISEASE OF THE AORTA AND ILIAC AND FEMORAL ARTERIES

Many of the techniques and benefits that are associated with endovascular grafting of aneurysmal disease can also be extended to the treatment of long-segment arterial occlusive disease. The unique advantages of eliminating a dissection of a previously operated site or avoiding surgery within a major body cavity constitute the essential goals of a successful endovascular graft procedure.

The earliest experience with the use of endovascular grafts for the treatment of clinically significant occlusive disease was reported by Volodos and colleagues[22] in Russia in 1986. Many of the ideas incorporated into Volodos's work had been anticipated by Dotter and colleagues at the time of his initial description of endovascular prostheses.[23] Broader clinical experience and technical advancements have only recently been attained, predominantly in the superficial femoral and aortoiliac circulations.[13, 24, 25]

Technique

Regardless of the device used, the techniques employed for endovascular grafting of occlusive vascular disease are relatively constant. The stenotic or occlusive lesion is first traversed by means of a recanalization guidewire. In stenotic lesions, the wire remains in the true vessel lumen. Recanalization of occluded vessels frequently results in the wire entering a layer of the arterial wall in a random fashion. A widened tract along the path of the recanalization wire is then created by balloon dilatation. Finally, the diffusely dilated vessel is "relined" with an endovascular graft, with fixation of the graft to the arterial wall by at least one intravascular stent (Fig. 18–4).

Most often in the management of long-segment aortoiliac disease, extending the graft across the inguinal ligament permitting termination within the femoral arteries is preferable (Fig. 18–5). This is consistent with time-tested principles and practices in the management of extensive aortoiliac disease using classic bypass techniques.[26]

Devices

European trials using the Cragg Endopro system (MinTek, Inc., Grand Bahama, The Bahamas) for treating aortoiliac and superficial femoral artery disease constitute one of the largest experiences with endovascular grafting of occlusive disease.[25] This system comprises a self-expanding nitinol metal stent encased in a thin-walled Dacron graft. The system, which has been used at the Montefiore Medical Center in New York, employs standard expanded polytetrafluoroethylene (ePTFE) grafts (IMPRA, Inc., Tempe, Ariz.; W. L. Gore and Associates, Flagstaff, Ariz.) that have been hand-sewn to a Palmaz balloon-expandable stent. The ideal attachment system and intravascular conduit for endovascular grafting of occlusive disease are not currently known. Special functional properties probably will be required of endovascular graft materials that will differ from those qualities presumed ideal for conduits used for standard extravascular use. The healing properties of endovascular grafts may also differ, with the porosity of the graft once again becoming a critical factor for graft incorporation.[27, 28]

Clinical Experience

The largest clinical series of patients with occlusive disease of the aortoiliac system use either ePTFE balloon-expand-

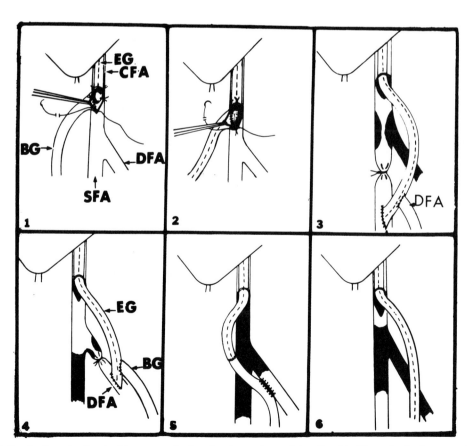

Figure 18–5. The free, distal end of the previously placed endovascular graft (see Fig. 18–4E) may be fixed to a suitable outflow vessel by one of these six techniques. BG, bypass graft; CFA, common femoral artery; DFA, deep femoral artery; EG, endovascular graft; SFA, superficial femoral artery.

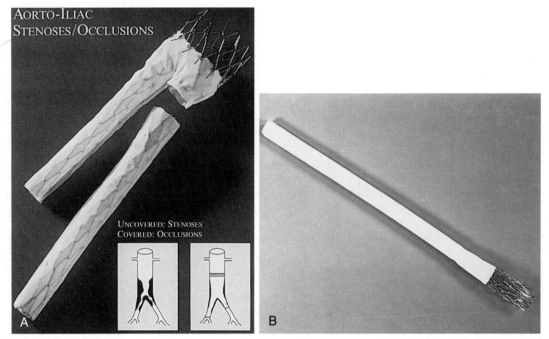

Figure 18–6. Endovascular grafts for the treatment of aortoiliac occlusive disease. *A,* MinTec (MinTec, Inc, Grand Bahama, The Bahamas) device for aortoiliac stenoses/occlusions is constructed of a nitinol frame (stent) covered externally with a thin-walled polyester graft. *B,* The endovascular graft used in the Montefiore experience employs a thin-walled, expanded polytetrafluoroethylene (ePTFE) graft and a Palmaz balloon-expandable stent.

able stent-grafts (the Montefiore system) or the Cragg Endopro system[29–31] (Fig. 18–6). These procedures are performed for long-segment disease of the aorta and iliac vessels (Fig. 18–7). In the Montefiore experience, the majority of endovascular reconstructions were carried out to supply arterial inflow to conventional infrainguinal bypasses.[32, 33] In this series, the primary patency rate at 2 years was 84% using a custom-fabricated device. Those grafts that are placed percutaneously (Cragg Endopro) do not permit reconstruction of the distal portion of the external iliac or femoral arteries. Restenosis at the level of the distal external iliac or femoral artery has been reported to occur in as many as 25% of patients within 18 months.[30] Doing most of the procedures for long-segment disease with a femoral artery exploration may therefore be preferable, permitting complete treatment of the external iliac artery and allowing for standard reconstruction of the femoral arteries (e.g., profundaplasty) or an infrainguinal bypass when necessary.[32, 34]

Endovascular stent-graft experience with superficial femoral artery occlusive disease is limited and includes principally the work of European investigators and small case series carried out in the United States.[30, 35, 36] The majority of this experience has been with the Cragg Endopro device. At the Montefiore Medical Center, the results obtained using ePTFE grafts combined with Palmaz stents to treat long, superficial femoral and popliteal artery occlusions have not been encouraging. Henry and colleagues[30] used the Cragg Endopro device to treat over 60 patients with infrainguinal disease. Unfortunately, in their series, primary patency for superficial femoral artery occlusive disease was 46% at 18 months. Additional work and device modifications are required before these techniques are adopted for small vessel reconstruction.

ENDOVASCULAR GRAFT REPAIR OF ILIAC AND PERIPHERAL ARTERY ANEURYSMS

Isolated aneurysms of the iliac arteries are relatively uncommon, accounting for only 2% to 7% of atherosclerotic aneurysms of the aortoiliac segment.[36–39] As with abdominal aortic aneurysms, iliac aneurysms may rupture, embolize, thrombose, or produce symptoms related to pressure on adjacent structures. Mortality rates after sudden rupture and emergent surgery for iliac artery aneurysms are as high as 33%.[40] However, because of the infrequent nature of these lesions, clear management guidelines have not been well defined for the asymptomatic patient.[41] Furthermore, the technical complexities of operating on vessels deep within the pelvis, especially after previous aortic surgery, have made standard elective surgical management of iliac aneurysms more difficult than that of aortic aneurysms. Alternative intravascular stents have been used in attempts to treat these aneurysms.[42–44] Though radiographic exclusion of flow from within the aneurysm after coil embolization has been demonstrated, continued growth and rupture of thrombosed and excluded lesions have been reported.[45–48]

Endovascular grafts have been used successfully to treat peripheral artery aneurysms primarily isolated to the iliac arteries[49–53] (Table 18–1, Fig. 18–8). Reported series are quite small, but early results with these aneurysm repairs have been encouraging. In the Montefiore series, endovascular grafts were successfully placed in 22 patients for the treatment of a total of 26 peripheral artery aneurysms.[49] Midterm follow-up of patients with common and internal iliac artery aneurysms remains favorable.[54] As with aortic

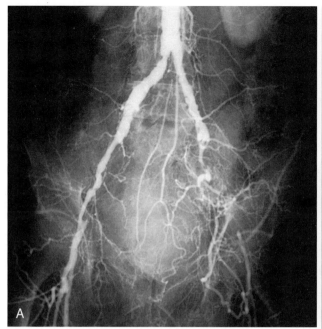

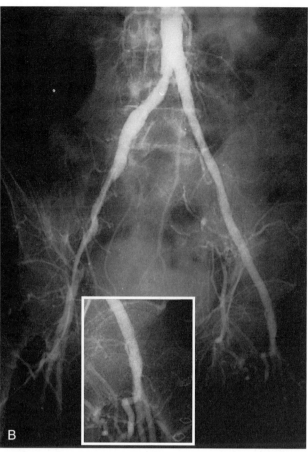

Figure 18–7. Arteriogram before *(A)* and after *(B)* endovascular graft treatment for occlusive disease of the aortoiliac system. *A,* The contralateral approach was used to recanalize this long segment left external iliac occlusion. *B,* After endovascular graft insertion, arterial continuity is reestablished.

TABLE 18–1

Endovascular Repair of Iliac, Popliteal, and Subclavian Artery Aneurysms

ANEURYSM LOCATION	ILIAC RECONSTRUCTION TECHNIQUE*	ANEURYSM SIZE (cm) PREOPERATIVELY/ POSTOPERATIVELY	COMPLICATIONS	HOSPITAL STAY (DAYS)	DURATION OF FOLLOW-UP (MO)
L CIA	A	4.2/4.2	—	12†	23‡
R CIA§	F	3.0/3.0	—	13†	29
R CIA	A	3.6/3.4	—	2	26
R IIA	E	5.2/5.0	—	4	21
R CIA		3.2/3.2			
R CIA	D	5.2/5.2	Transient colonic ischemia	12	20
R CIA§	F	5.0/4.9	Groin lymphocele	10†	18
L CIA		9.0/8.9			
R CIA	C	2.9/2.9	—	5	17
R CIA	C	3.4/3.4	Distal embolization; graft kink requiring stent	12	17
L CIA	B	4.4/4.5	—	3	16
R CIA	D	8.2/7.2	—	3	16
R IIA	E	4.7/4.5	—	2	16
R CIA		3.0/2.9			
R CIA	D	10.0/8.5	—	5	16
R CIA	E	3.0/3.0	—	2	14
R IIA		6.0/5.5			
L IIA	E	5.5/4.0	—	2	4
L CIA	A	4.0/3.0	Hematoma	4	4
R CIA	B	3.5/3.5	—	2	4
R CIA	B	4.0/4.0	—	3	2
R CIA	A	8.0/6.0	—	2	2
L CIA	B	4.5/4.5	—	3	2
L subclavian	—	3.0/3.0	—	2	13‖
L popliteal	—	4.0/4.0	—	—	12¶
L popliteal	—	3.5/3.0	—	5	36

*See Fig. 18–8.
†Extended hospital stay for additional therapy for unrelated medical illnesses.
‡Died of metastatic colon cancer with a patent graft.
§Concomitant abdominal aortic aneurysm.
‖Graft closed 6 weeks postprocedure without limb-threatening consequences.
¶Graft closed 6 days postprocedure and was converted to an open repair.
CIA, common iliac artery; IIA, internal iliac artery; L, left; R, right.

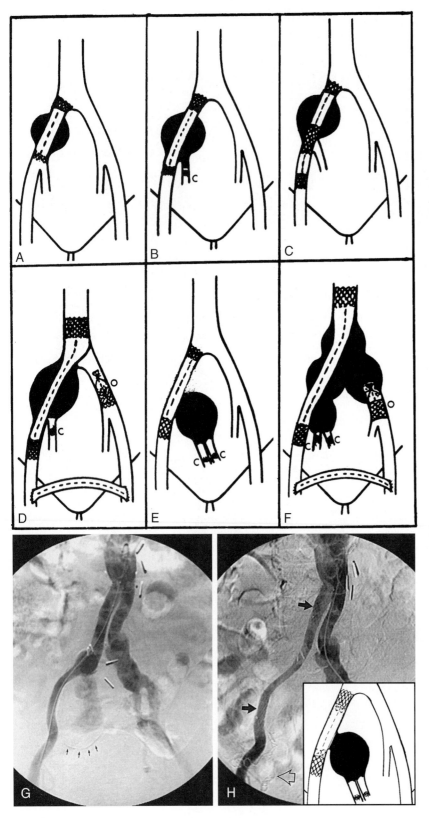

Figure 18–8. *A–F*, The varied techniques for treating iliac artery aneurysms. *A*, Localized common iliac artery aneurysm treated with stents anchoring the endovascular graft proximal and distal to the aneurysm. *B*, If the aneurysm of the common iliac artery extends to the hypogastric vessel, an occlusion coil (*c*) is usually placed at the internal iliac artery orifice before endovascular stent grafting to prevent retrograde flow from the hypogastric artery into the iliac aneurysm. *C*, Alternatively, retrograde flow into the aneurysm may be prevented by expansion of the graft across the hypogastric orifice or placement of an additional balloon expandable stent within the lumen of the graft, securing the graft material across the hypogastric artery orifice. *D*, When no aneurysm neck (normal iliac artery) is present within the cephalad portion of the aneurysm, the stented graft may be anchored to a normal portion of the distal aorta. A coil (*c*) may be placed in the proximal hypogastric artery to prevent retrograde flow from this vessel into the aneurysm. A covered "occluding" stent (*o*) is then positioned in the contralateral common iliac artery. A femorofemoral bypass is placed to reestablish vascular continuity. *E*, If a wide mouth opening to a hypogastric artery aneurysm is present, the anterior and posterior divisions of the hypogastric artery are individually coil embolized (*c*), and the endovascular graft is secured with a stent above and below the origin of the aneurysmal artery, functionally excluding it from the circulation. *F*, When the aorta and iliac arteries are involved in the aneurysmal process, all three aneurysms can be treated by modifications of the type F reconstruction. The branches of the aneurysmal iliac arteries are embolized preoperatively with coils (*c*). The proximal portion of the endovascular stented graft is then positioned immediately below the renal arteries. The distal part of the graft is brought down one iliac artery to below the distalmost extent of the aneurysms. The contralateral iliac artery is then occluded with an "occluding stent" (*o*), and a femorofemoral bypass is done to perfuse the opposite leg. In reconstruction techniques *B–E*, the second stent is responsible for fixing the distal portion of the graft to the arterial wall. The distal stent in these reconstructions may be eliminated by extending the endovascular graft to the common femoral artery (site of device insertion) and performing an endoluminal anastomosis before closure of the arteriotomy. *G*, Endovascular stent-graft treatment of an iliac artery aneurysm before graft insertion. *H*, After placement of a polytetrafluoroethylene (ePTFE) graft, the iliac aneurysm is excluded. *Open arrow*, coils; *closed arrows*, the proximal and distal stents. (*A–F*, From Marin ML, Veith FJ, Lyon RT, Cynamon J, Sanchez LA: Transfemoral endovascular repair of iliac artery aneurysms. Am J Surg 170:179–182, 1995.)

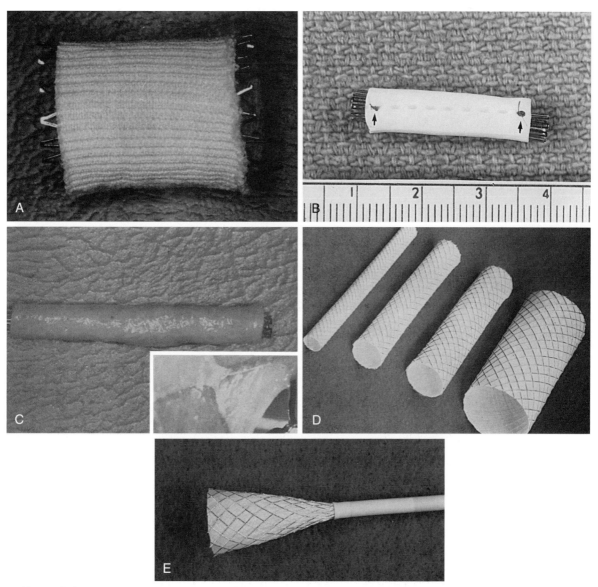

Figure 18–9. Endovascular covered stents. *A,* Polyester graft material may be used to cover a balloon expandable stent. These devices have been preferentially used by Parodi to treat traumatic lesions. *B,* Polytetrafluoroethylene may also function satisfactorily as a covering material for a balloon expandable stent. Two "U" stitches are used to attach the graft to the stent. *C,* An autogenous vein can be used to cover stents, creating a "biologic" stented graft. The collapsed stent-graft assumes a small profile, and the vein effectively covers the struts of the stent after its deployment *(insert). D,* The Corvita endovascular stented graft for arterial trauma. Polyurethane covers the braided wire mesh stent. *E,* The Corvita graft may be compressed to a very limited profile and inserted into a small delivery sheath, as seen here, with one half of the stent compressed inside the catheter. *(A,* From Parodi JC: Endovascular repair of abdominal aortic aneurysm and other arterial lesions. J Vasc Surg 21:549–557, 1995.)

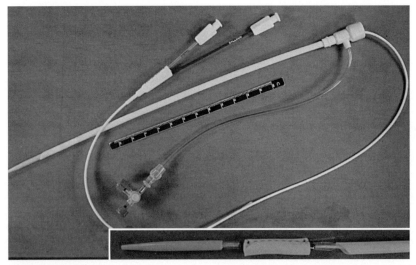

Figure 18–10. Delivery catheter system for the Corvita stent graft. A central "pusher" catheter ejects the self-expanding device out of the distal end of the catheter.

aneurysm treated by endovascular grafts, long-term success depends largely on the presence of healthy arterial tissue above and below the repair to which the endograft attaches.

Endovascular grafting for other peripheral artery aneurysms, including the popliteal and subclavian arteries, has been infrequent.[35, 55] Problems encountered with these devices are related to the small size of the access vessels, which are also frequently tortuous. Endovascular grafts must permit prosthesis bending while crossing joints to avoid compromise of graft function. Aneurysms of the iliac arteries may be treated by several different techniques, depending on the anatomic location of the lesion.[49–53]

ENDOVASCULAR GRAFTS FOR TRAUMA

Techniques and Devices

Transluminally placed stent-grafts for the treatment of traumatic arterial lesions represent another application of these unique devices that were first conceptualized by Dotter[2] in 1969. The first clinical application was performed by Volodos and colleagues using a Dacron graft and a self-expanding stent to repair a thoracic pseudoaneurysm.[7] Experimental and clinical experiences to date have been successful using several different devices for treating traumatic arterial lesions[14, 55, 56] (Fig. 18–9). However, the ideal composition of the external covering on the stent and the optimal stent for device fixation remain unclear.

At the Montefiore Medical Center, we have predominantly used the Palmaz balloon-expandable stent in conjunction with thin-walled ePTFE graft material to perform arterial repairs of pseudoaneurysms and arteriovenous fistulas (see Fig. 18–9B). The entire device was loaded into a 12-Fr delivery catheter for over-the-wire insertion either percutaneously or through an arterial cut-down.

In the United States, a phase I FDA trial of the Corvita stent-graft device (Corvita Corporation, Miami) for the treatment of arterial trauma began in 1997. This device is fabricated from a self-expanding stent of braided wire. The Corvita stent is covered with polyurethane fibers spun directly onto the wire stent (see Fig. 18–9D and E). One attractive feature of this device is that the stent-graft may be cut to the desired size with wire-cutting shears in the operating room before loading into a specially designed delivery sheath (Fig. 18–10).

Clinical Experience

Over a 3-year period at the Montefiore Medical Center, 12 patients had traumatic arterial lesions treated with stent-grafts (Table 18–2). In this initial experience, the age of the patients receiving these grafts ranged from 18 to 85 years. Ten patients were men. All endovascular graft repairs were performed from a remote site (Fig. 18–11). Seven injuries occurred as a result of gunshot wounds (Fig. 18–12). One patient with a knife wound, two patients with iatrogenic needle catheterization injuries, and two patients who had arterial trauma complications of gynecologic and spinal surgery were also included (Fig. 18–13). All injuries were associated with a pseudoaneurysm of variable size. In four instances the arterial injury formed a fistula to an injured adjacent vein. Coexisting injuries were present in seven patients. Stent-graft patency was 100%, with no early or late graft occlusions. In this series, one patient with a left axillary subclavian stent-graft developed a stent deformity secondary to compression at 12 months; this was treated with balloon angioplasty. This problem recurred within 3 months, and further dilatations were not attempted. This partially compressed stent device had not thrombosed during 2 years of follow-up. Mean follow-up for all stent grafts was 24 months, with a range of 2 to 38 months. Additional procedure-related complications affected one patient who had a subclavian pseudoaneurysm repaired with a stent-graft; this patient required a vein patch of a small brachial artery at the catheter insertion site at the conclusion of the procedure.

Stent Grafts for Arterial Trauma

SEX/AGE (YR)	MECHANISM OF INJURY	VESSEL(S) INVOLVED	PSEUDO-ANEURYSM	ARTERIOVENOUS FISTULA	ANESTHESIA	ASSOCIATED INJURIES	INJURY TO REPAIR TIME INTERVAL	STENT GRAFT LENGTH (cm)	ACCESS	HOSPITAL STAY (DAYS)	PATENCY (MO)	COMPLICATIONS
M/20	Bullet	LSFA LSFV	Yes	Yes	General	Soft tissue buttock	36 hr	3	LSFA percutaneous	5	38	None
M/28	Bullet	RSFA	Yes	No	Local	Left open femur fracture	12 hr	3	RSFA arteriotomy	9	36	None
M/22	Bullet	LSFA	Yes	No	Local	Soft tissue right thigh; left deep venous thrombosis	12 hr	3	LSFA arteriotomy	6	2*	None
M/24	Knife	LASA	Yes	No	General	Pneumothorax; hemothorax	4 hr	3	Left brachial arteriotomy	7	33	Stent compression
M/35	Bullet	RASA	Yes	No	Local	Brachial plexus	3 wk	3	Right brachial arteriotomy	4	29	None
F/78	Catheterization	RSA	Yes	No	Local	Hemothorax	24 hr	3	Right brachial arteriotomy	8 wk†	28	None
M/78	Catheterization	LCIA	Yes	No	Epidural	None	4 mo	2	LCFA arteriotomy	2	28	None
M/18	Bullet	RSA	Yes	Yes	Local	Hemothorax	48 hr	3	Right brachial artery	4	21	None
M/18	Bullet	RASA	Yes	No	Local	None	6 hr	3	Right brachial artery	3	12	None
M/22	Bullet	RASA	Yes	No	Local	Hemothorax	3 hr	3	Right brachial artery	6	12	None
F/85	Surgical trauma	RCIA	Yes	Yes	Local	None	8 yr	5‡	LCFA percutaneous	4	3	Distal emboli (treated with catheter suction thrombectomy)
M/52	Surgical trauma	RCIA	Yes	Yes	Local	None	3 yr	10§	RCFA arteriotomy	5	2	Groin hematoma

*Died 2 months postprocedure (homicide).
†Hospitalized for multiple medical problems.
‡Corvita stent graft.
§Two stents were used to anchor the ends of a piece of polytetrafluoroethylene graft.
F, female; LASA, left axillary subclavian artery; LCFA, left common femoral artery; LCIA, left common iliac artery; LSFA, left superficial femoral artery; LSFV, left superficial femoral vein; RCIA, right common iliac artery; RASA, right axillary subclavian artery; M, male.

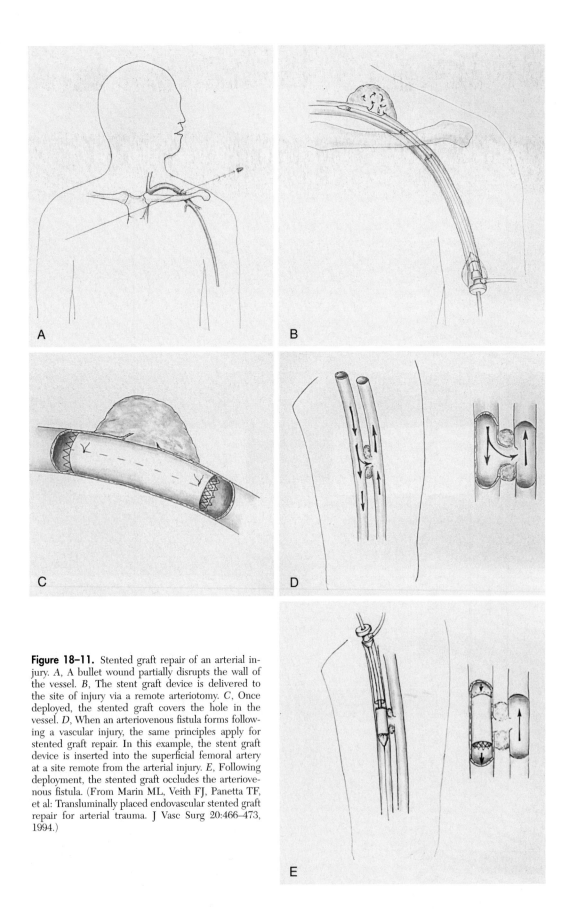

Figure 18–11. Stented graft repair of an arterial injury. *A,* A bullet wound partially disrupts the wall of the vessel. *B,* The stent graft device is delivered to the site of injury via a remote arteriotomy. *C,* Once deployed, the stented graft covers the hole in the vessel. *D,* When an arteriovenous fistula forms following a vascular injury, the same principles apply for stented graft repair. In this example, the stent graft device is inserted into the superficial femoral artery at a site remote from the arterial injury. *E,* Following deployment, the stented graft occludes the arteriovenous fistula. (From Marin ML, Veith FJ, Panetta TF, et al: Transluminally placed endovascular stented graft repair for arterial trauma. J Vasc Surg 20:466–473, 1994.)

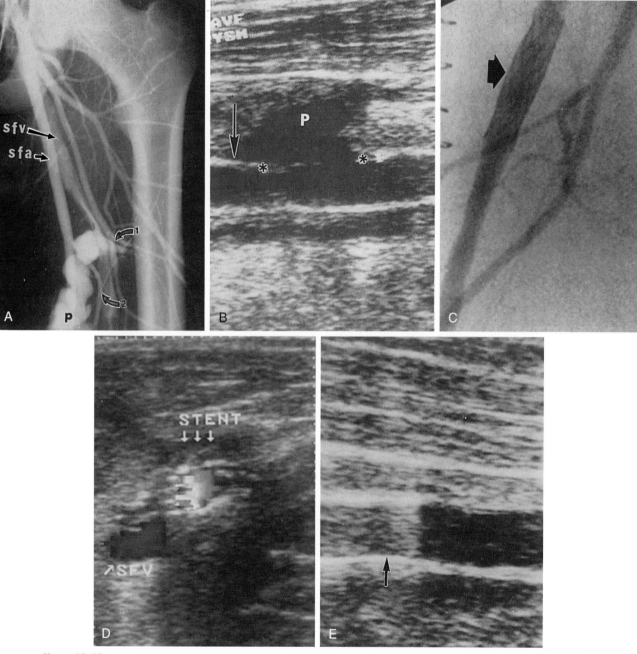

Figure 18–12. *A,* Femoral arteriogram after gunshot wound to the left thigh. An arteriovenous fistula associated with a large pseudoaneurysm is seen between the left superficial femoral artery (sfa) and the superficial femoral vein (sfv). p, pseudoaneurysm. *B,* Duplex ultrasonographic image of SFA depicted in *A.* Loss of the intimal stripe (arrow) and associated pseudoaneurysm (P) is seen. Arterial defect measures approximately 13 mm (distance between stars). *C,* Completion arteriogram demonstrates patency of the SFA, proper positioning of the stented graft (arrow), and no evidence of the arteriovenous fistula or extravasation. Metal clips were placed on the surgical drapes before the procedure to facilitate fluoroscopic localization of the arteriovenous fistula and proper placement of the stented graft. Transverse *(D)* and longitudinal *(E)* duplex ultrasonographic images of stented graft repair of the SFA after 3 months. *D,* Transverse image of artery and vein at the level of the stent can be identified with evidence of normal flow in arteries. *E,* Longitudinal duplex ultrasonogram identified stented graft within artery (arrow). Minimal changes in peak systolic velocities are appreciated between the native SFA and that portion of the vessel that is covered by the stented graft. (From Marin ML, Veith FJ, Panetta TF, et al: Percutaneous transfemoral stented graft repair of a traumatic femoral arteriovenous fistula. J Vasc Surg 18:298–301, 1993.)

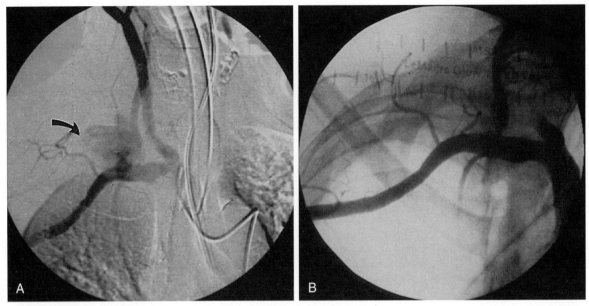

Figure 18–13. *A,* This arteriogram shows a large pseudoaneurysm of the subclavian artery (arrow) just distal to the right vertebral artery, which occurred after an attempted subclavian vein catheter insertion. *B,* Following stented graft placement through the right brachial artery, the pseudoaneurysm was excluded. Vertebral artery flow was preserved. (From Marin ML, Veith FJ, Panetta TF, et al: Transluminally placed endovascular stented graft repair for arterial trauma. J Vasc Surg 20:466–473, 1994.)

References

1. Taylor LM, Porter JM: Basic data related to clinical decision-making in abdominal aortic aneurysm. Ann Vasc Surg 1:502–504, 1980.
2. Dotter CT: Transluminally-placed coil spring endarterial tube grafts: Long term patency in canine popliteal artery. Invest Radiol 4:329–332, 1969.
3. Cragg A, Lund G, Rysavy J, et al: Non-surgical placement of arterial endoprosthesis: A new technique using nitinol wire. Radiology 147:261–263, 1983.
4. LeMolle GM, Spagna BM, Strong MD: Rigid intraluminal prosthesis for replacement of the thoracic and abdominal aorta. J Vasc Surg 1:22–26, 1984.
5. Balko A, Piasecki GJ, Shah DM, et al: Transfemoral placement of intraluminal polyurethane prosthesis for abdominal aortic aneurysm. J Surg Res 40:305–309, 1986.
6. Parodi JC, Palmaz JC, Barone HD: Transfemoral intraluminal graft implantation for abdominal aortic aneurysms. Ann Vasc Surg 5:491–499, 1991.
7. Volodos ML, Karpovich IP, Troyan VI, et al: Clinical experience of the use of a self-fixing synthetic prosthesis for remote endoprosthetics of the thoracic and the abdominal aorta and iliac arteries through the femoral artery and as intraoperative endoprosthesis for aortic reconstruction. Vasa Suppl 33:93–95, 1991.
8. Lazarus HM: Intraluminal graft device, system and method. US Patent No. 4,787,899 (1988).
9. Chuter TA, Green RN, Ouriel K, DeWeese JA: Infrarenal aortic aneurysm structure: Implications for transfemoral repair. J Vasc Surg 20:44–49, 1994.
10. Chuter TAN, Green RN, Ouriel K, et al: Transfemoral endovascular aortic graft placement. J Vasc Surg 18:185–197, 1993.
11. Moore WS: Endovascular grafting technique: A feasibility study. In Yao JST, Pearce WH (eds): Aneurysms: New Findings and Treatments. Norwalk, Conn, Appleton & Lange, 1993, pp 333–340.
12. Moore WS, Vescera CL: Repair of abdominal aortic aneurysm by transfemoral endovascular graft placement. Ann Surg 220:331–341, 1994.
13. Marin ML, Veith FJ, Cynamon J, et al: Transfemoral endovascular stented graft treatment of aorto-iliac and femoropopliteal occlusive disease for limb salvage. Am J Surg 168:156–162, 1994.
14. Parodi JC: Endovascular repair of abdominal aortic aneurysm and other arterial lesions. J Vasc Surg 21:549–557, 1995.
15. Quiñones-Baldrich WJ, Deaton DH, Mitchell RS, et al: Preliminary experience with the Endovascular Technologies bifurcated endovascular aortic prosthesis in a calf model. J Vasc Surg 22:370–381, 1995.
16. Moore WS, Rutherford RB (for the EVT Investigators): Transfemoral endovascular repair of abdominal aortic aneurysm: Results of the North American EVT phase 1 trial. J Vasc Surg 23:543–553, 1996.
17. Balm R, Eikelboom BC, May J, et al: Early experience with endovascular transfemoral aneurysm management (TEAM) in the treatment of aortic aneurysms. Eur J Vasc Endovasc Surg 11:214–220, 1996.
18. Moore WS, Brewster DC, Bernhard VM: Aorto-uni-iliac endograft for complex aortoiliac aneurysms compared with tube/bifurcation endografts: Results of the EVT/Guidant trials. J Vasc Surg 33(Suppl 2):S11–20, 2001.
19. Zarins CK, White RA, Schwarten DE, et al: AneuRx stent graft versus open surgical repair of abdominal aortic aneurysms: Multicenter prospective clinical trial. J Vasc Surg 29:292–308, 1999.
20. Zarins CK, White RA, Fogarty TJ: Aneurysm rupture after endovascular repair using the AneuRx stent graft. J Vasc Surg 31:960–970, 2000.
21. White GH, Yu W, May J, et al: Endoleak as a complication of endoluminal grafting of abdominal aortic aneurysms: Classification, incidence, diagnosis, and management. J Endovasc Surg 4:152–168, 1997.
22. Volodos NL, Shekhanin VE, Karpovich IP, et al: Self-fixing synthetic prosthesis for endoprosthetics of the vessels. Vestn Khir Im I I Grek 137:123–125, 1986.
23. Dotter CT, Buschmann RW, McKinney MK: Transluminal expandable nitinol coil stent grafting: Preliminary report. Radiology 147:259–260, 1983.
24. Cragg AH, Dake MD: Percutaneous femoropopliteal graft placement. Radiology 187:455–463, 1993.
25. Henry M, Amor M, Ethevenot G, et al: Initial experience with the Cragg Endopro System 1 for intraluminal treatment of peripheral vascular disease. J Endovasc Surg 1:31–43, 1994.
26. Moore WS, Cafferata HT, Hall AD, Blaisdell FW: In defense of grafts across the inguinal ligament: An evaluation of early and late results of aortofemoral bypass grafts. Ann Surg 168:207–214, 1968.

27. Marin ML, Veith FJ, Cynamon J, et al: Human transluminally placed endovascular stented grafts: Preliminary histopathologic analysis of healing grafts in aortoiliac and femoral artery occlusive disease. J Vasc Surg 21:595–604, 1995.
28. Ombrellaro MP, Stevens SL, Freeman MB, Goldman MH: Intra-arterial stented grafts: The effects of intraluminal placement on prosthetic graft healing. Surg Forum 46:373–377, 1995.
29. Marin ML, Veith FJ, Sanchez LA, et al: Endovascular repair of aortoiliac occlusive disease. World J Surg 20:679–686, 1996.
30. Henry M, Amor M, Henry I, et al: Endoluminal bypass grafting in leg arteries with the Cragg Endopro System 1: A series of 105 patients [abstract]. J Endovasc Surg 3:118, 1996.
31. Pernes JM, Auguste MA, Hovasse D, et al: Long iliac stenosis: Initial clinical experience with the Cragg endoluminal graft. Radiology 196:67–71, 1995.
32. Marin ML, Veith FJ, Sanchez LA, et al: Endovascular aortoiliac grafts in combination with standard infrainguinal arterial bypasses in the management of limb-threatening ischemia: Preliminary report. J Vasc Surg 22:316–325, 1995.
33. Wain RA, Veith FJ, Marin ML: Analysis of endovascular graft treatment for aortoiliac occlusive disease—what is its role based on midterm results. Ann Surg 230:145–151, 1999.
34. Wain RA, Lyon RT, Veith FJ, Marin ML: Alternative techniques for management of distal anastomoses of aortofemoral and iliofemoral endovascular grafts. J Vasc Surg 32:307–314, 2000.
35. Marin ML, Veith FJ, Cynamon J, et al: Initial experience with transluminally placed endovascular grafts for the treatment of complex vascular lesions. Ann Surg 222:449–469, 1995.
36. Diethrich EB, Papazoglou K: Endoluminal grafting for aneurysmal and occlusive disease in the superficial femoral artery: Early experience. J Endovasc Surg 2:225–239, 1995.
37. Nachbur BH, Inderbitzi RG, Bar W: Isolated iliac aneurysms. Eur J Vasc Surg 5:375–381, 1991.
38. McCready RA, Pairolero PC, Gilmore JC, et al: Isolated iliac artery aneurysms. Surgery 93:688–693, 1983.
39. Lowry SF, Kraft RO: Isolated aneurysms of the iliac artery. Arch Surg 113:1289–1293, 1978.
40. Richardson JW, Greenfield LJ: Natural history and management of iliac aneurysms. J Vasc Surg 8:165–171, 1988.
41. Sacks NPM, Huddy SPJ, Wegner T, Giddings AEF: Management of solitary iliac aneurysms. J Cardiovasc Surg 33:679–683, 1992.
42. Reuter SR, Carson SN: Thrombosis of a common iliac artery aneurysm by selective embolization and extraanatomic bypass. AJR Am J Roentgenol 134:1248–1250, 1980.
43. Michaels JA, McWhinnie D, Hands LJ, et al: Iliac aneurysm treated by percutaneous occlusion and femorofemoral crossover grafting. Br J Surg 81:37–38, 1994.
44. Vorwerk D, Gunther RW, Wendt G, Schurmann K: Ulcerated plaques and focal aneurysms of iliac arteries: Treatment with non-covered, self-expanding stents. AJR Am J Roentgenol 162:1421–1424, 1994.
45. Deb B, Benjamin M, Comeroto AJ: Delayed rupture of an internal iliac artery aneurysm following proximal ligation for abdominal aortic aneurysm repair. Ann Vasc Surg 6:537–540, 1992.
46. Kwaan JHM, Dahl RK: Fatal rupture after successful surgical thrombosis of an abdominal aortic aneurysm. Surgery 95:235–237, 1984.
47. Schanzer H, Papa MC, Miller CM: Rupture of surgically thrombosed abdominal aortic aneurysm. J Vasc Surg 2:278–280, 1985.
48. Cho SI, Johnson WC, Bush HL Jr, et al: Lethal complications associated with nonrestrictive treatment of abdominal aortic aneurysms. Arch Surg 117:1214–1217, 1982.
49. Marin ML, Veith FJ, Lyon RT, et al: Transfemoral endovascular repair of iliac artery aneurysms. Am J Surg 170:179–182, 1995.
50. Murphy KD, Richter GM, Henry M, et al: Aortoiliac aneurysms: Management with endovascular stent-graft placement. Radiology 198:473–480, 1996.
51. Rousseau H, Gieskes L, Joffre F, et al: Percutaneous treatment of peripheral aneurysms with the Cragg Endopro system. J Vasc Intervent Radiol 7:35–39, 1996.
52. Razavi MK, Dake MD, Semba CP, et al: Percutaneous endoluminal placement of stent-grafts for the treatment of isolated iliac artery aneurysms. Radiology 197:801–804, 1995.
53. Marin ML, Veith FJ, Panetta TF, et al: Transfemoral endoluminal stented graft repair of a popliteal artery aneurysm. J Vasc Surg 19:754–757, 1994.
54. Parsons RE, Marin ML, Veith FJ: Midterm results of endovascular stented grafts for the treatment of isolated iliac aneurysms. J Vasc Surg 30:915–921, 1999.
55. Marin ML, Veith FJ, Panetta TF, et al: Transluminally placed endovascular stented graft repair for arterial trauma. J Vasc Surg 20:466–473, 1994.
56. Rivera FJ, Palmaz JC, Encarnacion CE, et al: Aneurysm and pseudoaneurysm balloon expandable stent/graft bypass: Clinical experience [abstract]. J Vasc Intervent Radiol 5:19, 1994.

Questions

1. Community-based analysis reveals that conventional transabdominal repair of abdominal aortic aneurysm carries a mortality rate of
   (a) 1%
   (b) 2%
   (c) 5%
   (d) 10%
   (e) 15%

2. Complications seen with endovascular repair of abdominal aortic aneurysm include
   (a) perigraft leak
   (b) attachment system fracture
   (c) fever of unknown origin
   (d) wound infection
   (e) all of the above

3. Endovascular repair of abdominal aortic aneurysm is now considered a scientifically proven technique
   (a) true
   (b) false

4. The use of endovascular grafting is currently limited to aneurysms of the abdominal aorta
   (a) true
   (b) false

5. Attachment of endovascular graft to the native artery is accomplished with
   (a) balloon-expandable stents utilizing friction
   (b) self-expanding stents
   (c) self-expanding stents with hooks
   (d) balloon-seating stents with hooks
   (e) all of the above

Answers

1. d   2. e   3. b   4. b   5. e

19

Role of Sympathectomy in the Management of Vascular Disease and Related Disorders

Robert B. Rutherford

The concept of sympathetic denervation as therapy for arterial occlusive disease was first elaborated and tested by Leriche and Jaboulay in 1913.[1] Although their experience with periarterial sympathectomy was disappointing, Adson and Brown applied the technique of sympathetic ganglionectomy in 1925 to relieve debilitating lower extremity vasospasm with better long-term results. This ushered in an era in which sympathectomy was the only alternative to amputation for severe occlusive disease. Despite technical refinements over the next 40 years, clinical results remained variable and they spawned considerable debate over the value of sympathectomy in this setting. Better understanding of extremity pain syndromes and progress in direct arterial reconstructive surgery had largely eclipsed the prominent role of sympathectomy by the early 1960s. A growing body of experimental data supported the clinical impression that the beneficial effects of sympathectomy were usually short-lived and were palliative when applied for occlusive arterial disease. Current indications for upper or lower extremity sympathectomy are generally limited to patients with causalgic pain, hyperhidrosis, and *highly select* patients with vasospastic or distal arterial occlusive disease that is not amenable to drug or surgical therapy, respectively. Despite this limited application, properly selected patients are significantly benefited and vascular surgeons should know when and how to perform upper and lower extremity sympathectomy. In this chapter, the physiologic consequences, indications, techniques, and results of sympathectomy are discussed.

ANATOMIC AND PHYSIOLOGIC CONSIDERATIONS

The sympathetic nervous system comprises preganglionic and postganglionic neurons originating in the anteromedial columns of the thoracolumbar spinal cord. Regional sympathetic activity is the product of local reflex arcs between somatic afferent fibers and preganglionic efferent fibers. Central control of both segmental and systemic sympathetic activity is mediated through the spinothalamic tract, with important contributions from visceral nuclei in the pons and medulla. At a segmental level, preganglionic neurons primarily synapse with postganglionic neurons in paravertebral ganglia via white rami communicantes. A small percentage of preganglionic fibers bypass the paravertebral ganglia to form synapses in more peripherally located intermediate ganglia or cross over to innervate contralateral regions via conventional pathways.[2] Characteristically, preganglionic fibers that supply a specific region either synapse with multiple neurons in paravertebral ganglia or proceed more peripherally to synapse in intermediate ganglia, which are at a distance from their segmental source. Complete sympathetic denervation of an extremity, therefore, requires division of preganglionic fibers along their segmental origin, as well as excision of their corresponding relay ganglia and intercommunicating fibers.[3] The segmental innervation levels of the upper and lower extremity, as well as specific anatomic variations, are described in the sections on dorsal and lumbar sympathectomy.

The primary functions of the sympathetic nervous system are to prevent heat loss through reduction of superficial extremity blood flow and to modify basal organ functions in preparation for the demands of "fight or flight." Only the former need be considered here. Resting sympathetic activity primarily antagonizes the vasodilating influence of the parasympathetic nervous system on arteriolar resistance vessels, cutaneous precapillary sphincters, and capacitance venules. Local increases in sympathetic outflow cause decreased skin blood flow, piloerection, and sweating. Net extremity blood flow is reduced by sympathetic stimulation unless muscular activity increases perfusion by metabolic vasodilatation. These vasomotor effects are mediated by the constricting influence of norepinephrine on vascular smooth muscle. Thus, the primary vascular effect of increased sympathetic tone is a large reduction in cutaneous blood flow with lesser reductions in muscular blood flow that can be overcome by metabolic vasodilatation. Sympathectomy produces the *opposite* of these effects.

Complete sympathetic denervation of an extremity leaves the parasympathetics unopposed and thus causes a 40% to 100% increase in total resting blood flow in ischemic limb experiments.[4] The majority of this increased flow passes through cutaneous arteriovenous anastomoses with relatively modest changes in resting or exertional muscular perfusion.[5] Blood flow is redistributed to more peripheral parts to produce the characteristic warm, pink, and dry hand or foot. Maximal vasodilatation and increased extremity blood flow are noted immediately after sympathectomy. However, a progressive decline in resting vasodilatation usually begins within 1 week of denervation and results in minimal augmentation of flow by 6 months.[6] Explanations for this incremental recovery of baseline sympathetic vascular tone include incomplete sympathetic denervation, regeneration of severed fibers, and vascular receptor hypersensitivity to circulating catecholamines. Biochemical examination of recovery shows that the sensitivity of *extrasynaptic* α_2 receptors to exogenous norepinephrine is increased. However, decreases in both the concentration of *synaptic* α_1 receptors and the maximal vasoconstrictive response to norepinephrine have been demonstrated.[7, 8] These changes in the number and sensitivity of vascular smooth muscle α receptors seem to best explain the phenomenon of partial sympathetic tone recovery.

Despite the transient effects of sympathectomy on *resting* extremity blood flow, other effects, specifically the abolition of sweating and the vasoconstrictor response to cold, persist as long as the sympathectomy is anatomically complete.[9] This is also true of relief of certain types of extremity pain. Although objective assessment of symptom relief in both neuropathic and ischemic pain syndromes is difficult, aversive stimuli studies in cats have documented that sympathectomy produces enhanced tolerance of painful stimuli.[10] This pain tolerance lasts longer than the vasomotor effects of sympathectomy and may explain clinical observations of improved exercise performance in sympathectomized patients who have no objective increases in extremity blood flow.[11] Theories concerning this direct effect on pain thresholds suggest that sympathetic denervation decreases noxious stimulus perception by both decreasing tissue concentrations of norepinephrine and reducing spinal augmentation of pain stimulus transmission to cerebral centers.[12, 13] This role of sympathetic denervation in modulating pain perception is the most appealing explanation for this symptomatic relief.

Numerous reports of chronically ischemic extremities treated by sympathectomy alone have yielded controversial results. Both clinical and experimental studies indicate that the major circulatory effect of sympathectomy is increased distal skin blood flow. Using radioactively labeled microspheres, Cronenwett and colleagues[4] claimed that most of the increased skin blood flow is shunted through arteriovenous anastomoses and does not increase nutrient capillary perfusion. In contrast, Moore and Hall[14] showed that intra-dermal xenon clearance, and therefore cutaneous capillary blood flow, is significantly increased after lumbar sympathectomy. Measurements of tissue oxygen concentration before and after sympathectomy suggest that tissue oxygen supply is *not* augmented.[15] Despite these experimental results, several uncontrolled clinical experiences suggest that sympathectomy may sufficiently improve the oxygen supply-demand balance to allow ischemic ulcer healing in 35% to 62% of patients.[16–18] Unfortunately, none of these have been randomized prospective trials, and healing in a 20% to 30% range has been reported in the control groups of randomized trials of circulation-enhancing drugs like the prostanoids.[19]

Studies of blood flow distribution after sympathectomy have consistently shown that muscle perfusion is not improved. Using radioactively labeled microspheres, Rutherford and Valenta[20] noted that resting and exercise blood flow to muscle remains unchanged by sympathectomy in both normal and arterial-ligated extremities. This lack of responsiveness has been attributed to high intrinsic myogenic tone in muscle afferent arterioles, which compensates for decreases in sympathetic tone.[21] This experimental observation is consistent with the observed ineffectiveness of sympathectomy for claudication.[22] However, relief of rest pain due to distal ischemia has been noted after sympathetic denervation in 47% to 71% of patients.[16–18] This discrepancy between experimental and clinical observations requires explanation. Although relief of a causalgic component of "ischemic neuritis" has been suggested as the cause by some,[23] most feel that even small increments of improved perfusion, not measurable by clinical testing, could spell the difference in these marginal cases. Still, it is not necessary to invoke this explanation in view of the nonspecific effect of sympathectomy on pain perception. Thus, although a small fraction of patients may show improved blood flow, others may obtain relief because of the attenuating effects of sympathectomy on pain perception.

The influence of sympathetic denervation on resting *collateral blood flow* and vascular resistance has been studied in numerous experiments with both acute and chronic limb ischemia models. Dalessandri and colleagues[24] have shown in an acute canine limb ischemia preparation that sympathectomy causes a temporary but significant increase in collateral blood flow. This increase in flow around a complete arterial occlusion is thought to be caused by maximal vasodilatation in collateral channels that are not fully dilated by the metabolic stimuli of acute ischemia. This phenomenon of submaximal collateral vasodilatation has also been observed by Ludbrook[25] in 30% of patients with rest pain. After sympathectomy in this group, he observed an average 11% decrease in collateral vascular resistance with limb salvage in 42%. Although temporary, sympathectomy seems to relieve *inappropriate* vasoconstriction in the collateral blood vessels of an ischemic extremity. However, in the majority of patients with resting ischemia, regional metabolic factors dominate and cause maximal blood flow increases through existing and newly formed collateral channels.

In summary, sympathetic denervation temporarily increases blood flow to peripheral regions of the resting ischemic limb; however, much of this flow increase is nonnutrient arteriovenous shunt flow to the cutaneous circulation. Although debatable, skin capillary perfusion may be sufficiently increased to promote healing of small or superficial ischemic ulcers in selected patients with marginally inadequate perfusion. Persistent attenuation of ischemic or neuropathic pain perception is accomplished by reduction of noxious stimulus production peripherally and pain impulse transmission centrally. This effect probably explains the subjective pain relief observed in some patients who have no detectable flow improvement. Finally, increased muscular and collateral perfusion is observed in that small minority of patients who have significant limb ischemia associated with inappropriate vasoconstriction. Like its effect on sweating, the effect of sympathectomy on *abnormal* vasomotor tone is lasting. The latter is probably due to a reduction in the number and response of synaptic α receptors.

UPPER EXTREMITY SYMPATHECTOMY

Current indications for and technique of upper extremity sympathectomy are based on nearly a century of clinical experience. First used by Alexander in 1899 for epilepsy, dorsal sympathectomy has undergone multiple technical modifications to reduce its morbidity and maximize sympathetic denervation. Advice regarding the extent of ganglion resection has ranged from radical (stellate ganglion to T-5) to conservative (T-2 and Kuntz's nerve). Although the latter may indeed suffice for some indications, the author's experience indicates that clinically adequate upper extremity sympathectomy is best accomplished by resection of the T-2 and T-3 ganglia. T-4 should be included if the indication is hyperhidrosis and the axilla as well as the hand is involved. In terms of operative indications, long-term outcome analysis has shown that best results are achieved among patients with causalgia, hyperhidrosis, and vasospastic disorders complicated by digital ulceration.[26] Improved medical management of patients with Raynaud's disease has largely replaced dorsal sympathectomy as therapy for disabling digital vasospasm.[27] Patients with secondary Raynaud's phenomenon may be helped if small arteries are involved proximal to the digits, as in arterial embolism, but if the terminal digital arteries are involved, as in scleroderma, the response to sympathectomy is usually disappointing. Within this context, pertinent features of upper extremity sympathectomy are discussed.

Anatomic Features

Proper performance of thoracic dorsal sympathectomy requires appreciation of the anatomic variations in ganglion location and innervation patterns of the upper extremity. Preganglionic neurons supplying the face, neck, and upper extremity originate at the spinal cord levels of C-7 through T-5. Efferents from these levels form multiple synapses in the inferior cervical, stellate, and numbered thoracic ganglia. A direct fiber tract from the T-2 sympathectomy ganglion to the brachial plexus (the nerve of Kuntz) can be identified in most patients as a frequent variation in the relay chain between the spinal cord and upper extremity.[28] Other direct connections between the spinal cord and brachial plexus can be demonstrated with detailed dissection but are too variable to list. Similar variation in interganglionic connections are present at this level of the sympathetic nervous system and thus render complete upper extremity denervation difficult if not impossible.[29] With this fact in mind, most surgeons advocate resection of T-2 and T-3 ganglia as well as the nerve of Kuntz and other rami contributing directly to the brachial plexus at these levels.[30] Although providing less than 15% of upper extremity sympathetic innervation, the T-1 and inferior portion of the stellate ganglia make significant contributions to the eyes; therefore, complete resection of these ganglia substantially increases the risk of permanent Horner's syndrome. To eliminate the potential problem of partial sympathetic denervation, Roos[31] advocated selective division of rami from the stellate ganglion to the brachial plexus. Others, including the author, additionally resect only the lower tip, no more than the lower third of the stellate ganglion.

Operative Technique

A variety of chest, back, and axillary approaches have been used to gain open surgical exposure to the upper sympathetic ganglia. In fact, six distinct approaches have been described: three anterior (supraclavicular, infraclavicular, and high anterolateral thoracotomy), one dorsal, and two axillary (through a high interspace or the bed of a resected first rib). Critical review of reported series using each technique indicates that the latter two, the axillary transthoracic (Atkins[32]) and extrapleural axillary (Roos[31]) approaches to the stellate and upper thoracic ganglia, have the lowest complication rates and are recommended for most cases. Both techniques involve exposure of the posterior portion of the superior mediastinum through a transverse axillary incision. First-rib resection is recommended by Roos to facilitate both extrapleural retraction of the upper lung and identification of the sympathetic connections between the brachial plexus and higher ganglia. Similar exposure is obtained using the same incision with the transthoracic approach, by entering the chest through the third intercostal space and dividing the upper mediastinal pleura (Fig. 19–1). T-2 and T-3 ganglionectomy is performed by metal clip interruption and division of afferent and efferent fibers after the stellate ganglion has been identified on the neck of the first rib. Separation of the ganglia from adjacent intercostal vessels is facilitated by gentle traction on the T-2 ganglion and attached fibers with a right-angle clamp or nerve hook.

Transaxillary approaches are preferred because less dissection is required to fully visualize the target ganglia, and the incision is cosmetically acceptable. Major disadvantages of the transthoracic approach are the pain of a rib-spreading incision and frequent need for tube thoracostomy. Although preliminary first-rib resection in the extrapleural axillary approach is time-consuming in inexperienced hands, that time is compensated for by the simple closure. Fortunately, the first rib does not need to be divided as far posteriorly as it does for thoracic outlet syndrome, and it serves as a sure landmark for the stellate ganglion lying on its inner surface near its neck.

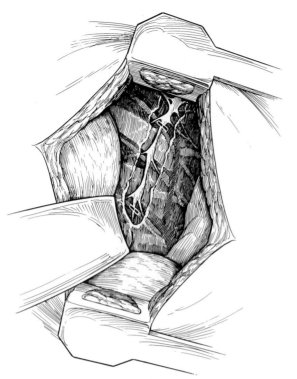

Figure 19–1. Transaxillary minithoracotomy through the second or third interspace provides good exposure of the upper thoracic sympathetic chain lying over the necks of the corresponding ribs. After opening the pleura, the segment of the chain from the lower tip of the stellate ganglion to T-3 is resected. (From Rutherford RB: Atlas of Vascular Surgery. Philadelphia, WB Saunders, 1993.)

The supraclavicular approach[33] poses the greatest risk of injury because numerous surrounding structures, including the phrenic nerve, subclavian artery, vertebral artery, thoracic duct, cupola of the lung, and brachial plexus, are encountered in gaining exposure of the sympathetic ganglia (Fig. 19–2). In addition, traction and dissection from above is more likely to cause Horner's syndrome. Most painful is

the posterior approach advocated by Cloward, because extensive paraspinal muscle division, laminectomy, and rib resection are required for visualization. Common to all approaches is the risk of injury to the thoracic duct, peripheral nerve roots, azygous vein, and intercostal arteries because of their proximity to the sympathetic chain. In my opinion, the overall risk of these technical complications is reduced by using the transaxillary approaches and remaining attentive to anatomic detail.

Thoracoscopic Sympathectomy

The thoracoscope is not a new idea, but the advent of new instrumentation and video systems has now made it practical for many purposes (e.g., division of pleural adhesions, lung biopsy, pleurodesis). Dorsal sympathectomy has been performed through a thoracoscope for a number of years in the United Kingdom and Australia. Early techniques use cautery to destroy the ganglion chains, but the advanced technology that laparascopic cholesystectomy and pelvic lymph node dissection have spawned has made precise excision of the upper thoracic sympathetic chain quite feasible. The technical details are important and are well described elsewhere.[34, 35] When dorsal sympathectomy is performed this way, it is safe and effective and *not* time-consuming.

After completion, a chest tube is placed in the viewing port and the two instrument ports are closed with one or two skin sutures. Chest pain is minimal and discharge on the first or second postoperative day is routine. This technical advance will likely impact willingness to apply sympathectomy for certain indications, such as hyperhidrosis and Raynaud's disease, for which the morbidity of operation was formerly an impediment. It should also limit the number of stellate blocks administered to causalgia or reflex sympathetic dystrophy patients before sympathectomy is performed. Numerous blocks are now unnecessary and even contraindicated, because the inflammation and scarring they cause make subsequent thoracoscopic sympathectomy

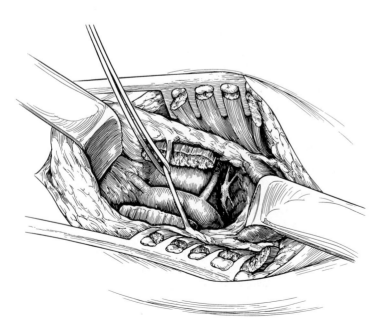

Figure 19–2. Through this right supraclavicular approach, the stellate ganglion is exposed just adjacent to and behind the vertebral artery, lying on the neck of the first rib. With further downward retraction, T2 and T3 can be exposed and resected with their rami and Kuntz's nerve using metal clips. (From Rutherford RB: Atlas of Vascular Surgery. Philadelphia, WB Saunders, 1993.)

difficult and dangerous, if not impossible. This approach is not feasible in those with previous thoracic operations, pulmonary infections, or diffuse pulmonary disease with severely impaired function, because such patients would not tolerate a *complete* pneumothorax using a Carlens' tube.

Results of Upper Extremity Sympathectomy

Assessment of the results of upper extremity sympathectomy requires categorization according to indications for the procedure. Additional factors warranting consideration are the duration of observation and technique of sympathectomy. With these factors in mind, the most successful indication for upper extremity sympathectomy is hyperhidrosis. Although a variety of ganglionectomy combinations have been performed for this condition, T-2, T-3, and T-4 ganglionectomy is sufficient. No short- or long-term failures have been reported, with maximal follow-up in one series of 7 years. Although never widely applied in North America, it remains popular in Europe.[26]

The prominent role of the sympathetic nervous system in perpetuating causalgic pain syndromes is unequivocal, despite the fact that the basic origin of this type of post-traumatic extremity pain remains conjectural. Confident diagnosis of causalgic extremity pain requires a history of antecedent trauma (although this may be relatively minor), associated vasomotor dysfunction, cutaneous hypersensitivity, and, usually, pain that is "burning" in character.[36] Consistent relief of the pain by sympathetic blockade increases that confidence immensely. Indeed, preoperative stellate ganglion blocks with local anesthetic have been advocated by Beurger and Smit[37] and me as routine to identify patients who will most likely benefit from surgical sympathectomy.[38] Sham blocks to identify the "suggestive" or hysterical patient have been recommended, but using local anesthetics of different duration (e.g., bupivacaine [Marcaine] and lidocaine [Xylocaine]) on consecutive blocks and requesting that the "blinded" patient make careful note of the duration of relief eliminates uncertainties about the validity of the response. Approximately 60% of these post-traumatic pain syndromes can be managed with serial blocks, physiotherapy, mild narcotics, tricyclic antidepressants, and anticonvulsants.[39] In the remainder, T-1 to T-3 ganglionectomy is required. Surgical results are excellent insofar as 75% to 100% of patients achieve permanent pain relief after up to 7 years of observation.[26, 37–41]

Retrospective assessment of the success of sympathectomy in relieving symptomatic episodic vasospasm is difficult because the pathologic definition of Raynaud's disease has undergone considerable revision. Although the classic distinction between the benign "disease" and the virulent "phenomenon" is usually not made in many series, one fact is clear: the results of sympathectomy for Raynaud's disease caused by collagen-vascular disease are disappointing. Characteristically, these patients suffer from progressive organic arterial disease that causes abnormal decreases in digital blood flow that are further aggravated by exposure to cold.[42] Sympathectomy initially prevents cold-induced ischemic attacks in 75% to 100% of these patients. Within 2 years, however, 80% to 94% of responders experience some recurrent symptoms because progression of the auto-immune vascular disease further reduces resting blood flow to the digits.[26, 37, 43–45]

Among a small number of patients with occlusive Raynaud's disease complicated by digital ulceration, however, sympathectomy allows healing of at least 75% of these lesions and prevents recurrent tissue loss even though cold-induced digital ischemia reappears.[26] Thus, sympathectomy may temporarily ameliorate symptoms and help with acute ulceration but generally does not prevent recurrent symptoms, because denervation does not affect the cause and course of the underlying vascular disease.

In contrast, occlusive Raynaud's disease caused by embolic or traumatic fibrotic lesions shows a more lasting and favorable response to sympathectomy. Abolition of cold-induced vasoconstriction in these patients reliably prevents digital ischemia because the lesions are discrete and the underlying disease is not progressive.[40, 46] Similarly, Raynaud's disease caused by thrombosis or subintimal fibrosis from chronic occupational trauma also responds to sympathetic denervation, and generally does not recur.[40, 46–48]

Raynaud's disease resulting from abnormal digital vasoconstriction without obstructing lesions has a more benign course than the occlusive variety. Although up to 33% of patients initially thought to be free of underlying disease may ultimately show signs of autoimmune vasculitis, true vasoconstrictive Raynaud's disease does not tend to be associated with digital ulceration.[42, 49] Treatment with α-adrenergic or calcium channel blocking agents provides symptomatic relief during the acute phase of the syndrome.[27, 50] Surgical sympathectomy, therefore, is not often indicated because medical management is sufficient or the symptoms are not sufficiently debilitating. Thoracoscopic sympathectomy may change this view. Unfortunately, among patients with Raynaud's phenomenon, surgery is least effective in those who need it the most, and vice versa. Clinical experience shows that sympathectomy can be justified by its overall benefit compared with risk only in patients with occlusive Raynaud's disease caused by occupational trauma, distal emboli, or autoimmune disease complicated by digital ulceration.[26, 27, 42, 46, 48]

Experience with sympathectomy in treating atherosclerotic disease of the upper extremity is limited insofar as this category accounts for only 5% to 7% of dorsal sympathectomies in most large series. Although initial symptomatic relief or healing of ischemic ulcers is obtained in 40% to 60% of patients, lasting improvement is not expected because of the diffuse distribution of upper extremity atherosclerotic lesions.[26, 27, 38] An exception would be those with embolism from proximal atherosclerotic ulcerated plaques or high-grade stenoses. Among patients with preoperative arteriograms, best results are obtained in those who have primarily distal occlusive lesions. Additionally, increased digital blood flow in response to sympathetic blockade helps to identify patients likely to respond to surgical sympathectomy.[37, 51] In general, however, progression of both proximal and distal occlusive disease militates against liberal use of sympathectomy for symptomatic arteriosclerotic disease of the upper extremity. In contrast to patients with atherosclerotic occlusive disease, those with Buerger's disease (thromboangiitis obliterans) of the upper extremity appear to benefit significantly from sympathectomy, particularly when it is performed endoscopically.[52]

A small proportion of patients in large series of cervicothoracic sympathectomy have causalgic pain after frostbite. Such patients also commonly have vasomotor instability and a small minority may have residual organic occlusive lesions. Complete and lasting relief of symptoms after sympathectomy has been reported in essentially all such patients with these refractory afflictions of the upper extremity.[26, 40] The small number of reported cases probably reflects the fact that the majority of these patients can be managed nonoperatively and have a geographic (in cold regions) predilection. However, sympathectomy is likely to be successful because the underlying disease process is self-limited in time and discrete in distribution.

Patient Selection Criteria

The presenting symptoms of patients under consideration for upper extremity sympathectomy are usually episodic hand pain, reactive color change, or digital ulceration. Preliminary evaluation of these patients should include a disease-oriented history and examination to identify concomitant peripheral vascular disease, collagen-vascular disease, antecedent trauma (isolated, occupational, or environmental), and evidence of tissue loss. Based on the presumed cause of the pain, further testing may include serologic tests or tissue biopsy to identify collagen-vascular disease as well as upper extremity and digital pressures and plethysmography to define the extent, severity, and level of occlusive disease, if present. Arteriography may be indicated to characterize both proximal and peripheral occlusive disease that is detected by segmental limb pressure measurements among those patients in whom therapeutic intervention is clearly needed.

Current Indications

Conditions most likely to permanently benefit from surgical sympathectomy are causalgia, hyperhidrosis, and Raynaud's disease caused by stable "occupational" digital thrombosis or arterial occlusions (e.g., traumatic subintimal fibrosis, emboli). Initially favorable responses can be expected in selected patients with Raynaud's disease complicated by digital ulcerations, distal atherosclerotic peripheral vascular disease, and Buerger's disease. In the last group, lasting benefit is found only in those who stop smoking. A trial of conservative treatment appropriate for the underlying disease is indicated for all patients. If medical measures (e.g., calcium channel blockers, cessation of smoking) fail, proper patient selection for most indications is improved by use of temporary stellate ganglion blocks to document the effectiveness of upper extremity sympathetic denervation. Among patients with vasospastic disease, abolition of cold-induced digital ischemia as monitored by digital pressures and plethysmography should be demonstrated before permanent sympathetic denervation. Ideally, several blocks should be done. Results indicating that sympathectomy will be efficacious are the following: (1) subjective relief of symptoms for a time period consistent with the duration of action of the local anesthetic, (2) greater than 50% increase in the amplitude of the digital plethysmographic tracing compared with baseline, and (3) abolition of the abnormally prolonged decline in the amplitude of digital plethysmographic tracings after ice water immersion. When systematically applied, these guidelines should improve both early and late results by objectively measuring the effects of sympathetic blockade.

Complications

Injury to the adjacent neurovascular and thoracic structures may occur in a small percentage of patients undergoing thoracic dorsal sympathectomy. Horner's syndrome is the complication of sympathetic denervation that creates the most concern, but its occurrence varies directly with the extent of stellate ganglion resection. When the lower one half is resected, 3% to 36% of patients experience temporary ptosis and miosis, with a 3% to 10% incidence of permanent Horner's syndrome.[26, 53] Even when the stellate ganglion is not completely resected, a 2% to 6% incidence of permanent Horner's syndrome has been reported. It should not occur if only the lower third, or the rami connecting with it, is resected. Significant postoperative neuralgia in the face, shoulder, or chest region occurs in 20% to 40% of patients.[41] The discomfort is temporary, usually lasting from 4 to 8 weeks, and requires only mild analgesics for pain relief. Unless forewarned, however, the patient may be convinced that this new discomfort outweighs the benefits of eliminating the preoperative symptoms. Significant changes in isolated pulmonary function parameters have been reported following T-2 to T-3 ganglionectomy by both intrapleural and extrapleural approaches. These changes consisted of a 15% to 20% reduction in total lung capacity and forced expiratory volume (in 1 second), but they resolved by the sixth postoperative month in all patients.[54] Operative mortality ranges from 0% to 4%, with deaths occurring secondary to the impact of surgical stress on underlying systemic disease rather than the consequences of sympathectomy itself.

Summary

Upper dorsal sympathectomy is best performed through a transaxillary incision with intrapleural or extrapleural visualization of the stellate and upper thoracic ganglia. It may also be performed using endoscopic instruments in selected patients with reduced postoperative pain, morbidity, and hospital stay. Adequate upper extremity sympathetic denervation for most indications is achieved by resection of the T-2 and T-3 ganglia alone. T-4 is also resected if cessation of axillary sweating is desired. The best indications for this procedure are hyperhidrosis, causalgia, and occupational or environmental digital pain syndromes. Less rewarding, but nonetheless occasionally justifiable, indications are Raynaud's disease with digital ulceration, symptomatic arteriosclerotic occlusive disease with primarily distal involvement, Buerger's disease, and distal thromboembolism. All patients should receive maximal appropriate medical therapy and those with vascular disease should have noninvasive definition of their digital perfusion before consideration of sympathectomy. Patient selection is improved by assessing symptomatic and digital perfusion responses to stellate ganglion blocks. Postoperative neuralgia and Horner's syndrome are the most common sequelae that affect patient satisfaction. The former is temporary; the latter can be minimized by restricting the extent of stellate ganglion resection.

LOWER EXTREMITY SYMPATHECTOMY

Primary indications for lumbar sympathectomy are similar to those of dorsal sympathectomy and include causalgia as well as the sequelae of distal arterial emboli and frostbite. Furthermore, a characteristic variant of causalgia after lumbar diskectomy has recently emerged as a valid indication for lumbar sympathetic denervation.[51] In terms of traditional indications, they are limited to identifying patients with "inoperable" arterial occlusive disease who can be reasonably expected to benefit. For the most part, the role of lumbar sympathectomy has become limited to threatened limbs with severe infrapopliteal occlusive disease because the limits of inoperability have been steadily reduced by newer reconstructive techniques. Its role as an adjunctive procedure to arterial reconstructions in patients with poor runoff or hypoplastic proximal or small-caliber distal arteries has been supported by past experience[55, 56] but can rarely be justified if it requires a separate incision, as for infrainguinal bypass. In addition, extended use in Europe of epidural sympathetic blockade has demonstrated its utility in improving early patency of difficult infrapopliteal bypasses.[57] However, this potential role for sympathetic blockade may be more easily fulfilled by perioperative dextran 40 infusions.[58] Thus, lumbar sympathectomy has become a well-standardized technique in search of more vascular indications.

Anatomic Considerations

Sympathetic outflow to the lower extremities originates in spinal cord segments T-10 to L-3. Preganglionic fibers from these segments form extensive synaptic connections in paravertebral ganglia from L-1 to S-3 to innervate the entire lower extremity and pelvic region. Sympathetic outflow to the lower extremity below the knee is primarily conveyed through the L-2 and L-3 ganglia. The remainder of the leg is supplied by ganglia from L-1 to L-4. Variations in the number and location of sympathetic ganglia are most common in the lumbar region, with the majority occurring at the L-1, L-4, and L-5 levels.[59] Overall, three lumbar ganglia are most commonly found, with fusion of the L-1 and L-2 ganglia accounting for the reduced number.[59] Crossover fibers occur in 15% of patients, with most leaving via the L-4 and L-5 ganglia.[60] Important structures adjacent to the lumbar ganglia are the ureter, lumbar vessels, genitofemoral nerve, aorta, and inferior vena cava. Operative injury to the inferior vena cava or its lumbar tributaries during right lumbar ganglionectomy primarily relates to their intimate association. Injuries to all adjacent structures, however, have been reported.[61]

Operative Technique

Access to the lumbar sympathetic chain is best achieved with a midabdominal oblique incision and extraperitoneal separation of the enclosed viscera from the underlying retroperitoneal structures. The ureter and gonadal vessels are reflected forward with the posterior peritoneum to expose the psoas muscle. The lumbar sympathetic chain is located medially over the transverse processes of the lumbar vertebrae, whereas the genitofemoral nerve lies more laterally over the midportion of the psoas (Fig. 19–3). Identification of the ganglia is facilitated by gently stroking or plucking them with the index finger and noting their characteristic "snap." Ganglion numbering is best done by distal dissection with identification of L-3 adjacent to a large (often crossing) lumbar vein or finding the L-4 ganglion in the deepening sulcus between the iliopsoas and pelvic muscles and then proceeding upward from these ganglia. Excision of the L-2 and L-3 ganglia is accomplished by metal clip application and division of all encountered rami interganglionic fibers. Inspection for lumbar vein bleeding and layered closure of the abdominal wall musculature complete the procedure.

Much like upper dorsal sympathectomy, clinically adequate sympathetic denervation is usually accomplished by excision of only two ganglia, L-2 and L-3. More complete resection has been advocated by Imparato[62] to reduce the possibility of incomplete denervation. Inclusion of the L-4 ganglion is considered necessary by some to remove crossover fibers; however, except for proximally located causalgic pain, L-1 ganglionectomy seems to add little and increases the risk of ejaculatory impotence in preclimacteric males.[63]

The high success rate with percutaneous sympathetic blockade using local anesthetic agents has promoted at-

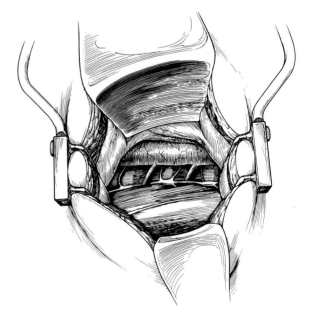

Figure 19–3. Retroperitoneal exposure of the right lumbar sympathetic chain from L-2 to L-4, lying next to the aorta of the transverse processes. The ureter has been retracted upward and the genitofemoral nerve lies laterally on the psoas muscle. As shown between L-3 and L-4, lumbar vessels may cross *in front of* the chain. (From Rutherford RB: Atlas of Vascular Surgery. Philadelphia, WB Saunders, 1993.)

tempts to achieve extended blockade by phenol neurolysis via the same approach. Using fluoroscopic confirmation with contrast injections adjacent to the L-1 to L-3 vertebrae, Sanderson[64] has shown that 80% of first injections are at the desired location. Second injections yielded complete lumbar sympathetic neurolysis in 90% of patients as determined by sudomotor and foot temperature testing. Although their successful percutaneous neurolysis rate was only 72%, Walsh and colleagues[65] demonstrated that the duration of sympathectomy using 10% phenol was identical to that of surgical denervation. Among 31 patients with successful neurolysis, 19 (61%) patients achieved symptomatic relief with signifcant increases in foot blood flow and skin temperature.

Experience with phenol lumbar sympathectomy in the United States is being gained but has not been convincing. Initial impressions are that this procedure produces less complete and less durable blockade than does surgical sympathectomy. Efforts to improve blockade by use of radiofrequency-heated probes with precision localization are still ongoing but to date this technique also appears to produce less complete or less durable sympathetic denervation.[66] Holiday and colleagues[67] compared surgical versus chemical sympathectomy in 70 patients with 76 limbs with chronic critical ischemia. Early success was significantly better for surgical sympathectomy (40% vs. 18%; $P = .01$). Late limb salvage rates were not statistically significantly different, probably because other factors affecting outcome reduced this advantage. Importantly, there was no mortality and morbidity was minimal. Further improvements in this approach may offer an alternative means of producing lasting lumbar sympathetic denervation without the morbidity (albeit now low) of a surgical procedure. However, until these techniques produce a reliably complete and lasting sympathetic denervation, they carry the disadvantage of seriously compromising the surgical procedure that can achieve this goal. Surgeons who have tried to perform lumbar sympathectomy through the scar and inflammatory tissue left in the wake of such attempts, including even too many lumbar anesthetic blocks, will attest to this.

As with dorsal sympathectomy, these considerations become even more important as endoscopic techniques come into play. These techniques are being applied to lumbar sympathectomy, although a literature review mainly shows initial experiences of only three to eight cases. Transperitoneal techniques appear to be yielding to a retroperitoneal approach using specially designed balloons inserted to dissect open the retroperitoneal space. This approach is understandably easier and safer on the left than on the right side, where the inferior vena cava overlies the sympathetic ganglia chain.

Results

Although Raynaud's disease has been reported to affect the lower extremities, use of lumbar sympathectomy for this condition has been limited in published reports. Application for frostbite is more common in colder climates. Comparison of sympathectomy outcomes with results of arterial

reconstruction for distal occlusive disease is difficult because prospective studies have not been done and reported patient groups are not comparable. Comparisons with nonoperative treatment or other nonreconstructive procedures (e.g., prostanoids, hyperbaric oxygen, or epidural spinal cord stimulation) have not been reported, but all studies report improvement in a minority of patients.[68] Review of later series allows some recommendations to be made because patient groups have been more uniformly categorized.

Ischemic Rest Pain

Critical assessment of the influence of lumbar sympathectomy on limb-threatening ischemia has previously been hampered by group variations in arteriographic extent of occlusive disease, criteria for determining operability, and magnitude of distal perfusion. Among patients with atherosclerotic arterial occlusions and Buerger's disease, primary indications for lumbar sympathectomy are limited to those who have inoperable disease complicated by rest pain or tissue loss. Experimental evidence indicates that muscular and nutrient blood flow are *not* significantly increased by sympathetic denervation of ischemic limbs. Clinical experience has shown, however, that nearly 80% of patients with an ankle-brachial index greater than 0.3, no evidence of neuropathy, and limited tissue loss obtain relief of their ischemic symptoms.[69] Although the criterion of an ankle-brachial index greater than 0.3 may seem arbitrary, it represents a marginal level of perfusion that may suffice to achieve limb salvage if slightly improved. Despite the known influence of sympathectomy on pain transmission that is independent of its circulatory effects, the selection criteria above define conditions in which sympathectomy results in sufficient improvement to prevent ischemic progression.

The primary importance of adequate arterial inflow, as determined by segmental limb pressure, was first recognized by Yao and Bergan.[70] In their retrospective review of unselected patients undergoing lumbar sympathectomy, no response was obtained in 90% of limbs with an ankle-brachial index less than 0.3. Additionally, Kim and colleagues[71] first noted the concomitant importance of intact sympathetic innervation by observing that diabetics with neuropathy rarely responded to sympathectomy. The authors theorized that many diabetics undergo "autosympathectomy" secondary to associated neuropathy; therefore, surgical sympathetic denervation in such patients could not further decrease sympathetic vascular tone in the affected extremity. Indirect confirmation of this theory was provided by histologic studies showing no difference in the number of periarterial sympathetic fibers in diabetics with and without previous lumbar sympathectomy.[72]

The increased blood flow requirements needed to heal deep ulcers or large areas of skin necrosis *cannot* be met by the small increases in perfusion afforded by sympathectomy. Tissue necrosis in most instances reflects a failure of both arterial inflow and local microcirculation that requires supranormal blood flow to meet the increased metabolic demands of healing. This tenet is indirectly supported by radionucleotide studies showing that small, uninfected lesions require at least a twofold increase in perfusion.[73] Large areas of tissue necrosis with infection therefore require perfusion increases that exceed the amount provided by sympathectomy alone. Thus, lumbar sympathectomy at best restores the delicate balance between blood flow supply and demand in essentially intact but chronically ischemic limbs.

Modern series favoring use of lumbar sympathectomy for rest pain in patients with inoperable arterial disease report symptomatic relief in 47% to 71% of unselected patients, with acute limb salvage rates of 60% to 94%.[16–18, 74] Best results were obtained by Perrson and colleagues[69] among 37 patients who had an ankle-brachial index greater than 0.3, no evidence of neuropathy, and limited tissue necrosis; 78% of this group enjoyed long-term relief of ischemic rest pain, and only 11% required amputation. Worst results were noted by Fulton and Blakely[75] among 17 unselected patients undergoing sympathectomy; only 6% of this group obtained relief, whereas 70% required early amputation. Although provocative, this latter older experience simply shows that disappointing results can be expected when limb-threatening ischemia is unselectively treated by sympathetic denervation.

Tissue Loss

Assessment of the results of lumbar sympathectomy for distal ischemic ulceration or gangrene is subject to the same limitations described for rest pain. Additionally, wound management technique is a variable requiring consideration when determining the efficacy of sympathectomy. Less impressive results than for rest pain are generally noted, with 35% to 62% of patients showing complete initial healing of the ischemic lesions or arrest of gangrene progression. In addition, both early and ultimate amputation rates were higher than the rest-pain group, with a range of 27% to 38%.[16–18, 74] Best results were again reported by Perrson and colleagues[69] among 22 patients who had adequate inflow, absent neuropathy, and no evidence of subcutaneous infection, 77% had ulcer healing and only 22% required ultimate amputation. Among patients who showed no healing, sympathectomy did not improve the amputation level required. Johnson and colleagues,[76] in 1998, reported a long-term follow-up of 10 patients with pedal ischemic necrosis, correlating successful outcome (healing and avoiding amputation) with perioperative cutaneous oxygen levels. The mean postoperative *increase* in partial pressure of capillary oxygen (Pco_2) in patients with successful outcome was 29 mm Hg compared with 5 mm Hg in those in whom sympathectomy failed to provide healing. Success was also predictable in those whose Pco_2 increased more than 20 mm Hg in response to changing limb position from the level to the dependent position.

Adjunct for Lower Extremity Arterial Reconstruction

The role of the sympathetic nervous system in mediating vasoconstrictor responses is well known; however, assessing the adjunctive utility of sympathetic denervation with arterial reconstruction has only been studied well in patients undergoing aortofemoral bypass. When added to proximal vascular reconstruction, sympathectomy increased total extremity blood flow by a factor of 1.55, decreased vascular resistance in the foot, and reduced the incidence of early graft thrombosis.[77–79] Long-term follow-up, however, disclosed no significant difference in the need for further infrainguinal reconstructive surgery, amputation rate, or incidence of graft limb thrombosis.

European evaluation of blood flow through femoropopliteal bypass grafts in the early postoperative period showed greater flow and lower early graft thrombosis rates in limbs subjected to surgical or chemical sympathetic denervation.[57, 80] Among patients with lumbar epidural anesthesia, Sandmann and colleagues[57] implanted electromagnetic flowmeters beyond the distal popliteal anastomosis and noted consistently higher flows than with conventional morphine analgesia. Although maximal blood flow peaked on the second postoperative day in both treatment groups, early graft thromboses were detected in the morphine control group within 4 days of operation. Similar enhancement of patency in small arterial anastomoses was noted by Casten and colleagues[81] in assessing the effect of lumbar sympathectomy in an arterial trauma model. Although early augmentation of graft flow seems advantageous, the chronic effects of sympathectomy on graft patency remain to be determined for infrainguinal reconstruction. The morbidity of an additional abdominal procedure, particularly a retroperitoneal dissection in a heparinized patient, seems greater than the potential benefits of high early graft patency. The use of perioperative dextran 40 infusion increases the early patency rate of difficult distal bypasses by threefold and may prove more practical than sympathectomy.[58]

Current Indications

Primary indications for lumbar sympathectomy are causalgia of any cause (including frostbite), symptomatic distal arterial emboli, and, in selected patients, inoperable distal arterial occlusive disease secondary to arteriosclerosis or Buerger's disease. Current determinations of inoperability differ with local expertise and availability of autogenous saphenous vein for infrapopliteal bypass grafting. In the rare circumstance when such revascularization procedures are not feasible or are inadvisable because of inadequate runoff or technical limitations, lumbar sympathectomy may be considered for patients with rest pain or ischemic ulceration who meet the following criteria: (1) ankle-brachial index greater than 0.3, (2) superficial tissue necrosis (confined to the forefoot or digits), (3) absent neuropathy on physical examination, (4) symptomatic relief or increased plethysmographic amplitude after lumbar sympathetic blockade, and (5) acceptable surgical risk for abdominal operation. Lumbar sympathectomy may also be used as an adjunct to improve early graft patency for more distal reconstructive procedures in patients with poor runoff or hypoplastic vessels, but other methods are preferable (e.g., dextran 40). The probability of the indications for sympa-

Stratification of Indications for Sympathectomy According to the Probability of Achieving Lasting Symptomatic Relief

INDICATION	DORSAL SYMPATHECTOMY	LUMBAR SYMPATHECTOMY
Best	Hyperhidrosis Causalgia Frostbite sequelae Raynaud's phenomenon caused by stable arterial occlusions (e.g., traumatic subintimal fibrosis, distal emboli)	Causalgia Frostbite sequelae Stable, small arterial occlusions (e.g., distal Buerger's atherosclerosis, arterial emboli) with Raynaud's or rest pain
Acceptable	Raynaud's syndrome with digital ulcerations or Distal arterial occlusions Buerger's disease	Inoperable, Buerger's or atherosclerotic arterial occlusions with limited tissue loss Adjunctive to aortofemoral arterial reconstruction
Contraindications	Uncomplicated Raynaud's disease	Claudication Diabetes with neuropathy

thectomy receiving lasting benefit are summarized for both dorsal and lumbar sympathectomy in Table 19–1.

Complications

The major morbidity of lumbar sympathectomy is preventable injury to adjacent structures (lumbar veins, aorta, inferior vena cava, and ureter). Attention to detail and adequate exposure render such injuries infrequent. Early recovery of sympathetic vascular tone ("fifth day phenomenon") and postoperative neuralgia occur in 20% to 50% of patients.[41, 63] This latter syndrome is self-limited and well treated with minor analgesics and rarely causes chronic morbidity. Similar lower extremity hyperesthetic states develop after phenol neurolysis but may last much longer. In patients with severe peripheral vascular disease, incomplete sympathectomy is difficult to distinguish clinically from progression of the underlying occlusive process. Mortality rates of 0% to 4% have been reported, with cardiac and pulmonary deterioration after operation the most common cause of death. Most of the deaths were reported in earlier studies. Proper perioperative monitoring should minimize patient deaths.

Summary

Lumbar sympathectomy currently has a limited role in the treatment of limb-threatening ischemia because direct revascularization techniques yield more consistent and far better results. L-2 and L-3 ganglionectomy provides sufficient denervation for most indications; L-4 resection is added when ablation of crossover innervation is desired. Best results are obtained when patients are selected according to threshold inflow criteria, absent neuropathy, limited or absent tissue necrosis, and favorable response to preoperative lumbar sympathetic blockade. Lumbar sympathectomy is indicated for truly operable occlusive disease complicated by rest pain or minor tissue loss and for causalgia. The most common complications of lumbar sympathectomy are temporary neuralgia and inadequate clinical improvement. Careful selection using the suggested criteria minimizes the latter.

References

1. Ewing M: The history of lumbar sympathectomy. Surgery 70:791–795, 1971.
2. Simeone FA: The lumbar sympathetic. Anatomy and surgical implications. Acta Chir Belg 76:17–26, 1977.
3. Ross JP: Surgery of the Sympathetic Nervous System. London, Bailliere, Tindall & Cox, 1958.
4. Cronenwett JL, Lindenauer SM: Hemodynamic effects of sympathectomy in ischemic canine hind limbs. Surgery 87:417–424, 1980.
5. Cronenwett JL, Zelenock GB, Whitehouse W Jr, et al: The effect of sympathetic innervation on canine muscle and skin blood flow. Arch Surg 118:420–424, 1983.
6. Simeone FA: Intravascular pressure, vascular tone and sympathectomy. [Presidential address, 16th Annual Meeting of Society for Vascular Surgery, Chicago, June 24, 1962.] Surgery 53:1, 1963.
7. Beran RD, Tsuru H: Functional and structural changes in rabbit ear artery after sympathetic denervation. Circ Res 49:478–485, 1981.
8. Bobik A, Anderson WP: Influence of sympathectomy on alpha 2 adrenoreceptor binding sites in canine blood vessels. Life Sci 33:331–336, 1983.
9. Barcroft H, Swan HJC: Sympathetic Control of Human Blood Vessels. London, Edward Arnold, 1952.
10. Petten CV, Roberts WJ, Rhodes DL: Behavioral test of tolerance for aversive mechanical stimuli in sympathectomized cats. Pain 15:177–189, 1983.
11. Courbier R, Reggi M, Jansserau JM: Evaluation of effectiveness of lumbar sympathectomy by non-invasive diagnostic techniques. J Cardiovasc Surg (Torino) 20:333–337, 1979.
12. Loh L, Nathan PW: Painful peripheral states and sympathetic blocks. J Neurol Neurosurg Psychiatry 41:664–671, 1978.
13. Melzack R, Wall PD: Pain mechanisms: A new theory. Science 150:971–979, 1965.
14. Moore WS, Hall AD: Effects of lumbar sympathectomy on skin capillary blood flow in arterial occlusive disease. J Surg Res 14:151–160, 1973.
15. Perry MO, Horton J: Muscle and subcutaneous oxygen tension: Measurements by mass spectrometry after sympathectomy. Arch Surg 113:176–178, 1978.
16. Collins GJ, Rich NM, Clagett GP, et al: Clinical results of lumbar sympathectomy. Am Surg 47:31–35, 1981.
17. Haimovici H, Steinman C, Karson IH: Evaluation of lumbar sympathectomy: Advanced occlusive arterial disease. Arch Surg 89:1089–1095, 1964.

18. Szilagyi DE, Smith RF, Scarpella JR, et al: Lumbar sympathectomy: Current role in the treatment of arteriosclerotic occlusive disease. Arch Surg 95:753–761, 1967.
19. Holcroft JW, Vassar MJ: Prostaglandins and their analogues: Experience in healing ischemic ulcers. Semin Vasc Surg 4:221–226, 1991.
20. Rutherford RB, Valenta J: Extremity blood flow and distribution: The effects of arterial occlusive, sympathectomy and exercise. Surgery 69:332–338, 1971.
21. Lindenauer SM, Cronenwett JL: What is the place of lumbar sympathectomy? Br J Surg 69(Suppl):532–533, 1982.
22. Enjalbert A: Effect of lumbar sympathectomy on the muscles. J Cardiovasc Surg (Torino) 20:295–300, 1979.
23. Owens JC: Indications for lumbar sympathectomy. In Dale WA (ed): The Management of Arterial Occlusive Disease. St Louis, Mosby–Year Book, 1971.
24. Dalessandri KM, Carson SN, Tillman P, et al: Effect of lumbar sympathectomy in distal arterial obstruction. Arch Surg 228:1157–1160, 1983.
25. Ludbrook J: Collateral arterial resistance in the human lower limbs. J Surg Res 6:423, 1966.
26. Welch E, Geary J: Current status of thoracic dorsal sympathectomy. J Vasc Surg 1:202–214, 1984.
27. Porter JM, Rivers SP, Anderson CJ, et al: Evaluation and management of patients with Raynaud's syndrome. Am J Surg 142:183–187, 1981.
28. Kuntz A: Distribution of the sympathetic rami to the brachial plexus: Its relation to sympathectomy affecting the upper extremity. Arch Surg 15:871–877, 1927.
29. Ray BS: Sympathectomy of the upper extremity: Evaluation of surgical methods. J Neurosurg 10:624–633, 1953.
30. Roos DB: Sympathectomy for the upper extremities. In Rutherford RB (ed): Vascular Surgery. Philadelphia, WB Saunders, 1984.
31. Roos DB: Transaxillary extrapleural thoracic sympathectomy. In Bergen JJ, Yao JST (eds): Operative Techniques in Vascular Surgery. New York, Grune & Stratton, 1980.
32. Atkins HJB: Preaxillary approach to the stellate and upper thoracic sympathetic ganglia. Lancet 2:1152, 1949.
33. Telford ED: The technic of sympathectomy. Br J Surg 23:448–459, 1935.
34. Ahn SS, Machleder HI, Concepcion B, Moore WS: Thoracoscopic cervicodorsal sympathectomy: Preliminary results. J Vasc Surg 20:511–519, 1994.
35. Josephs LG, Menzoian JO: Technical considerations in endoscopic cervicothoracic sympathectomy. Arch Surg 131:355–359, 1996.
36. Owens JC: Causalgia. Am Surg 23:636–640, 1957.
37. Beurger R, Smit R: Transaxillary sympathectomy (T2 to T4) for relief of vasospastic/sympathetic pain of upper extremities. Surgery 89:764–769, 1981.
38. Welling RE, Cranley JJ, Krause RJ, et al: Obliterative arterial disease of the upper extremity. Arch Surg 116:1593–1596, 1981.
39. Thompson JE: The diagnosis and management of post-traumatic pain syndromes (causalgia). Aust N Z J Surg 49:299–304, 1979.
40. Kirtley JA, Riddell DH, Stoney WS, et al: Cervicothoracic sympathectomy in neurovascular abnormalities of the upper extremity. Experience in 76 patients with 104 sympathectomies. Ann Surg 165:869–879, 1967.
41. Mockus M, Rutherford RB, Rosales C: Sympathectomy for causalgia: Patient selection and long-term results. Arch Surg 122:668–672, 1987.
42. Porter JM: Raynaud's syndrome and associated vasospastic conditions of the extremities. In Rutherford RB (ed): Vascular Surgery. Philadelphia, WB Saunders, 1984.
43. Baddely RM: The place of upper dorsal sympathectomy in the treatment of primary Raynaud's disease. Br J Surg 54:426–443, 1965.
44. Gifford EW Jr, Hines EA Jr, Craig VM: Sympathectomy for Raynaud's phenomenon: Followup study of 70 women with Raynaud's disease and 54 women with secondary Raynaud's phenomenon. Circulation 17:5–13, 1958.
45. Linder F, Jenal G, Assmus H: Axillary transpleural sympathectomy: Indication, technique and results. World J Surg 7:437–439, 1983.
46. Conn J Jr, Bergan JJ, Bell JL: Hypothenar hammer syndrome: Posttraumatic digital ischemia. Surgery 68:1122–1127, 1970.
47. Christophers AJ: Occupational aspects of Raynaud's disease: A critical historical survey. Med J Aust 2:730–733, 1972.
48. Montorsi W, Ghringhelli C, Annoni F: Indications and results of surgical treatment in Raynaud's phenomenon. J Cardiovasc Surg (Torino) 21:203–210, 1980.

49. Zweifler AJ, Trinkaus P: Occlusive digital artery disease in patients with Raynaud's phenomenon. Am J Med 77:995–1001, 1984.
50. Smith CR, Rodeffer RJ: Raynaud's phenomenon: Pathophysiologic features and treatment with calcium-channel blockers. Am J Cardiol 55:154B–157B, 1985.
51. Owens JG: Complications of sympathectomy. In Beebe HG (ed): Complications in Vascular Surgery. Philadelphia, JB Lippincott, 1973.
52. Komori K, Kowasaki K, Okasaki J, et al: Thoracoscopic sympathectomy for Buerger's disease of the upper extremities. J Vasc Surg 22:344–346, 1995.
53. Romeno A, Kurchin A, Rudich R, et al: Ocular manifestations after upper dorsal sympathectomy. Ann Ophthalmol 2:1083–1086, 1979.
54. Molno M, Shemesh E, Gordon D, et al: Pulmonary function abnormalities after upper dorsal sympathectomy: A comparison between the supraclavicular and transaxillary approaches. Chest 77:651–655, 1980.
55. DeLaurentis DA, Friedmann P, Wolferth CC Jr, et al: Atherosclerosis and the hypoplastic aortoiliac system. Surgery 83:27–37, 1978.
56. Satiani B, Liapis CD, Hayes JP, et al: Prospective randomized study of concomitant lumbar sympathectomy with aortoiliac reconstruction. Am J Surg 143:755–760, 1982.
57. Sandmann W, Kremer K, Wust H, et al: Postoperative control of blood flow in arterial surgery and results of electromagnetic blood flow measurement. Thorac Cardiovasc Surg 25:427–434, 1977.
58. Rutherford RB, Jones DN, Bergentz SE, et al: The efficacy of dextran-40 preventing early post-operative thrombosis following difficult lower extremity bypass. J Vasc Surg 1:765–773, 1984.
59. Yeager GH, Cowley RA: Anatomical observations on the lumbar sympathetics with evaluation of sympathectomies in organic peripheral vascular disease. Ann Surg 127:953–967, 1948.
60. Callow AD, Simeone FA: The Grimonster Symposium on the occasion of the 50th anniversary of the first lumbar sympathectomy. Arch Surg 113:295, 1978.
61. Rutherford RB: Complications of sympathectomy. In Towne JB, Bernhard VM (eds): Complications in Vascular Surgery, 2nd ed. New York, Grune & Stratton, 1984.
62. Imparato AM: Lumbar sympathectomy: Role in the treatment of occlusive arterial disease in the lower extremities. Surg Clin North Am 59:719–735, 1979.
63. Rutherford RB: Lumbar sympathectomy: Indications and technique. In Rutherford RB (ed): Vascular Surgery. Philadelphia, WB Saunders, 1984.
64. Sanderson CJ: Chemical lumbar sympathectomy with radiologic assessment. Ann R Coll Surg Engl 63:420–422, 1981.
65. Walsh JA, Glynn CJ, Cousins MJ, et al: Blood flow, sympathetic activity and pain relief following lumbar sympathetic blockade and surgical sympathectomy. Anesth Intensive Care 13:18–24, 1984.
66. Noe CE, Haynsworth RF Jr: Lumbar radiofrequency sympatholysis. J Vasc Surg 17:801–806, 1993.
67. Holiday FA, Barendregt WB, Slappendel R, et al: Lumbar sympathectomy in chronic critical ischema: Surgical, chemical, not at all? Cardiovasc Surg 7:200–202, 1999.
68. Dormandy J, Andreani D, Bell P, et al: Second European consensus document of chronic critical ischemia. Circulation 84(Suppl 5):IV-1–IV-26, 1991.
69. Persson AV, Anderson L, Rodberg FT Jr: Selection of patients for lumbar sympathectomy. Surg Clin North Am 65:393–403, 1985.
70. Yao JST, Bergan JJ: Predictability of vascular reactivity relative to sympathetic ablation. Arch Surg 107:676–681, 1973.
71. Kim GE, Igrahim IM, Imparato AM: Lumbar sympathectomy in end-stage arterial occlusive disease. Ann Surg 183:157–160, 1976.
72. Grove JH, Bauman FG, Riles TS, et al: Effect of surgical lumbar sympathectomy on innervation of arterioles in the lower limbs of patients with diabetes. Surg Gynecol Obstet 153:39–41, 1981.
73. Siegal ME, William GM, Giargiana FA Jr, et al: A useful objective criterion for determining the healing potential of an ischemic ulcer. J Nucl Med 21:993–998, 1975.
74. Walker PM, Johnston KW: Predicting the success of a sympathectomy: A prospective study using discriminant function and multiple regression analysis. Surgery 87:216–221, 1980.
75. Fulton RL, Blakely WR: Lumbar sympathectomy: A procedure of questionable value in the treatment of arteriosclerosis obliterans of the legs. Am J Surg 116:735–744, 1968.
76. Johnson WC, Watkins MT, Baldwin D, Hamilton J: Foot TcPO₂ re-

sponse to lumbar sympathectomy in patients with focal ischemic necrosis. Ann Vasc Surg 1998; 12:70–74, 1998.

77. Barnes RW, Baker WH, Shanik G, et al: Value of concomitant sympathectomy in aortoiliac reconstruction: Results of a prospective, randomized study. Arch Surg 112:1325–1330, 1977.

78. Collins GJ Jr, Rich HM, Anderson CA, et al: Acute hemodynamic effects of lumbar sympathectomy. Am J Surg 136:714–718, 1978.

79. Shanik GD, Ford J, Hayes AC, et al: Pedal vasomotor tone following

aortofemoral reconstructions: A randomized study of concomitant lumbar sympathectomy. Ann Surg 183:136–138, 1976.

80. Faenza A, Splare R, Lapilli A, et al: Clinical results of lumbar sympathectomy alone or as a complement to direct arterial surgery. Acta Chir Belg 76:101–107, 1977.

81. Casten DF, Sadler AH, Furman D: An experimental study of the effect of sympathectomy on patency of small blood vessel anastomoses. Surg Gynecol Obstet 115:462–466, 1962.

Questions

1. All of the following statements regarding the effects of sympathetic denervation are true except
   (a) increased extremity blood flow is primarily distributed through cutaneous arteriovenous anastomosis flow
   (b) partial recovery of resting vasomotor tone is mediated by increased sensitivity of extrasynaptic α_2 receptors to exogenous norepinephrine
   (c) sympathectomy produces maximal vasodilatation in an ischemic extremity 50% greater than that produced by local metabolic influences
   (d) sympathectomy is believed to enhance pain tolerance by decreasing tissue concentrations of norepinephrine and by reducing spinal transmission of impulses arising from noxious stimuli to peripheral nerves

2. Upper extremity sympathectomy produces worthwhile benefit for all of the following conditions except
   (a) causalgia
   (b) hyperhidrosis
   (c) distal emboli with Raynaud's phenomenon
   (d) Raynaud's syndrome caused by scleroderma

3. Horner's syndrome is most likely to follow
   (a) resection of T-2 and T-3 ganglia only
   (b) complete resection of the stellate ganglion
   (c) resection of the lower one third of the stellate ganglion
   (d) division of Kuntz's nerve

4. Which of the following techniques of thoracodorsal sympathectomy poses the greatest risk of injury to the phrenic nerve?
   (a) supraclavicular approach
   (b) axillary transthoracic approach
   (c) posterior approach
   (d) axillary extrapleural approach
   (e) thoracoscopic approach

5. Which of the following statements concerning Raynaud's disease secondary to nonocclusive vasospasm is true?
   (a) nearly all patients have recognizable signs of an associated collagen-vascular disease
   (b) symptom relief by surgical sympathectomy is ultimately required by the majority
   (c) up to 50% of patients develop signs of underlying collagen-vascular disease within 6 months of follow-up
   (d) the natural history follows a benign course with fewer than 50% of patients manifesting the stigmas of an associated collagen-vascular disease over 5 years of observation

6. Which is the most frequent complication following T-2, T-3, and T-4 sympathetic ganglionectomy for severe hyperhidrosis?
   (a) permanent Horner's syndrome
   (b) postoperative neuralgia
   (c) rebound vasospasm with cold sensitivity
   (d) recurrent hyperhidrosis

7. Which of the following criteria should be met before performing a lumbar sympathectomy in a diabetic patient with toe ulceration due to inoperable infrapopliteal arterial occlusive disease?
   (a) ankle-brachial index less than 0.3
   (b) ankle-brachial index greater than 0.3
   (c) absent neuropathy
   (d) limited tissue loss without associated infection

8. Which one of the following is not an indication for sympathectomy?
   (a) Raynaud's phenomenon after emboli to small vessels supplying the hand
   (b) intermittent claudication of the foot due to infrapopliteal occlusive disease
   (c) rest pain in a patient with inoperable arterial occlusions
   (d) post-frostbite causalgia

9. Crossover preganglionic sympathetic fibers most commonly exit the spinal axis at what level?
   (a) T-10 and L-1
   (b) L-2 and L-3
   (c) L-4 and L-5
   (d) S-1

10. The incidence of early postoperative thrombosis of distal bypass grafts has been demonstrably reduced by which of the following adjunctive measures?
    (a) dextran 40 infusions
    (b) temporary epidural block
    (c) lumbar sympathectomy
    (d) antiplatelet drugs

Answers

1. c   2. d   3. b   4. a   5. d   6. b   7. b, c, d   8. b   9. c   10. a, c, d

20

Thrombolytic Therapy for Vascular Disease

Niren Angle, Fernando E. Kafie, and William J. Quiñones-Baldrich

Thrombolytic therapy is an important modality in the current treatment of patients with peripheral vascular disease. Information is available from randomized clinical trials that compare thrombolytic therapy with traditional surgical options and thus provide important guidelines to patient selection. As a therapeutic intervention, lytic therapy may be the best alternative in certain clinical situations. On the other hand, it frequently serves as an adjunct to the overall care of patients with thrombotic complications of peripheral vascular disease.

The purpose of this chapter is to provide the reader with basic understanding of the fibrinolytic system and available agents. This information translates into guidelines that will help clinicians select patients who may benefit from thrombolytic therapy. Methods, dosages, complications, and new promising areas are discussed.

HISTORY

The fluidity of blood post mortem is an observation that dates to the Hippocratic school in the 4th century BC.[1] Almost 2000 years later, it was rediscovered by the Italian anatomist Malpighi.[2] In 1761, Morgagni[3] noted that blood does not retain its liquid state after death but frequently forms clots. This is followed by partial or complete reliquefaction.

In 1906, Morawitz[4] observed that postmortem blood destroyed fibrinogen and fibrin in normal blood. Thus, the presence of an active fibrinolysin was postulated. The term *fibrinolysis* had been coined by Dastre in 1893[5] to describe the disappearance of fibrin in unclottable blood obtained from dogs subjected to repeated hemorrhage. From the latter part of the 19th century until the present, intense investigation in this field has been attempted to elucidate the complex and vital functions of the fibrinolytic system. Its physiology, components, activators, and inhibitors are only partially understood. The role of the fibrinolytic system from the homeostatic point of view is fully appreciated.

Its potential, from the therapeutic standpoint, has emerged in the last few decades. Furthermore, results from prospective clinical trials are now available, providing guidelines to patient selection and therapy. Clearly, precise control of this system to favor resolution of a thrombotic process is on the frontier of clinical medicine. For the vascular specialist, this represents one of the most promising therapeutic modalities. Unfortunately, currently available agents lack the precise control necessary to avoid complications inherent to an overactive fibrinolytic system. Even so, in this era, thrombolytic therapy can be successfully used and, in some instances, is the preferential treatment.

THE FIBRINOLYTIC SYSTEM

The complex and intricate relationships between all components of the fibrinolytic system are not fully understood. Much progress has been made mostly owing to increased interest and recognition of the importance of the fibrinolytic system, both as a homeostatic system and as a therapeutic alternative. The concept of dynamic equilibrium was proposed by Astrup in 1958.[6] In a delicate balance, fibrinolysis breaks down fibrin that is continuously being deposited throughout the cardiovascular system. This is the result of limited activation of the coagulation system. This baseline fibrinolytic activity is probably under local and central control mechanisms. The feedback loop that prevents systemic fibrinolysis involves both inhibitors at the activator level and specific inhibitors of the proteolytic enzyme plasmin.

The final common pathway in the fibrinolytic system is the conversion of the proenzyme plasminogen to the active enzyme plasmin. Plasminogen is a glycoprotein produced by the liver. Full-sized plasminogen can be divided into a heavy N-terminal region that consists of five homologous but distinct triple disulfide-bonded domains (kringles) fused to a lighter catalytic C-terminal domain. At least four forms occur in plasma, based on variation of the N-terminal and the degree of glycosylation. The two main forms are labeled Glu-plasminogen and Lys-plasminogen.[7] Glu-plasminogen contains glutamic acid and exists in high concentrations in plasma. Lys-plasminogen, containing mostly lysin in the N-terminal, results from limited proteolysis of the Glu form, has a shorter half-life, and is found in higher concentrations in thrombus, most likely secondary to its higher affinity for fibrin.[8] A schematic view of the fibrinolytic system is presented in Figure 20–1.

The kringle portion of plasminogen is a nonprotease, or heavy chain, consisting of five homologous domains. These domains exhibit a high degree of sequence homology with each other and with domains found in prothrombin, (t-PA), urinary plasminogen activator, and factor XII. Kringle-4 shares homology with apolipoprotein A. The function of these kringles is thought to be of paramount importance in the binding of plasminogen and plasmin to fibrin, α_2-antiplasmin, and other macromolecules.[9, 10] In addition, the kringle portion of plasminogen has been implicated in mediating neutrophil adherence to endothelial cells.[11] On binding, conformational changes occur that transform a closed structure into an open structure. ϵ-Aminocaproic acid (EACA) and tranexamic acid will induce this change from the closed structure to the open structure. This change renders this plasminogen far more readily cleaved to the active enzyme plasmin by plasminogen activators. The open conformation also binds more readily to exposed lysine residues on the fibrin's surface. Concentrations of lysine analogs, such as tranexamic acid and aminocaproic acid, that actually promote the more active open conformation of Glu-plasminogen, will also prevent its binding to fibrin and therefore exhibit their antifibrinolytic effect.[12]

The primary substrates for the proteolytic activity of plasmin in circulation are fibrinogen and fibrin. Circulating fibrinogen is composed of three polypeptide chains known as the α, β, and γ chains. These chains are bonded together by disulfide bonds, which, in addition, are linked to a second identical chain, thus making fibrinogen a dimer of trimers. Thrombin, the common pathway of the coagulation cascade, removes several amino acid peptides from the end terminal of the α chain, the β chain (fibrinopeptide B), to form fibrin. As new sites are exposed, staggered polymerization is initiated.[7] Through catalysis by factor XIIIa, the domains are brought together and chemically cross-linked. Plasmin catalyzes the hydrolysis of these bonds, producing peptides that can be assayed in circulation. Specifically, those produced after the cleavage of fibrinogen consist of truncated polypeptides collectively known as X fragments. X fragments can be incorporated in both newly forming and existing thrombi, causing them to be more fragile. This has been proposed as an explanation of why fewer bleeding complications have not been observed with fibrin-specific fibrinolytic agents such as t-PA, compared with nonspecific agents. With t-PA being such a potent fibrinolytic activator, the accumulation of these X fragments may make existing thrombi more susceptible to its fibrinolytic action. Several fragments are specifically produced by the action of plasmin on fibrin, as opposed to fibrinogen. Unique fragments such as D dimers can be assayed, documenting fibrinolysis, as opposed to fibrinogenolysis.[13]

Plasmin is a relatively nonspecific protease and thus can hydrolyze many proteins found in plasma and extracellular spaces. Known targets of plasmin are factors V, VIII, and von Willebrand's factor.[1] Prothrombotic activity can be shown with the initial administration of fibrinolytic agents

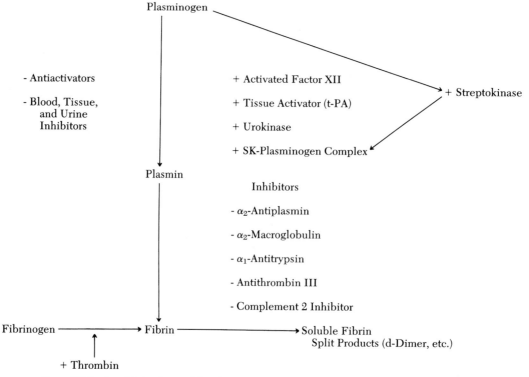

Figure 20–1. Simplified scheme of the fibrinolytic system with endogenous and exogenous activators.

(specifically, t-PA and streptokinase, which may relate to the release of fibrinopeptide A). Plasminogen can also cause the release of kinin from high-molecular-weight kininogen. It can also directly and indirectly activate prekallikrein, again inducing kinin formation.[14, 15] Plasmin can also attack protein components of basement membrane, as well as other active proteases within the matrix. These include fibronectin, collagen, and laminin.[7]

Activation of factor XII by various stimuli results in initiation of the coagulation cascade, conversion of prekallikrein to kallikrein and kinin (inflammatory response), and formation of plasmin from plasminogen. This intrinsic mechanism of activation is complemented by a second intrinsic pathway, not dependent on factor XII. The main pathway for plasminogen activation is known as the extrinsic system. Two activators are recognized in humans: urokinase-type plasminogen activator (u-PA) and t-PA. Their physiologic activity is controlled by inhibitors, mostly plasminogen activator inhibitor (PAI) type 1 (PAI-1) and PAI-3. These inhibitors control the activity of the activators in plasma and possibly at the cellular level. PAI-1 is synthesized in the liver and vascular endothelial cells and is normally present in trace amounts in plasma. When pharmacologic doses of these agents are administered, the inhibitor activity is suppressed. It is estimated that one third to one half of the initial pharmacologic dose of urokinase, for example, becomes inactivated shortly after administration.[11] Once plasminogen has been converted to plasmin, inhibitors of plasmin come into play. The main physiologic inhibitor of plasmin is α_2-antiplasmin. This protease inhibitor is a single-chain glycoprotein that inhibits plasminogen in two steps: a fast reversible binding step, followed by the formation of a covalent complex involving the active site of plasmin.[7] The half-life of this complex is approximately 12 hours.[16] Other inhibitors of plasmin include α_2-macroglobulin, protease nexin, and aprotinin. Protease nexin is a broad-spectrum inhibitor of serine proteinases, and inhibits, among others, trypsin, thrombin, urokinase, plasmin, and one- or two-chain t-PA. Once bound, these proteases are internalized via nexin receptors on the cell surface and rapidly degraded.[17] Aprotinin, also known as basic pancreatic trypsin inhibitor, has been isolated and purified and is sold under the name of Trasylol (Bayer, West Haven, Conn.). It is also a potent inhibitor of trypsin and kallikrein, in addition to plasmin. The use of bovine aprotinin to reduce postoperative bleeding after major surgery has been reported.[18, 19] In animal models, it has been shown to serve as an antidote to bleeding induced by administration of recombinant t-PA (rt-PA).[20] Since aprotinin inhibits plasmin and not the activator, it should work with other plasminogen activators.

This complex system is capable of maintaining a balanced equilibrium between clotting and lysis, such that blood fluidity is ensured. It is important to recognize that although plasmin is highly selective for fibrin, it also digests fibrinogen and other plasma proteins. Circulating plasmin inhibitors prevent this otherwise disordered lytic action and preclude free circulating plasmin under normal conditions. Other important biologic functions of the plasminogen-plasmin system have now been recognized. The actions of plasminogen activators are facilitated by the presence of receptors of plasminogen, u-PA, and t-PA on cell surfaces,

as well as in circulation. Expressions of these components have been observed in tissue cultures and in tissues. They are believed to be actively involved in biologic functions at the cellular level, such as embryogenesis, ovulation, neuron growth, muscle regeneration, wound healing, and angiogenesis, and in tumor growth and invasion.[21] It is now postulated that tumor cell invasion (as well as cell migration) and other important biologic processes are dependent on the plasminogen-plasmin system. Endothelial cells and smooth muscle cells that take an active role in thrombosis and in atherogenesis may involve the plasminogen-plasmin system and cellular receptors in the reparative process following vascular injury. The expression seems to be modulated by a variety of cytokines, including interleukin and tumor necrosis factor; hormones such as steroid; gonadotropins; and growth factors, including platelet-derived growth factor.[21] Focal proteolysis, accomplished by binding of these cellular receptors as part of the plasminogen-plasmin system, allows the migrating cell to penetrate its surrounding extracellular matrix. u-PA has also been found to be a growth stimulant and mitogenic for some tumor cells.[22–24] These findings suggest that proliferation of endothelial and smooth muscle cells during vascular repair and atherogenesis induces increased expression of u-PA in these cells. Both PAI-1 and PAI-2 are present on cell surfaces. Differences in distribution between u-PA and its inhibitor would allow proteolysis to occur at focal points where the activator is located. The inhibitor would allow a foothold for the cell, aiding in its movement.

The synthesis and release of PAI-1 by the endothelial and hepatic cells may be under control of plasma insulin. It has been suggested that insulin stimulates synthesis and release of PAI-1 from hepatocytes, while t-PA and PAI-1 are released simultaneously from endothelial cells because of an acute-phase response to chronic vascular disease and subsequently are rapidly inactivated by complex formation.[25] A link between lipoprotein metabolism and fibrinolytic function has been suggested by the demonstration of significant homology between the amino acid sequence of apolipoprotein A and the structure of plasminogen. Thus, a prothrombotic function by virtue of interference with the numerous physiologic functions of plasminogen has been suggested in patients with increased levels of apolipoprotein A. Apolipoprotein A has also been found to competitively inhibit the binding of plasminogen to fibrinogen and to the plasminogen receptor on endothelial cells.[26]

Plasma levels of both t-PA and PAI-1 exhibit circadian variations. t-PA activity is lowest in the early morning and highest in the afternoon. Plasma PAI activity peaks in the early morning and passes through a trough in the afternoon. Thus, overall, there is decreased fibrinolytic activity in the morning.[27–30] Differences in patterns have also been seen between men and women, suggesting a hormonal influence.[31] Furthermore, PAI activity has been noted to vary secondary to diet. Caffeine-containing beverages may enhance fibrinolytic activity. On the other hand, cigarette smoking induces an acute increase in t-PA; this increase in t-PA may deplete normal stores and thus paradoxically decrease fibrinolytic capacity.

From the foregoing discussion, it is evident that the fibrinolytic system (plasminogen-plasmin system) plays a vital role in biologic homeostasis. In addition, an increasingly pivotal role is seen in certain disease states, ranging from atherosclerosis to carcinogenesis.

From the therapeutic standpoint, drugs capable of converting plasminogen to plasmin achieve their lytic effect to a great extent by overwhelming circulating plasmin inhibitors and generating an abundance of plasmin (exogenous fibrinolysis). Circulating plasmin not only produces the desired fibrinolysis but also proceeds to digest circulating fibrinogen. A more desirable situation results in the activation of thrombus-bound plasminogen (endogenous fibrinolysis) by these agents. Thrombus-bound plasminogen is, to a certain extent, protected from circulating inhibitors and thus proceeds with fibrin digestion much more effectively. Current investigations are concentrated on producing agents with high affinity for thrombus-bound plasminogen and little activation of the circulating zymogen. Clinical experience to date has failed to demonstrate this theoretical benefit. With better understanding of the complexity of the fibrinolytic system, it is possible that these benefits can be realized.

FIBRINOLYTIC AGENTS

Agents capable of activating the fibrinolytic system can be divided into indirect and direct activators. Indirect activators include a long list of drugs capable of increasing fibrinolytic activity in vivo without direct in vitro activity on plasminogen. The mechanism of action is variable and has not been elucidated for most of these indirect agents.

From the therapeutic standpoint, chronic enhancement of the fibrinolytic activity is attractive but of unproved clinical value. Most indirect fibrinolytic drugs lose their effectiveness with time. Such is the case with nicotinic acid and epinephrine. Both cause an abrupt but transient increase in fibrinolytic activity by release of endothelial plasminogen activator. Thus, long-term administration is of no benefit.

Antidiuretic hormone (ADH) is capable of stimulating the fibrinolytic system at the expense of severe cardiovascular side effects. A more prolonged response without side effects has been observed with a synthetic analog of ADH, desmopressin acetate (DDAVP). Intranasal administration of this analog caused a plasminogen activator response with a half-life of over 6 hours.[32] The increased fibrinolytic response to DDAVP, however, seems to be clinically insignificant when compared with endothelial release of factor VIII and other important procoagulant effects, which have been clinically useful in managing patients with certain bleeding diatheses.

Steroids and diguanides (phenformin) are the most promising of these compounds. Stanozolol, for example, is an anabolic steroid capable of producing sustained stimulation of the fibrinolytic system for periods longer than 5 years with daily administration.[33] In a small clinical trial, Jarrett and colleagues[34] treated 16 patients who had chronic recurrent thrombophlebitis with stanozolol. Thirteen patients had no recurrences during short-term treatment (6 weeks). Renewed attacks were seen in five patients after discontinuation of therapy; these attacks were successfully relieved by the readministration of stanozolol and phenformin.[34]

Available evidence on indirect fibrinolytic agents is mostly anecdotal. The long-term benefits of an enhanced fibrinolytic system are open to speculation. In many cases, the increased fibrinolytic activity occurs in patients whose baseline activity is depressed. In others, no clinical benefit is observed despite a sustained drug effect. In addition, fibrinolytic capacity may be decreased by chronic stimulation, thus rendering the system incapable of adequately responding to a thrombotic stimulus.[10] Certainly, this is an area of promise that will require randomized controlled long-term studies to answer important questions on the value of chronic enhancement of fibrinolytic activity in vascular disease.

THROMBOLYTIC AGENTS

The use of thrombolytic agents has clearly resulted in significant improvement in the outcome of patients with acute cardiac ischemia or myocardial infarction. It has also resulted in a modification in the treatment algorithm for patients with peripheral arterial occlusion, and although an improvement in outcome with regard to limb salvage or mortality has not been demonstrated, it is clear that it represents an important option in the armamentarium of treatment for patients with vascular occlusive disease.

First-Generation Thrombolytic Drugs

The first generation of thrombolytic agents, namely streptokinase and urokinase, have been shown to be very effective at thrombolysis but are limited in their potency by the fact that they are not fibrin-specific. They also convert circulating plasminogen to plasmin, but because circulating plasminogen and plasminogen in the thrombus are in equilibrium, the plasminogen in the thrombus would be depleted, thus limiting the efficacy of the agent. This has been termed *plasminogen steal* and is thought to reduce clot lysis.

Streptokinase

Streptokinase is a single-chain nonenzymatic protein produced by β-hemolytic streptococci. Its discovery by Tillett and Garner[35] in 1933 revived the interest in fibrinolysis seen in the past seven decades. Early clinical experience was complicated by a multitude of pyrogenic and allergic reactions. This prompted manufacturers to refine the drug, achieving the currently purified product and a marked reduction in febrile and allergic reactions.

The mechanism of action of streptokinase is complex. It initially forms an equimolar complex with plasminogen to form a plasminogen activator. Thus, it requires plasminogen as a cofactor and a substrate. The initial reaction is species-specific, having excellent affinity for human and cat plasminogen, relatively poor affinity for dog and rabbit plasminogen, and no reaction with bovine proenzyme. Once the activator complex is formed, it is an excellent activator of all mammalian plasminogen. Besides converting uncomplexed plasminogen to plasmin, plasminogen within the activator complex is converted to plasmin, and during this conversion streptokinase undergoes rapid progressive degradation.

The kinetics of these reactions have been studied in vitro. In vivo, a more complicated series of reactions occurs. Infusion of streptokinase is followed initially by neutralization by circulating antistreptococcal antibodies. The remaining drug then combines with circulating plasminogen to form the activator complex. This then converts uncomplexed plasminogen to plasmin, which combines with any excess free streptokinase, is neutralized by circulating antiplasmins, or binds to preformed fibrin. The last produces the desired effect of thrombolysis. However, when activity is measured, two half lives are detected, one at 16 and one at 83 minutes, indicating that these complex interactions have a significant impact on the concentration and activity of the drug.

From the foregoing discussion, it is evident that precise control of thrombolysis is not possible because the dose-response relationship of streptokinase varies from patient to patient. Initially, clinical use was guided by titers of antistreptococcal antibodies and measurement of the various components or products of the system. This proved impractical, and current practice utilizes standardized dosages that achieve the desired effect in the great majority of cases. A potential drawback of this approach is the administration of excess amounts of drug that could utilize most of the circulating plasminogen to form activator complex. This may leave inadequate amounts of zymogen to convert to plasmin. This problem of exceeding plasminogen availability may be of importance during regional, rather than systemic, administration. Some investigators have combined streptokinase with plasmin administration, with improvement in measured parameters such as plasminogen level, fibrinogen level, and potential fibrinolytic capacity.[36] Similar results are obtained by intermittent rather than continued infusion of the drug. Unfortunately, the results of these noncontrolled trials have raised doubts as to the improved effectiveness of such regimens. For the average clinician, continuous infusion therapy remains the most practical method of administration.

Streptokinase has largely fallen out of favor, in part because of its immunogenicity, even in the refined form, as this results in fever, allergic reactions, and acquired drug resistance. A complex of streptokinase and acylated human plasminogen, called APSAC (*a*nisoylated *p*lasminogen *s*treptokinase *a*ctivator *c*omplex) or anistreplase, was developed in an attempt to solve some of the problems inherent to streptokinase. Although theoretically sound, clinical trials were unable to demonstrate any increase in efficacy or any decrease in antigenicity from the administration of APSAC.

Urokinase

Urokinase is a serine protease with direct activator activity, normally present in urine as a product of renal tubular cells. It was originally isolated by MacFarlane and Pilling in 1947.[37] Urokinase is present in varying molecular weights, with variability in its activity. Original purification was done from urine, yielding small amounts of the enzyme at a considerable cost. Current production uses human fetal kidney cell culture. This has reduced the cost considerably, making the drug available for clinical use.

Urokinase is nonantigenic, and its mechanism of action is much more direct compared with that of streptokinase. Urokinase cleaves plasminogen (its only known protein substrate), by first-order reaction kinetics, to plasmin. It is pH and temperature stable. The lack of circulating neutralizing antibodies and its direct mechanism of action allow for a predictable dose-response relationship. Although allergic reactions are rare, over the last few years febrile responses to drug administrations have become more common. It has been suggested that this may be related to interleukins still present in drug batches that have been recently manufactured. In the past, when drug usage was less common, aging of the drug actually allowed these interleukins to become inactive. These febrile reactions respond readily to antipyretics. Interestingly, urokinase does not contain any lysine binding sites and therefore does not have any fibrin-binding properties.[38] High-affinity receptors for urokinase, however, have been demonstrated in several cell types and postulated as a mechanism by which cells can invade intracellular matrix and play a role in other physiologic and pathologic processes.[39–41]

The activation of plasminogen by urokinase occurs by proteolysis of its substrate plasminogen. Once administered intravenously, urokinase is rapidly removed from circulation, mainly via hepatic clearance. It has been estimated that the half-life of urokinase in humans is on the order of 14 minutes. Urokinase will also react with other proteins, including fibrinogen. Urokinase is much more effective in cleaving the susceptible site in plasminogen when it is in the Lys form than in the Glu form. However, the activation reaction of the latter by urokinase may be enhanced by the presence of fibrin.[42] Administration of exogenous plasminogen may also accelerate thrombolysis by urokinase. In an experimental study, urokinase infusion was compared with urokinase infusion in clots laced with plasminogen. Lacing with plasminogen resulted in more rapid restoration of flow, when compared with urokinase infusion alone. The rate of clot dissolution was also significantly enhanced in the plasminogen-laced thrombi.[3] Thus, it appears that exhaustion of native plasminogen may be a limiting factor in clot dissolution, and thus provision of the zymogen during thrombolysis may improve the effectiveness of the drug. Recently completed randomized, prospective clinical trials have also helped improve patient selection. From the Surgery Versus Thrombolysis for Ischemia of the Lower Extremities (STILE) Trial (see later), patients with acute (less than 14 days) ischemia had lower amputation rates and shorter hospital stays with thrombolysis. Patients with ischemic symptoms of more than 14 days who were treated surgically had less ongoing or recurrent ischemia with lower morbidity. At 6 months of follow-up, there was an improved amputation-free survival in acutely ischemic patients (less than 14 days) treated with thrombolysis. However, patients with ischemic symptoms more than 14 days who were treated surgically had significantly lower major amputation rates. Thus, patients with acute ischemic events may benefit more from thrombolysis than from surgery. Importantly, this trial excluded patients with embolic occlusions, and thus information specific to that group of patients is lacking. In a subsequent analysis, patients with native arterial occlusions randomized within the STILE protocol were evaluated. A reduction in the predetermined surgical procedure was noted in 58% of patients with femoropopliteal occlusions and in 51% of patients with iliofemoral occlusions. However, at 1 year, the incidence of recurrent ischemia (64 vs. 35%, $P < .0001$) and major amputation (10 vs. 0%, $P = .0024$) was increased in patients randomized to lysis, compared with those randomized to surgical intervention. Factors that were associated with poor lytic outcome included femoropopliteal occlusion, the presence of diabetes, and critical ischemia. There was no difference in mortality at 1 year between lysis and surgery.

Controversy exists regarding the actual thrombolytic effect of urokinase when administered in vivo. Experimental studies have suggested exogenous fibrinolysis as the main pathway, with limited activation of plasminogen within the thrombus (endogenous fibrinolysis).[43] In vivo, however, laboratory findings in treated patients have shown a lesser fibrinogenolytic response, suggesting that plasminemia is reduced with urokinase administration when compared with streptokinase.[44] This implies a significant endogenous activity. In clinical practice, the results of urokinase therapy have paralleled those achieved with streptokinase, with a decreased incidence of bleeding complications suggested by several investigators.[45–47] Whereas major bleeding complications are seen in 15% to 20% of patients treated with streptokinase, such complications have been reported in only 5% to 10% of patients treated with urokinase. Thus, the benefits observed in laboratory changes and the reduced incidence of significant plasminemia with urokinase seem to translate into a decreased incidence of bleeding complications in clinical practice. Although the cost of urokinase remains high compared with that of streptokinase, when complications are taken into account, the cost of therapy for streptokinase and urokinase is comparable.[48]

Residual thromboplastic activity was detected in the early urokinase preparations[49] and may account for the initial hypercoagulable state reported by Kakkar and Scully.[50] At present, this does not appear to be a clinically significant problem.

The concept of oral fibrinolytic therapy has emerged as a possibility with oral urokinase administration. Toki and colleagues[51] administered 30,000 units of urokinase orally in a single capsule and demonstrated increased fibrinolytic activity in normal subjects, as evidenced by shortened euglobin lysis time and raised fibrin degradation products. The future of this type of intervention is open to speculation. From the peripheral vascular standpoint, chronic or perioperative administration could prove a useful adjunct.

Ironically, despite the record of safety and efficacy that urokinase had accrued over the years, the Food and Drug Administration (FDA) issued a halt to the release and use of urokinase, manufactured by Abbott Laboratories, on the grounds of deviations from the Current Good Manufacturing Practice (CGMP) guidelines of the FDA developed to prevent the manufacture of unsafe products. The FDA, upon inspection of Abbott's manufacturing facility in North Chicago in 1998, was concerned about the neonatal kidney cells that Abbott used as a source of urokinase.[52] They originated from Cali, Colombia and were obtained through a separate company. The population was thought to be at high risk for various diseases, including tropical diseases,

and although there were no documented cases of infectious transmission resulting from the use of urokinase administration, the FDA demurred on the point, stating that any connection between the drug and such cases might have gone unrecognized. Despite the objections and entreaties of the community of vascular practitioners, to date urokinase remains unavailable on the market and thus practitioners of vascular medicine remain deprived of a very useful and efficacious drug, with a very good therapeutic safety profile.

Second-Generation Thrombolytic Drugs

The second-generation agents are fibrin selective, in contrast to first-generation thrombolytic drugs that not only act on fibrin but also convert circulating plasminogen to plasmin. These agents were developed to avoid systemic depletion of circulating fibrinogen and plasminogen and the consequent systemic thrombolytic state; such agents are represented by tPA, or alteplase, and single-chain urokinase-type plasminogen activator (scu-PA), or pro-urokinase. It is, however, clear that t-PA is associated with a higher incidence of intracranial hemorrhage than streptokinase (0.7% vs. 0.5%, respectively);[53] the second-generation agents, therefore, have their own limitation.

Tissue Plasminogen Activator

t-PA is a naturally occurring enzyme present in all human tissues. Its concentration is variable, with high levels detected in the uterus and moderate amounts in the heart, skeletal muscle, kidney, ovary, lung, thyroid, pituitary, and lymph nodes. Scant amounts are found in the liver, spleen, brain, and testes.[54] t-PA is thought to originate from vascular endothelium, and, with the exception of liver and spleen, tissue concentration correlates with vascularity.

Isolation and purification of t-PA was initially hampered by inadequate sources and procedures. In 1979, Rijken and associates[55] were successful in obtaining 1 mg of t-PA from 5 kg of human uterine tissue. Recognizing the potential of this drug, investigators have concentrated on other sources.

At present, there are two main sources of t-PA. The Bowes melanoma cell line is uniquely efficient in producing large quantities of t-PA,[56] which was subsequently proved to be identical to uterine t-PA.[57] Another source has emerged from the use of recombinant DNA technology, with which efforts in the cloning and expression of the t-PA gene from the melanoma cell line have been successful. This product, known as rt-PA, seems as effective as melanoma t-PA, although further investigations are in progress.[58]

t-PA is a direct plasminogen activator. Its main advantage is its high affinity for thrombus-bound fibrin. In addition, the presence of fibrinogen enhances its efficiency in activation of plasminogen. Two types of t-PA are recognized, with a commercial preparation being a mixture of both types. A single-chain form is cleaved by plasminogen to yield two-chain t-PA. The one- and the two-chain forms of t-PA are comparable in activity, with the one-chain form being quickly converted to the two-chain type as lysis proceeds. Most of circulating t-PA is in the single-chain form. Its selective action promises to produce fewer systemic effects when compared with streptokinase or urokinase. The half-life of t-PA has been estimated to be between 4 and 7 minutes in vivo.[59] With its presumed nonantigenicity and high affinity for fibrin, t-PA theoretically should produce improved clinical results. However, recent randomized trials have failed to demonstrate significant clinical differences from other available agents.

When fibrin-selective agents are used for regional infusion, most of the thrombolytic effect is going to be secondary to fibrin-bound plasminogen. However, the importance of a fresh supply of plasminogen to maintain the fibrin-bound plasminogen pool has been emphasized. Experimental studies have suggested that clot lysis induced by activation of plasminogen is dependent on clot-associated plasminogen, which in turn depends on the concentration of plasminogen in plasma. Depletion of both will contribute to a lower frequency and rapidity of recanalization, which will be more noticeable with non–fibrin-selective agents, as compared with fibrin-selective agents, likely the result of the depletion of plasminogen that nonselective agents induce.[60]

Trials comparing rt-PA with streptokinase in patients with acute coronary thrombosis have failed to establish this more specific agent as a better thrombolytic agent. Systemic bleeding complications have been similar despite a milder homeostatic defect by laboratory evaluation in the rt-PA groups.[61] Questions still exist regarding proper dosage to achieve effective local lysis with minimal systemic effects.

t-PA may also bind and be activated on platelet surfaces.[62] Due to this binding to platelet receptors, platelets can direct t-PA action on their surface, leading to rapid cleavage of glycoprotein 1B and loss of platelet binding to von Willebrand's factor. This may explain why concentrations of t-PA achieved early in therapy may inhibit platelet aggregation.

In animal models of thrombolysis, it has been suggested that multiple bolus administration of t-PA has greater lytic efficacy than equal doses given as a single bolus or a continuous infusion.[63] This may have significant implications for clinical therapy, where protocols requiring continuous infusion of the agent have shown a greater incidence of bleeding complications than protocols where the drug is administered in bolus form. This may be explained by the accumulation of partially degraded fibrin (X fragments), which may increase the affinity of t-PA for plasminogen by about 17-fold.[7]

In a study in which 17 patients were infused with rt-PA, 0.1 mg/kg/hour, all patients demonstrated thrombolysis, with 16 showing improvement clinically.[64] More important, there were no systemic complications, with a mean fibrinogen drop of 42% of baseline. The infusion time was 1 to 6 hours, compared with the usual 48 to 72 hours necessary for streptokinase infusion. One patient died from an intracranial hemorrhage during postinfusion heparin therapy. Experience in randomized trials has suggested that a lower dose remains as effective, with decreased risk of bleeding. The recommended lower dose is 0.05 mg/kg/hour.[65]

Systemic complications may be more related to dose and method of administration than is the case with urokinase or streptokinase. It appears that t-PA is more potent and faster than currently available agents, perhaps because of its high fibrin affinity. In this regard, t-PA may be ideally suited for intraarterial administration, because a 4- to 6-hour trial could be followed by timely surgical intervention. In addition, intraoperative use could be a welcome adjunct to surgical embolectomy.

Pro-urokinase

Saruplase, also known as recombinant single-chain urokinase-type plasminogen activator (r-scu-PA) or pro-urokinase, is a prodrug produced from a naturally occurring, physiologic protease.[65] Pro-urokinase is a single-chain polypeptide of 411 amino acids that is converted by plasmin into an active, low-molecular-weight form of urokinase with 276 amino acids.[66] Administration of pro-urokinase causes decreases in α_2-antiplasmin and fibrinogen and an increase in fibrinogen degradation products. Pro-urokinase is highly effective in the conversion of Lys-plasminogen to plasmin. In contrast, it has little or no activity in the conversion of Glu-plasminogen to plasmin. Since Lys-plasminogen is present in high concentrations in thrombus, this gives pro-urokinase fibrin-specific properties. In addition, plasminogen that is absorbed in thrombus changes its configuration to a pseudo–Lys-plasminogen, which is also attacked by pro-urokinase, converting it to Lys-plasmin. Circulating prourokinase is very stable in plasma because of its resistance to plasma inhibitors and ionized calcium.[67] The fibrin-specificities of t-PA and prourokinase appear to rely on differing mechanisms. Whereas t-PA is fibrin clot–binding, the fibrin-selective properties of pro-urokinase are thought to be secondary to its preference for activation of Lys-plasminogen or Lys-like plasminogen substrate found in thrombus. This effect prolongs its half-life, which has been estimated to be several days. Such a prolonged half-life has theoretical advantages in clinical situations in which prolonged activity is desired. However, in peripheral arterial occlusions, if the regional infusion fails to produce the desired result and the patient must go to the operating room shortly following discontinuation of the infusion, this prolonged effect may be undesirable. At this time, there is no reported experience with such use. Many of the clinical trials utilizing this drug have been studies in patients with myocardial infarction, and in those trials the notable finding was the increased incidence of intracranial hemorrhage (0.9%).[68] The most recent trial was the PROACT II study, which evaluated intraarterial pro-urokinase for acute ischemic stroke.[69] Early intracranial hemorrhage with neurologic deterioration within 24 hours occurred in 10% of pro-urokinase and 2% of control patients. Although it is effective at thrombolysis, the increased bleeding risk has limited its widespread use. A phase II trial evaluating pro-urokinase versus urokinase for thrombolysis of acute peripheral arterial occlusion showed that pro-urokinase was associated with increased efficacy of thrombolysis and also an increased risk of bleeding complications at a dose of 8 mg/hour, whereas with a dose of 2 mg/hour of pro-urokinase, there was a slightly lower rate of thrombolysis, combined with a lower incidence of bleeding complications and fibrinogenolysis.[70]

Third-Generation Thrombolytic Drugs

The last few years have seen the development of a new generation of thrombolytic drugs, including mutant molecules of scu-PA and t-PA; chimeric plasminogen activators; conjugates of plasminogen activators with monoclonal antibodies against fibrin, platelets, or thrombomodulin; and plasminogen activators of animal and bacterial origin.[53]

Reteplase

Reteplase is a single-chain deletion mutant of alteplase, consisting of just the kringle-2 and protease domains.[71] Reteplase has a fivefold decrease in fibrin binding and a half-life of 14 to 18 minutes due to the aforementioned structural differences. Reteplase has less binding to endothelium and monocytes compared with t-PA, and this reduced binding results in increased circulating levels in the blood stream.[72] It catalyzes the cleavage of endogenous plasminogen to generate plasmin. The activation of plasminogen is stimulated in the presence of fibrin and is mediated by the kringle-2 domain.[10, 73] Plasmin then degrades the fibrin matrix of the thrombus, thus exerting its fibrinolytic action.

Reteplase has increasingly become the thrombolytic agent of choice in the treatment of peripheral vascular occlusion, given the disappearance of urokinase from the scene. Although it is being increasingly administered, published studies regarding its use in controlled trials are relatively few in number. There are two pilot studies that have evaluated the dosing regimen of reteplase in the treatment of myocardial infarction.[74, 75] These pilot studies demonstrated that reteplase gave significantly higher TIMI-3 flow rates at 60 and 90 minutes than did front-loaded alteplase. However, in two subsequent trials—the INJECT[76] and the GUSTO III[77] trials—despite the higher TIMI-3 flow rates, this did not translate into a lower mortality in the reteplase-treated patients (7.5% for reteplase and 7.2% for alteplase).[15] Reteplase has lower fibrin affinity and thus appears to penetrate thrombus effectively and activate fibrin-bound plasminogen within the clot, resulting in faster clot lysis. Thrombolytics may also cause platelet activation, and this may have been responsible for some of the previously noted lack of efficacy. The addition of glycoprotein IIb/IIIa inhibitors appears to increase the efficacy of thrombolytic agents and also the speed to lysis.

Tenecteplase

Tenecteplase (TNK-t-PA) is a t-PA mutant in which a threonine molecule (Thr[103]) is replaced by Asn, and the sequence Lys-His-Arg-Arg is changed to Ala-Ala-Ala-Ala. This confers high fibrin selectivity and prolongs the half-life to 15 to 19 minutes. It is very effective in arterial, platelet-rich thrombi, and is more resistant to plasminogen activator inhibitor. Again, all of the clinical trials with this drug have been in patients with myocardial infarction[78] and as such, the recommended dose emanating from these studies, 0.5 mg/kg, may not apply to peripheral arterial occlusions that require longer infusion protocols.

Staphylokinase

Staphylokinase is a plasminogen activator produced by certain strains of *Staphylococcus aureus* and was first described as having fibrinolytic properties in 1948.[79] The gene has been cloned from genomic DNA of a lysogenic strain of *S. aureus*. When exposed to a fibrin clot in human plasma, staphylokinase reacts with plasmin at the clot-plasma interface; this staphylokinase-plasmin complex activates thrombus-bound plasminogen and exerts its fibrinolytic activity. Any plasmin that is liberated from the clot is rapidly inactivated by α_2-antiplasmin. In this manner, plasminogen activation by staphylokinase is confined to the thrombus, and the collateral effects of fibrinogen depletion and serum plasminogen activation are minimized. Patients treated with staphylokinase do, however, develop neutralizing antibodies, the titers of which can remain elevated for several months.[80]

Immunofibrinolysis

In an attempt to develop fibrin-specific agents, monoclonal antifibrin antibodies have been bonded to urokinase or streptokinase, rendering these agents fibrin selective. These monoclonal antibodies do not appear to cross-react with fibrinogen and thus show marked increase in in vitro fibrinolysis compared with unmodified activator.[81] The clinical applicability of these agents remains to be determined. They may significantly alter the current approach to the management of thrombotic disease. Nevertheless, repeat therapy would require different monoclonal antibodies to prevent adverse immunologic reactions.

Summary

Most of the available clinical experience to date has been with streptokinase, urokinase, and, most recently, t-PA. The effectiveness and complication rates of each of these agents are discussed thoroughly under the specific sections dealing with the various clinical entities. Based on the experience to date, streptokinase seems to be a less desirable agent for use in peripheral vascular thrombosis, probably because of its complex mechanism of action, which translates into difficulty with dosage and complications in the clinical area.

Although fibrin selectivity has theoretical advantages, its clinical use so far has failed to demonstrate a significant benefit of such selectivity in the various protocols in which the drug has been tested. Specifically, the rate of bleeding complications with t-PA has been no different from that seen with streptokinase when it is used in the treatment of acute myocardial infarction. In fact, a slight increased incidence of intracranial bleeding was seen with t-PA. This may be due to its marked potency compared with other agents currently available. Regional administration of these

TABLE 20-1

Fibrinolytic Agents

	STREPTOKINASE	UROKINASE	TISSUE PLASMINOGEN ACTIVATOR
Source	β-Hemolytic streptococcus (nonenzymatic protein)	Fetal renal cell culture (enzyme)	Recombinant DNA technology (enzyme)
Mechanism	Streptokinase-plasminogen complex	Direct plasminogen activator	Direct plasminogen activator
Metabolism	Liver	Liver	Liver
Advantages	Low cost	Direct activator; no allergic reaction	Fibrin-selective direct activator; no allergic reaction
Disadvantages	Affected by antistreptococcus A,B; allergic reactions; complex mechanism of action	High cost	High cost
Systemic dosage	250,000 units IV 30 min loading; 100,000 units IV/hr	2000 units/lb IV 10 min loading; 2000 units/lb IV/hr	50 mg IV over 2 hr; may repeat 30–50 mg IV over 4–6 hr
Regional dosage	Low dose: 5000–10,000 units/hr High dose: 30,000–60,000 units/hr	30,000–50,000 units/hr 2000–4000 units/min for 1–2 hr, then 1000–2000 units/min	0.05–0.1 units kg/hr

IV, intravenously.

agents may realize the true benefit of their selective property. In addition to the proper method of infusion (systemic vs. regional), dosage may play an important role in realizing the clinical benefits of a fibrin-specific agent.

SYSTEMIC THROMBOLYTIC THERAPY

This section discusses systemic thrombolytic therapy for venous and peripheral arterial disease. Treatment of acute coronary thrombosis is specifically omitted.

Although systemic thrombolytic therapy has been used for peripheral arterial occlusions, results have been disappointing, with bleeding complications outweighing benefits obtained. Thus, systemic therapy is reserved for venous thromboembolic diseases. Local intraarterial administration prevents some of the systemic complications and is utilized for peripheral arterial and graft occlusion. Patient selection is probably the most important factor in obtaining good results with either modality (Table 20–1).

Patient Selection

During the course of systemic thrombolytic therapy, a systemic lytic state is achieved in which fibrin is lysed wherever it has been deposited throughout the body. Thus, hemostatic plugs are as vulnerable as the clot or thrombus for which therapy has been initiated. Selection of patients for systemic lytic therapy is based on the presence of an appropriate documented indication (see later) and careful evaluation for the presence of contraindications.

Contraindications to systemic therapy are listed in Table 20–2. Absolute contraindications are active internal bleeding and recent (within 2 months) cerebrovascular accident or other intracranial condition. Relative major contraindications include recent (fewer than 10 days) major surgery, trauma, obstetric delivery, organ biopsy, or puncture of a noncompressible vessel; recent gastrointestinal bleed; and severe hypertension. Relative minor contraindications (see Table 20–2) carry a higher risk of complications, but the

benefits of therapy may still outweigh the hazards. Peripheral embolization from a central source is a potential hazard of systemic lytic therapy. Therefore, valvular heart disease, atrial fibrillation, and previous history of emboli are relative contraindications to systemic lytic therapy. The presence of a mural thrombus is a relative contraindication to fibrinolytic therapy. The potential for peripheral embolization due to a fragmented mural thrombus may lead to devastating consequences. In patients with a thrombus in the left side of the heart demonstrable by echocardiography, we would preferentially consider alternative forms of treatment. It must be recognized, however, that lysis of ventricular thrombi with urokinase has been reported with success.[82]

TABLE 20-2

Contraindications to Systemic Lytic Therapy

Absolute

Active internal bleeding
Recent (< 2 mo) cerebrovascular accident
Intracranial pathologic condition

Relative Major

Recent (< 10 days) major surgery, obstetric delivery, or organ biopsy
Active peptic ulcer or GI disorder
Recent major trauma
Uncontrolled hypertension

Relative Minor

Minor surgery or trauma
Recent cardiopulmonary resuscitation
High likelihood of left heart thrombus (i.e., atrial fibrillation with mitral valve disease)
Bacterial endocarditis
Hemostatic defects (i.e., renal or liver disease)
Pregnancy
Diabetic hemorrhagic retinopathy

Streptokinase

Known allergy
Recent streptococcal infection
Previous therapy within 6 mo

GI, gastrointestinal.

Severe liver disease affects the metabolism of the drug, thus making the response unpredictable. During pregnancy, a systemic lytic state may precipitate abruptio placentae or may lead to hypofibrinogenemia in the fetus, with an increased risk of bleeding. Streptokinase is specifically contraindicated in patients with known allergy, previous therapy within 6 months, or recent streptococcal infection.

One of the most devastating complications of fibrinolytic therapy is intracranial hemorrhage. The incidence of this complication is on the order of 1% of treated patients in trials for acute myocardial infarction. The median time between the onset of clinical signs and the start of thrombolytic therapy ranges from 3 to 36 hours, with a mean of 16 hours. Mortality is high for this complication, with an estimated mortality of 66%. Factors predictive of intracranial hemorrhage by multivariate logistic regression analysis include oral anticoagulation prior to admission, body weight less than 70 kg, and age older than 65 years. An increased incidence of intracerebral hemorrhage has been observed in patients receiving higher doses of t-PA. In the Thrombosis in Myocardial Infarction (TIMI) trial,[83] 1.3% of patients receiving 150 mg of t-PA suffered an intracerebral hemorrhage, as opposed to 0.4% of patients receiving 100 mg of the drug. Interestingly, in the TIMI-II trial, patients who received immediate β-blockade as part of their regimen had no incidence of intracerebral hemorrhage when given 100 mg of t-PA, as compared with 0.5% in the group that did not receive β-blockade. This was not true, however, for the patients treated with 150 mg of t-PA. The mechanism by which β-blockers may protect against intracerebral bleeding is not established.[84]

In the STILE trial, patients were randomized to thrombolytic therapy with t-PA or urokinase versus surgery for the treatment of lower limb ischemia.[85] When evaluated by an intent-to-treat analysis, the incidence of life-threatening hemorrhage was 5.3% to 5.7%. When analyzed on a per-protocol basis, the incidence of this complication was 7.8% in the thrombolysis group. The incidence was similar in patients treated with t-PA and urokinase; these patients also received aspirin and heparin, which may have added to the risk. However, patients with bleeding complications did not receive more heparin or a higher dose of lytic agent; they appeared to respond differently to the therapy. At the end of the infusion, patients with bleeding complications had a significantly lower fibrinogen level than patients without hemorrhagic complications (188 mg/dL vs. 310 mg/dL, respectively). Measurement of fibrinogen level, along with the International Normalized Ratio and partial prothrombin time (PTT), may be helpful in guiding dose and duration of therapy.

Indications

Pulmonary Embolism

In 1968, a cooperative controlled randomized study to evaluate the use of urokinase in pulmonary embolism was initiated.[86] By 1970, 160 patients were entered and assigned to one of two therapeutic arms. Pulmonary angiography was performed on all patients before and after therapy, with lung scans repeated at 3, 6, and 12 months. The minimal eligibility was occlusion of at least one segmental pulmonary artery on angiography. Excluded from the trial were patients who had had recent operations or those with contraindications to heparin or thrombolytic therapy. Seventy-eight patients received anticoagulants alone (heparin, 75 units/pound loading dose, 10 units/pound/hour for 12 hours), and 82 received urokinase (2000 units/pound/hour for 12 hours). Following the 12-hour infusion, all patients received heparin for a minimum of 5 days to maintain a prolonged bleeding time.

The randomization produced reasonably good balance between the treatment groups. Urokinase therapy resulted in a significantly accelerated resolution of pulmonary emboli at 24 hours, as shown by pulmonary arteriograms, lung scans, and right-sided pressures. No significant differences in mortality or recurrence rate were observed. Patients receiving urokinase tended to respond better if they were younger (less than 50 years old), the embolus was recent (less than 48 hours old), or the embolus was large, especially if shock was present.

Bleeding complications were significant in both groups (heparin, 27%; urokinase, 45%). This high complication rate is likely the result of demands in the protocol for multiple, frequent invasive procedures, including cutdowns performed for pulmonary angiography. The study group concluded that further studies were indicated before specific therapeutic recommendations could be made.

In 1974, the second phase of this cooperative study was reported.[87] This study followed the same guidelines as in phase I, comparing 12 hours of urokinase therapy with 24 hours of urokinase therapy and 24 hours of streptokinase therapy. A group treated with heparin alone was not included because the protocol was almost identical to that in the phase I trial, which showed urokinase to be superior to heparin in clot resolution. Fifty-seven patients were given urokinase (2000 units/pound loading dose, 2000 units/pound/hour for 24 hours), and 61 patients received the same regimen for 12 hours. Fifty-eight patients received streptokinase (250,000 units loading dose, 100,000 units/hour for 24 hours).

As expected, the drop in plasminogen during therapy was steeper for patients receiving streptokinase, but otherwise the lytic effect was similar. Patients receiving 12 hours of urokinase infusion had a result nearly equivalent to those in the phase I trial receiving urokinase. No benefit was seen from 24 hours of urokinase over the 12-hour infusion. In patients with massive embolism, the greatest improvement was seen with 24-hour urokinase infusion, although the differences were not statistically significant. Streptokinase and urokinase yielded similar results, with small differences favoring urokinase. The study group concluded that all three regimens were more effective in accelerating resolution of pulmonary thromboemboli than heparin alone.

One of the major problems with the use of thrombolytic therapy for pulmonary embolism is that patients with pulmonary emboli usually have major contraindications to thrombolytic therapy. Such is the case with the occurrence of pulmonary embolism in the postoperative patient. In 1992, an experience with 13 patients treated for angiographically proven pulmonary embolism within 14 days of surgery was reported.[88] The protocol utilized urokinase,

2200 units/kg of body weight, injected directly into the clot through a catheter positioned in the pulmonary artery. A continuous infusion at the same dosage was then maintained for up to 24 hours, with the simultaneous administration of heparin at 500 units/hour. Fibrinogen level was maintained at less than 0.2 g/dL. No deaths or bleeding complications were seen, with complete lysis achieved in all patients. This selective therapy for pulmonary embolism may be appropriate for patients in the early postoperative period who suffer a major life-threatening pulmonary embolus.

The long-term results of patients randomized to the Urokinase Pulmonary Embolism Trial (UPET) study suggest the clinical importance of resolution of the obstructive process in the pulmonary circulation. Several patients from this study were reexamined at 7 years after the original pulmonary embolus. Those assigned initially to thrombolysis had significantly higher pulmonary capillary blood volumes and preservation of the normal pulmonary vasculature response to exercise at 7 years. In contrast, patients who had been treated with anticoagulants alone demonstrated a lower pulmonary capillary blood volume at 1 year and a markedly abnormal increase in pulmonary artery pressure and pulmonary vascular resistance when undergoing exercise testing during right heart catheterization.[89] These data suggest that initial management with thrombolysis can offer improved quality of life demonstrable years after the event.

More recently, rt-PA has been evaluated in the treatment of acute massive pulmonary embolism. In a multicenter trial, the intravenous administration of rt-PA was compared with intrapulmonary administration in 34 patients with massive pulmonary emboli.[90] All patients were systemically anticoagulated with heparin. Fifty milligrams of rt-PA were given over 2 hours, either intravenously or intrapulmonary, with an additional 22 patients receiving 50 mg over the subsequent 5 hours. No difference was noted between the intrapulmonary group and the intravenous administration group, and 7-hour administration was superior to a single infusion of 50 mg over 2 hours. In all groups, up to 38% resolution of the angiographically determined embolism occurred. A decline in the pulmonary arterial pressure was documented in all groups. Fibrinogen levels dropped significantly, with bleeding complications limited to puncture or operative sites, and in only four patients were blood transfusions required.[90]

In a separate trial, 36 patients with angiographically documented pulmonary emboli received 50 mg of rt-PA over 2 hours, followed by repeat arteriography and, if necessary, an additional 40 mg over 4 hours of rt-PA.[91] Thirty-four of 36 patients had angiographic evidence of clot lysis, with marked improvement in 24 of the 36. Two bleeding complications occurred, one related to a pelvic tumor and the other 8 days following coronary artery bypass surgery. Again, significant improvement in the clinical condition of these patients was documented.[91]

A randomized controlled trial of rt-PA versus urokinase in the treatment of acute pulmonary embolism was reported in 1988.[92] Forty-five patients were randomized to rt-PA, 100 mg over 2 hours, versus urokinase at systemic doses. At 2 hours, 82% of rt-PA patients had complete lysis, as opposed to 48% of patients receiving urokinase.

Eight of 23 urokinase patients required premature termination of the infusion because of bleeding complications. There was no difference in plasma fibrinogen level or improvement in lung scans between the two groups.[92]

In 1980, the NIH Consensus Development Conference[93] concluded that thrombolytic therapy results in greater improvement and normalization of the hemodynamic responses to pulmonary emboli than is observed with heparin alone. Lytic therapy may prevent permanent damage to the pulmonary vascular bed by lysing emboli and restoring pulmonary circulation to normal. The conference report also stated that although the incidence of bleeding complications in the trials discussed here was high, contemporary clinical experience suggested an incidence of around 5%, certainly within an acceptable range. The only thrombolytic agent currently approved by the FDA for use in the treatment of patients with pulmonary embolism is t-PA, given in a 100-mg dose over 2 hours. As stated above, there is no evidence of improved survival or outcomes in patients with pulmonary embolism that are hemodynamically stable. Tebbe and colleagues[94] evaluated the efficacy of reteplase, given as two 10-unit boluses 30 minutes apart, compared with t-PA in the 100-mg dose. There was no difference in clinical outcomes, complications, or mortality. The rates of stroke and intracranial hemorrhage were similar. However, reteplase resulted in reduction of pulmonary vascular resistance quicker than did t-PA. Although t-PA is the only currently approved agent for thrombolysis in pulmonary embolism, the newer third-generation thrombolytics agents offer certain advantages such as fibrin-specificity and faster onset of action. This having been said, it should be emphasized that there is no level I evidence that thrombolysis for the improvement of pulmonary embolism, except in cases of massive embolism with hemodynamic compromise, offers any survival advantage.

In current clinical practice, thrombolytic therapy should be considered in all patients with an established diagnosis of pulmonary embolism, any evidence (clinical or monitoring) of hemodynamic compromise, and no absolute contraindication to systemic lytic therapy. This excludes small pulmonary emboli with which, after the initial episode, the patient remains clinically stable. In the latter situation, the benefits of thrombolytic therapy over heparin alone are not clear.

It is important that the diagnosis of pulmonary emboli be well documented. We prefer pulmonary angiography because it remains the gold standard. If hemodynamic instability precludes obtaining pretreatment angiography, an alternative is to proceed with lytic therapy, which usually results in marked improvement within the hour. Angiography is then performed to help the clinician decide whether to continue therapy. If the angiogram confirms the diagnosis, the drug is continued for 12 to 24 hours, with hemodynamic response being assessed and depending on the presence or absence of complications or risk factors. Therapy beyond 24 hours does not seem to offer any benefit.

Under these guidelines, patients who are candidates for pulmonary embolectomy should have a trial of lytic therapy. Pulmonary embolectomy is then reserved for patients who fail or have an absolute contraindication to thrombolytic therapy.

Deep Venous Thrombosis

The goal of therapy for deep venous thrombosis (DVT) is the prevention of pulmonary embolism and of long-term sequelae characterized by the postphlebitic syndrome. Anticoagulation has been highly effective in achieving the former but ineffective in preventing valvular damage and, as a consequence, avoiding the postphlebitic syndrome. The incidence of such long-term complications can be as high as 90%.[95]

Several well-controlled randomized prospective studies have compared systemic lytic therapy with conventional heparin therapy in the treatment of DVT.[96–100] All concluded that dissolution of DVT with lytic therapy is faster and more complete than that observed with heparin alone. On the average, complete lysis was seen in 35% of patients, compared with 4% of those treated with heparin alone. At 3 to 6 months' follow-up, valve function was preserved in 7% of heparin-treated patients, compared with 50% of patients treated with thrombolytic agents. The incidence of pulmonary embolism was similar for both regimens, with no difference in mortality. Bleeding complications averaged 4% and 17% for heparin and lytic therapy, respectively. In one study, phlebography at a mean of 7 months following treatment suggested an improved outcome for patients treated with fibrinolytic agents. Normal venograms were found in 40% of streptokinase-treated patients, compared with 8% of those who had received heparin. Clinical symptoms were related to therapeutic results and previous thrombosis. Longer follow-up was reported by Arnesen and colleagues,[101] who phlebographically evaluated 35 patients at a mean observation period of 6.5 years after they randomly received streptokinase or heparin. Only seven patients had phlebographically normal veins, and all were in the streptokinase group. On clinical examination, 76% of patients in the streptokinase group had normal legs, compared with 33% of patients in the heparin group.[101] Contrasting results have been reported from a small prospective study in which 24 patients with major proximal DVT treated with heparin were compared with 25 patients similarly afflicted, treated with streptokinase.[102] After 2.5 years of follow-up, no major benefit was seen regarding hemodynamic status, as measured by foot volumetry, between the two groups. The authors questioned the validity of treatment with lytic therapy, given its inherent higher complication rate. In all of these studies, thrombi older than 3 to 5 days were less likely to respond.

Clinical experience with the use of t-PA in the treatment of DVT is limited. A randomized trial of rt-PA for the treatment of proximal DVT was carried out by Turpie and colleagues.[103] Twenty patients with proximal DVT were randomized to intravenous rt-PA (0.5 mg/kg) or placebo over 4 hours, following initiation of a therapeutic dose of intravenous heparin. Patients were randomized to rt-PA (0.5 mg/kg) or saline over 1 hour if repeat venography within 72 hours did not show complete lysis. Five of 10 patients treated with this protocol of rt-PA showed partial or complete lysis, compared with 1 of 10 patients treated with heparin. A systemic lytic effect was demonstrated by a drop in plasma fibrinogen and α_2-antiplasmin concentration, with positive fibrin degradation split products and elevated euglobulin lysis time. Thus, modest effectiveness

was seen in this study, similar to that achieved by urokinase or streptokinase. Long-term follow-up data on these patients are not available. Three other randomized trials have shown similar results.[104–106]

The concept of lytic therapy for DVT is attractive because it can relieve the obstructive process and may aid in the preservation of valvular function. These two features are established predictors of the development of the post-thrombotic syndrome.[107] The early reports of success with thrombolysis for DVT led to the development of a national multicenter registry for evaluation of catheter-directed thrombolysis for lower extremity DVT.[108] The early results in 473 patients were published in 1999 and demonstrated that the methods used to deliver the lytic agent (in this case, urokinase) affect the anatomic result. Attempts to lyse the thrombus by a pedal infusion were remarkably unsuccessful, with a failure rate of 80%. In contrast, catheter-directed lysis, with the agent laced directly into the clot, achieved substantial lysis in 83% of cases, and complete lysis in 33%. This experience is a strong argument for abandoning systemic infusion for thrombolysis, because the rates of lysis are not improved but the dose of the lytic agent administered is higher with systemic infusions. Major bleeding complications occurred in 11% of patients, most at the puncture site, and mortality was less than 1%. Comerota and colleagues[109] published a report evaluating health-related quality-of-life variables in patients with iliofemoral vein DVT treated with thrombolysis ($n = 68$) versus those treated with anticoagulation alone ($n = 30$). Patients treated with thrombolysis reported better overall physical functioning, less health distress, less stigma, and fewer post-thrombotic symptoms ($P < .05$ for each outcome measure).

It is reasonable to conclude that systemic thrombolytic therapy for DVT is as effective as heparin in preventing pulmonary embolic complications, with the added advantage of faster acute resolution in a significant number of patients. From the available studies, it appears that elimination of the obstructive component of DVT is better achieved with lytic therapy. Whether preservation of valve function is achieved by this more aggressive form of therapy remains uncertain. Clearly, with longer follow-up, more patients develop incompetent valves. This may result from minor valve damage progressing with time to a clinically significant problem. Nevertheless, it is difficult to ignore the significant improvement in the obstructive component of DVT, considering that the combination of obstruction and valvular incompetence will likely result in the most severe forms of postphlebitis syndrome. In view of this, should lytic therapy be offered to all patients with DVT? Clearly, the answer is no. When therapy is started beyond 5 days following the onset of symptoms, effectiveness is significantly decreased. The incidence of DVT is highest in postoperative patients, women during pregnancy or after childbirth, trauma victims, or after cerebrovascular accidents or spinal injury. Lytic therapy is contraindicated in these instances, as well as in septic thrombophlebitis. Prior episodes of thrombophlebitis are likely to have destroyed delicate vein valves, and thus the benefits of lytic therapy in recurrent attacks are uncertain. If clinical evidence of valve competence is present, an attempt to prevent further damage from a recurrent attack and resolve the obstructive component is a reasonable goal. In addition, lytic therapy seems to offer an advantage in more proximal thrombosis (i.e., popliteal vein or higher); thus treatment of isolated calf thrombi with lytic therapy is of questionable value.

From the foregoing discussion, it is evident that the impact of lytic therapy in DVT will be limited. However, patients suffering their first episode who have no contraindications and who receive treatment within 5 days of the onset of symptoms will likely benefit from systemic lytic therapy. As with pulmonary embolism, documentation of the diagnosis is essential before initiating thrombolytic therapy for DVT. It is our practice to obtain a venogram prior to lytic therapy. Repeat venography to assess the result is not necessary, although it is very helpful in instances in which clinical response is uncertain. Noninvasive studies are useful during therapy when an adequate clinical response is observed. The duration of therapy is guided by these studies but usually is no less than 3 days, unless complications require earlier discontinuation of the drug. Therapy beyond 5 days is rarely indicated and suggests resistance to lytic therapy. When using streptokinase, if no improvement is seen within the first 24 to 48 hours or a lytic state (see later in this section) is not documented within this time, switching to urokinase is recommended.

Phlegmasia cerulea dolens at onset causes massive iliofemoral thrombosis with limb-threatening venous outflow occlusion. The results of venous thrombectomy have been variable traditionally, with a significant incidence of rethrombosis and mortality, although more recent experience has been encouraging.[110, 111] A much more compelling argument can be made for the use of thrombolytic therapy in the treatment of phlegmasia cerulea dolens. There exists no real consensus on treatment for this entity, but the advent of catheter-directed thrombolysis presents an attractive and effective treatment option for this disease, which historically has resulted in a 20% to 40% mortality and a significant amputation rate in survivors.[112] Patel and colleagues[113] reported a case report of two patients with phlegmasia cerulea dolens treated with catheter-directed thrombolytic therapy and stenting that resulted in successful treatment without limb loss. Although this is a case report, it is one of many that demonstrate the feasibility and efficacy of this approach, and offers a real alternative to surgical thrombectomy for the treatment of phlegmasia cerulea dolens. Lytic therapy offers an important advantage over surgical thrombectomy; multiple peripheral thrombi not accessible to the catheter may be dissolved. In addition, a general anesthetic, frequently required for venous thrombectomy, is avoided. Although the experience with thrombolytic therapy in this entity is limited, of 14 reported cases, 13 were judged as having achieved excellent results with no mortality.[96, 114–116]

Axillary Vein Thrombosis

Axillary vein thrombosis (effort thrombosis) usually occurs in young individuals, and its sudden clinical manifestations lead the patient to seek early medical attention. This makes this entity ideally suited for thrombolytic therapy. Anticoagulation rarely leads to resolution and merely arrests the process, allowing for collateral drainage and amelioration of symptoms. This frequently leads to some degree of disability. Catheter-induced axillary subclavian vein thrombosis usually has a more gradual presentation, with slow progressive occlusion allowing for collateral venous drainage. The clinical presentation aids in the decision of whether to offer lytic therapy to a patient with catheter-induced axillosubclavian vein thrombosis. When symptoms have developed rapidly over the course of a few days, there is a good probability that the thrombotic material will be sensitive to lytic agents. A combination of infusion through the catheter and in the ipsilateral peripheral vein seems most effective. However, if symptoms have developed over weeks or months, they tend to be milder in nature and less responsive to fibrinolytic agents. This is likely a result of organization of the thrombotic material.

Both forms of axillary thrombosis have been successfully managed with lytic therapy[117–119] (Fig. 20–2). Either systemic or local low-dose infusion appears to be effective.[117] Local infusion requires that the catheter be lodged in thrombus; otherwise venous collaterals will decrease its effectiveness. A systemic lytic state is avoided in the majority of patients treated by local infusion.

Once complete resolution of the clot is achieved, repeat venography with the extremity in abduction and external rotation is recommended. If an underlying thoracic outlet compression is identified, surgical correction should be advised. In our own experience, this is best delayed for 2 to 3 months, during which the patient remains on oral anticoagulants. Early surgical intervention is associated with a higher incidence of rethrombosis, compared with delayed intervention. This may be secondary to remaining inflammatory changes that occur shortly after lysis of a thrombosed segment. After thoracic decompression, if a stenosis of the vein is identified, balloon dilatation has been successful in avoiding rethrombosis.[117]

Superior Vena Cava Thrombosis

Superior vena cava thrombosis is frequently the result of neoplastic, traumatic, or infectious processes in the mediastinum. In these instances, external compression or inflammation precludes successful resolution of the process with lytic agents. Thrombosis secondary to an indwelling catheter is usually a slow process, allowing for organization and fibrotic replacement of the clot. It is unlikely that this will respond to lytic therapy; surgical decompression may be an option in these patients. On the other hand, patients who develop rapidly progressive symptoms may respond to lytic therapy by dissolution of the most recently formed clot, which is likely to be sensitive to lysis.

In about 4% of cases, thrombosis is termed idiopathic. Successful resolution of idiopathic vena cava thrombosis has been reported with systemic thrombolytic therapy.[120]

Method

The goal of systemic administration of fibrinolytic agents is to establish a systemic lytic state. Once the diagnosis is documented by objective means and the patient deemed a suitable candidate for lytic therapy, informed consent

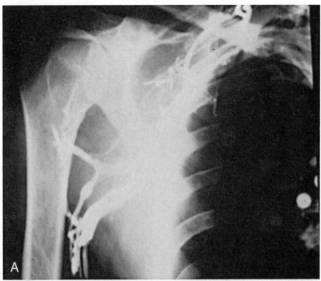

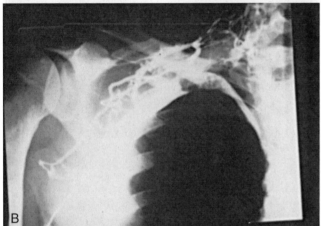

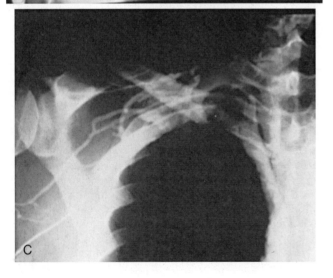

Figure 20–2. Venograms of a 28-year-old man with acute onset of pain and swelling in the right upper extremity. *A,* Ascending venogram confirms axillary vein thrombosis. Low-dose streptokinase infusion (10,000 units/hr) initiated. *B,* Twenty-four hours later, intraluminal thrombus is seen, with patency of the system. *C,* Forty-eight hours later, there is complete resolution of the occlusion.

should be obtained. Before infusion, fibrinogen level, thrombin time, prothrombin time (PT), PTT, hematocrit, and platelet count are obtained. If heparin has been given, it is discontinued. The agent is given intravenously. If streptokinase is chosen, 250,000 units are given over 30 minutes. This achieves a lytic state in 90% of the patients. A continuous infusion of 100,000 units/hour is then com-

menced and continued for the duration of therapy. We routinely administer 100 mg of hydrocortisone before streptokinase therapy, because it may prevent or ameliorate some of the allergic reactions. If urokinase is chosen, a loading dose of 2000 units/pound is given over 10 minutes, followed by a continuous infusion of 2000 units/pound/hour for the duration of therapy. Alternatively, 50 mg of rt-PA may be given over 2 hours. If a pulmonary artery catheter is present, the drug may be administered through the atrial port of the catheter. This is preferable to administration through the distal port of the catheter, which may be located in a branch of the pulmonary artery unrelated to the location of the occlusion. Thus, either peripheral vein administration or atrial administration through the proximal port of a Swan-Ganz catheter is preferable. As an alternative, the catheter used for pulmonary angiography may be lodged within the thrombus for regional infusion. High-dose regional therapy could then be utilized (see Native Vessel Occlusion later in this chapter). Invasive procedures are to be avoided, intramuscular injections are contraindicated, and bed rest is essential during therapy. Arterial blood gases are obtained only when necessary from the wrist and should be followed by at least 20 minutes of compression of the artery.

Three to 4 hours after commencing infusion, thrombin time (or PTT, if thrombin time is not available), fibrinogen level, and fibrin degradation product measurements are obtained. A lytic state is documented by a PTT that is twice normal and positive fibrin degradation products. Hematocrit is followed every 6 hours, with the other parameters measured on a daily basis. A drop in fibrinogen is expected and, in the absence of bleeding complications, is well tolerated. If a lytic state is not seen after the initial 4 hours, the hourly doses are increased. Conversely, if streptokinase is used, changing to urokinase may be beneficial.

Following completion of therapy (see Indications earlier in this section), the patient should receive anticoagulants. Usually 2 to 3 hours after discontinuation of the lytic agent heparin can be initiated at appropriate hourly doses without a loading dose. This is followed by warfarin in the conventional manner.

Complications

Bleeding is the most frequent and important complication of systemic lytic therapy. The incidence of major bleeding (requiring transfusions or discontinuation of the drug), as reported in the literature, varies from 7%[121] to as high as 45%.[86] Major bleeding occurs in an average of 15% of cases and correlates with the number and type of invasive procedures during therapy. Duration of therapy also seems to influence the incidence of bleeding.

Two broad categories of bleeding are observed. Superficial bleeding, seen at invasive sites, is frequently controlled with pressure. Avoidance of unnecessary procedures and preservation of an intact vascular system are the best preventive measures. Internal bleeding, usually seen in the gastrointestinal tract or the intracranial space, is frequently the result of poor patient selection. Internal bleeding should be suspected with unexplained drops in hematocrit. As a rule, any change in the neurologic status of a patient receiving fibrinolytic therapy is considered a complication of therapy, until proved otherwise. The infusion is discontinued immediately, and appropriate diagnostic and therapeutic measures instituted.

Superficial bleeding, which is controlled by local measures, can be tolerated in the final stages of therapy. Its

occurrence early in the infusion, or any significant bleeding requiring transfusion, should lead to discontinuation of therapy. The hemostatic defect is corrected by the administration of fresh-frozen plasma or cryoprecipitate. These two components are rich in fibrinogen and usually result in resolution of the lytic state. EACA administration (plasmin inhibitor) is rarely recommended and carries a significant risk of aggravating the process for which lytic therapy was instituted. Increasing the dose of streptokinase to decrease its proteolytic effect is scientifically correct but unnecessary. It is interesting to note that bleeding tends to occur in the lag period between termination of lytic therapy and anticoagulant administration.[56, 122] Thus, heparin administration should be delayed until the thrombin time or PTT is less than twice normal and initiated without a loading dose.

Laboratory parameters correlate poorly with the risk of bleeding. On the other hand, extremely low fibrinogen levels (less than 20% of baseline) in the presence of an otherwise minor bleeding complication do increase the chances of continued bleeding, requiring cessation of therapy. An alternative is to temporarily discontinue the drug, administer fresh-frozen plasma or cryoprecipitate, and restart the infusion several hours later.

Allergic reactions are not infrequent with streptokinase, although most are minor febrile episodes of no clinical consequence. Serious allergic reactions are extremely rare with the current preparations, and the few reported have responded well to conventional therapy.[93]

Pulmonary embolism can occur during treatment for DVT. The incidence appears to be similar to that seen with conventional heparin therapy. In the absence of other complications, continuation of lytic therapy is the treatment of choice. If recurrent emboli are observed, discontinuation of the fibrinolytic agent, heparin administration, and placement of a caval filter may be lifesaving.

INTRAARTERIAL THROMBOLYTIC THERAPY

The management of acute arterial and graft occlusions by the intraarterial local administration of fibrinolytic agents has emerged as an occasional alternative and, frequently, an adjunct to surgical therapy in a selected group of patients. Recently completed prospective, randomized clinical trials have helped establish the role of lytic therapy in the treatment of patients with peripheral vascular disease. Excellent results with low morbidity and mortality are now possible with modern vascular techniques. It is difficult to estimate the impact of intraarterial lytic therapy based on cases in which surgical management has traditionally been successful.

Emerging from the literature are a series of guidelines that have helped define the role of intraarterial lytic therapy. Unquestionably, patient selection is the most important factor in achieving good results with this nonoperative approach. As we gain experience in manipulating the fibrinolytic system, perhaps improvements in areas in which surgical results are poor will follow.

Patient Selection

As a rule, intraarterial fibrinolytic therapy should be considered when the surgical alternative carries a high morbidity or mortality, or when the surgical approach has traditionally yielded poor results. In patients with previous multiple vascular reconstructions, lytic therapy may offer an alternative to an otherwise difficult and unpredictable surgical intervention. In some cases, it may facilitate such an undertaking, thus serving as a true adjunct to surgical therapy.

In the early experience of intraarterial fibrinolytic therapy, low doses of the agent were administered close to the thrombus to minimize systemic effects. With a low-dose regimen, dissolution of intraarterial thrombi is a slow, gradual process, requiring 12 to 72 hours or longer to resolve. In patients in whom this method is chosen, the viability of the ischemic tissues should be assured. Otherwise, these patients are better managed surgically because prompt revascularization can be accomplished. Candidates for intraarterial lytic therapy must be able to tolerate ischemia for the duration of the infusion. However, with a high-dose regimen, restoration of forward flow frequently can be achieved in 2 to 6 hours, and thus the decision of whether to continue fibrinolytic infusion can be made in a timely fashion.

Cumulative experience in both retrospective and prospective analysis has helped define guidelines for patient selection. In a prospective study of 80 consecutive patients receiving intraarterial urokinase for acute (less than 14 days) ischemia, successful lysis was accomplished in 71% (57 patients).[123] Most of these, however, required additional adjunctive procedures to maintain patency, whereas only 28% of patients avoided the need for additional interventions. Prosthetic graft and native arterial occlusions responded equally well (78% and 72%, respectively), whereas vein graft occlusions were less likely to respond (53%). Diabetics fared significantly worse compared with nondiabetics. Most important, placement of the catheter within the substance of the thrombus and passage of the guidewire through the occlusive process were the best predictors of success. The location of the occlusion influenced the need for adjunctive procedures. Whereas 88% of aortoiliac and 82% of infrainguinal occlusions required adjunctive procedures, only 17% of upper extremity procedures required additional intervention. The investigators underscored the importance of patient selection, noting that unsuccessful thrombolysis not only delays revascularization but also increases the risk of bleeding complications.[123]

Absolute and relative contraindications to intraarterial fibrinolytic therapy are listed in Table 20–3. Approximately 50% of patients receiving low-dose intraarterial infusion of lytic drugs will develop a systemic lytic state. Thus, patients with active internal bleeding, recent cerebrovascular accidents (within 2 months), or intracranial lesions are not candidates for any form of fibrinolytic therapy.

Relative contraindications represent risk factors associated with a higher incidence of complications. Recent major surgery or trauma will increase significantly the risk of bleeding in the presence of a systemic lytic state. Individual judgment is required, but the presence of relative contraindications should not detract the clinician from utilizing regional lytic therapy if significant benefit is anticipated. These contraindications were discussed under Systemic Lytic Therapy earlier in this chapter.

Several cases of embolization to the ipsilateral extremity during intraarterial lytic therapy for occluded axillofemoral

TABLE 20–3

Contraindications to Intraarterial Fibrinolytic Therapy

Absolute

Intolerable ischemia
Active internal bleeding
Cerebrovascular accident within 3 mo
Intracranial pathologic condition

Relative

Recent major surgery or trauma
Minor GI bleeding
Severe hypertension
Valvular heart disease
Atrial fibrillation
Endocarditis
Coagulation disorders
Pregnancy
Minor surgery
Severe liver disease
Axillofemoral graft *or* knitted Dacron graft

Streptokinase

Known allergy
Recent streptococcal infection
Previous therapy within 6 mo

GI, gastrointestinal.

grafts have been reported.[123] The length of these grafts makes them unsuitable for lytic therapy, and thus surgical thrombectomy remains the therapy of choice. Dissolution of the fibrin layer that seals Dacron prostheses can occur with systemic absorption of the drug, leading to oozing through these porous prostheses. Discontinuation of therapy usually results in stabilization of the hematoma by the surrounding capsule.

Indications

Thrombosis after Percutaneous Angioplasty

Percutaneous angioplasty is now frequently performed in this country for stenotic arterial lesions in the iliac and femoral systems. Thrombosis after balloon angioplasty is relatively infrequent, but when it occurs, local thrombolytic therapy is highly effective in restoring patency. The onset of the occlusion is known and is usually within 24 hours of the dilatation; thus, the thrombotic material is fresh and highly sensitive to fibrinolysis. The underlying stenosis has been relieved by the angioplasty, and when thrombosis occurs immediately, it is a simple matter to change catheters so that proximal infusion is promptly initiated.

Over 80% of post–balloon dilatation thrombosis cases can be successfully treated with intraarterial lytic therapy.[124–126] The duration of therapy is short because the infusion is started early and the thrombotic material is fresh. Thus, thrombectomy of a friable, recently dilated artery can be avoided. If dilatation of an iliac lesion was performed through an ipsilateral puncture, there is risk of bleeding and pseudoaneurysm formation (Fig. 20–3). If patency was restored by the infusion, repair of the pseu-

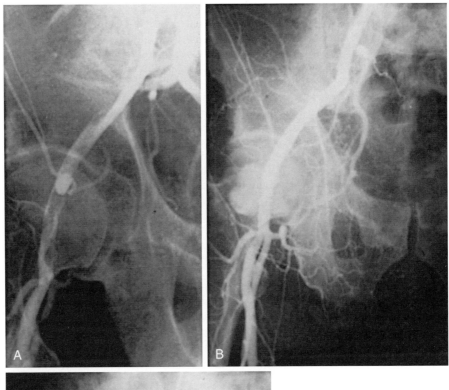

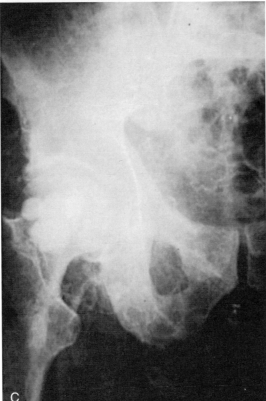

Figure 20–3. A 63-year-old man undergoing balloon angioplasty of a right external iliac stenosis. *A*, Postprocedural angiogram shows thrombosis of the dilated segment. *B*, After 12 hours of intraarterial streptokinase, there is complete resolution of the thrombus. *C*, A pseudoaneurysm is evident on angiography. Repair was limited to suture closure of perforation without the need for thrombectomy.

doaneurysm has been simplified to closure of the puncture site without embolectomy.

Native Vessel Occlusion

Acute occlusion of a native artery can be the result of thrombosis secondary to an underlying stenosis or embolization from a central source. In selecting patients for intraarterial lytic therapy, it is important to attempt to delineate the mechanism of occlusion. Lytic therapy appears to be more effective when applied to peripheral embolization.[123] Whereas 50% to 60% of thrombotic occlusions will resolve with thrombolytic therapy, around 80% of embolic occlusions will be effectively lysed. On the other hand, the surgical management of proximal lower extremity emboli by transfemoral embolectomy is highly successful, with low morbidity and mortality. In addition, some investigators have noted that emboli secondary to atrial fibrillation may have well-organized components and thus be resistant to fibrinolysis.[127] For these reasons, we prefer surgical embolectomy for proximal (iliac, femoral) emboli secondary to atrial fibrillation. If the embolus is secondary to a recent myocardial infarction (where the surgical risk is increased and the embolus is usually fresh clot), intraarterial fibrinolytic therapy should be considered. It must be kept in mind that the presence of mural thrombus in the ventricle, usually secondary to a recent myocardial infarction, is a relative contraindication to lytic therapy. Although the absence of such findings on echocardiography does not absolutely exclude the possibility, their presence, as demonstrated by an echocardiogram, should raise the level of concern in consideration of lytic therapy.

The management of multiple distal embolization must be individualized, depending on the viability of the extremity and the surgical risk. Intraarterial lytic therapy is a reasonable option in these patients when the extremity is viable and the anticipated surgical reconstruction difficult. If the ischemia is not well tolerated, we proceed with popliteal exploration, thrombectomy, and, on occasion, intraoperative lytic therapy (see later in this section).

The use of local fibrinolytic therapy for thrombotic arterial occlusions should be based on the anticipated difficulty, morbidity, and mortality of the surgical alternative. The success rate of fibrinolytic therapy alone in thrombotic occlusion is variable. Of 25 patients with atherosclerotic occlusion, Risius and associates[128] succeeded in treating 13 (52%); of these 13, only 4 required no further therapy, 3 had successful percutaneous transluminal angioplasty (PTA), and the remaining 6 required surgery or distal amputations. In 40 patients with thrombotic occlusions treated by Katzen and colleagues[125] with intraarterial lytic therapy, the outcomes of 32 (80%) were considered successful. No mention is made of other interventions in this group. Successful lysis was achieved by Graor and colleagues[124] in 25 (56%) of 45 patients with thrombotic arterial occlusions. Eighteen of these 25 patients required secondary procedures. Seventy-eight percent of patients whose thrombi were less than 30 days old were successfully lysed, compared with 37% of patients with older occlusions. This trend has been observed by others and confirmed by recently completed randomized prospective clinical trials (see later).

Careful analysis of the reported series reveals that although the lytic infusion may reestablish patency, additional procedures are often required. If surgical management becomes necessary, frequently this has been simplified because better preoperative planning is possible. Thus, if the ischemia is well tolerated, the anticipated surgical intervention complex, the occlusion fairly recent (within 2 weeks), and the patient at significant increased surgical risk, thrombolytic therapy seems justified. From the reported experience, long-term results will depend mainly on whether a correctable lesion is identified and on the location of the occlusion. Larger vessel occlusions resolved by intraarterial lytic therapy tend to do better, with an expected patency at 2 years of 60%. Superficial femoral and popliteal occlusions similarly treated, on the other hand, have a lower long-term patency of about 30% at 2 years.[129] If a correctable lesion is identified and appropriately treated, long-term results are significantly improved. Patencies as low as 20% at 2 years have been reported when no causative lesion was identified.[130]

There are specific instances in which surgical intervention has traditionally achieved poor results. Emboli or thrombosis of the popliteal artery with distal clot propagation or multiple tibial embolization carries a risk of amputation of 40%, despite prompt surgical embolectomy.[3, 131, 132] In patients with a viable extremity at presentation in whom no major runoff vessels are seen on angiography, a trial of local fibrinolytic therapy may improve these results. Surgical correction of the underlying lesion (stenosis or aneurysm) can be performed in a timely fashion. When severe ischemia precludes lytic therapy, we prefer to proceed with popliteal exploration and embolectomy. Intraoperative intraarterial infusion of lytic agents in an attempt to lyse clot inaccessible to the embolectomy catheter may improve results of embolectomy alone.

Thrombosis or embolization to the renal arteries is a promising area in which thrombolytic therapy may offer significant advantages over surgical intervention (Fig. 20–4). As a complication of myocardial infarction, an embolus to the renal artery carries an inordinate risk with surgical intervention. Capsular collaterals frequently maintain viability of the renal parenchyma to allow sufficient time for success with thrombolytic therapy. The material is sensitive to lysis, and the length of the occlusion is short. The reported experience is limited but has been highly successful.[125, 133] If a stenosis is uncovered during infusion, percutaneous dilatation or elective surgical repair may be undertaken, as deemed appropriate.

Acute mesenteric artery occlusion has been successfully treated by local intraarterial streptokinase infusion.[134] In contrast to the kidneys, the bowel is exquisitely sensitive to ischemia and reperfusion. It is difficult to assess clinically the tolerance to ischemia on presentation and during therapy. We have attempted lytic therapy in four patients with emboli to the mesenteric circulation as a complication of an acute myocardial infarction. Two patients required laparotomy and bowel resection. In one, no further revascularization was necessary. The other necessitated embolectomy and second-look laparotomy. The third patient had complete resolution of symptoms, avoiding laparotomy

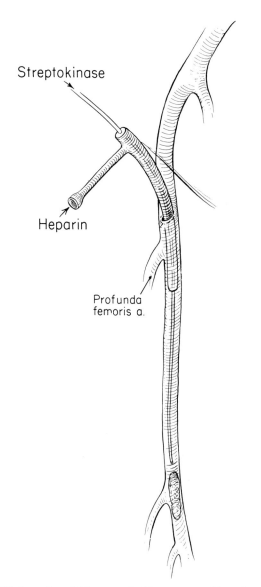

Figure 20–4. Preferred delivery method for intraarterial lytic therapy for distal lower extremity occlusions. Low-dose heparin is infused through the coaxial system to avoid upstream thrombus.

altogether (Fig. 20–5). The fourth patient required laparotomy without bowel resection or need for revascularization. The fourth case underscores the difficulty in clinical follow-up during this type of nonoperative approach. If lytic therapy is elected for acute mesenteric ischemia, any deterioration in the overall clinical status, persistent acidosis, or sepsis should mandate emergency exploration. Otherwise, frequent angiographic assessment, as often as every 6 hours, is advisable. Failure to show progress during these intervals should trigger early, rather than delayed, exploration.

Acute Graft Occlusion

Acute occlusion of an arterial graft frequently leads to recurrent symptoms and, on occasion, limb-threatening ischemia. Thrombectomy, with or without revision, achieves excellent results in prosthetic grafts and variable results in

autogenous vein grafts.[135] Autogenous vein grafts frequently require extensive revision and replacement. Intraarterial thrombolytic therapy, on the other hand, has been highly unsuccessful in resolving prosthetic graft occlusions. Of 25 patients with prosthetic graft occlusions treated with local lytic therapy by Sussman and coworkers,[123] only six were successful, five of which required surgical correction of the offending lesion. In the 17 failures, amputation followed in 12 patients. In the experience reported by Van Breda and colleagues,[132] of 19 patients with 20 prosthetic graft occlusions, only 4 patients were managed nonoperatively, 2 of whom required PTA. Despite this, lytic therapy was considered beneficial because it allowed elective surgery in 12 patients and improvement in the surgical risk in an additional two patients. An adjunctive role for lytic therapy was proposed. Although achieving successful lysis in 7 of 10 polytetrafluoroethylene (PTFE) grafts with thrombolytic therapy, Graor and associates[124] noted that surgical revision was required in most of these patients. In view of the excellent results obtained with surgical thrombectomy, one must seriously question the value of thrombolytic therapy in the management of prosthetic graft occlusions.

The results obtained with lytic therapy in the management of occluded autogenous grafts have been somewhat more gratifying. In the experience of Perler and colleagues,[136] occluded vein grafts were more susceptible to lytic therapy than were PTFE grafts. This experience is shared by others.[137] Graor and coworkers,[124] however, observed a similar response between PTFE and vein grafts, reporting a 75% success rate in vein grafts occluded for less than 14 days. Taking into account the variable results with surgical thrombectomy in the management of occluded autologous grafts, a trial of lytic therapy, when the event has been recent, is an attractive alternative. However, in our experience, long saphenous vein grafts to tibial vessels in the lower third of the leg or ankle appear to be less responsive to lytic therapy. This may have to do with limited supplies of plasminogen in these very low-flow grafts. Nevertheless, even in unsuccessful attempts, at op-

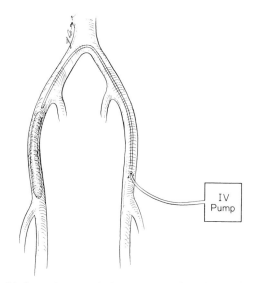

Figure 20–5. Preferred method of intraarterial lytic therapy for proximal (*iliac, common femoral*) occlusions. If possible, the catheter tip should be within the thrombus.

eration it is not unusual to find liquefied, thickened blood in the graft, thus minimizing the need for mechanical thrombectomy. The operation may actually be limited to removal of the most distal occlusive material and revision of an identified lesion. Retrieving an occluded vein graft in these circumstances is possible with minimal mechanical trauma to the endothelium.

We take into account several factors when deciding whether to use lytic therapy for an occluded graft. Certainly, surgical risk must be assessed. Infrequently, surgery is avoided altogether. If delaying surgical intervention allows for improvement of the overall risk, lytic therapy should be considered. If little improvement is expected, it is preferable to proceed with thrombectomy in a timely fashion. When dealing with a prosthetic graft occlusion, thrombectomy remains the therapy of choice. In patients in whom multiple previous reconstructions make a surgical approach less desirable, a trial of lytic therapy is a reasonable option; however, one must realize that the chances of success without eventual surgical correction are low. The management of an occluded vein graft differs, in that the results of surgical thrombectomy are less predictable. Thus, if the ischemia is well tolerated, a trial of lytic therapy may help restore patency of the vein graft. Correction of the causative lesion may then be undertaken without the need for thrombectomy of the graft. This can be accomplished percutaneously if the lesion is less than 0.5 cm in length, or preferably surgically for longer lesions. Long-term results of this approach tend to correlate with preocclusion history of the bypass. Grafts that fail within the first year after implantation fare worse than those that have been patent for longer periods. Thus, an early failure of a vein bypass graft in which a complex lesion is identified may be best treated with a new reconstruction if autogenous tissue is available. Failure of a vein graft beyond 1 year may be best treated with a trial of lytic therapy and correction of the causative lesion.

Results of Randomized Trials in Peripheral Vascular Disease

Despite a multitude of retrospective reviews of the results of thrombolytic therapy in the management of thrombotic complications of peripheral arterial disease, the precise role of this form of therapy could not be clearly established. For this reason, several investigators embarked in prospective, randomized trials comparing surgery versus thrombolysis for ischemia of the lower extremities.

The largest trial to date (STILE) randomized 393 patients with either native arterial or bypass graft occlusion to either optimal surgical therapy or intraarterial, catheter-directed thrombolysis with either rt-PA or urokinase.[138] Outcomes were analyzed on an intention-to-treat basis to maintain statistical validity. rt-PA was given at 0.05 mg/kg/hour for up to 12 hours, or urokinase at 250,000-unit bolus injection, followed by 4000 units/minute for 4 hours, then 2000 units/minute for up to 36 hours. End points measured included death, ongoing or recurrent ischemia, major amputation, and major morbidity. Additional end points included reduction in surgical procedure, clinical outcome classification, length of hospitalization, and outcome by

duration of ischemia. The randomization produced equivalent groups in terms of risk factors and comorbid conditions. A monitoring committee terminated the study prior to its anticipated patient recruitment because a significant primary end point occurred in the first interim analysis. Failure or inability to place the catheter in the thrombolytic group occurred in 28% of patients who were randomized, and these were considered treatment failures. A significant benefit of surgical therapy compared with thrombolysis occurred at 30 days, primarily because of a reduction in ongoing or recurrent ischemia. Clinical outcome classification at 30 days was similar. Stratification by duration of ischemia suggested that patients with ischemia of less than 14 days' duration had lower amputation rates with thrombolysis and shorter hospital stays. Patients with ischemia of longer duration (more than 14 days) who were treated surgically had less ongoing or recurrent ischemia and trends toward lower morbidity. At 6 months, there was an improved amputation-free survival in acutely ischemic patients treated with thrombolysis. However, chronically ischemic patients who were treated surgically had lower major amputation rates. Fifty-five percent of patients treated with thrombolysis had a reduction in the magnitude of their surgical procedure. No difference between rt-PA and urokinase was noted, with fibrinogen depletion being a predictor of hemorrhagic complications. The investigators concluded that surgical revascularization of patients with less than 6 months' duration of ischemic symptoms was more effective and safer than catheter-directed thrombolysis. Crossover to surgical treatment from the thrombolytic group probably accounted for the clinical outcomes being similar in both groups at 30 days. Patients who had less than 14 days' duration of ischemia who were treated with thrombolysis had an improved amputation-free survival compared with patients who underwent surgical treatments. Of concern was the 28% of patients in the thrombolytic arm, who in reality did not receive thrombolytic therapy because of failure to place the catheter within the thrombus. Subsequent analysis revealed that even if these patients were eliminated from the analysis as failures in the thrombolytic arm, the results and conclusions did not change.

Further analysis of those patients within the STILE study[139] who had native, nonembolic arterial thrombosis has been completed. Two hundred thirty-seven patients with lower extremity ischemia due to iliofemoral or superficial femoropopliteal native artery occlusion, with symptomatic deterioration within 6 months, were randomized to either thrombolytic therapy or surgical revascularization. Prior to randomization, the optimal surgical procedure was determined for subsequent comparison with eventual outcome. For patients randomized to lytic therapy, the catheter could be properly positioned and the lytic agent delivered in 78% of patients. Thus, 22% of patients did not receive lytic therapy within the lytic therapy group due to inability to position the catheter. A reduction in the subsequent surgical procedure performed occurred in 58% of patients with femoropopliteal occlusions and in 51% of patients with iliofemoral occlusions. rt-PA and urokinase were equally effective and safe, but lysis time was shorter with rt-PA compared with that with urokinase (8 vs. 24 hours, respectively). At 1 year, the incidence of recurrent ischemia was significantly higher in patients treated with thrombolytic therapy compared with those treated with surgery (64 vs. 35%, respectively). Major amputation rates were also higher in the thrombolytic therapy group, with 10% of patients eventually requiring a major amputation in the thrombolytic arm of the study versus no patients in the surgical therapy arm. Factors that were associated with poor lytic outcome included femoropopliteal occlusion, diabetes, and the presence of critical ischemia. There was no difference in mortality observed at 1 year between the surgical and lytic therapy groups. The investigators concluded that surgical revascularization for lower extremity native arterial occlusions was more effective and durable than thrombolysis. A reduction in the planned surgical procedure occurred for the majority of patients treated with thrombolysis. However, long-term outcome was inferior, particularly in those patients with femoropopliteal occlusions, diabetes, or critical ischemia.

A prospective, randomized comparison of thrombolytic therapy with operative revascularization in the initial management of acute peripheral arterial ischemia was performed in a single institution and published in 1994.[140] In this study, patients with limb-threatening ischemia of less than 7 days' duration were randomly assigned to intraarterial, catheter-directed urokinase therapy or operative intervention. If an anatomic lesion was unmasked by the thrombolytic infusion, this was treated with either balloon angioplasty or surgery. Primary end points included limb salvage and survival. One hundred fourteen patients were randomized; 57 received thrombolytic therapy, and an equal number were randomized to surgery. Thrombolytic therapy resulted in dissolution of occluding thrombus in 70% of patients in the lytic group. Cumulative limb salvage was similar in the two treatment groups at 12 months (82%). Cumulative survival, however, was significantly improved in patients randomized to thrombolysis (84% vs. 58% at 12 months). Mortality differences appeared to be primarily due to an increased frequency of in-hospital cardiopulmonary complications in the surgical arm. The benefits of thrombolysis appeared to be accomplished without significant differences in the duration of hospitalization and with a modest increase in hospital cost (median, $15,672 vs. $12,253). Intraarterial thrombolytic therapy was associated with the reduction of in-hospital cardiopulmonary complications and therefore improved patient survival. Based on these results and to further elucidate the possible impact of thrombolytic therapy on 1-year survival, a multicenter, randomized, prospective trial comparing thrombolysis or peripheral arterial surgery (TOPAS) was carried out.[141] Phase I of this trial was designed as a dose-ranging trial to evaluate the safety and efficacy of three doses of recombinant urokinase in comparison with surgery. Two hundred thirteen patients who had acute lower extremity ischemia of less than 14 days' duration were prospectively randomized to one of two groups. The first group received one of three dosages of recombinant urokinase (2000, 4000, or 6000 IU/minute for 4 hours, then 2000 IU/minute for a maximum of 48 hours). The second group underwent surgical revascularization. When success was accomplished with thrombolytic therapy, this was followed by either surgical or endovascular intervention when a lesion responsible for the occlusion was recognized. Follow-up on an intent-to-treat basis was carried out to 1 year. The most effective dosage of recombinant urokinase was found to be 4000 IU/minute. This accomplished complete thrombolysis in 35 (71%) of the 49 patients who were randomized to this dosage within the lytic therapy group. Mean infusion time was 23 hours. Patients who received 2000 IU/minute had a 67% success rate, whereas patients who were randomized to the highest dosage (6000 IU/minute) had a 60% success rate. Hemorrhagic complications were 2%, 13%, and 16% in the 4000-, 2000-, and 6000-IU/minute groups, respectively. When comparing the 4000-IU/minute group within the thrombolytic arm with the surgical group, the 1-year mortality rate was similar (14% vs. 16%, respectively), and amputation-free survival was not statistically different (75% vs. 65%, respectively). Again, patients treated with lytic therapy had a decrease in the planned surgical procedure that was statistically significant. The investigators concluded that recombinant urokinase is most effective at 4000 IU/minute. Thrombolytic therapy and surgical therapy had similar rates of survival and limb salvage.

From the foregoing results, it is evident that in patients with relatively acute ischemia, thrombolytic therapy is an important and effective treatment, with results that compare favorably with those of surgery. Considerable judgment is required in patient selection, which should take into account not only the duration of the ischemia but also the complexity of the anticipated surgical intervention, the presence of contraindications to thrombolytic therapy, and the tolerance of the limb to ischemia. Furthermore, the number of vein grafts included in these trials was not sufficient to allow specific recommendations. However, retrospective information would suggest that the long-term outcome of thrombolytic therapy in the management of thrombosed vein grafts is best when the vein graft has failed late (more than 1 year) and when a specific lesion can be identified and corrected after completion of the lytic infusion.

Hemodialysis Access

Thrombosed arteriovenous fistulas can be successfully managed by intragraft administration of fibrinolytic agents. Usually the diagnosis is established early, as the patient notices the absence of a thrill, and thus the thrombotic material is very sensitive to lysis. Administration is by direct puncture because there are no collaterals to dilute the effect of the agent. It is usually best to lace the intragraft thrombus with the lytic agent and then proceed with high-dose intragraft administration. Of 46 arteriovenous fistulas, Graor and colleagues[125] were successful in treating 40 (87%); both PTFE and vein fistulas were equally responsive. Thrombi older than 4 days were less susceptible to lysis (29%). Unfortunately, most patients required surgical revision of the venous anastomosis, and thus lytic therapy served as a temporizing intervention. In some patients, however, this would allow for better preoperative preparation and elective, rather than urgent, operation.

A new method of opening thrombosed grafts is the use of heparinized saline delivered by pulse-spray technique, followed by balloon maceration. A relatively underappreciated but well-documented phenomenon resulting from pulse-spray pharmacomechanical thrombolysis of clotted hemodialysis access grafts is that of pulmonary embolism. The introduction of pulse-spray pharmacomechanical thrombolysis in the treatment of thrombosed grafts allowed for successful lysis of the graft but on a quicker time scale and with a smaller dose of lytic agent. The pulse-spray can be done with heparinized saline or with a thrombolytic agent. A prospective, randomized double-blinded study to evaluate the incidence of pulmonary embolism following the use of this technique revealed that although pulmonary embolism occurred in both groups as documented by lung perfusion scan, the incidence was 18.2% with the use of urokinase and 64.3% with the use of heparinized saline ($P = .04$).[142] All of the patients, it should be noted, were asymptomatic.

Many studies have attempted to perform cost-benefit analysis with regard to thrombolysis versus surgical thrombectomy. The most common reason for dialysis graft failure is a lesion, usually neointimal hyperplasia, at the venous anastomosis. The interventional techniques allow thrombolysis and identification of the underlying anatomic lesion. This can be treated with attempted balloon angioplasty, and although successful in many cases, it usually requires a surgical revision at some point in the future.

Acute Stroke

The FDA, in June 1996, approved t-PA as a safe and effective treatment for acute stroke, if given within 3 hours of the onset of symptoms.[143] Following this, there has been a proliferation of large clinical trials testing the efficacy of antiplatelet and antithrombotic treatment regimens. The approval of the use of intravenous t-PA was based on the results of the National Institute of Neurological Disorders and Stroke Recombinant Tissue Plasminogen Activator Stroke Study (NINDS rt-PA stroke study), in which 624 patients with ischemic stroke were treated with 0.9 mg/kg of t-PA within 3 hours of the onset of symptoms.[144] Of the t-PA group, 31% to 50% had complete or near-complete recovery at 3 months, compared with 20% to 38% of the placebo group. This benefit prevailed for 1 year. However, there was an incidence of symptomatic brain hemorrhage of 6.4% in the t-PA group versus 0.6% in the placebo group. The mortality rates were similar between groups. The presence of a mass effect or a greater severity of initial neurologic deficit presented an increased risk of hemorrhage. The beneficial effect of t-PA was not observed in three other large trials (the European Cooperative Acute Stroke Study I, II, and the alteplase thrombolysis for acute noninterventional therapy in ischemic stroke—the ATLANTIS trial).[145-147] However, patients in these three trials were treated much later (14% treated within 3 hours) than those in the NINDS rt-PA study (622/624 enrolled within 3 hours, and 48% treated within 90 minutes).

There have been two large randomized trials evaluating intraarterial thrombolytic therapy for stroke. The Prolyse in Acute Cerebral Thromboembolism II (PROACT II) trial evaluated patients with angiographically documented occlusion of the middle cerebral artery or a first-order branch.[148] By 2 hours, there was partial or complete lysis in 67% of patients in the pro-urokinase group compared with 18% in the heparin-only group ($P<.001$). The primary outcome measure analyzed was the ability of patients to live independently 3 months after the stroke. The percentage of patients able to attain this end point was 40% in the pro-urokinase group and 25% in the heparin group ($P<.05$). Intracerebral hemorrhage with neurologic deterioration occurred in 10% of patients in the pro-urokinase group and in 2% in the heparin group ($P = .06$). This was the first trial to show a clinical benefit from the use of intraarterial thrombolysis of a middle cerebral artery occlusion. To date, there are no randomized, controlled trials comparing the efficacy of intravenous thrombolytics with intraarterial thrombolytics. It is, however, clear that at this time, thrombolytic therapy for acute ischemic stroke can no longer be considered experimental, as it has been shown to have clinical benefit, provided patient selection is strictly in

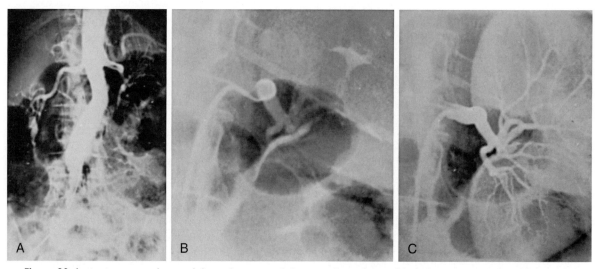

Figure 20–6. *A,* Aortogram showing left renal artery embolus. *B,* After 1 hour of high-dose intraarterial urokinase, there is partial clearing and improved perfusion to left kidney. *C,* Complete clearance of embolus after 3 hours of high-dose intraarterial urokinase.

accordance with criteria set forth in the trials and in the NINDS guidelines.

Method

Consideration of thrombolytic therapy should begin prior to the initial angiographic needle puncture. The approach is chosen so as to maximize access to the occlusion and minimize morbidity. Arterial punctures distal to the presumed occlusion are avoided. Sites where bleeding may cause serious morbidity (axillary, translumbar) are avoided. When the suspected occlusion is at a superficial femoral artery or below (strong femoral pulse), we prefer an antegrade ipsilateral puncture (Fig. 20–6). When the suspected occlusion is at the femoral level or above, a contralateral puncture with passage of the catheter around the aortic bifurcation is preferred (Fig. 20–7). Infusions in the upper extremities or aortic branches are carried out through a transfemoral approach. End-hold catheters are used for infusion, with the tip into the thrombus. If this is not possible, there should be no large branches between the catheter tip and the occlusion. When the infusion is at the popliteal level or below, small (3-Fr) catheters are used through a coaxial system to prevent upstream clot formation (Fig. 20–8). A flush heparin infusion is maintained through the coaxial catheter.

The dosage chosen will partly depend on the length and volume of thrombus and the location and clinical importance of the vascular territory. Small-volume, short thrombi in important territories (i.e., renal) are better treated with high-dose infusions aimed at rapid fibrinolysis. Excellent results have been reported using high-dose urokinase (4000 units/minute, followed after initial recanalization with 1000 to 2000 units/minute).[149] These authors recommended creation of a channel into the thrombus with the angiographic guidewire. In fact, passage of the guidewire through the occlusion is a prognostic indicator as to the response to fibrinolytic infusion. Failure to pass the guidewire through the occlusion implies either plaque or well-organized thrombus, which may be resistant to fibrinolysis. On the other hand, easy passage of the guidewire through the occlusion not only establishes a channel in which the fibrinolytic agent will have the opportunity to concentrate but also implies soft, lysable thrombi. Lacing the thrombus with 50,000 units of urokinase, so that the agent is distributed within the thrombus itself, and then retrieval of the catheter for infusion are frequently practiced and seem to be effective. When prolonged infusion is deemed necessary because of the amount of thrombus, switching to a low-dose regimen (streptokinase, 5000 to 10,000 units/hour; urokinase, 30,000 to 50,000 units/hour) is appropriate, with angiography carried out within 12 to 16 hours to assess progress. From the accumulated experience, it appears that bleeding complications correlate most with duration of therapy, rather than with total dosage of the agent. Thus, high-dose, short-term infusions are better tolerated than long-term, low-dose infusions. Therefore, it is preferable to infuse higher doses of the agent if the duration of therapy can be shortened.

Duration of the infusion is guided by periodic angiographic and clinical monitoring but should rarely exceed

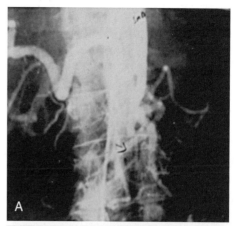
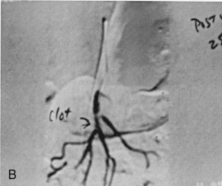
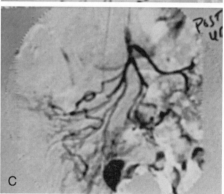

Figure 20–7. *A,* Selective superior mesenteric artery angiogram showing occlusion of distal tree. *B,* Partial clearing of embolus after 250,000 units of intraarterial urokinase administered over 1 hour. *C,* Complete resolution of superior mesenteric artery occlusion after 2 hours (500,000 units) of urokinase intraarterial therapy.

96 hours. When high-dose infusion is used, it is best to keep the patient in the radiology suite and repeat angiography as often as every 30 minutes. For low-dose infusion, the patient is monitored in an intensive care unit, and angiography is repeated daily or sooner, depending on the clinical response.

Before initiating therapy, baseline fibrinogen, thrombin time, PTT, and fibrin degradation product measurements are obtained. These are repeated 12 hours after commencing the infusion and then daily. It is expected that the fibrinogen level will drop and fibrin degradation products will become positive. Prolongation of the PTT or thrombin time suggests a systemic lytic state and will occur in about 50% of patients. Although specific parameters do not corre-

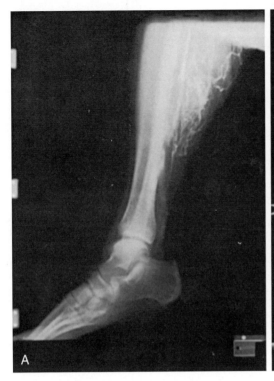
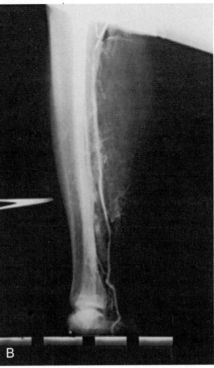

Figure 20–8. *A,* Intraoperative completion angiogram after popliteal embolectomy. Note absence of runoff vessels to the foot. *B,* Repeat angiogram after intraoperative infusion of streptokinase, 60,000 units; heparin, 1000 units over 30 minutes through the same catheter used for angiography. Note remarkable improvement in runoff.

late with the risk of bleeding, the presence of the systemic lytic state does increase such risk. If good progress is being made by the infusion, a low fibrinogen value (less than 50% of baseline) or evidence of a lytic state in the absence of bleeding complications is tolerated and therapy is continued. In the absence of a systemic lytic state when little progress is evident, the dosage is increased and the result reassessed. Therapy should be discontinued if there is no improvement in any 24-hour interval, persistent or worsening ischemia, or a major bleeding complication.

The administration of heparin during regional thrombolytic therapy is advocated by most investigators. Clearly, in patients with profound ischemia found to have very low flow in the extremity and in instances in which pericatheter thrombus formation would be significant (such as when 3 to 4 cm of the catheter is into a vessel with low or no flow), concomitant heparin administration should be strongly considered. Heparin administration may also be useful in increasing thrombolysis and minimizing the adverse consequences of a potential episode of distal clot migration or embolization. Heparin therapy, however, may increase the incidence and severity of pericatheter bleeding during lytic therapy and may increase the risk of distant bleeding.

Heparin administration is usually through a continuous infusion to maintain a prolonged PTT at 1.5 to 2.0 times control. A bolus infusion before initiation of continuous therapy is used when there is acute severe ischemia or when low-flow states are identified in the ipsilateral system or around the catheter. When using a coaxial system, a lower dose of heparin may be administered through the larger catheter, usually 500 units/hour. It is important that the PTT not exceed 60 seconds at the time of catheter and sheath removal. Heparin may then be restarted without a bolus.

When emergency surgery is required, the lytic agent is discontinued and fresh-frozen plasma administered if the fibrinogen level is below 100 mg/dL. The half-life of these agents is very short and thus usually not a problem in this setting.

Complications

As with any form of lytic therapy, bleeding is the most feared and frequent complication of low-dose fibrinolytic therapy. The risk of major bleeding (requiring cessation of therapy or blood transfusions) ranges from 5% to 15% when appropriate precautions are observed.[124, 149] Bleeding is usually related to systemic effects of the drug, and management was discussed under Systemic Lytic Therapy earlier in this chapter.

Considering that high-risk patients may be preferentially treated by this nonsurgical approach, the incidence of bleeding with intraarterial lytic therapy must be considered. The most recent experience seems to indicate that the risk of bleeding correlates more with duration than with actual total dosage. It is therefore preferable to utilize higher-dose protocols, especially in circumstances in which a short occlusion is being treated. Although specific coagulation parameters do not correlate with the risk of bleeding, the presence of a systemic lytic state increases this risk. It is important to document whether systemic effects of the drug are present because such knowledge helps determine the most appropriate course of action. Systemic effects are heralded by a 50% drop in fibrinogen from baseline, a prolongation of the thrombin time to two times normal (or higher), or both. If significant progress is being made, continuation of therapy is warranted, despite systemic fibrinolysis. If, on the other hand, no significant improvement is noted within the last interval, reassessment should be made, weighing the risks and benefits of the alternatives.

Treatment of hemorrhagic complications depends on the severity of and the progress made during lytic therapy. A small amount of oozing around the catheter entry site, without hematoma formation during the final stages of the infusion, can be controlled locally, keeping the patient under close observation until therapy is completed. The same situation in the early stages of the infusion, when more than 12 to 24 hours of therapy are anticipated, should lead to discontinuation of the drug. Development of a significant hematoma or bleeding at a remote site warrants cessation of therapy. Fibrinogen should be replaced by the administration of fibrinogen-rich components, such as cryoprecipitate or fresh-frozen plasma. This usually suffices because the half-life of both urokinase and streptokinase is short.

Distal embolization occurs more frequently than is clinically appreciated. Continuation of therapy is preferable, with perhaps a temporary increase in the hourly dose. When severe ischemia is seen as the result of distal emboli, discontinuation of lytic therapy with prompt surgical embolectomy is indicated.

Several cases of embolization to the ipsilateral extremity have been reported during intraarterial lytic therapy for occlusion of axillofemoral grafts.[124] The length of these grafts makes them unsuitable for lytic therapy, and thus surgical thrombectomy remains the therapy of choice.

Allergic reactions to streptokinase were discussed under Systemic Lytic Therapy. Routine administration of 100 mg of intravenous hydrocortisone may prevent some of these reactions and is recommended.

Pseudoaneurysm formation is rare but may occur secondary to bleeding from an arterial puncture site. Surgical repair is recommended.

Intracranial bleeding is a recognized complication of any form of lytic therapy. Any change in the neurologic status of the patient during therapy should be viewed as related to the fibrinolytic agent until proved otherwise. Bleeding from an unrecognized intracranial lesion must be ruled out. Lytic therapy should be discontinued while evaluation is proceeding.

Fatal pulmonary emboli have been reported during intraarterial fibrinolytic therapy.[126] A possible mechanism for this complication implies decreased venous circulation in the ischemic extremity, with clot formation, partial lysis, and eventual pulmonary embolization. This is a rare occurrence. Treatment options include cessation of lytic therapy with heparinization or switching to systemic intravenous lytic therapy. If the latter is chosen, leaving the intraarterial catheter in place may decrease the risk of bleeding through the arterial puncture site.

Conversion of an ischemic myocardial infarction into a hemorrhagic infarct as a complication of fibrinolytic therapy has been reported.[126] The relationship between lytic therapy and the few reported cases is unclear. Deterioration of cardiac function in the presence of an acute myocardial infarction during fibrinolytic therapy should lead the clinician to consider this possibility. Therapy should be discontinued until the cause of the cardiac decompensation is determined.

INTRAOPERATIVE THROMBOLYTIC THERAPY

Approximately 30% of lower extremity embolectomies are incomplete, with remaining intravascular defects demonstrable by completion angiography.[150] Experimental studies suggest that the true incidence may be as high as 80%.[151] The idea of removing the bulk of thrombus surgically and lysing any remaining defects is attractive from the therapeutic standpoint. Alternatives include repeat embolectomy with the balloon catheter,[152] irrigation in an attempt to flush the residual clot,[153] passage of Dormia catheters,[154] and distal exploration. All these will further injure the endothelium and thus increase its thrombogenicity. Certain endovascular procedures, such as endoscopy, atherectomy, or dilatations, may also temporarily increase the thrombogenicity of these vessels, leading to early thrombosis. Further mechanical manipulation is likely to result in further injury and thus is unlikely to solve the problem. For these reasons, controlled chemical intraoperative fibrinolysis may be a welcome alternative in the treatment of these complications. When dealing with delayed intervention in the presence of a thrombotic process, propagation of clot into the branches of the arterial tree may be most difficult to retrieve. Once these clots lose their integrity with the parent thrombus, enzymatic dissolution may be the only alternative.

Bleeding complications secondary to intraarterial fibrinolytic therapy are the result of prolonged infusions necessary to lyse extensive thrombus. The potential for intraoperative or perioperative lytic therapy was suggested by several investigators.[155–157] Common to all these observations was the lack of bleeding complications. There are several advantages to the intraoperative use of lytic agents when compared with the percutaneous method. First, the bulk of the thrombus has been surgically removed, and thus there is a decrease in the amount of lysis required. Second, a higher concentration of the agent, with control of inflow (and therefore circulation time), can be accomplished. Finally, infusion within the thrombus or adjacent to it is theoretically unnecessary, and repeat embolectomy with reassessment of the intervention can be done with repeated infusions, as necessary.

In 1985, we reported our initial experience with five patients in whom intraoperative infusions of 20,000 to 100,000 units of streptokinase were successful in restoring adequate circulation to limbs still threatened after embolectomy.[158] We have now extended this experience to 23 infusions in 22 patients.[159] In 17 of these patients, both preinfusion and postinfusion arteriograms were available; improvement following lytic therapy was seen in 13 patients (76%). Only one of these reconstructions rethrombosed in the postoperative period. All of the four patients without angiographic improvement suffered rethrombosis. Thus, it appears that preinfusion and postinfusion arteriography has prognostic significance, implying that failure to improve after intraoperative infusion of the lytic agent suggests a high likelihood of failure; therefore, alternative methods of reconstruction need to be considered at the time of surgery.

Bleeding is the most feared complication of intraoperative lytic therapy. In our experience, of 23 patients in whom lytic infusions were carried out intraoperatively, five had hematomas. All of the hematomas occurred in patients who were fully heparinized postoperatively. Among 12 patients who were not heparinized after surgery, there were no bleeding complications. Thus, bleeding after intraoperative lytic therapy is secondary to aggressive antithrombotic and anticoagulation regimens rather than to the lytic therapy itself.

Clinical experience to date is summarized in Table 20–4. Five additional clinical series have been reported since our initial report.[122, 165–167] Cohen and colleagues[122] performed 13 infusions by bolus of 25,000 to 250,000 units of streptokinase. Eight (61%) of the infusions were successful. Five bleeding complications occurred, one of them resulting in death secondary to retroperitoneal bleeding during aortoiliac reconstruction. This suggests that caution should be exercised with intraoperative use of lytic agents during major abdominal or retroperitoneal surgery. Norem and associates[166] reported their experience with 19 infusions of 50,000 to 200,000 units of streptokinase by bolus injection. They followed the infusion with repeat embolectomy and were able to retrieve additional thrombus in each instance. Two wound hematomas occurred in the postoperative period. Heparin was maintained following surgery at low doses (200 to 500 units/hour). With this regimen, bleeding complications appeared to have been minimized. In a report from Spain, investigators studied 66 femoropopliteal or distal acute arterial occlusions by means of arteriography and Doppler imaging before and after surgery. Patients were prospectively evaluated after either mechanical thromboembolectomy as a single technique ($n = 35$) or

thromboembolectomy plus 250,000 IU of urokinase administered over 30 minutes intraarterially at the completion of thromboembolectomy ($n = 31$). Intraoperative angiography revealed residual thrombus in 30% of patients and unsuspected arterial lesions in 34%. Recurrence of thrombosis was associated with residual thrombus and amputation. Patients who received the intraoperative thrombolytic infusion had higher ankle-arm indices postoperatively than did those who underwent mechanical thromboembolectomy alone. Amputations and the need for distal revascularization were not different between the two groups, although quantitatively the results were better in the lytic group than in the group receiving mechanical thromboembolectomy alone (failure rate, 9.68% vs. 22.86%). There were no bleeding complications with routine intraoperative use of lytic therapy after mechanical thromboembolectomy.

Our preferred technique for intraoperative infusion of fibrinolytic agents consists of a drip infusion of the agent without occlusion of the inflow. Experimental evidence suggests that maintenance of blood flow in the system during administration of fibrinolytic agents enhances their effectiveness. This can be accomplished by insertion of a cannula distal to the arteriotomy after repair of the latter. We prefer urokinase, 250,000 units dissolved in 100 mL of saline, delivered over 30 minutes. On the basis of our original experimental study, we continue to recommend the addition of heparin to the infusate at 1 to 4 units/mL.[151] Preinfusion and postinfusion arteriography is recommended to document the effectiveness of the agent. Failure to show improvement in the postinfusion angiogram would suggest a high likelihood of failure and consideration of alternative management. More recently, the use of an

TABLE 20-4

Results of Intraoperative Regional Fibrinolytic Therapy

REFERENCE	CASES (N)	DRUG DOSE AND METHOD	SUCCESSFUL (%)	COMPLICATIONS	REMARKS
Cohen et al.[122]	13	SK: 25,000–250,000 units by bolus	61	5 rethromboses; 5 bleeding complications; 1 death after retroperitoneal surgery	2 renal infusions, 1 partly successful; death related to retroperitoneal bleeding
Norem et al.[161]	19	SK: 50,000–200,000 units by bolus	100	2 wound hematomas	All patients underwent repeat embolectomy; postoperative heparin in low doses (200–500 units/hr)
Parent et al.[162]	28	SK: 50,000–150,000 units by bolus UK: 35,000–150,000 units by bolus	88	Bleeding 11%; compartment syndrome 21%; 2 deaths	Deaths not related to lytic therapy; 2 bleeding complications in 2 patients after retroperitoneal surgery
Comerota et al.[160]	38	SK: Maximum 50,000 units UK: Maximum 150,000 units by bolus 2 patients; isolated limb—UK: 1,000,000 units	74	1 wound hematoma; 5 deaths	Deaths not related to lytic agent
Quiñones-Baldrich et al.[158]	23	SK: 60,000–100,000 units UK: 250,000–375,000 units plus heparin 1–4 units/ml Gravity infusion over 30 min	74	6 rethromboses; 5 wound hematomas	All wound hematomas in patients fully heparinized postoperatively

SK, streptokinase; UK, urokinase.

isolated limb perfusion with an extracorporeal pump has shown promise in further enhancing the effectiveness of the lytic agent.[163]

Urokinase appears to be a safer agent for intraoperative use. Allergic reactions are not seen. The mechanism of action is direct, and the risk of plasminogen depletion, as may occur with streptokinase, is eliminated. The best method and the appropriate dosage, however, have not been determined. The logistic advantages of bolus infusion are obvious. Nevertheless, a slow infusion has the theoretical advantage of providing a constant amount of the drug while plasminogen is being supplied by the collateral circulation. Bolus infusion, although achieving a high concentration of the agent rapidly, is likely to be washed out, and thus the effect may be very short-lived. An experimental study was carried out in our laboratory to further elucidate the best method of infusion. In addition to bolus infusion and slow 30-minute infusion, we included a group of animals in which the limb was isolated with a proximal tourniquet and the artery and vein connected to an extracorporeal pump. Angiographic results were significantly improved by the use of the isolated limb perfusion technique with simi-

lar doses of urokinase.[163] In addition, maintenance of inflow during the slow infusion appeared to improve results compared with when inflow was occluded. However, these were not statistically significant, probably due to the number of animals studied. Thus, isolated limb perfusion with extracorporeal pump support of the extremity during revascularization may enhance fibrinolytic activity and improve the efficacy of drug delivery. Clinical experience with this technique to date is promising but limited.

The high selectivity for fibrin of t-PA and the positive early results with relatively short-term infusion suggest that this is a promising agent for intraoperative use. To date, there are no reports of intraoperative use of t-PA.

In summary, we do not hesitate to proceed with an intraoperative fibrinolytic infusion when faced with either residual thrombus inaccessible to the balloon catheter or persistent ischemia after restoration of flow. Although the best method of delivery and most appropriate dosage have not been fully determined, reported clinical experience has allowed guidelines that permit the clinician to obtain the benefits of fibrinolytic infusion in these difficult cases with both safety and efficacy.

References

1. Gross R: Fibrinolyse and Thrombolyse. Panorama, September 1962:4.
2. Malpighi M: De polypo cordis. Opera omnia, p 2. Ludg Batav, 1687, p 311.
3. Morgagni JB: De sedivus et causis morborum per anatomen indagatis, 2nd ed. 1761. Translated by Alexander B: The Seats and Causes of Diseases Investigated by Anatomy, vol 3, book 4. London, Millar, 1769.
4. Morawitz P: Über einige postmortale Blutveränderungen. Beitr Chem Physiol Pathol 8:1, 1906.
5. Dastre A: Fibrinolyse dans le sang. Arch Physiol Norm Pathol 5:661, 1893.
6. Astrup T: The haemostatic balance. Thromb Diath Haemost 2:347, 1958.
7. Henkin J, Marcotte P, Yang H: The plasminogen-plasmin system. Prog Cardiovasc Dis 34:135–164, 1991.
8. Kwaan HC: Hematologic aspects of thrombolytic therapy. In Comerota AJ (ed): Thrombolytic Therapy. Orlando, Fla, Grune & Stratton, 1988.
9. Sugiyama N, Iwamoto M, Abiko A: Effects of kringles derived from human plasminogen on fibrinolysis in vitro. Thromb Res 47:459–468, 1987.
10. Wiman B, Lijnen HR, Collen D: On the specific interaction between the lysine-binding sites in plasminogen and complementary sites in α_2-antiplasmin and in fibrinogen. Biochim Biophys Acta 579:142–154, 1979.
11. Lo SK, Ryan TJ, Gilboa N, et al: Role of catalytic and lysine-binding sites in plasmin-induced neutrophil adherence to endothelium. J Clin Invest 84:793–801, 1989.
12. Thorsen S: Differences in the binding to fibrin of native plasminogen and plasminogen modified by proteolytic degradation influence of omega-aminocarboxylic acids. Biochim Biophys Acta 393:55–65, 1975.
13. Rylatt DB, Blake LE, Cottis DA, et al: An immunoassay for human d-dimer using monoclonal antibodies. Thromb Res 31:767, 1983.
14. Burrowes CE: Activation of human prekallikrein by plasmin. Fed Proc 30:451, 1971.
15. Powell JR, Castellino FJ: Amino acid sequence analysis of the asparagine-288 region of the carbohydrate variants of human plasminogen. Biochemistry 22:923–927, 1983.
16. Collen D, Wiman B: Turnover of antiplasmin, the fast-acting plasmin inhibitor of plasma. Blood 53:313–324, 1979.
17. Low DA, Baker JB, Koonce WC: Released protease nexin regulates

cellular binding, internalization, and degradation of serine proteases. Proc Natl Acad Sci USA 78:2340–2344, 1981.
18. Royston D: Review paper: The serine antiprotease aprotinin (Trasylol™): A novel approach to reducing postoperative bleeding. Blood Coagul Fibrinolysis 1:55–69, 1990.
19. Verstraete M: Clinical applications of inhibitors of fibrinolysis. Drugs 29:236–261, 1985.
20. Clozel JP, Banken L, Roux S: Aprotinin: An antidote for recombinant tissue-type plasminogen activator (rt-PA) active in vivo. J Am Coll Cardiol 16:507–510, 1990.
21. Kwaan HC: The biologic role of components of the plasminogen-plasmin system. Prog Cardiovasc Dis 34:309–316, 1992.
22. Kirchheimer JC, Wojta J, Christ G, et al: Proliferation of a human epidermal tumor cell line stimulated by urokinase. FASEB J 1:125–218, 1987.
23. Kirchheimer JC, Wojta J, Christ G, et al: Mitogenic effect of urokinase on malignant and unaffected adjacent human renal cells. Carcinogenesis 9:2121–2123, 1988.
24. Rabbani SA, Desjardins J, Bell AW, et al: An aminoterminal fragment of urokinase isolated from a prostate cancer cell line (PC-3) is mitogenic for osteoblast-like cells. Biochem Biophys Res Commun 173:1058–1064, 1990.
25. Juhan-Vague I, Alessi MC, Joly P, et al: Plasma plasminogen activator inhibitor-1 in angina pectoris. Influence of plasma insulin and acute-phase response. Arteriosclerosis 9:362–367, 1989.
26. Wiman B, Hamsten A: Impaired fibrinolysis and risk of thromboembolism. Prog Cardiovasc Dis 34:179–192, 1991.
27. Andreotti F, Davies GJ, Hackett DR, et al: Major circadian fluctuations in fibrinolytic factors and possible relevance to time of onset of myocardial infarction, sudden cardiac death and stroke. Am J Cardiol 62:635–637, 1988.
28. Grimaudo V, Hauert J, Bachmann F, et al: Diurnal variation of the fibrinolytic system. Thromb Haemost 59:495–499, 1988.
29. Angleton P, Chandler WL, Schmer G: Diurnal variation of tissue-type plasminogen activator and its rapid inhibition. Circulation 79:101–106, 1989.
30. Chandler WL, Trimble SL, Loo S-C, Mornin D: Effect of PAI-1 levels on the molar concentrations of active tissue plasminogen activator (t-PA) and t-PA/PAI-1 complex in plasma. Blood 76:930–937, 1990.
31. Urano T, Sumiyoshi K, Nakamura M, et al: Fluctuation of tPA and PAI-1 antigen levels in plasma: Difference in their fluctuation patterns between male and female. J Thromb Res 60:55–62, 1990.

32. Mannucci PM, Rota L: Plasminogen activator response after DDAVP: A clinical fibromycological study. Thromb Res 20:69, 1980.

33. Walker ID, Davidson JF: Long term fibrinolytic enhancement with anabolic steroid therapy: A five year study. In Davidson JF, Rowan RM, Samama MM, Desnoyers PC (eds): Progress in Chemical Fibrinolysis and Thrombolysis, vol 3. New York, Raven Press, 1978, pp 491–500.

34. Jarrett PE, Moreland M, Browse NL: Idiopathic recurrent superficial thrombophlebitis: Treatment with fibrinolytic enhancement. BMJ 1:933, 1977.

35. Tillett WS, Garner RL: The fibrinolytic activity of hemolytic streptococci. J Exp Med 58:485, 1933.

36. Kakkar VV, Sagar S, Lewis M: Treatment of deep vein thrombosis with intermittent streptokinase and plasminogen infusion. Lancet 2:674, 1975.

37. MacFarlane RG, Pilling J: Fibrinolytic activity of normal urine. Nature 159:779, 1947.

38. Lijnen HR, Zamarron C, Blaber M, et al: Activation of plasminogen by pro-urokinase. I. mechanism. J Biol Chem 261:1253–1258, 1986.

39. Barnathan ES, Kuo A, Rosenfeld L, et al: Interaction of single-chain urokinase-type plasminogen activator with human endothelial cells. J Biol Chem 265:2865–2872, 1990.

40. Behrendt N, Ronne E, Plough M, et al: The human receptor for urokinase plasminogen activator. NH$_2$-terminal amino acid sequence and glycosylation variants. J Biol Chem 265:6453–6460, 1990.

41. Nykjaer A, Petersen CM, Christensen EI, et al: Urokinase receptors in human monocytes. Biochim Biophys Acta 1052:399–407, 1990.

42. Watahiki Y, Takeda Y, Takeda A: Kinetic analyses of the activation of Glu-plasminogen by urokinase in the presence of fibrin, fibrinogen or its degradation products. Thromb Res 46:9–18, 1987.

43. Feissinger JN, Aiach M, Capron L, et al: Effect of local urokinase on arterial occlusion of lower limbs. Thromb Haemost 45:230, 1981.

44. McNicol GP, Gale SB, Douglas AS: In vitro and in vivo studies of a preparation of urokinase. BMJ 1:909, 1963.

45. Belkin M, Belkin B, Bucknam CA, Straub JJ, Lowe R: Intraarterial fibrinolytic therapy: Efficacy of streptokinase versus urokinase. Arch Surg 121:769, 1986.

46. Tennant SN, Dixon J, Venable TC, et al: Intracoronary thrombolysis in patients with acute myocardial infarction: Comparison of the efficacy of urokinase versus streptokinase. Circulation 69:756, 1984.

47. Van Breda A, Katzen BT, Deutsch AS: Urokinase versus streptokinase in local thrombolysis. Radiology 165:109, 1987.

48. Graor RA, Young JR, Risius B, Ruschhaupt WF: Comparison of cost effectiveness of streptokinase and urokinase in the treatment of deep vein thrombosis. Ann Vasc Surg 1:524, 1987.

49. Fletcher AP, Alkjaersig N, Sherry S, et al: The development of urokinase as a thrombolytic agent. Maintenance of a sustained thrombolytic state in man by intravenous infusion. J Lab Clin Med 65:713, 1965.

50. Kakkar VV, Scully MF: Thrombolytic therapy. Br Med Bull 34:191, 1978.

51. Toki N, Sumi H, Sasaki K, et al: Oral administration of high molecular weight urokinase in human subjects and in an experimental dog model. In Davidson JF, Nilsson IM, Astedt B (eds): Progress in Fibrinolysis, vol 5. Edinburgh, Churchill Livingstone, 1981.

52. Ouriel K: Urokinase and the US Food and Drug Administration. J Vasc Surg 30:957–958, 1999.

53. Verstraete M: Third-generation thrombolytic drugs. Am J Med 109:52–58, 2000.

54. Albrechtsen OK: The fibrinolytic agents in saline extracts of human tissues. Scand J Clin Lab Invest 10:91, 1958.

55. Rijken DC, Wijngaards G, Zaal-DeJong M, et al: Purification and partial characterization of plasminogen activator from human uterine tissue. Biochim Biophys Acta 580:140, 1979.

56. Collen D: Human tissue type plasminogen activator: From the laboratory to the bedside [editorial]. Circulation 72:18, 1985.

57. Rijken DC, Collen D: Purification and characterization of the plasminogen activator secreted by human melanoma cells in culture. J Biol Chem 156:7035, 1981.

58. Collen D, Stassen JM, Marafine BJ Jr, et al: Biological properties of human tissue type plasminogen activator obtained by expression of recombinant DNA in mammalian cells. J Pharmacol Exp Ther 231:146, 1984.

59. Sherry S: Tissue plasminogen activator (t-PA): Will it fulfill its promise? N Engl J Med 313:1014, 1985.

60. Stoughton J, Ouriel K, Shortell CK, et al: Plasminogen acceleration of urokinase thrombolysis. J Vasc Surg 19:298–305, 1994.

61. TIMI Study Group: The Thrombolysis in Myocardial Infarction (TIMI) Trial. Phase I findings. N Engl J Med 312:932, 1985.

62. Gao S, Morser J, McLean K, et al: Differential effect of platelets on plasminogen activation by tissue plasminogen activator, urokinase, and streptokinase. Thromb Res 58:421–433, 1990.

63. Klabunde RE, Burke SE, Henkin J: Enhanced lytic efficacy of multiple bolus injections of tissue plasminogen activator in dogs. Thromb Res 58:511–517, 1990.

64. Graor RA, Risius B, Young JR, et al: Peripheral artery and bypass graft thrombolysis with recombinant human tissue type plasminogen activator. Circulation 72(Suppl 3):III–15, 1985.

65. Ross AM: New plasminogen activators: A clinical review. Clin Cardiol 22:165–171, 1999.

66. Stringer KA: Biochemical and pharmacologic comparison of thrombolytic agents. Pharmacotherapy 16:119S–126S, 1996.

67. Pannell R, Gurevich V: Pro-urokinase: A study of its stability in plasma and of a mechanism for its selective fibrinolytic effect. Blood 67:1215–1223, 1986.

68. Tebbe U, Michels R, Adgey J, et al: Randomized, double-blind study comparing saruplase with streptokinase therapy in acute myocardial infarction: The COMPASS Equivalence Trial. Comparison Trial of Saruplase and Streptokinase (COMASS) Investigators. J Am Coll Cardiol 31:487–493, 1998.

69. Furlan A, Higashida R, Wechsler L, et al: Intraarterial prourokinase for acute ischemic stroke. The PROACT II study: A randomized controlled trial. Prolyse in Acute Cerebral Thromboembolism. JAMA 282:2003–2011, 1999.

70. Ouriel K, Kandarpa K, Schuerr DM, et al: Prourokinase versus urokinase for recanalization of peripheral occlusions, safety and efficacy: The PURPOSE trial. J Vasc Interv Radiol 10:1083–1091, 1999.

71. Kohnert U, Randolph R, Verheijen JH, et al: Biochemical properties of the kringle 2 and protease domains are maintained in the refolded t-PA deletion variant BM06.022 by synthetic inhibitors and substrates. Protein Sci 1:1007–1013, 1992.

72. Hajjar KA: The endothelial cell tissue plasminogen activator receptor. Specific interaction with plasminogen. J Biol Chem 266:21962–21970, 1991.

73. Jmazrtin U, Bader R, Bohm E, et al: Boehringer Mannheim 06.22: A novel recombinant plasminogen activator. Cardiovasc Drug Rev 11:299–311, 1993.

74. Smalling RW, Bode C, Kalbfleisch J, et al, and the RAPID Investigators: More rapid, complete, and stable thrombolysis with bolus administration of reteplase compared with alteplase infusion in acute myocardial infarction. Circulation 91:2725–2732, 1995.

75. Bode C, Smalling RW, Berg G, et al, for the RAPID II Investigators: Randomized comparison of coronary thrombolysis achieved with double-bolus reteplase and front-loaded, accelerated alteplase in patients with acute myocardial infarction. Circulation 94:891–898, 1996.

76. International Joint Efficacy Comparison of Thrombolytics: Randomized, double-blinded comparison to reteplase double-bolus administration with streptokinase in acute myocardial infarction (INJECT): Trial to investigate equivalence. Lancet 346:329–336, 1995.

77. The Global Use of Strategies to Open Occluded Coronary Arteries (GUSTO III) Investigators: A comparison of reteplase with alteplase for acute myocardial infarction. N Engl J Med 337:1118–1123, 1997.

78. Giugliano RP, Cannon CP, McCabe CH, et al: Lower dose heparin with thrombolysis is associated with lower rates of intracranial hemorrhage: Results from TIMI 10B and ASSENT I. Circulation 96:535, 1997.

79. Lack CH: Staphylokinase: An activator of plasma protease. Nature 161:559–560, 1948.

80. Vanderschueren S, Collen D, Van de Werf F: A pilot study on bolus administration of recombinant staphylokinase for coronary artery thrombolysis. Thromb Haemost 76:541–544, 1996.

81. Bode C, Matsueda G, Haber E: Targeted thrombolysis with a fibrin specific antibody urokinase conjugate. Circulation 72:111–192, 1985.

82. Kremer P, Fiebig R, Tilsner V, et al: Lysis of left ventricular thrombi with urokinase. Circulation 72:112, 1985.

83. Gore JM, Sloan M, Price TR, et al: Intracranial hemorrhage, cerebral infarction, and subdural hematoma after acute myocardial infarction and thrombolytic therapy in the thrombolysis in myocardial

infarction study: Thrombolysis in Myocardial Infarction (TIMI), Phase II, pilot and clinical trial. Circulation 83:448–459, 1991.

84. Gore JM: Prevention of severe neurologic events in the thrombolytic era. Chest 100(Suppl 4):124S–130S, 1992.

85. The STILE Investigators: Results of a prospective randomized trial evaluating surgery versus thrombolysis for ischemia of the lower extremity. Ann Surg 220:251–268, 1994.

86. National Heart and Lung Institute Cooperative Study Group: Urokinase Pulmonary Embolism Trial: Phase I results. JAMA 214:2163, 1970.

87. National Heart and Lung Institute Cooperative Study Group: Urokinase-Streptokinase Embolism Trial: Phase II results. JAMA 229:1606, 1974.

88. Molina JE, Hunter DW, Yedlicka JW, Cerra FB: Thrombolytic therapy for postoperative pulmonary embolism. Am J Surg 163:375–381, 1992.

89. Sharma GVRK, Folland ED, McIntyre KM, et al: Long-term hemodynamic benefit of thrombolytic therapy in pulmonary embolic disease [abstract]. J Am Coll Cardiol 15:65A, 1990.

90. Verstraete M, Miller AH, Bounameaux H, et al: Intravenous and intrapulmonary recombinant tissue type plasminogen activator in the treatment of acute massive pulmonary embolism. Circulation 77:353, 1988.

91. Goldhaber SZ, Markis JE, Meyerovitz MF, et al: Acute pulmonary embolism treated with tissue plasminogen activator. Lancet 2:886, 1986.

92. Goldhaber SZ, Kessler CM, Heit J, et al: A randomized controlled trial of recombinant tissue plasminogen activator versus urokinase in the treatment of acute pulmonary embolism. Lancet 2:293–298, 1988.

93. NIH Consensus Development Conference: Thrombolytic therapy in treatment. BMJ 1:1585, 1980.

94. Tebbe U, Graf A, Kamke W, et al: Hemodynamic effects of double bolus reteplase versus alteplase infusion in massive pulmonary embolism. Am Heart J 138:39–44, 1999.

95. Berni GA, Bandyk DF, Zierler RE, et al: Streptokinase treatment of acute arterial occlusion. Ann Surg 198:185, 1983.

96. Arnesen H, Heilo A, Jakobson E: A prospective study of streptokinase and heparin in the treatment of deep vein thrombosis. Acta Med Scand 203:457, 1978.

97. Kakkar VV, Flanc C, Howe CT: Treatment of deep vein thrombosis. A trial of aspirin, streptokinase, and arvin. BMJ 1:806, 1969.

98. Marder VJ, Soulen RL, Atichartakarn V, et al: Quantitative venographic assessment of deep vein thrombosis in the evaluation of streptokinase and heparin therapy. J Lab Clin Med 89:1018, 1977.

99. Porter JM, Seaman AJ, Common HH, et al: Comparison of heparin and streptokinase in the treatment of venous thrombosis. Am Surg 41:511, 1975.

100. Tsapogas MJ, Peabody RA, Wu KT, et al: Controlled study of thrombolytic therapy in deep vein thrombosis. Surgery 74:873, 1973.

101. Arnesen H, Hoiseth A, Ly B: Streptokinase or heparin in the treatment of deep vein thrombosis: Follow-up results of a prospective study. Acta Med Scand 211:65, 1982.

102. Kakkar VV, Lorenz D: Hemodynamic and clinical assessment after therapy for deep vein thrombosis: A prospective study. Am J Surg 140:54, 1985.

103. Turpie GG, Jay RM, Carter CJ, Hirsh J: A randomized trial of recombinant tissue plasminogen activator for the treatment of proximal deep vein thrombosis [abstract]. Circulation 72:193, 1985.

104. Verhaeghe R, Besse P, Bounameaux H, et al: Multi-center pilot study of the efficacy and safety of systemic rt-PA administration in the treatment of deep vein thrombosis of the lower extremities and/or pelvis. Thromb Res 55:5–11, 1989.

105. Goldhaber SZ, Meyerovitz MF, Green D, et al: Randomized controlled trial of tissue plasminogen activator in proximal deep venous thrombosis. Am J Med 88:235–240, 1990.

106. Marder VJ, Brenner B, Totterman S, et al: Comparison of dosage schedules of rt-PA in the treatment of proximal deep vein thrombosis. J Lab Clin Med 119:485–495, 1992.

107. Johnson BF, Manzo RA, Bergelin RO, et al: Relationship between the changes in the deep venous system and the development of the post-thrombotic syndrome after an acute episode of lower limb deep vein thrombosis: A one-to-six year follow-up. J Vasc Surg 21:307–312, 1995.

108. Mewissen MW, Seabrook GR, Meissner MH, et al: Catheter-directed thrombolysis for lower extremity deep venous thrombosis: Report of a National Multicenter Registry. Radiology 211:39–49, 1999.

109. Comerota AJ, Throm RC, Mathias SD, et al: Catheter-directed thrombolysis for iliofemoral deep venous thrombosis improves health-related quality of life. J Vasc Surg 32:130–137, 2000.

110. Alemany J, Marsal T: Early and late results in the surgical treatment of phlegmasia cerulea dolens. Vasc Surg July/Aug:271, 1987.

111. Shionoya S, Yamada I, Sakurai T, et al: Thrombectomy for acute deep vein thrombosis: Prevention of postthrombotic syndrome. J Cardiovasc Surg 30:484, 1989.

112. Robinson DL, Teitelbaum GP: Phlegmasia cerulea dolens: Treatment by pulse-spray and infusion thrombolysis. AJR Am J Roentgenol 160:1288–1290, 1993.

113. Patel NH, Plorde JJ, Meissner M: Catheter-directed thrombolysis in the treatment of phlegmasia cerulea dolens. Ann Vasc Surg 12:471–475, 1998.

114. Elliot MS, Immelman EJ, Jeffrey P, et al: The role of thrombolytic therapy in the management of phlegmasia cerulea dolens. Br J Surg 66:422, 1979.

115. Paquet KJ, Popov S, Egli H: Richtlinien und Ergebnisse der konsequenten fibrinolytischen Therapie der Phlegmasia caerulea dolens. Dtsch Med Wochenschr 16:903, 1970.

116. Roberts WM: Some clinical problems in patients undergoing thrombolytic therapy. S Afr Med J 50:243, 1976.

117. Druy EM, Trout HH, Giordano JM, et al: Lytic therapy in the treatment of axillary and subclavian vein thrombosis. J Vasc Surg 2:821, 1985.

118. Rubenstein M, Greger WP: Successful streptokinase therapy for catheter induced subclavian vein in thrombosis. Arch Intern Med 140:1370, 1980.

119. Wilson JJ, Lesk D, Newman H: Subclavian-axillary vein thrombosis: Successful treatment with streptokinase. Can Med Assoc J 130:891, 1984.

120. Herrera JL, Wilis SM, Williams TH: Successful streptokinase therapy of acute idiopathic superior vena cava thrombosis. Am Heart J 102:1063, 1981.

121. Elliot MS, Immelman EJ, Jeffrey P, et al: A comparative randomized trial of heparin vs streptokinase in the treatment of acute proximal venous thrombosis. An interim report of a prospective trial. Br J Surg 66:838, 1979.

122. Cohen LH, Kaplan M, Bernhard VM: Intraoperative streptokinase: An adjunct to mechanical thrombectomy in the management of acute ischemia. Arch Surg 121:708, 1986.

123. Sussman B, Dardik H, Ibrahim IM, et al: Improved patient selection for enzymatic lysis of peripheral arterial and graft occlusions. Am J Surg 148:244, 1984.

124. Graor RA, Risius B, Denny KM, et al: Local thrombolysis in the treatment of thrombosed arteries, bypassed grafts, and arteriovenous fistulas. J Vasc Surg 2:406, 1985.

125. Katzen BT, Edwards KC, Albert AS, et al: Low dose direct fibrinolysis in peripheral vascular disease. J Vasc Surg 1:718, 1984.

126. Sicard GA, Schier JJ, Totty WG, et al: Thrombolytic therapy for acute arterial occlusion. J Vasc Surg 2:65, 1985.

127. Taylor LM, Porter JM, Bauer GM, et al: Intraarterial streptokinase infusion for acute popliteal and tibial arterial occlusion. Am J Surg 147:583, 1984.

128. Risius B, Zelch MG, Graor RA, et al: Catheter directed low dose streptokinase infusion: A preliminary experience. Radiology 150:349, 1984.

129. McNamara TO, Bomberger RA: Factors affecting initial and six months patency following high dose intraarterial urokinase thrombolysis. Am J Surg 152:709, 1986.

130. Gardiner GA, Harrington DP, Koltun W, et al: Salvage of occluded arterial bypass grafts by means of thrombolyses. J Vasc Surg 9:426, 1989.

131. Porter JM, Taylor LM: Current status of thrombolytic therapy. J Vasc Surg 2:239, 1985.

132. Van Breda A, Robinson JC, Feldman L, et al: Local thrombolysis in the treatment of arterial graft occlusions. Vasc Surg 1:103, 1984.

133. Cronan JJ, Dorfman GS: Low dose thrombolysis: A non-operative approach to renal artery occlusion. J Urol 130:757, 1983.

134. Pillari G, Doscher W, Fierstein J, et al: Low dose streptokinase in the treatment of celiac and superior mesenteric artery occlusion. Arch Surg 118:1340, 1983.

135. Hargrove WC, Berkowitz HD, Freiman DB, et al: Recanalization of totally occluded femoral popliteal vein grafts with low dose streptokinase infusion. Surgery 92:890, 1982.

136. Perler BA, White RI, Ernst CB, et al: Low dose thrombolytic therapy for infrainguinal graft occlusions: An idea whose time has passed? J Vasc Surg 2:799, 1985.

137. Hargrove WC, Berkowitz HD, Freiman DB, et al: Treatment of acute peripheral arterial and graft thrombosis with low dose streptokinase. Surgery 92:981, 1982.

138. The STILE Investigators: Results of a prospective randomized trial evaluating surgery versus thrombolysis for ischemia of the lower extremity. Ann Vasc Surg 220:251–268, 1994.

139. Weaver FA, Comerota AJ, Youngblood M, et al: Surgical revascularization versus thrombolysis for nonembolic lower extremity native artery occlusions: Results of a prospective randomized trial. J Vasc Surg 24:513–523, 1996.

140. Ouriel K, Shortell CK, DeWeese JA, et al: A comparison of thrombolytic therapy with operative revascularization in the initial treatment of acute peripheral arterial ischemia. J Vasc Surg 19:1021–1030, 1994.

141. Ouriel K, Veith FJ, Sasahara AA: Thrombolysis or peripheral arterial surgery: Phase I results. Topas Investigators. J Vasc Surg 23:64–73, 1996.

142. Kinney TB, Valji K, Rose SC, et al: Pulmonary embolism from pulse-spray pharmacomechanical thrombolysis of clotted hemodialysis grafts: Urokinase versus heparinized saline. J Vasc Interv Radiol 11:1143–1152, 2000.

143. Activase, alteplase recombinant for acute ischemic stroke: Efficacy supplement. Peripheral and Central Nervous System Drug Advisory Committee Meeting, Bethesda, Md, June 1996.

144. The National Institute of Neurological Disorders and Stroke rt-PA Stroke Study Group: Tissue plasminogen activator for acute ischemic stroke. N Engl J Med 333:1581–1587, 1995.

145. Hacke W, Kaste M, Fieschi C, et al: Intravenous thrombolysis with recombinant tissue plasminogen activator for acute hemispheric stroke. JAMA 274:1017–1025, 1995.

146. Hacke W, Kaste M, Fieschi C, et al: Randomised, double-blind placebo controlled trial of thrombolytic therapy with intravenous alteplase in acute ischaemic stroke (ECASS II). Lancet 352:1245–1251, 1998.

147. The NINDS t-PA Stroke Study Group: Intracerebral hemorrhage after intravenous t-PA for ischemic stroke. Stroke 28:2109–2118, 1997.

148. Furlan A, Higashida R, Weschler L, et al: Intraarterial prourokinase for acute ischemic stroke: The PROACT II study: A randomized controlled trial. JAMA 282:2003–2011, 1999.

149. McNamara TO, Fischer JR: Thrombolysis of peripheral arterial and graft occlusions: Improved results using high dose urokinase. AJR Am J Roentgenol 144:769, 1985.

150. Plecha FR, Pories WJ: Intraoperative angiography in the immediate assessment of arterial reconstruction. Arch Surg 105:802, 1972.

151. Quiñones-Baldrich WJ, Ziomek S, Henderson T, et al: Intraoperative fibrinolytic therapy: Experimental evaluation. J Vasc Surg 4:229, 1986.

152. Satiani B, Gross WS, Evans WE: Improved limb salvage after arterial embolectomy. Ann Surg 118:153–157, 1978.

153. Green RM, DeWeese JA, Rob CG: Arterial embolectomy before and after the Fogarty catheter. Surgery 77:24–33, 1975.

154. Greep JM, Aleman PJ, Jarrett F, Bast TJ: A combined technique for peripheral arterial embolectomy. Arch Surg 105:869–874, 1972.

155. Chaise LS, Comerota AJ, Soulen RL, et al: Selective intraarterial streptokinase therapy in the immediate postoperative period. JAMA 247:2397, 1982.

156. Feissinger JN, Vayssiarirat M, Juillet Y, et al: Local urokinase in arterial thromboembolism. Angiology 31:715, 1980.

157. Tsapogas MJ: The role of fibrinolysis in the treatment of arterial thrombosis. Experimental and clinical aspects. Ann R Coll Surg Engl 24:293, 1964.

158. Quiñones-Baldrich WJ, Zierler RE, Hiatt JC: Intraoperative fibrinolytic therapy: An adjunct to catheter thromboembolectomy. J Vasc Surg 2:319, 1985.

159. Quiñones-Baldrich WJ, Baker JD, Busuttil RW, et al: Intraoperative infusion of lytic drugs for thrombotic complications of revascularization. J Vasc Surg 10:408, 1989.

160. Comerota AJ, White JV, Grosh JD: Intraoperative intraarterial thrombolytic therapy for salvage of limbs in patients with distal arterial thrombosis. Surg Gynecol Obstet 160:283, 1989.

161. Norem RF, Short DH, Kerstein MD: Role of intraoperative fibrinolytic therapy in acute arterial occlusion. Surg Gynecol Obstet 167:87–91, 1988.

162. Parent III FN, Bernhard VM, Pabst TS, et al: Fibrinolytic treatment of residual thrombus after catheter embolectomy for severe lower limb ischemia. J Vasc Surg 9:153, 1989.

163. Quiñones-Baldrich WJ, Colburn MD, Gelabert HA, et al: Isolated limb perfusion with extracorporeal pump increases effectiveness of lysis by urokinase. J Surg Res 57:344–51, 1994.

Questions

1. Streptokinase and urokinase have the following similarities:
   1. both are bacterial products
   2. both are enzymes
   3. both are highly fibrin-specific
   4. both are direct fibrinolytic agents
      (a) 1, 2, 3
      (b) 1, 3
      (c) 2, 4
      (d) 4 only
      (e) none of the above

2. Increasing the dose of streptokinase to decrease its lytic effect
   (a) is indicated when bleeding occurs during therapy
   (b) is a predictable response
   (c) is scientifically correct but unnecessary
   (d) increases the risk of bleeding
   (e) none of the above

3. Tissue plasminogen activator
   (a) is a nonenzymatic protein
   (b) has fibrinolytic activity in plasminogen-free media
   (c) is highly antigenic
   (d) is mainly an exogenous fibrinolytic activator
   (e) none of the above

4. A patient with deep vein thrombosis of the femoral system
   1. is a candiate for lytic therapy if the thrombosis is recent and is the first episode
   2. may be treated with low-dose local lytic therapy
   3. has about a 50% to 60% chance of failure to clear completely with lytic therapy
   4. is at higher risk of pulmonary embolism with lytic therapy than with heparin
      (a) 1, 2, 3
      (b) 1, 3
      (c) 2, 4
      (d) 4 only
      (e) none of the above

5. Intraarterial lytic therapy
   (a) is initiated with a loading dose
   (b) is highly effective in graft thrombosis
   (c) is highly effective in postdilatation thrombosis
   (d) can be safely administered in patients after a stroke
   (e) usually prevents a systemic lytic state

6. The dose of urokinase is
   (a) guided by plasminogen levels
   (b) 2000 units/kg/hour without a loading dose
   (c) 2000 units/kg/hour with a loading dose of 2000 units/kg over 10 minutes

(d) 2000 units/pound/hour
(e) none of the above

7. Pulmonary emboli
   (a) may be a complication of lytic therapy
   (b) require at least 72 hours of systemic lytic therapy to completely resolve
   (c) can be effectively treated by streptokinase, 2000 units/kg/hour
   (d) should always be treated with systemic thrombolytic therapy
   (e) none of the above

8. Complications of thrombolytic therapy are
   (a) due to the antigenicity of the agent
   (b) due to plasminemia
   (c) reduced by avoidance of invasive procedures
   (d) sometimes treated by increasing the dose
   (e) all of the above

9. Intraoperative thrombolytic therapy
   1. is contraindicated because bleeding results from systemic absorption
   2. may improve the results of incomplete thrombectomy
   3. is done by intravenous administration of the agent
   4. should include heparin in the infusate
   (a) 1, 2, 3
   (b) 1, 3
   (c) 2, 4
   (d) 4 only
   (e) none of the above

10. Streptokinase administration
   (a) results in a drop in plasminogen
   (b) is contraindicated in patients who have received streptokinase any time in the past
   (c) is more effective than urokinase when given intraarterially
   (d) results in a predictable lytic response
   (e) none of the above

Answers

1. d   2. c   3. e   4. b   5. c   6. d   7. a   8. e   9. c   10. a

21

Evaluation of Cardiac Risk in the Patient with Vascular Disease

Michael Belkin, Anthony D. Whittemore, Magruder C. Donaldson, and John A. Mannick

Successful arterial reconstruction in patients with atherosclerotic cardiovascular disease requires initial recognition and subsequent management of the underlying systemic disease process. The increased prevalence of concurrent manifestations of atherosclerosis in vascular surgical patients has been repeatedly documented in the literature. The Framingham Study is one of the earliest reports demonstrating that patients with claudication harbor a significantly higher incidence of coronary artery disease, as well as cerebrovascular and hypertensive disease, than does a nonclaudicating population.[1] Approximately 50% of patients undergoing a variety of peripheral vascular procedures have clinically overt cardiac disease, and an additional 20% have clinically silent but highly significant myocardial ischemia.[2–5] Routine coronary angiography carried out in one of the larger reported series documented a 31% incidence of severe but surgically correctable coronary disease in patients with aortic aneurysms.[3] Similar findings were demonstrated in 26% of patients with cerebrovascular disease and 21% of those with lower limb ischemia.

Myocardial infarction remains the most common source of perioperative morbidity and mortality after a variety of arterial reconstructions.[4, 5] Cardiac morbidity has been most extensively studied in patients undergoing aneurysm repair because the initially compromised myocardium is maximally stressed by aortic clamping, declamping, and attendant fluid shifts. The marked reduction in operative mortality from the initial 20% rate noted in the early 1960s to the current mortality figure, consistently less than 5%, is undoubtedly multifactorial.[4–8] Vast improvements in our understanding of hemodynamics, perioperative fluid administration, monitoring techniques, anesthetic management, cardiologic support, autotransfusion, and management of sepsis have all contributed to the current excellent results (Table 21–1). The primary cause of postoperative death in the vascular surgical population, however, remains cardiac. Further reduction in mortality figures, if realistically achievable at all, requires the identification of high-risk groups and appropriate alterations in management according to more specific stratification. To this end, a plethora of clinical risk parameters and laboratory procedures have emerged with which to evaluate a patient's cardiac status in an effort to minimize the considerable morbidity associated with impaired myocardial performance in patients undergoing vascular reconstruction.

CLINICAL RISK PARAMETERS
Coronary Artery Disease

Although patients with angina pectoris are at higher risk of postoperative cardiac complications than those without,

TABLE 21–1

Operative Mortality Rate for Repair of Intact Abdominal Aortic Aneurysms

YEAR	AUTHORS	NO. OF PATIENTS	30-DAY OPERATIVE MORTALITY RATE (%)
1980	Whittemore et al	110	0
1981	Crawford et al	140	1.4
1981	Brown et al	422	2.4
1983	Hertzer	206	3.4
1985	Ruby et al	227	1.3
1989	Johnston et al	666	4.8
1990	Golden et al	500	1.6

Data from Golden MA, Whittemore AD, Donaldson MC, Mannick JA: Selective evaluation and management of coronary artery disease in patients undergoing repair of abdominal aortic aneurysms. Ann Surg 212:415–423, 1990.

clinically overt angina is not an independent predictor of postoperative cardiac complications distinct from other clinical manifestations of impaired cardiac function.[9] The significant clinical parameters available from history, physical, and routine electrocardiogram (ECG) that are of predictive value for postoperative myocardial infarction consist of age greater than 70 years, mitral insufficiency, ventricular ectopy in excess of 5 beats per minute, poorly controlled congestive failure, and recent antecedent myocardial infarction.[9] The evaluation and management of patients with angina, however, remain highly controversial. This controversy is founded in the recent marked reduction in postoperative incidence of cardiac events and (1) differing methods of patient selection, (2) variable criteria used to define postoperative myocardial infarction (50% of which are entirely silent), and (3) evidence that preliminary coronary bypass reduces the number of postoperative cardiac events after noncardiac surgery.[5–10]

Little argument exists that patients with unstable, crescendo, or nocturnal angina require urgent coronary angiography and appropriate therapy as indicated. This course is dictated with or without contemplated vascular surgery, and in the event that such patients warrant emergent attention to an expanding abdominal aortic aneurysm or critical limb ischemia, simultaneous procedures directed toward both critical issues have been successfully carried out.[5] On the other end of the spectrum of coronary disease, as many as 20% of our vascular surgical population harbor clinically silent but significant coronary artery disease, yet major vascular procedures may be undertaken without inordinate risk of postoperative cardiac events, if modern principles of management are employed.[4, 5] The results of this policy are illustrated in Table 21–1, which represents the cardiac morbidity associated with 500 aneurysm repairs using our clinical method of risk stratification. The most controversial patients with ischemic heart disease remain those with chronic stable angina as defined by New York Heart Association Class II. These patients sustain the highest risk of cardiac events in our experience. Current efforts at risk stratification are directed primarily toward this group.

The single most significant predictor for postoperative cardiac complications is recent myocardial infarction. Several reports from the early 1970s document postoperative mortality rates ranging from 50% to 80% resulting from postoperative reinfarction. Patients operated on within 3 months of a myocardial infarction sustained a risk of reinfarction or cardiac death approaching 30%. Noncardiac procedures carried out 3 to 6 months after infarction were associated with a 15% incidence of recurrent infarction, and after 6 months the reinfarction rate finally stabilized at 5%.[9–14] Contrary to earlier reports, no significant difference in risk imposed by transmural compared with subendocardial infarctions exists.[10] Improvements in the perioperative management of these patients, however, have reduced the reinfarction rate to less than 10% within 3 months of infarction and to less than 5% for those undergoing noncardiac procedures between 3 and 6 months.[15, 16] Although further improvements have been made in management of patients who have sustained an infarction in the immediate postoperative period, delaying elective vascular reconstruction for 3 to 6 months after antecedent myocardial infarction is prudent in an effort to minimize cardiac morbidity.[17] Emergent situations requiring immediate vascular reconstruction may be carried out but require maximal intensive monitoring and management to reduce the added associated risk.

Congestive Heart Failure

Patients with severe congestive heart failure, clinically evident by a third heart sound or significant jugular venous distention, incur a 25% to 30% risk of pulmonary edema, in sharp contrast to a 2% incidence for those without a prior history of congestive failure.[9, 18] The incidence of cardiogenic pulmonary edema correlates with the functional classification as outlined by the New York Heart Association. Of critical importance, however, is that the perioperative mortality rate correlates with the degree of congestive failure present at the time of operation, rather than with the severity of failure by history. Satisfactory preoperative control of poorly compensated congestive heart failure has therefore resulted in a substantial reduction in the overall risk of cardiac morbidity and mortality. Maximal therapy may require the use of vigorous diuresis with fluid restriction, which is invariably associated with some degree of intravascular hypovolemia. Allowing sufficient time for reequilibration before surgery is advisable so that the vasodilatation associated with anesthesia is better tolerated. Conversely, under urgent circumstances, judicious diuresis should be used to control the failure, and anesthetic technique should be adjusted to minimize sudden vasodilatation.

Arrhythmia

Significant risk of perioperative cardiac morbidity has been repeatedly associated with preoperative arrhythmia, particularly with frequent premature ventricular contractions.[9, 10] The ischemic or congestive complications in this group, however, relate primarily to the underlying coronary artery or myocardial disease rather than to the arrhythmia itself.[19] Prophylactic pharmacologic control of the arrhythmia is usually unnecessary unless it results in ischemic changes or deterioration of myocardial function. For instance, intravenous antiarrhythmic agents would be appropriate perioperatively for patients with a history of ventricular tachyarrhythmia associated with hypotension. In most instances, however, the chronic antiarrhythmic regimen should be continued through the morning of surgery and subsequent perioperative therapy dictated by the hemodynamic significance of the specific arrhythmia.

Of particular concern are patients with complete heart block who are at increased risk of cardiac morbidity in excess of that imposed by their underlying myocardial disease.[20] These individuals are less able to augment cardiac output in response to peripheral vasodilatation or myocardial depression induced by anesthetic agents or to successfully compensate for a wide variation in peripheral resistance and left ventricular filling pressure, particularly during major aortic surgery. Individuals with chronic heart block should probably be provided with a pacemaker before surgery.[21]

The management of patients with chronic bifascicular block has been controversial. Although little evidence shows that such individuals progress to complete heart block during the perioperative period, a significant number of patients indeed progress during evolution of an acute myocardial infarction.[9] Appropriate monitoring usually identifies such individuals before sudden hemodynamic decompensation, and appropriate pacing is instituted as necessary. Because approximately 5% of patients with established bifascicular block develop complete heart block on an annual basis, syncope unexplained by history in these individuals may warrant the insertion of a pacing wire. Even with pacemaker backup, however, these individuals remain at increased risk of perioperative myocardial events, primarily from their underlying myocardial disease rather than from the specific conduction defect.

Valvular Disease

Cardiac morbidity associated with valvular disease also reflects the degree of resultant myocardial decompensation. Asymptomatic patients and those with a mild degree of functional limitation (New York Heart Association Class II) require no particular preoperative therapy beyond routine antibiotic prophylaxis for endocarditis. Patients with critical stenosis and significant physical limitations, however, are at substantial risk of sudden decompensation and death.[22, 23] Preoperative cardiac catheterization should therefore be carried out in those patients with aortic valve stenosis associated with angina, syncopal episodes, or significant congestive failure.[24] Preliminary aortic valve replacement should be seriously considered for critical aortic stenosis, and intensive hemodynamic perioperative monitoring should be employed in those with symptomatic but noncritical lesions. Similar principles should apply to patients with mitral stenosis. Valvular insufficiency resulting in significant aortic or mitral regurgitation also increases the risk of postoperative cardiac morbidity associated with severe congestive failure. Valve replacement is not usually necessary unless failure cannot be adequately controlled.

Optimal management of patients with prosthetic valves who require chronic anticoagulation has not been firmly established. A significant increase in the number of thromboembolic events has not been documented when anticoagulants are withheld during the immediate perioperative period.[25, 26] Although chronic anticoagulation is usually withheld to minimize the incidence of hemorrhagic complications in patients undergoing noncardiac surgery, most bleeding can be ultimately controlled, whereas the sequelae of a single thromboembolic event may be irrevocable. Therefore, considering some form of anticoagulation during the preoperative period, especially in those patients with prosthetic valves known to be particularly thrombogenic, is not unreasonable. Chronic anticoagulation with warfarin is discontinued approximately 3 days before surgery, during which time the patient should be heparinized. Intravenous dextran is often administered during the immediate postoperative period to provide some coverage until heparin therapy or oral anticoagulation can be reinstituted safely.

CLINICAL RISK ASSESSMENT

Scoring Systems

Initial attempts to stratify risk using clinical criteria focused on the independent parameters of prior myocardial infarction, angina, congestive heart failure, arrhythmia, and valvular disease. Several clinical scoring systems have since been developed in an attempt to provide multivariate assessment of cardiac risk.[9, 27–30] One of the earliest and perhaps most rigorous of such systems is the Goldman Cardiac Risk Index,[9] which documented the particularly ominous predictive value of poorly controlled congestive heart failure and recent myocardial infarction as previously mentioned. A variety of clinical parameters were assigned a relative value based on association with postoperative myocardial events observed in retrospective analysis of surgical patients (Table 21–2). Goldman then developed a cardiac risk index derived from the total point score number of independent variables and relative points. As might be anticipated, patients in risk classes III and IV with the highest number of points sustained the higher incidence of postoperative cardiac complications (Table 21–3). Although proved reliable in some series, the index does not accurately reflect current management of even the most severe manifestations of coronary artery disease as demonstrated by Rivers and coworkers, who found that patients in risk index class IV sustained a 33% incidence of cardiac complications, significantly lower than the 78% that would have been predicted by the Goldman Cardiac Risk Index.[17] None of Rivers' patients, however, underwent surgery of the magnitude required for aortic reconstruction.

A variety of additional clinical scoring systems have been devised, including Dripps-ASA Score,[27] Cooperman's Equation,[30] Detsky Modified Risk Index,[28] and Eagle's Clinical Markers.[29] These clinical indicators have not proved

T A B L E 2 1 - 2

Computation of Multifactorial Index Score to Estimate Cardiac Risk in Noncardiac Surgery

FACTORS	POINTS
S_3 gallop or jugular venous distention on preoperative physical examination	11
Transmural or subendocardial myocardial infarction in the previous 6 months	10
Premature ventricular beats, more than 5/min, documented at any time	7
Rhythm other than sinus or presence of premature atrial contractions on last preoperative electrocardiogram	7
Age >70 years	5
Emergency operation	4
Intrathoracic, intraperitoneal, or aortic site of surgery	3
Evidence for important valvular aortic stenosis	3
Poor general medical condition*	3

*As evidenced by electrolyte abnormalities (potassium, <3.0 mEq/L; HCO_3, <20 mEq/L); renal insufficiency (blood urea nitrogen, >50 mg/dL; creatinine, >3.0 mg/dL); abnormal blood gases (PO_2, aspartate transaminase or signs on physical examination of chronic liver disease); or any condition that has caused the patient to be chronically bedridden.

Data from Goldman L: Cardiac risks and complications of noncardiac surgery. Ann Surg 198:780–791, 1983.

Incidence of Cardiac Complications after Noncardiac Surgery in 1001 Patients Classified According to Risk Index

RISK CLASS	INDEX POINTS	FATAL (%)	NONFATAL (%)
I	0–5	0.7	0.2
II	6–12	5	2
III	13–25	11	2
IV	26	2	56

Data from Goldman L: Cardiac risks and complications of noncardiac surgery. Ann Surg 198:780–791, 1983.

convincingly accurate as demonstrated by Lette and associates,[31] who found none of the systems of reliable predictive value. Most of the data used to derive these systems were obtained retrospectively and have become outdated by the dramatic advances in medical and anesthetic management of the impaired myocardium; none account for silent ischemia.

Ejection Fraction

The ejection fraction derived by multigated radionuclide ventriculography has also proved of equivocal predictive value.[32–36] Although Pasternack and coworkers[33] documented a 17% incidence of postoperative myocardial infarction in patients undergoing aneurysm repair with an ejection fraction below 40%, significantly greater than the 3.4% incidence found in patients with an ejection fraction in excess of 40%, most reports attest to the lack of specificity for this derived parameter. This is not surprising, because the ejection fraction is an estimate of the efficiency of ventricular function at a single point in time and therefore may not reflect the severity of associated ischemic coronary artery disease.

Exercise Stress Tests

The exercise tolerance test has been widely used to provoke evidence of myocardial ischemia but is subject to several limitations with respect to vascular surgical patients.[37–41] Approximately one third of such patients cannot successfully complete the standard examination, which has been proved a useful predictor only when patients achieve 85% of their predicted maximal heart rate (PMHR).[37–39] Up to 70% of patients cannot achieve their PMHR. Furthermore, results do not necessarily correlate with the relative severity of coronary atherosclerosis subsequently documented on arteriography, particularly in patients without a significant prior cardiac history.[39–41] In a large proportion of vascular surgical patients, the exercise tolerance test provides equivocal results and cannot be relied on for accurate stratification of patients most likely to benefit from coronary arteriography.

Coronary Angiography

The uncertainties with regard to the predictive value of clinical scoring systems, ejection fraction, and exercise stress tests in patients with coronary artery disease prompted some institutions to adopt a policy of routine coronary angiography.[3, 42] Patients subsequently determined to harbor severe surgically reconstructable disease, such as left main or severe triple-vessel atherosclerosis, would then undergo preliminary coronary artery bypass before vascular reconstruction. Hertzer and associates[3] documented severe but operable coronary disease in 25% of 1000 consecutive angiograms carried out in vascular surgical patients. Up to 20% of such individuals had no significant history of myocardial ischemia. Subsequent coronary artery bypass in nearly 25% of the entire group was associated with a 5.3% operative mortality rate before the planned vascular reconstruction. Although only one of those who survived the coronary bypass died of the subsequent vascular procedure, routine preliminary coronary arteriography for patients with stable angina is probably not justified, because the mortality associated with catheterization and subsequent bypass may be significantly greater than the risks of the same complications occurring from the anticipated noncardiac procedure alone.[3, 40, 43] Additional means are necessary to substratify the group of patients with stable angina who can benefit from more vigorous evaluation. Coronary angiography is usually reserved at present for those patients whose risk of myocardial ischemia is determined by other parameters.

Myocardial Scintigraphy

A variety of thallium imaging techniques have been developed and have shown potential for identifying those patients most likely to benefit from initial cardiac intervention.[44, 45] After an initial dose of radioactive thallium chloride, the relative distribution of thallium can be documented with a gamma scintillation camera. A normally perfused segment of myocardium shows a homogeneous distribution. In contrast, areas of myocardial ischemia or scar appear as initial defects (Fig. 21–1). A second image taken 3 to 4 hours later may demonstrate redistribution within an area that initially appeared as a defect, compatible with viable but relatively ischemic myocardium (Fig. 21–2). A persistent defect suggests antecedent infarction.

Although thallium has been the agent of choice for myocardial perfusion imaging, other agents have gained widespread acceptance and offer advantages over thallium. The most popular new perfusion agent is ^{99m}Tc-sestamibi.[46] Sestamibi allows estimation of cardiac ejection fraction via a first-pass technique. It has a long myocardial residence time and generates a higher count density than thallium, resulting in superior quality images. The kinetics of uptake and excretion also facilitate more rapid completion of the study than is possible with thallium imaging.

Both exercise and intravenous dipyridamole in conjunction with thallium imaging are equally effective in inducing relative vasodilatation and increased blood flow to normally perfused myocardium, which, in turn, provide increased uptake and more rapid clearance of thallium. Regions of

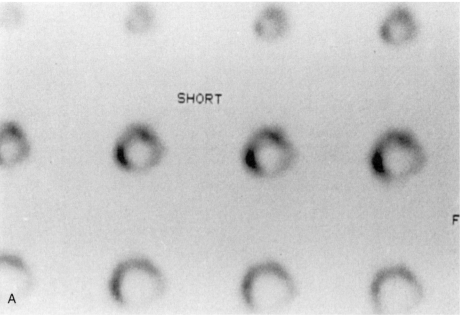

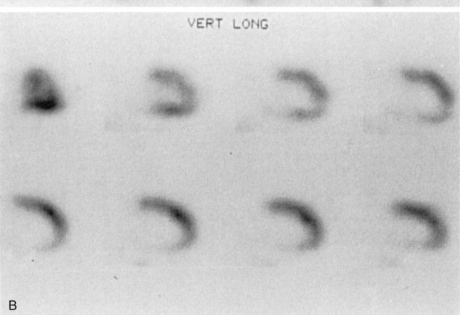

Figure 21-1. Initial images of myocardium after intravenous injection of dipyridamole and radioactive thallium demonstrate perfusion defects of inferior and lateral segments on short axis (A) and inferior segment on vertical axis (B).

myocardium supplied by significantly stenotic vessels, however, show relatively decreased or delayed thallium uptake, enhancing overall sensitivity. As is the case with treadmill exercise tolerance tests, a large proportion of vascular patients cannot satisfactorily sustain the exercise required for successful imaging. The dipyridamole-thallium scan has therefore become most widely used. Intravenous adenosine has a more rapid onset of action than does dipyridamole, but it is associated with a higher incidence of adverse reactions and its use remains primarily investigational.[47]

As summarized by Yeager,[48] dipyridamole-thallium scanning has proved to be a sensitive and specific predictor for angiographically significant coronary disease and perioperative cardiac events associated with vascular surgery, including both myocardial infarction and cardiac death. More specifically, redistribution of initial defects appears more predictive for perioperative events than fixed defects. In contrast, fixed defects are more ominous with respect to long-term survival. The dipyridamole-thallium scan is not, however, uniformly reliable, because persistent defects determined as "fixed" at 3 hours may redistribute on further delayed gamma scan. Second, a significant gray zone exists in distinguishing persistent defects from minimal redistribution on scans or after reinjection of thallium.[49] The fact that some defects initially perceived as "fixed" but subsequently proved to reflect viable myocardium by delayed scans or by reinjection may account for the unanticipated higher incidence of cardiac complications in patients with fixed deficits reported in some series.[50]

Experience suggests that dipyridamole-thallium imaging combined with appropriate clinical parameters may be useful in identifying those patients most likely to benefit from preliminary treatment of coronary artery disease.[51–53] Several authors have addressed the issue of quantitative differ-

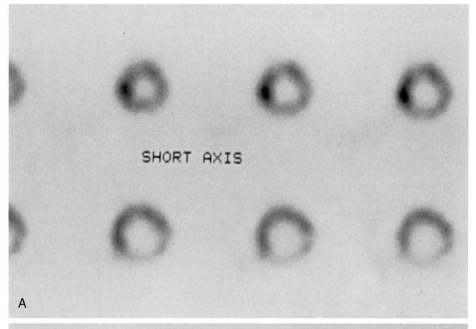

SHORT AXIS

A

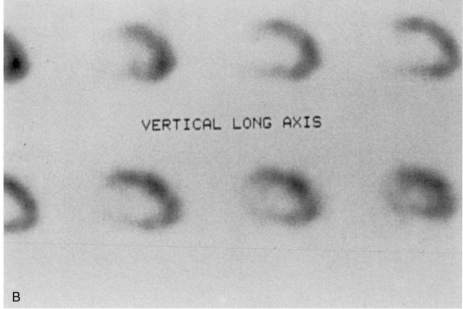

VERTICAL LONG AXIS

B

Figure 21–2. Delayed image subsequently demonstrates reperfusion of the inferior and lateral segments, suggestive of myocardium at risk for ischemia.

ences in thallium redistribution. Although Eagle and coworkers[51] and Cambria and coworkers[53] recommend invasive cardiac evaluation in those patients with multiple redistribution defects, Lette and coworkers[52] have developed a means of quantifying multiple redistribution defects that is perhaps even more precise. In a relatively small group of 125 patients undergoing elective vascular surgery, quantitative indices were developed using data derived from dipyridamole-thallium scans. The myocardium was divided into six anatomic regions and the degree of reversibility scaled from 0 to 3. The number of segments affected and the degree of reversibility in each of the six anatomic regions are added to provide a "Summed Reversibility Index" (SRI). An SRI greater than 4 placed patients at high risk of postoperative cardiac events; 85% of such individuals so classified sustained postoperative events in

spite of intensive postoperative monitoring and antianginal medication. In contrast, only 5% of patients classified as intermediate risk (SRI less than 4) sustained cardiac events.

Although prior attempts to correlate the extent of reversibility with cardiac risk have provided equivocal results, this particular method of quantitation proved reliable in this study. Although this study's end points were limited to cardiac death and infarction (and results may have been different if expanded to include all cardiac events), these two end points do seem the most significant. This study supports the contention that patients of intermediate risk with a limited number of reversible deficits can undergo surgery with minimal morbidity, whereas those in the high-risk group with multiple redistribution zones may require more aggressive coronary evaluation.

In contrast to these retrospective studies, which have

suggested that the dipyridamole-thallium imaging technique is a sensitive test for identifying patients at risk of ischemic cardiac events after major vascular surgery, two prospective studies document a more limited usefulness for this study. Mangano and associates[54] studied a group of 60 patients who underwent double-blind dipyridamole-thallium imaging before major vascular surgery. In that study, no association existed between redistribution defects and adverse cardiac events. Fifty-four percent (7 of 13) of adverse events occurred in patients without redistribution defects, whereas the relative risk for patients with redistribution defects to have an adverse event was only 1.5 ($P = 43$). In another prospective double-blind trial of 457 patients undergoing abdominal aortic surgery after dipyridamole-thallium imaging, Baron and associates[55] found no predictive value to the test. The relative risk of adverse cardiac events was 1.1 for patients with redistribution defects and 1.5 for patients with fixed perfusion defects.

Ambulatory Holter Monitoring

Ambulatory Holter monitoring seems a relatively simple and inexpensive means of documenting myocardial ischemia.[56–58] Our prospective study of 176 patients undergoing a variety of vascular reconstructions demonstrated its potential in defining a group of patients at highest risk of postoperative cardiac events.[56] All but one of these events occurred in patients with positive ambulatory Holter evidence for myocardial ischemia. All but one were entirely clinically silent. These results were similar to those reported by Pasternack and coworkers,[57] who found that 75% of their patients showed silent ischemic changes. Mangano and coworkers[58] have also proved a significant correlation between preoperative ambulatory Holter changes and postoperative events in univariate analysis, but postoperative ischemic changes proved more highly predictive in multivariate analysis. Although further investigation is ongoing, perhaps some combination of ambulatory Holter monitoring and quantitative dipyridamole-thallium scans will allow us to inexpensively and noninvasively determine those patients at highest risk of cardiac ischemia and most likely to benefit from invasive coronary evaluation and treatment.

THE CURRENT ROLE OF CARDIAC EVALUATION

Despite attempts to refine and improve the predictive value of clinical scoring systems, myocardial contractility measurements, stress testing, and myocardial scintigraphy, these methods of evaluation all have limitations. Recognition of these limitations and the gradual but steady decreases in cardiac morbidity and mortality after vascular surgery procedures have led some authors to question the use of preoperative attempts at cardiac risk evaluation. Taylor and associates[59] reported only a 3.9% myocardial infarction rate (less than 1% cardiac mortality) after 534 vascular operations with no routine cardiac evaluation other than history, physical examination, and electrocardiogram. Only 5.8% of patients suspected to have severe symptomatic coronary artery disease had further cardiac evaluation,

and only three patients underwent prophylactic coronary bypass surgery before the planned vascular operation. These authors argued that cardiac screening is unnecessary and cost ineffective when applied to the general vascular surgery population.

In a decision-analysis study, Mason and associates[60] focused on a population of vascular surgery patients who had no or mild angina symptoms and a positive dipyridamole-thallium scan. The authors found that subjecting these patients to coronary arteriography and coronary artery intervention led to higher expense and morbidity than did proceeding directly to vascular surgery. Nonetheless, the authors predicted that morbidity and mortality would be lower with coronary arteriography if vascular surgery was canceled or modified in patients with severe inoperable coronary artery disease.

Although the great majority of patients can be "gotten through" vascular surgical procedures with acceptably low morbidity and mortality, few would argue the merits of identifying the presence and significance of coronary artery disease in preoperative patients. Although few patients require coronary arteriography and even fewer any form of coronary revascularization, the recognition of coronary artery disease allows optimal short- and long-term care. Optimization of preoperative medical management, perioperative invasive monitoring, and long-term risk factor modification are all facilitated by an accurate cardiac evaluation. On our service, we currently actively modify our perioperative management based on preoperative ambulatory cardiac ischemic monitoring results. Patients often show silent myocardial ischemia at a certain heart rate threshold. Perioperative oral and intravenous β-blockade are then directed at maintaining the heart rate below that threshold value.

Recently, the merits of perioperative β-blockade have been established in two trials. Mangano and colleagues compared the effects of atenolol versus placebo on survival and overall cardiac morbidity in a double-blinded randomized trial in patients undergoing noncardiac surgery. Overall mortality was significantly lower in atenolol patients at 6 months (0% vs. 8%, P < 0.001), 12 months (3% vs. 14%, P = 0.005), and 24 months (10% vs. 21%, P = 0.019).[65] More recently, more dramatic effects of β-blockade on perioperative morbidity and mortality were demonstrated by Poldermans and associates.[66] In this study, patients undergoing vascular surgery who were identified as high-risk candidates by clinical criteria and dobutamine echocardiography were randomly assigned to receive standard care instead of perioperative β-blockade, with bisoprolol starting one week before surgery. Treatment with bisoprolol significantly reduced perioperative mortality (3.4% vs. 17%, P < 0.02) and nonfatal myocardial infarction (0% vs. 17%, P < 0.001). These dramatic results have led some authorities to focus attention less on preoperative risk stratification and more on routine perioperative β-blockade when no contraindications exist.[67]

CONCLUSION

The fact that patients without clinically overt coronary disease can undergo major vascular reconstructive procedures safely without further evaluation and with perhaps an irreducible minimum of postoperative cardiac fatalities has been repeatedly documented in the literature.[5, 51–53, 59, 61–63] In contrast, patients with severe coronary disease manifest by unstable angina, ischemic congestive failure, or recent myocardial infarction probably benefit from invasive cardiac evaluation and either preliminary coronary intervention or an alternate vascular procedure of lesser magnitude.[5, 63] Should indications for vascular reconstruction be urgent or emergent, simultaneous coronary reconstruction may well reduce the increased risk of cardiac morbidity associated with urgent procedures.[5, 59] What remains uncertain is the best course of action for patients with clinically evident but stable coronary disease.

Clinical scoring systems and most noninvasive laboratory methods have proved unreliable predictors of myocardial ischemic events.[51, 53, 64] Perhaps a more precise method of substratification of this group of patients lies in quantification of redistribution zones on dipyridamole-thallium scans as an initial screening device.[52, 53] Quantitative dipyridamole-thallium scan using a summed reversibility index in conjunction with preoperative ambulatory monitoring may well allow us to expeditiously identify those patients with the highest degree of susceptibility to postoperative myocardial ischemia and cardiac fatality. Although the overall minimal mortality currently associated with most vascular reconstructions may represent an irreducible minimum, the persistently higher rate observed in patients with overt coronary disease justifies further effort.

References

1. Kannel WB, Skinner JJ Jr, Schwartz MJ, et al: Intermittent claudication: Incidence in the Framingham Study. Circulation 41:857, 1970.
2. Hertzer NR, Young JR, Kramer JR, et al: Routine coronary angiography prior to elective aortic reconstruction: Results of selective myocardial revascularization in patients with peripheral vascular disease. Arch Surg 114:1336–1344, 1979.
3. Hertzer NR, Beven EG, Young JR, et al: Coronary artery disease in peripheral vascular patients. A classification of 1000 coronary angiograms and results of surgical management. Ann Surg 199:223–233, 1984.
4. Brown OW, Hollier LH, Pairolero PC, et al: Abdominal aortic aneurysm and coronary artery disease: A reassessment. Arch Surg 116:1484–1488, 1981.
5. Golden MA, Whittemore AD, Donaldson MC, Mannick JA: Selective evaluation and management of coronary artery disease in patients undergoing repair of abdominal aortic aneurysms. Ann Surg 212:415–423, 1990.
6. DeBakey ME, Crawford ES, Cooley DA, et al: Aneurysm of the abdominal aorta: Analysis of results of graft replacement therapy one to eleven years after operation. Ann Surg 160:622–639, 1964.
7. Voorhees AB Jr, McAllister FF: Long-term results following resection of arteriosclerotic abdominal aortic aneurysms. Surg Gynecol Obstet 117:355–358, 1963.
8. Szilagyi DE, Smith RF, DeRusso FJ, et al: Contribution of abdominal aortic aneurysmectomy to prolongation of life. Ann Surg 164:678–697, 1966.
9. Goldman L, Caldera DL, Nussman SR, et al: Multifactorial index of cardiac risk in noncardiac surgical procedures. N Engl J Med 297:845–850, 1977.
10. Goldman L, Caldera DL, Southwick FS, et al: Cardiac risk factors and complications in noncardiac surgery. Medicine 57:357, 1978.
11. Tarhan S, Moffitt EA, Taylor WF, et al: Myocardial infarction after general anesthesia. JAMA 220:1451, 1972.
12. Rose SD, Corman LC, Mason DT: Cardiac risk factors in patients undergoing noncardiac surgery. Med Clin North Am 63:1271, 1979.
13. Portal RW: Elective surgery after myocardial infarction. BMJ 284:843, 1982.
14. Steen PA, Tinker JH, Tarhan S: Myocardial reinfarction after anesthesia and surgery. JAMA 239:2566, 1978.
15. Wells PH, Kaplan JA: Optimal management of patients with ischemic heart disease for non-cardiac surgery by complementary anesthesiologist and cardiologist interaction. Am Heart J 102:1029, 1981.
16. Rao TLK, El-Etr AA: Myocardial reinfarction following anesthesia in patients with recent infarction. Anesth Analg 60:271, 1981.
17. Rivers SP, Scher LA, Gupta SK, Veith FJ: Safety of peripheral vascular surgery after recent acute myocardial infarction. J Vasc Surg 11:70–76, 1990.
18. Goldman L: Cardiac risks and complications of noncardiac surgery. Ann Surg 198:780–791, 1983.
19. Schulze RA Jr, Rouleau J, Rigo P, et al: Ventricular arrhythmias in the late hospital phase of acute myocardial infarction: Relation to left ventricular function detected by gated cardiac blood pool scanning. Circulation 52:1006, 1975.
20. Lyons C: Cardiac arrhythmias as a predictable surgical risk. Surgery 35:292, 1954.
21. Wolf MA, Braunwald E: General anesthesia and noncardiac surgery in patients with heart disease. In Braunwald E (ed): Heart Disease. Philadelphia, WB Saunders, 1980.
22. Skinner JF, Pearce ML: Surgical risk in the cardiac patient. J Chronic Dis 17:54, 1964.
23. Chambers DA: Anesthesia for the patient with acquired valvular heart disease. In Kaplan JA (ed): Cardiac Anesthesia. New York, Grune & Stratton, 1979, p 197.
24. Perlroth MG, Hultgren HN: The cardiac patient and general surgery. JAMA 232:1279, 1975.
25. Tinker JH, Tarhan S: Discontinuing anticoagulant therapy in surgical patients with cardiac valve prostheses. JAMA 239:738, 1978.
26. Katholi RE, Nolan SP, McGuire LB: Living with prosthetic heart valves: Subsequent noncardiac operations and the risk of thromboembolism or hemorrhage. Am Heart J 92:162, 1976.
27. Dripps RD, Lamont A, Eckenhoff JE: The role of anesthesia in surgical mortality. JAMA 178:261–266, 1961.
28. Detsky AS, Abrams HB, Forbath N, et al: Cardiac assessment of patients undergoing noncardiac surgery: A multifactorial risk index. Arch Intern Med 146:2131–2134, 1986.
29. Eagle KA, Singer DE, Brewster DC, et al: Dipyridamole-thallium scanning in patients undergoing vascular surgery. JAMA 257:2185–2189, 1987.
30. Cooperman M, Pflug B, Martin EW Jr, Evans WE: Cardiovascular risk factors in patients with peripheral vascular disease. Surgery 84:505–509, 1978.
31. Lette J, Waters D, Lassande J, et al: Postoperative myocardial infarction and cardiac death. Ann Surg 211:84–90, 1990.
32. Pasternack PF, Imparato AM, Bear G, et al: The value of radionuclide angiography as a predictor of perioperative myocardial infarction in patients undergoing abdominal aortic aneurysm resection. J Vasc Surg 1:320–325, 1984.
33. Pasternack PF, Imparato AM, Riles TS, et al: The value of the radionuclide angiogram in the prediction of perioperative myocardial infarction in patients undergoing lower extremity revascularization procedures. Circulation 72:13–17, 1985.
34. Kazmers A, Cerqueira MD, Zierler RE: The role of preoperative radionuclide ejection fraction in direct abdominal aortic aneurysm repair. J Vasc Surg 8:128–136, 1988.
35. McCann RL, Wolfe WG: Resection of abdominal aortic aneurysm in patients with low ejection fractions. J Vasc Surg 10:240–244, 1989.
36. Franco CD, Goldsmith J, Veith FJ, et al: Resting gated pool ejection fraction a poor predictor of perioperative myocardial infarction in patients undergoing vascular surgery for infrainguinal bypass grafting. J Vasc Surg 10:656–661, 1989.
37. Cutler BS, Wheeler HB, Paraskos JA, Cardullo PA: Applicability and interpretation of electrocardiographic stress testing in patients with peripheral vascular disease. Am J Surg 141:501–506, 1981.
38. Arous EJ, Baum PL, Cutler BS: The ischemic exercise test in patients with peripheral vascular disease: Implications for management. Arch Surg 119:780–783, 1984.

39. McPhail N, Calvin JE, Shariatmadar A, et al: The use of preoperative exercise testing to predict cardiac complications after arterial reconstruction. J Vasc Surg 7:60–68, 1988.

40. Goldman L: Cardiac risks and complications of noncardiac surgery. Ann Intern Med 98:504, 1983.

41. Gage AA, Bhayana JN, Balu V, et al: Assessment of cardiac risk in surgical patients. Arch Surg 112:1488–1492, 1977.

42. Hertzer NR, Young JR, Drawer JR, et al: Routine coronary angiography prior to elective aortic reconstruction: Results of a selective myocardial revascularization in patients with peripheral vascular disease. Arch Surg 114:1336–1344, 1979.

43. Kennedy JW, Kaiser GC, Fisher LD, et al: Clinical and angiographic predictors of operative mortality from the collaborative study in coronary artery surgery. Circulation 63:793–801, 1981.

44. Boucher CA, Brewster DC, Darling RC, et al: Determination of cardiac risk by dipyridamole-thallium imaging before peripheral vascular surgery. N Engl J Med 312:389–394, 1985.

45. Cutler BS, Leppo JA: Dipyridamole thallium 201 scintigraphy to detect coronary artery disease before abdominal aortic surgery. J Vasc Surg 5:91, 1987.

46. Berman DS, Kiat H, Maddahi J: The new ^{99m}Tc myocardial perfusion imaging agents: ^{99m}Tc-sestamibi and ^{99m}Tc-teboroxine. Circulation 84(Suppl I):I-7–I-21, 1991.

47. New ways to scan the myocardium [medical letter]. Med Lett Drugs Ther 33:87, 1991.

48. Yeager RA: Basic data related to cardiac testing and cardiac risk associated with vascular surgery. Ann Surg 4:193–197, 1990.

49. Dilsizian V, Rocco TP, Freedman NMT, et al: Enhanced detection of ischemic but viable myocardium by the reinjection of thallium after stress-redistribution imaging. N Engl J Med 323:141–146, 1990.

50. McEnroe CS, O'Donnell TF, Yeager A, et al: Comparison of ejection fraction and Goldman risk factor analysis to dipyridamole-thallium 201 studies in the evaluation of cardiac morbidity after aortic aneurysm surgery. J Vasc Surg 11:497–504, 1990.

51. Eagle KA, Coley CM, Newell JB, et al: Combining clinical and thallium data optimizes preoperative assessment of cardiac risk before major vascular surgery. Ann Intern Med 110:859–866, 1989.

52. Lette J, Waters D, Lassonde J, et al: Multivariate clinical models and quantitative dipyridamole-thallium imaging to predict cardiac morbidity and death after vascular reconstruction. J Vasc Surg 14:158–169, 1991.

53. Cambria RP, Brewster DC, Abbott WM, et al: The impact of selective use of dipyridamole-thallium scans and surgical factors on the current morbidity of aortic surgery. J Vasc Surg 15:43–51, 1992.

54. Mangano DT, London MJ, Tubau JF, et al: Dipyridamole thallium-201 scintigraphy as a preoperative screening test: A reexamination of its predictive potential. Circulation 84:493–502, 1991.

55. Baron JF, Mundler O, Bertrand M, et al: Dipyridamole-thallium scintigraphy and gated radionuclide angiography to assess cardiac risk before abdominal aortic surgery. N Engl J Med 330:663–669, 1994.

56. Raby KE, Goldman L, Creager MA, et al: Correlation between preoperative ischemia and major cardiac events after peripheral vascular surgery. N Engl J Med 321:1296–1300, 1989.

57. Pasternack PF, Grossi EA, Baumann FG, et al: The value of silent myocardial ischemia monitoring in the prediction of perioperative myocardial infarction in patients undergoing peripheral vascular surgery. J Vasc Surg 10:617–625, 1989.

58. Mangano DT, Browner WS, Hollenberg M, et al: Association of perioperative myocardial ischemia with cardiac morbidity and mortality in men undergoing noncardiac surgery. N Engl J Med 323:1781–1788, 1990.

59. Taylor LM Jr, Yeager RA, Moneta GL, et al: The incidence of perioperative myocardial infarction in general vascular surgery. J Vasc Surg 15:52–61, 1992.

60. Mason JJ, Owens DK, Harris RA, et al: The role of coronary angiography and coronary revascularization before noncardiac vascular surgery. JAMA 273:1919–1925, 1995.

61. Perry MO, Calcagno D: Abdominal aortic aneurysm surgery: The basic evaluation of cardiac risk. Ann Surg 208:738–742, 1988.

62. Mackey WC, O'Donnell TF Jr, Callow AD: Cardiac risk in patients undergoing carotid endarterectomy: Impact on perioperative and long-term mortality. J Vasc Surg 11:226–234, 1990.

63. Hollier LH: Cardiac evaluation in patients with vascular disease: Overview: A practical approach. J Vasc Surg 15:726–729, 1992.

64. Bunt TJ: The role of a defined protocol for cardiac risk assessment in decreasing perioperative myocardial infarction in vascular surgery. J Vasc Surg 15:626–634, 1992.

65. Mangano DT, Layug EL, Wallace A, Tateo I: Effect of atenolol on mortality and cardiovascular morbidity after noncardiac surgery. N Engl J Med 335:1713–1720, 1996.

66. Poldermans D, Boersma E, Bax JJ, et al: The effect of bisoprolol on perioperative mortality and myocardial infarction in high-risk patients undergoing vascular surgery. N Engl J Med 341:1789–1794, 1999.

67. Lee TH: Reducing cardiac risk in noncardiac surgery. N Engl J Med 341:1838–1840, 1999.

Review Questions

1. The most significant predictor of a postoperative cardiac complication is
   (a) uncontrolled congestive heart failure
   (b) symptoms of angina
   (c) a positive dipyridamole-thallium stress test
   (d) a recent myocardial infarction

2. Most retrospective studies have found that symptoms of stable angina
   (a) increase perioperative risk for myocardial complication by 20%
   (b) should be evaluated by coronary arteriography before elective vascular surgery
   (c) do not greatly affect operative risk for perioperative complications after vascular surgery
   (d) increase perioperative risk by 50%

3. The following statement is true concerning exercise-thallium stress testing
   (a) exercise-thallium imaging has proven as accurate as dipyridamole-thallium imaging studies
   (b) exercise-thallium imaging is limited in that approximately one third of patients are unable to achieve sufficient exercise for accurate testing
   (c) both
   (d) neither

4. Two recent prospective evaluations of the accuracy of dipyridamole-thallium stress imaging have concluded that
   (a) a normal dipyridamole-thallium stress test confers a low perioperative risk for myocardial complications
   (b) a positive dipyridamole-thallium stress test confers a high risk for perioperative complications
   (c) both
   (d) neither

5. The increased perioperative risk for myocardial infarction after a recent myocardial infarction plateaus
   (a) after 1 month
   (b) after 3 months
   (c) after 6 months
   (d) never

6. Most well-documented clinical scoring systems for operative risk have
   (a) proved to be reproducible from institution to institution
   (b) not proved to be reproducible from institution to institution
   (c) remained valid despite improvements in anesthetic and perioperative management
   (d) generally performed well when applied to prospective populations of patients

7. When routine coronary arteriography was applied preoperatively to peripheral vascular surgery patients
   (a) significant coronary artery disease was identified only in patients with significant clinical histories
   (b) severe, operable coronary artery disease was identified in 10% of patients
   (c) severe, operable coronary artery disease was identified in 25% of patients
   (d) the combined morbidity and mortality of coronary artery interventions and vascular surgery was proved to be less than if coronary arteriograms had not been done

8. For an exercise stress test to be accurate, the patient must
   (a) exercise for 12 minutes
   (b) exercise to the point that sustained S-T depression of 1 mm is achieved
   (c) achieve 85% of his or her predicted maximal heart rate
   (d) none of the above

9. Randomized prospective trials have demonstrated that
   (a) routine application of stress testing followed by selective coronary arteriography lowers the incidence of perioperative myocardial complications
   (b) routine application of stress testing followed by selective coronary arteriography does not influence the perioperative myocardial infarction rate
   (c) routine application of stress testing and selective coronary arteriography improves long-term patient survival
   (d) none of the above

Answers

1. d   2. c   3. c   4. d   5. c   6. b   7. c   8. c   9. d

22

Vascular Grafts: Characteristics and Rational Selection of Prostheses

William M. Abbott and Michael E. Landis

Most medical historians trace the advent of modern vascular surgery to the work of Alexis Carrel,[1] who was one of four surgeons to have won the Nobel prize in this field. His work included a description of autogenous venous grafting in dogs. Since then, both vascular surgeons and scientists have sought better vascular grafts with only partial success. Although current synthetic prosthetic grafts yield good results in aortoiliac reconstructive surgery, the best results in peripheral small vessel reconstruction are still achieved only with venous autografts. The greater saphenous vein is the conduit of choice for small vessel reconstruction and most closely approaches the characteristics of the ideal vascular graft. However, 20% or more of current candidates for infrainguinal reconstruction have insufficient or unsuitable autogenous vein.[2] The saphenous vein may have been used during previous vascular procedures or may be inadequate due to chronic disease. In these circumstances, the vascular surgeon must be aware of all graft choices available and the relative advantages and disadvantages of each. Furthermore, although autogenous vein is currently the best conduit, it is *not* a perfect arterial substitute. It is considered the gold standard, but it is a tarnished one.

This chapter reviews the relevant characteristics of the normal human artery and those of an ideal vascular graft, which, unfortunately, does not currently exist. A brief overview of the autogenous and various prosthetic grafts available follows. Some conduits that are no longer in use are presented for their historical and scientific interest. A brief description of some of the more promising research initiatives in vascular graft development also is given. Recommendations for the most appropriate grafts for specific procedures are made based on published results from our and other institutions.

THE NORMAL ARTERY

An artery is much more than the inert conduit it was considered to be until the 1970s. For this reason, prosthetic grafts have fallen far short of the durability of native artery. The longevity of native arteries in terms of their ability to remain patent and free from aneurysmal change is measured in decades, whereas that of prosthetic grafts is generally measured in years. The functional characteristics of large elastic arteries such as the aorta differ from those of the medium-sized muscular arteries, such as the carotid, and must be taken into account when either designing or choosing a prosthetic graft.

An artery is composed of three layers: the intima, the media, and the adventitia. The intima is the inner layer and is composed of endothelium, *extracellular matrix*, and the internal elastic lamina. The endothelium, in addition to forming a smooth lining, is biologically active, and in addition to providing a vasoregulatory function, modulates the humoral and cellular coagulation systems by imparting a negative (hydrophobic) charge, and by actively secreting antithrombotic agents.[3] The media consists of layers of smooth muscle cells oriented in both longitudinal and circumferential directions that are surrounded by a basal lamina and fibers of collagen and elastin. The media contributes to the strength and durability of the artery, but its main role is control over elasticity and vessel diameter. Vasoconstriction or relaxation allows for regionalization of blood flow by varying the diameter of the vessel lumen. The adventitia, long thought to be an inert, nonfunctional structure, contains the vasa vasorum and a collagenous matrix whose main function is to provide tensile strength to the artery.

CONCEPT OF THROMBOREACTIVITY

For the purpose of this chapter, *a vascular prosthesis is* defined as a man-made or man-altered device meant to replace a blood vessel. In common vascular surgical usage, this term is not usually applied to living autogenous conduits. Any prosthesis placed into the arterial system enters a thromboreactive state that can be defined in terms of intensity and duration. Depending on that state, as well as a number of other host variables (e.g., low flow due to poor runoff), the graft either remains patent or occludes. Graft thromboreactivity and the parameters that influence it vary over the life of the implant in early (weeks), intermediate (weeks to months), and long-term (years) time frames. Although thromboreactivity is most intense immediately after implantation, in most current prostheses it persists at a lower level forever.

CHARACTERISTICS OF AN IDEAL PROSTHETIC GRAFT

A vascular prosthetic graft may be composed of manufactured material, or it may be of biologic (i.e. tissue) origin. An ideal vascular prosthetic graft would have characteristics that minimize both the intensity and duration of the thromboreactive state. Specifically, such a graft would be impermeable, thromboresistant, compliant, biocompatible, durable, resistant to infection, easy to sterilize, easy to implant, readily available, and cost-effective.[4] This ideal has yet to be achieved.

Impermeability to blood is obviously important, although this characteristic is somewhat at odds with the need for sufficient permeability or porosity to allow graft incorporation and healing. *Thromboresistance*, the ability of the graft surface to tolerate blood contact without activating platelets or the humoral coagulation cascade, is vital and is related to several factors, including graft surface reactivity with blood, ionic charge, porosity, and compliance relative to that of the adjacent native artery. *Compliance*, defined as volume change per unit of pressure change, is important. Considerable data have shown that compliance or compliance mismatch is an important contributor to thrombosis.[5, 6] *Biocompatability* is necessary because significant tissue reaction may promote thrombosis, loss of graft integrity, and graft failure. A prosthetic graft must be *durable* enough to obviate the need for future replacement due to dilatation, aneurysm formation, or rupture. *Resistance to infection* and *sterility* are necessary to lessen the incidence of graft infection. A graft should have handling characteristics—strength, flexibility, suture retention, and ease of suturing—that make it *easy to implant*. The graft should be *readily available* for both elective and emergent use. Finally, in this era of increasingly limited health care resources, the graft must be relatively *cost-effective*, with the cost of the graft measured against the operative time required to implant it and freedom from complications that require secondary or revision intervention.

Of all the arterial grafts currently in use, venous autografts most closely meet these specifications and are thus discussed first.

AUTOGENOUS VEIN GRAFTS

Anatomy

The greater saphenous vein, the one most commonly used for arterial reconstruction, consists of a monolayer of endo-

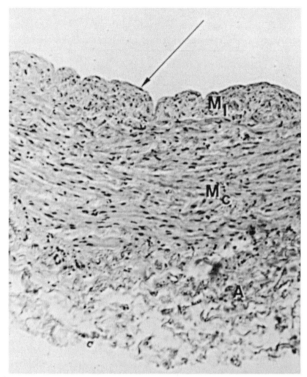

Figure 22–1. Normal human saphenous vein. Intimal structures (*arrow*) include endothelium and scant subendothelial connective tissue. Medial structures composed of an inner layer of longitudinally arranged smooth muscle (M_l) and an outer region of circumferentially oriented smooth muscle (M_c). Adventitial structures appear as a loose collection of connective tissue (A) with occasional vasa vasorum. (From Stanley JC, Burkel WE, Lindenauer SM, et al: Biologic and Synthetic Vascular Prostheses. New York, Grune and Stratton, 1982.)

thelium, basement membrane, a media composed of two layers of smooth muscle cells, and an adventitia, which is the thickest layer of the vein wall[7] (Figs. 22–1 and 22–2). The wall of normal veins is considerably thinner than that of arteries, and although many vein walls are thickened at harvest as a result of chronic venous disease, the vein may still be usable as an arterial conduit.

The anatomy of the greater saphenous vein is important to the vascular surgeon, and anatomic variation can affect the success of the vein harvest and its performance as a graft. The greater saphenous vein originates in the dorsum of the foot and ascends anterior to the medial malleolus. It follows a superficial course on the anteromedial aspect of the tibia, and at the level of the knee lies 8 to 10 cm below the medial edge of the patella. The greater saphenous vein is duplicated in an estimated 8% of patients.[8] Lower extremity veins contain valves, which are more numerous distally and less numerous proximally. Perforating veins tend to occur in the midthigh at the level of the adductor hiatus, just above the knee joint, and midway between the knee and the ankle.[9]

The lesser saphenous vein runs in a slightly oblique course from behind the lateral malleolus to the popliteal vein. It may be used as an autograft, but its length is markedly shorter and its diameter is significantly smaller than those of the greater saphenous vein.

The cephalic vein is 50 cm long, and although often quite thin, may be an acceptable alternative as an auto-

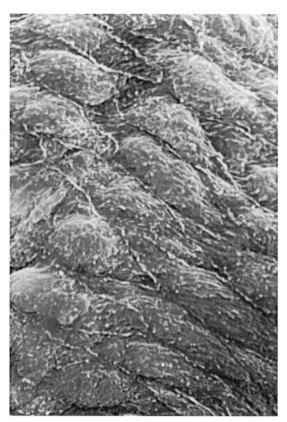

Figure 22–2. Normal vein lumen, showing characteristic endothelial cell surface (SEM, ×30).

graft.[10] In practice, the suitability of a vein for use as a conduit is quite variable and often is not predictable in advance of the operation. The suitability of any autogenous vein is best determined by preoperative venous mapping by duplex scan.

Arterialization

After implantation as an arterial conduit, autogenous veins undergo morphologic changes in response to the hemodynamic forces of the arterial circulation. These changes begin immediately after implantation, continue over time, and (in some cases) may become detrimental to the performance of the graft. This process is known as arterialization, originally described by Carrel.[1] In most cases, arterialization is a normal and salutary adaptive response of the vein to the new arterial environment. In a smaller cohort, it becomes a pathologic response variably termed *intimal hyperplasia*. Distinct internal and external elastic laminae appear,[11] and smooth muscle cells migrate into the intima where they proliferate, become hypertrophic, and produce extracellular matrix. In intimal hyperplasia, this process becomes uncontrolled and leads to progressive narrowing of the entire graft, or focal narrowing. In either instance, it accounts for a significant percentage of early (within 1 year) graft occlusion.[12, 13] Focal hyperplasia is thought to represent an aggravated response to local injury and typically occurs at sites of valve lysis, or in perianastomotic regions.[14] Diffuse hyperplasia is poorly understood.

Intimal hyperplasia occurs in approximately 11% to 33% of vein grafts in peripheral reconstructions, with 75% developing within the first year.[15] This problem is being investigated at both the hemodynamic and cellular levels. Data from our laboratory have implicated anastomotic flow disturbances and compliance mismatch in the development of anastomotic neointimal hyperplasia.[16, 17] Hyperhomocysteinemia has been shown to be associated with the development of preexisting intimal hyperplasia in veins and subsequent vein graft failure.[18] Clowes and colleagues[19] investigated the interaction between endothelium and smooth muscle cells extensively at the cellular and cytokine levels, and developed a multifactorial theory of smooth muscle cell proliferation.

Since the cause of intimal hyperplasia is poorly understood, no effective prophylaxis or treatment measure exists. It is probably the number one unsolved problem in vascular surgery, with the lack of a satisfactory prosthesis a close second. Several animal studies have shown promising results in inhibition of intimal hyperplasia, including external beam irradiation, adenoviral-mediated gene transfer of nitric oxide synthase and other vasoactive peptides, L-arginine supplementation, and matrix metalloproteinase inhibition. Unfortunately, these therapies have had as yet minimal clinical application, and their utility remains to be determined.[20–23]

Vein Harvest: Surgical Technique

Several techniques may be employed by the vascular surgeon to minimize damage to the vein from harvest and arterialization. Basic surgical principles of precise, atraumatic dissection with delicate tissue handling are important to minimize endothelial and vessel wall damage. Venous branches should be ligated well away from the vein wall to minimize endothelial crimping. The spasm induced by operative dissection, in conjunction with chronic changes from venous disease, may render many veins alarmingly small. However, with gentle dilatation, most veins enlarge sufficiently to allow their use as a conduit (3.5–4.0 mm minimum internal diameter) in the view of most vascular surgeons.[9, 24] Care should be taken when distending the vein, because high pressure (greater than 300 mm Hg) may produce marked transmural damage and lead to early graft failure.[25] Papaverine infusion may be helpful in ameliorating vein spasm. Clamp injury may cause fibrosis and stenosis, leading many surgeons to prefer atraumatic, broad-based clamps. Storage solutions for the vein have been shown to endanger endothelial integrity, with several studies demonstrating decreased cytotoxicity and permeability with the use of a cold cardioplegia solution (U.W. organ preservation or Bretschneider's HTK solution) or heparinized whole blood.[26, 27] Whatever storage solution is chosen, it is important that it be kept cold.

Three general methods are used for saphenous vein preparation: the *in situ* technique, which leaves the vein in its normal anatomic position; the *reversed* technique, which moves the vein from its native location; and the *nonreversed* translocation technique. The last also moves the vessel from its normal anatomic position, but, as with the in situ technique, it requires valve lysis. Regardless of the bypass technique used, the technique of vein harvest and preparation does affect the performance of the graft. Careful, gentle harvesting and handling increase the early and late patency of vein grafts, whereas vein damage caused by careless technique increases the incidence of early graft failure due to technical problems, and late failure due to hyperplastic or degenerative changes in the vein.

If the in situ or nonreversed translocation technique is used, extreme care should be taken when lysing valves. Several problems can result from improper valve lysis, such as inadvertent injury to the vessel wall. This can lead to perioperative failure from an intimal flap or early failure from neointimal hyperplasia. Missed valves or incomplete lysis of valve leaflets may also cause early graft failure.[28] Even properly lysed valves can cause late focal stenosis.

If the reversed technique is used, limiting the amount of time the graft spends outside the body results in less ischemia to the vein. If necessary, the graft should be kept in a chilled isotonic solution such as cold autologous heparinized blood.[28]

Vein grafts are susceptible to a number of complications. Aneurysm formation may occur in up to 12% of infrainguinal bypass grafts.[29] Atherosclerosis, extremely rare in the venous circulation, may occur in 7% to 15% of transplanted veins[30] and may be related to smoking and uncontrolled hyperlipidemia.[14] Neointimal hyperplasia, focal stenosis from valve injuries and missed valves, aneurysmal change, and graft atherosclerosis account for a significant number of early and late failures.[31] Careful technique can minimize but cannot eliminate these problems.

Results

Infrainguinal bypass grafts using autogenous vein yield the highest patency rates in the most recent literature. Five-year primary patency rates of 72% to 82% have been reported for femoropopliteal bypasses.[32, 33] For infrapopliteal bypass, 5-year patency rates of 59% to 69% and limb salvage rates of 90% have been reported.[34, 35] Interestingly, results do not appear to be significantly different for in situ, reversed, or nonreversed translocation techniques. Primary patency rates with arm vein and lesser saphenous vein are lower, in the range of 40% to 50% at 5 years, but still considerably higher than those for prosthetic grafts.[36, 37]

ARTERIAL AUTOGRAFTS

Medium-sized muscular arteries possess an important characteristic that renders them particularly amenable to auto-transplantation as free grafts—their vasa vasorum originate from small arterial branches and remain intact if harvested carefully.[38] For these reasons, arterial autografts approach the characteristics of the ideal vascular graft more closely than do vein grafts, and should be the gold standard. Unfortunately, few arteries are suitable as autografts. In certain situations, common, internal, and external iliac segments may be harvested as a bypass graft, and replaced with a prosthetic graft. Alternatively, an occluded iliofemoral segment that has been bypassed can be harvested and, after endarterectomy, used as a bypass conduit. From these

sites, segments of graft from 10 to 20 cm in length may be obtained.[38]

Arterial autografts are particularly attractive conduits for use in children because their growth rate is proportional to that of the other vessels of the arterial system.[39] They are particularly advantageous in renal artery reconstruction.[29] Another potential use of arterial autografts is in an infected tissue bed, where a prosthetic graft would not be appropriate owing to the danger of graft infection.[40]

The use of splenic arterial autografts for extra-anatomic renovascular reconstruction is an accepted and efficacious means of treating renovascular disease.[41] The internal mammary artery is also used in a similar manner, and its superior patency compared with vein grafts in the coronary artery bypass graft (CABG) (84% and 53%, respectively, at 10 years) illustrates the better patency rates that may be obtained with arterial autografts.[42]

Results

In properly selected patients, arterial autografts can provide excellent results. In the report of Stoney and colleagues[43] of renal revascularization in children, late patency was 100%, grafts were noted to grow normally, and only a single instance of graft dilatation was noted. Cambria and coworkers,[41] in a review of 52 splenorenal bypass grafts, noted an early and late patency of greater than 90% at 5 years.

ALLOGRAFTS

Arterial and venous allografts were used extensively in the early days of aortic reconstruction[44] for both aneurysmal and occlusive disease. Aortic segments, harvested from cadavers, were stored in various preservative solutions at 4°C, frozen or freeze-dried. These grafts suffered from the twin disadvantages of nonviability and tissue antigenicity. Enthusiasm for the use of large vessel allografts subsequently waned when reports were published showing a high rate of graft calcification and aneurysm formation.[45, 46] As textile grafts for aortic reconstruction became available, the use of allografts all but disappeared. Several recent reports in the literature, however, have recommended the use of cadaveric arterial allografts for in situ replacement of infected abdominal aortic grafts,[47–49] and for thoracic aortic graft replacement in the presence of endocarditis.[50] Unpublished work from our own laboratory shows that cryopreservation actually decreases the manifestation of rejection of arterial allografts (W.B. Abbott, personal personal communication, 10/98).

Efforts directed at obtaining a useful small vessel allograft have been similarly disappointing. Cadaveric human saphenous vein allografts were implanted in the 1960s in patients with unsuitable autogenous vein, but follow-up showed poor long-term patency.[51] Cryopreservation of human saphenous vein using dimethyl sulfoxide (DMSO) has resulted in viable vein grafts.[52–54] Unfortunately, viable allografts are antigenic and capable of stimulating a rejection response. Cryopreserved vein allografts are still under investigation, and a phase I study using cryopreserved venous valved segments to treat chronic venous insufficiency suggests that this may be a therapeutic option in selected individuals.[55]

Two studies of 115 cryopreserved vein grafts implanted in the infrageniculate position showed a poor patency rate compared with that of autogenous vein and recommended the use of this graft only in infected fields when autogenous vein was not available.[56] Arterial allografts also have been used for infrainguinal reconstruction, but they too have been shown to have relatively poor patency, with a primary patency rate of only 35% at 3 years noted in a recent study from Great Britain and Ireland.[57] There is an increasing use of cryopreserved superficial femoral vein grafts for dialysis because they may be more resistant to infection than expanded polytetrafluoroethylene (ePTFE). The role of immunosuppressive drugs and the use of anticoagulation in conjunction with these grafts are still under investigation. In a prospective clinical trial, Carpenter and Tomaszewski[58] found that vein allograft failure was not eliminated by low-dose azidothymidine immunosuppressive therapy. Unless the results of future studies show a clear advantage of these grafts over existing, available conduits, their expense may preclude their use.

The Human Umbilical Cord Vein Allograft

The human umbilical vein (HUV) allograft is of interest because of the relatively large experience surgeons have acquired with it since it was first implanted more than 40 years ago.[59] Disappointing short-term patency results led to a loss of interest in this graft, but Dardik and colleagues[60, 61] have revised it by stabilization with glutaraldehyde instead of dialdehyde starch. Glutaraldehyde seemingly produces better cross-linking of collagen, resulting in a graft that is purportedly not only stronger but also less antigenic. After fixation, the graft was encased in a Dacron mesh to add strength, because early animal studies demonstrated a significant incidence of HUV graft dilatation without mesh.[62]

As with other preserved allografts (with the exception of cryopreserved saphenous veins), the HUV graft is not viable after fixation and is essentially a musculocollagenous tube. Thus, any potential advantage of the HUV graft over synthetic prosthetic grafts in terms of late patency is related to the surface characteristics of its inner layer and its compliance.

The majority of HUV graft experience has been in infrainguinal reconstruction. Because autogenous greater saphenous vein is the conduit of choice for these procedures,[2, 34] the clinical efficacy of HUV grafts lies in their ability to provide a better conduit than synthetic grafts for infrainguinal reconstruction in those patients for whom autogenous greater saphenous vein is not an option.[2] One factor limiting the potential usefulness of HUV is the greater technical difficulty involved in handling, tunneling, and anastomosing the graft, compared with that of either autogenous vein or other prosthetic grafts.[63] Suturing is tedious owing to the thickness of the graft and because care must be taken to include both the basement membrane and the outer Dacron mesh in the suture line. HUV grafts are also friable and prone to mural dissection if not handled gently.

Results

In 1988, Dardik and coworkers[64] published the largest series of HUV graft experiences in a report describing 907 bypasses, half of which were to tibial vessels. Five-year patency rates were 53% for femoropopliteal reconstruction, 26% for femorotibial reconstruction, and 28% for femoroperoneal reconstruction.[64] Several studies have demonstrated no significant difference in patency between HUV and ePTFE grafts in infrainguinal reconstruction,[65–68] although two randomized prospective studies have shown superior patency of HUV for femoropopliteal bypasses.[69, 70] Results published in 1999 demonstrated 5-year patency rates of up to 67%, confirming the potential utility of HUV grafts.[71] The most serious drawback of the HUV graft is its tendency to degenerate. Late graft dilatation and aneurysm formation reportedly occur in up to 57% of HUV grafts.[72–74] (Fig. 22–3). Although the incidence of clinically significant aneurysm formation requiring graft salvage or replacement is lower,[75] this is a significant enough problem, in the opinion of most vascular surgeons, to make it an unacceptable conduit.

XENOGRAFTS

Interest in the use of animal tissue for vascular grafts dates to the 1950s, when bovine carotid arteries were enzymatically digested with ficin to remove antigenic cellular material and then tanned with dialdehyde starch.[76] This graft was used clinically as a femoropopliteal graft, and over the next decade considerable experience was gained with it. Unfortunately, its late patency was no better than that of synthetic grafts,[77, 78] with 5-year patency rates of 40% to 50% in the above-knee position. The incidence of aneurysm formation has been reported at 3% to 6%, but it is probably much higher. Infection rates were 3% to 7%.[77] Thus, use of these xenografts in infrainguinal bypasses ceased, although they continued to be somewhat useful in angioaccess for hemodialysis, with high patency and low infection rates.[79] More recent experience with ePTFE for angioaccess has limited the applicability of xenografts for this purpose.[80]

Sawyer and colleagues[81] developed another modification of the tanning process using carboxylated collagen, which resulted in a negatively charged, glutaraldehyde-tanned (NCGT) graft. This graft is a bovine carotid xenograft used for infrainguinal reconstruction. In the authors' initial report, 146 NCGT grafts were implanted in 108 patients with a 5-year patency rate of 67%. Four percent of grafts developed aneurysms.[81] Although this report was encouraging, long-term follow-up has not been forthcoming.

The Solcograft-P, a bovine carotid artery graft undergoing a totally different chemical fixation process, was developed in Europe.[82] Although its handling properties were excellent and its early results were outstanding, this graft was voluntarily withdrawn from clinical use after a late incidence of aneurysm was noted.[83]

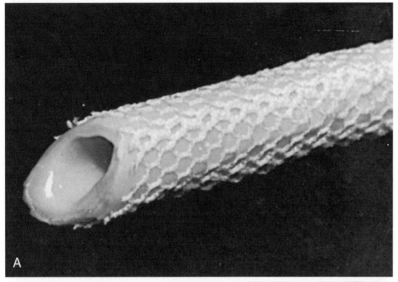

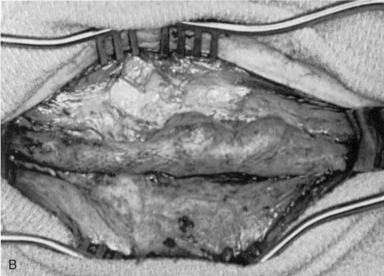

Figure 22–3. Human umbilical vein graft with surrounding Dacron mesh, prior to implantation (*A*), and aneurysmal segment 5 years after implantation (*B*).

Results

Results with commercially available xenografts have been too poor to recommend their clinical use at this time. Poor patency and graft degeneration continue to plague xenografts. Research into better fixation methods continues, however, because this type of graft offers the real advantage of being a biologic graft in nearly unlimited supply. New grafts of bovine origin preserved by a unique photofixation process are currently under investigation. Short-term results in a canine model undergoing infrainguinal reconstructive procedures show comparable patency to polytetrafluoroethylene (PTFE) in the common femoral artery and no evidence of degenerative changes.[84] This approach must await further information.

SYNTHETIC GRAFTS

The concept of constructing grafts from synthetic materials was developed in 1952 when Voorhees, then a surgical resident, and others observed that a silk thread in the atrium of a dog (being used for another study) was not only tolerated without ill effect but had become coated with a smooth endothelial-like layer.[85] Because of this phenomenon, Vorhees and colleagues speculated that arterial conduits fashioned of synthetic fabric would become similarly coated with a nonthrombogenic pseudointima. The first fabric grafts were made using polymers from the plastics industry. The first grafts, made of Vinyon-N,[85] were implanted in the aortic position in dogs and found to be well tolerated, patent, and "incorporated" in the sense that they underwent ingrowth of fibroblasts from the surrounding tissue into the interstices of the graft. This laboratory success led to successful implantation in 18 patients.[86]

It soon became apparent that the early textile grafts lost tensile strength over time, and a search was carried out for materials that would maintain strength and be resistant to dilatation. Rayon and nylon were tried, but were unsatisfactory. Silk, although popular in China, has never been adequately evaluated in the United States. However, two textile grafts, polyethylene terephthate (polyester or Dacron) and polytetrafluoroethylene (PTFE or Teflon), were found

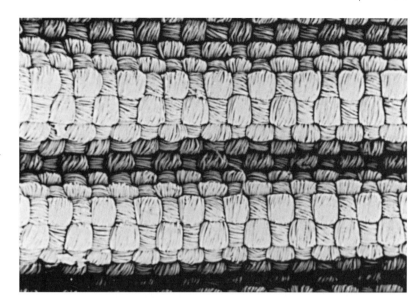

Figure 22–4. Woven crimped Dacron graft with interlaced network of threads (SEM, ×30).

to retain nearly all their strength long after implantation,[87] and interest was concentrated on these materials. PTFE is no longer available in textile form, but is common in its extruded form, which is discussed later.

Dacron (Polyester) Grafts

Dacron grafts are textile grafts composed of yarn, which is either woven or knitted to form the fabric. Braiding, once tried, is no longer used for synthetic grafts. Each method imparts different physical characteristics to the fabric. In *woven grafts*, weaving interlaces threads in both the warp (longitudinally oriented) and weft (transversely oriented) directions (Fig. 22–4). These grafts are tighter and less porous than knitted grafts and have little stretch in any direction. They are relatively impermeable, fairly stiff, and very strong. They usually do not need preclotting and have little tendency toward late dilatation. They also take longer to become incorporated owing to lower porosity.[88] Tradi-

tionally, woven Dacron grafts were recommended for situations in which hemostasis without time-consuming preclotting was desirable. The development of impregnated grafts has eliminated these advantages.

Early woven grafts, in addition to being quite stiff, were prone to fraying and actually required heat sealing of their cut ends to prevent suture pullout. These problems led to the development of *knitted graft*, in which the yarn is also oriented in either the warp or weft direction (Fig. 22–5). Knitted grafts are generally more porous than woven grafts, which is believed to promote faster and more complete healing and incorporation[87] (Fig. 22–6). Knitted grafts also have superior handling. However, because they are more porous, they require preclotting to prevent blood loss through the graft. Preclotting seals the interstices of the graft with fibrin, and, by coating the lumen of the graft, is thought to render the flow surface less thrombogenic.[89] A four-step method was described by Yates and colleagues.[90] However, the advent of coated grafts (described later) has made this largely of historical interest.

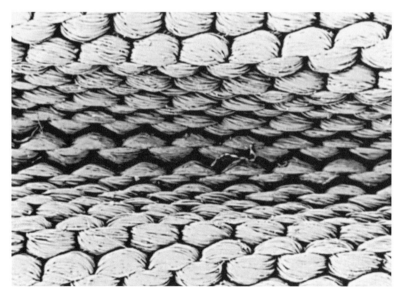

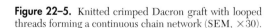

Figure 22–5. Knitted crimped Dacron graft with looped threads forming a continuous chain network (SEM, ×30).

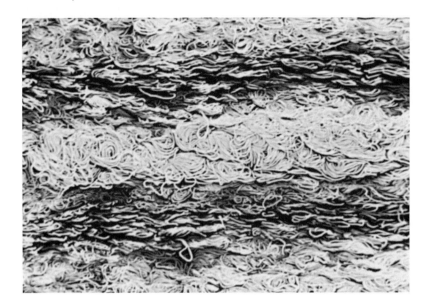

Figure 22–6. Inner capsule of chronically implanted knitted Dacron graft (longitudinal section, ×300).

Many modifications to Dacron prostheses deserve discussion. Crimping adds flexibility and elasticity to the graft, and enables it to be tunneled around bends without kinking. It also adds circumferential "memory," providing a more circular cut end to facilitate suturing of the anastomosis. Although crimping imparts better handling characteristics, it also adds the potential disadvantage of greater surface area and an uneven inner graft surface. This may disturb laminar flow, encourage fibrin deposition, and increase the thrombogenicity of the graft.[91] Many of the advantages of crimping can now be obtained with externally supported rings or coils, which do not interfere with the internal flow surface of the graft.

Another modification is the addition of velour finishes to either knitted or woven Dacron grafts. Velour fabrics have loops of yarn extending upward at a right angle to the fabric's surface [91–94] (Fig. 22–7). Grafts initially had velour on their outer surface, later on their inner surface, and sometimes on both surfaces. Velour was thought to improve the compliance and handling characteristics of Dacron grafts as well as improve the efficiency of preclotting, which would allow the use of more porous knitted grafts. An external surface of velour theoretically allows faster incorporation by encouraging ingrowth of fibroblasts. These advantages, however, have not resulted conclusively in better graft patency or durability. Concerns about excess fibrin formation on the luminal surface have limited their use.[89]

The latest development is impregnation of the interstices. Impregnation was originally developed to allow bonding of active substances, such as antibacterial agents, to the graft. A byproduct of the impregnation process was the realization that knitted Dacron grafts, when coated with a bioresorbable material, maintained their superior handling and incorporation characteristics without the need for preclotting.[95–99] Three different coatings were initially available in the United States: albumin, gelatin, and collagen. Albumin grafts, however, have been withdrawn. Polymer coatings are currently under investigation. The Vantage graft, designed for infrainguinal reconstruction, has a light collagen inner surface and a light velour outer surface,

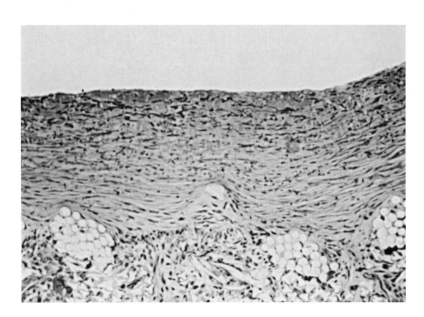

Figure 22–7. Knitted velour crimped Dacron graft with loops of Dacron extending upward from the surface (SEM, ×30).

with microcrimping that provides longitudinal give. The major advantage of these grafts is the time saved in the operating room. In a prospective, randomized trial comparing the long-term performance of the different coating materials in knitted Dacron aortobifemoral prostheses, no significant advantage was seen with any one material. Primary and secondary patency rates at 5 years were 92% and 94% to 98%, respectively.[92] The major disadvantage of these grafts is their expense; they cost approximately twice the price of standard Dacron grafts. This may be a considerable disadvantage in the current economic environment, although most surgeons feel that the operative time saved overcomes this factor. Currently, the overwhelming number of grafts implanted in the Western world are coated.

The most common concern about Dacron grafts is dilatation. Knitted grafts are more likely to dilate over time than woven grafts, with increases in size of 23% to 94% reported. The clinical significance of the dilatation is, however, unclear.[100] Graft dilatation may be an etiologic factor in the development of anastomotic aneurysms.[101] For this reason, the vascular surgeon should anticipate a dilatation of up to 20% and *undersize* knitted Dacron grafts accordingly. Monitoring these grafts with periodic imaging studies is also prudent.[102]

Other potential complications of Dacron grafts include loss of compliance, atherosclerotic change, and perigraft seroma formation.[103, 104] Seroma formation without graft infection, caused by a failure of graft incorporation, occurs in less than 1% of cases. This complication usually necessitates graft replacement.[105] Graft infection occurs in 2% of cases.[106] Several investigations of antibiotic-coated grafts are under way to determine whether binding antibiotic molecules to the graft or to the coating of impregnated grafts decreases the incidence of graft infection. In a study to determine whether the routine use of antibiotic-bonded, gelatin-coated Dacron grafts in extra-anatomic reconstruction decreased the incidence of graft infection, early results showed no significant advantage.[107] Experimental studies continue.

Results

Dacron grafts have the highest patency in large vessel reconstruction (e.g., aortoiliac grafts). Late patency of 85% to 96% has been reported for aortofemoral reconstruction using Dacron grafts.[108] Patency rates for above-knee femoropopliteal grafts are inferior to those for vein and similar to those for PTFE, ranging from 57% to 71% in four large studies.[109–112] Patency below the knee is quite poor, as is true for all prosthetic grafts. When used in extra-anatomic vascular reconstruction, assisted primary patency rates of 50% at 5 years have been reported.[113]

Expanded Polytetrafluoroethylene Grafts

ePTFE is a polymer of carbon and fluorine that was originally developed for industrial use by W.L. Gore in 1969.[114] ePTFE is not a textile graft but rather an extruded material that is originally impermeable. After forcible expansion, ePTFE becomes semipermeable (Fig. 22–8) because the resulting material is composed of solid nodes of PTFE with interconnecting fibrils. The micropores lie between the fibrils (Fig. 22–9), and graft porosity is an important determinant of healing. Golden and colleagues[115] showed complete luminal endothelial cell coverage of ePTFE grafts with an internodal distance of 60 μm. Low-porosity (10–30 μm) and high-porosity (90 μm) grafts were associated with incomplete or focal endothelial cell loss. PTFE is actually more porous than textile grafts, but permeability to water and blood is less due to the hydrophobicity of the material.[116] The first clinical application of ePTFE as an arterial bypass graft was reported in 1976,[117] and the graft rapidly gained popularity for many infrainguinal, extra-anatomic, and angioaccess procedures.

ePTFE offers the advantages of strength, resistance to significant dilatation, ability to be implanted without preclotting, and amenability to thrombectomy with a balloon catheter. ePTFE grafts may be more resistant to infection than textile grafts, possibly because the smoother surface of the graft makes bacterial adherence difficult.[118] ePTFE grafts also have less platelet deposition and decreased activation of the complement cascade, theoretically making the graft less thrombogenic.[119, 120]

The main disadvantage of ePTFE is its stiffness. The

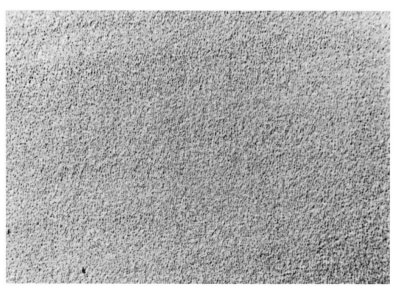

Figure 22–8. Expanded PTFE graft with homogenous surface characteristic of extruded manufacturing process (SEM, ×30).

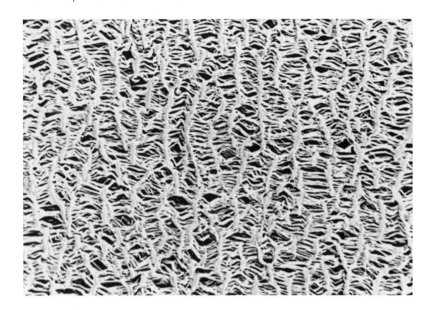

Figure 22–9. Expanded PTFE graft at higher magnification (SEM, ×300), revealing circumferentially oriented nodes of PTFE connected by smaller fibrils.

material is less compliant than textile grafts, a characteristic that may contribute to its tendency to form anastomotic aneurysms[121–123] and may increase the incidence of neointimal hyperplasia, a common cause of late graft failure.[12] Another disadvantage of ePTFE is the higher incidence of needle-hole bleeding owing to the "memory" of the material. Needle-hole bleeding is annoying but can generally be controlled with the use of ePTFE suture and topical hemostatic agents.[124]

Early PTFE grafts were prone to dilatation. Thus the original ePTFE graft was strengthened with a solid PTFE outer wrapping.[125] Currently, two grafts (W.L. Gore and Baxter) have this wrapping. These grafts are not entirely ePTFE, but rather a composite of ePTFE and a perforated sheet of Teflon. Grafts made by other companies have solved the dilatation problem with other modifications.[126] These grafts (Impra, Atrium) are composed entirely of ePTFE.

Several modifications of ePTFE grafts have been developed. *Thin-walled PTFE grafts* still have the outer wrap of solid PTFE, but are thinner, allowing for a larger luminal diameter with the same external diameter. They also have better handling characteristics. *Stretch PTFE grafts* have greater longitudinal elasticity because of the process of "microcrimping." Stretch grafts are more conformable and forgiving of imprecision in graft length. They also have less needle-hole bleeding. No data, however, indicate that either stretch grafts or thin-walled grafts offer superior patency or durability, and they are more expensive than standard ePTFE.[127]

Another common modification is that of external supporting rings or coils that prevent graft compression. These are particularly helpful when the graft is tunneled across the knee or in extra-anatomic positions. Although rings may be valuable in axillofemoral grafts, the efficacy of external supports has not been definitively documented.[128]

ePTFE initially became popular in femoropopliteal bypass grafts because of reports suggesting that the early patency rate of ePTFE was similar to that of vein grafts above the knee.[117, 129] Longer follow-up, however, revealed that the late patency of ePTFE in the above-knee popliteal position was inferior to results obtained with vein.[130] Five-year primary patency rates for above-knee PTFE grafts range from 34% to 58%, with secondary patency rates of up to 79% reported.[130, 131]

Patency rates for below-knee bypass with ePTFE were more discouraging. One randomized trial comparing saphenous vein and ePTFE for tibial bypasses showed 4-year patency rates of 49% for vein versus 12% for ePTFE.[34] Better results were seen when ePTFE was used for below-knee femoropopliteal bypass in patients with claudication, with primary and secondary patency rates of 58% and 73%, respectively.[131] The poor patency rates of ePTFE grafts used below the knee may be improved with postoperative anticoagulation. In one trial, a 4-year patency rate of 37% was attained for patients given warfarin postoperatively.[132] The use of vein cuffs (Fig. 22–10) also improves the patency rates of ePTFE in below-knee vessels[133, 134] and may be related to a reduction in compliance mismatch or an

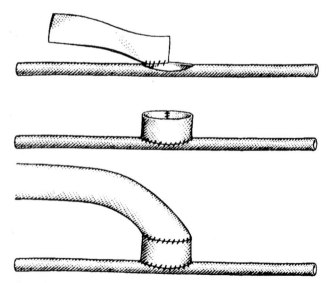

Figure 22–10. Anastomosis of a 6-mm PTFE graft to a small-caliber artery incorporating an interposition vein cuff. From Beard JD: Hemodynamics of the interposition vein cuff. Br J Surg 73: 823; 1986.

alteration in the shear stress flow patterns at the distal anastomosis.[5, 135] A recent study has shown a 5-year primary patency rate of 58% and a limb salvage rate of 80% for these composite grafts.[136]

Given the poor long-term patency rates of prosthetic material in distal reconstruction, all reasonable routes of autogenous conduit, including arm vein, composite-sequential grafting, short-segment grafting, and combined catheter-directed and surgical therapy, should be considered first. If these options are not available, the use of a synthetic conduit may be considered. ePTFE or Dacron grafts are probably equally appropriate. A study from our institution demonstrated a superior patency rate for Dacron in both the above-knee and below-knee positions.[111] However, a recent prospective, randomized trial comparing a knitted Dacron polyester graft impregnated with collagen with a thin-walled, reinforced ePTFE graft to the above-knee popliteal artery showed no statistical difference between groups (62% and 57%, respectively). Patency rates in both groups were inferior in patients receiving smaller (5–6 mm) grafts, and in younger patients who smoked.[112]

Aortic grafts made of ePTFE have had modest use over the last 10 years. A prospective evaluation of the graft noted an absence of significant graft dilatation or late anastomotic aneurysms.[137] Other authors have noted superior patency and lower complication rates with ePTFE aortofemoral grafts,[138–140] although they are not currently accepted as superior to Dacron bifurcated grafts. One group thought that patency rates were better in smaller vessels with ePTFE and recommended that these grafts be used in patients with small iliac and femoral vessels.[141]

In addition to aortic and infrainguinal reconstruction, common uses for ePTFE include carotid-subclavian, axillofemoral, axilloaxillary, aortorenal, and femorofemoral bypass.[142–144] ePTFE is particularly useful for extra-anatomic tunneling, because its relative stiffness makes it resistant to kinking and its smooth surface easy to use in thrombectomy. It is also the material of choice for angioaccess in hemodialysis patients with renal failure, showing surprising resistance to infection.[145, 146] Finally, ePTFE has been used in reconstruction of the inferior vena cava[147] and in patch angioplasty of the carotid and femoral arteries.

Results

Most vascular surgeons believe there is a role for prosthetic grafts in infrainguinal reconstruction. Prosthetic grafts offer the advantages of shorter operative time and smaller incisions, advantages that may be crucial in selected patients. Patency rates for above-knee femoropopliteal reconstruction range from 38% to 65% in large series, similar to results for Dacron grafts.[148–151] Patency rates below the knee are poor, but are improved with the addition of an interposition vein cuff at the distal anastomosis.[133, 134, 136] In aortofemoral reconstructions, ePTFE and Dacron graft patency rates do not appear to be different, although some data suggest that ePTFE grafts may have a lower incidence of late complications.[137, 140] When used for extra-anatomic bypass or hemodialysis access, ePTFE patency rates appear similar to those of Dacron. Most surgeons, however, prefer ePTFE in these locations because of the handling characteristics of the graft, its resistance to external compression, and ease of use in thrombectomy.[144, 152]

FUTURE CONCEPTS

The development of a better vascular prosthesis was until recently an active area of research in vascular surgery. However, significant redirection has occurred toward endovascular devices, which we believe is shortsighted. The development of new, less thrombogenic prosthetic graft materials (both biologic and synthetic), the modification of existing materials with nonthrombogenic coatings, and the prevention of neointimal hyperplasia still remain important unsolved issues.

Endothelial Seeding

Unfortunately, endothelial cell resurfacing of prosthetic grafts, which occurs partially or completely in many animal models, does not occur in humans except for several centimeters in both directions from the anastomoses of the graft.[153] As yet, no flow surface has been developed that has the antithrombotic properties of endothelium. Endothelial cells in ePTFE-seeded grafts remain functional, and have been shown to express factor VIII and thrombomodulin, and to activate protein C.[154]

One avenue that has been pursued is the in vitro seeding of prosthetic grafts with autologous endothelial cells extracted from other tissue beds. Cells were originally harvested mechanically or by enzymatic digestion of adipose tissue.[155] More recently, seeding for prosthetic grafts has been done with endothelial cells cultured from external jugular or cephalic veins,[156] or from an immortalized human dermal endothelial cell line.[157] Data in humans have shown that seeded grafts maintain viable endothelial cells and exert an antiplatelet effect not seen in unseeded grafts.[158–160] In a phase II study by Deutsch and colleagues,[156] the 5-year patency rate of a fibrin glue precoated ePTFE graft was 66% for above-knee grafts and 76% for below-knee grafts, results comparable with those of vein grafts.

Several problems still may limit widespread clinical application of this technology. Methods of obtaining cells in sufficient quantity are not perfected. Cell culture increases the number of cells available, but seeding may take several weeks, obviously a considerable logistic handicap when grafting is performed for limb salvage or in other emergency situations. Implantation techniques are still problematic, with the loss of a significant number of cells when the graft is exposed to flow.[161] Newer methods of improving endothelial cell adherence have been developed that significantly increase the cell retention rate.[162–164] Although clinical applicability at present is limited, early results show this to be a promising technique for the near future.

Surface-Modified Grafts

The concept of modifying a prosthetic graft with a surface-active substance is not new. Gott and coauthors[165] described the technique of bonding heparin to prosthetic conduits in 1963. Considerable experimental work has been done regarding the durability of heparin bonding, and studies with animal models have revealed that heparin bonded to PTFE grafts is not associated with increased intraoperative blood loss[166] and is effective at reducing thrombosis.[167, 168] As yet, heparin bonding has not been effective clinically at preventing prosthetic graft failure. Interest has also focused on the possibility of impregnating thrombolytic substances such as tissue plasminogen activator, which in one study decreased the thrombogenicity of prosthetic grafts in an animal model.[169] A Biolite, or pyrolytic carbon-coated Dacron graft, has recently been shown to enhance endothelial cell growth.[170]

Polyurethanes

Polyurethanes are a family of synthetic polymers whose compliance closely approximates that of native arteries. They have been under investigation in various forms since 1960.[171] Polyurethanes have compliance characteristics more favorable than those of ePTFE or Dacron and are much less thrombogenic, making them potentially attractive for synthetic grafts. Animal studies to date have shown only moderate success, with patency rates not appreciably different from those of other synthetic grafts.[172, 173] Durability and structural integrity remain issues, with poly(ester)urethanes and poly(ether)urethanes subject to hydrolytic and oxidative degradation. Short-term results with a second-generation poly(carbonate)urethane graft show it to have improved biodurability.[174] Continued research in polymer development is needed.

Fibrocollagenous Tubes

For several decades, investigators worked on the concept of fibrocollagenous tube formation; that is, an autogenous or heterologous tube may be formed over a mandril implanted in a tissue bed. Poor long-term patency and stability with all of these conduits suggest that this is not an area worthy of further investigation.

Bioresorbable Polymeric Grafts

Because the biomechanical effects of the current prosthetic grafts are the cause of a significant number of late graft failures, considerable research has focused on the concept of developing a prosthetic graft that would be completely resorbed over time, leaving only autogenous tissue that would be nonantigenic and less thrombogenic.[175] Animal studies have shown that a polyglactin prosthesis made from a polyglycolic acid copolymer is absorbed over several months, leaving a "vessel" consisting of collagen, myofibroblasts, and an endothelial-like surface.[176] Dilatation and aneurysm formation were a problem, however. Short-term results in an animal study with a new copolymer graft of polyglactin and polyhydroxyalkanoate implanted in the thoracic aorta show no evidence of dilatation and mechanical properties approaching that of the native artery.[177] Further work with different compounds continues, with the goal of developing a graft resistant to intimal hyperplasia and with the physiologic characteristics of native vessels.

Photodynamic Fixation Techniques

Another area of research interest involves a method of biologic graft fixation by photodynamic treatment. The current unsatisfactory results of biologic prosthetic grafts are the result of graft thrombosis, degeneration, and dilatation. Photodynamic therapy (PDT) is a method of tissue preservation without conventional chemical fixation that may result in a more stable graft. One process involves perfusing an artery with photosensitizing agents such as methylene blue or chloroaluminum sulfonated phthalocyanine, dyes that selectively absorb light energy at a specific wavelength.[178] This process leads to the production of reactive oxygen species, which induces an apoptotic, noninflammatory decellularization of the treated vessel segment.[178, 179]

Animal studies have shown that PDT inhibits the development of intimal hyperplasia in the body of vein grafts.[180] Intimal hyperplasia was seen, however, at the anastomoses and thought to be secondary to proliferating smooth muscle cells from the adjacent native artery. In a clinical study to evaluate the effects of adjuvant endovascular PDT after percutaneous angioplasty of the femoral artery, there was no evidence of thrombosis or restenosis (as determined by duplex ultrasonography) at 6 months.[181] LaMuraglia and colleagues[182] studied PDT-treated allografts in animals and found that PDT inhibited allograft rejection and aneurysmal dilatation. One effect of PDT is that it cross-links proteins in the extracellular matrix, which theoretically may strengthen the vessel. Protein cross-linking also may mask antigenic epitopes of the extracellular matrix, making it a novel technique for the development of a vascular xenograft. Studies investigating the short-term patency and compliance of PDT-treated xenografts are encouraging, and further modifications of this promising technique continue.

Bioengineered Blood Vessels

The poor patency of small-caliber (less then 4 mm) grafts has stimulated research into the development of bioengineered blood vessels. Huynh and colleagues[183] have developed a collagen biomaterial graft derived from porcine intestinal submucosa and bovine collagen, which when implanted into rabbits serves as a scaffold for infiltration of host smooth muscle and endothelial cells. Short-term results with these grafts show that they are patent and without evidence of thrombosis at 13 weeks. Niklason and associates[184] have created a functional artery in vitro by seeding bovine and porcine smooth muscle and endothelial cells on a biodegradable polyglycolic acid scaffold under pulsatile conditions (Fig. 22–11). These bioengineered vessels are histologically similar to native arteries and display contractile responses to serotonin, endothelin-1, and prostaglandin $F_{2\alpha}$. Studies investigating the short-term patency of this promising technique continue.

The AMVP (acellular matrix vascular prosthesis) is a new concept graft that uses stepwise enzymatic and detergent extraction of arteries, leaving a tissue framework of structural proteins.[185] When used as a coronary artery bypass allograft in canines, these biografts showed no inflammation and minimal cellular repopulation at 6 months.[186] This process is in current clinical use to produce a stentless porcine aortic valve xenograft (Cryolife-O'Brien), with good results.[187]

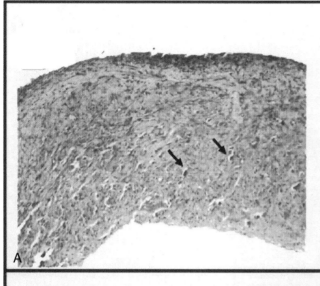

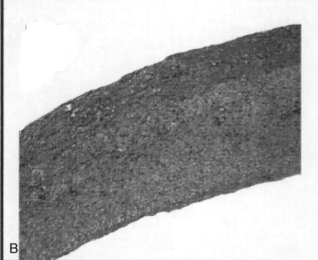

Figure 22–11. Hematoxylin and eosin stain of bioengineered graft, *A*, Autologous porcine vessel, preimplantation; polymer remnants are indicated (*arrows*). *B*, Explanted autologus vessel with intact wall structure containing loosely organized smooth muscle cells. The inflammatory response is minimal and polymer remnants are no longer visible. (From Niklason LE: Functional arteries grown in vitro. Science 284: 492; 1999.)

CURRENT RECOMMENDATIONS

At the beginning of the 21st century, few absolutes exist in graft selection for a particular reconstruction. Above all, the goals of the procedure must be clearly defined. The choice of a conduit to treat a patient with rest pain or a nonhealing ischemic ulcer may be different if the bypass is required emergently for limb salvage. In determining the most appropriate graft for an operation, the vascular surgeon must consider the following: the hemodynamic environment (inflow, outflow, blood pressure), the presence of systemic or graft bed infection, the patient's ability to tolerate lengthy surgery and the need and ability to tolerate chronic anticoagulation, the patient's overall health status, and the patient's projected life span. These factors must be balanced against the performance characteristics of the various available grafts. For these reasons, a graft that is

optimal for one patient may not be the best choice for another. The following general recommendations, however, offer choices that are applicable in most circumstances.

Aortic Reconstruction

Prosthetic large vessel grafts have been implanted in many hundreds of thousands of patients and have shown good patency and durability. The choice of a textile or nontextile synthetic aortic prosthesis depends on several factors.

For operations in which significant hemorrhage, systemic anticoagulation, or extensive dissection is anticipated (such as thoracic aortic reconstructions and ruptured abdominal aortic aneurysms), a coated or woven Dacron graft or PTFE graft may be the best choice, because preclotting is not necessary.

For elective abdominal aneurysm repair, knitted Dacron grafts are routinely employed by many surgeons. Standard grafts require preclotting, whereas the coated grafts do not. The newer ePTFE aortic grafts are also a valid choice. As more data become available, the relative resistance of these grafts to dilatation in comparison with textile grafts may be revealed as a significant advantage.

Infrainguinal Reconstruction

If available, autogenous ipsilateral saphenous vein is clearly the conduit of choice for infrainguinal reconstruction. For infrapopliteal target vessels, the difference in patency between vein and prosthetic conduits is even greater.

Some authors advocate the preferential use of prosthetic conduits for grafting to the above-knee popliteal artery, with the rationale that although the patency of vein may be superior to prosthetic grafts, it is not markedly so, particularly for patients with claudication. Many of these patients will die of coronary disease before occlusion of their graft. Further, those patients requiring additional, more distal peripheral reconstruction or a CABG would have autogenous vein available.[188–190] Unfortunately, this argument would result in an increased number of total operations and reoperations being performed, a position difficult to justify. Certainly, the initial use of prosthetic grafts in selected patients is appropriate.

For all target vessels below the knee, autogenous vein is preferable. When it is not available, the alternative is less attractive. Before the acceptance of PTFE as a conduit, Dacron grafts were popular in this situation. The lack of need for preclotting helped PTFE become the more popular prosthetic conduit; however, this advantage ceased with the availability of coated grafts. Certainly, in patients without usable vein who are undergoing limb salvage procedures, PTFE conduits can provide limb salvage in a third or more of patients, as shown by Veith and associates.[24] The good short-term patency rates of prosthetic grafts may also allow an adequate window for healing of a transmetatarsal amputation. The addition of a vein cuff at the distal anastomosis should be considered, especially when using small-diameter (less than 6 mm) grafts. Considering the cost of rehabilitation and the total cost of primary amputation (similar to the cost of distal bypass), the use of a prosthetic graft may be superior to primary amputation in patients with limb-threatening ischemia.

The use of any biologic graft, although intuitively appealing, is currently not justified. HUV allografts were used previously in the lower extremity, but problems with late degeneration have made their use rare, despite some data suggesting their patency may be better when used below the knee and in poor runoff situations.[191] The use of cryopreserved veins should be reserved for limb-threatening ischemia for extremely distal bypass or in infected fields, when autogenous vein is not available.

Extra-Anatomic and Angioaccess Procedures

ePTFE has become the graft of choice for most extra-anatomic reconstructions. The advantages in these situations include a lower incidence of hematoma formation from graft leakage and the resistance of ePTFE to kinking. ePTFE grafts are also amenable to catheter thrombectomy, an important consideration in axillofemoral or axilloaxillary grafts. Depending on the patient's habitus and the length of the subcutaneous tunnel, externally supported grafts may be helpful.

For angioaccess in patients receiving hemodialysis in which arteriovenous fistulas are not feasible or have failed, ePTFE grafts have become the conduit of choice. They are easy to implant, resistant to infection, amenable to revision, and tolerate multiple punctures with a low incidence of pseudoaneurysm formation.[192]

Acknowledgments

We thank Dr. James Stanley for permission to use graphic materials from his chapter in previous editions of this book.

References

1. Carrel A, Guthrie CG: Uniterminal and biterminal venous transplantations. Surg Gynecol Obstet 2:226, 1906.
2. Taylor LM, Edwards JM, Porter JM: Present status of reversed vein bypass grafting: Five year results of a modern series. J Vasc Surg 11:193, 1990.
3. Jaff EA: Biology of Endothelial Cells. Boston, Martinus Nijhoff, 1984.
4. Scales JT: Tissue reactions to synthetic materials. Proc R Soc Med 46:647, 1953.
5. Abbott WM, Megerman J, Hasson JE, et al: Effect of compliance mismatch on vascular graft patency. J Vasc Surg 5:376, 1987.
6. Walden R, L'Italien GJ, Megerman J, Abbott WM: Matched elastic properties and successful arterial grafting. Arch Surg 10:1166–1169, 1980.
7. Milroy CM, Scott DJ, Beard JD, et al: Histologic appearance of the long saphenous vein. J Pathol 159:311, 1989.
8. Thompson H: The surgical anatomy of the superficial and perforating veins of the lower limb. Ann R Coll Surg Engl 61:198, 1979.
9. Shah DM, Chang BB, Leopold PW, et al: The anatomy of the greater saphenous venous system. J Vasc Surg 3:273–283, 1986.
10. Kakkar VV: The cephalic vein as a peripheral vascular graft. Surg Gynecol Obstet 128:551, 1969.
11. Leather RP, Karmody AM: The in situ saphenous vein for arterial bypass. In Staley JC (ed): Biologic and Synthetic Vascular Prostheses. New York, Grune & Stratton, 1982, pp 351–364.
12. Sottiurai VA, Yao JST, Flinn WR, et al: Intimal hyperplasia and neointima: An ultrastructural analysis of thrombosed grafts in humans. Surgery 93:809, 1983.
13. Spray TL, Roberts WC: Fundamentals of clinical cardiology: Changes in saphenous veins used as aortocoronary bypass grafts. Am Heart J 94:500, 1977.
14. Szilagyi DE, Elliott JP, Hageman JH, et al: Biologic fate of autogenous vein implants as arterial substitutes: Clinical, angiographic and histopathologic observations in femoropopliteal operations for atherosclerosis. Ann Surg 178:232, 1973.
15. Bandyk DF: Essentials of graft surveillance. Semin Vasc Surg 6:92, 1993.
16. Abbott WM, Wieland S, Austen WG: Structural changes during preparation of autogenous venous grafts. Surgery 76:1031, 1974.
17. Hasson JE, Wiebe DH, Sharefkin JB, Abbott WM: Migration of adult human vascular endothelial cells: Effect of extracellular matrix proteins. Surgery 100:384, 1986.
18. Beattie DK, Sian M, Greenhalgh RM, Davies AH: Influence of systemic factors on pre-existing intimal hyperplasia and their effect on the outcome of infrainguinal reconstruction with vein. Br J Surg 86:1441, 1999.
19. Clowes AW, Clowes MM, Fingerle J, Reidy MA: Regulation of smooth muscle cell growth in injured artery. J Cardiovasc Pharmacol 14:512, 1989.
20. Schafer U, Micke O, Dorszewski A, et al: External beam irradiation inhibits neointimal hyperplasia after injury-induced arterial smooth muscle cell proliferation. Int J Radiat Oncol Biol Phys 42:617, 1998.
21. Shears LL 2nd, Kibbe MR, Murdock AD, et al: Efficient inhibition of intimal hyperplasia by adenovirus-mediated inducible nitric oxide synthase gene transfer to rats and pigs in vivo. J Am Coll Surg 187:295, 1998.
22. LeTourneau T, Van Belle E, Corseaux D, et al: Role of nitric oxide in restenosis after experimental balloon angioplasty in the hypercholesterolemic rabbit: Effect on neointimal hyperplasia and vascular remodeling. J Am Coll Cardiol 33:876, 1999.
23. Porter KE, Loftus IM, Peterson M, et al: Marimastat inhibits neointimal thickening in a model of human vein graft stenosis. Br J Surg 85:1373, 1998.
24. Veith FJ, Moss CM, Sprayregen S, et al: Preoperative saphenous venography in arterial reconstructive surgery of the lower extremity. Surgery 85:253, 1979.
25. Adcock OT Jr., Adcock GL, Wheeler JR, et al: Optimal techniques for harvesting and preparation of reversed saphenous autogenous vein grafts for use as arterial substitutes: A review. Surgery 96:886, 1984.
26. Schaeffer U, Tanner B, Strohschneider T, et al: Damage to arterial and venous endothelial cells in bypass grafts induced by several solutions used in bypass surgery. Thorac Cardiovasc Surg 45:168, 1997.
27. Welz A, Stadtmuller A, Schaffer U, et al: Cytotoxicity of various crystalloid solutions to the endothelial cells of autologous grafts. Thorac Cardiovasc Surg 39:236, 1991.
28. Donaldson, MC, Mannick JA, Whittemore AD: Causes of primary graft failure after in situ saphenous vein bypass grafting. J Vasc Surg 15:150, 1992.
29. DeWeese JA, Rob CG: Autogenous venous grafts ten years later. Surgery 82:775, 1977.
30. Stanley JC, Graham LM, Whitehouse WM, et al: Autogenous saphenous vein as an arterial graft: Clinical status. In Stanley JC (ed): Biologic and Synthetic Vascular Prostheses. New York, Grune & Stratton, 1982, pp 333–349.
31. Fuchs JCA, Mitchener JS III, Hagen P-O: Postoperative changes in autologous vein grafts. Ann Surg 188:1, 1978.
32. Watelet J, Soury P, Menard JF, et al: Femoropopliteal bypass: In situ or reversed saphenous vein? Ten-year results of a randomized study. Ann Vasc Surg 11:510, 1997.
33. Donaldson MC, Mannick JA, Whittemore AD: Femoral-distal bypass with in-situ saphenous vein: Long term results using the Mills valvulotome. Ann Surg 213:457, 1991.
34. Veith FJ, Gupta SK, Ascer E, et al: Six year prospective multicenter

randomized comparison of autologous saphenous vein and expanded PTFE in infrainguinal reconstruction. J Vasc Surg 3:107, 1986.

35. Luther M, Lepantalo M: Infrainguinal reconstructions: Influence of surgical experience on outcome. Cardiovasc Surg 6:351, 1998.

36. Harward TRS, Coe D, Flynn TC, Seeger JM: The use of arm vein conduits during infrageniculate arterial bypass. J Vasc Surg 3:104, 1986.

37. Calligaro KD, Syrek JR, Dougherty MJ, et al: Use of arm and lesser saphenous vein compared with prosthetic grafts for infrapopliteal arterial bypass: Are they worth the effort? J Vasc Surg 26:919, 1997.

38. Ehrenfeld WK, Stoney RJ, Wylie EJ: Autogenous arterial grafts. In Stanley JC (ed): Biologic and Synthetic Vascular Prostheses. New York, Grune & Stratton, 1982, pp 291–309.

39. Kreitman B, Riberi A, Jimeno MT, Metras D: Experimental basis for autograft growth and viability. J Heart Valve Dis 4:379, 1995.

40. Ehrenfeld WK, Wibur BG, Olcott CN, et al: Autogenous tissue reconstruction in the management of infected prosthetic grafts. Surgery 85:82, 1979.

41. Cambria RP, Brewster DC, L'Italien GJ, et al: The durability of different reconstructive techniques for atherosclerotic renal artery disease. J Vasc Surg 20:76, 1994.

42. Grondin CM, Campeau L, Lesperance J, et al: Comparison of late changes in internal mammary artery and saphenous vein grafts in two consecutive series of patients 10 years after operation. Circulation 70(Suppl 1):1, 1984.

43. Stoney RJ, DeLuccia N, Ehrenfeld WK, et al: Aortorenal arterial autografts: Longterm assessment. Arch Surg 116:1416, 1981.

44. Gross RE, Hierwitt ES, Bill AH Jr, et al: Preliminary observations on the use of human arterial grafts in the treatment of certain cardiovascular defects. N Engl J Med 239:578, 1948.

45. Szilagyi DE, McDonald RT, Smith RF, et al: Biologic fate of human arterial homografts. Arch Surg 75:506, 1957.

46. Deterling RA, Clauss RH: Long term fate of aortic arterial homografts. J Cardiovasc Surg (Torino) 11:35, 1970.

47. Kieffer E, Bahnini A, Kishas F, et al: In situ allograft replacement of infected infrarenal aortic prosthetic grafts: Results in 43 patients. J Vasc Surg 17:349, 1993.

48. Locati P, Novali C, Socrati AM, et al: The use of arterial allografts in aortic graft infections. A three year experience on eighteen patients. J Cardiovasc Surg (Torino) 39:735, 1998.

49. Nevelsteen A, Feryn T, Lacroix H, et al: Experience with cryopreserved arterial allografts in the treatment of prosthetic graft infections. Cardiovasc Surg 6:378, 1998.

50. Carrel T, Pasic M, Jenni R, et al: Reoperations after operation on the thoracic aorta: Etiology, surgical techniques, and prevention. Ann Thorac Surg 56:259, 1993.

51. Oschner JL, Lawson JD, Eskind SJ, et al: Homologous veins as an arterial substitute: Long term results. J Vasc Surg 1:306, 1984.

52. Selke FW, Meng RC, Rossi NP: Cryopreserved saphenous vein homografts for femoral-distal vascular reconstruction. J Cardiovasc Surg (Torino) 30:836, 1989.

53. Fujtani RM, Bassiouny HS, Gewertz BL, et al: Cryopreserved saphenous vein allogenic homografts: An alternative conduit in lower extremity arterial reconstruction in infected fields. J Vasc Surg 15:519, 1992.

54. Walker PJ, Mitchell RS, McFadden PM, et al: Early experience with cryopreserved saphenous vein allografts as a conduit for complex limb-salvage procedures. J Vasc Surg 18:561, 1993.

55. Dalsing MC, Raju S, Wakefield TW, Taheri S: A multicenter, phase I evaluation of cryopreserved venous valve allografts for the treatment of chronic deep venous insufficiency. J Vasc Surg 30:854, 1999.

56. Martins RS 3rd, Edwards WH, Mulherin JL Jr., et al: Cryopreserved saphenous vein allografts for below-knee extremity revascularization. Ann Surg 219:664, 1994.

57. Albertini JN, Barral X, Branchereau A, et al: Vascular Surgical Society of Great Britain and Ireland: Mid-term results of arterial allograft below-knee bypasses for limb salvage. Br J Surg 86:701, 1999.

58. Carpenter JP, Tomaszewski JE: Immunosuppression for human saphenous vein allograft bypass surgery: A prospective randomized trial. J Vasc Surg 26:32, 1997.

59. Nabseth DC, Wilson JT, Tan B, et al: Fetal arterial heterografts. Arch Surg 81:929, 1960.

60. Dardik H, Baier RE, Meenaghan M, et al: Morphologic and biophysical assessment of long-term human umbilical cord vein implants used as vascular conduits. Surg Gynecol Obstet 154:17, 1982.

61. Dardik H, Ibrahim IM, Dardik I: Modified and unmodified umbilical vein allograft and xenografts employed as arterial substitutes: A morphologic assessment. Surg Forum 26:286, 1975.

62. Dardik I, Dardik H: The fate of human umbilical cord vessels used as interposition arterial grafts in the baboon. Surg Gynecol Obstet 140:567, 1975.

63. Dardik H: Technical aspects of umbilical bypass to the tibial vessels. J Vasc Surg 1:916, 1984.

64. Dardik H, Miller N, Dardik A, et al: A decade of experience with the glutaraldehyde tanned umbilical cord vein graft for revascularization of the lower limb. J Vasc Surg 7:336, 1988.

65. Rutherford RB, Jones DN, Bergentz SE, et al: Factors affecting the patency of infrainguinal bypass. J Vasc Surg 8:236, 1988.

66. Johnson WC, Squires JW: Axillo-femoral (PTFE) and infrainguinal revascularization (PTFE and umbilical vein). J Cardiovasc Surg (Torino) 32:344, 1991.

67. McCollum C, Kenchington G, Alexander C, et al: PTFE or HUV for femorpopliteal bypass: A multicentre trial. Eur J Vasc Surg 5:435, 1991.

68. Alders GJ, Van Vroonhoven TJM: PTFE versus HUV in above-knee femoropopliteal bypass: Six year results in a randomized clinical trial. J Vasc Surg 16:816, 1992.

69. Eickhoff JH, Broome A, Ericsson BF, et al: Four year's results of a prospective randomized clinical trial comparing polytetrafluoroethylene and modified human umbilical vein for below-knee femoropopliteal bypass. J Vasc Surg 6:506, 1987.

70. Aalders FJ, van Vroonhoven TJM: Polytetrafluoroethylene versus human umbilical vein in above-knee femoropopliteal bypass: Six year results of a randomized clinical trial. J Vasc Surg 16:816, 1992.

71. Wengerter K: Biological vascular grafts. Semin Vasc Surg 12:46, 1999.

72. Hasson JE, Newton WD, Waltman AC, et al: Mural degeneration in the glutaraldehyde-tanned umbilical vein graft: Incidence and implications. J Vasc Surg 4:243, 1986.

73. Julien S, Gill F, Guidoin R, et al: Biologic and structural evaluation of 80 surgically excised human umbilical vein grafts. Can J Surg 32:101, 1989.

74. Karkow WS, Cranley JJ, Cranley RE, et al: Extended study of aneurysm formation in umbilical vein grafts. J Vasc Surg 4:486, 1986.

75. Dardik H: Umbilical vein graft for atherosclerotic lower extremity occlusive disease. In Ernst CB, Stanley JC (eds): Current Therapy in Vascular Surgery. St Louis, Mosby–Year Book, 1995, pp 484–487.

76. Rosenberg N, Gaughran ERL, Henderson J, et al: The use of segmental arterial implants prepared by enzymatic modification of heterologous blood vessels. Surg Forum 6:242, 1956.

77. Rosenberg N, Thompson JE, Keshishian JM, et al: The modified bovine arterial graft. Arch Surg 111:222, 1976.

78. Dale WA, Lewis MR: Further experiences with bovine arterial grafts. Surgery 80:711, 1976.

79. Brems J, Castenada M, Garvin PJ: A five year experience with the bovine heterograft for vascular access. Arch Surg 121:941, 1986.

80. Enzler MA, Rajmon T, Lachat M, Largiader F: Long-term function of vascular access for hemodialysis. Clin Transplant 10:511, 1996.

81. Sawyer PN, Fitzgerald J, Kaplitt MJ, et al: Ten year experience with the negatively charged glutaraldehyde-tanned vascular graft in peripheral vascular surgery: Initial multicenter trial. Am J Surg 154:533, 1987.

82. Schroder A, Imig H, Peiper U, et al: Results of a bovine collagen vascular graft (Solcograft-P) in infrainguinal positions. Eur J Vasc Surg 2:315, 1988.

83. Guidoin R, Domurado D, Coutue J, et al: Chemically processed bovine heterografts of the second generation as arterial substitutes: A comparative evaluation of three commercial prostheses. J Cardiovasc Surg (Torino) 30:202, 1989.

84. Mozami N, Argenziano M, Williams M, et al: Photo-oxidized bovine arterial grafts: Short-term results. ASAIO J 44:89, 1998.

85. Voorhees AB Jr., Jaretzke AL, Blakemore AH: Use of tubes constructed from Vinyon-N cloth in bridging arterial defects. Ann Surg 135:332, 1952.

86. Blakemore AH, Voorhees AB Jr.: The use of tubes constructed from Vinyon-N cloth in bridging arterial defects: Experimental and clinical. Ann Surg 140:324, 1954.

87. Fry WJ, DeWeese MS, Kraft RO, et al: Importance of porosity in arterial prostheses. Arch Surg 88:36, 1964.

88. Snyder RW, Botzko KM: Woven, knitted, and externally supported

Dacron vascular prostheses. In Stanley JC (ed): Biologic and Synthetic Vascular Prostheses. New York, Grune & Stratton, 1982, pp 485–508.

89. Goldman M, McCollum CN, Hawker RJ, et al: Dacron arterial grafts: The influence of porosity, velour, and maturity on thrombogenicity. Surgery 92:947, 1982.

90. Yates SJ, Barros D'Sa AA, Berger K, et al: The preclotting of porous arterial prostheses. Ann Surg 188:611–622, 1978.

91. Kenney DA, Sauvage LR, Woud SJ, et al: Comparison of noncrimped, externally supported (EXS), and crimped nonsupported Dacron prostheses for axillofemoral and above-knee femoropopliteal bypass. Surgery 92:931, 1982.

92. Meister RH, Schweiger H, Lang W: Knitted double-velour Dacron prosthesis in aortobifemoral position—long-term performance of different coating materials. Vasa 27:236, 1998.

93. Lindenauer SM, Weber TR, Miller TA, et al: Velour vascular prosthesis. ASAIO J 20:314, 1974.

94. Hall CW, Liotta D, Ghidoni JJ, et al: Velour fabrics applied to medicine. J Biomed Mater Res 1:179, 1967.

95. Reigel MM, Hollier LH, Pairolero PC, et al: Early experience with a new collagen-impregnated aortic graft. Ann Surg 54:134, 1988.

96. Canadian Multicenter Hemashield Study Group: Immunological response to collagen-impregnated vascular grafts: A randomized prospective study. J Vasc Surg 12:741, 1990.

97. Kottke-Marchant K, Anderson JM, Umennura Y, et al: Effects of albumin coating on the in vitro compatability of Dacron arterial prostheses. Biomaterials 110:147, 1989.

98. Fleischlag JD, Moore WS: Clinical experience with a collagen-impregnated knitted Dacron vascular graft. Ann Vasc Surg 4:449, 1990.

99. Jones RA, Zieir G, Schoen FJ, et al: A new sealant for knitted Dacron prostheses: Minimally cross-linked gelatin. J Vasc Surg 4:414, 1988.

100. Blumberg RM, Gelfand ML, Barton ED, et al: Clinical significance of aortic graft dilation. J Vasc Surg 14:175, 1991.

101. Claggett GP, Salander JM, Eddleman WL, et al: Dilation of knitted Dacron aortic prostheses and anastomotic false aneurysms: Etiologic considerations. Surgery 93:9, 1983.

102. Nunn DB, Freeman MH, Hodgins PC: Postoperative alterations in size of Dacron aortic grafts: An ultrasonic evaluation. Ann Surg 189:741, 1979.

103. Clark RE, Apostolous S, Kardesw JL: Mismatch of mechanical properties as a cause of arterial prostheses thrombosis. Surg Forum 27:298, 1976.

104. Paes E, Vollmar JF, Mohr W, et al: Perigraft reaction: Incompatability of synthetic vascular grafts? New aspects of clinical manifestation, pathogenesis, and therapy. World J Surg 12:750, 1988.

105. Blumenberg RM, Gefland ML, Dale WA: Perigraft seromas complicating arterial grafts. Surgery 97:194, 1985.

106. White JV, Benvenisty AI, Reemstma K, et al: Simple methods for direct antibiotic protection of synthetic vascular grafts. J Vasc Surg 1:372, 1984.

107. Braithwaite BD, Davies B, Heather BP, Earnshaw JJ: Early results of a randomized trial of rifampicin-bonded Dacron grafts for extraanatomic vascular reconstruction. Joint Vascular Research Group. Br J Surg 85:1378, 1998.

108. Szilagyi DE, Smith RF, Elliott JP, et al: Long-term behavior of a Dacron arterial substitute. Ann Surg 162:453, 1965.

109. EI-Massry S, Saad E, Sauvage L, et al: Femoropopliteal bypass with externally supported knitted Dacron grafts: A follow-up of 200 grafts for one to twelve years. J Vasc Surg 19:487, 1994.

110. Rosenthal D, Evans D, McKinsey J, et al: Prosthetic above-knee femoropopliteal bypass graft for intermittent claudication. J Cardiovasc Surg (Torino) 31:462, 1990.

111. Prevec WC, Darling RC, L'Italien GJ, et al: Femoropopliteal reconstruction with knitted non-velour Dacron versus expanded PTFE. J Vasc Surg 16:60, 1992.

112. Abbott WM, Green RM, Matsumoto T, et al: Prosthetic above-knee femoropopliteal bypass grafting: Results of a multicenter randomized prospective trial. Above-knee Femoropopliteal Study Group. J Vasc Surg 25:19, 1997.

113. Johnson WC, Lee KK: Comparative evaluation of externally supported Dacron and polytetrafluoroethylene prosthetic bypasses for femorofemoral and axillofemoral arterial reconstructions. Veterans Affairs Cooperative Study #141. J Vasc Surg 30:1077, 1999.

114. U.S. Patent 3,962,153 (June 8, 1976 to W.L. Gore and Associates): Very highly stretched polytetrafluoroethylene and process therefore. 1976, pp 1–24.

115. Golden MA, Hanson SR, Kirkman TR, et al: Healing of polytetrafluoroethylene arterial grafts is influenced by graft porosity. J Vasc Surg 11:838, 1990.

116. Matsumoto H, Hasegawa T, Fuse K: A renovascular prosthesis for a small caliber artery. Surgery 74:518, 1973.

117. Campbell DC, Brooks DH, Webster MW, et al: The use of expanded microporous polytetrafluoroethylene for limb salvage: A preliminary report. Surgery 79:485, 1976.

118. Bandyk DF, Bergamini TM, Kinney EV, et al: In situ replacement of vascular prostheses infected by bacterial biofilms. J Vasc Surg 13:575, 1991.

119. Senfield NA, Connolly R, Ramberg K, et al: The systemic activation of platelets by Dacron grafts. Surg Gynecol Obstet 166:454, 1988.

120. Shepard AD, Gelfand JA, Callow AD, O'Donnell TF Jr.: Complement activation by synthetic vascular prostheses. J Vasc Surg I:829, 1984.

121. Abbott WM, Cambria RP: Control of physical characteristics (elasticity and compliance) of vascular grafts. In Stanley JC (ed): Biologic and Synthetic Vascular Prostheses. New York, Grune & Stratton, 1982, pp 189–220.

122. Walden R, L'Italien G, Megerman J, et al: Matched elastic properties and successful arterial grafting. Arch Surg 115:1166, 1980.

123. Mehigan DG, Fitzpatrick B, Browne HI, Boucher-Hayes DJ: Is compliance mismatch the major cause of anastamotic arterial aneurysms? Analysis of 42 cases. J Cardiovasc Surg (Torino) 26:147, 1985.

124. Miller CM, Sangiolo P, Jacobson JH II: Reduced anastamotic bleeding using new sutures with a needle-suture diameter of one. Surgery 101:156, 1987.

125. Campbell CD, Brooks DH, Webster MW, et al: Aneurysm formation in expanded polytetrafluoroethylene prostheses. Surgery 79:491, 1976.

126. Hanel KC, McCabe C, Abbott WM, et al: Current PTFE grafts: A biomechanical scanning electron, and light microscopic evaluation. Ann Surg 195:456, 1982.

127. Gupta SK, Veith FJ, Kram HB, et al: Prospective randomized comparison of ringed and non-ringed PTFE femoropoliteal bypass grafts: A preliminary report. J Vasc Surg 13:162, 1991.

128. Harris JE, Taylor LM, McConnell DB, et al: Clinical results of axillofemoral bypass using externally supported polytetrafluoroethylene. J Vasc Surg 12:416, 1990.

129. Veith FJ, Moss CM, Fell SC, et al: Comparison of expanded PTFE and vein grafts in lower extremity arterial reconstructions. J Cardiovasc Surg (Torino) 19:341, 1978.

130. Archie JP Jr.: Femoropopliteal bypass with either adequate ipsilateral reversed saphenous vein or obligatory polytetrafluoroethylene. Ann Vasc Surg 8:475, 1994.

131. Allen BT, Reilly JM, Rubin BG, et al: Femoropopliteal bypass for claudication: Vein vs. PTFE. Ann Vasc Surg 10:178, 1996.

132. Flinn WR, Rohrer MJ, Yao JST, et al: Improved long-term patency of infragenicular polytetrafluoroethylene grafts. J Vasc Surg 7:685, 1985.

133. Raptis S, Miller JH: Influence of vein cuff on polytetrafluoroethylene grafts for primary femoropopliteal bypass. Br J Surg 82:487, 1995.

134. Stonebridge PA, Prescott RJ, Ruckley CV: Randomized trial comparing infrainguinal polytetrafluoroethylene bypass grafting with and without vein interposition cuff at the distal anastamosis. The Joint Vascular Research Group. J Vasc Surg 26:543, 1997.

135. Zwolak RM, Adams MC, Clowes AW: Kinetics of vein graft hyperplasia: Association with tangential stress. J Vasc Surg 5:126, 1987.

136. Bastounis E, Georgopoulos S, Maltezos C, et al: PTFE-vein composite grafts for critical limb ischaemia: A valuable alternative to all-autogenous infrageniculate reconstructions. Eur J Vasc Endovasc Surg 18:127, 1999.

137. Corson JD, Baraniewski HM, Shah DM, et al: Large diameter expanded polytetrafluoroethylene grafts for infrarenal aortic aneurysm surgery. J Cardiovasc Surg (Torino) 31:702, 1990.

138. Avramov S, Petrovic P, Fabri M: Bifurcated grafts (Dacron vs. PTFE) in aortoiliac reconstruction: Five years follow-up. J Cardiovasc Surg (Torino) 28:33, 1987.

139. Lord RSA, Nash PA, Raj PT, et al: Prospective randomized trial of polytetrafluoroethylene and Dacron aortic prostheses, I: Perioperative results. Ann Vasc Surg 3:248, 1988.

140. Cintora I, Pearce DE, Cannon JA: A clinical survey of aortobifemoral bypass using two inherently different graft types. Ann Surg 208:625, 1988.

141. Burke PM Jr., Herman JB, Cutler BS: Optimal grafting methods for the smaller abdominal aorta. J Cardiovasc Surg (Torino) 28:420, 1987.

142. Campbell CD, Brooks DH, Siewers RD, et al: Extraanatomic bypass with expanded polytetrafluoroethylene graft. Surg Gynecol Obstet 148:525, 1979.

143. Haimov M, Giron F, Jacobson JH II: The expanded polytetrafluoroethylene graft: Three years experience with 362 grafts. Arch Surg 114:673, 1979.

144. Chang JB: Current status of extraanatomic bypasses. Am J Surg 152:202, 1986.

145. Palder SB, Kirkman BL, Whitemore AD, et al: Vascular access for hemodialysis: Patency rates and results of revision. Ann Surg 202:235, 1985.

146. Raju S: PTFE for hemodialysis access: Techniques for insertion and management of complications. Ann Surg 206:666, 1987.

147. Gloviczki P, Pairolero PC, Cherry KJ, et al: Reconstruction of the vena cava and its primary tributaries: A preliminary report. J Vasc Surg 11:373, 1990.

148. Quinones-Baldrich WJ, Prego AA, Ucelay-Gomez R, et al: Long term results of infrainguinal revascularization with PTFE: A ten-year experience. J Vasc Surg 16:209, 1992.

149. Gupta SK, Veith FJ, Ascer E, et al: Cost factors in limb-threatening ischemia due to infrainguinal atherosclerosis. Eur J Vasc Surg 2:151, 1988.

150. Taylor RS, Lob A, McFarland RJ, et al: Improved techniques for polytetrafluoroethylene bypass grafting: Long-term results using anastamotic vein patches. Br J Surg 79:348, 1992.

151. Wright JG: A randomized prospective clinical trial of the Taylor patch [letter]. J Vasc Surg 23:376, 1996.

152. Connolly JE, Kwan JHM, Brownell D, et al: Newer developments of extraanatomic bypass. Surg Gynecol Obstet 158:415, 1984.

153. Berger K, Sauvage LR, Rao AM, et al: Healing of arterial prostheses in man: Its incompleteness. Ann Surg 175:118, 1972.

154. Hedeman JPP, Verhagen HJ, Heijnen-Snyder GJ, et al: Thrombomodulin activity of fat-derived microvascular endothelial cells seeded on expanded polytetrafluoroethylene. J Vasc Res 36:91, 1999.

155. Herring M, Gardner A, Glover J: A single-stage technique for seeding vascular grafts with autogenous endothelium. Surgery 84:498, 1978.

156. Deutsch M, Meinhart J, Fischlein T, et al: Clinical autologous in vitro endothelialization of infrainguinal ePTFE grafts in 100 patients: A 9-year experience. Surgery 126:847, 1999.

157. Robinson KA, Candal FJ, Scott NA, Ades EW: Seeding of vascular grafts with an immortalized human dermal microvascular endothelial cell line. Angiology 46:107, 1995.

158. Herring MB, Baughmon S, Glover JL: Endothelium develops on seeded arterial prosthesis: A brief clinical report. J Vasc Surg 2:727, 1985.

159. Ortenwall P, Wadenvick H, Kutti J, et al: Reduction in deposition of indium-111–labeled platelets after autologous endothelial cell seeding of Dacron aortic bifurcation grafts in humans: A preliminary study. J Vasc Surg 6:17, 1987.

160. Ortenwall P, Wadenvick H, Risberg B: Reduced platelet deposition on seeded versus unseeded segments of expanded polytetrafluoroethylene grafts: Clinical observations after a six month follow-up. J Vasc Surg 10:374, 1989.

161. Rosenman JE, Kempczinski RF, Pearce WH, et al: Kinetics of endothelial cell seeding. J Vasc Surg 2:778, 1985.

162. Seeger JM: Improved endothelial cell seeding efficiency with cultured cells and fibronectin coated grafts. J Surg Res 38:641, 1985.

163. Bhattacharya V, McSweeney PA, Shi Q, et al: Enhanced endothelialization and microvessel formation in polyester grafts seeded with CD34(+) bone marrow cells. Blood 95:581, 2000.

164. Sugarwarsa Y, Miyata T, Sato O, et al: Rapid postincubation endothelial retention by Dacron grafts. J Surg Res 67:132, 1997.

165. Gott VL, Whiffen JD, Dutton RC: Heparin bonding on colloidin graphite surfaces. Science 142:1927, 1963.

166. Becquemin JP, Riff Y, Kovarsky S, et al: Evaluation of a polyester collagen-coated heparin bonded vascular graft. J Cardiovasc Surg (Torino) 38:7, 1997.

167. Esquivel CO, Bjork C-G, Bergentz S-E, et al: Reduced thrombogenic characteristics of expanded polytetrafluoroethylene and polyurethane arterial grafts after heparin bonding. Surgery 95:102, 1984.

168. Walpoth BH, Rogulenko R, Tikhvinskaia E, et al: Improvement of patency rate in heparin-coated small synthetic grafts. Circulation 98:II319, 1998.

169. Greco RS, Kim HC, Denetz AP, Harvey RA: Patency of a small vessel prosthesis bonded to tissue plasminogen activator and iloprost. Ann Vasc Surg 9:140, 1995.

170. Bernex F, Mazzzzucotelli JP, Roudiere JL, et al: In vitro endothelialization of carbon-coated Dacron vascular grafts. Int J Artif Organs 15:172, 1992.

171. Dryer B, Akutsu T, Kolff WJ: Aortic grafts of polyurethane in dogs. J Appl Physiol 15:18, 1960.

172. Geeraert AJ, Callaghan JC: Experimental study of selected small calibre arterial grafts. J Cardiovasc Surg (Torino) 18:155, 1977.

173. Cronenwett JL, Zelenock GB: Alternative small arterial grafts. In Stanley JC (ed): Biologic and Synthetic Vascular Prostheses. New York, Grune & Stratton, 1982, pp 595–620.

174. Greisler HP: Arterial regeneration over absorbable prostheses. Arch Surg 177:1425, 1982.

175. Edwards A, Carson RJ, Szycher M, Bowald S: In vitro and in vivo biodurability of a compliant microporous vascular graft. J Biomater Appl 13:23, 1998.

176. Greisler HP, Endean ED, Klosak JJ, et al: Polyglactin 910/polydioxanone biocomponent totally resorbable vascular prostheses. J Vasc Surg 7:697, 1988.

177. Shum-Tim D, Stock U, Hrkach J, et al: Tissue engineering of autologous aorta using a new biodegradable polymer. Ann Thorac Surg 68:2298, 1999.

178. Chandrasekar NR, L'Italien G, Warnock DF, et al: Compliance and the effects of photodynamic therapy of arteries. Surg Forum 34:351, 1993.

179. Moore MA, Bohachevsky IK, Cheung DT, et al: Stabilization of pericardial tissue by dye-mediated photooxidation. J Biomed Mater Res 28:611, 1994.

180. LaMuraglia GM, Klyachkin ML, Adili F, Abbott WM: Photodynamic therapy of vein grafts: Suppression of intimal hyperplasia of the vein graft but not the anastomosis. J Vasc Surg 21:882, 1995.

181. Jenkins MP, Buonaccorsi GA, Raphael M, et al: Clinical study of adjuvant photodynamic therapy to reduce restenosis following femoral angioplasty. Br J Surg 86:1258, 1999.

182. LaMuraglia GM, Adili F, Schmitz-Rixen T, et al: Photodynamic therapy inhibits experimental allograft rejection: A novel approach for the development of vascular prostheses. Circulation 92:1919, 1995.

183. Huynh T, Abraham G, Murray J, et al: Remodeling of an acellular collagen graft into a physiologically responsive neovessel. Nat Biotechnol 17:1083, 1999.

184. Niklason LE, Gao J, Abbott WM, et al: Functional arteries grown in vitro. Science 284:489, 1999.

185. Wilson GJ, Yeger H, Klement P, et al: Acellular matrix allograft small caliber vascular prostheses. ASAIO J 36:M340, 1990.

186. Wilson GJ, Courtman DW, Klement P, Lee JM, Yeger H: Acellular matrix: A biomaterials approach for coronary artery bypass and heart valve replacement. Ann Thorac Surg 60:S353, 1995.

187. O'Brien MF, Gardner MA, Garlick RB, et al: The Cryolife-O'Brien stentless aortic porcine xenograft valve. J Card Surg 13:376, 1998.

188. Edwards JM, Taylor LM, Porter JM: Treatment of failed lower extremity bypass grafts with new autogenous vein bypass grafting. J Vasc Surg 11:136, 1990.

189. Budd JS, Langdon I, Brenan J, Bell PRF: Above-knee prosthetic grafts do not compromise the ipsilateral long saphenous vein. Br J Surg 78:1379, 1991.

190. Brewster DC, LaSalle AJ, Robison JE, et al: Femoropopliteal graft failures: Clinical consequences and success of secondary reconstructions. Arch Surg 118:1043, 1983.

191. Robinson JG, Brewster DC, Abbott WM, Darling RC: Femoropopliteal and tibioperoneal artery reconstruction using human umbilical vein. Arch Surg 118:1039, 1983.

192. Raju S: PTFE grafts for hemodialysis access: Techniques for insertion and management of complications. Ann Surg 206:666, 1987.

Questions

1. In general, grafts of biologic origin
   - (a) have patency rates superior to synthetics
   - (b) handle better than synthetics
   - (c) have all had problems with structural degeneration
   - (d) (b) and (c)
   - (e) (a), (b), and (c)

2. Coatings of fabric vascular prostheses
   - (a) improve healing
   - (b) increase resistance to infection
   - (c) decrease cost
   - (d) all of the above
   - (e) none of the above

3. Autogenous long saphenous veins
   - (a) have ideal performance characteristics
   - (b) never develop aneurysms
   - (c) sometimes occlude due to diffuse intimal hyperplasia
   - (d) have superior results when used in situ
   - (e) all of the above

4. Neointimal hyperplasia causes graft failure as a result of hypertrophy of
   - (a) endothelial cells
   - (b) collagen fibers
   - (c) smooth muscle cells
   - (d) elastic fibers
   - (e) macrophages

5. The following statement(s) is/are true
   - (a) in humans, synthetic prostheses do not completely spontaneously resurface with endothelial cells
   - (b) endothelial cell seeding is a useful technique in humans that awaits widespread application
   - (c) adequate endothelial cell function in a graft enhances its patency
   - (d) (a) and (c)
   - (e) (b) and (c)

6. At implantation, the endothelium of cryopreserved human saphenous vein allografts is
   - (a) present but not viable
   - (b) viable but not antigenic
   - (c) viable but antigenic
   - (d) not viable but antigenic
   - (e) not present

7. The advantage of using expanded polytetrafluoroethylene (ePTFE) compared with Dacron grafts for above-knee femoropopliteal bypass is
   - (a) better patency
   - (b) lower cost
   - (c) less bleeding
   - (d) lesser anastomotic intimal hyperplasia
   - (e) none of the above

8. Dacron is a
   - (a) nontextile synthetic graft
   - (b) nontextile extruded graft
   - (c) textile synthetic graft
   - (d) textile biologic graft
   - (e) nontextile biologic graft

9. The main disadvantage of ePTFE is its
   - (a) stiffness
   - (b) high compliance
   - (c) high porosity
   - (d) low porosity
   - (e) tendency toward early aneurysm formation

10. Compared with woven uncoated Dacron grafts, knitted uncoated Dacron grafts are
    - (a) less stiff and more porous
    - (b) more stiff and more porous
    - (c) more stiff and less porous
    - (d) less stiff and less porous
    - (e) equally stiff and more porous

Answers

1. c   2. e   3. c   4. c   5. d   6. c   7. e   8. c   9. a   10. a

23

Thoracoabdominal Aortic Aneurysms

Nicholas J. Morrissey, Ian N. Hamilton, Jr., and Larry H. Hollier

Since the first successful thoracoabdominal aortic aneurysm (TAAA) repair by Etheredge and associates in 1955,[1] care of the TAAA patient has undergone significant improvements. These improvements have resulted from a refinement of risk assessment, improved diagnostic capabilities, an expansion of anesthetic and intraoperative support, the evolution of surgical techniques, and a multimodality approach to the prevention of perioperative complications.[2, 3] Together, these efforts have led to a dramatic reduction in the overall complication rate associated with TAAA repair over more than 40 years. However, TAAA repair remains a formidable procedure associated with serious complications at rates exceeded by few other procedures. Further insight into the etiology of these complications, as well as refinements in preoperative assessment, surgical technique, and postoperative care, will allow a continued reduction in the morbidity and mortality associated with TAAA repair.

CLASSIFICATION

Aneurysms of the thoracoabdominal aorta may be classified by their extent and their causes. In 1986, Dr. E. Stanley Crawford and colleagues[4] classified TAAAs based on the extent of aortic involvement (Fig. 23–1). This classification may be properly applied to aortic aneurysms of all causes, including, but not limited to, degenerative or dissected aneurysms or those resulting from Marfan's or Ehlers-Danlos syndrome. Type I aneurysms involve all or most of the descending thoracic aorta and the upper abdominal aorta but do not involve the aorta below the level of the renal arteries. Type II aneurysms involve all or most of the descending thoracic aorta and all or most of the abdominal aorta. Type III aneurysms involve the distal half or less of the descending thoracic aorta and varying segments of the abdominal aorta. Type IV aneurysms involve all or most of the abdominal aorta, including the segment from which the visceral vessels arise.

The Crawford classification has advanced the surgical treatment of TAAA because it has permitted a standardized reporting of aneurysm extent, allowing an appropriate stratification of risk and comparison between type of aneurysm and treatment groups. The Crawford classification has also promoted the evaluation and application of specific treatment modalities based on the extent of TAAA.[5] Similarly, the Crawford classification has allowed a type-specific determination of neurologic deficit as well as morbidity and mortality associated with TAAA repair (Tables 23–1 and 23–2).

Aortic dissection, whether developing into aortic aneurysm or not, has also been classified by numerous authors based on the extent of aortic involvement.[6] The most widely used classification system has been that of DeBakey and coworkers[7] (Fig. 23–2). DeBakey and associates classified aortic dissection into three basic types related to anatomic and pathologic features. Types I and II involve the ascending aorta, whereas type III involves the descending aorta. Type I and type II dissections are differentiated from one another in that type I dissections extend beyond the

TABLE 23–1

Reported Average Incidence of Postoperative Neurologic Deficits by Crawford Classification of Thoracoabdominal Aortic Aneurysms (TAAAs)

	TYPE I (%)	TYPE II (%)	TYPE III (%)	TYPE IV (%)
Nondissecting TAAA	13	31	7	4
Dissecting TAAA	20	34	15	11

Modified from Panneton JM, Hollier LH: Nondissecting thoracoabdominal aortic aneurysms: Part I. Ann Vasc Surg, 9:503–514, 1995; Panneton JM, Hollier LH: Dissecting descending thoracic and thoracoabdominal aortic aneurysms: Part II. Ann Vasc Surg 9:596–605, 1995.

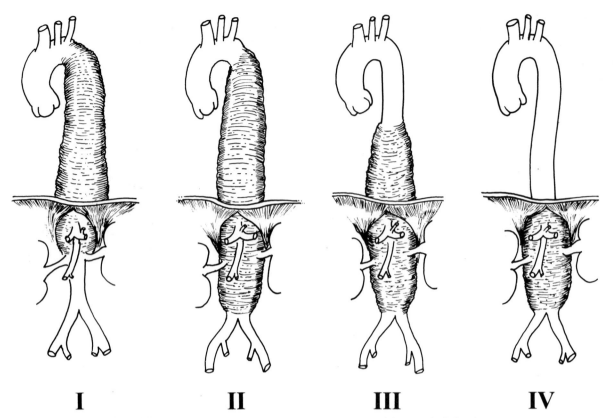

I II III IV

Figure 23–1. Types I–IV thoracoabdominal aortic aneurysms of the Crawford classification.

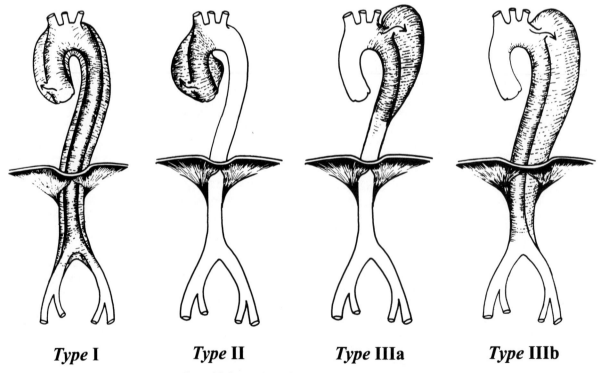

Type I *Type* II *Type* IIIa *Type* IIIb

Figure 23–2. DeBakey classification of aortic dissection.

TABLE 23-2

Reported Incidence of Operative Mortality Associated with Thoracoabdominal Aortic Aneurysms (TAAAs)*

CAUSE	NONDISSECTING TAAA (MEDIAN %)†	DISSECTING TAAA (AVERAGE %)
Pulmonary complication	38	—
Respiratory failure	—	19
Myocardial infarction	37	—
Cardiac‡	—	44
Renal failure	27	18
Hemorrhage	14	27
Sepsis	19	20
Pulmonary embolism	8	6
Stroke	8	5

*Several series reported multiple causes of death; therefore, the total percentage is >100%.

†Median has been used due to the wide variance in reporting of nondissecting TAAA data.

‡Myocardial infarction, low cardiac output, or arrhythmia.

Modified from Panneton JM, Hollier LH: Nondissecting thoracoabdominal aortic aneurysms: Part I: Ann Vasc Surg 9:503–514, 1995; Panneton JM, Hollier LH: Dissecting descending thoracic and thoracoabdominal aortic aneurysms: Part II. Ann Vasc Surg 9:596–605, 1995.

aortic arch. DeBakey type III aortic dissections do not involve the ascending aorta or the aortic arch. They may be subdivided into type IIIa (dissecting process limited to the descending thoracic aorta) and type IIIb (dissecting process extending below the diaphragm). A DeBakey type IIIb dissection corresponds to a type I or II TAAA with regard to the extent of aortic involvement by the dissecting process.

Over the past 30 years, a more functional approach to the classification of aortic dissection has emerged (Fig. 23–3). These systems are based on whether the ascending aorta is involved without regard to the site of the primary intimal tear. If the ascending aorta is involved, the dissection is termed a Stanford "type A,"[8] Najafi "anterior,"[9] University of Alabama "ascending,"[10] or Massachusetts General Hospital "proximal"[11] aortic dissection. If the ascending aorta is not involved, then it may be referred to as a "type B," "posterior," "descending," or "distal" aortic dissection, respectively (see Fig. 23–3). Combining these five classification systems allows us to see that DeBakey types I and II aortic dissections are synonymous with type A, anterior, ascending, and proximal. These forms of aortic dissection may be associated with complications (cardiac tamponade, acute aortic regurgitation, or coronary artery dissection or occlusion) that require cardiac surgical procedures (ascending aorta replacement, aortic arch replacement, aortic valve replacement or suspension, or coronary artery reimplantation), which are beyond the scope of this chapter. However, DeBakey types IIIa and IIIb aortic dissections, which are synonymous with type B, posterior, descending, and distal aortic dissections, may acutely or chronically degenerate into descending thoracic aortic aneurysms or TAAAs. From the viewpoint of the vascular surgeon, we prefer the Stanford classification because it is simple yet functional and clearly delineates the surgical approach required.

Aortic dissections that are detected within 14 days of the onset of the process are classified as acute, whereas those diagnosed beyond 2 weeks are termed chronic.[6] Although aortic dissection, whether acute or chronic, may require intervention or surgical treatment for reasons other than aneurysmal expansion, we have limited our discussion of aortic dissection to those that are aneurysmal and involve the descending thoracic or abdominal aorta, or both, thus qualifying as Crawford types I through IV TAAAs (Table 23–3).

ETIOLOGY

Atherosclerotic medial degenerative disease (82%) and aortic dissection (17%) together account for over 95% of all reported cases of TAAA.[12] Marfan's and Ehlers-Danlos syndromes, mycotic aneurysm, and Takayasu's aortitis are less frequent causes. The importance of establishing a proper diagnosis for aneurysmal disease lies in the unique natural history and treatment requirements for each type of TAAA.[13–15]

Patients with nondissecting (includes degenerative, Marfan's, Ehlers-Danlos, and others) and dissecting TAAA have different associated risk factors that influence their natural history, treatment, and long-term survival (Table 23–4). Both groups of patients with TAAA have a high incidence of associated hypertension. However, patients with degenerative aneurysms tend to have a higher incidence of coronary artery disease, chronic renal insufficiency, cerebrovascular disease, and peripheral vascular disease than patients with dissecting aneurysms. These patterns of coexistent disease significantly influence the risk of perioperative morbidity (Table 23–5) and mortality (see Table 23–2), as well as the overall risk-benefit ratio of TAAA repair.

NATURAL HISTORY

The judgment that goes into the decision to offer or withhold surgery from a patient diagnosed with a TAAA demands an understanding of the natural history of the aneurysm as well as an assessment of the patient's overall risk for surgery. In 1982, Bickerstaff and coworkers[16] noted a 2-year actuarial survival rate of 28.7% in patients with untreated thoracic and thoracoabdominal aneurysms. In

TABLE 23-3

Extent of Aortic Involvement by Crawford Classfication of Thoracoabdominal Aortic Aneurysms (TAAAs)

	TYPE I (%)	TYPE II (%)	TYPE III (%)	TYPE IV (%)
Nondissecting TAAA	23	23	26	28
Dissecting TAAA	32	48	14	6

Modified from Panneton JM, Hollier LH: Nondissecting thoracoabdominal aortic aneurysms: Part I. Ann Vasc Surg 9:503–514, 195; Panneton JM, Hollier LH: Dissecting descending thoracic and thoracoabdominal aortic aneurysms: Part II. Ann Vasc Surg 9:596–605, 1995.

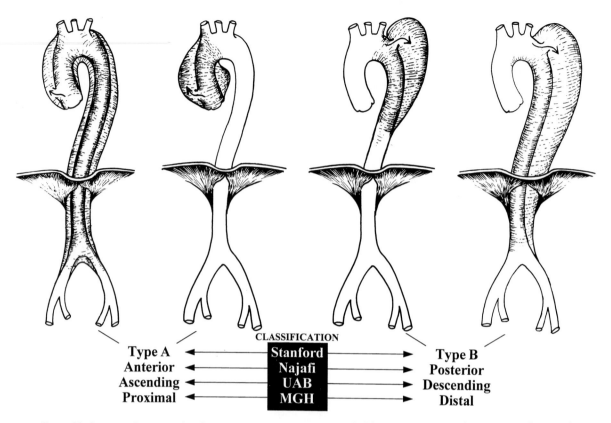

Figure 23–3. Aortic dissection classification systems. UAB, University of Alabama; MGH, Massachusetts General Hospital.

TABLE 23–4

Reported Incidence of Associated Risk Factors Associated with Thoracoabdominal Aortic Aneurysms (TAAAs)

RISK FACTOR	NONDISSECTING TAAA (MEDIAN %)*	DISSECTING TAAA (AVERAGE %)
Smoking	80	—
Hypertension	70	83
Coronary artery disease	35	19
Chronic obstructive pulmonary disease	35	25
Visceral occlusive disease	25	—
Chronic renal failure	20	9
Marfan's syndrome	—	6
Congestive heart failure	—	5
Cerebrovascular disease	15	—
Stroke	—	4
Peripheral vascular disease	15	—
Diabetes mellitus	5	3

*Median data have been used due to the wide variance in reporting of nondissecting TAAA data.

Modified from Panneton JM, Hollier LH: Nondissecting thoracoabdominal aortic aneurysms: Part I. Ann Vasc Surg 9:503–514, 1995; Panneton JM, Hollier LH: Dissecting descending thoracic and thoracoabdominal aortic aneurysms: Part II. Ann Vasc Surg 9:596–605, 1995.

TABLE 23–5

Reported Incidence of Postoperative Complications Following Thoracoabdominal Aortic Aneurysm (TAAA) Repair

COMPLICATION	NONDISSECTING TAAA (AVERAGE %)	DISSECTING TAAA (AVERAGE %)
Respiratory insufficiency	32	12
Pulmonary infection	12	—
Tracheotomy	—	9
Renal dysfunction	21	18
Need for dialysis	7	6
Paraplegia/paresis	13	25
Myocardial infarction	11	—
Cardiac*	—	7
Reoperation for bleeding	7	7
Stroke	3	4
Gastrointestinal bleeding	7	3
Pulmonary embolism	—	1

*Myocardial infarction, low cardiac output, or life-threatening arrhythmia.

Modified from Panneton JM, Hollier LH: Nondissecting thoracoabdominal aortic aneurysms: Part I. Ann Vasc Surg 9:503–514, 1995; Panneton JM, Hollier LH: Dissecting descending thoracic and thoracoabdominal aortic aneurysms: Part II. Ann Vasc Surg 9:596–605, 1995.

1986, Crawford and DeNatale[17] published the results of 94 patients with unoperated-on TAAA whose cases were followed over a 25-year period. This report was a mixture of dissected and nondissected TAAAs demonstrating a 2-year survival of 24%, with 52% of all deaths resulting from aneurysm rupture. For comparison, in a contemporary review, 605 patients underwent surgery for TAAA repair by Crawford and coworkers[4] with a 71% 2-year survival rate.

However, the degenerative and dissecting TAAAs differ not only in their etiology and associated risk factors but also in their natural history. In the series of Bickerstaff and coworkers, the 5-year survival for patients with dissecting aneurysms not operated on was 7%, whereas the survival for those with nondissecting aneurysms not operated on was 19.2%. Here we noted that rupture was also a major cause of death.[16] Cambria and colleagues,[18] in 1995, reported on the natural history of 57 patients with degenerative, nondissecting TAAA with a 37-month follow-up. In this series, rupture was the second most frequent cause of death, preceded only by cardiopulmonary disease. The overall risk of rupture with nonoperative treatment was 12% at 2 years and 32% at 4 years. In patients with aneurysms greater than 5 cm, the risk of rupture increased to 18% at 2 years. The authors reported a repair-free survival rate of 52% at 2 years and 17% at 5 years. In contrast, the authors noted a survival rate of 50% at 5 years after TAAA repair in a contemporary series of patients.

The natural history of acute and chronic aortic dissection should similarly be considered separately, just as the natural history of degenerative and dissecting aortic aneurysms should. Among patients with aortic dissection, those with acute dissection have a higher mortality than those with chronic dissection.[19] Subset analysis of a mixed population of type B dissecting aneurysms reveals the percentage of deaths from aortic rupture to be 83% in acute type B dissecting aneurysms, as opposed to 56% in chronic type B dissecting aortic aneurysms.[20] Additionally, the 1- and 5-year survival rates of surgically treated patients with acute type B aortic dissection are 56% and 48% versus 78% and 59%, respectively, in surgically treated patients with chronic type B aortic dissections.[19] Furthermore, dissections with a patent false lumen have a higher complication rate than those with partial or complete thrombosis of the false lumen.[21] High flow rates within a patent false lumen and retrograde flow proximal to the left subclavian artery also have been associated with higher complication and mortality rates.[22] These data emphasize the importance of fully assessing the etiology and anatomy of a TAAA in determining a patient's treatment plan. The natural history of degenerative TAAA is different from that of both acute and chronic dissecting TAAA. An evaluation of each individual patient's risk for death from aortic aneurysm rupture compared with an estimate of his or her operative risk provides the database necessary for the best overall treatment plan and long-term survival (Table 23–6).

PRESENTATION

Degenerative TAAAs and dissecting type B aortic aneurysms are asymptomatic at the time of diagnosis in 43% and 15% of patients, respectively.[12, 23] Although the asymp-

TABLE 23–6

Late Survival After Thoracoabdominal Aortic Aneurysm (TAAA) Repair

SURVIVAL TIME (YR)	NONDISSECTING TAAA (%)	DISSECTING TAAA (%)
1	80	74
5	61	50
10	33	—

Modified from Panneton JM, Hollier LH: Nondissecting thoracoabdominal aortic aneurysms: Part I. Ann Vasc Surg 9:503–514, 1995; Panneton JM, Hollier LH: Dissecting descending thoracic and thoracoabdominal aortic aneurysms: Part II. Ann Vasc Surg 9:596–605, 1995.

tomatic TAAA may be found during a routine history and physical examination, more commonly, abdominal ultrasonography, computed tomography (CT) scan, or magnetic resonance (MR) imaging (MRI) performed in the course of a seemingly unrelated workup reveals an incidental aortic aneurysm.

Degenerative TAAAs and dissecting type B aortic aneurysms have a symptomatic presentation in 57% and 85% of patients, respectively.[12, 23] The most frequent complaint in both types is pain. As an aneurysm increases in size, it may compress or erode adjacent structures along the course of the aorta, resulting in chest, back, flank, or abdominal pain. Compression of organs and structures adjacent to a large aneurysm can result in a variety of signs and symptoms. Stretching of the recurrent laryngeal nerve may result in hoarseness; left lung or bronchial compression may have onset with dyspnea, wheezing, cough, or recurrent pulmonary infections; esophageal compression may cause dysphagia; and duodenal stretching from an underlying aneurysm can produce partial small bowel obstruction. Ureteral obstruction may result from an enlarging abdominal or iliac component of a TAAA, especially if the aneurysm has an inflammatory component.[24] Erosion of a large TAAA into the lung, esophagus, duodenum, or renal collecting system may lead to fistula formation with "herald" or life-threatening hemorrhage in the form of hemoptysis, hematemesis, hematochezia, melena, or hematuria. Erosive fistula formation into the inferior vena cava may appear with an abdominal bruit, widened pulse pressure, edema, and heart failure. Degenerative TAAA may rarely manifest with paralysis resulting from vertebral body erosion with spinal cord compression, spinal artery thrombosis, or embolization.

Dissecting type B aortic aneurysms are more commonly symptomatic than are degenerative TAAAs and may include all previously mentioned presentations. The pain of acute aortic dissection is described as an excruciating, ripping, or tearing chest or intrascapular pain that may radiate into the flank, abdomen, or legs as the dissection progresses distally. The vascular complications resulting from aortic dissection are not rare and include renal ischemia (12%), visceral ischemia (9%), acute leg ischemia (9%), and paraplegia or paraparesis (3%).

Rupture as a manifestation of TAAA occurs with equal frequency (9%) in both atherosclerotic degenerative and dissecting type B aortic aneurysms.[12, 23] TAAAs rupture with equal frequency within the thoracic and abdominal aortic segments.[25] Rarely, rupture occurs into the lung, tracheobronchial tree, or esophagus. Thoracic rupture appears with chest, back, or shoulder pain, whereas abdominal rupture manifests with generalized abdominal, left flank, left shoulder, or back pain. The majority of patients suffering from a ruptured TAAA die outside the hospital. Of patients admitted with rupture, 25% are hypotensive and 55% of these patients suffer a cardiac arrest before operation.[25]

DIAGNOSIS

The modalities available for the diagnosis of and preoperative planning for TAAA include chest radiographs, angiography, CT, and transesophageal echocardiography (TEE).

Chest film findings associated with TAAA are typically nonspecific but abnormal in the majority of patients. Findings may be erroneously reported as aortic tortuosity or dilatation; mediastinal widening and displacement of intimal calcifications are less frequently noted (Fig. 23–4). Additionally, chest film findings associated with leaking or ruptured thoracic aortic aneurysms may include pleural effusion or pleural hematoma.

Conventional aortography has been the historical gold standard for the evaluation of the aorta and its branches. In that regard, aortography remains the single best study for evaluating aortic branch vessels for aneurysm, dissection, or stenosis (Fig. 23–5). However, aortography is the most invasive of all diagnostic techniques, requires nephrotoxic iodinated contrast agents, and does not evaluate nonperfused or thrombosed areas of aortic aneurysms. There-

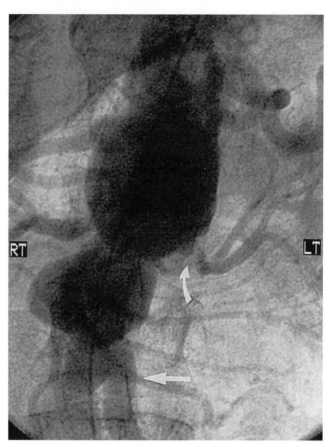

Figure 23–5. Aortogram demonstrating left renal artery stenosis (*curved arrow*) in a patient with a type III thoracoabdominal aortic aneurysm (TAAA) 2 years after infrarenal TAAA repair (*straight arrow*).

fore, the entire size and extent of a TAAA may not be fully ascertained using aortography alone.

CT and CT angiography provide excellent delineation of the aorta, including aneurysm diameter, type and extent of dissection, thrombus characteristics (Fig. 23–6), evidence of aneurysm leak, branch vessel anatomy (Fig. 23–7), venous anatomy and anomalies, and abnormalities of adjacent mediastinal, retroperitoneal, and abdominal organs. Helical or spiral CT with options for three-dimensional reconstruction provides additional information about aortic branch vessel anatomy (Fig. 23–8). However, CT angiography also requires the use of nephrotoxic intravenous contrast agents, and exposures must be appropriately timed with the intravenous bolus to adequately evaluate branch arteries.

MRI with options for arterial enhancement, three-dimensional reconstruction, and cardiovascular imaging with cine–MR angiography (MRA) now enable us to define the entire extent of aortic aneurysms and dissections while avoiding nephrotoxic intravenous contrast materials.[26] MRI, MRA, and cine-MRA are user independent, have a large field of view, have multiplane and three-dimensional capabilities, lack ionizing radiation, and do not require critical timing of contrast infusion or image acquisition. The evaluation of aortic branch vessels with MR techniques is generally equal to that of CT; however, it is slightly inferior to conventional arteriography. MR technology—specifically cine-MRA—also has the ability to detect cardiac wall mo-

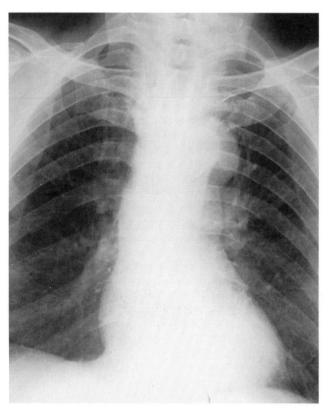

Figure 23–4. Chest radiograph read as tortuous aorta with wide mediastinum in a patient with a 9-cm aortic aneurysm.

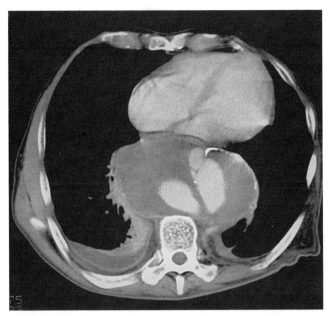

Figure 23–6. Computed tomography angiogram of a large dissecting thoracoabdominal aortic aneurysm with three separately perfused lumina and circumferential laminated thrombus.

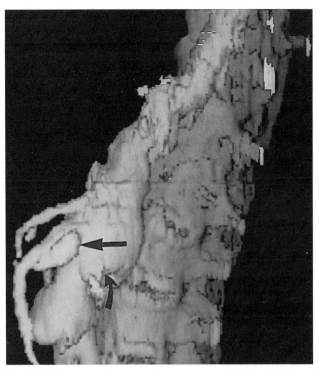

Figure 23–8. Computed tomography angiogram with three-dimensional reconstruction of a thoracoabdominal aortic aneurysm demonstrating a superior mesenteric artery aneurysm *(straight arrow)* and dissection onto the origin of the left renal artery causing stenosis *(curved arrow)*.

tion abnormalities and valvular disease with nearly as much accuracy as echocardiography (Fig. 23–9). However, MR technology has certain limitations. It cannot be offered to patients with implanted electronic devices such as pacemakers, and previously placed metallic surgical clips create artifact that can obscure anatomic detail. MR cannot be performed on unstable patients, and mechanical ventilation makes high-quality image acquisition difficult. Patients suffering from claustrophobia require sedation preceding MR examination.

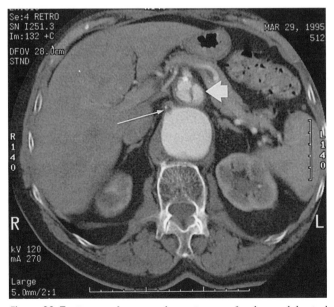

Figure 23–7. Computed tomography angiogram of a thoracoabdominal aortic aneurysm demonstrating a dissecting aneurysm of the superior mesenteric artery *(thick arrow)* and right renal artery stenosis *(thin arrow)*.

TEE can be safely and rapidly performed at the patient's bedside or in the operating room. It provides information on myocardial performance, cardiac valvular function, and the presence of pericardial effusion or tamponade, and it provides excellent anatomic information on the ascending and descending thoracic aorta. It does not require intravenous contrast and can be performed rapidly at a reasonable cost. The disadvantages of TEE include its limitation in visualizing portions of the aortic arch and proximal brachiocephalic vessels and its inability to evaluate the infradiaphragmatic aorta.

In addition to the anatomic assessment of the aneurysm itself, a complete preoperative evaluation of the patient's concomitant risk factors is mandatory for successful outcome following TAAA repair. After a thorough history and physical examination, routine preoperative studies usually include a baseline chest radiograph; electrocardiogram; arterial blood gases; complete blood count; complete serum chemistry profile, including liver function tests and electrolytes; urinalysis; platelet count; and prothrombin time, partial thromboplastin time, and fibrinogen levels.

All patients undergo thorough cardiac evaluation, including cardiac stress testing, to detect possible coronary artery disease (CAD), and B mode ultrasonography to assess valvular competence. (Aortic valvular insufficiency is a relative contraindication to proximal clamping of the descending thoracic aorta unless shunt or pump bypass techniques are employed.) If significant CAD is shown to be present by stress testing, coronary angiography is performed.

Carotid artery duplex ultrasound scanning is routinely performed as part of the preoperative assessment. Severe

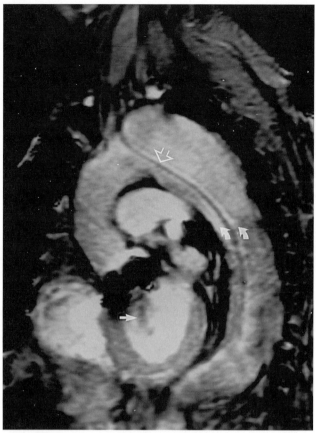

Figure 23–9. Cine magnetic resonance angiogram of a type B dissection demonstrating perfusion of the true and false lumina (*curved arrows*), dissection flap (*open arrow*), and aortic insufficiency (*small arrow*) in a patient with prior aortic valve replacement.

carotid artery disease with stenosis greater than 70% diameter reduction is treated by carotid endarterectomy prior to elective TAAA repair. Additionally, the patient's nutritional status should be assessed preoperatively. Those patients found to be in a catabolic state or negative nitrogen balance should have attempts made to place them into a positive nitrogen balance if this does not delay surgery inappropriately. Patients found to be fit for surgery undergo preoperative hydration, mechanical bowel preparation, bathing with antimicrobial soap, and type and cross-matching for 6 units of packed red blood cells, 6 units of fresh-frozen plasma, and 12 units of platelets.

TREATMENT

Anesthetic support has become increasingly critical to the successful performance of TAAA repair. The anesthesiology service is responsible for the placement of a double-lumen endotracheal tube with bronchoscopic positioning and assistance with the placement of a Swan-Ganz catheter, radial arterial line, and an intrathecal catheter for the drainage of cerebrospinal fluid (CSF) and continuous monitoring of CSF pressure.[2, 27] Additionally, two large-bore central venous catheters are placed for volume infusions, and a high thoracic epidural catheter is placed for perioperative analgesia, the attenuation of the catecholamine stress re-

sponse,[28] enhanced cardioprotection, and hemodynamic stability.[29] TEE is helpful in determining cardiac volume status, intraoperative cardiac valvular function, and, most important, the early detection of myocardial ischemia as evidenced by cardiac wall motion abnormalities.

Distal aortic perfusion techniques have been associated with a decrease in the incidence of serious morbidity and mortality following TAAA repair.[5, 30, 31] Options available for the performance of distal aortic perfusion during TAAA repair include the use of passive shunt techniques (temporary axillary-to-femoral artery graft or Gott shunt) or one of two techniques of pump perfusion (left atrial-to-femoral artery or femoral vein-to-femoral artery bypass). The perfusionist is intimately involved in the performance of the procedure when distal aortic pump perfusion (DAPP) is utilized. The perfusionist may also be responsible for the operation of the red blood cell salvage-washing and rapid-infusion devices (Cell Saver and R.I.S., Haemonetics Corp., Braintree, Mass.). This may be a shared responsibility with the anesthesia service. The coordination of the procedure demands frequent communication between the surgical, anesthesia, and perfusion teams.

After the appropriate tubes, lines, and monitoring devices have been placed, the patient is positioned in a right lateral decubitus position, allowing the hips to fall into a near supine position. This provides access to the left ilio-femoral vessels for DAPP techniques. The skin is widely prepared with povidone-iodine solution and meticulous placement of adhesive iodinated plastic drapes. The thoracoabdominal incision is made in the fourth or fifth intercostal space for a type I or high type II TAAA or in the seventh to ninth intercostal space for type III or type IV TAAA.[2] The abdominal incision is then carried down the midline or paramedian line from the fourth intercostal incision or made obliquely across the abdomen from the seventh or ninth intercostal incision. Additional exposure may be gained by excising a rib or transecting the posterior portion of the rib above and below the intercostal incision. Proper preoperative planning usually prevents the need for a double thoracotomy, which may be associated with an increased risk of postoperative pulmonary complications. The abdominal exposure is continued in a retroperitoneal plane posterior to the left kidney. The diaphragm is divided in a circumferential fashion with marking sutures placed on the edges of the divided diaphragm to facilitate closure. The crus of the diaphragm is divided to the left of the aorta. The proximal portions of the visceral and renal arteries are identified, and control of the superior mesenteric and renal arteries is obtained to allow these vessels to be snared after placement of selective visceral and renal perfusion catheters (Fig. 23–10). These catheters originate from a Y connection in the arterial perfusion line and provide oxygenated blood to the cannulated mesenteric and renal arteries, thus decreasing the overall ischemic time and subsequent ischemia-related complications. Additional thoracic exposure involves the division of the inferior pulmonary ligament and dissection of the mediastinal pleura overlying the normal aortic segment proximal to the aneurysm.

For type I and type II TAAA, the proximal clamp may need to be applied on the distal aortic arch between the origin of the left common carotid and left subclavian arte-

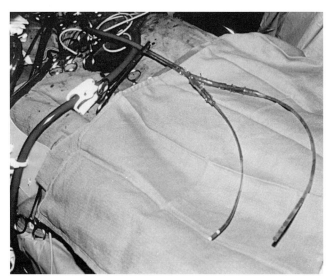

Figure 23–10. Selective perfusion catheters from the divided arterial perfusion line are used with distal aortic pump perfusion to maintain superior mesenteric and renal artery blood flow during visceral aortic reconstruction.

ries. Dissection at this level should be performed with great care, protecting the left phrenic, vagus, and recurrent laryngeal nerves. We incorporate the techniques of staged aortic clamping and sequential anastomoses with DAPP during the performance of the proximal aortic and intercostal anastomoses. Therefore, an additional segment of mediastinal pleura is dissected overlying a segment of mid- to distal descending thoracic aorta, allowing aortic control at this level as the anatomy of the aneurysm permits. All intraperitoneal viscera must be carefully retracted medially and to the patient's right, avoiding splenic or pancreatic injury.

Before and during aortic cross-clamping, CSF should be withdrawn as needed to maintain a CSF pressure of less than 10 mm Hg. The patient's core temperature is allowed to passively drift down to 32°C to 34°C. Additionally, intravenous steroids, mannitol, and thiopental (or, more frequently, propofol) are administered before aortic clamping.

Our distal aortic perfusion technique of choice involves femoral vein-to-femoral artery pump perfusion utilizing heparin-coated circuitry (Duraflow II, Bentley Laboratories, Baxter Healthcare Corp., Irvine, Calif.; or Carmeda Bioactive Surface, Medtronic Cardiopulmonary, Anaheim, Calif.), including a hollow-fiber membrane oxygenator and heat exchanger with a heparin-coated centrifugal pump (Sarns Delphin, Sarns 3-M Healthcare, Ann Arbor, Mich.; or Bio-Medicus Bio-Pump, Medtronic Bio-Medicus Inc., Eden Prairie, Minn.). This system has been shown to function safely without any clot formation, with maintenance of activated clotting times (ACTs) greater than 180 seconds.[30] Therefore, full systemic heparinization is not required, and we administer only a low initial bolus dose of heparin (50 IU/kg) before aortic cross-clamping. Next, the left iliac artery and the vena cava at the level of the right atrium are cannulated via the left common femoral artery and vein, respectively. Using staged sequential aortic clamping, the mid- to distal descending thoracic aorta is

clamped, after which the proximal aortic clamp is placed, and then the proximal segment of the aneurysm is opened longitudinally. A high proximal aortic pressure (150 to 170 mm Hg) is maintained to maximize perfusion through collateral vessels while DAPP is instituted for lower body, renal, mesenteric, lumbar, and lower intercostal artery perfusion at this time. In most instances, no attempt is made to control back-bleeding from intercostal arteries in the opened segment of aorta, because they are to be reimplanted after completion of the proximal anastomosis. Autologous shed blood salvaging systems using the combination of a red blood cell salvage-washing device and the heparin-coated cardiotomy suction system from the perfusion pump are used to retrieve blood from back-bleeding vessels. The proximal aorta is often transected to avoid the development of aortoesophageal fistula associated with endoaneurysmorrhaphy at this level. Large intercostal arteries in the vicinity of the proximal anastomosis are preserved via incorporation into a posterior tongue of aortic wall as part of an oblique anastomosis. This proximal anastomosis is performed with a properly sized, low-porosity, collagen-impregnated Dacron graft (Hemashield, Meadox, Oakland, N.J.) and sutured with a running 0 polypropylene (Prolene) suture (Ethicon, Summerville, N.J.) on a V7 needle. Felt strip reinforcement of the proximal aortic anastomosis is helpful in obtaining a hemostatic suture line with dissections and friable atheromatous aortic tissue.

After completing the proximal anastomosis, the proximal clamp is moved onto the graft, and flow is restored to any reimplanted intercostal arteries. Additional large intercostal arteries are reimplanted as separate cuffs onto the posterior aspect of the graft using the Carrel patch technique. In some cases of aortic dissection, intercostal arteries may be hidden from view by the intimal flap of the dissection (Fig. 23–11). This flap should be excised and all intercostal arteries exposed so that they may be reimplanted if technically feasible. Occasionally, in extensive or dissecting aneu-

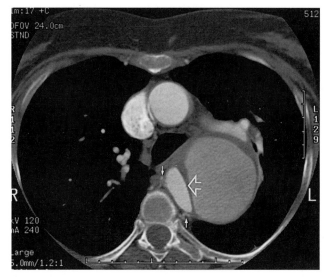

Figure 23–11. Computed tomography angiogram of a dissecting thoracoabdominal aortic aneurysm in which the dissection flap *(open arrow)* has hidden the orifices of two intercostal arteries *(small arrows).* The septum should be excised and the intercostal arteries reimplanted or oversewn.

rysms with multiple patent intercostal arteries, two separate cuffs of arteries will need to be reimplanted. Each cuff of intercostal arteries is sequentially reperfused by moving the proximal clamp distally on the graft, thus restoring flow to the spinal cord as soon as possible.

Next, an infrarenal portion of aorta or, alternatively, the common iliac arteries are clamped for distal control. The remaining section of the aneurysmal aorta is opened longitudinally posterior to the orifice of the left renal artery. The orifices of the celiac, superior mesenteric, and renal arteries are inspected. Significant atherosclerotic osteal lesions are treated by endarterectomy. The perfusion catheters from the divided arterial line are then brought onto the field, and the superior mesenteric and right renal arteries are selectively cannulated and perfused (Fig. 23–12). Likewise, perfusion cooling of the left renal artery or selective perfusion with the divided arterial line is performed at this time. The visceral vessels are then reimplanted into the side of the graft using the Carrel patch technique. Generally we try to reimplant the celiac, superior mesenteric, and right renal arteries as a single cuff; however, if the origins of the renal vessels are closely approximated to the visceral vessels, all may be reimplanted as a single cuff. Occasionally, separate grafts may be used to revascularize renal or mesenteric vessels, especially if aortic dissection has extended into the branch vessels.

In patients with aortic dissection, the ostia of the visceral and renal vessels may contain the flap or septum of the dissection process such that a single cuff reimplantation of these dissected vessels may lead to perfusion of both a true and false lumen, risking mesenteric and renal ischemia postoperatively (Fig. 23–13). In these situations, separate grafts may be presutured to the straight aortic graft, allowing independent reimplantation of individual visceral and renal vessels in an end-to-end fashion beyond the point of dissection. After completing the visceral and renal

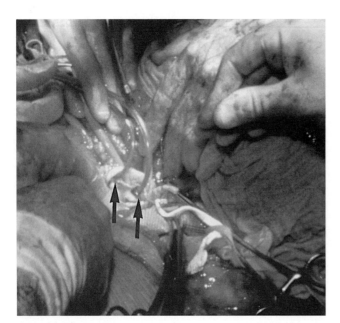

Figure 23–12. Selective visceral perfusion catheters in the superior mesenteric and right renal arteries (arrows) during a type II thoracoabdominal aortic aneurysm repair.

reimplantation, reperfusion of these vascular beds may lead to activation of the complement, kallikrein, fibrinolytic, and coagulation cascades, causing hypotension, metabolic acidosis, and risking the development of coagulopathy and disseminated intravascular coagulation (DIC). Selective visceral perfusion during the period of visceral aortic reconstruction decreases the period of ischemia to these critical vascular beds and may reduce this risk of ischemia-reperfusion–associated complications. Cambria and coworkers[32] have demonstrated that perfusion of the mesenteric bed during aortic cross-clamping resulted in shorter mesenteric ischemia time and a decrease in the rise of end-tidal CO_2 following reperfusion of the visceral vessels. The aortic clamp should be released slowly while blood and crystalloid solutions are rapidly infused. Additionally, sodium bicarbonate, mannitol, fresh-frozen plasma, and platelets are routinely administered concomitantly with aortic declamping.

Next, the distal aortic anastomosis is performed. At times, this needs to be carried out to the common iliac arteries, as dictated by aneurysm anatomy. Internal iliac artery perfusion should be assured after completion of the distal anastomosis to decrease the risk of lower spinal cord or lumbosacral nerve root ischemic injury.[33] After backbleeding and flushing the final distal anastomosis and femoral artery cannula, the pump perfusion system with heat exchanger may be used to rapidly raise the patient's body temperature, decreasing the risk of hypothermia-associated coagulopathy. When cardiac indices and systemic and pulmonary blood pressure have stabilized, protamine is administered based on ACT to help counteract the anticoagulant effect that may result from mesenteric reperfusion. All heparin-coated circuitry should be removed from the patient before protamine is given. Our approach to distal aortic perfusion (DAP) is based on a thorough knowledge of available techniques and is a choice based on individual patient characteristics. We have increased our experience with the use of a right axillary-femoral arterial bypass as a method of DAP. It can be performed quite easily and it can be left in place in a subcutaneous tunnel, obviating the need to dismantle it at the end of the procedure.

After completing each anastomosis, adequate hemostasis must be ensured. Likewise, adequate perfusion to each of the branch vessels must be verified. If fibrinolysis is suspected, an infusion of an antifibrinolytic agent is started and continued up to 24 hours postoperatively. The wall of the aneurysm is closed tightly over the entire length of the graft. If coverage is incomplete, Gore-Tex (W.L. Gore & Associates, Inc., Flagstaff, Ariz.) membrane is used to provide full coverage of the aortic graft (Fig. 23–14). This provides tamponade against oozing and prevents graft erosion into adjacent viscera or lung. Fibrin glue may be injected into the space between the graft and the Gore-Tex membrane for additional hemostasis. After achieving hemostasis throughout the operative field, the diaphragm is reapproximated with interrupted mattress sutures. Two chest tubes are used to drain the costophrenic sulcus and the apex of the left chest. Abdominal and retroperitoneal drainage is generally avoided. The chest and abdomen are closed with multiple layers in standard fashion. The patient is transferred directly to the surgical intensive care unit for close observation.

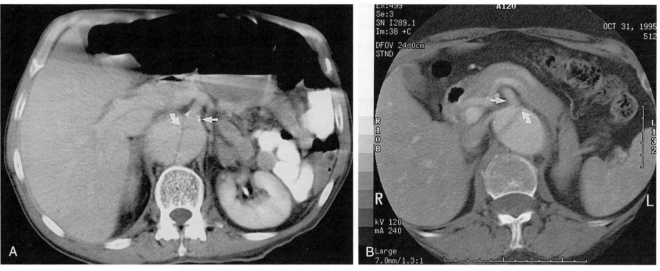

Figure 23–13. Computed tomography scans of two different dissecting thoracoabdominal aortic aneurysms demonstrating the proximity of the dissecting flap *(curved arrows)* to the orifice of the superior mesenteric artery *(straight arrows)*.

POSTOPERATIVE CARE

In the immediate postoperative period, maintaining hemo-dynamic stability and adequate oxygenation decreases the likelihood of myocardial ischemia, tachycardia, stroke, renal failure, or paraplegia. If rewarming is not complete, hypo-thermia must be corrected with warmed intravenous fluids and inhaled gases and a warming blanket. Blood pressure and cardiac indices are continuously monitored and main-tained within the patient's normal preoperative level with crystalloid, colloid, and appropriate blood products. Arterial blood gases, coagulation studies, hemoglobin, and serum electrolytes are frequently monitored and maintained within normal ranges. Inotropic support may be required in the first few hours postoperatively; however, it is discon-tinued as soon as adequate volume loading has led to hemodynamic stability. The patient is maintained on a low-dose dopamine infusion (2 to 3 μg/kg/minute) to enhance renal vasodilatation for the first 24 to 48 hours, and lactated

Ringer's solution is infused at a rate to replace urine output on a milliliter-per-milliliter basis for the first 12 to 24 hours.

The patient is maintained on a ventilator, and weaning is started only on the following postoperative day, as dic-tated by arterial blood gases and evidence of appropriate pulmonary function. Maintenance fluid is decreased daily from the initial rate of 125 mL/hour (plus urinary replace-ment) to 60 mL/hour by the third postoperative day. Grad-ual weaning from the ventilator is ideally timed with the mobilization of third-space fluid. Furosemide may be given at this point to assist with fluid mobilization and minimize the associated pulmonary congestion. Careful monitoring of serum potassium is important at this time, because rapid diuresis may deplete potassium levels and result in cardiac arrhythmias. The chest tubes are removed when drainage has decreased to less than 100 to 200 mL/day, which is generally between the second and fifth postoperative day. CSF pressure monitoring is continued up to 3 days postop-eratively while CSF pressure is maintained at 10 mm Hg

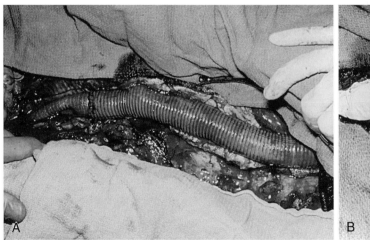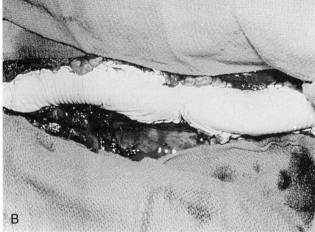

Figure 23–14. *A*, Operative photograph demonstrating thoracoabdominal aortic aneurysm (TAAA) graft, which cannot be covered with residual aneurysm wall. *B*, Operative photograph demonstrating the use of a Gore-Tex membrane to provide full coverage of a TAAA graft.

or less to decrease the risk of delayed-onset neurologic injury. Cephalosporin antibiotics are continued at least until the intrathecal lumbar catheter is removed. Cytoprotective agents or histamine blockers are used for ulcer prophylaxis until the resolution of postoperative ileus, at which time enteral feeding should be started.

POSTOPERATIVE COMPLICATIONS AND THEIR PREVENTION

Although it has become a much safer procedure than in years past, TAAA repair is still associated with complication rates that are exceeded by those of few other procedures. These rates are a reflection of the systemic nature of the arterial diseases affecting the aorta and multiple other organ systems accounting for a significant incidence of comorbidities. Furthermore, the procedure itself requires entrance into both the thoracic and abdominal or retroperitoneal regions, creates an ischemia-reperfusion phenomenon in several organ systems with risk for cellular injury, may be associated with large fluid shifts and significant blood loss, and is generally associated with a prolonged operative time. Cumulatively, these factors help explain the postoperative complication rates associated with TAAA repair (see Table 23–5). However, the pulmonary, cardiac, renal, neurologic, and hemorrhagic complication rates associated with TAAA repair have been consistently improved. We employ a multimodality approach to the prevention of perioperative morbidity and mortality associated with this procedure.

Evidence for the role of mesenteric ischemia-reperfusion in the development of systemic morbidity after thoracoabdominal aneurysm repair continues to accumulate. The production of proinflammatory cytokines by the mesentery following ischemia-reperfusion has been demonstrated experimentally.[34, 35] The mesenteric release of these cytokines results in pulmonary injury in a mouse model.[36] In another series of animal studies, inhibition of certain proinflammatory cytokines (i.e., tumor necrosis factor-α) can attenuate the systemic effects of mesenteric ischemia–reperfusion.[37, 38] In the clinical setting, it has been shown that longer periods of mesenteric ischemia lead to higher complication rates following repair of thoracoabdominal aneurysms.[39] Further analysis of the systemic effects of cytokine production by the mesentery after transient ischemia may lead to improvements in outcomes after thoracoabdominal aortic operations.

Pulmonary Complications

Pulmonary insufficiency, need for tracheotomy, or prolonged ventilator dependency is the most common complication associated with TAAA repair. The high incidence of respiratory morbidity is related to the prevalence of preoperative chronic obstructive pulmonary disease, the frequency of tobacco use, the deleterious impact of a thoracophrenolaparotomy on respiratory mechanics, intraoperative lung manipulation and barotrauma, and increases in pulmonary microvascular permeability following ischemia-reperfusion.[40, 41] Prolonged postoperative ventilator dependency places the patient at increased risk of pneumonia, sepsis, and death. Svensson and collaborators[42] showed a decrease in hospital survival from 98% to 83% and a decreased long-term survival at 12 months from 96% to 71% in patients with postoperative respiratory failure following TAAA repair.

Efforts to minimize the overall pulmonary-related complication rate following TAAA repair should be targeted at the preoperative, intraoperative, and postoperative phases of care. Preoperative pulmonary management includes encouraging the cessation of smoking, antibiotic treatment for any existing bronchitis, bronchodilator treatment, aggressive pulmonary physiotherapy, preoperative instruction in the use of incentive spirometry, and epidural analgesia for postoperative pain relief. Additionally, systemic corticosteroid therapy may be considered for patients with marginal lung function.[43] Intraoperatively, double-lumen tracheal intubation with full collapse of the left lung provides exposure of the descending thoracic aorta and minimizes pulmonary trauma from the combination of lung manipulation, compression, and pulmonary barotrauma, which may result from lung overexpansion following thoracoprenolaparotomy.

The ischemia-reperfusion phenomenon associated with TAAA repair is responsible for local organ injury,[44, 45] as well as for injury to remote organs, including the lungs.[40] This injury pattern appears to be a neutrophil-dependent increase in microvascular permeability[46, 47] that may be preventable in part or in whole through the use of free radical scavengers[40] and minimizing the ischemic interval through the use of DAPP and selective visceral perfusion.[48–50] With the implementation of this pulmonary protocol, including meticulous attention to pulmonary hygiene, Swan-Ganz data, serial blood gas determinations, and transcutaneous oxygen monitoring, gradual weaning from the ventilator is tolerated in the majority of patients, ensuring a successful extubation.

Cardiac Complications

Cardiac complications are the next most common cause of perioperative morbidity and mortality following TAAA repair. Preoperative cardiac evaluation with resting and stress electrocardiograms, as well as stress echocardiography for the assessment of valvular and ventricular function, proves invaluable in stratifying cardiac risk and determining the need for preoperative coronary angiography. Patients with angina, wall motion abnormalities on stress echocardiography, and abnormal redistribution on dipyridamole-thallium scans are at increased risk for perioperative myocardial infarction due to increases in left ventricular afterload associated with thoracic aorta cross-clamping. Anatomic cardiac evaluation in the form of coronary angiography should be performed as indicated based on the findings of the history, physical examination, and functional cardiac evaluation. In elective circumstances, these moderate- and high-risk patients should first undergo myocardial revascularization with percutaneous transluminal coronary angioplasty or coronary artery bypass grafting.

Other measures used to minimize the risk of myocardial ischemia include preoperative admission to an intensive care unit with Swan-Ganz and arterial monitoring and optimization of myocardial performance using antianginal and inotropic medications. Intraoperative measures recommended to decrease cardiac morbidity include cardiovascular anesthesia, TEE, continued Swan-Ganz and arterial hemodynamic monitoring, and epidural analgesia.[29, 43] Additionally, we use DAPP during periods of aortic cross-clamping in types I and II TAAA to control proximal hypertension and minimize elevations in left ventricular afterload. This is achieved by increasing pump flow rates such that preoperative pulmonary artery diastolic or left ventricular end-diastolic pressures are maintained during aortic cross-clamping. The resultant left ventricular protection decreases the risk of perioperative myocardial infarction and pulmonary insufficiency.[51] Poldermans and coworkers,[52] in 1999, demonstrated that perioperative β-blockade using bisoprolol resulted in a significant reduction in cardiovascular morbidity and mortality after vascular surgery in high-risk patients. The combination of DAPP and CSF drainage permits the safe administration of intravenous sodium nitroprusside to control proximal aortic blood pressure, providing additional myocardial protection. Sodium nitroprusside may be given under these circumstances without risking a decrease in spinal cord perfusion pressure that may otherwise result from a steal phenomenon when sodium nitroprusside is given in the absence of distal aortic perfusion.[31, 53, 54]

Renal Complications

Patients with preoperative renal insufficiency are at increased risk of operative mortality, postoperative renal dysfunction, neurologic deficits, and late death following TAAA repair.[12, 23] Postoperative renal failure is also a significant predictor of early death following TAAA repair. The two major determinants of postoperative renal failure include the extent of preexisting renal dysfunction and the duration of intraoperative renal ischemia.

Existing renal function may be preserved by minimizing or avoiding diagnostic studies requiring nephrotoxic contrast agents and adjusting or replacing medications such as angiotensin-converting enzyme inhibitors, which may exacerbate renal insufficiency. In patients with elevated serum creatinine, MRA may be used to assess aortic anatomy with selective use of CT angiography or conventional aortography for the evaluation of specific branch vessel anatomy not clearly seen with MRA. Renal artery stenosis should be specifically looked for and treated at the time of TAAA repair. Any contrast studies performed should be preceded by intravenous hydration, mannitol, and furosemide, and consideration given to renal dose dopamine infusion during and after the procedure. Serum creatinine levels should be closely monitored following contrast studies, and elective procedures should be delayed until renal function returns to baseline.

Immediate preoperative intravenous volume expansion and intraoperative mannitol administration should precede aortic cross-clamping. Distal aortic pump perfusion with selective renal perfusion techniques is associated with a decrease in postoperative renal insufficiency,[55] as is renal perfusion using cold (4°C) Collins solution.[56] Postopera-

tively, low-dose intravenous dopamine at 2 to 3 μg/kg/minute is used as a renal vasodilator until the patient enters a diuretic phase with mobilization of third-space fluid.

Neurologic Complications

The reported incidence of neurologic injury following TAAA repair averages 13% for nondissecting TAAA and is even higher for dissecting type B TAAA.[12, 23] Preoperative variables predictive of neurologic deficit following TAAA repair include prior proximal aortic aneurysm repair and the presence of aortic dissection.[23] Classically, the presence of aortic dissection has been considered a predictor of neurologic morbidity after TAAA repair.[4, 23, 57, 58] A recent analysis of 660 patients by Coselli and colleagues[59] suggested that chronic dissection was not a risk factor for postoperative neurologic deficit. This series emphasized the aggressive reattachment of intercostal and lumbar arteries, selective use of atriodistal bypass, and passive moderate hypothermia. Neurologic complications occurred in 5.5% of patients without dissection and in 5.0% of patients with dissection. Paraplegia occurred in 19% of patients who manifested acute dissection. The authors concluded that acute but not chronic dissection was a risk factor for the development of postoperative neurologic complications.[59] Intraoperative variables predictive of neurologic deficit include the duration of aortic cross-clamping, the extent of aorta replaced, and the oversewing of intercostal arteries. Postoperative hypotension and hypoxia have similarly been shown to consistently place the patient at risk for delayed-onset neurologic deficit.[60, 61]

The pathophysiology of neurologic injury following TAAA repair is dictated by the severity of the ischemic insult, the degree of reperfusion injury, and spinal cord neuronal metabolism. Our multimodality approach toward the prevention of neurologic injury is targeted at these three variables (Fig. 23–15).

Spinal cord perfusion pressure is equivalent to the difference between the anterior spinal artery pressure and CSF pressure (or venous pressure, whichever is greater).[62] Therefore, maintaining a spinal cord perfusion pressure that minimizes or eliminates ischemia may be achieved by increasing the spinal cord mean arterial pressure, decreasing the CSF pressure, or both. Our approach to increasing the spinal cord perfusion includes the maintenance of a high proximal aortic blood pressure (150 to 170 mm Hg) to maximize collateral blood flow. Additionally, DAPP provides oxygenated blood flow to unopened portions of the distal aorta, including the lower intercostal, lumbar, and pelvic arteries, whereas the technique of staged clamping and sequential anastomosis is used to perform proximal aortic procedures. We routinely reimplant all major patent intercostal arteries with a single or multicuff Carrel patch technique. Some surgeons have advocated oversewing of all patient intercostal and lumbar vessels to minimize clamp time and reduce neurologic complications.[57] Most series, however, demonstrate significant reduction in postoperative neurologic deficits when reimplantation of patient intercostal vessels in certain critical regions is performed.[63] Reattachment of patent arteries between the T-8–L-1 level appeared to be most crucial.[63, 64]

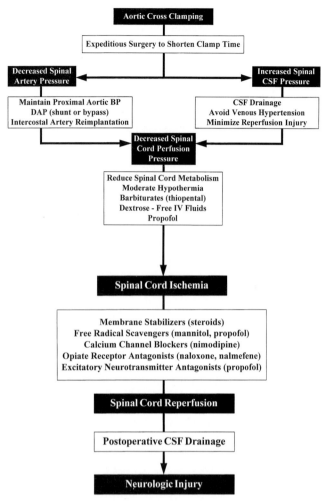

Figure 23–15. Schematic diagram of the pathophysiologic cascade of events leading to neurologic injury (*black boxes*) and the multimodality approach aimed at preventing neurologic injury (*white boxes*) during and after thoracoabdominal aortic aneurysm repair.

We and other authors have demonstrated the clinical benefit of CSF drainage to lower the CSF pressure, thus maximizing spinal cord perfusion pressure for any mean arterial blood pressure.[3, 27, 65] We place an intrathecal catheter at the lumbar level immediately preceding the operation. This catheter is connected to an external drainage system (EDMS, Pudenz-Shulte Medical Corp., Goleta, Calif.), which allows monitoring of CSF pressure and automatic overflow drainage of CSF whenever the pressure rises above 10 mm Hg. Similarly, other investigators have recently shown a statistically significant decrease in the incidence of neurologic injury associated with TAAA repair with a combination of DAPP and CSF drainage.[5, 31] Safi and associates[31] demonstrated a total neurologic complication rate of 9% for the treatment group (DAPP, moderate hypothermia, and CSF drainage) versus 19% for a control group. Subset analysis demonstrated a neurologic complication rate for patients with type II TAAA of 13% in the treatment group versus 41% in the control group. Furthermore, in patients with aortic clamp times longer than 45 minutes, the neurologic complication rate was 13% in patients treated with the multimodality approach versus

39% in control patients.[31] A recent randomized, prospective trial demonstrated significant reduction of neurologic complications with the use of CSF drainage.[66]

The restoration of blood flow to a spinal cord having suffered any ischemic time period risks a reperfusion injury. Many investigators have demonstrated the ability to modulate this reperfusion injury with free radical scavengers, antioxidants, monoclonal antibodies, excitatory neurotransmitter antagonists, opiate receptor antagonists, and calcium channel blockers.[67–73] Our protocol, which attempts to minimize the reperfusion injury, is aimed at eliminating or minimizing the initial ischemic insult. We modulate the reperfusion injury through the administration of steroids as membrane stabilizers and the free radical scavenger mannitol before aortic clamping and again preceding intercostal artery reperfusion. Experimental studies have demonstrated that apoptosis occurs in spinal motor neurons after transient aortic occlusion.[74] Pharmacologic inhibitors of such programmed cell death are currently being investigated. Such agents may in the future be included in the multimodality approach to spinal cord protection.

The last component of our multimodality approach to spinal cord protection is aimed at lowering the neuronal metabolic rate during the period of aortic cross-clamping. We achieve this by allowing the patient's temperature to drift passively to 32°C to 34°C, providing moderate systemic hypothermia beneficial for both spinal cord and renal protection. We have administered barbiturate in the form of thiopental sodium to further decrease the spinal cord metabolic rate. We have substituted the intravenous anesthetic agent propofol for thiopental owing to its ability to reduce central nervous system metabolic requirements for oxygen[75] while maintaining cerebral oxygenation and autoregulation.[76] Furthermore, propofol has been shown to be a free radical scavenger with excellent central nervous system distribution.[77, 78] This may translate into enhanced central nervous system protection from ischemic injury. All intravenous fluids are dextrose-free.[79] We do not recommend the use of local spinal cord cooling through infusion of cooling solutions into the epidural space because we are aware of acute deaths from brain stem infarction that occurred in several centers attendant on the use of that technique.

Hemorrhagic Complications

Perioperative bleeding complications, including coagulopathy and reoperation for bleeding, are associated with significant morbidity and mortality. Reoperation for bleeding is a predictor of early death after TAAA repair. Svensson and colleagues[58] demonstrated a mortality rate of 25% in patients undergoing reoperation for bleeding following TAAA repair. Others have found an associated mortality rate as high as 58% attributable to perioperative bleeding in patients after TAAA repair.[18] In a review of the literature, the average incidence of reoperation for bleeding after TAAA repair in both dissected and nondissected aneurysms was 7%. Additionally, hemorrhage as a cause of early death has an incidence of 14% in nondissected, and 27% in dissected TAAA.[12, 23] Reoperation for bleeding has also been shown to be associated with an increased risk of postoperative myocardial infarction and renal failure.[65]

The etiology of bleeding associated with TAAA repair is multifactorial. It may be related to the existence of preoperative coagulopathy, inadequate surgical hemostasis, hypothermia, DIC, hemodilution, fibrinolysis, anticoagulation, the use of extracorporeal circulation, or mesenteric ischemia and reperfusion.

Up to 39% of patients with large aortic aneurysms, including TAAA, have a significant elevation of fibrin split products preoperatively, and 4% of patients have a clinical presentation of DIC with extensive bruising, petechiae, and ecchymosis on physical examination.[80] The cause of preoperative coagulopathy in these patients is the exposed subintima and the aneurysm itself, which result in coagulation factor consumption as well as a subsequent fibrinolysis.[81] The treatment for these patients is aneurysmectomy; however, their preoperative coagulopathy and increased risk of intraoperative bleeding should be appreciated and treated with infusion of platelets and fresh-frozen plasma both before and during TAAA repair.

Bleeding complications resulting from improper surgical hemostasis are preventable. TAAA repair requires an extensive field of dissection as well as multiple anastomotic suture lines. We use electrocautery for the majority of our dissection and limit the dissection only to the areas of necessity. Our suture lines are usually reinforced with felt strips.

We allow passive moderate hypothermia of 32°C to 34°C to enhance neurologic and renal protection; however, if the temperature continues to drift downward, platelet function and the enzymatic cascades of the coagulation system are negatively affected, placing the patient at risk for hypothermia-associated coagulopathy. We use an in-line heater in the extracorporal circulation circuit to actively rewarm the patient following the completion of all aortic anastomoses. Additionally, inhalation gases and intravenous fluids are warmed. In the intensive care department, rewarming continues with the addition of a warm air recirculating blanket.

Besides preoperative effects on coagulation factors, it has become increasingly clear that supraceliac aortic clamping can itself affect the balance of the coagulation and fibrinolytic systems.[48, 49, 82] Gertler and coworkers[83] demonstrated a decrease in clotting factors and an increase in fibrinolytic activity after placement of the supraceliac clamp. Illig and colleagues[84] also demonstrated the occurrence of a primary fibrinolytic state soon after supraceliac clamping. Whether this results from mesenteric ischemia-reperfusion or hepatic ischemia with resulting poor clearance of tissue plasminogen activator, it appears clear that supraceliac aortic clamping results in an overall state of hypocoagulability and fibrinolysis. Further clinical and experimental studies have demonstrated that mesenteric perfusion during cross-clamping can attenuate this coagulopathy. In addition, the use of antifibrinolytic agents such as aprotinin or ε-aminocaproic acid (Amicar) may be helpful in alleviating the effect of fibrinolysis. Aggressive correction of coagulopathy postoperatively with factor replacement, antifibrinolytics, platelets, and restoration of physiologic temperature is mandatory to avoid reoperation for ongoing bleeding.

The use of extracorporeal circulation (ECC) for distal aortic perfusion may in itself contribute to the development of hemorrhagic complications. Through the use of heparin-coated circuitry, which reduces the amount of systemic heparinization needed, femorofemoral DAPP may be performed safely as long as the ACT is maintained for longer than 180 seconds. In addition, the heparin-coated circuitry increases the biocompatibility of the ECC system, decreasing the activation of the complement, kininogen, fibrinolytic, and coagulation pathways. The use of heparin-coated circuitry in the performance of femoral vein-to-femoral artery DAPP during TAAA repair has been associated with decreased heparin and protamine requirements, fewer anticoagulation bleeding complications, less bleeding and hemolysis, and reduced transfusion requirements, as compared to uncoated circuitry.[30]

CLINICAL RESULTS

Efficacy of any specific surgical technique is difficult to establish because our current technique has evolved over many years and the various aspects of the procedure have been modified as additional research findings have suggested ways of improvement. Nevertheless, it is useful to tabulate the overall results in a given practice because they provide the surgeon and the patient with a general estimate of risk. Over the past 21 years, the senior author (L.H.H.) has undertaken surgical repair of 265 TAAAs using routine intercostal reimplantation as the major effort to reduce neurologic deficit. During the past 16 years, CSF drainage has been added to the protocol. Over the past 11 years, use of a shunt or pump bypass has been added for types I and II TAAAs. Since the routine addition of the latter, we have seen no incidence of postoperative paraplegia, though transient paraparesis was occasionally noted. Moreover, since the additional use of selective visceral perfusion, we have had no intraoperative deaths. Tables 23–7 and 23–8 summarize our overall morbidity and mortality associated with TAAA repair and include both elective and ruptured aneurysms.

ENDOVASCULAR APPROACH TO THORACOABDOMINAL AORTIC ANEURYSMS

The treatment of abdominal aortic aneurysms by endovascular placement of stent-grafts represents a significant advance in the management of these lesions. The technique has undergone rapid improvements since its introduction in 1991. The application of endovascular therapy to thoracic and thoracoabdominal aneurysms has progressed less quickly owing to a number of anatomic limitations. The need for a 20-mm proximal neck for stent attachment limits the number of lesions that are amenable to endovascular grafting. The use of carotid-subclavian transposition can create a proximal aortic neck of sufficient length to overcome this limitation. In addition, newer devices have bare proximal stents which can be placed across the subclavian orifice to improve fixation in the case of shorter proximal necks. The major limitation of stent-grafting for TAAA is

TABLE 23-7

Mortality with Thoracoabdominal Aortic Aneurysms (TAAAs)

	TYPE OF TAAA				
	I	II	III	IV	Total
Patients (n)	40	74	78	73	265
or deaths (n [%])	5 (12.5)	2 (2.7)	2 (2.6)	0	9 (3.4)
30-day death (n [%])	2 (5.0)	4 (5.4)	5 (6.4)	1 (1.4)	12 (4.5)
Total (n [%])	7 (17.5)	6 (8.1)	7 (8.9)	1 (1.4)	21 (7.9)

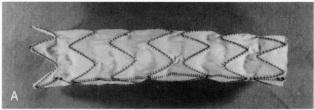
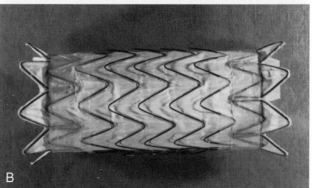

Figure 23–16. Examples of stent-grafts available for treatment of thoracic aortic aneurysms. *A*, The Talent thoracic endoprosthesis (World Medical Corporation, Sunrise, Fla.) and *(b)* the Gore Excluder Thoracis endoprosthesis (WL Gore and Associates, Flagstaff, Az).

the involvement of aortic segments that contain the origins of renal and visceral vessels. The use of composite techniques comprised of transabdominal or retroperitoneal replacement of aneurysmal abdominal aorta followed by placement of a stent-graft to exclude the descending thoracic aneurysm holds promise for expanding the application of this technique to more complex lesions. The inability to reimplant large patent intercostal arteries during endovascular stent-graft placement raises concern for postoperative paraplegia.

Early Results

The earliest devices for excluding thoracic aortic aneurysms were "homemade." Commercially produced stent-grafts designed specifically for TAAA are currently in clinical trials. These devices include the Talent thoracic system (World Medical, Sunrise, Fla.) and the Gore Excluder thoracic endoprosthesis (W.L. Gore & Associates, Inc., Flagstaff, Az.) which are shown in Figure 23–16. The results of endovascular stent-grafting for descending thoracic aneurysms in a series of 103 high-risk patients have recently been published.[85] The authors reported a mortality rate of 9%, and an early endoleak rate of 24%. Other major complications included stroke in 7%, paraplegia or paraperesis in 3%, myocardial infarction in 2%, and pulmonary complications in 12% of patients. There was a tendency toward higher paraplegia rates in patients with simultaneous abdominal and descending thoracic aneurysms. The high incidence of stroke was believed to be due to manipulation of catheters and sheaths in and around the aortic arch and its branches. At least one case of delayed-

onset paraplegia has been reported after stent-graft repair of a descending thoracic aortic aneurysm.[86] Another series of 25 high-risk patients has recently been reported. There was a 20% 30-day mortality rate and three conversions to open repair. Three patients developed neurologic deficits.[87]

In our own experience with endovascular repair of approximately 50 thoracic and thoracoabdominal aneurysms, we have also seen complications such as endoleak and delayed-onset paraparesis. Our ongoing experience has uncovered other complications. Delayed onset of back pain has been noted to occur in 8% of cases. In all of these cases, complete exclusion of the lesion without evidence of endoleak was demonstrated angiographically. This symptom may be related to muscle ischemia due to intercostal artery thrombosis. The development of clinically significant pleural effusion occurred in 10% of patients; some of whom required thoracentesis. In one patient, thoracentesis needed to be repeated. The etiology of this is unclear but may represent an inflammatory reaction due to stent compression of the aortic wall. Figure 23–17 demonstrates the case of a man who presented with a contained rupture of a descending thoracic aneurysm. The angiogram shows a penetrating ulcer in the descending aorta and the CT scan reveals fluid around the aorta indicating contained rupture. An intraoperative angiogram and follow-up CT scan demonstrate exclusion of the aneurysm with the stent-graft. As experience with this technology expands, we can expect a larger role for endovascular therapy in thoracic and abdominal aneurysm disease.

CONCLUSIONS

Care of the patient with a TAAA has been an evolutionary process in which past techniques have undergone improvement and reapplication, whereas other techniques have

TABLE 23-8

Neurologic Deficit with Thoracoabdominal Aortic Aneurysms (TAAA)

	TYPE OF TAAA				
	I	II	III	IV	Total
Patients (n)	40	74	78	73	265
Paraplegic or paraparesis (n [%])	3 (7.5)	4 (5.4)	4 (5.1)	1 (1.4)	12 (4.5)
Deficit at discharge (n [%])	1 (2.5)	3 (4.1)	1 (1.3)	0 (0)	5 (1.9)

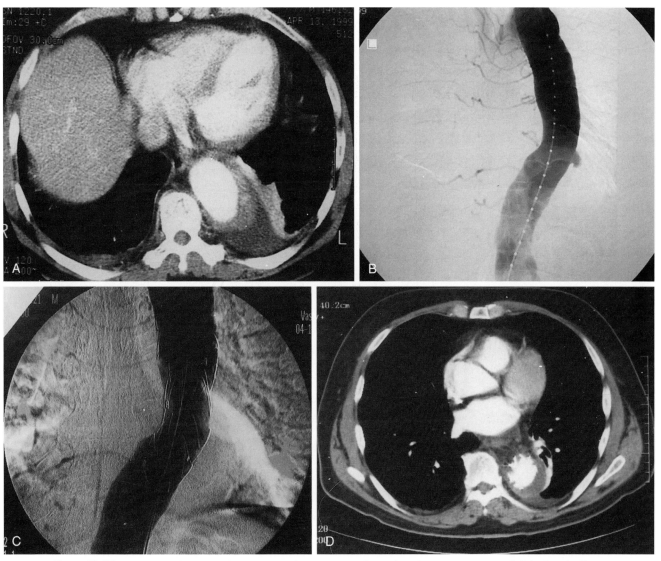

Figure 23–17. *A,* Computed tomography (CT) scan demonstrates a descending thoracic aneurysm with left pleural effusion indicating contained rupture. *B,* Preoperative angiogram illustrates penetrating ulcer of descending thoracic aorta. *C,* Intraoperative angiogram shows exclusion of the aneurysm with a stent-graft. *D,* Postoperative CT scan indicates successful exclusion of descending thoracic aneurysm without endoleak.

been newly introduced or discarded. Although all of the complexities of the pathophysiology of TAAA repair are not fully understood, research has greatly improved our knowledge over the past 10 years. Continued research efforts are necessary to provide a more thorough understanding of these processes, enabling us to further refine risk assessment, incorporate useful surgical and perioperative support techniques, and expand the multimodality prevention of perioperative complications. We hope this will allow a continued reduction in the morbidity and mortality associated with this most formidable of vascular surgical procedures. Perhaps the ability to treat TAAA from remote access sites using endovascular techniques will further reduce the morbidity and mortality associated with these aneurysms. The applicability of this technology to such complex lesions and its durability have yet to be demonstrated and must await further study.

ACKNOWLEDGMENT

We thank and acknowledge Mr. James Green for the original artwork appearing in this chapter.

References

1. Etheredge SN, Yee J, Smith JV, et al: Successful resection of a large aneurysm of the upper abdominal aorta and replacement with homograft. Surgery 38:1171–1181, 1955.
2. Hollier LH: Technical modifications in the repair of thoracoabdominal aortic aneurysms. In Greenhalgh RM (ed): Vascular Surgical Techniques. London, WB Saunders, 1989, pp 144–151.
3. Hollier LH, Money SR, Naslund TC, et al: Risk of spinal cord dysfunction in patients undergoing thoracoabdominal aortic replacement. Am J Surg 164:210–214, 1992.
4. Crawford ES, Crawford JL, Safi HJ, et al: Thoracoabdominal aortic aneurysms: Preoperative and intraoperative factors determining immediate and long-term results of operations in 605 patients. J Vasc Surg 3:389–404, 1986.
5. Safi HJ, Bartoli S, Hess KR, et al: Neurologic deficit in patients at high risk with thoracoabdominal aortic aneurysms: The role of cerebral spinal fluid drainage and distal aortic perfusion. J Vasc Surg 20:434–443, 1994.
6. Miller DC: Acute dissection of the descending thoracic aorta. Chest Surg Clin North Am 2:347–378, 1992.
7. DeBakey ME, Henley WS, Cooley DA, et al: Surgical management of dissecting aneurysms of the aorta. J Cardiovasc Surg 49:130–149, 1965.
8. Daily PO, Trueblood HW, Stinson EB, et al: Management of acute aortic dissections. Ann Thorac Surg 10:237–247, 1970.
9. Meng RL, Najafi H, Javid H, et al: Acute ascending aortic dissection: Surgical management. Circulation 64(Suppl 2):II-231–234, 1981.
10. Appelbaum A, Karp RB, Kirklin JW: Ascending vs descending aortic dissections. Ann Surg 183:296–300, 1976.
11. Doroghazi RM, Slater EE, DeSanctis RW, et al: Long-term survival of patients with treated aortic dissection. J Am Coll Cardiol 3:1026–11034, 1984.
12. Panneton JM, Hollier LH: Nondissecting thoracoabdominal aortic aneurysms: Part I. Ann Vasc Surg 9:503–514, 1995.
13. Coselli JS, LeMaire SA, Buket S: Marfan syndrome: The variability and outcome of operative management. J Vasc Surg 21:432–443, 1995.
14. Cikrit CF, Miles JH, Silver D: Spontaneous arterial perforation: The Ehlers-Danlos specter. J Vasc Surg 5:248–255, 1987.
15. Hollier LH, Money SR, Creely B, et al: Direct replacement of mycotic thoracoabdominal aneurysms. J Vasc Surg 18:477–485, 1993.
16. Bickerstaff LK, Pairolero PC, Hollier LH, et al: Thoracic aortic aneurysms: A population-based study. Surgery 92:1103–1108, 1982.
17. Crawford ES, DeNatale RW: Thoracoabdominal aortic aneurysm: Observations regarding the natural course of the disease. J Vasc Surg 3:578–582, 1986.
18. Cambria RA, Gloviczki P, Stanson AW, et al: Outcome and expansion rate of 57 thoracoabdominal aortic aneurysms managed nonoperatively. Am J Surg 170:213–217, 1995.
19. Fann JI, Miller C: Basic data underlying clinical decision making: Aortic dissection. Ann Vasc Surg 9:311–323, 1995.
20. Pressler V, McNamara JJ: Thoracic aortic aneurysm: Natural history and treatment. J Thorac Cardiovasc Surg 79:489–498, 1980.
21. Ergin MA, Phillips RA, Galla JD, et al: Significance of distal false lumen after type A dissection repair. Ann Thorac Surg 57:820–825, 1994.
22. Erbel R, Oelert H, Meyer J, et al: Effect of medical and surgical therapy on aortic dissection evaluated by transesophageal echocardiography: Implications for prognosis and therapy. Circulation 87:1604–1615, 1993.
23. Panneton JM, Hollier LH: Dissecting descending thoracic and thoracoabdominal aortic aneurysms: Part 2. Ann Vasc Surg 9:596–605, 1995.
24. Pennell RC, Hollier LH, Lie JT, et al: Inflammatory abdominal aortic aneurysms: A thirty year review. J Vasc Surg 2:859–869, 1985.
25. Crawford ES, Hess KR, Cohen ES, et al: Ruptured aneurysm of the descending thoracic and thoracoabdominal aorta. Ann Surg 213:417–426, 1991.
26. Dupuy DE, Hollier LH: Cine magnetic resonance angiography. In Greenhalgh RM (ed): Vascular Imaging for Surgeons. London, WB Saunders, 1995, pp 31–40.
27. McCullough JL, Hollier LH, Nugent M: Paraplegia after thoracic aortic occlusion: Influence of cerebrospinal fluid drainage. Experimental and early clinical results. J Vasc Surg 7:153–160, 1988.
28. Smeets HJ, Kievit J, Dulfer FT, vanKleef JW: Endocrine-metabolic response to abdominal aortic surgery: A randomized trial of general anesthesia versus general plus epidural anesthesia. World J Surg 17:601–606, 1993.
29. Kirno K, Friberg P, Grzegorczyk A, et al: Thoracic epidural anesthesia during coronary artery bypass surgery: Effects on cardiac sympathetic activity, myocardial blood flow and metabolism, and central hemodynamics. Anesth Analg 79:1075–1081, 1994.
30. von Segesser LK, Killer I, Jenni R, et al: Improved distal circulatory support for repair of descending thoracic aortic aneurysms. Ann Thorac Surg 56:1373–1380, 1993.
31. Safi HJ, Hess KR, Randel M, et al: Cerebral spinal fluid drainage and distal aortic perfusion: Reducing neurologic complications in repair of thoracoabdominal aortic aneurysm types I and II. J Vasc Surg 23:223–228, 1996.
32. Cambria RP, Davison JK, Giglia JS, Gertler JP: Mesenteric shunting decreases visceral ischemia during thoracoabdominal aneurysm repair. J Vasc Surg 27:745–749, 1998.
33. Gloviczki P, Cross SA, Stanson AW, et al: Ischemic injury to the spinal cord or lumbosacral plexus after aorto-iliac reconstruction. Am J Surg 162:131–136, 1991.
34. Bathe OF, Chow AWC, Phang PT: Splanchnic origin of cytokines in a porcine model of mesenteric ischemia-reperfusion. Surgery 123:79–88, 1998.
35. Tamion F, Richard V, Lyoumi S, et al: Gut ischemia and mesenteric synthesis of inflammatory cytokines after hemorrhagic or endotoxic shock. Am J Physiol 273:G314–G321, 1997.
36. Welborn MB III, Douglas WG, Abouhamze Z, et al: Visceral ischemia-reperfusion injury promotes tumor necrosis factor and interleukin-1 dependent organ injury in the mouse. Shock 6:171–176, 1996.
37. Yao YM, Sheng ZY, Yu Y, et al: The potential etiologic role of tumor necrosis factor in mediating multiple organ dysfunction in rats following intestinal ischemia-reperfusion injury. Resuscitation 29:157–168, 1995.
38. Yao YM, Bahrami S, Redl H, Schlag G: Monoclonal antibody to tumor necrosis factor-α attenuates hemodynamic dysfunction secondary to intestinal ischemia/reperfusion in rats. Crit Care Med 24:1547–1553, 1996.
39. Vermeulen EG, Blankenstein JD, van Urk H: Is organ ischemia a determinant of the outcome of operations for suprarenal aortic aneurysms? Eur J Surg 165:441–445, 1999.
40. Paterson IS, Klausner JM, Goldman G, et al: Pulmonary edema after aneurysm surgery is modified by mannitol. Ann Surg 210:796–801, 1989.
41. Klausner JM, Paterson IS, Mannick JA, et al: Reperfusion pulmonary edema. JAMA 261(7):1030–1035, 1989.
42. Svensson LG, Hess KR, Coselli JS, et al: A prospective study of respiratory failure after high risk surgery on thoracoabdominal abdominal aorta. J Vasc Surg 14:271–282, 1991.
43. Hallett JW Jr, Bower TC, Cherry KJ Jr, et al: Selection and preparation of high-risk patients for repair of abdominal aortic aneurysms. Mayo Clin Proc 69:763–768, 1994.
44. Murphy ME, Kolvenbach R, Aleksis M, et al: Antioxidant depletion in aortic crossclamping ischemia: Increase of the plasma α-tocopheryl quinone/α-tocopherol ratio. Free Radic Biol Med 13:95–100, 1992.
45. Tan S, Gelman S, Wheat JK, Parks DA: Circulating xanthine oxidase in human ischemia reperfusion. South Med J 88:479–482, 1995.
46. Seekamp A, Mulligan MS: Role of 2 integrins and ICAM-1 in lung injury following ischemia-reperfusion of rat hind limbs. Am J Pathol 143:464–472, 1993.
47. Seekamp A, Mulligan MS, Till GO, Ward PA: Requirements for neutrophil products and L-arginine in ischemia-reperfusion injury. Am J Pathol 142:1217–1226, 1993.
48. Cohen JR, Angus L, Asher A, et al: Disseminated intravascular coagulation as a result of supraceliac clamping: Implications for thoracoabdominal aneurysm repair. Ann Vasc Surg 1:552–557, 1987.
49. Cohen JR, Schroder W, Leal J, Wise L: Mesenteric shunting during thoracoabdominal aortic clamping to prevent disseminated intravascular coagulation in dogs. Ann Vasc Surg 2:261–267, 1988.
50. Kazui M, Andreoni KA, Williams GM, et al: Visceral lipid peroxidation occurs at reperfusion after supraceliac aortic cross-clamping. J Vasc Surg 19:473–477, 1994.
51. Hug HR, Taber RE: Bypass flow requirements during thoracic aneu-

rysmectomy with particular attention to the prevention of left heart failure. J Thorac Cardiovasc Surg 57:203–213, 1969.

52. Poldermans D, Boersma E, Bax JJ, et al: The effect of bisoprolol on perioperative mortality and myocardial infarction in high risk patients undergoing vascular surgery. Dutch Echocardiographic Cardiac Risk Evaluation Applying Stress Echocardiography Study Group. N Engl J Med 341:789–794, 1999.

53. Simpson JI, Eide TR, Schiff GA, et al: Effect of nitroglycerin on spinal cord ischemia after thoracic aortic cross-clamping. Ann Thorac Surg 61:113–117, 1996.

54. Cernaianu AC, Olah A, Cilley JH Jr, et al: Effects of sodium nitroprusside on paraplegia during cross-clamping of the thoracic aorta. Ann Thorac Surg 56:1035–1038, 1993.

55. Kazui T, Komatsu S, Yokoyama H: Surgical treatment of aneurysms of the thoracic aorta with the aid of partial cardiopulmonary bypass: An analysis of 95 patients. Ann Thorac Surg 43:622–627, 1987.

56. Gloviczki P, Toomey BJ, Panneton JM: Visceral and spinal cord protection during repair of thoracoabdominal aortic aneurysms: The Mayo Clinic experience. In Weimann S (ed): Thoracic and Thoracoabdominal Aortic Aneurysm. Bologna, Monduzzi Editore, 1994, pp 189–198.

57. Acher CW, Wynn MM, Hoch JR, et al: Combined use of cerebrospinal fluid drainage and naloxone reduces the risk of paraplegia in thoracoabdominal aneurysm repair. J Vasc Surg 19:236–248, 1994.

58. Svensson LG, Crawford ES, Hess KR, et al: Experience with 1509 patients undergoing thoracoabdominal aortic operations. J Vasc Surg 17:357–370, 1993.

59. Coselli JS, LeMaire SA, Poli de Figueiredo L, Kirby RP: Paraplegia after thoracoabdominal aortic aneurysm repair: Is dissection a risk factor? Ann Thorac Surg 63:28–36, 1997.

60. Moore WM Jr, Hollier LH: The influence of severity of spinal cord ischemia in the etiology of delayed-onset paraplegia. Ann Surg 213:427–432, 1991.

61. Hill AB, Kalman PG, Johnston KW, et al: Reversal of delayed-onset paraplegia after thoracic aortic surgery with cerebrospinal fluid drainage. J Vasc Surg 20:315–317, 1994.

62. Hollier LH: Protecting the brain and spinal cord. J Vasc Surg 5:524–528, 1987.

63. Svensson LG, Hess KR, Coselli JS, Safi HJ: Influence of segmental arteries, extent, and atriofemoral bypass on postoperative paraplegia after thoracoabdominal aortic operations. J Vasc Surg 20:255–262, 1994.

64. Safi HJ, Miller CC III, Carr C, et al: Importance of intercostal artery reattachment during thoracoabdominal aortic aneurysm repair. J Vasc Surg 27:58–66, 1998.

65. Hollier LH, Symmonds JB, Pairolero PC, et al: Thoracoabdominal aortic aneurysm repair. Analysis of postoperative morbidity. Arch Surg 123:871–875, 1988.

66. Coselli JS, LeMaire SA, Schmittling ZC, Koksoy C: Cerebrospinal fluid drainage in thoracoabdominal aortic surgery: Results of a prospective, randomized trial. Semin Vasc Surg 13:308–314, 2000.

67. Granke K, Hollier LH, Zdrahal P, Moore W: Longitudinal study of cerebral spinal fluid drainage in polyethylene glycol–conjugated superoxide dismutase in paraplegia associated with thoracic aortic cross-clamping. J Vasc Surg 13:615–621, 1991.

68. Coles JC, Ahmed SN, Mehta HU, Kaufmann JCE: Role of free radical scavenger in protection of spinal cord during ischemia. Ann Thorac Surg 41:551–556, 1986.

69. Wisselink W, Money SR, Crockett DE: Ischemia-reperfusion injury of the spinal cord: Protective effect of the hydroxyl radical scavenger dimethylthiourea. J Vasc Surg 20:444–450, 1994.

70. Clark WM, Madden KP, Rothlein R, Zivin JA: Reduction of central nervous system ischemic injury by monoclonal antibody to intracellular adhesion molecule. J Neurosurg 75:623–627, 1991.

71. Madden KP, Clark WM, Marcoux FW, et al: Treatment with conotoxin, an "N-type" calcium channel blocker, in neuronal hypoxic-ischemic injury. Brain Res 537:256–262, 1990.

72. Fowl RJ, Patterson RB, Gewirtz RJ, Anderson DK: Protection against postischemic spinal cord injury using a new 21-aminosteroid. J Surg Res 48:597–600, 1990.

73. Yum SW, Faden AI: Comparison of the neuroprotective effects of the N-methyl-D-aspartate antagonist MK-801 and the opiate-receptor antagonist nalmefene in experimental spinal cord ischemia. Arch Neurol 47:277–281, 1990.

74. Sakurai M, Hayashi T, Abe K, et al: Delayed and selective motor neuron death after transient spinal cord ischemia: A role of apoptosis. J Thorac Cardiovasc Surg 115:1310–1315, 1998.

75. Smith I, White PF, Nathanson M, Gouldson R: Propofol: An update on its clinical use. Anesthesiology 81:1005–1043, 1994.

76. Newman MF, Murkin JM, Roach G, et al: Cerebral physiologic effects of burst suppression doses of propofol during nonpulsatile cardiopulmonary bypass. CNS Subgroup of McSPI. Anesth Analg 81:452–457, 1995.

77. Murphy PG, Bennett JR, Myers DS, et al: The effect of propofol anaesthesia on free radical–induced lipid peroxidation in rat liver microsomes. Eur J Anaesthesiol 10:261–266, 1993.

78. Shyr MH, Tsai TH, Tan PP, et al: Concentration and regional distribution of propofol in brain and spinal cord during propofol anesthesia in the rat. Neurosci Lett 184:212–215, 1995.

79. LeMay DR, Neal S, Zelenock GB, D'Alecy LG: Paraplegia in the rat induced by aortic cross-clamping: Model characterization and glucose exacerbation of neurologic deficit. J Vasc Surg 6:383–390, 1987.

80. Fisher DF, Yawn DH, Crawford ES: Preoperative disseminated intravascular coagulation caused by abdominal aortic aneurysm. Arch Surg 118:1252–1255, 1983.

81. Thompson RW, Adams DH, Cohen JR: Disseminated intravascular coagulation caused by abdominal aortic aneurysm. J Vasc Surg 4:184–186, 1986.

82. Godet G, Samama CM, Ankri A, et al: Mécanismes et prédiction des complications hémorragiques au cours de la chirurgie des anévrysmes de l'aorte thoracoabdominale. Ann Fr Anesth Reanim 9:415–422, 1990.

83. Gertler JP, Cambria RP, Brewster DC, et al: Coagulation changes during thoracoabdominal aneurysm repair. J Vasc Surg 24:936–945, 1996.

84. Illig KA, Green RM, Ouriel K, et al: Primary fibrinolysis during supraceliac aortic clamping. J Vasc Surg 25:244–251, 1997.

85. Dake MD, Miller DC, Mitchell RS, et al: The first generation of endovascular stent-grafts for patients with descending thoracic aortic aneurysms. J Thorac Cardiovasc Surg 116:689–704, 1998.

86. Kasirajan K, Dolmatch B, Ouriel K, Clair D: Delayed onset of ascending paralysis after thoracic aortic stent graft deployment. J Vasc Surg 31:196–199, 2000.

87. Greenberg R, Resch T, Nyman U, et al: Endovascular repair of descending thoracic aortic aneurysms: An early experience with intermediate-term follow-up. J Vasc Surg 31:147–156, 2000.

Questions

1. The Crawford classification of thoracoabdominal aortic aneurysms
   (a) is based upon the extent of aortic involvement
   (b) applies to degenerative and dissected aneurysms
   (c) designates thoracoabdominal aortic aneurysms as type I through type IV
   (d) allows comparison between aneurysm type and treatment groups
   (e) all of the above

2. Each of the following classification systems describes aortic dissections except

   (a) DeBakey
   (b) Crawford
   (c) Stanford
   (d) Najafi
   (e) University of Alabama
   (f) Massachusetts General Hospital

3. Which of the following is the most common etiology of thoracoabdominal aortic aneurysms?
   (a) atherosclerotic medial degenerative disease
   (b) dissection
   (c) Marfan's syndrome

(d) Ehlers-Danlos syndrome

(e) Takayasu's aortitis

4. Assign a number (1 = shortest expected survival through 5 = longest expected survival) to each of the following 6-cm thoracoabdominal aortic aneurysms
   (a) repaired, nondissecting
   (b) not operated, nondissecting
   (c) ruptured
   (d) repaired, dissecting
   (e) not operated, acute, dissecting

5. The most accurate diagnostic modality for the diagnosis of a thoracoabdominal aortic aneurysm is
   (a) physical examination
   (b) ultrasonography
   (c) computed tomography
   (d) angiography
   (e) transesophageal echocardiography

6. The preoperative evaluation of patients being considered for thoracoabdominal aortic aneurysm repair should include which of the following systems?
   (a) respiratory
   (b) cardiac
   (c) renal
   (d) peripheral vascular
   (e) coagulation
   (f) all of the above

7. Pulmonary complications following thoracoabdominal aortic aneurysm repair may be reduced by
   (a) maximizing preoperative pulmonary function
   (b) epidural anesthesia/analgesia
   (c) reducing the ischemia-reperfusion phenomenon
   (d) minimizing pulmonary trauma
   (e) all of the above

8. The following modalities may be cardioprotective during thoracoabdominal aortic aneurysm repair except
   (a) epidural anesthesia/analgesia
   (b) supranormal left ventricular end-diastolic pressures
   (c) indicated preoperative myocardial revascularization
   (d) sodium nitroprusside
   (e) distal aortic perfusion

9. Preoperative renal insufficiency in patients with a thoracoabdominal aortic aneurysm is associated with an increased risk of
   (a) operative mortality
   (b) postoperative renal dysfunction
   (c) neurologic deficits
   (d) late death
   (e) all of the above

10. Variables predictive of neurologic deficit following thoracoabdominal aortic aneurysm repair include
    (a) prior proximal aortic aneurysm repair
    (b) aortic dissection
    (c) duration of aortic cross-clamping
    (d) extent of aorta replaced
    (e) oversewing intercostal arteries
    (f) all of the above

11. Techniques shown to reduce the incidence of neurologic deficit following thoracoabdominal aortic aneurysm repair include the following except
    (a) cerebrospinal fluid drainage
    (b) moderate hypothermia
    (c) distal aortic perfusion
    (d) reducing the ischemia-reperfusion phenomenon
    (e) hyperglycemia

Answers

1. e   2. b   3. a   4. a-5,   5. c   6. f   7. e   8. b   9. e   10. f   11. e
                          b-3,
                          c-1,
                          d-4,
                          e-2

24

Aneurysms of the Aorta and Iliac Arteries

Jerry Goldstone

Aneurysms of the abdominal aorta are a common condition. The incidence (the number of new cases) of this entity has been estimated at between 30 and 66 per 1000 persons, and since 1970 it has tripled. Unfortunately, the age-specific death rate from ruptured aneurysms has also increased. The increasing incidence has been noted in the United States as well as other Western countries and appears to be real and not merely a reflection of the increasing age of the population and improved diagnostic methods.[1-4] The incidence and prevalence (the number of existing cases) vary, depending on the population studied, being lowest in unselected groups and higher in patient groups with other atherosclerotic lesions (Table 24–1).[5-10] In a study at Massachusetts General Hospital, abdominal aortic aneurysms were found in 2% of 24,000 consecutive autopsies.[5] In a more recent autopsy series from Malmö, Sweden, abdominal aortic aneurysms were found in 4.3% of men and 2.1% of women.[6] The frequency of aneurysms increases steadily in men older than 55 years, reaching a peak of 5.9% at 80 to 85 years. In women, there is a continuous increase after 70 years of age, reaching a peak of 4.5% at age greater than 90 years. In community screening programs, the prevalence in males 65 to 74 years old ranges from 2.7% to 3.4%, whereas in elderly hypertensive men and women, the prevalence has been found to be from 10.7% to 12%.[11, 12]

Abdominal aortic aneurysms have a propensity for sudden rupture and death. Approximately 15,000 deaths per year are due to abdominal aortic aneurysm, making this the 13th leading cause of death in the United States. It is the 10th leading cause of death in men. The importance of this condition is obvious. The only way to reduce the death rate is to identify and treat these lesions before they rupture.

There is disagreement as to what constitutes an aneurysm. The ad hoc committee on reporting standards of the Society for Vascular Surgery (SVS) and the International Society for Cardiovascular Surgery (ISCVS) (North American Chapter) has defined an *aneurysm* as a permanent localized dilatation of an artery with increase in diameter of greater than 50% (1.5 times) its normal diameter.[13] However, the normal value for an artery depends on several factors, including age, sex, and blood pressure, and the aortic diameter steadily increases with age. Thus, the normal infrarenal aortic diameter in a 75-year-old person can vary from 12.4 mm in a small woman to 27.6 mm in a large man.[14] The normal sizes of the aorta in males and females are listed in Table 24–2.[14] Generalized dilatation of an artery, frequently present in patients with aneurysms, but with increased diameter of less than 50% of normal is termed *ectasia*, whereas *arteriomegaly* represents diffuse enlargement of the arterial tree but not large enough to meet the criteria for aneurysm.[15] In some patients with abdominal aortic aneurysms, the entire aortoiliofemoral

TABLE 24–1

Incidence of Abdominal Aortic Aneurysms (%)

Autopsy	1.5–3.0
Unselected patients screened by ultrasonography	3.2
Selected patients with CAD	5.0
Selected patients with PVD	10.0
Patients with femoral or popliteal aneurysms	50.0

CAD, coronary artery disease; PVD, peripheral vascular disease.

TABLE 24–2

Normal Diameter of Human Aorta*

	11th RIB	SUPRARENAL	INFRARENAL	BIFURCATION
Male	26.9 ± 3.9	23.9 ± 3.9	21.4 ± 3.6	18.7 ± 3.3
Female	24.4 ± 3.4	21.6 ± 3.1	18.7 ± 3.3	17.5 ± 2.5

*All measurements in millimeters, plus or minus standard error.
Data from Steinberg CR, Morton A, Steinberg I: Measurement of the abdominal aorta after intravenous aortography in health and arteriosclerotic peripheral vascular disease. AJR 95:703, 1965.

arterial tree is arteriomegalic or ectatic. Thus, an aorta of any given diameter may be merely dilated, ectatic, or an aneurysm, depending on the size of the normal aorta above the dilated segment.

Aneurysms of the infrarenal aorta are by far the most common arterial aneurysms encountered in clinical practice. They occur from three to seven times more frequently than thoracic aneurysms. Men are affected more than women by a ratio of 4:1.[8] Other aneurysms frequently coexist in patients with aortic aneurysms, including common or internal iliac aneurysms (20%–30%) and femoropopliteal aneurysms (in about 15% of patients). Conversely, popliteal aneurysms are markers of abdominal aortic aneurysms. Aortic aneurysms can be found in about 8% of patients who are diagnosed with a unilateral popliteal aneurysm but in up to 50% of patients who have bilateral popliteal aneurysms. In at least one group of patients with carotid atherosclerosis, there was a 10% incidence of abdominal aortic aneurysm, and in another group of patients with tortuous internal carotid arteries, a 40% incidence of aortic aneurysms was found.[16, 17] Aortic aneurysms are found in 1.5% to 3.0% of ultrasound-screened British males older than 60 years. Aortic aneurysms have also been detected by ultrasound screening in 8.8% of male smokers older than 65 years who have peripheral vascular occlusive disease. Screening appears to be cost-effective in selected patient groups such as these.[18]

Cigarette smoking also correlates with the presence of aortic aneurysms, there being an 8:1 preponderance of aneurysms in smokers compared with nonsmokers. Hypertension is another common accompanying condition, factor in up to 40% of patients with aortic aneurysms. All of these associations have implications regarding the cause of aneurysms.

ETIOLOGY/PATHOGENESIS OF AORTIC ANEURYSMS

There are several well known but uncommon causes of true abdominal aortic aneurysm, including cystic medial necrosis, dissection, Ehlers-Danlos syndrome, and syphilis. Most aortic aneurysms, however, are associated with atherosclerosis, and this has traditionally been considered the primary etiology. This concept has been seriously challenged in recent years by new information that indicates the participation of several factors in addition to atherosclerosis.[19] One observation casting doubt on atherosclerosis as the sole cause of aortic aneurysms is that most patients with aneurysmal disease do not have occlusive vascular disease involving the aortoiliofemoral segments.[20, 21] It has been estimated that no more than about 25% of aortic aneurysms are associated with significant occlusive disease.[22] Also, induction of aneurysms in animals fed an atherogenic diet has not been predictable, although regression of experimental atheromata has led to aneurysm formation in monkeys. These plus several other observations indicate that atherosclerosis is either a coincidental or facilitating process rather than the primary etiology.

Biochemical studies have shown decreased quantities of both elastin and collagen in the wall of aneurysms.[23–26] Elastin depletion is complete early in aneurysm develop-

ment. This has been correlated with the histopathologic features of a thin, dilated wall with replacement and fragmentation of the elastin in the media by a much thinner layer of collagen. This thinned wall usually contains calcium as well as atherosclerotic lesions, rendering the wall brittle. Laminated thrombus lines the lumen concentrically, resulting in a nearly normal flow channel (Figs. 24–1 through 24–3). Elongation of aneurysms occurs as they enlarge, causing them to become bowed and tortuous.[21] It is believed that it is the weakening and fragmentation of the elastic lamellas (elastin) that permits vessels to lengthen excessively and become tortuous. Thus, failure of elastin to provide sufficient retractive force in the circumferential, as well as in the longitudinal, direction allows for the increased diameter and length, respectively, of aneurysms.

The aortic wall is made up of lamellar units that consist of collagen (mainly types I and III) and elastin, as well as vascular smooth muscle cells. There are more lamellar units in the thoracic than in the abdominal aorta, and there is a further abrupt decrease below the renal arteries. Mature elastin and collagen are the major structural proteins responsible for the integrity of the aortic wall. Collagen makes up about 25% of the wall of an atherosclerotic aorta but only 6% to 18% of an aneurysmal aortic wall. In addition, the fragmentation of the elastin and the overall thinning of the wall contribute to its weakening.[21] The large loss of elastin is one of the most consistent biochemical and histochemical findings in human aortic aneurysms.[27]

These well-established histologic features have prompted a search for nonatherogenic mechanisms that disrupt collagen and elastin in the aortic wall. Several investigators have found excessive collagenase (MMP-1,2,3) activity in the wall of aneurysmal aortas, and others have found increased elastase (MMP-9) activity. These are members of a family of matrix metalloproteases that are now thought to play an essential role in aneurysm formation. Increased activity of other matrix proteases in aneurysmal aortic tissue has also been reported, as has an increased leukocyte-derived elastase in the blood of smokers with aneurysms. Deficiencies in antiproteases, such as several tissue inhibitors of metalloprotease (TIMP) and α_1-antitrypsin, have also been described. The latter is one of the most important natural antagonists to elastase. This may explain the association of aortic aneurysm rupture and chronic obstructive pulmonary disease (emphysema patients with reduced α_1-antitrypsin levels).[28] Another factor is the chronic inflammatory infiltrate that occurs in the outer layers of aneurysmal aortas, consisting of macrophages and T and B lymphocytes. There are also increased levels of IgG and IgM that are not seen in association with aging or with occlusive aortic lesions. These inflammatory cells are believed to interact in some as yet unexplained way with the connective tissue cells and matrix proteins in the pathogenesis of aneurysms.[29, 30] Most of the research has focused on the aortic media, but the role of the adventitia in aneurysm formation has recently been investigated. Normally, the adventitia is thought to limit maximum aortic diameter. Topical application of elastase to the adventitia leads to aneurysm formation in experimental animals solely due to degradation of elastin.[31]

Although not all of the studies of this type are conclusive, it is now generally agreed that an imbalance between

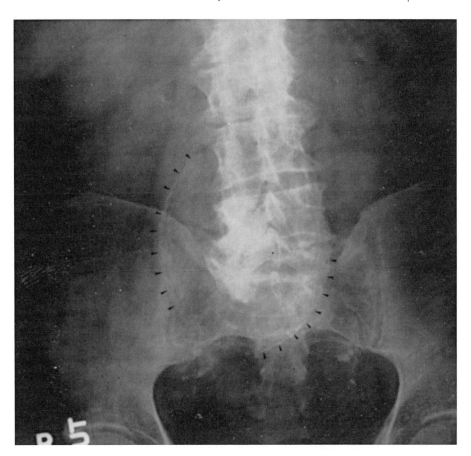

Figure 24–1. Plain abdominal radiograph showing large aortic aneurysm with calcified rim (*arrowheads*).

aortic wall proteases and antiproteases is an important factor in the pathogenesis of human abdominal aortic aneurysms. This imbalance causes degradation of extracellular matrix and loss of structural integrity of the aortic wall and

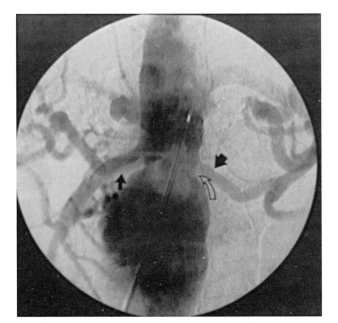

Figure 24–2. Digital subtraction aortogram of large juxtarenal aneurysm. This angled view allows identification of short infrarenal neck (*open arrow*) and origins of both renal arteries (*dark arrows*).

is largely responsible for the extensive remodeling of the aorta that occurs during aneurysm formation.

There is also considerable evidence that there is a genetic susceptibility to aortic aneurysm formation.[32, 33] Several investigators have discovered genetically linked enzyme deficiencies that are associated with aneurysms in experimental animals. For example, Tilson and coworkers have shown that a deficiency in the copper-containing enzyme lysyl oxidase is the cause of aortic aneurysms in a strain of mice.[34, 35] Lysyl oxidase is important in collagen and elastin cross-linking. Furthermore, this enzyme defect is sex chromosome–linked. In addition, several reports of familial clustering of abdominal aneurysms support the notion of a genetic predisposition to this disease.[36–39] Approximately 20% to 29% of patients with abdominal aneurysms have a first-order relative with the same condition.[38] The age- and sex-adjusted increased risk is 11.6 times, according to one report. Female siblings are at particularly high risk. The genetic pattern of increased susceptibility has not been worked out. Available evidence supports both X chromosome–linked and autosomal dominant patterns of inheritance.

Hemodynamic (mechanical) factors may also play a role in aneurysm development. The abdominal aorta is subjected to large pulsatile stresses as a result of its tapering geometry, relatively increased stiffness, and the reflected pressure waves from the peripheral vessels. Reductions in the number of elastic lamellae and the virtual lack of vasa vasorum in the media of the distal abdominal aorta may also be factors favoring aneurysmal formation in this seg-

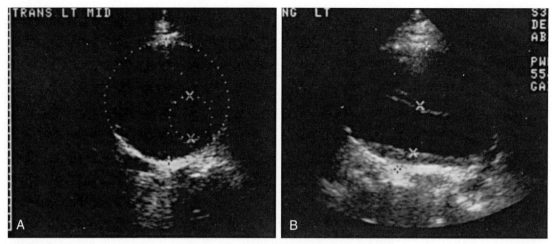

Figure 24–3. *A*, B mode ultrasound scan showing large aortic aneurysm measuring 74.7 mm in diameter and mural thrombus creating smaller lumen (26.4 mm) (*transverse view*). *B*, B mode ultrasound scan in same patient showing large aortic aneurysm, mural thrombus, and nearly normal flow channel (*longitudinal view*).

ment of the arterial tree by making the aorta structurally less well adapted to handle the increased hemodynamic stresses that occur there.[22]

In summary, contemporary concepts of aortic aneurysm development and growth must incorporate two distinctly different pathophysiologic processes: (1) elastin fragmentation as the critical structural defect required for aneurysm *formation*, and (2) collagen deposition and degradation governing aneurysm *enlargement*. Many other processes interact with these to produce the clinical features that are so well recognized. So, for the present, these aneurysms should be referred to as degenerative or nonspecific rather than atherosclerotic. They account for more than 90% of abdominal aortic aneurysms.

Once an aneurysm develops, regardless of the cause, its enlargement is governed by physical principles, especially Laplace's law. This law describes the relationship between the tangential stress (T) tending to disrupt the wall of a sphere and the radius (R) and transmural pressure (P): T = PR. Thus, for a given transmural pressure, the wall tension is proportional to the radius. Once dilatation of the aorta has started, Laplace's law explains why aortic enlargement is enhanced. It also explains why large aneurysms are more prone to rupture than small ones and why hypertension is an important risk factor for rupture. Using Laplace's law, tripling the aortic radius from 2 to 6 cm results in a 12-fold increase in wall tension, and when this tension exceeds the tensile strength of the collagen in the aortic wall, disruption occurs.

CLINICAL MANIFESTATIONS

From 70% to 75% of all infrarenal abdominal aortic aneurysms are asymptomatic when first detected.[37] This most often occurs during a routine physical examination or during an imaging study performed for some other reason (i.e., upper gastrointestinal series, barium enema, intravenous pyelogram, lumbosacral spine radiographs, or abdominal computed tomography or ultrasound examination). Occasionally, an aneurysm is first discovered during an unrelated abdominal operation.

Abdominal aortic aneurysms may cause symptoms as a result of rupture or expansion, pressure on adjacent structures, embolization, dissection, or thrombosis.[40, 41] Compression of adjacent bowel can cause early satiety and even nausea and vomiting. Virtually any type of abdominal, flank, or back pain can be caused by an aneurysm. This fact often leads to delays in diagnosis. Abdominal or back pain is the most common symptom, occurring in up to one third of patients. Large aneurysms can actually erode the spine and cause severe back pain even in the absence of rupture.

The abrupt onset of severe pain in the back, flank, or abdomen is characteristic of aneurysmal *rupture* or *expansion*. It is not certain why pain is produced by an expanding but unruptured (intact) aneurysm. The best explanation is sudden stretching of the layers of the aortic wall with pressure on adjacent somatic sensory nerves or overlying peritoneum. Tenderness of the palpated aneurysm suggests that abdominal symptoms are arising from the aneurysm. In most surgical series, symptomatic but unruptured aneurysms make up from 6% to nearly 40% of cases (average of five series totaling 311 patients: 13.7%). The determination of the timing of surgical treatment is made more difficult in these cases.

Ruptured aneurysms comprise between 20% and 25% of most series. The presence of an aneurysm is known in about 25% to 33% of patients before rupture. The nature of symptoms and their time course vary, depending on the nature of the rupture.[42–44] Small tears of the aneurysmal sac may result in a small leak that at least temporarily seals with minimal blood loss. This is usually followed within a few hours by frank rupture, which produces a catastrophic medical emergency. Rupture most frequently occurs through the posterolateral aortic wall into the retroperitoneal space and less commonly through the anterior wall into the free peritoneal cavity. The incidence of this latter type of rupture is higher than indicated in most surgical series, because most of these patients die before reaching the hospital. Rarely, an abdominal aortic aneurysm ruptures into the inferior vena cava or one of the iliac veins, producing an aortocaval (or aortoiliac) fistula, or into the gastrointestinal tract, producing a primary aortoenteric fistula.

The classic clinical manifestations of ruptured aortic aneurysm consist of mid- or diffuse abdominal pain, shock, and a pulsatile abdominal mass. The pain may be more prominent in the back or flank, or it may radiate into the groin or thigh. Because the most frequent site of rupture is the left posterolateral wall, pain is more commonly felt on the left side. It tends to be severe and steady. The severity of the shock varies from mild to profound, depending on the amount of blood loss. Abdominal distention is common, often preventing palpation of the pulsatile abdominal mass. The duration of symptoms may vary from a few minutes to more than 24 hours. Although aneurysm rupture is usually an acute catastrophic event, it can be contained for prolonged periods. These *chronic ruptures* have masqueraded as radicular compression, symptomatic inguinal hernia, femoral neuropathy, and even obstructive jaundice. It is thought that chronic contained ruptures eventually progress to free ruptures, and they should, therefore, be treated surgically on an urgent basis.[45]

The pain of an expanding but intact aneurysm may closely mimic that of a ruptured one. It tends to be severe, constant, and unaffected by position. The signs of hypovolemia are absent because hypotension and shock do not usually occur in the absence of actual rupture.

The diverse and nonspecific nature of the pain caused by expanding and leaking aneurysms all too often leads to errors in diagnosis, delays in finally establishing the correct diagnosis, and catastrophic rupture in the midst of a diagnostic procedure. Occasionally, a patient with a contained rupture arrives in the emergency room with angina pectoris from blood loss and reflex tachycardia and is rapidly transported to a coronary care unit without the abdominal examination that would identify the true cause of the chest pain. Most diagnostic errors such as these are due either to failure to palpate the expansile, pulsatile epigastric mass or to consider ruptured aneurysm as a possibility.

DIAGNOSTIC METHODS

Careful physical examination can detect most large aneurysms. Except in thin patients, an abdominal aortic aneurysm must be about 5 cm in diameter to be detectable on a routine physical examination. Thus, aneurysms palpated in obese patients are large. The reported accuracy in establishing the correct diagnosis by physical examination alone ranges between 30% and 90%. However, even when an aneurysm is detected, determination of its size by palpation is imprecise. Obesity, ascites, and patient uncooperativeness impair aneurysmal detection by physical examination. On the other hand, tumors or cystic lesions adjacent to the aorta, unusual aortic tortuosity, and excessive lumbar lordosis can all lead to a diagnosis of abdominal aortic aneurysm when none is present. The expansile nature of a pulsatile mass is a key element in deciding whether it is an aneurysm.

Although physical examination detects most large aneurysms, more objective methods are available to measure size and identify smaller aneurysms. Size determination is especially important, because it is the most important criterion of rupture and often determines management decisions. Plain abdominal and lateral spine radiographs can establish the diagnosis of 67% to 75% of abdominal aortic aneurysms by detecting a fine rim of calcium representing the aortic wall (see Fig. 24–1). Unfortunately, accurate determination of maximal aortic size is possible in only about two thirds of these cases. Therefore, a negative or inadequate plain film cannot be relied on to exclude the diagnosis of aortic aneurysm.

Imaging Modalities for Abdominal Aortic Aneurysms

Several imaging modalities are now widely available for establishing the presence of an aortic aneurysm and accurately determining its size.[46] These include ultrasonography, CT, and MRI.

Real-time, *B mode ultrasonography* is available in most hospitals and clinics. It employs no ionizing radiation, provides structural detail of vessel walls and atherosclerotic plaques, and can accurately measure aneurysm size in longitudinal as well as cross-sectional directions (three-dimensional) (see Fig. 24–3). Compared with intraoperative measurements, ultrasonic measurements are accurate to within ± 5 mm. Many studies have documented the ability of B mode ultrasonography to establish the diagnosis and accurately determine the size of abdominal and peripheral aneurysms.[47–49] Ultrasonography has not been as useful for imaging the thoracic or suprarenal aorta because of the overlying air-containing lung. Similarly, it has been less reliable in defining the relationship between abdominal aortic aneurysms and the renal arteries. Although use of a transesophageal ultrasound transducer can largely avoid this problem, this is not practical for routine evaluation of abdominal aortic disease. Because ultrasonography can obtain images in longitudinal, transverse, and oblique projections, it can be especially helpful in differentiating a tortuous aorta from an aneurysm.

Ultrasonography requires considerable skill on the part of the technician to obtain a satisfactory image, and interpretation can sometimes be difficult. The images are also impaired by obesity, intestinal gas, or barium in the bowel. The overlying bowel gas often interferes with evaluation of the iliac arteries. The major advantages of ultrasonography are its wide availability, its painlessness and absence of known side effects, its lack of ionizing radiation, its relatively low cost, and its ability to image vessels in longitudinal as well as cross-sectional planes. The studies can be performed quickly and at the bedside. In addition, the portability of ultrasound machines is advantageous for the emergency room evaluation of suspected ruptured aneurysms. Emergency room ultrasonography can establish the presence of an aneurysm in most cases, but it is not nearly as accurate in demonstrating rupture. These factors make ultrasonography the modality of choice for the initial evaluation of pulsatile abdominal or peripheral masses and for follow-up surveillance of aneurysms to determine increase in size.

CT employs ionizing radiation to obtain cross-sectional images of the aorta and other body structures. CT images provide reliable information about the size of the entire aorta, including the thoracic aorta, so the extent as well as the size of an aneurysm can be accurately measured. Mod-

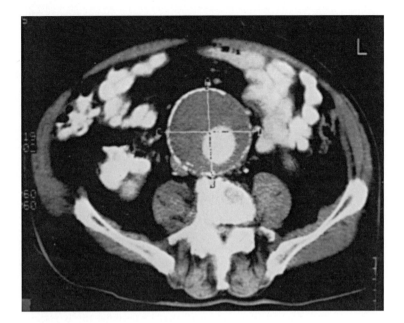

Figure 24–4. Computed tomography scan of abdomen showing large calcified abdominal aortic aneurysm (82.7 mm in diameter).

ern CT scanners possess sufficient spatial resolution to allow identification of celiac, superior mesenteric, renal, and iliac arteries and their relationship to the aneurysm as well as adjacent organs. Major venous structures, including anomalies, can also be identified by CT.[49] The administration of intravenous contrast allows evaluation of the size of the aortic lumen, the amount and location of mural thrombus, and, in the presence of dissection, differentiation of the true from the false lumen (Fig. 24–4). Contrast-enhanced CT scans are also useful for assessing the retroperitoneum and can identify retroperitoneal hematoma (aneurysmal rupture) and the periaortic fibrosis associated with inflammatory aneurysms.[50-53]

CT images are degraded by patient motion and the presence of metallic surgical clips. CT scanning requires more time and is more expensive than ultrasonography and only provides images in one (transverse) plane, but it gives more information about other abdominal and retroperitoneal structures than ultrasound. One of the most helpful uses of CT is to define the relationship of an aneurysm to the renal artery origins. Depending on the thickness of each CT slice and the distance between slices, this is not always accurate, especially when there is buckling of the aorta to the extent that the superior border of the aneurysm ascends anterior to the aorta. Many of the limitations of conventional CT scans are avoided by spiral or helical CT scans, which have emerged as an excellent technique to image the abdominal aorta and its branches.[54, 55] Scan times are extremely short and slices as thin as 2 to 3 mm can be obtained. This allows three-dimensional reconstruction of the overlapping cross-sectional images, producing a CT angiography (CTA) scan (Fig. 24–5). Spiral CT is quicker and is associated with less radiation exposure than aortography, but it requires a relatively large volume of intravenously administered contrast. Since the reconstructed three-dimensional images can be rotated in space and viewed from any projection, CTA is an excellent method of determining the often complex relationships between the aorta, its branches, and the aneurysm. Overall, spiral CT scans are currently the most useful imaging method

for evaluation of the abdominal aorta and have nearly obviated the need for aortography in the evaluation of aneurysmal disease. This technique has also become an almost essential component of the process of determining suitability for and size of endograft treatment of aneurysms.

MRI has also proved to be a useful imaging modality for evaluation of aortic aneurysms[51, 56] (Fig. 24–6). MRI employs radiofrequency energy and a strong magnetic field to produce images in longitudinal, transverse, and coronal planes. MRI instruments are not as widely available as ultrasound or CT scanners, and interpretation of the images requires considerable experience and skill. The spatial resolution has significantly improved, but the presence of

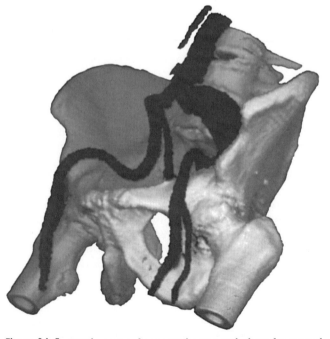

Figure 24–5. Spiral computed tomography scan with three-dimensional reconstruction showing large left common iliac aneurysm, as viewed from inferior oblique projection.

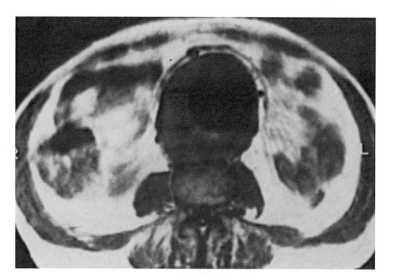

Figure 24–6. Magnetic resonance image of large abdominal aortic aneurysm showing eccentric mural thrombus and flow channel.

metallic surgical clips, cardiac pacemakers, and monitoring equipment makes MRI impossible to perform. Also, these studies are more expensive and require more time than either CT or ultrasonography scans. Nevertheless, MRI clearly distinguishes arteries and veins from viscera and other surrounding tissue. MR imaging of aortic aneurysms has excellent agreement with ultrasound and CT images in determining aortic diameter, and MRI is better at demonstrating involvement of branch vessels. This is especially true for the renal arteries. Some authors have reported visualization of the renal arteries in more than 90% of cases.[51] Other advantages of MRI over CT are the lack of ionizing radiation, its ability to obtain multiplane images, and the relatively large field of image. In addition, it is not necessary to use toxic contrast agents for MRI scans to achieve intravascular enhancement; however, paramagnetic contrast agents, such as gadolinium, can improve the images of vascular structures.

MRI instruments are able to quantitate blood flow and reconstruct images to look like conventional angiograms (MR angiography [MRA]).[46] These techniques are becoming routinely available, and magnetic resonance (MR) may become the only imaging method necessary for most patients with aortic disease of any type. However, at present, adequate visualization of aortic branch arteries is not as frequently achieved with MRA as with CT angiography, and a significant number of patients cannot complete MR scans because of claustrophobia.

Objective documentation of the size should probably be accomplished with one of these imaging modalities in all patients with suspected abdominal aortic aneurysm. Each method can measure the diameter accurately. An initial scan can be used for comparison with subsequent scans to determine aneurysmal enlargement. For routine situations, ultrasonography is probably the method of choice because of its widespread availability, lower cost, and lack of ionizing radiation. When there is suspicion of suprarenal or thoracoabdominal aortic involvement or dissection, MR imaging or CT is preferable. For pre-operative planning, a multiplanar study with three-dimensional reconstruction (CTA, MRA) is usually indicated to clearly delineate the aneurysm, aortic branch vessels, and neighboring struc-

tures. This is especially true if treatment by endografting is being considered.

For symptomatic aneurysms, MR imaging and CT also have the advantage over ultrasonography because of their better ability to identify contained rupture. CT and MR imaging probably have equally superior capability to demonstrate unexpected features such as venous anomalies, perianeurysmal fibrosis, and horseshoe kidney, although the ureters are not easily identified by MR imaging.

Aortography

The limitations of aortography for the diagnosis and evaluation of aortic aneurysms, like those of plain film roentgenograms, are well known. Because the nearly always present mural thrombus tends to reduce the aneurysmal lumen size toward normal, aortography is not a reliable method to determine the diameter of an aneurysm or even to establish its presence. With better imaging methods now routinely available, aortography has little use as a *diagnostic method* for abdominal aortic aneurysms. However, it may be useful in the preoperative evaluation of some patients with aneurysms.[57, 58] It can define the extent of an aneurysm, especially suprarenal and iliac involvement, and also the associated arterial lesions involving renal and visceral vessels, as well as distal occlusive lesions (Table 24–3; see also Fig. 24–2). Although many of these associated lesions are readily detectable and then manageable intraoperatively, preoperative identification of such lesions is useful in planning operative strategy, especially if complex anatomy is suspected. It must be emphasized that aortography used in this way is not a diagnostic study used to determine presence or size of an abdominal aneurysm.

There are risks associated with aortography, including potential renal toxicity from the large contrast volumes that are sometimes required to adequately fill a large aneurysm and the branch vessels. In addition, manipulation of a retrograde catheter through the laminated mural thrombus risks distal embolization, and there is always the possibility of local complications at the arterial puncture site through which the angiographic catheter is introduced. The use of

Angiographically Detected Lesions Associated with Abdominal Aortic Aneurysms

FINDINGS	TOTAL PATIENTS	NUMBER	(%)
Suprarenal extension	680	46	6.7
Renal stenosis/occlusion	763	138	18.0
Accessory/multiple renal artery	680	92	13.5
Celiac/superior mesenteric artery stenosis	628	87	13.8
Iliofemoropopliteal stenosis/occlusion	680	298	43.5
Iliofemoropopliteal aneurysm	680	243	34.2

Collected data from Rich NM, Clagett GP, Salander JM, et al: Role of arteriography in the evaluation of aortic aneurysms. In Bergan JJ, Yao JST (eds): Aneurysms: Diagnosis and Treatment. New York, Grune & Stratton, 1982, pp 233–241; Gaspar MR: Role of arteriography in the evaluation of aortic aneurysms. The case against. In Bergan JJ, Yao JST (eds): Aneurysms: Diagnosis and Treatment. New York, Grune & Stratton, 1982, pp 243–254.

digital subtraction angiographic techniques has lessened but not eliminated these risks. Aortography should be performed very selectively in patients with aneurysms for the following indications:[59] (1) clinical suspicion of visceral ischemia, (2) occlusive iliofemoral vascular lesions, (3) severe hypertension or impaired renal function in a patient in whom a concomitant renal artery stenosis would be repaired if discovered, (4) suspicion of presence of a horseshoe kidney, (5) suspicion of suprarenal or thoracoabdominal aneurysm, and (6) the presence of femoral or popliteal aneurysms. With the evolution and availability of MRI, MRA, and spiral CT, it is now possible to obtain information similar to that available from aortography, with fewer complications.

RISK OF ANEURYSM RUPTURE

As noted earlier, the majority of abdominal aortic aneurysms are now discovered in asymptomatic patients or during an evaluation for an unrelated problem. Aneurysms are being discovered at a smaller size than when the original studies on their natural history were first published by Estes, Wright, Szilagyi, and others.[60–62] Most aneurysms detected in screening programs are small (<5.0 cm). Even though aneurysms can cause symptoms and serious consequences from thrombosis and distal embolization, rupture is the most important risk, and the size of an aneurysm is the most important factor that determines the risk of rupture. In general, the risk of rupture correlates directly with size: the larger the aneurysm, the greater the risk of rupture. For example, the *yearly* risk of rupture for abdominal aortic aneurysms[5, 28, 63, 64] between 4.0 and 5.4 cm in size is about 0.5% to 1.0% and increases to 6.6% for aneurysms between 6.0 and 7.0 cm and to 19% for aneurysms larger than 7.0 cm in diameter.[5, 64, 65] Calculated as 5-year rupture rates, these figures become 5%, 33%, and 95%, respectively. The steepness of a curve plotting this type of data increases sharply at a diameter of about 6 cm, and this led to earlier recommendations to defer elective aneurysm repair until an aneurysm reached this size. More contem-

porary data, obtained from objective imaging studies, were interpreted as showing that aneurysm rupture risk begins to increase at a diameter of 5.0 cm, and this led to the SVS-ISCVS guidelines adoption of this size as the important surgical decision point.[66] However, even though still smaller aneurysms can and occasionally do rupture, this recommendation may need to be revised in light of data from two randomized, controlled clinical trials that studied survival in patients with asymptomatic abdominal aortic aneurysms that were between 4.0 and 5.4 to 5.5 cm in diameter. These studies were the United Kingdom (UK) Small Aneurysm Trial, published in 1998, and the Veterans Administration sponsored ADAM (Aneurysm Detection and Management) trial (unpublished as of this writing).[67, 68] These two trials were quite similar in design, size, and results. The rupture rate for aneurysms in these trials was 0.5% to 1.0% per year, and neither trial showed a difference in long-term survival, the primary end point, between patients allocated to early operation or ultrasonography or CT surveillance. The 6-year survival in both groups was 64% in the UK and about 70% in the ADAM trial. Even though 61% of those randomized to surveillance in both studies ultimately underwent aneurysm operations, for enlargement or symptoms, long-term survival was not improved by early operation. Furthermore, delaying operation for these small aneurysms was not associated with increased operative or late mortality. These data are consistent with those from older, nonrandomized studies.[69–71] For example, the population-based data from Rochester, Minnesota, showed a mean enlargement rate for aneurysms less than 5.0 cm diameter of only 0.32 cm/year, and after 5 years of observation, no aneurysm less than 5.0 cm ruptured.[72]

Cronenwett and associates[28] have shown that chronic obstructive pulmonary disease and systolic hypertension were predictors of increased risk of rupture of small abdominal aneurysms. In a subsequent study, they found that the rate of enlargement of small aneurysms was unpredictable, but either increased systolic or decreased diastolic pressure (i.e., increased pulse pressure) was associated with an increased rate of aneurysm expansion.[73] In this study, there was considerable variability in the rate of aneurysm enlargement even though the average rate of expansion was 0.4 cm/year in anteroposterior dimensions and 0.5 cm/year in lateral dimensions. Large aneurysms enlarge more rapidly than small ones. There are some data that suggest that the expansion rate of large aneurysms can be diminished by β-adrenergic blockade (propranolol).[74] Other studies have shown that aneurysms are frequently elliptical rather than round and that aneurysmal expansion is initially more rapid in the lateral direction. It is interesting to recall that most frequently the site of aneurysm rupture is in the lateral wall.

In a review of four series, including their own, Cronenwett and coworkers[73] described the outcome of 378 patients with small aortic aneurysms initially treated nonoperatively. After an average follow-up of 31 months, 27% of the patients were alive with intact aneurysms, 29% had died of other causes, 39% had had elective aneurysm operations because their aneurysm diameter reached 5 to 6 cm, and 4% had suffered aneurysm rupture or acute expansion leading to emergency operation. Overall, there was a mean

5-year survival of 54% in these patients, somewhat less than the 6-year survival rate of 64% in the UK Small Aneurysm Trial and the greater than 70% 6-year survival rate in the ADAM trial.[70–74]

In light of these more recent studies, autopsy studies showing high rates of rupture of small aneurysms must be viewed with caution. Some have shown that 23.4% of aneurysms between 4.1 and 5.0 cm rupture, and the same is true for up to 10% of aneurysms less than 4 cm in diameter.[5] Data such as these have led surgeons to recommend operation for almost all aortic aneurysms in good-risk patients. However, autopsy studies underestimate aneurysm size owing to the lack of a distending blood pressure, and several more recent studies on living patients demonstrate a rupture rate of about 1% per year for aneurysms less than 5.0 cm in diameter.[5]

There is little debate about the appropriateness of elective aneurysm surgery for patients with large aneurysms (>6 cm in diameter) because of the high risk of rupture and associated mortality when rupture occurs.

It must be emphasized that although the risk of aneurysm rupture correlates most closely with aneurysm size, and the average rate of aneurysmal enlargement is known (0.4–0.5 cm/year), it is impossible to predict when a small aneurysm may rupture in any given patient.[75] Although the harmlessness of a small, asymptomatic abdominal aortic aneurysm is deceptive, coronary artery disease, and not rupture, is the most frequent cause of death in patients with small aneurysms.

RISKS OF SURGICAL TREATMENT

The natural history of untreated abdominal aortic aneurysms is well documented. This is especially true now for those aneurysms that are 5.5 cm or less in diameter. Since the first report of successful surgical resection and graft replacement of an infrarenal aortic aneurysm in 1952, there have been a large number of publications documenting the operative and long-term survival after surgical treatment. There has been a steady improvement in operative results for elective operations. Several large, contemporary series have reported operative mortality rates of between 0.9% and 5% for university medical centers and only slightly higher rates for community hospitals.[75–92] The 1.8% operative mortality in the ADAM trial compares favorably with these (Table 24–4). This improvement in surgical results has occurred despite the fact that more patients are being operated on who are older and have more severe comorbid conditions. Preoperative detection and treatment of significant cardiac disease have been important factors.

Operative mortality in this range (<5%) justifies elective repair, even for relatively small aneurysms in good-risk patients.[66] Most of the deaths, even in elective operations, occur in so-called high-risk patients. Chronologic age is not as important as physiologic age in assessing operative risk, so patients should not be denied elective operation based solely on age. Even octogenarians can undergo elective aneurysm surgery with low morbidity and mortality rates.[80] Most vascular surgeons have successfully treated ruptured aneurysms in patients previously rejected for elective operation because they were "too old."

The major risks for elective abdominal aortic aneurysm resection are similar to those for other major intraabdominal operations and include adequacy of cardiopulmonary and renal function. High-risk patients are those with unstable angina or angina at rest, cardiac ejection fraction less than 25% to 30%, congestive heart failure, serum creatinine greater than 3 mg/dL, and pulmonary disease manifested by room air Po_2 of less than 50 mm Hg or elevated Pco_2 or both. A substantial percentage of these high-risk patients die of ruptured aneurysm and not from the diseases that led to their categorization as high risk. With intensive perioperative monitoring and support, aneurysm resection has been carried out even in these high-risk patients with operative mortality of less than 6% by Hollier and colleagues[93] and others.[74, 77, 87] Thus, even in high-risk patients, large abdominal aneurysms should be considered

TABLE 24-4

Operative Mortality and Late Survival of Elective Surgical Treatment of AAA

REFERENCE	PATIENTS (n)	AGE (yr)*	MORTALITY (%)†	5-YEAR SURVIVAL (%)‡
DeBakey et al, 1964[79]	1332	—	7	58
Levy et al, 1966[84]	100	64	17	34
Szilagyi et al, 1966[59]	401	—	15	49
May et al, 1968[85]	135	—	13	49
Baker and Roberts, 1970[86]	240	63	9	54
Stokes and Butcher, 1973[87]	87	—	3	60
Hicks et al, 1975[88]	225	67	8	60
O'Donnell et al, 1976[89]	63	82	5	70
Whittemore et al, 1980[74]	110	68	0	84
Crawford et al, 1981[90]	860	66	5	63
Reigel et al, 1987[91]	499	76	3	66
Bernstein et al, 1988[92]	123	71	1	72
UK Small AAA 1998[67]	563	69	5.8	64
Adam Trial 2001[68]	569	68	1.8	70

*Mean.
†Operative mortality.
‡Cumulative.
AAA, Abdominal aortic aneurysm.

for elective treatment, if the appropriate support facilities are available. It is in this group, however, that endovascular repair can be expected to have the most significant improvement over standard open aneurysm repair.

The use of endoluminally placed stent-grafts to treat aortic aneurysms has become a clinical reality. More than 20,000 patients have been treated worldwide in this manner. Two stent-graft and deployment systems were approved for general clinical use by the United States Food and Drug Administration (FDA) in 1999, and several others are in various stages of clinical testing. A very large number of clinical and experimental studies on this subject have been published, and carefully audited information that included 3 years of follow-up data are now available. The consistent findings are that 40% to 60% of patients with abdominal aortic aneurysms are anatomically suitable for endoluminal repair and that it can be accomplished with mortality rates equal to or lower than those for open surgical repair and morbidity rates that are clearly lower than those of open surgical repair. The length of hospital stay is shortened and patient satisfaction and surgeon enthusiasm are high. However, there is a small but disturbing incidence of endoleak, failure of the aneurysm sac to shrink, device slippage, device structural failure, and even late aneurysm rupture. Because of these late complications and problems, patients with these implants require close monitoring with CT or other studies every 6 to 12 months indefinitely. Most of the devices in current use are second generation, and continued improvement in ease of insertion, size, and durability can be expected. Because of lingering uncertainties about long-term results, there is no consensus about which patients and which aneurysms are best treated in this manner. For these reasons, at the present time, the indications for endoluminal repair should be considered as the same for open surgical repair in terms of aneurysm size and expected longevity. This topic is covered in detail in Chapter 18.

In spite of widespread elective aneurysm treatment programs, the incidence of aneurysm rupture has not decreased. A substantial percentage (50%) of patients whose aneurysms rupture die before reaching a medical facility.[69, 70] Another 24% arrive at a hospital alive but die before a definitive operation can be performed. Thus, operative mortality figures underestimate the true significance of aneurysmal rupture. The overall mortality from ruptured aneurysms, as reported in two large community-based studies, ranges from 74 to more than 90%.

The operative results for ruptured aneurysms are not nearly as favorable and have not generally improved over the years as have the results of elective aneurysm operations.[94-97] Although there are a few series with better results, overall, nearly 50% of patients die after being operated on for rupture. The nature of the rupture influences the results. Less than 10% of patients presenting in shock with free intraperitoneal rupture survive. In contrast, stable patients with small contained leaks have a better than 80% survival rate.

The factors contributing to failure in the treatment of ruptured abdominal aortic aneurysm have been reviewed by Hiatt and associates.[94] The four most important were failure to perform elective aneurysmectomy in patients with known aneurysms; errors in diagnosing rupture when it occurred, leading to delay in operation; technical errors committed during the operation (all venous injuries); and undue delays in induction of anesthesia. These are all realistically preventable. Other series have also attempted to identify factors leading to death after aortic aneurysm rupture. Repeatedly, delays in performing the surgery and the total volume of blood transfused are found to be important.[95, 96] Preoperative cardiac arrest, female gender, age of 80 years or older, massive blood loss, or ongoing major transfusion requirements were predictors of 90% to 100% mortality in Johansen's series, which included a very efficient transport and resuscitation response.[97] Encouraging early results from endovascular treatment of ruptures have been recently reported, with 92% of patients surviving. If these results are sustainable and reproducible, they will represent the most significant advance in the treatment of this highly lethal entity in several decades. Some of the differences in operative mortality between various reports are due in part to inconsistencies in patient categorization by considering all forms of rupture together. Many of these series also fail to separate patients with unruptured but symptomatic aneurysms who undergo emergency operations. The operative morbidity and mortality for this group are intermediate between elective, asymptomatic patients and those with frank rupture, averaging 16% to 19%.[28, 72] It has been postulated that the reason for this increased mortality is the omission of thorough preoperative evaluation and preparation necessitated by the emergency operation.

LATE SURVIVAL

It is accepted that the commonest cause of death among patients with large abdominal aortic aneurysm is rupture and that elective surgical repair prevents rupture and is associated with excellent perioperative survival rates. The next question that must be answered is: What is the long-term outlook for survivors? Is life prolonged by aneurysmectomy? After all, this is the primary objective of the detection and management of this condition. Several long-term studies using life-table methods have revealed 5-year survival rates ranging from 49% to 84% (averaging 61%) (see Table 24–4).[98-101]

Although these data are far more encouraging than those for the survival of patients not undergoing operation, they do not equal the survival expected for the normal age-matched population. For example, Johnson and coworkers[99] reported a 50% survival of 7.4 years for patients surviving elective operative treatment for abdominal aneurysm, whereas the age-adjusted figure for the United States general population was 15.7 years, and that for North Carolina was 14.5 years. These authors could not identify any influence of age on operative mortality, although it affected late mortality, as one would expect. Most of the excess late mortality could be attributed to coronary artery disease. This has led some centers to pursue an aggressive coronary evaluation and treatment protocol before elective aortic aneurysm operations.[102]

Several large surveys have shown that the safety of vascular surgical procedures in patients who have had previous coronary revascularization is comparable with that of patients with no evidence of ischemic cardiac disease, but this has not been evaluated by randomized clinical trials,[103–107] and it has been estimated, based on data from the Canadian Aneurysm Study, that aggressive cardiac treatment only increases the 5-year survival by 5% to 10%.[108]

ASSESSMENT OF CARDIAC RISK

Approximately 30% to 40% of patients with aortic aneurysms have no clinically evident coronary artery disease (e.g., no angina pectoris, no history of myocardial infarction, normal electrocardiogram [ECG], normal exercise stress test). However, there is a high prevalence (50%) of angiographically documented severe coronary artery disease in patients in whom coronary disease is clinically suspected (about 50% of the total).[102, 107] The prevalence is still 20% in patients in whom the traditional clinical indicators of coronary disease are absent. Coronary artery disease is responsible for at least 50% to 60% of all perioperative and late deaths after operations on the abdominal aorta.[109, 110] The incidence of fatal myocardial infarction after elective abdominal aortic aneurysm surgery has been reported to be as high as 4.7%, and nonfatal infarction occurs in up to 16% of patients.

It is possible to identify the high-risk cardiac patient using clinical assessment, exercise stress testing, radionuclide angiography (multiple gated scan), echocardiography, dipyridimole-thallium scanning, continuous portable electrocardiographic Holter monitoring, and coronary angiography.[109, 111, 112] The problem is in deciding which patients need cardiac screening before aneurysm surgery.[113] Clinical factors predictive of increased risk for postoperative cardiac complications include a history of previous myocardial infarction, congestive failure, angina pectoris, abnormal preoperative ECG, diabetes mellitus, and advanced age.[111] Dipyridamole (or dobutamine- or adenosine-) thallium myocardial scanning has replaced exercise stress testing for these elderly patients in many hospitals. It identifies areas of myocardium that are reversibly ischemic and is quite sensitive for identifying patients likely to have a perioperative cardiac complication, but unfortunately its specificity is relatively low.[114, 115] Determination of left ventricular ejection fraction by radionuclide angiography identifies patients with poor ventricular function. Although ejection fraction less than 30% has been associated with increased cardiac complications in some series, it does not predict postoperative myocardial infarction or death. Continuous portable ECG monitoring of vascular surgical patients for silent ischemia associated with ST-T segment changes has been shown to correlate with postoperative myocardial infarction in some series, but additional studies are needed to verify the value of this technique. Routine preoperative screening of all aortic aneurysm patients with coronary angiography is not feasible or prudent, even though Hertzer has reported a nearly fivefold increase in operative mortality (5.1%) in aneurysm patients with suspected coronary disease, compared with those with no (1.1% mortality) or corrected (0.44% mortality) coronary artery disease.[102, 103] Late survival was also better in the groups with no or corrected coronary artery disease. Despite these data, no solid data have proved that there is decreased perioperative mortality or increased long-term survival for patients undergoing prophylactic coronary revascularization before aortic aneurysm repair. Furthermore, no single means exists to accurately predict perioperative cardiac risk after aortic aneurysmorrhaphy, but this is an area of intensive current research.

Each of the modalities discussed has its own usefulness as well as limitations. Older patients with congestive heart failure, active angina pectoris, previous myocardial infarction, or markedly abnormal noninvasive cardiac studies deserve thorough cardiac evaluation before elective aortic aneurysm surgery. Younger patients without overt cardiac disease and with normal ECG readings probably do not need this type of evaluation. The difficult decisions are in patients who fall between these two extremes (about 50% of the total), in whom unexpected coronary events still occur.[116] Because the ultimate objective of a cardiac evaluation is to identify and correct dangerous coronary artery lesions, the results of the subsequent interventions (i.e., coronary artery bypass grafting, percutaneous transluminal angioplasty) in the appropriate hospital must be considered and balanced against the relatively low myocardial infarction rates that can be achieved in patients who do not undergo coronary revascularization. Overall, preliminary myocardial revascularization before aortic aneurysm repair should be truly necessary in only about 10% to 20% of patients.

INDICATIONS FOR ABDOMINAL AORTIC ANEURYSM REPAIR

The objectives of surgical treatment of abdominal aortic aneurysm are to relieve symptoms, if present, prevent rupture (thereby prolonging life), and restore arterial continuity. These goals are best accomplished when operations are performed electively under optimal conditions. The natural history (unoperated) of abdominal aortic aneurysms and the excellent results currently achievable for surgical treatment justify a vigorous diagnostic and therapeutic approach.

Emergent operation is indicated for almost all patients with known or suspected *rupture*, regardless of the size of the aneurysm or age of the patient. There are obvious exceptions to this approach. The coexistence of another fatal illness, such as metastatic cancer, may be sufficient reason for choosing a nonoperative approach. Emergent or urgent operation is also indicated for *symptomatic aneurysms* in the absence of signs of rupture. It is frequently impossible to determine whether an aneurysm has in fact ruptured or is just expanding. Although CT and MRI scans can be relied on to detect the presence of periaortic blood in most cases, the absence of this finding should not lead to unnecessary delays in operating, because actual rupture can occur at any time. In addition, these imaging units are frequently located in areas of hospitals where close monitoring of the patient is difficult.

Elective aneurysm repair should be recommended for *asymptomatic patients* with aneurysms 5.5 cm or larger in diameter who are acceptable operative risks and who have an estimated life expectancy of 2 years or more. Elective operation should also be considered for smaller aneurysms, less than 5.5 cm in maximum diameter, in good-risk patients, especially if they are hypertensive or live in a remote area where proper medical care would not be readily available should signs and symptoms of rupture develop. Aneurysms between 4.0 and 5.5 cm in diameter that have shown documented enlargement of more than 0.5 cm in less than 6 to 12 months by serial imaging studies should also be treated surgically. Enlargement at this rate suggests an unstable, changing aortic wall.

High-risk patients (those who are very old or who have nonreconstructible coronary disease, poor left ventricular function with congestive heart failure, renal failure, or severe obstructive lung disease) with small aneurysms should be observed until the aneurysm becomes symptomatic or large. High-risk patients with large aneurysms require thorough evaluation for the condition that puts them in the high-risk category.[74, 93] Frequently, such evaluations fail to substantiate the original degree of presumed risk, and it has been reported that fewer than 50% of these patients die of the disease for which they were initially denied aneurysm repair.

Because of excessively high operative mortality in some very high-risk patients with large abdominal aneurysms, several surgeons proposed extra-anatomic bypass in conjunction with induced thrombosis of the aneurysm.[117] Thrombosis of the aneurysm, it was argued, would eliminate the risk of rupture, and the extra-anatomic bypass would lower operative mortality by avoiding the risks of a major intra-abdominal operation and aortic cross-clamping. Unfortunately, nonresective therapy has not been as successful as originally hoped. Rupture still occurs in about 20% of patients so treated, and operative mortality has been more than 10%, a figure far in excess of the mortality reported in similar but highly selected groups of patients subjected to conventional aneurysm operations.[93, 118–120] Fortunately, this nonresective form of surgical therapy for abdominal aneurysms is being abandoned, even by some of its earlier proponents. Endoluminal stent-grafting has become the treatment of choice for these very high risk patients when they have suitable anatomy.

OPERATIVE TECHNIQUE

Incision and Exposure

There are three options for the incision for abdominal aortic aneurysm operations. The *full-length midline incision* provides access to the entire abdominal cavity, including the supraceliac aorta and iliac arteries; is rapid to make and close; and provides the fewest limitations. For the treatment of supra- or pararenal aneurysms, medial-visceral rotation can be added and usually provides adequate exposure of the entire suprarenal segment of the abdominal aorta. This maneuver involves mobilization, from lateral to medial, of the left colon, the spleen, and the pancreas in what is normally an avascular plane. Significant splenic injury requiring splenectomy occurs about 25% of the time when this is done, and there is an increased risk of pancreatic injury.

A *wide transverse incision*, extending from flank to flank

and curved either above or below the umbilicus, depending on the aortic and iliac pathology, also provides excellent exposure for aortic aneurysm repair and is the preference of many surgeons. It is more time consuming to create and close than a midline incision and is said to be stronger, although proof of superiority in terms of wound dehiscence is lacking. Transverse incisions are less painful and therefore interfere less with respiratory function postoperatively because they cut across fewer intercostal nerves.

Both of these incisions offer wide access to the peritoneal cavity and the retroperitoneum and its contents. They permit a thorough abdominal exploration that should be performed as a preliminary step in all elective operations, because there is a significant incidence of coexisting pathology, including colon tumors and gallstones.

Retroperitoneal exposure of the aorta can also be achieved through an *oblique incision* extending from the left 11th intercostal space to the edge of the rectus abdominus muscle.[121–123] For this, the patient is placed in a semilateral position but with the hips allowed to rotate back to the supine position, which allows access to both femoral arteries. Through this retroperitoneal exposure, the suprarenal aorta can be controlled if necessary, but access to the right iliac artery is often very limited, especially if the aortic aneurysm is large or if there is a large right iliac aneurysm. Among the advantages claimed for the retroperitoneal approach are less postoperative respiratory compromise, lower intravenous fluid volume requirements, less intraoperative hypothermia, a shorter period of postoperative ileus, and avoidance in many cases of the need for postoperative nasogastric intubation. Although it has been perceived that these patients generally "do better" than those operated on through a midline incision, when the two incisions were compared in prospective studies, no significant important differences were found.[121–123] One major disadvantage of the retroperitoneal approach is that the contents of the peritoneal cavity are not available for inspection. Nevertheless, many surgeons prefer this approach for elective aneurysm operations, and some even use it for ruptured aneurysms that are contained because of the ability to achieve rapid control of the upper abdominal aorta in this way.[124]

The choice of incision is a matter of personal preference. Factors to consider in making this choice include the extent of the aneurysm, the status of the iliac arteries, the degree of obesity and pulmonary disease, previous abdominal operations, the necessity to inspect intraperitoneal structures (especially in patients with atypical symptoms), and the speed with which aortic control must be attained. Surgeons should be familiar with all three approaches to be able to take advantage of each when appropriate. Transperitoneal or retroperitoneal exposure of the aorta through small incisions, with or without laparoscopic assistance, has been successfully used to treat aortic aneurysms by several surgical groups, and completely laparoscopic procedures have also been accomplished. The special instruments, vascular clamps, and retractors necessary to accomplish this have been developed and are being improved. Turnipseed and colleagues compared 50 patients who had aortic aneurysms or occlusive disease treated via minimal incisions with 50 similar patients treated using a long midline incision. The minimal incision technique was as safe and effective as the standard incision and was associated with reduced intensive care unit and total hospital length of stay, reduced morbidity, and reduced costs. It was more cost-efficient than either the standard incision or endoluminal stent-grafting techniques.[125] Completely laparoscopic aneurysm repair has also been performed.[126]

Extensive perioperative monitoring is indicated for patients undergoing abdominal aortic aneurysm repair.[74, 127] This has contributed significantly to the improved results reported in large series of electively treated patients. Monitoring usually includes continuous recording of ECG, intra-arterial pressure, body temperature, urine output, and central venous or pulmonary artery pressures. In high-risk patients, especially if the aorta will be cross-clamped above the renal arteries, transesophageal two-dimensional echocardiographic monitoring of left ventricular function may be superior to measurements of pulmonary artery pressure for evaluation of intravascular volume status.[128] Various blood components should be monitored as well, including arterial oxygen and carbon dioxide content and pH, plasma glucose, electrolytes, and coagulation parameters and factors. Monitoring the clotting system is especially important in ruptured aneurysms and in other cases in which there has been a need to infuse large volumes of blood and blood products or a supraceliac clamp has been used. The use of autotransfusion is routine in some places to minimize the amount of homologous blood transfusion. Unfortunately, its use has not been found to be cost-effective in randomized trials. For elective operations, patients should be encouraged to donate their own blood for autologous transfusion in the perioperative period.

When midline or transverse incisions are used, the aorta is exposed by a retroperitoneal incision that should be kept slightly to the right of the midline. The duodenum must be carefully reflected laterally along with the rest of the small bowel. The left renal vein usually marks the cephalad extent of the dissection unless the aneurysm extends to (juxtarenal aneurysm) or involves the renal arteries (pararenal aneurysm). In either of these situations, suprarenal aortic clamping is necessary, and the left renal vein should be thoroughly mobilized so that it can be retracted cephalad or caudad to facilitate adequate exposure of the pararenal aorta.[129, 130] It is sometimes necessary to divide the left renal vein. This is usually well tolerated if the left adrenal and gonadal veins are not ligated, but there is an increased risk of sustained elevation in serum creatinine, a temporary reduction of left renal function, and increased retroperitoneal bleeding. Reanastomosis of the transected renal vein avoids these but is not always necessary.[131]

Distally, the dissection should avoid the fibroareolar tissue overlying the left common iliac artery because it contains branch vessels of the inferior mesenteric artery and the autonomic nerves that control sexual function in men. If the common iliac arteries are relatively normal (i.e., not aneurysmal, stenotic, or heavily calcified), they can be clamped and a straight tube graft used for the aortic replacement. Significant disease of the common iliac arteries makes a bifurcated graft preferable. Control of the iliac arteries in these situations is best achieved by mobilizing the external and internal iliac arteries and clamping them individually. Particular care must be paid in this location to avoid injury to accompanying posterior venous

structures, as well as the ureters, which cross anterior to the common iliac bifurcation. Every effort should be made to ensure antegrade perfusion in at least one hypogastric artery to minimize the risk of postoperative ischemia of the left colon as well as buttock claudication. This sometimes requires construction of end-to-side anastomoses between the graft limbs and the external iliac artery when anastomosis to the common iliac is not possible.

Aneurysm Repair

Regardless of the extent of the aortic aneurysm, the proximal graft anastomosis should be made as close as possible to the renal arteries to prevent recurrent aortic pathology. The degree of disease in the iliac arteries determines the distal extent of the graft. In some series, up to 80% of patients were successfully treated with a straight tube graft, although in the experience of others, only about one third of patients had suitable anatomy for this approach. There does not appear to be a significant incidence of subsequent iliac aneurysm formation when tube grafts are used in the presence of normal-sized or slightly enlarged iliac arteries.

The choice of graft material, polyester (knitted or woven) or expanded polytetrafluoroethylene (PTFE), is a controversial but relatively unimportant issue. There is no proven superiority of any one graft type used for aortic replacement. Most surgeons find knitted grafts easier to handle, and knitted grafts sealed with collagen or gelatin do not require preclotting and are gaining in popularity. For ruptured aneurysms, nonporous grafts are clearly preferable because of savings in time and interstitial blood loss. Many surgeons routinely use woven polyester or extruded PTFE grafts for elective aneurysm repair for the same reason.

Systemic heparin is nearly universally administered during the occlusive phase of elective aneurysm operations, because most surgeons believe its use provides an added margin of safety from distal thrombosis. The distal clamps should be applied before the proximal aortic clamp to prevent distal embolization. The aorta is opened longitudinally and either partially or completely transected at the site of the proximal anastomosis. If there is a very short or no infrarenal neck (juxtarenal aneurysm), temporary proximal aortic clamping above the renal arteries is required for an infrarenal repair (see Fig. 24–2). The proximal anastomosis can be done with a continuous or interrupted suture technique; the former is quicker. If the aorta is especially weak or friable, the sutures can be supported with Teflon-felt pledgets or strips.

The distal anastomoses can be end to end or end to side, depending on their location and the status of the common and internal iliac arteries. All mural thrombus and atheroma should be débrided from the aneurysm wall. Several studies have shown a surprisingly high incidence of positive bacterial cultures of this material, in from 10% to 15% to 40% of patients. The significance of these positive cultures is unknown, but most of them have been due to coagulase-negative *Staphylococcus* species, an organism commonly found in aortic graft infections.[129] Back-bleeding lumbar vessels can be the source of significant blood loss and should be suture-ligated from within the aortic sac. If the inferior mesenteric artery is patent and actively back-bleeding, it can also be ligated within the aneurysm sac, but if back-bleeding is meager, the vessel should be preserved and reassessed after distal flow is reestablished, especially if internal iliac flow is compromised. Reimplantation of the inferior mesenteric artery is relatively easy to perform when necessary, with use of the Carrel patch technique.

All anastomoses should be constructed with permanent synthetic sutures. Braided polyester and monofilament polypropylene or PTFE are the most commonly used. Theoretical fears about late fracture of polypropylene sutures have not been substantiated in clinical practice. If suprarenal clamping is necessary, the clamp should be moved onto the graft and below the renal arteries as soon as possible to minimize renal ischemia after ensuring that the proximal anastomosis is secure. The distal anastomoses can then be constructed as indicated by the iliac artery disease. It is sometimes easier to control iliac artery back-bleeding by the use of intraluminal balloon catheters and to oversew the common iliac arteries from within the opened aortic or iliac aneurysms or both. In unusual circumstances, external iliac disease necessitates making the distal anastomosis to the common femoral artery.

Declamping hypotension is now an unusual event in elective aortic aneurysm surgery. It is essential to maintain excellent communication with the anesthesiology team so that depth of anesthesia and blood and fluid replacement can be adjusted in anticipation of lower extremity reperfusion. Even though the graft and native vessels are flushed and back-bled before reestablishing distal flow, it is preferable to reestablish flow first into one hypogastric artery to minimize the chances of distal embolization to the leg. Before abdominal closure, adequacy of lower extremity and left colon perfusion should be ensured by direct inspection or noninvasive instrumentation. The graft should be insulated from the overlying bowel by careful closure of the aneurysm sac over the graft. This is sometimes impossible when the aneurysm is small, and in these situations, rotation of a flap of the aneurysm wall or use of a vascularized omental pedicle can be employed to separate the graft from the duodenum.

It is beyond the scope of this chapter to discuss all of the technical details that might be encountered in the course of the surgical treatment of an aortic aneurysm. The principles outlined here are generally applicable for most cases. If additional vascular procedures are required, such as renal or visceral artery reconstruction, appropriate modifications in technique are required.[133] The introduction and widespread clinical use of endovascular aortic aneurysm repair makes this a promising treatment modality, especially in high-risk patients.[134, 135] Straight and bifurcated endoprostheses have been successfully implanted so that coexisting or isolated iliac artery aneurysms are also treatable with these methods. This is discussed in more detail earlier in this chapter and in Chapter 18.

Repair of Ruptured Aneurysm

For ruptured aneurysms, the first priority is to control the hemorrhage by gaining proximal control of the aorta.

Resuscitation is best done in the operating room rather than in the emergency department. Usually, it is better to have the patient prepared and draped, with the surgical team ready to make a rapid entry into the abdomen, before induction of anesthesia. The induction of anesthesia in these circumstances is often associated with sudden and severe hypotension when the tamponade effects and reflex vasoconstriction are relieved by relaxation of the abdominal wall. The reintroduction of the practice of proximal balloon occlusion using a catheter inserted via the upper extremity is based largely on avoiding this phenomenon. The availability of high-quality digital fluoroscopy in the operating room makes this feasible. If the rupture is contained, proximal aortic control is best achieved at the level of the supraceliac aorta through the lesser omentum. The hematoma can then be entered and the clamp repositioned distally after the aortic neck is identified. The hematoma usually makes this portion of the dissection relatively easy, but caution must be exercised to avoid injury to major venous structures, because this is one of the commonest causes of excessive hemorrhage and subsequent death. If there is a free intraperitoneal rupture, the aorta can be quickly compressed at the diaphragm with an assistant's hand or a commercial compression device without formally dissecting this area. An infrarenal clamp or an intraluminal occluding balloon catheter can be substituted as soon as possible. After bleeding is controlled, adequate blood and volume replenishment should be achieved before attempting to restore flow to the lower extremities. Heparin is unnecessary and should be avoided in ruptured aneurysms because bleeding and coagulopathy are frequently associated with the shock, hypothermia, and massive blood loss and replacement that occur. The proper use of blood and blood products, including platelets and fresh-frozen plasma, is essential for survival of these patients.

COMPLICATIONS OF AORTIC ANEURYSM REPAIR

Survival after aortic aneurysm surgery was discussed earlier in this chapter. Mortality ranges from 0% to 3% for patients with uncomplicated aneurysms operated on electively to more than 80% for patients with rupture, hypotension, and oliguria. The most frequent cause of death is myocardial dysfunction, usually ischemic in origin. Nonfatal myocardial infarction is also fairly common after even elective aortic aneurysm repair, occurring in from 3.1% to 16% (average, 6.9%) of patients in reported series.[8] The varying incidence is due to differing criteria used to define myocardial infarction and possibly to differing protocols for evaluating and treating coronary artery disease preoperatively.

Several other major complications can occur during or after aortic aneurysm operations. *Hemorrhage* is a constant threat, most often from injury to iliac or lumbar veins. It can be severe and extremely difficult to control, especially if it involves the left common iliac vein, where it passes beneath the right common iliac artery. Extreme care must be taken when mobilizing the iliac arteries, especially if they are aneurysmal, in which case they are especially likely to be adherent to the underlying veins. Injury to the left renal vein or one of its tributaries is also associated with brisk bleeding. This is particularly likely when there are venous anomalies such as a retroaortic left renal vein or a circumaortic venous collar. These venous anomalies can usually be identified preoperatively if a CT scan has been performed. Intraoperatively, they should be suspected when, during cephalad dissection of the aortic neck, either a small or no left renal vein is encountered in its usual location crossing anterior to the aorta. Postoperative hemorrhage can occur in any patient, and hemodynamic instability and evidence of continued blood loss should lead to early reexploration of the abdomen.

Declamping hypotension is not as frequent or severe a problem as it once was. Better understanding of its physiology, more aggressive management of intravascular volume, and better monitoring and anesthetic techniques have all contributed to the reduction in the incidence and seriousness of this problem. The surgeon can help to minimize this condition by giving the anesthesiologist advance notification of plans to restore distal perfusion and then doing it gradually. Despite these precautions, declamping hypotension can still be a serious problem, especially in the setting of a ruptured aneurysm in a cold, hypovolemic patient with poor cardiac performance.

Renal failure is another serious but now infrequent complication. At one time, 3% to 12% of operative deaths after elective abdominal aortic aneurysm operations and an even higher percentage after emergency operations for rupture were attributable to acute renal failure.[136] Renal failure or less severe degrees of renal functional impairment can occur even when there is no hypotension and the proximal aortic clamp has been infrarenal in location. The etiology of renal dysfunction in these situations is poorly understood but is thought to involve reflex renal vasoconstriction and intrarenal redistribution of blood flow. Atheromatous embolization from clamping or manipulation of the perirenal aorta is also a potential contributing factor, as is temporary suprarenal clamping when it is required. Sometimes, the large contrast load of an aortogram or CT scan performed 1 or 2 days preoperatively can cause renal dysfunction that only becomes apparent postoperatively. Mannitol and/or loop diuretics are commonly administered before aortic cross-clamping to increase urine output and prevent renal failure. Although this seems reasonable, studies have shown that intraoperative urine volume does not predict postoperative renal function.[137] Renal failure due to acute tubular necrosis is much more common after operations for ruptured aortic aneurysms, occurring in 21% of survivors of operation in one series. Unfortunately, the mortality associated with this complication still ranges from 50% to 70% despite the use of acute hemodialysis and adequate nutritional support.

Technical injury to the bowel or ureters can cause catastrophic infectious complications involving the newly implanted prosthetic graft. This is most likely to occur when there are adhesions from previous operations or the structures are in an unusual position (i.e., the ureters displaced anteriorly and laterally by the aneurysm). Such injuries should be meticulously repaired and the area irrigated with antibiotic solution. Ureteral injuries should be stented. In some situations, nephrectomy is the safest course to avoid possible graft contamination.

Gastrointestinal complications of a functional nature regularly occur after conventional aortic aneurysm surgery. Ileus is the rule for at least 2 to 3 days after transperitoneal surgery. Typically, gastric and colonic ileus persists longer than small bowel ileus. Occasionally, duodenal obstruction persists for longer periods of time. The presence of hematoma and edema in the vicinity of the proximal anastomosis is thought to contribute to this problem. Postoperative pancreatitis is relatively common, as determined by elevation of serum amylase, although clinically apparent pancreatitis is unusual. The pancreas can be injured by retractors, however, and a few patients have serious consequences from these seemingly minor injuries.

The most serious gastrointestinal complication is ischemia of the left side of the colon and the rectum. The incidence of ischemic colitis after aortic reconstruction is about 2% (range 0.2% to 10%).[138] It is three to four times more common after operations for aortic aneurysm than after operations for occlusive disease, and the incidence is several times higher in patients studied prospectively with colonoscopy after sustaining a ruptured aneurysm. Ligation of a patent inferior mesenteric artery in the presence of inadequate collateral circulation to the sigmoid colon and rectum is thought to be an important pathophysiologic mechanism, but the inferior mesenteric artery is already occluded in the majority of patients with abdominal aneurysms. Improper ligation of the inferior mesenteric artery too far away from the wall of the aneurysm can contribute to this complication by interfering with collateral blood supply to the rectosigmoid.[139] Postoperative hypotension and hemodynamic instability are significant contributory factors. Therefore, it is important to maintain antegrade perfusion in at least one internal iliac artery after arterial reconstruction for aortic aneurysm. Even though most patients with occlusion of both internal iliac arteries and the inferior mesenteric artery have adequate colonic perfusion, postoperative hypotension, bowel distention, and mesenteric vessel compression by hematoma can all contribute to postoperative colonic ischemia.

Postoperative colonic ischemia can involve the mucosa only, which usually causes a transient, mild form of ischemic colitis, or it can involve mucosa and muscularis, which may result in fibrous healing and stricture formation. The most severe and dreaded form is transmural ischemia, which occurs in more than 60% of the reported cases.[140] The clinical manifestations of bowel ischemia depend on the severity of ischemia. Diarrhea, especially if it is bloody, is one of the earliest manifestations and usually begins within 48 hours of operation. It is an indication for colonoscopy to assess the status of the colonic mucosa. Other findings indicative of bowel gangrene and peritonitis may be present and demand prompt reoperation, resection of all compromised bowel, and creation of appropriate stomas. During bowel resection, efforts should be made to isolate the underlying aortic prosthesis from the surgical field, although this is usually impossible, setting the stage for subsequent prosthetic infection. If the graft becomes grossly contaminated, it should be removed and lower extremity perfusion restored by axillofemoral bypass. Less severe degrees of colonic ischemia can be managed nonoperatively, although subsequent correction of a colonic stricture may be required. A high index of suspicion of this complication must be maintained to detect and treat it in a timely fashion.

The mortality for postoperative colon ischemia following aortic aneurysm surgery is about 50% overall but increases to 90% when full-thickness colonic gangrene and peritonitis occur. Preoperative evaluation of the blood supply to the colon and intraoperative assessment of colonic perfusion by Doppler or inferior mesenteric artery back-pressure measurements may help to identify patients at highest risk for this disatrous complication so that preventive measures (i.e., inferior mesenteric artery reimplantation) can be taken.

Paraplegia due to *spinal cord ischemia*, a well-recognized complication of thoracoabdominal aneurysm repair, is a rare event after operations confined to the infrarenal aorta, with only slightly more than 50 cases reported. Szilagyi and coworkers[141] noted an incidence of 0.2% in more than 3000 aortic operations, and it occurred 10 times more frequently in patients with ruptured aneurysms. This suggests that hypotension is a contributing factor in most cases, even though injury to an unusually located arteria magna radicularis (artery of Adamkiewicz) to the spinal cord may be the primary event. Pelvic hypoperfusion associated with internal iliac artery occlusion is an important contributing factor in some patients. This emphasizes again the importance of maintaining perfusion of at least one hypogastric artery. Unfortunately, this complication is not preventable, predictable, or treatable. Although the severity of the clinical manifestations varies and approximately 50% of affected survivors recover some neurologic function, there is a 50% mortality associated with this complication.

Ischemia of the lower extremities can also occur after aortic aneurysm surgery. This may be due to embolization of dislodged mural thrombus or atherosclerotic plaque from the aneurysm itself, thrombosis of a vessel due to distal stasis, creation of an intimal flap, or crushed atherosclerotic plaque. The use of heparin during the occlusive phase of aneurysm repair does not prevent the embolic events from occurring but may limit the propagation of thrombus and should prevent formation of stasis thrombi in the distal vascular beds. Before closing the abdomen, the surgeon must be satisfied with the perfusion status of the lower extremities.

Microembolization can also occur, resulting in small patchy areas of ischemia, usually on the plantar aspect of the feet. Pedal pulses are usually still palpable in this situation. Colloquially, this is known as "trash foot," and if recognized intraoperatively, the passage of small balloon catheters can sometimes retrieve at least some of the atheromatous debris. Lumbar sympathectomy may also be beneficial in limiting or preventing full-thickness tissue loss.

An abdominal compartment syndrome has been recognized as an unusual but important cause of renal and respiratory failure, especially after operations for ruptured aneurysms. Manifested by massive abdominal distention, oliguria, and difficulty maintaining adequate ventilation, it is an indication for prompt reexploration of the abdomen to relieve the intraabdominal pressure. The usual finding is massive visceral edema, and deliberate abdominal wall hernia must be created for its treatment. This syndrome may be preventable by mesh-assisted delayed abdominal closure.

Infection involving the prosthetic graft used to restore aortic continuity occurs in from less than 1% to about 6% of patients. It is more common after treating ruptured aneurysms. It may be associated with graft-enteric fistula, which is more common after surgery for aortic aneurysm than after surgery for aortic occlusive disease. These infections usually become manifest months to years after graft implantation and are discussed in detail in Chapter 38.

UNUSUAL PROBLEMS ASSOCIATED WITH ABDOMINAL AORTIC ANEURYSMS

Several anatomic and pathologic conditions can complicate the management of abdominal aortic aneurysms and adversely affect the outcome.

Venous Anomalies

There are several anomalies of the inferior vena cava and left renal vein that are important in aortic surgery. They were found in 2.8% of nearly 1400 aortic operations in one series and are potential sources of serious, unexpected hemorrhage. Many of these can be identified on preoperative CT scans.[142] The inferior vena cava may be entirely on the left side (without situs inversus) or may be duplicated, with one on each side of the aorta. Double vena cava is estimated to occur in up to 3% of patients, but the isolated left-sided vena cava occurs in only 0.2% to 0.5%.[143, 144] An isolated left-sided vena cava usually crosses obliquely in front of the aorta and may be joined by a short, immobile right renal vein. It can also cross from left to right behind the aorta. These anomalies can be especially troublesome if the aorta is approached retroperitoneally from the patient's left side. Near the neck of an aortic aneurysm, these anomalously positioned veins are prone to injury. Sometimes a crossing left inferior vena cava must be divided to enable satisfactory handling of the proximal aortic anastomosis. With a duplicated inferior vena cava, the left-sided one can be ligated if necessary, but care must be exercised to ensure that adequate venous drainage of the adrenal gland and left kidney is provided.

A retroaortic left renal vein, either alone or in association with an anterior vein in the usual location, is another rare anomaly that can lead to exsanguinating hemorrhage if it is injured during dissection or clamping of the aortic neck.[145] The incidence of this anomaly is 1.8% to 2.4%. As mentioned earlier, when the surgeon cannot find the left renal vein in its usual preaortic location, he or she should assume that it is retroaortic and limit dissection in that area. Great care must be taken when applying the aortic cross-clamp to avoid tearing these posterior veins. If such a vein is injured, transection of the aorta is usually required to expose it well enough to control the bleeding.

Circumaortic venous collar is more common, occurring in up to 8.7% of cases.[146] This anomaly is even more prone to injury, because the anterior component can be normal in size, leading the surgeon to disregard the possibility of a second, posterior renal vein.

Inflammatory Aneurysm

Nearly 5% of abdominal aortic aneurysms are associated with a dense, inflammatory, fibrotic reaction in the retroperitoneum that incorporates adjacent structures.[147, 148] This appears to be a distinct clinicopathologic entity of uncertain etiology, although an autoimmune basis has been proposed. It is characterized histologically by marked thickening of the adventitia and media (in contrast to other aortic aneurysms, which have a thinned, attenuated medial layer). Both layers are infiltrated with a prominent acute and chronic inflammatory reaction that includes giant cells. The majority of the inflammatory cells are activated T lymphocytes. The desmoplastic inflammatory reaction involves the duodenum in 90% of cases, the inferior vena cava and left renal vein in more than 50%, and the ureters in about 25%.[149] These aneurysms tend to be large, and most patients are symptomatic (pain) in the absence of rupture. A majority of the patients have an elevated erythrocyte sedimentation rate of uncertain significance and many have an elevated C-reactive protein and have lost weight. The diagnosis can be suspected on the CT scan, where the periaortic fibrous tissue can be easily seen obliterating tissue planes, and a typical halo effect of this tissue appears after intravenous contrast administration. MRI also shows a characteristic appearance of inflammatory aneurysm consisting of several concentric rings surrounding the aortic lumen. Either of these imaging techniques can establish the presence of an inflammatory aneurysm in a high percentage of cases. Published reports have pointed out several advantages of the left-sided retroperitoneal approach for these lesions, and establishing this diagnosis preoperatively makes possible the selection of this technique. In cases of ureteric involvement, the ureters are pulled medially and may be obstructed (again, in contrast to other large aneurysms, which tend to push the ureters laterally). At laparotomy, the diagnosis can be immediately established by recognition of the dense, shiny, white, highly vascular reaction in the retroperitoneum, centered over the aortic aneurysm. Once the lesion is recognized, the usual maneuvers of aneurysmorrhaphy should be modified to avoid injury to adherent structures, especially the duodenum. The aorta should be exposed cephalad to the renal vein or at the diaphragm and opened without dissecting the duodenum off the wall. Concomitant ureterolysis is seldom necessary because the inflammatory reaction usually resolves postoperatively. Ureteral catheterization is a useful adjunct, however, and helps to avoid intraoperative ureteral injury. Although the transfusion requirements and operative mortality are slightly higher than for noninflammatory aneurysms, the long-term outlook for these patients is comparable with that for patients with ordinary abdominal aortic aneurysms, and the usual criteria for recommending elective operation should be applied, because these aneurysms can rupture despite their very thick anterior wall.[150]

Horseshoe Kidney

Horseshoe kidney occurs in 1:400 to 1:1000 of the general population. Its association with abdominal aortic aneurysm is rare, but it complicates graft replacement because the kidney mass is usually fused anterior to the aorta, the collecting system and ureters are medially displaced, and there are frequently multiple renal arteries arising from the aorta, including the aneurysmal part or the iliac arteries or both.[151, 152] The renal blood supply is anomalous in 80% of cases, and it has been estimated that it requires some form of surgical correction in most of them.[153] Preoperative arteriography is essential for the proper evaluation of these renal arteries, but unless it is performed as a matter of routine, it is not usually considered unless the diagnosis is suspected from an intravenous pyelogram or CT or ultrasound scan. The isthmus of a horseshoe kidney seldom needs to be or should be divided, because the aortic graft can be passed behind it. If renal arteries arise from the aneurysm, they can be reimplanted into the graft as a Carrel patch. If horseshoe kidney is recognized preoperatively, a left retroperitoneal approach allows easier management of the multiple and accessory renal arteries.

Associated Intraabdominal Pathology and Concomitant Surgical Procedures

Occasionally, there are stenotic atherosclerotic lesions in aortic branches that require surgical correction at the time of aortic aneurysm repair. This most often involves the renal arteries in patients with renovascular hypertension or impaired renal function.[154, 155] Rarely, chronic visceral ischemia necessitates concomitant visceral artery repair and aneurysmorrhaphy. In most series, the morbidity and mortality of combined procedures exceed those of elective aneurysm repair alone, so caution is urged in the performance of purely prophylactic procedures in this setting.

Malignant tumors are unexpectedly found in 4% to 5% of patients undergoing operation for abdominal aneurysm. Most of these are colonic. Because operating on the colon converts a clean into a contaminated procedure, with its potential for prosthetic graft infection, the decision is not always easy regarding how to treat each lesion (aneurysm, colon mass). It is sometimes difficult to distinguish cancer from inflammatory lesions intraoperatively. In addition, most vascular surgeons do not employ a formal bowel preparation for patients undergoing elective aortic aneurysm surgery. For these reasons, unless there are compelling reasons for treating the colonic lesion (perforation, obstruction, hemorrhage), the aneurysm procedure should be completed and the colon left alone. The colonic lesion can then be properly evaluated and treated postoperatively. Generally, it is possible to perform an elective colon operation sooner after an aortic aneurysm repair than the opposite, especially if there has been a septic complication (common after colon surgery but rare after aortic surgery).

The presence of asymptomatic gallstones is a far more common condition found unexpectedly in 5% to 20% of patients undergoing aortic surgery. Several series have been published attesting to the safety of concomitant cholecystectomy and aortic repair.[156, 157] A major impetus for this philosophy is the postulated high incidence of postoperative cholecystitis in such patients who have only their aortic pathology treated. In the series reported by String,[156] there was only one documented late graft infection in 34 patients who underwent combined procedures. However, the follow-up was rather short, especially when one considers the usual long intervals between aortic grafting and the first manifestations of graft infection. In addition, the incidence of positive cultures from bile of patients with cholelithiasis is as high as 33%. As with colonic lesions, performance of elective cholecystectomy, which could possibly lead to contamination of a newly implanted aortic prosthesis, should not be performed in conjunction with vascular grafting operations.[157, 158] The consequences of infection of the aortic graft are so grave that the risk of performing elective cholecystectomy is unjustified for an elective operation. The advent of laparoscopic cholecystectomy has made this less of an issue because of the relatively benign nature of this procedure, which can be safely performed either shortly before or after aortic aneurysm repair, if necessary.

Aortocaval Fistula

Abdominal aortic aneurysms can rupture into the inferior vena cava or iliac veins. This is the most frequent cause of aortocaval fistula and occurs in 0.2% to 1.3% of patients with typical, nonspecific abdominal aortic aneurysms.[159, 160] The incidence is at least twice as high in cases of ruptured aneurysm. Approximately 5% to 10% of spontaneous aortocaval fistulas occur in conjunction with other etiologies, such as mycotic aneurysm and the Ehlers-Danlos and Marfan syndromes. The most frequent site of fistulization is the distal aorta at or just above the confluence of the iliac veins. Almost all aortocaval fistulas are symptomatic, and impaired renal function is common. Hemodynamically, there is typically a hyperdynamic, high-output state (tachycardia, decreased diastolic blood pressure, and cardiac dilatation) which can quickly progress to medically refractory congestive heart failure. Abdominal and/or back pain is present in more than 80% of patients, and most have a palpable mass; 75% have an audible bruit, but only about 25% have a palpable thrill. Venous hypertension can affect the gastrointestinal and urinary tracts as well as the lower extremities, and lower gastrointestinal tract bleeding and hematuria are common.

Despite these protean manifestations, the diagnosis of aortocaval fistula is usually not made clinically. Aortography is the best diagnostic modality, although the fistulas can sometimes be documented by CT, MRI, or ultrasound scans. The natural history of aortocaval fistula is progressive cardiac decompensation and death. Surgical correction offers the only hope for survival and should be undertaken promptly. A conventional infrarenal aortic aneurysm operation with oversewing of the fistula from within the opened aorta cures the fistula. Hemodynamic improvement is immediate, and renal function usually recovers rapidly. Nevertheless, reported mortality rates have been between 22% and 51%, largely as a result of blood loss, cardiac decompensation, and pulmonary embolism.[158]

MYCOTIC AORTIC ANEURYSMS

Mycotic aneurysm refers to an aneurysm of infectious although not necessarily fungal etiology. The term *mycotic* is derived from the mushroom-shaped false aneurysm of the arterial wall that is typically found. These aneurysms usually occur as a consequence of bacterial or septic emboli lodging at a point on the intimal surface of an artery of sufficient quantity to produce a locally invasive infection spreading to become a transmural arteritis. Although this can occur in normal arteries, it more commonly affects large, major atherosclerotic vessels and their branches. A septic embolus may also lodge in vasa vasorum and initiate a necrotic process in the arterial wall. A third mechanism is arterial invasion from a septic focus adjacent to a major artery. Traumatic contamination of an artery has replaced endocarditis as the most common etiology, often as a result of drug abuse.[161]

In the largest collective review of mycotic aneurysms, the abdominal aorta was the second most frequent site of involvement (31%), exceeded only by the femoral artery (38%).[159] Chan and associates[162] have reported a series of 22 mycotic aortic aneurysms out of a series of 2585 patients, an incidence of 0.85%. Coincident with the change in etiology, there has been a change in the bacteriology of mycotic aneurysms, with *Salmonella* species declining, whereas *Staphylococcus* species are increasing. However, together these are still the most frequently cultured organisms from aortic mycotic aneurysms.[163] The predilection for the infrarenal abdominal aorta probably relates to the frequent occurrence of atherosclerotic plaques in this location.

Most patients are diagnosed with a nonspecific febrile illness of variable duration, and many do not have a palpable aneurysm. Only about one third have abdominal pain. The triad of abdominal pain, fever, and a pulsatile abdominal mass should suggest the diagnosis of mycotic aneurysm. Leukocytosis is a common finding, but only about 50% have positive blood cultures. Mycotic aneurysms are often detected by CT scans performed for evaluation of undiagnosed fever. They appear as a mass located on one side of the aorta rather than a circumferential enlargement.[161, 163] They enhance with intravenously administered contrast, but the significance of this can be difficult to appreciate. Angiography demonstrates the characteristic lobulated saccular aneurysm, which may be multiple and contiguous. These are false aneurysms, contained by compressed periaortic tissue. The aneurysm wall tends to be thin and friable and associated with contiguous lymphadenopathy and obvious inflammation. Blood clot of varying age is present both within and outside the aneurysmal sac because there is a high incidence of rupture, although it is usually contained. Periaortic abscess may also be present. The opening between the aorta and the aneurysm tends to be irregular or ragged.

Mycotic aneurysms are a fulminant infectious process and must be treated vigorously and promptly.[162, 164–166] Control of clinical sepsis does not appear to be necessary for successful surgical treatment, and delays in operative intervention are associated with aneurysmal rupture. Proper antibiotic therapy must be combined with resection of the infected arterial segments, débridement of all adjacent necrotic tissue, and arterial reconstruction. Control of infection by antibiotics does not prevent rupture of the aneurysm, and excision is mandatory and should be carried out promptly. Many of these aneurysms involve the upper abdominal aorta, where it is not always possible to avoid use of prosthetic arterial grafts. In situ prosthetic replacement is necessary when renal or visceral perfusion would be compromised by aortic excision. For the infrarenal aorta, if the intraoperative Gram stains are negative and there is no periaortic purulence, in situ prosthetic grafting is also the procedure of choice. It should be followed with 6 to 8 weeks of specific antibiotic therapy, and, in the case of *Salmonella* infections, probably lifelong antibiotics. When there is frank periaortic pus and/or a positive Gram stain of an infrarenal mycotic aneurysm, management can be either aortic débridement and ligation or extra-anatomic bypass and a shorter course of antibiotics, or alternatively by the in situ grafting technique described previously. Recent data tend to favor the in situ method. Using these principles, Crawford's group has reported an operative survival rate of 86%, with only one recurrent infection.[162]

ILIAC ARTERY ANEURYSMS

Common iliac artery aneurysms occur in continuity or association with abdominal aortic aneurysms in 16% to 20% of patients. As isolated lesions, they are very uncommon, accounting for only 1% to 2% of all aneurysms involving the aortoiliac segments and being identified in only 0.03% of autopsies.[167–171] The etiology of the vast majority is nonspecific or multifactorial and they therefore occur in association with atherosclerosis in the atherosclerosis age group. However, they have developed during pregnancy in the absence of atherosclerosis, and several other etiologies have been recognized. Mycotic and traumatic iliac aneurysms have been reported, the latter usually after lumbar disc or hip surgery. Other even less frequent etiologies include cystic medial necrosis, dissection, Takayasu's disease, the Marfan and Ehlers-Danlos syndromes, and Kawasaki's disease.

Most isolated iliac aneurysms involve the common iliac (70%) or internal iliac (20%) arteries. Isolated external iliac artery aneurysms are extremely rare. Multiple iliac aneurysms occur in the majority of patients. In the Richardson and Greenfield series, two or more vessels were involved in 67% of patients.[172] These aneurysms are bilateral in about 33% of patients. Because most occur in association with atherosclerosis, the average age at diagnosis is around 69 years, and the male-to-female ratio is 7:1. The left and right sides are equally involved.

The clinical presentation of iliac aneurysms is variable and often obscure. Because they are in the pelvis, they are difficult to palpate on physical examination unless they are quite large. The majority, 50% to 67% in recent reviews, are symptomatic even in the absence of rupture. Symptoms are caused mainly by pressure on adjacent pelvic structures (e.g., urinary tract, lower gastrointestinal tract, lumbosacral nerves, pelvic veins).[173] Thus, lower abdominal, flank, and groin pain are the most common. Because these are not usually symptoms attributable to the arterial system, delays in diagnosis occur frequently. Diagnosis is usually made based on an imaging study that was performed to look for the cause of the symptoms or for an unrelated condition. Both CT and ultrasonography are highly reliable for these lesions, and there is excellent correlation between CT and ultrasound measurements. As with aortic aneurysms, arteriography documents the presence of most iliac aneurysms but frequently underestimates size because of the presence of laminated thrombus. Other studies occasionally useful in making the diagnosis are barium enema, proctosigmoidoscopy, cystoscopy, and plain x-ray films.

Even though iliac artery aneurysms are difficult to detect by routine physical examination, large ones can be palpated on abdominal, rectal, or pelvic examinations. Common iliac aneurysms are generally more easily felt abdominally, whereas internal iliac aneurysms are more easily felt rectally.

In most reports, iliac aneurysms tend to be quite large when diagnosed, which probably accounts for the high incidence of symptoms and rupture. In Shuler and Flanigan's collected review, the average size was 8.5 cm, and the incidence of rupture was 51%.[169] In Krupski's more recent report, the average size was 5.6 cm, with a 29% rupture rate.[174]

There are no prospective studies of isolated iliac artery aneurysms, but the natural history of large ones appears to be unfavorable. The reported high rate of rupture within a few months of diagnosis probably reflects large aneurysm size at the time of diagnosis. Not surprisingly, operative mortality in patients with ruptured aneurysms ranges from 25% to 56%, with an average of 40%. In contrast, the operative mortality for elective operations is much better, averaging 10% to 11%. The outlook for smaller aneurysms does not appear to be so poor. In Santilli's series of 47 isolated iliac aneurysms, the average size was 2.3 cm, and the only rupture was an aneurysm larger than 5.0 cm.[175] The average rate of enlargement in this series was 0.12 to 0.26 cm/year, with larger aneurysms expanding at a greater rate than smaller ones. No patient developed symptoms with an aneurysm smaller than 4.0 cm. These and other data suggest that isolated common iliac aneurysms smaller than 3.0 cm can be followed with semiannual ultrasound or CT scans, with minimal risk of symptom development or rupture. Aneurysms 3.5 to 4.0 cm diameter or greater should be repaired, even if asymptomatic. Symptomatic iliac aneurysms should be repaired regardless of size. The same size guidelines should be used for internal and external iliac aneurysms because so few data are available about these less common lesions. Common iliac aneurysms associated with aortic aneurysms appear to behave in a similar manner, but it seems prudent to deal with aneurysms larger than about 2.0 to 2.5 cm at the time of aortic aneurysm repair using a bifurcated graft. Smaller iliac arteries can be left in place with very low probability that they will enlarge enough to become clinically significant.

The advent of stent grafts has added another option to the treatment of common iliac aneurysms. The standard treatment is graft replacement, and because the external iliac is almost never aneurysmal, the operation can be confined to the abdomen. Bilateral common iliac aneurysms necessitate use of an aortoiliac bifurcation prosthesis. Small internal iliac aneurysms can be treated with catheter-based techniques by injecting coils and other thrombogenic materials into the aneurysm and its branches. Alternatively, they can be treated by endoaneurysmorrhaphy. They should not be treated by simple ligation of the neck because they will remain pressurized via collaterals, which enable further enlargement.

The long-term prognosis of iliac aneurysms after treatment has not been well documented. Nachbur reported a 55% 5-year survival for patients with ruptured iliac aneurysms.[176] It is reasonable to expect the survival rates to be similar to those for the treatment of aortic aneurysms.

References

1. Bickerstaff LK, Hollier LH, Van Peenen HJ, et al: Abdominal aortic aneurysm: The changing natural history. J Vasc Surg 1:6, 1984.
2. Castelden W, Mercer J: Abdominal aortic aneurysms in western Australia: Descriptive epidemiology and patterns of rupture. Br J Surg 72:109, 1985.
3. Melton L, Bickerstaff L, Hollier LH, et al: Changing incidence of abdominal aortic aneurysms: A population based study. Am J Epidemiol 120:379, 1984.
4. Norman PE, Castleden WM, Hockey RL: Prevalence of abdominal aortic aneurysm in Western Australia. Br J Surg 78:1118, 1991.
5. Darling RC, Messina CR, Brewster DC, Ottinger LW: Autopsy study of unoperated aortic aneurysms. Circulation 56(Suppl 2):161, 1977.
6. Bengtsson H, Sonesson B, Bergqvist D: Incidence and prevalence of abdominal aortic aneurysms, estimated by necropsy studies and population screening and ultrasound. Ann N Y Acad Sci 800:1, 1996.
7. Thurmond AS, Semler JH: Abdominal aortic aneurysm. Incidence in a population at risk. J Cardiovasc Surg 27:457, 1986.
8. Taylor LM, Porter JM: Basic data related to clinical decision-making in abdominal aortic aneurysms. Ann Vasc Surg 1:502, 1980.
9. Graham LM, Zelenock GB, Whitehouse WM, et al: Clinical significance of atherosclerotic femoral artery aneurysms. Arch Surg 155:502, 1980.
10. Vermilion BD, Kimmins SA, Pace WG, Evans WE: A review of 147 popliteal aneurysms with long-term follow-up. Surgery 90:1009, 1981.
11. Bengtsson H, Bergqvist D, Ekberg O, Janzon L: A population based screening of abdominal aortic aneurysms (AAA). Eur J Vasc Surg 5:53, 1991.
12. Scott RAP, Ashton HA, Kay DN: Abdominal aortic aneurysm in 4237 screened patients: Prevalence, development and management over 6 years. Br J Surg 78:1122, 1991.
13. Johnston KW, Rutherford RB, Tilson MD, et al: Suggested standards for reporting on arterial aneurysms. J Vasc Surg 13:452, 1991.
14. Steinberg CR, Morton A, Steinberg I: Measurement of the abdominal aorta after intravenous aortography in health and arteriosclerotic peripheral vascular disease. AJR 95:703, 1965.
15. Hollier LH, Stanson AW, Gloviczki P, et al: Arteriomegaly: Classifications and morbid implications of diffuse aneurysmal disease. Surgery 93:700, 1983.
16. Bengtsson H, Ekberg O, Aspelin P, et al: Abdominal aortic dilatation in patients operated on for carotid artery stenosis. Acta Chir Scand 154:441, 1988.
17. Mukherjee D, Mayberry JC, Inahara T, Greig JD: The relationship of the abdominal aortic aneurysm to the tortuous internal carotid artery. Is there one? Arch Surg 124:955, 1989.
18. Wolfe YG, Otis SM, Schwend RB, Bernstein EF: Screening for abdominal aortic aneurysms during lower extremity arterial evaluation in the vascular laboratory. J Vasc Surg 22:417, 1995.
19. Cohen J: Pathogenesis of aortic aneurysms. Perspect Vasc Surg 3:103, 1990.
20. Tilson DM, Stansel HC: Differences in results for aneurysm vs. occlusive disease after bifurcation grafts. Results of 100 elective grafts. Arch Surg 107:1173, 1980.
21. Dobrin PB: Pathophysiology and pathogenesis of aortic aneurysms. Current concept. Surg Clin North Am 69:687, 1989.
22. Zarins CK, Glagov S: Aneurysms and obstructive plaques: Differing local responses to atherosclerosis. In Bergan JJ, Yao JST (eds): Aneurysms: Diagnosis and Treatment. New York, Grune & Stratton, 1982, pp 61–82.
23. Busuttil RW, Abou-Zamzam AM, Machleder HI: Collagenase activity of the human aorta: Comparisons of patients with and without abdominal aortic aneurysms. Arch Surg 115:1373, 1980.
24. Busuttil RW, Heinrich R, Flesher A: Elastase activity: The role of elastase in aortic aneurysm formation. J Surg Res 32:214, 1982.
25. Dobrin PB, Baker WH, Gley WC: Elastolytic and collagenolytic studies of arteries: Implications for the mechanical properties of aneurysms. Arch Surg 119:405, 1984.
26. Dobrin PB, Baker WH, Schwarcz TH: Mechanisms of arterial and aneurysmal tortuosity. Surgery 104:568, 1988.
27. Cohen J, Mandell C, Chang JB, Wise L: Elastin metabolism of the infrarenal aorta. J Vasc Surg 7:210, 1988.
28. Cronenwett JL, Murphy TF, Zelenock GB, et al: Actuarial analysis of variables associated with rupture of small aortic aneurysms. Surgery 98:472, 1985.
29. Louwrens H, Pearce WH: Role of inflammatory cells in aortic aneurysms. In Yao JST, Pearch WH (eds): Aneurysms. New Findings and Treatments. East Norwalk, CT, Appleton & Lange, 1994, pp 11–23.
30. Dobrin PB, Baumgartner N, Anidjar S, et al: Inflammatory aspects of experimental aneurysms. Effect of methylprednisolone and cyclosporine. Ann N Y Acad Sci 800:74, 1996.
31. White JV, Mazzacco SL: Formation and growth of aortic aneurysms induced by adventitial elastolysis. Ann N Y Acad Sci 800:97, 1996.
32. Majumder PP, St. Jean PL, Ferrell RE, et al: On the inheritance of abdominal aortic aneurysm. Am J Hum Genet 48:164, 1991.
33. Verloes A, Sakalihasan N, Limet R, Koulischer L: Genetic aspects of abdominal aortic aneurysm. Ann N Y Acad Sci 800:44, 1996.
34. Tilson MD, Seashore MR: Human genetics of the abdominal aortic aneurysm. Surg Gynecol Obstet 158:129, 1984.
35. Tilson MD: Decreased hepatic copper levels: A possible chemical marker for the pathogenesis of aortic aneurysms in man. Arch Surg 117:1212, 1982.
36. Tilson MD: Generalized arteriomegaly: A possible predisposition to the formation of abdominal aortic aneurysms. Arch Surg 116:1030, 1981.
37. Collin J, Walton J: Is abdominal aortic aneurysm familial? Br Med J 299:493, 1989.
38. Johansen K, Koepsell T: Familial tendency for abdominal aortic aneurysms. JAMA 256:1934, 1986.
39. Clifton, MA: Familial abdominal aortic aneurysms. Br J Surg 64:765–766, 1977.
40. Szilagyi DE: Clinical diagnosis of intact and ruptured abdominal aortic aneurysms. In Bergan JJ, Yao JST (eds): Aneurysms: Diagnosis and Treatment. New York, Grune & Stratton, 1982, pp 205–215.
41. Sterpetti AV, Feldhaus RJ, Schultz RD, Blair EA: Identification of abdominal aortic aneurysm patients with different clinical features and clinical outcomes. Am J Surg 156:466, 1988.
42. Lawrie GM, Crawford ES, Morris GC Jr, Howell JF: Progress in the treatment of ruptured abdominal aortic aneurysm. World J Surg 4:653, 1980.
43. Rutherford RB, McCroskey BL: Ruptured abdominal aortic aneurysms. Special considerations. Surg Clin North Am 69:859, 1989.
44. Bower TC, Cherry KJ Jr, Pairolero PC: Unusual manifestations of abdominal aneurysms. Surg Clin North Am 69:745, 1989.
45. Moran KT, Persson AV, Jewell ER: Chronic rupture of abdominal aortic aneurysms. Am Surg 55:485, 1989.
46. Goldstone J: Vascular imaging techniques. In Rutherford RB (ed): Vascular Surgery, 3rd ed. Philadelphia, WB Saunders Company, 1989, pp 119–128.
47. Quill DS, Colgan MP, Summer DS: Ultrasonic screening for the detection of abdominal aortic aneurysms. Surg Clin North Am 69(4):713, 1989.
48. Bluth EI: Ultrasound of the abdominal aorta. Arch Intern Med 144:377, 1984.
49. Gomes MN, Choyke PL: Pre-operative evaluation of abdominal

aortic aneurysms: Ultrasound or computed tomography? J Cardiovasc Surg 28:159, 1987.

50. Greatorex RA, Dixon AK, Flower CDR, Pulvertaft RW: Limitations of computed tomography in leaking abdominal aortic systems. Br Med J 297:284, 1988.
51. Amparo EG, Hoddick WK, Hricak H, et al: Comparison of magnetic resonance imaging and ultrasonography in the evaluation of abdominal aortic aneurysms. Radiology 154:451, 1985.
52. Clayton MJ, Walsh JW, Brewer WH: Contained rupture of abdominal aortic aneurysms: Sonographic and CT diagnosis. AJR 138:154, 1982.
53. Weinbaum FI, Dubner S, Turner JW, et al: The accuracy of computed tomography in the diagnosis of retroperitoneal blood in the presence of abdominal aortic aneurysm. J Vasc Surg 6:11, 1987.
54. Gomes MN, Davros WJ, Zeman RK: Preoperative assessment of abdominal aortic aneurysm. The value of helical and three-dimensional computed tomography. J Vasc Surg 20:367–375, 1994.
55. Raptopoulos V, Rosen MP, Kent KC, et al: Sequential helical CT angiography of aorto-iliac disease. AJR 166:1347, 1996.
56. Lee JKT, Ling D, Heiken JP, et al: Magnetic resonance imaging of abdominal aneurysms. AJR 143:1197, 1984.
57. Rich NM, Clagett GP, Salander JM, et al: Role of arteriography in the evaluation of aortic aneurysms. In Bergan JJ, Yao JST (eds): Aneurysms: Diagnosis and Treatment. New York, Grune & Stratton, 1982, pp 233–241.
58. Friedman SG, Kerner BA, Krishnasastry KV, et al: Abdominal aortic aneurysmectomy without preoperative angiography: A prospective study. N Y State J Med 90(1):176, 1990.
59. Gaspar MR: Role of arteriography in the evaluation of aortic aneurysms. The case against. In Bergan JY, Yao JST (eds): Aneurysms: Diagnosis and Treatment. New York, Grune & Stratton, 1982, pp 243–254.
60. Estes JE Jr: Abdominal aortic aneurysm: A study of 102 cases. Circulation 2:258, 1950.
61. Wright IS, Urdenata E, Wright B: Re-opening the case of the abdominal aortic aneurysm. Circulation 13:754, 1956.
62. Szilagyi DE, Smith RF, De Russo FJ, et al: Contribution of abdominal aortic aneurysmectomy to prolongation of life. Ann Surg 164:678, 1966.
63. Bernstein EF, Chan EL: Abdominal aortic aneurysm in high risk patients: Outcome of selective management based on size and expansion rate. Ann Surg 200:255, 1984.
64. Szilagyi DE, Elliott JP, Smith RF: Clinical fate of the patient with asymptomatic abdominal aortic aneurysm and unfit for surgical treatment. Arch Surg 104:600, 1972.
65. Foster JH, Bolasny BL, Gobbel WG, Scott HW: Comparative study of elective resection and expectant treatment of abdominal aortic aneurysm. Surg Gynecol Obstet 129:1, 1969.
66. Hollier LH, Taylor LM, Ochsner J: Recommended indications for operative treatment of abdominal aortic aneurysms. Report of a subcommittee of the Joint Council of the Society for Vascular Surgery and the North American Chapter of the International Society for Cardiovascular Surgery. J Vasc Surg 15:1046, 1992.
67. UK Small Aneurysm Trial Participants: Mortality results for randomized controlled trial of early elective surgery or ultrasonographic surveillance for small abdominal aortic aneurysms. Lancet 352:1649, 1998.
68. ADAM trial. Unpublished data.
69. Glimaker H, Holmberg L, Elvin A, et al: Natural history of patients with abdominal aortic aneurysm. Eur J Vasc Surg 5:125, 1991.
70. Johansson G, Nydahl S, Olofsson P, Swedenborg J: Survival in patients with abdominal aortic aneurysms. Comparison between operative and nonoperative management. Eur J Vasc Surg 4:497, 1990.
71. Walsh AKM, Briffa N, Nash JR, Callum KG: The natural history of small abdominal aortic aneurysms: An ultrasound study. Eur J Vasc Surg 4:459, 1990.
72. Nevitt MP, Ballard DJ, Hallett JW Jr: Prognosis of abdominal aortic aneurysms. N Engl J Med 321:1009, 1989.
73. Cronenwett JL, Sargent SK, Wall MH, et al: Variables that affect the expansion rate and outcome of small abdominal aortic aneurysms. J Vasc Surg 11:260, 1990.
74. Gadowski GR, Pilcher DB, Ricci MA: Abdominal aortic aneurysm expansion rate: Effect of size and beta-adrenergic blockade. J Vasc Surg 19:727, 1994.
75. Crawford ES, Saleh SA, Babb JW III, et al: Infrarenal abdominal aortic aneurysm. Factors influencing survival after operation performed over a 25 year period. Ann Surg 193:699, 1981.
76. Pilcher DB, Davis JH, Ashileoga T, et al: Treatment of abdominal aortic aneurysm in an entire state over 7½ years. Ann J Surg 139:487, 1980.
77. Pairolero PC: Repair of abdominal aortic aneurysms in high-risk patients. Surg Clin North Am 69:755, 1989.
78. Hertzer NR, Avellone JC, Farrel CJ, et al: The risk of vascular surgery in a metropolitan community. J Vasc Surg 1:13, 1984.
79. DeBakey ME, Crawford ES, Cooley DA, et al: Aneurysm of abdominal aorta. Analysis of results of graft replacement therapy one to eleven years after operation. Ann Surg 169:622, 1964.
80. Robson AK, Currie IC, Poskitt KR, et al: Abdominal aortic aneurysm repair in the over eighties. Br J Surg 76:1018, 1989.
81. Vasko JS, Spencer FC, Bahnson HT: Aneurysm of the aorta treated by excision: Review of 237 cases followed up to seven years. Am J Surg 105:793, 1963.
82. Cannon JA, Van De Water J, Barker WF: Experience with the surgical management of 100 consecutive cases of abdominal aortic aneurysm. Am J Surg 106:128, 1963.
83. Voorhees AB, McAllister FF: Long term results following resection of arteriosclerotic abdominal aortic aneurysms. Surg Gynecol Obstet 117:355, 1963.
84. Levy JF, Kouchoukos NT, Walker WB, Butcher HR: Abdominal aortic aneurysmectomy: A study of 100 cases. Arch Surg 92:498, 1966.
85. May AG, DeWeese JA, Frank I, et al: Surgical treatment of abdominal aortic aneurysms. Surgery 63:711, 1968.
86. Baker AG, Roberts B: Long-term survival following abdominal aortic aneurysmectomy. JAMA 212:445, 1970.
87. Stokes J, Butcher HR: Abdominal aortic aneurysms: Factors influencing operative mortality and criteria of operability. Arch Surg 107:297, 1973.
88. Hicks GL, Eastland MW, DeWeese JA, et al: Survival improvement following aortic aneurysm resection. Ann Surg 181:863, 1975.
89. O'Donnell TF, Darling RC, Linton RR: Is 80 years too old for aneurysmectomy? Arch Surg 111:1250, 1976.
90. Crawford ES, Saleh SA, Babb JW III, et al: Infrarenal abdominal aortic aneurysm: Factors influencing survival after operations performed over a 25-year period. Ann Surg 193:699, 1981.
91. Reigel MM, Hollier LH, Kazmier FJ, et al: Late survival in abdominal aortic aneurysm patients: The role of selective myocardial revascularization on the basis of clinical systems. J Vasc Surg 5:222, 1987.
92. Bernstein EF, Dilley RB, Randolph HF III: The improving long term outlook for patients 70 years of age with abdominal aortic aneurysms. Ann Surg 207:318, 1988.
92. Bernstein EF, Dilley RB, Randolph HF III: The improving long abdominal aortic aneurysm in the high-risk patient: A plea for aneurysms. Ann Surg 207:318, 1988.
93. Hollier LH, Reigel MM, Kozmier FJ, et al: Conventional repair of abdominal aortic aneurysm in the high-risk patient: A plea for abandonment of nonresective treatment. J Vasc Surg 3:712–717, 1986.
94. Hiatt JCG, Barker WF, Machleder HI, et al: Determinants of failure in the treatment of ruptured abdominal aortic aneurysms. Arch Surg 119:1264, 1984.
95. Fielding JWL, Black J, Ashton F, Slaney G: Ruptured aortic aneurysms: Postoperative complications and their aetiology. Br J Surg 72:487, 1984.
96. Donaldson MC, Rosenberg JM, Bucknam CA: Factors affecting survival after ruptured abdominal aortic aneurysm. J Vasc Surg 2:564, 1985.
97. Johansen K, Kohler RT, Nicholls SC, et al: Ruptured abdominal aortic aneurysm. The Harborview experience. J Vasc Surg 13:240, 1991.
98. Burnham SJ, Johnson G Jr, Gurri JA: Mortality risks for survivors of vascular reconstructive procedures. Surgery 92:107, 1982.
99. Johnson G Jr, Gurri JA, Burnham SJ: Life expectancy after abdominal aortic aneurysm repair. In Bergan JJ, Yao JST (eds): Aneurysms: Diagnosis and Treatment. New York, Grune & Stratton, 1982, pp 279–285.
100. Hollier LH, Plate G, O'Brien PC, et al: Late survival after abdominal aortic aneurysm repair. Influence of coronary artery disease. J Vasc Surg 1:290, 1984.

101. Hertzer NR: Fatal myocardial infarction following abdominal aortic aneurysm resection: 343 patients followed 6–11 years postoperative. Ann Surg 190:667, 1980.
102. Hertzer NR: Clinical experience with pre-operative coronary angiography. J Vasc Surg 2:510, 1985.
103. Hertzer NR, Young JR, Bevan EG, et al: Late results of coronary bypass in patients with infra-renal aortic aneurysms. The Cleveland Clinic Study. Ann Surg 205:360, 1987.
104. Crawford ES, Morris GC Jr, Howell JF, et al: Operative risk in patients with previous coronary artery bypass. Ann Thorac Surg 26:215, 1978.
105. Ruby ST, Whittemore AD, Couch NP, et al: Coronary artery disease in patients requiring abdominal aortic aneurysm repair. Selective use of a combined operation. Arch Surg 201:758, 1985.
106. Reul G Jr, Cooley DA, Duncan MJ, et al: The effect of coronary bypass on the outcome of peripheral vascular operation in 1093 patients. J Vasc Surg 3:788, 1986.
107. Bevan EG: Routine coronary angiography in patients undergoing surgery for abdominal aortic aneurysm and lower extremity occlusive disease. J Vasc Surg 3:682, 1986.
108. Johnston KW: Canadian study of the late results of abdominal aortic aneurysm repair. In Yao JST, Pearce WH (eds): Aneurysms. New Findings and Treatments. East Norwalk, CT, Appleton & Lange, 1994, pp 79–87.
109. Yeager RA, Moneta GL: Assessing cardiac risk in vascular surgical patients: Current status. Perspect Vasc Surg 2:18, 1989.
110. Blomberg PA, Ferguson IA, Rosengarten DS, et al: The role of coronary artery disease in complications of abdominal aortic aneurysm repair. Surgery 101:150, 1987.
111. Goldman L: Cardiac risks and complications of non-cardiac surgery. Ann Surg 198:780, 1983.
112. Golden MA, Whittemore AD, Donaldson MC, Mannick JA: Selective evaluation and management of coronary artery disease in patients undergoing repair of abdominal aortic aneurysms: A 16-year experience. Ann Surg 212:415, 1990.
113. Cambria RP, Eagle K: Cardiac screening before abdominal aortic aneurysm surgery: A reassessment. Semin Vasc Surg 8:93, 1995.
114. McPhail NV, Ruddy TD, Calvin JE, et al: A complication of dipyridamole-thallium imaging and exercise testing in the prediction of post-operative cardiac complications in patients requiring arterial reconstruction. J Vasc Surg 10:51, 1989.
115. Boucher CA, Brewster DC, Darling RC, et al: Determination of cardiac risk by dipyridamole-thallium imaging before peripheral vascular surgery. N Engl J Med 312:389, 1985.
116. Cheitlin MD: Finding the high-risk patient with coronary artery disease. JAMA 259:2271–2277, 1988.
117. Karmody AM, Leather RP, Goldman M, et al: The current position of non-resective treatment for abdominal aortic aneurysm. Surgery 94:591–597, 1983.
118. Schwartz RA, Nichols WK, Silver D: Is thrombosis of the infrarenal abdominal aortic aneurysm an acceptable alternative? J Vasc Surg 3:448–455, 1986.
119. Cho SI, Johnson WC, Buch HL Jr, et al: Lethal complications associated with nonresective treatment of abdominal aortic aneurysms. Arch Surg 117:1214–1217, 1982.
120. Inahara T, Beary GL, Mukherjee D, Egan JM: The contrary position to the nonresective treatment for abdominal aortic aneurysm. J Vasc Surg 2:42–48, 1985.
121. Sicard GA, Allen BJ, Munn JS, Anderson CB: Retroperitoneal vs. transperitoneal approach for repair of abdominal aortic aneurysms. Surg Clin North Am 69:795–806, 1989.
122. Cambria RP, Brewster DC, Abbott WM, et al: Transperitoneal versus retroperitoneal approach for aortic reconstruction. A randomized, prospective study. J Vasc Surg 11:314–325, 1990.
123. Cambria RP, Brewster DC: Advantages of the retroperitoneal approach for aortic surgery: Fact or fancy? Perspect Vasc Surg 3:52–69, 1990.
124. Chang BB, Shan DJ, Paty PS, et al: Can the retroperitoneal approach be used for ruptured abdominal aortic aneurysms? J Vasc Surg 11:326–330, 1990.
125. Turnipseed WD: A less-invasive minilaparotomy technique for repair of aortic aneurysms and occlusive disease. J Vasc Surg 33:431, 2001.
126. Dion Y-M, Gracia CR, Hassen BEK: Totally laparoscopically abdominal aortic aneurysm repair. J Vasc Surg 33:181, 2001.
127. Goldstone J: Intraoperative monitoring in aortic surgery. In Bergan JJ, Yao JST (eds): Arterial Surgery. New Diagnostic and Operative Techniques. Orlando, FL, Grune & Stratton, 1988, pp 257–271.
128. Roizen MF, Beaupre PN, Albert RA, et al: Monitoring with two-dimensional transesophageal echocardiography. J Vasc Surg 1:300, 1984.
129. Budden J, Hollier LH: Management of aneurysms that involve the juxtarenal or suprarenal aorta. Surg Clin North Am 69:837, 1989.
130. Allen BT, Anderson CB, Rubin BG, et al: Preservation of renal function in juxtarenal and suprarenal abdominal aortic aneurysm repair. J Vasc Surg 17:948, 1993.
131. AbuRhama AF, Robinson PA: The risk of ligation of the left renal vein in resection of the abdominal aortic aneurysm. SG & O; 173:33, 1991.
132. Macbeth GA, Rubin JR, McIntyre KE, et al: The relevance of arterial wall microbiology to the treatment of prosthetic graft infections. Graft infection vs. arterial infection. J Vasc Surg 1:754, 1984.
133. Schwarcz TH, Flanigan DP: Repair of abdominal aortic aneurysms in patients with renal, iliac, or distal arterial occlusive disease. Surg Clin North Am 69:845, 1989.
134. Moore WS, Rutherford RB: Transfemoral endovascular repair of abdominal aortic aneurysms: Results of the North American EVT phase 1 trial. J Vasc Surg 23:543, 1996.
135. Parodi JC: Endovascular repair of abdominal aortic aneurysms and other arterial lesions. J Vasc Surg 21:549, 1996.
136. Castronuovo JJ Jr, Flanigan DP: Renal failure complicating vascular surgery. In Bernhard VM, Towne JB (eds): Complications in Vascular Surgery, 2nd ed. Orlando, FL, Grune & Stratton, 1985, pp 259–273.
137. Alpert RA, Roizen MF, Hamilton WK, et al: Intraoperative urinary output does not predict postoperative renal function in patients undergoing abdominal aortic revascularization. Surgery 95:707, 1984.
138. Ernst CB, Hagihara PF, Daughorty ME, et al: Ischemic colitis incidence following abdominal aortic reconstruction: A prospective study. Surgery 80:417, 1976.
139. Ernst CB: Prevention of intestinal ischemia following abdominal aortic reconstruction. Surgery 93:102, 1983.
140. Schroeder T, Christofferson JK, Anderson J, et al: Ischemic colitis complicating reconstruction of the abdominal aorta. Surg Gynecol Obstet 160:299, 1985.
141. Szilagyi DE, Hagemen JH, Smith RF, et al: Spinal cord damage in surgery of the abdominal aorta. Surgery 83:38, 1978.
142. Calligaro KD, DeLaurentis DA, Dougherty MJ: Venous anomalies encountered during abdominal aortic surgery. In: Caligaro KD, Dougherty MD, Hollie L (eds): Diagnosis and Treatment of Aortic and Peripheral Arterial Aneurysms. Philadelphia, WB Saunders, 1999, pp 183–192.
143. Bartle EJ, Pearce WH, Sun JH, et al: Infrarenal venous anomalies and aortic surgery. J Vasc Surg 6:590–593, 1987.
144. Giordano JM, Trout HH: Anomalies of the inferior vena cava. J Vasc Surg 3:924–928, 1986.
145. Brener BJ, Darling C, Frederick PL, et al: Major venous anomalies complicating abdominal aortic surgery. Arch Surg 108:160, 1974.
146. Kunkel JM, Weinstein ES: Preoperative detection of potential hazards in aortic surgery. Perspect Vasc Surg 2:1, 1989.
147. Goldstone J, Malone JM, Moore WS: Inflammatory aneurysms of the abdominal aorta. Surgery 83:425, 1978.
148. Goldstone J: Inflammatory aneurysms of the abdominal aorta. Semin Vasc Surg 1:165, 1988.
149. Crawford JL, Stowe CL, Safitt J, et al: Inflammatory aneurysms of the aorta. J Vasc Surg 2:113, 1985.
150. Pennell RC, Hollier LH, Lie JT, et al: Inflammatory abdominal aortic aneurysms: A thirty year review. J Vasc Surg 2:859, 1985.
151. Conelly TL, McKinnon W, Smith RB III, et al: Abdominal aortic surgery and horseshoe kidney. Arch Surg 115:1459, 1980.
152. Starr DS, Foster WJ, Morris GC Jr: Resection of abdominal aortic aneurysm in the presence of horseshoe kidney. Surgery 89:387, 1981.
153. Hollis HW, Rutherford RB: Abdominal aortic aneurysms associated with horseshoe or ectopic kidneys. Techniques of renal preservation. Semin Vasc Surg 1:148, 1988.
154. Tarazi RY, Hertzer NR, Bevan EG, et al: Simultaneous aortic reconstruction and renal revascularization: Risk factors and late results in 89 patients. J Vasc Surg 5:707, 1987.
155. Stewart MT, Smith RB III, Fulenwider JT, et al: Concomitant renal

revascularization in patients undergoing aortic surgery. J Vasc Surg 2:400, 1985.

156. String ST: Cholelithiasis and aortic reconstruction. J Vasc Surg 1:664, 1984.

157. Ouriel K, Ricotta JJ, Adams JT, DeWeese JA: Management of cholelithiasis in patients with abdominal aortic aneurysms. Ann Surg 198:717, 1983.

158. Goldstone J, Effeny DJ: Prevention of arterial graft infection. In Bernhard VM, Towne JB (eds): Complications in Vascular Surgery, 2nd ed. Orlando, FL, Grune & Stratton, 1985, pp 487–498.

159. Alexander JJ, Imbebo AL: Aorta-vena cava fistula. Surgery 105:1, 1989.

160. Baker WH, Sharzer LA, Ehrenhaft JL: Aortocaval fistula as a complication of aortic aneurysms. Surgery 72:933, 1972.

161. Brown SL, Busuttil RW, Baker JD, et al: Bacteriologic and surgical determinants of survival in patients with mycotic aneurysms. J Vasc Surg 1:541, 1984.

162. Chan FY, Crawford ES, Coselli JS, et al: In situ prosthetic graft replacement for mycotic aneurysms of the aorta. Ann Thorac Surg 47:193, 1989.

163. Parson R, Gregory J, Palmer DL: *Salmonella* infections of the abdominal aorta. Rev Infect Dis 5:227, 1983.

164. Reddy DJ, Lee RE, Oh HK: Suprarenal mycotic aortic aneurysm: Surgical management and follow-up. J Vasc Surg 3:917, 1986.

165. Muller BT, Wegener OR, Grabitz K, et al: Mycotic aneurysms of the thoracic and abdominal aorta and iliac arteries: Experience with anatomic and extra-anatomic repair in 33 cases. J Vasc Surg 33:106, 2001.

166. Scher LA, Brenner BJ, Goldenkranz RJ, et al: Infected aneurysms of the abdominal aorta. Arch Surg 115:975, 1980.

167. Lawrence PF, Lorenzo-Rivero S, Lyon JL: The incidence of iliac, femoral, and popliteal aneurysms in hospitalized patients. J Vasc Surg 22:409, 1995.

168. Brunkwall J, Bergentz SE: Solitary iliac aneurysms. In Yao JST and Pearce WH (eds): Aneurysms. New Findings and Treatments. Norwalk, CT, Appleton and Lange, 1994, pp 459–473.

169. Schuler JJ, Flanigan DP: Iliac artery aneurysms. In Bergan JJ, Yao JST (eds): Aneurysms: Diagnosis and Treatment. New York, Grune & Stratton, 1982, pp 469–485.

170. Lowry SF, Kraft RO: Isolated aneurysms of the iliac artery. Arch Surg 113:1289, 1978.

171. McCready RA, Pairolero PC, Gilmore JC, et al: Isolated iliac artery aneurysms. Surgery 93:688, 1983.

172. Richardson JW, Greenfield LJ: Natural history and management of iliac aneurysms. J Vasc Surg 8:165, 1988.

173. Marino R, Mooppan UMM, Zein TA, et al: Urologic manifestations of isolated iliac artery aneurysms. J Urol 137:232, 1987.

174. Krupski WC, Selzman CH, Florida R, et al: Contemporary management of isolated iliac artery aneurysms. J Vasc Surg 28:1, 1998.

175. Santilli SM, Wernsing SE, Lee ES: Expansion rates and outcomes for iliac artery aneurysms. J Vasc Surg 31:114, 2000.

176. Nachbur BH, Inderbitzi RGC, Bär W: Isolated iliac aneurysms. Eur J Vasc Surg 5:375, 1991.

Review Questions

1. Factors considered to be involved in the pathogenesis of abdominal aortic aneurysms include all of the following except
   (a) heredity
   (b) atherosclerosis
   (c) enzyme deficiencies
   (d) enzyme excess
   (e) hormones

2. The incidence of abdominal aortic aneurysm is highest among patients with
   (a) femoral aneurysm
   (b) aortoiliac occlusive disease
   (c) thoracic aortic aneurysm
   (d) bilateral popliteal aneurysm
   (e) isolated iliac artery aneurysm

3. The risk of rupture of infrarenal abdominal aortic aneurysms
   (a) increases with increasing size of the aneurysm
   (b) increases with increasing age of the patient
   (c) is negligible for aneurysms less than 6.0 cm in diameter
   (d) is not affected by blood pressure
   (e) is related to plasma lipoprotein levels

4. The most common cause of late death following surgical treatment of abdominal aortic aneurysm is
   (a) renal failure
   (b) respiratory failure
   (c) myocardial ischemia
   (d) graft infection
   (e) malignancy

5. The true mortality for ruptured abdominal aortic aneurysms, including prehospital deaths, is approximately
   (a) 15%
   (b) 30%
   (c) 50%
   (d) 60%
   (e) 90%

6. Which of the following is true when the surgeon fails to see the left renal vein during exposure of an abdominal aortic aneurysm?
   (a) the dissection should be extended above the superior mesenteric artery
   (b) the neck of the aneurysm should be thoroughly mobilized
   (c) the inferior mesenteric vein should be carefully preserved
   (d) the surgeon can relax because the left renal vein is probably congenitally absent
   (e) extra care must be paid to the application of the aortic cross-clamp

7. Aortocaval fistulas
   (a) are usually infectious in origin
   (b) are usually symptomatic
   (c) usually occur just below the left renal vein
   (d) all of the above
   (e) none of the above

8. Which of the following statements is/are true about complications of aortic aneurysm repair?
   (a) colon ischemia is associated with a mortality rate of about 50%
   (b) renal failure does not occur if the aortic cross-clamp is totally infrarenal
   (c) paraplegia occurs only with suprarenal clamping
   (d) myocardial dysfunction is now an uncommon cause of postoperative death
   (e) the use of autotransfusion devices has greatly reduced the degree of postoperative hemorrhage

9. All of the following statements are true about inflammatory aneurysms except
   (a) they have thick fibrous walls
   (b) they are frequently associated with abdominal tenderness in the area of the aneurysm
   (c) they require CT scanning for definitive preoperative diagnosis
   (d) they frequently rupture
   (e) they are frequently associated with ureteral obstruction

10. All of the following statements about iliac artery aneurysms are true except
    (a) asymptomatic aneurysms should be 2.5 cm in diameter for repair
    (b) most are associated with or are an extension of infrarenal abdominal aortic aneurysms
    (c) most isolated iliac aneurysms manifest symptoms before rupture
    (d) they may be diagnosed by digital examination of the vagina and rectum
    (e) most can be palpated by abdominal examination

Answers

1. e   2. d   3. a   4. c   5. e   6. e   7. b   8. a   9. d   10. a

25

Aneurysms of the Peripheral Arteries

D. Preston Flanigan

Peripheral arterial aneurysms are distinctly less common than aortic aneurysms but nevertheless can cause significant morbidity. Although occasionally these lesions may lead to death, the most common serious complication is usually end-organ loss or dysfunction. For the purposes of this chapter, peripheral aneurysms include the upper extremity arteries distal to and including the subclavian artery, the lower extremity arteries distal to and including the femoral artery, and the extracranial carotid arteries. Mycotic aneurysms affecting these vessels are also included.

NONMYCOTIC PERIPHERAL ANEURYSMS

Incidence and Etiology

Overall, the most common cause of nonmycotic peripheral aneurysms is atherosclerosis. However, when based on location, this is not true for all peripheral aneurysms. In general, all peripheral aneurysms can be considered rare. In descending order, the relative frequency of these aneurysms is probably popliteal, femoral, subclavian and axillary, and carotid. More reports on distal aneurysms involving the brachial, radial, ulnar, profunda femoris, and tibial and peroneal arteries are limited to small series or case reports. Although true aneurysms have been reported in these areas,[1, 2] for the most part forearm and hand aneurysms are secondary to trauma or are mycotic in origin.[3]

Age and sex distribution is dependent on cause. Atherosclerotic aneurysms tend to occur primarily in men over 50 years of age. Aneurysms due to trauma are also more common in men but occur at a younger age. Aneurysms secondary to thoracic outlet syndrome are most commonly seen in middle-aged women (75%).

Extracranial Carotid Artery Aneurysms

The rarity of extracranial carotid aneurysms is demonstrated by numerous publications reporting institutional experiences with aneurysm patients. Of 2300 aneurysms reported from Baylor University, only seven were extracranial carotid aneurysms.[4] In 30 years at Johns Hopkins, only 12 such aneurysms were seen.[5] Only eight carotid aneurysms were noted by Houser and Baker[6] after performing 5000 cerebral arteriograms. The largest single series of patients with true extracranial carotid aneurysms was reported by McCollum and colleagues.[7] In their series, 37 aneurysms were seen over a 21-year period. Zhang and associates[8] reported 66 extracranial carotid aneurysms of which 28 were true, nonmycotic aneurysms.[8]

Currently, the common carotid artery is the artery most often affected. This is followed by the internal carotid artery, the external carotid artery rarely being involved.[9]

The most common cause of extracranial carotid aneurysms is atherosclerosis. These aneurysms tend to be fusiform in nature and are almost always associated with arterial hypertension. Most of the patients also have evidence of generalized atherosclerosis.[9] Another cause of carotid aneurysm is trauma, both blunt and penetrating.[10] False aneurysms of the carotid artery have occurred after carotid endarterectomy.[11] Rarer causes include cystic medial necrosis, Marfan's syndrome, fibromuscular dysplasia, medial arteriopathy, granulomatous disease, radiation, and congenital defects.[10]

Subclavian and Axillary Aneurysms

Aneurysms of the subclavian and axillary arteries are also rare. In 1982, Hobson and colleagues[12] reviewed the world literature on the subject and found only 195 aneurysms in these locations. This accounts for only 1% of all peripheral aneurysms. Of the 195 cases, 88% involved the subclavian artery. Subclavian and axillary aneurysms are rarely due to atherosclerosis, with this cause accounting for only 15% of the aneurysms. Thoracic outlet syndrome is primarily responsible for the majority of subclavian artery aneurysms (74%), whereas crutch trauma accounts for most of the

TABLE 25-1

Etiology of Subclavian/Axillary Aneurysms

ETIOLOGY	SUBCLAVIAN	AXILLARY	TOTAL
Thoracic outlet syndrome	127	1	128
Crutch trauma	—	13	13
Atherosclerosis	24	5	29
Pseudoaneurysm	5	2	7
Blunt trauma	2	—	2
Fibromuscular dysplasia	—	2	2
Dissection	—	1	1
Other	13	—	13
Total	171	24	195

cases of axillary aneurysms (54%). Other, rarer causes have also been reported (Table 25–1).

Forearm and Hand Aneurysms

True aneurysms in the forearm and hand are quite rare. During a 10-year period, only 10 such patients were treated at the University of Chicago.[2] Half of true aneurysms in these areas are associated with occupational or recreational trauma. Most forearm and hand pseudoaneurysms are secondary to penetrating trauma,[3] whereas most true aneurysms in these locations are secondary to blunt trauma.[13]

Femoral and Popliteal Artery Aneurysms

Femoral and popliteal artery aneurysms are grouped together because of their similar etiology, similar clinical behavior, and frequent association.

Aside from trauma and rare degenerative and congenital disorders, femoral and popliteal aneurysms are almost exclusively atherosclerotic in origin.[14, 15] Together, these two types of aneurysms account for more than 90% of peripheral aneurysms.[16] Femoral aneurysms may involve the common femoral artery in the groin, but occasionally these aneurysms may be limited to the superficial femoral artery in the midthigh. These latter lesions are not unusual and are often seen in patients with arteriomegaly or "aneurysmosis."

Dent and coworkers[17] have shown an association between popliteal and femoral aneurysms and other aneurysms of atherosclerotic origin. Most commonly, these associated aneurysms are located in the aortoiliac vessels, but more rarely they involve the renal, splanchnic, and brachiocephalic vessels. Of patients with at least one peripheral aneurysm, 83% had multiple aneurysms. Of patients with a common femoral aneurysm, 95% had a second aneurysm, 92% had an aortoiliac aneurysm, and 59% had bilateral femoral aneurysms. Of patients with a popliteal aneurysm, 78% had a second aneurysm, 64% had an aortoiliac aneurysm, and 47% had bilateral popliteal artery aneurysms.

Natural History

As with aortic aneurysms, peripheral aneurysms can be asymptomatic or may lead to significant complications. Un-

like aortic aneurysms, which tend to rupture, peripheral aneurysms most commonly thrombose or give rise to arterial emboli.

Extracranial Carotid Artery Aneurysms

Central neurologic events are very common in these patients. Rhodes and colleagues[9] reported that 13 of the 19 carotid aneurysms in the University of Michigan series had amaurosis fugax, transient ischemic attacks, stroke, or vague neurologic symptoms such as dizziness. Most of these symptoms are thought to be secondary to embolization. Cranial nerve compression leads to local neurologic dysfunction and can include facial pain (fifth cranial nerve), oculomotor palsies (sixth cranial), auricular pain (11th cranial), and hoarseness (10th cranial). Horner's syndrome can also be seen from compression of the sympathetic chain. As cervical carotid aneurysms enlarge, they can cause dysphagia, cranial nerve compression, and pain. Hemorrhage has also been seen as a complication of these aneurysms; however, rupture is uncommon.

Subclavian and Axillary Artery Aneurysms

Only 10% of patients with known subclavian or axillary aneurysms are asymptomatic.[12] Good natural history studies are not available, probably because of the small number of patients with this problem. Because 90% of patients are symptomatic at the time of presentation, the likelihood of complications subsequently occurring in asymptomatic aneurysms appears great. The primary complication seen with subclavian and axillary aneurysms is embolization (68%).[12] Thrombosis and rupture are rare but have been reported.[12, 18]

Forearm and Hand Aneurysms

At onset the most common signs and symptoms of aneurysms in the forearm and hand are mass and pain. Distal embolization occurs in roughly one third of these patients.[2]

Femoral and Popliteal Artery Aneurysms

The natural history of femoral and popliteal aneurysms not operated on shows a high incidence of thromboembolic events. Tolsted and coauthors[19] reported a 43% rate of thrombosis in conservatively managed femoral aneurysms, and in Cutler and Darling's series,[20] 47% presented with major complications. In the series of Szilagyi and colleagues[14] popliteal aneurysms, only 32% of those managed conservatively remained without complication at 5 years. Vermilion and colleagues[15] studied 26 popliteal aneurysms an average of 3 years and demonstrated that eight (31%) patients suffered limb-threatening complications, with two patients requiring major amputation and two patients left with rest pain. Rupture of femoral or popliteal aneurysms has only rarely been reported. Profunda femoris aneurysms are particularly prone to rupture, with rates of 50% being reported.[1] Popliteal aneurysms rupture, on occasion, into the popliteal vein.[21] Less catastrophic complications include pain secondary to tibial nerve compression and popliteal vein thrombosis secondary to popliteal vein compression.

Diagnosis

Most peripheral aneurysms can be diagnosed by simple palpation of the artery in question. More sophisticated studies such as ultrasonography, computed tomography (CT) scans, and arteriography augment the diagnosis and allow for better preoperative planning.

Extracranial Carotid Artery Aneurysms

The most common manifestation of carotid aneurysms is a palpable pulsatile, submandibular, lateral neck mass or a mass appearing in the tonsillar fossa. The former presentation is most often seen with common carotid aneurysms, whereas appearance in the tonsillar fossa is more often seen with internal carotid artery aneurysms. Because of the variability in the location of the carotid bifurcation, the presentation can be only a rough guide to the artery involved. The differential diagnosis includes kinked or redundant carotid arteries, enlarged lymph nodes, salivary gland tumors, branchial cleft cysts, cystic hygromas, and carotid body tumors. When the diagnosis is not clear, CT scanning with contrast injection is usually diagnostic. Arteriography further aids in elucidating the diagnosis and is required for proper preoperative planning. Carotid duplex ultrasound scanning may also be helpful.

Subclavian and Axillary Artery Aneurysms

The most common signs and symptoms at onset of subclavian and axillary artery aneurysms are secondary to distal embolization (68%). Other signs and symptoms include tissue loss, claudication, pain, and evidence of brachial plexus compression (Table 25–2).

When the aneurysm is secondary to thoracic outlet syndrome, it often cannot be palpated. Aneurysms secondary to atherosclerosis tend to be larger and are palpable in two thirds of patients at the time of presentation.[18] A bruit may be present in the subclavian fossa or in the axilla. Small punctate cyanotic lesions affecting the fingers and palm

TABLE 25–2

Clinical Findings in Subclavian/Axillary Artery Aneurysms

FINDING	NUMBER	PERCENT
Asymptomatic	20	10
Claudication	9	5
Pain	36	18
Brachial plexus palsy	24	12
Tissue loss	20	10
Embolization	136	68

that are painful and occur suddenly are often present as a result of distal embolization. Rarely, embolization causes large axial artery occlusion. This event usually requires immediate embolectomy but may lead to claudication if the initial ischemia does not precipitate the need for immediate medical attention. With chronic small embolization, the distal radial and ulnar pulses may not be palpable due to buildup of embolic material. Repeated embolization may be associated with distal digital ulceration or tissue loss and severe pain. Many patients have vague shoulder pain on presentation. Rupture produces severe shoulder pain radiating into the upper arm and lower neck.

When all types of subclavian and axillary aneurysms are considered, only 16% can be palpated.[12] Occasionally, ultrasonography can be applied in the diagnosis of subclavian artery aneurysms, but the bony cage of the thoracic outlet may preclude adequate exposure in some patients. CT scanning is also able to demonstrate subclavian and axillary aneurysms. However, because in most cases the diagnosis should be suspected on the basis of history and physical examination, arteriography is the most useful test, because it is also needed preoperatively for proper planning of the operative procedure.

Forearm and Hand Aneurysms

Forearm (and especially hand) aneurysms are most often diagnosed by palpation of a pulsatile mass. These aneurysms can also be diagnosed by ultrasound or CT scanning, but nonpalpable aneurysms generally are found on arteriography in patients being studied for embolization.

Femoral and Popliteal Artery Aneurysms

The diagnosis of femoral and popliteal aneurysms is usually made by palpation. This is particularly easy in the case of femoral aneurysms because of their superficial nature. Popliteal aneurysms are suspected in any patient in whom the popliteal pulse is widened and very easily felt. Femoral and popliteal aneurysms should be considered in any patient with an acute arterial occlusion in the leg or with embolic disease affecting the foot and lower leg. Many popliteal aneurysms are calcified and can be detected by plain radiographs of the popliteal fossa. Both femoral and popliteal aneurysms are easily diagnosed by ultrasound scanning. CT scanning is particularly accurate in making the diagnosis (Fig. 25–1). Despite the presence of mural thrombus, arteriography usually confirms the diagnosis and is necessary for proper operative planning. The status of the runoff vessels visualized arteriographically is particularly important for patients with popliteal aneurysms.

Indications for Operation

Unlike aortic aneurysms, for which size is the main determinant of the need for surgery, the presence of a peripheral aneurysm is often all that is required to suggest the need for operative correction. As with patients with aortic aneurysms, the decision to operate on a patient with a periph-

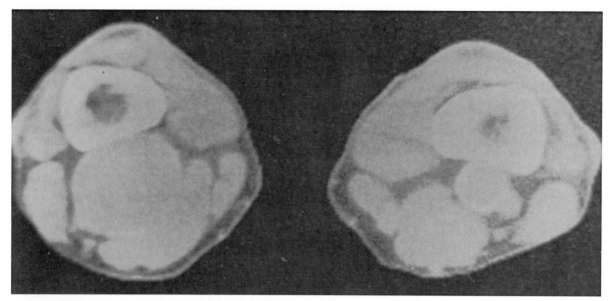

Figure 25–1. A computed tomography scan showing obvious right popliteal artery aneurysm and smaller left popliteal artery aneurysm.

eral aneurysm must be tempered by the overall medical condition of the patient so that the risk of operation is considerably less than the risk of the natural history of the disease.

Extracranial Carotid Artery Aneurysms

The indication for operation in a patient with a cervical carotid artery aneurysm is usually the presence of the aneurysm. Because patients with this condition are rarely seen when asymptomatic, most patients are operated on for the relief of symptoms. The high incidence of cranial nerve compression and central nervous system events in untreated patients, however, justifies surgery for asymptomatic carotid aneurysms as well (68% in Rhodes and colleagues' series).[9] This finding is common in nearly all reported studies, and the point is not a controversial one.[22–24]

Subclavian and Axillary Artery Aneurysms

Generally speaking, the presence of a subclavian or axillary aneurysm is an indication for surgery. The anticipated natural history would indicate that these lesions are both life- and limb-threatening.[18] As is the case with carotid aneurysms, most patients are symptomatic at the time of presentation and have clear indications for surgical intervention. Some controversy exists regarding the small fusiform poststenotic subclavian dilatation often seen with thoracic outlet compression of the subclavian artery. The natural history of this lesion, if not resected at the time of thoracic outlet decompression, is not well established. In the four patients with subclavian artery aneurysms in Pairolero and colleagues' series[18] who had only thoracic outlet decompression, no subsequent thromboembolic events occurred during follow-up.

Femoral and Popliteal Artery Aneurysms

The presence of a femoral or popliteal aneurysm is generally thought to be an indication for surgery. This recommendation is based on the high incidence of thromboembolic complications associated with these lesions as detailed above. Size is generally not used in assessing risk from these aneurysms, because even small aneurysms in these locations give rise to serious complications.[25]

Treatment

Only two primary objectives exist in the surgical management of peripheral aneurysms: exclusion of the aneurysm and restoration of arterial continuity. In most cases, both objectives can be achieved. In some inaccessible aneurysms, however, exclusion alone must be accepted because restoration of arterial continuity may not be possible.

Extracranial Carotid Artery Aneurysms

The techniques applied to the management of extracranial carotid aneurysms are ligation (or angiographic occlusion), endoaneurysmorrhaphy, resection with primary anastomosis, resection with graft replacement, or stent-grafting.

The preferred treatment is resection with primary anastomosis or graft replacement. Redundancy of the carotid artery is not uncommon when an aneurysm is present. In such cases, resection of the aneurysm with mobilization of the carotid artery and primary anastomosis is sometimes quite easily accomplished (Fig. 25–2). This technique is most applicable to internal carotid artery aneurysms. An alternative technique for flow restoration after resection of an internal carotid artery aneurysm is to divide the distal external carotid artery and perform an end-to-end anastomosis between the proximal external carotid and the distal

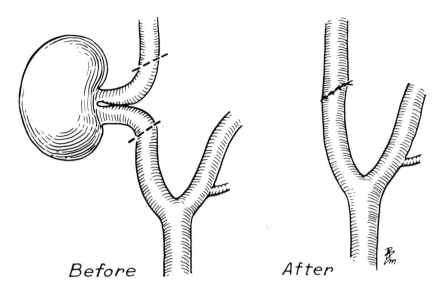

Figure 25–2. Method of end-to-end repair of a redundant internal carotid artery after aneurysm resection. (From Trippel OH, et al: Extracranial carotid aneurysms. In Bergan JJ, Yao JST [eds]: Aneurysms. New York, Grune & Stratton, 1982, pp 493–503.)

Before   *After*

internal carotid arteries. Aneurysm of the external carotid artery is rare and can be resected without the need to restore arterial continuity. Aneurysms of the carotid bifurcation usually require resection with graft replacement between the common and internal carotid arteries. When the internal carotid is redundant, it can be mobilized and anastomosed end to end to the common carotid artery. In both these latter cases the external carotid is usually ligated. Aneurysms involving the common carotid artery can usually be treated by resection and primary anastomosis or graft replacement. All of the above procedures can usually be performed through a standard neck incision as is used for carotid endarterectomy.

The need for an indwelling carotid artery shunt is no better understood for aneurysm patients than it is for patients undergoing carotid endarterectomy. If the use of a shunt is desired, shunting can be accomplished in most patients. In patients undergoing resection with primary anastomosis, a shunt can be inserted into the open ends of the arteries to be anastomosed after opening of the aneurysm. If a graft is to be used, the shunt is placed through the graft before performing any anastomosis and is inserted into the arterial ends after opening the aneurysm.

Aneurysms that involve the distal cervical internal carotid artery are often inaccessible by standard techniques. In some patients, mandibular subluxation or transection allows application of the above-mentioned methods of repair.[26] Alternative approaches are often required for high internal carotid lesions, however. In some patients, high fusiform aneurysms can be treated by aneurysmorrhaphy with an indwelling shunt for flow continuity and as a method of distal arterial control. In many cases, distal lesions must be treated by ligation or balloon occlusion with use of angiographic techniques. Unfortunately, acute occlusion of the internal carotid artery in these patients is associated with high neurologic morbidity. Stroke rates from 30% to 60% have been reported after this procedure; half of the patients who had sustained a stroke died as a result.[10] This morbidity and mortality clearly approaches the morbidity and mortality secondary to the natural history of the disease.

One way to select patients who may safely undergo carotid ligation is to measure carotid stump pressure. This can be done at surgery, but the preoperative knowledge of this pressure allows better operative planning. The carotid stump pressure can also be measured by temporary balloon occlusion at the time of arteriography with use of an endhole balloon catheter,[27] or it can be assessed by carotid compression maneuvers during the measurement of ocular pressures that use Gee oculopneumoplethysmograph.[28] Stump pressures in excess of 70 mm Hg appear safe for patients undergoing carotid ligation. Because many strokes occurring after carotid ligation are not present immediately after the procedure but rather occur hours to days later, these patients should be maintained on heparin anticoagulation for 7 to 10 days postoperatively.

When stump pressure measurements indicate that carotid ligation is not safe, the performance of an extracranial-to-intracranial bypass with use of the ipsilateral superficial temporal artery has been suggested.[26] Because this procedure is usually only necessary for high internal carotid lesions, the ipsilateral external carotid artery is usually preserved, thus allowing adequate inflow into the superficial temporal artery.

More recently, stent-grafts have been used in a few patients. Early results are good, but a larger experience with longer follow-up is required to determine the appropriateness of this technique.[29, 30]

Subclavian and Axillary Artery Aneurysms

The approach to the surgical treatment of subclavian and axillary aneurysms depends on the cause, size, and location of the aneurysm and the status of the distal circulation. Except in cases of small, asymptomatic subclavian artery aneurysms secondary to thoracic outlet syndrome (for which thoracic outlet decompression alone may be adequate), the aneurysm should be excluded and arterial continuity restored if possible. Proximal and distal ligation of these aneurysms has been reported. Although tissue loss does not usually occur after this procedure, claudication is not uncommon.[18]

When a symptomatic or large asymptomatic subclavian

aneurysm is present as a result of thoracic outlet syndrome, repair of the aneurysm should be accompanied by thoracic outlet decompression. Although this combined technique has been reported through an axillary approach, I prefer the supraclavicular approach, which allows safe control of the artery, although the thoracic outlet decompression is more involved. Hobson and colleagues[12] recommended performing the aneurysm repair through the supraclavicular approach combined with a transaxillary approach to the first rib.

Atherosclerotic and traumatic distal subclavian artery aneurysms or pseudoaneurysms can be managed with a supraclavicular approach. When the aneurysm is proximal enough that proximal control cannot be safely obtained through this approach, a median sternotomy (right side) or a left-sided thoracotomy (left side) is needed, usually in combination with the supraclavicular approach. Midsubclavian lesions can often be managed through a supraclavicular approach with medial clavicular resection.

Primary anastomosis is usually not possible, and graft replacement is required. This is most commonly performed as an interposition graft using either saphenous vein or prosthetics. Prosthetics are more commonly used because of the size of the subclavian artery. The vertebral artery should be preserved when possible. In patients with a dominant contralateral vertebral artery, this may not be necessary.

High-risk patients with proximal aneurysms who are thought too frail to undergo a major procedure can be treated with distal ligation and axilloaxillary bypass. Alternatively, stent-grafting can be applied to carefully selected high-risk patients, but long-term results are not yet known.[31, 32]

Management of axillary artery aneurysms often may be accomplished through the axillary approach. In many patients, proximal control must be obtained through an infraclavicular approach. With more proximal lesions or lesions involving both the subclavian and axillary arteries, a combined supraclavicular and infraclavicular approach must be used. Aneurysms involving the axillary artery are often intimately involved with the cords of the brachial plexus, and resection may be hazardous. When symptoms of brachial plexus compression are present, resection and interposition grafting may be indicated. For smaller lesions, however, proximal and distal ligation combined with bypass can be performed, thus avoiding dissection around the brachial plexus.

When subclavian and axillary aneurysms are complicated by embolization and ischemia, revascularization of the arm may be required in combination with aneurysm repair. This is usually accomplished by autogenous vein bypass from proximal to the aneurysm to the most appropriate distal artery. In this situation, the aneurysm can either be ligated, if appropriate, or resected.

Forearm and Hand Aneurysms

Aneurysms of the forearm arteries may be treated by ligation if the remaining vessels provide adequate collateral circulation to the hand. More often, however, vein interposition grafting is performed because it is simple to accomplish. Aneurysms of vessels in the hand tend to be less well collateralized, and vein graft repair is usually necessary.[2]

Femoral and Popliteal Artery Aneurysms

The treatment of femoral artery aneurysms is usually resection and graft interposition. Because of the size of the common femoral artery, a prosthetic graft is preferred. When the profunda femoris artery is involved, the graft may be sewn end to end to the superficial femoral artery, and the origin of the profunda implanted into the side of the graft. When femoral aneurysms are being treated concomitantly with an inflow or outflow procedure, it is still best, in most cases, to replace the common femoral artery with an interposition graft. Inflow or outflow grafts are then anastomosed to the interposition graft in an end-to-side fashion (Fig. 25–3). Repair of profunda femoris

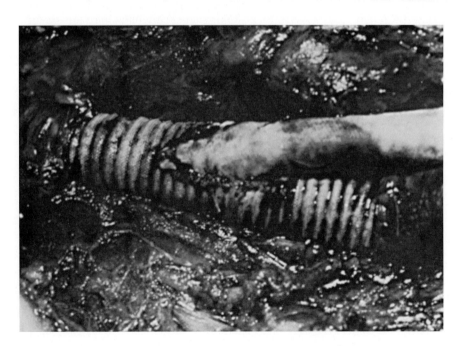

Figure 25–3. Concomitant repair of femoral aneurysm followed by prosthetic femoropopliteal bypass.

aneurysms is dictated by the patency of the superficial femoral artery and how distal the aneurysm is located in the profunda femoris artery. Approximately 50% of profunda femoris aneurysms can be safely ligated, whereas 50% require reestablishing arterial continuity.[1]

Superficial femoral and popliteal aneurysms are preferably bypassed rather than resected. In most cases, this means an above-knee to below-knee bypass using autogenous vein through a medial approach. In some patients, the popliteal aneurysm may extend proximally into the superficial femoral artery. In these patients, the proximal anastomosis can be made to the common femoral artery or, more commonly, to the midsuperficial femoral artery proximal to the adductor canal.

Reports are now beginning to be published on the use of femoropopliteal stent grafts for the treatment of popliteal aneurysms. The procedure is technically achievable, but accurate assessment of results has not yet been accomplished.[33, 34]

When extensive embolization leading to obliteration of the outflow tract of the popliteal artery has occurred, popliteal-to-tibial or popliteal-to-peroneal bypass is required. This should be performed with use of autogenous vein.

When popliteal aneurysms are large enough to cause symptomatic compression of the surrounding nerve and vein, consideration should be given to resection of the aneurysm with interposition grafting. The risk of damage to these structures is greater, but if this is not done, many patients remain symptomatic postoperatively. This procedure is best performed through a posterior approach as long as both anastomoses are within the limitations of the operative field.

When patients show severe ischemia due to thromboembolic complications of popliteal artery aneurysms, the degree of arterial occlusion is often so great that no outflow vessel is patent. Many of these patients, especially in late stages, also have thrombosis of the microcirculation. In such patients, bypass is often either not possible or is subject to a high failure rate due to poor runoff. The use of preoperative or intraoperative thrombolytic therapy provides patent runoff in most of these patients, thereby allowing succesful bypass.[35] In patients at especially high surgical risk, thrombolytic therapy alone has been used with success.[36, 37]

Results of Therapy

Because most patients with peripheral aneurysms do not have occlusive disease, the results of reconstructive vascular procedures are usually excellent. In some cases, however, embolization from the aneurysm can lead to obliteration of some or all of the outflow tract, leading to poor results.

Extracranial Carotid Artery Aneurysms

The small number of patients in reports assessing the results of surgical therapy for carotid aneurysm makes the calculation of morbidity and mortality statistics somewhat unreliable. Most reports, however, have indicated that

these procedures can be performed with safety. In Rhodes and colleagues' series[9] from Michigan, 1 of 19 aneurysm operations resulted in a stroke, which was thought to be due to intraoperative embolization. No operative death occurred. Excision of large and distal aneurysms is associated with an increased incidence of cranial nerve injury. Long-term results are sparsely reported but, when reported, have been excellent. All investigators agree that the results of surgery are vastly superior to the natural history of the disease.[9, 10, 22–24]

Subclavian and Axillary Artery Aneurysms

The results of surgery for subclavian and axillary aneurysms are similar to those for upper extremity reconstruction for occlusive disease.[18, 38] Pairolero and colleagues[18] showed that 18 of 18 patients undergoing aneurysm resection with restoration of arterial continuity retained patent reconstructions during an average 9.2-year follow-up. This is most likely due to the lack of distal occlusive disease. Patients with obliteration of their radial and ulnar arteries, however, have a high failure rate after arm revascularization.[38] This latter point further emphasizes the need for early surgical intervention in these patients.

Forearm and Hand Aneurysms

Both ligation in the presence of adequate collateral circulation and vein graft repair are quite successful in the treatment of forearm and hand aneurysms. Clark and coworkers[2] reported 100% patency at 7 years for vein graft repairs in the forearm and hand.

Femoral and Popliteal Artery Aneurysms

When femoral and popliteal aneurysms are treated before complications arise, the results are excellent. The 18 asymptomatic patients with femoral aneurysms in Cutler and Darling's series[20] all had excellent early and late results (no graft occlusions). However, of the 45 symptomatic patients with femoral aneurysms, four had amputations and 17 remained symptomatic despite therapy. In Lilly and colleagues' series[39] of 48 popliteal aneurysms, the 5-year patency rate for reconstructions for asymptomatic lesions was 91% compared to 54% for symptomatic lesions. These differing results were directly related to the status of the tibial runoff vessels. In a series of 51 popliteal aneurysms reported by Shortell and colleagues,[40] results were dependent on the clinical presentation and the status of the runoff vessels. Patients with limb-threatening ischemia had a graft patency rate of 69% at 1 year, whereas all electively performed grafts were patent at 1 year. After 3 years, runoff dictated patency, as grafts with good runoff had a patency rate of 89%, whereas poor runoff was associated with a 3-year patency rate of only 30%. Numerous, more recent reports of large series of popliteal aneurysms have confirmed these earlier results.[41–44]

Because of the vastly inferior results of therapy once thromboembolic complications have occurred, attention has been focused on the reestablishment of runoff preoperatively through the use of thrombolytic therapy.[35] Although no prospective randomized studies have been carried out, most reports indicate good success in improving runoff and suggest improved limb salvage when preoperative thrombolytic therapy is employed. Varga and colleagues[35] in 1994 performed a retrospective multicenter study of 200 popliteal aneurysms and concluded that intraarterial thrombolytic therapy clearly improved preoperative runoff in patients with limb-threatening ischemia.

Hoelting and associates[36] described 24 patients with acute ischemia secondary to popliteal artery aneurysm thrombosis. Nine patients were treated with preoperative thrombolysis and underwent successful bypass. Six of these patients achieved complete lysis. For three patients, lysis was incomplete but established sufficient runoff that successful bypass could be performed. Furthermore, the authors reviewed the literature and demonstrated an amputation rate of approximately 27% in 455 patients treated with bypass alone compared to approximately 20% in 14 patients in whom only thrombolytic therapy was used. However, in 30 patients in whom thrombolytic therapy was combined with bypass, no limb was lost.

Dawson and colleagues[45] compared operative and nonoperative approaches to 71 popliteal aneurysms. Thromboembolic complications developed in 57% of asymptomatic popliteal aneurysms over a mean follow-up period of 5 years. In aneurysms studied a full 5 years, the complication rate was 74%. In comparison, patients operated on had graft patency and limb salvage of 64% and 95%, respectively, at 10-year follow-up.

Dawson and colleagues also revealed a high risk of subsequent aneurysm development in these patients. At 5-year follow-up, 32% of patients developed additional aneurysms, and at 10 years, 49% had new aneurysms.[45]

The above reports strongly support the early surgical treatment of asymptomatic popliteal aneurysms and underscore the need for careful follow-up of these patients for the development of new aneurysms.

MYCOTIC ANEURYSMS

Mycotic aneurysms are considered separately because they generally have a different cause, affect arteries in a different distribution, require different treatment, and have poorer outcomes than bland aneurysms. Despite the term *mycotic*, mycotic aneurysms are considered to be any true or false aneurysm that is infected.

Etiology

Numerous classifications for mycotic aneurysms have been proposed and are nicely described by Moore and Malone[46] and Wilson and colleagues.[47] Patel and Johnston[48] indicated that the source of infection must be either endogenous or exogenous. Endogenous sources include embolism, septicemia, or direct extension; exogenous sources include trauma and iatrogenic injury. They further suggested that classifications be based on the preexisting status of the

artery: normal, atherosclerotic, aneurysmal, or prosthetic. Any classification must consider these factors.[48]

Normal axial arteries are seldom infected primarily, but clumps of bacteria or fungi may lodge in smaller vessels and cause transmural necrosis and aneurysm formation. Normal, larger arteries can be infected, however, by organisms lodging in the vasa vasorum. Arteries that are diseased with atherosclerosis or aneurysm, and prosthetic grafts, are subject to local invasion by circulating organisms. The process is similar to that described earlier in that infection leads to arterial wall weakening and subsequent aneurysm formation. Infection may spread to arterial walls from outside the vessel through direct contact with abscesses, wound infections, salivary glands, and the like. Exogenous sources of arterial infections include diagnostic and therapeutic catheterizations, penetrating trauma, and drug abuse. Graft infections may also lead to infected pseudoaneurysm formation, usually as a result of disruption of an anastomosis.

Mycotic aneurysms have been reported in essentially all arteries. The location of mycotic aneurysms is primarily a result of the cause. Mycotic aneurysms secondary to bacterial endocarditis favor the superior mesenteric artery, followed by the aorta and femoral arteries. Those mycotic aneurysms that occur after trauma most commonly involve the extremities. Mycotic aneurysms occurring as a result of infection of already present atherosclerotic aneurysms commonly affect the aorta and femoral and popliteal arteries. Those secondary to atherosclerosis alone involve the aorta and superficial femoral arteries as well as other common atherosclerotic sites. Those secondary to catheters and drug abuse involve the brachial, radial, and most commonly, the femoral arteries. For unknown reasons, *Salmonella* species favor the infrarenal aorta.

The organisms most commonly involved in mycotic aneurysms differ depending on the source of the organism. When bacterial endocarditis is the source, *Streptococcus* and *Staphylococcus* prevail. *Salmonella, Staphylococcus,* and *Escherichia coli* are the most common organisms causing mycotic aneurysms secondary to bacteremia. Mycotic aneurysms secondary to direct extension of infections are predominantly caused by *Salmonella, Staphylococcus, Mycobacterium,* and fungi.[46] *Staphylococcus aureus* and *E. coli* are the most common organisms seen in mycotic aneurysms secondary to trauma (all types).[49]

In the preantibiotic era, most mycotic aneurysms were secondary to bacterial endocarditis and syphilis. Today, most mycotic aneurysms are probably secondary to trauma (including drug abuse, surgery, and arterial catheterization). This change is most likely due to the use of antibiotic therapy for endocarditis, the significant decrease in the prevalence of syphilis, the increasing use of diagnostic catheterization, the increase in violent trauma, and widespread drug abuse. In my experience, these forces have now made common femoral artery mycotic aneurysms the most common type currently encountered.

Natural History

Once established, the natural course of a mycotic aneurysm is to enlarge and eventually rupture in most known cases.

Occasionally, spontaneous thrombosis may occur with resolution of the septic process; however, the thrombosed aneurysm may serve as a continuing septic focus. Septic emboli arising from the aneurysm are not uncommon and can lead to miliary abscesses and septic arthritis.

Diagnosis

Patients with mycotic aneurysms may show catastrophic illness or insidious disease. Most patients have some combination of fever, malaise, weight loss, chills, night sweats, pain, leukocytosis, positive downstream blood cultures, and elevated sedimentation rate. A history of trauma or a recent infectious disease usually exists. When the aneurysm is superficial, as most peripheral aneurysms are, it can be palpated in 90% of patients.[50] The aneurysm may appear bland but, more commonly, shows signs of erythema, warmth, and tenderness. Particularly large aneurysms may also show skin necrosis and risk of imminent rupture (Fig. 25–4). Petechial lesions in the skin may be seen distal to the aneurysm when embolization has occurred. Many patients show rupture on presentation.

The diagnosis of mycotic aneurysm is often deduced by combining the findings of history and physical examination with test findings. In some patients, the history and physical examination may be sufficient (see Fig. 25–4; this patient had a retained polyester chimney left attached to her right femoral artery after removal of an intra-aortic balloon catheter). In other patients, the diagnosis is made by the finding of sepsis and an aneurysm in a patient in whom no other septic focus can be found.

Ultrasound and CT scans may be used to visualize mycotic aneurysms. CT scans have the advantage of being able to more clearly demonstrate surrounding fluid or gas, a finding consistent with infection. Gallium scans and radioactively tagged white blood cell scans are usually positive with mycotic aneurysms. Arteriography is usually required in preoperative planning, except in emergency situations, and usually demonstrates a saccular aneurysm or pseudoaneurysm (Fig. 25–5).

Treatment

The indication for treatment of a mycotic aneurysm is its presence. Antibiotic therapy, guided by culture results when available, should be used in all patients. Antibiotics alone are not sufficient, and surgical removal of the mycotic aneurysm is required in nearly all cases. Basic surgical principles dictate that all infected tissue must be removed and adequate circulation must remain or be provided when possible.

Extracranial Carotid Artery Mycotic Aneurysms

As noted earlier, cervical carotid aneurysms are rare. Therefore, cervical carotid mycotic aneurysms are extremely rare. In 1988, Jones and Frusha[51] reviewed the English-language literature and found only 23 bacteriologically proven cases. In 1991, Jebara and colleagues[52] noted an additional four cases.

Treatment of these lesions requires complete excision of the artery, under antibiotic coverage, and débridement of all infected tissue. Vascular reconstruction should be avoided if possible, because reconstruction in an infected field yields less than optimal results.[53] Patients should be selected for arterial ligation based on carotid stump pressure as described above. Heparin should be continued for 7 to 10 days postoperatively when ligation is employed. If ligation is not safe, then reconstruction using autogenous vein is the treatment of choice. In Jones and Frusha's review, the overall mortality rate was 23%. The death rate was 27% in the ligation group compared to 11% in the grafted group. Extracranial-intracranial bypass has not been reported in these patients.[51]

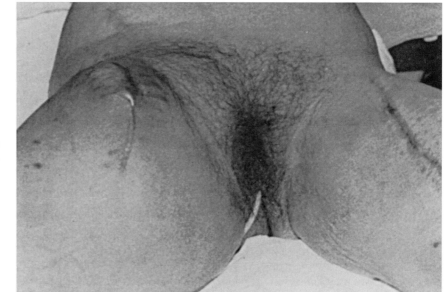

Figure 25–4. Mycotic aneurysm in the right side of the groin with overlying skin necrosis and imminent rupture.

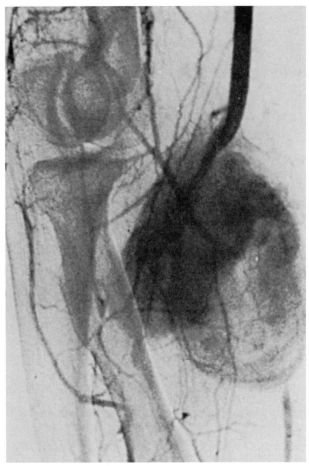

Figure 25–5. Arteriogram of a mycotic popliteal artery aneurysm.

Subclavian and Axillary Artery Mycotic Aneurysms

Mycotic aneurysms in the subclavian-axillary area are also quite rare and usually the result of trauma and drug abuse. The approach to the subclavian artery depends on the side and distal and proximal extent of the aneurysm as mentioned above for bland aneurysms in this location. In this location, complete excision of the aneurysm may be too risky in view of the proximity of the brachial plexus and subclavian vein. Successful treatment with arterial ligation and incision and drainage of the aneurysm has been reported.[54] Proximal subclavian artery ligation usually does not lead to the need for revascularization.

Axillary mycotic aneurysms are usually palpable. The principles of management of subclavian mycotic aneurysms probably apply to axillary lesions. Axillary artery ligation may be associated with ischemia more often, however, and extra-anatomic bypass may be required in some patients. This can usually be performed in clean tissue planes about the shoulder with use of autogenous vein.

Forearm and Hand Artery Mycotic Aneurysms

Treatment of mycotic aneurysms in the forearm and hand follows the general guidelines for other mycotic aneurysms.

Arterial ligation with aneurysm excision is generally all that is required. In the rare situation in which distal ischemia might occur, autogenous revascularization in clean planes is required.

Femoral and Popliteal Artery Mycotic Aneurysms

The treatment of infected groin aneurysms has evolved through several stages. Although most of these lesions are secondary to trauma and drug abuse, the principles applied to the management of groin mycotic aneurysms secondary to other causes should probably be the same in most cases.

Several options are available, including remote bypass followed by aneurysm resection, aneurysm resection followed by remote bypass if needed, aneurysm resection alone, or aneurysm resection with in situ autogenous reconstruction.

Initial obturator bypass followed by aneurysm resection usually requires the use of prosthetic material, because most of these patients are drug addicts whose saphenous veins have been destroyed. Reddy and colleagues[49] showed this approach to be associated with a 100% graft infection rate in drug addicts. In other patients, vein is often available and this approach is preferred. Buerger and Feldman[55] reported that revascularization is not effective in reducing the amputation rate after aneurysm resection in drug addicts (17% in their series) and may occasionally be fatal. In Buerger and Feldman's series, the same amputation rate was achieved without any death when aneurysm excision and ligation alone was used.[55]

Reddy and colleagues[49] obtained a similar amputation rate (19%) with excision and ligation. They reported that excision and ligation of only one of the three femoral arteries in the groin can be performed without limb loss, but when the common femoral bifurcation is involved, thus necessitating the ligation of all three vessels, the amputation rate is very high. They suggested that, as an alternative in these latter patients, immediate autogenous vein reconstruction with sartorius muscle flap coverage may be used when adequate débridement can be performed to control sepsis. Using this approach, they reported a 9% amputation rate without mortality. Reddy and colleagues[49] found that, even in drug addicts, satisfactory saphenous vein usually exists in the thigh for femoral artery reconstruction. A 1999 report by Benjamin and coworkers[56] demonstrated successful treatment of mycotic aneurysms using deep leg veins when larger-sized conduits were required. Ligation and excision with postoperative observation to assess the need for subsequent revascularization did not yield satisfactory results in the series of Reddy and colleagues.[49]

Mycotic aneurysms involving the popliteal artery are uncommon, and few guidelines are provided in the vascular surgical literature. In my experience, aneurysm excision with in situ autogenous interposition grafting has worked well. Most of these patients have normal tibial artery runoff facilitating long-term patency, and the readily available soft tissue coverage afforded by the muscles in the popliteal space facilitates healing of the surgical wound without complication.

References

1. Tait WF, Vohra RK, Carr HMI, et al: True profunda femoris aneurysms: Are they more dangerous than other atherosclerotic aneurysms of the femoropopliteal segment? Ann Vasc Surg 5:92–95, 1991.
2. Clark FT, Mass DP, Bassiouny HS, et al: True aneurysmal disease in the hand and upper extremity. Ann Vasc Surg 5:276–281, 1991.
3. Flinn WR, Yao JST, Bergan JJ: Aneurysms of secondary and tertiary branches of major arteries. In Bergan JJ, Yao JST (eds): Aneurysms. New York, Grune & Stratton, 1982, pp 449–467.
4. Beall AC, Crawford ES, Cooley DA, et al: Extracranial aneurysms of the carotid artery: Report of seven cases. Postgrad Med 32:93, 1962.
5. Reid MR: Aneurysms in the Johns Hopkins Hospital. Arch Surg 12:1, 1926.
6. Houser OW, Baker HL Jr: Fibromuscular dysplasia and other uncommon diseases of the cervical carotid artery: Angiographic aspects. AJR 104:201, 1968.
7. McCollum CH, Wheeler WG, Noon GP, et al: Aneurysms of the extracranial carotid artery: Twenty-one years' experience. Am J Surg 137:196, 1979.
8. Zhang Q, Duan SJ, Xin XW et al: Management of extracranial carotid artery aneurysms: 17 years' experience. Eur J Endovasc Surg 18:162–165, 1999.
9. Rhodes EL, Stanley JC, Hoffman CL, et al: Aneurysms of extracranial carotid arteries. Arch Surg 111:3 39, 1976.
10. Goldstone J: Aneurysms of the extracranial carotid artery. In Rutherford RE (ed): Vascular Surgery. Philadelphia, WB Saunders, 1984, pp 1279–1287.
11. Ehrenfeld WK, Hays RJ: False aneurysm after carotid endarterectomy. Arch Surg 104:2 88, 1972.
12. Hobson RW II, Israel MR, Lynch TO: Axillo-subclavian arterial aneurysms. In Bergan JJ, Vito JST (eds): Aneurysms. New York, Grune & Stratton, 1982, pp 435–447.
13. Gray RJ, Stone WM, Fowl RJ, et al: Management of true aneurysms distal to the axillary artery. J Vasc Surg 28:606–610, 1998.
14. Szilagyi DE, Schwartz RL, Reddy DJ: Popliteal arterial aneurysms. Their natural history and management. Arch Surg 116:724, 1981.
15. Vermilion ED, Kinunmns SA, Pace WC, et al: A review of one hundred forty-seven popliteal aneurysms with long-term follow-up. Surgery 90:1009, 1981.
16. Evans WE, Vermilion ED: Popliteal and femoral aneurysms. In Rutherford RB (ed): Vascular Surgery. Philadelphia, WB Saunders, 1984, pp 814–827.
17. Dent TL, Lindenaur SM, Ernst CE, et al: Multiple arteriosclerotic arterial aneurysms. Arch Surg 105:338, 1972.
18. Pairolero PC, Walls JT, Payne WS, et al: Subclavian-axillary artery aneurysms. Surgery 90:757, 1981.
19. Tolstedt GE, Radke HM, Bell JW: Late sequelae of arteriosclerotic femoral aneurysms. Angiology 12:601, 1961.
20. Cutler BS, Darling RC: Surgical management of arteriosclerotic femoral aneurysms. Surgery 74:764, 1973.
21. Reed MIC, Smith EM: Popliteal aneurysm with spontaneous arteriovenous fistula. J Cardiovasc Surg 32:482–484, 1991.
22. Faggioli G, Freyrie A, Stella A, et al: Extracranial internal carotid artery aneurysms: Results of a surgical series with long-term follow-up. J Vasc Surg 23:587–595, 1996.
23. Rosset E, Roche PH, Magnan PE, et al: Surgical management of extracranial internal carotid artery aneurysms. Cardiovasc Surg 2:567–572, 1994.
24. Coffin O, Maiza D, Galateau-Salle F, et al: Results of surgical management of internal carotid artery aneurysm by the cervical approach. Ann Vasc Surg 11:482–490, 1997.
25. Poirier NC, Verdant A: Popliteal aneurysm: Surgical treatment is mandatory before complications occur. Ann Chir 50:613–618, 1996.
26. Stoney RJ, Qvarfordt PC: Accessible and inaccessible aneurysms of the extracranial carotid artery. In Moore WS (ed): Surgery for Cerebrovascular Disease. New York, Churchill Livingstone, 1987, pp 567–577.
27. Mathis JM, Barr J, Yonas H, et al: Temporary balloon test occlusion of the internal carotid artery: Experience in 500 cases. AJNR 16:749–754, 1995.
28. Gee W, Mehigan JT, Wylie EJ: Measurement of collateral cerebral hemispheric blood pressure by ocular pneumoplethysmography. Am J Surg 130:121, 1975.
29. Beregi JP, Prat A, Willoteaux S, et al: Covered stents in the treatment of peripheral arterial aneurysms: Procedural results and midterm follow-up. Cardiovasc Interv Radiol 22:13–19, 1999.
30. Hurst RW, Haskal ZJ, Bagley LJ, et al: Endovascular stent treatment of cervical internal carotid artery aneurysms with parent vessel preservation. Surg Neurol 50:313–317, 1998.
31. Szeimies U, Kueffer G, Stoeckelhuber B, et al: Successful exclusion of subclavian aneurysms with covered nitinol stents. Cardiovasc Interv Radiol 21:246–249, 1998.
32. Baudier JF, Justesen P, Astrup M, et al: Endovascular treatment of subclavian artery aneurysm. Ugeskr Laeger 161:1774–1775, 1999.
33. Muller-Hulsbeck S, Link J, Schwarzenberg H, et al: Percutaneous endoluminal stent and stent-graft placement for treatment of femoropopliteal aneurysms: Early experience. Cardiovasc Interv Radiol 22:96–102, 1999.
34. van Sambeek MR, Gussenhoven EJ, van der Lugt A, et al: Endovascular stent-grafts for aneurysms of the femoral and popliteal arteries. Ann Vasc Surg 13:247–253, 1999.
35. Varga ZA, Locke-Edmunds JC, Baird RN, et al: Multicenter study of popliteal aneurysms. J Vasc Surg 20:171–177, 1994.
36. Hoelting T, Paetz B, Richter GM, Allenberg JR: The value of preoperative lytic therapy in limb-threatening acute ischemia from popliteal artery aneurysm. Am J Surg 168:227–231, 1994.
37. Greenberg R, Wellander E, Nyman U, et al: Aggressive treatment of acute limb ischemia due to thrombosed popliteal aneurysms. Eur J Radiol 28:211–218, 1998.
38. Gross WS, Flanigan DP, Kraft RO, et al: Chronic upper extremity ischemia: Etiology, manifestations, and treatment. Arch Surg 84:417, 1978.
39. Lilly MP, Flinn WR, McCarthy WJ et al: The effect of distal arterial anatomy on the success of popliteal aneurysm repair. J Vasc Surg 7:653, 1988.
40. Shortell CK, DeWeese JA, Ouriel IC, Green EM: Popliteal artery aneurysms: A 25 year experience. J Vasc Surg 14:771–779, 1991.
41. Sarcina A, Bellosta R, Luzzanil L, et al: Surgical treatment of popliteal artery aneurysm. A 20-year experience. J Cardiovasc Surg (Torino) 38:347–354, 1997.
42. D'Angelo F, Gatti S, Pace M, et al: Aneurysm of the popliteal artery. A case contribution of a 15-year surgical experience. Minerva Cardioangiol 44:499–509, 1996.
43. Davidovic LB, Lotina SI, Kostie DM, et al: Popliteal artery aneurysms. World J Surg 22:812–817, 1998.
44. Duffy ST, Colgan MP, Sultan S, et al: Popliteal aneurysms: A ten year experience. Eur J Vasc Surg 16:218–222, 1998.
45. Dawson I, van Bockel H, Brand R, Terpstra JL: Popliteal artery aneurysms: Long-term follow-up of aneurysmal disease and results of surgical treatment. J Vasc Surg 13:398–407, 1991.
46. Moore WS, Malone JM: Mycotic aneurysms. In Bergan JJ, Yao JST (eds): Aneurysms. New York, Grune & Stratton, 1982, pp 581–595.
47. Wilson SE, Wagenen PV, Passaro E Jr: Arterial infection. Curr Probl Surg 15:1519, 1978.
48. Patel S, Johnston KW: Classification and management of mycotic aneurysms. Surg Gynecol Obstet 144:691, 1977.
49. Reddy DJ, Smith RF, Elliot JP, et al: Infected femoral artery false aneurysms in drug addicts: Evolution of selective vascular reconstruction. J Vasc Surg 3:7–18, 1986.
50. Anderson CE: Mycotic aneurysms. In Rutherford RE (ed): Vascular Surgery. Philadelphia, WB Saunders, 1984, pp 835–847.
51. Jones TR, Frusha JD: Mycotic cervical carotid artery aneurysms: A case report and review of the literature. Ann Vasc Surg 2:373, 1988.
52. Jebara VA, Acar C, Dervanian P, et al: Mycotic aneurysms of the carotid arteries: Case report and review of the literature. J Vasc Surg 14:215–219, 1991.
53. Howell HS, Baruraao T, Craziano J: Mycotic cervical carotid aneurysm. Surgery 81:357–359, 1977.
54. Miller CM, Sangiuolo P, Schanzer H: Infected false aneurysms of the subclavian artery: A complication in drug addicts. J Vasc Surg 1:684, 1984.
55. Buerger F, Feldman AJ: Infected groin aneurysms from heroin addiction. In Bergan JJ, Yao JST (eds): Aneurysms. New York, Gruue & Stratton, 1982, pp 643–655.
56. Benjamin ME, Cohn EJ Jr, Purtill WA, et al: Arterial reconstruction with deep leg veins for the treatment of mycotic aneurysms. J Vasc Surg 30:1004–1015, 1999.

Questions

1. Subclavian artery aneurysms are most commonly caused by
   (a) atherosclerosis
   (b) thoracic outlet syndrome
   (c) fibromuscular dysplasia
   (d) trauma

2. The most common complication of subclavian artery aneurysms is
   (a) rupture
   (b) pain secondary to nerve compression
   (c) embolization
   (d) thrombosis

3. Most carotid artery aneurysms are identified because of
   (a) rupture of the aneurysm
   (b) a mass in the neck
   (c) neurologic complications
   (d) a swishing sound heard in the patient's ipsilateral ear

4. Which of the following statements is true regarding femoral and popliteal artery aneurysms?
   (a) these aneurysms should only be repaired when they become very large and cause pain from adjacent nerve compression
   (b) these aneurysms are rarely associated with other peripheral aneurysms
   (c) these aneurysms are particularly dangerous because of a high incidence of distal embolization or aneurysm thrombosis
   (d) long-term surgical results in the treatment of femoral and popliteal aneurysms are not dependent on the degree of arterial occlusive disease distal to the aneurysm

5. The most common cause of peripheral aneurysms is
   (a) atherosclerosis
   (b) infection
   (c) trauma
   (d) connective tissue disorders

6. Which of the following peripheral aneurysms is most likely to rupture?
   (a) popliteal
   (b) carotid
   (c) profunda femoris
   (d) axillary

7. For a patient showing ischemia secondary to thrombosis of a popliteal aneurysm and occlusion of the popliteal outflow tract, the best initial treatment is
   (a) thrombolytic therapy
   (b) thrombectomy and bypass
   (c) observation
   (d) sympathectomy

8. The most common cause of mycotic aneurysm is
   (a) trauma
   (b) bacterial endocarditis
   (c) direct extension of adjacent infections
   (d) food poisoning

9. Popliteal aneurysms
   (a) are frequently bilateral
   (b) are commonly associated with abdominal aortic aneurysms
   (c) rarely rupture
   (d) all of the above

10. Carotid artery aneurysms
    (a) most commonly involve the internal carotid artery
    (b) are more common than subclavian artery aneurysms
    (c) require surgical repair in most patients
    (d) none of the above

Answers

1. b   2. c   3. c   4. c   5. a   6. c   7. a   8. a   9. d   10. c

26

Splanchnic and Renal Artery Aneurysms

James C. Stanley, Louis M. Messina, and Gerald B. Zelenock

Aneurysms of the visceral branches of the abdominal aorta are being recognized with increasing frequency. More than 3400 splanchnic and renal aneurysms have been described in the English-language literature, of which over half have been reported during the past 25 years. Splanchnic aneurysms are approximately two and a half times more common than renal aneurysms. These aneurysms are best addressed individually because of the marked variability in their biologic character and clinical importance.

SPLANCHNIC ARTERY ANEURYSMS

Splanchnic artery aneurysms are an uncommon but important vascular disease (Table 26–1). Nearly 22% of these aneurysms have been reported to appear as surgical emergencies, including 8.5% that have resulted in the patient's death.[1] The major splanchnic vessels involved with these macroaneurysms, in decreasing order of frequency, include the splenic, hepatic, superior mesenteric, celiac, gastric-gastroepiploic, jejunal-ileal-colic, pancreaticoduodenal-pancreatic, and gastroduodenal arteries (see Table 26–1A and B). The clinical relevance and treatment of splanchnic artery aneurysms have become well defined during the past three decades.[2–10]

Splenic Artery Aneurysms

Splenic artery aneurysms account for 60% of all reported splanchnic artery aneurysms.[10, 11] The frequency of splenic artery aneurysms in the general population approaches the 0.78% incidence noted in nearly 3600 consecutive abdominal arteriographic studies performed for reasons other than suspected aneurysmal disease.[11] Women are nearly four times more likely than men to develop these aneurysms, in all likelihood because of hormonal-related events associated with many of these lesions.

Three distinct, preexisting conditions are suspected to contribute to the development of splenic artery aneurysms.

The first is medial fibrodysplasia, usually a cause of hypertension secondary to renal artery involvement. Blood pressure elevations in these patients may also contribute to aneurysmal formation. The coexistence of renal artery medial fibrodysplasia and splenic artery aneurysms has only been identified in women. Approximately 2% of patients with medial fibrodysplasia of the renal artery have splenic artery aneurysms. Second are the deleterious effects of increased splenic blood flow and the altered levels of reproductive hormones on elastic vascular tissue that accompany repeated pregnancies. Approximately 40% of women harboring these lesions are grand multiparas, having completed six or more pregnancies. Third, portal hypertension with splenomegaly has been associated with splenic artery macroaneurysms in nearly 10% of patients.[11, 12] This may reflect the greater splenic blood flow,[13, 14] as well as elevated estrogen activity associated with cirrhosis. There has been an increased recognition of these aneurysms in patients subjected to orthotopic liver transplantation.[15–17] Aneurysms in these latter patients are multiple in nearly 90% of cases, affect women more often than men, and appear directly related to the transplant patient's antecedent portal hypertension.[17]

Although certain splenic artery aneurysms exhibit arteriosclerotic disease, the typical calcific advanced arteriosclerotic changes in many of these aneurysms are more likely a secondary event, rather than a primary etiologic process. Inflammatory disease, such as chronic pancreatitis and penetrating trauma, are less common causes of these aneurysms. Splenic microaneurysms are usually associated with generalized vasculitis, such as polyarteritis nodosa, and are of less clinical importance than extraparenchymal macroaneurysms.

Most splenic artery aneurysms associated with arterial fibrodysplasia, multiple pregnancies, or portal hypertension are saccular and occur at vessel branchings (Fig. 26–1). These are true aneurysms, not false aneurysms. It is at arterial branchings that discontinuities exist in the internal elastic lamina of normal vessels, and subsequent degenera-

TABLE 26-1A

Splanchnic Artery Macroaneurysms

ANEURYSM LOCATION	FREQUENCY WITHIN SPLANCHNIC CIRCULATION (%)	MALE-FEMALE RATIO	CONTRIBUTING FACTORS
Splenic artery	60	1:4	Medial degeneration; arterial fibrodysplasia; multiple pregnancies; portal hypertension; chronic pancreatitis with arterial erosion by pseudocysts
Hepatic artery	20	2:1	Medial degeneration; blunt and penetrating liver trauma; infection related to intravenous substance abuse
Superior mesenteric artery	5.5	1:1	Infection related to bacterial endocarditis, often associated with nonhemolytic streptococci and more recently with intravenous substance abuse; medial degeneration
Celiac artery	4.0	1:1	Medial degeneration
Gastric and gastroepiploic arteries	4.0	3:1	Periarterial inflammation; medial degeneration
Jejunal, ileal, and colic arteries	3.0	1:1	Medial degeneration; connective tissue diseases
Pancreaticoduodenal, pancreatic, and gastroduodenal arteries	1.5	4:1	Pancreatitis-related arterial necrosis and arterial erosion by pseudocysts (60% of gastroduodenal, 30% of pancreaticoduodenal artery aneurysms); medial degeneration

tive effects involving elastic tissue, as occur with pregnancy, are apt to produce aneurysmal changes at these sites. Aneurysms unrelated to portal hypertension are multiple 20% of the time. On the other hand, splenic artery aneurysms associated with pancreatitis usually involve the main splenic artery and tend to be solitary (Fig. 26–2).

Curvilinear or signet-ring calcifications in the left upper quadrant of radiographs are often evidence of the presence of a splenic artery aneurysm. However, diagnosis in contemporary times usually results from arteriographic demonstration of the aneurysm during studies being undertaken for some other disease state. Ultrasonography, computed tomography (CT) scanning, and magnetic resonance imaging (MRI) are useful in recognizing these lesions and are often helpful in identifying bleeding aneurysms.[10, 18] These noninvasive studies are particularly valuable for following size changes in asymptomatic aneurysms.

Left upper quadrant or epigastric pain occurs in a minority of all reported individuals with splenic artery aneurysms, with some form of abdominal discomfort affecting approximately 20% of those patients in an earlier report.[11] In a 1996 review of 83 cases that included many single case reports, 46% of patients had abdominal pain and 25% presented in shock.[6] However, it is important to note that individual case reports often are spectacular and not likely to be representative of the usual clinical course.

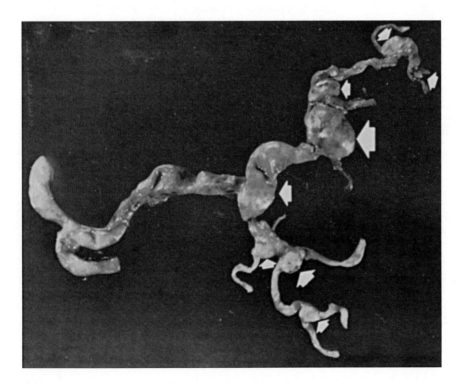

Figure 26–1. Multiple splenic artery aneurysms (*arrows*) occurring at each bifurcation of the distal artery in a grand multipara. (From Stanley JC, Thompson NW, Fry WJ: Splanchnic artery aneurysms. Arch Surg 101:689–697, 1970.)

TABLE 26-1B

Splanchnic Artery Macroaneurysms

ANEURYSM LOCATION	FREQUENCY OF REPORTED RUPTURE	SITE OF RUPTURE	MORTALITY WITH RUPTURE	USUAL TREATMENT OPTIONS
Splenic artery	2% (bland aneurysms)	Intraperitoneal within lesser sac; intragastric with pancreatitis-related inflammatory aneurysms	25% bland and unassociated with pregnancy; during pregnancy 70% maternal, 75% fetal	Splenectomy; aneurysm exclusion or excision without splenectomy
Hepatic artery	20%	Intraperitoneal and biliary tract with equal frequency	35%	Aneurysmectomy with and without hepatic artery reconstruction; hepatic territory resection; transcatheter aneurysm obliteration
Superior mesenteric artery	Uncommon (thrombosis more common)	Intraperitoneal and retroperitoneal	50%	Aneurysmectomy with superior mesenteric artery reconstruction; ligation if collateral circulation is adequate
Celiac artery	13%	Intraperitoneal	50%	Aneurysmectomy with celiac artery reconstruction; ligation if circulation is adequate
Gastric and gastroepiploic arteries	90%	Intraperitoneal (30%); intestinal tract (70%)	70%	Aneurysm excision with involved gastric tissue; ligation if extramural
Jejunal, ileal, and colic arteries	30%	Intestinal tract common; intraperitoneal uncommon	20%	Aneurysm excision with involved intestine; ligation if extramural
Pancreaticoduodenal, pancreatic, and gastroduodenal arteries	75% inflammatory 50% noninflammatory	Intestinal tract (85%); intraperitoneal (15%)	50%	Aneurysm ligation within false aneurysms (pseudocyst-related); pancreatic resection; ligation if extrapancreatic

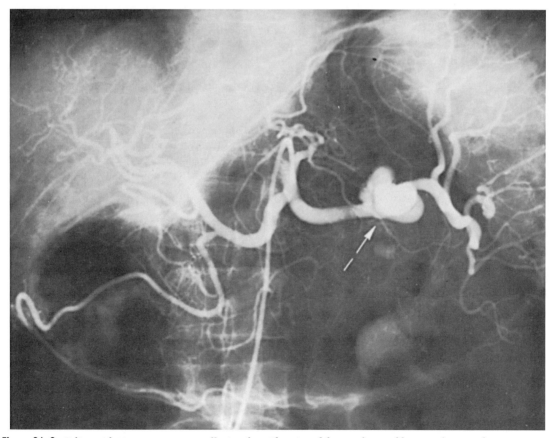

Figure 26–2. Solitary splenic artery aneurysm affecting the midportion of the vessel, caused by arterial erosion from a pancreatic pseudocyst in an alcoholic patient. (From Stanley JC, Frey CF, Miller TA, et al: Major arterial hemorrhage. A complication of pancreatic pseudocysts and chronic pancreatitis. Arch Surg 111:435–440, 1976.)

Bleeding from a ruptured splenic artery aneurysm is usually initially contained within the lesser sac. Eventually, free hemorrhage into the peritoneal cavity occurs and causes vascular collapse. This "double-rupture" phenomenon is often referred to in discussions of splenic artery aneurysms but is, in fact, relatively uncommon. Pancreatitis-related aneurysms are often a source of intestinal hemorrhage after erosion of a pseudocyst into an adjacent artery and subsequently into the stomach or pancreatic ductal system.[19–23] Arteriovenous fistula formation from rupture of a splenic artery aneurysm into the adjacent splenic vein is a rare but recognized cause of gastrointestinal hemorrhage from esophageal varices due to left-sided portal hypertension.[24]

The risk of splenic artery aneurysm rupture relates to its etiology. Rupture of bland aneurysms occurs in less than 2% of cases.[11] Contrary to earlier misconceptions, rupture has been just as likely to occur when the aneurysm is calcified, occurs in a normotensive patient, or affects the very elderly. Bland aneurysms in liver transplant recipients appear to be nearly twice as likely to rupture than those in other patients.[15, 17]

Nearly 95% of aneurysms first recognized during pregnancy have ruptured.[25–28] Maternal mortality in these cases approaches 70%, and fetal mortality exceeds 75%. However, these figures are misleading in that most women develop aneurysms during the course of repeated pregnancies. Although the rupture rate during pregnancy reported in the literature is very high, many splenic artery aneurysms in pregnant women are likely to go unrecognized without rupture. Nevertheless, splenic artery aneurysms diagnosed during pregnancy, even though asymptomatic, are a serious potential threat to the health of the mother and fetus.

The operative mortality from rupture of a splenic artery aneurysm in the past has been 25%.[8] Thus, it would seem prudent to undertake elective operative intervention for asymptomatic splenic artery aneurysms when the risk of operative death is less than 0.5%. This latter figure represents the product of the 25% mortality and the 2% rupture rate of bland aneurysms. Even if the mortality rate accompanying rupture is greater, elective intervention should be undertaken only in good-risk patients.

Splenectomy for splenic artery aneurysms was the most common form of surgical therapy in the past.[6, 10, 11] With contemporary recognition of the immunologic importance of splenic preservation, even in the aged, simple ligature obliteration or excision of these aneurysms appears preferable to splenectomy.[29] This would clearly be appropriate in the management of most proximal and many distal splenic artery aneurysms. In selected cases this may be undertaken by a laparoscopic approach.[30, 31] Percutaneous transcatheter embolization of splenic artery aneurysms may represent a reasonable alternative to an open operative intervention.[3, 32–34]

Certain splenic artery aneurysms embedded in the pancreas are best treated by distal pancreatectomy. Other aneurysms, especially false aneurysms associated with pseudocyst erosion into the adjacent artery, are most easily treated by incision of the aneurysmal sac and ligation from within of the entering and exiting vessels.[22] Pancreatic resection in the latter cases must be individualized and usually depends on the degree of associated pancreatic inflammation and the general condition of the patient.[35]

Hepatic Artery Aneurysms

Hepatic artery aneurysms account for 20% of all reported splanchnic artery aneurysms,[10, 36, 37] although they appear to be more common in contemporary practice.[6] Men are twice as likely to be affected as women, although sex differences appear to be less significant in more recent times.[6, 38] Nontraumatic and nonmycotic aneurysms are most often discovered during the sixth decade of life.

Two facts regarding the etiology of hepatic artery aneurysms are noteworthy. First, arteriosclerosis represents a secondary event rather than an actual cause of these aneurysms. Second, with increasing societal violence in the form of both penetrating as well as blunt liver injury, there has been a marked increase in the number of reported traumatic aneurysms. In fact, nearly 50% of recently reported hepatic artery aneurysms have been false aneurysms of intrahepatic arterial branches.[6] Iatrogenic false aneurysms secondary to biliary tract operative trauma remain very uncommon. However, iatrogenic false aneurysms associated with percutaneous and therapeutic biliary tract procedures are relatively common.[6] Mycotic aneurysms secondary to intravenous drug abuse–related sepsis and endocarditis is another contemporary cause of these aneurysms. Surprisingly, nearly 17% of hepatic artery aneurysms reported from 1985 to 1995 were associated with liver transplantation.[6] Connective tissue arteriopathies, such as periarteritis nodosa, have also been incriminated as a cause of occasional macroaneurysms involving the hepatic vessels.[39] Hepatic artery aneurysms are usually solitary, being extrahepatic in nearly 80% of cases and intrahepatic in 20%. In general, these aneurysms are fusiform when less than 2 cm in diameter and saccular when larger (Fig. 26–3).

Most hepatic artery aneurysms in contemporary times have been recognized as incidental findings during arteriography, CT scans, or ultrasonography for other illnesses.[6, 40, 41] Very few nontraumatic hepatic artery aneurysms are symptomatic, but when such is the case, they characteristically produce right upper quadrant and epigastric pain. Acute expansion of hepatic artery aneurysms can cause severe abdominal discomfort, similar to that of pancreatitis. Large aneurysms have been reported to cause obstructive jaundice.[42] However, most hepatic artery aneurysms are too small to compress the biliary ducts. Similarly, these lesions rarely manifest as pulsatile abdominal masses. Trauma-related aneurysms, because of the very nature of abdominal injury, are often associated with pain.

The reported incidence of rupture of hepatic artery aneurysms in contemporary times is close to 20%, but the true incidence may be considerably less. Overall mortality rates attending aneurysm rupture have been reported to be approximately 35%, although recent experience suggests a lesser mortality rate.[6] Bleeding from ruptured hepatic artery aneurysms occurs equally into the biliary tract or into the peritoneal cavity. In the case of the former, hemobilia, manifest by biliary colic, hematemesis, and jaundice, is often evident.[43, 44] Chronic gastrointestinal hemorrhage is

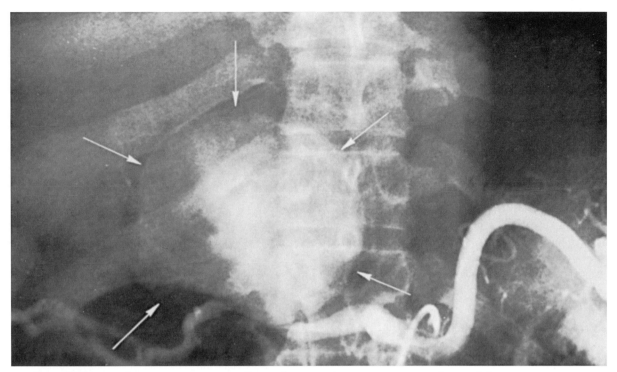

Figure 26–3. Large hepatic artery aneurysm affecting the proximal artery in a patient with an underlying connective tissue disorder. (From Stanley JC, Whitehouse WM Jr: Aneurysms of splanchnic and renal arteries. In Bergan JJ, Yao JST [eds]: Surgery of the Aorta and Its Body Branches. Orlando, Grune & Stratton, 1979, pp 497–519.)

an uncommon sequela of aneurysm rupture into the biliary tract. Intraperitoneal bleeding occurs most often with false aneurysms caused by periarterial inflammatory processes eroding into the hepatic vessels.

Common hepatic artery aneurysms have been most often treated by aneurysmectomy or aneurysm exclusion, without arterial reconstruction.[6, 36] Simple ligation is usually undertaken if temporary operative occlusion of the aneurysmal artery does not cause obvious hepatic ischemia. The extensive collateral circulation to the liver and the ability of portal venous flow to increase, in most cases, usually provide adequate liver blood flow despite interruption of the proximal hepatic artery. If compromised liver blood flow becomes apparent after hepatic artery occlusion, direct vascular reconstruction must be undertaken with either prosthetic or autologous grafts.

Hepatic ischemia is most likely to accompany treatment of aneurysms involving the more distal hepatic artery. Casual ligation of extrahepatic branches to control bleeding from intrahepatic aneurysms may cause liver necrosis.[36] Because of this potential complication, hepatic territory resection for intrahepatic aneurysms may be appropriate therapy in selected patients. Percutaneous transcatheter obliteration of the aneurysm with balloons, coils, or thrombogenic particulate matter may be a reasonable alternative to surgical intervention.[6, 32, 45–47] It must be recognized that transcatheter embolization may be unsuccessful initially, and repeated embolization or surgical therapy may subsequently be required in these patients.[37, 48] Although endograft exclusion of hepatic artery aneurysms has not been reported, it has been used to repair rupture of the hepatic artery and may prove useful in selected patients with these aneurysms.[49]

Superior Mesenteric Artery Aneurysms

Aneurysms of the proximal superior mesenteric artery are the third most common splanchnic artery aneurysm, accounting for 5.5% of these lesions.[10] Men are affected nearly twice as often as women.[6] Mycotic aneurysms secondary to bacterial endocarditis are a common lesion affecting this vessel.[6, 50] Nonhemolytic streptococci and a variety of pathogens associated with parenteral substance abuse account for these latter lesions. Superior mesenteric artery aneurysms also have been related to medial degeneration, periarterial inflammation, and trauma. Arteriosclerosis, when present, has been considered a secondary event rather than an etiologic process. Superior mesenteric artery aneurysms have been recognized most often during arteriographic studies for other diseases. A majority of reported superior mesenteric artery aneurysms have been symptomatic.[6] In these patients, abdominal discomfort varied from mild to severe pain, and, in many, was suggestive of intestinal angina.

Rupture of superior mesenteric artery aneurysms is unusual,[51] and aneurysmal dissection is uncommon.[52] The fact is that gastrointestinal hemorrhage associated with these aneurysms usually reflects their acute occlusion and bleeding from areas of intestinal infarction.[8] The unique location of these aneurysms near the origins of the inferior pancreaticoduodenal and middle colic arteries effectively isolates the distal mesenteric circulation should aneurysmal dissection or occlusion occur. It is in this setting that profound intestinal ischemia occurs, because the usual collateral network from the adjacent celiac and inferior mesenteric arterial circulations is lost.

Aneurysmectomy or simple ligation of vessels entering and exiting a superior mesenteric artery aneurysm may necessitate intestinal revascularization by means of an aortomesenteric graft or some other bypass. However, such has been accomplished infrequently. Because of the potential for graft infection if bowel ischemia is present, autologous vein grafts are favored over prosthetic conduits for these reconstructions.

Ligation of superior mesenteric artery aneurysms without arterial reconstruction may prove possible in certain cases.[6, 10] This is especially true in treatment of aneurysms associated with prior arterial obstruction in patients who have developed an adequate collateral circulation to their midgut structures.[10] Surprisingly, ligation and aneurysmorrhaphy have been the most commonly reported means of managing these superior mesenteric artery lesions.[53–55] Doppler assessment of blood flow along the intestine's antimesenteric border assists in defining the adequacy of collateral vessels in these circumstances.

Celiac Artery Aneurysms

Celiac artery aneurysms account for 4% of all splanchnic artery aneurysms.[10] Men and women appear equally affected.[56] Half of the celiac artery aneurysms encountered before 1950 had an infectious cause. More recently, most aneurysms have been associated with medial defects. Arteriosclerosis is a frequent finding, but, as in the case of other splanchnic artery aneurysms, it is considered a secondary process. Celiac artery aneurysms are usually saccular, affecting the distal trunk of this vessel (Fig. 26–4), with some evolving from poststenotic dilatations due to preexisting occlusive disease or entrapment of the proximal artery by the median arcuate ligament.

Most contemporary celiac artery aneurysms have been asymptomatic or have been associated with vague abdominal discomfort.[6, 56] Antemortem diagnoses usually result from these aneurysms having been recognized as incidental findings during ultrasonography, angiography, or CT for other diseases. Rupture has been reported to affect 13% of these aneurysms and carries a mortality of 50%.[56] In contrast to this more contemporary experience are previously published rupture rates of greater than 80%.[57] Celiac artery aneurysm rupture usually causes exsanguinating hemorrhage, first into the lesser space and then into the general peritoneal cavity. Aneurysmal rupture rarely occurs into the gastrointestinal tract.

Operative treatment of all celiac artery aneurysms is recommended, unless prohibitive surgical risks exist.[56] In the presence of acute expansion or rupture, these lesions are best approached through a thoracoabdominal incision. Most nonruptured aneurysms may be treated through an abdominal approach. Aneurysmectomy with arterial reconstruction of the celiac trunk is the preferred treatment for most celiac artery aneurysms. However, exclusion of an aneurysm with ligation of the branches entering and exiting the aneurysm can be performed in selected patients.[6, 56, 58, 59] If simple ligature is undertaken, the foregut collateral blood flow to the liver must first be documented to be sufficient to prevent hepatic necrosis. If such is not the case, hepatic revascularization is mandatory. An aortoceliac

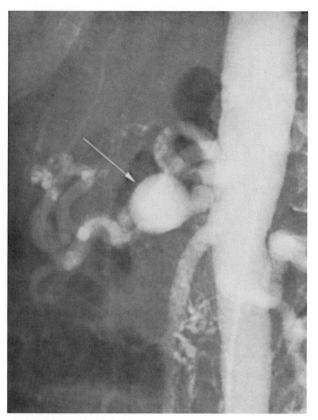

Figure 26–4. Celiac artery aneurysm affecting the distal trunk of the vessel. (From Whitehouse WM Jr, Graham LM, Stanley JC: Aneurysms of the celiac, hepatic, and splenic arteries. In Bergan JJ, Yao JST [eds]: Aneurysms. Diagnosis and Treatment, New York, Grune & Stratton, 1981, pp 405–415.)

or aortohepatic artery bypass under these circumstances is usually undertaken with an autologous vein or prosthetic graft. Successful outcomes of surgical therapy in contemporary times have been reported in greater than 90% of patients with celiac artery aneurysms treated operatively.[56]

Gastric and Gastroepiploic Artery Aneurysms

Gastric and gastroepiploic artery aneurysms account for 4% of splanchnic artery aneurysms.[10] Gastric artery aneurysms are 10 times more common than are gastroepiploic artery aneurysms. Men are three times more likely than women to have these aneurysms. The majority of these perigastric lesions affect patients older than 50 years of age. Most of these aneurysms are solitary and are acquired either as a result of periarterial inflammation or medial degeneration. Arteriosclerosis, when present, is a secondary accompaniment of these lesions.

Surprisingly few gastric or gastroepiploic artery aneurysms have been asymptomatic when initially recognized.[10, 60] In fact, these perigastric aneurysms usually manifest as emergencies without preceding symptoms.[10, 61, 62] Rupture occurred in greater than 90% of reported cases, with gastrointestinal bleeding being twice as common as intraperitoneal hemorrhage. That rupture of these aneurysms may

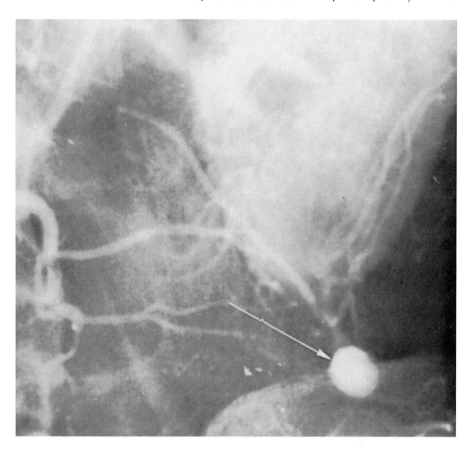

Figure 26–5. Ileal artery branch aneurysm. (From Stanley JC, Whitehouse WM Jr: Aneurysms of splanchnic and renal arteries. In Bergan JJ, Yao JST [eds]: Surgery of the Aorta and Its Body Branches. New York, Grune & Stratton, 1979, pp 497–519.)

be catastrophic is emphasized by the reported 70% mortality of such an event.[8]

Surgical treatment of gastric and gastroepiploic artery aneurysms does not involve vascular reconstructive surgery.[10, 60] Intramural gastric aneurysms require excision with the involved portion of the stomach. Extramural aneurysms should be treated by arterial ligation alone, with or without aneurysm excision. In selected cases laparoscopic resection may be appropriate.[63] These perigastric aneurysms are very small, and a search for them is often tedious if preoperative localization has not been established by arteriographic studies.[8, 22]

Jejunal, Ileal, and Colic Artery Aneurysms

Aneurysms of the jejunal, ileal, and colic arteries account for 3% of splanchnic artery aneurysms.[10] They are usually recognized in patients older than 60 years of age, with men and women affected equally. Multiple aneurysms have been reported in 10% of cases. Acquired medial defects are responsible for most lesions, and arteriosclerosis, present in 20% of these aneurysms, is considered a secondary event rather than a causative process. Multiple aneurysms occasionally evolve as a result of infected emboli associated with subacute bacterial endocarditis,[64] or result from periarteritis nodosa as well as other connective tissue diseases.[65]

Most of the reported aneurysms have been symptomatic, with the majority exhibiting abdominal pain.[6, 66] Nevertheless, many aneurysms are undoubtedly asymptomatic,

being recognized as incidental findings during arteriography for gastrointestinal bleeding[67] (Fig. 26–5). Although the majority of reported intestinal branch aneurysms have ruptured, actual rupture rates are probably close to 30%. Aneurysms of ileal branches are more apt to rupture, with jejunal branch aneurysm rupture being relatively rare.[68] Rupture is associated with a mortality of approximately 20%,[10] and is frequently a cause of gastrointestinal hemorrhage. Although rupture into the mesentery or the free peritoneal cavity is uncommon, these small mesenteric branch aneurysms are more apt to cause abdominal apoplexy than any other splanchnic artery aneurysm.

Operation for intestinal branch aneurysms entails arterial ligation, with or without aneurysmectomy, for extraintestinal lesions. Intramural aneurysms or those associated with bowel infarction necessitate resection of the involved segment of intestine. In selected patients transcatheter embolization is appropriate, but intestinal necrosis with perforation or stricture formation is a recognized complication of such therapy.[69] Aneurysms of the inferior mesenteric artery are quite rare and knowledge of their clinical importance is anecdotal at best.[6, 70]

Pancreaticoduodenal, Pancreatic, and Gastroduodenal Artery Aneurysms

Pancreatic and pancreaticoduodenal artery aneurysms account for 2%, and gastroduodenal artery aneurysms represent an additional 1.5% of all splanchnic artery aneu-

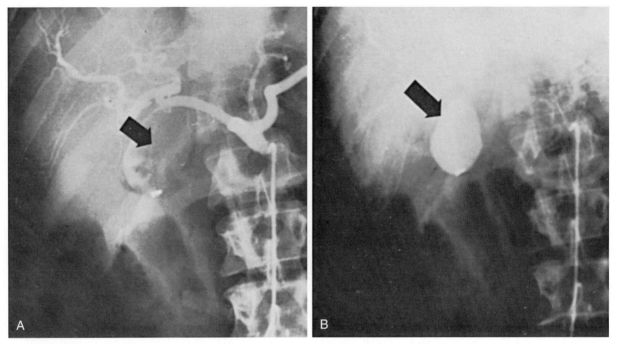

Figure 26–6. Gastroduodenal aneurysm associated with arterial erosion by an adjacent infected pancreatic pseudocyst. *A,* Early-phase selective celiac arteriogram. *B,* Late-phase arteriogram with contrast collection in the false aneurysm.

rysms.[10] Men are four times as likely as women to exhibit pancreaticoduodenal and gastroduodenal artery aneurysms, with sex differences being more notable with the former aneurysms compared to the latter. Most patients with these lesions are older than 45 years of age. These peripancreatic aneurysms, in general, are the most difficult to treat of all splanchnic artery aneurysms.[22, 71–76]

The most common cause of these aneurysms is pancreatitis-related vascular necrosis or vessel erosion by an adjacent pancreatic pseudocyst (Fig. 26–6). Medial degenerative and traumatic lesions are less common, and arteriosclerosis is invariably a secondary, not a causative, process. Lastly, pancreaticoduodenal artery aneurysms have been increasingly recognized to evolve as an apparent consequence of excessive blood flow within the collateral vessels of patients having celiac artery stenoses.[77–81] Although less well recognized, gastroduodenal artery aneurysms may develop for the same reason in cases of superior mesenteric artery stenosis.[82]

The vast majority of patients with these aneurysms experience epigastric pain and discomfort.[7, 10] This may be due to underlying pancreatic disease in that approximately 50% of gastroduodenal and 30% of pancreaticoduodenal artery aneurysms are pancreatitis-related. Asymptomatic aneurysms of these arteries are unusual. Arteriography is necessary to confirm the existence of these lesions. CT scanning and MRI are of increasing importance in recognizing these aneurysms, and are helpful in detecting the presence of rupture or associated pancreatic lesions.

Gastroduodenal and pancreaticoduodenal aneurysm rupture has been described in more than half the reported cases.[6, 10, 79] Bleeding in these circumstances has been reported in 75% of inflammatory and 50% of noninflammatory lesions. The site of hemorrhage may be the stomach, the biliary tract, or the pancreatic ductal system. Hemor-rhage into the peritoneal cavity is less common, affecting approximately 15% of these aneurysms. Overall, mortality rates with rupture approach 25%,[6] and, in the case of true pancreaticoduodenal artery aneurysms, approach 50%.

Operative intervention is mandatory in all but the poorest risk patient with a gastroduodenal, pancreaticoduodenal, or pancreatic arterial aneurysm.[6, 22, 71, 72, 83, 84] Surgical treatment of pancreatitis-related false aneurysms is often best accomplished by arterial ligation from within the aneurysmal sac rather than extra-aneurysmal arterial ligation. Extensive dissection about the pancreas in this setting is hazardous. If a pancreatic pseudocyst or abscess has eroded into an artery and caused a false aneurysm, some form of drainage procedure may need to accompany ligature control of the affected vessel. Pancreatic resections, including distal pancreatectomy or pancreaticoduodenectomy, may be the safest therapy in selected patients.[22, 85] Transcatheter embolization and electrocoagulation have been employed in very high-risk patients to ablate certain aneurysms.[78, 86–88] Unfortunately, rebleeding and late aneurysmal rupture with such therapy can occur and restrict its universal use.[78, 89] In those patients with coexistent celiac artery occlusion, the affected artery may be an important collateral vessel and simple operative ligature or transcatheter embolic occlusion may result in foregut ischemia and should be undertaken cautiously.

RENAL ARTERY MACROANEURYSMS

Renal artery aneurysms represent an uncommon vascular disease (Table 26–2). Although our understanding of these aneurysms is reasonably well defined, controversy still persists concerning their clinical importance.[90–98] This relates, in part, to the fact that complications of these aneurysms

TABLE 26-2

Renal Artery Macroaneurysms

LESION	MALE-FEMALE RATIO	CONTRIBUTING FACTORS	FREQUENCY OF REPORTED RUPTURE	MORTALITY WITH RUPTURE	USUAL TREATMENT OPTIONS
Renal artery aneurysm	1:1.2	Medial degeneration; arterial fibrodysplasia; hypertension	3% (bland aneurysms)	10% (bland aneurysms); during pregnancy 45% maternal, 85% fetal	Aneurysmectomy with renal artery reconstruction; nephrectomy for ruptured aneurysms
Renal artery dissection	10:1	Blunt abdominal trauma; intraarterial catheterization; medial degeneration	Uncommon (thrombosis more common)	Undefined	Renal artery reconstruction

have been overestimated in reports that usually describe operative experiences rather than population-based experiences.[98, 99] Discussion of these lesions must take into consideration the differences between true and dissecting aneurysms of the renal artery.

Renal Artery Aneurysms

The incidence of true renal artery aneurysms approaches 0.1%, a figure derived from the 0.09% frequency of these aneurysms in approximately 8500 patients subjected to arteriographic studies for nonrenal disease.[97] Women are more likely than men to have renal artery aneurysms. However, when aneurysms in patients having renal arterial dysplasia are excluded, there is no sex predilection. That the right renal artery is more likely to develop aneurysms than the left may reflect the fact that dysplastic disease is known to more commonly affect the right renal artery.[97]

Most renal artery aneurysms are saccular (Fig. 26–7). Seventy-five percent are located at primary or secondary renal artery bifurcations. Most aneurysms have diameters of less than 1.5 cm. Intraparenchymal aneurysms occur in fewer than 10% of cases.

Renal artery aneurysms usually appear to be caused by a medial degenerative process.[97] In many instances, these aneurysms appear to be part of medial fibroplasia[92, 97] (Fig. 26–8). Systemic arterial hypertension may contribute to certain of these aneurysms. Arteriosclerosis, with hemorrhage, calcium deposition, collections of cholesterol, and necrotic cellular debris within a matrix of fibrous tissue, affects a third of these aneurysms. However, similar changes of the adjacent renal artery are very uncommon and the former findings are thought to represent a secondary event rather than a primary process. Importantly, arteriosclerosis in some but not all aneurysms in the same patient suggests a nonarteriosclerotic cause of these lesions.[97]

Evidence exists that both congenital and acquired factors contribute to the evolution of most renal artery macroaneurysms. In this regard, deficiencies in the internal elastic lamina of muscular arteries appear to be congenital, but the reported increase in aneurysm appearance with increasing age indicates the presence of acquired factors. Microaneurysms secondary to necrotizing arteritides, such as polyarteritis nodosa, are usually small, although some of these lesions may become relatively large.[100]

The majority of renal artery aneurysms are asymptomatic.[97] Some authors have suggested that few of these aneurysms ever cause serious clinical complications.[92, 98, 99] Nevertheless, aneurysmal expansion or renal infarction from dislodged thrombus may occasionally account for symptoms attributed to these lesions. Hematuria and abdominal bruits, when present in these cases, are unlikely to be related to aneurysmal disease. Similarly, because they are small, very few aneurysms present as pulsatile masses on physical examination.

Rupture represents the most serious complication attending renal artery aneurysms.[101] Such an event is likely to affect fewer than 3% of cases. Mortality with rupture has been reported to be approximately 10% in the past,

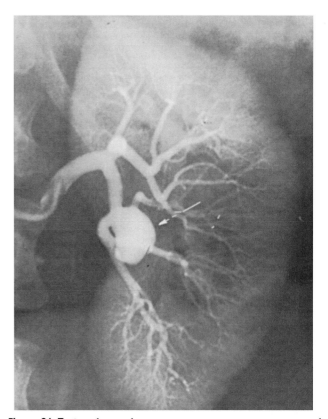

Figure 26–7. Saccular renal artery aneurysm occurring at a segmental branching. (From Stanley JC, Whitehouse WM Jr: Renal artery macroaneurysms. In Bergan JJ, Yao JST [eds]: Aneurysms. Diagnosis and Treatment. New York, Grune & Stratton, 1981, pp 417–431.)

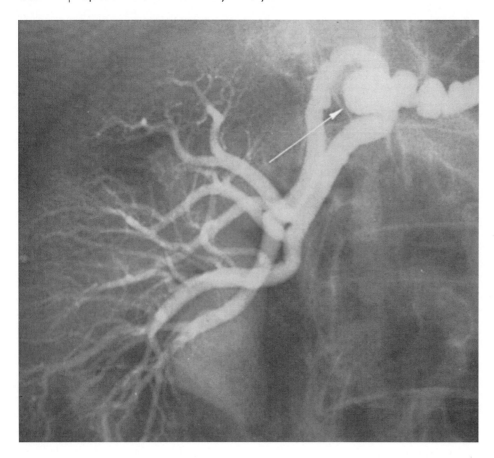

Figure 26–8. Renal artery macroaneurysm affecting the primary bifurcation of a vessel exhibiting medial fibrodysplasia. (From Stanley JC, Whitehouse WM Jr: Renal artery macroaneurysms. In Bergan JJ, Yao JST [eds]: Aneurysms. Diagnosis and Treatment. New York, Grune & Stratton, 1981, pp 417–431.)

but has been less common in recent times.[101] However, loss of the kidney is almost inevitable with aneurysm rupture. It has been suggested that aneurysms of less than 1.5 cm in diameter, calcified aneurysms, and those occurring in normotensive patients are not likely to rupture, but such has not proved to be the case.

Renal artery aneurysm rupture during pregnancy is an exception regarding the life-threatening nature of these lesions.[102–106] Rupture in this setting does not appear related to patient age, presence of hypertension, or parity. Aneurysm rupture in pregnancy has caused nearly an 85% fetal mortality and resulted in approximately a 45% maternal mortality. The affected kidney has been salvaged in nearly 20% of surviving women.

The cause-effect association of renal artery aneurysms with elevated arterial blood pressure is controversial.[95, 107–109] It is possible that aneurysmal thrombus may embolize or propagate and occlude a distal artery, thereby producing renal ischemia and renovascular hypertension.[94, 97] Extensive atheromatous disease within large aneurysmal sacs may predispose to thrombotic events, yet small nonarteriosclerotic aneurysms also have been recognized as the source of distal cortical embolization. Aneurysmal compression, or twisting and narrowing of adjacent arteries, has been proposed as an additional cause of renovascular hypertension, but such is very uncommon. However, intrinsic stenotic disease adjacent to an aneurysm, which is not always evident on preoperative arteriograms, may be the cause of secondary hypertension in many of these cases. Determination of renal–systemic renin indices in hypertensive patients with isolated renal artery aneurysms may better define the presence or absence of renin-mediated blood pressure elevations.

Indications for operative treatment of renal artery macroaneurysms have become better defined.[91, 97] Certainly, all symptomatic patients with suspected aneurysmal expansion should be subjected to operation. Similarly, aneurysms coexisting with functionally important renal artery stenoses are best treated operatively. Surgical therapy is also warranted for aneurysms that contain thrombus if distal embolization is evident. Because of the potential for catastrophic rupture during pregnancy, operative therapy is recommended for aneurysms in all women of childbearing age who might conceive in the future.

Surgical therapy is directed at elimination of the aneurysm without loss of the kidney or compromise of normal renal blood flow.[94, 97, 110] An exception exists in the management of ruptured aneurysms, in which kidney salvage may be impossible and nephrectomy may be the only logical therapy.[101, 105] Large aneurysms of the main renal artery may often be excised with simple primary repair of the artery. Excision of smaller aneurysms usually necessitates an angioplastic vein patch arterial closure or implantation of the involved artery into an adjacent uninvolved artery. In situ renal artery reconstructions with autogenous saphenous vein (or internal iliac artery grafts for bifurcation aneurysms) for aneurysms associated with functionally important stenoses are perhaps the most common means of treating patients with these particular lesions. In selected instances, ex vivo repairs are appropriate.[111, 112] Partial nephrectomy may be necessary for intraparenchymal aneurysms. These latter lesions and occasional aneurysms of extrarenal arteries may be treated by transcatheter embolization.[94, 113] Endovascular exclusion of true renal artery aneurysms is not possible in most patients because of the usual location of these lesions at arterial bifurcations. Patients not subjected to operation must be followed carefully with serial CT scans or arteriography. Particular attention should be directed to controlling hypertension in patients not subjected to surgical therapy.

Renal Artery Dissections

Isolated dissections of the renal arteries are usually classified as those due to blunt abdominal trauma or intraluminal catheter-induced injury and those occurring spontaneously.[114, 115] All forms of dissections may be associated with false aneurysm formation (Fig. 26–9). Men are 10 times more likely than women to exhibit dissections of the renal artery.[116] The right renal artery is much more often affected than the left. This may reflect increased physical stresses on this artery because of greater ptosis of the right kidney compared with the left. Approximately one third of renal artery dissections are bilateral.

Two primary mechanisms contribute to renal artery dissections due to blunt abdominal trauma. The first is displacement of the kidney during deceleration, with marked stretching of the vascular pedicle. In these circumstances, fracture of the intima, which is the least elastic arterial wall component, leads to subintimal dissections. The second relates to direct trauma of the renal artery over the unyielding posteriorly located vertebral bodies. Medial hemorrhage and false aneurysm formation may occur in this setting. Renal artery injury during arteriography appears to be a very uncommon but important cause of dissections. In one large series, only four renal artery, catheter-related dissections were encountered among more than 11,000 abdominal arteriographic examinations, including more than 2200 selective renal arteriograms.[114]

The second major category of renal artery dissections is that associated with spontaneous vessel wall disruption. Surprisingly, spontaneous dissections affect the renal arteries more than any other peripheral artery. They usually appear related to coexistent renovascular disease. Spontaneous dissections have been reported in 0.5% of patients having renal artery dysplasia.[114]

Spontaneous dissections are most apt to extend within the outer media. This is in contrast to the subintimal and inner medial location of most traumatic dissections. In certain instances, these spontaneous dissections have been attributed to rupture of abnormal vasa vasorum. Under such circumstances the dissecting mural hematoma may increase vessel wall ischemia and further compromise its integrity. Spontaneous renal artery dissections most often originate in the proximal vessels and terminate at first-order branchings.

Pain, hematuria, and elevated blood pressure are frequent manifestations of acute renal artery dissections, regardless of their cause.[114] Chronic manifestations of these

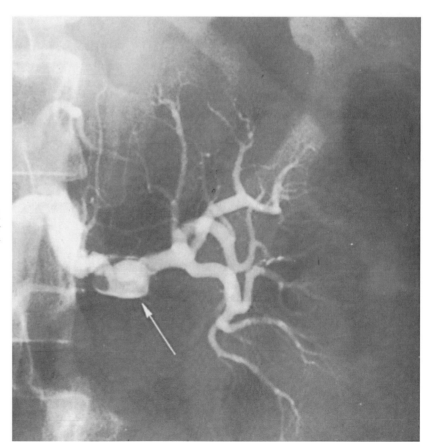

Figure 26–9. Renal artery dissection with associated false aneurysm. (From Gewertz BL, Stanley JC, Fry WJ: Renal artery dissections. Arch Surg 112:409–414, 1977.)

dissections are often associated with compromised renal function and renovascular hypertension. Delayed rupture is uncommon. An incorrect initial clinical diagnosis is common, occurring in nearly 60% of patients with renal artery dissections.[114] Intravenous urography, often with tomography, may be useful in establishing the presence of renal ischemia in these cases, but the accuracy of this study is limited. Because prompt diagnosis may improve the results of surgical therapy, intravenous urography should be deferred in favor of prompt arteriography. Criteria for arteriographic diagnosis of renal artery dissections include (1) luminal irregularities with aneurysmal dilatation or saccular dissections associated with segmental stenoses; (2) the predilection of dissections to extend distally to the first renal artery bifurcation; (3) cuffing at branchings causing a "rolled-down sock" appearance; and (4) variable degrees of reversibility documented by serial studies.

Kidney preservation is of prime importance in patients exhibiting renal artery dissections. This is particularly relevant given the fact that renal artery disease involves the contralateral kidney in half the patients exhibiting spontaneous dissections.[114] Arterial reconstructions using autogenous saphenous vein or hypogastric artery may be complex, and ex vivo repairs are appropriate in selected cases. Dissections secondary to severe blunt trauma usually necessitate emergent arterial reconstructions. Delayed repair becomes necessary when hypertension persists or renal function deteriorates. Some physicians have taken a cautious nonsurgical approach toward managing traumatic dissections because operation in the acute setting often results in nephrectomy. Treatment using an endovascular stent has appeal, but still remains an unproven therapy.[117] In contrast, spontaneous dissecting aneurysms should all be subjected to surgical therapy once hemodynamically significant stenoses or occlusions are recognized as causing renovascular hypertension or deterioration in renal function.[114, 116]

References

1. Stanley JC: Abdominal visceral aneurysms. In Haimovici H (ed): Vascular Emergencies. New York, Appleton-Century-Crofts, 1981, pp 387–397.
2. Busuttil RW, Brin BJ: The diagnosis and management of visceral artery aneurysms. Surgery 88:619–630, 1980.
3. Carr SC, Pearce WH, Vogelzang RL, et al: Current management of visceral artery aneurysms. Surgery 120:627–633, 1996.
4. Graham JM, McCollum CH, DeBakey ME: Aneurysms of the splanchnic arteries. Am J Surg 140:797–801, 1980.
5. Rokke O, Sondenaa K, Amundsen SR, et al: Successful management of eleven splanchnic artery aneurysms. Eur J Surg 163:411–417, 1997.
6. Shanley CJ, Shah NL, Messina LM: Common splanchnic artery aneurysms: Splenic, hepatic and celiac. Ann Vasc Surg 10:315–322, 1996.
7. Shanley CJ, Shah NL, Messina LM: Uncommon splanchnic artery aneurysms: Pancreaticoduodenal, gastroduodenal, superior mesenteric, inferior mesenteric and colic. Ann Vasc Surg 10:506–515, 1996.
8. Stanley JC, Thompson NW, Fry WJ: Splanchnic artery aneurysms. Arch Surg 101:689–697, 1970.
9. Wagner WH, Allins AD, Treiman RL, et al: Ruptured visceral artery aneurysms. Ann Vasc Surg 11:342–347, 1997.
10. Zelenock GB, Stanley JC: Splanchnic artery aneurysms. In Rutherford RB (ed): Vascular Surgery, 5th ed. Philadelphia, WB Saunders, 2000, pp 1369–1382.
11. Stanley JC, Fry WJ: Pathogenesis and clinical significance of splenic artery aneurysms. Surgery 76:889–909, 1974.
12. Puttini M, Aseni P, Brambilla G, Belli L: Splenic artery aneurysms in portal hypertension. J Cardiovasc Surg 23:490–493, 1982.
13. Nishida O, Moriyasu F, Nakamura T, et al: Hemodynamics of splenic artery aneurysm. Gastroenterology 90:1042–1046, 1986.
14. Ohta M, Hashizume M, Ueno K, et al: Hemodynamic study of splenic artery aneurysm in portal hypertension. Hepatogastroenterology 41:181–184, 1994.
15. Ayalon A, Wiesner RH, Perkins JD, et al: Splenic artery aneurysms in liver transplant patients. Transplantation 45:386–389, 1988.
16. Bronsther O, Merhav H, Van Thiel D, Starzl TE: Splenic artery aneurysms occurring in liver transplant recipients. Transplantation 52:723–756, 1991.
17. Kobori L, van der Kolk MJ, de Jong KP, et al: Splenic artery aneurysms in liver transplant patients. Liver Transplant Group. J Hepatol 27:890–893, 1997.
18. Martin KW, Morian JP Jr, Lee JK, Scharp DW: Demonstration of a splenic artery pseudoaneurysm by MR imaging. J Comput Assist Tomogr 9:190–192, 1985.
19. de Vries JE, Schattenkerk ME, Malt RA: Complications of splenic artery aneurysm other than intraperitoneal rupture. Surgery 91:200–204, 1982.
20. Harper PC, Gamelli RL, Kaye MD: Recurrent hemorrhage into the pancreatic duct from a splenic artery aneurysm. Gastroenterology 87:417–420, 1984.
21. Stabile BE, Wilson SE, Debas HT: Reduced mortality from bleeding pseudocysts and pseudoaneurysms caused by pancreatitis. Arch Surg 118:45–51, 1983.
22. Stanley JC, Frey CF, Miller TA, et al: Major arterial hemorrhage. A complication of pancreatic pseudocysts and chronic pancreatitis. Arch Surg 111:435–440, 1976.
23. Wager WH, Cossman DV, Treiman RL, et al: Hemosuccus pancreaticus from intraductal rupture of a primary splenic artery aneurysm. J Vasc Surg 19:158–164, 1994.
24. Brothers TE, Stanley JC, Zelenock GB: Splenic arteriovenous fistula: Review of the literature with four new case reports. Int Surg 80:189–194, 1995.
25. Angelakis EJ, Bair WE, Barone JE, Lincer RM: Splenic artery aneurysm rupture during pregnancy. Obstet Gynecol 48:145–148, 1993.
26. MacFarlane JR, Thorbjarnason B: Rupture of splenic artery aneurysm during pregnancy. Am J Obstet Gynecol 95:1025–1037, 1966.
27. O'Grady JP, Day EJ, Toole AL, Paust JC: Splenic artery aneurysm rupture in pregnancy. A review and case report. Obstet Gynecol 50:627–630, 1977.
28. Vassalotti SB, Schaller JA: Spontaneous rupture of splenic artery aneurysm in pregnancy. Report of first known antepartum rupture with maternal and fetal survival. Obstet Gynecol 30:264–268, 1967.
29. Taylor JL, Woodward DA: Splenic conservation and the management of splenic artery aneurysm. Ann R Coll Surg Engl 69:179–180, 1987.
30. Arca MJ, Gagner M, Beniford BT, et al: Splenic artery aneurysms: Methods of laparoscopic repair. J Vasc Surg 30:184–188, 1999.
31. Hashizume M, Ohta M, Ueno K, et al: Laparoscopic ligation of splenic artery aneurysm. Surgery 113:352–354, 1993.
32. Baker KS, Tisnado J, Cho SR, Beachley MC: Splanchnic artery aneurysms and pseudoaneurysms: Transcatheter embolization. Radiology 163:135–159, 1987.
33. McDermott VG, Shlansky-Goldberg R, Cope C: Endovascular management of splenic artery aneurysms and pseudoaneurysms. Cardiovasc Intervent Radiol 17:179–184, 1994.
34. Waltman AC, Luers PR, Athanasoulis CA, Warshaw AL: Massive arterial hemorrhage in patients with pancreatitis. Complementary roles of surgery and transcatheter occlusive techniques. Arch Surg 121:439–443, 1986.
35. de Perrot M, Buhler L, Schneider PA, et al: Do aneurysms and pseudoaneurysms of the splenic artery require different surgical strategy? Hepatogastroenterology 46:2028–2032, 1999.
36. Iseki J, Tada Y, Wada T, Nobori M: Hepatic artery aneurysm. Report of a case and review of the literature. Gastroenterol Jpn 18:84–92, 1983.

37. Guida PM, Moore SW: Aneurysm of the hepatic artery. Report of five cases with a brief review of the previously reported cases. Surgery 60:299–310, 1966.

38. Lumsden AB, Mattar SG, Allen RC, Bacha EA: Hepatic artery aneurysms: The management of 22 patients. J Surg Res 60:345–350, 1996.

39. Parangi S, Oz MC, Blume RS, et al: Hepatobiliary complications of polyarteritis nodosa. Arch Surg 126:909–912, 1991.

40. Athey PA, Sax SL, Lamki N, Cadavid G: Sonography in the diagnosis of hepatic artery aneurysms. AJR Am J Roentgenol 147:725–727, 1986.

41. Kibbler CC, Cohen DL, Cruicshank JK, et al: Use of CAT scanning in the diagnosis and management of hepatic artery aneurysm. Gut 26:752–756, 1985.

42. Lal RB, Strohl JA, Piazza S, et al: Hepatic artery aneurysm. J Cardiovasc Surg 30:509–513, 1989.

43. Harlaftis NN, Akin JT: Hemobilia from ruptured hepatic artery aneurysm: Report of a case and review of the literature. Am J Surg 133:229–232, 1977.

44. Stauffer JT, Weinman MD, Bynum TE: Hemobilia in a patient with multiple hepatic artery aneurysms: A case report and review of the literature. Am J Gastroenterol 84:59–62, 1989.

45. Kadir S, Athansoulis CA, Ring EJ, Greenfield A: Transcatheter embolization of intrahepatic arterial aneurysms. Radiology 134:335–339, 1980.

46. Okazaki M, Higashihara H, Ono H, et al: Percutaneous embolization of ruptured splanchnic artery pseudoaneurysms. Acta Radiol 32:349–354, 1991.

47. Thibodeaux LC, Deshmukh RM, Hearn AT, et al: Management options for hepatic artery aneurysms. Ann Vasc Surg 9:285–288, 1995.

48. Salam TA, Lumsden AB, Martin LG, Smith RB: Nonoperative management of vascular aneurysms and pseudoaneurysms. Am J Surg 164:215–219, 1992.

49. Bürger T, Halloul Z, Meyer F, et al: Emergency stent-graft repair of a ruptured hepatic artery secondary to local postoperative peritonitis. J Endovasc Ther 7:324–327, 2000.

50. Friedman SG, Pogo GJ, Moccio CG: Mycotic aneurysm of the superior mesenteric artery. J Vasc Surg 6:87–90, 1987.

51. Blumenberg RM, David D, Skovak J: Abdominal apoplexy due to rupture of a superior mesenteric artery aneurysm: Clip aneurysmorrhaphy with survival. Arch Surg 108:223–226, 1974.

52. Cormier F, Ferry J, Artru B, et al: Dissecting aneurysms of the main trunk of the superior mesenteric artery. J Vasc Surg 15:424–430, 1992.

53. DeBakey ME, Cooley DA: Successful resection of mycotic aneurysm of superior mesenteric artery: Case report and review of the literature. Am Surg 19:202–212, 1953.

54. Geelkerken RH, van Bockel JH, de Roos WK, Hermans J: Surgical treatment of intestinal artery aneurysms: Eur J Vasc Surg 4:563–567, 1990.

55. Olcott C, Ehrenfeld WK: Endoaneurysmorrhaphy for visceral artery aneurysms. Am J Surg 133:636–639, 1977.

56. Graham LM, Stanley JC, Whitehouse WM Jr, et al: Celiac artery aneurysms: Historical (1745–1949) versus contemporary (1950–1984) differences in etiology and clinical importance. J Vasc Surg 2:757–764, 1985.

57. Shumacker HB Jr, Siderys H: Excisional treatment of aneurysm of celiac artery. Ann Surg 148:885–889, 1958.

58. Hertzer NR, Mullally PH: Celiac artery aneurysmectomy with hepatic artery ligation. Arch Surg 104:337–339, 1972.

59. Parfitt J, Chalmers RTA, Wolfe JHN: Visceral aneurysms in Ehlers-Danlos syndrome: Case report and review of the literature. J Vasc Surg 31:1248–1251, 2000.

60. Funahashi S, Yukizane T, Yano K, et al: An aneurysm of the right gastroepiploic artery. J Cardiovasc Surg 38:385–388, 1997.

61. Jacobs PPM, Croiset van Ughelen FAAM, Bruyninckx CMA, Hoefsloot F: Haemoperitoneum caused by a dissection aneurysm of the gastroepiploic artery. Eur J Vasc Surg 8:236–237, 1994.

62. Witte JT, Hasson JE, Harms BA, et al: Fatal gastric artery dissection and rupture occurring as a paraesophageal mass: A case report and literature review. Surgery 107:590–594, 1990.

63. Uchikoshi F, Sakamoto T, Imabunn S, et al: Aneurysm of the right gastroepiploic artery: A case report of laparoscopic resection. Cardiovasc Surg 1:550–551, 1993.

64. Trevisani MF, Ricci MA, Michaels RM, Meyer KK: Multiple mesenteric aneurysms complicating subacute bacterial endocarditis. Arch Surg 122:823–824, 1987.

65. Selke FW, Williams GB, Donovan DL, Clarke RE: Management of intra-abdominal aneurysms associated with periarteritis nodosa. J Vasc Surg 4:294–298, 1986.

66. Sarcina A, Bellosta R, Magnaldi S, Luzzani L: Aneurysm of the middle colic artery—case report and literature review. Eur J Vasc Endovasc Surg 20:198–200, 2000.

67. Bleichrodt RP, Smulders TAE, Schreuder F, et al: Aneurysms of the jejunal artery. J Cardiovasc Surg 25:376–377, 1984.

68. Diettrich NA, Cacioppo JC, Ying DPW: Massive gastrointestinal hemorrhage caused by rupture of a jejunal branch artery aneurysm. J Vasc Surg 8:187–189, 1988.

69. Naito A, Toyota N, Ito K: Embolization of a ruptured middle colic artery aneurysm. Cardiovasc Intervent Radiol 18:56–58, 1995.

70. Graham LM, Hay MR, Cho KJ, Stanley JC: Inferior mesenteric artery aneurysms. Surgery 97:158–163, 1985.

71. Eckhauser FE, Stanley JC, Zelenock GB, et al: Gastroduodenal and pancreaticoduodenal artery aneurysms: A complication of pancreatitis causing spontaneous gastrointestinal hemorrhage. Surgery 88:335–355, 1980.

72. Gadacz TR, Trunkey D, Kieffer RF: Visceral vessel erosion associated with pancreatitis. Case reports and a review of the literature. Arch Surg 113:1438–1440, 1978.

73. Gangahar DM, Carveth SW, Reese HE, et al: True aneurysm of the pancreaticoduodenal artery: A case report and review of the literature. J Vasc Surg 2:741–742, 1985.

74. Spanos PK, Kloppedal EA, Murray CA: Aneurysms of the gastroduodenal and pancreaticoduodenal arteries. Am J Surg 127:345–348, 1974.

75. Taheri SA, Mueller G: Surgical approach and review of literature on gastroduodenal aneurysm: A case report. Angiology 36:895–898, 1985.

76. Verta MJ Jr, Dean RH, Yao JST, et al: Pancreaticoduodenal artery aneurysms. Ann Surg 186:111–114, 1977.

77. Chiou AC, Josephs LG, Menzoian JO: Inferior pancreaticoduodenal artery aneurysm: Report of a case and review of the literature. J Vasc Surg 17:784–789, 1993.

78. de Perrot M, Berney T, Deleaval J, et al: Management of true aneurysms of the pancreaticoduodenal arteries. Ann Surg 229:416–420, 1999.

79. Iyomasa S, Matsuzaki Y, Hiei K, et al: Pancreaticoduodenal artery aneurysm: A case report and review of the literature. J Vasc Surg 22:161–166, 1995.

80. Quandalle P, Chambon JP, Marache P, et al: Pancreaticoduodenal artery aneurysms associated with celiac axis stenosis: Report of two cases and review of the literature. Ann Vasc Surg 4:540–545, 1990.

81. Suzuki K, Kashimura H, Sato M, et al: Pancreaticoduodenal artery aneurysms associated with celiac axis stenosis due to compression by medial arcuate ligament and celiac plexus. J Gastroenterol 33:434–438, 1998.

82. Gouny P, Fukui S, Aymard A, et al: Aneurysm of the gastroduodenal artery associated with stenosis of the superior mesenteric artery. Ann Vasc Surg 8:281–284, 1994.

83. Coll DP, Ierardi R, Kerstein MD, et al: Aneurysms of the pancreaticoduodenal arteries: A change in management. Ann Vasc Surg 12:286–291, 1998.

84. Granke K, Hollier LH, Bowen JC: Pancreaticoduodenal artery aneurysms: Changing patterns. South Med J 83:918–921, 1990.

85. Pitkaranta P, Haapiainen R, Kivisaari L, Schroder T: Diagnostic evaluation and aggressive surgical approach in bleeding pseudoaneurysms associated with pancreatic pseudocysts. Scand J Gastroenterol 26:58–64, 1991.

86. Mandel SR, Jaques PF, Mauro MA, Sanofsky S: Nonoperative management of peripancreatic arterial aneurysms. A 10-year experience. Ann Surg 205:126–128, 1987.

87. Thakker RV, Gajjar B, Wilkins RA, Levi AJ: Embolization of gastroduodenal artery aneurysm caused by chronic pancreatitis. Gut 24:1094–1098, 1983.

88. Vujic I, Anderson MC, Meredith HC, Cullon JW: Successful embolization of the dorsal pancreatic artery to control massive upper gastrointestinal hemorrhage. Ann Surg 46:184–186, 1980.

89. Lina JR, Jaques P, Mandell V: Aneurysm rupture secondary to transcatheter embolization. AJR 132:553–556, 1979.

90. Bulbul MA, Farrow GA: Renal artery aneurysms. Urology 40:124–126, 1992.

91. Dzinich C, Gloviczki P, McKusick MA, et al: Surgical management of renal artery aneurysm. Cardiovasc Surg 1:243–247, 1993.

92. Henriksson C, Lukes P, Nilson AE, Pettersson S: Angiographically discovered, non-operated renal artery aneurysm. Scand J Urol Nephrol 18:59–62, 1984.

93. Hubert JP JR, Pairolero PC, Kazmier FJ: Solitary renal artery aneurysm. Surgery 88:557–565, 1980.

94. Hupp T, Allenberg JR, Post K, et al: Renal artery aneurysm: Surgical indications and results. Eur J Vasc Surg 6:477–486, 1992.

95. Martin RS III, Meacham PW, Ditesheim JA, et al: Renal artery aneurysm: Selective treatment for hypertension and prevention of rupture. J Vasc Surg 9:26–34, 1989.

96. Stanley JC: Renal artery aneurysms and dissections. In Vieth FJ (ed): Current Critical Problems in Vascular Surgery, vol 3. St Louis, Quality Medical, 1991, pp 311–319.

97. Stanley JC, Rhodes EL, Gewertz BL, et al: Renal artery aneurysms: Significance of macroaneurysms exclusive of dissections and fibrodysplastic mural dilations. Arch Surg 110:1327–1333, 1975.

98. Tham G, Ekelund L, Herrlin K, et al: Renal artery aneurysms. Natural history and prognosis. Ann Surg 197:348–352, 1983.

99. Henriksson C, Bjorkerud S, Nilson AE, Pettersson S: Natural history of renal artery aneurysm elucidated by repeated angiography and pathoanatomical studies. Eur Urol 11:244–248, 1985.

100. Smith DL, Wernick R: Spontaneous rupture of a renal artery aneurysm in polyarteritis nodosa: Critical review of the literature and report of a case. Am J Med 87:464–467, 1989.

101. Schorn B, Falk V, Dalichau H, Mohr FW: Kidney salvage in a case of ruptured renal artery aneurysm: Case report and literature review. Cardiovasc Surg 1345:134–136, 1997.

102. Cohen JR, Shamash FS: Ruptured renal artery aneurysms during pregnancy. J Vasc Surg 6:51–59, 1987.

103. Cohen SG, Cashdan A, Burger R: Spontaneous rupture of a renal artery aneurysm during pregnancy. Obstet Gynecol 39:897–902, 1972.

104. Dayton B, Helgerson RB, Sollinger HW Acher CW: Ruptured renal artery aneurysm in a pregnant uninephric patient: Successful ex vivo repair and autotransplantation. Surgery 107:708–711, 1990.

105. Lacroix H, Bernaerts P, Nevelsteen A, Hassens M: Ruptured renal artery aneurysm during pregnancy: Successful ex situ repair and autotransplantation. J Vasc Surg 33:188–190, 2001.

106. Schoon IM, Seeman T, Niemand D, et al: Rupture of renal arterial aneurysm in pregnancy. Acta Chir Scand 154:593–597, 1988.

107. Cummings KB, Lecky JW, Kaufman JJ: Renal artery aneurysms and hypertension. J Urol 109:144–148, 1973.

108. Ruberti U, Miani S, Scorza R, et al: Aneurysms of the renal artery. Int Angiol 6:407–414, 1987.

109. Soussou ID, Starr DS, Lawrie GM, Morris GM Jr: Renal artery aneurysm: Long-term relief of renovascular hypertension by in situ operative correction. Arch Surg 114:1410–1415, 1979.

110. Mercier C, Piquet P, Piligian F, Ferdani M: Aneurysms of the renal artery and its branches. Ann Vasc Surg 1:321–327, 1986.

111. Bugge-Asperheim B, Sdal G, Flatmark A: Renal artery aneurysm. Ex vivo repair and autotransplantation. Scand J Urol Nephrol 18:63–66, 1984.

112. Dubernard JM, Martin X, Gelet A, Mongin D: Aneurysms of the renal artery: Surgical management with special reference to extracorporeal surgery and autotransplantation. Eur Urol 11:26–30, 1985.

113. Centenera LV, Hirsch JA, Choi IS, et al: Wide-necked saccular renal artery aneurysm: Endovascular embolization with the Guglielmi detachable coil and temporary balloon occlusion of the aneurysm neck. J Vasc Interv Radiol 9:513–516, 1998.

114. Gewertz BL, Stanley JC, Fry WJ: Renal artery dissections. Arch Surg 112:409–414, 1977.

115. Reilly LM, Cunningham CG, Maggisano R, et al: The role of arterial reconstruction in spontaneous renal artery dissection. J Vasc Surg 14:468–479, 1991.

116. Edwards BS, Stanson AW, Holley KE, Sheps SG: Isolated renal artery dissection: Presentation, evaluation, management and pathology. Mayo Clin Proc 57:564–571, 1982.

117. Mali WP, Geyskes GG, Thalman R: Dissecting renal artery aneurysm: Treatment with an endovascular stent. AJR Am J Roentgenol 153:623–614, 1989.

Questions

1. Which of the following represents the reported ranking of splanchnic artery aneurysms in order of decreasing frequency?
   (a) splenic, hepatic, superior mesenteric (artery) (SMA), celiac
   (b) hepatic, splenic, celiac, SMA
   (c) intestinal, celiac, hepatic, splenic
   (d) splenic, hepatic, celiac, SMA

2. Splenic artery aneurysms
   (a) are more common in women than men
   (b) tend to be saccular and occur at vessel branchings
   (c) may exhibit a "double-rupture" phenomenon
   (d) all of the above

3. Hepatic artery aneurysms
   (a) account for 20% of reported splanchnic artery aneurysms
   (b) often appear with obstructive jaundice
   (c) have ruptured in 20% of reported cases with approximately a 50% mortality accompanying rupture
   (d) are twice as likely to rupture into the biliary tract as the peritoneal cavity

4. Aneurysms of the SMA
   (a) are the fifth most common splanchnic artery aneurysm, accounting for 2.5% of all such aneurysms
   (b) are commonly mycotic in origin
   (c) affect men twice as often as women
   (d) have ruptured in 12% of reported cases

5. Celiac artery aneurysms
   (a) are best treated by simple ligation with or without aneurysmectomy
   (b) are rarely diagnosed before rupture in contemporary times
   (c) are associated with a 50% mortality when they do rupture
   (d) are more likely to affect women than men

6. Jejunal, ileal, and colic artery aneurysms
   (a) are most commonly due to atherosclerosis
   (b) occur most commonly in women
   (c) when multiple tend to be associated with subacute bacterial endocarditis or periarteritis nodosa
   (d) carry a risk of rupture of 30%

7. Renal artery aneurysms
   (a) are demonstrated in 0.1% of patients undergoing angiography for nonrenal indications
   (b) tend to be fusiform and occur at branchings of the main renal artery
   (c) are usually caused by atherosclerosis
   (d) cause hypertension in approximately 15% of cases

8. Ruptured renal artery aneurysms
   (a) usually appear with hematuria
   (b) carry a mortality approaching 10%
   (c) are most commonly treated by arterial reconstruction
   (d) are more likely to occur with noncalcified than calcified lesions

9. Renal artery aneurysms may be associated with hypertension due to
   (a) depulsatile blood flow beyond the aneurysm
   (b) common compression of adjacent veins
   (c) intrinsic stenotic disease adjacent to the aneurysm
   (d) contralateral release of renal renin

10. Spontaneous dissections of the renal artery
    (a) are a rare form of arterial dissection
    (b) occur most often in women
    (c) are bilateral in a third of cases
    (d) rarely require surgical therapy

Answers

1. d   2. d   3. a   4. b   5. c   6. c   7. a   8. b   9. c   10. c

27

Aortoiliac Occlusive Disease

Michael Belkin, Anthony D. Whittemore, Magruder C. Donaldson, and John A. Mannick

Arteriosclerotic occlusive disease of the abdominal aorta and iliac arteries is a common cause of ischemic symptoms in the lower extremities of middle-aged and elderly patients in the Western world. Although not as common as occlusive disease of the femoropopliteal arterial system, with which it may be combined, aortoiliac occlusive disease may be more disabling because of the greater number of muscle groups subjected to diminished perfusion. The initial manifestation of occlusive disease of the distal aorta or iliac arteries is intermittent claudication with symptoms involving muscles of the thigh, hip, and buttock, as well as the calf. Because the calf muscles are usually the only muscle groups affected by intermittent claudication caused by superficial femoral artery occlusion, the involvement of more proximal muscles in the symptom complex may help to distinguish aortoiliac occlusive disease from femoropopliteal occlusive disease. Unfortunately, a sizable minority of patients with aortoiliac disease complain only of calf claudication. In addition to claudication, male patients with aortoiliac occlusive disease may complain of difficulty in achieving and maintaining an erection because of inadequate perfusion of the internal pudendal arteries. The Leriche syndrome consists of the manifestations of aortoiliac occlusive disease in the male and includes claudication of the muscles of the thigh, hip, and buttocks; atrophy of the leg muscles; impotence; and diminished femoral pulses.[1]

Aortoiliac occlusive disease per se is rarely the cause of ischemia at rest or ischemic tissue loss, except by embolization. The collateral circulation that develops around the occlusive process in the aorta and iliac arteries is usually rich and sufficient to supply the lower extremities with adequate quantities of arterial blood to ensure good resting tissue perfusion. However, arteriosclerotic plaques in the aorta and iliac arteries may cause the so-called blue toe syndrome (i.e., microembolization of arteriosclerotic debris to the terminal vessels in the foot).[2-5] Such symptoms may occur in a patient who otherwise appears to have adequate distal arterial supply, including, in some instances, palpable pedal pulses. Under these circumstances, a search must be made by angiography for a proximal source of microembolization.

When aortoiliac occlusive disease is combined with femoropopliteal occlusive disease, a finding more common in elderly patients, resting ischemia may result.[6] As in any arterial system, tandem lesions in the arteries supplying the extremities are more significant than single lesions.

The risk factors for aortoiliac occlusive disease are those for atherosclerosis in general and include cigarette smoking, hypertension, elevated serum cholesterol, and diabetes.[7-18] In our experience, patients reporting symptoms of claudication caused by aortoiliac occlusive disease are on average nearly a decade younger than those complaining of claudication on the basis of superficial femoral artery occlusion. However, patients with ischemia at rest from the combination of aortoiliac and femoropopliteal occlusive disease are in general in the seventh decade of life and are not notably younger than those who develop ischemic rest pain from femoropopliteal disease.

The initial lesions of aortoiliac occlusive disease in most patients appear to begin at the terminal aorta and the proximal portions of the common iliac arteries or at the bifurcations of the common iliacs (Fig. 27–1). The lesions then progress proximally and distally. Approximately one third of the patients we have operated on for symptomatic aortoiliac disease have had disease at the origin of the profunda femoris arteries in the groin and more than 40% have had superficial femoral artery occlusions. The natural history of aortoiliac occlusive disease is one of slow progression.[19, 20] The ultimate anatomic result of progressive aortoiliac atherosclerosis is variable but may progress to occlusion of the distal abdominal aorta with progression of the thrombus up to the level of the renal arteries (Fig. 27–2). Although occlusion of the terminal aorta, once it occurs, may remain stable for years, it does not always have a benign course, as indicated in the report by Starrett and Stoney.[21] They observed that more than one third of a series of patients with aortic occlusion went on to show thrombosis of the renal arteries over a period of 5 to 10 years (Fig. 27–3). However, Reilly and colleagues[22] later suggested that the renal arteries remain patent; no instances of thrombosis occurred in 21 patients followed up with arteriography after a mean of 27.7 months.

Variants in the pattern of aortoiliac occlusive disease

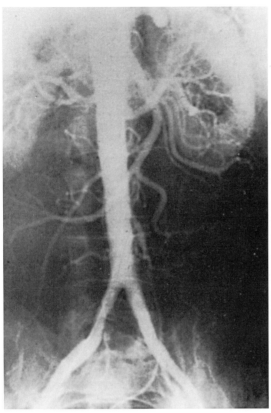

Figure 27–1. The earliest manifestations of aortoiliac occlusive disease are evident in the terminal aorta and proximal common iliac vessels.

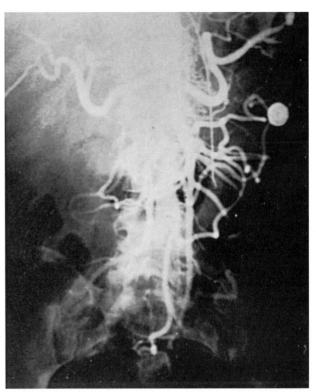

Figure 27–3. The end result of aortoiliac occlusive disease consists of total aortic thrombosis, which may include the origins of the renal arteries.

Figure 27–2. Aortoiliac occlusive disease results in a variable degree of collateral-ization shown as a discrete channel from a lumbar to the deep iliac circumflex ar-tery (A) and as a multiplicity of small vessels that supply the hemorrhoidal and gluteal arteries that reconstitute the fem-oral vessels via iliac and femoral circum-flex arteries (B).

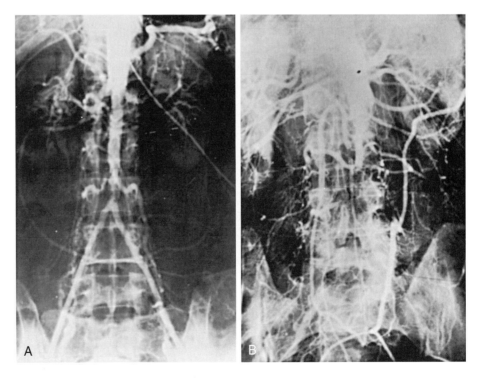

occur, including relatively circumscribed occlusive lesions of the midabdominal aorta described in early middle-aged women who are heavy cigarette smokers (Fig. 27–4). Although the upper abdominal aorta is ordinarily spared in patients with aortoiliac occlusive disease, a minority of such patients have marked involvement of this aortic segment, with occlusive disease of the origins of the major visceral vessels and renal arteries (Fig. 27–5).

DIAGNOSIS

The diagnosis of aortoiliac occlusive disease is ordinarily easily made on the basis of the patient's symptoms. Complaints of high claudication, with or without accompanying sexual dysfunction in the male, certainly suggest this disease process. Claudication symptoms, however, must be distinguished from symptoms of nerve root irritation caused by spinal stenosis or intervertebral disk herniation, which may be associated with activity and relieved by sitting or lying down in some individuals.[23] These patients can ordinarily be distinguished quite easily from patients with true claudication by the fact that their symptoms are produced as much by standing still as by walking, and by the typical sciatic distribution of the pain.

The patient with intermittent claudication on the basis of aortoiliac disease ordinarily has lower extremities that appear healthy and well perfused at rest, although the muscles may be somewhat atrophic from disuse. Dimin-

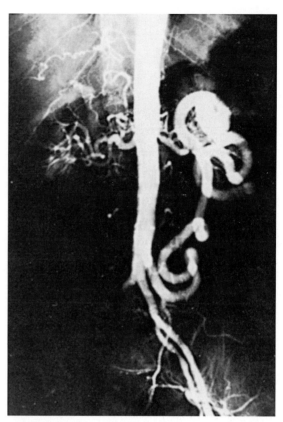

Figure 27–5. A large meandering mesenteric artery associated with total superior mesenteric artery celiac occlusion, renal artery stenosis, complete occlusion of the right common iliac, and distal left external iliac stenoses with a single patent hypogastric. End-to-side proximal anastomosis may best preserve both mesenteric and pelvic circulation.

ished or even absent femoral pulses are often a principal clue to the level of the occlusive process. Bruits heard in the groins can also call attention to proximal occlusive lesions. However, stenotic lesions at the origins of the superficial femoral or profunda femoris arteries can also cause femoral bruits. Easily palpable pedal pulses at rest may be found in patients with severe claudication from aortoiliac occlusive disease, even when the femoral pulses are barely discernible. This reflects the rich collateral circulation that is ordinarily present in such patients.

Segmental Doppler pressures at all levels in the lower extremity are ordinarily lower than the brachial pressure. If no accompanying superficial femoral occlusive disease exists, no impressive gradient occurs between the high thigh pressure and the ankle pressures; however, disabling symptoms may occur in patients with aortoiliac disease who have resting ankle pressures in the near-normal range and a normal ankle-brachial pressure index. Thus, in evaluating these patients, repeating the pressure measurements after a period of graded exercise is often wise.[24] A marked fall in ankle pressure immediately after exercise occurs if the patient's symptoms are on the basis of significant aortoiliac occlusive disease. More sophisticated Doppler waveform analysis or the use of a pulse volume recorder may reveal patterns suggestive of proximal occlusive lesions.[25–27] We have, however, found resting and postexercise Doppler pressure measurements satisfactory for the evaluation of the vast majority of patients.

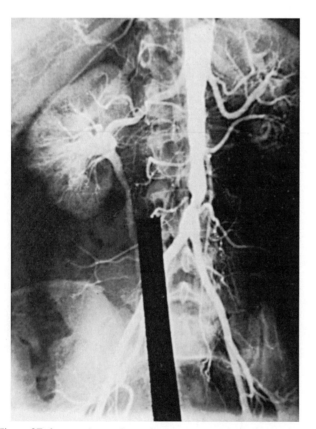

Figure 27–4. Aortoiliac occlusive disease may consist of a short segment circumferential lesion, especially common in younger females. Such a lesion may be amenable to localized endarterectomy.

The indications for surgery in symptomatic aortoiliac occlusive disease are disabling claudication and ischemia at rest manifested by rest pain in the foot, ischemic ulceration, or pregangrenous skin changes. Patients with aortoiliac disease and ischemia at rest ordinarily have accompanying femoropopliteal disease unless the ischemic lesions are the result of microemboli, as noted earlier.

PREOPERATIVE EVALUATION

Preoperative evaluation of the patient with aortoiliac occlusive disease includes a careful evaluation of any accompanying cardiac and pulmonary disease. In our experience, approximately 40% of patients with symptomatic aortoiliac occlusive disease have clear-cut clinical and electrocardiographic evidence of coronary artery disease. Symptomatic unstable coronary artery disease in such individuals clearly demands investigation, including cardiac catheterization and coronary angiography in many cases. If coronary artery reconstruction is indicated, this procedure should clearly be done first and the aortoiliac occlusive disease repaired as a second procedure. Patients with mild or stable coronary artery disease can ordinarily undergo aortoiliac reconstruction without great risk. Elderly patients with severe cardiopulmonary disease, who are not good candidates for coronary artery reconstruction, are probably best managed by extra-anatomic bypass procedures of lesser magnitude than formal aortoiliac or aortofemoral reconstruction. Patients with severe restrictive pulmonary disease may require a period of preoperative preparation, which includes bronchodilators, broad-spectrum antibiotics, and abstinence from cigarette smoking.

Angiography, an essential part of preoperative evaluation in the patient with symptomatic aortoiliac disease, can, in a surprising number of instances, be performed by the retrograde Seldinger technique using the femoral approach.[28] When this is not possible, studies by the translumbar or transaxillary route are performed.[29, 30] The goal of the radiographic examination is to provide views of the entire abdominal aorta in two planes to demonstrate unexpected lesions of the celiac axis or superior mesenteric artery origins, to provide anteroposterior and oblique views of the pelvis to define any iliac artery lesions in more than one plane, and to demonstrate possible lesions at the origins of the profunda femoris arteries. Views should also be obtained of the vessels in the thighs, at the knees, and in the calves to demonstrate associated femoropopliteal occlusive disease and the quality of the runoff. At the time of angiography, obtaining pull-back pressures across iliac artery lesions of doubtful significance is very useful, because this technique can demonstrate directly whether such lesions are likely to interfere with flow. Measurements should be taken at rest and after papaverine injection or during a period of reactive hyperemia after tourniquet ischemia to mimic the hemodynamic situation that occurs during exercise.[31] Intraarterial digital subtraction angiography has become quite useful for evaluation of the aortoiliac arterial segment. This technique has the advantage of the use of very small amounts of contrast medium and good resolution of the vessels studied.

Increasing experience with magnetic resonance arteriography has documented a high degree of accuracy for the evaluation of infrainguinal arterial occlusive disease.[32] Nonetheless, accurate diagnosis of aortoiliac disease has often proved problematic with current technology.[33]

AORTOFEMORAL BYPASS GRAFT

History

During the past 15 years, the aortofemoral bypass graft has become the preferred method of treatment of symptomatic aortoiliac occlusive disease and has, to a considerable degree, supplanted a more limited aortoiliac bypass in the hands of most surgeons. The 5% to 8%, 30-day operative mortality rate for this procedure prevalent in the early 1970s has been reduced in our own experience to less than 2% over the past 15 years, a level consistent with reports from other surgeons and similar to that observed in patients undergoing elective abdominal aortic aneurysm repair.[34–40] Arterial insufficiency of the lower extremities is a manifestation of a systemic process that results in clinically evident coronary artery disease in approximately 50% of these patients.[41–43] Reduced operative mortality has been observed and is associated with a concomitant reduction in the number of early cardiac deaths. The improved perioperative management of the patient with a diseased heart has resulted from a number of factors, which include selective employment of preliminary cardiac surgery for certain individuals, sophisticated pharmacologic management of the damaged myocardium, and more precise perioperative fluid management tailored to the individual patient's myocardial reserve.[40]

Initial aortobifemoral graft limb patency rates now approach 100%, and the 5-year patency is greater than 80% in a number of recent reports.[34, 35, 37, 44, 45] Long-term patency has also improved to an anticipated 75% at 10 years.[34] A number of refinements of operative technique may be responsible for the low incidence of graft limb thrombosis in recent years. The more prevalent use of the aortobifemoral graft as opposed to an aortoiliac bypass or extended aortoiliofemoral endarterectomy has negated the effect of unsuspected or progressive atherosclerosis in the external iliac vessels. Meticulous avoidance of graft limb redundancy and an awareness of the desirability of compatibility of the diameter of the graft limb and the vessel into which it is implanted have also probably helped to maintain long-term patency.

Surgical Procedures

The knitted Dacron prosthesis is the standard graft material used by most surgeons with experience in aortoiliac reconstruction. This material, with or without a velour construction, may provide a more stable pseudointima than woven prostheses.[46, 47] An important factor contributing to improved results has undoubtedly been the recognition of the critical role played by the deep femoral artery in providing sustained patency of the aortofemoral graft limb.[34, 37, 48, 49] The current practice of extending the distal anastomosis down over the origin of the profunda femoris to ensure an adequate outflow tract has been widely accepted and is undoubtedly important in patients with tandem superficial femoral occlusions and in patients with stenosis of the profunda origin. We have found, however, that if extensive profundaplasty or profunda endarterectomy is necessary, this vessel is better closed with an autogenous tissue patch of saphenous vein or endarterectomized superficial femoral artery than if the surgeon attempted to make a long profunda femoris patch with the distal end of an aortofemoral prosthesis.[48]

The incidence of graft infection has been minimized with preoperative and intraoperative antibiotics.[34, 50–52] Aortoenteric fistulas can be prevented by closure of retroperitoneal tissue and the posterior parietal peritoneum over the graft and proximal suture line to prevent erosion of the graft into the duodenum.[34, 53, 54] The abandonment of the use of silk sutures in favor of permanent prosthetic suture material has undoubtedly helped to reduce the incidence of false aneurysm formation.

A good deal of controversy remains as to the proper method of performing the proximal anastomosis of an aortobifemoral graft.[34, 55, 56] Most surgeons probably favor the end-to-end technique of proximal anastomosis with transection of the aorta between clamps about 1 to 2 inches below the renal arteries and oversewing or stapling the distal end (Fig. 27–6). This permits an endarterectomy or

thrombectomy of the proximal aortic stump under direct vision prior to constructing the anastomosis. It also has the advantage of not requiring flow to be reestablished in the more distal aorta, where arteriosclerotic plaque and mural thrombus may have been loosened by application of the distal clamp. This may have advantages in avoiding intraoperative emboli to the lower extremities.

The end-to-end technique has also been claimed by some authors to reduce the incidence of aortoduodenal fistulas because the end-to-end anastomosis does not project anteriorly as does an end-to-side aortofemoral reconstruction. Unfortunately, such controlled studies as are available do not indicate that the end-to-end technique gives results significantly superior to the end-to-side techniques. Therefore, we have taken the position that the end-to-end technique is probably more appropriate for those patients who will not suffer any hemodynamic disadvantage from interruption of forward flow in the abdominal aorta. This technique also appears desirable for those patients who have already suffered complete aortic occlusion. The end-to-side technique (Fig. 27–7) is reserved for those individuals who would lose perfusion of an important hypogastric or inferior mesenteric artery if forward flow in the aorta were sacrificed at the time of surgery.[55] Arteriographic studies in patients with indications for an end-to-side anastomosis are shown in Figures 27–5 and 27–8.

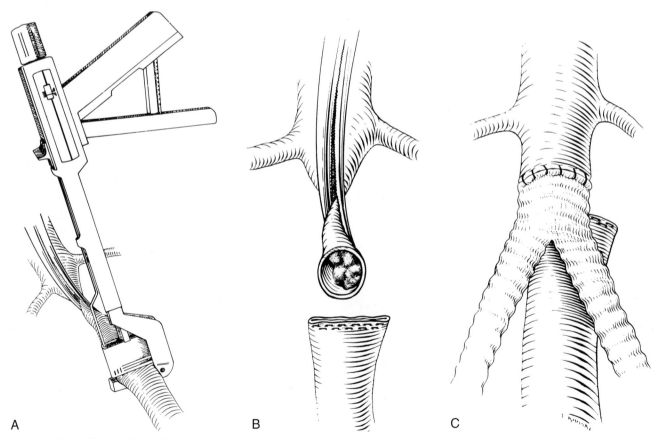

A   B   C

Figure 27–6. End-to-end proximal anastomosis for aortofemoral reconstruction may be initiated with the infrarenal aortic cross clamp placed in anterior/posterior direction with minimal dissection as close to the origin of the renal arteries as possible. The aorta is then stapled or occluded with a second clamp just proximal to the origin of the inferior mesenteric artery, as illustrated (*A*). After transection of the infrarenal aorta and complete thromboendarterectomy of the proximal infrarenal aortic cuff (*B*), end-to-end anastomosis is completed with continuous 3-0 polypropylene suture (*C*).

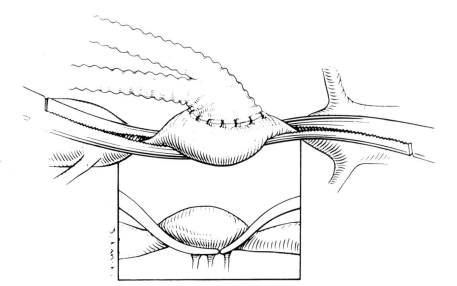

Figure 27–7. End-to-side proximal anastomosis for aortofemoral reconstruction is required to preserve antegrade pelvic perfusion in situations where retrograde perfusion from distal femoral anastomoses is doubtful. The infrarenal aorta is occluded proximal to the origin of the inferior mesenteric artery and just distal to the origin of the renal arteries. After longitudinal arteriotomy and thorough thromboendarterectomy, if required, the anastomosis is constructed using continuous polypropylene suture.

Although aortofemoral reconstruction has the potential of restoring potency to males with sexual dysfunction on the basis of inadequate hypogastric artery perfusion,[55, 56] surgical dissection in the area of the terminal aorta and proximal left common iliac artery can also cause difficulty with both erection and ejaculation by interfering with the autonomic nervous plexus, which sweeps over these vessels. In performing aortofemoral bypass grafting, therefore, we have chosen to confine the dissection of the aorta to the area between the renal arteries and the inferior mesenteric artery. The aorta is exposed anteriorly and laterally, without

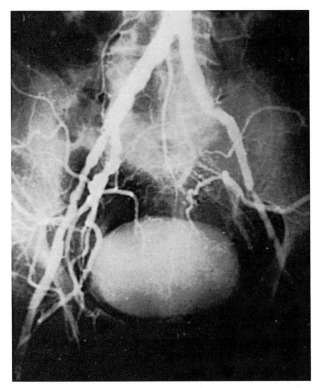

Figure 27–8. Diffuse aortoiliac disease with left hypogastric occlusion and minimal left pelvic collateralization may warrant end-to-side proximal anastomosis to preserve right hypogastric system.

distorting the vessel, to avoid embolization of arteriosclerotic debris. After systemic heparinization, the distal clamp is placed proximal to the inferior mesenteric artery and then the aorta is cross-clamped below the renal arteries where the aortic wall is likely to be considerably less diseased. The aorta is divided transversely and the distal end beveled and oversewn.

In the case of an end-to-side anastomosis, the longitudinal aortotomy is placed high up near the renals in the more normal aorta, and great care is taken to remove all loose debris and mural thrombus from the lumen in the excluded aortic segment. At completion of an end-to-side anastomosis, great care is also given to adequate back-flushing of all loosened debris and clot from the distal aorta before forward flow is reestablished. In performing either type of proximal anastomosis, a short stem of a graft is sutured to the aorta with a running suture of 3-0 polypropylene. Knitted Dacron prostheses are invariably used and the size is selected so that the limb diameter corresponds to the diameter of the patient's common femoral arteries. The average prosthesis size used for males is 14 × 7 mm or, in larger individuals, 16 × 8 mm. For females, the most commonly used sizes are 12 × 6 mm and 13 × 6.5 mm. After completion of the proximal anastomosis, the limbs are tunneled retroperitoneally into the groins. On the left, the tunnel ordinarily passes beneath the sigmoid mesentery and into the groin in a rather lateral channel that avoids trauma to the nerve plexuses at the terminal aorta. On the right, the tunnel is made along the course of the right common iliac artery beneath the ureter. In the groins, end-to-side anastomoses are fashioned in the distal common femoral with 5-0 polypropylene. The anastomoses are carried down into the profunda femoris arteries for a short distance if any evidence exists of incipient stenosis of the origins of these vessels or if the superficial femorals are occluded. The end of the graft thus acts as a patch, widening the orifice of the profunda femoris.

Despite significant advances in laparoscopic general surgery, applications of this new technique to vascular surgery have been few. However, several authors have applied laparoscopic techniques to aortofemoral reconstruction.

Whether performed completely via the laparoscopic approach or through limited incisions with laparoscopic-assisted dissection, the procedure has proved time-consuming and technically challenging.[57, 58] As the technology evolves and intracorporeal anastamotic techniques are refined, however, the role of laparoscopic aortofemoral bypass will expand and become clearer.

Results

Although excellent results have been achieved with aortoiliac endarterectomy for occlusive disease, this operation, even in the hands of enthusiasts, is now confined to those individuals whose disease ends distally near the bifurcation of the common iliac arteries[34] (Fig. 27–9; also see Fig. 27–4). Endarterectomy of the external iliac is tedious and unrewarding for most surgeons. At present, little evidence suggests that endarterectomy is superior to a properly performed aortofemoral bypass graft in terms of the early or late results. In our practice, aortoiliac endarterectomy is confined to a minority of individuals who appear to have principally aortic disease with little involvement of the iliac arteries. This group of patients is characteristically early middle-aged women with occlusive disease of the midabdominal aorta, which ends at the aortic bifurcation or in the proximal portions of the common iliac arteries. We have avoided aortoiliac endarterectomy in males because of concern over interference with the autonomic nerves at the terminal aorta and proximal left common iliac artery.

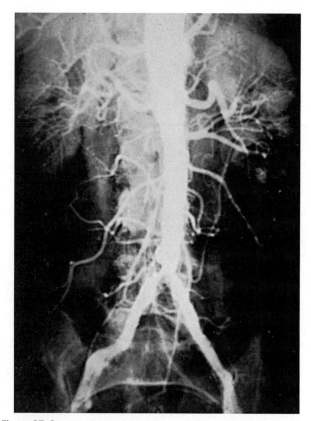

Figure 27–9. Aortoiliac occlusive disease with significant lesion confined to the origin of the right common iliac artery, amenable to either local endarterectomy or percutaneous transluminal angioplasty.

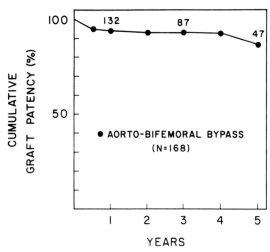

Figure 27–10. For 168 aortobifemoral graft limbs inserted in 84 consecutive patients, the 5-year cumulative patency was 86%.

Our results with aortofemoral bypass grafting are illustrated in Figure 27–10. The 5-year cumulative patency of 86% is comparable with that reported in a number of other studies.[34, 35, 37, 44] Thirty-day operative mortality was slightly less than 1%. This low mortality rate undoubtedly reflects careful patient selection as well as improved operative management and anesthetic technique. However, because aortoiliac occlusive disease is rarely life-threatening, (although it may be limb-threatening), we prefer to treat high-risk patients with procedures of lesser magnitude.

Although most authors have reported excellent patency rates after aortofemoral bypass, several subgroups with inferior results have been identified. Younger patients and those with small aortas have proved more vulnerable to late graft failure. A study of aortofemoral reconstructions in 73 patients younger than 50 years of age[56] documented a 50% primary patency rate 5 years after bypass. In that study, patients with aortas less than 1.8 cm wide had significantly lower patency rates (6-year patency of 20%) than did those with aortas greater than 1.8 cm (6-year patency of 60%).

Although the excellent graft patency rates for aortofemoral bypass grafts do not necessarily reflect functional results, approximately 95% of patients are initially rendered asymptomatic or improved, and after 5 years about 80% remain in this category.[37, 44] A study from the United Kingdom[59] indicated that of patients fully employed before aortobifemoral bypass, 85% returned to full employment an average of 4 months after surgery, and more than 50% of those not previously employed returned to work after bypass. Other studies have documented a more sobering functional outcome after successful aortofemoral arterial reconstruction. One study,[60] employing the SF-20 questionnaire, found that, after aortobifemoral bypass, patients had decrements in physical and role function and general health perception similar to those of patients with congestive heart failure or recent myocardial infarction. Clearly, more functional outcome analysis is necessary after treatment of aortoiliac occlusive disease.

The 5-year cumulative survival rate for patients undergoing aortofemoral bypass grafting remains some 14%

lower than that anticipated for a normal age-corrected population. However, nearly 80% survive 5 years, whereas less than 50% survive 10 years.[42]

Concomitant Distal Reconstructions

When patients have threatened limb loss from a combination of aortoiliac and femoropopliteal occlusive disease, repair of the proximal or inflow lesions is necessary to permit salvage of the extremity. However, whether concomitant distal reconstructions, such as a femoropopliteal bypass, should be performed at the time of the initial operation is not always clear. Results reported in the literature and our own experience suggest that in the majority of patients with ischemia at rest, on the basis of combined aortoiliac and femoropopliteal disease, repair of the aortoiliac occlusive disease and restoration of normal perfusion to the profunda femoris arteries achieves limb salvage in the vast majority (probably 80%) of patients.[49, 61] However, in those patients, particularly individuals with diabetes, who have extensive tissue necrosis of the skin of the forefoot or heel, restoration of pulsatile flow in the foot may be necessary to achieve healing. Under these circumstances, we believe that a combination of both proximal and distal reconstructive procedures may be necessary at the initial operation. The combined procedure has the disadvantage of increasing the operating time and surgical trauma in a group of patients who are likely to be elderly with a high incidence of coronary artery disease; however, with modern anesthetic management and a two-team operative approach, this combined reconstruction can be performed safely and within a reasonable period of time.

ALTERNATIVES FOR THE HIGH-RISK PATIENT

Although transabdominal arterial reconstruction for aortoiliac occlusive disease can be performed successfully with low morbidity and mortality in many patients, less extensive procedures may be preferable in patients who are high risks for major surgery under general anesthesia. In such patients, distal aortic and proximal iliac arterial occlusions may be treated by axillofemoral bypass grafts, which are discussed subsequently.[62–66] If the occlusive disease is limited to one common, or external, iliac artery, alternatives to axillofemoral bypass are warranted in poor-risk individuals because use of the patent iliac system as an origin for a bypass permits a shorter graft segment and affords better long-term patency. The femorofemoral bypass is an example of such a procedure.[67] However, an anatomically similar procedure, the iliofemoral graft, has received little attention in the literature.

Ilioiliac and Iliofemoral Bypass Grafts

We have reviewed our experience with 94 patients undergoing ilioiliac or iliofemoral bypass grafting from 1982 to 1992. Poor-risk patients, particularly those with severe cardiopulmonary impairment, who had no important occlusive disease in the aorta or in the proximal segment of at least one common iliac artery, were considered for reconstruction using a patent common or external iliac artery for the proximal anastomosis (ses Fig. 27–5). The iliac site for anastomosis has several technical advantages, including exposure through an oblique suprainguinal, "renal transplant" incision, which is quite simple technically, even in obese patients. The graft is more deeply placed and therefore more cushioned than in the femorofemoral position. Ilioilial grafts are shorter than femorofemoral grafts, and no disturbance of inguinal lymph nodes or lymphatics occurs. The femoral artery on the donor side is left undisturbed for later use as the origin for a distal bypass, if indicated.

The mean age of the 94 patients undergoing ilioiliac or iliofemoral bypass was 60 years, and 26% had diabetes mellitus. Forty-one percent had clear-cut clinical and electrocardiographic evidence of coronary artery disease, and 43% had significant hypertension. Fifty-eight percent of the patients were operated on for claudication and 42% for limb salvage. Twenty-three patients had ilioilial grafts and 71 patients had iliofemoral grafts. Fifty-seven iliounifemoral grafts and 14 iliobifemoral grafts were performed.

In patients subjected to iliac arterial reconstruction, the patent iliac arterial segment was exposed extraperitoneally through a curvilinear incision parallel to and above the inguinal ligament, identical to the approach for renal transplantation. Limited iliac endarterectomy was necessary in a few instances. Separate vertical groin incisions were made to expose the common femoral arteries. For ilioiliac bypass, symmetrical incisions were made to expose the iliac vessels and the graft was positioned in the retroperitoneum (Fig. 27–11A). The grafts to the femoral arteries were placed under the inguinal ligament (see Fig. 27–11B and C). For patients undergoing bilateral iliofemoral reconstruction, the crossover limb was placed from the iliofemoral graft retroperitoneally in the iliac fossa or, in a few cases, subcutaneously to the contralateral femoral artery (see Fig. 27–11C).

The 30-day operative mortality for these procedures was zero. The 4-year cumulative patency for the ilioiliac grafts (23 limbs) was 96%; that for the iliofemoral grafts (91 limbs) was 72%. The 4-year patency for iliobifemoral grafts (28 limbs) was 72%, and for iliounifemoral grafts (63 limbs), 71% (Fig. 27–12). When both the superficial and deep femoral arteries were patent, the cumulative patency rate for iliofemoral grafts was higher (85%) at 4 years than when only the deep femoral artery was patent (62%). Demonstration of a statistically significant difference in late patency between aortofemoral grafts and iliofemoral grafts was not possible, although the aortofemoral grafts had numerically superior 4- and 5-year patencies. We thus believe that the iliofemoral bypass is an adequate substitute for aortofemoral bypass in certain elderly and poor-risk individuals who have their proximal occlusive disease confined largely to the external iliac arteries or to one iliac system.

Femorofemoral Bypass Graft

In patients whose occlusive disease is confined to one iliac artery and whose aorta and contralateral iliac system are

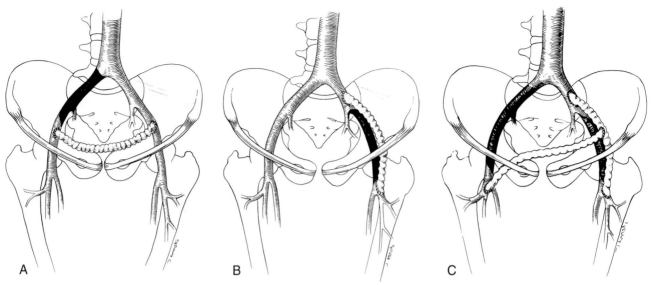

Figure 27–11. A patent common or external iliac artery may be used as a donor vessel for (A) ilioiliac, (B) iliofemoral, or (C) iliobifemoral bypasses in appropriate patients who would otherwise require axillofemoral reconstruction.

free of hemodynamically significant lesions, the femoro-femoral bypass is often employed. Brief and coworkers,[68] Plecha and Pories,[69] Vetto,[67] and our own group[65] have demonstrated that these operations yield quite satisfactory long-term results (60% to more than 80% 5-year patency). Failure of these grafts because of progressive worsening of proximal atherosclerosis has been uncommon. Such worsening may be retarded by increased flow through the donor iliac system, which is required to supply both the lower extremities with blood. Berguer and coworkers[70] have reported experimental support for this hypothesis by demonstrating in animals that intimal hyperplasia correlates inversely with blood flow and shear stress. However, experimental results yielding the opposite conclusion have also been reported.[71]

The femorofemoral graft is particularly applicable to high-risk patients because it can be performed easily under epidural or spinal anesthesia. The two common femoral arteries are exposed through short vertical groin incisions. The groin incisions are connected by a subcutaneous suprapubic tunnel created by blunt dissection on the deep fascia. We prefer to have the graft form a **C** configuration, with the anastomoses placed in the distal common femoral arteries and the graft traveling proximally up through the suprapubic tunnel and down to the opposite common femoral (Fig. 27–13). Over the past 15 years, we have had experience with femorofemoral grafts in 53 patients. Sixty percent of these were operated on for limb salvage and 40% for disabling claudication. The average age of these patients was 61 years. Forty-one percent had clinical evidence of coronary artery disease, 33% were diabetic, and 44% had significant hypertension. One postoperative mortality occurred in this group of patients, from a pulmonary

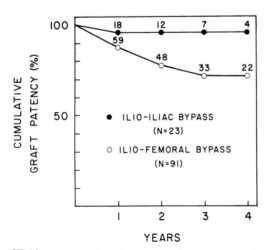

Figure 27–12. Using a patent iliac vessel as the donor artery, the 4-year cumulative graft patency for 23 ilioiliac grafts was 96%, whereas the patency for 91 iliofemoral graft limbs was 72%.

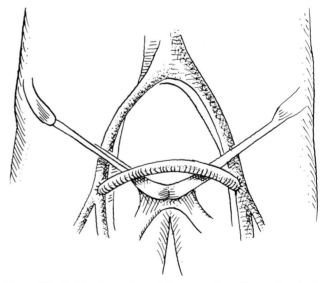

Figure 27–13. The femorofemoral bypass graft is illustrated with the preferred **C** configuration of the subcutaneous tunnel constructed well above the pubis.

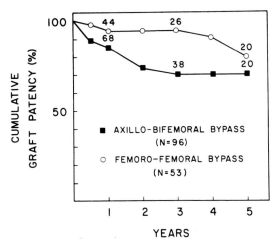

Figure 27–14. The 4-year cumulative graft patency for 53 femorofemoral grafts was 80%, and the patency for 48 axillobifemoral grafts (96 limbs) was 70%.

embolus. The 5-year cumulative graft patency was 80% (Fig. 27–14). The late patency rate is not statistically significantly different from that achieved with aortofemoral bypass in our hands, but it is slightly numerically inferior.

The reasonably good long-term results, the ease of performance, and the low morbidity associated with the femorofemoral bypass suggest that it might logically be employed in good-risk as well as poor-risk patients who have their proximal occlusive disease confined to one iliac arterial segment. Although arguing against this point of view is difficult, the fact that the groins have been operated on and the common femoral arteries dissected during the course of performing a femorofemoral graft makes an aortobifemoral reconstruction in such individuals technically more difficult if progression of proximal disease causes return of symptoms or late failure of the femorofemoral bypass. Therefore, in good-risk patients with evidence of arteriosclerotic disease in the aorta or in the patent iliac system, we recommend aortobifemoral bypass at the outset in an attempt to avoid the need for possible future reoperation.

Axillofemoral Bypass Graft

In very elderly and high-risk patients who are in danger of limb loss from a combination of aortoiliac and femoropopliteal occlusive diseases and whose proximal occlusive lesions involve the aorta and proximal iliac arteries, the axillofemoral bypass graft is the logical alternative to aortoiliac reconstruction or primary amputation. Extra-anatomic reconstruction may also prove useful for patients with multiple prior abdominal procedures, multiple adhesions, or previous pelvic irradiation. Intraabdominal sepsis, not infrequently resulting from an infected aortic graft, is another common indication. If an axillofemoral graft is chosen for such individuals, the axillobifemoral graft is preferred to the axillounifemoral graft because several reports, beginning with that of LoGerfo and colleagues,[64] show that the axillobifemoral graft has a decidedly better 5-year cumulative patency.[66] The probable reason for this finding is that

the axillobifemoral graft has approximately double the flow rate in its axillary limb as has the axillounifemoral graft.

In constructing an axillobifemoral graft, the first portion of the axillary artery is exposed by an incision placed beneath the clavicle on the side selected for the proximal anastomosis (Fig. 27–15). We ordinarily split the pectoralis major and divide the pectoralis minor muscle to provide better operative exposure and more space for the graft as it emerges from the axilla into the subcutaneous plane. The common femoral arteries are exposed through bilateral short groin incisions.

A DeBakey tunneling instrument can then be passed from the infraclavicular incision laterally to a subcutaneous plane in the midaxillary line. The curve in the tunneler is used to direct the tunnel anteriorly above the iliac crest and then in front of the inguinal ligament into the ipsilateral groin incision. A Dacron or polytetrafluoroethylene prosthesis, usually 8 mm in diameter, is attached to the tunneling instrument and is drawn back through the tunnel into the axillary incision for anastomosis with the first portion of the axillary artery. A side limb is attached to the graft in the ipsilateral groin incision just proximal to the anastomosis with the common femoral artery. The side limb is then passed through a subcutaneous suprapubic tunnel into the opposite groin in a manner similar to that used for a femorofemoral graft.

Because neither the thoracic nor the abdominal cavity is "entered" in performing an axillofemoral graft, this procedure usually does not interfere with the patient's ability to breathe, cough, or take oral feedings. On the first post-

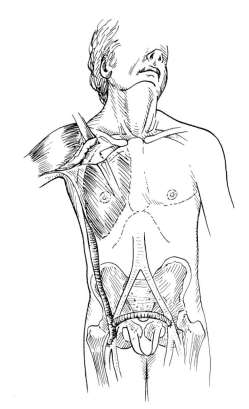

Figure 27–15. Subcutaneous axillobifemoral bypass graft completed with proximal anastomosis to the right axillary artery, right distal anastomosis to the common and deep femoral arteries, and extension of the prosthesis with side limb to left common femoral artery.

operative day, most patients are ambulatory and on a regular diet. From 1982 to 1992 we performed axillobifemoral grafts electively in 48 poor-risk patients for symptomatic aortoiliac occlusive disease. All but two of these patients were operated on for limb salvage from a combination of far-advanced aortoiliac and femoropopliteal disease. The 5-year cumulative graft patency in this group of patients was 70% (see Fig. 27–14). Although this figure is not completely discouraging, it is statistically significantly inferior to the results achieved with aortofemoral bypass grafting during the same time period. We therefore believe that axillofemoral grafts should be offered only to poor-risk individuals in danger of limb loss and should not be used for the treatment of symptoms of claudication alone.

When axillofemoral grafts do fail, they can frequently be reopened by thrombectomy under local anesthesia if the patient presents himself or herself promptly after graft thrombosis has occurred. About 25% of grafts thrombectomized in this fashion go on to long-term patency.[64] Thus, the functional good results achieved with axillobifemoral grafting may be somewhat higher than the 70% graft patency figure would indicate.

Patency rates associated with axillofemoral reconstruction range from a low of 30% to a high of 85%.[72, 73] The reasons for this extraordinary variability are in large part explained by patient selection, indication, and status of the outflow vessels. Extra-anatomic reconstruction for nonocclusive disease, as is the case for patients with intraabdominal sepsis or an infected aneurysm repair, achieves better patency rates than operation primarily for occlusive disease. Patients with claudication fare better than those requiring limb salvage because of inherent outflow restriction in the latter group. In similar fashion, patients who undergo simultaneous distal femoropopliteal reconstruction show better results than those whose infrainguinal disease is not addressed. Finally, in some series, axillobifemoral grafts sustain a significantly better 5-year patency than do unilateral reconstructions. Flow through the descending axillary limb in bilateral reconstructions is twice that of axillounilateral grafts, perhaps explaining the improvement in some series. Other investigators have found no significant difference whatsoever between bilateral and unilateral reconstructions, again, in all probability, reflecting patient selection and status of outflow.

Thus, the most favorable results achieved as reported by Harris and colleagues[73] in 1990 are an 85% patency rate after 4 years in a group of 76 patients, 26% of whom were operated on for nonocclusive disease, 20% of whom underwent simultaneous outflow reconstruction, and all of whom had axillobifemoral grafts. This series was also carried out in a single institution using a technique that has been standardized for many years. Similar excellent 5-year patency and limb salvage rates of 74% and 89%, respectively, were reported by Passman and colleagues.[74] These authors believe that more liberal application of the axillobifemoral bypass is warranted. In contrast, a less favorable patency rate (29%) was reported by Donaldson and colleagues[72] for 72 patients managed in several institutions by a group of 30 surgeons operating on patients with predominately occlusive disease. Finally, many authors have reported secondary patency rates, either exclusively or in addition to primary rates, which further confuses the statistics. These series show clearly that the secondary patency rate is significantly better than the primary, attesting to the fact that up to 25% of axillobifemoral grafts require subsequent thrombectomy to maintain patency.

Descending Thoracic Aorta-to-Femoral Artery Bypass

The descending thoracic aorta may be used as an inflow source for bypass to the femoral arteries.[75, 76] Although seldom indicated as a primary procedure, this bypass offers a durable alternative after aortic failure, aortic graft infection, or other problems that necessitate avoidance of the abdominal aorta. We generally expose the thoracic aorta through a sixth or seventh interspace incision. A 10-mm synthetic graft is tunneled through the diaphragm at the posterior pleural reflection and down through the retroperitoneal space to the left groin. We usually make a small lateral flank incision to facilitate safe tunneling through the retroperitoneum. The descending thoracic aorta is generally of good quality and is usually clampable with a partially occluding clamp. The procedure is completed with a femorofemoral bypass. Relatively few reports focusing on this procedure are available in the literature. McCarthy and colleagues[75] achieved a 100% 4-year patency rate with 21 thoracic aorta-to-femoral artery bypasses, whereas Criado and Keagy[76] reported an 83% 6- to 8-year secondary graft patency rate.

PERCUTANEOUS TRANSLUMINAL ANGIOPLASTY

Percutaneous catheter dilatation of atheromatous vascular stenoses was introduced by Dotter and Judkins in 1963.[77] However, this technique did not become widely applied until Gruntzig designed and developed the double-lumen balloon catheter for percutaneous transluminal angioplasty in the early 1970s. In the Gruntzig technique, the balloon catheter is inserted into a stenotic arterial region with the Seldinger technique and is expanded to a fixed diameter. In one of Gruntzig's original reports in 1977,[78] percutaneous dilatation was attempted in 41 patients with isolated iliac artery stenosis and proved to be initially successful in 90%.

Early success is not necessarily sustained, as evidenced by the lower 50% to 60% 5-year success rate reported by Johnston and coworkers[79] among 684 iliac angioplasties carried out in Toronto between 1978 and 1986. If initial technical failures are excluded, however, success rates improve by 10% to 15% as confirmed in a randomized prospective multicenter trial reported by Wilson and coworkers.[80] This study demonstrated that successful results were sustained for 3 years in 73% of dilated iliac lesions, not significantly different from the 82% success rate observed with conventional surgery. Success rates for percutaneous transluminal angioplasty are maximal when indicated for claudication resulting from common iliac stenosis with excellent runoff (75%) and minimal when carried out for critical ischemia caused by external iliac occlusion with poor runoff (19%).

This technique has been very useful in the initial management of patients with symptomatic short segmental iliac stenoses (see Fig. 27–9). High-risk patients with appropriate lesions can be palliated effectively without undergoing anesthesia and major surgery. Even in good-risk patients, percutaneous transluminal angioplasty has an advantage as initial therapy for symptomatic lesions in that it does not in any way jeopardize future surgical approach to the aorta or iliac arteries if the angioplasty ultimately fails.

The application of intraluminal stents has broadened the number of iliac lesions amenable to balloon angioplasty. Whether employed secondarily to correct a technically inadequate angioplasty (e.g., a dissection of residual stenosis) or primarily to open a long-segment occlusion, stents have increased the technical success rates of percutaneous angioplasty. A review of 230 iliac Palmaz stent placements in 184 patients followed up with angiography at 6 months confirmed an 86% 4-year primary patency rate.[86] Most restenotic lesions were successfully treated with follow-up angioplasty.

The cost-effectiveness of a successful procedure is unquestionable, because patients may be discharged from the hospital the day after dilatation. Effective use of transluminal angioplasty can be achieved only through a cooperative effort on the part of both angiographers and vascular surgeons. Such cooperation is important with regard to proper patient selection, appropriate combination or staging of procedures, and prompt treatment of complications.

References

1. Leriche R, Morel A: The syndrome of thrombotic obliteration of the aortic bifurcation. Ann Surg 127:193, 1948.
2. Crane C: Atherothrombotic embolism to lower extremities in arteriosclerosis. Arch Surg 94:96, 1967.
3. Karmody AM, Powers SR, Monaco VJ, et al: "Blue toe" syndrome. Arch Surg 111:1263, 1976.
4. Moldveen-Geronimus M, Merriam JC Jr: Cholesterol embolization: From pathological curiosity to clinical entity. Circulation 35:946, 1967.
5. Williams GM, Harrington D, Burdick J, White RI: Mural thrombus of the aorta. Am Surg 194:737, 1981.
6. Brewster DC, Perier BA, Robison JG, et al: Aortofemoral graft for multilevel occlusive disease: Predictors of success and need for distal bypass. Arch Surg 117:1593, 1982.
7. Ballantyne D, Lawrie TDV: Hyperlipoproteinemia and peripheral vascular disease. Clin Chim Acta 47:269, 1973.
8. Cox FC, Rifking B, Robinson J, et al: Primary hyperlipoproteinaemias in myocardial infarction. In Peeters H (ed): Protides of the Biological Fluids, vol 19. New York, American Elsevier, 1972, p 279.
9. Doyle JT, Dawber TR, Kannel WB, et al: The relationship of cigarette smoking to coronary heart disease: The second report of the combined experience of the Albany, N.Y., and Framingham, Mass., studies. JAMA 190:886, 1964.
10. Greenhalgh RM, Rosengarten DS, Mervant I, et al: Serum lipids and lipoproteins in peripheral vascular disease. Lancet 2:947, 1971.
11. Kannel WB, Castelli WP, Gordon T, et al: Serum cholesterol lipoproteins and the risk of coronary heart disease. Ann Intern Med 74:1, 1971.
12. Kannel WB, Dawber TR, Friedman GD, et al: Risk factors in coronary artery disease. Ann Intern Med 61:888, 1964.
13. Oberman A, Harlan WR, Smith M, et al: The cardiovascular risk: Associated with different levels and types of elevated blood pressure. Minn Med 52:1283, 1969.
14. Paterson D, Slack J: Lipid abnormalities in male and female survivors of myocardial infarction and their first degree relatives. Lancet 1:393, 1972.
15. Paul O: Physical inactivity: The associated cardiovascular risk. Minn Med 52:1327, 1969.
16. Sirtori CR, Biasi G, Vercellio G, et al: Diets, lipids and lipoproteins in patients with peripheral vascular disease. Am J Med Sci 268:325, 1974.
17. Strong JP, Eggen DA: Risk factors and atherosclerotic lesions. In Jones RJ (ed): Atherosclerosis: Proceedings of the Second International Symposium. New York, Springer-Verlag, 1970, pp 355–364.
18. Vogelberg KH, Berchtold P, Berger H, et al: Primary hyperlipoproteinemias as risk factors in peripheral artery disease documented by arteriography. Atherosclerosis 22:271, 1975.
19. Boyd AM: The natural course of arteriosclerosis of the lower extremities. Proc R Soc Med 55:591, 1962.
20. Imparato AM, Kim G, Davidson T, et al: Intermittent claudication: Its natural course. Surgery 78:795, 1975.
21. Starrett RW, Stoney RJ: Juxta-renal aortic occlusion. Surgery 76:890, 1974.
22. Reilly LM, Sauer L, Weinstein ES, et al: Infrarenal aortic occlusion: Does it threaten renal perfusion or function? J Vasc Surg 11:216–225, 1990.
23. Karayannacos PE, Yashon D, Vasko JS: Narrow lumbar spinal canal with "vascular" syndromes. Arch Surg 111:803, 1976.
24. Raines JK, Darling RC, Both J, et al: Vascular laboratory criteria for the management of peripheral vascular disease of the lower extremities. Surgery 79:21, 1976.
25. Darling RC, Raines JK, Brener BJ, et al: Quantitative segmental pulse volume recorder: A clinical tool. Surgery 72:873, 1972.
26. Winsor T, Sibley AE, Fisher EK, et al: Peripheral pulse contours in arterial occlusive disease. Vasc Dis 5:61, 1968.
27. Yao JST: Haemodynamic studies in peripheral arterial disease. Br J Surg 57:761, 1970.
28. Seldinger SE: Catheter replacement of needle in percutaneous arteriography: New technique. Acta Radiol 39:368, 1953.
29. Plug MH, Westra D: Complications in catheterization of the axillary artery. Radiol Clin Biol 42:510, 1973.
30. McAfee JG, Wilson JKV: A review of the complications of translumbar aortography. AJR Am J Roentgenol 75:956, 1956.
31. Udoff EJ, Barth KH, Harrington DP, et al: Hemodynamic significance of iliac artery stenosis: Pressure measurements during angiography. Radiology 132:289, 1979.
32. Itoch JR, Tullis MJ, Kennell TW, et al: Use of magnetic resonance angiography for the preoperative evaluation of patients with infrainguinal arterial occlusive disease. J Vasc Surg 23:792, 1996.
33. Baum RA, Rutter CM, Quinn SF, et al: Multicenter trial to evaluate vascular magnetic resonance angiography of the lower extremity. JAMA 274:875, 1995.
34. Brewster DC, Darling RC: Optimal methods of aortoiliac reconstruction. Surgery 84:739, 1978.
35. Crawford ES, Bomberger RA, Glaeser DH, et al: Aortoiliac occlusive disease: Factors influencing survival and function following reconstructive operation over a twenty-five-year period. Surgery 90:1055, 1981.
36. DeBakey ME, Crawford ES, Cooley DA, et al: Surgical considerations of occlusive disease of the abdominal aorta and iliac and femoral arteries: Analysis of 803 cases. Am Surg 148:306, 1958.
37. Malone JM, Moore WS, Goldstone J: The natural history of bilateral aortofemoral bypass grafts for ischemia of the lower extremities. Arch Surg 110:1300, 1975.
38. Moore WS, Caferata HT, Hall AD, et al: In defense of grafts across the inguinal ligament: An evaluation of early and late results of aortofemoral bypass grafts. Ann Surg 168:207, 1968.
39. Perdue GD, Long WD, Smith RB III: Perspective concerning aortofemoral arterial reconstruction. Ann Surg 173:940, 1971.
40. Whittemore AD, Clowes AW, Hechtman HB, et al: Aortic aneurysm repair: Reduced operative mortality associated with maintenance of optimal cardiac performance. Ann Surg 192:414, 1980.
41. Kannel WB, Skinner JJ Jr, Schwartz MJ, et al: Intermittent claudication: Incidence in the Framingham study. Circulation 41:857, 1970.
42. Malone JM, Moore WJ, Goldstone J: Life expectancy following aortofemoral arterial grafting. Surgery 81:551, 1977.
43. McAllister FF: The fate of patients with intermittent claudication managed non-operatively. Am J Surg 132:593, 1976.

44. Mozersky DJ, Summer DS, Strandness DE: Long-term results of reconstructive aortoiliac surgery. Am J Surg 123:503, 1972.

45. Whittemore AD, Mannick JA: The ischemic leg. In McLean LD (ed): Advances in Surgery. St. Louis, Mosby–Year Book, 1981, p 293.

46. Cooley DA, Wukasch DC, Bennett JG, et al: Double velour knitted Dacron grafts for aortoiliac vascular replacements. Paper presented at Vascular Graft Symposium, National Institutes of Health, Bethesda, Md, November 5, 1976.

47. Yates SG, Barros D'Sa AA, Berger K, et al: The preclotting of porous arterial prosthesis. Ann Surg 188:611, 1978.

48. Malone JM, Goldstone J, Moore WS: Autogenous profundaplasty: The key to long-term patency in secondary repair of aortofemoral graft occlusion. Ann Surg 188:817, 1978.

49. Morris GC Jr, Edwards W, Cooley DA, et al: Surgical importance of profunda femoris artery. Arch Surg 82:32, 1961.

50. Kaiser AB, Clayson KR, Mulherin JL, et al: Antibiotic prophylaxis in vascular surgery. Ann Surg 188:283, 1978.

51. Lindenaver SM, Fry WJ, Schaub G, et al: The use of antibiotics in the prevention of vascular graft infections. Surgery 62:487, 1967.

52. Szilagyi DE, Smith RF, Elliott JP, et al: Infection in arterial reconstruction with synthetic grafts. Ann Surg 176:321, 1972.

53. Knox GW: Peripheral vascular anastomotic aneurysms. Ann Surg 183:120, 1976.

54. Stoney RJ, Albo EJ, Wylie EJ: False aneurysms occurring after arterial grafting operations. Am J Surg 110:153, 1965.

55. Pierce GE, Turrentine M, Stringfield S, et al: Evaluation of end-to-side v end-to-end proximal anastomosis in aortobifemoral bypass. Arch Surg 117:1580, 1982.

56. Valentine RJ, Hansen ME, Myers SI, et al: The influence of sex and aortic size on late patency after aortofemoral revascularization in young adults. J Vasc Surg 21:296, 1995.

57. Ahn SS, Hiyama DT, Rudkin GH, et al: Laparoscopic aortobifemoral bypass. J Vasc Surg 26:128, 1997.

58. Said S, Mall J, Peter F, Muller JM: Laparoscopic aortofemoral bypass grafting: Human cadaveric and initial clinical experiences. J Vasc Surg 29:639, 1999.

59. Waters KJ, Proud G: Return to work after aortofemoral bypass surgery. BMJ 2:556, 1977.

60. Scheider JR, McHorney CA, Malenka DJ, McDaniel MD, Walsh DB, Cronenwett JL: Functional health and well-being in patients with severe atherosclerotic peripheral vascular occlusive disease. Ann Vasc Surg 7:419, 1993.

61. Royster TS, Lynn R, Mulcare RJ: Combined aortoiliac and femoropopliteal occlusive disease. Surg Gynecol Obstet 143:949, 1976.

62. Blaisdell FW, Hall AD, Lim RC Jr, et al: Aortoiliac substitution utilizing subcutaneus grafts. Ann Surg 172:775, 1970.

63. Eugene J, Goldstone J, Moore WS: Fifteen year experience with subcutaneous bypass grafts for lower extremity ischemia. Ann Surg 186:177, 1977.

64. LoGerfo FW, Johnson WC, Carson JD, et al: A comparison of the late patency rates of axillobilateral femoral and axillounilateral femoral grafts. Surgery 81:33, 1977.

65. Maini BS, Mannick JA: Effect of arterial reconstruction on limb salvage. Arch Surg 113:1297, 1978.

66. Mannick JA, Williams LE, Nabseth DC: The late results of axillofemoral grafts. Surgery 68:1038, 1970.

67. Vetto RM: The treatment of unilateral iliac artery obstruction with a transabdominal, subcutaneous, femorofemoral graft. Surgery 52:342, 1962.

68. Brief DK, Brener FJ, Alpert J, Parsonnet V: Cross-over femorofemoral grafts followed up five years or more. Arch Surg 110:1294, 1975.

69. Plecha FR, Pories WJ: Extra-anatomic bypasses for aortoiliac disease in high risk patients. Surgery 80:480, 1976.

70. Berguer R, Higgins RF, Reddy DJ: Intimal hyperplasia: An experimental study. Arch Surg 115:332, 1980.

71. Towne JB, Quinn K, Salles-Cunha S, et al: Effect of increased arterial blood flow on localization and progression of atherosclerosis. Arch Surg 117:1469, 1982.

72. Donaldson MC, Louras JC, Bucknam CA: Axillofemoral bypass: A tool with a limited role. J Vasc Surg 3:757, 1986.

73. Harris EJ, Taylor LM, McConnell DB, et al: Clinical results of axillobifemoral bypass using externally supported polytetrafluoroethylene. J Vasc Surg 12:416–421, 1990.

74. Passman MA, Taylor LM, Moneta GL, et al: Comparison of axillofemoral and aortofemoral bypass for aortoiliac occlusive disease. J Vasc Surg 23:263, 1996.

75. McCarthy WJ, Mesh CL, McMillan WD, et al: Descending thoracic aorta-to-femoral artery bypass: Ten years' experience with a durable procedure. J Vasc Surg 17:336, 1993.

76. Criado E, Keagy BA: Use of the descending thoracic aorta as an inflow source in aortoiliac reconstruction: Indications and long term procedure. Ann Vasc Surg 8:38, 1994.

77. Dotter CT, Judkins MD: Transluminal treatment of arteriosclerotic obstruction: Description of a technique and a preliminary report of its application. Circulation 30:654, 1964.

78. Gruntzig A: Die perkutane transluminale Rekanalisation chronischer Arterienverschlüsse mit einer neuen Dilatationstechnik. Baden-Baden, Germany, G Witzstrock Verlag, 1977.

79. Johnston KW, Rae M, Hogg-Johnston SA, et al: Five year results of a prospective study of percutaneous transluminal angioplasty. Ann Surg 206:403, 1987.

80. Wilson SE, Wolf GL, Cross AP, et al: Percutaneous transluminal angioplasty versus operation for peripheral arteriosclerosis. J Vasc Surg 9:1–8, 1989.

81. Henry M, Amor M, Ethevenot G, et al: Palmaz stent placement in iliac and femoropopliteal arteries: Primary and secondary patency in 310 patients with 2–4-year follow-up. Radiology 197:167, 1995.

Questions

1. Symptoms of the Leriche syndrome include all of the following except
   (a) claudication of the thigh and buttocks
   (b) rest pain of the feet
   (c) impotence
   (d) diminished femoral pulses

2. Blue toe syndrome is usually characterized by
   (a) severe claudication symptoms
   (b) absence of distal palpable pulses
   (c) palpable pedal pulses
   (d) severe tibial artery occlusive disease

3. Patients with isolated aortoiliac occlusive disease
   (a) generally do not suffer from ischemic rest pain
   (b) often have relatively normal ankle-brachial indices at rest
   (c) frequently have palpable pedal pulses
   (d) all of the above
   (e) none of the above

4. Advantages of the end-to-end technique for proximal anastomosis of an aortobifemoral bypass graft include all of the following except
   (a) decreased incidence of aortoduodenal fistulas
   (b) more complete endarterectomy of the proximal aortic stump
   (c) more complete preservation of pelvic blood flow
   (d) decreased incidence of distal atheroemboli

5. The end-to-side technique for aortobifemoral bypass grafts is preferred in patients with
   (a) extremely calcified infrarenal aortas
   (b) occluded inferior mesenteric arteries
   (c) common iliac artery occlusions
   (d) external iliac artery occlusions

6. Reported results of aortobifemoral bypass surgery suggest
   (a) 5-year cumulative patency rates of greater than 80%
   (b) poor patency rates for those patients with small (less than 1.8 cm) aortas

(c) significant decrements in physical and social role function despite successful bypass

(d) all of the above

7. The patency rates of axillobifemoral bypass grafts are most affected by
   (a) patient status
   (b) choice of prosthetic conduit
   (c) quality of the outflow bed
   (d) unilateral versus bilateral graft configuration

8. Success rates for percutaneous transluminal angioplasty of the iliac arteries are better for
   (a) common iliac than for external iliac lesions
   (b) for patients with claudication rather than rest pain
   (c) stenotic rather than occlusive lesions
   (d) all of the above

9. The use of intraluminal stents for iliac angioplasty
   (a) should be used as an adjunct for all iliac angioplasty
   (b) should be reserved for only technical failures of primary balloon angioplasty
   (c) has broadened the number of iliac lesions amenable to balloon angioplasty
   (d) has had no significant impact on the primary patency of iliac angioplasty

10. Concomitant inflow and infrainguinal revascularization is indicated
    (a) in all cases with complete superficial femoral artery occlusion
    (b) for patients with severe rest pain
    (c) for patients with extensive tissue necrosis
    (d) for diabetics

Answers

1. b   2. c   3. d   4. c   5. d   6. d   7. c   8. d   9. c   10. c

28

Femoral-Popliteal-Tibial Occlusive Disease

Evan C. Lipsitz and Frank J. Veith

Arteriosclerosis may involve the femoral arteries; the popliteal artery; any of the infrapopliteal arteries, including their terminal branches; or any combination of these arteries. This involvement generally begins early in adult life and progresses slowly to the point where a flow-reducing stenosis or occlusion occurs in one or more of the arteries below the inguinal ligament. As the average age of the population increases, the number of individuals with this hemodynamically significant infrainguinal arteriosclerosis also increases. This chapter deals with the present status of treatment for arteriosclerotic occlusive disease of the femoral, popliteal, and tibial arterial systems.

Obviously, this disease is associated in varying degrees with arteriosclerotic involvement elsewhere in the body, and this fact must constantly be considered when making therapeutic decisions in afflicted patients. This consideration guides the surgeon correctly to a lesser intervention or operation that maintains function rather than one that restores a normal circulation. The generalized and slowly progressive nature of the disease process and the imperfect results of all interventional treatments should also deter any who might be unwisely tempted to treat asymptomatic or minimally disabling arteriosclerotic occlusive lesions of the lower extremities. In management of the increasingly common entity of infrainguinal arteriosclerosis, diagnostic and therapeutic restraint and the desire to minimize risks and avoid doing harm must be paramount principles if the disease is not producing major functional impairment or tissue necrosis. On the other hand, despite the advanced age and poor generalized condition of the afflicted population, aggressive intervention for both diagnosis and treatment is justified if there is substantial threat of limb loss as a result of the disease process.

CLINICAL PRESENTATION

The reserve of the human arterial system is enormous. Hemodynamically significant stenoses or major artery occlusions can exist in the infrainguinal arterial tree with no or only minimal symptoms. This is particularly true if collateral pathways are normal or the patient's activity level is limited by coronary arteriosclerosis or other disease processes. Accordingly, the most common manifestation of a short segmental occlusion of the superficial femoral artery, the most common site of major arteriosclerotic involvement below the inguinal ligament, is mild intermittent claudication. Similarly, this lesion is often totally asymptomatic, as is usually the case if only one or two tibial arteries are occluded without other significant lesions. Thus the usual patient with severe disabling intermittent claudication or tissue necrosis has multiple sequential occlusions or so-called combined segment disease with hemodynamically significant lesions at the aortoiliac level and the superficial femoral and popliteal level, or either or both of these combined with severe infrapopliteal disease.[1]

Staging

Patients with hemodynamically significant infrainguinal arteriosclerosis may be classified into one of five stages depending on their clinical presentation as indicated in Table 28–1. Patients in stages III and IV are those whose limbs may be considered imminently threatened, although some patients with mild ischemic rest pain may remain stable for many years, and an occasional patient with a small patch of gangrene or an ischemic ulcer experiences healing with aggressive local wound care and close observation. With the exception of these few patients, invasive diagnostic procedures such as angiography are easily justified for those with stage III and IV disease, which is usually associated with disease at several levels.

Rest pain as an isolated symptom in patients with infrainguinal arteriosclerosis can be difficult to evaluate unless it is accompanied by other findings. Many patients with significant arterial lesions have pain at rest from causes other than arteriosclerosis, such as arthritis or neuritis.

TABLE 28-1

Staging of Infrainguinal Arteriosclerosis with Hemodynamically Significant Stenosis or Occlusions

STAGE	PRESENTATION	INVASIVE DIAGNOSTIC AND THERAPEUTIC INTERVENTION
0	No signs or symptoms	Never justified
I	Intermittent claudication (>1 block); no physical changes	Usually unjustified
II	Severe claudication (<½ block); dependent rubor; decreased temperature	Sometimes justified; not always necessary; may remain stable
III	Rest pain, atrophy, cyanosis, dependent rubor	Usually indicated but may do well for long periods without revascularization
IV	Nonhealing ischemic ulcer or gangrene	Usually indicated

Such pain is not improved by a revascularization procedure. Significant ischemic rest pain must be associated not only with decreased pulses but also with other objective manifestations of ischemia such as atrophy, decreased skin temperature compared with the other extremity, marked rubor, and relief of pain with dependency. In some patients with rest pain of complex origin, a noninvasive laboratory and angiographic evaluation may be necessary before the predominant cause of the symptom can be determined and appropriate treatment instituted. Every patient with pain at rest and decreased pulses is not a candidate for angiography and an arterial bypass. Some of these patients experience relief through appropriate treatment of comorbid conditions such as gout or osteoarthritis. Others can be well managed with simple analgesics and reassurance that the limb is not in jeopardy. Such reassurance generally suffices for patients with stage I disease and those with stage II disease who are elderly (older than 80 years old) or at high risk because of intercurrent disease or atherosclerotic involvement of other organs such as the heart, the kidneys, or the brain.

This conservative approach to patients with stage I involvement from infrainguinal arteriosclerosis is becoming increasingly widespread, albeit not universally so.[2] Conservatism appears to be clearly justified by the numerous reports of the benignancy and slow progression of stage I disease to more advanced stages.[3-5] Without treatment, 10% to 15% of patients in stage I improve over 5 years, and 60% to 70% do not progress over the same period. The 10% to 15% who do worsen are, in our opinion, best treated with a primary operation or other therapeutic intervention *after* their disease progresses. We further believe that this conservative approach to stage I disease is justified by the greater surgical difficulty encountered when

a procedure for claudication fails in the early or remote postoperative period and the patient then has a threatened limb, a situation that we have observed all too frequently.

The fact that some patients in stage II and a few in stage III or IV may remain stable and easily managed without intervention for protracted periods of 1 or more years justifies a cautiously conservative nonoperative approach to selected patients in these stages. This often requires frequent visits to the involved physician so that the patient and the progress of ischemia can be assessed. Moreover, this conservative approach is particularly indicated if the patient is elderly and a poor surgical risk from a systemic and a local point of view. An example of this would be an octogenarian with intractable congestive heart failure in whom a difficult distal small vessel bypass would be required to alleviate stage III signs and symptoms. Close observation can and often should be the preferred management for such patients for several months or even years; however, we would not hesitate to revascularize these patients when their rest pain became intolerable or when they developed a small progressive patch of gangrene.[1, 6]

Impact of Newer Interventional Treatments on Threshold for Therapy

The relative simplicity of percutaneous balloon angioplasty alone or in combination with other newer endovascular treatments (atherectomy devices, stents, and endovascular grafts) has prompted some physicians to recommend lowering of the therapeutic thresholds for the treatment of infrainguinal atherosclerosis. Some surgeons, radiologists, and particularly cardiologists new to the peripheral vascular field and armed with these new techniques and devices have used them routinely to treat stage I and even stage 0 disease detected incidentally during physical examination or coronary arteriography. This practice is to be condemned at this time for many reasons. Most important, the mid- and long-term results of these newer treatments remain totally unknown. Even if they are successful immediately, they can initiate a healing process in the artery that causes late failure or, worse, an acceleration of the occlusive process and, ultimately, net harm to the patient. Therefore, they subject patients to risks they may not fully appreciate. Practitioners should not usually treat these relatively early, minimally symptomatic lesions before more is known about these newer high-tech treatments. Although they are all exciting and interesting to patients and physicians alike and although they may prove to be safe and effective, this has not yet been shown. Accordingly, no justification exists to lower the threshold for intervening in patients with infrainguinal arteriosclerosis. This fact should be communicated freely to patients to offset the unjustified marketing efforts of uninformed practitioners.

Differential Diagnosis

Intermittent claudication, or pain brought on by exertion and relieved by rest, is a fairly distinct symptom and usually a manifestation of arteriosclerotic occlusive disease. Mild calf claudication can be produced by a significant stenotic lesion in the iliac, superficial femoral, or popliteal arteries. An occasional patient describes claudication as a sense of heaviness, weakness, or fatigue in the limb without pain, and such patients may be mistakenly diagnosed as having neuromuscular disorders. Sometimes claudication-like symptoms can be produced by lesions compressing the lower spinal cord or cauda equina.[7, 8] Such *pseudoclaudication* is most often produced by spinal stenosis and can easily be suspected when peripheral pulses are normal. Occasionally, neurologic problems coexist with arterial occlusive disease, making an exact determination of the cause of the patient's symptoms a difficult challenge for the neurologist and the vascular surgeon. In such circumstances, angiography and computed tomography (CT) or magnetic resonance imaging (MRI) of the lumbar spine and myelography may be necessary.

Some of the difficulties that can be encountered in differentiating pain at rest from true *ischemic rest pain* have already been discussed. Similar difficulties can be encountered in determining the primary cause of ulcerating lesions in the ankle region and on the foot. The typical *venous ulcer* occurs in a setting of chronic venous disease, is associated with stasis changes and normal arterial pulses, is usually relatively painless, and heals with elevation and compressive measures. The typical *arterial* or *ischemic ulcer* is far more painful and is associated with other manifestations of ischemia. It usually has a more necrotic base and is located at an area of chronic pressure or trauma, such as over the malleoli or the bunion area. Both conditions may be improved by hospitalization, bed rest, and local care. Differential diagnosis is usually only difficult when chronic venous and arterial disease coexist. Venous evaluations, including duplex scanning, plethysmography, and sometimes venography in addition to arteriography, may be required to completely evaluate these patients. In some patients, the primary cause of the ulcer can be determined only when arterial reconstruction produces healing after a period of intense conservative management has failed to do so.

When a patient has a gangrenous (black) or pregangrenous (blue) toe, several causes other than progression of chronic arteriosclerotic occlusive disease must be considered. *Local infection* can be the sole or a major contributing cause of a toe lesion. This is particularly common in diabetics. If foot pulses or noninvasive tests of arterial function are normal, the gangrenous condition can be presumed to result from local arterial or arteriolar thrombosis secondary to infection. Radical local *excision* and drainage of all involved tissue plus antibiotics usually results in a healed foot. Diagnosis is more difficult when infection coexists with arterial occlusive disease. Noninvasive studies and arteriography are usually required to determine whether the treatment should consist of excision and drainage alone or in combination with an arterial reconstruction. Decision making under these conditions can be among the most difficult in vascular surgery.

Black or blue toes may also occur as the result of embolic processes. Such emboli may originate from the heart, a proximal aneurysm, or any proximal atherosclerotic lesion. In the last circumstance, small cholesterol, platelet, or fibrin emboli may lodge in interosseous or digital arteries. Peripheral pedal pulses may be normal, and spontaneous improvement of the resulting blue toe often occurs. This sequence of events has been termed the "blue toe syndrome," and its pathogenesis is thought to be analogous to that of transient ischemic attacks from atherosclerotic disease at the carotid bifurcation.[9] If a single dominant arterial lesion can be identified by noninvasive means or angiography (or both), it should be treated by endarterectomy or, more commonly, by an appropriate bypass. However, in our experience, identifying a single lesion in the arterial tree of these patients has been difficult, and we have usually operated only after the patients have experienced multiple embolic episodes.

When ischemia develops suddenly, the possibility of a major embolus from the heart or a proximal aneurysm must be considered. In such circumstances, angiography is indicated even if limb viability is not in question, because major emboli should be removed as soon as they are identified. In the last several decades, with the significant improvements in the prevention and treatment of rheumatic heart disease, almost all patients we have evaluated with major arterial emboli and acute occlusions have had them superimposed on extensive arteriosclerosis. Even with angiography, *which we employ routinely in such cases,* the diagnosis and treatment of embolic disease is difficult and the results imperfect.[10] The only certain diagnostic feature of embolic occlusion is multiplicity. Furthermore, the location of the embolus may be atypical, and the vascular surgeon treating a presumed embolus in the presence of extensive arteriosclerosis must be prepared to perform an extensive arterial reconstruction or bypass even if the operation is undertaken soon after the acute event.[10]

Because of these facts and because acute thrombosis sometimes cannot be differentiated in any way from an embolus, complete preoperative angiography should be mandatory in any suspected embolic occlusion of the lower extremity in a patient who could have arteriosclerosis. Exploration of the distal popliteal artery is usually the best surgical approach in patients with severe ischemia due to an acute occlusion of the popliteal or distal superficial femoral arteries,[11] although use of intraarterially administered lytic agents may have significant therapeutic advantages in the management of acute thromboembolic occlusions of native lower extremity arteries, especially those with some underlying atherosclerosis.[12] Moreover, the care and surgical treatment of such cases should only be undertaken by an experienced vascular surgeon. A more complete discussion of the management of acute thromboembolic arterial occlusions appears in Chapter 36.

PATIENT EVALUATION

Local Factors and Extremity Physical Examination

As already indicated, the findings on physical examination of the involved extremity contribute to the staging of the atherosclerotic process and provide a rough guide to whether diagnostic or therapeutic intervention is justified and needed. Physical findings such as discoloration, swelling, erythema, and localized tenderness can provide evidence of the presence and extent of infection in the involved foot. As a general rule, the extent of infection and necrosis deep to the skin is greater than one might expect from an examination of the skin. Reexamination after a short period of soaking to soften the epidermis and dried exudate may be helpful in revealing purulent collections and subcutaneous necrosis. Exploration of suspicious areas can sometimes be carried out without anesthesia if the patient has diminished sensation from diabetic neuropathy. If not, such exploration and necessary débridement should be performed in the operating room under appropriate anesthesia.

A thorough initial examination of a patient with suspected infrainguinal arterial disease is required and is helpful in ascertaining the nature and extent of previous arterial surgery and ipsilateral saphenous vein harvest as well as evidence of associated chronic disease. In evaluating an ischemic limb, particular attention must be given to careful inspection of the heel and between the toes, where unsuspected ischemic ulcers or infection may be present. A flashlight is extremely helpful in this regard. The uninvolved extremity must also be examined carefully. Because of the symmetry of atherosclerosis, the opposite extremity may harbor unsuspected ischemic lesions. Moreover, such findings as coolness and bluish discoloration are far more meaningful if they are asymmetrical, because cool dusky extremities may sometimes be present without significant arterial disease.

Pulse examination in the lower extremities of a patient with suspected ischemia is extremely important. It requires considerable experience and must be performed with care. The strength of a pulse as assessed by an experienced examiner is a valuable semiquantitative assessment of the arterial circulation at that level. Pulses are graded from 0 to 4+, and a pulse cannot be described as "plus or minus" or "questionable." The latter indicates an incomplete examination. A 0 pulse cannot be felt. A 1+ pulse is definitely present but definitely diminished. Both 2+ and 3+ are normal intensities, and 4+ is an abnormally strong pulse, as with an aneurysm or aortic insufficiency. If a pulse is 2+ on one side and 3+ on the opposite side, the 2+ is a decreased pulse, and arterial pressure at that site is probably diminished (unless the 3+ pulse is due to an aneurysm).

In examining a patient with diminished pulses, counting the pulse to an assistant who is palpating the patient's radial pulse helps to ensure that the examiner is not feeling his or her own pulse or spurious muscular activity. Before one describes a pulse as being absent, considerable time and effort must be expended and ectopic localization of pulses, such as the lateral tarsal artery pulse, must be examined. In this era of frequently performed noninvasive arterial tests, the value of a carefully performed and recorded pulse examination cannot be overemphasized. An accurate pulse examination predicts both the pattern of infrainguinal disease and the treatment required to relieve the symptoms. It also provides a basis for comparison if subsequent disease progression occurs.

For example, if a patient with a gangrenous toe lesion has a pedal pulse, local treatment without reconstructive arterial surgery is almost always the correct approach to achieve a healed foot. If a patient with an ischemic foot lesion has a normal popliteal pulse but no pedal pulses, some form of infrapopliteal or small vessel bypass is almost always the correct approach. If a patient with an ischemic foot lesion has a normal ipsilateral femoral pulse without distal pulses, some form of infrainguinal arterial reconstruction, hopefully a femoropopliteal bypass, is the correct approach. If such a patient has a diminished femoral pulse, often with an associated bruit, some form of proximal arterial reconstruction or angioplasty above the inguinal ligament is almost certainly required.

Systemic Factors

Systemic factors that are important in the patient who is a candidate for interventional treatment for infrainguinal arteriosclerosis include all those in the history, physical examination, and routine laboratory tests that might indicate major organ failure. Most important are evidence of heart disease, diabetes, renal disease, hypertension, chronic pulmonary disease, and atherosclerotic involvement of the cerebral circulation. All these intercurrent diseases, if present, require appropriate medical management before, during, and after diagnostic and therapeutic interventions so that risks are minimized. A detailed discussion of this management is beyond the scope of this chapter. However, because all patients with infrainguinal arteriosclerosis also have some degree of coronary involvement and because myocardial infarction is the principal cause of operative as well as late mortality in this group of patients, some details of cardiac evaluation and management should be mentioned. Evidence of myocardial ischemia and congestive heart failure should be sought. Noninvasive cardiac stress tests after exercise or infusion of intravenous agents such as dipyridamole or dobutamine may be useful for screening. If marked abnormalities or severe angina pectoris is present, some patients should be subjected to coronary arteriography and aortocoronary bypass before treatment of the limb ischemia. Patients with recent myocardial infarctions and those in congestive heart failure should have a Swan-Ganz catheter inserted and have their fluid and volume replacement optimized before, during, and after operation on the basis of appropriate cardiac output and pressure measurements.[13] Renal function must be monitored repetitively after any angiographic procedure, because transient renal failure is common. If detected and appropriately treated, this is almost always reversible and rarely a serious problem.

Noninvasive Vascular Laboratory Tests

Although the nature and value of noninvasive laboratory tests are discussed in depth in Chapter 13, several relevant points should be made here regarding their role in patients with infrainguinal arteriosclerosis. In the early stages, in which interventional measures are not required, segmental arterial pressures and pulse-volume recordings provide an objective and semiquantitative assessment of the circulation and help to confirm the diagnosis made by the history and physical examination, including a careful pulse examination. These tests also provide a baseline for future comparison and serve as a rough index of the localization of occlusive lesions and the degree of ischemia in the foot. However, the correlation is not absolute. Flat ankle and forefoot wave tracings with ankle pressures less than 35 mm Hg may not be associated with foot lesions or serious symptoms. In addition, decreased thigh waveforms and pressures may be entirely due to disease below the inguinal ligament as well as aortoiliac disease. The differentiation between these two types of lesions can only be made by femoral pulse examination and direct pressure measurements. The exact localization and definition of these lesions can be made using duplex scanning, and there has been a great deal of interest in planning infrainguinal revascularizations on the basis of duplex arterial mapping alone,[14, 15] but angiography, often in two planes, may be necessary. In some circumstances, screening duplex arterial mapping supplemented by limited intraoperative arteriography provides an excellent road map and also minimizes contrast, cost, and preoperative hospitalization. We have been using this approach with increasing frequency and good results.

Noninvasive testing can be extremely helpful in predicting when a toe amputation or local procedure on the foot has virtually no chance of healing. A flat-line forefoot tracing with an ankle pressure below 50 mm Hg indicates that a toe amputation or other foot operation for an ischemic lesion will not heal without prior revascularization. Because these tests do not evaluate the severity or extent of infection, the opposite is not always true. Good forefoot pulse waves and ankle pressures do not guarantee healing of foot operations, although they suggest it will occur if infection can be eliminated. Furthermore, a gray zone of intermediate values exists in which the noninvasive tests are of limited value and a therapeutic trial of a local foot procedure is justified and appropriate.

Angiographic Evaluation

As in other areas of vascular surgery, proper high-quality *arteriography* is still essential to make the most accurate diagnosis of infrainguinal arteriosclerosis, to determine whether a therapeutic intervention is possible and justified by its risk, and to allow planning of the optimal form that this intervention should take.[5] Adequate arteriography also defines the localization and extent of arteriosclerotic involvement in the infrarenal aorta and iliac arteries, although for optimal accuracy it may have to be supplemented by direct pressure measurements taken at the time of arteriography or operation.

To provide adequate information, the arterial tree from the renal arteries to the forefoot should be well visualized in continuity, preferably by the transfemoral route. This is generally possible only if a long film changer, multiple exposures, large boluses of contrast, and other technical modifications described elsewhere[16] are employed. Oblique views may be required to visualize completely the origin and proximal portion of the deep femoral artery. Good preoperative distal artery visualization is, in our opinion, the key to performing optimal bypass surgery on arteries in the foot and lower leg. Reactive hyperemia, digitally augmented views, and delayed films may be necessary to achieve the needed visualization. Although others have advocated intraoperative arteriography to achieve this end,[17] we have found it less effective and rarely necessary. Magnetic resonance (MR) angiography can provide preoperative evaluation of patent distal leg and foot arteries without the need for dye injection and arterial catheterization.[18, 19] Although this technique is becoming more widely available, it is expensive and of variable quality in different centers.[20]

Saphenous venography and, more recently, *duplex ultrasonography* have also been helpful in planning long bypasses.[21, 22] They may show a vein defect preoperatively and thereby spare the patient and the surgeon the needless effort of harvesting a saphenous vein that cannot be used. These techniques are particularly indicated in patients who have undergone prior bypasses, because many of these patients have had their veins used or inadvertently injured at their first operation. However, neither method is totally accurate, and surgical exploration is the only way to assess vein quality with certainty.

TREATMENT: PRINCIPLES, PROCEDURES, AND JUDGMENTAL ISSUES

In general, our approach, which is detailed in subsequent paragraphs, represents the most aggressive effort for limb salvage in patients with severe infrainguinal arteriosclerosis. Patients who have ischemic foot lesions or pain but who can be treated successfully by aortofemoral, femorofemoral, or axillofemoral bypass alone are excluded from the following discussion, even though many of them have infrainguinal arteriosclerosis in addition to their more proximal disease.

General Considerations

According to our aggressive approach to patients whose limbs are threatened because of infrainguinal arteriosclerosis, limb salvage should be considered and attempted if feasible, unless gangrene extends into the deeper tissues of the tarsal region of the foot or the patient has severe organic mental syndrome with inability to ambulate, communicate, or provide self-care.[1, 6] Patients in the latter categories should undergo primary below- or above-knee amputation. Primary above-knee amputation should also be employed if a patient with foot gangrene is unable to stand or walk because of long-standing severe flexion contractures.

Medical Considerations

As expected, these patients have a high incidence of other arteriosclerotic manifestations and more than 60% have diabetes mellitus.[6] The mean age is older than 70 years, and the number of patients older than 80 years is rapidly increasing. Many have suffered documented myocardial infarctions, some are in uncompensated congestive heart or renal failure, some have had myocardial infarctions within 3 weeks of presentation,[6, 23] and some have concurrent carcinomas.[2]

The general plan of medical management is to achieve maximal improvement of cardiac, renal, and diabetic status before proceeding with arteriographic examination and operation. In some instances, the urgency of the ischemic situation, coupled with progressive infection in the foot, makes it necessary to perform the angiographic examination and intervention before ideal medical control can be achieved. In these patients, the decision to proceed is made jointly by the surgeon, the internist, and the patient. Almost without exception, age, medical status, incurable malignancy, and a contralateral amputation are not considered absolute contraindications to arterial reconstruction.[1, 6]

Surgical Considerations and Criteria for Reconstructability

Femoropopliteal Bypass

Patients whose limbs are clearly threatened and who have undergone arteriographic examination should undergo femoropopliteal bypass when the superficial femoral or popliteal artery is occluded and the patent popliteal artery segment distal to the occlusion has luminal continuity, on arteriographic examination, with any of its three terminal branches. This is true even if one or more of these branches ends in an occlusion anywhere in the leg. Even if the popliteal artery segment into which the graft is to be inserted is occluded distally, femoropopliteal bypass to this *isolated segment*[24] may be the procedure of choice in selected patients. If the isolated popliteal segment is less than 7 cm in length, or if extensive gangrene or infection in the foot is present, a femoral-to-popliteal-to-distal artery bypass or *sequential bypass* is sometimes performed, in one or two stages.[25, 26] All femoropopliteal bypasses can be classified on the basis of their relationship to the knee joint and runoff from the popliteal artery, as determined radiographically by previously described criteria.[26] However, all angiographic evaluations of popliteal runoff are imperfect and correlated in only a limited way with outflow resistance and bypass patency.[27]

Infrapopliteal Bypass

Bypasses to arteries beyond the popliteal (small vessel or tibial bypasses) are performed only when femoropopliteal bypass is not deemed possible or appropriate, according to the foregoing criteria. These small vessel bypasses are performed to the posterior tibial, the anterior tibial, or the peroneal arteries, in that order of preference. A tibial artery is generally used only if its lumen runs without obstruction into the foot, although short vein bypasses to isolated tibial artery segments and other disadvantaged outflow tracts have been performed and have remained patent over 4 years.[28–31] A peroneal artery is usually used if it is continuous with one or two of its terminal branches, which then run into the foot. Absence of a plantar arch and vascular calcification *are not* considered contraindica-

tions to a reconstruction.[6, 28, 29] Some patients require a bypass to an artery or arterial branch in the foot.[1, 6, 28–31] Very few patients fail to have in their leg or foot an artery that meets these requirements; therefore, less than 1% of our patients are now considered unreconstructible on the basis of angiographic findings.[1]

With both femoropopliteal and small vessel bypasses, a stenosis of less than 50% of the diameter of the vessel is acceptable at or distal to the site chosen for the distal anastomosis. Although every effort is made to find the most disease-free segment of artery to use for the distal anastomosis, this may be tempered by the advisability of using the most proximal patent segment possible to shorten the length of the bypass. For example, we believe that a mildly diseased proximal popliteal artery should be used for a distal anastomosis in preference to a nondiseased distal popliteal artery.

The common femoral artery has been generally used as the site of origin for all bypasses to the popliteal and more distal arteries. However, since 1976, we have also used as inflow sites the superficial femoral, popliteal, or tibial arteries when these vessels were relatively undiseased or vein length was limited.[28, 32, 33] The superficial femoral and popliteal arteries are now used preferentially if possible; that is, if no proximal luminal stenosis exists in excess of 40% of the cross-sectional diameter.

Axillopopliteal Bypass

Axillopopliteal bypass is used only when amputation is imminent and a more standard arterial reconstruction is not feasible because of groin infection, previous operative scarring, or extensive bilateral arteriosclerotic involvement of the iliac and femoral arterial systems.[34, 35]

Profundaplasty

Endarterectomy of the origin and proximal portion of the deep femoral artery is most valuable for salvaging threatened limbs when it is combined with some form of inflow operation, such as an aortofemoral or axillofemoral bypass.[36] As an isolated procedure in patients whose limbs are threatened because of infrainguinal arteriosclerosis, we have found profundaplasty to be of little value. Perhaps it is occasionally justified as the sole procedure if the patient has rest pain without necrosis *and* a tight stenosis or occlusion of the deep femoral artery with a demonstrable pressure gradient across the lesion at operation. In practice we have used a short vein bypass to the distal deep femoral artery more frequently than an isolated profundaplasty.

Graft Material

Until 1976, reversed autologous saphenous vein (ASV) grafts were clearly the graft material of choice, with a variety of polyester fabric grafts serving as the alternative material if the vein was unavailable. Tubular expanded polytetrafluoroethylene (PTFE) grafts became available in 1976 and were first used only when ipsilateral saphenous vein was unavailable or unusable. Promising early and intermediate results with this material in femoropopliteal bypasses[37–39] prompted liberalization of the indications for its use in this operation to include patients whose probable life expectancy is less than 3 years, and some surgeons, after adequately analyzing their results, still advocate the preferential use of PTFE grafts for femoropopliteal bypass to the above-knee segment.[40]

In 1986, we completed, with Drs. Bergan, Bernhard, Yao, Flinn, Towne, and others, a cooperative, randomized, prospective study comparing ASV with PTFE grafts in all infrainguinal bypass operations.[41, 42] ASV and PTFE grafts were compared in 845 infrainguinal bypass operations, 485 to the popliteal artery and 360 to infrapopliteal arteries. Life-table primary patency rates for randomized PTFE grafts to the popliteal artery paralleled those for randomized ASV grafts to the same level for 2 years and then became significantly different (4-year patency of 68% ± 8% [± SE] for ASV versus 47% ± 9% for PTFE, P <.025). Four-year patency differences were not statistically significant for randomized above-knee grafts (61% ± 12% for ASV versus 38% ± 13% for PTFE, P >.25), but were for randomized below-knee grafts (76% ± 9% for ASV versus 45% ± 11% for PTFE, P <.05). Four-year limb salvage rates after bypasses to the popliteal artery for critical ischemia did not differ for the two types of randomized grafts (75% ± 10% for ASV versus 72% ± 10% for PTFE, P >.025). Although primary patency rates for randomized PTFE grafts and obligatory PTFE grafts to the popliteal artery were significantly different (P <.025), 4-year limb salvage rates were not (70% ± 10% versus 68% ± 20%, P <.25). Primary patency rates at 4 years for infrapopliteal bypasses with randomized ASV were significantly better than those with randomized PTFE (49% ± 10% versus 12% ± 7%, P <.001). Three-and-one-half-year limb salvage rates for infrapopliteal bypasses with both randomized grafts (57% ± 10% for ASV and 61% ± 10% for PTFE) were better than those for obligatory infrapopliteal PTFE grafts (38% ± 11%, P <.01). These results fail to support the routine preferential use of PTFE grafts for either femoropopliteal or more distal bypasses. However, this graft may be used preferentially in selected poor-risk patients for femoropopliteal bypasses, particularly those that do not cross the knee. In addition, although every effort should be made to use autologous vein for infrapopliteal bypasses, a PTFE distal bypass is a better option than a primary major amputation. Recent reports have shown improved results for femorotibial bypasses using PTFE grafts with or without distal anastomotic vein patches. The best reported primary patency rates of these grafts at 5 years with a distal anastomotic vein patch are 54% ± 10%.[43] A recent report of distal PTFE grafts without a distal vein patch reported 5-year secondary patency rates of 43% ± 10% and limb salvage rates of 66% ± 8%.[44]

Although we believe that PTFE grafts are the best currently available alternative arterial prosthetic if the ipsilateral ASV is not available for femoropopliteal bypass or if no vein is available for infrapopliteal bypasses, other grafts have also been used with some success. The tanned umbilical vein graft has received the greatest attention, and patency rates similar to those of PTFE grafts have been reported in both the femoropopliteal and infrapopliteal positions.[45] A number of randomized comparisons of the two grafts have been completed. However, many of these studies were flawed or yielded inconclusive differences. In addition, reports of a high incidence of aneurysmal degeneration occurring in umbilical vein grafts after even a few years are worrisome and suggest that this graft be used with caution even though the manufacturers have strengthened the external polyester fabric mesh.[46]

Another alternative prosthetic that may have some usefulness in infrainguinal bypasses is the polyester fabric graft. A 1992 retrospective study by Pevec and colleagues[47] suggested that these grafts can have excellent results when used as a femoropopliteal conduit. In addition, externally supported grafts may also be useful for infrapopliteal bypasses.[48] Polyester fabric and PTFE grafts have been compared in a randomized, prospective fashion as conduits for femoropopliteal bypasses to arterial segments above the knee.[49] At 5 years, no significant difference was evident in primary or secondary patency rates.

At present, use of any new prosthetic grafts *in preference* to ipsilateral ASV is clearly wrong until appropriate randomized prospective studies comparing the prosthetic graft with vein have been completed. Many surgeons succumb to the temptation of finding a rationale to use a prosthetic graft preferentially. We believe this temptation must be resisted and encourage randomized study of all promising new prosthetic grafts before they are used preferentially. Sixty percent to eighty percent of patients have a usable vein if a real effort is made to find it.[18, 50] On the other hand, many patients do not have an adequate autologous vein, and use of a prosthetic graft is far better than an unwise attempt to use a small (<3.0 mm in distended diameter), fibrotic, or otherwise inadequate autologous vein.[50–53] These considerations should be kept in mind when evaluating the "all-autologous policy" espoused by some capable vascular surgeons.[54] As more and more secondary operations become necessary to save limbs, the proportion of patients who do not have an adequate autologous vein conduit will increase. In such patients, a prosthetic (PTFE) graft yields better results than ill-advised use of a poor or intrinsically diseased vein.

In Situ versus Reversed Saphenous Vein Grafts

The in situ saphenous vein graft was described as an infrainguinal arterial conduit by Hall in 1962.[55] It has several theoretical advantages over the more commonly used reversed saphenous vein graft, although the technique is demanding and requires elimination of all venous valves and occlusion of branches. Leather and coworkers[56] devised methods for rendering the venous valves incompetent, and the Albany group[57] and Gruss and coworkers[58] of Germany popularized the use of in situ vein grafts for infrainguinal arterial reconstructions. Recently, a number of claims have been made regarding the superiority of in situ vein grafts to reversed vein grafts, particularly for tibial and peroneal bypasses. Although better endothelial preservation may be possible with in situ veins and although they may offer advantages when long bypasses with small veins are required, superior patency rates in comparable situations have never been proved. Comparisons using historical controls are not valid.

In a multicenter, prospective, randomized comparison of in situ and reversed vein grafts that we carried out with Gregor Shanik of Dublin and Peter Harris of Liverpool and others,[59] no significant differences were evident in the primary patency, secondary patency, and limb salvage rates between the two groups. Moreover, many of the striking results that can be accomplished with in situ vein grafts can also be successfully accomplished with reversed vein grafts.[28] This includes the use of small-caliber veins to disadvantaged outflow tracts (Figs. 28–1, 28–2, and 28–3). In addition, many patients who have autologous vein suitable for an *ectopic* reversed vein graft do not have a vein suitable for an in situ graft. Patients without any remaining major superficial vein in the ipsilateral lower extremity but with a good vein in the opposite leg or an arm are one example. Thus, until the superiority of in situ grafts is clearly documented by adequately controlled studies, we will adhere to the belief that the technical perfection of the operation and the commitment of surgeons and their colleagues to the limb salvage goal are far more important

in achieving good results than whether the vein graft is in the reversed or in situ position.

Taylor and colleagues[60] published their results with infrainguinal reversed vein bypasses and claimed that reversed vein grafts were better than in situ grafts. However, more than 20% of the patients whom these authors included in their cases were operated on for indications other than limb salvage. Thus their claims of superiority for reversed vein grafts are based on data without comparable, concurrent controls, the same defect that they noted in the reports of others who claimed that the in situ technique gave superior results. Thus, the question of which type of vein graft is better remains an unanswered one that requires further study. We have recently noted extremely poor late patency rates for long reversed vein grafts less than 3.5 mm in diameter and short vein grafts less than 3.0 mm in diameter.[52, 53] Because similar poor patency has not been reported in small-diameter in situ grafts,[61] the in situ technique may be superior in patients whose vein is less than 3.0 mm in distended diameter.

Upper Extremity Veins

The cephalic and basilic veins from the upper extremities have been advocated for use as a graft when lower extremity autologous vein is unavailable. Although the work of Schulman and Bradley[62] and many others suggest that arm veins are inferior to the saphenous vein in infrainguinal bypasses, other observations indicate that the cephalic vein can be used with good success in lower extremity arterial reconstructions.[63–65] However, arm veins are more thin-walled and more difficult to work with than the saphenous vein. Moreover, in our experience arm veins can have frequent fibrotic, recanalized segments from previous trauma and venipunctures. When several healthy segments are joined to form a composite graft, poorer patency results. This is in part due to intrinsic disease in the venous conduit. Intraoperative angioscopy is very useful in evaluating these veins[66] with discarding of severely diseased segments that may appear normal on external inspection. In addition, aggressive surveillance is necessary to discover and potentially correct the vein graft lesions that more commonly develop in these conduits.[54]

On this basis and because of the high degree of symmetry in infrainguinal arteriosclerosis, we believe use of a prosthetic graft in the femoropopliteal position is presently justified if the ipsilateral saphenous vein is unsuitable or unavailable. However, for infrapopliteal bypasses, every effort should be made to find usable autogenous vein. In this regard, lesser saphenous veins, accessory saphenous veins, and veins from the opposite thigh and upper extremities may all be useful, and we use them in that order of preference.

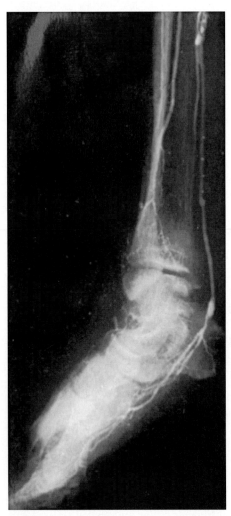

Figure 28–1. Arteriogram performed on patient 3 years after posterior tibial-to-posterior tibial bypass. The plantar arch is incomplete. (From Veith FJ, Ascer E, Gupta SK, et al: Tibiotibial vein bypass grafts: A new operation for limb salvage. J Vasc Surg 2:552–557, 1985.)

Operative Technique

All operations are performed with the patient under light general, spinal, or epidural anesthesia. Care is taken to protect the opposite heel by placing a small pillow under the Achilles tendon. The arterial blood pressure is moni-

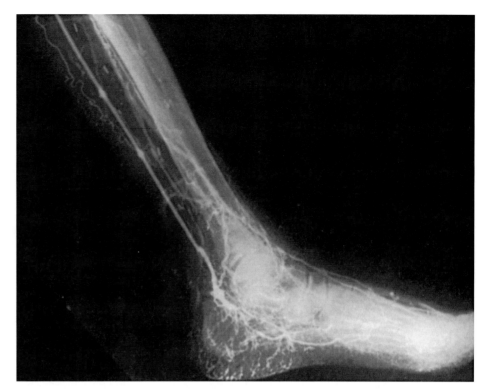

Figure 28–2. Intraoperative arteriogram after bypass from tibioperoneal trunk to the posterior tibial artery at its bifurcation in the foot. Note small size of vein graft and intact plantar arch. (From Veith FJ, Ascer E, Gupta SK, et al: Tibiotibial vein bypass grafts: A new operation for limb salvage. J Vasc Surg 2:552–557, 1985.)

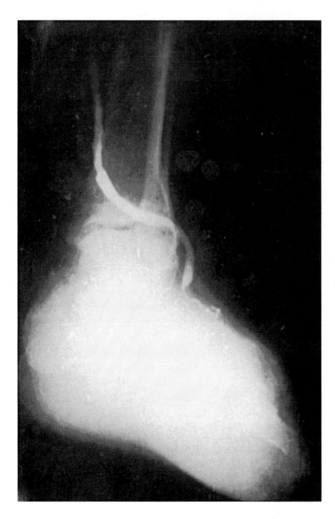

Figure 28–3. Postoperative arteriogram after bypass to the lateral tarsal artery, which appears to end in a total occlusion. There is also no patent plantar arch. (From Veith FJ, Ascer E, Gupta SK, et al: Tibiotibial vein bypass grafts: A new operation for limb salvage. J Vasc Surg 2:552–557, 1985.)

tored by a radial artery catheter. Surgical techniques are detailed elsewhere,[35, 38, 67] and illustrated in Figures 28–4 and 28–5. Vessels are occluded with a minimum of force and distortion. We have found tourniquet occlusion, as recommended by Bernhard and colleagues,[68] to also be very useful during the creation of the distal and sometimes proximal anastomosis. Anastomoses are meticulously constructed with continuous 6-0 polypropylene sutures, with particular care to take small, evenly spaced bites of all layers of the vessel wall and to exclude all adventitia from

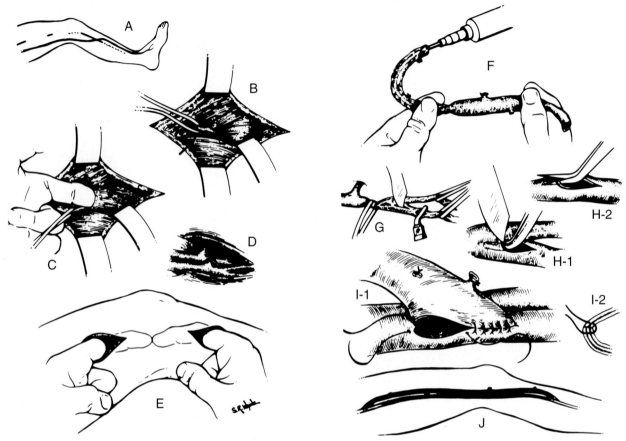

Figure 28–4. Small vessel bypass in the upper and middle thirds of the leg. This may be performed to the tibioperoneal trunk, the posterior tibial artery, or the peroneal artery using a medial approach below the knee joint to gain access to these vessels. The anterior tibial artery requires an additional anterior incision (shown in Fig. 28–5). A, In heavy lines, the position of the incisions required to perform bypasses from the femoral artery to the tibioperoneal trunk or the peroneal or posterior tibial arteries in the upper third of the leg. The upper incision provides access to the common or superficial femoral artery. The above-knee incision allows tunneling under the sartorius muscle and along the course of the popliteal vessels behind the knee. The dashed extension to the lower incision provides access to the posterior tibial and peroneal arteries in the middle third of the leg. If the saphenous vein is to be used, all incisions should be placed over the vein as shown by the double line, and access to deeper structures obtained when needed by raising thick flaps.

B, The below-knee incision opened through the skin, subcutaneous fat, and deep fascia of the popliteal space. The gastrocnemius muscle is retracted posteriorly. The more superficial popliteal vein is encircled with a Silastic loop to facilitate dissection of the underlying popliteal artery (*arrow*), which can be seen disappearing deep to the fibers of the soleus muscle. C, A finger or right-angle clamp being placed deep to the soleus muscle before cutting it at its origin from the fibrous band that attaches to the back of the tibia. This exposes the origin of the anterior tibial artery and its accompanying vein or veins. D, Division of these veins allows further retraction of overlying veins and exposure of the tibioperoneal trunk and its terminal branches. E, Tunnels are fashioned by finger dissection.

F, Details of vein preparation using a long (6-inch) cannula to permit the vein to be distended in segments so that leaks can be controlled and recanalized segments detected. G, Elevation of the arteries by Silastic vessel loops and the beginning of the scalpel incision in the artery. In this view, only the taut Silastic loops are required to control bleeding, except for the posterior tibial artery, which also has a microvascular clip applied to it. H, Placement of a mosquito clamp to facilitate extension of the initial opening in the artery (1). Alternatively, a microvascular scissors may be used to extend the arteriotomy if the vessel is thin walled and normal (2). I, Details of the anastomotic suturing, which is begun at the distal end and continued to the midportion of each side of the anastomosis of the artery and the saphenous vein graft. Equal bites of all layers of each vessel are included in each stitch, which is always placed under direct vision. F, Completed graft in place. If more distal exposure of the posterior tibial or peroneal arteries is required, further separation of the soleus muscle from the posterior surface of the tibia and its overlying muscles provides access to the neurovascular bundles. Careful dissection of the veins with ligation of crossing branches provides access to the more deeply placed arteries. These can be dissected free, taking great care to preserve all branches, so that an appropriate segment of artery can be elevated and controlled to perform the distal anastomosis. (From Veith FJ, Gupta SK: Femoral-distal artery bypasses. In Bergan JJ, Yao JST [eds]: Operative Techniques in Vascular Surgery. New York, Grune & Stratton, 1980, pp 141–150.)

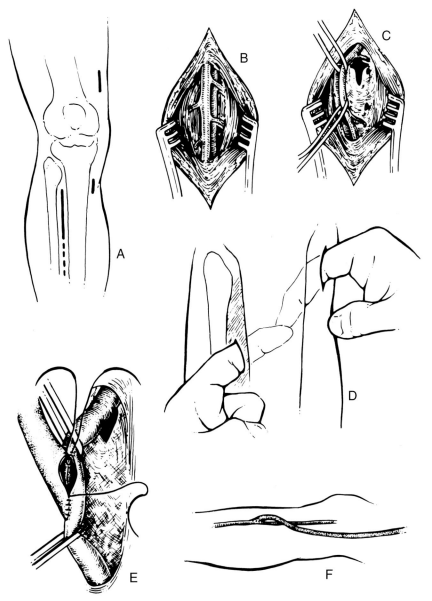

Figure 28–5. Bypass to the anterior tibial artery in the upper and middle thirds of the leg. *A,* This requires an anterolateral incision in the leg midway between the tibia and fibula over the appropriate segment of patent artery. Additional small medial incisions are also required for tunneling. *B,* The anterior incision is carried through the deep fascia, and the fibers of the anterior tibial muscle and the long extensors of the toes are separated to reveal the neurovascular bundle. Mobilization of accompanying veins with division of branches allows visualization of the anterior tibial artery, which can then be carefully mobilized. *C,* After the artery is freed, it is elevated and retracted along with the accompanying veins by Silastic loops. This permits further posterior dissection, which allows the interosseous membrane to be visualized and incised in a cruciate fashion. *D,* Careful blunt finger dissection from this anterior approach and from the popliteal fossa via the medial incision facilitates creation of a tunnel without injuring the numerous veins in the area. Alternatively, the tunnel for the bypass may be placed lateral to the knee in a subcutaneous plane. *E,* By elevating the anterior tibial artery, a meticulous distal anastomosis can be constructed as already described. *F,* The resulting graft in place. (From Veith FJ, Gupta SK: Femoral-distal artery bypasses. In Bergan JJ, Yao JST [eds]: Operative Techniques in Vascular Surgery. New York, Grune & Stratton, 1980, pp 141–150.)

the anastomotic lumen. Intraoperative angiographic examination is performed after most small vessel bypasses, but only if special problems are encountered after a femoropopliteal bypass. Although many vascular surgeons think of completion angiography as a panacea, it is not. Defects can be overlooked or not visualized because the proximal portion of the reconstruction is not included on the film. Moreover, "pseudodefects" may be visualized and may prompt time-consuming, needless, and potentially harmful further manipulation.[69] Intraoperative fluoroscopy is a very useful adjunct to infrainguinal bypass surgery.[70] After introduction of a small diagnostic catheter, the graft, both anastomoses, and the runoff vessels can be carefully evaluated in multiple planes with minimal contrast, enhancing the accuracy of the study.[71] In addition, intraoperative duplex scanning can be an additional adjunct to evaluate the hemodynamics of the arterial tree and bypass graft immediately after completion of the procedure.[72] Both techniques allow prompt diagnosis and correction of any problems.

Bypasses to Ankle or Foot Arteries

For many years, our group has advocated the effectiveness of performing bypasses to arteries near the ankle or in the foot in patients who have no usable patent artery for distal bypass insertion at a more proximal level.[6, 28] With adequate preoperative arteriography, these very distal arteries can usually be visualized if they are patent. Indeed, visualization of such arteries and using them for bypass insertion has been a major factor in reducing the proportion of patients whose arterial disease was so distal that they were "unsuitable for an attempt at limb salvage" or inoperable. Although our advocacy of these very distal perimalleolar and inframalleolar bypasses was at first greeted with skepticism, these procedures are now being performed and advocated widely. Excellent results have been reported for perimalleolar and inframalleolar bypasses to major arteries.[28, 29, 32] In addition, bypasses to the plantar and tarsal branches of pedal arteries can be successfully performed[30, 31] (Fig. 28–6; see also Figs. 28–1, 28–2, and 28–3).

Perioperative and Postoperative Drug Treatment

All patients receive prophylactic antibiotic treatment with 1 g of cefazolin preoperatively and postoperatively, if necessary. All receive heparin, 100 to 150 units/kg, during periods of vascular occlusion, and adequate anticoagulation is ensured by following activated clotting times (ACTs) intraoperatively.

Based on the experimental observations of Oblath and colleagues,[73] all patients receive perioperative antiplatelet therapy. This generally consists of 325 mg of aspirin given one to three times daily, with or without the addition of a more potent agent, such as clopidogrel. Therapy is begun 48 hours before operation and continued for several weeks.[4] After this period, one of these drugs, usually aspirin, is continued indefinitely if possible.

Management of Foot Lesions

Approximately 75% of our patients have gangrenous or necrotic foot or toe lesions.[1, 6] Small (less than 2 cm²), uninfected gangrenous lesions on the toe or foot are not treated. Larger gangrenous lesions and any area of infection associated with necrosis is usually extensively débrided at the end of any arterial reconstruction. These débridements often require excision of one or more toes and frequently consist of a partial (medial or lateral) transmetatarsal amputation. An attempt is made to excise enough bone so that overhanging skin and soft tissue is present. These wounds are usually left open, and drying of the soft tissues is prevented by placing a normal saline wet dressing on the wound. Subsequent débridement of foot lesions is often required on the ward or in the operating room. This is performed to remove all infected or necrotic tissue and exposed cartilage without regard for anatomic landmarks.

Performing multiple secondary operative procedures is sometimes necessary, particularly in diabetic patients, to achieve a healed foot. Skin grafts are used to cover large cutaneous defects but are placed only when the wound is rendered entirely clean and granulating by débridement and frequent dressing changes. In some patients, particularly those with extensive foot gangrene or infection and a femoropopliteal bypass that is inserted into an isolated popliteal artery segment, achieving healing at the metatarsal or even tarsal level is impossible, and below-knee amputation is required even though the bypass is patent. In some similar instances, foot healing has been obtained by performing a secondary bypass to an artery distal to the popliteal segment.[26] However, in the occasional patient with extensive infection and necrosis, a healed foot cannot be obtained even with straight-line arterial flow into pedal arteries. This is particularly common in patients with end-stage renal disease and diabetes.[75]

Reoperation

Host patients whose bypasses thrombose in the first month after operation undergo reoperation. The techniques employed have been described in detail elsewhere.[76]

Intraoperative fluoroscopy is a very useful adjunct to the performance of graft and arterial thrombectomy and for complete evaluation of the graft inflow and outflow vessels.[70, 77] It significantly improves intraoperative evaluation and surgical manipulations compared with static intraoperative angiography.

Vein grafts that failed immediately after operation usually require interposition of a segment of PTFE[78] or total

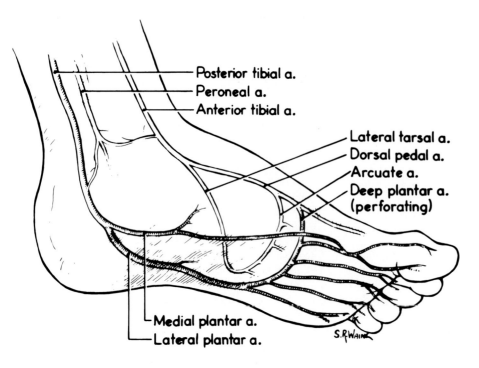

Figure 28–6. Named arteries in the ankle region and foot. Any of the main arteries or their branches, if patent, may be approached surgically and used as the distal outflow for a limb salvage bypass. (From Ascer E, Veith FJ, Gupta SK: Bypasses to plantar arteries and other tibial branches: An extended approach to limb salvage. J Vasc Surg 8:434–441, 1988.)

replacement with this material, although in our experience an occasional thrombectomized vein graft remains patent if no causative lesion is present.

Patients whose bypasses thrombose after the first postoperative month are considered for aggressive reoperation, and femoral angiography is usually performed; however, the patients are subjected to reoperation only if the bypass failure is associated with a renewed threat to limb viability. If the patient has originally undergone operation elsewhere and details of the first operation are not known or the distal anastomosis is at or below the knee joint, a totally new bypass is usually performed. This is best accomplished using a variety of unusual approaches that permit access to infrainguinal arteries via unscarred, uninfected tissue planes.[76, 78, 79] These approaches include a direct approach to the distal two thirds of the deep femoral artery[80, 81] (Figs. 28–7 and 28–8), lateral approaches to the popliteal artery above and below the knee,[82] and medial or lateral approaches to all three of the infrapopliteal arteries. In addition to permitting dissection in virginal tissue planes, these unusual access routes facilitate the use of shorter grafts, which enable the surgeon to use the patient's remaining segments of good vein when his or her ipsilateral greater saphenous vein has been used or injured by the primary operation.

If the surgeon elects to salvage an old PTFE graft, which may be appropriate if the original distal anastomosis was above the knee and the patient's veins are poor as determined by venography or duplex ultrasonography, appropriate surgical techniques are critical to obtaining a favorable outcome.[76, 79] The prior distal incision is opened, and the distal end of the graft, the distal anastomosis, and the proximal and distal artery are dissected free. The graft is opened with a longitudinal incision to within a few millimeters of its distal tip (Fig. 28–9). The graft is then thrombectomized by passage of balloon catheters, best performed under fluoroscopic control.[71] This technique allows the evaluation of the contour of the thrombectomy balloon for a potential lesion and its location. In addition, catheter-wire techniques can be used to advance a thrombectomy catheter safely in patients in whom this catheter is difficult to advance.

Thrombus is gently removed from the distal anastomosis under direct vision, and balloon catheters are passed proximally and distally in the artery using extreme gentleness and care. If no disease or defect is seen within the anastomotic lumen, the opening in the graft is closed and a complete fluoroscopic evaluation of the inflow, graft, and outflow vessels is performed. If no lesion is found, the operation is terminated. If intimal hyperplasia or other disease is noted at or just distal to the anastomosis, the opening in the graft is extended across its toe and down the artery to a point beyond the disease. A patch graft is placed to close this opening, and a completion study is performed. If graft thrombosis has resulted from progression of arteriosclerosis proximal or distal to an anastomosis, an appropriate graft extension is constructed after removing all clot. Failed below-knee PTFE femoropopliteal and small vessel bypasses can be similarly managed but are probably best treated by performance of an entirely new

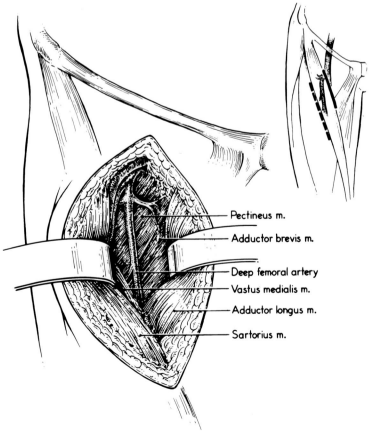

Figure 28–7. Incisions and anatomy for direct approaches to the distal two thirds of the deep femoral artery. (From Nunez A, Veith FJ, Collier P, et al: Direct approach to the distal portions of the deep femoral artery for limb salvage bypasses. J Vasc Surg 8:576–581, 1988.)

Pectineus m.
Adductor brevis m.
Deep femoral artery
Vastus medialis m.
Adductor longus m.
Sartorius m.

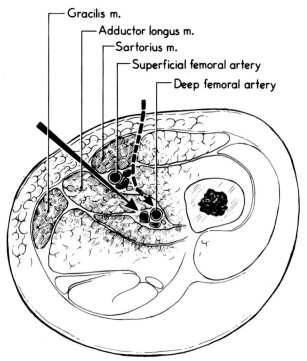

- Gracilis m.
- Adductor longus m.
- Sartorius m.
- Superficial femoral artery
- Deep femoral artery

Figure 28–8. Cross-sectional anatomy for direct approaches to the distal two thirds of the deep femoral artery. (From Nunez A, Veith FJ, Collier P, et al: Direct approach to the distal portions of the deep femoral artery for limb salvage bypass. J Vasc Surg 8:576–581, 1988.)

bypass, preferably with vein and using previously undissected arteries, if possible. Thrombolytic therapy can be used to salvage a thrombosed graft, but its role in the treatment of these patients is still under evaluation. Early results suggest that lysis of a prosthetic graft leads to only a 25% 6-month patency rate after the intervention.[83] If a treatable lesion is found, the results are better, with a 6-month patency rate of 80%.[83]

Failing Graft Concept

Intimal hyperplasia, progression of proximal or distal disease, or lesions within the graft itself can produce signs and symptoms of hemodynamic deterioration in patients with a prior arterial reconstruction without producing concomitant thrombosis of the bypass graft.[84–86] We have referred to this condition as a "failing graft" because, if the lesion is not corrected, graft thrombosis will almost certainly occur.[85] The importance of this failing graft concept lies in the fact that many difficult lower extremity revascularizations can be salvaged for protracted periods by relatively simple interventions if the lesion responsible for the circulatory deterioration and diminished graft blood flow can be detected before graft thrombosis occurs.

We have now been able to detect more than 250 failing grafts and to correct the lesions before graft thrombosis has occurred. The majority of these grafts were vein grafts, but approximately one half were prosthetic grafts.[87] Invariably the corrective procedure is simpler than the secondary operation required if the bypass had gone on to thrombose. Some lesions responsible for the failing state could be remedied by percutaneous transluminal angioplasty (PTA), although many required a vein patch angioplasty, a short bypass of a graft lesion, or a proximal or distal graft extension. Some of the transluminal angioplasties of these lesions failed and required a second reintervention; others remained effective in correcting the responsible lesion, as documented by arteriography more than 2 to 5 years later. If the failing graft is a vein bypass, detection of the failing state permits accurate localization and definition of the responsible lesion by arteriography and salvage of any undiseased vein. In contrast, if the graft is permitted to thrombose, the responsible lesion may be difficult to identify; the vein may be difficult or impossible to thrombectomize; and the patient's best graft, the ipsilateral greater saphenous vein, may have to be sacrificed, rendering the secondary operation even more difficult and more likely to

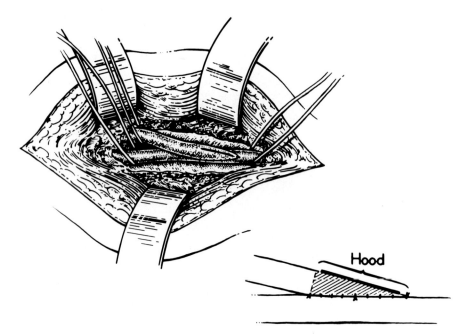

Hood

Figure 28–9. Technique for a reoperation in which graft salvage will be attempted. Control of the artery proximal and distal to the anastomosis must be obtained. The opening in the graft is placed so that the interior of the anastomosis can be visualized.

fail with associated limb loss. Most important, the results of reinterventions for failing grafts, in terms of both continued cumulative patency and limb salvage rates, have been far superior to the results of reinterventions for grafts that have thrombosed and failed.[85–88]

This difference in results, together with the ease of reintervention for failing grafts, mandates that surgeons performing infrainguinal bypass operations monitor their patients closely in the postoperative period and indefinitely thereafter. Ideally, noninvasive laboratory tests, including duplex studies, should be performed with similar frequency.[88] If the patient has any recurrence of symptoms or the surgeon detects *any* change in peripheral pulse examination or other manifestations of ischemia, the circulatory deterioration must be confirmed by noninvasive modalities and *urgent arteriography.* If a lesion is detected as a cause of the failing state, it is corrected urgently by PTA or operation. Surgical reconstruction is the treatment of choice for failing vein graft lesions,[89–91] but single lesions less than 1.5 cm in length with grafts more than 3.0 mm in diameter yield reasonable results after successful PTA.[91] The role of stents and atherectomy devices for these lesions is still under investigation.

Role of Angioplasty

Opinions regarding the usefulness of angioplasty differ considerably, and its exact role in the treatment of infrainguinal arteriosclerosis is still somewhat controversial. Our own[92] and others'[93, 94] experience suggests that with appropriate patient selection and in skilled hands, the complication rate is low. Moreover, when complications or failure of PTA do occur, they can generally be well treated by relatively simple surgical procedures with little if any increased patient morbidity or mortality.[92]

On this basis, we presently attempt a PTA on any patient with sufficiently severe disease and ischemia (usually stage III or IV) to warrant intervention and in whom the procedure is deemed suitable. Patients with stage III or IV ischemia who have a hemodynamically significant segmental iliac stenosis and infrainguinal arteriosclerosis generally have a PTA, with or without stent placement, of the iliac lesion as their first therapeutic intervention. If the PTA is unsuccessful, a bypass to the femoral level is performed. If the PTA is successful, further arterial intervention, usually some form of infrainguinal bypass, is performed only if the ischemia is unrelieved and a healed foot cannot be obtained. We do not hesitate to perform a bypass distal to an iliac artery treated by PTA, and subsequent experience has borne out the effectiveness of this approach.[1, 6, 95, 96]

PTA is also used as the primary therapeutic intervention in patients without hemodynamically significant iliac artery disease who have a short (5-cm) segmental stenosis of the superficial femoral or popliteal artery, if this lesion is judged hemodynamically significant on the basis of pulse examination or noninvasive testing. In slightly less than half of our cases treated by angioplasty, some form of direct arterial surgery has also been required, usually for bypass of a second lesion distal to the one successfully treated by angioplasty.[1, 6] PTA has also been effective in the treatment of stenotic lesions in tibial arteries and stenoses developing

in or proximal or distal to a still-functioning vein or PTFE graft.[1, 85, 94, 97] After reviewing our data for infrainguinal PTA we narrowed our indications for its use. Only focal isolated stenotic lesions less than or equal to 1.5 cm in length are being treated with angioplasty because of poor results in other lesions. The role of atherectomy, stents, and endovascular grafts for infrainguinal disease has been less promising but is still under evaluation.[98, 99] The successful subintimal recanalization of both femoropopliteal and crural segments was reported by Bolia and colleagues[100] and by London and associates[101] with encouraging results.

RESULTS OF TREATMENT

Arteriosclerotic involvement is generally less, both in regard to extent and multiplicity of lesions, in patients with intermittent claudication than in those who have a threatened limb. Not surprisingly, short-term and long-term patency results of infrainguinal arterial bypasses performed for intermittent claudication are generally better than those done for limb salvage, and this difference has been documented by virtually every author who evaluated results on the basis of operative indications.[50, 102] Because we believe that femoropopliteal bypass should rarely be performed for intermittent claudication and that the other infrainguinal bypasses should never be performed for this indication alone, we restrict our discussion of results to operations performed because of severe ischemic rest pain, a nonhealing ulcer, or gangrene. However, femoropopliteal bypasses for truly disabling claudication are justified by their good results and low risk rate,[2] provided the patient is informed of the risks of intervention. In our experience, when patients are so informed, they usually opt for a trial of noninterventional treatment before considering other options.

Results of infrainguinal bypasses clearly vary with the training, technical skill, and commitment of the surgeon. These operations are demanding and should be performed only by surgeons doing them regularly and, more important, by surgeons with the skill and commitment to reoperate successfully should a bypass fail in the early or late postoperative period. In deciding whether these operations and an aggressive approach to limb salvage are, in fact, justified in a given setting, vascular surgeons should continually examine their own results to see if they are good enough to justify continued application of these sometimes difficult operations in these often brittle patients.

Operative Mortality

The 30-day mortality for all patients undergoing infrainguinal arterial reconstructions for threatened limbs ranges from 2% to 6%.[1, 6, 76, 103] Operative mortality is slightly greater for infrapopliteal and axillopopliteal bypasses than for femoropopliteal bypasses, probably because the former operations are required in patients with more advanced generalized as well as lower extremity disease. The principal cause of death from these operations is myocardial infarction.

These low operative mortalities contrast with the high late-death rates reflected in Figure 28–10, which shows

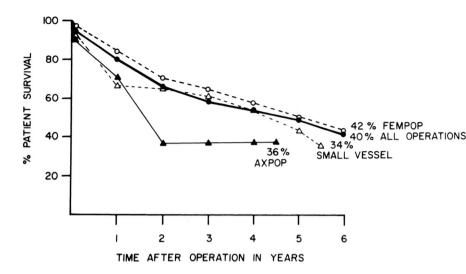

Figure 28–10. Cumulative life-table patient survival rates after 318 femoropopliteal (FEMPOP), 204 small vessel (infrapopliteal), and 29 axillopopliteal (AXPOP) bypasses. Fifty-two percent of all patients undergoing all reconstructive arterial operations for limb-threatening infrainguinal arteriosclerosis died within 5 years. (From Veith FJ, Gupta SK, Samson RH, et al: Progress in limb salvage by reconstructive arterial surgery combined with new or improved adjunctive procedures. Ann Surg 194:386–400, 1981.)

that only 48% of all patients who had arterial reconstructions were alive 5 years later. Almost all late deaths were unrelated to the original operation, most being due to concurrent arteriosclerotic events, chiefly myocardial infarction. These findings again reflect the advanced stage of generalized arteriosclerosis present in these patients.

Limb Salvage

When the aggressive approach already outlined for the management of patients whose limbs are threatened by infrainguinal arteriosclerosis was used and when only those patients who had organic mental syndrome and extensive local gangrene were excluded, 96% of patients underwent arteriographic examination.[6] Ninety-four percent of patients who underwent arteriography were suitable candidates for some form of arterial revascularization procedure. With recent technical advances, only 1% to 2% of patients undergoing arteriography do not have some patent distal artery suitable for use in an attempt at revascularization, and most of these are patients who underwent previous failed operations.[1]

Immediate Limb Salvage

Defined as relief of ischemia and healing of ischemic lesions for 1 month after the first revascularization procedure, immediate limb salvage was achieved in 86% of patients in whom revascularization was possible.[6] This immediate limb salvage rate was calculated by subtracting from the number of patients who could undergo revascularization procedures those patients who died or whose arterial reconstructive operation or angioplasty failed irretrievably within 1 month of the primary procedure and those patients who required major amputations despite a successful revascularization procedure. Multiple local operations and prolonged hospitalizations were required to achieve foot healing in 7% of our patients. Heel and forefoot gangrene did not preclude ultimate limb salvage, although they could, if extensive, contribute to the need for prolonged periods of hospitalization. Even when the initial

procedure attempted to achieve limb salvage failed immediately, the involved extremity could often be saved by promptly performing some secondary procedure.[1, 6, 86] This was particularly common if a PTA was technically unsuccessful or failed to improve the arterial supply to the foot.[1, 6, 92]

Late Limb Salvage

The cumulative limb salvage rates for all patients having arterial reconstructive operations are shown in Figure 28–11. Sixty-six percent of the patients who survived 5 years after a reconstructive arterial operation below the inguinal ligament for limb salvage had an intact limb up to that time. The limb salvage rates were better after femoropopliteal bypass than after a small vessel bypass or an axillopopliteal bypass (P <.25) (Fig. 28–12). Even though all operations were performed because the limb was threatened, limb salvage rates (see Fig. 28–12) could not be equated to bypass patency rates (Fig. 28–13). In some patients, gangrene and infection had been healed by the original operation, and the limb remained intact when the bypass thrombosed; moreover, in many instances when the limb was rethreatened, bypass patency could be restored by appropriate reoperation. This was particularly common if the original procedure had been a femoropopliteal bypass.[76] On the other hand, limb salvage rates could be rendered lower than bypass patency rates if a major amputation was required despite a patent arterial reconstruction, which is most common in patients with end-stage renal disease.[75]

Patency of Arterial Reconstructive Operations

Older cumulative life-table patency rates for reconstructive arterial operations are shown in Figure 28–13. More recent patency rates have improved somewhat and continue to be significantly better for femoropopliteal bypasses than for small vessel or axillopopliteal bypasses (P <.01). Our small vessel bypass patency rate was not affected by age, sex,

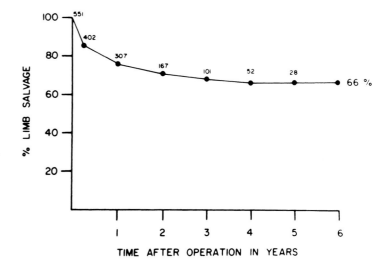

Figure 28–11. Cumulative life-table limb salvage rates of all patients undergoing reconstructive arterial operations for limb-threatening infrainguinal arteriosclerosis. The number with each point indicates the number of cases observed with intact limbs for that length of time. (From Veith FJ, Gupta SK, Samson RH, et al: Progress in limb salvage by reconstructive arterial surgery combined with new or improved adjunctive procedures. Ann Surg 194:386–400, 1981.)

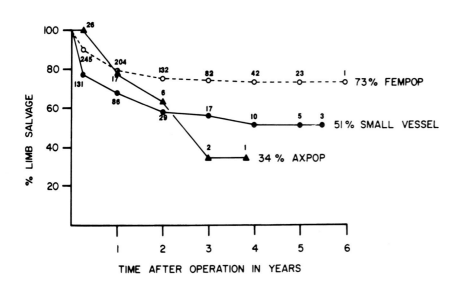

Figure 28–12. Cumulative life-table limb salvage rates of 318 femoropopliteal (FEMPOP), 204 small vessel (infrapopliteal), and 29 axillopopliteal (AXPOP) bypasses performed for limb-threatening infrainguinal arteriosclerosis. The number with each point indicates the number of cases observed with intact limbs for that length of time. (From Veith FJ, Gupta SK, Samson RH, et al: Progress in limb salvage by reconstructive arterial surgery combined with new or improved adjunctive procedures. Ann Surg 194:386–400, 1981.)

Figure 28–13. Cumulative life-table patency rates of 318 femoropopliteal (FEMPOP), 204 small vessel (infrapopliteal), and 29 axillopopliteal (AXPOP) bypasses performed for limb-threatening infrainguinal arteriosclerosis. The number with each point indicates the number of cases observed to be patent for that length of time. (From Veith FJ, Gupta SK, Samson RH, et al: Progress in limb salvage by reconstructive arterial surgery combined with new or improved adjunctive procedures. Ann Surg 194:386–400, 1981.)

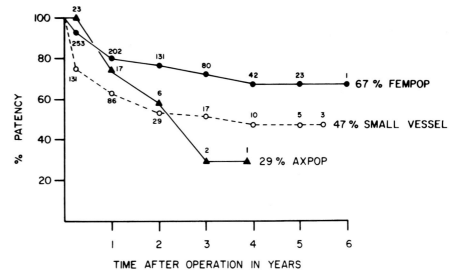

hypertensive or diabetic status, or previous ipsilateral bypass. In contrast to reports from other groups, an incomplete plantar arch, a heavily calcified bypass insertion site, an unusable saphenous vein, and a very low ankle pressure did not preclude long-term success, although these factors were associated with a somewhat higher early failure rate.[1, 6]

Results

Several reports have documented better late limb salvage and bypass patency results than those presented. Although some of these apparently improved results may reflect more refined surgical and management techniques, these more optimistic reports have generally included only patients operated on by a particular surgical technique, such as reversed vein bypass or in situ vein bypass. Because these techniques, although ideal, are not applicable to all patients with a threatened lower extremity, the older statistics that are presented above probably are still representative of the overall results that can be achieved in an entire group of patients undergoing lower limb arterial reconstruction to save an extremity. Moreover, some articles with favorable late bypass patency results are actually reporting secondary patency figures that are achievable with a more aggressive policy of detecting and reintervening on failing bypasses, and some reports include results on substantial numbers of patients undergoing operation for intermittent claudication. Thus, although reports of results may be real, much of the success may be due to patient selection and differences in the methods of reporting or analyzing results.

Angioplasty Durability

Eleven percent of our iliac angioplasties and 8% of our femoropopliteal angioplasties were initially unsuccessful. If one considers the durability of those angioplasties that were initially successful, cumulative life-table patency at 4 years was 78% for the iliac angioplasties but significantly less for femoropopliteal procedures. The use of stents has improved the results of iliac angioplasty, but their role for infrainguinal lesions is still unclear. Femoropopliteal angioplasties are reserved for single stenotic lesions less than or equal to 1.5 cm in length. Surgical techniques are used for more extensive lesions and angioplasty failures. This approach resulted in protracted limb salvage in more than 70% of cases. We continue to regard PTA, when performed by a committed radiology-surgery team, as an important part of an aggressive approach to salvaging limbs.[1] However, 81% of patients with threatened limbs require operative treatment at some point in their course; only 19% can be treated by PTA alone.[1]

Reoperations

Our policy of performing a graft thrombectomy on all thrombosed small vessel and axillopopliteal bypasses, if and when the thrombosis was associated with a threat to the limb, has not resulted in any operative deaths, but has generally been unrewarding. The majority of these reoperated grafts rethrombosed within a few days, weeks, or months. In occasional instances (approximately 10% of such cases), patency was restored and persisted more than 3 years.

Thus, our present policy for the treatment of failed small vessel bypass if the limb is rethreatened is to perform an entirely new bypass to another segment, not operated on, of an infrapopliteal artery. Our results with such secondary small vessel bypasses have not differed greatly from those of primary procedures, although others have not had a similar experience.

The results of aggressive reoperation for failed vein and nonvein *femoropopliteal bypasses* have been surprisingly good.[1, 6, 76, 86, 104, 105] In our series of 318 femoropopliteal bypasses, 13 failed *during the first month after operation,* and all were treated by reoperation. One postoperative death and two late deaths occurred among the patients with patent bypasses, 3 and 14 months after operation. Eight of the 10 other bypasses were patent for 2 to 44 months (mean, 25 months). The ninth patient had a viable limb 26 months after the original operation, although the graft subsequently rethrombosed 1 year ago, and the 10th patient also had a viable limb 4 months after the original operation, although her graft reoccluded 2 months after her reoperation.

Thirty-nine of our femoropopliteal bypasses failed *more than 1 month after operation* and were considered for aggressive reoperation. A conservative approach to a failed bypass that did not place the limb in jeopardy was justified by the continued viability for 2 to 72 months of all eight limbs in this category. Reoperation was performed in the remaining 31 patients with threatened limbs. In 28 patients, bypass patency was reestablished for at least 2 months. In 20 patients, graft patency persisted until death or the present. The range of patency after reoperation in this group of 20 patients is 2 to 48 months, with a mean of over 17 months, although seven patients required a secondary reoperation to maintain bypass patency and limb viability. Sixteen grafts have remained open more than 1 year after reoperation. Only 8 of the 39 patients in whom late graft occlusion occurred ultimately required a major amputation, and in all but two instances this could be successfully performed below the knee. One of the 31 patients died within 1 month of the reoperation.

The sustained effectiveness of appropriate reoperations when limb salvage femoropopliteal bypasses fail in the early or late postoperative period is illustrated by Figure 28–14, which shows that reoperation increased overall patency rates by 15% at 5 years. When the same calculations were applied to 440 cases with longer periods of follow-up, this difference between primary and secondary patency rates at 5 years fell to 8%. Limb salvage rates are, of course, similarly increased by effective reoperations. The efficacy of such reoperations in maintaining durable patency is further shown by the cumulative life-table 4- to 6-year patency rate of 56% for our 44 femoropopliteal bypasses requiring reoperation for thrombosis. Limb salvage rates were even higher. Similar patency rates and limb salvage rates have also been achieved by Whittemore and colleagues,[86] who employed reoperations in the management of a group of patients with failed vein femoropopliteal

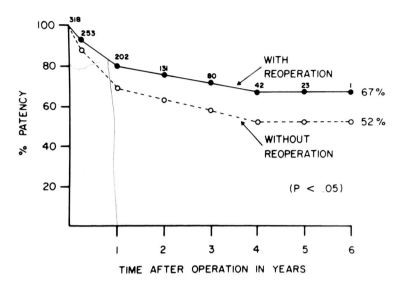

Figure 28–14. Cumulative life-table patency rates of 318 femoropopliteal bypasses performed for limb salvage. The upper curve was calculated without regard to whether a reoperation was required to maintain patency. The lower curve was calculated on the basis of time to first bypass occlusion even if reoperation restored patency. The number with each point indicates the number of cases observed to be patent for that length of time. (From Veith FJ, Gupta SK, Samson RH, et al: Progress in limb salvage by reconstructive arterial surgery combined with new or improved adjunctive procedures. Ann Surg 194:386–400, 1981.)

bypasses and threatened limbs. Whittemore's group, our group, and many other groups have found that detection of *failing* reconstructions *before* graft thrombosis has occurred permits simpler corrective measures to be used and results in much better long-term graft patency and limb salvage rates.[78, 84–87, 91, 106]

Although Craver and his colleagues[107] showed many years ago that reoperation for early postoperative thrombosis of femoropopliteal vein grafts was associated with poor long-term patency rates, we have found this not to be the case with PTFE bypasses above the knee,[76] and Whittemore and associates[86] have reported similar protracted successes after reoperation for failure of saphenous vein femoropopliteal grafts. Appropriate use of intraoperative angiography and other technical details of these reoperations are important in achieving the reported good results. In both series, surgical clot removal from thrombosed vein and PTFE grafts sometimes allows these conduits to be used effectively for protracted periods if all other lesions encroaching substantially on the lumen are corrected or bypassed.[76, 86]

Lytic Agents

A number of reports have advocated the use of intraarterially administered streptokinase, urokinase, and tissue plasminogen activator (t-PA) to restore patency to thrombosed infrainguinal grafts. Although these agents may ultimately prove to be useful to treat failed grafts and to detect the cause of failure, PTA or surgical graft revision is almost always required to correct the lesion causing thrombosis. In patients showing acute ischemia and a closed graft, urokinase has been successfully used as with other patients with acute ischemia.[12] Early reports suggest that these agents can restore patency in 70% to 90% of grafts but short-term results are very poor if a treatable lesion is not found.[83] Moreover, the long-term efficacy of such combined procedures remains to be demonstrated, and in most patients we still believe that a totally new bypass is the best treatment for a thrombosed graft that is associated with limb-threatening ischemia.

Arteriographic Outflow Characteristics of the Popliteal Artery and Patency

With significant numbers of patients now receiving follow-up for 5 years or more, patency rates of femoropopliteal bypasses inserted into popliteal artery segments that appeared on arteriograms to be occluded at both ends were not significantly different from those of bypasses inserted into popliteal arteries that appeared to be continuous with one or more of their main terminal branches. These results support the use of femoropopliteal bypass to isolated segments of popliteal artery in selected patients.[26, 108] This appears to be true even when the absence of a usable saphenous vein makes it necessary to use a PTFE graft. A major disadvantage is the high incidence of continued threat to the limb despite a patent bypass. This is particularly common if extensive gangrene or infection in the foot is present.[26] In such circumstances, a femoral-to-popliteal-to-small vessel bypass or sequential bypass is indicated, and the distalmost portion of this complex bypass is best performed with autologous vein if it is available in any of the patient's extremities.[25, 26, 109, 110]

Relationship of Position of Anastomosis to Patency

In our hands, femoropopliteal bypass patency was not significantly influenced solely by the position of the distal anastomosis relative to the knee joint. This was true with both PTFE and vein grafts. Other patient-related factors are probably more important in determining patency than the location of the popliteal anastomosis. These factors are not controlled in any study comparing above-knee and below-knee results, thereby rendering the comparisons meaningless in terms of selecting the best level of popliteal artery to use if it is patent above and below the knee in a given patient.

Amputation Level

When major amputation was required after a revascularization procedure had been performed, every effort was made to perform it at the below-knee level. This was possible in all 18 patients who required amputation despite a patent bypass, in 90% of patients who required a major amputation when a femoropopliteal bypass occluded, in 69% of patients who required a major amputation after a failed small vessel bypass, and in 30% of major amputations required after thrombosis of an axillopopliteal bypass.[6] The operative mortality rate for these secondary amputations was 4%.

ANALYSIS OF COST-BENEFIT RATIO OF AGGRESSIVE EFFORTS AT LIMB SALVAGE

Our results indicate that more than 98% of patients whose limbs are threatened because of infrainguinal arteriosclerosis have a distribution of occlusive and stenotic arterial lesions that is suitable for reconstructive arterial surgery, which can relieve the ischemia at least partially and salvage the limb. The results also show that obtaining immediate limb salvage is possible in more than 85% of the patients in whom revascularization is possible, with an operative mortality rate of less than 4% and a low morbidity rate despite the existence in many patients of local and systemic factors that might, in the past, have precluded attempts at revascularization and limb salvage. These factors include advanced age, recent congestive heart failure or myocardial infarction, concurrent malignancy, extensive forefoot or heel gangrene, a contralateral amputation, an isolated popliteal artery segment, absence of usable saphenous vein, and the presence of a popliteal pulse with three-vessel occlusive disease in the upper, middle, and lower thirds of the leg. In the last circumstance, a bypass to a target artery at the ankle or foot level may still be feasible.

The fact that limbs can now be saved in such circumstances is of interest. Alone, it does not mean that limb salvage attempts, which may require multiple operations and prolonged periods of hospitalization to obtain a healed foot, are justified in this group of patients, whose life expectancy is known to be poor. Is the cost-benefit ratio such that attempts at limb salvage are worthwhile in these patients?

This is a difficult question to answer with certainty because, in part, the answer depends on one's philosophy and perspective and on subjective factors such as quality of life and the ability to live and function independently. However, certain objective parameters are relevant. Among these are the durability of limb salvage in surviving patients and the longevity of the patients. Figure 28–10 is an index of patient longevity. Figure 28–11 is a measure of the durability of limb salvage in surviving patients. Of the 48% of patients who survived 5 years after operation, two thirds retained their limb at least that long. Of every 100 patients who underwent operation, 68 lived at least 1 year after operation with an intact limb, and 54 lived at least 2 years with a viable, usable extremity. Moreover, of the 52% of the patients who died within 5 years, 88% (81% to 95%) retained the salvaged limb until they died (Fig. 28–15). Both we and almost all of our patients believe that these benefits outweigh the risks and costs of an aggressive attempt at limb salvage, even if this attempt entails a lengthy period of hospitalization with several operative procedures to achieve a healed foot. Similar conclusions have been reached by Reichle and Tyson,[103] Maini and Mannick,[111] and Perdue,[112] Bartlett,[104] and Auer[113] and their colleagues in their analyses of patients with limb-threatening ischemia.

A case can also be made for performing a primary below-knee amputation in some or all of these patients, and relatively rapid rehabilitation may be achieved with such a procedure.[114, 115] However, our experience has shown that older, poor-risk patients do not ambulate easily or quickly with a below-knee prosthesis.[116] Such patients may never walk and, if they do, may require 2 or 3 months of institutional training to learn. For some patients, limb salvage offers the only opportunity for them to care for themselves, maintain their independence, and avoid permanent admission to an institution. Furthermore, in many patients the opposite limb soon becomes threatened be-

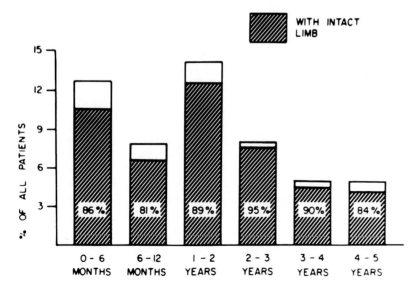

Figure 28–15. Percentage of all patients who underwent limb salvage attempts and who died in the various intervals after operation. The cross-hatched areas indicate the proportion of these patients who died without losing their previously threatened limb. (From Veith FJ, Gupta SK, Samson RH, et al: Progress in limb salvage by reconstructive arterial surgery combined with new or improved adjunctive procedures. Ann Surg 194:386–400, 1981.)

cause of the symmetry of the disease process, and salvage of at least one limb is critical for the patient to maintain independence. Finally, the point has been made that unsuccessful attempts at limb salvage result in a high incidence of loss of the knee.[50, 115, 117] Our data fail to confirm this except after failed axillopopliteal bypass, a procedure performed in patients with the most advanced disease. Thus, we believe that limb salvage should be attempted if suitable vessels for revascularization are present, unless the patient has severe organic mental syndrome or gangrene and infection proximal to the midfoot.

Economic Impact of Limb Salvage

The dollar cost of an aggressive approach to salvage limbs is high, with a mean cost of $19,000 for femoropopliteal bypass and $29,000 for small vessel bypass. These figures include all physician, hospital, and rehabilitation costs, including those of reoperations. On the other hand, the mean total cost of below-knee amputation, which in 26% of our patients resulted in failed rehabilitation with a need for chronic institutional care or professional assistance at home, was $27,000. Thus, limb salvage surgery is expensive but no more so than the less attractive alternative of amputation.[118] In the new climate of decreasing medical expenses, many of these patients are being treated successfully with significantly shorter hospital stays and decreased costs.

NEW DEVELOPMENTS

Clearly, all the principles and practices outlined thus far describe our present attitudes toward the treatment of a complex disease process. As we have tried to point out, many of these attitudes are controversial. More important, they are all in a state of constant evolution. As more data and newer methods become available, our attitudes and those of others interested in the problems of femoral-popliteal-tibial arteriosclerosis should and will change. In this section we describe briefly some of the new developments that have the greatest likelihood of leading to future therapeutic improvements.

Improvements in Diagnostic Techniques

Noninvasive arterial evaluations, including duplex scanning,[72] MR angiography,[18, 19] and helical CT scanning, are rapidly improving and may become the initial diagnostic modality for patients with aortoiliac and infrainguinal aneurysmal and occlusive disease, but further refinements are needed before these techniques can replace diagnostic arteriography. Intravascular ultrasonography is another diagnostic modality being developed to better assess the extent of arterial disease and to evaluate immediate results after interventions.[119–121]

Improvements in Endovascular Devices

Angioplasty has been successfully used for the treatment of stenotic iliac lesions and the results have improved further with use of intravascular stents.[122] The role of infrainguinal angioplasty has been limited, and to date the use of stents has not significantly improved results. However, stents are being used for selected lesions in the femoral and popliteal arterial segments. Atherectomy has been successfully used in the coronary circulation, but the results for infrainguinal disease to date have been very poor.[123, 124]

A further development is the use of endovascular grafts. These have been successfully used for the treatment of a variety of arterial lesions with early success.[125] The role of the evolving techniques in the treatment of infrainguinal disease is still unclear.

New Developments in Tibial and Pedal Bypasses

Since 1981, because of some of the promising results already discussed, we have been evaluating other procedures to simplify or extend the limits of operability for limb salvage. Some of these procedures show sufficient promise to deserve mention.

Tibiotibial bypasses are an extension of our concept of using more distal arteries as bypass origins than were previously thought optimal.[32] All these distal origin procedures allow shorter segments of saphenous vein to be used, shorten operative time, avoid dissection in obese or infected groins, and may have superior patency. We have now performed more than 80 distal vein bypasses to the lower third of the leg or foot using the infrapopliteal (tibial) arteries as inflow sites.[28, 29] Many of these grafts remained patent more than 4 years despite their insertion into isolated tibial artery segments and the fact that they were performed with saphenous veins 2.5 to 3.0 mm in smallest diameter (see Figs. 28–1, 28–2, and 28–3).

Small vessel bypasses to blind tibial artery segments have been performed in some patients facing imminent amputation. These operations have been done in patients in whom no other procedures were possible because of the arterial anatomy or local infection in the foot. Again, vein grafts were used. Several of these bypasses have remained patent over 2 years and many otherwise unsalvageable limbs have been saved.[28]

Use of heavily calcified tibial arteries for distal bypass insertion sites has been possible with a variety of techniques that include crushing of the involved artery and intraluminal occlusion to permit incision and suture placement. Acceptable early and midterm patency has resulted.[6] Small vessel bypasses to plantar and tarsal arterial branches can be achieved successfully in patients with patent pedal arches with acceptable long-term patency and excellent limb salvage results.[30, 31]

Minimally Invasive Adjunctive Techniques for Lower Extremity Vein Bypasses

Less invasive techniques are being developed for the performance of in situ and reversed saphenous vein bypasses.

The use of long flexible valvulotomes, angioscopic visualization,[126, 127] coil occlusion techniques for side branches,[128, 129] and endoscopic subcutaneous vein dissection and harvesting[130] may allow the performance of these lower extremity bypasses through minimal incisions, allowing diminished pain, fewer local complications, and decreased hospital stays for some patients.

Intraoperative Adjunctive Techniques and Procedures

The intraoperative use of fluoroscopy has added a new dimension to the options of the vascular surgeon. Diagnostic arteriography can be performed before and after a bypass procedure. Graft and arterial thrombectomies can be performed using catheter-guidewire techniques to improve success and safety.[71] The greater saphenous vein can be evaluated for in situ bypasses. Proximal and distal arterial lesions can be treated using balloon angioplasty[131] with or without the addition of intravascular stents. And finally, fluoroscopy allows the performance of complex procedures, such as endovascular grafting, that require the combined use of interventional and standard surgical techniques.[125] Angioscopy, duplex scanning, and intravascular ultrasonography are being increasingly used to improve the results of intraoperative procedures.

References

1. Veith FJ, Gupta SK, Wengerter KR, et al: Changing arteriosclerotic disease patterns and management strategies in lower limb–threatening ischemia. Ann Surg 212:402–414, 1990.
2. Donaldson MC, Mannick JA: Femoropopliteal bypass grafting for intermittent claudication: Is pessimism warranted? Arch Surg 115:724–727, 1980.
3. Boyd AM: The natural course of arteriosclerosis of the lower extremities. Proc R Soc Med 55:591–593, 1962.
4. Coran AG, Warren R: Arteriographic changes in femoropopliteal arteriosclerosis obliterans: A five year follow-up study. N Engl J Med 274:643–645, 1966.
5. Imparato AM, Kim GE, Davidson T, Crowley JG: Intermittent claudication: Its natural course. Surgery 78:795–797, 1975.
6. Veith FJ, Gupta SK, Samson RH, et al: Progress in limb salvage by reconstructive arterial surgery combined with new or improved adjunctive procedures. Ann Surg 194:386–401, 1981.
7. Goodreau JJ, Greasy JK, Flanigan DP, et al: Rational approach to the differentiation of vascular and neurogenic claudication. Surgery 84:749–757, 1978.
8. Kavanaugh GJ, Svien HJ, Holman CB, Johnson RM: "Pseudoclaudication" syndrome produced by compression of the cauda equina. JAMA 206:2477–2481, 1968.
9. Karmody AM, Powers SR, Monaco VJ, Leather RP: Blue toe syndrome: An indication for limb salvage surgery. Arch Surg 111:1263–1268, 1976.
10. Haimovici HC, Moss CM, Veith FJ: Arterial embolectomy revisited. Surgery 78:409–411, 1975.
11. Gupta SK, Samson RH, Veith FJ: Embolectomy of the distal part of the popliteal artery. Surg Gynecol Obstet 153:254–258, 1981.
12. Ouriel K, Shortell CK, DeWeese JA, et al: A comparison of thrombolytic therapy with operative revascularization in the initial treatment of acute peripheral arterial ischemia. J Vasc Surg 19:1021–1030, 1994.
13. Whittemore AD, Clowes AW, Hechtman HB, Mannick JA: Aortic aneurysm repair: Reduced operative mortality associated with maintenance of optimal cardiac performance. Ann Surg 192:414–420, 1980.
14. Ascher E, Mazzariol F, Hingorani A, et al: The use of duplex ultrasound arterial mapping as an alternative to conventional arteriography for primary and secondary infrapopliteal bypasses. Am J Surg 178:162–165, 1999.
15. Wain RA, Berdejo GL, Del Valle WN, et al: Can duplex scan arterial mapping replace contrast arteriography as the test of choice before infrainguinal revascularization? J Vasc Surg 29:100–107, 1999.
16. Sprayregen S: Principles of angiography. In Haimovici H (ed): Vascular Surgery, Principles and Techniques. New York, McGraw-Hill, 1976, pp 39–66.
17. Flanigan DP, Williams LR, Keifer T, et al: Prebypass operative arteriography. Surgery 92:627–633, 1982.
18. Owen RS, Carpenter JP, Baum RA, et al: Magnetic resonance imaging of angiographically occult runoff vessels in peripheral arterial occlusive disease. N Engl J Med 326:1577–1581, 1992.
19. Carpenter JP, Owen RS, Baum RA, et al: Magnetic resonance angiography of peripheral runoff vessels. J Vasc Surg 16:807–815, 1992.
20. Hoch JR, Tullis MJ, Kennell TW, et al: Use of magnetic resonance angiography for the pre-operative evaluation of patients with infrainguinal arterial occlusive disease. J Vasc Surg 23:792–800, 1996.
21. Sapala JA, Szilagyi DE: A simple aid in greater saphenous phlebography. Surg Gynecol Obstet 140:265–266, 1975.
22. Veith FJ, Moss CM, Sprayregen S, Montefusco CM: Preoperative saphenous venography in arterial reconstructive surgery of the lower extremity. Surgery 85:253–255, 1979.
23. Rivers SP, Scher LA, Gupta SK, Veith FJ: Safety of peripheral vascular surgery after recent myocardial infarction. J Vasc Surg 11:17–35, 1967.
24. Mannick JA, Jackson BT, Coffman JD: Success of bypass vein grafts in patients with isolated popliteal artery segments. Surgery 61:17–35, 1967.
25. Flinn WR, Flanigan DP, Verta MJ, et al: Sequential femoral-tibial bypass for severe limb ischemia. Surgery 88:357–365, 1980.
26. Veith FJ, Gupta SK, Daly V: Femoropopliteal bypass to the isolated popliteal segment: Is polytetrafluoroethylene graft acceptable? Surgery 89:296–303, 1981.
27. Ascer E, Veith FJ, Morin B, et al: Components of outflow resistance and their correlation with graft patency in lower extremity arterial reconstructions. J Vasc Surg 1:817–825, 1984.
28. Veith FJ, Ascer E, Gupta SK, et al: Tibiotibial vein bypass grafts: A new operation for limb salvage. J Vasc Surg 2:552–557, 1985.
29. Lyon RT, Veith FJ, Marsan BU, et al: Eleven-year experience with tibiotibial bypass: An unusual but effective solution to distal tibial artery occlusive disease and limited autologous vein. J Vasc Surg 20:61–69, 1994.
30. Ascer E, Veith FJ, Gupta SK: Bypasses to plantar arteries and other tibial branches: An extended approach to limb salvage. J Vasc Surg 8:434–441, 1988.
31. Sanchez LA, Schwartz ML, Veith FJ: Bypass surgery into plantar vessels: An effective extension of limb salvage surgical techniques. Perspect Vasc Surg 7:47–55, 1994.
32. Veith FJ, Gupta SK, Samson RH, et al: Superficial femoral and popliteal arteries as inflow site for distal bypasses. Surgery 90:980–990, 1981.
33. Wengerter KR, Yang PM, Veith FJ, et al: A twelve-year experience with the popliteal-to-distal artery bypass: The significance and management of proximal disease. J Vasc Surg 15:143–151, 1992.
34. Gupta SK, Veith FJ, Ascer E, et al: Five year experience with axillopopliteal bypass for limb salvage. J Cardiovasc Surg 26:321–324, 1985.
35. Veith FJ, Moss CM, Daly V, et al: New approaches in limb salvage by extended extraanatomic bypasses and prosthetic reconstructions to foot arteries. Surgery 84:764–774, 1978.
36. Towne JB, Bernhard VM, Rollins DL, Baum PL: Profundaplasty in perspective: Limitations in the long-term management of limb ischemia. Surgery 90:1037–1046, 1981.
37. Campbell CD, Brook DH, Webster MW, et al: Expanded microporous polytetrafluoroethylene as a vascular substitute: A two-year follow-up. Surgery 85:177–183, 1979.

38. Gupta SK, Veith FJ: Three year experience with expanded polytetra-fluoroethylene arterial grafts for limb salvage. Am J Surg 140:214–217, 1980.

39. Veith FJ, Moss CM, Fell SC, et al: Comparison of expanded polytet-rafluoroethylene and autologous saphenous vein grafts in high risk arterial reconstructions for limb salvage. Surg Gynecol Obstet 147:749–752, 1978.

40. Quiñones-Baldrich WJ, Busuttil RW, Baker JD, et al: Is the preferential use of polytetrafluoroethylene grafts for femoropopliteal bypass justified? J Vasc Surg 8:219–228, 1988.

41. Bergan JJ, Veith FJ, Bernhard VM, et al: Randomization of autogenous vein and polytetrafluoroethylene grafts in femoral-distal reconstruction. Surgery 92:921–930, 1982.

42. Veith FJ, Gupta SK, Ascer E, et al: Six year prospective multicenter randomized comparison of autologous saphenous vein and expanded polytetrafluoroethylene grafts in infrainguinal arterial reconstructions. J Vasc Surg 3:104–114, 1986.

43. Taylor RS, Loh A, McFarland RJ, et al: Improved technique for polytetrafluoroethylene bypass grafting: Long-term results using anastomotic vein patches. Br J Surg 79:348–354, 1992.

44. Parsons RE, Suggs WD, Veith FJ, et al: Polytetrafluoroethylene bypasses to infrapopliteal arteries without cuffs or patches: A better option than amputation in patients without autologous vein. J Vasc Surg 23:347–356, 1996.

45. Dardik H, Baier RE, Meenaghan M, et al: Morphologic and biophysical assessment of long term human umbilical cord vein implants used as vascular conduits. Surg Gynecol Obstet 154:17–26, 1982.

46. Cranley JJ, Karkow WS, Hafner CD, Flanagan LD: Aneurysmal dilatation in umbilical vein grafts. In Bergan JJ, Yao JST (eds): Reoperative Arterial Surgery. Orlando, Fla, Grune & Stratton, 1986, pp 343–358.

47. Pevec WC, Darling RC, L'Italien GJ, Abbott WM: Femoropopliteal reconstruction with knitted non-velour Dacron vs expanded polytet-rafluoroethylene. J Vasc Surg 16:60–65, 1992.

48. Kenney AD, Sauvage LR, Wood SJ, et al: Comparison of non-crimped, externally supported (EXS) and crimped, nonsupported Dacron prosthesis for axillofemoral and above knee femoropopliteal bypasses. Surgery 92:931–946, 1982.

49. Green RM, Abbott WM, Matsumoto T, et al: Prosthetic above knee femoropopliteal grafting: Five year results of a randomized trial. J Vasc Surg 31:417–425, 2000.

50. Szilagyi DE, Hageman JH, Smith RF, et al: Autogenous vein grafting in femoropopliteal atherosclerosis. The limits of its effectiveness. Surgery 86:836–851, 1979.

51. Szilagyi DE, Smith RF, Elliot JP, Hageman JH: The biologic fate of autogenous vein implants as arterial substitutes: Clinical, angiographic and histopathologic observations in femoropopliteal operations for atherosclerosis. Ann Surg 178:232–244, 1973.

52. Wengerter KR, Gupta SK, Veith FJ, et al: Critical vein diameter for infrainguinal arterial reconstructions. J Cardiovasc Surg (Torino) 28:109, 1987.

53. Wengerter KR, Veith FJ, Gupta SK: Influence of vein size (diameter) on infrapopliteal reversed vein graft patency. J Vasc Surg 11:525–531, 1990.

54. Kent KC, Whittemore AD, Mannick JA: Short-term and mid-term results of an all autologous tissue policy for infrainguinal reconstruction. J Vasc Surg 9:107–114, 1989.

55. Hall KV: The great saphenous vein used "in-situ" as an arterial shunt after extirpation of the vein valves. Surgery 51:492–495, 1962.

56. Leather RP, Shah DM, Karmody AM: Infrapopliteal bypass for limb salvage: Increased patency and utilization of the saphenous vein used "in situ." Surgery 90:1000–1008, 1981.

57. Leather RP, Shah DM, Chang BB, et al: Resurrection of the in situ vein bypass: 1000 cases later. Ann Surg 205:435–442, 1988.

58. Gruss JD, Bartels D, Vargas H, et al: Arterial reconstruction for distal disease of the lower extremities by the in situ vein graft technique. J Cardiovasc Surg (Torino) 23:231–234, 1982.

59. Wengerter KR, Veith FJ, Gupta SK, et al: Prospective randomized multicenter comparison of in situ and reversed vein infrapopliteal bypasses. J Vasc Surg 12:189–199, 1991.

60. Taylor LM, Edward JM, Porter JM: Present status of reversed vein bypass: Five year results of a modern series. J Vasc Surg 11:207–215, 1990.

61. Towne JB, Schmidt DD, Seabrook GR, Bandyk DF: The effect of vein diameter on early patency and durability of in situ bypass grafts. J Cardiovasc Surg (Torino) 30:64, 1989.

62. Schulman ML, Bradley MR: Late results and angiographic evaluation of arm veins as long bypass grafts. Surgery 92:1032–1041, 1982.

63. Harris RW, Andros G, Dulana LB, et al: Successful long-term limb salvage using cephalic vein bypass grafts. Ann Surg 200:785–794, 1984.

64. Londrew GL, Bosher LP, Brown PW, et al: Infrainguinal reconstruction with arm vein, lesser saphenous vein and remnants of greater saphenous vein: A report of 257 cases. J Vasc Surg 20:451–457, 1994.

65. Sesto ME, Sullivan TM, Hertzer NR, et al: Cephalic vein grafts for lower extremity revascularization. J Vasc Surg 15:543–549, 1992.

66. Stonebridge PA, Miller AM, Tsoukas A, et al: Angioscopy of arm vein infrainguinal bypass grafts. Ann Vasc Surg 5:170–175, 1991.

67. Veith FJ, Gupta SK: Femoral-distal artery bypasses. In Bergan JJ, Yao JST (eds): Operative Techniques in Vascular Surgery. New York, Grune & Stratton, 1980, pp 141–150.

68. Bernhard VM, Boren CH, Towne JB: Pneumatic tourniquet as a substitute for vascular clamps in distal bypass surgery. Surgery 87:709–713, 1980.

69. Marin ML, Veith FJ, Panetta TF, et al: A new look at intraoperative completion arteriography: Classification and management strategies for intraluminal defects. Am J Surg 166:136–140, 1993.

70. Wain RA, Veith FJ: Use of digital cine-fluoroscopy and catheter-directed techniques to improve and simplify standard vascular procedures. Surg Clin North Am 79:489–506, 1999.

71. Marin ML, Veith FJ, Panetta TF, et al: A new look at intraoperative completion arteriography: Classification and management strategies for intraluminal defects. Am J Surg 166:136–140, 1993.

72. Bandyk DF, Kaebnick, Bergamini TM, et al: Hemodynamics of in situ saphenous vein arterial bypass. Arch Surg 123:477–482, 1988.

73. Oblath RW, Buckley FO, Green RM, et al: Prevention of platelet aggregation and adherence to prosthetic vascular grafts by aspirin and dipyridamole. Surgery 84:37–44, 1978.

74. Creager MA: Results of the CAPRIE trial: Efficacy and safety of clopidogrel. Clopidogrel versus aspirin in patients at risk of ischemic events. Vasc Med 3:257–260, 1998.

75. Sanchez LA, Goldsmith JG, Rivers SP, et al: Limb salvage surgery in end stage renal disease: Is it worthwhile? J Cardiovasc Surg (Torino) 33:344–348, 1992.

76. Veith FJ, Gupta SK, Ascer E, et al: Improved strategies for secondary operations on infrainguinal arteries. Ann Vasc Surg 4:85–93, 1990.

77. Parsons R, Marin ML, Veith FJ, et al: Fluoroscopically assisted thromboembolectomy: An improved method for treating acute occlusions of native arteries and bypass grafts. Ann Vasc Surg 10:201–210, 1996.

78. Sanchez LA, Suggs WD, Marin ML, et al: The merit of polytetra-fluoroethylene extensions and interposition grafts to salvage failing infrainguinal vein bypasses. J Vasc Surg 23:329–335, 1996.

79. Veith FJ, Ascer E, Nunez A, et al: Unusual approaches to infrainguinal arteries. J Cardiovasc Surg (Torino) 28:58, 1987.

80. Nunez A, Veith FJ, Collier P, et al: Direct approach to the distal portions of the deep femoral artery for limb salvage bypasses. J Vasc Surg 8:576–581, 1988.

81. Bertucci WR, Marin MD, Veith FJ: Posterior approach to the deep femoral artery. J Vasc Surg 29:741–744, 1999.

82. Veith FJ, Ascer E, Gupta SK, Wengerter KR: Lateral approach to the popliteal artery. J Vasc Surg 6:119–123, 1987.

83. McNamara TO, Bomberger RA: Factors affecting initial and 6-month patency rates after intraarterial thrombolysis with high-dose urokinase. Am J Surg 152:709–711, 1986.

84. O'Mara CS, Flinn WR, Johnson ND, et al: Recognition and surgical management of patent but hemodynamically failed arterial grafts. Ann Surg 193:467–476, 1981.

85. Veith FJ, Weiser RK, Gupta SK, et al: Diagnosis and management of failing lower extremity arterial reconstructions. J Cardiovasc Surg (Torino) 25:381–384, 1984.

86. Whittemore AD, Clowes AW, Couch NP, Mannick JA: Secondary femoropopliteal reconstruction. Ann Surg 193:35–42, 1981.

87. Sanchez L, Gupta SK, Veith FJ, et al: A ten-year experience with one hundred fifty failing or threatened vein and polytetrafluoroethylene arterial bypass grafts. J Vasc Surg 14:729–738, 1991.

88. Bandyk DF, Cata RF, Towne JB: A low flow velocity predicts failure of femoro-popliteal and femoro-tibial bypass grafts. Surgery 98:799–809, 1985.

89. Perler BA, Osterman FA, Mitchell SE, et al: Balloon dilatation vs

surgical revision of infrainguinal autogenous vein graft stenoses: Long term follow-up. J Vasc Surg 14:729–738, 1991.

90. Whittemore AD, Donaldson MC, Polak JF, Mannick JA: Limitations of balloon angioplasty for vein graft stenosis. J Vasc Surg 14:340–345, 1991.

91. Sanchez LA, Suggs WD, Marin ML, et al: Is percutaneous balloon angioplasty appropriate in the treatment of graft and anastomotic lesions responsible for failing vein bypasses? Am J Surg 168:97–101, 1994.

92. Samson RH, Sprayregen S, Veith FJ, et al: Management of angioplasty complication, unsuccessful procedures and early and late failures. Ann Surg 199:234–240, 1984.

93. Gruntzig A, Kumpe DA: Technique of percutaneous transluminal angioplasty with the Gruntzig balloon catheter. AJR Am J Roentgenol 132:547–552, 1979.

94. Ring EJ, Alpert JR, Frieman DB, et al: Early experience with percutaneous transluminal angioplasty using a vinyl balloon catheter. Ann Surg 191:438–442, 1980.

95. Alpert JR, Ring EJ, Freiman DB, et al: Balloon dilatation of iliac stenosis with distal arterial surgery. Arch Surg 115:715–717, 1980.

96. Kadir S, Smith GW, White RI Jr, et al: Percutaneous transluminal angioplasty as an adjunct to the surgical management of peripheral vascular disease. Ann Surg 195:786–795, 1982.

97. Bandyk DF, Johnson BL, Gupta AK, Esses GE: Nature and management of duplex abnormalities encountered during infrainguinal vein bypass grafting. J Vasc Surg 24:430–436, 1996.

98. Ahn SS, Concepcion B: The current status of peripheral atherectomy. Eur J Vasc Endovasc Surg 10:133–135, 1995.

99. Lampmann LE: Stenting in the femoral superficial artery: An overview. Eur J Radiol 29:276–279, 1999.

100. Bolia A: Percutaneous intentional extraluminal (subintimal) recanalization of crural arteries. Eur J Radiol 28:199–204, 1998.

101. London NJ, Srinivasan R, Naylor AR, et al: Subintimal angioplasty of femoropopliteal artery occlusions: The long-term results. Eur J Vasc Surg 8:148–155, 1994.

102. DeWeese JA, Robb CG: Autogenous venous grafts ten years later. Surgery 82:775–784, 1977.

103. Reichle FA, Tyson R: Comparison of long-term results of 364 femoropopliteal or femorotibial bypasses for revascularization of severely ischemic lower extremities. Ann Surg 182:449–455, 1975.

104. Bartlett ST, Olinde AJ, Flinn WR, et al: The reoperative potential of infrainguinal bypass: Long-term limb and patient survival. J Vasc Surg 5:170–179, 1987.

105. Boontje AH: Occlusion of femoropopliteal bypasses (Biograft). J Cardiovasc Surg (Torino) 25:385–390, 1984.

106. Sanchez LA, Suggs WD, Veith FJ, et al: Is surveillance to detect failing polytetrafluoroethylene bypasses worthwhile? Twelve-year experience with ninety-eight grafts. J Vasc Surg 18:981–990, 1993.

107. Craver JM, Ottinger LW, Darling RC, et al: Hemorrhage and thrombosis as early complications of femoropopliteal bypass grafts: Causes, treatment and prognostic implications. Surgery 74:839–845, 1973.

108. Davis RC, Davies WT, Mannick JA: Bypass vein grafts in patients with distal popliteal artery occlusion. Am J Surg 129:421–425, 1975.

109. DeLaurentis DA, Friedman P: Arterial reconstruction above and below the knee: Another look. Am J Surg 121:392–397, 1971.

110. Edwards WS, Gerety E, Larkin J, Hoyt TW: Multiple sequential femoral tibial grafting for severe ischemia. Surgery 80:722–728, 1976.

111. Maini BS, Mannick JA: Effect of arterial reconstruction on limb salvage: A ten-year appraisal. Arch Surg 113:1297–1304, 1978.

112. Perdue GD, Smith RB, Veazey CR, Anslery JD: Revascularization for severe limb ischemia. Arch Surg 115:168–171, 1980.

113. Auer AI, Hurley JJ, Binnington HB, et al: Distal tibial vein grafts for limb salvage. Arch Surg 118:597–602, 1983.

114. Hobson RW, Lynch TG, Jamil Z, et al: Results of revascularization and amputation in severe lower extremity ischemia: A five-year clinical experience. J Vasc Surg 2:205–213, 1985.

115. Stoney RJ: Ultimate salvage for the patients with limb-threatening ischemia: Realistic goals. Am J Surg 136:228–232, 1978.

116. Suggs WD, Yuan JG, Parsons RE, et al: Functional outcome after infrainguinal bypass: A justification for limb salvage surgery. Presented at the Peripheral Vascular Surgery meeting, Chicago, June 7–8, 1996.

117. Ramsburgh SR, Lindenauer SM, Weber IR, et al: Femoropopliteal bypass for limb salvage surgery. Surgery 81:453–458, 1977.

118. Gupta SK, Veith FJ, Samson RH, et al: Cost analysis of operations for infrainguinal arteriosclerosis. Circulation 66(Suppl 2):II–9, 1982.

119. Tabbara M, White R, Cavaye D, Kopchock G: In vivo comparison of intravascular ultrasonography and angiography. J Vasc Surg 14:496–504, 1991.

120. Waller BF, Pinkerton CA, Slack JD: Intravascular ultrasound: A histological study of vessels during life: The new "gold standard" for vascular imaging. Circulation 85:2305–2310, 1992.

121. Van Sambeek MRHM, Qureshi A, Van Lankeren W, et al: Discrepancy between stent deployment and balloon size used assessed by intravascular ultrasound. Eur J Vasc Endovasc Surg 15:57–61, 1998.

122. Palmaz JC, Laborde JC, Rivera FJ, et al: Stenting of the iliac arteries with the Palmaz stent: Experience from a multicenter trial. Cardiovasc Intervent Radiol 15:291–297, 1992.

123. Myers KA, Denton MJ, Devine TJ: Infrainguinal atherectomy using the transluminal endarterectomy catheter: Patency rates and clinical success for 144 procedures. J Endovasc Surg 1:61–70, 1994.

124. The Collaborative Rotablator Atherectomy Group (CRAG): Peripheral atherectomy with the Rotablator: A multicenter report. J Vasc Surg 19:509–515, 1994.

125. Marin ML, Veith FJ, Cynamon J, et al: Initial experience with transluminally placed endovascular grafts for the treatment of complex vascular lesions. Ann Surg 222:449–469, 1995.

126. White GH, White RA, Kopchok GE: Intraoperative video angioscopy compared to arteriography during peripheral vascular operations. J Vasc Surg 6:488–495, 1987.

127. White GH, White RA, Kopchok GE, Wilson SE: Angioscopic thromboembolectomy: Preliminary observations with a recent technique. J Vasc Surg 7:318–325, 1988.

128. Rosenthal D: Improved endovascular techniques for in situ vein bypass. In Veith FJ (ed): Current Critical Problems in Vascular Surgery, vol 6. St Louis, Quality Medical Publishing, 1994, pp 130–132.

129. Rosenthal D, Arous EJ, Friedman SG, et al: Endovascular-assisted versus conventional in situ saphenous vein bypass grafting: Cumulative patency, limb salvage, and cost results in a 39-month multicenter study. J Vasc Surg 31:60–68, 2000.

130. Lumsden AB, Eaves FF: Subcutaneous, video-assisted saphenous vein harvest. Perspect Vasc Surg 7:43–55, 1994.

131. Fogarty TJ, Chin A, Shoor PM, et al: Adjunctive intraoperative arterial dilatation: Simplified instrumentation technique. Arch Surg 116:1391–1398, 1981.

Questions

1. Which of the following statements concerning arterial emboli is generally *not* true?
   - (a) the only certain way to diagnose an embolic occlusion is the demonstration that the occlusive process is multifocal
   - (b) emboli are often associated with moderate or severe atherosclerosis
   - (c) the treatment of emboli is generally simple and results are almost uniformly good
   - (d) angiography is usually indicated for lower extremity emboli
   - (e) emboli can be effectively removed even after several days

2. Bypasses to arteries below the popliteal should be performed for limb salvage with polytetrafluoroethylene (PTFE) grafts
   - (a) when no acceptable autologous vein is present in the involved lower extremity
   - (b) only when no autologous vein is available in any of the patient's four extremities
   - (c) in no circumstances
   - (d) only to the posterior tibial artery
   - (e) none of the above

3. Heavily calcified incompressible tibial arteries are unsuitable for use in limb salvage arterial bypasses. True or false?

4. Studies have clearly shown that in situ vein bypasses are uniformly superior to reversed vein bypasses. True or false?

5. The standard arteriogram for femoropopliteal occlusive disease should visualize all arteries from the renals to the forefoot. True or false?

6. Preferential use of PTFE grafts for above-knee femoropopliteal bypass is justified in patients whose life expectancy is less than
   (a) 1 year
   (b) 2 years
   (c) 3 years
   (d) 4 years
   (e) none of the above

7. Bypass to a tibial artery at the ankle level or in the foot is indicated for disabling intermittent claudication

(a) occasionally
(b) almost never
(c) rarely
(d) infrequently
(e) very infrequently

8. Toe amputation or foot débridement should never be combined with an arterial revascularization. True or false?

9. The presence of pedal pulses is evidence of sufficiently good circulation in the foot that a toe amputation for infection is likely to heal. True or false?

10. Patients who have had an infrainguinal bypass that fails and who again have a threatened limb have a poor chance of having the foot saved by a secondary revascularization. True or false?

Answers

1. c   2. b   3. False   4. False   5. True   6. b   7. b   8. False   9. True   10. False

29

Renovascular Disease

Kimberley J. Hansen and Richard H. Dean

Although hypertension has been recognized for centuries, the importance of its identification and treatment has been appreciated only during the past 150 years. Most commonly, hypertension is a silent process and is manifested only by its sequelae: acceleration of atherogenesis and associated cardiovascular morbid and mortal events. Uncommonly, the hypertension may be so severe that the elevated pressure itself produces vessel wall injury and the clinical picture of malignant hypertension. Although most physicians appreciate the potentially lethal nature of this malignant variety and the importance of its control, physician apathy toward the merits of aggressive diagnostic evaluation and management of asymptomatic patients with less severe hypertension continues and limits population-wide contemporary treatment of this disorder.

Richard Bright of Guy's Hospital, London,[1] called attention to the association of hypertension and renal disease in 1836. He observed the apparent association between hardness of the pulse, "dropsy," albuminuria, and granular shrunken kidneys. This is especially remarkable, because the modern sphygmomanometer was not described until 1896. Although Bright's observation stimulated much interest in the kidney, 70 years passed before Tigerstedt and Bergman,[2] in 1898, discovered a renal pressor substance in the rabbit. They called this crude extract "renin." Confirmation of a renovascular source of hypertension, however, awaited Goldblatt's classic experiment.[3] In 1934, he and his coworkers showed that constriction of the renal artery produced atrophy of the kidney and hypertension in the dog. After this documentation of a renovascular origin for hypertension, many patients were treated by nephrectomy on the basis of hypertension and a small kidney on intravenous pyelography. Curiously, the presence of renal artery occlusive disease was rarely documented in any of these patients.

Dissatisfaction with the results of this form of treatment prompted Smith,[4] in 1956, to review 575 cases treated in this manner. He found only a 26% cure of hypertension by nephrectomy using these criteria. This led him to suggest that nephrectomy should be limited to strict urologic indications. Two years previously, however, Freeman[5] performed an aortic and bilateral renal artery thromboendarterectomy on a hypertensive patient with resultant

resolution of hypertension. This was the first cure of hypertension by renal revascularization.

DeCamp and Birchall,[6] Morris and colleagues,[7] and others[8, 9] soon followed with additional descriptions of relief of hypertension by renal revascularization. Concomitant with these reports, aortography began to be widely used. During the late 1950s, many centers were demonstrating renal artery stenosis in hypertensive patients by aortography and then performing either aortorenal bypass or thromboendarterectomy. Nevertheless, by 1960, investigators had noted that revascularization in hypertensive individuals with renal artery stenosis was associated with reduction of blood pressure in less than 50% of patients. General pessimism followed regarding the merits of operative treatment of hypertension.

As this experience pointed out, the coexistence of renal artery stenosis and hypertension does not establish a causal relationship. Many normotensive patients, especially those older than the age of 50 years, have renal artery stenosis. Obviously, special studies are required to establish the functional significance of renal artery lesions. The most recent era in the history of operative treatment of renovascular hypertension (RVH) began with the introduction of meaningful tests of split renal function by Howard and Conner[10] and by Stamey and colleagues.[11] Furthermore, the work of Page and Helmes[12] and others[13–15] in the identification of the renin-angiotension system of blood pressure control added a new dimension to our understanding of RVH. With the later addition of accurate methods of measuring plasma renin activity, the physician now can accurately predict which renal artery lesion is producing RVH. Our experience has shown that if the split renal function studies or renal vein renin assays are positive, one can expect a good response in blood pressure after successful operation in over 95% of cases.[16]

The prevalence of RVH, the necessity of its identification, and the value of interventional management, however, remain poorly defined. In addition, contemporary reports have emphasized the relationship between renovascular disease (RVD) and renal insufficiency.[17–19] The term *ischemic nephropathy* has been adopted to describe this relationship. By definition, ischemic nephropathy reflects severe occlusive disease of the extraparenchymal renal artery in combination with excretory renal insufficiency. In 1962, Morris and associates[20] reported on eight azotemic patients with global renal ischemia who had improved blood pressure and renal function after renal revascularization. This early report and others that followed suggested that ischemic nephropathy could mediate renal insufficiency that was rapidly progressive, contributing to end-stage renal disease (ESRD). In this chapter, diagnostic studies and methods of management of the respective causes of RVD, RVH, and ischemic nepropathy are reviewed, with emphasis placed on the current status of their value and results of their use.

PATHOLOGY

Occlusive lesions of the renal artery can be divided into two main groups: atherosclerotis and fibromuscular dysplasia. Atherosclerosis of the renal artery is not peculiar; the pathogenesis parallels atherosclerotic lesions elsewhere, with cholesterol-rich lipid deposition and intimal thickening. Later, this "atheroma" may undergo central degeneration and even calcification. Atheromas typically occur at or near the renal artery ostium (Fig. 29–1), are most commonly found on the left, and account for about 70% of patients with RVH. Often, arteriographic evidence exists of asymptomatic simultaneous involvement of the abdominal aorta and its bifurcation. Occasionally, the renal artery stenosis is only one manifestation of severe end-stage generalized atherosclerosis. Like atherosclerosis elsewhere, angiographic findings pathognomonic for a hemodynamically

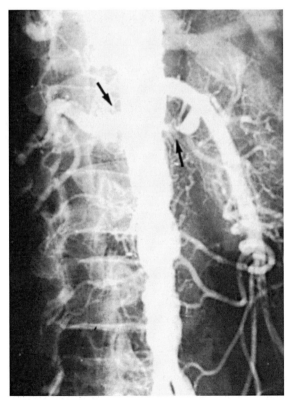

Figure 29–1. Arteriogram showing typical appearance of atherosclerotic renal artery stenosis located at the origin of the vessel (*arrow*).

significant lesion include poststenotic dilatation and the presence of collateral vessels.

Fibromuscular dysplasia of the renal artery encompasses a variety of hyperplastic and fibrosing lesions of the intima, media, or adventitia. They are most frequently seen in young women. This is of no predictive value, however, because fibrodysplastic lesions can be found at any age and in either sex. Medial fibroplasia is the most common lesion; the right renal artery is more commonly affected than the left, but bilateral involvement is present in the vast majority of patients. The basic cause of medial fibroplasia remains unknown, but its frequent occurrence in multiple arteries suggests a systemic arteriopathy. Embryologic variations, hormonal influences, autoimmune mechanisms, and even recurrent trauma during youth have been suggested as possible causative factors. None of these explanations are adequate, however, and the evidence in their support remains mostly conjectural.

Based on the angiographic appearance of fibromuscular disease, several methods of categorization have been suggested. To establish a uniform terminology, Harrison and McCormack[21] combined their experience and developed a classification of these lesions correlating the histologic and angiographic appearance. Depending on the layer predominantly involved, lesions may either be intimal, medial, or adventitial. Clinically, however, it may be difficult to segregate individual lesions into one of their respective categories. The most common variety of fibromuscular dysplasia is medial fibroplasia with mural aneurysms (Fig. 29–2). This variety accounts for about 70% of all renal artery dysplasias. It often involves long segments of the renal artery and its branches, producing a characteristic "string-of-beads" appearance angiographically. Less commonly, the dysplastic lesions may be a single mural stenosis (Fig. 29–3) consistent with intimal fibroplasia or perimedial dysplasia.

PATHOPHYSIOLOGY

The kidney, by its influence on circulating plasma volume as well as on modulation of vasomotor tone, is a dominant site of blood pressure regulation. To examine the pathophysiology of RVH, reviewing the normal homeostatic activities of the kidney in regulation of blood pressure is appropriate.

Renin-Angiotensin-Aldosterone System

The renin-angiotensin-aldosterone system is a complex feedback mechanism normally acting to maintain a stable blood pressure and blood volume under varying conditions. Richly innervated modified smooth muscle cells located along the afferent arterioles in juxtaposition to the renal glomerulus (juxtaglomerular apparatus) are sensitive monitors of perfusion pressure. Diminished perfusion pressure stimulates these cells to release renin, a proteolytic enzyme. Renin, in turn, interacts with an α-globulin (angiotensinogen) manufactured in the liver to produce angiotensin I. Angiotensin I, an inactive and labile decapeptide, is converted to the potent vasoconstrictor angiotensin II by con-

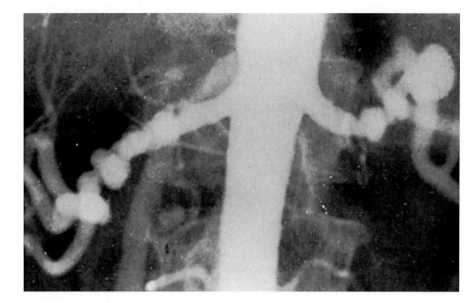

Figure 29–2. Arteriogram demonstrating typical "string-of-beads" appearance of medial fibromuscular dysplasia with microaneurysm.

verting enzyme abundant in the lungs and other tissues. In addition to its potent vasoconstrictor properties, angiotensin II through its conversion to angiotensin III also increases blood pressure by stimulation of aldosterone release from the zona glomerulosa of the adrenal cortex. This, in turn, increases plasma volume by increasing sodium and water resorption in the renal tubules. Through these actions of angiotensin II and III, blood pressure, plasma volume, and plasma sodium content are increased. In addition, the adjacent cells of the distal convoluted tubule (macula densa) may play a role by acting as sensors of sodium concentration in the distal tubules and exerting a positive feedback mechanism on renin release. As these mechanisms increase perfusion pressure in the juxtaglo-

merular cells, further renin production and release are suppressed, and blood pressure is modulated within a narrow range. This scheme is a simplistic representation of a very complex mechanism.

Many intermediate steps remain unknown. The role of prostaglandins in the regulation of renin release remains unsettled. Their action in blood pressure control, and specifically the part they play in RVH, is the focus of intensive investigation. In addition, a variety of angiotensin peptides with salt-wasting and volume-reducing properties exist that probably mediate blood pressure control. These and other components of the renin-angiotensin axis have been described at the tissue level in almost every organ system studied. "Local" renin-angiotensin production may modulate both end-organ effects of RVH as well as other chronic manifestations.

Cause of Hypertension (Two Forms)

Potentially, two forms of hypertension may be produced by the development of RVD: (1) renin-dependent hypertension and (2) volume-dependent hypertension. Through the mechanisms just described, decreased perfusion activates the renin-angiotensin-aldosterone axis of vasoconstriction and volume expansion. Current information regarding the nature of RVH suggests that a functionally significant unilateral renal artery stenosis activates both the angiotensin II–mediated increase in peripheral resistance and blood pressure as well as aldosterone-mediated volume expansion. When the contralateral renal artery and kidney are normal, the feedback mechanisms in the normal kidney produce a natriuresis and compensatory reduction in circulating plasma volume. In this scheme, an angiotensin II–vasoconstrictive source of hypertension is created.

In contrast, when the contralateral renal artery or kidney is also diseased, this compensatory diuresis is lost and volume expansion occurs, producing an angiotensin-aldosterone–mediated, volume-dependent hypertension. Modification of renal perfusion by renal revascularization can

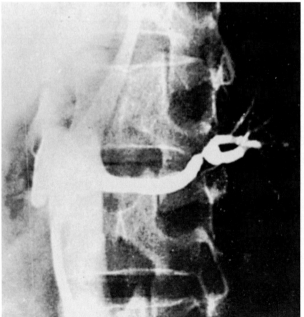

Figure 29–3. Appearance of single mural fibromuscular dysplastic lesion on arteriogram.

effectively diminish or abolish the underlying mechanism producing either of these varieties of RVH.

PREVALENCE OF RENOVASCULAR HYPERTENSION

RVH is generally thought to account for 5% to 10% of the hypertensive population. Tucker and Labarthe[22] have suggested an even lower prevalence. Likewise, Shapiro and colleagues[23] have suggested that the identification and successful operative treatment of RVH in patients over the age of 50 years is so unlikely that diagnostic investigation for a correctable cause in that group should be undertaken only when hypertension is severe and uncontrollable. Estimates of the prevalence of hypertension in the United States from all causes range from 60 to 80 million people, and it may be present in 10% to 15% of the adult population.

Indeed, the incidence of RVH is undoubtedly low in this general hypertensive population if all patients with even mild hypertension are included. Because RVH tends to produce relatively severe hypertension, its prevalence in the large subpopulation of mildly hypertensive patients (diastolic blood pressure less than 105 mm Hg) is probably negligible. In contrast, however, it is a frequent cause of hypertension in the smaller group of severely hypertensive people. In our experience, the presence of severe hypertension at the two extremes of life carries the highest probability of being RVH. Our review of the causes of hypertension in 74 children admitted for diagnostic evaluation over a 5-year period showed that 78% of the children younger than 5 years of age had a correctable renovascular origin (Table 29–1).[24] In 1996, one center screened 629 hypertensive adults older than 50 years of age for RVD (Table 29–2). Overall, 25% of subjects demonstrated significant renal artery disease. However, 52% of those older than 60 years whose diastolic pressure was greater than 110 mm Hg had significant renal artery stenosis or occlusion. When serum creatinine was elevated in conjunction with this age and blood pressure, 71% of subjects demonstrated hemodynamically significant renovascular disease.

From these data, viewing hypertensive patients as a homogeneous group with respect to the prevalence of RVH is inappropriate. Rather, the probability of finding RVH correlates with patient age, the severity of hypertension, and the pressure of associated renal insufficiency. Accordingly, the search for RVH should be directed to the subset

TABLE 29–1

Classification of Hypertension in 74 Children

	0–5 YR	6–10 YR	11–15 YR	16–20 YR
Total no. of children	9	9	29	27
Essential	1	5	24	21
Correctable	8 (78%)	4 (44%)	5 (17%)	6 (22%)

From Lawson JD, Boerth RK, Foster JH, et al: Diagnosis and management of renovascular hypertension in children. Arch Surg 112:1307, 1977.

TABLE 29–2

Renal Duplex Sonography in 629 New Hypertensive Adults

	RENAL VASCULAR DISEASE		
	Present (%)	Absent (%)	TOTAL
All patients	154 (24)	475 (76)	629 (100)
>60 yr + DBP ≥ 110 mm Hg	98 (52)	91 (48)	189 (30)
DBP ≥ 110 mm Hg + SCr ≥ 2.0 mg/dL	53 (71)	22 (29)	75 (12)

DBP, diastolic blood pressure; SCr, serum creatinine.

of patients who have the more severe degree of hypertension, especially when severe hypertension is associated with renal insufficiency. However, severity of hypertension is based on its level without medication interference and does not refer to the difficulty of control by drug therapy.

CHARACTERISTICS OF RENOVASCULAR HYPERTENSION

Because of the relative infrequency of RVH in the entire hypertensive population, many reports have focused on the value of demographic factors, physical findings, and screening tests to discriminate between essential hypertension (EH) and RVH. Most frequently quoted as discriminate factors suggesting the presence of RVH and a need for further study are recent onset of hypertension, young age, lack of family history of hypertension, and the presence of an abdominal bruit. The most complete study comparing the clinical characteristics of patients with RVH to those with EH was the Cooperative Study of Renovascular Hypertension.[25] In that study, the prevalence of certain clinical characteristics in 339 patients with EH was compared with their prevalence in 175 patients with RVH secondary to atherosclerotic lesions (91 patients) and fibromuscular dysplasia (84 patients). Although the prevalence of several characteristics is significantly different when RVH is compared with EH, none of the characteristics has sufficient discriminant value to be used to exclude patients from further diagnostic investigation for RVH. Certainly, the finding of an epigastric bruit in a young white female with malignant hypertension is strongly suggestive of a renovascular origin of the hypertension. The absence of such criteria, however, does not exclude the presence of RVH, and such criteria should not be used to eliminate patients from further diagnostic study.

In a review of the first 200 patients with RVH treated in our center, 64% had family histories of hypertension, 46% had no audible abdominal bruit, and ages ranged from 5 to 80 years (mean, 56 years).[26] Because RVH can be secondary to any of several processes affecting the renal artery and because each of these diseases has its own clinical characteristics, the use of demographic or physical findings such as age, abdominal bruit, and duration of hypertension to exclude patients from study inappropriately excludes patients with RVH from further evaluation. Therefore, one should base the decision for diagnostic study on the severity of hypertension. Mild hypertension has a minimal chance of being renovascular in origin. In contrast, the more severe the hypertension, the higher the probability that it is from a correctable cause. With this in mind, we submit all patients with diastolic blood pressures greater than 105 mm Hg who would be acceptable operative candidates to evaluation for a correctable origin of hypertension.

DIAGNOSTIC EVALUATION

The selection and appropriate sequence of diagnostic studies in the evaluation of hypertensive patients remain ill-defined. The general evaluation of all hypertensive patients should include a careful medical history, physical examination, serum electrolytes and creatinine determination, and an electrocardiogram. Electrocardiography is important to gauge the extent of secondary myocardial hypertrophy or associated ischemic heart disease. Serum electrolytes and serial serum potassium determinations can effectively exclude patients with primary aldosteronism if potassium levels are greater than 3.0 mg/dL. One must remember, however, that hypokalemia is often due to salt-depleting diets and previous diuretic therapy. Finally, estimation of renal function is mandatory. Preexisting renal disease may reduce renal function and cause hypertension. Conversely, renal dysfunction may reflect RVD, that is, ischemic nephropathy.

Screening Studies

Identification of a noninvasive screening test that accurately identifies all patients with RVD that might require interventional management remains an elusive goal. Prior methods such as peripheral plasma renin activity, rapid sequence intravenous pyelography, and saralasin infusion are examples of tests that have been abandoned. Screening studies are basically one of two types: functional studies or anatomic studies. Of the functional type, isotope renography continues to be proposed as a valuable screening test, yet the methods employed are continuously modified with the hope of improving the sensitivity and specificity. The newest versions of isotope renography consist of renal scans performed before and after exercise or captopril infusion. Of these, only captopril renal scanning (CRS) has gained widespread use and acceptance as a screening tool. Anatomic screening studies include renal duplex sonography and arteriography.

Captopril Renal Scanning

To grasp the basis of CRS one must understand some of the components of renal excretory physiology and the importance of the renin-angiotensin system in maintenance of homeostasis. Glomerular filtration is governed partially by the relative tone of the afferent and efferent arterioles. During periods recognized by the juxtaglomerular apparatus of reduced blood pressure (e.g., proximal renal artery stenosis), increased renin is released that ultimately leads to an increase in the level of angiotensin II. Angiotensin II acts predominantly to constrict the efferent arteriole to maintain renal glomerular perfusion pressure and filtration. When an angiotensin II–converting enzyme inhibitor such as captopril is given in this circumstance, an acute reduction in the amount of angiotensin II occurs. This in turn leads to a reduction in constriction of the efferent arteriole and a decrease in the glomerular filtration pressure (GFR). Therefore, CRS is a study that is composed of a baseline renogram and a repeat renogram performed after a dose of captopril. A test is considered positive when a normal baseline scan becomes abnormal after captopril administration, either by an increase in the time to peak activity to more than 11 minutes or by a normal glomerular filtration ratio between the two sides increasing to greater than 1.5:1 (Fig. 29–4). In experienced hands this study is reported to be highly reliable.[27] Unfortunately, it is less reliable when significant parenchymal disease is present. For that reason, we have not relied on its results to stop workup in azotemic patients.

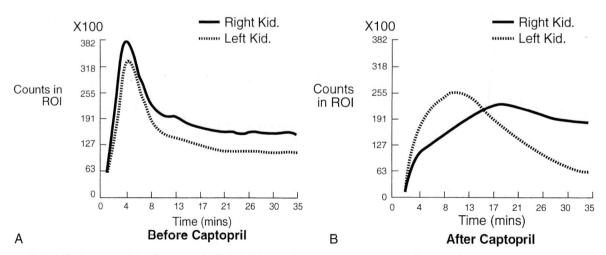

Figure 29–4. Captopril renal scintigraphy before (A) and after (B) captopril ingestion demonstrates the positive finding of a slowing of the rate of isotope clearance and time to peak radioactivity after captopril.

TABLE 29-3

Doppler Velocity Criteria for B-Scan Defects

Defect	Criteria
<60% diameter-reducing RA defect	RA-PSV from entire RA < 2.0 m/sec
≥60% diameter-reducing RA defect	Focal RA-PSV ≥ 2.0 m/sec and distal turbulent velocity waveform
Occlusion	Doppler-shifted signal from renal artery B-scan image
Inadequate study for interpretation	Failure to obtain Doppler samples from entire main renal artery

RA, renal artery; RA-PSV, renal artery peak systolic velocity.
From Hansen KJ, Tribble RW, Reaves SW, et al: Renal duplex sonography. Evaluation of clinical utility. J Vasc Surg 12:227–236, 1990.

Renal Duplex Sonography

Through continued improvements in probe design and duplex sonographic technology, imaging and Doppler shift interrogation of deep abdominal vasculature have been introduced as a screening method to identify and quantify visceral and renal artery occlusive disease. Our clinical experience with its use has centered on evaluation of RVD. We have evaluated the role of duplex sonography as an initial surface screening test, as an intraoperative study to confirm the technical success of reconstructive procedures, and as a postoperative surveillance method to follow progression of disease and stability of reconstructions.

Technically successful studies, defined as a complete main renal artery interrogation from aortic origin to renal hilum, should be obtained in almost 95% of cases. These results are ensured by proper patient preparation and method of examination. Details of the conduct of the procedure are covered elsewhere.[28]

Renal duplex sonography (RDS) criteria for critical renal artery stenosis are depicted in Table 29–3. Assuming that renal artery peak systolic velocity (RA-PSV) varies with the degree of renal artery stenosis and aortic PSV (i.e., inflow), most authors[29–32] have advocated the ratio of RA-PSV to aortic PSV (the renal-aortic ratio) to define critical renal artery stenosis. In contrast, we have found no relationship between RA-PSV and aortic PSV in the presence or absence of disease (Fig. 29–5). Focal RA-PSV of 2 m/second or more in combination with distal poststenotic turbulence correlates highly with the angiographic presence of 60% or greater diameter-reducing stenosis of the renal artery.[28] In 122 kidneys with single renal arteries with renal angiography for comparison, RDS correctly identified 67 of 68 kidneys with normal and less than 60% renal artery steno-

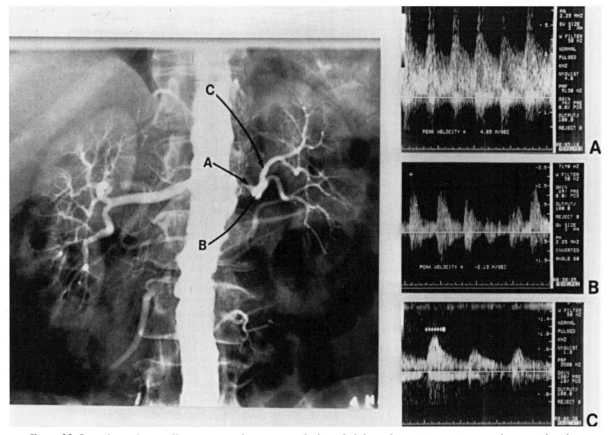

Figure 29–5. Radiographic cut-film angiogram demonstrating high-grade left renal artery stenosis. *A*, Doppler spectral analysis at the site of stenosis demonstrating focal increase in RA-PSV (4.6 m/sec). *B*, Distal spectral analysis demonstrating turbulent waveform-decreased RA-PSV with ragged spectral envelope and spontaneous bidirectional signals. *C*, Spectral analysis several vessel diameters distal to stenosis demonstrating return of nearly normal waveform.

sis, and 35 of 39 kidneys with 60% to 99% renal artery stenosis. All 15 renal artery occlusions were correctly identified by failure to obtain a Doppler-shifted signal from an imaged renal artery. Using this method and criteria for interpretation, RDS was 93% sensitive and 98% specific.

Renal Arteriography

Controversy continues over the use of aortography and renal arteriography in the routine screening of hypertensive individuals. Some believe these should be reserved for select groups of patients. We do not share this conservative view and proceed with arteriography in circumstances summarized in the previous section.

Although intraarterial digital subtraction angiography is used in many centers to evaluate the renal arteries, we have continued to use standard cut-film arteriography. In our experience, adequate assessment of the renal vasculature and juxtarenal aorta requires multiple injections when intraarterial digital subtraction angiography is used. A single midstream flush aortogram requires no more contrast material than is required for multiple intraarterial digital subtraction studies. In addition, standard arteriography provides information concerning cortical thickness and renal length, as well as improved clarity for interpretation of the renal artery anatomy. The fact that arteriography in patients with severe renal insufficiency, especially those with concomitant diabetes mellitus, can aggravate renal failure is recognized widely. Nevertheless, we believe that this risk is justified in patients with severe or accelerated hypertension and in those with positive RDS results. In these circumstances, the potential benefit derived from the identification and correction of a functionally significant renovascular occlusive lesion exceeds the risk of arteriography. In fact, we have not had a single patient placed on permanent dialysis as a result of contrast-related renal failure.

Both aortography and selective renal arteriography using multiple projections may be necessary to adequately examine the entire renal artery. The proximal third of the left renal artery usually courses anteriorly, the middle third transversely, and the distal third posteriorly, whereas the right renal artery pursues a more consistent posterior course. Lesions in the renal artery that are coursing anteriorly or posteriorly are frequently not seen or may appear insignificant in an anteroposterior (AP) aortogram. Oblique aortography or oblique selective renal arteriography projects these portions of the vessels in profile and reveals the stenosis. Figure 29–6 shows how the delicate septal lesions of fibromuscular dysplasia may be unrecognizable or appear insignificant in the AP projection, whereas in the oblique projection the true severity is demonstrated.

Functional Studies

Two tests, renal vein renin assays and split renal function studies, have proved valuable in confirming the functional significance of renal artery stenosis. Neither has great value, however, when severe bilateral disease or disease in the renal artery supplying a single kidney is present. In

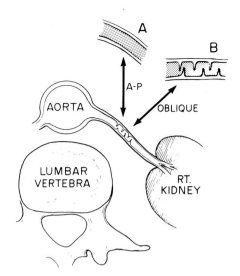

Figure 29–6. Graphic illustration of how the septa of fibromuscular dysplasia can be missed. *A,* When the vessel is viewed with an anteroposterior arteriogram, the septa are masked by the overlying dye column. *B,* They are demonstrated by oblique projection placing the direction of the vessel in a perpendicular direction and the septa parallel to the direction of the x-ray.

these circumstances, the decision for operation is based on the severity of hypertension and the degree of renal insufficiency. Further, urologically performed split renal function studies are no longer done in any center studying patients with RVH. Therefore, the reader is referred to earlier texts describing their use historically.[33, 34]

Renal Vein Renin Assays

When a unilateral obstructive lesion is found by renal arteriography, its functional significance should be evaluated. Most centers now rely solely on renal vein renin assays (RVRAs) to establish the diagnosis of RVH. The unfortunate consequence of this trend is that one must presume that all patients with RVH have lateralizing RVRAs. Results of evaluation of this study in our center underscore the fallacy of this presumption. Many factors affect the results of the RVRA that, if not properly managed, lead to erroneous results.

The effect of antihypertensive medications and unrestricted sodium intake on renin release, and thereby the RVRA, is widely recognized. Many antihypertensive medications, especially those that function through β-adrenergic blockade, suppress renin output and can lead to false nonlateralization of the RVRA. Before one can consider that no drug interference in the release of renin is occurring, all such medications must be withheld for at least 5 days or, preferably, 2 weeks before the RVRA. Similar effects on renin levels are seen when sodium intake is not restricted. For this reason, the patient must be on no more than a 2-g sodium diet for at least 2 weeks before the study. The preparation of patients for RVRA in our center is summarized in Table 29–4.

The technical aspects of performing the RVRA cannot be overemphasized. The left renal vein contains not only renal venous effluent but also adrenal, gonadal, and lumbar

TABLE 29–4

Patient Preparation for Renal Vein Renin Assays

1. Chronic salt restriction (2-g sodium diet)
2. Discontinue all antihypertensive drugs except diuretics for at least 5 days before the study
3. Oral furosemide (40 mg) diuresis the night before the study
4. Nothing by mouth for 8 hr before the study
5. Strictly flat bed rest for 4 hours before and during the study
6. Prestudy sedation with intramuscular diazepam (Valium) (5 mg)

venous effluent. Misplacement of the venous catheter into the origin of one of the nonrenal branches or sampling in the proximal renal vein where a mixture from these other sources is present may dilute the renin activity coming from the kidney. This leads to erroneously low measurements of renin activity and produces a false interpretation of the RVRA.

The time of sampling the two renal veins for renin activity is also a potential source of error in the RVRA. In studies performed with a single catheter, several minutes may elapse between sampling the two renal veins as the catheter is switched from one side to the other. Furthermore, catheter manipulation and patient discomfort may affect renin release. Not surprisingly, therefore, when the single catheter is employed, both false-positive and false-negative renal vein renin ratios are frequent.

Several methods of stimulating renin release have been suggested. These include tilting the patient to the upright posture during the study, stimulation with intravenous hydralazine hydrochloride, and, more recently, nitroprusside stimulation. Although all of these methods increase renin release, they also increase false-positive determinations and reduce the reliability of the RVRA to unacceptable levels.

Vaughn and colleagues[35] stressed the importance of expressing the RVRA in relation to the systemic renin activity rather than simply evaluating the ratio of renin activity between the two renal veins. In patients with RVH secondary to unilateral renal artery stenosis, one should find hypersecretion of renin from the ischemic kidney and suppression of renin secretion from the normal kidney. Through application of this hypothesis, Stanley and Fry[36] have shown a statistically significant difference in the renal–systemic renin indices in patients who were cured of RVH by operation compared with those who were only improved. Although this method has appeal as a predictor of the extent of benefit, its value in patients with bilateral renal artery lesions is limited. Because both lesions may be producing RVH, both this method and renal vein renin ratios have reduced validity as predictors of response to operation. Furthermore, the risk of hypertension is more directly related to its severity rather than to its absolute presence or absence. If one bases the decision for operative management solely on whether absolute cure is expected, many patients who would receive the benefit of reduction in severity of hypertension to a mild, easily controlled level would be dropped from consideration as operative candidates. Therefore, this method of RVRA interpretation should be considered only as an additional predictive tool

and not as an alternative to the evaluation of renal vein renin ratios.

RVRAs also may be spuriously unrevealing in patients with accessory or segmental renal artery stenosis if renal venous sampling is limited to the main renal vein. Because recognition of renin hypersecretion depends on sampling the ischemic areas of the kidneys, selective segmental venous sampling must be done in these patients. When segmental sampling is required, the renin activity from the segment sampled is compared with the simultaneously collected contralateral main renal vein sample to calculate the renal vein renin ratio.

THERAPEUTIC OPTIONS

Identification of the optimal method of treating patients with RVH remains an elusive goal. Advocates of drug therapy, operative management, and, more recently, percutaneous transluminal angioplasty (PTA) separately defend their viewpoints with selective data from the literature to strengthen their argument. A majority of the medical community still only evaluates patients for RVH when medications are not tolerated and hypertension remains severe and uncontrolled. Currently, no prospective study compares medical therapy with surgical intervention in a randomized fashion. The study by Hunt and Strong[37] is the most informative study currently available to assess the comparative value of drug therapy and operation. In their study, they compared the results of operative treatment in 100 patients with the results of drug therapy in 114 similar patients. After 7 to 14 years of follow-up, 84% of the patients in the group undergoing operation were alive compared with 66% in the drug therapy group. Furthermore, of the 84% of patients alive in the group undergoing operation, 93 were cured or significantly improved, whereas 16 (21%) of the patients alive in the drug therapy group required operation for uncontrollable hypertension. Another seven patients remained uncontrolled without operation. Death during follow-up was twice as common in the medically treated group. These differences were statistically significant ($P < .01$) in both patients with atherosclerotic lesions and those with fibromuscular lesions of the renal artery.

Additional information influencing the decision for operative management of RVH in the atherosclerotic patient is the anatomic and renal function changes that occur during drug therapy. We have reported the results of serial renal function studies that were performed on 41 patients with RVH secondary to atherosclerotic renal artery disease who had been randomly selected for nonoperative management[38] (Table 29–5). In 19 patients, serum creatinine levels increased between 25% and 50%. The GFRs dropped between 25% and 50% in 12 patients. Fourteen patients (37%) lost more than 10% of renal length. In four patients (12%), a significant stenosis progressed to total occlusion. Seventeen patients (41%) had deterioration of renal function or loss of renal size that led to operation. One patient required removal of a previously reconstructable kidney. Of the 17 patients with deterioration, 15 had acceptable blood pressure control during the period of nonoperative observation. Therefore, we believe that progressive deterio-

TABLE 29-5

Frequency of Severe Deterioration in Parameters of Renal Function During Drug Therapy

PARAMETER	PATIENTS MONITORED	MEAN FOLLOW-UP	FAILURE EVENT	NO. AFFECTED	PERCENTAGE AFFECTED
Renal length	38	33 mo	≥10% decrease	14	37
Serum creatinine	41	25 mo	≥100% increase	2	5
Glomerular filtration rate or creatinine clearance	30	19 mo	≥50% decrease	1	3
Totals	41			17	41

From Dean RH, Kieffer RW, Smith BM, et al: Renovascular hypertension. Arch Surg 116:1408, 1981.

ration of renal function in nonoperatively treated patients with atherosclerotic renal artery stenosis and RVH is indicated, even in the presence of blood pressure control with drugs.

The detrimental changes that occur during drug therapy and the current excellent results of operative management[16] argue for the merits of renal revascularization in the treatment of RVH. Our indications for operative management of RVH have been outlined in detail elsewhere.[39] Nevertheless, in brief, all patients with severe, difficult-to-control hypertension should be considered for operation. This includes patients with complicating factors such as branch lesions or extrarenal vascular disease and patients with associated cardiovascular disease that would be improved by blood pressure reduction.

Young patients with moderate hypertension and no complicating diseases who have an easily correctable atherosclerotic or fibromuscular main renal artery stenosis also are candidates for operation. The chance for cure of moderate hypertension is quite good in such patients who have no complicating factors. Whether drug control is ever as good as the complete cure of hypertension remains to be determined. In fact, one might argue that reduction in the driving pressure of blood flow across the stenosis by successful drug therapy might accelerate deterioration in renal function by further reducing renal perfusion.

Finally, no clear evidence shows that age, type of lesion (whether atherosclerotic or fibromuscular), duration of hypertension, or the presence of bilateral lesions by themselves has proven value as a determinant of operative risk or likelihood of successful operative management. Therefore, these factors should not be used as deterrents to such management.

Preoperative Preparation

Antihypertensive medications are reduced during the preoperative period to the minimum necessary for blood pressure control. Frequently, patients requiring large doses of multiple medications for control have significantly reduced requirements while hospitalized and placed at bed rest. If continued therapy is required, vasodilators (e.g., nifedipine) in combination with selective β-adrenergic blockade (e.g., atenolol) are the drugs of choice. Little effect occurs on hemodynamics when these agents are combined with anesthesia. If the patient's diastolic blood pressure exceeds

120 mm Hg, the pressure must be brought under control and operative treatment must be postponed until this is accomplished. If blood pressure has been difficult to control, we have transferred the patient to the intensive care unit, where intravenous nitroprusside therapy with continuous intraarterial monitoring of blood pressure is instituted for the 24 hours before operation. Similarly, if the patient has a significant history of heart disease, pulmonary artery wedge pressure and cardiac performance are monitored to maintain optimal cardiac hemodynamics and recognize and correct adverse changes before they become clinically significant.

Operative Techniques

A variety of operative techniques have been used to correct renal artery stenoses. From a practical standpoint, three basic operations have been most frequently utilized: aortorenal bypass, thromboendarterectomy, and reimplantation. Bypass is most versatile. Endarterectomy has particular application to artificial atherosclerosis, especially when renal-type arteries are involved. When the renal artery is sufficiently redundant, reimplantation is technically easiest and has particular application in children (Fig. 29–7).

Certain measures and maneuvers are applicable to almost all renal arterial operations. Mannitol, 12.5 g, is administered intravenously early in the operation. Just before renal artery cross-clamping, heparin, 100 units/kg, is given intravenously and systemic anticoagulation is verified by activated clotting time. Protamine is rarely required for reversal of the heparin at the end of the reconstruction.

Mobilization and Dissection

Through a midline xiphoid-to-pubis incision, the posterior peritoneum overlying the aorta is incised longitudinally and the duodenum is reflected to the patient's right to expose the left renal artery. By extending the posterior peritoneal incision to the left along the inferior border of the pancreas, an avascular plane behind the pancreas can be entered (Fig. 29–8) to expose the entire renal hilum on the left.

This exposure is of special significance when distal lesions must also be managed. The left renal artery lies behind the left renal vein. In some cases, the vein can be

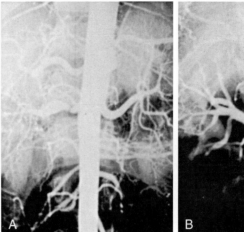

Figure 29–7. Preoperative *(A)* and postoperative *(B)* arteriograms in a 5-year-old child who underwent right renal artery reimplantation.

retracted cephalad to expose the artery; in other cases, caudal retraction of the vein provides better access. Usually, the gonadal and adrenal veins, which enter the left renal vein, must be ligated and divided to facilitate exposure of the artery. Frequently, a lumbar vein enters the posterior wall of the left renal vein, and it can be avulsed easily unless special care is taken while mobilizing the renal vein. The proximal portion of the right renal artery can be exposed through the base of the mesentery by ligating two or more pairs of lumbar veins and retracting the left renal vein cephalad and the vena cava to the patient's right. However, the distal portion of the right renal artery is best exposed by mobilizing the duodenum and right colon medially (Fig. 29–9). Then the right renal vein is mobilized and usually retracted cephalad to expose the artery.

When bilateral renal artery lesions are to be corrected and when correction of a right renal artery lesion or bilateral lesions is combined with aortic reconstruction, we modify these exposure techniques. First, we extend the base of the mesentery exposure to allow complete evisceration of the entire small bowel and the right and transverse portions of the colon; in this exposure, the posterior peritoneal incision begins with division of the ligament of Treitz and proceeds along the base of the mesentery to the cecum

and then up the lateral gutter to the foramen of Winslow (Fig. 29–10). Second, we extend the incision to the left along the inferior border of the pancreas to enter a retropancreatic plane, thereby exposing the aorta to a point above the superior mesenteric artery. Through this modified exposure, simultaneous bilateral renal endarterectomies, aortorenal grafting, or renal artery attachment to the aortic graft can be performed with wide visualization of the entire area.

One other technique that we sometimes use is partially dividing both diaphragmatic crura as they pass behind the renal arteries to their paravertebral attachment. By this partial division of the crura, the aorta above the superior mesenteric artery is easily visualized and can be mobilized for suprarenal cross-clamping.

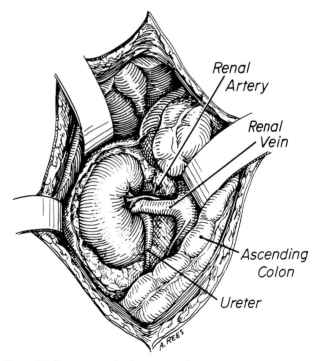

Figure 29–9. Drawing of reflection of right colon and duodenum to the left to expose the distal right renal artery.

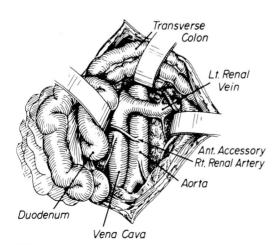

Figure 29–8. Exposure of the retroperitoneum through the base of the mesentery.

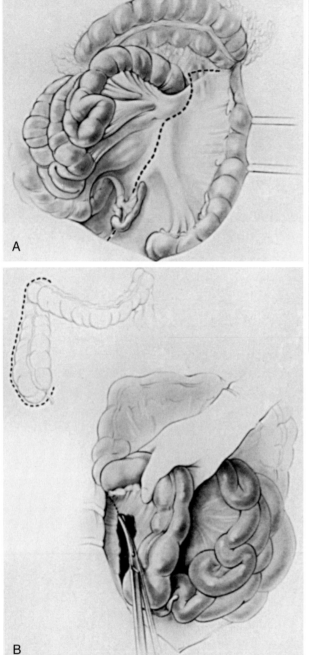

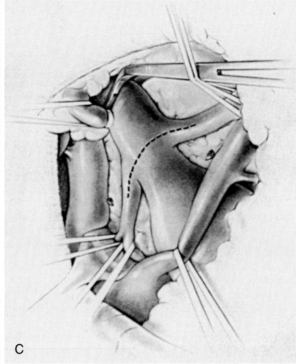

Figure 29–10. Drawing of evisceration for bilateral renal artery exposure. Incision begins at base of mesentery *(A)* and continues around the cecum and up the right lateral mesocolon peritoneal reflection *(B)*. With the use of this technique, the entire small bowel and right side of the colon are eviscerated for exposure of the entire juxtarenal aorta and both renal arteries *(C)*.

Aortorenal Bypass

Three types of graft are usually available for aortorenal bypass: autologous saphenous vein, autologous hypogastric artery, and synthetic prosthesis. The decision as to which graft should be used depends on a number of factors. We use the saphenous vein preferentially. However, if it is small (less than 4 mm in diameter) or sclerotic, the hypogastric artery or a synthetic prosthesis may be preferable. A thin-walled 6-mm polytetrafluoroethylene graft is quite satisfactory when the distal renal artery is of large caliber.

When an end-to-side renal artery bypass is used, the anastomosis between the renal artery and the graft is done first. Silastic slings can be used to occlude the renal artery

distally. This method of vessel occlusion is especially applicable to this procedure. In contrast to vascular clamps, these slings are essentially atraumatic to the delicate renal artery. The absence of clamps in the operative field is also advantageous. Furthermore, when tension is applied to the slings, they lift the vessel out of the retroperitoneal soft tissue for more accurate visualization.

The length of the arteriotomy should be at least three times the diameter of the renal artery to guard against late suture-line stenosis. A 6-0 or 7-0 monofilament polypropylene suture material is employed with loop magnification.

After the renal artery anastomosis is completed, the occluding clamps and slings are removed from the artery and a small bulldog clamp is placed across the vein graft adjacent to the anastomosis. The aortic anastomosis is then done. First, an ellipse of the anterolateral aortic wall is removed, and then the anastomosis is performed. If the graft is too long, kinking of the vein and subsequent thrombosis may result. If any element of kinking or twisting of the graft occurs after both anastomoses are completed, the aortic anastomosis should be taken down and redone after appropriate shortening or reorientation of the graft. In most instances, an end-to-end anastomosis between the graft and the renal artery provides a better reconstruction. This is especially true for combined aortorenal reconstruction. In this circumstance, the renal artery graft is attached to the Dacron aortic graft before its insertion. After the aortic graft is attached and flow is restored to the distal extremities, the renal artery can be transected and attached to the end of the saphenous vein graft without interrupting aortic flow.

Thromboendarterectomy

Thromboendarterectomy is used only for atherosclerotic renal artery stenosis. It is not applicable in fibromuscular disease. Transaortic endarterectomy of bilateral main renal artery lesions has been strongly advocated by Wylie and colleagues.[40] In this procedure, the proximal aortic clamp must usually be placed above the superior mesenteric artery. If it is placed below this artery, it seriously compromises the exposure of the orifices of the renal arteries. Visualization of the distal end of the renal artery endarterectomy is facilitated by inversion of the renal artery into the aorta. Alternatively, a transrenal endarterectomy uses a transverse aortotomy, carrying the incision across the stenoses and into each renal artery. By this method, the entire endarterectomy can be performed under direct vision with Dacron patch closure (Fig. 29–11).

Extra-anatomic Bypasses

Extra-anatomic procedures have received increased use and popularity as an alternative method of renal revascu-

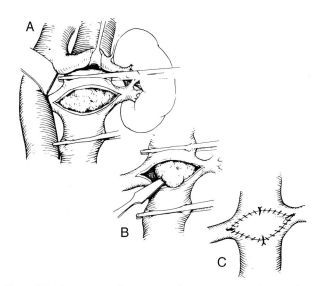

Figure 29–11. Drawing of arteriotomy for transaortic renal artery thromboendarterectomy.

larization for the high-risk patient.[41] We do not believe that these procedures are equivalent to direct reconstructions, but they are useful in a highly selective subgroup of high-risk patients.

Hepatorenal Bypass

A right subcostal incision is usually used to perform the hepatorenal bypass. The hepatoduodenal ligament is incised, and the common hepatic artery both proximal and distal to the gastroduodenal artery origin is encircled. Next, the descending duodenum is mobilized by Kocher's maneuver, the inferior vena cava is identified, the right renal vein is identified, and the right renal artery is encircled where it is found, either immediately cephalad or caudad to the renal vein.

A greater saphenous vein graft is usually used to construct the bypass. The hepatic artery anastomosis of the vein graft can be placed at the site of the amputated stump of the gastroduodenal artery or proximal to this branch when it must be saved as a collateral for gut perfusion. After completion of this anastomosis, the renal artery is transected and brought anterior to the vena cava for anastomosis end to end to the graft.

Splenorenal Bypass

Splenorenal bypass can be performed through a midline or a left subcostal incision. The posterior pancreas is mobilized by reflecting the inferior border cephalad. When the retropancreatic plane has been entered, the splenic artery can be mobilized from the left gastroepiploic artery to the level of its branches. The left renal artery is exposed as described earlier. After the splenic artery has been completely mobilized, it is divided distally, spatulated, and anastomosed end to end to the transected renal artery.

Ex Vivo Reconstruction

Ex vivo management is necessary in patients with fibromuscular dysplasia and aneurysms or stenoses involving renal artery branches, patients with fibromuscular dysplasia, renal artery dissection, and branch occlusion, patients with congenital arteriovenous fistulas of renal artery branches requiring partial resection, and patients with degeneration of previously placed grafts to the distal renal artery. Several methods of ex vivo hypothermic perfusion and reconstruction are available. A midline xiphoid-to-pubic incision is used for most renovascular procedures and is preferred when autotransplantation of the reconstructed kidney or combined aortic reconstructions are to be performed. An extended flank incision made parallel to the lower rib margin and carried to the posterior axillary line is used for complex branch renal artery repairs and is our preferred approach for ex vivo reconstructions without autotransplantation. The ureter is always mobilized but left intact, and an elastic sling or noncrushing clamp is placed around it to prevent collateral perfusion, inadvertent rewarming, or continued blood loss through the ureter.

TABLE 29-6

Electrolyte Solution* for ex vivo Repair

COMPOSITION		IONIC CONCENTRATION		ADDITIVES AT TIME OF USE TO 930 mL OF SOLUTION
Component	Amount (g/L)	Electrolyte	Concentration (mEq/L)	
K_2HPO_4	7.4	Potassium	115	50% dextrose: 70 mL
KH_2PO_4	2.04	Sodium	10	Sodium heparin: 2000 units
KCl	1.12	Phosphate (HPO_4^{2-})	85	
$NaHCO_3$	0.84	Phosphate ($H_2PO_4^-$)	15	
		Chloride	15	
		Bicarbonate	10	

*Electrolyte solution for kidney preservation supplied by Travenol Labs, Inc, Deerfield, Ill.

After the kidney is mobilized and the vessels divided, the kidney is placed on the abdominal wall and perfused with a renal preservation solution. Continuous perfusion during the period of total renal ischemia is possible with complex perfusion pump systems, and may be superior for prolonged renal preservation during storage periods. However, simple intermittent flushing with a chilled preservation solution provides equal protection during the shorter periods (2 to 3 hours) required for ex vivo dissection and complex renal artery reconstructions. For intermittent flushing, we refrigerate the preservative overnight, add the additional components (Table 29–6) immediately before use to make up a liter of solution, and hang the chilled (5°C to 10°C) solution on an intravenous stand to provide gravitational perfusion pressure of at least 2 m. Five hundred milliliters of solution are flushed through the kidney immediately after its removal from the renal fossa. As each anastomosis is completed, an additional 150 to 200 mL of solution is flushed through the kidney, a procedure that also shows any leaks at the suture line.

Surface hypothermia is used to maintain constant hypothermia during ex vivo renal artery reconstruction. Our method of surface hypothermia consists of the following steps. We place 2-L bottles of normal saline solution in ice slush overnight. When we remove the kidney, we place it in a watertight plastic sheet from which excess saline solution can be suctioned away and place laparotomy pads over the kidney, keeping it cool and moist by a constant drip of the chilled saline solution. With this technique, we can maintain renal core temperatures of 10°C to 15°C throughout the period of ischemia.

We do not believe that autotransplantation to the iliac fossa is necessary for most ex vivo reconstructions, even though it is the accepted method for reattachment of the ex vivo reconstructed renal artery. Autotransplantation of the reconstructed kidney to the iliac fossa was borrowed from the renal transplant surgeon without thought being given to the significant difference between the two patient populations. Reduction in the magnitude of the operative exposure, manual palpation of the transplanted kidney, potential use of irradiation for episodes of rejection, and ease of removal when treatment of rejection has failed are all historical and practical reasons for placing the transplanted kidney into the recipient's iliac fossa, but none of these advantages apply to the patient's requiring ex vivo reconstruction.

Rather, the factors most important in this patient are related to improving the predictability of permanent patency after revascularization. Because many ex vivo procedures are performed in relatively young patients, the durability of operation should be measured in terms of decades. For this reason, attachment of the kidney to the iliac arterial system within or below sites that are highly susceptible to significant atherosclerotic occlusive disease subjects the repaired vessels to disease that may, in time, threaten their patency. Furthermore, subsequent management of peripheral vascular disease may be complicated by the presence of the autotransplanted kidney. Finally, if the kidney is replaced in the renal fossa and the renal artery graft is properly attached to the aorta at a proximal infrarenal site, the result should mimic that of the standard aortorenal bypass and thus carry a high probability of technical success and long-term durability.

For replacement of the kidney in its original site, Gerota's capsule must be removed from the kidney during mobilization. Before transection of the renal vein begins, a large vascular clamp is placed to partially occlude the vena cava where it is entered by the renal vein. An ellipse of vena cava containing the entrance site of the renal vein is then excised, and the kidney is removed for ex vivo perfusion and reconstruction (Fig. 29–12). When the renal artery–graft anastomoses are completed and the kidney is replaced in its bed, the ellipse of vena cava is reattached (Fig. 29–13). This technique protects against stenosis of the renal vein anastomosis as a result of technical error. The renal artery graft is then attached to the aorta in the standard manner.

Nephrectomy

Nephrectomy is a procedure that should be limited to a subgroup of patients with RVH in whom the kidney responsible for the hypertension has nonreconstructable vessels and negligible residual excretory function. In these circumstances, nephrectomy can provide benefit in control of hypertension while not diminishing overall excretory function. In all other circumstances in which significant residual excretory renal function is present, the price of nephrectomy (loss of functioning renal mass) is greater than the potential benefit. This extreme conservatism for the role of nephrectomy is based on the knowledge that

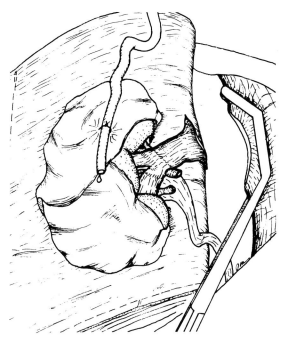

Figure 29–12. Drawing of mobilized kidney and divided renal artery and vein for ex vivo repair. Note that a partial occlusion clamp is used on the lateral vena cava to excise an ellipse that includes the origin of the renal vein.

unacceptable frequency of technical failures, and the low rate of favorable blood pressure response to operation. Certainly, the literature adequately documents the fact that poorly performed operations in poorly selected patients result in an infrequent favorable blood pressure response. Current results of operative intervention in centers experienced with management of RVH, however, underscore the predictability of success. Although our cumulative experience spans over 30 years and includes the operative management of over 1200 patients, review of the results of a recent series of 200 consecutive patients exemplifies current experience.[26] The evolution of the patient population seeking management is shown by comparing this group with the first 122 patients reported by the senior author over 30 years ago (Table 29–7).

During a 54-month period,[26] atherosclerotic RVD was the predominant pathologic condition, accounting for 78% of patients, 83% of renal artery lesions repaired, and 100% of the operative (3.1%) and follow-up patient mortality rates (17.1%). Despite the frequent need for extensive vascular repair (69%) superimposed on diffuse or extreme atherosclerotic disease (ASD) (85%) and organ-specific damage (94%), beneficial hypertension response was observed in 90% of patients with atherosclerotic RVD. Note that the contemporary group is considerably older and

more than 35% of patients with atherosclerotic lesions develop contralateral severe lesions during follow-up. Such lesions place the patient at risk of clinically severe renal failure and recurrent hypertension. This is of even greater importance in children, among whom 50% of those who initially show a unilateral lesion subsequently develop contralateral disease.

EFFECT OF OPERATION ON HYPERTENSION

Most of the controversy surrounding the role of operative treatment of RVH relates to the risk of operation, the

TABLE 29–7

Comparison of Surgical Experience over Time

	1961–1972*	1987–1991†
No. of patients	122	200
Mean age (yr)		
NAs RVD	33	38
As RVD	50	62
Duration of hypertension (yr)		
NAs RVD	4.6	11.2
As RVD	5.1	15.0
Renal artery disease (%)		
NAs RVD	35	21
As RVD	65	79
Renal artery repair (%)		
Unilateral	80	60
Bilateral	20	40
Combined‡	13	32
Renal insufficiency (%)		
Not dependent on dialysis	8	65
Dependent on dialysis	0	6
Graft failure (%)	16	3
Hypertension response (%)		
NAs RVD		
Cured	72§	43
Improved	24§	49
As RVD		
Cured	53§	15
Improved	36§	75

*Data from Foster JH, Dean RH, Pinkerton JA, et al: Ten years experience with the surgical management of renovascular hypertension. Ann Surg 177:755, 1973.
†Data from Hansen KJ, Starr SM, Sands RE, et al: Contemporary surgical management of renovascular disease. J Vasc Surg 16:319–333, 1992.
‡Combined aortic repair for occlusive or aneurysmal disease.
§Hypertension response excluding technical failures.
As, atherosclerotic; NAs, nonatherosclerotic; RVD, renovascular disease.

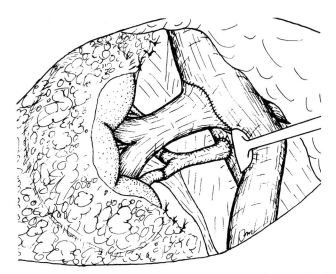

Figure 29–13. Drawing of the reimplanted kidney with arterial and venous attachments completed. The envelope of Gerota's fascia is reattached to secure the kidney in its original position.

more diffusely atherosclerotic than the patients treated in the earlier era.

Among patients with nonatherosclerotic RVD, 92% had a beneficial hypertension response; however, only 43% were considered cured, a figure below cure rates reported from earlier surgical series.[28, 42] This difference may be explained by the number of older patients, the number of patients with uncorrected contralateral lesions, and the duration of hypertension in many of these patients with nonatherosclerotic RVD. In contrast to the blood pressure results obtained in the entire group, patients younger than 55 years of age who had all anatomic renal artery lesions corrected and who had been hypertensive for less than 5 years had a cure rate of 68% and an improvement rate of 32%. This response rate is comparable with results from earlier reports.

Although operation was accomplished in the nonatherosclerotic RVD group without death and with minimal morbidity (8.5%), the operative (3.1%) and later (17.1%) mortality among 157 patients with atherosclerotic RVD was high. Twenty-six of 32 operative and late deaths occurred in patients considered to have extreme atherosclerotic disease. The presence of near end-stage renal insufficiency (mean estimated glomerular filtration rate [EGFR] 13.7 mL/minute) accounted for this significant association with follow-up death. Furthermore, follow-up death was significantly influenced by renal function response to operation and progression to dependence on dialysis. Patients with extreme disease but improved EGFR after operation demonstrated improved survival and decreased risk of eventual dependence on dialysis compared with patients with no change in EGFR. These differences were both significant and independent. Nevertheless, the low actuarial survival among patients with extreme atherosclerotic RVD (49% at 48 months) raises the question of whether death within this group was actually accelerated by operation. Because no parallel patient group with extreme atherosclerotic RVD was medically managed, data to provide an answer to this question are lacking.

EFFECT OF RENAL REVASCULARIZATION ON ISCHEMIC NEPHROPATHY

Little information is available regarding the incidence, prevalence, spectrum of clinical presentations, or natural history of ischemic nephropathy. Nevertheless, circumstantial evidence suggests that it may be a more common cause of progressive renal failure in the atherosclerotic age group (45 years or older) than previously recognized. In a 1988 report, 73% of end-stage renal disease patients were in the atherosclerotic age group.[43] In a report by Mailloux and colleagues,[44] a presumed renovascular cause of ESRD increased in frequency from 6.7% for the period 1978 to 1981 to a frequency of 16.5% for the period 1982 to 1985. The median age at onset of ESRD for that group was the oldest of all groups, falling in the seventh decade of life.

To improve our understanding of ischemic nephropathy we undertook a retrospective review of data collected during a 42-month period from 58 consecutive patients with ischemic nephropathy who were admitted to our center for

operative management.[45] We examined the rate of decline in their renal function during the period before intervention and the impact of operation on their outcome. Their ages ranged from 22 years to 79 years (mean, 69 years). Based on serum creatinine values, immediate preoperative EGFR ranged from 0 to 46 mL/minute (mean 23.85 ± 9.76 mL/minute). Patients with at least three sequential measurements for calculations of EGFR changes during the 6 months before operation ($n = 50$) and the first 12 months after operation ($n = 32$) were used to describe the preoperative rate of decline in EGFR and the impact of operation on this decrease in the operative survivors. In addition, comparative analyses of data from patients with unilateral versus bilateral lesions and patients classified as having improvement in EGFR versus no improvement after operation were performed. Comparison of the immediate preoperative EGFR with the immediate postoperative EGFR for the entire group showed significant improvement in response to operation (Fig. 29–14). Likewise, the rate of deterioration in EGFR for the total group was improved after operation (Fig. 29–15). A similar improvement in the rate of deterioration in EGFR was seen in the subgroup of patients who received an immediate improvement in EGFR in response to operation (Fig. 29–16).

From this review we found that site of disease (unilateral or bilateral), the anatomosis status of the distal renal artery, and the rate of deterioration in renal function were significant predictors of benefit to renal function by operation. Conversely, unilateral disease, absence of severe hypertension, and diffuse branch vessel occlusive disease were negative predictors of such benefit.

The data presented in this retrospective review argue that ischemic nephropathy is a rapidly progressive form of renal insufficiency. The effect of renal revascularization on renal function, however, was heterogeneous. Nevertheless, the frequency of both retrieval of renal function and slow-

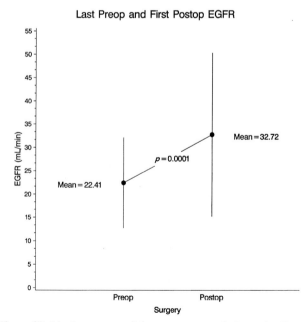

Figure 29–14. Comparison of the mean estimated glomerular filtration rate (EGFR) immediately before and at least 1 week after operation. The p value for the differences is determined using t test for unpaired data.

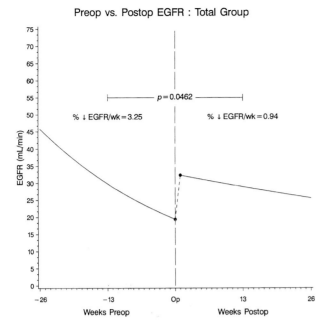

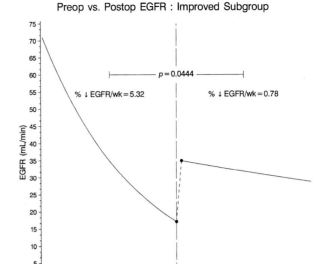

Figure 29–15. Graphic depiction of the percentage deterioration of EGFR per week for the entire group during the 6 months before ($n = 50$) and after ($n = 32$) operation. The immediate effect of operation on the estimated glomerular filtration rate (EGFR) is also depicted. The p values for differences are determined using t test for unpaired data. Note the improvement in the slope of decline in EGFR after operation.

Figure 29–16. Graphic depiction of the percentage deterioration of estimated glomerular filtration rate (EGFR) per week during the 6 months before ($n = 23$) and after ($n = 25$) operation in the group of patients who received at least a 20% improvement in EGFR following operation. The immediate effect of operation on EGFR in this group is also depicted. The p values for differences are determined using t test for unpaired data. Note the improvement in the slope of decline in EGFR after operation in this group.

ing of the rate of its deterioration during follow-up was gratifying and encourages enthusiasm for the continued study of the role of operation in properly selected patients. Most important, the results argue that a carefully controlled prospective randomized trial comparing operation with medical therapy is necessary to confirm the value of operation in patients with controlled hypertension. Only through this method could one accurately clarify the role of operation in dialysis-free survival among patients with ischemic nephropathy.

Our experience underscores the rapidity of the deterioration in renal function in patients with ischemic nephropathy and the potential benefit of operation on both GFR and its rate of deterioration in this subset of patients. Nevertheless, the risk associated with operation is not inconsequential. This risk and the rate of survival must be

placed in context with the probability of survival without operation. In a study of the duration of survival after the institution of dialysis, Mailloux and coworkers[44] found that ESRD caused by uncorrected RVD was associated with the most rapid rate of death during follow-up. In their study, patients with RVD had a median survival after the initiation of dialysis of only 27 months and a 5-year survival rate of only 12%. This equates with a death rate in excess of 20% per year. In this regard, we have recently reported our experience with 20 patients who were dialysis dependent at the time of operation. No operative deaths occurred in this group and 16 (80%) (Table 29–8) were rendered free of dialysis postoperatively.[46] Their life table survival curve is shown in Figure 29–17. Survival in those rendered

TABLE 29-8

Immediate and Late Function Response versus Site of Disease

DIALYSIS STATUS	UNILATERAL ($n = 4$) NO. OF PATIENTS (%)	BILATERAL ($n = 16$) NO. OF PATIENTS (%)	TOTAL ($n = 20$) NO. OF PATIENTS (%)
Immediate result°			
Dependent	3 (75)	1 (6)	4 (20)
Independent	1 (25)	15 (94)	16 (80)
Late result†			
Dependent	3 (75)	3 (19)	6 (30)
Independent	1 (25)	13 (81)	14 (70)

°$P = .01$, significant at the 0.05 alpha level after controlling for multiple comparisons.
†$P = .06$.

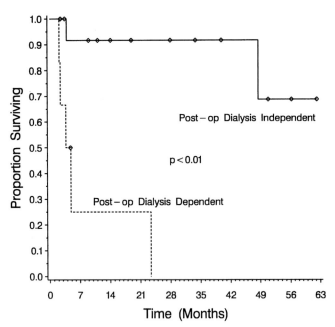

Figure 29–17. Product limit estimate of patient survival according to dialysis status after operation (*n* = 20).

dialysis independent was excellent. Those not freed from dialysis by operation had a death rate during follow-up similar to those in Mailloux's group who were not submitted to operation.

LATE FOLLOW-UP RECONSTRUCTIONS

From our experience with the operative management of RVH, 1- to 23-year follow-up sequential angiography of 198 reconstructions is available for evaluation (Table 29–9). Five saphenous vein grafts and two hypogastric autografts have undergone aneurysmal dilatation. Only one of these, a hypogastric autograft, has required replacement (Fig. 29–18). The remaining six have stabilized, and the patients have remained cured of hypertension. Aneurysmal dilatation of autogenous grafts (vein or artery) has occurred only in the young children in our experience. This suggests that the immature saphenous vein is particularly susceptible to this phenomenon. For this reason, we prefer the normal hypogastric artery as the conduit of choice for this group. In the two instances of autogenous arterial graft aneurysmal

TABLE 29-9

Sequential 1- to 23-Year Follow-up Arteriography (198 Reconstructions)

STATUS	NO. OF GRAFTS	PERCENTAGE
No adverse change	174	88%
Aneurysmal dilatation	7	3.5%
Stenosis	10	5.0%
Occlusion	4	2.0%
False aneurysm	3	1.5%

degeneration, fibromuscular dysplasia of the donor hypogastric artery was identified in retrospective microscopic evaluation.

Ten grafts developed suture-line or midgraft stenoses requiring revision from 1 to 8 years after the initial operation (Fig. 29–19). Four patients had graft occlusions during follow-up and probably represent missed graft stenoses that progressed to occlusion. Three grafts required correction of aortic anastomotic false aneurysms of Dacron grafts in two patients 8 and 20 years postoperatively. The remaining grafts (88%) had no untoward changes and continued patency of the reconstruction during follow-up (Fig. 29–20).

Follow-up angiography also showed progression of mild to moderate contralateral renovascular disease in 38% of patients. This is most important in children, in whom 7 of 15 with fibromuscular dysplasia had bilateral involvement.[24] Only three of these seven children had the contralateral disease demonstrated at the time of the initial evaluation and operation. The remaining four children had documentation of the development and progression of contralateral disease subsequently. This occurrence of subsequent contralateral stenosis has led us to perform nephrectomy in children only if blood pressure is uncontrollable and revascularization is impossible. Because the longest follow-up was only 10 years, the true incidence of subsequent contralateral disease requires additional longitudinal follow-up.

EFFECT OF BLOOD PRESSURE RESPONSE ON LONG-TERM SURVIVAL

Because the rationale for management of hypertension of any cause is to decrease long-term cardiovascular morbidity and improve event-free survival, we reviewed the outcome

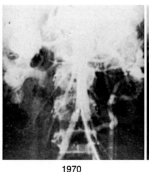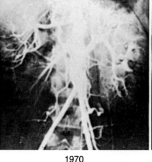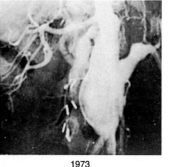

1970
PRE-OP

1970
POST-OP

1973
POST-OP

Figure 29–18. Sequential follow-up arteriograms of a 10-year-old child who underwent a hypogastric autograft to the left renal artery and an iliac vein autograft to the superior mesenteric artery. Ultimately, both grafts required replacements.

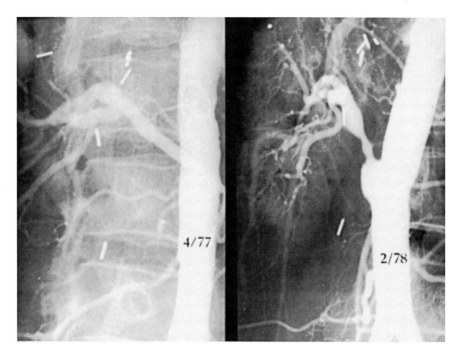

Figure 29–19. Postoperative arteriograms showing fibrous narrowing of the saphenous vein graft secondary to subendothelial fibroblastic proliferation.

of 71 patients who underwent operative management of RVH from 15 to 23 years previously.[47] Complete follow-up was available in 66 of the 68 patients who survived operation. Comparison of the initial blood pressure response after operation (1 to 6 months postoperatively) with the blood pressure status at the time of death or current date (up to 23 years later) showed that the effect of operative treatment is maintained over long-term follow-up (Fig. 29–21). In those patients who required repeat renovascular operation for recurrent RVH during follow-up, the majority of the operations were performed for the management of contralateral lesions that had progressed to functional significance (i.e., produced RVH).

Assessment of the effect of blood pressure response on late survival produced results that are not surprising. Although the subgroup of nonresponders is small, they experienced a significantly more rapid death rate during

follow-up than did those patients who had a blood pressure response to operation (Fig. 29–22). This confirms the validity of the premise that inadequate management of RVH leaves the patient at higher risk of early death from cardiovascular events. The presence of angiographically diffuse atherosclerosis at the time of evaluation and operation was predictive of a more rapid rate of death during follow-up (Fig. 29–23).

This difference in subsequent death rate was present, even though comparison between patients with diffuse atherosclerotic disease and focal atherosclerotic disease (ASF) was undertaken only in patients experiencing a significant blood pressure response. In view of the suggestion by some physicians that the presence of diffuse disease precludes a high rate of blood pressure response to operation, we stress that no significant difference occurred in frequency of response between the ASF (80%) and ASD (77%) groups in

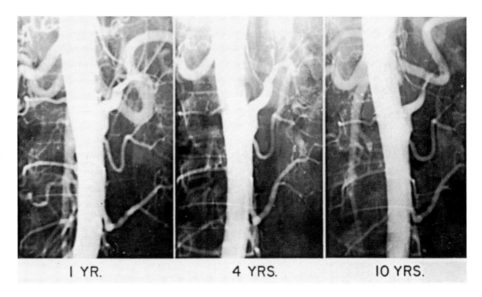

Figure 29–20. Sequential follow-up arteriograms after autogenous vein aortorenal bypass showing its long-term durability.

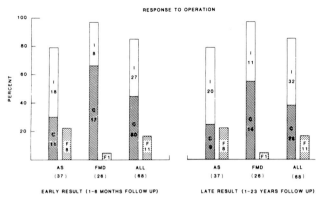

Figure 29-21. Comparison of initial benefit with late blood pressure response in the respective types of lesions. AS, arteriosclerotic lesion; FMD, fibromuscular dysplasia.

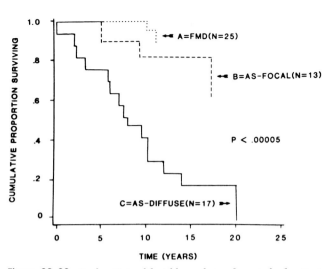

Figure 29-23. Kaplan-Meier life table analysis of survival of patients benefited from operation by type and stage of disease, with 55 patients cured or improved (deaths from cardiovascular causes). FMD, fibromuscular dysplasia; AS-DIFFUSE, diffuse atherosclerosis; AS-FOCAL, focal atherosclerosis.

this study. In addition, although the presence of ASD was associated with a more rapid death rate, it does not preclude the probability of a longer survival in this subgroup compared with a similar group of patients who either did not undergo operation or received no blood pressure benefit from such intervention. Furthermore, if one considers that ASD is only a later stage of ASF, the fact that the end point of clinically significant disease, namely, death from cardiovascular events, arrives sooner when one begins follow-up or removes a risk factor that causes its acceleration later in its natural history is not surprising.

In contrast to the group described above, the contemporary group of 534 patients managed by us during the past decade do not demonstrate improved event-free survival in association with beneficial blood pressure response to operation.[48] Although there are a number of theoretical explanations for this observed difference, renal function response among contemporary patients demonstrates a significant and independent association with follow-up survival. Global renal disease treated with complete renal

artery repair after rapid decline in renal function provides the best opportunity for improved glomerular filtration. Patients with renal function both unimproved and worsened remain at increased risk for eventual dialysis dependence. In the contemporary population, progression to dialysis dependence is the single strongest risk factor for follow-up death.

PERCUTANEOUS TRANSLUMINAL ANGIOPLASTY

The introduction of the alternative interventional modality PTA by Gruntzig and colleagues[49] in 1978 led to a new era in the management of patients with renal artery stenosis. This technique employs the principle of coaxial dilatation of the vessel by inflation of a balloon-tipped catheter that has been introduced across the stenotic renal artery lesion. The stenotic lesion is disrupted, and, by stretching the vessel wall itself, portions of the media are disrupted as well, leaving the vessel at a greater diameter than its dimension before dilatation. The increased luminal diameter is primarily created by disruption of the intima, the atherosclerotic or fibrodysplastic lesion, and dilatation of the less diseased arterial wall. Early reports of the results of this technique showed that stenotic renal arteries frequently could be dilated successfully with immediate improvement in levels of hypertension in patients with RVH.

By reviewing the reported experience with PTA and the observations from the operative management of unsuccessful PTA, one can formulate indications for the preferential use of each procedure in the treatment of RVH. Reported experience with PTA of medial fibroplasia shows results similar to those of open surgical repairs. Beneficial blood pressure responses have been reported to be as high as 100% after PTA in properly selected patients, and although vessel perforation, hemorrhage, and branch occlusions have been reported, their incidence has been less than 5%.[50] One would anticipate that such complications would be

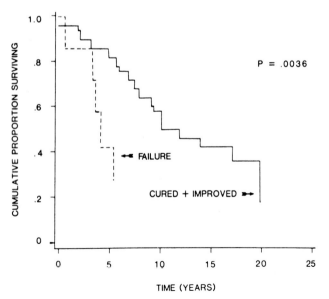

Figure 29-22. Kaplan-Meier life table analysis: survival by response to operation in 37 arteriosclerotic patients (deaths from cardiovascular causes).

TABLE 29–10

Percutaneous Transluminal Angioplasty with Renal Artery Stent Placement for Ostial Atherosclerotic Renal Artery Stenosis

SOURCE (YR)	PATIENTS WITH OSTIAL LESIONS (n)	PATIENTS WITH RENAL DYSFUNCTION (n)	FUNCTION RESPONSE			HYPERTENSION			RESTEN-OSIS (%)
			Improved (%)	Unchanged (%)	Worsened (%)	Cured (%)	Improved (%)	Failed (%)	
Rees et al. (1991)[54]	28	14	36	36	29	11	54	36	39
Hennequin et al., (1994)[55]	7	2	0	50	50	0	100	0	43
Raynaud et al. (1994)[56]	4	3	0	33	67	0	50	50	33
MacLeod et al. (1995)[57]	22	13	15	85		0	31	69	20
van de Ven et al. (1995)[58]	24	NR	33	58	8	0	73	27	13
Blum et al (1997)[59]	68	20	0	100	0	16	62	22	17
Total	153	52	13	73	14	9	59	32	23

NR, not reported.

most likely in patients with diffuse fibromuscular dysplasia affecting both the distal main renal artery and its branches. The cure rate after PTA of fibromuscular dysplasia when the procedure is performed by experienced interventionalists ranges from 37% to 51%.[51] We believe that fibromuscular dysplasia extending to the branch level is best managed primarily by an open operative approach and that PTA should be reserved for the subgroup of medial dysplastic lesions that are clearly limited to the main renal artery.

Stenotic lesions occurring in children are usually discrete narrowings and therefore would appear ideal for PTA. However, the stenotic area is commonly a congenital narrowing of the entire vessel wall and is predominantly composed of elastic tissue. When such a vessel is submitted to PTA, the original diameter returns after dilatation or, if the vessel has been overdistended, rupture of the entire vessel wall is likely. Therefore, we believe that PTA is an inappropriate method of intervention in children with renal artery stenosis and that success is best achieved by operative correction.

Finally, a review of series reporting results with PTA for atherosclerotic lesions dramatizes the frequency of failure with this lesion as well. Early reports by Miller and colleagues,[52] in 1985, noted that only 45% of ostial and mixed lesions were improved after 6 months; Sos and colleagues[51] reported only a 14% benefit rate when bilateral ostial lesions were treated. These results show that PTA alone has little value in the treatment of this variety of lesion, for one must accept the risks of cholesterol embolization, vessel thrombosis, and loss of renal function while expecting only a minimal chance for prolonged benefit.

Endoluminal stenting of the renal artery was first introduced in the United States in 1988 as part of a multicenter trial with 263 patients.[53] During this same period, the Palmaz stent (Johnson & Johnson Interventional Systems, Warren, NJ) and Wallstent (Medinvent, Lausanne, Switzerland; Schneider, Minneapolis) were being used in Europe. Although currently no stent has been approved for renal use in the United States, the most common indications for use seem to be (1) elastic recoil of the vessel immediately after angioplasty, (2) dissection after angioplasty, and (3) restenosis after angioplasty. In the multicenter trial, improvement or cure in hypertension was seen in 61% of patients at 1 year. After follow-up of less than 1 year, angiographic restenosis occurred in 32.7% of patients.

These results remain inferior compared with contemporary surgical results.[26]

Table 29–10 summarizes single-center reports with renal function and angiographic follow-up after treatment of ostial atherosclerosis by PTA in combination with endoluminal stents.[54–59] These studies differ in regard to criteria for ostial lesions, evaluation of the clinical response to intervention, and parameters for significant restenoses. Despite these differences, these cumulative results provide the best available estimates of early hypertension response, change in renal function, and primary patency. From these data, immediate technical success was observed in 99% of patients and beneficial blood pressure response (cured and improved) was observed in 68%. However, only 13% of patients with renal insufficiency demonstrated improved excretory renal function, whereas 14% of patients were worse after intervention. During angiographic follow-up ranging from 5.8 to 16.4 months, restenosis was observed in 13% to 39% of patients. Based on available data, percutaneous angioplasty with stenting of ostial atherosclerosis appears to yield blood pressure, renal function, and anatomic results that are inferior compared with contemporary surgical results.[60] Moreover, no studies to date have examined long-term renal function results after either primary or secondary PTA with or without stents. For these reasons, we believe that operation remains the initial treatment of choice for patients with ostial renal artery atherosclerosis, especially when hypertension is present in combination with renal insufficiency.

To summarize, experience with the liberal use of PTA has helped to clarify its role as one of the therapeutic options in the treatment of RVH, but the data now accumulated argue for its selective application. In this regard, PTA of nonorificial atherosclerotic lesions and medial fibrodysplastic lesions limited to the main renal artery yields results comparable with those of operation if carried out by persons experienced in the technique. In contrast, the use of PTA for the treatment of congenital stenotic lesions, fibrodysplastic lesions involving renal artery branches, and ostial atherosclerotic lesions in association with ischemic nephropathy is associated with inferior results and with increased risk of complications. We believe that operation remains the initial treatment of choice for patients in these groups, although the type of interventional therapy for RVH must always be individualized.

References

1. Bright R: Cases and observations illustrative of renal disease accompanied with the secretion of albuminous urine. Guys Hosp Rep 1:388, 1836.

2. Tigerstedt R, Bergman PG: Niere und Kreislauf. Scand Arch Physiol 8:223, 1898.

3. Goldblatt H: Studies on experimental hypertension. J Exp Med 59:347, 1934.

4. Smith HW: Unilateral nephrectomy in hypertensive disease. J Urol 76:685, 1956.

5. Freeman N: Thromboendarterectomy for hypertension due to renal artery occlusion. JAMA 157:1077, 1973.

6. DeCamp PT, Birchall R: Recognition and treatment of renal arterial stenosis associated with hypertension. Surgery 43:134, 1958.

7. Morris GC Jr, Cooley DA, Crawford ES, et al: Renal revascularization for hypertension: Clinical and physiologic studies in 32 cases. Surgery 48:95, 1960.

8. Hurwitt ES, Seidenburg B, Hainovoco H, et al: Splenorenal arterial anastomosis. Circulation 14:537, 1956.

9. Luke JC, Levitan BA: Revascularization of the kidney in hypertension due to renal artery stenosis. Arch Surg 79:269, 1959.

10. Howard JE, Conner TB: Use of differential renal function studies in the diagnosis of renovascular hypertension. Am J Surg 107:58, 1964.

11. Stamey TA, Nudelman IJ, Good PH, et al: Functional characteristics of renovascular hypertension. Medicine (Baltimore) 40:347, 1961.

12. Page IH, Helmes OM: A crystalline pressor substance (angiotensin) resulting from the reaction between renin and renin activator. J Exp Med 71:29, 1940.

13. Braun-Menendez E, Fasciolo JC, Lelois LF, et al: La substancia hypertensora de la sangre del rinon, isquemiado. Rev Soc Argent Biol 15:420, 1939.

14. Lentz KE, Skeggs LT Jr, Woods KR, et al: The amino acid composition of angiotensin II and its biochemical relationship to hypertension. Int J Exp Med 104:183, 1956.

15. Tobian L: Relationship of juxtaglomerular apparatus to renin and angiotensin. Circulation 25:189, 1962.

16. Dean RH: Operative management of renovascular hypertension. In Bergan JJ, Yao JST (eds): Surgery of the Aorta and Its Body Branches. New York, Grune & Stratton, 1979, p 377.

17. Dean RH, Englund R, Dupont WD, et al: Retrieval of renal function by revascularization. Study of preoperative outcome predictors. Ann Surg 202:367, 1985.

18. Novick AC, Pohl MA, Schreiber M, et al: Revascularization for preservation of renal function in patients with atherosclerotic renovascular disease. J Urol 129:907, 1983.

19. Zinman L, Libertino JA: Revascularization of the chronic totally occluded renal artery with restoration of renal function. J Urol 228:517, 1977.

20. Morris GC Jr, DeBakey ME, Cooley DA: Surgical treatment of renal failure of renovascular origin. JAMA 182:609, 1962.

21. Harrison EG Jr, McCormack LJ: Pathologic classification of renal arterial disease in renovascular hypertension. Mayo Clin Proc 46:161, 1971.

22. Tucker RM, Labarthe DR: Frequency of surgical treatment for hypertension in adults at the Mayo Clinic from 1973 through 1975. Mayo Clin Proc 52:549, 1977.

23. Shapiro AP, Perez-Stable E, Scheib ET, et al: Renal artery stenosis and hypertension. Am J Med 47:175, 1969.

24. Lawson JD, Boerth RK, Foster JH, et al: Diagnosis and management of renovascular hypertension in children. Arch Surg 112:1307, 1977.

25. Simon N, Franklin SS, Bleifer KH, Maxwell MH: Clinical characteristics of renovascular hypertension. JAMA 220:1209, 1972.

26. Hansen KJ, Starr SM, Sands RE, et al: Contemporary surgical management of renovascular disease. J Vasc Surg 16:319–331, 1992.

27. Meier GH, Sumpio B, Black HR, Gusberg RJ: Captopril renal scintigraphy: An advance in the detection and treatment of renovascular hypertension. J Vasc Surg 11:770–777, 1990.

28. Hansen KJ, Tribble RW, Reavis S, et al: Renal duplex sonography: Evaluation of clinical utility. J Vasc Surg 12:227–236, 1990.

29. Norris CS, Pfeiffer JS, Rittgers SE, Barnes RW: Noninvasive evaluation of renal artery stenosis and renovascular disease. J Vasc Surg 1:192–201, 1984.

30. Kohler TR, Zierler RE, Martin RL, et al: Noninvasive diagnosis of renal artery stenosis by ultrasonic duplex scanning. J Vasc Surg 4:450–456, 1986.

31. Taylor DC, Kettler MD, Moneta GL, et al: Duplex ultrasound scanning in the diagnosis of renal artery stenosis: A prospective evaluation. J Vasc Surg 7:363–369, 1988.

32. Barnes RW: Utility of duplex scanning of the renal artery. In Bergan JJ, Yao JST (eds): Arterial Surgery: New Diagnostic and Operative Techniques. Orlando, Fla, Grune & Stratton, 1988, pp 351–366.

33. Dean RH: Renovascular hypertension. Curr Probl Surg 22:6–67, 1985.

34. Dean RH, Rhamy RK: Split renal function studies in renovascular hypertension. In Stanley JC, Ernst CB, Fry WJ (eds): Renovascular Hypertension. Philadelphia, WB Saunders, 1984, pp 135–145.

35. Vaughn ED, Buhler FR, Larach JH, et al: Renovascular hypertension: Renin measurements to indicate hypersecretion and contralateral suppression, estimate renal plasma flow, and score for surgical curability. Am J Med 55:402, 1973.

36. Stanley JC, Fry WJ: Surgical treatment of renovascular hypertension. Arch Surg 112:1291, 1977.

37. Hunt JC, Strong CG: Renovascular hypertension. Mechanisms, natural history and treatment. Am J Cardiol 32:562, 1973.

38. Dean RH, Kieffer RW, Smith BM, et al: Renovascular hypertension. Arch Surg 116:1408, 1981.

39. Dean RH: Indications for operative management of renovascular hypertension. J S C Med Assoc 73:523–525, 1977.

40. Wylie EJ, Perloff DL, Stoney RJ: Autogenous tissue revascularization techniques in surgery for renovascular hypertension. Ann Surg 170:416, 1969.

41. Moncure AC, Brewster DC, Darling RC, et al: Use of the splenic and hepatic arteries for renal revascularization. J Vasc Surg 3:196, 1986.

42. Foster JH, Dean RH, Pinkerton JA, et al: Ten years experience with the surgical management of renovascular hypertension. Ann Surg 177:755, 1973.

43. Eggers PW: Effect of transplantation on the Medicare end-stage renal disease program. N Engl J Med 318:223–229, 1988.

44. Mailloux LU, Bellucci AG, Mossey RT, et al: Predictors of survival in patients undergoing dialysis. Am J Med 84:855–862, 1988.

45. Dean RH, Tribble RW, Hansen KJ, et al: Evolution of renal insufficiency in ischemic nephropathy. Ann Surg 213:446–456, 1991.

46. Hansen KJ, Thomason RB, Craven TE, et al: Surgical management of dialysis-dependent ischemic nephropathy. J Vasc Surg 21:197–211, 1995.

47. Dean RH, Krueger TC, Whiteneck JM, et al: Operative management of renovascular hypertension: Results after 15-23 years follow-up. J Vasc Surg 1:234, 1984.

48. Hansen KJ, Deitch JS, Oskin TC, et al: Renal artery repair: Consequence of operative failures. Ann Surg 227:678–690, 1998.

49. Gruntzig A, Vetter W, Meier B, et al: Treatment of renovascular hypertension with transluminal dilatation of a renal artery stenosis. Lancet 1:801, 1978.

50. Tegtmeyer CJ, Kellum D, Ayers C: Percutaneous transluminal angioplasty of the renal artery: Results and long-term follow-up. Radiology 153:77–84, 1984.

51. Sos TA, Pickering TG, Sniderman K, et al: Percutaneous transluminal renal angioplasty in renovascular hypertension due to atheroma of fibromuscular dysplasia. N Engl J Med 309:274–279, 1983.

52. Miller GA, Ford KK, Braun SD, et al: Percutaneous transluminal angioplasty vs. surgery for renovascular hypertension. AJR Am J Roentgenol 144:447–450, 1985.

53. Bacharach JM, Graor RA, et al: Utility of stenting for osteal renal artery stenosis. Presented at the 1994 Meeting of the Society of Vascular Surgery and International Society of Cardiovascular Surgery. Seattle, June 4–8, 1994.

54. Rees CR, Palmaz JC, Beck GJ, et al: Palmaz stent in atherosclerotic stenoses involving the ostia of the renal arteries: Preliminary report of a multicenter study. Radiology 507–514, 1991.

55. Hennequin LM, Joffre FG, Rousseau HP, et al: Renal artery stent placement: Long-term results with the Wallstent endoprosthesis. Radiology 191:713–719, 1994.

56. Raynaud AC, Beyssen BM, Turmel-Rodrigues LE, et al: Renal artery stent placement: Immediate and midterm technical and clinical results. J Vasc Interv Radiol 5:849–858, 1994.

57. MacLeod M, Taylor AD, Baxter G, et al: Renal artery stenosis man-

aged by Palmaz stent insertion: Technical and clinical outcome. J Hypertens 13:1791–1795, 1995.

58. Van de Ven PJG, Beutler JJ, Kaatee R, et al: Transluminal vascular stent for ostial atherosclerotic renal artery stenosis. Lancet 346:672–674, 1995.

59. Blum U, Krummer B, Flogel P, et al: Treatment of ostial renal artery stenoses with vascular endoprostheses after unsuccessful balloon angioplasty. N Engl J Med 336:459–465, 1997.

60. Hansen KJ, Starr SM, Sands RE, et al: Contemporary surgical management of renovascular disease. J Vasc Surg 16:319, 1992.

Questions

1. Which test is most sensitive for identification of all hypertensive patients who might have renovascular hypertension?
   (a) isotope renography
   (b) rapid sequence intravenous pyelography
   (c) arteriography
   (d) peripheral plasma renin activity

2. Which test is most specific (accurate) in confirming the presence of renovascular hypertension?
   (a) demonstration of collaterals by renal arteriography
   (b) lateralization (1.5:1) of renal venous renin assays
   (c) absence of function on rapid sequence intravenous pyelography
   (d) elevation of peripheral plasma renin activity
   (e) presence of severe renal artery stenosis in a patient with hypertension

3. What endogenous pressor substance causes elevation of blood pressure in patients with renovascular hypertension?
   (a) angiotensinogen
   (b) renin
   (c) angiotensin I
   (d) prostaglandin E_2
   (e) angiotensin II

4. Which of the factors listed is *not* a marker predictive of renal function retrieval by renal revascularization?
   (a) low volume with hypoconcentration of creatinine in urine from the affected kidney
   (b) normal intrarenal vessels on arteriography
   (c) hyperconcentration of nonreabsorbable solutes in the urine of the affected kidney
   (d) normal glomeruli and tubules on microscopic evaluation of renal biopsy
   (e) none of the above

5. Which operative technique is *never* an acceptable method for treatment of an orificial renal artery occlusion?
   (a) thromboendarterectomy
   (b) saphenous vein aortorenal bypass
   (c) synthetic graft aortorenal bypass
   (d) renal artery reimplantation
   (e) none of the above

6. In regard to long-term durability, which material is the most desirable for renal revascularization in children?
   (a) normal saphenous vein
   (b) expanded polytetrafluoroethylene
   (c) normal hypogastric artery
   (d) artery Dacron
   (e) none of the above

7. What is the apparent incidence of progressive loss of renal function in kidneys of patients treated medically for renovascular hypertension secondary to atherosclerotic renal artery stenosis?
   (a) less than 10%
   (b) 10% to 20%
   (c) greater than 40%
   (d) greater than 60%
   (e) greater than 80%

8. What percent technical success rate should be expected as an acceptable result when performing renal revascularization?
   (a) less than 50%
   (b) 50% to 70%
   (c) 70% to 80%
   (d) 80% to 90%
   (e) greater than 90%

9. Which factor most frequently determines the likelihood of long-term maintenance of initially successful blood pressure reduction by operative management of renovascular hypertension?
   (a) graft material used for aortorenal bypass
   (b) progression of contralateral disease
   (c) development of stenosis of graft anastomosis
   (d) development of new lesions beyond the bypass in the kidney operated on
   (e) none of the above

10. Which of the following does *not* have an adverse effect on the accuracy of renal venous renin assay results?
   (a) diuretic therapy
   (b) salt loading
   (c) β-adrenergic response blockers (e.g., Inderal)
   (d) intravascular volume expansion
   (e) sequential sampling of the two renal veins

Answers

1. c   2. b   3. e   4. a   5. e   6. c   7. c   8. e   9. b   10. a

30

Visceral Ischemic Syndromes

Lewis B. Schwartz, James F. McKinsey, and Bruce L. Gewertz

Although the causal relationship between acute mesenteric vascular occlusion and intestinal gangrene had been known for centuries, it was not until 1895 that the first successful case of preoperative recognition and treatment by intestinal resection was reported by J.W. Elliott.[1] Recognition of the chronic form soon followed, with the term "angina abdominis" applied by Goodman[2] to illustrate the similarities to the newly described "angina pectoris." Indisputable evidence was provided in 1936 by J.E. Dunphy,[3] then a surgical resident at the Peter Bent Brigham Hospital in Boston, who described the clinical course of a 47-year-old man with weight loss and periumbilical pain out of proportion to the findings on physical examination. The patient died suddenly in the hospital and postmortem examination revealed chronic mesenteric disease with fresh thrombus completely occluding the celiac trunk. Dunphy reviewed 12 other deaths from mesenteric vascular occlusion and found an antecedent history of chronic recurrent abdominal pain in seven.

The first successful reports of mesenteric revascularization appeared in 1958.[4] In that year, Shaw and Maynard from the Massachusetts General Hospital reported two cases of superior mesenteric artery (SMA) thrombosis superimposed upon atherosclerotic occlusive disease. Both patients were treated by SMA thromboendarterectomy and survived. The surgeons made the astute observation that although the responsible atherosclerotic lesions involved all three mesenteric arteries, they were confined to their proximal segments, such that vascular reconstruction was technically feasible.[4]

Since that time, intestinal ischemic disorders have been recognized as uncommon but clinically important causes of abdominal pain. Although their incidence is estimated at only a few cases per 100,000 population, their lethal nature requires vigilance and a high index of clinical suspicion to avoid catastrophe. This chapter reviews the pathophysiology, clinical presentation, and treatment of intestinal ischemic disorders.

VASCULAR ANATOMY

The mesenteric circulation consists primarily of three branches of the abdominal aorta (Fig. 30–1): the celiac axis (CA), the SMA, and the inferior mesenteric artery (IMA). Their multiple branch points and interconnections form a rich anastomotic network, such that compromise of two of the three major arteries is usually required for the development of chronic ischemic symptoms. Knowledge of the normal and variant anatomy is essential for surgical diagnosis and revascularization.

Celiac Axis

The CA supplies the stomach, liver, spleen, portions of the pancreas, and the proximal duodenum. It originates from the ventral portion of the abdominal aorta, near the level of T-12–L-1, between the diaphragmatic crura. Its origin is encased in the median arcuate ligament, a dense fibrous portion of the central posterior diaphragm draped across the aortic hiatus. In most patients, the CA branches soon after its origin into the common hepatic, splenic, and left gastric arteries. In 1% of cases, the SMA arises from the CA as well, forming a common celiacomesenteric trunk.

The hepatic artery is usually the first branch of the CA. It may also arise from the SMA (the so-called replaced right hepatic artery) in about 12% of cases. Additional variants include the "replaced common hepatic artery" (about 2.5%) and direct origin of the common hepatic artery from the aorta (about 2%). The common hepatic artery gives rise to the right gastric artery and the gastroduodenal artery, which further divides into the right gastroepiploic and superior pancreaticoduodenal arteries. The remaining proper hepatic artery gives rise to the cystic, right hepatic, and left hepatic arteries, which respectively serve the gallbladder, the right and caudate hepatic lobes, and the middle and left hepatic lobes.

The second branch of the CA is the splenic artery. Its first named branch is the dorsal pancreatic artery supplying the posterior body and tail of the pancreas. Just before entering the splenic hilum, the splenic artery gives rise to the left gastroepiploic artery and multiple short gastric arteries, providing blood flow to the gastric fundus.

The final branch of the CA is the left gastric artery. It courses cephalad and to the left to supply the gastric cardia and fundus along the lesser curvature of the stomach,

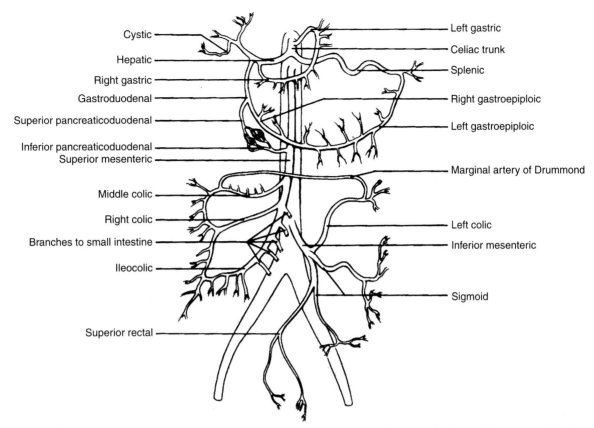

Figure 30–1. The mesenteric circulation. (From Schwartz LB, Davis RD Jr, Heinle JS, et al: The vascular system. In Lyerly HK, Gaynor JW Jr [eds]: The Handbook of Surgical Intensive Care, 3rd ed. St. Louis, Mosby Year Book, 1992, p 287.)

joining centrally with the right gastric artery from the hepatic artery. In approximately 12% of the population, the left hepatic artery originates from the left gastric artery.

Superior Mesenteric Artery

The SMA arises from the aorta just distal to the CA at the level of L-1–L-2. It passes behind the neck of the pancreas, in front of the uncinate process, and over the third portion of the duodenum. Its first branch, the inferior pancreatico-duodenal artery, courses superiorly to join the superior pancreaticoduodenal artery (from the gastroduodenal) and forms the proximalmost collateral pathway with the CA. The central branches of the SMA supply the midgut from the ligament of Treitz to the mid-transverse colon. These include the middle colic (serving the proximal two thirds of the transverse colon), right colic (mid- and distal ascending colon), and ileocolic (distal ileum, cecum, appendix, and proximal ascending colon).

Inferior Mesenteric Artery

The IMA arises from the left side of the aorta 8 to 10 cm distal to the SMA at the level of L3. It travels caudad and to the left before dividing into the left colic and sigmoid arteries. The IMA supplies the distal third of the transverse colon, the descending and sigmoid colon, and the proximal rectum. It has anastomotic communications with the left

branch of the middle colic from the SMA, and portions of the middle and inferior rectal arteries from the internal iliac.

Collateral Circulation

The mesenteric circulation has a redundant collateral network that serves to maintain perfusion even with compromise of the proximal main channels. The CA and SMA communicate primarily via the superior and inferior pancreaticoduodenal arteries (via the gastroduodenal artery). The SMA and IMA communicate via the centrally located *arc of Riolan* (often referred to as the *meandering mesenteric artery*), as well as by the multiple communications at the periphery of the colon called the *marginal arteries of Drummond*. In addition to these collateral pathways, muscular branches of the aorta may contribute to intestinal perfusion, including the lumbar intercostal arteries, internal mammary arteries (via the deep epigastric arteries), middle sacral artery, and internal iliac arteries (via collaterals between the inferior and superior rectal arteries). Because of this plentiful collateral network, it is understandable that in most instances of gradual occlusion at least two of the three major mesenteric orifices must be blocked to produce the clinical syndromes of chronic intestinal ischemia. In contrast, sudden occlusion of one widely patent vessel can cause acute ischemia because collaterals may be underdeveloped.

ACUTE ISCHEMIA

Pathophysiology

There are four primary etiologies for acute mesenteric ischemia (AMI): *embolization* to the SMA (roughly 50% of all cases); *thrombosis* of a preexistent atherosclerotic lesion at the origin of the vessel (20%); *nonocclusive mesenteric ischemia* (20%); and *mesenteric venous thrombosis* (10%).[5, 6] In earlier series, the phenomenon of nonocclusive mesenteric ischemia was not well appreciated and, hence, frequently misdiagnosed as acute venous occlusion. For example, Cokkinis[7] reported in 1935 that acute mesenteric venous thrombosis accounted for the majority of cases of AMI.

Other unusual arteropathies, such as Takayasu's arteritis, fibromuscular dysplasia, and polyarteritis nodosa, may first present with intestinal ischemia. Isolated dissections of the SMA also have been reported,[8] although the more common mechanism is extension of dissections of the descending thoracic aorta into the SMA and CA.[9, 10]

If untreated, intestinal ischemia commonly leads to intestinal infarction. Tissue loss may result from both hypoxia during flow interruption and reperfusion injury once intestinal arterial blood flow is restored. Reperfusion injury is principally mediated by the activation of the enzyme xanthine oxidase and the recruitment and activation of circulating neutrophils (PMNs).[11, 12] In the presence of oxygen and hypoxanthine (a byproduct of adenosine triphosphate metabolism), xanthine oxidase produces oxygen-derived free radicals that cause severe local tissue injury through lipid peroxidation, membrane disruption, and increased microvascular permeability.[13] PMNs are attracted to reperfused tissue by the local secretion of cytokines (tumor necrosis factor-α, interleukin-1, platelet-derived growth factor) by ischemic endothelium.[14-16] Subsequent rolling, adherence, and activation of the PMNs in the microcirculation result in the secretion of myeloperoxidase, collagenases, and elastases that can further injure the already ischemic and vulnerable tissue.[17-19] The activation of the inflammatory cascade may also have systemic effects, with cardiac, pulmonary, and other organ system dysfunction.[20]

Acute Mesenteric Arterial Embolism

Most mesenteric arterial emboli originate from left atrial or ventricular mural thrombi or cardiac valvular lesions. These thrombi are usually associated with cardiac dysrhythmias such as atrial fibrillation or hypokinetic regions from previous myocardial infarctions. The majority of mesenteric emboli lodge in the SMA because of its high basal flow and near-parallel course to the abdominal aorta. Only 15% of SMA emboli remain impacted at the origin of the vessel. The majority of emboli progress distally 3 to 10 cm to the tapered segment of the SMA just past the origin of the middle colic artery (Fig. 30–2). A substantial fraction (10%–15%) of mesenteric emboli are associated with concurrent emboli to another arterial bed.[21] Intestinal ischemia due to embolic arterial occlusion can be compounded by reactive mesenteric vasoconstriction, which further reduces collateral flow and aggravates the ischemic insult.

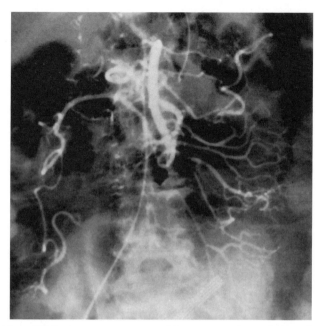

Figure 30–2. Anteroposterior view of the aorta revealing embolic occlusion of the proximal superior mesenteric artery (SMA). Note the normal-appearing proximal jejunal arterial branches then an abrupt cutoff of the SMA. (From McKinsey JF, Gewertz BL: Acute mesenteric ischemia. Surg Clin North Am 77:307–318, 1997.)

Acute Mesenteric Arterial Thrombosis

Thrombosis of the SMA or the CA is usually associated with preexisting arterial lesions. When carefully questioned, many of these patients have histories consistent with chronic mesenteric ischemia (CMI) including postprandial pain, weight loss, "food fear," bloating, and early satiety. By far the most common underlying lesion is an atherosclerotic plaque that slowly progresses to a critical stenosis over years until the residual lumen suddenly thromboses during a period of low flow. Unlike embolic occlusions, thrombosis of the SMA generally occurs flush with the aortic origin of the vessel.

As noted previously, an unusual cause of AMI is aortic dissection involving the origins of the visceral vessels. The intimal flap of the dissection can exclude, compress, or extend into the visceral vessels, resulting in acute thrombosis. The symptoms of bowel ischemia may be masked by the pain associated with the aortic dissection, leading to a delay in diagnosis and treatment. Acute mesenteric ischemia following coronary artery bypass grafts (CABGs) is very rare but highly lethal, with mortality rates as high as 70%. As would be expected, ischemia occurs in patients with severely stenotic mesenteric vessels that occlude during the nonpulsatile perfusion of extracorporeal bypass.[22, 23]

Nonocclusive Mesenteric Ischemia

Mesenteric ischemia unassociated with anatomic arterial or venous obstruction can occur during periods of low cardiac output. Such low-flow states can result from cardiac failure, sepsis, or administration of α-adrenergic agents or digitalis compounds. Although less common, mesenteric vasospasm can also follow elective revascularization procedures for chronic SMA occlusion in which vasoconstriction of small and medium-sized vessels is precipitated by early enteral feeding.[24] The older mean age of the population has produced a number of people with severe medical problems at risk for this type of mesenteric ischemia. The diagnosis is made at the time of angiography. Radiographic criteria suggesting the diagnosis include (1) narrowing of the origins of multiple branches of the SMA; (2) alternate dilatation and narrowing of the intestinal branches—the "string-of-sausages sign"; (3) spasm of the mesenteric arcades; and (4) impaired filling of the intramural vessels.[25] The mortality of this specific subset of patients is relatively high irrespective of treatment owing to the underlying serious medical conditions and the frequent delays in diagnosis.[26]

Mesenteric Venous Thrombosis

Mesenteric venous thrombosis (MVT) refers to thrombosis of the veins draining the intestine (inferior mesenteric, superior mesenteric, splenic, and portal veins). The obstruction in venous return leads to edema, distention, and eventual infarction of affected segments. *Primary* MVT is idiopathic, although given the improved understanding of predisposing conditions, the number of patients in this category is diminishing. Patients in whom an etiologic event is identified are said to have *secondary* MVT. These factors include a myriad of clinical syndromes, including trauma, surgery, cancer, cirrhosis, pancreatitis, and dehydration, and increasingly recognized hypercoagulable syndromes such as polycythemia vera, thrombocytosis, protein C and S deficiency, antithrombin III deficiency, antiphospholipid antibody syndrome, and factor V Leiden mutation (activated protein C resistance).[27]

Patients with MVT have a somewhat different presentation from those who have ischemia due to arterial obstruction; the onset of symptoms may be insidious and the findings more subtle. Pain out of proportion to the physical examination is still an essential feature. The test of choice to confirm the diagnosis is contrast-enhanced computed tomography (CT), although duplex scanning and magnetic resonance imaging (MRI) are gaining popularity. Thrombus is located in the superior mesenteric vein in 70% of patients, with portal and inferior mesenteric vein thrombus found in about 30%.[28]

Symptomatic acute MVT is a lethal disease with a 30-day mortality of about 25% and a 3-year survival of 35%.[28] Patients with evidence of chronic thrombosis fare somewhat better, because collateral venous channels form to augment intestinal venous drainage.

Clinical Presentation and Diagnosis

AMI can appear *precipitously* with decompensation over hours or *insidiously* with progression over days. Classic symptoms of AMI include sudden abdominal pain out of proportion to the physical examination, with gut emptying at the onset of pain. The subacute pattern of mesenteric ischemia is characterized by a more gradual development of vague abdominal signs and symptoms. These include less intense and nonspecific abdominal pains with nausea, vomiting, and changes in bowel habits. The abdomen may become distended but still have active bowel sounds.

Predictably, physical signs intensify as the syndrome progresses. In the early phases, signs of peritoneal irritation such as abdominal guarding and rebound are absent. As the bowel becomes more ischemic, necrosis progresses from the mucosal layers to the seromuscular layers. After full-thickness bowel infarction, the abdomen is often grossly distended with absent bowel sounds and exquisite tenderness to palpation. Bowel infarction can impart a feculent odor to the breath.

Ancillary laboratory evaluations often reveal an increase in hemoglobin and hematocrit consistent with hemoconcentration. There is a marked leukocytosis with a predominance of immature white blood cells (left shift). Although no specific laboratory findings are diagnostic, serum levels of amylase, lactic dehydrogenase, creatine phosphokinase, and alkaline phosphatase, singly or severally, are often elevated along with a metabolic acidosis with a persistent base deficit.[29] Unfortunately, most of these abnormalities do not develop until after bowel necrosis has occurred.

Plain abdominal radiographs are used to exclude other potential causes of abdominal pain rather than confirm the diagnosis of AMI. In fact, completely normal plain abdominal films are seen in more than 25% of patients with mesenteric ischemia.[30] Subtle signs of AMI on plain abdominal films include a dynamic ileus and distended air-filled loops of bowel. Bowel wall thickening from submucosal edema or hemorrhage can be prominent, especially in cases of acute MVT. In advanced stages, pneumatosis of the bowel wall and portal vein gas portend an extremely poor prognosis.

Barium contrast evaluations of the upper and lower gastrointestinal tracts are contraindicated because residual intraluminal contrast can limit visualization of the mesenteric vasculature during diagnostic angiography. On the rare occasion when barium studies are performed in a patient with gradual development of abdominal pain, the submucosal edema and hemorrhage of intestinal ischemia are manifest by thickening of the bowel wall, strictures, or ulcerations.

Duplex ultrasonography may be of some benefit in visualizing flow in the SMA and CA. With expert technical assistance, these tests can document proximal stenoses in the SMA or CA or complete occlusion of these vessels.[31] In recent series, color Doppler ultrasonography has been shown to be a valuable screening tool for AMI, which is far more specific than clinical evaluation alone.[32, 33] Unfortunately, a significant percentage of patients at risk for mesenteric ischemia have dilated air-filled loops of bowel that make ultrasonography difficult if not impossible.

CT of the abdomen and pelvis can delineate subtle changes consistent with subacute bowel ischemia such as focal or segmental bowel wall thickening.[34] Thrombus within the mesenteric veins or the lack of opacification of the veins after intravenous contrast is often seen in MVT.[35] Nonenhancement of the arterial vasculature with timed intravenous contrast injections can be noted in acute mesenteric arterial thrombosis or embolization. CT scans can also vividly demonstrate pneumotosis or portal vein gas.

Recent advances in contrast-enhanced and cine phase

magnetic resonance angiography have allowed better visualization of the visceral vasculature and may, in the future, have a more important role in the diagnosis of AMI.[36] Specifically, when MRI is coupled with magnetic resonance oximetry, both anatomic and physiologic information regarding the mesenteric circulation can be obtained.[37]

Despite these aforementioned developments, the definitive diagnostic study remains mesenteric angiography. Angiography requires multiple views for adequate assessment of the vessels at risk. The origins of the CA and the SMA can only be visualized by lateral views, whereas the more distal CA and SMA distributions are best viewed through anteroposterior projections. Selective cannulation of the origins of the CA and SMA is often required to completely define the anatomy and pathophysiology. Thorough aortography is also needed to evaluate potential inflow and outflow sites for bypass grafts, as well as to clarify the extent and location of other atherosclerotic lesions in the iliac artery and the IMA.

In patients suffering from nonocclusive ischemia, angiography usually reveals multiple areas of narrowing and irregularity in major branches. The small and medium-sized arterial branches may be decreased or absent, and the vasculature is diffusely pruned with an absent submucosal "blush." In mesenteric venous thrombosis, selective angiograms may demonstrate reflux of contrast material back into the aorta due to extremely slow flow and heightened outflow resistance. A prolonged arterial phase with accumulation of contrast and thickened bowel walls is also characteristic. In extreme cases, angiographic contrast may extravasate into the bowel lumen, indicative of active bleeding. The definitive diagnosis of mesenteric venous thrombosis is made during the venous phase; either a filling defect is noted within the portal vein or, in more severe cases, the entire venous phase is absent.

Treatment Options

Initial treatment of patients with AMI includes volume resuscitation, correction of acidosis, and administration of appropriate antibiotics. Heparin anticoagulation should be started immediately to prevent further propagation of thrombus. A urinary catheter, as well as a peripheral arterial catheter, should be placed for monitoring intravascular volumes and hemodynamic status. A nasogastric tube should be placed to decrease the chance of aspiration.

Mesenteric angiography should be performed immediately. As noted earlier, such studies are diagnostic and have the potential to be therapeutic in selected cases. In highly selected patients with early diagnosis of SMA embolus unassociated with bowel necrosis, some authors have advocated a trial of thrombolytic therapy.[38, 39] Such treatment should be strictly limited to patients with abdominal pain for less than 8 hours without signs of peritoneal irritation. If lysis is not evident within 4 hours of commencing high-dose thrombolytic therapy, or if peritoneal signs develop, the infusion should be discontinued and immediate surgical exploration performed.

An increasing number of case reports have detailed the use of percutaneous angioplasty to dilate significant atherosclerotic plaques of the SMA that are unmasked by thrombolytic therapy.[40–42] Owing to the variable angle of the origin of the SMA from the aorta, placement and removal of the angioplasty catheter and stent placement may be more difficult than lower extremity angioplasties.[10] Restenosis rates range from 25% to 50% in the limited series reported to date.[40, 41]

When an aortic dissection involves the origin of one or more of the visceral vessels, endovascular repairs have been attempted through stent placements[43, 44] and balloon fenestration of the dissection septum.[45] Although such minimally invasive treatments are quite attractive, they are currently limited by the frequent rapid onset of ischemic symptoms, inability to gain access to the dissection channel, or the need for surgical repair of an associated aortic aneurysm.

Irrespective of cause, most patients with acute arterial occlusion require early surgical exploration and reestablishment of mesenteric flow to prevent or minimize bowel infarction. A generous midline incision should be made and the extent of mesenteric ischemia and necrosis assessed. If the entire small bowel is frankly gangrenous, enterectomy with lifelong hyperalimentation is the only option. In many instances, patient preferences and family consultation may argue for simple abdominal closure with terminal pain relief as a more appropriate choice. If bowel infarction is not profound, surgical revascularization should be performed.

To achieve adequate exposure, the transverse colon is retracted superiorly and the fourth portion of the duodenum mobilized to the ligament of Treitz. The SMA is identified by palpation of the root of the mesentery. If the etiology of mesenteric ischemia is an embolus, a more proximal SMA pulse is often noted. The SMA is encircled at or just distal to the level of obstruction (Fig. 30–3A), and a transverse arteriotomy is made. Balloon-tipped embolectomy catheters are inserted retrograde, and the embolus is extracted (Fig. 30–3B). Embolectomy catheters should also be passed distally to ensure that no fragmentation of the clot or discontinuous thrombosis has occurred. Transverse arteriotomies are closed primarily with interrupted fine monofilament sutures to ensure that the vessel is not stenosed (Fig. 30–3C). If a longitudinal arteriotomy is required, closure is best accomplished with a vein patch. Appropriately selected longitudinal arteriotomies can also be used for distal anastomoses of bypass grafts if thrombectomies are unsuccessful in obtaining arterial inflow.

When flow is restored, the bowel is reinspected for persistent regions of ischemia. Segments that previously demonstrated equivocal viability may improve with revascularization and resection may be avoided; lengths of bowel that are obviously nonviable must be removed. Bowel continuity can be restored primarily, or stomas may be exteriorized if the patient is unstable. In most instances, a "second-look" operation should be performed at 24 to 36 hours to assess the cumulative effects of reperfusion. Planning for this reexploration allows the surgeon to minimize the amount of bowel primarily resected as well as to ensure that the final bowel anastomoses are performed with viable bowel.

The management of SMA thrombosis due to underlying atherosclerotic lesions is more challenging because simple surgical thrombectomy is unlikely to be durable.[46] The

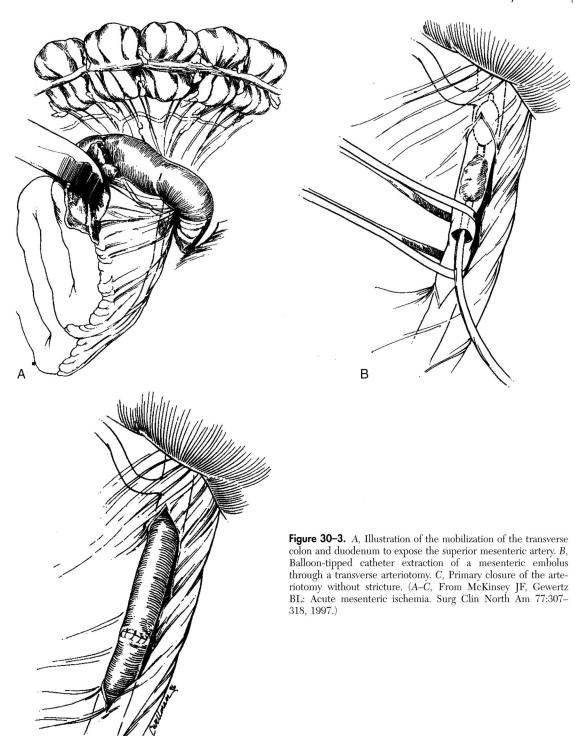

A

B

C

Figure 30–3. *A,* Illustration of the mobilization of the transverse colon and duodenum to expose the superior mesenteric artery. *B,* Balloon-tipped catheter extraction of a mesenteric embolus through a transverse arteriotomy. *C,* Primary closure of the arteriotomy without stricture. (*A–C,* From McKinsey JF, Gewertz BL: Acute mesenteric ischemia. Surg Clin North Am 77:307–318, 1997.)

proximal SMA should be opened through a longitudinal arteriotomy. If thrombectomy is temporarily successful, an intraarterial shunt is placed while the exposures needed for definitive revascularization are performed. The longitudinal arteriotomy in the SMA can serve as the distal anastomotic site for both antegrade bypasses originating in the supraceliac aorta or retrograde bypasses from the infrarenal aorta or iliac vessels. If there is a high likelihood of bowel resection, an autologous conduit should be used for the bypass conduit.

In syndromes of nonocclusive ischemia, the primary therapy is selective arterial administration of vasodilating agents such as papaverine. Such treatment must be coupled with the cessation of α-agonists or other vasoconstrictors. Heparin should also be administered to prevent thrombosis in the cannulated vessel, but the drug must be infused through a peripheral intravenous catheter to avoid precipitation when mixed with papaverine. If a patient demonstrates signs of continued bowel ischemia or necrosis, as evidenced by rebound tenderness or guarding, surgical exploration is required. All necrotic bowel should be resected while arterial infusions of vasodilators continue. Room temperature should be elevated and the bowel kept in moist laparotomy pads to minimize vasoconstriction during exploration. Most patients should undergo a second-look operation in 24 to 48 hours to reassess bowel viability.

The surgical treatment of MVT is restricted to fluid resuscitation, correction of any underlying coagulopathy, and resection of nonviable bowel. Unfortunately, venous thrombectomy is of limited durability and has not proved effective in most instances. The extent of bowel resection should be generous, and repeat exploratory laparotomy is often required to ensure that adequate bowel resection has been performed. Because many patients succumb despite these measures, a more aggressive stance toward early surgical thrombectomy or fibrinolysis has been advocated by some.[47, 48] The risks of these maneuvers are considerable, however, and intervention should be reserved for patients who do not improve with conventional therapy.

Although the detection of frankly necrotic bowel is not difficult, the determination of viability in the marginally perfused bowel is more challenging. Simple indicators of viability include visible peristalsis as well as a pink and normal color of the serosa. Along with palpation of the distribution of the SMA for arterial pulsations, Doppler ultrasonography can be used to further evaluate arterial signals within the vascular arcades. If any question remains, the bowel should be reassessed at a minimum of 30 minutes after revascularization. Administration of intravenous fluorescein followed by illumination with a Wood's ultraviolet light will confirm perfusion of the bowel. The primary limitation of fluorescein is that it is eventually absorbed in fat; therefore, it can only be administered once before it diffuses throughout all tissue and loses its specificity. Unfortunately, no combination of tactics is sufficiently sensitive or specific for error-free evaluation of bowel viability.[49]

Long-term patient outcomes after acute intestinal ischemia are strongly dependent on the timeliness of diagnosis, the underlying lesion, and the associated cardiovascular status. In a comprehensive report by Klempnauer and colleagues[50] of 90 patients suffering from intestinal ischemia, 31 patients survived and were discharged from the hospital. Cumulative 5-year survival was about 50% (16/31). Mortality was greatest during the first year after the incident. The worst survival (20% at 5 years) was seen in patients who suffered mesenteric arterial thrombosis, and the best survival was seen in patients with emboli or nonocclusive ischemia (about 70%). Only one patient who survived the first episode of arterial thrombosis died because of recurrent bowel ischemia. Remarkably, 8 of the 15 surviving patients returned to work.

CHRONIC MESENTERIC ISCHEMIA

In contrast to the varied causes of AMI, CMI is a result of end-stage atherosclerosis in more than 90% of cases. Risk factors parallel those of atherosclerosis in general, including a positive family history, smoking, hypertension, and hypercholesterolemia. Interestingly, in most series, there is a slight female preponderance, and nearly 50% of patients have a history of prior cardiovascular surgery.[51] Nonatherosclerotic causes of CMI include thrombosis associated with thoracoabdominal aneurysm, aortic coarctation, aortic dissection, mesenteric arteritis, fibromuscular dysplasia, neurofibromatosis, middle aortic syndrome, Buerger's disease, and extrinsic celiac artery compression by the median arcuate ligament.

Clinical Presentation

The sine qua non of CMI is postprandial abdominal pain. It is characteristically dull and crampy, occurring primarily in the epigastrium or midabdomen. The discomfort results from activation of visceral afferent nerves that respond to distention and ischemia but that poorly localize pain. The pain occurs 15 to 45 minutes after eating, with increasing severity according to the size and nature of the meal. The temporal relationship between pain and food ingestion often leads to "food fear," another classic but not invariable complaint.

Weight loss is the second classic symptom of CMI. Although malabsorption can contribute to malnutrition in severe cases, most weight loss is simply due to the patient's fear of eating. Many patients become so emaciated that they undergo extensive evaluations for occult neoplasms.

Other, less common symptoms of CMI include diarrhea, nausea and vomiting, and constipation. The variability in signs and symptoms is due, in part, to the region of the gut affected. Foregut ischemia (CA distribution) is usually accompanied by nausea, vomiting, and bloating, whereas, midgut ischemia (SMA) causes classic postprandial abdominal pain and weight loss. The infrequent findings of constipation, occult blood in the stool, and ischemic colitis on colonoscopic biopsy may signify hindgut (IMA) involvement. The lack of specificity of signs and symptoms of this syndrome often leads to delay in diagnosis, and it is common for affected patients to have undergone a myriad of interventions, including antacid or antireflux therapy, cholecystectomy, hysterectomy, and adhesiolysis.

The findings on physical examination are also nonspecific, but the astute clinician can recognize several clues indirectly suggesting the diagnosis. Unexplained weight loss and emaciation alone should arouse suspicion of the syndrome. Manifestations of atherosclerosis in other vascular beds is common, including a cervical or peripheral bruit, decreased peripheral pulses, or signs of chronic lower extremity ischemia. An abdominal bruit can be heard in up to 70% of affected patients.

Diagnosis

Routine laboratory evaluation is rarely helpful, although malnutrition may be accompanied by hemoconcentration, immunoincompetence, hypoalbuminemia, hypoproteinemia, or hypocholesterolemia. More specific tests for panmalabsorption, such as stool fat content, D-xylose tolerance, or vitamin B_{12} absorption, may be positive but are nonspecific. Plain abdominal films may reveal aortic or arterial calcification suggesting mesenteric atherosclerosis. Additional imaging studies, such as endoscopy, gastrointestinal

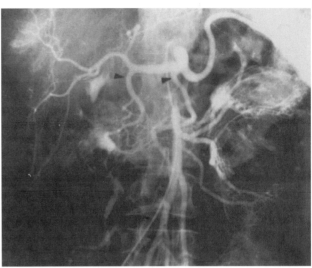

Figure 30–4. Chronic mesenteric ischemia in a 67-year-old woman who had undergone antrectomy, vagotomy, and cholecystectomy and who presented with nausea, vomiting, and a 40-pound weight loss. Anteroposterior arteriogram with direct celiac injection showing critical stenosis of the celiac (*large arrow*) with distal reconstitution of an occluded superior mesenteric artery (*small arrow*). (From Schwartz LB, Gewertz BL: Chronic mesenteric arterial occlusive disease: Clinical presentation and diagnostic evaluation. In Perler BA, Becker GL [eds]: Vascular Intervention: A Clinical Approach. New York, Thieme Medical, 1998, p 522).

contrast examination, and CT, rarely establish the diagnosis but are useful in excluding more common clinical syndromes.

Ultrasonography has added a new dimension to the diagnostic evaluation of patients with suspected CMI. The ability to screen patients with chronic abdominal pain without incurring the risk of contrast arteriography has been a significant advance in the identification of affected patients. Predictive values in excess of 80% have been documented using peak systolic velocity criteria of greater than 275 cm/second for the SMA and greater than 200 cm/second for the CA.[52, 53] The test is highly operator-dependent, however, and independent confirmation of accuracy is necessary for each noninvasive vascular test laboratory employing this technique.

For positive or equivocal ultrasound examinations, diagnostic arteriography is required for more exact lesion localization and for planning revascularization. A complete examination consists of both anteroposterior and lateral aortic views, as well as selective injections of the CA, SMA, and IMA (Fig. 30–4). Occlusion of two or three of the main trunks is generally required for development of the CMI syndrome (Fig. 30–5). Significant mesenteric occlusive disease combined with the development of large collateral vessels is essentially pathognomonic (Fig. 30–6). CA occlusion by the median arcuate ligament is also readily demonstrated by contrast arteriography, and may be responsible for CMI in younger patients[54] (Fig. 30–7).

Treatment Options

As there is no effective medical therapy for CMI, its treatment is focused on the mechanical relief of occlusive lesions and restoration of blood flow. Percutaneous transluminal mesenteric angioplasty (PTMA) with or without intraluminal stenting has been championed by some, although current experience is limited.[27, 55] Early results have been encouraging, with technical success in up to 80% of cases and relief of symptoms and weight gain in the majority. However, restenosis has been problematic, occurring in

30% to 50% of cases, which compares unfavorably with surgical revascularization.

Surgical revascularization remains the treatment of choice for CMI. Early reports emphasized single-vessel reconstruction using autologous vein and a retrograde approach with bypass grafts originating from the infrarenal aorta.[56, 57] Although this procedure avoids supraceliac aortic dissection and clamping, the geometry of a retrograde bypass is theoretically unfavorable, with the potential for compression by the overlying abdominal viscera. In the modern era, antegrade bypass using grafts originating in the supraceliac aorta has become the preferred surgical technique.[58]

Proper patient selection for mesenteric revascularization is critical to optimize results. Other common gastrointestinal disorders should be excluded and the diagnosis of CMI made certain. Concurrent extracranial carotid and coronary artery disease should be detected and treated appropriately. Medical or percutaneous treatment for myocardial ischemia is preferred, because patients with CMI are at increased risk for intestinal infarction during and after coronary artery revascularization.

Although hypoproteinemia with serum albumin of less than 3.0 mg/dL frequently accompanies CMI, postponement of operative therapy in order to nourish the patient is rarely helpful. The risk of intestinal infarction during the preoperative period is significant and often associated with catastrophic results. In patients with life-threatening malnutrition, consideration should be given to endovascular therapy as a temporizing measure before surgical reconstruction.

Antegrade Bypass

Aorto-celiac-mesenteric bypass is best performed through a transperitoneal approach. After a thorough exploration of the abdomen, attention is directed toward exposure of the distal thoracic aortic inflow source. This portion of the aorta is usually spared from atherosclerosis. The triangular ligament of the left lobe of the liver is divided, and moist laparotomy packs are inserted to protect the liver paren-

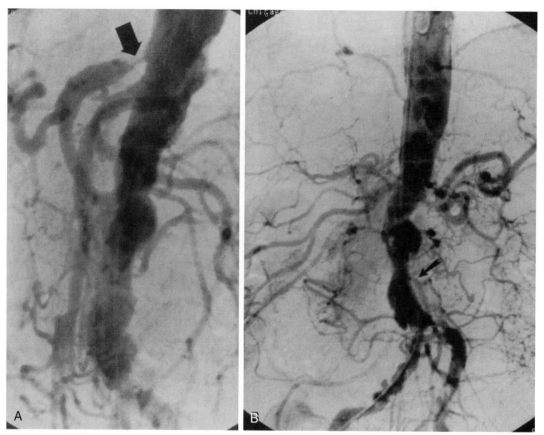

Figure 30–5. Chronic mesenteric ischemia in a 78-year-old woman who had undergone coronary artery bypass and carotid endarterectomy and who presented with claudication, 30-pound weight loss, and postprandial pain. *A*, Lateral aortogram showing critical CA stenosis (*arrow*). *B*, Anteroposterior aortogram showing severe infrarenal aortic disease and critical inferior mesenteric artery stenosis (*arrow*). (From Schwartz LB, Gewertz BL: Intestinal ischemic disorders. In Yao JST, Pearce WH [eds]: Modern Trends in Vascular Surgery. Appleton and Lange, 1999, pp 347–367.)

chyma. Although exposure is greatly facilitated by the use of self-retaining retractor systems, care should be taken to avoid the excessive force that can be easily produced by their mechanical advantage. The lesser sac is entered by division of the gastrohepatic ligament. The esophagus is retracted to the left, and final aortic exposure is achieved by division of the diaphragmatic crura and median arcuate ligament. This allows isolation of 8 to 10 cm of the distal thoracic aorta without division of the diaphragm.

The mesenteric arterial branches are next identified. The origin of the CA is already substantially exposed during the aortic dissection. Dissection along its length is continued until a soft patent distal target is appreciated (usually within the distal CA before its branching). Following this, the operative field is temporarily shifted to the midabdomen by lifting and superiorly displacing the transverse colon. The small bowel and the fourth portion of the duodenum are retracted to the right. The SMA is palpated in the small bowel mesentery as the vessel courses from the retroperitoneum at the inferior margin of the pancreas. The peritoneal membrane is incised, and a suitable segment is isolated. Blunt dissection is used to develop a tunnel behind the pancreas on the left side of the aorta.

Intravenous heparin (100 units/kg) and mannitol (25 g) are administered. A longitudinal incision in the aorta is made and additional arterial wall removed as needed. A bifurcated Dacron or polytetrafluoroethylene graft (typi-

cally 14 × 7 mm) is delivered to the field. Proximal aortic followed by distal CA anastomosis is performed and the viscera reperfused. SMA anastomosis is performed last, after the second limb of the graft is tunneled beneath the pancreas (Fig. 30–8). An alternative but equally effective technique involves sequential bypass using a single 8-mm Dacron graft[58–60] (Fig. 30–9).

Retrograde Bypass

Mesenteric bypass grafts originating from the infrarenal aorta or iliac arteries ("retrograde bypass") were the first techniques used in surgical correction of mesenteric arterial lesions.[6] This approach offers the advantages of limited dissection and avoidance of supraceliac aortic occlusion. Despite these features, retrograde bypass has been used less frequently in recent years. Results from a number of clinical series suggest (but do not prove) that retrograde bypass is less durable than its antegrade counterpart.[61, 62] This is presumed to be due to the tendency for SMA grafts to kink or twist when the viscera are returned to their normal anatomic positions. Although the use of "stiffer" prosthetic conduits and meticulous technique can improve orientation of these reconstructions, retrograde bypass should be considered a third option to be used only after antegrade bypass and aortomesenteric endarterectomy are

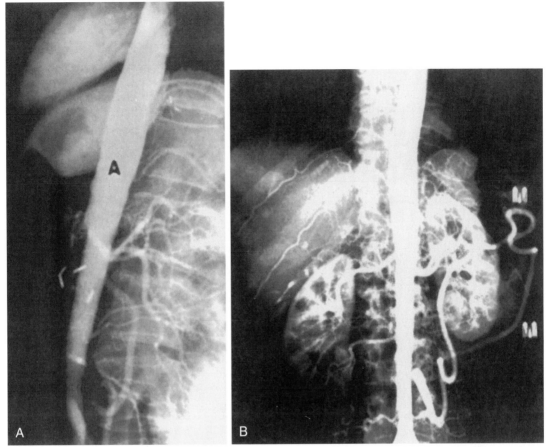

Figure 30–6. Chronic mesenteric ischemia in a 67-year-old woman with postprandial abdominal pain and 30-pound weight loss. A, Anteroposterior aortogram (early phase) showing occlusion of celiac and SMA along with critical stenosis of the IMA origin (*asterisk*). Note the presence of a meandering mesenteric artery (*arrow*). B, Anteroposterior aortogram (late phase) showing reconstitution of the SMA (*arrow*) via collaterals. (From Schwartz LB, Gewertz BL: Chronic mesenteric arterial occlusive disease: Clinical presentation and diagnostic evaluation. In Perler BA, Becker GL [eds]: Vascular Intervention: A Clinical Approach. New York, Thieme Medical, 1998, p 521.)

not feasible. Specific indications for retrograde bypass currently include (1) emergency revascularization in patients undergoing laparotomy for AMI, (2) inaccessible supraceliac aorta due to previous surgery or subphrenic inflammation, (3) severe cardiac disease with contraindications to supraceliac aortic occlusion, and (4) the need for simultaneous infrarenal aortic and mesenteric revascularization.

Retrograde mesenteric bypass begins with exposure of the most proximal suitable segment of the SMA as it exits from beneath the pancreas. The more proximal the anastomosis in the SMA, the less likely kinking will occur because the graft will lie geometrically parallel to the aorta. The mesentery is then returned to its normal position as the graft is pulled taut to lie adjacent to the aorta. A soft portion of the aorta or iliac artery is located and the proximal anastomosis is performed; a fair amount of tension must be maintained on the graft to avoid laxity and kinking when the abdomen is closed (Fig. 30–10).

Access to the CA is problematic with this approach; therefore, celiac revascularization is usually performed via anastomosis to the common hepatic artery or, less commonly, the splenic artery. The common hepatic anastomosis (distal anastomosis) is performed in an end-to-side fashion at 90 degrees. After the Kocher maneuver, the graft can be tunneled behind the duodenum and head of the pancreas, en route to the infrarenal aorta. In this position, torsion and kinking are minimized. When the less robust splenic artery is used, grafts are tunneled behind the tail of the pancreas and anterior to the left renal vein.

Outcomes of Surgical Treatment

A review of collected series of the surgical treatment of CMI during the 1980s and 1990s reveals an overall operative mortality rate of 6%, with 20% of patients sustaining major complications.[63] Although documentation of nearly 500 cases appears in the literature, these mostly represent small case series, and the rarity of the syndrome implies that few institutions have extensive experience. Most clinicians agree that recurrence is less likely if more than one vessel is revascularized. This concept was first championed by Robin and colleagues[48] who noted differential recurrence rates corresponding to the number of vessels treated. Subsequent reports confirmed this finding,[64, 65] making complete revascularization the standard.

Although many clinicians report excellent symptomatic relief after surgical revascularization for CMI, only a few

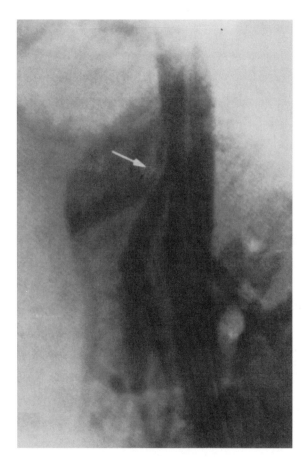

Figure 30–7. Median arcuate compression syndrome. Lateral aortogram in a 27-year-old woman with postprandial abdominal cramping, bloating, and occasional nausea and vomiting. Note the compression of the CA and superior mesenteric artery (*arrow*). Her twin sister had similar complaints and arteriographic findings. (From Bech F, Loesberg A, Rosenblum J, et al: Median arcuate ligament compression syndrome in monozygotic twins. J Vasc Surg 19:935, 1994.)

Figure 30–8. Aorta/carotid artery/superior mesenteric artery bypass using bifurcated Dacron graft. (From Zarins CK, Gewertz BL: Atlas of Vascular Surgery. New York, Churchill Livingstone, 1989, p 109.)

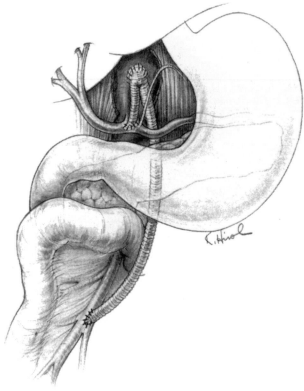

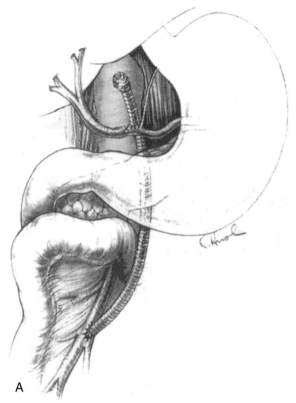

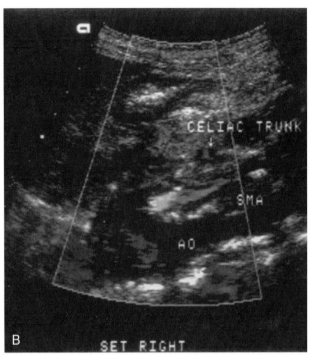

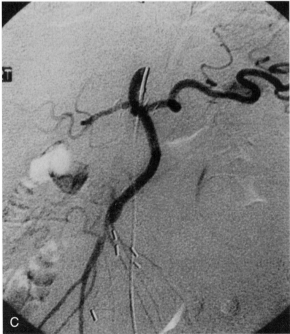

Figure 30–9. Sequential aorto-CA-SMA bypass using 8-mm Dacron graft. *A,* Drawing of the reconstruction. *B,* Postoperative duplex scan with color flow mapping showing patent bypass graft (*large arrow*) from aorta (AO) to celiac trunk and SMA. *C,* Postoperative angiogram showing patent sequential reconstruction. (Modified from Zarins CK, Gewertz BL: Atlas of Vascular Surgery. New York, Churchill Livingstone, 1989, p 109; and Moawad J, McKinsey JF, Wyble CW, et al: Current results of surgical therapy for chronic mesenteric ischemia. Arch Surg 132:616, 1997.)

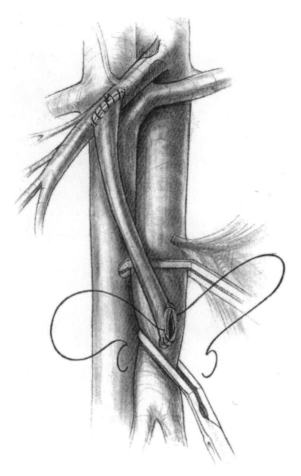

Figure 30–10. Retrograde infrarenal aorto-SMA bypass using autologous vein. (From Zarins CK, Gewertz BL: Atlas of Vascular Surgery. New York, Churchill Livingstone, 1989, p 107.)

have rigorously examined graft patency.[58, 66, 67] McMillan and coworkers[66] used duplex scans and arteriography to document patency of grafts in 25 patients undergoing mesenteric bypass. Their series included 16 treated for CMI and 9 treated for AMI in whom the perioperative morbidity was predictably higher. Considering the 22 patients who survived for more than 1 month, graft patency after a mean of 35 months was 89%. The success rates of retrograde and antegrade grafts were indistinguishable, as were the outcomes of prosthetic or autogenous vein reconstructions. It was noted that two of the three patients experiencing

occluded grafts were asymptomatic, emphasizing that patency cannot be inferred from clinical criteria alone.

Expected results in the modern era are typified by the University of Chicago experience with 24 consecutive patients undergoing mesenteric revascularizations over a 10-year period.[58] All patients had significant SMA involvement and 21 also had lesions of the CA. Seventeen antegrade and seven retrograde bypasses were performed. Calculated 5-year primary patency, documented by duplex scans or arteriography or both, was 78%, and 5-year patient survival by life table analysis was 71% (Fig. 30–11).

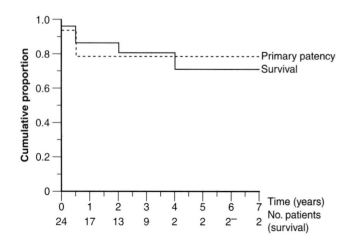

Figure 30–11. Symptom-free survival ($n = 24$) and primary patency ($n = 19$) in patients undergoing surgical revascularization for chronic mesenteric ischemia. Calculation was done using the life table method. Number of patients per interval shown at the bottom. (Modified from Moawad J, McKinsey JF, Wyble CW, et al: Current results of surgical therapy for chronic mesenteric ischemia. Arch Surg 132:616, 1997.)

References

1. Elliot J: The operative relief of gangrene of intestine due to occlusion of the mesenteric vessels. Ann Surg 1:9–23, 1895.
2. Goodman EH: Angina abdominis. Am J Med Sci 155:524–528, 1918.
3. Dunphy JE: Abdominal pain of vascular origin. Am J Med Sci 192:109–113, 1936.
4. Shaw RS, Maynard EP III: Acute and chronic thrombosis of the mesenteric arteries associated with malabsorption. N Engl J Med 258:874–878, 1958.
5. Kairaluoma MI, Karkola P, Heikkinen D, et al: Mesenteric infarction. Am J Surg 133:188–193, 1977.
6. Stoney RJ, Cunningham CG: Acute mesenteric ischemia. Surgery 114:489–490, 1993.
7. Cokkinis A: Mesenteric Venous Occlusion. London, Bailliere, Tindall, 1935.
8. Vignati PV, Welch JP, Ellison L, Cohen JL: Acute mesenteric ischemia caused by isolated superior mesenteric artery dissection. J Vasc Surg 16:109–112, 1992.
9. Cambria RP, Brewster DC, Gertler J, et al: Vascular complications associated with spontaneous aortic dissection. J Vasc Surg 7:199–209, 1988.
10. Chopra PS, Grassi CJ: Superior mesenteric artery angioplasty with the TEG wire: Usefulness and technical difficulties. J Vasc Interv Radiol 3:523–526, 1992.
11. Parks DA, Granger DN: Ischemia-induced vascular changes: Role of xanthine oxidase and hydroxyl radicals. Am J Physiol 245:G285–289, 1983.
12. Parks DA, Granger DN: Contributions of ischemia and reperfusion to mucosal lesion formation. Am J Physiol 250:G749–753, 1986.
13. Del Maestro RF, Bjork J, Arfors KE: Increase in microvascular permeability induced by enzymatically generated free radicals. I. In vivo study. Microvasc Res 22:239–254, 1981.
14. Ali MH, Schlidt SA, Hynes KL, et al: Prolonged hypoxia alters endothelial barrier function. Surgery 124:491–497, 1998.
15. Marcus BC, Wyble CW, Hynes KL, Gewertz BL: Cytokine-induced increases in endothelial permeability occur after adhesion molecule expression. Surgery 120:411–416 [discussion 416–417], 1996.
16. Marcus BC, Hynes KL, Gewertz BL: Loss of endothelial barrier function requires neutrophil adhesion. Surgery 122:420–426 [discussion 426–427], 1997.
17. Korthuis RJ, Anderson DC, Granger DN: Role of neutrophil-endothelial cell adhesion in inflammatory disorders. J Crit Care 9:47–71, 1994.
18. Korthuis RJ, Granger DN: Reactive oxygen metabolites, neutrophils, and the pathogenesis of ischemic-tissue/reperfusion. Clin Cardiol 16:119–126, 1993.
19. Sisley AC, Desai T, Harig JM, Gewertz BL: Neutrophil depletion attenuates human intestinal reperfusion injury. J Surg Res 57:192–196, 1994.
20. Tullis MJ, Brown S, Gewertz BL: Hepatic influence on pulmonary neutrophil sequestration following intestinal ischemia-reperfusion. J Surg Res 66:143–146, 1996.
21. Kaleya RN, Sammartano RJ, Boley SJ: Aggressive approach to acute mesenteric ischemia. Surg Clin North Am 72:157–182, 1992.
22. Schutz A, Eichinger W, Breuer M, et al: Acute mesenteric ischemia after open heart surgery. Angiology 49:267–273, 1998.
23. Klempnauer J, Grothues F, Bektas H, Wahlers T: Acute mesenteric ischemia following cardiac surgery. J Cardiovasc Surg (Torino) 38:639–643, 1997.
24. Gewertz BL, Zarins CK: Postoperative vasospasm after antegrade mesenteric revascularization: A report of three cases. J Vasc Surg. 14:382–385, 1991.
25. Siegelman SS, Sprayregen S, Boley SJ: Angiographic diagnosis of mesenteric arterial vasoconstriction. Radiology 112:533–542, 1974.
26. Deehan DJ, Heys SD, Brittenden J, Eremin O: Mesenteric ischaemia: Prognostic factors and influence of delay upon outcome. J R Coll Surg Edinb 40:112–115, 1995.
27. Schwartz LB, Gewertz BL: Mesenteric ischemia. Surg Clin North Am 77:275–507, 1997.
28. Rhee RY, Gloviczki P, Mendonca CT, et al: Mesenteric venous thrombosis: Still a lethal disease in the 1990s. J Vasc Surg 20:688–697, 1994.
29. Graeber GM, Cafferty PJ, Reardon MJ, et al: Changes in serum total creatine phosphokinase (CPK) and its isoenzymes caused by experimental ligation of the superior mesenteric artery. Ann Surg 193:499–505, 1981.
30. Smerud MJ, Johnson CD, Stephens DH: Diagnosis of bowel infarction: A comparison of plain films and CT scans in 23 cases. AJR 154:99–103, 1990.
31. Harward TR, Smith S, Seeger JM: Detection of celiac axis and superior mesenteric artery occlusive disease with use of abdominal duplex scanning. J Vasc Surg 17:738–745, 1993.
32. Danse EM, Van Beers BE, Goffette P, et al: Diagnosis of acute intestinal ischemia by color Doppler sonography. Color Doppler sonography and acute intestinal ischemia. Acta Gastroenterol Belg 59:140–142, 1996.
33. Danse EM, Laterre PF, Van Beers BE, et al: Early diagnosis of acute intestinal ischaemia: Contribution of colour Doppler sonography. Acta Chir Belg 97:173–176, 1997.
34. Klein HM, Lensing R, Klosterhalfen B, et al: Diagnostic imaging of mesenteric infarction. Radiology 197:79–82, 1995.
35. Rosen A, Korobkin M, Silverman PM, et al: Mesenteric vein thrombosis: CT identification. AJR Am J Roentgenol 143:83–86, 1984.
36. Li KC: MR angiography of abdominal ischemia. Semin Ultrasound CT MR 17:352–359, 1996.
37. Li KC: Magnetic resonance angiography of the visceral arteries: Techniques and current applications. Endoscopy 29:496–503, 1997.
38. McBride KD, Gaines PA: Thrombolysis of a partially occluding superior mesenteric artery thromboembolus by infusion of streptokinase. Cardiovasc Intervent Radiol 17:164–166, 1994.
39. Rivitz SM, Geller SC, Hahn C, Waltman AC: Treatment of acute mesenteric venous thrombosis with transjugular intramesenteric urokinase infusion. J Vasc Interv Radiol 6:219–223 [discussion 224–228], 1995.
40. Hallisey MJ, Deschaine J, Illescas FF, et al: Angioplasty for the treatment of visceral ischemia. J Vasc Interv Radiol 6:785–791, 1995.
41. Levy PJ, Haskell L, Gordon RL: Percutaneous transluminal angioplasty of splanchnic arteries: An alternative method to elective revascularisation in chronic visceral ischaemia. Eur J Radiol 7:239–242, 1987.
42. VanDeinse WH, Zawacki JK, Phillips D: Treatment of acute mesenteric ischemia by percutaneous transluminal angioplasty. Gastroenterology 91:475–478, 1986.
43. Slonim SM, Nyman UR, Semba CP, et al: True lumen obliteration in complicated aortic dissection: Endovascular treatment. Radiology 201:161–166, 1996.
44. Yamakado K, Takeda K, Nomura Y, et al: Relief of mesenteric ischemia by Z-stent placement into the superior mesenteric artery compressed by the false lumen of an aortic dissection. Cardiovasc Intervent Radiol 21:66–68, 1998.
45. Slonim SM, Nyman U, Semba CP, et al: Aortic dissection: Percutaneous management of ischemic complications with endovascular stents and balloon fenestration. J Vasc Surg 23:241–251 [discussion 251–253], 1996.
46. Whitehill T, Rutherford R: Acute mesenteric ischemis caused by arterial occlusions: Optimal management to improve survival. Semin Vasc Surg 3:149–155, 1990.
47. Poplausky MR, Kaufman JA, Geller SC, Waltman AC: Mesenteric venous thrombosis treated with urokinase via the superior mesenteric artery. Gastroenterology 110:1633–1635, 1996.
48. Robin P, Gurel Y, Lang M, et al: Complete thrombosis of mesenteric vein occlusion with recombinant tissue-type plasminogen activator. Lancet 1:1391, 1988.
49. Ballard JL, Stone WM, Hallett JW, et al: A critical analysis of adjuvant techniques used to assess bowel viability in acute mesenteric ischemia. Am Surg 59:309–311, 1993.
50. Klempnauer J, Grothues F, Bektas H, Pichlmayr R: Long-term results after surgery for acute mesenteric ischemia. Surgery 121:239–243, 1997.
51. Schwartz LB, Gewertz BL: Chronic mesenteric arterial disease: Clinical presentation and diagnostic evaluation. In Perla BA, Becker GJ (eds): Vascular Intervention: A Clinical Approach. New York, Thieme Medical 1998, pp 517–524.
52. Moneta GL, Lee RW, Yeager RA, et al: Mesenteric duplex scanning: A blinded prospective study. J Vasc Surg 17:79–84 [discussion 85–86], 1993.
53. Nicoloff AD, Williamson K, Moneta GL, et al: Duplex ultrasonogra-

phy in evaluation of splanchnic artery stenosis. In Schwartz LB, Gewertz BL (eds): Mesenteric Ischemia. Philadelphia, WB Saunders, 1997, pp 339–355.

54. Bech F, Loesberg A, Rosenblum J, et al: Median arcuate ligament compression syndrome in monozygotic twins. J Vasc Surg 19:934–958, 1994.

55. Allen RC, Martin GH, Rees CR, et al: Mesenteric angioplasty in the treatment of chronic intestinal ischemia. J Vasc Surg 24:415–421 [discussion 421–423], 1996.

56. Hildebrand HD, Zierler RE: Mesenteric vascular disease. Am J Surg 139:188–192, 1980.

57. Crawford ES, Morris GC Jr, Myhre HO, Roehm JO Jr: Celiac axis, superior mesenteric artery, and inferior mesenteric artery occlusion: Surgical considerations. Surgery 82:856–866, 1977.

58. Moawad J, McKinsey JF, Wyble CW, et al: Current results of surgical therapy for chronic mesenteric ischemia. Arch Surg 132:613–618 [discussion 618–619], 1997.

59. Wolf YG, Berlatzky Y, Gewertz BL: Sequential configuration for aorto-celiac-mesenteric bypass. Ann Vasc Surg 11:640–642, 1997.

60. Geroulakos G, Tober JC, Anderson L, Smead WL: Antegrade visceral revascularisation via a thoracoabdominal approach for chronic mesenteric ischaemia. Eur J Vasc Endovasc Surg 17:56–59, 1999.

61. Rapp JH, Reilly LM, Qvarfordt PG, et al: Durability of endarterectomy and antegrade grafts in the treatment of chronic visceral ischemia. J Vasc Surg 3:799–806, 1986.

62. Johnston KW, Lindsay TF, Walker PM, Kalman PG: Mesenteric arterial bypass grafts: Early and late results and suggested surgical approach for chronic and acute mesenteric ischemia. Surgery 118:1–7, 1995.

63. Schwartz LB, Moawad J, Gewertz BL: Mesenteric ischemia. In Corson JD, Williamson RN (eds): Surgery. London, Mosby–Year Book, (in press).

64. Zelenock GB, Graham LM, Whitehouse WM Jr, et al: Splanchnic arteriosclerotic disease and intestinal angina. Arch Surg 115:497–501, 1980.

65. McAfee MK, Cherry KJ Jr, Naessens JM, et al: Influence of complete revascularization on chronic mesenteric ischemia. Am J Surg 164:220–224, 1992.

66. McMillan WD, McCarthy WJ, Bresticker MR, et al: Mesenteric artery bypass: Objective patency determination. J Vasc Surg 21:729–740 [discussion 740–741], 1995.

67. Kihara TK, Blebea J, Anderson KM, et al: Risk factors and outcomes following revascularization for chronic mesenteric ischemia. Ann Vasc Surg 13:37–44, 1999.

31

Extracranial Cerebrovascular Disease: The Carotid Artery

Wesley S. Moore

HISTORICAL REVIEW

The development of surgery on the extracranial cerebrovascular circulation was dependent on three principal factors: (1) recognition of the pathologic relationship between extracranial cerebrovascular disease and subsequent cerebral infarction, (2) the introduction of cerebral angiography to identify lesions before the patient's death, and (3) the development of vascular surgical techniques that could be applied to the extracranial vessels once the anatomic patterns of disease were understood and described.

The earliest report linking cervical carotid artery disease to stroke is credited to Savory,[1] who in 1856 described a young woman with left monocular symptoms in combination with a right hemiplegia and dysesthesia. Postmortem examination demonstrated an occlusion of the cervical portion of the left internal carotid artery together with bilateral subclavian artery occlusions. In 1875, Gowers[2] reported a similar case, and subsequent reports of individual cases were made by Chiari[3] in 1905, Guthrie and Mayou[4] in 1908, and Cadwater[5] in 1912. By 1914, Ramsay Hunt,[6] in an important publication, emphasized the relationship between extracranial carotid artery disease and stroke. He also described the phenomenon of intermittent cerebral symptoms associated with partial occlusion and used the term "cerebral intermittent claudication" as a characterizing analogy. Hunt also pointed out that the clinicopathologic observations in patients with stroke were hampered by the fact that routine autopsies did not include examination of the cervical carotid arteries (as is often the case today because of the desire to maintain access to the external carotid artery for the mortician). He emphasized that no examination of cerebral infarction can be considered complete without examination of the neck vessels.[6]

The next major step in the evolution of the management of extracranial cerebrovascular disease came with the development of carotid angiography by Moniz[7] in 1927. By 1937, Moniz and colleagues[8] had described four cases of internal carotid occlusion diagnosed by angiography. In 1938, Chao and colleagues[9] added two more cases, and by 1951, Johnson and Walker[10] had collected from the world literature a total of 101 cases of occlusion of the cervical carotid artery diagnosed by angiography. In spite of these early observations, the medical world was still slow to appreciate the relationship between extracranial cerebrovascular disease and cerebral symptoms, as emphasized by the fact that when cerebral angiography came into common use for neurologic diagnosis in the 1950s and 1960s, only the intracranial vessels were included on films. The area of the carotid bifurcation was seldom looked at. By the late 1950s, patients were still commonly admitted with a hemiplegia and diagnosed as having a "middle cerebral artery thrombosis" without considering the carotid bifurcation as a source of the problem.

The next major steps in the evolution of understanding came from reports by C. Miller Fisher[11, 12] in 1951 and 1954. Fisher reemphasized the relationship between extracranial arterial occlusive disease and cerebral symptoms. He also pointed out that the lesion could either be total occlusion or stenosis. His most important observation, however, was that the disease was often quite localized to a short segment of the carotid artery, and he predicted that surgical correction might be possible if patients could be identified in the early stages of the clinical syndrome. Fisher stated that "It is even conceivable that some day vascular surgery will find a way to bypass the occluded portion of the artery during the period of ominous fleeting symptoms. Anastomosis of the external carotid artery or one of its branches with the internal carotid artery above the area of narrowing should be feasible."

The surgical phase of understanding and management of extracranial cerebrovascular disease probably began in 1951, but it was actually not reported in the literature until 1955. This early report by Carrea and colleagues[13] from Buenos Aires described their experience with the management of a patient with carotid artery stenosis. They resected the diseased internal carotid artery and performed an anastomosis between the external carotid artery and the distal internal carotid as predicted earlier by Fisher. In 1953, Strully and coworkers[14] attempted a thromboendarterectomy of a totally thrombosed internal carotid artery. This was unsuccessful, but the authors suggested that thromboendarterectomy should be technically feasible before thrombosis as long as the internal carotid artery was patent distally. The first carotid endarterectomy was probably performed by DeBakey and colleagues[15] in an operation done on August 7, 1953, but it was not actually written up until 1959 and was then subsequently reviewed in 1975.[16] The report that was most important in calling the world's attention to the feasibility of carotid artery reconstruction came from Eastcott and associates[17] who published their experience in *The Lancet* in November 1954. Their operation was performed on May 19, 1954, on a patient who was having hemispheric transient ischemic attacks (TIAs) with demonstrable disease at the carotid bifurcation; they used direct, end-to-end anastomosis between the common carotid artery and the internal carotid artery distal to the atherosclerotic lesion.

Although operations on the carotid artery were in the early phase of development, surgical attack was also considered feasible on occlusive lesions of the major arch vessels. In 1956, Davis and colleagues[18] reported their experience with endarterectomy of the innominate artery performed on a patient on March 20, 1954. In 1957, Warren and Triedman[19] reported the second case.

By this time, the stage was set for explosive development of the aggressive surgical approach to managing extracranial cerebrovascular disease as a means of preventing or treating cerebral infarction.

Thompson,[20] in his 1996 Willis lecture, related in great detail the history of surgery to prevent stroke. Those interested in the definitive history will be rewarded by reading this excellent paper.

NATURAL HISTORY OF EXTRACRANIAL ARTERIAL OCCLUSIVE DISEASE

Therapy aimed at prevention of cerebral infarction must be compared with the natural history of the disease process. The prognosis of a patient with extracranial arterial occlusive disease differs depending on the presence or absence of symptoms. When a permanent neurologic deficit is present, the outlook worsens, thus underscoring the importance of prevention. A thorough understanding of the natural history of the disease is essential to formulating a rational and effective therapeutic program. The physician needs to be familiar with the expected results of each available option. This implies that no one alternative is applicable to all situations and that individualization is the key to effective prevention.

Approximately 500,000 people become new stroke victims in the United States each year. In 200,000 of these cases, death follows, but at any one time, around 1 million stroke victims are alive and disabled. In 1976, the annual direct and indirect cost of stroke was estimated at $7,363,784,000.[21] Twenty-five years later, with inflation and the accelerating cost of medical care, this cost has probably quadrupled. The incalculable morbidity of the affected

individual adds further to the magnitude of this problem. Prevention remains the most plausible alternative.

The initial mortality of an ischemic stroke ranges from 15% to 33%.[22–24] Survivors remain at an inordinately high risk of subsequent stroke, estimated between 4.8% and 20% per year.[25, 26] This implies that half of the patients will experience a second event within 5 years.[23, 27, 28] The average recurrent stroke rate reported in the literature is between 6% and 12% each year. The most common cause of death in patients with extracranial arterial occlusive disease is myocardial infarction. In an analysis of 535 stroke victims, however, the leading cause of death was recurrent stroke, as opposed to the expected myocardial mortality.[26]

Since 1973, public health statistics have documented an accelerating decline in stroke mortality.[29] This has led to the erroneous assumption that a decline has also occurred in stroke incidence, which is not the case.

In 1989, Wolf and colleagues[30] reported the epidemiologic data from the Framingham Study to the 14th International Joint Conference on Stroke and Cerebral Circulation. They reviewed the experience from three successive decades, beginning in 1953. A decline in stroke fatality in both men and women was observed. However, the 10-year prevalence of stroke actually rose, and the incidence of stroke rose in men from 5.7% to 7.6% to 7.9%, without any apparent change in women. The authors postulated that falling case fatality rates might have resulted from changes in diagnostic criteria, a lessening in stroke severity, or improved care of stroke patients.[30]

Harmsen and colleagues[31] reviewed the experience of stroke incidence and fatality in Göteborg, Sweden, between 1971 and 1987. They noted that the stroke incidence remained the same during that interval but that the stroke fatality rate declined in both sexes. This was more marked for intracerebral hemorrhage and subarachnoid hemorrhage than for infarction. They concluded that the decline in stroke fatality rates might have been related to decreases in smoking habits or better management of blood pressure. They had no explanation as to why no corresponding decline in stroke incidence occurred.[31]

Finally, Modan and Wagener[32] examined the epidemiologic aspects of stroke based upon death certificate information available from the National Center for Health Statistics compressed mortality file for all 50 states and the District of Columbia for the period 1968 to 1988. They noted a decline in stroke mortality that continued through the 1970s and 1980s, whereas morbidity remained constant and possibly even increased. They noted similar morbidity and mortality rates in both sexes. They concluded that the observed decrease in stroke mortality rates resulted from an improved survival rather than a decline in incidence.[32]

A variety of reasons for decline in stroke mortality have been postulated, including the more aggressive treatment of hypertension. No one has suggested that the decline of stroke mortality might have been related to the increasing use of carotid endarterectomy. Figure 31–1 compares the declining incidence in stroke mortality with the accelerating incidence of carotid endarterectomy. Although this is not proof of a relationship, neither should a possible relationship be discounted.

Two clinical syndromes deserve special emphasis because of their dismal natural history. *Stroke in evolution,*

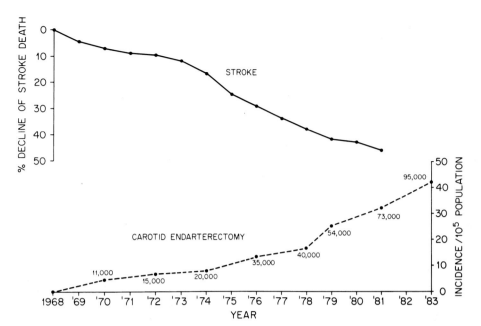

Figure 31-1. The declining incidence of stroke-related death from 1968 to 1981 is compared with the accelerating frequency with which carotid endarterectomy was performed during the same time interval.

also known as progressing stroke or incomplete stroke, is an acute neurologic deficit of modest degree that within hours or days progresses to a major cerebral infarct. This can happen in a sequential series of acute exacerbations or in a pattern of waxing and waning in signs and symptoms over hours or days, with incomplete recovery eventually leading to a major fixed neurologic deficit. *Crescendo transient ischemic attacks (TIAs)* is the pattern that allows complete recovery between ischemic events, suggesting repeated frequent embolization from a point arterial source in the affected territory.

In a review of the literature, Mentzer and colleagues[33] identified 263 reported cases of stroke in evolution managed conservatively. Twenty-three percent had complete resolution or mild neurologic deficit on follow-up. Sixty-two percent had a moderate to severe deficit in the early recovery phase. The overall mortality was 14.5%. In their own series, 26 patients showed stroke in evolution that was treated conservatively. Mortality was 15%, but, more important, 66% suffered moderate to severe permanent neurologic deficit, with only five patients recovering completely or experiencing only mild neurologic dysfunction. These results are compared with a series of 17 patients operated on emergently for stroke in evolution. None had worsening of the preoperative neurologic deficit, four (24%) remained unchanged, and 12 (70%) had complete recovery.[33]

In 1972, Millikan[34] reviewed the natural history of patients with progressing stroke. Of 204 patients, 12% were normal at 14 days, 7% had developed moderate to severe neurologic deficits, and 14% had died. Thus, stroke in evolution treated conservatively carries a poor prognosis. More than half of the patients develop a severe permanent neurologic deficit within a few days of the onset, and around 15% die as a result. Only 10% to 20% recover full or partial neurologic function.[34]

Patients who experience TIAs are also at a higher risk of developing a stroke. In the Mayo Clinic population study,[35] 118 patients with TIAs were monitored as a control group without therapy. The stroke rates at 1, 3, and 5 years were 23%, 37%, and 45%, respectively. Most permanent deficits occurred during the first year. This represents a 16-fold increased risk of stroke compared with an age- and sex-adjusted population. The Oxfordshire project[36] reported an actuarial risk of stroke during the first year after the onset of TIAs to be 11% to 16%. For each subsequent year, the rate was 5% to 9% per year. Some series[37, 38] have reported lower figures, but the average reported in the literature is on the order of 30% to 35% at 5 years, or 10% the first year and 6% each year thereafter.

Finally, Toole,[39] in his Willis lecture, reminded us that a surprising frequency of cerebral infarction that occurs in TIA patients goes unrecognized by either patient or physician. These lesions are now identified by better neuroimaging techniques, and one question is whether TIAs are actually small strokes.[39] If a TIA is actually a small stroke, the implied benignity of TIA must be reexamined. Thus, it may be equally important to prevent TIA because it may be a small stroke. This consideration is further strengthened by the observations of Grigg and colleagues,[40] who correlated cerebral infarction and atrophy as a function of TIAs and percentage stenosis. They graded carotid stenosis in symptomatic patients from A (no stenosis) to E (occlusion). In patients with amaurosis fugax, the incidence of cerebral infarction rose from 2% in patients with stenosis grades A, B, and C to 40% in grade D and 58% in grade E. The incidence of atrophy increased in parallel from 10% in grade A to 30% in grade E.

The natural history of asymptomatic patients with significant extracranial or arterial occlusive disease is most difficult to predict accurately. Most studies that have addressed this problem have used the presence of a cervical bruit as the sole criterion for inclusion. This inevitably includes patients without significant occlusive disease and omits others without cervical bruit but with high-risk lesions in their extracranial circulation.

As noninvasive studies develop, detection of hemodynamically significant lesions in the carotid system improves.

Kartchner and McRae[41] monitored for a mean of 24 months 1130 patients who either were asymptomatic or had nonhemispheric symptoms. Of 303 patients with hemodynamically significant lesions, 11.9% had strokes at 2 years. The group with negative noninvasive studies had a much lower stroke rate, on the order of 3% over the same follow-up period. Busuttil and colleagues[42] noted an unfavorable trend toward higher stroke rates in asymptomatic patients with hemodynamically significant lesions in the carotid bifurcation.

In a report by Roederer and colleagues,[43] 167 asymptomatic patients with cervical bruits were monitored with serial duplex scanning regardless of the degree of the stenosis at the time of presentation. During follow-up, 10 patients became symptomatic. The development of symptoms was accompanied by disease progression in 80% of patients. By life-table analysis, the annual rate of symptom occurrence was 4%; however, the presence of progression graded at 80% stenosis was highly correlated with either the development of total occlusion of the internal carotid artery or new symptoms. Thus, 89% of the symptoms were preceded by progression of the lesion to a greater than 80% stenosis. Progression of a lesion to more than 80% stenosis was an important warning observation because it carried a 35% risk of ischemic symptoms or internal carotid occlusion within 6 months and a 46% risk at 12 months. Conversely, only 1.5% of the lesions that remained in a less than 80% stenosis category developed such a complication. These data suggest that careful follow-up with repeated noninvasive evaluation is of great assistance in determining the appropriate management of the asymptomatic carotid lesion.[43]

In an analysis of 294 asymptomatic and nonhemispheric patients submitted to cerebrovascular testing, Moore and colleagues[44] found a 15% stroke incidence during the first 2 years in patients with a greater than 50% stenosis. This was compared with a 3% incidence at 2 years in patients with a 1% to 49% stenosis. The difference was found to be statistically significant ($P < 0.05$). The 5-year cumulative stroke incidence was 21% with greater than 50% stenosis, 14% with 1% to 49% stenosis, and 9% in patients without noninvasive evidence of carotid artery disease.[44]

Chambers and Norris[45] monitored a group of 500 asymptomatic clinical patients with noninvasive studies and clinical evaluation. They identified two high-risk groups: those with stenosis greater than 75% and those who showed disease progression between studies. For patients with a greater than 75% stenosis, the 1-year neurologic event rate (TIA and stroke) was 22%. The 1-year stroke rate alone was 5%. In a later publication,[46] the authors continued to note that neurologic events correlated with increasing percentage stenosis as well as disease progression between test intervals. In the study viewed over 5 years, the annual average neurologic event rate was 10% to 15%, with the highest event rate occurring within the first year of diagnosis. Finally, the incidence of silent cerebral infarction as documented on computed tomographic (CT) scan was studied in the same patient population. The authors noted a 10% incidence of cerebral infarction among patients with mild (35% to 50%) stenosis, 17% with moderate (50% to 75%) stenosis, and 30% in patients with severe (greater than 75%) stenosis. The authors concluded that silent cerebral infarction might be an indication for carotid endarterectomy in asymptomatic patients.[47]

Although the natural history of the asymptomatic carotid stenosis remains controversial, studies using serial noninvasive cerebrovascular testing have concluded that an increased risk of stroke exists ipsilateral to a 50% or greater carotid artery stenosis. These lesions appear to carry a risk of subsequent stroke on the order of 4% per year. In addition, progression of the disease carries an even higher risk of stroke, with lesions of greater than 80% stenosis carrying a 35% risk of subsequent symptoms or carotid occlusion at 2 years.

Other studies have suggested that the composition of the plaque influences the stroke risk of carotid artery lesions. In one analysis, 297 patients with carotid stenosis greater than 75% at the time of initial study were at higher risk than peers without significant narrowing or development of symptoms ipsilateral to the lesion.[48] Even those patients with less than 75% stenosis were at greater risk if the associated plaque was less organized (i.e., soft). This was determined by B mode ultrasonography, by which plaques were classified as dense, calcified, or soft. A definite trend toward higher risk was seen in plaques of lower density. Only 10% of those patients with calcified plaque in significantly stenotic vessels developed symptoms, whereas 92% of patients with soft plaques and tight stenosis developed symptoms within the first 3 years of follow-up.[48] The morphology of the atherosclerotic plaque, as documented by B mode ultrasonography, is emerging as one of the more important factors associated with embolic potential and stroke risk. Two studies have concluded that a heterogeneous plaque carries an increased risk of stroke and is a variable independent from carotid stenosis alone.[49, 50]

The embolic potential of ulcerated carotid lesions has been well documented.[51–53] Patients who experience symptoms from these probably have the same prognosis as patients with occlusive lesions. Whether the former patient group responds more favorably to platelet antiaggregants remains to be determined. Moore and coworkers[54] first pointed out the fact that asymptomatic patients with significant ulceration in a carotid plaque in the absence of stenosis appeared to be at a higher risk of stroke. In a subsequent report, they expanded their series to 153 patients with asymptomatic nonstenotic ulcerative lesions in the carotid bifurcation. Patients with deep (B) or complex (C) ulcerations received follow-up and were found to have a stroke rate of 4.5% and 7.5% each year, respectively.[55] Other reports have suggested a similar stroke risk for complex ulcerations in the carotid bulb. However, a much lower stroke risk was reported for deep ulcerations, with no significant added risk of stroke observed in these patients. Controversy still exists about deep ulceration without complex morphology. However, agreement exists that complex ulcerations in the carotid bulb do increase the risk of stroke in asymptomatic patients.[56]

The presence of an asymptomatic hemodynamically significant stenosis may increase the risk of stroke during major surgery. Kartchner and McRae[57] reported their experience with 234 patients, 41 of whom had evidence of significant carotid artery stenosis by oculoplethysmography. Seven postoperative strokes developed in the group with positive criteria (17%), whereas postoperative cerebral infarction developed in 2 (1%) of 192 patients with negative noninvasive studies. The mechanisms of stroke and the territory involved were not specifically reported. This high incidence of permanent neurologic deficits led the authors to conclude that prophylactic carotid endarterectomy should be considered in patients with hemodynamically significant carotid stenosis who are undergoing a major cardiovascular procedure.[57]

Other series have reported results to the contrary.[58–61] Using noninvasive vascular evaluation and, in one series, angiography, patients with 50% or greater stenosis in the carotid bifurcation were compared with patients who had lesser degrees of stenosis undergoing cardiovascular surgery. No increased incidence of perioperative strokes was found in patients with positive criteria. Most of these investigators, however, have excluded preocclusive stenosis in their considerations. Lesions of 90% or greater stenosis were excluded from these series and subjected to prophylactic endarterectomy before cardiovascular operation.

Cardiac surgeons have long been concerned about the presence of carotid stenosis in a patient who will be undergoing bypass with a decrease in pump perfusion pressure, believing that a corresponding and unacceptable drop in cerebral blood flow will occur. In fact, the opposite occurs. Von Reutern and colleagues[62] used transcranial Doppler ultrasonography to study middle cerebral artery blood flow before and during cardiopulmonary bypass in patients with and without carotid artery disease. Surprisingly, middle cerebral artery blood flow actually increased during cardiopulmonary bypass. Although the increase was not as great in patients with carotid artery disease, it was clearly an increase over baseline. This observation should dispel the concern about a potential drop in cerebral blood flow in patients with carotid stenosis while on the pump.

Patients with a combination of severe carotid stenosis and symptomatic coronary artery disease represent a cohort that is at high risk of death, myocardial infarction, and stroke. Brener and colleagues[63] carried out an extensive literature review that examined complications associated with different treatment strategies. Patients who underwent staging with carotid endarterectomy first had a high cardiac morbidity and mortality. Patients who had coronary bypass first had a higher stroke morbidity. The data suggested that combined or simultaneous coronary artery bypass grafting (CABG) and carotid endarterectomy might reduce overall morbidity and mortality. However, evidence from retrospective reviews was not sufficiently compelling to make a definitive recommendation.[63] Consensus exists that this is an appropriate topic for a prospective randomized trial.

The natural history of extracranial arterial occlusive disease cannot be complete without including the natural history of frequently associated conditions such as coronary artery disease, hypertension, and diabetes. Myocardial infarction remains the most frequent cause of death in these patients. Including these variables in the equation when one is formulating a treatment plan for a particular patient is therefore important. The goal of therapy should be the prevention of a permanent neurologic deficit. When deciding on the most effective way to achieve this, one must consider the life expectancy of the patient and the inherent risk of each particular form of therapy.

PATHOLOGY OF EXTRACRANIAL ARTERIAL OCCLUSIVE DISEASE

The pathology of cerebrovascular disease of extracranial origin can be divided into flow-restrictive lesions and lesions with embolic potential. Each of these can be further subdivided into occlusive or aneurysmal lesions. All entities that have been described as etiologic in extracranial disease fall within these categories.

Atherosclerosis

By far the most common lesion found in patients with extracranial cerebrovascular disease is an atherosclerotic plaque in the carotid bifurcation. This can produce symptoms by reducing blood flow to the hemisphere supplied or, more commonly, by releasing embolic material. Emboli can be made up of clot, platelet aggregates, or cholesterol debris.

The carotid bifurcation appears to be susceptible to the development of atherosclerotic plaques.[64] Frequently, severe changes at the carotid bifurcation occur with minimal or no changes present in the common or internal carotid artery.[65] Several investigators have proposed conflicting theories based on hemodynamic observations in various models. High shear stress and fluctuations in shear stress,[66] disordered or turbulent flow, flow separation, and high and low flow velocity have all been implicated.[67–70] Which of these mechanisms is responsible for plaque formation is not known. Zarins and colleagues[71] used a model of the human carotid bifurcation under steady flow and compared its hemodynamics with those of cadaver specimens. They concluded that carotid lesions localize in regions of low flow velocity and flow separation rather than in regions of high velocity and increased shear stress. They used their model to explain the propensity of the outer wall of the carotid sinus opposite the flow divider to develop atherosclerotic plaques (Fig. 31–2). This may have further clinical implications in that an enlarged carotid bulb after endarterectomy may create a region of reduced flow velocity with increased boundary layer separation that may favor recurrent plaque deposition.

Once the initial intimal injury is produced by these forces, platelet deposition, smooth muscle cell proliferation, and the slow accumulation of lipoproteins are involved in the reparative process (Fig. 31–3). These eventually lead to plaque formation, which further alters the hemodynamics of the system and favors further injury.

The contribution of platelets to atheroma formation may be of several types.[72] Platelets may adhere to one another, to the diseased vessel, or both. This can lead to thrombus formation. This process may narrow the vessel lumen, or it may dislodge, resulting in distal embolization. Vasoactive substances stored in granules within the platelet may be released, causing vasospasm and further contributing to compromise of the arterial lumen. The platelet's interaction with collagen, exposed in an injured intima, may include elaboration of a smooth muscle growth factor that can lead to intimal thickening. The activation of enzymes in platelets, by their contact with collagen, initiates the production of highly active prostaglandins. The production of throm-

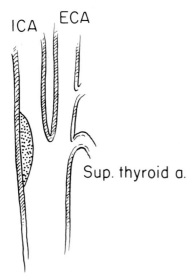

Figure 31-2. The common carotid artery bifurcation; the most common site for atherosclerotic plaque deposition is located on the wall opposite the divider. ECA, external carotid artery; ICA, internal carotid artery.

boxane A_2 represents the final common pathway of platelet response to diverse stimuli.[73] This substance is a potent stimulant of platelet aggregation and a powerful vasoconstrictor and is believed important in the pathophysiology of plaque formation and/or symptoms from an already established atheroma.

Hemorrhage into a plaque may also play a significant role in the development of symptoms from an atherosclerotic lesion. Imbalances in wall tension secondary to asymmetrical deposition of plaques can lead to the sudden development of plaque fracture and intraplaque hemorrhage.[74] These can lead to sudden expansion of the atheroma with acute restriction of flow or breakdown of the intimal surface and concomitant embolization. An alternative mechanism for sudden intraplaque hemorrhage may be

related to an increase in neovascularity within the plaque substance. Hypertension may be responsible for precipitating rupture of neovascular vessels, leading to intraplaque hemorrhage and expansion.[75] This process may be responsible for a large number of symptomatic lesions. In a prospective evaluation[76] of 79 atheromatous plaques removed from 69 patients undergoing carotid endarterectomy, 49 of 53 (92.5%) symptomatic patients had evidence of intramural hemorrhage. In contrast, only 7 of 26 (27%) asymptomatic patients showed recent or acute intraplaque hemorrhage. Rupture of an atherosclerotic plaque with intraluminal release of atheromatous debris has also been correlated with acute stroke and internal carotid occlusion in an autopsy study.[77]

Fibromuscular Dysplasia

Fibromuscular dysplasia is a nonatherosclerotic process that affects medium-sized arteries. It was first described in the carotid artery in 1964,[78] and since then it has been recognized as a cause of cerebrovascular symptoms.[79] It may also affect the intracranial arteries, and around 30% of patients with cervical involvement have associated intracranial aneurysms.[80] Up to 65% of patients have bilateral disease,[80] and 25% have associated atherosclerotic changes.[81]

Four histologic types of fibromuscular dysplasia have been described:[82]

1. *Intimal fibroplasia* accounts for about 5% of cases and affects both sexes equally. It usually appears as long tubular stenoses in young patients and as focal stenoses in older patients. It results from an accumulation of irregularly arranged subendothelial mesenchymal cells with a loose matrix of connective tissue. Medial and adventitial structures are always normal.
2. *Medial hyperplasia* is a rare form of the disease that produces focal stenoses. The intima and adventitia re-

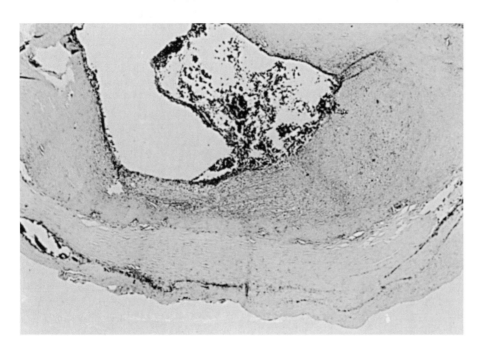

Figure 31-3. Microscopic section of an atherosclerotic plaque removed from the carotid bifurcation. Notice the fibrointimal proliferation with cholesterol cleft formation. Thrombotic material is adherent to the luminal surface of the plaque.

main normal, whereas the media shows excess smooth muscle.

3. *Medial fibroplasia* is the most common pattern of fibromuscular dysplasia, accounting for most, if not all, internal carotid involvement. It may appear as a focal stenosis or multiple lesions with intervening aneurysmal outpouchings. Histologically, the disease is limited to the media, with replacement of smooth muscle by compact fibrous connective tissue. The inner media may show accumulation of collagen and ground substance separating disorganized smooth muscle cells. Gradation of these changes correlates with the severity of the lesion. Mural dilatations and microaneurysms are common.

4. *Perimedial dysplasia* is characterized by accumulation of elastic tissue between the media and the adventitia. It affects renal arteries and is associated with macroaneurysms.

Fibromuscular dysplasia preferentially affects long arteries with few primary branches. Hormonal effects on medial tissue, mechanical stresses on the vessel wall, and unusual distribution of the vasa vasorum in these arteries seem to play an etiologic role.[82] The fact that women are most commonly affected (92% of cases)[81] and some experimental evidence[83] support a possible role of hormones in this process. The normal paucity of vasa vasorum in long nonbranching arterial segments such as the extracranial carotid artery and the renal artery in the appropriate hormonal environment may predispose to mural ischemia and the initiation of the fibroplastic process. Experimental evidence supports this concept.[84]

The exact cause of symptoms is controversial. Thromboembolism from clot or platelets, or both; decreased flow due to a critical stenosis or a series of noncritical narrowings; intracranial involvement with or without aneurysm formation; and hypertension have been implicated.[81]

Coils and Kinks of the Extracranial Arteries

Coils and kinks of the extracranial system on occasion have been associated with fibromuscular dysplasia.[81] More commonly, these are due to embryologic events and changes that occur in the aging process. Neurologic manifestations from these have been reported in children[85] and in adults.[86–88] Embryologically, the internal carotid artery is derived from the third aortic arch and the dorsal aortic root. In its early stages, a normally occurring kink is straightened as the heart and great vessels descend in the mediastinum. Failure of this process may account for the occurrence of coils and loops in children and for its bilaterality in about 50% of cases.[88]

In adults, kinking of the extracranial vessels is almost always associated with atherosclerosis. In the aging process, loss of elasticity of the vessel wall occurs, which, in combination with lateral stresses, causes elongation between fixed points, the skull and the thoracic inlet. This produces bowing, with eventual formation of coils and kinks. Between 5% and 16% of patients submitted for angiographic evaluation have coiling or kinking of one of the extracranial vessels.[86, 88] The kinking of the artery is more likely to

produce symptoms due either to flow reduction or to concomitant plaque formation with distal embolization. Kinking is considered as an angle of less than 90 degrees between arterial segments (Fig. 31–4). Flow restriction is unlikely to exist in the absence of this configuration. This acute angulation is more likely to occur when the head is turned to the ipsilateral side.[85] In other cases, contralateral rotation, neck flexion, and extension may exaggerate the abnormality to markedly reduce flow. A history of TIAs associated with head motion should lead the clinician to suspect the presence of kink. Abnormal pulsations in the neck, sometimes suggesting an aneurysmal dilatation, may be present on physical examination. Secondary arteriosclerotic changes may occur because of abnormal flow patterns that predispose to plaque formation and ulceration, accounting for the development of neurologic symptoms. Rarely is the vertebral circulation affected by a kink.[86]

Aneurysms

Aneurysms of the carotid artery can cause neurologic symptoms by several mechanisms. Thrombosis and rupture are rare, but embolization is a frequent event.[89] Pressure of cranial nerves can be seen when expansion is rapid, but more frequently this is associated with acute dissection.

Most extracranial aneurysms are secondary to atherosclerosis. Internal elastic lamina disruption and medial thinning are frequent histologic findings.[90] Two types are recognized: fusiform and saccular. Fusiform aneurysms are the most common. These are frequently bilateral and are associated with other arterial aneurysms. Saccular aneurysms are often unilateral and tend to involve the common or internal arteries more often. They may also have a congenital, degenerative, or traumatic origin.[91] Atherosclerotic aneurysms of the extracranial circulation are almost always associated with hypertension.[90]

Trauma is a frequent cause of carotid aneurysms. These are usually saccular and most commonly result from blunt rather than penetrating injury. Hyperextension and rotation of the neck cause compression of the internal carotid artery on the transverse process of the atlas.[92] An intimal injury is produced that frequently leads to thrombosis but that may also produce aneurysmal dilatation.[90]

Mycotic aneurysms are rare. Syphilis and peritonsillar abscess were once common causes of these aneurysms.[93] *Staphylococcus aureus* is the responsible organism at present.

False aneurysms of the carotid artery may form after penetrating injury, but the most frequent cause at present is previous carotid surgery. They are more common after patch closure of the artery than after primary closure.[89] Disruption of the suture line by infection, suture failure, and technical error are believed to be responsible for their formation. False aneurysms can expand, thrombose, rupture, or lead to distal embolization. The diagnosis is an indication for surgical repair.

Acute dissection of the carotid artery with or without aneurysm formation is another cause of neurologic events resulting from abnormalities in the extracranial circulation. It can occur secondary to atherosclerosis, fibromuscular dysplasia, or cystic medial necrosis.[94] A history of trauma

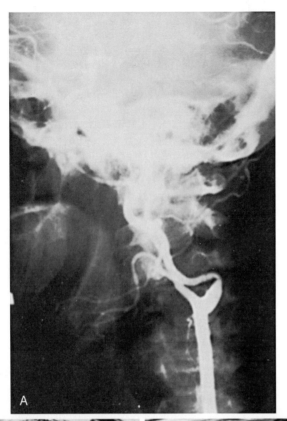

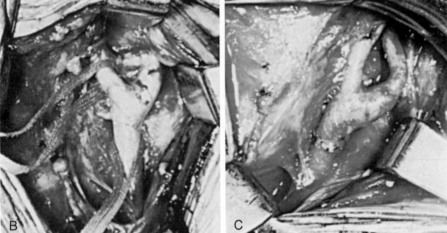

Figure 31–4. *A,* Selective left carotid arteriogram demonstrating kink of the internal carotid artery. Note the angulation of less than 90 degrees and the paucity of contrast material beyond the kink. *B,* Operative appearance of the internal carotid artery kink. *C,* Operative appearance of the internal carotid artery after connection of the kink by mobilization and segmental resection of the common carotid artery. The carotid bifurcation is pulled down and an end-to-end anastomosis is constructed.

may or may not be present. On gross inspection, a sharply demarcated transition between the normal color and size of the carotid artery and the dark-blue and cylindrical dilatation in the dissected segment is noted.[95] More commonly, the internal carotid artery is affected, and frequently the end of the dissection is not surgically accessible. A double lumen is usually present, with the dissection occurring in the outer layers of the media. Smooth muscle cells are widely separated, and degeneration and fragmentation of the internal elastic membrane occur.[95] The most frequent presentation is a sudden onset of temporal headache or cervical pain associated with a neurologic or visual deficit or Horner's syndrome. The acute expansion may cause compression of cranial nerves IX, X, XI, or XII, with concomitant dysfunction.[94] Horner's syndrome is thought

to be secondary to disruption of periadventitial sympathetic fibers. The carotid artery is far more frequently affected than the vertebral. Only a few cases of the latter have been reported, with involvement of the segment between C-1 and C-2 noted consistently.[94]

Takayasu's Arteritis

In 1908, Takayasu[96] described ocular changes in a 21-year-old woman with nonspecific arteritis. These consisted of a peculiar capillary flush with rustlike arteriovenous anastomoses around the papilla and blindness due to cataracts. Similar cases were later described with the absence of pulses in the arm. Since then, Takayasu's arteritis has been recognized as a cause of neurologic symptoms secondary to a nonspecific inflammatory process of unknown cause segmentally affecting the aorta and its main branches. The end result of this process is a constriction or occlusion and occasional aneurysm formation of the affected vessels secondary to marked fibrosis and thickening of the arterial wall.[97] Originally thought to be rare in this hemisphere, many cases of atypical coarctations of the aorta and other unusual lesions of its main branches are now well recognized as Takayasu's arteritis. This explains the many eponyms given to this syndrome.[98]

Four varieties of the disease are recognized.[99] In type 1, the involvement is localized to the aortic arch and its branches. Type 2 does not have arch involvement; the lesions are confined to the descending and abdominal aorta. Type 3 has features of both, and type 4 describes any of the above with involvement of the pulmonary artery. In a retrospective study of 107 patients,[99] 84% were female, and 80% were aged 11 to 30 years.

Two phases of the disease are recognized. In the acute or prepulseless stage, systemic symptoms of a nonspecific nature are present. Skin rashes, fever, myalgia, arthralgias, pleuritis, generalized weakness, and other nonspecific symptoms develop, making the diagnosis difficult. These may resolve and go unrecognized by the patient or physician until months or years later, when the second, or occlusive, stage evolves. Then, symptoms of obstruction of the main aortic branches develop. These lesions are not easily managed by endarterectomy. This makes bypass surgery the treatment of choice.

Other forms of arteritis, specifically giant cell arteritis, can cause neurologic symptoms because of extra- or intracranial involvement. Patients are older than those with Takayasu's arteritis, and both sexes appear to be equally affected.[98] Systemic symptoms are usually present. Tenderness over the carotid or other affected areas may occur.[100] The histologic picture is characteristic, with changes confined to the media, where a large number of giant cells interspersed with lymphocytes are seen. Early diagnosis is important because corticosteroid therapy may abort the latter stages of the process.[100]

Radiation Therapy Injury

External cervical radiation therapy is now recognized as a cause of accelerated atherosclerotic changes in the extracranial circulation. Experimentally,[101] atherosclerotic lesions similar to the naturally occurring one can be produced in the abdominal aorta in dogs by x-ray and electron beam radiation. Injury to the endothelial cell, ground substance, elastic lamina, and smooth muscle appear to alter the vessel wall, increasing its permeability to circulating lipids and impairing its ability to repair elastic tissue, leading to formation of a plaque characterized by fibrosis, fatty infiltration, and intimal destruction.[102] These changes may occur months to years after completion of therapy. Lesions occur in locations unusual for atherosclerosis (Fig. 31–5). Blowout of the affected carotid may occur, but it is more frequent when surgery is combined with radiation in treating cervical malignancies. Hyperlipidemia and hypercholesterolemia appear to predispose patients receiving radiation

therapy to the development of these accelerated changes.[103] Endarterectomy of the affected segments is somewhat more difficult but can be carried out safely.[102, 104]

Moritz and colleagues[105] reported their experience with 53 patients who had undergone radiation therapy to the neck an average of 28 months previously and compared them with 38 patients who did not have radiation and served as a control group. Thirty percent of the radiated group had moderate to severe lesions of the carotid bifurcation, as detected by duplex scanning, in contrast to only 6% of the control group. Five patients in the radiated group were symptomatic. The authors concluded that patients who receive carotid radiation should undergo follow-up periodic duplex scanning of the carotid arteries.[105]

Recurrent Carotid Stenosis

Recurrent carotid stenosis has been reported to occur in a range from 1% to 21%[106–111] and may yield an incidence of hemodynamically significant stenosis as high as 32% after 7 years.[106] This can lead to neurologic symptoms by producing emboli or restricting flow. The most common lesion developing within the first 2 years after surgery is myointimal fibroplasia. Histologically, a concentric lesion occurs with no calcium or lipid deposits. Dense accumulation of collagen and mucopolysaccharides surrounds cellular elements. These substances are produced by the myointimal cell in the normal healing process. An accelerated production seems responsible for the development of the fibroplastic lesion leading to stenosis of the lumen. An endarterectomy plane is almost impossible to develop.

The morphologic characteristics of the early (less than 2 years) restenosis suggest a lower risk of stroke when compared with arteriosclerotic lesions of similar degree.[112] In addition, regression of stenosis documented by noninvasive tests has been reported. Thus, controversy exists as to management of early recurrent stenosis after carotid endarterectomy.[113] In the asymptomatic stage, a restenosis documented by successive noninvasive testing should lead the surgeon to consider surgical intervention if progression of persistent stenosis to greater than 80% of the diameter occurs. Recurrent symptoms are certainly an indication for reoperation unless a different cause is suspected. Interestingly, Bernstein and colleagues[114] showed an inverse correlation between a greater than 50% recurrent stenosis and late stroke and death. Their data suggested that patients with early recurrent stenosis had a better long-term prognosis than those who did not develop recurrent stenosis.[114]

When a stenotic lesion develops more than 2 years after carotid endarterectomy, atherosclerosis is usually the causative process. Injury to the vessel by vascular clamps may play a role. Elevated serum cholesterol has a statistically significant association with recurrent carotid stenosis.[107]

These lesions probably carry the same stroke risk as primary arteriosclerotic lesions in the carotid bifurcation. Recommendation for reoperation thus is based on the known risk factors of similar primary arteriosclerotic lesions.

Some investigators have suggested that patch closure at the time of the initial carotid endarterectomy may prevent

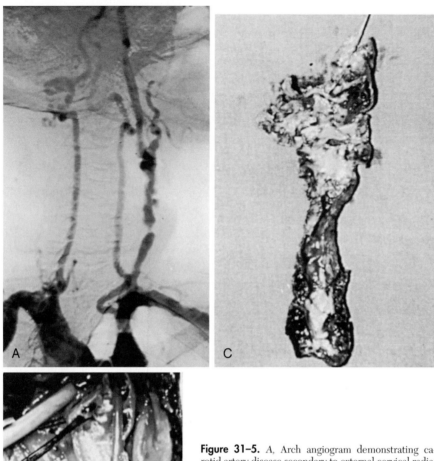

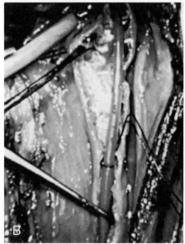

Figure 31–5. *A,* Arch angiogram demonstrating carotid artery disease secondary to external cervical radiation. Note complete occlusion of the right common carotid artery. Multiple stenoses are in the left common carotid artery, an unusual site for primary atherosclerosis. *B,* Operative appearance of the lesion secondary to external radiation. *C,* Intimectomy specimen of the lesion produced by external cervical radiation.

recurrent stenosis. Several prospective randomized studies, either completed or in progress, suggest a lower incidence of restenosis with the use of patch angioplasty.[108, 115–118] The most compelling argument in favor of patch closure comes from a prospective study by Abu Rahma and colleagues.[119] The authors identified 74 patients with bilateral carotid stenoses in need of bilateral operation—one side was closed primarily and the opposite side closed with patch angioplasty. In this manner, demographic and patient characteristics were controlled. The incidence of ipsilateral stroke for primary closure was 4% versus 0% in the patch group. Primary closure had a 22% incidence of recurrent stenosis versus 1% in the patch group (P < .003). Primary closure had an 8% incidence of internal carotid artery occlusion versus 0% in the patch group. Restenosis requiring reoperation was 14% in the primary closure group versus 1% in the patch group. In a life-table analysis, the 24-month freedom from recurrence was 75% in the primary closure group versus 98% in the patch group.[119] A significant benefit of patch angioplasty appears to be a reduction in technical end-point problems. Therefore, patching may be equally important in preventing occurrence as well as preventing recurrence. The same objective can be achieved by preventing or correcting technical errors at the time of operation when identified with completion angiography. Data obtained from experimental hemodynamic studies suggest that an enlarged bulb that would follow after patch closure of an endarterectomy site may predispose to areas of low shear stress and therefore recurrent disease. For this reason, it is important not to overenlarge the bulb when using a patch. Overenlargement may be responsible for a higher incidence of recurrence after vein patch angioplasty (9%) versus prosthetic patch angioplasty (2%). However, both were superior to primary closure (34%) in a randomized study.[120] The benefit of patch closure was also seen in a retrospective analysis of other data from the Asymptomatic Carotid Atherosclerosis Study (ACAS). The study examined the incidence of recurrence for three time intervals: within 3 months of operation (residual disease), 3 to 18 months (myointimal hyperplasia), and 18 to 60 months (recurrent atherosclerosis). The use of patch angioplasty reduced the overall risk of restenosis from 21.2% to 7.1%.[121] Factors associated with early recurrence include incomplete intimectomy (occurrence), the use of distal tacking sutures, female sex, continued cigarette smoking, and primary closure of an anatomically small internal carotid artery.[122–124]

Many clinicians routinely prescribe aspirin preoperatively as well as postoperatively. This is done with the hope and expectation that embolic events from platelet aggregates can be reduced or eliminated. Clinicians hoped that aspirin would reduce the incidence of myointimal hyperplasia by reducing platelet adhesion or aggregation and would interfere with the platelet release reaction. Unfortunately, the carotid artery, like other areas of arterial reconstruction, has not been shown to benefit. A prospective, randomized, placebo-controlled trial has failed to show any benefit of aspirin in preventing early carotid restenosis.[125]

PATHOGENETIC MECHANISMS OF TRANSIENT ISCHEMIC ATTACKS AND CEREBRAL INFARCTION

In reviewing the mechanisms for TIA and cerebral infarction, emphasis is placed on those events related to disease in the extracranial vessels. Hemorrhagic stroke is excluded. Cerebral ischemic events related to hypertension and cardiac emboli are briefly reviewed because of their importance in the differential diagnosis and workup of the symptomatic patient. Finally, from a pathogenetic standpoint, the difference between TIA and fixed deficit is a matter of degree, duration, and presence of actual infarction. The mechanisms of occurrence are essentially the same. Therefore, for purposes of discussion, we use the general inclusive term "ischemic event."

Arterial Thrombosis

When an atherosclerotic plaque expands to produce a critical reduction in blood flow, the vessel ultimately undergoes thrombosis. In the case of the internal carotid artery, if this column of thrombus stops at the ophthalmic artery and remains stable, and if collateral circulation is sufficient via the circle of Willis, the thrombotic event may be entirely asymptomatic (Fig. 31–6). If the thrombus propagates beyond the ophthalmic artery to occlude the middle cerebral artery (Fig. 31–7), however, or if small thrombi rather than a thrombotic column form and are subsequently carried to the intracranial vessels by continuous blood flow (Fig. 31–8), then the patient experiences cerebral symptoms that can vary from transient ocular or hemispheric events to a profound hemiplegia, depending on the extent of propagated thrombus or embolus. In addition, if the collateral circulation to the circle of Willis is poor, the sudden loss

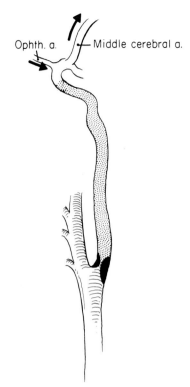

Figure 31–6. A thrombus occurring distal to an occlusive lesion of the internal carotid artery. Notice the column thrombus stops short of the ophthalmic artery, with maintenance of patency of the middle cerebral artery.

of flow through a diseased internal carotid artery may incite a precipitous drop in flow to the hemisphere, resulting in ischemic infarction as a consequence of inadequate proximal blood flow.

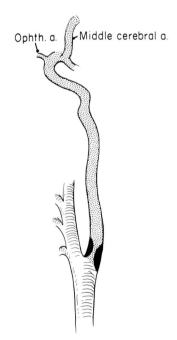

Figure 31–7. In this instance, the thrombus that develops secondary to an occlusive atherosclerotic lesion of the internal carotid artery progresses beyond the ophthalmic artery to involve the middle cerebral artery.

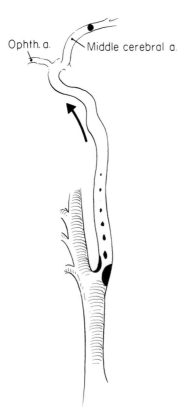

Ophth. a.　Middle cerebral a.

Figure 31–8. Emboli released from a plaque strategically placed at the origin of the internal carotid artery can pass into the middle cerebral artery and lodge in the terminal branch. This results in either a temporary or a permanent neurologic deficit in the distribution appropriate to the arterial occlusion.

Flow-Related Ischemic Events

Although flow-related ischemia used to be considered the most common cause of transient ischemic events, it is actually a rather rare occurrence. Transient drops in hemispheric blood flow or the development of a chronic low-flow state can be responsible for nonspecific symptoms of lightheadedness, presyncope, or intellectual deterioration.[1, 126] It must also be recognized that other causes of these symptoms exist that are nonvascular and probably more frequent.

The collateral blood flow to the brain, via the circle of Willis, is an extremely efficient system. Multiple patients have been described who have bilateral internal carotid artery occlusion, perhaps combined with occlusion of the vertebral artery, but were totally asymptomatic from a central neurologic point of view. Experience obtained performing carotid endarterectomy under local anesthesia has shown that only about 10% of patients experience neurologic symptoms when the carotid artery is clamped.[53] This 10% can have symptoms on the basis of compromised blood flow when the stenosis progresses or goes on to complete occlusion. Another circumstance that can produce symptoms of global ischemia is simultaneous stenosis or occlusion in more than one extracranial vessel; for example, a carotid occlusion on one side combined with a high-grade stenosis in the contralateral carotid artery. Under these circumstances, transient drops in blood pressure,

perhaps posturally related, can produce either global or focal ischemic symptoms. Rarely, patients with unilateral carotid occlusion may have a downstream vascular bed that is marginally perfused. Postural changes under these circumstances can also produce focal ischemia and result in a flow-related TIA. Under these conditions, a patient would be a good candidate for extracranial-to-intracranial bypass grafting.

Flow-restricting lesions in the vertebral arteries or in major vessels proximal to the vertebral origin, such as the innominate or subclavian artery, can produce symptoms related to hypoperfusion in the posterior circulation. One of the most dramatic anatomic observations is the so-called subclavian steal syndrome. If a stenosis or occlusion of the subclavian artery is present proximal to the vertebral artery takeoff, the pressure drop distal to the obstruction causes its branches to serve as sources of collateral blood flow by reversing the normal flow direction. The branches now contribute to the flow of the main trunk rather than receiving flow from the proximally affected artery. The vessels that contribute to collateral blood flow of the distal subclavian artery by reversing flow include the vertebral artery. Under these circumstances, the vertebral artery not only is deprived of the usual antegrade flow but also actually siphons off blood flow from the basilar artery circulation because of flow reversal. This siphoning off of blood may be entirely without symptoms if abundant sources of inflow from the other vertebral artery or from the anterior circulation exist. On the other hand, if the opposite vertebral artery is small or occluded, a deficiency in basilar artery flow may be present that results in symptoms of basilar artery insufficiency. These symptoms may first appear or become exaggerated if the demand for flow in the affected subclavian artery increases, such as results from doing active exercise of the arm (Fig. 31–9).

Cerebral Emboli

The most common causes of cerebral ischemic events are embolic phenomena, primarily arterial in origin and secondarily from cardiac sources. The emboli of arterial origin occur as a consequence of morphologic change present on the luminal surface of a critical artery.[52, 53, 127, 128] These changes most often are associated with atheromatous plaques but can also occur with other lesions such as fibromuscular dysplasia. When an irregular surface producing turbulence exists, a stimulus for platelet aggregation is present. If the platelet aggregates become large enough and embolize to an important vessel in the brain, symptoms occur. If the platelet aggregates break up quickly from mechanical forces or from the effect of arterial prostacyclin, the symptoms are transient. If the embolic fragment persists, however, it can lead to focal infarction (Fig. 31–10).

An atherosclerotic plaque may undergo central degeneration or softening. When this occurs, bleeding into the plaque substance may also occur, leading to sudden plaque expansion[49, 75, 110, 129] with intraluminal rupture, or the plaque may spontaneously rupture into the lumen, discharging its contents into the arterial stream. The plaque contents consist of degenerative atheromatous debris, in-

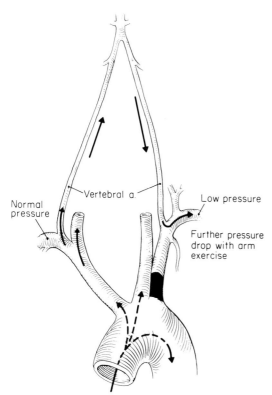

Figure 31–9. The mechanism of the subclavian steal syndrome. Note the occlusion in the origin of the left subclavian artery. This produces a pressure gradient with reversal of blood flow in the left vertebral artery, producing a siphoning or steal from the basilar artery.

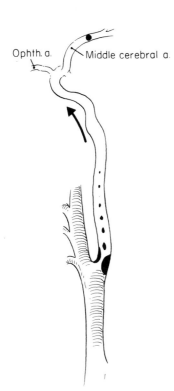

Figure 31–10. An embolic fragment in the middle cerebral artery. If this persists, it will lead to focal infarction. If the fragment breaks up and distributes itself through the microcirculation, the ischemic event will be transient.

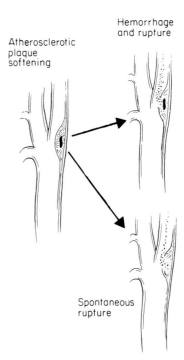

Figure 31–11. An atherosclerotic plaque undergoing central softening. Spontaneous hemorrhage may occur into the center of the plaque, producing rupture and discharge of embolic fragments, or the plaque may spontaneously rupture as a result of hydrostatic forces, releasing necrotic, embolic debris.

cluding various mixtures of cholesterol crystals, calcific material, or thrombotic remnants. If the atherosclerotic plaque is located at a critical point, such as the origin of the internal carotid artery, considerable likelihood exists that embolic atheromatous fragments will be carried to important vascular beds of the brain, producing either transient or permanent neurologic events (Fig. 31–11). These events are considered primary embolic events of atherosclerotic plaque origin.

After the plaque has ruptured, a defect is left behind that is called an ulcer (Fig. 31–12). Further primary emboli can continue to escape from the raw ulcerated surface, or the ulcer itself may serve as a focal point for thrombus or platelet aggregate material to form. These platelet or thrombotic aggregates may secondarily dislodge, owing to blood flow turbulence, and embolize to the brain (Fig. 31–13). Thus, the embolic material from an atherosclerotic

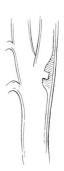

Figure 31–12. Following evacuation of an atherosclerotic plaque, a defect or ulcer is left behind.

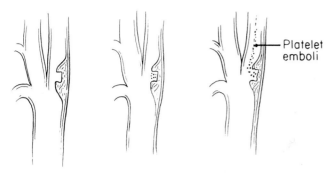

Figure 31-13. The ulcerated lesion within an atheromatous plaque can serve as a nidus for platelet aggregate or thrombotic material. These aggregates can secondarily embolize from the ulcer crypt.

plaque can consist of atheromatous debris, platelet aggregates, or blood clot. The emboli of arterial origin can be primary, occurring with plaque rupture or occurring on thrombogenic arterial plaque surfaces,[128, 130] or secondary, having developed within ulcerative lesions from previous plaque rupture.[131]

Embolic events may produce the more dramatic focal neurologic events that are immediately appreciated by the patient, or the embolic fragments may travel to more silent areas of the brain, in which case the results are more subtle and appreciated on a chronic basis, such as cerebral atrophy or multi-infarct dementia.[132, 133] The use of transcranial Doppler ultrasonography has provided more objective evidence of emboli from carotid plaques by discerning discrete noise as an embolic particle passes a point of Doppler insonation.[134] Finally, the occurrence of TIAs in a hemisphere distal to a carotid occlusion raises the question of the relationship of decreased flow to arterial border zones. Experimental data, however, have demonstrated that emboli originating from a contralateral carotid artery can cross through the circle of Willis and produce focal infarcts in the hemisphere distal to a carotid occlusion.[135] Thus the contralateral patent carotid artery should always be considered a possible source of emboli when a patient with a carotid occlusion begins to experience symptoms in the hemisphere distal to the occlusion.

Emboli can also occur from cardiac sources, which include aortic valvular disease, mitral valve prolapse, cardiac arrhythmias, and mural thrombus after myocardial infarction. More recently, atherosclerotic plaques of the ascending aorta, as seen with transesophageal echocardiography, have been identified as another source of cerebral embolization.[136–138]

Lacunar Infarction

Focal areas of cerebral necrosis occurring in the basal ganglia, internal capsule, or pons have been described as a consequence of end-vessel occlusive disease involving the lenticulostriate or thalamoperforant arteries. The underlying cause is related to uncontrolled hypertension, and the resulting neurologic deficit is often clinically identified as a pure motor or pure sensory stroke.[139] Although descriptions of this phenomenon date back to the early 1900s, its cur-

rent understanding and popularity are due to the efforts and writings of C. Miller Fisher.[140]

The clinical picture may often be confused with arterial-arterial emboli in that antecedent TIAs may have occurred. The differential diagnosis is best made by the very focal neurologic deficit seen clinically and the typical anatomic location as seen on the CT brain scan. Evidence now shows that the so-called lacunae may, in fact, be the consequence of emboli of arterial origin.[141–144] Thus, the presence of symptoms with imaging of a deep white matter infarct does not rule out atheromatous plaque from carotid bifurcation as a cause of the event.

CLINICAL SYNDROMES OF EXTRACRANIAL ARTERIAL OCCLUSIVE DISEASE

Extracranial arterial occlusive disease may result in varying symptoms or in other instances may be completely asymptomatic. A thorough history must be obtained, because this alone may provide clues as to the specific nature of the event in question. Often, one discovers that symptoms exist that the patient has ignored. A complete review of symptoms is mandatory, because this in itself may alter the therapeutic alternatives available. Risk factors for atherosclerosis should be specifically recorded.

Patients can be classified into three categories: asymptomatic patients, patients with TIAs, and patients with cerebral infarction. Asymptomatic patients represent that group in which a hemodynamically significant lesion or a nonocclusive ulcerated arteriosclerotic plaque in the extracranial circulation has been discovered in the absence of transient or permanent neurologic symptoms. The presence or absence of a bruit in the cervical area should not be a criterion for inclusion in this category. It should be recorded as a general marker of a patient at high risk of atherosclerosis.[145]

In an analysis of 1287 patients with cervical bruits, less than one third of the carotid lesions with bruits proved to be hemodynamically significant by noninvasive criteria.[41] The fact that significant lesions can occur in the absence of a bruit and vice versa is important. The available data on the natural history of asymptomatic bruits cannot be applied to patients with these lesions. This group of patients is usually discovered by angiography in studying other conditions or by noninvasive studies carried out because of the presence of a bruit or screening before major surgical procedures. Because of what is known of the natural history of these lesions, as discussed later, therapeutic intervention in the asymptomatic stage may be beneficial.

The two categories of symptomatic patients with extracranial arterial occlusive disease are discussed separately.

Transient Ischemic Attacks

General Considerations

TIAs are defined as temporary focal neurologic deficits lasting no more than 24 hours, with complete recovery.

The event is caused by ischemia in the territory of the brain supplied by a particular artery or branch. Clinically, symptoms are of sudden onset, without aura, and resolution is often within minutes. When symptoms last longer than 6 hours, a permanent abnormality is more likely, although it may not be clinically detectable.[146] Because of its territorial nature, symptoms tend to be stereotyped. Disappearance of symptoms is swift, ordinarily taking only a few minutes.[147] The frequency of attacks is variable. The patient may experience only one episode or multiple attacks, with variable symptom-free intervals. The most common cause of these transient territorial deficits is extracranial arterial occlusive lesions. The pathology of these lesions has been discussed. Other important causes in the differential diagnosis include heart disease; hematologic disorders such as systemic lupus erythematosus, hyperglobulinemia, polycythemia and sickle cell disease; disseminated intravascular coagulation; subacute bacterial endocarditis; paroxysmal embolism; and several rare connective tissue disorders such as pseudoxanthoma elasticum and Ehlers-Danlos syndrome.[146] Migraine, especially when associated with transient neurologic deficit, can be confused with a TIA. A history of migraine in the family, the throbbing quality of the headache, and its occurrence on recovery from the neurologic deficit can be helpful in the differential diagnosis.

An important concept when evaluating patients with symptoms suggestive of TIA is that the symptoms secondary to emboli from a point source such as the extracranial circulation are the same with every attack. In contrast, patients whose emboli are from the heart tend to have variable symptoms.

Because only about 9% of patients with TIAs are seen by a physician during an attack,[148] the history remains the main factor in establishing the diagnosis. In this regard, family members may be extremely helpful.

Two important syndromes deserve mention. Occasionally, a patient experiences frequent repeated attacks of a specific neurologic deficit without the interval allowing time for complete recovery. If the deficit is the same with each attack and no deterioration in function is seen, this is known as crescendo TIAs. If progressive deterioration is seen with each successive attack, a stroke in evolution may be present. In any case, evaluation must proceed on an emergency basis. If a surgically correctable lesion is present and the neurologic deficit is not dense (no loss of consciousness or dense hemiparesis), serious consideration should be given to proceeding with emergency operation.

Carotid Artery Transient Ischemic Attacks

Manifestations of a transient ischemic episode in the territory of the carotid artery include deficits in areas supplied by the anterior and middle cerebral arteries. In older individuals, both anterior cerebral arteries and posterior arteries may be supplied by one carotid artery.[146]

Ischemia in a cerebral hemisphere often produces contralateral symptoms. Motor dysfunction can include weakness, paralysis, or clumsiness of one or both limbs contralateral to the affected hemisphere. Sensory alterations include numbness, loss of sensation, or paresthesia in the opposite side of the face or in one or both limbs. When examined during an attack, this sensory loss may not be objectively demonstrable.[148]

Ninety-five percent of patients have a dominant left hemisphere. Both receptive and motor aphasia can occur. When the former is present, the patient or family may interpret it as confusion. Dysarthria may occur as a function of the nondominant hemisphere, but when it is present as the sole symptom, it is more common in vertebrobasilar TIAs. Other functions of the nondominant side include inattention to the patient's own person and environment on the contralateral side.[146] Loss of function of these areas may also be interpreted as confusion.

Transient visual loss (amaurosis fugax) or blurring of vision in the ipsilateral eye is one of the most reliable symptoms of carotid artery TIAs.[149] This may be described as a curtain coming down (altitudinal) or as quadrant field defects. Conjugate eye deviation, as occurs in seizures or completed strokes, is not seen. Homonymous hemianopsia in combination with any of the above-mentioned symptoms suggests carotid TIAs. This is the result of ischemia in the area of the optic radiation emanating from the optic chiasm. This produces loss of vision in the ipsilateral temporal visual field and the contralateral nasal visual field. When TIAs occur secondary to carotid artery disease, these visual field defects usually are limited to a quadrant corresponding to the distribution of the optic radiation. When hemianopsia is complete, it cannot be distinguished from a vertebrobasilar TIA.[146]

Ischemic optic neuropathy is a condition characterized by blindness and is associated with giant cell arteritis in about 10% of cases. In the other 90% of cases, it has been labeled idiopathic. Berguer[150] found a significant correlation between extracranial occlusive disease and idiopathic optic neuropathy. In fact, of 20 symptomatic eyes examined, significant extracranial arterial occlusive disease was found in 12 (60%). An embolic mechanism was suggested as the cause of the optic nerve infarct. A more severe form is seen in patients with very severe extracranial disease, usually occlusion on one side and a high degree of stenosis on the other. These patients develop an ischemic ophthalmopathy characterized by neovascularization of the iris. The term "rubeosis" has been used to characterize this entity. This suggests that patients with idiopathic optic neuropathy not found to be secondary to giant cell arteritis should undergo extracranial vascular evaluation.[150]

Convulsions can occur but are more suggestive of a completed or hemorrhagic stroke. When sensory or motor symptoms are present, they appear all at one time, without a march suggestive of focal seizure activity.[147] A combination of symptoms may carry more reliability than a single symptom alone. In right carotid artery TIA, the combination of ipsilateral visual loss and any contralateral arm symptoms has an increased relationship. In left carotid TIA, diagnostic reliability is increased when language disturbance is combined with right face or extremity weakness or sensory loss.[149]

Altered consciousness or syncope can occur, but as the only symptom it is extremely rare and more often is associated with other illnesses such as cardiac arrhythmias.[146] Other symptoms that represent difficulty in the initial evaluation are dizziness, amnesia, or confusion and impaired vision with alteration in consciousness. These, without other more specific symptoms, are not to be considered as manifestations of TIAs, because they occur most often with other illnesses.

Vertebrobasilar System Transient Ischemic Attacks

Transient ischemia of the area in the brain supplied by the vertebrobasilar system can occur owing to flow restriction or emboli from lesions in the vertebral or basilar arteries. Emboli from other sources may also affect this system.

An occlusive lesion at the origin of the subclavian artery can cause vertebrobasilar symptoms as the affected arm is exercised and reversal of flow occurs in the vertebral circulation. This subclavian steal is often accompanied by exertional pain in the arm of the affected side.[146]

Alternating hemipareses or hemisensory symptoms in repetitive attacks and bilateral circumoral sensory symptoms associated with unilateral arm or leg weakness or ataxia are highly suggestive of vertebrobasilar TIAs. Symptoms may change from one side to the other with different attacks and may even involve all four limbs at one time. Drop attacks, or falling precipitously to the ground without premonitory symptoms, occur in less than 4% of patients.[149] In this syndrome, loss of consciousness is absent or so brief that the patient remembers striking the ground, a feature not present in syncope or seizure.[146]

Equilibratory gait or postural disturbance not associated with vertigo can occur. Complete or partial loss of vision in both homonymous fields or homonymous hemianopsia alone is highly suggestive. Vertigo alone, when not associated with other of the above specific symptoms, should not be considered indicative of TIA. When it occurs in clear relationship to focal weakness of the face, arm, or leg or to ataxia or to persistent diplopia, the existence of TIA is likely. Tinnitus is not a feature of vertigo of a vertebrobasilar TIA and is suggestive of labyrinthine vertigo. Single occurrences of bilateral visual blurring, dysarthria, hoarseness, diplopia, dysphasia, confusion, hiccups, vomiting, loss of consciousness, and vital sign alteration may be manifestations of vertebrobasilar TIAs. These symptoms have so many other causes, however, that the diagnosis is uncertain unless they occur in combination or with additional signs of focal brain stem or posterior hemisphere dysfunction.

Cerebral Infarction

A completed cerebral infarction with or without a clinically apparent neurologic deficit can be another manifestation of extracranial arterial occlusive disease. The specific deficits that are clinically detectable are the same as those discussed as manifestations of TIAs.

Estimating accurately what percentage of all strokes are secondary to lesions in the extracranial circulation is difficult. Available studies differ in population, criteria for diagnosis, and therapeutic approach, and thus the estimates range from 15% to 52%.[151, 152] Extracranial vascular lesions play a major role in the occurrence of cerebral infarction.

Approximately 50% of these events are preceded by TIAs, thus providing a clue to diagnosis.[153]

Lacunar infarcts, emboli from a cardiac source, intracerebral or intracranial bleeding, and some hematologic disorders as causes of stroke should be included in the differential diagnosis. Cerebrospinal fluid examination, electroencephalography (EEG), echocardiograms, Holter monitors, and brain CTs are helpful adjuncts in reaching etiologic explanation. Angiography should be considered, because noninvasive studies do not exclude ulcerative lesions in the extracranial circulation that may be responsible for the embolic infarction.

Identification of a cause of the stroke is essential, because these patients remain at high risk of developing a subsequent cerebral infarction.

ROLE OF THE VASCULAR LABORATORY

The vascular laboratory from the standpoint of method, accuracy, and interpretation is covered in detail in Chapter 14. The role of the vascular laboratory in the evaluation of patients with suspected cerebrovascular disease has been disputed by some and perhaps misused by others. The vascular laboratory has an ever-increasing role of importance for evaluating patients with cerebrovascular disease. In this section, we endeavor to review its current application.

Asymptomatic Patients

Patients without symptoms may come to our attention as possible candidates for extracranial cerebrovascular disease because of the presence of one or more associated risk factors (cigarette smoking, hypertension, diabetes mellitus, coronary artery disease, or peripheral vascular disease) or by the presence of a bruit heard over the carotid artery bifurcation. The occurrence of a preocclusive carotid stenosis in the past could be ascertained only by proceeding with carotid angiography, yet the incidence of finding a lesion of significance by angiographic screening was only 20% to 30%. That means that 70% of the suspect population were subjected to costly and needless hospitalization, plus the risk and discomfort of angiography. Currently, with the available vascular laboratory modalities, the presence or absence of a hemodynamically significant lesion can be ascertained in an inexpensive, noninvasive manner with an accuracy of greater than 95%.

Symptomatic Patients

Patients may show territorial neurologic events typical of carotid artery or vertebrobasilar disease, or they may have symptoms that are entirely nonspecific or atypical. In the case of the patient with nonspecific symptoms, such as "dizzy spells," these symptoms may be related to global ischemic events as a consequence of decreased blood flow associated with multiple extracranial occlusive lesions, or they may be due to a myriad of disorders unrelated to cerebrovascular disease. The vascular laboratory serves as an effective screen for these patients and can result in avoiding many negative and hence useless angiograms.

Angiography used to be considered mandatory for the workup of symptomatic patients. This is no longer true. Duplex scanning in a qualified laboratory may provide definitive information necessary for both medical and surgical management. For this reason, a carefully performed duplex scan has now become a critical part of the evaluation of symptomatic patients. Contrast angiography is now limited to patients in whom symptoms are not explained by findings on duplex scanning. In addition, the preoperative baseline data from the vascular laboratory are extremely helpful in following patients immediately after operation as well as in the late follow-up interval. A conversion from a positive to a negative test after operation is expected. If this does not occur, a technical problem is suggested that may require investigation and management. Also, an abnormal study 6 months or a year after surgery in a patient who had a normal study after operation alerts the surgeon to the possibility of recurrent stenosis, often before the onset of symptoms. Finally, the importance of obtaining baseline data on the opposite, asymptomatic carotid artery should not be overlooked. Late strokes that occur in patients who have undergone successful carotid endarterectomy are most often related to the side not operated on. Early identification of progression on the contralateral side permits earlier intervention as a means of preventing contralateral stroke.

BRAIN SCANS AND ANGIOGRAPHY

The advent of CT and magnetic resonance imaging (MRI) for head scanning has been a benefit in the evaluation of patients with cerebrovascular disease and has virtually eliminated the use of radionuclide scanning. Intracranial space-occupying lesions such as neoplasms, vascular malformations, or subdural hematomas enter into the differential diagnosis of patients with even the most convincing symptoms of transient cerebral ischemia. CT and MRI scanning are quick, noninvasive means of ruling out alternative abnormalities during patient workup.

The patient who presents with a TIA may have actually suffered a small cerebral infarction. CT or MRI scanning identifies an unsuspected cerebral infarction and establishes a baseline status before operation. The advance knowledge that a small infarction exists is helpful information with respect to intraoperative and postoperative management.

Although head scanning may not currently be routine in a preoperative workup, it should become a standard part of evaluation of the symptomatic patient. MRI is replacing CT in some centers. It does not require ionizing radiation or contrast. It can identify acute cerebral infarction sooner than CT and can image smaller infarcts than CT. Finally, newer acquisition programs have enabled magnetic resonance to be used to reconstruct cervical and intracranial arterial anatomy, so-called magnetic resonance angiography (MRA).

Those patients who show a clinically overt cerebral in-

farction should have a CT or MRI scan to document infarct size and to differentiate between an ischemic and hemorrhagic infarction. A hemorrhagic infarction is promptly visible on CT scan, whereas an ischemic infarction may take several days of evolution before its low-density character is visualized. CT scan data are necessary in decisions concerning the proper timing of operation after acute stroke in patients who have experienced a good neurologic recovery. In fact, of 245 patients with persistent neurologic deficits seen by Dosick and colleagues,[154] 171 were found to have negative CT scans. Appropriate carotid lesions were found in 110 (64%) of this group. All 110 patients underwent carotid endarterectomy within 14 days of the initial onset of their neurologic deficits. The perioperative morbidity was 0.9%. These investigators concluded that angiography and carotid endarterectomy may be safely performed when indicated in patients with negative CT scans within the first 2 weeks after a prolonged neurologic deficit.[154]

The EEG has generally not been considered helpful in the workup of patients with cerebrovascular disease, with the exception of ruling out seizure disorder in the differential diagnosis. However, a new application of cerebral electrical activity, so-called computerized brain mapping, is of value. This modality utilizes 32 electrodes (rather than the 16 used with EEG) arranged over both hemispheres. The data are digitized and color-coded. The information is computer-analyzed, and hard-copy–integrated data are generated. In a recent report comparing CT, MRI, and brain mapping, brain mapping was more sensitive in identifying small areas of cortical dysfunction.[155] Aortocranial angiography has been the cornerstone of diagnosis in the workup of patients with suspected cerebrovascular disease. *The angiogram is a preoperative study.* An angiogram should not be ordered unless the patient and surgeon are prepared to proceed promptly with operation. No place exists for the use of angiography as a routine database item unless the information obtained is going to be used for therapeutic decision making. Noninvasive studies are now sophisticated enough for diagnosis. The angiogram should be used to confirm the presence of a surgically accessible lesion and a satisfactory distal vascular bed.

The extent of angiographic visualization required for proper evaluation in patients with cerebrovascular disease is controversial. The options include (1) visualization of the aortic arch and extracranial vessels in two oblique views, (2) selective injection of both common carotid arteries in anteroposterior and lateral projections to obtain both extracranial and intracranial carotid visualization, (3) combined arch and selective carotid angiograms, (4) the possible addition of subclavian-vertebral angiography for both extracranial and intracranial visualization, (5) digital intravenous or intraarterial subtraction angiography, and (6) no angiography at all, relying solely on noninvasive testing.

Although aortocranial angiography remains the gold standard for identification of both extracranial and intracranial cerebrovascular disease, there are an increasing number of institutions around the world that are electing to forego angiography provided that preoperative noninvasive testing is of diagnostic quality and correlates with the clinical presentation of the patient. Noninvasive testing, primarily carotid duplex scanning, perhaps supplemented with information from MRA or CT angiography, can clearly identify patients with carotid bifurcation disease. MRA or CT can perhaps more accurately define the percentage of stenosis than data from contrast angiography, because the contrast angiogram almost inevitably underestimates the percentage of stenosis. Noninvasive testing, however, cannot accurately define carotid ulceration independent of carotid stenosis. However, the definition of carotid ulceration, even with angiography, is limited. A recent correlation between the preoperative angiogram and inspection of the plaque at the time of operation was performed in the first 540 patients entered into the North American Symptomatic Carotid Endarterectomy Trial (NASCET).[156] The sensitivity and specificity for detecting ulcerated plaques was 45.9% and 74.1%, respectively. The positive predictive value for identifying an ulcer was 71.8%.[156] Thus, even the gold standard of angiography appears imperfect in making or ruling out the diagnosis of ulceration. One possible explanation for missing ulceration is that it may be filled with thrombus when the angiogram is performed.

The routine preoperative use of angiography has been questioned in the literature. This remains a controversial issue, but the practice has clearly increased in those centers that have validated, certified vascular laboratories.[157]

The benefit of performing carotid endarterectomy without angiography is that angiography carries a significant risk to the workup of patients with extracranial arterial occlusive disease. In the ACAS,[158, 159] the neurologic morbidity and mortality was 1.2% for angiography alone. This is almost equal to the risk of operation. Although some express the opinion that this complication was abnormally high, all patients had been prescreened with ultrasonography and had documented hemodynamically significant lesions. Therefore, this represents a select, high-risk group of patients for angiography. Thus, with improved techniques of imaging the carotid bifurcation, there has been increasing acceptance of noninvasive imaging as the sole substitute for preoperative angiography in patients scheduled for carotid endarterectomy. This change in opinion began with the use of improved-quality duplex scanning. It continues with the use of MRA. Finally, recognizing the limitations of both of these techniques, the most recent suggestion has been to combine duplex scanning and MRA for preoperative assessment. When clear agreement exists between the two techniques, this appears to be a safe substitute for contrast angiography. On the other hand, when conflicting information occurs, or if the noninvasive study is unsatisfactory, or if the clinical picture is unexplained by noninvasive imaging, the selective use of contrast angiography is clearly indicated.[160–171]

SURGICAL CONSIDERATIONS AND TECHNIQUE

Anesthesia and Hemodynamic Monitoring

Patients about to undergo cerebrovascular surgery are probably best managed under general anesthesia. Although some surgeons still prefer to do carotid endarterectomy under local or cervical block anesthesia,[172] general anesthe-

sia has the advantage of reducing the cerebral metabolic demand of the brain and increasing cerebral blood flow. General anesthesia also provides good airway control, reduced patient anxiety, and a quiet surgical field.

Intraoperative blood pressure control and oxygenation are particularly critical during periods of arterial clamping. These parameters are best monitored with an arterial line, usually placed in the radial artery. The judicious use of nitroprusside or vasopressors by the anesthesiologist to maintain blood pressure in the patient's optimal physiologic range is of paramount importance.

Two primary options are available to monitor cerebral perfusion as might be required, particularly during trial clamping of the carotid artery before a decision to use an internal shunt. These options are the measurement of internal carotid artery back-pressure[173, 174] and the intraoperative use of EEG.[175] Although controversy exists as to which is more effective, excellent results have been reported with both techniques. EEG with CT brain mapping is a sensitive and accurate means of identifying patients who require shunting.[155, 176] A new technique, that of somatosensory evoked potentials, has been investigated and does not appear to be as sensitive as EEG.[177] Finally, proponents of no monitoring exist, some advocating the routine use of an intraluminal shunt,[178] and others advocating routine operation without a shunt but done in an expeditious manner.[179, 180] The literature currently supports either selective shunting based on clinical and monitoring criteria or routine shunting. The consensus is that either of these techniques provides the safest operation with the best outcome.[181, 182]

The argument in favor of selective shunting is that because only 15% of patients actually require an intraluminal shunt, as judged by observation of operations carried out under local anesthesia, why expose the other 85% of patients to the risks of an internal shunt, which include (1) possible air or atheroma embolisms, (2) scuffing or dissection of distal intima, (3) difficulty with end-point visualization, and (4) risk of leaving an intimal flap that may lead to thromboembolic complications? The arguments in favor of the routine use of an intraluminal shunt are that (1) with routine use, operator facility with the technique is increased and less likelihood of incurring complications exists, and (2) the presence of the intraluminal shunt acts as a stent that can aid in the closure of the internal carotid portion of the arteriotomy.

The criteria for mandatory shunting based on back-pressure measurement, as originally described by Moore and colleagues,[173, 174] include patients who have had a prior cerebral infarction on the side of operation (regardless of back-pressure value) or patients without a prior cerebral infarction but with a back-pressure of 25 mm Hg or less who are otherwise neurologically intact. The EEG criteria for shunt use include a loss of amplitude or slowing of rhythm during trial clamping of the carotid artery.

Carotid Bifurcation Endarterectomy

Indications

The indications for carotid endarterectomy have undergone considerable review and analysis. Data based on retrospective reviews, results of prospective randomized trials, and committee discussion based on expert opinion have been brought together to define the current indications for carotid endarterectomy.[183–185]

More recently, the Stroke Council of the American Heart Association convened a consensus conference on the indications for carotid endarterectomy. These two reports constitute the most up-to-date agreement concerning indications.[186, 187] The ad hoc committee recognized four categories: (1) proven—the strongest indication, usually supported by results of prospective randomized trials; (2) acceptable but not proven—a good indication for operation supported by promising but not scientifically certain data; (3) uncertain—data insufficient to define the risk-benefit ratio; (4) proven inappropriate—current data adequate to show that the risk of surgery outweighs any benefit.

The recommendations are further stratified by the symptomatic or asymptomatic status of the patient. Finally, the risk of operation based on the comorbid condition of the patient and the individual surgeon's track record is taken into account. Based on this classification, the general indication for carotid endarterectomy can be classified as follows: For symptomatic good-risk patients with a surgeon whose surgical morbidity and mortality is less than 6%:

A. Proven indications
   1. One or more TIAs in last 6 months and a carotid stenosis greater than or equal to 70%
   2. Mild stroke with carotid stenosis greater than or equal to 70%
B. Acceptable but not proven
   1. TIAs in past 6 months and a stenosis of 50% to 69%
   2. Progressive stroke and stenosis greater than or equal to 70%
   3. Mild or moderate stroke in past 6 months and a stenosis of 50% to 69%
   4. Carotid endarterectomy ipsilateral to TIAs and a stenosis greater than or equal to 70%, combined with required coronary bypass grafting
C. Uncertain indicators
   1. TIAs with stenosis less than or equal to 50%
   2. Mild stroke with stenosis less than or equal to 50%
   3. Symptomatic acute carotid thrombosis
D. Proven inappropriate
   1. Moderate stroke with stenosis less than or equal to 50%, not receiving aspirin
   2. Single TIA, stenosis less than or equal to 50%, not receiving aspirin
   3. High-risk patient with multiple TIAs, stenosis less than or equal to 50%, not receiving aspirin
   4. High-risk patient, mild or moderate stroke, stenosis less than or equal to 50%, not receiving aspirin
   5. Global ischemic symptoms with stenosis less than or equal to 50%
   6. Acute internal carotid dissection, asymptomatic, receiving heparin

For asymptomatic good-risk patients treated by a surgeon whose surgical morbidity-mortality rate is less than 3%, the indications for carotid endarterectomy are:

A. Proven
   1. Stenosis greater than or equal to 60% (following ACAS publication)

B. Acceptable but not proven
   1. None defined
C. Uncertain
   1. High-risk patient or surgeon with a morbidity-mortality rate greater than 3%, combined carotid-coronary operations, or nonstenotic ulcerative lesions
D. Proven inappropriate
   1. Operations with a combined stroke morbidity-mortality rate greater than or equal to 5%

The Stroke Council of the American Heart Association has updated this report and reaffirmed the indications.[188]

Technique

After the induction of satisfactory anesthesia and the placement of appropriate access and monitoring lines, the patient is positioned supine on the operating table with the head turned away from the side of operation. The neck is moderately extended on the shoulders. The head of the table is flexed about 10 degrees to reduce venous pressure, which minimizes bleeding. I prefer a longitudinal incision placed along the anterior border of the sternocleidomastoid muscle and centered over the carotid bifurcation. This incision can be extended proximally to the sternal notch for more proximal exposure of the common carotid artery and distally to the mastoid process for extensile exposure of the internal carotid artery, when needed. The dissection plane is maintained along the anterior border of the sternocleidomastoid muscle, which permits anterior mobilization of the tail of the parotid gland rather than the bloody division of its substance, with risk of salivary fistula. The sternocleidomastoid muscle is mobilized off the carotid sheath, and self-retaining retractors are placed. The jugular vein is visualized through the carotid sheath, and the sheath is open along the anterior border of the vein. The vein is mobilized until the large tributary, the common facial vein, is identified. The common facial vein, when present, is a relatively constant landmark for the carotid bifurcation. The common facial vein is divided between ligatures. In the case of a high carotid bifurcation, particular care must be taken to make sure that the hypoglossal nerve is not lurking behind the common facial vein, because this may lead to its inadvertent injury. Once the common facial vein is divided, the jugular vein can be mobilized laterally off the carotid bifurcation, providing excellent exposure. The vagus nerve usually lies in the posterior portion of the carotid sheath, but on occasion may spiral anteriorly. Particular care must be taken to watch for this anomalous course to avoid nerve injury. Another anomaly is the occasional presence of a nonrecurrent laryngeal nerve that comes directly off the vagus on the way to innervate the vocal cord. This nerve can cross anterior to the carotid artery and may be mistaken for a part of the ansa hypoglossi, resulting in mistaken division and cord paralysis. This anomaly most often occurs on the right side of the neck, but it has also been seen on the left side.

The common carotid artery is mobilized for sufficient length to get proximal to the atheromatous lesion as well as to provide sufficient length in case an internal shunt is required. When the dissection approaches the area of the

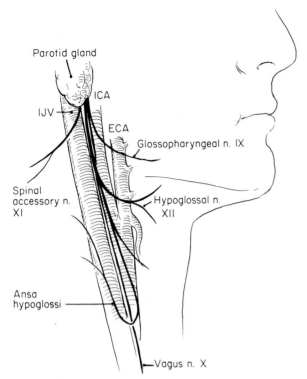

Figure 31–14. The anatomic relationship between the carotid bifurcation and the cranial nerves in the neck. Note the intimate relationship between the hypoglossal nerve and the upper portion of the internal carotid artery (ICA). ECA, external carotid artery; IJV, internal jugular vein.

Once the carotid artery has been sufficiently mobilized, 5000 units of heparin are administered systemically.

If the decision has been made to selectively shunt the patient based on back-pressure criteria, a 22-gauge needle is connected to rigid pressure tubing and hooked up to an arterial pressure transducer. The tubing is flushed with saline, and a zero-pressure level is obtained adjacent to the carotid bifurcation. The needle is carefully bent at a 45-degree angle and inserted into the common carotid artery so that the axis of the distal needle is parallel with the axis of the artery and lies freely within the lumen. The free carotid artery pressure is measured and compared with the radial artery pressure to ensure accurate reading. When the patient's blood pressure is stable and at the optimal level, the common carotid artery is clamped proximal to the needle, and the external carotid artery is also clamped, thus permitting the reading of the internal carotid artery back-pressure (Fig. 31–15). If the back-pressure is greater than 25 mm Hg, the internal carotid artery is clamped and the needle withdrawn. If the pressure is less than 25 mm Hg, the clamps on the common and external carotid arteries are temporarily removed, the needle withdrawn, and preparations made for the use of an internal shunt.

With the common, external, and internal carotid arteries clamped, an arteriotomy is made on the lateral portion of the common carotid artery with a No. 11 blade and is extended toward the plaque and up the internal carotid artery with Potts scissors. The arteriotomy is extended as far as necessary up the internal carotid artery to get beyond the plaque and to expose relatively normal artery. An intimectomy plane is then established between the diseased intima and the internal elastic lamina, attempting to leave the circular medial fibers attached to the arterial adventitia. This facilitates getting a clean distal end point. The proximal end point is obtained by sharply dividing the plaque. The intimectomy surface is copiously irrigated with heparinized saline solution so as to visualize all bits of debris and facilitate their removal.

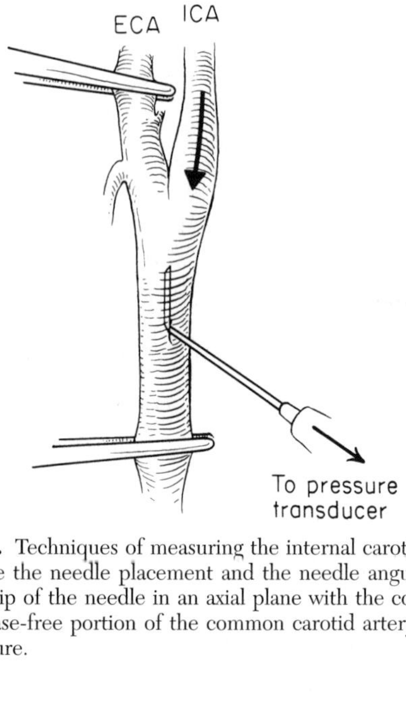

carotid bifurcation, it may be necessary to inject a local anesthetic in the area of the carotid bifurcation to block the nerve to the carotid body to prevent or reverse reflex bradycardia. The external and internal carotid arteries are then mobilized for sufficient length to get completely beyond the atheromatous plaque and to a point where the vessels are completely normal circumferentially. When mobilizing the internal carotid artery, particular care must be taken to avoid injury to the hypoglossal nerve (Fig. 31–14).

In the case of a high bifurcation or an extensive lesion, mobilizing the internal carotid artery for its maximum extracranial length may be necessary. Several maneuvers are available to gain additional length. The first and most important maneuver is to extend the skin incision all the way up to the mastoid process, with complete mobilization of the sternocleidomastoid muscle toward its tendinous insertion on the mastoid process. Care must be taken to avoid injury to the spinal accessory nerve (cranial nerve XI) which enters the substance of the sternocleidomastoid muscle at that level. The posterior belly of the digastric muscle comes into view. This muscle can be mobilized anteriorly or, if necessary, divided with impunity, giving additional exposure of the internal carotid artery. If further exposure is needed, the limiting structures are the styloid process and the ramus of the mandible. The styloid process, after suitable preparation, can be divided with bone rongeurs, and the mandible can be displaced anteriorly. Techniques have also been described for dividing the ramus of the mandible to gain additional exposure, but I have not found this maneuver necessary.

Figure 31–15. Techniques of measuring the internal carotid artery back-pressure. Note the needle placement and the needle angulation so as to maintain the tip of the needle in an axial plane with the common carotid artery. A disease-free portion of the common carotid artery is chosen for arterial puncture.

The arteriotomy can be closed primarily or with patch angioplasty. Evidence suggests that female patients, patients with small internal carotid arteries, and patients who continue to smoke are at increased risk of recurrent carotid stenosis.[122, 123] The use of patch angioplasty in these patients may reduce the risk of recurrent stenosis. Trial results indicate that routine use of a prosthetic patch results in the lowest rate of recurrent stenosis.[119–121] Patch angioplasty should be routinely used when the indication for operation is recurrent stenosis.

Flow is established first to the external and then to the internal carotid artery. I recommend the use of routine completion angiography. There is a 5% to 8% incidence of unsuspected technical error associated with carotid endarterectomy. This is best documented with completion angiography.[189, 190] Completion angiography is used, primarily, to identify technical error involving the internal carotid artery. Intimal flaps in the external carotid artery occur more commonly but are considered to be of no consequence. We reported three cases of postoperative stroke secondary to intimal flaps in the external carotid artery. Clot formed, propagated retrograde, and then embolized up the internal carotid artery.[191] For this reason, we advocate correction of intimal flaps of the external as well as the internal carotid artery.

An alternative method to completion angiography is the use of intraoperative duplex scanning. In a report, Lipski and colleagues[192] showed that the incidence of residual disease and perioperative neurologic complications was statistically significantly reduced in patients who had completion duplex scanning compared with a control group who did not undergo completion imaging. Furthermore, the use of completion duplex scanning identified technical problems and led to their prompt correction in 9 of 39 patients.

Internal Carotid Artery Dilatation

Indications

Internal carotid artery dilatation is uniquely applicable to fibromuscular dysplasia of the carotid artery. It is a major technical advance in simplifying the surgical correction of this lesion.

Technique

The carotid bifurcation is exposed in the usual manner. The internal carotid artery is exposed for maximal length so that dilatation can be carried out under visual and palpable control. Heparin is administered systemically, and the artery is clamped. A vertical arteriotomy, approximately 1 cm in length, is made in the carotid bulb, adjacent to the internal carotid artery. Coronary artery dilators are introduced and gently passed toward the base of the skull. I usually start with a 2-mm dilator and progress at 0.5-mm increments to a 4-mm dilator. The surgeon has a sensation of intraluminal septal "popping" as the dilator is passed to the base of the skull. Back-bleeding is allowed to occur after each passage (Fig. 31–16). On completion, the arteriotomy is closed, blood flow is restored, and a completion

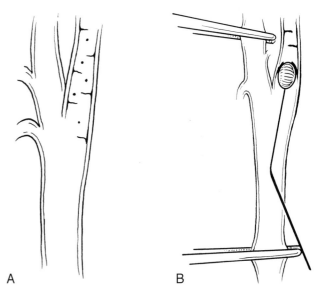

Figure 31–16. *A*, The septated lesion of fibromuscular dysplasia. This kind of irregularity leads to symptoms from platelet aggregation and embolization. *B*, A coronary dilator is introduced through a small arteriotomy and advanced up the internal carotid artery. The olive tip of the dilator disrupts the small septa of the fibromuscular dysplastic segment. With an open arteriotomy, opportunity for back-bleeding occurs, which flushes any residual intimal segments or platelet aggregates.

angiogram is obtained to ensure adequate dilatation. As an alternative, intraoperative balloon angioplasty of the affected segment of the internal carotid artery may be carried out. This technique is probably safer because traction injury to the intima is avoided. Assistance from a radiologist familiar with balloon angioplasty may be very helpful. The intraoperative use, through an open arteriotomy, avoids the possibility of forward embolization from the angioplasty site. After the balloon angioplasty is completed, vigorous back-bleeding of the vessel is allowed to retrieve any debris loosened by the dilatation. As with progressive dilatation of the vessel, completion angiography is highly recommended to ensure an adequate technical result. I do not favor percutaneous balloon dilatation of fibromuscular dysplastic segments of the extracranial vessels.

On occasion, the surgeon may not be sure that the dilator has been advanced fully to the base of the skull. Under these circumstances, obtaining a plain x-ray film with the dilator in place and comparing that film with the preoperative angiogram to ensure that the dilator has been passed sufficiently far distally is helpful.

Correction of Kinking of the Internal Carotid Artery

Indications

This procedure is indicated by (1) symptomatic kinking of the internal carotid artery and (2) excessive redundancy of the internal carotid artery after mobilization of that vessel for endarterectomy.

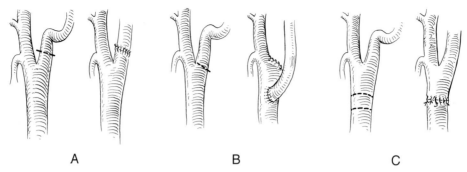

Figure 31–17. *A,* A kink of the internal carotid artery can be repaired by segmental resection of the redundant portion of the internal carotid artery and direct end-to-end anastomosis. *B,* The redundant internal carotid artery can be straightened by dividing it at its origin and moving it proximally to the common carotid artery for end-to-side anastomosis. *C,* The kinked internal carotid artery can be straightened by mobilization of the carotid bifurcation, resection of a segment of the common carotid artery, and direct end-to-end anastomosis, resulting in straightening of the kinked vessel.

Technique

Redundancy of the internal carotid artery can be corrected in a variety of ways, including (1) resection of the redundant internal carotid artery with end-to-end anastomosis, (2) division of the internal carotid artery with reimplantation onto the proximal common carotid artery, and (3) resection of a segment of the common carotid artery, thus permitting the redundant internal carotid artery to straighten when the carotid bifurcation is brought down for end-to-end anastomosis (Fig. 31–17).

In my experience, the easiest repair is resection of a segment of the common carotid artery, because the anastomosis is the easiest to perform. This requires mobilization of the external carotid artery to move the entire bifurcation proximally.

External Carotid Endarterectomy

Indications

External carotid endarterectomy is indicated (1) in the case of TIAs from embolization or flow reduction and (2) for correction of significant stenosis or ulceration before extracranial-to-intracranial bypass grafting.

Technique

The carotid bifurcation is dissected out in the usual manner. The internal carotid artery distal to the obstructed plaque is carefully examined because on occasion the vessel may still be patent, thus permitting a standard endarterectomy to be performed with restoration of blood flow to the internal carotid artery. If the internal carotid artery is confirmed to be occluded, it is divided flush with the carotid bifurcation. An arteriotomy is positioned on the posterior lateral aspect of the common carotid artery so that its distal extension passes through the divided orifice of the internal carotid artery and onto the external carotid artery, beyond the atherosclerotic plaque in that vessel. An endarterectomy is then performed. The arteriotomy may be closed primarily, leaving a smooth, tapered transition

from the common carotid to the external carotid artery (Fig. 31–18). If the external carotid artery is particularly small, use of a patch may be necessary and is probably preferable. The patch may be of prosthetic material, a vein, or a segment of the occluded internal carotid artery that has been resected and opened. This serves nicely as autogenous arterial patch.

Postoperative Care

The first 12 hours are the most critical in management of the patient after cerebrovascular reconstruction. In addition to the usual management of a patient recovering from a general anesthetic, the most important factors are observation of the patient's neurologic status, blood pressure control (either hypotension or hypertension must be appropriately treated), and close wound observation. An expanding hematoma should be identified early and the patient promptly returned to the operating room.

Although intensive care monitoring used to be routine, now only a small percentage of patients actually require an intensive care unit. The majority of patients can be sent to a regular room if they are neurologically intact and hemodynamically stable in the recovery room. Most patients can be safely discharged the next morning. This

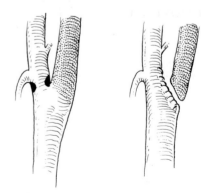

Figure 31–18. An external carotid endarterectomy can be performed by removing the occluded internal carotid artery and continuing the arteriotomy past the stenotic lesion. This permits end-arterectomy under direct vision and primary closure, leaving a smooth taper between the common and the external carotid artery.

method of case management has materially reduced hospital cost.[193–195]

Our practice is to resume antiplatelet drugs. One adult aspirin per day is recommended. If this is not tolerated, dipyridamole (Persantine) or clopidogrel (Plavix) can be used. The rationale for the continued use of antiplatelet drugs is to prevent platelet aggregation and embolization from the new intimectomy site, as well as to serve as prophylaxis in the case of residual, unoperated atherosclerotic plaques in other critical cerebral vessels.

COMPLICATIONS AFTER CAROTID ENDARTERECTOMY

Few vascular operations are as well tolerated as uncomplicated carotid endarterectomy. The operative trauma, blood loss, and recovery period are minimal after a successful reconstruction. On the other hand, the benefits of the procedure, especially in asymptomatic patients, can be negated by a high complication rate. The justification for surgical repair requires that the morbidity of the procedure be kept to a minimum. Possible intraoperative and postoperative complications, their prevention, and their management are discussed.

Intraoperative Complications

One of the most important steps in the prevention of intraoperative problems is adequate preoperative preparation of the patient. Hypertensive patients should have their blood pressure well controlled before the procedure. Patients must be well hydrated, especially if an angiographic procedure has been done within 24 to 48 hours or if they have been on chronic diuretic therapy. Their myocardial status must be ascertained by careful history, electrocardiography, and other studies as indicated. The use of nitrates during the procedure should be considered in patients with coronary artery disease.

Intraoperative monitoring includes electrocardiographic and frequent or continuous blood pressure readings. I routinely use an intraarterial line to obtain continuous readouts and promptly recognize fluctuations in the patient's blood pressure. The use of Swan-Ganz catheters should be considered in selected patients.

Hypertension and Hypotension

Hypertension and hypotension are frequent during and immediately after carotid endarterectomy. Bove and colleagues[196] found significant hypertension in 19% and hypotension in 28% of 100 consecutive carotid endarterectomies and reported a 9% incidence of neurologic deficits in this group, as opposed to no neurologic morbidity in normotensive patients. This fact, plus the deleterious effects on myocardial function, underscores the importance of early recognition and immediate treatment of extremes of blood pressure. Taking into account the minimal trauma and blood loss that occur during carotid endarterectomy, other

factors must play a role in the development of this fluctuation. Some investigators[197] have found a significant increase in the incidence of this problem in chronically hypertensive patients not well controlled preoperatively. The interference with the baroreceptor mechanisms at the carotid sinus may contribute to postoperative blood pressure fluctuations. The postendarterectomy bulb, which is now distensible, may also play a role.[198] Increased cerebral renin production during carotid cross-clamping has been implicated in the development of postendarterectomy hypertension.[199] In a retrospective study of 100 patients, we found a correlation between the use of halogenated fluorocarbon general anesthesia and the development of postendarterectomy hypertension.[200] In a subsequent study we demonstrated correlation between cranial norepinephrine levels in jugular venous blood, and not renin, in patients who developed postoperative hypertension.[201]

Bradycardia during carotid manipulation usually responds to the local injection of 0.5% lidocaine (Xylocaine) in the soft tissues around the nerve to the carotid sinus. Failure of this maneuver to restore normal heart rate and blood pressure should be followed by immediate investigation and correction of other possible causes. Ranson and colleagues[202] suggested that an uncorrected preoperative deficit in intravascular volume is a critical factor in the development of hypotension and bradycardia. Blocking the reflex arch by the administration of atropine sulfate while volume deficits are corrected frequently returns the blood pressure to within normal limits. If no response is seen after this, the use of vasoconstrictor agents should be considered, and they should be routinely available for immediate administration. Use of these drugs can be deleterious to myocardial function in the presence of hypovolemia.[146, 203] My preference has been the use of dopamine hydrochloride titrated by an infusion pump.

Hypertension during or after endarterectomy should also be promptly treated. My preference is the use of sodium nitroprusside by infusion pump. It is usually started in normotensive patients when the systolic blood pressure is above 160 mm Hg and in chronically hypertensive patients, above 180 mm Hg. It is titrated to keep the systolic levels between 140 and 160 mm Hg, respectively. In any case, diastolic pressure is kept below 100 mm Hg. The need for intravenous antihypertensive therapy usually lasts less than 24 hours. In patients with essential hypertension, oral medications are restarted within that period.

Technical Complications

Technical problems during the procedure can be avoided by careful dissection and adherence to a proven established routine. The occurrence of intimal flaps at the distal end point of the endarterectomized segment usually results from incomplete removal of the plaque or too deep a plane of dissection in the media. Several steps must be taken to ensure that no distal intimal flap develops. Careful angiographic assessment and gentle palpation of the internal carotid reveals the distal end of the plaque. The arteriotomy should be carried beyond this point. If a shunt is to be inserted, this becomes of critical importance.[204] Only in this manner can the lesion be completely removed under direct vision. As the endarterectomy is carried distally in the internal carotid artery, the most superficial plane in the media that allows complete removal of the plaque should be chosen. In this manner, a tapered end is almost always encountered, and tacking sutures are virtually never required. The use of intraoperative completion angiograms is encouraged so that distal end-point defects are recognized and corrected before completion of the procedure.

Emboli during or after carotid endarterectomy are probably the most frequent cause of a neurologic deficit seen after the procedure. Intraoperatively, these can occur during artery mobilization or shunt insertion or after arteriotomy closure. Care should be taken in the distal insertion of the shunt so that it is done beyond the end of the lesion, as previously mentioned. Failure to do this results in fragmentation of the plaque with embolization or elevation and wrinkling of the intima. Allowing the shunt to back-bleed freely ensures adequate position and removal of all air. I prefer proximal insertion with the shunt fully clamped so that slow, careful release allows immediate reclamping if any air or debris is seen flowing through the shunt.

After the endarterectomy is completed, the area should be free of any loose fragments. Careful irrigation with heparinized saline ensures this. Before completion of the arteriotomy closure, the internal, external, and common carotid arteries should be allowed to bleed freely. When completed, flow should be established to the external carotid artery first to ensure that any debris that may be present preferentially goes to this system.

Emboli in the immediate postoperative period in the absence of an intimal flap or other technical error are likely to be from fibrin and platelet aggregates formed in the endarterectomized segment. Antiplatelet agents such as aspirin or dextran 40 may prevent such occurrences.

Occasionally, when the procedure is completed, one finds that a kink is now present in the endarterectomized portion of the internal carotid artery. If the angle between the segments is less than 90 degrees, flow restriction may occur, and disturbances that promote recurrent stenosis are likely. Many times this can be anticipated when an elongated or coiled artery is present before the endarterectomy. I do not feel comfortable when this situation develops, and in severe cases, I prefer to correct the problem by some angioplastic procedure. My preference is resection of a segment of the common carotid with pull-down and primary anastomosis (see Fig. 31–17C). Ligation and division of the external carotid artery are rarely required, because dissection of the trunk and main branches allows sufficient mobility to correct the kink. Ligation and division of the nerve of Herring and surrounding bifurcation tissues are always necessary.

A carotid-cavernous sinus fistula is a feared complication of embolectomy with balloon catheters of the internal carotid artery. On the rare occasions when it is necessary, several maneuvers should be attempted before the use of balloon catheters. The clot should be carefully separated from the intima and gently pulled down. The internal carotid back-pressure is sometimes helpful in this process, and shunting the external circulation may make the difference necessary to extract the clot. If the use of balloon catheters becomes necessary, they should never be inserted beyond the proximal intracranial portion of the artery, and forcefulness is to be condemned. Although perforating the carotid artery intracranially with the balloon catheter is possible, the most common mechanism of injury that creates a carotid-cavernous sinus fistula is that of traction with the balloon catheter. This shearing force creates a transverse tear in that portion of the intracranial carotid that is intimately adherent to the cavernous sinus and fixed to the petrous portion of the skull. Therefore, traction on the inflated balloon catheter should be gentle. Fluoroscopic guidance may be helpful. Failure of these maneuvers makes abandonment of the procedure mandatory and requires consideration of an extracranial-to-intracranial bypass.

Cranial Nerve Injury

Peripheral cranial nerve injury is another source of morbidity after carotid endarterectomy. In a prospective analysis, Hertzer and colleagues[205] found a 16% incidence of cranial nerve dysfunction after this procedure. Only 60% of injuries were symptomatic. The rest would have gone unnoticed by the patient or physician had further detailed examination been omitted. A similar overall incidence was found by Evans and colleagues[206] on clinical grounds, but when speech pathologists were added as part of the evaluation team, the incidence increased to 39%, mostly related to superior laryngeal and recurrent laryngeal dysfunction. The great majority of these deficits were temporary, and when evaluation was repeated in 6 weeks, the incidence was between 1% and 4%. These injuries can be avoided with careful dissection, the principle being to stay in the plane of the artery and to be familiar with the anatomy of the area, including well-recognized anomalies (Fig. 31–19).

The *hypoglossal nerve* is almost always visualized during carotid endarterectomy. It can be seen descending along the course of the internal carotid, then crossing the external carotid in a more superficial plane. Mobilization of this nerve is necessary only when a high bifurcation is present or when the lesion extends high in the internal carotid. This is accomplished by careful division of small veins that tent the nerve downward. A branch of the external carotid to the sternocleidomastoid muscle is frequently present and requires division. The ansa hypoglossi can frequently be retracted medially, but on occasion it requires division as it comes off the hypoglossal nerve. Traction or retractor injury to the hypoglossal nerve should be avoided. Clinically, the deficit is manifested by deviation of the tongue to the ipsilateral side. Speech, deglutition, and mastication problems have been reported.[205]

The *spinal accessory nerve* is rarely seen during this dissection but on high dissections is seen entering the sternocleidomastoid muscle superiorly. It can be left attached and retracted with the muscle, but care should be taken not to compress it with the retractor.

The *vagus nerve* is always seen, usually posterolateral to the carotid artery, between the latter and the jugular vein. On occasion, it lies anteromedial to the artery. Keeping the dissection close to the artery prevents injury to this nerve. The recurrent laryngeal nerve usually lies within the trunk of the vagus at this level, but a nonrecurrent laryngeal

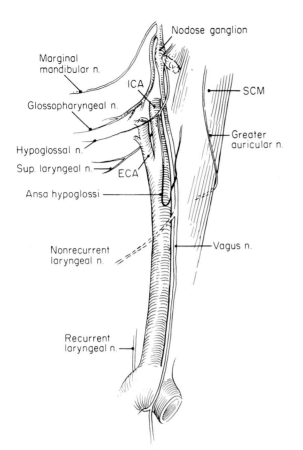

Figure 31–19. The surgical anatomy and relationship of structures encountered during exposure of the carotid bifurcation. ECA, external carotid artery; ICA, internal carotid artery; SCM, sternocleidomastoid muscle.

nerve on occasion traverses posterior to the common carotid artery. Injury to these structures can be asymptomatic or manifested by hoarseness. The asymptomatic injury gains significance when bilateral staged reconstructions are planned. On the other hand, hoarseness in the postoperative period is due to vocal cord paresis in about half of the patients.[205] This underscores the importance of laryngoscopic examination in reaching a specific diagnosis. When staged bilateral carotid endarterectomy is planned, routine laryngoscopic visualization of the vocal cords is highly recommended. Detection of a paralyzed vocal cord mandates delaying the procedure until recovery is complete. If vocal cord paralysis is permanent, appropriate precautions should be taken to avoid bilateral injury, and perioperative airway management should be given special consideration.

The *superior laryngeal nerve* leaves the inferior ganglion of the vagus (nodose ganglion) and courses behind the internal carotid artery, bifurcating into an internal and an external branch. The internal branch is sensitive to the larynx, and the external innervates the inferior constrictor and cricothyroid muscles. The latter is responsible for the quality of voice, specifically the higher pitches. Injury to the external laryngeal nerve can be avoided by again keeping the dissection close to the arterial wall, specifically when controlling the superior thyroid artery.

The *glossopharyngeal nerve* is usually not seen in the dissection but can be injured when dissections are carried

high, especially those requiring division of the digastric muscles.[207, 208] This nerve courses posterior to the high portion of the internal carotid artery and can be injured with the application of a vascular clamp that includes other tissues than the artery itself. Again, dissection close to the arterial wall is the key in prevention. Clinically, the dysfunction is evident when tasks requiring oral pharyngeal muscle activity, mostly deglutition, are examined. Horner's syndrome may be produced by injury to the ascending sympathetic fibers in the area of the glossopharyngeal nerve.

The *cervical branch of the facial nerve* lies beneath the platysma, inferior to the angle of the jaw. In some patients, this nerve sends branches to the mandibular branch, and its injury produces sagging of the ipsilateral corner of the lower lip. The marginal mandibular branch can itself be injured when the incision is carried too close to the jaw. Both of these injuries can be prevented by curving the upper portion of the incision toward the mastoid process.[204] Self-retaining retractors should be carefully placed in this area.

The greater auricular nerve courses deep to the platysma over the sternocleidomastoid muscle at an angle toward the ear in the upper portion of the dissection. Its division should be avoided but is frequently necessary in high dissections. Numbness of the ear lobe is the usual consequence, although, surprisingly, some patients have no complaints after its deliberate division.

The *parotid gland* lies in the superior portion of the incision anterior to the sternocleidomastoid muscle. Again, curving the incision toward the mastoid process prevents injury in high dissections. Troublesome bleeding and the risk of a parotid fistula can be prevented by this maneuver.

Postoperative Complications

On completion of the operation, if done under general anesthesia, the patient is awakened in the operating room. A gross neurologic examination is performed. If no deficit is found, the patient is transferred to the recovery room, where a more detailed examination is performed.

Stroke is the most feared complication of carotid endarterectomy. In experienced hands, this occurs in between 1% and 3% of patients, depending on the indication for the procedure.[209] Most of the low rates of stroke have been reported from specialized centers. Unfortunately, pooled data from community surveys have shown rates of combined stroke morbidity and mortality ranging from 6.5% to 21%.[210–212] Because carotid endarterectomy is a prophylactic operation employed to prevent stroke, these higher complication rates erase most benefits and are clearly unacceptable. A committee of the Stroke Council of the American Heart Association reviewed this problem and set standards for upper acceptable limits of stroke and death as a function of indication for operation. Thus, for patients undergoing carotid endarterectomy for asymptomatic carotid stenosis, the combined operative stroke morbidity and mortality should not exceed 3%; for TIA as an indication, 5%; for prior stroke as an indication, 7%; and for recurrent carotid stenosis, 10%.[213] A mechanism for individual surgeon audit was described and recommended.

TIAs in the first postoperative week have been reported with a frequency as high as 8%. When a neurologic deficit is found on awakening the patient, the main question to be resolved regards patency of the internal carotid artery. If a completion angiogram is obtained and no abnormalities are seen, the event is likely to be embolic, and immediate reoperation would be of no benefit. If no angiographic data are available, patency of the vessel should be assessed by noninvasive means.[214] If occlusion is suggested, immediate reoperation may reverse the deficit.[215] If the vessel appears patent by noninvasive tests, the surgeon needs to determine whether the emboli occurred during the operation or whether a source is now present in the operated segment. This is also the case in a patient who is neurologically intact and who develops an event in the ipsilateral hemisphere hours or days after surgery. Once patency is evidenced by noninvasive means, immediate angiography is indicated. Reoperation is necessary if a significant defect or any clot is present. Otherwise, conservative therapy with anticoagulation or antiplatelet agents or both is warranted. This excludes a patient experiencing repeated or progressive neurologic events, in whom immediate reoperation should be considered. Other factors inevitably influence the decision to reoperate or observe the patient. The difficulty of the initial reconstruction, the patient's general status, and the availability and reliability of ancillary facilities affect this difficult decision (see algorithm in Fig. 31–20).

Mortality after carotid endarterectomy has declined significantly as the incidence of postoperative stroke has diminished. Pulmonary problems, renal insufficiency, and sepsis are extremely unusual complications owing to the nature of this procedure. Myocardial infarction remains the most frequent cause of death in the early postoperative period, more so in patients with suspected coronary artery disease.[216] Because of this, preoperative assessment is of paramount importance. Postoperatively, electrocardiographic monitoring for the first 24 hours and a 12-lead electrocardiographic tracing should be obtained. Any suspicion of a myocardial event should be investigated and treated aggressively.

Wound infections after carotid endarterectomy are extremely rare. Routine use of prophylactic antibiotics for 24 hours during the perioperative interval is recommended.

Taking into account that the procedure is done under full heparinization and that many patients have received platelet antiaggregates preoperatively, the incidence of wound bleeding is low. In Thompson's personal series,[209] reoperation for this problem was required in 0.7% of 1022 patients.

Large cervical hematomas may form, and reoperation and drainage should be strongly considered in the otherwise stable patient. The routine use of a Silastic drain may reduce the incidence of this complication. Rarely does bleeding occur from the suture line. More often, a diffuse ooze is present requiring reversal of anticoagulation. In any case, drainage of the hematoma and correction of its cause prevents chronic draining wounds, infection, and the rare occurrence of pseudoaneurysm formation. The latter is more frequent when closure is performed with a patch.[209]

Headache after carotid endarterectomy is not unusual. It may be associated with a neurologic deficit, in which case a CT scan should be performed. In the majority of cases, however, it runs a self-limited course and is probably related to altered autoregulatory dysfunction of the cerebral circulation. The use of propranolol (Inderal) has been effective in treating troublesome headache.

Complications after carotid endarterectomy may be prevented by careful patient preparation, meticulous technique, and adherence to a rational, well-established routine. An uneventful operation is the best way to effectively change the natural history of extracranial arterial occlusive disease.

RESULTS OF SURGICAL TREATMENT FOR EXTRACRANIAL ARTERIAL OCCLUSIVE DISEASE

The most frequently performed operation for extracranial arterial occlusive disease is endarterectomy of the carotid

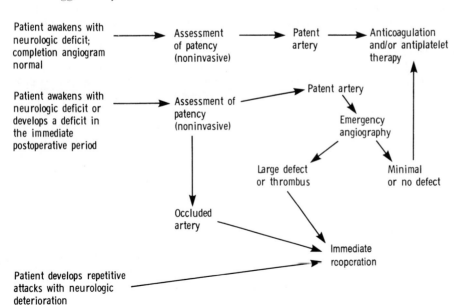

Figure 31–20. Algorithm that can be applied to the management of the patient who awakens with postoperative neurologic deficit after carotid endarterectomy.

bifurcation. As experience is gained with this procedure, results have improved, and in experienced hands it can be done with morbidity and mortality rates well below the Stroke Council guidelines. In recommending this procedure, the results of the particular surgeon or institution are to be considered, because a higher morbidity and mortality may negate any beneficial effects of surgery.

The first multi-institutional study that compared surgical and medical treatment in a prospectively randomized fashion came from the joint study on extracranial arterial occlusion,[217] in which 1225 symptomatic patients with extracranial arterial occlusive disease were randomly allocated to receive either medical or surgical therapy. Long-term survival of as long as 42 months was better in the surgically treated group with unilateral carotid stenosis who were experiencing TIAs or cerebral infarction with minimal residual deficit. The neurologic morbidity in 316 patients who were identified as having hemispheric TIAs as an indication for inclusion in the study was evaluated. The incidence of cerebral infarction at 42 months was reduced in the surgical group. Recurrent TIAs or cerebral infarction usually affected the side not operated on in the surgical patients, in contrast to the medically treated group, in whom neurologic events chiefly occurred in the distribution of the symptomatic artery at the time of randomization. The differences were statistically significant. The combined postoperative morbidity and mortality in the surgically treated group was around 8%, which is considered high by today's standards. This may have affected the results of this study in favor of medical therapy.

The preoperative neurologic status of the patient does affect the immediate postoperative results. Asymptomatic patients fare better than patients with TIAs, and the latter, in turn, have lower morbidity than patients with a completed stroke. Rothwell and colleagues[218] reviewed 25 studies and performed a meta-analysis. The combined perioperative risk of death and stroke was 3.0% to 3.5% compared with 5.18% for symptomatic patients. These differences were consistent across all studies and indicate that operation on asymptomatic patients is safest. In fact, late results may be similarly affected. Bernstein and colleagues[219] reported a series of 456 carotid endarterectomies monitored for between 1 and 11 years, with an average follow-up of 45.3 months. Asymptomatic patients that were operated on had a 1.6% incidence of TIAs and 3.2% incidence of stroke on late follow-up. Those operated on because of TIAs had a 19.5% and 5.2% incidence of recurrent TIAs or stroke, respectively. Patients with a permanent neurologic deficit preoperatively had an incidence of TIAs of 7.9%, and 11.0% developed a stroke on late follow-up.

Similar results were reported by Hertzer and Arison[220] in 329 patients monitored for a minimum of 10 years after carotid endarterectomy. The cumulative incidence of stroke by the life-table method was 24% at 10 years after operation. Only 10% of patients sustained strokes that clearly involved the ipsilateral cerebral hemisphere. Hypertension, preoperative stroke as an indication, and patients with recognized contralateral carotid stenosis had a much higher incidence of stroke on long-term follow-up. Contralateral hemispheric strokes occurred in 36% of patients with uncorrected contralateral lesions, compared with 8% of those who had elective bilateral reconstruction. This difference

was statistically significant. Patients undergoing elective myocardial revascularization had a significant increase in long-term survival when compared to patients with uncorrected coronary artery disease. These results suggest that the annual incidence of late stroke, specifically involving the cerebral hemisphere ipsilateral to previous carotid repair, is 1.1%, a figure within the expected range for the normal population. Stroke in the subset of patients with bilateral carotid arterial disease was five times more common in the contralateral than in the ipsilateral cerebral hemisphere. Therefore, staged contralateral endarterectomy should be seriously considered in patients with documented but otherwise asymptomatic advanced contralateral carotid stenosis.[220]

Analysis of the available surgical series with long-term follow-up reveals that a successfully performed carotid endarterectomy places the patient at a significantly lower risk of stroke. The results of the various available surgical series are summarized in Table 31–1 according to the indications for operation.[221-230] Asymptomatic patients have a 1.2% per year stroke risk, including perioperative morbidity and mortality. Patients whose indication for endarterectomy is TIAs have an initial perioperative morbidity and mortality of about 3%, with a long-term risk of stroke of 2% per year. Patients whose indication for operation is cerebral infarction have a higher perioperative morbidity, averaging about 5%. Long-term results suggest that these patients have an annual stroke rate of approximately 4% per year. The average recurrence of TIAs is on the order of 8% to 10% at 5 years for all indications. These results represent a clear improvement over the natural history of the disease, including the use of antiplatelet drugs; however, they do underscore the importance of maintaining the operative stroke rate at acceptable levels for the various indications. A higher figure negates the early and late beneficial results of surgical therapy.

The results of carotid endarterectomy for nonhemispheric symptoms are less predictable. In a series of 107 patients subjected to carotid endarterectomy, the initial perioperative morbidity and mortality were similar to those in patients with specific indications for operation. Carotid endarterectomy was successful in ameliorating symptoms in patients with nonhemispheric symptoms who had greater than 60% diameter reduction of the carotid artery and classic symptoms of vertebrobasilar insufficiency.[231] The same series of 61 patients was updated by Ricotta and colleagues.[232] They compared the results of their cohort of patients with nonhemispheric symptoms to the remainder of their series. Follow-up lasted a mean of 42.3 months. The perioperative stroke rate was 4.9%. Survival was 85.3% at 3 years and 64.9% at 5 years. Stroke-free survival was 77.1% at 3 years and 63.4% at 5 years. During follow-up, 11 patients (18%) developed recurrent nonhemispheric symptoms. These results were not different from the cohort of 553 patients. The authors concluded that carotid endarterectomy provided long-term benefit in this group of patients.[232]

The use of complete cerebral angiography can also be very helpful in selecting patients. The presence of a posterior communicating artery suggests that the anterior circulation may be a major contributor to the vertebrobasilar system. Its presence suggests that removal of a hemody-

TABLE 31-1

Results of Carotid Endarterectomy According to the Indication for Operation

INDICATION	AUTHORS	NO. OF PATIENTS	FOLLOW-UP	OPERATIVE Morbidity (%)	OPERATIVE Mortality (%)	RECURRENT TIAs IPSILATERAL (%)	STROKE Ipsilateral (%)	STROKE Contralateral (%)
Asymptomatic	Thompson et al.[178]	132	55.1 mo	1.2	0	0.75	4.7°	NS
	Sergeant et al.[221]	43	6.48 mo	2.3	2.3	0	0	0
	Moore et al.[222]	72	6–180 mo	0	0	2.7	5.6†	2.7
	Bernstein et al.[223]	87‡	43 mo	NS§	0	NS	6.3‖	NS
	Hertzer & Arison[220]	126	10–14 yr	NS	NS	NS	9§§	7§§
	Lord[224]	226	30–144 mo	2.6	1.1	NS	0.4	1.1
TIA	Bernstein et al.[223]	370°°	12–132 mo	NS	0	19.5††	5.2	NS
	DeWeese et al.[225]	103	60-mo minimum	6.0	0.97	18.4¶	7.7#	10.6
	Thompson et al.[226]	293	To 156 mo	2.7	1.4	16.3	4.7	0.6
	Takolander et al.[227]	142	5-yr actuarial	4.9	1.8	14.7	6.5	4.0
	Hertzer & Arison[220]	123	10–14 yr	NS	NS	NS	6§§	9§§
Stroke	Thompson et al.[226]	217	Up to 156 mo	5.0	7.4		8.2	NS
	Eriksson et al.[228]	55	21-mo avg	3.7	3.7		3.8	NS
	Bardin et al.[229]	127	56-mo avg	3.9	3.1		20	NS
	Takolander et al.[227]	60	5-yr actuarial	4.9	5.9	11.6‖	10	NS
	McCullough et al.[230]	50	41-mo avg	3.4	1.7		3.3	NS
	Hertzer & Arison[220]	80	10–14 yr	NS	NS	NS	6§§	13

°Side of stroke not specified; three strokes were fatal.
†Two patients suffered transient postoperative deficits with complete recovery.
‡Number of procedures; exact number of patients not specified.
§Perioperative stroke rate of 3% in the entire series of 370 patients.
‖Side of neurologic event not specified; risk of stroke at 5 years by life-table analysis.
¶Includes patients with nonterritorial symptoms.
#Includes operative morbidity.
°°Total number of patients in series, including TIA patients.
††Territory affected not specified.
§§Does not include perioperative strokes.
TIAs, transient ischemic attacks; NS, not specified; avg, average.

namically significant lesion in the carotid territory would be beneficial in alleviating posterior circulation systems.

In the absence of significant extracranial carotid artery disease, direct vertebral artery reconstruction is the procedure of choice for patients with vertebrobasilar systems secondary to extracranial occlusive disease. The results with direct vertebral artery reconstruction have been good, although the experience is not as extensive as that with carotid artery surgery. In a series of 109 vertebral artery operations, Imparato[233] reported an operative mortality of 3%. Other complications included temporary hemidiaphragm paralysis and Horner's syndrome. Two thromboses of the reconstruction occurred. No perioperative strokes occurred. Long-term follow-up revealed a stroke incidence of 1.5% per year of follow-up. No controlled series on the natural history of these patients is available for comparison.[233]

The experience with external carotid revascularization has been limited, and, therefore, long-term results are not available. In a series of 42 external carotid artery reconstructions, O'Hara and colleagues[234] reported no early morbidity or mortality when the operation was limited to external carotid artery endarterectomy and patch angioplasty. When the procedure was combined with bypass to the external carotid artery or with an extracranial-to-intracranial bypass, however, a 33% incidence of stroke was observed. No neurologic symptoms have occurred in 25 (60%) of the entire series on follow-up ranging from 1 to 72 months (mean, 27 months). These authors concluded

that external carotid artery endarterectomy can be performed with acceptable risks and long-term effectiveness. When the reconstruction involves bypass to the external carotid artery or extracranial-to-intracranial bypass, a higher operative risk can be expected.[234] A similar note of caution was expressed by Halstuk and colleagues,[235] describing 49 external carotid revascularization procedures performed in 36 patients. Indications included ipsilateral TIAs, amaurosis fugax, and a preparatory procedure in anticipation of extracranial-to-intracranial bypass. Twenty patients had preoperative strokes. Twenty-nine patients underwent unilateral external carotid endarterectomy, with the remaining patients undergoing other procedures in addition to the external revascularization. The incidence of postoperative strokes within 8 days of external carotid revascularization was 13.8%. One operative death occurred, for a mortality rate of 2.7%. Long-term follow-up ranging from 1 to 75 months (mean, 29 months) revealed a 14.2% incidence of late neurologic ischemic events. Three of these were TIAs, one was a reversible ischemic neurologic deficit, and one patient had a stroke 50 months after his initial operation. These results suggest caution in recommending external carotid artery surgery, especially when the revascularization is to involve more than just endarterectomy with patch closure.[235]

The perioperative use of aspirin in patients undergoing carotid endarterectomy reduces the risk of stroke and death up to 6 months. Lindblad and associates[236] carried out a prospective randomized trial comparing carotid endarterec-

TABLE 31-2

The Effect of Perioperative Use of Aspirin

TIME AFTER OPERATION	COMPLICATION	CEA PLUS ASA, PATIENTS (n [%])	CEA WITHOUT ASA, PATIENTS (n [%])
1 wk	Stroke	0	7 (6)
30 days	Stroke	2 (1.7)	11 (9.6)
6 mo	Stroke	2 (1.7)	11 (9.6)
30 days	Mortality	0.8	4.3
6 mo	Mortality	3–4	6

ASA, acetylsalicylic acid; CEA, carotid endarterectomy.

tomy in patients with and without aspirin. Their results are summarized in Table 31–2.

CURRENT STATUS OF THE PROSPECTIVE RANDOMIZED TRIALS

In spite of the fact that retrospective data analysis clearly demonstrates the superiority of carotid endarterectomy over medical management with respect to stroke prevention, a number of well-meaning critics point out that retrospective data analysis can be misleading. Retrospective studies compare surgical results with available natural history data. The natural history of a particular disease process can change, often for the better, leaving the basis of comparison invalid. Likewise, retrospective reviews are often performed in centers of excellence, where surgical complication rates may be lower than the actual risk of operation as judged by analyzing community results. For this reason, several prospective randomized trials were initiated in North America and Europe. The objective of the trials was to scientifically evaluate the efficacy (or lack thereof) of carotid endarterectomy in preventing stroke for a variety of indications when compared with a true control group. The trials can be generally categorized into two major classifications: asymptomatic and symptomatic carotid artery disease.

Three asymptomatic trials have completed their data acquisition and reported results. These are as follows: (1) the Veterans Administration Asymptomatic Carotid Stenosis Study; (2) the Carotid Surgery Versus Medical Therapy in Asymptomatic Carotid Stenosis Study (CASANOVA); and (3) ACAS. The European Asymptomatic Carotid Surgery Trial (ACST) represents a fourth study that is still in progress. Three symptomatic trials have been completed. These are as follows: (1) the NASCET; (2) the Medical Research Council (MRC) European Carotid Surgery Trial (ECST); and (3) the Veterans Administration Symptomatic Trial.

Asymptomatic Trials

Veterans Administration Asymptomatic Carotid Stenosis Study

Ten Veterans Administration (VA) medical centers entered into a prospective randomized trial designed to test the hypothesis that carotid endarterectomy plus best medical management (aspirin and risk factor control) would result in fewer TIAs than treatment with best medical management alone. The design of the study was published in 1986.[237] Angiography was performed in 713 patients, of whom three (0.4%) sustained a neurologic deficit.[238]

Four hundred forty-four patients were randomized over a 54-month interval. Two hundred eleven carotid endarterectomies were performed in the surgical group, who received aspirin therapy. Two hundred thirty-three patients were treated with aspirin alone. The study spanned a total of 8 years. The 30-day mortality rate was 1.9%, and the incidence of stroke was 2.4%. The combined stroke and mortality rate was 4.3%.[239]

The results were positive for the surgery group in the hypothesis being tested. The data analysis demonstrated that all neurologic events in any distribution including the study artery combined with deaths showed a total event number of 30 in the carotid endarterectomy group, which represented 14.2% of the population. This included all deaths, strokes, TIAs, and amaurosis. For the patients treated medically, a total of 55 events occurred, for an event rate of 23.6%. This difference is statistically significant ($P < .006$). When the data were analyzed for deaths plus ipsilateral events only, a total of 21 events occurred, for an incidence of 10% in the carotid endarterectomy group, in contrast to 46 events for an incidence of 19.7% in the medically treated group. Once again, this difference was statistically significant ($P < .002$). Although the study was not designed to look at stroke alone with respect to a difference in event rate, this was done retrospectively. A total of 10 strokes occurred in the carotid endarterectomy group ipsilateral to the study artery, for an incidence of 4.7%. A total of 20 strokes occurred in the study artery distribution in the medically treated group, for an incidence of 8.6%. This difference fell just short of statistical significance ($P = .056$), probably due to small sample size. No difference occurred in survival rate between the surgically treated and medically treated groups. This is not surprising, because the major cause of death in this patient group is myocardial infarction, and prevention of stroke is unlikely to have a beneficial effect on reducing fatal myocardial infarction. The absence of difference of survival between the surgically treated and medically treated groups should not be considered a negative factor when interpreting data results inasmuch as the objective of operation is to maintain the patient stroke-free during the patient's remaining lifetime.[240]

The Carotid Surgery Versus Medical Therapy in Asymptomatic Carotid Stenosis Study

CASANOVA was a multi-institutional European study designed to test the hypothesis that asymptomatic patients with stenosis greater than 50% but less than 90% would have fewer strokes and deaths when treated with surgery plus aspirin and dipyridamole than a comparable group of patients treated with aspirin and dipyridamole alone. The end points were stroke and death. TIA was not considered an end point. Four hundred ten patients were randomly allocated to two groups. Group A, 206 patients, was the surgical group. Group B, 204 patients, was the control group. Patients with high-grade stenosis, 90% or greater, were excluded from the study and presumably operated on preferentially. The surgery group underwent unilateral operation if a unilateral lesion was present or bilateral operations if bilateral lesions were present. Unfortunately, the medical group also had significant indication for operation as well. If a patient randomized to medical management was found to have bilateral stenoses, surgery was done on the more affected side. If during the course of follow-up a progression of the medically randomized lesion to 90% or greater occurred, surgery was performed. In the medically managed group, if the patient developed bilateral stenoses that exceeded 50%, one artery was operated on. Finally, if patients in the medically managed group developed the onset of TIAs, the patient was allowed to cross over and receive operation.

Unfortunately, from the standpoint of data analysis, none of these events were considered end points. Furthermore, the design of the study was "intent to treat." That means that even though the patients were allowed to cross over to operation, the patients were still analyzed as if they were being treated medically alone. As a result, 216 carotid endarterectomies were performed on 204 patients in the surgical group and 118 operations were performed on 206 patients in the so-called medical group. Not surprisingly, when the study was completed, no difference was apparent between group A and group B. Group A experienced 22 end points, for an incidence of 10.7%, and group B experienced 23, for an incidence of 11.3%. The authors concluded that surgery is not recommended for patients with asymptomatic carotid stenosis of less than 90%. Unfortunately, this conclusion is unjustified because of serious flaws in study design and data analysis.

First of all, high-risk patients (those with 90% stenosis or greater) were excluded from the randomization process. Second, patients with bilateral stenosis in the medical group received operation on the tighter (presumably higher-risk) lesion but were still considered medically managed for purposes of analysis. Patients in the medical group were allowed to cross over to surgery if they developed a 90% stenosis of the study artery, bilateral stenoses 50% or greater, or the onset of TIAs. When they crossed over to surgery, they were not considered end points or treatment failures but continued to be analyzed as if they were managed medically. The net result was that 118 high-risk lesions were removed from the medical group and treated surgically but continued to be analyzed as if they were treated medically. This study was invalidated by a flawed design and method of statistical analysis. If any information is to be gained from this study, it might be that patients selectively treated with carotid endarterectomy did as well as those routinely treated with carotid endarterectomy. That is, patients with 90% carotid stenosis, bilateral carotid stenoses, disease progression, or onset of TIAs were selected for operation in contrast to applying routine operation to all patients with carotid artery stenosis. Unfortunately, when this interpretation is applied, we are missing the important control group, which would be those patients who received no operation at all, to determine whether selective or routine carotid endarterectomy is any better than no operation.[241]

The Asymptomatic Carotid Atherosclerosis Study

The ACAS is the largest of the trials of asymptomatic carotid stenosis. This is a prospective randomized trial consisting of 34 centers in North America and sponsored by the National Institutes of Health (NIH). The hypothesis that was tested was that carotid endarterectomy plus aspirin and risk factor control results in fewer TIAs, strokes, and deaths than aspirin and risk factor control alone.

The design of the study was published in 1989.[242] It was a prospective randomized trial. Initially, 1500 patients were to be randomized when TIA was indicated as an end point. After criticism of the VA study, the protocol was amended to have stroke and death as the end points. The Data Safety and Monitoring Committee (DSMB) of the NIH gave permission to increase the sample size from 1500 to 1800 patients.

In December 1994, the DSMB called a halt to the study and informed the investigators, and subsequently the public, that an end point had been reached in favor of carotid endarterectomy.[243] The full report was published in the *Journal of the American Medical Association*.[158] One thousand, six hundred sixty-two patients with diameter-reducing lesions of 60% or greater (as measured by angiography using the North American method) were randomly allocated to receive carotid endarterectomy plus best medical management, including aspirin; the control group received best medical management alone. After a mean follow-up of 2.7 years (4657 patient-years of observation), the aggregate risk over 5 years for ipsilateral stroke, any perioperative stroke, and death was 5.1% for surgical patients and 11% for patients treated medically. The results of surgery, including perioperative morbidity and mortality, reduced the risk of death and stroke by 5.9% absolutely and yielded a 53% risk reduction. This difference was highly significant.

The beneficial effect of surgery in the asymptomatic patient was due in large part to the low 30-day perioperative stroke morbidity and mortality. Before the study began, the surgical management committee for ACAS established criteria to audit prospective surgeons who wished to participate in the study.[244] Validation of the audit method was possible on conclusion of the study. Eight hundred twenty-five patients were randomized to surgery. The stroke morbidity and mortality within 30 days of randomization was 2.3%. However, this included a stroke morbidity and mortality of 1.2% for preoperative angiography. Because of the intent-to-treat design, the angiographic complications were credited to surgery. Of the 724 patients who actually had carotid endarterectomy, mortality was 0.14%, and stroke rate was 1.38%. Thus, the true 30-day stroke morbidity and mortality was 1.52%.[159]

The Asymptomatic Carotid Surgery Trial

A group of European investigators, headed by a team from the United Kingdom, have embarked on yet another trial. However, included in their trial are methods designed to try to identify a higher-risk group of patients. At this time, patient entry is still in progress, and no results are available.[245]

Symptomatic Trials

The North American Symptomatic Carotid Endarterectomy Trial

The NASCET study is a large prospective trial carried out in North America and designed to test the hypothesis that symptomatic patients (TIA or prior mild stroke) with ipsilateral carotid stenosis (30% to 99%) have fewer fatal and nonfatal strokes after carotid endarterectomy than patients treated with medical management alone, including aspirin. Investigators anticipated that approximately 3000 patients would be randomly allocated to receive either medical or surgical management and monitored for a minimum of 5 years. The NASCET study also was stratified to study two subsets of patients as a function of their degree of carotid occlusive disease. The first patient subset included those with 70% to 99% stenosis, and the second subset included patients with more moderate lesions ranging from 30% to 69%.[246] Included in the design of the trial and required by the granting institution (NIH) is the establishment of an oversight committee. The responsibility of the oversight committee is to review the results of the data from time to time and to call a halt to the study if during the course of the study a clear difference should appear between the two groups.

On February 25, 1991, a clinical alert was issued by the oversight committee, who reported that a clear difference had developed between the two groups, which indicated that carotid endarterectomy was superior to medical management in the high-grade stenosis category (70% to 99%). No clear difference had yet occurred in the moderate stenosis group (30% to 69%), and the latter continues to enter patients for randomization.

In the high-grade stenosis category, 295 patients received medical management and 300 patients received surgical management. Sixteen of the medically treated patients (5.4%) actually crossed over to surgery. Once again, because of the "intent-to-treat" analysis design, these patients continue to be analyzed as if they were managed medically in spite of the fact that they had operation. Crossovers become important if the group that they are leaving is in fact a disadvantaged group, as is the case in this study.

The 30-day operative morbidity and stroke mortality for patients managed surgically was 5.0%. The analysis at the end of 18 months of follow-up, which was the basis of the oversight committee's calling a halt to this arm of the study, is as follows. In the surgical group including the perioperative morbidity and mortality at the end of 18 months, a 7.0% incidence of fatal and nonfatal strokes occurred. In the medical group, a 24% incidence of fatal and nonfatal strokes occurred. The difference was highly statistically significant ($P < .001$). This represents an absolute reduction in risk of 17% in favor of surgical management and a relative risk reduction of 71% comparing surgical management with medical management by the end of 18 months.

A surprising finding occurred when the mortality rates were analyzed. To date, no study has shown that carotid endarterectomy patients enjoy greater longevity than those treated medically. However, at the end of 18 months, the mortality rate among the medically treated group was 12%

in contrast to the 5% rate for the surgically treated group. Once again these differences were statistically significant ($P < .01$). This indicates a relative mortality risk reduction of 58% in favor of carotid endarterectomy. Further analysis demonstrated that for every 10% increase in percentage stenosis between 70% and 99%, a progressive increase occurred in morbidity and mortality in the control group.[231, 247] The NASCET investigators reported their results in the moderate stenosis group (30% to 69%) in 1998.[248] They demonstrated a beneficial effect of surgery in the 50% to 69% group but not in those patients with less than 50% stenosis. The 30-day mortality and disabling stroke rate was 2.7% and the nondisabling stroke rate was 4.0% for a total of 6.7%. The 5-year rate for ipsilateral stroke in the surgical group was 15.7% compared to 22% for patients treated medically. Thus 15 patients would need to undergo carotid endarterectomy to prevent one stroke over a 5-year interval.[248]

Medical Research Council European Carotid Surgery Trial

The ECST is a large, multicenter European trial of symptomatic patients with carotid artery disease that was carried out over a 10-year interval and reported at approximately the same time as the NASCET study. It confirmed the results reported to date of the NASCET study: 2518 patients were randomized over a 10-year interval, providing a mean follow-up of 3 years. This trial stratified their data into three groups, including mild stenosis (10% to 29%), moderate stenosis (30% to 69%), and severe stenosis (70% to 99%). In the mild stenosis category, no apparent benefit was evident for carotid endarterectomy compared with the risk of operation. However, in the severe stenosis category, a highly significant benefit in favor of operation was evident. Carotid endarterectomy, in spite of an upfront 7.5% risk of death and stroke in the perioperative interval, resulted in a sixfold reduction in subsequent strokes in a 3-year interval. This difference was highly statistically significant ($P < .0001$).[249]

One interesting and important difference has come to light between NASCET and ECST; they have different methods of measuring carotid stenosis. The European method is

$$\% \text{ stenosis} = \frac{1 - R}{B} \times 100$$

where R is minimal residual lumen diameter through the stenosis, and B is the projected diameter of the carotid bulb; this cannot actually be visualized because it is occupied by plaque. Therefore, an imaginary line is drawn to outline what is believed to be the bulb. NASCET uses a method common in North America and first described in the VA asymptomatic trial:

$$\% \text{ stenosis} = \frac{1 - R}{D}$$

where D is the diameter of the normal internal carotid artery where the walls become parallel. The result of this

Comparison of Carotid Stenosis by European and North American Methods

PERCENT STENOSIS, EUROPEAN	PERCENT STENOSIS, NORTH AMERICAN
60%	18%
70%	40%
80%	61%
90%	80%

Data from Eliasziw M, Smith RF, Singh N, et al: Further comments on the measurements of carotid stenosis from angiograms. Stroke 25:2445–2449, 1994.

difference is most apparent at the moderate stenosis, where the European method would appear to greatly overestimate the percent stenosis. Eliasziw and colleagues[250] compared the same angiograms using the European and North American methods. Their findings are partly summarized in Table 31–3.

The differences are somewhat startling. Because the ECST trial found significant benefit of carotid endarterectomy in patients with stenosis of 60% to 90%, as such, they have corroborated the results in the NASCET moderate stenosis group. The ECST study reported no benefit of surgery in the 30% to 69% group as measured by the European method. This is not surprising, because a 69% ECST stenosis is only a 40% stenosis as measured by the North American method.[251]

Veterans Administration Symptomatic Trial

The VA symptomatic trial is a prospective randomized trial designed to test the hypothesis that patients with greater than 50% ipsilateral internal carotid stenosis who were experiencing symptoms, including transient cerebral ischemia and mild stroke, would have fewer neurologic events, including cerebral infarction or crescendo TIAs, in the vascular distribution of the study artery after carotid endarterectomy plus best medical management versus best medical management alone. This study was just getting under way when the results of the ECST and NASCET studies were reported and therefore was brought to a halt earlier than anticipated. Nonetheless, 189 patients with symptomatic carotid stenoses were randomly allocated to receive either medical or surgical management. When the results were analyzed with a mean follow-up of 11.9 months, 7.7% of the patients randomized to surgical care had experienced stroke or crescendo TIA during the perioperative or follow-up interval. In contrast, those patients randomized to medical management alone experienced a 19.4% incidence of stroke or crescendo TIA. This difference was statistically significant ($P = .01$). The benefit of operation became apparent within 2 months of randomization when compared with the medically managed control group.[252]

ALTERNATIVES TO SURGICAL THERAPY

The pathophysiology in the development of a stroke from an extracranial lesion has been discussed. The rationale for current medical therapy has evolved from an attempt to alter factors responsible for the development of symptoms secondary to extracranial arterial occlusion. At present, two forms of therapy are considered the mainstays in the medical management of this disease. Antiplatelet agents and anticoagulation are the principal therapeutic alternatives in the medical management of these patients.

Any form of therapy aimed at stroke prevention must include control of commonly associated conditions such as hypertension, diabetes, arrhythmias, and coronary artery disease. Cigarette smoking is also a major independent risk factor for development of carotid bifurcation disease and stroke.[253–255] Any approach to medical control of stroke risk must begin with advice to the patient to stop smoking.

Anticoagulation, mainly with Coumadin (warfarin sodium), has been evaluated in several reports in an attempt to determine whether its use significantly altered the natural history of extracranial arterial lesions. Baker and associates[256] reported a randomized prospective study in patients who had TIAs treated with Coumadin. On follow-up, those treated with anticoagulation had a significant reduction in the number of TIAs when compared with control patients. A favorable trend for fewer strokes was noted in the treated group, although the difference in the incidence of cerebral infarction between treated and control patients was not statistically significant.

A reduction in stroke rate was observed in a retrospective study in the community of Rochester, Minnesota, regarding the use of anticoagulants in cerebral ischemia.[35] In this study, the net probability of having a stroke within 5 years was around 20% for those patients treated with anticoagulants. Although this compares favorably with the probability in untreated controls (40%), it represents a significant risk when compared with other forms of available therapy.

Two reports from Sweden have also shown a reduction in the development of TIAs and stroke in patients treated with anticoagulants. The study by Link and colleagues[257] showed a higher incidence of stroke when anticoagulants were discontinued, and thus long-term therapy was recommended. In the second study, by Terent and Anderson,[258] patients treated with anticoagulants showed an increased mortality rate. Unacceptably serious bleeding complications were also seen in this group. Finally, a meta-analysis of 16 randomized studies of anticoagulation failed to show any benefit in patients suffering from TIA or ischemic stroke compared with untreated control groups. However, evidence does suggest that patients with thrombosis in evolution may benefit from anticoagulation.[259]

The available evidence indicates that although reduced, the incidence of stroke and recurrent TIAs in patients treated with anticoagulants remains high compared with that of other forms of available therapy. The need for long-term administration with its concomitant increased risk of complications makes anticoagulant therapy less desirable.

Antiplatelet agents, mainly aspirin, have been advocated for use in patients with extracranial arterial occlusive disease. The rationale for this therapy is based on available evidence that platelets play a major role in the pathophysiology of this disease. At present, seven double-blind, randomized, prospective studies compare the use of platelet antiaggregants with placebo in treating patients who suffered cerebral ischemia secondary to extracranial atherosclerosis. In the Canadian Cooperative Study Group,[260] 585 patients who evidenced cerebral ischemia of extracranial origin were prospectively randomized into four treatment regimens. Each regimen was taken four times daily and consisted of a 200-mg capsule of sulfinpyrazone plus placebo, a placebo tablet plus 325 mg of aspirin, both active drugs, or both placebos. Follow-up from 12 to 57 months revealed no statistically significant reduction in TIAs, stroke, or death for patients on sulfinpyrazone. Aspirin reduced risk for continuing ischemic episodes, strokes, or death by 19%. When analysis was restricted to stroke or death alone, the risk reduction increased to 31%, and when male patients were analyzed, the reduction was even higher. No statistically significant differences in stroke or death rate were found among female patients taking any of the four regimens. Considering this observation literally, the probability of stroke in men taking aspirin was in excess of 5% each year and in women, higher than 8% each year.[261] Platelet antiaggregants reduce the incidence of stroke in patients with extracranial lesions. The question still remains if this reduction equals that achieved by other forms of available therapy.

In 1972, a double-blind, randomized, prospective trial of aspirin versus placebo was started in several American centers and continued for 37 months.[262] Sixty percent of these patients had operable lesions in the extracranial territory. The treatment group received 10 grains of aspirin twice daily. At 6 months of follow-up, a statistically significant difference in favor of aspirin was seen when death, cerebral or retinal infarction, and TIAs were grouped together. When each group was considered separately, the difference did not achieve statistical significance. Patients for whom a decision was made to proceed with endarterectomy were also assigned to a randomized, double-blind trial of aspirin during the postoperative period. The results of this trial constitute a separate report.[263] Life-table analyses of these end points at 24 months did not reveal a statistically significant difference in favor of aspirin. When non–stroke-related deaths were eliminated, a significant difference in favor of aspirin emerged. A favorable trend was also noted when the occurrence of TIAs within the first 6 months of follow-up was taken into consideration. In the placebo group, eight brain infarcts occurred among eight patients, reaching an end point in the first 24 months. Eight patients also reached an end point in the aspirin group; however, only two of these suffered a neurologic event.

These two studies showed a favorable trend toward a reduction in the stroke rate among patients receiving aspirin as treatment for symptomatic lesions in the extracranial circulation. In the first, aspirin was used as the principal form of therapy, whereas in the second, aspirin was an adjunct to surgical therapy. In the surgically treated group, the absolute level of cases having an unfavorable outcome was about half the percentage of unfavorable cases in those treated medically only (11.3% vs. 2%). This differential may reflect the independent favorable effect of surgery.

Two other studies have evaluated the use of aspirin in a randomized, controlled, prospective fashion. In a study from France,[264] 604 patients with arteriothrombotic cerebral ischemic events referable to the carotid or vertebro-

basilar circulation were entered in a double-blind, randomized clinical trial comparing aspirin 1 g/day, aspirin 1 g/day plus dipyridamole (225 mg/day), and placebo. The comparison of placebo and aspirin groups showed a significant reduction ($P < .05$) of cerebral infarction in the aspirin group. Overall, 66 patients of the entire group suffered a cerebral infarction during the trial. This corresponds to a cumulative stroke rate for the placebo group of 18% and a rate of 10.5% for each of the aspirin groups. No significant difference in the aspirin plus dipyridamole group was found. Thus, the incidence of stroke per year was on the order of 6% for placebo versus 3% per year for the treatment groups. This represents, again, a 50% reduction in the stroke risk.[264] In the dipyridamole-aspirin trial in cerebral ischemia, the American-Canadian Cooperative Study Group[265] found no difference between the stroke risk in patients receiving aspirin or aspirin plus dipyridamole in the prevention of stroke during long-term follow-up. Interestingly, the stroke rate reported in patients treated with either aspirin or aspirin plus dipyridamole was on the order of 20% at 5 years. This yields a 4% per year stroke risk, which is not dissimilar to the lower rates reported in natural history studies.[265]

In 1983, a Danish cooperative study[266] comparing the outcomes of patients with extracranial occlusive disease treated with aspirin or placebo was reported. No favorable influence of aspirin could be determined in the prevention of ischemic attacks. Unfortunately, only 203 patients were monitored, which is probably insufficient to achieve any statistically valid data. This study has been criticized and probably suffers from type II statistical error.[267]

The objective of any treatment regimen for carotid artery disease should be the reduction of stroke risk. Although each of the prospective randomized trials of antiplatelet agents showed a trend toward stroke risk reduction, none achieved statistical significance with regard to that parameter. Only when the end points of TIA, stroke, and nonfatal and fatal myocardial infarction were lumped together did a statistically significant benefit in favor of aspirin emerge. Individual studies always lacked sufficient numbers of patients to show a reduction of stroke risk in favor of aspirin. A statistical technique known as meta-analysis permits the combination of patients from the various series. In doing this, the best that could be shown is a 15% stroke risk reduction in favor of aspirin, and this still failed to achieve statistical significance.[268]

The antiplatelet drug ticlopidine hydrochloride was compared with aspirin in a multicenter prospective randomized trial[269] of 3069 patients with recent transient or mild persistent focal cerebral or retinal ischemia. The 3-year event rate for nonfatal stroke or death from any cause was 17% for ticlopidine and 19% for aspirin. The rates of fatal and nonfatal stroke at 3 years were 10% for ticlopidine and 13% for aspirin. The authors concluded that ticlopidine was somewhat more effective than aspirin in preventing stroke in their study population but that the risks of side effects were greater.[269]

Failures of antiplatelet therapy in the treatment of symptomatic carotid artery disease have been reported.[270] Caution should be used in patients who receive platelet antiaggregants as primary therapy for this disease. Partial disappearance of their symptoms should be considered a failure and alternative forms of treatment considered. Patients who experience complete relief of symptoms should be monitored carefully with annual noninvasive studies. Progression of the lesion may be obscured because of suppression of symptoms by the therapy. In a recent review of 27 aspirin failures requiring urgent operation,[270] 12 of the surgical specimens showed fresh hemorrhage in the atherosclerotic plaque. Whether this was induced or aggravated by aspirin cannot be concluded. This incidence of fresh hemorrhage in an endarterectomy specimen appears high when compared with the findings in elective cases. Finally, good evidence suggests that aspirin is of no benefit to the asymptomatic patient with respect to subsequent neurologic events. Cote and colleagues[271] carried out a prospective randomized trial in asymptomatic patients with carotid stenosis of at least 50%. One hundred patients received aspirin, and 184 patients received placebo. The median follow-up was 2.3 years. The annual rates for vascular events were 11% in the placebo group and 10.7% in the aspirin group.

A 1995 report[272] described the use of lovastatin in an attempt to modify carotid plaques. In patients who were in the 60th to 90th percentile of low-density lipoprotein cholesterol levels, lovastatin appeared to slow the rate of plaque progression. No evidence existed of plaque regression.

In conclusion, the available forms of medical management produce a reduction in the stroke rate in patients with significant atherosclerotic lesions of the extracranial circulation. This reduction does not appear to be as significant as that achieved by successful carotid endarterectomy. Medical treatment for symptomatic extracranial arterial disease should thus be reserved for patients with limited life expectancy or unidentified or surgically inaccessible lesions or for those who are poor surgical candidates.

NEW AND CONTROVERSIAL TOPICS IN CEREBROVASCULAR DISEASE

Carotid Endarterectomy for Acute Stroke

Emergent operation after acute stroke was used early in the history of endarterectomy. Because of several reports indicating the risk of converting an ischemic cerebral infarction into a hemorrhagic cerebral infarction, this procedure was abandoned. In reviewing those reports, several factors are common to the patients who experienced those complications. These include patients being operated on with massive cerebral infarction and in obtunded states, patients in whom an attempt was made to open an occluded internal carotid artery several days to weeks after thrombosis, and patients being operated on with severe hypertension in whom the hypertension was inadequately controlled.[273]

Later evidence suggested improved results if carotid artery surgery is delayed for at least 5 weeks after the acute event. Of 49 carotid endarterectomies done for acute cerebral infarction, 27 were performed within 5 weeks and 22 were done between 5 and 20 weeks after the acute neurologic event. The latter group showed no morbidity or mortality, whereas patients undergoing early operation had an 18.5% incidence of new postoperative neurologic deficits. The authors concluded that an unstable situation during the early phase of stroke contraindicated endarterectomy. No details as to the preoperative degree of neurologic deficit or recovery in these patients were available.[274] Following these guidelines, Dosick and colleagues[154] noted a 21% incidence of recurrent stroke during the 4- to 60-week observation interval. This led these authors to select their patients on the basis of CT scans, proceeding with surgery if the CT scans were negative. One hundred ten patients underwent early endarterectomy after a persistent neurologic deficit with negative CT scans. No patient suffered a neurologic deficit in the territory of the operated artery and no patient died. A similar experience was reported in 28 patients with small fixed neurologic deficits undergoing endarterectomy an average of 11 days from the onset of symptoms. Whittemore and colleagues[275] reported one postoperative death in this small group of patients and no new perioperative neurologic deficits. They recommended proceeding with endarterectomy early in this select group of patients with small cerebral infarct.

In general, surgical intervention during the acute phase of a stroke is contraindicated. If the patient has a dense neurologic deficit, loss of consciousness, or cardiovascular instability, clearly surgery is not indicated. However, if the patient has a mild to moderate deficit and is fully conscious and otherwise stable, carotid endarterectomy of the responsible lesion can be undertaken soon after the patient has reached a plateau in recovery. This may be days or weeks after the onset of the event. In the small group of patients in whom a clinically unstable lesion exists, manifested by crescendo TIAs or stroke in evolution, emergent endarterectomy should be strongly considered.

Crescendo Transient Ischemic Attacks and Stroke in Evolution

Crescendo TIAs and stroke in evolution used to be considered contraindications to operation. I initially reported my experience with a select group of patients in whom stroke in evolution or crescendo TIA patients were acutely studied with angiography. If an unstable condition such as a free-floating thrombus or a propagating thrombus in the presence of a distally patent internal carotid artery was identified, these patients were taken promptly to the operating room for operation. The net result in a series of approximately 25 patients was no deaths and essentially a return to a normal neurologic status, in contrast to the natural history of stroke in evolution, which has approximately an 80% expected mortality.[276]

A similar experience was reported by Mentzer and colleagues[33] with 17 patients operated on emergently for stroke in evolution. None had worsening of the preoperative neurologic deficit, four (24%) remained unchanged, and 12 (70%) had complete recovery. One death occurred, for a 6% operative mortality. This compared favorably with a parallel nonrandomized group of 26 patients with stroke in evolution treated conservatively. The medical group showed 15% mortality, but more important, 17 patients (66%) suffered moderate to severe permanent neurologic deficit. In this report, the collated operative results reported in the literature in 90 cases were presented. After successful endarterectomy, 55% were improved, 25% had no change, and 10% were worse. A 10% mortality for the collated experience was reported. Thus, surgical intervention in the presence of stroke in evolution carries a significantly increased risk of both perioperative stroke and death. However, the results of surgical therapy are considerably better than the natural history of the untreated condition. A specific goal for surgical intervention must be identified by preoperative angiography. Indications for emergent endarterectomy include the presence of an unstable condition such as a free-floating thrombus or propagating thrombus in the presence of a distally patent internal carotid artery. Exclusion by the use of CT scan of other associated conditions that could appear as stroke in evolution is highly recommended.

More recently, a derivative report from the VA symptomatic trial identified crescendo TIAs as a surgical imperative.[277]

Possible Deleterious Effect of Antiplatelet Drugs

In patients with asymptomatic carotid bifurcation plaques or with minimal plaques and TIAs whom the physician elects to treat with antiplatelet drugs, instances have been reported of a progression, more rapid than expected, of the atheromatous lesion to near-total occlusion. Operation at that time has indicated a high degree of intraplaque hemorrhage. The antiplatelet drugs may precipitate intraplaque hemorrhage, with a progression of the lesion more rapid than anticipated.[270] A subsequent report compared plaque histopathology with the preoperative use of antiplatelet drugs. Those patients taking antiplatelet drugs had an 80.1% incidence of multiple intraplaque hemorrhage in contrast to a 19.7% incidence of intraplaque hemorrhage in patients not receiving antiplatelet drugs.[278]

Balloon Angioplasty

Carotid balloon angioplasty with stenting has been used with increasing frequency in multiple centers worldwide. Anecdotal reports provide conflicting data with respect to safety and efficacy. The first large series was reported by Diethrich and colleagues.[279] Between April 1993 and September 1995, 110 nonconsecutive patients underwent treatment using balloon angioplasty and stenting in accord with an approved protocol in a single institution. It is important to note that 72% of the patients treated were asymptomatic. There were seven periprocedural (in-hospital) strokes for an incidence of 6.4%. There were two in-hospital deaths for an incidence of 1.8%. This brings the combined stroke morbidity and mortality, in hospital, to 8.2%. Two patients undergoing stented angioplasty went on to occlusion within 30 days.[279] Roubin and colleagues[280] reported their experience with 74 patients undergoing placement of 210 stents in 152 vessels. They reported one death and nine in-hospital strokes, for a periprocedural stroke morbidity and mortality of 14%.[280] These and several other anecdotal reports prompted a multidisciplinary group of physicians to write an editorial expressing concern about the proliferation of this procedure without proof of its safety and efficacy. They recommended that a prospective trial comparing stented balloon angioplasty with carotid endarterectomy be carried out.[281] The CREST (Carotid

Revascularization–Endarterectomy versus Stent Trial) trial, approved and funded by the National Institute of Neurological Diseases and Stroke of the NIH, with additional financial support from the Guidant Corporation, is now underway. At the time of this writing, four patients have been randomized. The trial is well designed and should provide accurate data with regard to safety, efficacy, and the role of angioplasty in the management of patients with extracranial cerebrovascular disease compared with the gold standard of carotid endarterectomy.

Asymptomatic Carotid Ulceration

Not uncommonly, a large, nonstenotic, ulcerative lesion in a contralateral carotid artery is discovered incidentally at the time that the ipsilateral symptomatic carotid artery is being studied by angiography. A decision of whether to operate on this ulcerative lesion has often been questioned. We have carried out two retrospective reviews of patients with identified nonstenotic ulcerative lesions that have been monitored without treatment. We observed that the medium or large ulcerative lesions carried a significant stroke risk, usually not preceded by warning TIAs.[54] In the most recent study, the risk of stroke in patients being monitored expectantly with large ulcerative lesions was approximately 7.5% each year of follow-up after initial identification.[55] I currently recommend that medium "B" and large "C" ulcers, when identified incidentally, undergo prophylactic repair.

Tandem Lesions

Not uncommonly, one discovers a stenosis of the origin of the internal carotid artery in conjunction with a significant lesion of the carotid siphon. The question is often raised whether operating on the carotid artery alone is justified, if the siphon lesion is larger than the lesion of the internal carotid artery. Several reports now indicate that even though tandem lesions exist, the embolic potential of the atherosclerotic plaque at the carotid bifurcation greatly outweighs the thrombotic or embolic risk of the lesion in the carotid siphon.[282] My practice is to operate on the carotid bifurcation lesion in symptomatic patients in spite of the presence of a siphon lesion.[283] A retrospective review was reported in which the perioperative morbidity, mortality, and late results were compared in patients undergoing carotid endarterectomy with and without angiographically documented intracranial arterial occlusive disease. No difference occurred in results between the two groups. The perioperative stroke rate was 1.9% versus 1.8%; mortality was 0.5% versus 0.7%; and the 3-, 5-, and 10-year stroke rates were 93% versus 92%, 87% versus 90%, and 79% versus 85%, respectively.[284]

Combined Carotid and Coronary Occlusive Disease

The carotid-coronary area is particularly controversial and depends on whether symptoms exist in either vascular bed. In patients with symptomatic coronary artery disease in whom an asymptomatic carotid stenosis is found, it is difficult to know whether the carotid artery should be fixed first, followed by coronary artery bypass; whether both lesions should be fixed simultaneously; or whether surgery for the carotid artery lesion should be put off until after coronary artery bypass. The literature is controversial on this subject, and we are continuing to individualize patients depending on which lesion appears to be most critical. For example, if a patient has triple coronary artery disease with unstable angina and an asymptomatic carotid stenosis, we usually recommend that the coronary artery surgery be performed first and that the carotid lesion be evaluated after recovery. On the other hand, if the patient has relatively stable angina and has symptomatic carotid artery disease or a preocclusive (>90%) stenosis, operating on the carotid artery first and then managing the coronary artery lesions a few days later may well be wise. Finally, if the patient has both symptomatic carotid artery disease and unstable angina, a simultaneous, combined approach would appear justified.

Intellectual Testing and Improvement with Carotid Endarterectomy

After carotid endarterectomy, patients and their families often report that the patient appears intellectually brighter and is able to carry out tasks that have been alien for quite some time. Numerous attempts have been made to quantitate this intellectual improvement, usually without success. We must be careful not to regard intellectually impaired patients as being routine candidates for carotid endarterectomy, because the majority of those patients are suffering from organic brain disease rather than compromised blood flow.

Extracranial-to-Intracranial Bypass Grafting

The technical ability to connect an extracranial arterial branch such as the temporal artery to a cortical branch of the middle cerebral artery has been developed over the past 15 years. To determine whether extracranial-to-intracranial (EC-IC) bypass surgery would benefit patients with symptomatic atherosclerotic disease of the internal carotid artery, an international randomized trial[285] was begun in 1977 and completed in 1982: 1377 patients with recent hemispheric strokes, retinal infarction, or TIAs who had arterial narrowing or occlusion of the ipsilateral carotid artery or middle cerebral artery were randomized. Of these, 714 were assigned to best medical care and 663 were assigned to the surgical group. An EC-IC arterial bypass was performed, with a patency rate on long-term follow-up of 96%. The 30-day surgical mortality was 6.6%, with a stroke morbidity of 2.5%. Nonfatal and fatal strokes on long-term follow-up occurred both more frequently and earlier in patients treated with EC-IC bypass. Survival analysis comparing the two groups for major strokes and all deaths for ipsilateral ischemic strokes demonstrated a similar lack of benefit from surgery. Reduction in the number of TIAs was noted in 77% of the surgical patients. An equal number (80%) of the medical patients also showed reduction or disappearance of TIAs. In all parameters studied, EC-IC bypass failed to improve the results of medical therapy. The large number of patients with long-term follow-up, the uniformity of the disease process in the population studied, the randomization method (which produced a balanced treatment group), the presence of complete and accurate records of all entry and event dates, and the achievement of effective anastomosis with acceptably low morbidity and mortality suggest that this conclusion is not only statistically powerful but clinically significant.[285]

Magnetic Resonance Angiography

In the continuing quest to find a substitute for invasive contrast angiography, the use of MRI of the vascular system has been developed: so-called magnetic resonance angiography. Various computer programs for postprocessing of MR images to delineate the vascular system are under active development. To date, excellent imaging of the cervical and intracranial vessels has been achievable. However, several limitations of MRA have been identified. In several instances, the MR image suggested total occlusion when contrast angiograms showed a patent vessel with a string sign. MRA also tends to overcall percentage stenosis, making minimal lesions look like hemodynamically significant lesions. Finally, MRA cannot delineate surface irregularity or ulceration.[286–288]

References

1. Savory WS: Case of a young woman in whom the main arteries of both upper extremities and of the left side of the neck were throughout completely obliterated. Med Chir Trans Lond 39:205–219, 1856.
2. Gowers WR: On a case of simultaneous embolism of central retinal and middle cerebral arteries. Lancet 2:794, 1875.
3. Chiari M: Ueber das Verhalten des tei lungs-winkels der Carotis communis bei der Endarteritis chronica deformans. Verh Dtsch Ges Pathol 9:326–330, 1905.
4. Guthrie LG, Mayou S: Right hemiplegia and atrophy of left optic nerve. Proc R Soc Med 1:180, 1908.
5. Cadwater WB: Unilateral optic atrophy and contralateral hemiplegia consequent on occlusion of the cerebral vessels. JAMA 59:2248, 1912.
6. Hunt JR: The role of the carotid arteries in the causation of vascular lesions of the brain, with remarks on certain special features of the symptomatology. Am J Med Sci 147:704–713, 1914.
7. Moniz E: L'encéphalographie artérielle: Son importance dans la localisation des tumeurs cérébrales. Rev Neurol (Paris) 2:72–90, 1927.
8. Moniz E, Lima A, de Lacerda R: Hémiplégies par thrombose de la carotide interne. Proc Med 45:977–980, 1937.
9. Chao WH, Kwan ST, Lyman RS, et al: Thrombosis of the left internal carotid artery. Arch Surg 37:100–111, 1938.
10. Johnson HC, Walker AE: The angiographic diagnosis of spontaneous thrombosis of the internal and common carotid arteries. J Neurosurg 8:631–659, 1951.
11. Fisher M: Occlusion of the internal carotid artery. Arch Neurol Psychiatry 65:346–377, 1951.
12. Fisher M: Occlusion of the carotid arteries. Arch Neurol Psychiatry 72:187–204, 1954.
13. Carrea R, Molins M, Murphy G: Surgical treatment of spontaneous thrombosis of the internal carotid artery in the neck: Carotid-caroti-

deal anastomosis: Report of a case. Acta Neurol Latinoam 1:71–78, 1955.

14. Strully KJ, Hurwitt ES, Blankenberg HW: Thromboendarterectomy for thrombosis of the internal carotid artery in the neck. J Neurosurg 10:474–482, 1953.

15. DeBakey ME, Crawford ES, Cooley DA, et al: Surgical considerations of occlusive disease of innominate, carotid, subclavian, and vertebral arteries. Ann Surg 149:690–710, 1959.

16. DeBakey ME: Successful carotid endarterectomy for cerebrovascular insufficiency: Nineteen-year follow-up. JAMA 233:1083, 1975.

17. Eastcott HHG, Pickering GW, Rob C: Reconstruction of internal carotid artery in a patient with intermittent attacks of hemiplegia. Lancet 2:994–996, 1954.

18. Davis JB, Grove WJ, Julian OC: Thrombic occlusion of the branches of the aortic arch, Martorell's syndrome: Report of a case treated surgically. Ann Surg 144:124–126, 1956.

19. Warren R, Triedman LJ: Pulseless disease and carotid artery thrombosis. N Engl J Med 257:685–690, 1957.

20. Thompson JE: The evolution of surgery for the treatment and prevention of stroke: The Willis lecture. Stroke 27:1427–1434, 1996.

21. Adelman SM: Economic impact. In McDowell FM (ed): Report on the National Survey of Stroke (American Heart Association monograph number 75). Stroke 12:1, 1981.

22. Mohr JP, Caplan LR, Meski JW, et al: The Harvard Cooperative Stroke Registry: A prospective registry. Neurology 28:754, 1978.

23. Sacco RL, Wolf PA, Kannel WB, McNamara PM: Survival and recurrence following stroke: The Framingham Study. Stroke 13:290, 1982.

24. Soltero I, Lin K, Cooper R, et al: Trends in mortality from cerebrovascular diseases in the United States, 1960 to 1975. Stroke 9:549, 1978.

25. Enger E, Boysen S: Longterm anticoagulant therapy in patients with cerebral infarction: A controlled clinical study. Acta Med Scand Suppl 438:1–61, 1965.

26. Robinson RW, Demirel M, LeBeau RJ: Natural history of cerebral thrombosis. 9–19 year follow-up. J Chronic Dis 21:221, 1968.

27. Schmidt EV, Smirnov VE, Ryabova VS: Results of the seven-year prospective study of stroke patients. Stroke 19:942–949, 1988.

28. Swedish Cooperative Study: High-dose acetylsalicylic acid after cerebral infarction. Stroke 18:325–334, 1987.

29. Klag MJ, Whelton PK, Seidler AJ: Decline in US stroke mortality demographic trends and antihypertensive treatment. Stroke 20:14–21, 1989.

30. Wolf PA, O'Neal A, D'Agostino RB, et al: Declining mortality, not declining incidence of stroke: The Framingham Study. Stroke 20:29, 1989.

31. Harmsen P, Tsipogianni A, Wilhelmsen L: Stroke incidence rates were unchanged, while fatality rates declined, during 1971–1987 in Göteborg, Sweden. Stroke 23:1410–1415, 1992.

32. Moden B, Wagener DK: Some epidemiologic aspects of stroke: Mortality/morbidity trends, age, sex, race, socioeconomic status. Stroke 23:1230–1236, 1992.

33. Mentzer RM Jr, Finkelmeier BA, Crosby JK, Wellons HA Jr: Emergency carotid endarterectomy for fluctuating neurologic deficits. Surgery 89:60, 1981.

34. Millikan CH: Discussion. In McDowell FH, Brennan RW (eds): Cerebral Vascular Diseases (Transactions of the Eighth Princeton Conference on Cerebral Vascular Disease). New York, Grune & Stratton, 1973, p 209.

35. Whisnant JP, Matsumoto M, Elveback LR: The effects of anticoagulant therapy on the prognosis of patients with transient cerebral ischemic attacks in a community. Rochester, Minnesota, 1965–1969. Mayo Clin Proc 48:844, 1973.

36. Dennis M, Bamford J, Sandercock P, Warlow C: Prognosis of transient ischemic attacks in the Oxfordshire Community Stroke Project. Stroke 21:848–853, 1990.

37. Hass WK, Jonas S: Caution falling rock zone: An analysis of the medical and surgical management of threatened stroke. Proc Inst Med 33:80, 1980.

38. Loeb C, Priano A, Albana C: Clinical features and long-term follow-up of patients with reversible ischemic attacks. Acta Neurol Scand 57:471, 1978.

39. Toole JF: The Willis Lecture: Transient ischemic attacks, scientific method, and new realities. Stroke 22:99–104, 1991.

40. Grigg MJ, Papadakis K, Nicolaides AN, et al: The significance of cerebral infarction and atrophy in patients with amaurosis fugax and transient ischemic attacks in relation to internal carotid artery stenosis. A preliminary report. J Vasc Surg 7:215–222, 1988.

41. Kartchner MM, McRae LP: Noninvasive evaluation and management of the asymptomatic carotid bruit. Surgery 82:840, 1977.

42. Busuttil RW, Baker JD, Davidson RK, Machleder HI: Carotid artery stenosis: Hemodynamic significance and clinical course. JAMA 245:1438, 1981.

43. Roederer GO, Langlois YE, Jager KA, et al: The natural history of carotid arterial disease in asymptomatic patients with cervical bruits. Stroke 15:605–613, 1984.

44. Moore DJ, Miles RD, Gooley NA, Summer DS: Non-invasive assessment of stroke risk in asymptomatic and non-hemispheric patients with suspected carotid disease: Five year follow-up of 294 unoperated and 81 operated patients. Ann Surg 202:491–504, 1985.

45. Chambers BR, Norris JW: Outcome in patients with asymptomatic neck bruits. N Engl J Med 315:860–865, 1986.

46. Norris JW, Zhu CZ, Bornstein NM, Chambers BR: Vascular risks of asymptomatic carotid stenosis. Stroke 22:1485–1490, 1991.

47. Norris JW, Zhu CZ: Silent stroke and carotid stenosis. Stroke 23:483–485, 1992.

48. Johnson JM, Kennelly MM, Decesare D, et al: Natural history of asymptomatic carotid plaque. Arch Surg 120:1010–1012, 1985.

49. Langsfeld M, Gray-Weale AC, Lusby RJ: The role of plaque morphology and diameter reduction in the development of new symptoms in asymptomatic carotid arteries. J Vasc Surg 9:548–557, 1989.

50. Sterpetti AV, Schultz RD, Feldhaus RJ, et al: Ultrasonographic features of carotid plaque and the risk of subsequent neurologic deficits. Surgery 104:652–660, 1988.

51. Madison FE, Moore WS: Ulcerated atheroma of the carotid artery: Arteriographic appearance. AJR Am J Roentgenol 107:530, 1969.

52. Moore WS, Hall AD: Ulcerated atheroma of the carotid artery: A cause of transient cerebral ischemia. Am J Surg 116:237, 1968.

53. Moore WS, Hall AD: Importance of emboli from carotid bifurcation in pathogenesis in cerebral ischemia attacks. Arch Surg 101:708, 1970.

54. Moore WS, Boren C, Malone JM, et al: Natural history of nonstenotic asymptomatic ulcerative lesions of the carotid artery. Arch Surg 113:1352, 1978.

55. Dixon S, Pais SO, Raviola C, et al: Natural history of nonstenotic, asymptomatic ulcerative lesions of the carotid artery: A further analysis. Arch Surg 117:1493, 1982.

56. Harward TRS, Kroener JM, Wickbom IG, et al: Natural history of asymptomatic ulcerative plaques of the carotid bifurcation. Am J Surg 146:208, 1983.

57. Kartchner MM, McRae LP: Guidelines for non-invasive evaluation of asymptomatic carotid bruits. Clin Neurosurg 28:418–428, 1981.

58. Barnes RW, Liebman PR, Marszalek PP, et al: Natural history of asymptomatic carotid disease in patients undergoing cardiovascular surgery. Surgery 90:1075–1083, 1981.

59. Breslau PJ, Fell G, Ivey TD, et al: Carotid arterial disease in patients undergoing coronary artery bypass operations. J Thorac Cardiovasc Surg 82:765–767, 1981.

60. Furlan AJ, Craciun AR: Risk in stroke during coronary artery bypass graft surgery in patients with internal carotid artery disease documented by angiography. Stroke 16:797–799, 1985.

61. Turnipseed WD, Berkoff HA, Belzer FO: Post-operative stroke in cardiac and peripheral vascular disease. Ann Surg 192:365–368, 1980.

62. Von Reutern G-M, Hetzel A, Birnbaum D, Schlosser V: Transcranial Doppler ultrasonography during cardiopulmonary bypass in patients with severe carotid stenosis or occlusion. Stroke 19:674–680, 1988.

63. Brener BJ, Hermans H, Eisenbud D, et al: The management of patients requiring coronary bypass and carotid endarterectomy. In Moore WS (ed): Surgery for Cerebrovascular Disease, 2nd ed. Philadelphia, WB Saunders, 1996, pp 278–287.

64. Schwartz CJ, Mitchell JRA: Observations on localization of arterial plaques. Circ Res 11:63, 1962.

65. Heath D, Smith P, Harris P, Winson M: The atherosclerotic human carotid sinus. J Pathol 110:49, 1973.

66. Caro CG, Fitzgerald JN, Schroter RC: Atheroma and arterial wall shear: Observation, correlation and proposal of a shear-dependent mass transfer mechanism for atherogenesis. Proc R Soc Lond B Biol Sci 117:109, 1971.

67. Balasubramanian K, Giddens DP, Maybon RS: Steady flow at the carotid bifurcation. In Schneck DJ (ed): Biofluid Mechanics, vol 6. New York, Plenum Press, 1980, p 475.

68. Ferguson GG, Roach MR: Flow conditions at bifurcations as determined in glass models with reference to the focal distribution of vascular lesions. In Bergel DH (ed): Cardiovascular Fluid Dynamics, vol 2. New York, Academic Press, 1972.

69. Fox JA, Hugh AE: Static zones in the internal carotid artery: Correlations with boundary layer separation and stasis in mobile flows. Br J Radiol 43:370, 1976.

70. LoGerfo FW, Nowak MD, Quist WC, et al: Flow studies in a model carotid bifurcation. Arteriosclerosis 1:235, 1981.

71. Zarins CK, Giddens DB, Glagov S: Atherosclerotic plaque distribution and flow velocity profiles in the carotid bifurcation. In Bergan JJ, Yao JDT (eds): Cerebrovascular Insufficiency. New York, Grune & Stratton, 1982, p 19.

72. Salzman EW: Platelet-vessel interactions in cerebrovascular disease: The role of prostaglandins in cerebrovascular insufficiency. In Bergan JJ, Yao JST (eds): Cerebrovascular Insufficiency. New York, Grune & Stratton, 1983, p 31.

73. Meyers KM, Seachord CL, Holmsen H, et al: The dominant role of thromboxane formation in secondary aggregation of platelets. Nature 282:331, 1979.

74. Born BGR: Arterial thrombosis and its prevention. In Hayase S, Murao S (eds): Proceedings of the Eighth World Congress of Cardiology, Tokyo. Amsterdam, Excerpta Medica, 1978, p 81.

75. Fryer JA, Myers PC, Appleberg M: Carotid intraplaque hemorrhage: The significance of neovascularity. J Vasc Surg 63:341–349, 1987.

76. Lusby RJ, Ferrell LD, Wylie EJ: The significance of intraplaque hemorrhage in the pathogenesis of carotid arteriosclerorosis. In Bergan JJ, Yao JST (eds): Cerebrovascular Insufficiency. New York, Grune & Stratton, 1983, p 41.

77. Ogata J, Masuda J, Yutani C, Yamguchi T: Rupture of atheromatous plaque as a cause of thrombotic occlusion of stenotic internal carotid artery. Stroke 21:1740–1745, 1990.

78. Palubinskas AJ, Ripley HR: Fibromuscular hyperplasia in extrarenal arteries. Radiology 82:451, 1964.

79. Patman RD, Thompson JE, Talkington CM, et al: Natural history of fibromuscular dysplasia of the carotid artery. Stroke 1:135, 1980.

80. Osborn AG, Anderson RE: Angiographic spectrum of cervical and intracranial fibromuscular dysplasia. Stroke 8:617, 1977.

81. Effeney DJ, Ehrenfeld WK, Stoney RJ, et al: Fibromuscular dysplasia of the internal carotid artery. World J Surg 3:179, 1979.

82. Stanley JC, Gewertz BL, Bove EL, et al: Arterial fibrodysplasia: Histopathologic character and current etiologic concepts. Arch Surg 110:561, 1975.

83. Ross R, Klebanoff SJ: Fine structural changes in uterine smooth muscle and fibroblasts in response to estrogen. J Cell Biol 32:155, 1967.

84. Nakata Y: An experimental study on the vascular lesions caused by obstruction of the vasa vasorum. Jpn Circ J 31:275, 1967.

85. Sarkari NBS, Palms JM, Bickerstaff ER: Neurological manifestations associated with internal carotid loops and kinks in children. J Neurol Neurosurg Psychiatry 33:194, 1973.

86. Metz H, Murray-Leslie RM, Bannister RG, et al: Kinking of the internal carotid artery in relation to cerebrovascular disease. Lancet 1:424, 1961.

87. Quattlebaum JK Jr, Upson ET, Neville RL: Strokes associated with elongation and kinking of the internal carotid artery. Ann Surg 150:824, 1959.

88. Vannix RS, Joergenson EJ, Carter R: Kinking of the internal carotid artery: Clinical significance and surgical management. Am J Surg 134:82, 1977.

89. Busuttil RW, Davidson RK, Foley KT, et al: Selective management of extracranial carotid arterial aneurysms. Am J Surg 140:85, 1980.

90. Rhodes EL, Stanley JC, Hoffman GL, et al: Aneurysms of extracranial carotid arteries. Arch Surg 111:339, 1976.

91. Kaupp HA, Haid SP, Juraj MN, et al: Aneurysms of the extracranial carotid artery. Surgery 72:946, 1972.

92. Boldrey E, Maass L, Miller E: The role of atlantoid compression in the etiology of internal carotid thrombosis. J Neurosurg 13:127, 1956.

93. Smith RF, Szilagyi DE, Colville JM: Surgical treatment of mycotic aneurysms. Arch Surg 85:663, 1962.

94. Bradac GB, Kaernbach A, Bolk-Weischedel D, Finck GA: Spontaneous dissecting aneurysm of cervical cerebral arteries: Report of six cases and review of the literature. Neuroradiology 21:149, 1981.

95. Ehrenfeld WK, Wiley EJ: Spontaneous dissection of the internal carotid artery. Arch Surg 111:1294, 1976.

96. Takayasu M: Case with unusual changes of the central vessels of the retina. Acta Soc Ophthalmol Jpn 12:554, 1908.

97. Nasu T: Pathology of pulseless disease: Systematic study and critical review of 21 autopsy cases reported in Japan. Angiology 14:225, 1962.

98. Lande A, Berkmen YM: Aortitis: Pathologic, clinical and arteriographic review. Radiol Clin North Am 14:219, 1976.

99. Lupi-Herrera E, Sanchez-Torres G, Marcushamer J, et al: Takayasu's arteritis. Clinical study of 107 cases. Am Heart J 93:94–103, 1977.

100. Hamrin B, Jousson N, Landberg T: Involvement of large vessels in polymyalgia arteritica. Lancet 1:1193, 1965.

101. Lindsay S, Entenman C, Ellis EE, Geraci CL: Aortic arteriosclerosis in the dog after localized aortic irradiation with electrons. Circ Res 10:61, 1962.

102. Silverberg GD, Britt RH, Goffinet DR: Radiation-induced carotid artery disease. Cancer 41:132, 1978.

103. McCready RA, Hyde GE, Bevins BA, et al: Radiation-induced arterial injuries. Surgery 93:306–312, 1983.

104. Levinson SA, Close MB, Ehrenfeld WK, Stoney RJ: Carotid artery occlusive disease following external cervical irradiation. Arch Surg 107:395–397, 1973.

105. Moritz MW, Higgins RF, Jacobs JR: Duplex imaging and incidence of carotid radiation injury after high-dose radiotherapy for tumors of the head and neck. Arch Surg 125:1181–1183, 1990.

106. DeGrotte RD, Lynch JG, Jamil Z, Hobson RW II: Carotid restenosis: Long term non-invasive follow-up after carotid endarterectomy. Stroke 18:1031–1036, 1987.

107. Hertzer NR, Martinez BD, Benjamin SP, Beven EG: Recurrent stenosis after carotid endarterectomy. Surg Gynecol Obstet 149:360–364, 1979.

108. Hertzer NR, Beven EG, O'Hara PJ, Krajewski LP: A prospective study of vein patch angioplasty during carotid endarterectomy. Ann Surg 206:628–635, 1987.

109. Lees CD, Hertzer NR: Postoperative stroke and late neurologic complications after endarterectomy. Arch Surg 116:1561, 1981.

110. Stoney RJ, String ST: Recurrent carotid stenosis. Surgery 80:705–710, 1976.

111. Zierler RE, Bandyk DF, Thiele BL, Strandness DE Jr: Carotid artery stenosis following endarterectomy. Arch Surg 117:1408–1415, 1982.

112. O'Donnell TF Jr, Callew AD, Scott G, et al: Ultrasound characteristics of recurrent carotid disease: Hypothesis explaining the low incidence of symptomatic recurrence. J Vasc Surg 2:26–41, 1985.

113. Nicholls SC, Phillips DJ, Bergelin RO, et al: Carotid endarterectomy: Relationship of outcome to early restenosis. J Vasc Surg 2:375–381, 1985.

114. Bernstein EF, Torem S, Dolley RB: Does carotid restenosis predict an increased risk of late symptoms, stroke, or death? Ann Surg 212:629–636, 1990.

115. Awad IA, Little JR: Patch angioplasty in carotid endarterectomy — advantages, concerns, and controversies. Stroke 20:417–422, 1989.

116. Curley S, Edwards WS, Jacob TP: Recurrent carotid stenosis after autologous tissue patching. J Vasc Surg 6:350–354, 1987.

117. Eikelboom BC, Ackerstaff RGA, Hoeneveld H, et al: Benefits of carotid patching: A randomized study. J Vasc Surg 7:240–247, 1988.

118. Lord RSA, Raj TB, Stary DL, et al: Comparison of saphenous vein patch, polytetrafluoroethylene patch, and direct arteriotomy closure after carotid endarterectomy, pt 1: Perioperative results. J Vasc Surg 9:521–529, 1989.

119. Abu Rahma AF, Robinson PA, Saiedy S, et al: Prospective randomized trial of bilateral carotid endarterectomies: Primary closure versus patching. Stroke 30:1185–1189, 1999.

120. Abu Rahma AF, Robinson PA, Saiedy S, et al: Prospective randomized trial of carotid endarterectomy with primary closure and patch angioplasty with sapherous vein, jugular vein, and polytetrafluoroethylene: Long-term follow-up. J Vasc Surg 27:222–232, 1998.

121. Moore WS, Kempczinski RF, Nelson JJ, Toole JF: Recurrent carotid stenosis: Results of this asymptomatic carotid atherosclerosis study. Stroke 29:2018–2025, 1998.

122. Salvian A, Baker JD, Machleder HI, et al: Cause and noninvasive detection of restenosis after carotid endarterectomy. Am J Surg 146:29–34, 1983.

123. Gelabert HA, El-Massry S, Moore WS: Carotid endarterectomy with primary closure does not adversely affect the rate of recurrent stenosis. Arch Surg 129:648–654, 1994.

124. Petrik PV, Gelabert HA, Moore WS, et al: Cigarette smoking accel-

erates carotid artery intimal hyperplasia in a dose-dependent manner. Stroke 26:1409–1414, 1995.

125. Hansen F, Lindblad B, Persson NH, Bergqvist D: Can recurrent stenosis after carotid endarterectomy be prevented by low-dose acetyl salicylic acid? A double blind, randomized and placebo-controlled study. Eur J Vasc Surg 7:380–385, 1993.

126. Crawford ES, De Bakey ME, Blaisdell FW, et al: Hemodynamic alteration in patients with cerebral arterial insufficiency before and after operation. Surgery 48:76, 1960.

127. Gunning AJ, Pickering GW, Robb-Smith AHT, Russell RR: Mural thrombosis of the internal carotid artery and subsequent embolism. Q J Med 33:155–195, 1964.

128. Hertzer NR, Beven EG, Benjamin SP: Ultramicroscopic ulcerations and thrombi of the carotid bifurcation. Arch Surg 112:1394–1042, 1977.

129. Imparato AM, Riles TS, Gorstein F: The carotid bifurcation plaque: Pathology findings associated with cerebral ischemia. Stroke 10:238–245, 1979.

130. Edwards JH, Kricheff II, Riles T, Imparato A: Angiographically undetected ulceration of the carotid bifurcation as a cause of embolic stroke. Radiology 132:369–373, 1979.

131. Sterpetti AV, Hunter WJ, Schultz RD: Importance of ulceration of carotid plaque in determining symptoms of cerebral ischemia. J Cardiovasc Surg (Torino) 32:154–158, 1991.

132. Loeb C, Gandolfo C, Bino G: Intellectual impairment and cerebral lesions in multiple cerebral infarcts. Stroke 19:560–565, 1988.

133. Zukowski AJ, Nicolaides AN, Lewis RJ, et al: The correlation between carotid plaque ulceration and cerebral infarction seen on CT scan. J Vasc Surg 1:782–786, 1984.

134. Siebler M, Sitzer M, Steinmetz H: Detection of intracranial emboli in patients with symptomatic extracranial stroke 23:1652–1654, 1992.

135. Tietjen GE, Futrell N, Garcia JH, Millikan C: Platelet emboli in rat brain cross when the contralateral carotid artery is occluded. Stroke 22:1053–1058, 1991.

136. Amarenco P, Cohen A, Baudrimont M, Bousser MG: Transesophageal echocardiographic detection of aortic arch disease in patients with cerebral infarction. Stroke 23:1005–1009, 1992.

137. Amarenco P, Cohen A, Tzourio C, et al: Atherosclerotic disease of the aortic arch and the risk of ischemic stroke. N Engl J Med 331:1474–1479, 1994.

138. Stone DA, Hawke MW, La Monte M, et al: Ulcerated atherosclerotic plaques in the thoracic aorta are associated with cryptogenic stroke: A multiphase transesophageal echocardiographic study. Am Heart J 130:105–108, 1995.

139. Mohr JP: Lacunes. Stroke 13:3–11, 1982.

140. Fisher CM: Pure motor hemiplegia of vascular origin. Arch Neurol 13:30–44, 1965.

141. Pullicino P, Nelson RF, Kendall BE, Marshall J: Small deep infarcts diagnosed on computed tomography. Neurology 30:1090–1096, 1980.

142. Bladin PF, Berkovic SF: Striatocapsular infarction: Large infarcts in the lenticulostriate arterial territory. Neurology 34:1423–1430, 1984.

143. Bamford JM, Warlow CP: Evolution and testing of the lacunar hypothesis. Stroke 19:1074–1082, 1988.

144. Horowitz DR, Tuhrim S, Weinberger JM, Rudolph SJ: Mechanisms in lacunar infarction. Stroke 23:325–327, 1992.

145. Heyman A, Wilkinson WE, Heyden S, et al: Risk of stroke in asymptomatic persons with cervical arterial bruits: A population study in Evans County, Georgia. N Engl J Med 302:838, 1980.

146. Reinmuth OM: Transient ischemic attacks. Curr Neurol 1:166, 1978.

147. Heyman A, Leviton A, Millikan CK, et al: XI. Transient focal cerebral ischemia: Epidemiological and clinical aspects. Stroke 5:277, 1974.

148. Price TR, Gotshall RA, Poskanzer DC, et al: Cooperative study of hospital frequency and character of transient ischemic attacks, VI: Patients examined during an attack. JAMA 238:2512, 1977.

149. Futty DE, Conneally M, Dyken ML, et al: Cooperative study of hospital frequency and character of transient ischemic attacks, V: Symptom analysis. JAMA 238:2386, 1977.

150. Berguer R: Idiopathic ischemic syndrome of the retina and optic nerve and their carotid origin. J Vasc Surg 2:649–653, 1985.

151. Mohr JP: Transient ischemic attacks and the prevention of stroke. N Engl J Med 299:93, 1978.

152. Pessin MS, Duncan GW, Mohr JP, Poskanzer DC: Clinical and angiographic features of carotid transient ischemic attacks. N Engl J Med 296:358, 1977.

153. Yatsu SM, Coull BM: Stroke. Curr Neurol 3:159, 1981.

154. Dosick SM, Whalen RC, Gale SS, Brown OW: Carotid endarterectomy in the stroke patient: Computerized axial tomography to determine timing. J Vasc Surg 2:214–219, 1985.

155. Ahn SS, Jordan SE, Nuwer MR, et al: Compared electroencephalographic topographic brain mapping—A new and accurate monitor of cerebral circulation and function for patients having carotid endarterectomy. J Vasc Surg 8:247–254, 1988.

156. Strefler JY, Eliasziw M, Fox AJ, et al: Angiographic detection of carotid plaque ulceration: Comparison with surgical observations in a multicenter study. [North American Symptomatic Carotid Endarterectomy Trial]. Stroke 25:1130–1132, 1994.

157. Moore WS, Ziomek S, Quiñones-Baldrich WJ, et al: Can clinical evaluation and non-invasive testing substitute for arteriography in the evaluation of carotid artery disease? Am Surg 208:91–94, 1988.

158. The Executive Committee for the Asymptomatic Carotid Atherosclerosis Study: Endarterectomy for asymptomatic carotid artery stenosis. JAMA 273:1421–1428, 1995.

159. Moore WS, Young B, Baker WH, et al: Surgical results: A justification of the surgeon selection process for the ACAS Trial. J Vasc Surg 23:323–328, 1996.

160. Blackshear WM, Connar RG: Carotid endarterectomy without angiography. J Cardiovasc Surg (Torino) 23:477, 1982.

161. Sandmann W, Hennerici M, Nullen H, et al: Carotid artery surgery without angiography: Risk or progress? In Greenhalgh RM, Rose FC (eds): Progress in Stroke Research II. London, Pitman, 1983, pp 447–461.

162. Ricotta JJ, Holen J, Schenk E, et al: Is routine angiography necessary prior to carotid endarterectomy? J Vasc Surg 1:96–102, 1984.

163. Crew JR, Dean M, Johnson JM, et al: Carotid surgery without angiography. Am J Surg 148:217–220, 1984.

164. Walsh J, Markowitz I, Kerstein MD: Carotid endarterectomy for amaurosis fugax without angiography. Am J Surg 152:172–174, 1986.

165. Marshall WG, Kouchoukos NT, Murphy SF, Pelate C: Carotid endarterectomy based on duplex scanning without preoperative arteriography. Circulation 78(Suppl 1):I-1–I-5, 1988.

166. Moore WS, Ziomek S, Quiñones-Baldrich WJ, et al: Can clinical evaluation and noninvasive testing substitute for arteriography in the evaluation of carotid artery disease? Ann Surg 208:91–94, 1988.

167. Gelabert HA, Moore WS: Carotid endarterectomy without angiography. Surg Clin North Am 70:213–223, 1990.

168. Ranaboldo C, Davies J, Chant A: Duplex scanning alone before carotid endarterectomy: A five-year experience. Eur J Vasc Surg 5:415–419, 1991.

169. Wagner WH, Treiman RL, Cossman DV, et al: The diminishing role of diagnostic arteriography in carotid artery disease: Duplex scanning as definitive preoperative study. Ann Vasc Surg 5:105–110, 1991.

170. Gertler JP, Cambria RP, Kistler JP, et al: Carotid surgery without arteriography: Non-invasive selection of patients. Ann Vasc Surg 5:253–256, 1991.

171. Chervu A, Moore WS: Carotid endarterectomy without angiography: Personal series and review of the literature. (Presented SVS/ISCVS Breakfast Session, June 1992) Ann Vasc Surg 8:296–302, 1994.

172. Connolly JE: Carotid endarterectomy in the aware patient. Am J Surg 150:159, 1985.

173. Moore WS, Hall AD: Carotid artery back pressure. Arch Surg 99:702, 1969.

174. Moore WS, Yee TM-I, Hall AD: Collateral cerebral blood pressure: An index of tolerance to temporary carotid occlusion. Arch Surg 106:520, 1973.

175. Baker JD, Gluecklich B, Watson CW, et al: An evaluation of electroencephalographic monitoring for carotid surgery. Surgery 78:787–794, 1975.

176. Elmore JR, Eldrup-Jorgensen J, Leschey WH, et al: Computerized tomographic brain mapping during carotid endarterectomy. Arch Surg 125:734–738, 1990.

177. Kearse LA Jr, Brown EN, McPeck K: Somatosensory evoked potentials sensitivity relative to electroencephalography for cerebral ischemia during carotid endarerectomy. Stroke 23:498–505, 1992.

178. Thompson JE, Patman RD, Talkington CM: Asymptomatic carotid bruit: Long term outcome of patients having endarterectomy compared with unoperated controls. Ann Surg 188:308, 1978.

179. Baker WM, Dorner DB, Barnes RW: Carotid endarterectomy: Is an indwelling shunt necessary? Surgery 82:321, 1977.

180. Whitney DG, Kahn EM, Estes JW, Jones CE: Carotid surgery without a temporary indwelling shunt: 1,917 consecutive procedures. Arch Surg 115:1393–1399, 1980.

181. Archie JP Jr: Technique and clinical results of carotid stump back-

pressure to determine selective shunting during carotid endarterectomy. J Vasc Surg 13:319–327, 1991.

182. Halsey JH Jr: Risks and benefits of shunting in carotid endarterectomy. Stroke 23:1583–1587, 1992.

183. Matchar DB, Goldstein LB, McCory DC, et al: Carotid endarterectomy: A literature review and ratings of appropriateness and necessity. Rand GRA-05, 1992.

184. Moore WS, Mohr JP, Najafi H, et al: Carotid endarterectomy: Practice guidelines. Report of the ad hoc committee to the joint council of the Society for Vascular Surgery and the North American Chapter of the International Society for Cardiovascular Surgery. J Vasc Surg 15:469–479, 1992.

185. Moore WS: Current status of carotid endarterectomy for stroke prevention. West J Med 159:37–43, 1993.

186. Moore WS, Barnett HJ, Beebe ME, et al: Guidelines for carotid endarterectomy: A multidisciplinary consensus statement from the ad hoc committee, American Heart Association. Stroke 26:188–201, 1995.

187. Moore WS, Barnett HJ, Beebe ME, et al: Guidelines for carotid endarterectomy: A multidisciplinary consensus statement from the ad hoc committee, American Heart Association. Circulation 91:566–579, 1995.

188. Biller J, Feinberg WM, Lastaldo JE, et al: Guidelines for carotid endarterectomy: A statement for health care professionals from a special writing group of the Stroke Council, American Heart Association. Stroke 29:554–562, 1998.

189. Blaisdell FM, Lim R Jr, Hall AD: Technical results of carotid endarterectomy: Arteriographic assessment. Am J Surg 114:239, 1967.

190. Gaspar MR, Movius HJ, Rosental JJ: Routine intraoperative arteriography in carotid artery surgery. J Cardiovasc Surg (Torino) Spec No: 477–481, 1973.

191. Moore WS, Martello JY, Quiñones-Baldrich WJ, Ahn SS: Etiologic importance of the intimal flap of the external carotid artery in the development of post–carotid endarterectomy stroke. Stroke 21:1497–1502, 1990.

192. Lipski DA, Bergamini TM, Garrison RN, Fulton RL: Intraoperative duplex scanning reduces the incidence of residual stenosis after carotid endarterectomy. J Surg Res 60:317–320, 1996.

193. O'Brien MS, Ricotta JJ: Conserving resources after carotid endarterectomy: Selective use of the intensive care unit. J Vasc Surg 14:796–800, 1991.

194. Hoyle RM, Jenkins JM, Edwards WH Sr, et al: Case management in cerebral revascularization. J Vasc Surg 20:396–401, 1994.

195. Hirko MK, Morasch MD, Burke K, et al: The changing face of carotid endarterectomy. J Vasc Surg 23:622–627, 1996.

196. Bove EL, Fry WJ, Gross WS, Stanley JC: Hypotension and hypertension as consequences of baroreceptor dysfunction following carotid endarterectomy. Surgery 85:633–637, 1979.

197. Towne JB, Bernard VM: The relationship of postoperative hypertension to complications following carotid endarterectomy. Surgery 88:375, 1980.

198. Angell-James JE, Lumley JSP: The effects of carotid endarterectomy on the mechanical properties of the carotid sinus and carotid sinus nerve activity in atherosclerotic patients. Br J Surg 61:805, 1974.

199. Smith BL: Hypertension following carotid endarterectomy: The role of cerebral renin production. J Vasc Surg 1:623–627, 1984.

200. Skydell JL, Machleder HI, Baker JD, et al: Incidence and mechanism of post-carotid endarterectomy hypertension. Arch Surg 122:1153–1155, 1987.

201. Ahn SS, Marcus DR, Moore WS: Post-carotid endarterectomy hypertension: Associated with elevated cranial norepinephrine. J Vasc Surg 9:351–350, 1989.

202. Ranson JHC, Imparato AM, Clauss RH, et al: Factors in the mortality and morbidity associated with surgical treatment of cerebrovascular insufficiency. Circulation 39(Suppl 1):I269–I274, 1969.

203. Riles TL, Koppleman I, Imparato AM: Myocardial infarction following carotid endarterectomy: A review of 683 operations. Surgery 85:249, 1979.

204. Matsumoto GH, Cossman D, Callow AD: Hazards and safeguards during carotid endarterectomy: Technical consideration. Am J Surg 133:485, 1977.

205. Hertzer NR, et al: A prospective study of the incidence of injury to the cranial nerve during carotid endarterectomy. Surg Gynecol Obstet 151:781, 1980.

206. Evans WE, Mendelowitz DS, Liapis C, et al: Motor speech deficit following carotid endarterectomy. Am Surg 196:461–464, 1982.

207. Bryant MF: Complications associated with carotid endarterectomy. Am Surg 42:665, 1976.

208. Verta MJ Jr, Applebaum EL, McCluskey DA, et al: Cranial nerve injuring during carotid endarterectomy. Ann Surg 185:192–195, 1977.

209. Thompson JE: Complications of endarterectomy and their prevention. World J Surg 3:155, 1979.

210. Brott T, Thalinger K: The practice of carotid endarterectomy in a large metropolitan area. Stroke 15:950–955, 1984.

211. Brott TG, Labutta RJ, Kempczinski RF: Changing patterns in the practice of carotid endarterectomy in a large metropolitan area. JAMA 225:2609–2612, 1986.

212. Easton JD, Sherman DG: Stroke and mortality rate in carotid endarterectomy: 228 consecutive operations. Stroke 8:565–568, 1977.

213. Beebe HG, Clagett GP, DeWeese JA, et al: Assessing risk associated with carotid endarterectomy. Stroke 20:314–315, 1989.

214. Sundt TM Jr, Houser DW, Sharbrough FW, Messick JM Jr: Carotid endarterectomy. Results, complications, and monitoring techniques. Adv Neurol 16:97, 1977.

215. Kwaan JHM, Connelly JE, Sharefkin JB: Successful management of early stroke after carotid endarterectomy. Ann Surg 190:676, 1979.

216. Hertzer NR, Lees CD: Fatal myocardial infarction following carotid endarterectomy: 335 patients followed 6-11 postoperative years. Ann Surg 194:212–218, 1981.

217. Bauer RB, Meyer JS, Fields WS, et al: Joint study of extracranial arterial occlusion, III: Progress report of controlled study of long-term survival in patients with and without operation. JAMA 208:509–518, 1969.

218. Rothwell PM, Slattery J, Warlow CP: A systematic comparison of the risks of stroke and death due to carotid endarterectomy for symptomatic and asymptomatic stenosis. Stroke 25:266–269, 1996.

219. Bernstein EF, et al: Influence of preoperative factors on late neurologic events after carotid endarterectomy. In International Vascular Symposium Programs and Abstracts. New York, Macmillan, 1981, p 460.

220. Hertzer NR, Arison R: Cumulative stroke and survival ten years after carotid endarterectomy. J Vasc Surg 2:661–668, 1985.

221. Sergeant PT, Derom F, Berzsenyi G, et al: Carotid endarterectomy for cerebrovascular insufficiency: Long-term follow-up of 141 patients followed for up to 16 years. Acta Chir Belg 79:309–316, 1980.

222. Moore WS, Boren C, Malone JM, et al: Asymptomatic carotid stenosis: Immediate and long term results after prophylactic endarterectomy. Am J Surg 138:228, 1979.

223. Bernstein EF, Humber PB, Collins GM, et al: Life expectancy and late stroke following carotid endarterectomy. Ann Surg 198:80, 1983.

224. Lord RSA: Later survival after carotid endarterectomy for transient ischemic attacks. J Vasc Surg 1:512, 1984.

225. DeWeese JA, Rob CG, Satran R, et al: Results of carotid endarterectomy for transient ischemic attacks—five years later. Ann Surg 178:258–264, 1973.

226. Thompson JE, Austin BJ, Patman RD: Carotid endarterectomy for cerebrovascular insufficiency: Long-term results in 592 patients followed up to 13 years. Ann Surg 172:663, 1970.

227. Takolander RJ, Bergentz SE, Ericsson BF: Carotid artery surgery in patients with minor stroke. Br J Surg 70:13, 1983.

228. Eriksson SE, Link H, Alm A, et al: Results from eighty-eight consecutive prophylactic carotid endarterectomy in cerebral infarction and transitory ischemic attacks. Acta Neurol Scand 63:209, 1981.

229. Bardin JA, Bernstein EF, Humber PB, et al: Is carotid endarterectomy beneficial in prevention of recurrent stroke? Arch Surg 117:1401, 1982.

230. McCullough JL, Mentzer RM, Harman PK, et al: Carotid endarterectomy after a completed stroke: Reduction in long term neurologic deterioration. J Vasc Surg 2:7, 1985.

231. Ouriel K, et al: Carotid endarterectomy for nonhemispheric symptoms: Predictors of success. J Vasc Surg 1:331–345, 1984.

232. Ricotta JJ, O'Brien MS, DeWeese JA: Carotid endarterectomy for non-hemisphere ischemia: Long-term follow-up. Cardiovasc Surg 2:561–566, 1994.

233. Imparato AM: Vertebral arterial reconstruction: A nineteen year experience. J Vasc Surg 2:626–634, 1985.

234. O'Hara PJ, Hertzer NR, Beven EG: External carotid revascularization: Review of a ten year experience. J Vasc Surg 2:709–714, 1985.

235. Halstuk KS, Baker WH, Littooy FN: External carotid endarterectomy. J Vasc Surg 1:398–402, 1984.

236. Lindblad B, Persson NH, Takolander R, Bergqvist D: Does low-dose acetylsalicylic acid prevent stroke after carotid surgery? A

double-blind, placebo-controlled randomized trial. Stroke 24:1125–1128, 1993.

237. Veterans Administration: A Veterans Administration Cooperative Study: Role of carotid endarterectomy in asymptomatic carotid stenosis. Stroke 17:534–539, 1986.

238. Hobson RW, Song IS, George AM, Weiss DG: Results of arteriography for asymptomatic carotid stenosis. Stroke 20:135, 1989.

239. Towne JB, Weiss DG, Hobson RW: First phase report of cooperative Veterans Administration asymptomatic carotid stenosis study—operative morbidity and mortality. J Vasc Surg 11:252–259, 1990.

240. Hobson RW, Weiss DG, Fields WS, et al: Efficacy of carotid endarterectomy for asymptomatic carotid stenosis. N Engl J Med 328:221, 1993.

241. The CASANOVA Study Group: Carotid surgery vs medical therapy in asymptomatic carotid stenosis. Stroke 22:1229–1235, 1991.

242. The Asymptomatic Carotid Artery Stenosis Group: Study design for randomized prospective trial of carotid endarterectomy for asymptomatic atherosclerosis. Stroke 20:844–849, 1989.

243. Clinical advisory: Carotid endarterectomy for patients with asymptomatic internal carotid artery stenosis. Stroke 25:523–524, 1994.

244. Moore WS, Vescera CL, Robertson JT, et al: Selection process for surgeons who wished to participate in the Asymptomatic Carotid Atherosclerosis Study. Stroke 22:1353–1357, 1991.

245. Haddiday AM, Thomas D, Mansfield A: The Asymptomatic Carotid Surgery Trial (ACST): Rationale and design. Eur J Vasc Surg 8:703–710, 1994.

246. North American Symptomatic Carotid Endarterectomy Trial (NASCET) Steering Committee: North American Symptomatic Carotid Endarterectomy Trial: Methods, patient characteristics, and progress. Stroke 22:711–720, 1991.

247. North American Symptomatic Carotid Endarterectomy Trial Collaborators: Beneficial effect of carotid endarterectomy in symptomatic patients with high-grade carotid stenosis. N Engl J Med 325:445–453, 1991.

248. Barnett MJM, Taylor DW, Eliasziw M, et al: Benefit of carotid endarterectomy in patients with symptomatic moderate or severe stenosis. N Engl J Med 339:1415–1425, 1998.

249. European Carotid Surgery Trialists' Collaborative Group: MRC European Carotid Surgery Trial: Interim results for patients with severe (70–99%) or with mild (0–29%) carotid stenosis. Lancet 337:1235–1243, 1991.

250. Eliasziw M, Smith RF, Singh N, et al: Further comments on the measurements of carotid stenosis from angiograms. Stroke 25:2445–2449, 1994.

251. Endarterectomy for moderate symptomatic carotid stenosis: Interim results from the MRC European Carotid Surgery Trial. Lancet 347:1591–1593, 1996.

252. Maybert MR, Wilson SE, Yatsu F, et al: Carotid endarterectomy and prevention of cerebral ischemia in symptomatic carotid stenosis. JAMA 266:3289, 1991.

253. Wolf PA, D'Agostino RB, Kannel WB, et al: Cigarette smoking as a risk factor for stroke: The Framingham Study. JAMA 259:1025–1029, 1988.

254. Whisnant JP, Homer D, Ingall TJ, et al: Duration of cigarette smoking is the strongest predictor of severe extracranial carotid artery atherosclerosis. Stroke 21:707–714, 1990.

255. Dempsey RJ, Moore RW: Amount of smoking independently predicts carotid artery atherosclerosis severity. Stroke 23:693–696, 1992.

256. Baker RN, Schwartz WS, Rose AS: Transient ischemic strokes: A report of a study of anticoagulant therapy. Neurology 16:841, 1964.

257. Link H, Lebram G, Johansson I, Radberg C: Prognosis in patients with infarction and TIA in carotid territory during and after anticoagulant therapy. Stroke 10:529, 1979.

258. Terent A, Anderson B: The outcome of patients with transient ischemic attacks and stroke treated with anticoagulants. Acta Med Scand 208:359, 1980.

259. Jonas S: Anticoagulant therapy in cerebrovascular disease: Review and meta-analysis. Stroke 19:1043–1048, 1988.

260. The Canadian Cooperative Study Group: A randomized trial of aspirin and sulfinpyrazone in threatened strokes. N Engl J Med 299:53, 1978.

261. Whisnant JP: The Canadian trial of aspirin and sulfinpyrazone in threatened strokes. Am Heart J 99:129, 1980.

262. Fields WS, Lemak NA, Frankowski RF, Hardy RJ: Controlled trial of aspirin in cerebral ischemia. Stroke 8:301, 1977.

263. Fields WS, et al: Controlled trial of aspirin in cerebral ischemia, pt 2: Surgical group. Stroke 9:309, 1978.

264. Bousser MD, et al: AICLA controlled trial of aspirin and dipyridamole in the secondary prevention of arteriothrombotic cerebral ischemia. Stroke 14:5–14, 1983.

265. The American Canadian Cooperative Study Group: Persantine-aspirin trial in cerebral ischemia. Part 2: End point results. Stroke 16:405, 1985.

266. Sorenson PS, Pedersen H, Marquardsen J, et al: Acetylsalicylic acid in the prevention of stroke in patients with reversible cerebral ischemic attacks: A Danish cooperative study. Stroke 14:15–22, 1983.

267. Dyken ML: Editorial. Stroke 14:2–4, 1983.

268. Sze PC, Reitman D, Pincus MM, et al: Antiplatelet agents in the secondary prevention of stroke: Meta-analysis of the randomized control trials. Stroke 19:436–442, 1988.

269. Hass WK, Easton D, Adams MP Jr, et al: A randomized trial comparing ticlopidine hydrochloride with aspirin for the prevention of stroke in high-risk patients. N Engl J Med 321:501–507, 1989.

270. Carson SN, et al: Aspirin failure in symptomatic arteriosclerotic carotid artery disease. Surgery 90:1084, 1981.

271. Cote R, Battista RM, Abrahamowicz M, et al: Lack of effect of aspirin in asymptomatic patients with carotid bruits and substantial carotid narrowing. Ann Intern Med 123:649–655, 1995.

272. Probstfield JL, Magrite SE, Byington RP, et al: Results of the primary outcome measure and clinical events from the Asymptomatic Carotid Artery Progression Study. Am J Cardiol 76:47C–53C, 1995.

273. Wylie EJ, Hein MF, Adams JE: Intracranial hemorrhage following surgical revascularization for treatment of acute strokes. J Neurosurg 21:212–215, 1964.

274. Giordano JM, et al: Timing carotid arterial endarterectomy after stroke. J Vasc Surg 2:250, 1985.

275. Whittemore AD, Ruby ST, Couch NP, et al: Early carotid endarterectomy in patients with small fixed neurologic deficits. J Vasc Surg 1:795, 1984.

276. Goldstone J, Moore WS: Emergency carotid artery surgery in neurologically unstable patients. Arch Surg 111:1284, 1976.

277. Wilson SE, Mayberg MR, Yatsu F, Weiss DG: Crescendo transient ischemic attacks: A surgical imperative. J Vasc Surg 17:49–55, 1993.

278. Abu Rahma AF, Boland JP, Robinson P, Delanio R: Antiplatelet therapy and carotid plaque hemorrhage and its clinical implications. J Cardiovasc Surg 31:66–70, 1990.

279. Diethrich EB, Ndiaye M, Reid DB: Stenting in the carotid artery: Initial experience in 110 patients. J Endovasc Surg 3:42–46, 1996.

280. Roubin GS, Yadev S, Iyer SS, Vitek J: Carotid stent-supposed angioplasty: A neurovascular intervention to prevent stroke. Am J Cardiol 78:8–12, 1996.

281. Beebe MG, Archie JP, Baker WH, et al: Concern about safety of carotid angioplasty. Stroke 27:197–198, 1996.

282. Schuler JJ, et al: The effect of carotid siphon stenosis on stroke rate, death, and relief of symptoms following elective carotid endarterectomy. Surgery 92:1058–1067, 1982.

283. Moore WS: Does tandem lesion mean tandem risk in patients with carotid artery disease? J Vasc Surgery 7:454–455, 1988.

284. Mackey WC, O'Donnell JF Jr, Callow AD: Carotid endarterectomy in patients with intracranial vascular disease: Short-term risk and long-term outcome. J Vasc Surg 10:432–438, 1989.

285. The EC/IC Bypass Study Group: Failure of extracranial-intracranial arterial bypass to reduce the risk of ischemic stroke: Results of an international randomized trial. N Engl J Med 313:1191–1200, 1985.

286. Wilkerson DK, Keller I, Mezich R, et al: The comparative evaluation of three-dimensional magnetic resonance for carotid artery disease. J Vasc Surg 14:803–811, 1991.

287. Mattle HP, Kent KC, Adelman RR, et al: Evaluation of the extracranial carotid arteries: Correlation of magnetic resonance angiography, duplex ultrasonography, and conventional angiography. J Vasc Surg 13:838–845, 1991.

288. Wiles TS, Eidelman EM, Litt AW, et al: Comparison of magnetic resonance angiography, conventional angiography, and duplex scanning. Stroke 23:341–346, 1992.

Questions

1. The most common cause of perioperative neurologic deficits after carotid endarterectomy is
   (a) thrombosis of the repair
   (b) lack of cerebral perfusion
   (c) tandem lesions in the carotid system
   (d) low cardiac output
   (e) none of the above

2. Carotid endarterectomy for asymptomatic disease
   1. is now a proved indication for stenosis 60% or greater, as documented by angiography
   2. carries the lowest perioperative morbidity and mortality
   3. should be considered when progression to 80% stenosis is documented
   4. may prevent stroke, which is the most common initial manifestation of asymptomatic carotid disease
   (a) 1, 2, 3
   (b) 1, 3
   (c) 2, 4
   (d) 4 only
   (e) 1, 2, 3, and 4

3. Tandem lesions in the intracranial carotid system
   (a) carry a similar stroke risk compared with a carotid bifurcation lesion
   (b) carry a lower stroke risk than a similar extracranial bulb lesion
   (c) carry a higher risk than a similar extracranial bulb lesion
   (d) should deter the surgeon from recommending bifurcation endarterectomy
   (e) are more frequently the source of symptoms when combined intra- and extracranial disease is present

4. The following is/are true about fibromuscular dysplasia
   1. best described as an atherosclerotic process affecting medium-sized arteries
   2. 30% of patients with cervical involvement may have intracranial aneurysms
   3. medial hyperplasia is the most common type affecting the carotid system
   4. most commonly affects women, suggesting a hormonal factor
   (a) 1, 2, 3
   (b) 1, 3
   (c) 2, 4
   (d) 4 only
   (e) none of these

5. Kinks of the carotid artery
   (a) are frequently the cause of cerebrovascular symptoms
   (b) may be congenital
   (c) never cause symptoms
   (d) frequently require excision and grafting for repair
   (e) are rarely associated with atherosclerosis

6. Transient ischemic attacks (TIAs)
   1. carry a 40% risk of stroke over 5 years when secondary to extracranial arterial occlusive disease
   2. are always secondary to platelet emboli
   3. may be a manifestation of lacunar infarction
   4. as a manifestation of cardiac emboli are usually stereotyped with similar symptoms with each occurrence
   (a) 1, 2, 3
   (b) 1, 3
   (c) 2, 4
   (d) 4 only
   (e) 1, 2, 3, and 4

7. The use of an internal shunt during carotid endarterectomy
   (a) is necessary in approximately 50% of patients
   (b) may be predicted based on angiographic findings
   (c) carries no added risk
   (d) all of the above
   (e) none of the above

8. External carotid endarterectomy
   (a) carries significant risks when combined with extracranial-intracranial bypass
   (b) rarely requires patch closure
   (c) frequently relieves amaurosis, but rarely relieves hemispheric TIAs
   (d) all of the above
   (e) none of the above

9. Stroke in evolution
   1. may be a manifestation of lacunar infarction
   2. suggests an unstable process in which urgent evaluation and therapy are indicated
   3. has a 10% mortality with surgical therapy
   4. should be treated with prompt medical therapy in view of the increased risk of surgery
   (a) 1, 2, 3
   (b) 1, 3
   (c) 2, 4
   (d) 4 only
   (e) none of these

10. The following is/are true regarding carotid endarterectomy for acute stroke
   1. the risks of surgical intervention during the acute phase of a stroke are high; therefore, surgery is never indicated
   2. if a CT scan done within 12 hours of the event is negative, endarterectomy can be safely performed
   3. level of consciousness, hypertension, and severity of the deficit should not influence timing of surgical intervention
   4. if the patient shows continuous recovery without deterioration, endarterectomy may be safely performed once a plateau has been reached
   (a) 1, 2, 3
   (b) 1, 3
   (c) 2, 4
   (d) 4 only
   (e) none of these

Answers

1. e   2. e   3. b   4. c   5. b   6. b   7. e   8. a   9. a   10. d

32

Reconstruction of the Supraaortic Trunks and Vertebrobasilar System

Ramon Berguer

The supraaortic trunks (SATs) are those segments of the neck arteries ascending through the mediastinum that begin at the arch of the aorta and end short of the carotid bifurcation and of the origin of the vertebral arteries. The trunks as defined carry the entire blood supply to the head and upper extremities. The vertebrobasilar system is composed of the two vertebral arteries and the basilar artery and its branches to the brain stem, cerebellum, and occipital lobes.

Occlusive disease of the SATs may result in symptoms of hemispheric (carotid) distribution or in manifestations of vertebrobasilar ischemia or in both. In addition, proximal subclavian disease may result in ischemia of the hand by hypoperfusion or embolization. Vertebrobasilar ischemia may be secondary to poor inflow through both carotids and vertebral arteries, to a reversal of blood flow in the vertebral arteries caused by a proximal subclavian artery occlusion (subclavian steal), to a reversal of both carotid and vertebral artery flow from an innominate artery occlusion, and to embolization from proximal subclavian or vertebral arteries.

Vertebral artery occlusive disease may, by restricting inflow into the basilar artery, result in vertebrobasilar ischemia. The latter is more likely if compensatory flow from the carotid system is not available because of internal carotid occlusion or because of the absence of a well-developed posterior communicating artery.

The SATs are involved by atherosclerosis in the late years of life. This results in the development of plaques that may obstruct flow or embolize. Aneurysmal atherosclerotic disease of the SATs is rare. In other latitudes, the SATs are a common site for arteritis of the Takayasu type, usually in younger individuals. Traumatic and mycotic aneurysms of the SATs are uncommon but life-threatening conditions.

The incidence of atherosclerotic disease is lower in the trunks than in the more distal vessels (internal carotid and vertebral artery origins). However, the extensive study of extracranial arterial disease reported by Hass and colleagues[1] showed that one third of the patients in the joint study of extracranial arterial occlusion undergoing arteriography had a severe lesion involving one or more of the SATs. The morphology of the atherosclerotic lesions of the SATs is also less well-known than that of the plaques found in the internal carotid. This is partly due to the fact that for years the SATs were not routinely visualized during arteriography of the cerebral vessels. In addition, they are not easily accessible to ultrasonic examination, which has given us important morphologic information in other areas, notably in the carotid bifurcation. Because we have limited knowledge of the natural history of these lesions, the facts on which we draw our surgical indications are partly inferred. In addition, SAT lesions are often found in individuals who already have carotid or vertebral artery disease, a situation that confuses the identification of the offending lesion.

Stenosing lesions of the SATs are usually located at the origin of these vessels and often involve more than one artery. Because these plaques are located in the ostia, they are often continuous with plaques of atheroma extending over the dome of the aortic arch. Outlining the lesions of the SATs by arteriography requires an arch injection, preferably in two projections (right and left posterior oblique). If the anatomic circumstances permit, the arteriographic study should also include selective injections of both common carotid and subclavian arteries (four-vessel arteriogram). The high incidence of concomitant carotid and vertebral artery lesions makes it mandatory to outline the entire extra- and intracranial circulation. The use of arteriographic intraarterial digital techniques has brought a substantial improvement in that lesser volumes of contrast material are now needed for these studies.

SYMPTOMS

Patients with occlusive disease of the SATs may show symptoms of carotid, basilar, and upper extremity arterial ischemia. The traditional belief was that in SAT lesions, the mechanism for the production of cerebral symptoms is restriction of blood flow rather than microembolization, but, in fact, no pathologic evidence supports this view. In stenosing lesions of the subclavian artery, both mechanisms—hypoperfusion and embolization—are observed. In patients with SAT disease, the hemispheric symptoms are the same as those seen in internal carotid artery disease: hemisensory or motor deficits and amaurosis fugax from either embolization or hypoperfusion. Likewise, the symptoms of vertebrobasilar ischemia from proximal subclavian or vertebral artery disease are due to hypoperfusion or embolization (see later in this chapter).

Obliteration of the SATs is suggested by absent pulses in the neck (subclavian, carotid) or arm (axillary, brachial), in one or both sides, and the recording of an unequal or abnormally low pressure in the upper extremities. Waveforms recorded by Doppler tracings are dampened in those vessels whose origins are stenosed or occluded. Bruits may or may not be present. In patients with subclavian steal, a pulse lag may be felt between both radial arteries or, more precisely, a pulse wave delay of greater than 30 msec may be measured by recording simultaneously both brachial artery waveforms.[2] Claudication of the arm or digital artery embolization, or both, may be present in subclavian artery disease.

A computed tomography scan of the brain is an essential part of the workup of these patients. It often reveals clinically unsuspected cerebral infarctions.

In symptomatic vertebral (or basilar) artery occlusive disease the patient shows any combination of the following symptoms: dizziness, vertigo, diplopia, perioral numbness, blurring of vision, tinnitus, ataxia, bilateral sensory deficits, and drop attacks. In the evaluation of these patients, the mechanism that triggers the symptom must be sought. Patients with orthostatic hypotension have vertebrobasilar symptoms when they stand abruptly after sitting or lying down. A recording of their blood pressure immediately after standing up shows a drop in systolic pressure greater than 20 mm Hg. This mechanism is particularly common in diabetic patients with sympathetic paralysis and loss of venomotor tone because they pool a substantial amount of blood in their legs on standing.

The presence of vertebrobasilar ischemia related to turning of the neck suggests osteophytic compression on the vertebral arteries or inner ear disease. In general, in patients with labyrinthine disorders, symptoms appear with brief, head-shaking motions. Patients who develop symptoms by extrinsic compression of the vertebral arteries usually require a few seconds with the neck rotated maximally in a particular direction to develop symptoms. In addition to orthostatism and osteophytic compression, other conditions are capable of causing vertebrobasilar ischemia and must be ruled out. The most common are inappropriate antihypertensive medication, cardiac arrhythmias, anemia, brain tumors, and subclavian steal.

INDICATIONS

No databank exists for the atherosclerotic lesions of the SATs comparable with that available for internal carotid artery disease. We know from arteriograms and postmortem studies that they are less frequently involved by atherosclerotic disease than the carotid bifurcations. On the other hand, we generally do not have the ability to use ultrasonography to define the composition of these plaques. The specimens obtained at operation show degenerative features similar to those seen in carotid plaques: surface thrombus, ulceration, and intraplaque hemorrhage. Because most operations to reconstruct the SAT are bypasses rather than endarterectomies, few specimens are available for pathologic study. One may infer that the same pathologic mechanisms that operate in carotid artery plaques take place in these SAT lesions. Until more precise information is available, use of criteria similar to those that we follow in carotid disease to advance guidelines for surgical treatment appears reasonable. These criteria are to be tempered by the fact that the risk of surgical reconstruction of the SATs is generally higher than that of carotid endarterectomy.

Our indications for surgical repair of lesions of the SATs are (1) lesions encroaching on more than 70% of the diameter or plaques with ulceration or surface irregularities in patients with appropriate symptoms (ipsilateral carotid or vertebrobasilar); (2) the same lesions plus ipsilateral internal carotid disease for which an endarterectomy is indicated (the operation should correct both); (3) the same lesions plus a nonacute ipsilateral hemispheric infarction (overt or silent); and (4) preocclusive (>90% cross-sectional area loss) lesions in asymptomatic patients who are good surgical risks and have more than 5 years of life expectancy. This last indication is arbitrary albeit reasonable.

The primary indication for reconstructing a vertebral artery is to treat vertebrobasilar ischemia. Vertebral artery occlusive disease is a frequent anatomic finding in individuals who do not have symptoms of vertebrobasilar ischemia. Conversely, many systemic causes of vertebrobasilar ischemia are not related to vertebral artery disease. Therefore, the indication for reconstructing a vertebral artery must be based on the strong anatomic and clinical presumption that the symptom (vertebrobasilar ischemia) is secondary to the anatomic lesion (occlusive disease of the vertebral arteries).

Vertebrobasilar ischemia may be due to stenosis or occlusion of the vertebral or basilar arteries, causing hypoperfusion of the territory. This is the so-called low-flow ("hemodynamic") mechanism. These patients often have repetitive transient ischemic attacks (TIAs) triggered by positional or postural mechanisms. Although their risk for stroke is lower than for patients with carotid disease, they may suffer serious traumatic injuries due to loss of balance. Ischemia of the vertebrobasilar territory may also be due to microembolization. Contrary to popular views in the neurologic literature, an estimated one third of vertebrobasilar ischemic episodes are caused by embolization from plaques or mural lesions of the vertebral arteries.[3] These patients are at high risk for infarctions in the brain stem, cerebellum, and occipital lobes. The mechanism here is microembolization from a plaque in the proximal subclavian or vertebral arteries or from a lesion in the wall of the vertebral artery secondary to repetitive trauma from an osteophyte or intramural dissection.

In patients with low-flow symptoms of ischemia in the vertebrobasilar territory, the surgical indication rests on the assumption that the basilar artery is not receiving adequate inflow from the vertebral arteries.

Because two vertebral arteries usually supply the basilar artery, the presence of a normal vertebral artery contraindicates an operation on its opposite regardless of the anatomic condition of the latter (in low-flow symptoms). A vertebral artery of normal caliber emptying into a basilar artery is enough to supply appropriately the basilar territory. This means that for a lesion in the vertebral arteries to be considered significant, not only must it be severe (>75% stenosis), but the opposite vertebral artery must be equally diseased, hypoplastic, or absent.

Our approach to the patient with vertebrobasilar ischemia is first to determine whether any of the clinical conditions listed earlier as capable of producing these symptoms are present. If so, they should be corrected. If symptoms persist after treatment, an arteriogram is indicated. If the arteriogram shows a lesion that fulfills the anatomic criteria listed previously and the operation appears technically feasible, a reconstruction of the vertebral arteries is indicated.

In patients with vertebrobasilar ischemia secondary to *embolization*, the indication for surgery rests on the demonstration of the embologenic lesion, regardless of the condition of the opposite vertebral artery.

TECHNIQUES FOR RECONSTRUCTION OF THE SUPRAAORTIC TRUNKS

The main decision in reconstruction of the SATs is whether to do the repair through the chest or through the neck. Cervical repairs are traditionally done by means of a bypass between a good donor vessel and the diseased one. Most of these bypasses run transversely either between vessels on the same side of the neck (carotid and subclavian) or across the neck (remote bypasses). Bypass procedures between the ipsilateral carotid and subclavian arteries are being partially superseded by translocation procedures that present the advantage of a single arterial anastomosis without the need for a saphenous vein or a prosthetic tube. Transthoracic or axial repairs require a midsternotomy for the direct approach to these vessels. The lesions are rarely dealt with by endarterectomy and, commonly, by a bypass from the ascending aorta.

The choice between transthoracic (axial) and cervical (transverse) repairs can be made using the following general guidelines. Axial repairs are preferred in younger patients who have innominate artery lesions or multiple lesions (usually innominate and left common carotid). They are also the natural choice for patients in whom a simultaneous coronary bypass operation is indicated. In patients with atherosclerotic disease of the SATs and coronary arteries, repairing concomitant severe lesions of the first segment of the left subclavian artery is advisable even though no symptoms may occur from the stenosis of this vessel. This repair later permits a myocardial revascularization using the left internal mammary artery.

Cervical repairs are preferred in older patients, in those who are at high risk of thoracotomy, and in those who have had previous transsternal procedures. Cervical repair is the choice for all single arterial lesions (other than the innominate artery).

Cervical Repairs

In the early 1970s, techniques for revascularization of the SATs consisting of a transverse bypass between a donor and a recipient (diseased) vessel became popular. The insertion of a bypass between the carotid and subclavian arteries, although described in 1957,[4] became popular in the 1970s. These bypasses were tended between the midportion of the carotid artery and the second (retroscalene) or third portions of the subclavian artery. In some cases, the carotid artery acted as the donor vessel and the bypass corrected a blockage of the first portion of the subclavian artery. In others, the subclavian artery was the donor vessel to bypass a common carotid artery lesion. The theoretical concern that when the carotid artery was the donor vessel these bypasses might divert too much flow into the subclavian and reduce distal carotid flow did not materialize. In subclaviocarotid bypasses, in which the anastomosis to the carotid artery is of the end-to-side type, the possibility exists of proximal embolization (from the diseased proximal common carotid) or of extension of the proximal thrombus across the end-to-side anastomosis. Because of this, we advocate end-to-end anastomosis (see later) into the common carotid artery.

Carotosubclavian bypasses became the standard operation for the correction of subclavian steal syndrome in the 1970s. When use of the carotid as the donor vessel was not deemed advisable (because it was the only carotid artery patent or because of significant disease in the common carotid artery), the correction of subclavian steal was achieved with bypasses tended between both subclavian or both axillary arteries. These remote subclaviosubclavian and axilloaxillary bypasses became known by the awkward name of "extra-anatomic" operations. Although they have the advantage of avoiding a thoracotomy and of carrying a lower operative mortality, they do not have the same long-term patency rates achieved by axial reconstructions. In the case of axilloaxillary bypasses, the graft crosses in front of the sternum, giving a poor cosmetic result and being liable to external compression as well as interfering with a midsternotomy possibly required for coronary revascularization later on.

Many of the cervical bypasses done in the 1970s used saphenous vein as a preferred graft material. There was fear of embolization from the "neointima" of prosthetic tubes and doubts about their patency rates. However, saphenous veins also presented specific problems. They were not always available, and, often, gross mismatches in caliber occurred between the vein and the recipient arteries. In addition, the length involved in these remote bypasses brought the possibility of axial rotation or of compression or kinking of the vein graft with rotation of the neck. Because of these difficulties, many surgeons explored prosthetic substitutes as the preferred material for these remote neck bypasses. The long-term results observed make them preferable to saphenous vein because they provide a good caliber match and their patency rates are excellent,[5] no doubt as a result of the high flow rates usually measured in these vessels.

Anatomic Indications for Cervical Repairs

Innominate Artery Occlusion or Stenosis

A variety of cervical techniques are available for the correction of innominate artery stenosis or occlusion. Subclavio-subclavian and axilloaxillary bypasses can supply the right carotid by retrograde flow in the subclavian or axillary artery. Uncommonly, the needed supply to the right common carotid or right subclavian may be derived through a remote bypass from the left subclavian artery. Carotocarotid bypasses are technically feasible, but for this particular indication, they probably represent an unnecessary risk, because both carotid systems are severely hypotensive during insertion of the bypass into the donor left common carotid artery (unless shunted).

If the innominate artery lesion is suspected to be embolizing, or if it presents a grossly irregular surface or large ulcerations, its distal portion should be ligated at the completion of the procedure. This may not be possible using a supraclavicular approach. A complex solution to this need is an end-to-end anastomosis between the proximal subclavian and the proximal right common carotid artery, with ligation of the proximal carotid stump and then revascularization of the middle or distal third of the right subclavian through a remote bypass from the other side of the neck.

In general, I prefer to do axial reconstructions (see later) in all innominate artery lesions.

Common Carotid Artery Occlusion or Stenosis

The common carotid can be revascularized by means of a subclaviocarotid bypass with the distal anastomosis being end to end to avoid embolization from the diseased proximal common carotid artery. Even in those cases in which the entire carotid system on one side is not visualized on the arteriogram, one must consider the possibility of the carotid bifurcation being intact, with retrograde flow from the external carotid perfusing the internal carotid artery. Delayed subtracted films may show this late opacification. Duplex imaging is an expedient way to show patency of the bifurcation and its branches. In these circumstances, usually an additional plaque exists at the origin of the internal carotid artery that needs to be cleared by endarterectomy. After amputation of the distal common carotid artery, the carotid bulb is opened posteriorly and the endarterectomy of the internal carotid is done. At the completion of the endarterectomy, the bypass from the subclavian artery is anastomosed to this spatulated bulb in an end-to-end fashion, supplying both external and internal carotid arteries.

An alternative method (Fig. 32–1) is to open the bifurcation as is usually done for an endarterectomy, clear the plaque in the distal common and proximal internal carotid arteries, and do an end-to-side anastomosis of the bypass to the arteriotomy as an "on-lay" patch. This end-to-side anastomosis is functionally transformed into an end-to-end

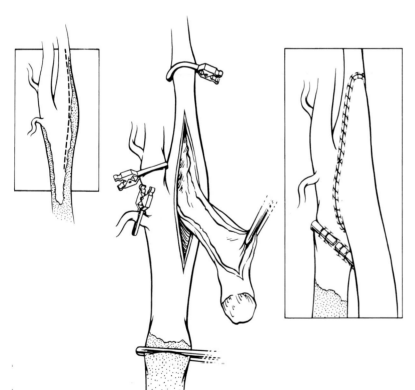

Figure 32–1. A method for anastomosing the limb of a graft to an endarterectomized carotid bulb. The occlusion of the common carotid artery immediately below the anastomosis transforms it into a functional end-to-end junction.

junction by ligation of the common carotid artery below the anastomosis, in the soft segment created by endarterectomy of the distal portion of the common carotid artery.

A third method, and the one I use preferentially for the anastomosis of a subclaviocarotid graft to a patent but diseased carotid bifurcation, is to divide the distal common carotid artery 1 cm below its bifurcation, do an eversion endarterectomy of the bifurcation, and anastomose the bypass to the distal rim of common carotid artery.

If the common carotid artery is stenosed at its origin and its midportion is free of disease, transposition of the midportion of the common carotid artery to the subclavian artery is a better procedure than a subclaviocarotid bypass. It requires only one anastomosis and no prostheses. On occasion, a thrombosed common carotid artery with a patent bifurcation can be thrombectomized after dividing it close to its origin and doing an eversion endarterectomy. The distal portion of the endarterectomy is terminated under direct vision through the standard arteriotomy used for internal carotid endarterectomy. After endarterectomy, the common carotid is reimplanted into the second portion of the subclavian. Subclaviocarotid bypasses and transposition of the carotid into the subclavian are easier on the right side, where the subclavian artery is more accessible.

In those cases in which the ipsilateral subclavian artery is not a suitable donor vessel, a common carotid artery lesion may be corrected by means of a carotocarotid bypass. This operation is traditionally done by placing a bypass between both carotids in front of the airway. I prefer to use the shorter retropharyngeal route (see later in this chapter).

Subclavian Artery Occlusion

Most operations on the proximal subclavian artery are done to correct a symptomatic subclavian steal or an emboligenous lesion of the proximal subclavian, or to revascularize the subclavian before an internal mammary transposition to the coronary arteries. Carotosubclavian bypass is a proven operation to correct this situation. When the subclavian lesion is a source of embolization, the prevertebral subclavian artery must be ligated at the time of the bypass. My preference for the last decade has been to use a direct transposition of the subclavian artery (prevertebral portion) into the common carotid artery. Although the operation is slightly more complex technically, it involves only one anastomosis and excludes the diseased proximal subclavian as well.

Description of Techniques for Cervical Repair

Carotosubclavian or Subclaviocarotid Bypass and Carotid (or Subclavian) Transposition

The approach is through a supraclavicular incision dividing the clavicular head of the sternocleidomastoid. The dissection is first lateral to the jugular vein, which is retracted medially. The prescalene fat pad is entered and the scalenus anticus exposed. The subclavian artery may be isolated behind the scalenus anticus (second portion) or lateral to it (third portion) if a bypass is planned. In the first case, the phrenic nerve is isolated from the surface of the latter and, after division of the scalenus anticus, the subclavian artery is exposed. The site chosen for anastomosis of the bypass is usually lateral to the thyrocervical trunk. Alternatively, the subclavian artery may be exposed in the third segment without dividing the scalenus anticus muscle.

The dissection is then moved medial to the jugular vein and the common carotid artery is exposed. A suitable site is selected for the anastomosis of the graft to the carotid artery. In the case of carotosubclavian bypass for subclavian steal, the vein graft or prosthetic tube is anastomosed to the side wall of the carotid artery and then passed under the jugular vein into proximity of the subclavian artery (Fig. 32–2). Both anastomoses are end to side.

If the bypass is intended to revascularize the common carotid artery, the subclavian artery anastomosis is done first and the graft is then tunneled under the jugular vein and anastomosed end to end to the common carotid artery or to the bifurcation (Fig. 32–3), ligating the proximal carotid stump. Another alternative is to do an end-to-side anastomosis to the common carotid artery and ligate the common carotid artery immediately proximal to the anastomosis, which makes it functionally an end-to-end anastomotic junction. This is necessary to avoid proximal embolization from the proximal common carotid artery or extension of the thrombus from there into the distal common carotid artery.

Other than in cases of common carotid artery occlusion the bypass technique between the carotid and subclavian arteries is seldom used. The transposition of one of these vessels into the other (Fig. 32–4) is a better surgical solution in that only one artery-to-artery anastomosis is necessary. The long-term patency rates are superb. The drawbacks are some increased technical difficulty and the

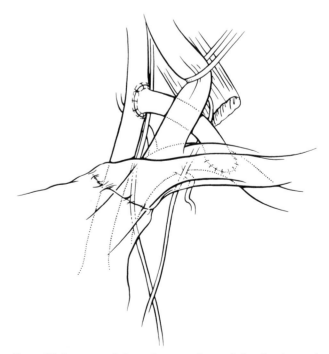

Figure 32–2. Carotosubclavian bypass graft tunneled under the jugular vein.

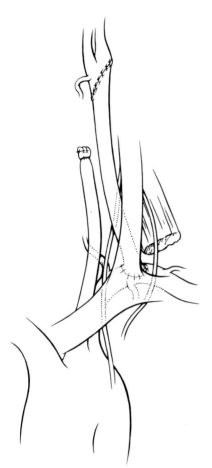

Figure 32–3. A bypass from the left subclavian artery to the left carotid bifurcation.

possibility of mediastinal bleeding from improper handling of the stump of the left subclavian artery. The transposition operation is particularly easy when the common carotid artery is the one being transposed; once freed, the common carotid, which has no branches, moves about the neck with ease. The translocation of the subclavian artery into the common carotid may be difficult on the left side, where the subclavian artery may have a deep location and where the vertebral artery may take a low origin. In cases in which this low origin interferes with good proximal control of the short first portion of the subclavian, we have divided both the vertebral artery at its origin and the subclavian artery low in the neck (distal to it) and reimplanted the subclavian artery into the common carotid artery and, separately, the vertebral artery into either one of the two vessels. When transposing the subclavian artery, care must be taken to assure proper position of the vertebral artery in the planned anastomosis. Excessive length in the vertebral artery, once the subclavian artery is freed and moved upward, may cause kinking of this vessel and its thrombosis. Although some have advocated division of the left internal mammary artery to facilitate the transposition, we believe this to be unwise, because it negates the possibility of a later myocardial revascularization using the internal mammary artery.

Subclaviosubclavian Bypass

The incision is supraclavicular on both sides, and the second or third portions of the subclavian are approached in the manner described earlier. The tunnel connecting the two subclavian arteries is made behind the sternocleidomastoid, staying as low as possible to protect the graft behind the upper edge of the manubrium. Care is taken to avoid any axial rotation of the graft when tunneling across the neck.

Axilloaxillary Bypass

The axillary arteries are exposed between the sternal and clavicular heads of the pectoralis major. Removal of part or all of the pectoralis minor from the coracoid process improves exposure of the axillary artery. The graft is tunneled under the sternal part of the pectoralis major and through presternal subcutaneous tissue into the opposite axillary artery (Fig. 32–5). Both anastomoses are end to side.

Carotocarotid Bypass

This technique is used to revascularize a common carotid artery whose origin in the mediastinum is involved by disease. One carotid acts as donor vessel to the other. Because exposure of the common carotid arteries is a reasonably simple procedure, carotocarotid bypass is a good technique to revascularize one common carotid trunk when the other one is healthy and the ipsilateral subclavian artery is not suitable as a donor vessel. The bypass between both common carotid arteries lies low in the midline, partially

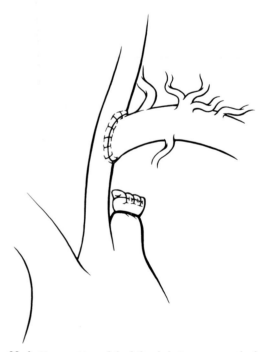

Figure 32–4. Transposition of the left subclavian artery to the left common carotid artery.

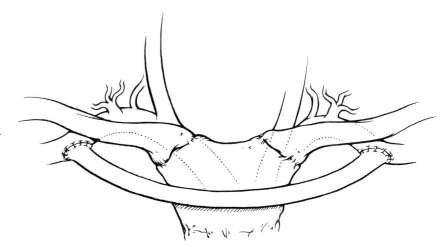

Figure 32–5. An axilloaxillary bypass.

hidden by the upper edge of the manubrium. Although these grafts make a rather lengthy loop and take off from the donor site at an oblique angle, their patency rate is excellent, provided the donor vessel is free of disease. These bypasses are sometimes cosmetically poor and, as mentioned previously, the grafts run a lengthy trajectory to link two vessels that anatomically are only four finger-breadths apart. We prefer to run the bypass between both carotids through the retropharyngeal space (Fig. 32–6), which is a much shorter and therefore better path. The tunnel for the bypass is behind the pharynx and in front of the prevertebral lamina. This space is loose and admits easily a good-sized prosthesis without any pharyngeal compression.[6]

The distance between both carotids in the retropharyngeal space is short enough that it permits the direct reimplantation of one carotid into the other without a graft (Fig. 32–7). This procedure has the disadvantage of requiring clamping of both common carotid arteries simultaneously, and because of this, it is one of the few instances in which the protection of a shunt may be required to perfuse a clamped (donor) common carotid artery.

Axial Repairs

Endarterectomy was the first technique reported in reconstruction of the innominate artery[7]; it was later formally described and perfected by Wylie and his group.[8] Innominate endarterectomy has the appeal of being a true anatomic reconstruction and of avoiding the need for a pros-

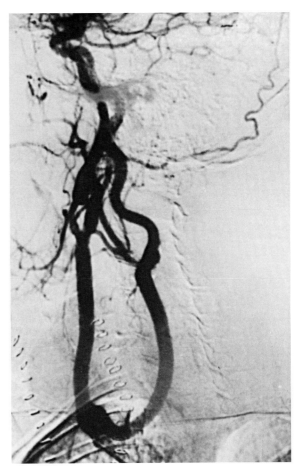

Figure 32–7. A direct transposition of the left carotid artery to the right common carotid artery using the retropharyngeal route. (From Berguer R: The short retropharyngeal route for arterial bypasses across the neck. Ann Vasc Surg 1:127–129, 1986.)

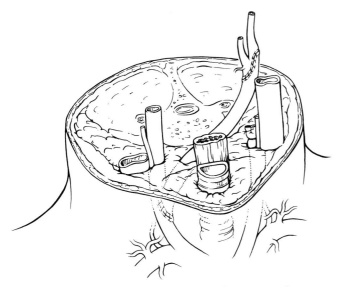

Figure 32–6. Cross-section of the neck showing the trajectory of a caroto-carotid bypass through the retropharyngeal space.

thesis. Its main drawback is the difficulty of clamping the origin of the innominate artery without occluding the left common carotid artery or damaging the plaque that may be present about the ostium of the latter. A common origin for the innominate and left common carotid is present in 17% of individuals. In addition, the left common carotid artery is a branch of the innominate in another 8% of individuals. In either of these two instances, a clamp placed at the origin of the innominate artery results in severe hemispheric ischemia. When an innominate endarterectomy is done in a patient who has a common ostium for the innominate and left common carotid arteries, a temporary shunt from the ascending aorta to the left common carotid artery is mandatory. Additional difficulties may be encountered in terminating satisfactorily the endarterectomy in the aortic wall, where tacking sutures are often required. Finally, about half of the patients we see with symptomatic innominate artery stenosis have severe lesions of either the left common carotid or left subclavian artery. These concomitant lesions cannot be treated by endarterectomy using the transsternal approach.

We prefer to use a bypass from the ascending aorta to correct innominate and other associated lesions that may be present. The technique of bypass from the ascending aorta was introduced by DeBakey and associates.[9]

The approach to the vessels in the mediastinum is through a midsternotomy (Fig. 32–8). If the right carotid needs to be reached, the sternotomy is prolonged through a short incision that follows the right anterior edge of

the sternocleidomastoid. After dividing the sternum, the innominate vein is dissected and the thymic veins are ligated. The thymus is separated through its midline. The thymus must be preserved to be used as tissue interposed between the graft and the sternum at the time of closure. The ascending aorta is approached below the innominate vein, opening the pericardial sac. The dissection continues over the origin of the innominate artery and onto its bifurcation. During dissection of the innominate bifurcation, care is taken not to injure the recurrent nerve near the origin of the right subclavian artery.

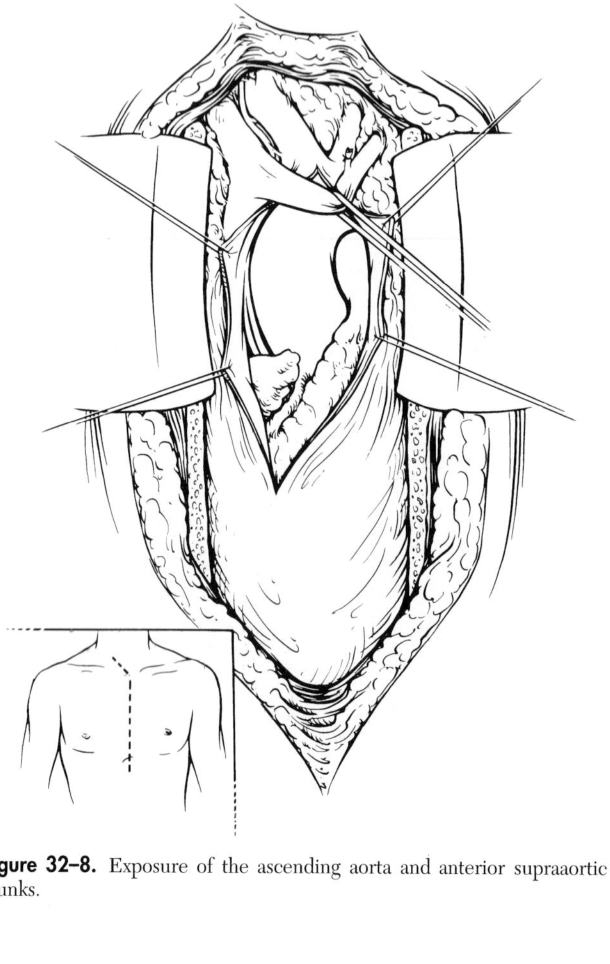

Partial Midsternotomy

Today, we prefer to approach the anterior SATs through a ministernotomy, which involves only the upper three sternal segments. The manubrium is divided down to the interspace between its third and fourth segments. At that point, a small notch toward the right with the oscillating saw results in a subperiosteal fracture when the sternal spreader is placed. If the right carotid system is to be approached, we make a small prolongation of the midline incision that follows the anterior edge of the sternal mastoid upward for about 2 inches.

The advantages of this midsternotomy is that the chest cage remains stable in its lower half, postoperative pain is noticeably reduced, and the chances for sternal instability are lessened.

Bypass from the Ascending Aorta

If the intent is to replace the innominate artery with a bypass, the first inch of the right subclavian and right common carotid arteries is exposed. More often, however, one and sometimes both carotid bifurcations need to be exposed to be revascularized. This is done by dissecting anterior to the sternocleidomastoid in the same manner as is done for a carotid endarterectomy. After obtaining control of the right subclavian and common carotid arteries, an appropriate prosthetic tube is selected for the bypass. We use a 10-mm polytetrafluoroethylene (PTFE) or Dacron fabric tube; it matches the caliber of the innominate artery, requires only a moderate amount of aortic wall to be excluded, and does not occupy much space in the anterior mediastinum.

The proximal end of the prosthesis is beveled, and the patient is prepared for exclusion clamping of the proximal aorta. Secure clamping requires the use of nitroglycerin to reduce the systemic pressure to about 110 mm Hg systolic. The exclusion clamp is placed on the proximal aorta (Fig. 32–9). With the clamp secured, the aorta is opened, and the beveled end of the graft is anastomosed to the ascending aortotomy with continuous 3–0 polypropylene suture. To avoid air embolization, the patient is then placed in the Trendelenburg position and, with the distal end of the graft pinched between the fingers, the proximal anastomosis is vented and tested. If found satisfactory, a proximal clamp is placed immediately above the anastomosis, and the table is returned to the horizontal position.

The patient is then systemically heparinized. Occluding

Figure 32–8. Exposure of the ascending aorta and anterior supraaortic trunks.

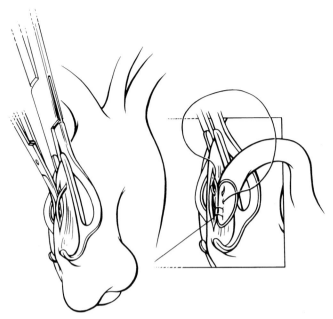

Figure 32–9. Exclusion clamping of the ascending aorta and anastomosis of the main prosthesis to the aortotomy.

clamps are placed first in the proximal right carotid and subclavian arteries and in the proximal portion of the innominate artery. The innominate artery is divided proximal to its bifurcation and prepared for anastomosis. The bypass graft, which runs over the innominate vein, is cut to appropriate length and anastomosed to the innominate artery with continuous 5–0 polypropylene suture. The graft and the distal vessels are bled before completing the anastomosis, and flow is reestablished first into the right subclavian and then into the right common carotid artery. The proximal stump of the innominate artery is closed with a continuous double running suture and an additional proximal ligature.

In those cases in which additional arteries need to be revascularized (usually the left common carotid), an additional 8-mm PTFE or Dacron side branch is anastomosed at an appropriate angle to the 10-mm main prosthesis after the proximal suture line is completed. Adding side branches as needed before the distal anastomosis is done avoids having to reclamp the innominate portion of the bypass after having established flow through it. With the side branch anastomosed and excluded, one can maintain perfusion in the right carotid (and vertebral) artery while the left carotid anastomosis is being done (Fig. 32–10).

In multiple replacements of the SATs, the main bypass is the one supplying the right-sided trunk (innominate or right carotid and right subclavian). From this trunk emerge the branches supplying the left carotid or left subclavian artery or both (Fig. 32–11).

Innominate Endarterectomy

The technique of endarterectomy of the innominate artery requires a midsternotomy and the same approach to the ascending aorta described previously. The innominate ar-

tery is dissected. The innominate vein crosses the innominate artery and is retracted either superiorly or inferiorly to provide the best exposure. The patient is systemically heparinized and the carotid and subclavian clamps are placed first. A J clamp is placed about the origin of the innominate artery, taking care not to involve the origin of the left common carotid artery in this exclusion clamping (Fig. 32–12). Enough rim of the aortic wall surrounding the origin of the innominate artery is included in the exclusion clamp to be able to properly terminate the endarterectomy and, as is often necessary, tack the edge of the intima to the aortic arch wall after removing the plaque. The endarterectomy plane is most obvious in the midportion of the innominate artery and should be at the level of the internal elastic membrane (superficial). Sometimes, the endarterectomy has to be carried out beyond the bifurcation of the innominate artery and into one of its branches because of ostial lesions at the origin of the subclavian or common carotid arteries.

The closure of the arteriotomy may require a patch. Before the closure is completed, the patient is placed in the Trendelenburg position, the distal and proximal arteries are bled into the wound, and flow is reestablished by removing first the subclavian, then the aortic, and finally the common carotid clamp.

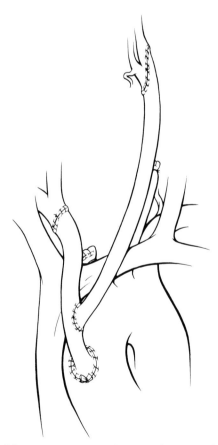

Figure 32–10. A common pattern for revascularization of the anterior supraaortic trunks (SATs): the main prosthetic (10-mm) replaces the innominate artery, and an 8-mm side branch supplies the left carotid system.

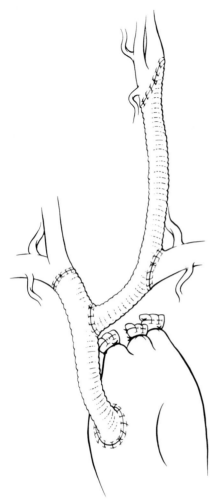

Figure 32–11. Revascularization of all three supraaortic trunks completed by transposing the left subclavian to the prosthetic that replaces the left carotid system.

Results and Complications of Reconstruction of the Supraaortic Trunks

Transthoracic reconstructions are generally done in younger patients with multiple vessel involvement. Cervical repairs are done in older patients, less likely to tolerate a thoracotomy, who have single-vessel disease.

Comparing the results of the thoracic and cervical approach in the experience published in the literature is difficult because the groups of patients for whom a transthoracic or a cervical repair are advised are different. In addition to age and anatomic extent of disease, other considerations weigh in the choice of the approach, such as pulmonary function, previous coronary artery bypass surgery, and life expectancy.

Our experience with reconstruction of the SATs from 1982 to 1998 encompasses 282 cases, including 182 cervical repairs and 100 transthoracic repairs (Table 32–1). The most frequent indication for a cervical repair in our practice is previous myocardial revascularization or single-trunk disease (carotid or subclavian artery). Innominate artery lesions are operated on through the chest.

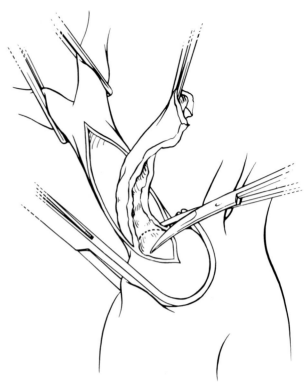

Figure 32–12. Endarterectomy of the innominate artery ends proximally at the level of the aortic arch. The intima of the latter is later affixed to the endarterectomized wall of the innominate artery by a continuous monofilament suture to avoid retrograde dissection when flow is reestablished.

Operative mortality for transthoracic repair may range from 3% to 19%,[10, 11] with most authors reporting series of 20 to 40 patients and some smaller series reporting no mortality.[12] Increasing experience, refinement in anesthesia and perioperative care, and better patient selection have brought down the mortality of transthoracic repair from 10% to 5% in the reports from the Baylor group[11, 12] and from 10% to 3.8% from the first to the second half of our experience.

In the literature, the mortality for cervical repairs has been considered lower than for thoracic repairs and has been reported between 0% and 4%. In our series, the stroke and TIA morbidity in patients undergoing cervical repair has been 3.8%. These patients undergoing cervical repair are among the highest risk patients in the group with cerebrovascular disease. Patients who have had previous myocardial revascularization procedures and those with severe pulmonary disease are more likely to undergo a cervical operation.

TABLE 32–1

Repair of Supraaortic Trunks

	PERIOD	NO. OF PATIENTS	TIA/STROKE (%)	DEATHS (%)
Cervical	1982–1998	182	3.8	0.5
Thoracic	1981–1996	100	8.0	8.0

TIA, transient ischemic attack.

The higher morbidity shown in our earlier experience with cervical reconstructions dropped dramatically. Over the last decade, we have switched operative techniques and noted a fall in operative complications and an increase in patency rates. Whereas a decade ago we often did subclaviocarotid and carotosubclavian grafts, today, most of these reconstructions are done by direct transposition of one vessel to the other. The improvement in patency rates and the decrease in reoperations has been substantial. The patency rate for transposition procedures has been 100%.

Likewise, the techniques for transthoracic reconstruction have been refined and extended. Endarterectomy of the innominate artery is a rare operation. In addition, we attempt to revascularize the left subclavian artery in patients who may later be candidates for myocardial revascularization. In the last 8 years, the mortality and morbidity of cervical and transthoracic repair have been almost equal. This may be a reflection of our selection of patients, which has changed. Table 32–1 shows the incidence of death and stroke after cervical and transthoracic repair in our entire series.

The most frequent and serious complication reported after either cervical or transthoracic repair of the SATs is myocardial infarction.[5, 13] The second most frequent complication is stroke, which may develop during the operation or after 3 to 4 days. The latter may be hemorrhagic and is probably related to hyperperfusion and regional hypertension. In our experience, stroke has been a more frequent complication than myocardial infarction. Perioperative strokes are more common in patients with multiple intra- and extracranial involvement.[11] Some may be due to technical mishaps resulting in distal embolization. Clamping time ischemia may be the cause of some operative strokes, and the usual cerebral protection methods have been reported by different authors. We do not use shunts in repair of SATs, with the rare exception listed under the description of carotocarotid bypass and in the rare patient with a left carotid arising as a branch of the innominate in whom an endarterectomy of the latter is indicated. In the latter case, we use a temporary aorto–left carotid shunt.

Technical problems may cause peri- or postoperative bleeding, which can be severe and life-threatening. Suture line bleeding, aortic wall tears from clamp or suture injury, and bleeding from a ligated arterial stump may result in serious operative bleeding or severe mediastinal compression postoperatively.

Postoperative graft thrombosis and infections are rare. The long-term outcome of these patients is largely determined by their atherosclerotic disease. Ten-year survival is approximately 50%[13–15] for both groups, cervical and transthoracic repairs. Myocardial infarction is the most common cause of death during follow-up.

The long-term patency of these reconstructions is excellent.[14] Cumulative primary patency rates at 10 years are 82% and 88% for cervical and thoracic repairs.[16, 17] Transpositions, however, have the best patency rate of all cervical repairs, which has been 100% in our series. Saphenous veins fare worse than synthetics in cervical repairs; axial rotation, caliber mismatch, kinking, and intimal hyperplasia probably account for this.

In conclusion, cervical reconstruction is indicated in patients who have had previous myocardial revascularization and in those with single lesions of the common carotid or subclavian arteries. In this last group, our preference today is to use transposition techniques between the carotid or subclavian or, if the midline needs to be crossed, a retropharyngeal bypass. These techniques using short (retropharyngeal) bypasses or no bypasses at all have outstanding patency rates that contrast with the poor patency rates reported for the conventional "extra-anatomic" bypasses. The transthoracic approach is favored for patients with multiple-vessel disease. It may be done in conjunction with coronary artery bypass grafts. This approach should be confined to centers with experience in these techniques, where the operative mortality is similar to that obtained in cervical repairs.[14]

RECONSTRUCTION OF THE VERTEBROBASILAR SYSTEM

Two types of vertebral artery reconstructions are done: reconstructions of its proximal segment for stenosing disease of the ostium and distal vertebral reconstructions for compression or thrombosis of the intraspinal portion of this artery.

Reconstruction of the Proximal Vertebral Artery

Although the first reconstructions of the vertebral arteries were endarterectomies,[18–20] this technique is seldom used today. Vertebral artery bypass was advocated in the 1970s.[21] Today, most proximal vertebral artery lesions are dealt with by transposition[22] of the artery into the neighboring common carotid artery. The appeal of this operation is that it consists of one anastomosis and does not require a vein graft (needed for bypass) or dissection of the subclavian artery (needed for endarterectomy) (Fig. 32–13).

The operation is done through a supraclavicular incision. The approach is between the bellies of the sternocleidomastoid muscles. The vertebral artery is isolated below the vertebral vein, dissected from its origin up to the point where it disappears under the longus colli, and freed from the overlying sympathetic ganglion or crossing sympathetic fibers. After clearing the adventitia of the chosen transposition site in the posterolateral wall of the common carotid artery, the patient is heparinized and the vertebral artery is divided above the stenotic area, with its proximal stump. The distal segment of the artery is swung into the common carotid artery (Fig. 32–14). A small arteriostomy is made in the common carotid wall with an aortic punch, and the vertebral artery is translocated to this orifice in end-to-side fashion using 6–0 or 7–0 polypropylene suture and an open-type anastomosis.

In a few instances, this technique is not possible. The most common problems encountered are a contralateral common or internal carotid artery occlusion or a short first segment of the vertebral artery entering the cervical spine through the transverse process of C-7 rather than that of C-6. In the first instance, when the opposite common or internal carotid artery is occluded, clamping of the re-

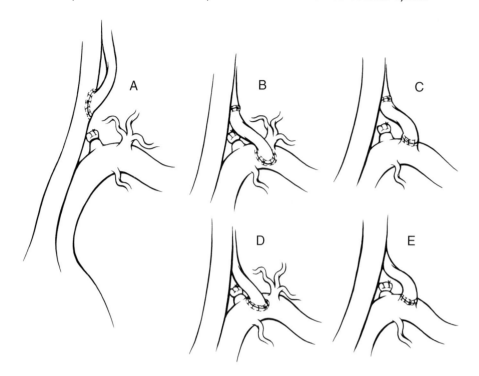

Figure 32–13. Common techniques for reconstruction of the proximal vertebral artery. *A*, Transposition of the proximal vertebral artery to the common carotid artery. *B*, Bypass from the subclavian to the proximal vertebral artery. *C*, Subclaviovertebral bypass taking origin in the amputated stump of the thyrocervical trunk. *D*, Transposition of the vertebral artery to another subclavian site. *E*, Transposition of the vertebral artery to the stump of the thyrocervical trunk.

maining ipsilateral common carotid artery to transpose the vertebral artery to it carries severe risk of brain ischemia. In this situation, a subclavian-to-vertebral bypass is preferred. If the vertebral artery is too short to be brought easily to the common carotid artery wall, it can also be bypassed from the subclavian artery with use of a saphenous vein graft.[21] The bypass takes origin from the subclavian artery lateral to the thyrocervical trunk and is anastomosed end to end to the vertebral artery below the longus colli muscle. This procedure does not require any type

of shunting. The most frequent complications are partial Horner's syndrome from manipulation (or injury) of the intermediate or stellate ganglia overlying the vertebral artery and an occasional lymphocele from injury to, or inappropriate ligature of, the main or accessory thoracic ducts.

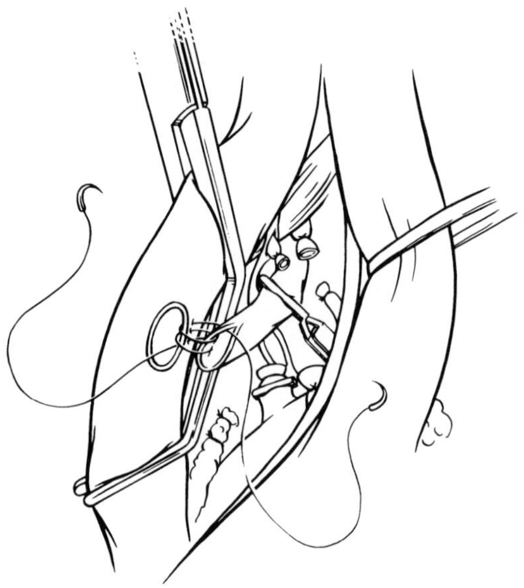

Reconstruction of the Distal Vertebral Artery

Regardless of the level below C-2 at which the external compression or the occlusive process takes place, the distal vertebral artery is reconstructed at the space between the C-1 and C-2 transverse processes. This is the widest gap between transverse processes in the neck and is also the segment where the vertebral artery is often maintained patent by collaterals from the occipital artery, even though the proximal segment of the artery may be occluded.[23, 24]

The operation is done through an incision similar to that used for carotid endarterectomy. Exposure of the vertebral artery at this level requires dissecting posterior to the jugular vein and identifying the spinal accessory nerve and the levator scapulae muscle. The levator is cut and the transverse course of the anterior ramus of the C-2 nerve is exposed. The artery lies below the ramus and is perpendicular to it. The ramus is cut and the artery is exposed. Dissection of the vertebral artery is made difficult by the plexus of veins that surrounds it.

Once the artery is isolated (Fig. 32–15), it can be reconstructed in several ways. The classic reconstruction is a bypass from the common carotid artery to the distal vertebral artery immediately below the transverse process of C-1 using autogenous vein (Fig. 32–16). This requires dissection of the common carotid below the bifurcation and the availability of a saphenous vein with a size matching that of the vertebral artery. Once the end-to-side anastomosis

Figure 32–14. Technique for transposing the left vertebral artery to the left common carotid artery. The thoracic duct is seen doubly ligated. The proximal vertebral artery stump has been clipped and suture ligated. The sympathetic chain left intact is now seen behind the distal segment of the vertebral artery as the latter is brought to the common carotid artery for its anastomosis.

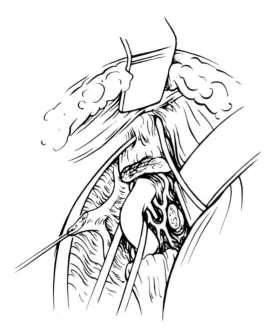

Figure 32–15. The vertebral artery is isolated between the transverse process of C1 and C2. The anterior ramus of the C2 nerve has been divided and is pulled out of the field by a stay suture. The artery has been dissected away from the surrounding vertebral plexus, which is now seen behind it.

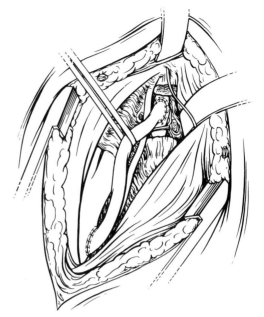

Figure 32–16. A completed common carotid to distal vertebral artery bypass graft. A metal clip occludes the distal vertebral artery immediately below the anastomosis, making the latter a functional end-to-end junction.

of the vein graft to the vertebral artery is completed, the latter is ligated immediately below the anastomosis to avoid embolization from its proximal segment.

Another alternative is to use the external carotid artery (or, in rare cases, the occipital artery) to revascularize the distal vertebral artery (Fig. 32–17). The external carotid is skeletonized and transposed below the jugular vein, anastomosing it end to end to the distal vertebral artery. The appeal of this procedure is that it does not require clamping of the internal carotid supply and that the caliber match between the distal external carotid artery and the vertebral artery is usually good. This choice obviously requires the

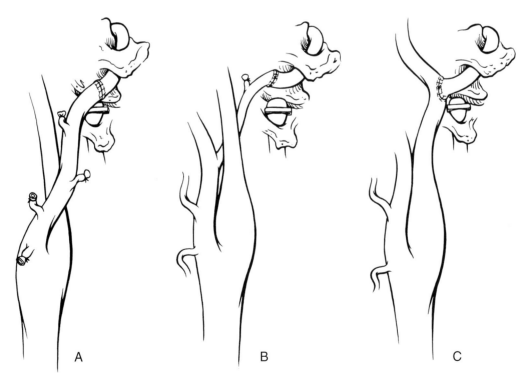

A   B   C

Figure 32–17. Alternative methods of reconstruction of the distal vertebral artery. *A,* External carotid transposition to the distal vertebral artery. *B,* Occipital artery transposition to the distal vertebral artery. *C,* Transposition of the distal vertebral artery to the distal internal carotid artery.

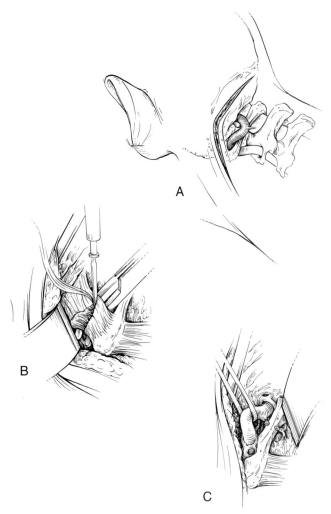

Figure 32–18. *A,* Incision to approach the suboccipital segment of the vertebral artery. *B,* Division of the obliquus capitis superior. *C,* The looped artery is lifted from the underlying lamina of C1. A descending muscular branch has been ligated and divided. (From Berguer R: Revascularization of the vertebral arteries. In Nyhus LM, Baker RJ, Fischer JE [eds]: Mastery of Surgery. Boston, Little, Brown, 1996.)

over the lamina of the atlas. The approach is posterior through a racquet-shaped incision, with the patient in the "park bench" position (Fig. 32–18). The semispinalis, splenius, and longus capitis muscles are cut and the sternomastoid is deinserted from the mastoid process. The transverse process of C-1 is identified and the obliquus capitis superior muscle is cut. The artery rests on the posterior lamina of the atlas covered by a dense plexus of veins and tethered by one or two muscular branches, which are divided. The vein bypass is anastomosed end to side. The distal cervical internal carotid artery can be isolated after dissecting away the vagus and hypoglossal nerve trunks that cover it posteriorly. The bypass is anastomosed end to side to the distal cervical internal carotid artery (Fig. 32–19). In some patients, the problem is extrinsic compression of the vertebral artery between the occipital ridge and the posterior lamina of C-1. In this situation, once the vertebral artery is dissected (using the suboccipital approach described earlier), a laminectomy is done. A bypass will only be needed under very rare circumstances.

Results and Complications of Reconstructions of Vertebral Arteries

The risks and patency rates of vertebral artery operations are different for proximal and distal repairs.[25] Proximal reconstructions are technically easier. Distal reconstructions are more demanding and lengthier procedures.

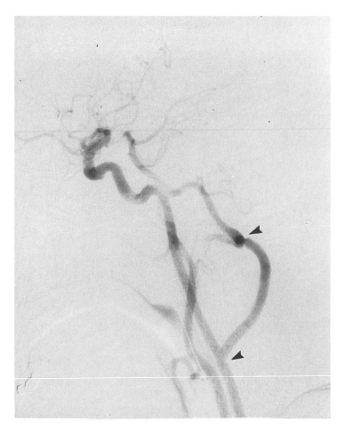

Figure 32–19. Postoperative arteriogram showing a bypass from the cervical internal carotid artery to the suboccipital vertebral artery (*arrowheads*) before its entry into the foramen magnum.

external carotid and, for that matter, the carotid bifurcation to be free of atherosclerotic disease. We have used this type of operation most often in individuals who have external compression or occlusion of the vertebral artery by osteophytes during neck rotation. These patients are generally younger and free of disease in the carotid bifurcation.

A third solution is translocation of the distal segment of the vertebral artery into the internal carotid artery by means of an end-to-side anastomosis. This, again, has the appeal of a limited dissection and the lack of need of a vein graft. The shortcoming is that one needs to clamp the internal carotid artery for the end-to-side anastomosis. This technique should not be used in patients in whom the opposite internal carotid artery is severely diseased or occluded.

A few patients have a diseased vertebral artery above the level of C-1. In these patients, the reconstruction is done in the distal-most segment of the extracranial vertebral artery before it penetrates the dura mater as it courses

Among patients undergoing isolated proximal or distal vertebral artery reconstruction, the 10-year survival rates are 84% and 82%, respectively. We have done 252 proximal vertebral artery reconstructions with a combined mortality and morbidity of 0.9%. The cumulative secondary patency rate for proximal reconstructions has been 92% at 10 years.

In 117 distal vertebral reconstructions, the combined mortality and morbidity has been 3.4%, four times higher than that found in proximal repairs. Kieffer and colleagues,[26] in a larger series, reported a 2.4% mortality. In the last 8 years, the combined morbidity and mortality rates for proximal and distal reconstructions have been 0% and 1.5%, respectively.

Postoperative thrombosis of a proximal reconstruction is rare. We have seen this complication in 3 of 252 cases. In all three cases, a short vertebral artery (entering at C-7) could not be repaired by a standard vertebral-to-carotid transposition, and subclavian-vertebral or carotid-vertebral bypass was done. In one case, tension at the anastomotic line, and in two others, a kink in an interposition vein graft, resulted in postoperative thrombosis. All patients underwent reoperation and thrombectomy, and the technical flaw was corrected. Patency remained after 3, 5, and 7 years.

Other complications of proximal reconstruction have been an occasional lymphocele and a partial Horner's syndrome from manipulation or injury to the lower cervical sympathetics. In one case of distal reconstruction, we noted an injury to the spinal accessory nerve.

Postoperative thrombosis of distal vertebral artery reconstructions has been more frequent. We have seen it in 4 of 117 distal reconstructions. The causes were faulty anastomoses or inadequate vein grafts. Thrombectomy and the insertion of a new graft reestablished patency in two of the four failures.

Presenting symptoms of vertebrobasilar ischemia have been relieved in 83% of patients.[21, 24] Among survivors, the 5-year protection rate from stroke has been 97%.

References

1. Hass WK, Fields WS, North RR, et al: Joint study of extracranial arterial occlusion, II: Arteriography, techniques, sites, and complications. JAMA 203:961–968, 1968.
2. Berguer R, Higgins RF, Nelson R: Noninvasive diagnosis of reversal of vertebral flow. N Engl J Med 301:1349–1351, 1980.
3. Caplan L, Tettenborn B: Embolism in the posterior circulation. In Berguer R, Caplan L (eds): Vertebrobasilar Arterial Disease. St. Louis, Quality Medical, 1992.
4. Lyons C, Gailbraiter G: Surgical treatment of atherosclerotic occlusion of the internal carotid artery. Ann Surg 146:487–494, 1957.
5. Criado FJ: Extrathoracic management of aortic arch syndrome. Br J Surg 69(Suppl):S45–S51, 1982.
6. Berguer R: The short retropharyngeal route for arterial bypass across the neck. Ann Vasc Surg 1:127–129, 1986.
7. David JB, Grove WJ, Julian OC: Thrombotic occlusion of the branches of the aortic arch, Martorell's syndrome: Report of a case treated surgically. Ann Surg 144:124–126, 1956.
8. Carlson RE, Ehrenfeld WK, Stoney RJ, Wylie EJ: Innominate artery endarterectomy: A 16-year experience. Arch Surg 112:1389–1393, 1977.
9. DeBakey ME, Morris GC, Jordan GL, et al: Segmental thrombo-obliterative disease of branches of aortic arch. JAMA 166:988, 1958.
10. Brewster DC, Moncure AC, Darling RC, et al: Innominate artery lesions: Problems encountered and lessons learned. J Vasc Surg 2:99–112, 1985.
11. DeBakey ME, Crawford ES, Cooley DA, et al: Surgical considerations of occlusive disease of the innominate, carotid, subclavian and vertebral arteries. Ann Surg 149:690–710, 1959.
12. Thompson BW, Read RC, Campbell GS: Operative correction of proximal blocks of the subclavian or innominate arteries. J Cardiovasc Surg (Torino) 21:125–130, 1980.
13. Crawford ES, Stowe CL, Powers RW Jr: Occlusion of the innominate, common carotid, and subclavian arteries: Long term results of surgical treatment. Surgery 94:781, 1983.
14. Zelenock GB, Cronenwett JL, Graham LM, et al: Brachiocephalic arterial occlusions and stenoses: Manifestations and management of complex lesions. Arch Surg 120:370–376, 1985.
15. Vogt DP, Hertzer NR, O'Hara PJ, et al: Brachiocephalic arterial reconstruction. Ann Surg 196:541–552, 1982.
16. Berguer R, Morasch MD, Kline RA, et al: Cervical reconstruction of the supra-aortic trunks: A 16-year experience. J Vasc Surg 29:239–248, 1999.
17. Berguer R, Morasch MD, Kline RA: Transthoracic repair of innominate and common carotid artery disease: Immediate and long-term outcome for 100 consecutive surgical reconstructions. J Vasc Surg 27:34–42, 1998.
18. Moore WS, Malone JM, Goldstone J: Extrathoracic repair of branch occlusions of the aortic arch. Am J Surg 132:249–257, 1976.
19. Cate WR, Scott HW: Cerebral ischemia of central origin: Relief by subclavian vertebral artery thromboendarterectomy. Surgery 45:19, 1959.
20. Imparato AM, Lin JPT: Vertebral artery reconstruction: Internal plication and vein patch angioplasty. Ann Surg 166:213–221, 1967.
21. Natali J, Maraval M, Kieffer E: Surgical treatment of stenosis and occlusion of the carotid and vertebral arteries. J Cardiovasc Surg (Torino) 13:4–15, 1972.
22. Berguer R, Bauer RB: Vertebral artery reconstruction: A successful technique in selected patients. Ann Surg 193:441, 1981.
23. Roon AJ, Ehrenfeld AJ, Cooke PB, et al: Vertebral artery reconstruction. Am J Surg 138:29–36, 1980.
24. Berguer R: Distal vertebral artery bypass: Technique, the "occipital connection" and potential uses. J Vasc Surg 2:621, 1985.
25. Berguer R, Flynn LM, Kline RA, Caplan L: Surgical reconstruction of the extracranial vertebral artery: Management and outcome. J Vasc Surg 31:9–18, 2000.
26. Kieffer E, Rancurel G, Richard T: Reconstruction of the distal cervical vertebral artery. In Berguer R, Bauer RB (eds): Vertebrobasilar Arterial Occlusive Disease. New York, Raven Press, 1984, p 265.

Questions

1. In patients with a retroesophageal right subclavian artery the following associated anomalies are expected or are likely to occur
   1. nonrecurrent right inferior laryngeal nerve
   2. thoracic duct emptying on the right side
   3. common trunk as origin of both common carotid arteries
   4. right vertebral artery arising from the right common carotid artery
   5. left vertebral artery arising from the left common carotid artery
      (a) 1, 3, 4, 5
      (b) 2, 3, 4, 5

    (c) 1, 2, 3, 4
    (d) all of the above

2. The most efficient operation to correct a severe stenosis of the origin of a vertebral artery is
    1. subclavian-to-vertebral-artery autogenous vein bypass
    2. transposition of vertebral artery to the common carotid artery
    3. endarterectomy and patch of the origin of the vertebral artery
    4. balloon angioplasty of the stenotic origin
    (a) 1
    (b) 2

    (c) 3
    (d) 4

3. Vertebrobasilar ischemia may be the result of
    1. a hemodynamically significant lesion of the vertebral artery
    2. a hemodynamically significant lesion of the basilar artery
    3. microembolization from a vertebral artery lesion
    4. microembolization from a subclavian artery plaque
    5. microembolization from a dissected vertebral artery
    (a) 1, 3, 4, 5
    (b) 1, 3, 5
    (c) 1, 2, 5
    (d) all of the above

Answers

1. c   2. b   3. d

33

Vascular Disease of the Upper Extremity and the Thoracic Outlet Syndromes

Herbert I. Machleder

The upper extremities are subject to a variety of unique intrinsic arterial and venous disorders, as well as the peripheral manifestations of systemic collagen vascular diseases. The extensive use of the upper extremities for venous and arterial vascular access additionally results in a host of problems requiring recognition and management by the vascular surgical specialist.

Patients developing arterial insufficiency of the upper extremities generally demonstrate one of three different clinical patterns: (1) attacks of Raynaud's disease symptoms, (2) digital ischemia and gangrene, or (3) crampy pain with exercise, often referred to (with disregard for the word origin) as claudication. The uniformity of clinical symptoms belies the multiplicity of underlying diseases, which range from relatively simple cases of trauma to complex autoimmune and connective tissue disorders. This complexity of underlying disease requires a methodical approach to ensure expeditious diagnosis and an effective therapeutic plan.

A peculiar blanching and cyanosis of the fingertips characterizes upper extremity vascular insufficiency. Raynaud put it rather succinctly in the introduction to his second treatise on vasospastic syndromes affecting the upper extremity:

> In the slight cases the ends of the fingers and toes become cold, cyanosed, and livid, and at the same time more or less painful. In grave cases the area affected by cyanosis extends upwards for several centimeters above the roots of the nails; . . . finally, if this state is prolonged for a certain time, we see gangrenous points appear on the extremities; the gangrene is always dry, and may occupy the superficial layers of the skin from the extent of a pin's head up to the end of a finger, rarely more.[1]

The initial evaluation should enable differentiation of arterial and venous obstruction, recognition of chronologic elements of obstructive phenomena (such as repetitive events versus a single isolated and progressive event), and whether the ischemic symptom is related to vasospasm or true arterial occlusion. It is also important to recognize at the outset whether the vascular manifestations in the upper extremity are symmetric, part of a generalized process, or confined to an isolated event in the affected extremity.

Raynaud's phenomenon, which is characteristic of the early onset of many types of vascular occlusive phenomena, is generally quite evident to the patient and is noticed as a blanching of a single digit, perhaps symmetrically disposed to both upper extremities, usually precipitated by a drop in temperature, which may, however, be quite slight (of only several degrees' magnitude). The blanching becomes cadaveric in appearance, and the finger becomes numb. Then within seconds to minutes—occasionally longer—the blanching is replaced by a mottled, deeply cyanotic, and ruborous appearance. The return of capillary filling is generally accompanied by dysesthesia and, occasionally, frank burning pain. The symptom may spread to other digits as time progresses and in fact may involve the entire hand unilaterally or both hands symmetrically. Occasionally, this sequence of events can be seen in traumatic situations, which, although not specifically linked to temperature changes, may well be exacerbated by exposure to cold.

VASCULAR EXAMINATION OF THE UPPER EXTREMITY

The initial examination of the upper extremity should begin with *inspection* for color changes; areas of gangrene; discoloration such as blanching, cyanosis, and livido reticularis; or areas of erythema. A note should be made of abnormal distention of veins, particularly related to positional changes of the upper extremity. Ordinarily, prominent veins on the dorsum of the hand and antecubital fossa should be flat as the arms reach the cardiac position. Observation of marked collateral vessels, particularly around the shoulder, should be noted, particularly if they are asymmetric. When venous obstruction is suspected, measurement of recumbent venous pressure in an antecubital vein can be easily done with a spinal manometer filled with saline.

Palpation should follow inspection, involve the carotid arteries bilaterally, and look for prominent pulsations in the supraclavicular area, as well as assess the axillary, brachial, radial, and ulnar pulses. The Allen test should be performed routinely in assessing the arterial competence of the palmar arch. The test is performed in the following manner, evaluating one hand at a time. With the patient facing the examiner, palmar surface of the hand up, both the radial and ulnar arteries are compressed. The examiner's thumb is placed on the arteries, and the remaining digits are placed along the back of the patient's wrist. The arteries are compressed while the patient clenches his or her fist to evacuate blood from the hand. When the hand is opened, the palm has a pale, mottled appearance. Radial artery compression is released first, whereupon prompt color or even reactive hyperemia should appear on the entire palmar surface of the hand. In the presence of radial artery occlusion, the pallor remains and mottling continues. When there is insufficient collateral flow across the palmar arch, only the radial portion of the hand will be perfused, and the ulnar part of the hand will remain blanched and mottled. When the ulnar artery is then released, color will return to the ulnar aspect of the hand. The examiner next repeats the test by compressing the radial and ulnar artery with the thumbs while the patient clenches his or her hand and then opens it, revealing the blanched, mottled appearance. Compression is then released from the ulnar artery, and again, if normal, prompt blushing of the hand or even reactive hyperemia should occur. In the event of ulnar artery occlusion, the hand remains white and mottled; if there is insufficient collateral circulation across the palmar arch, perfusion of only the ulnar aspect of the hand will be apparent. The test is then repeated on the contralateral extremity. When properly performed, this test is extremely accurate, with a high degree of sensitivity and specificity.

Auscultation is an important part of upper extremity examination and should begin in the supraclavicular fossa. Subclavian bruits often begin just lateral to the palpable carotid pulse at the base of the neck and radiate toward the acromioclavicular joint and below the middle third of the clavicle toward the axilla. Auscultation should be done bilaterally with the arm in the neutral position and then with Adson's maneuver. Auscultation should then be performed with the diaphragm of the stethoscope placed just beneath the middle third of the clavicle as the arm is gradually brought into the abducted and externally rotated position. This is done while the examiner palpates the radial pulse, and if obliteration of the radial pulse occurs, careful auscultation should then be augmented by moving the stethoscope laterally in the infraclavicular area, then medially in the supraclavicular area in an attempt to detect any site of compressive occlusion. Bruits in this area are typically obliterated over a few degrees of the abduction

and external rotation arc, and the maneuver must be performed slowly so that the point of maximum bruit can be ascertained. Placing the arm in a full abducted and externally rotated position may totally obliterate the pulse, and the bruit may be overlooked.

The bell and diaphragm of the stethoscope should be used to auscultate over any abnormal group of veins or angiomatous malformation. Arteriovenous fistulas are often identified in this manner, and this technique is highly accurate in identifying this type of lesion.

VASCULAR LABORATORY DIAGNOSIS

Noninvasive vascular testing can be used to further document disorders that may be suggested by symptoms or subtle physical findings. The systolic pressure should be measured at the brachial artery and at the radial or ulnar artery with the patient supine and the arm in the neutral position. This is done by placing the blood pressure cuff around the upper arm in a manner identical to that used in assessing the standard blood pressure, with auscultation for Korotkoff sounds. During the vascular examination, the clinician uses the Doppler flow detector to assess the exact point of initiation of systolic flow. The flow detector is placed over the antecubital brachial artery, and the pressure cuff is inflated until arterial signals are obliterated. Pressure is slowly released, and the pressure is noted when the initial thumping arterial sound resumes (Fig. 33–1). By doing this first over the brachial artery and then over the radial and ulnar arteries with the cuff moved to the forearm, segmental pressures can be recorded that may further indicate a site of obstruction, if this should be the case. If thoracic outlet obstruction is a possibility, the test should be repeated with the patient in the sitting position. It is difficult to elicit vascular compressive signs of thoracic outlet compression when the patient is recumbent.

The sensitivity of all tests must be well recognized by the examiner, and it should be specifically understood that reductions of cross-sectional area in an artery less than 75% or reductions of cross-sectional diameter less than 50% rarely result in a pressure drop unless specific measures are used to reduce peripheral resistance and increase flow rates (such as reactive hyperemia or specific ergometric testing).

A specific and detailed history of positional characteristics that bring on symptoms of arterial or venous obstruc-

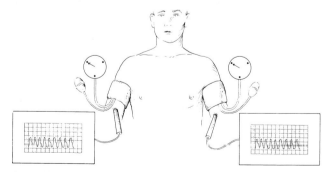

Figure 33–1. Use of the Doppler flow detector for the determination of brachial artery pressures.

tion must be documented and these positions used when a variety of arterial and venous tests are performed. The extensive collateralization of the upper extremity may lead to a paucity of signs and symptoms in the patient at rest in the face of severe disability when specific muscle groups are called on during work or recreational activity.

As in the lower extremity, the more distal the obstruction (especially in the presence of tandem lesions), the more severe the pressure drop appreciated peripherally. Occasionally, differences of up to 15 mm Hg between the two upper extremities may be within the normal range and can be accounted for by the extreme sensitivity of the upper extremity vessels to sympathetic innervation and minute changes in peripheral resistance. In general, an occlusion at the level of the subclavian artery results in a pressure drop of between 30 and 40 mm Hg. When evaluating upper extremity pressures that are symmetric, particularly in the face of other evidence of vascular insufficiency, an ankle-brachial index should be assessed in an attempt to recognize symmetric occlusions of the major aortic branches, as may occur in some varieties of arteritis. When suspicion is high, oculopneumoplethysmography can also be used in an attempt to assess the true central arterial pressure in the event of symmetric subclavian occlusive disease.

The presence of an abnormal Allen test on the initial examination should always be further assessed by measuring segmental pressures with the probe placed over the radial as well as the ulnar artery in an attempt to establish the level of occlusive disease. In more sophisticated testing, small finger cuffs can be used to assess individual digital artery pressures. This can be done either with a Doppler flow probe or with a mercury strain gauge or digital photoplethysmograph.

The significant reactivity of the digital vessels to sympathetic stimulation should alert the examiner to changes in ambient temperature as well as changes in the patient's apprehension during the examination. Insensitivity to these factors may often give rise to results that in retrospect become difficult to interpret. Furthermore, many individuals have a dramatic response to smoking, which may last from 1 to 8 hours after even a single cigarette. Before embarking on these sensitive arterial evaluations, the history of recent smoking must be noted.

Digital plethysmography can be useful in differentiating proximal from distal arterial obstructive phenomena, and the effect of reactive hyperemia on the pulse wave pattern also differentiates primary Raynaud's disease from Raynaud's phenomenon, which is associated with collagen vascular diseases. When vasodilatation is effected, either by immersing the hand in warm water or applying a cuff to maintain ischemia for 5 minutes, patients with primary vasospastic syndromes demonstrate a normal return of pulse volume and curve characteristics. Those with collagen diseases, however, have vascular obstructive phenomena secondary to intimal proliferation or deposition of immune complexes and fixed lesions that demonstrate minimal, if any, change after reactive hyperemia. These tests are extremely useful in assessing the potential response to vasodilating or sympatholytic therapies.[2]

In addressing the upper extremity arterial circulation, the examiner should become familiar with normal and abnormal Doppler signals, which are obtained from peripheral vessels. The ordinary signal is described as triphasic but can be appreciated only by assiduous listening to establish a good baseline for recognition. Although tracings can be subjected to more sophisticated analysis, this should rarely be necessary in all but the most extensive of upper extremity vascular evaluations. The normal high-frequency short burst of systolic flow, followed by a short, low-pitched diastolic component, is easily recognized and can be detected in other peripheral vessels that clinically do not seem involved in the disease process. The abnormal flow sound is usually described as monophasic, of lower frequency and longer duration, and more undulant in quality. At times, it approaches the venous signal, which can be used as a reference. Segmental auscultation with the Doppler flowmeter can often reveal the site of obstruction without more sophisticated testing.

The need for sequential performance of these tests cannot be overemphasized, because Allen's test often identifies an obstruction in the radial or ulnar artery, whereas nondirectional Doppler assessment may reveal a relatively normal flow pattern in both vessels. The flow, however, may well be reversed in the obstructed vessel because of the extensive collateralization across the palmar arch. It should be quite obvious that Allen's test, although based on a visual interpretation, can be further documented by performance using the Doppler flow detector to assess signal changes during compression.

Some specific noninvasive assessment procedures aid in the diagnosis of *venous obstruction*. The presence of swelling should be documented by segmental girth measurements. Occasionally, there is distention of the superficial veins and mild cyanosis. Patient complaints generally are of heaviness and pressure or a distensive feeling with exercise. Although venous collateral vessels develop rapidly and extensively, symptoms abate slowly, if at all, and are particularly exacerbated by exercise (Fig. 33–2). Edema, present from primary lymphatic obstruction, may occasionally be difficult to differentiate from venous obstruction but often

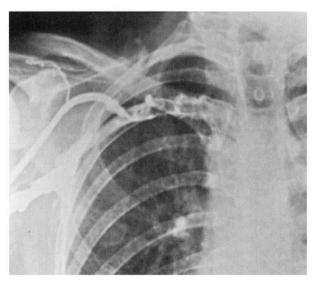

Figure 33–2. Axillosubclavian vein thrombosis characteristic of Paget-Schroetter syndrome or effort thrombosis variant of thoracic outlet compression syndrome. Note the collateral vessels and intraluminal thrombus.

can be clarified by measurement of antecubital vein pressures using the saline-filled manometer.

Flow in the upper extremity is paradoxically related to venous flow in the lower extremity, and this fact must be kept in mind when assessing upper extremity venous outflow. Often, outflow in the upper extremities is decreased with deep inspiration related to changes in intrathoracic pressure. The upper extremity venous return tends to be more pulsatile than that demonstrated in the lower extremities. Velocity changes in the antecubital and axillary veins can be assessed with the Doppler flowmeter, much as they can in the lower extremities when these important differences are kept in mind.

Surgically constructed arteriovenous fistulas are dealt with in more detail in Chapter 34. However, several characteristics should be appreciated, referable to the previously described examinations. The arterial flow distal to a surgically constructed arteriovenous fistula may well be retrograde in the artery distal to the fistula. Additionally, flow in the distal vein of a side-to-side arteriovenous fistula is commonly reversed so that the flow is traveling in a distal direction. Dramatic augmentation of flow is appreciated in the donor artery to the arteriovenous fistula. Compression of the fistula generally restores normal flow patterns in the distal, arterial, and venous vessels.[3]

SMALL VESSEL OCCLUSION IN THE UPPER EXTREMITY

Gangrene of the digits of the upper extremity is most often secondary to small arterial occlusive disease. Nevertheless, in somewhat less than half of the patients with this presentation, a proximally obstructing or embolizing lesion can be found and must be looked for carefully. A majority of these gangrenous manifestations are due to occlusions of the proper digital vessels or of major vessels of the palmar arch. In ascertaining the underlying cause of these small arterial occlusions, one must take into account a host of local phenomena as well as a large array of systemic diseases that may have other manifestations but that appear primarily with digital gangrene. Digital gangrene is rarely associated with primary Raynaud's disease, and an underlying occlusive process generally will be identified if a meticulous evaluation is undertaken.

The so-called group of *collagen vascular diseases* manifest themselves by deposition of immune complexes in the intimal and subintimal surfaces of small vessels. Additionally, obliterative proliferative processes characterize selective diseases such as scleroderma and diabetes. The fact that digital ischemia may precede systemic manifestations of these diseases adds to the difficulty of the initial diagnosis and emphasizes the need for a logical approach, which may have to be repeated on occasion during the evolution of a patient's disease.[4, 5] Certain patients with digital ischemia may be subject to hypersensitivity associated with increase in circulating catecholamines or release of other humeral elements (e.g., prostaglandins, serotonin). These manifestations have been reviewed by Bauer and associates.[6] The response to cigarette smoking, particularly in men who have been suspected of suffering from Buerger's disease, is characteristic of this group of patients. The process of gangrene in the fingers is quite different from that of necrosis, which is a wet suppurative process. Fingertip gangrene is more often a process of desiccation and mummification, which was meticulously described by Raynaud.

The presence of digital gangrene in the young patient without evidence of atherosclerosis or aneurysmal disease, and particularly in the presence of normal upper extremity segmental pressures, should indicate the possibility of a generalized collagen vascular disease as the most likely etiology for the digital ischemic changes. Thoracic outlet arterial compression with poststenotic dilatation and aneurysm formation is uncommon but nevertheless must be suspected. Axillobrachial aneurysms of atherosclerotic origin are extremely uncommon but must also be considered in these types of lesions. Industrial trauma, induced by the use of vibrating equipment (e.g., jackhammers, laboratory tools), or exposure to heavy metals should be investigated. Occupational exposure, such as the particular use of tools and the use of the hand in pounding, often indicates the source of the traumatic occlusion. This is particularly pertinent where the hamate process of the wrist occludes the ulnar artery in a well-described but infrequently recognized hypothenar hammer syndrome.

Many authors have emphasized that the presence of gangrene is unlikely in vasospastic disorders, and in the vast majority of cases, areas of actual digital occlusive processes are identified.

Arteriography is useful in excluding proximal lesions, although it rarely demonstrates specific changes that may be characteristic of certain of the arteritides (Fig. 33–3). The serologic tests that form the basis for the diagnostic workup in these patients include serum protein electrophoresis, cold agglutinins, rheumatoid factor, VDRL (Venereal Disease Research Laboratory), Hep2, antinuclear antibodies, antinative DNA antibodies, total hemolytic complement, extractable nuclear antibody, complement (C3,C4), immunoglobulin electrophoresis, cryoglobulin, cryofibrinogen, direct Coombs' test, HBsAb hepatitis B antibodies, and HBsAg hepatitis B antigen. In cases in which skin biopsy is performed, immunofluorescence staining is extremely helpful. Collagen vascular diseases may also be documented by plain x-ray films of the hands, which dem-

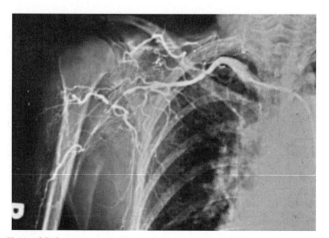

Figure 33–3. Typical pattern of axillosubclavian arterial occlusive disease seen in giant cell arteritis.

onstrate distal phalangeal tuft reabsorption and evidence of soft tissue atrophy with particular loss of pulp dimensions on the palmar surface of the distal phalanges. Evidence of skin atrophy and shiny tenseness or calcinosis of the skin are also extremely valuable diagnostic findings. When a diagnosis can be made early, scleroderma is the most common entity manifesting with digital ischemia.

A pragmatic approach to this problem is justifiable, given that the definitive diagnosis may not be made during the early periods of significant symptoms. Medical therapy should be initiated either systemically or locally. The most effective systemic medications have been methyldopa (Aldomet), reserpine, guanethidine, and phenoxybenzamine. More recently, agents such as nifedipine have been proved useful in relief of arterial spasm and associated digital ischemia.

Medical management includes avoidance of cold exposure, use of gloves, and discontinuation of tobacco use. Pharmacologic therapy for nonrelated disorders must be reviewed to eliminate medications that may aggravate peripheral vasospasm, such as propranolol or ergot preparations for migraine. Calcium channel blockers are currently the primary pharmacologic agents for the treatment of digital vasospasm, ischemia, and gangrene. Nifedipine in 10-mg doses may be used up to four to six times per day. Peripheral edema, dizziness, headache, and fatigue often limit the use of this important drug before a sustained digital effect can be achieved. Diltiazem at a dose of 30 mg twice a day, given alone or as a supplement to nifedipine, has been reported to be effective.[7]

When episodes of ischemia or Raynaud's symptoms are infrequent and do not require long-term sustained treatment, sublingual nifedipine is rapid in onset, with fewer side effects. The nongeneric drug, Procardia (Pfizer, Parsippany, NJ), must be used. The 10-mg capsule is perforated with an 18-gauge needle, and two or three drops are placed sublingually by the patient.

We avoid the use of topical antibiotics because the vehicle often leads to maceration of otherwise desiccated tissue. An occasional case of suppuration can be effectively combated with systemic antibiotics. Patients are advised to avoid cold and to use gloves during all possible episodes of exposure. During the winter, we have patients carry a camping-type pocket hand warmer for additional protection. Patients who are refractory to these therapeutic measures or whose digital ischemia is exacerbated while they are on optimal medical therapy for the systemic collagen vascular disease often respond to dorsal cervical sympathectomy. Periods of spontaneous remission are quite common, and extensive progression of these gangrenous lesions is extremely unusual, although partial digital amputation is occasionally necessary. Sympathectomy, although not demonstrably superior to conservative therapy, has the advantage of avoiding long-term exposure to potent vasodilating drugs and a host of side effects that may be associated with their use. Nevertheless, the frequent effectiveness of conservative therapy must be emphasized.

ARTERIOGRAPHY

Arteriography can be useful in the diagnosis and assessment of vascular disorders of the upper extremity, but it plays a much less prominent role than in vascular disorders of the visceral or lower extremity vessels. The transfemoral route is preferred, particularly to enable visualization of the proximal aortic vessels and to avoid the need to traverse a potentially diseased axillosubclavian vessel. Upper extremity arteriography with meglumine diatrizoate (60%) is generally perceived as painful by most patients, and premedication is useful, as is the addition of lidocaine to the angiographic solution. The use of tolazoline (Priscoline) or nitroglycerin assists in magnification views of the digital vessels, particularly when one is looking for small, clearly occlusive processes.

Proximal arterial aneurysms and atherosclerotic occlusive disease as well as ulcerating plaques are generally well identified radiographically. Thoracic outlet compression is infrequently identified, particularly when the procedure is performed with the patient in the supine position. The use of digital intravenous angiography, which allows the patient to be radiographed in the sitting position, demonstrates a much higher yield of arterial compression lesions, correlating much more closely with the clinical findings (Fig. 33–4). Arteriography and venography in the upper extremities should be performed in the neutral position, with the arm at the patient's side, and in the "stress" position, with the upper arm at right angles to the chest. We often perform the positional exposures with the patient's hand behind the head. If this is not done, many of the compressive abnormalities at the thoracic outlet are missed. This is true for both arterial and venous compressive abnormalities.

Proximal subclavian occlusion with subclavian steal phenomena and retrograde flow in the vertebral artery is easily demonstrated angiographically. This lesion should be suspected whenever there is a pressure discrepancy greater than 40 mm Hg in contralateral brachial artery pressure.

Some arteriographic findings that are specific to various collagen vascular diseases have been well documented: In general, the lesions occur bilaterally, and the vessels show evidence of obstruction without evidence of calcium in the vessel wall or in the body of the lesion. Atherosclerotic changes are generally absent. The arterial lumen is smoothly narrowed, with a smooth reduction in the caliber of the vessel above the thrombosed segment. Lesions may be totally occlusive or may show a stringlike appearance (Fig. 33–5). Multiple segmental occlusive lesions occur predominantly in the forearm and hand, with sites of predilection in the cubital arch, palmar arch, and digital arteries. Collateral circulation is generally less well developed than in arteriosclerotic vascular occlusive disease. This collateralization is primarily through the vasa vasorum of the thrombosed segment, giving a winding corkscrew appearance of the fine vessels that accompany the occluded segment. The small, attenuated terminal digital branches have often been described as having the appearance of a "tree root."[8]

Characteristics of Takayasu's arteritis are generally confined to the proximal great vessels of the aortic arch, with solitary or multiple segmental narrowings of a tapered configuration. Linear calcifications in aneurysm formation are also often seen. Giant cell arteritis, on the other hand, generally is manifest by long, smooth stenotic segments alternating with areas of relatively normal or dilated seg-

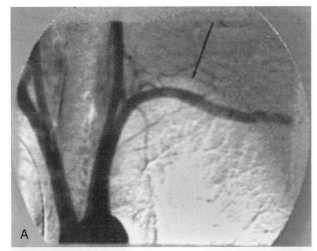

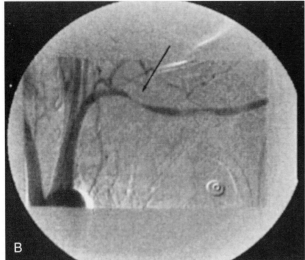

Figure 33–4. Digital intravenous axillosubclavian angiogram performed (A) in the supine and (B) in the sitting position to demonstrate thoracic outlet compressive changes (*arrows*) seen frequently only in the sitting position.

ments. The occlusive process is generally smooth and tapered, with absence of irregular plaques and ulcerations. Distinction between giant cell arteritis and Takayasu's arteritis is often difficult to establish, particularly in the upper extremity.

Magnification views of the hand during arteriography, particularly if augmented by hand cooling, hand warming, or injection of intraarterial vasodilating drugs, such as papaverine or nitroglycerin, can differentiate between Raynaud's phenomenon, which is generally associated with segmental occlusions, and Raynaud's disease, which is generally identifiable only by a vasospastic hypersensitivity. The angiographic characteristics of arterial vasospasm are marked delay in flow, a threadlike appearance, and tapered areas of occlusion relieved subsequently by injection of vasodilating drugs or hand warming.

Arteriography is very useful in the identification and assessment of arteriovenous malformation. When adequate to enable morphologic identification of arteriovenous malformations, it requires large volumes of contrast material injected at rapid rates, and often the true extent of the lesion is not be evident unless selective arterial injections are used.

Acquired arteriovenous fistulas often have an associated false aneurysm, and although the fistula itself may not be demonstrable owing to extremely high flow rates, the immediate filling of the adjacent vein is a reliable diagnostic finding. Ordinarily, the proximal artery may be dilated, tortuous, and even aneurysmal and often shows atherosclerotic change. The proximal veins are generally dilated as well. Transcatheter embolization is useful in palliation and, occasionally, in the cure of these symptomatic and destructive lesions. A number of critical aspects of transcatheter embolization have been identified, including preservation of the feeding vessels, in contradistinction to the previous practice of feeding vessel obliteration. The feeding vessel offers access to the nidus, or central portion, of the arteriovenous malformation, which must be extensively occluded, and thrombosis must be initiated if successful obliteration is to be accomplished. Obliteration of the feeding vessels without prior thrombosis of the central nidus leads only to rapid reformation of the arteriovenous malformation. A host of embolic materials have been developed, but the essential facet is careful subselective arteriography and central lesion embolization. In general, embolization is followed by pain, fever, and elevated creatinine phosphokinase. Fibrin split products may be transiently elevated, and patients in whom this occurs require hospitalization, sedation, and parenteral analgesics. Low-grade fever may persist for several weeks, although most symptoms resolve within 3 to 7 days. Embolization may require several staged procedures, and the therapy should always be considered palliative, with the potential for additional therapy necessary over time.

AFFLICTIONS OF THE MAJOR VASCULAR STRUCTURES OF THE UPPER EXTREMITY

About 50% of cases of acute arterial insufficiency of the upper extremity are secondary to embolization, and of the

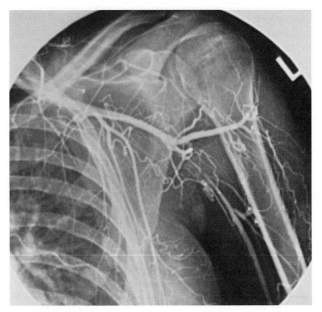

Figure 33–5. Intimal dissection and occlusion of the axillobrachial artery at the level of the brachial plexus cords. This lesion is best repaired by reverse vein grafting, care being taken to avoid entrapment of brachial plexus elements.

remainder, 25% are the result of primary arterial thrombosis and 25% are iatrogenic in origin. The vast majority of embolic arterial occlusions in the upper extremity are of cardiac origin, but brachiocephalic aneurysmal disease occasionally results in embolic episodes.

The diagnosis of upper extremity ischemia is quite straightforward. The triad of symptoms—pain, paresthesias, and pallor—is generally accompanied by a loss of radial and ulnar pulse and diminished segmental pressures on noninvasive testing. Surprisingly, atherosclerotic occlusive disease, which is so prominent in the lower extremities, afflicts the upper extremity less commonly in the occlusive process. The mortality rate in patients with arterial embolization to the upper extremities is about 25%, primarily attributable to recurrence and repetition of the embolic process into additional arterial distributions, particularly cerebrovascular, renal, and mesenteric.

Diagnostic and therapeutic measures must be prompt in episodes of acute upper extremity embolization. It has been documented that patients successfully treated within 12 hours of the embolic episode have excellent long-term results. After 12 hours, only approximately 25% of the patients have normal return of function and vascular integrity. The exact 12-hour time period may not be critical, but it does emphasize the problem of delay and the relative ineffectiveness of rapid collateral revascularization.[9, 10]

Two modes of therapy may well provide satisfactory results in the treatment of this problem. The most efficacious has been the immediate administration of continuous intravenous heparin with careful monitoring of the thromboplastin time. Intravenous heparin can be discontinued for a short time to allow angiographic investigation but can be maintained during arterial embolectomy, which is ideally performed through the antecubital fossa. The embolectomy should be carried out promptly, and careful observation should then be instituted for development of compartment syndrome. This compressive hydrostatic change occurs less frequently than in the lower extremities but nevertheless must be managed promptly by fasciotomy when it is recognized.

Selected cases, particularly in patients who represent poor operative risks, may be managed with fibrinolytic therapy, which is best carried out when initiated within 36 hours of the embolic event. Experience has grown with direct intraarterial fibrinolytic therapy, which can immediately follow angiographic diagnosis and localization of the lesion.[11]

Although urokinase has been used effectively, its recent availability has been limited. In January of 1999 the Center for Biologic Evaluation and Research, a branch of the United States Public Health Service, issued an advisory indicating that the Food and Drug Administration recommends that the available urokinase, Abbokinase, be reserved for only those situations in which a physician has considered the alternatives and determined that the use of Abbokinase is critical to the care of a specific patient in a specific situation. This recommendation was made in response to a possible deviation from the Current Good Manufacturing Practice regulations designed to help assure product safety.[11A] Experience is now accumulating with recombinant tissue-plasminogen activator (r-tPA).

Trauma to the brachial vessels generally carries a poor prognosis secondary to the commonly associated nerve injury (see Fig. 33–5). Lateral arterial repair and suture, or end-to-end anastomosis, is generally satisfactory in low-velocity missle and stab wounds. As in other areas of the body, high-velocity missle injury generally requires resection of the damaged artery to avoid recurrent thrombosis secondary to more extensive intimal damage. Reversed interposition vein graft is the most satisfactory reconstructive material and should be the graft of choice in the upper extremity.

When signs of ischemia accompany an upper extremity fracture, fracture reduction should be done as a primary maneuver, and reassessment of arterial integrity should be done promptly. In the presence of residual signs of ischemia, abnormal segmental arterial pressures, or incomplete return of pulses, arteriographic investigation is advisable. Although spasm can occur with torsion and traction on upper extremity arteries, there is generally a fairly prompt remission and restitution of normal pulses. We have rarely encountered spasm of a magnitude sufficient to cause a fall in segmental arterial pressures when assessed with the Doppler flowmeter and blood pressure cuff. A pressure drop in the range of 20 to 30 mm Hg lasting more than 30 minutes should be considered an indication of arterial occlusion, and the proper diagnostic and therapeutic steps should be instituted promptly. The consequence of delaying treatment in this type of ischemia in the upper extremity is a Volkmann-type ischemic contraction, which often may develop insidiously in the presence of minimal signs of arterial insufficiency. This difficult problem is particularly characteristic in children who have suffered a supracondylar fracture, when meticulous attention may not have been paid to concomitant arterial insufficiency.

Humeral fractures and shoulder dislocation are also associated with axillobrachial artery occlusions, and the basic principles of arterial reassessment after fracture reduction are advisable. False aneurysms of the brachial vessels may develop in instances of humeral fracture, even in the presence of distal arterial integrity. These generally appear as a pulsatile mass, occasionally associated with extensive hematoma and ecchymosis. In the absence of acute neurovascular compression, delayed repair has been satisfactory in these cases.

With the extensive use of the upper extremity for arterial blood pressure monitoring, sampling of arterial blood gases, and creation of an arteriovenous fistula for dialysis, 25% of episodes of upper extremity ischemia arise as a consequence of these diagnostic and therapeutic necessities. The incidence of radial and ulnar artery occlusion after percutaneous arterial cannulation is in the range of 30%.[12] The lowest incidence of complications has been reported with polytetrafluoroethylene (Teflon) 20-gauge or smaller catheters. Catheters of other materials and larger sizes have a significantly higher complication rate.

In general, the more disastrous complications of radial or ulnar artery occlusion occur in patients with an incomplete palmar arch or other anatomic abnormalities that lead to poor perfusion. Although most instances of thrombosis may be totally asymptomatic, it is incumbent on the physician to perform Allen's test before using the radial or ulnar arteries for diagnostic or therapeutic procedures.

Brachial artery catheterization is a well-documented

cause of upper extremity ischemia. The absence of a pulse or a persistent drop in segmental pressures lasting more than 30 minutes to 60 minutes should indicate the likelihood of occlusion and suggest the need for further diagnostic studies and operative therapy. Occlusion at the brachial level may be asymptomatic at rest but is accompanied by a significant degree of ischemic arm symptoms with exercise and work-related activities.[13]

Axillary cannulation has become a particularly popular method of angiographic study, and it is exceedingly important to be aware of the neurologic complications that occasionally accompany this particular site of access. Postcannulation bleeding tends to be confined to the axillary sheath and often leads to neurologic impairment. The patient who has a neurologic deficit after axillary artery cannulation, particularly in the distribution of the median nerve, should undergo surgical exploration for decompression of the hematoma. Failure to decompress this area often leads to permanent neurologic impairment.

It should be evident that careful arterial assessment of the upper extremity, as outlined earlier in this chapter, should always be undertaken before axillofemoral grafting procedures or other extraanatomic bypasses that use the axillosubclavian vessels. This prevents the uncommon but serious complications of upper extremity ischemia that occasionally result from these increasingly popular reconstructive procedures.[14]

Aneurysms of the axillobrachial vessels are relatively uncommon. Although tortuous subclavian vessels often are suspected of being aneurysmal at the time of clinical assessment, the diagnosis is rarely sustained after angiographic investigation. Nevertheless, when these infrequent abnormalities are encountered, the treatment of choice is excision and interposition vein graft reconstruction.

In episodes of acute embolization or thrombosis with ischemia, we have used intraarterial thrombolytic agents (primarily urokinase) as well as intravenous infusion of prostaglandin E_1. These measures can serve as an effective bridge to subacute and chronic maintenance therapy. Pentoxifylline at 400 mg given three times per day has been shown to be effective (by clinical observation) in improving the capillary circulation in some of our patients with upper extremity digital ischemia.

High-dose local infusion of urokinase by a transarterial catheter has been effective in the lysis of intraarterial thrombi. This technique can be used intraoperatively to more effectively remove thrombotic material from the very vasoactive vessels of the upper extremities, thus avoiding the trauma of repetitive passage of a balloon embolectomy catheter. An infusion of 250,000 units of urokinase dissolved in 100 mL of normal saline can be given over a 30-minute period. If the patient is not systemically heparinized, 1000 units of heparin can be added to the infusate. If there is any clinical or radiographic evidence of vasospasm, 30 mg of papaverine can be infused via the same catheter.[15]

In July of 1999, Zoon,[15A] writing for the Food and Drug Administration branch of the Department of Health and Human Services, indicated that their inspection process revealed "numerous significant deviations from the current good manufacturing practice regulations in the production of urokinase from human neonatal kidney cells. Between January and July of 1999, questions remained regarding the screening of donors of the human neonatal kidney cells. Lots of in-process bulk harvest were found to contain three separate strains of reovirus and one instance of mycoplasma."

As of July 14, 1999, many questions still remained and urokinase was still not readily available.[12] Other approved thrombolytic agents are discussed in the section on Venous Insufficiency.

Recent advances in the diagnosis and management of arterial disorders of the upper extremity have been recently described and reviewed by Gelabert and Machleder.[15B]

VENOUS INSUFFICIENCY OF THE UPPER EXTREMITY

Although thoracic outlet compression can lead to axillosubclavian vein thrombosis, the vast majority of venous occlusive processes result from trauma or iatrogenic injury.

Long-term intravenous alimentation, upper extremity intravenous access for therapy, or procedures such as central venous pressure monitoring and Swan-Ganz monitoring may result in axillosubclavian thrombotic episodes. It is important to recognize that chronic axillosubclavian vein thrombosis may be an indolent and relatively silent process and is infrequently associated with symptoms in the upper extremity. During the course of monitoring and therapy using the upper extremity veins, the more serious illness for which the patient is being treated or monitored may overshadow subtle signs of progressive axillosubclavian thrombosis. Whenever this problem has been looked at prospectively, however, the incidence of venous thrombosis in the major upper extremity veins approaches 25% and is significant perhaps when repetitive subclavian vein catheterizations might be required in the course of a long or recurrent illness. Heparin therapy rarely leads to lysis but may prevent extension of thrombosis when the problem is recognized and cannulas have been removed. Thrombolytic therapy with streptokinase or urokinase may prove efficacious, but good controlled studies in the upper extremity have not yet been satisfactorily documented. Reports of successful surgical therapy by either thrombectomy or interposition grafting do not demonstrate any superiority over conservative management, and the failure rate is sufficiently high that enthusiastic recommendation of surgical intervention cannot be supported.

Spontaneous, or effort-related, thrombosis of the axillosubclavian vein is a disabling disorder of young, otherwise healthy, individuals. This type of thrombosis was described independently over 100 years ago by Paget in England and Von Schroetter in Germany. In 1949, Hughes analyzed 320 cases of spontaneous upper extremity venous thrombosis collected from the medical literature. He recognized the first two descriptions by naming the entity the "Paget-Schroetter syndrome."[16] Over the course of subsequent investigations, it has come to be understood that, in contrast to the apparent spontaneous nature of the event, there is an underlying chronic venous compressive anomaly at the thoracic outlet (see Fig. 33–2). The subclavius muscle tendon can be demonstrated to be the site of obstruction in many cases in which intermittent obstruction is

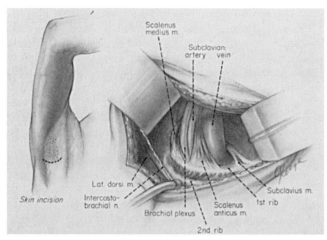

Figure 33–6. View of thoracic outlet structures from the transaxillary approach to first rib resection. (From Machleder HI [ed]: Vascular Disorders of the Upper Extremity, 2nd ed. Mt. Kisco, NY, Futura Publishing Company, 1989.)

present but has not yet led to thrombosis. Pulmonary embolism from axillosubclavian vein thrombosis has been well documented, and deaths from pulmonary embolism from these sources have also been recorded in the surgical literature.

Studies of a relatively large group of patients have shown the value of immediate catheter-directed thrombolytic therapy with urokinase followed by a period of anticoagulation to allow the acute phlebitic process to subside. Patients are then treated by transaxillary first rib resection to relieve the external compression. In patients with long-standing compression of the vein, stricture and fibrosis may result. This can be treated with transvenous balloon angioplasty after the external compressive elements have been removed. With this course of therapy, an excellent functional result can be expected.[17–19]

Alternative thrombolytic agents have been approved by the Food and Drug Administration, although they have not been extensively used for axillosubclavian vein thrombosis:

streptokinase, alteplase, anistreplase, and reteplace.[19A] There are anecdotal reports that suggest that these drugs can be used successfully in treatment of patients with Paget-Schroetter syndrome.

Although additional studies have validated the staged, multidisciplinary approach, there have been successful reports of immediate surgical decompression following thrombolytic therapy. These cases have been insufficient thus far to result in a publication available for general review.[19B]

THORACIC OUTLET COMPRESSION

Thoracic outlet compression syndrome can be associated with a constellation of neurologic or vascular symptoms. The vascular compressive phenomena in this entity are much more apt to be demonstrable on clinical and currently available objective tests.[20] The first rib generally forms the floor of the axillary canal through which the neurovascular structures traverse. The superior portion of this canal is formed by the clavicle and the subclavius muscle. Structures that enter the thoracic outlet canal and can cause symptoms of neurovascular compression include the scalenus anticus muscle, which inserts on the first rib between the axillary artery and vein, and the subclavius muscle tendon, which inserts at the medial border of the costochondral junction of the first rib and, as has been mentioned previously, often compresses the subclavian vein. Most laterally, the scalenus medius muscle has insertions to the first rib that are closely associated with the cords of the brachial plexus (Fig. 33–6). A host of fibrocartilaginous congenital bands have been described in this area. Many are perhaps rudimentary insertions of incompletely formed cervical ribs. Complete cervical ribs often insert on the first rib and occasionally are accompanied by an area of hyperostosis or even a fairly well-developed joint structure. Minor trauma, which may alter the rather close tolerances of the thoracic outlet by upsetting the musculoskeletal balance, leads to the thoracic outlet compression syndrome (Figs. 33–7 and 33–8). Developmental anomalies

Figure 33–7. Typical hypertrophy of the subclavius tendon and associated exostoses seen at the subclavius and scalenus anticus insertions to the first rib (visualized from the transaxillary surgical approach). The vein is compressed in the most medial area of the thoracic outlet. (From Kunkel JM, Machleder HI: Treatment of Paget-Schroetter syndrome: A staged multidisciplinary approach. Arch Surg 124:1153–1158, 1989.)

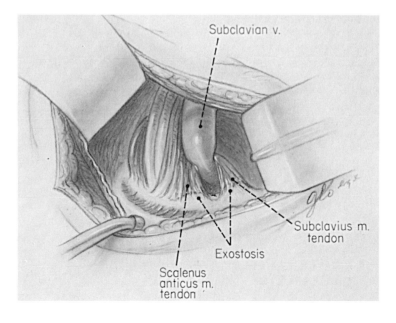

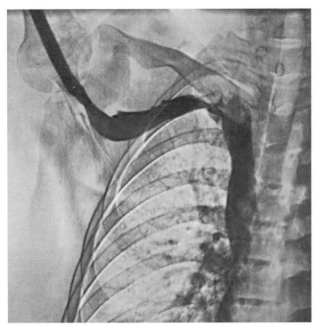

Figure 33–8. Typical venographic picture of axillosubclavian compression at the thoracic outlet that eventually leads to thrombosis and the acute clinical presentation.

occur frequently in the thoracic outlet area and can become clinically significant and symptomatic under certain circumstances of discrete or cumulative trauma. Abnormal muscle attachments or supernumerary muscles become symptomatic in particular industrial or recreational settings, particularly when there is hypertrophy or increased muscle contraction. These developmental anomalies have been studied and reported.[21]

Recent studies focusing on careful histochemical and morphometric analysis of the anterior scalene muscle have opened a new area for investigating the causes of neurovascular compression at the thoracic outlet. This research has been particularly useful in demonstrating the changes that occur in post-traumatic neurogenic thoracic outlet compression syndrome and often appear in the absence of obvious structural abnormalities.

Vertebrate skeletal muscle is composed of several distinctive muscle fiber types, each having different morphologic, metabolic, and contractile characteristics that are distinguishable by specific histochemical staining methods. Despite a high degree of specialization, these fibers retain the capacity for accommodating changes in demand and patterns of stimulation, responding with alterations in basic biochemical elements.

Human skeletal muscle usually comprises predominantly type 2, quick-reacting fibers, which have low oxidative enzyme capacity. A smaller percentage of slow tonic-contracting type 1 fibers, characterized by greater oxidative capacity, complete the complement. These latter fibers (type 1) are common to postural muscle groups. Anterior scalene muscle demonstrates type 1 fiber predominance, which indicates that this muscle is, at the outset, uniquely structured in fiber composition to sustain protracted periods of tonic contraction.

Striking increases in type 1 fiber composition and selec-tive hypertrophy of the type 1 fiber system occur in patients with post-traumatic thoracic outlet compression syndrome. The anterior scalene muscle in these patients demonstrates an extraordinary adaptive transformation and recruitment response in the type 1 fiber system, possibly reflecting chronic increased tone or motor neuron stimulation. It seems likely that in post-traumatic thoracic outlet syndrome, stretch injury to the muscle initiates a response of muscle contraction or denervation and reinnervation, compromising the interscalene triangle (between anterior and middle scalene muscles) and constricting the brachial plexus, to both accentuate and perpetuate the neurovascular compressive phenomenon.

Symptoms may be predominantly ulnar or medial in distribution and occasionally involve both nerve groups. Numbness, weakness, and paresthesias, particularly when the arms are in the abducted and externally rotated position, are characteristic. Common activities such as combing the hair, reaching or working with arms overhead, and even automobile driving when hands are placed on top of the steering wheel bring on symptoms. Patients generally seek therapy when symptoms become quite severe or when they occur in association with occupational requirements. Clinical findings are most useful in diagnosis and include reduction or obliteration of radial pulse with thoracic outlet maneuvers such as the costoclavicular, the scalenus anticus, the Adson, and the abduction-external rotation maneuvers. These maneuvers often reproduce symptoms or result in a subclavian bruit.

Progress has been made in facilitating the objective evaluation of neurogenic thoracic outlet compression by defining the role and usefulness of the somatosensory evoked response.[22, 23] The most characteristic abnormality found in patients with neurogenic thoracic outlet compression syndrome is a reduction in the amplitude of the ulnar nerve response at the N9, the Erb point, or the brachial plexus recording electrode. This dampening of the N9 amplitude can be accentuated, or the potential completely ablated, by placing the arm in the abducted and externally rotated position, which is the most symptomatic position for patients with thoracic outlet compression syndrome. Criteria for performing and interpreting sensory evoked potential testing have been established in a recent preoperative and postoperative study of patients undergoing surgical correction of neurovascular compression at the thoracic outlet.[24]

Objective tests are useful for the diagnosis of thoracic outlet compression and can include

1. Cervical spine x-ray films for assessment of arthritic or degenerative changes and presence of cervical ribs
2. Chest x-ray film to identify apical lung pathology and superior sulcus tumor
3. Nerve conduction studies and electromyography to delineate the possible significance of neuroforaminal or cervical disk disease, as well as median nerve compression at the carpal tunnel or ulnar nerve compression at the cubital or Guyon tunnel; these studies are very helpful in those patients with the "double crush syndrome," in which there are multiple sites of peripheral nerve compression
4. F-wave studies and somatosensory evoked responses to evaluate the brachial plexus

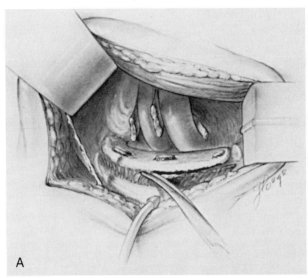

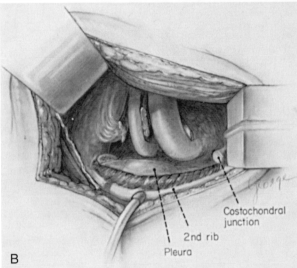

Figure 33–9. Steps in transaxillary first rib resection. *A*, Division of subclavius, scalenus anticus, and scalenus medius tendons as well as initial incision of the intercostal muscle. *B*, Relationship of structures after removal of first rib.

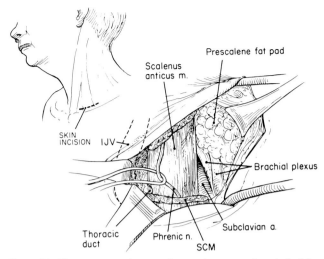

Figure 33–10. Transcervical approach to scalenectomy for relief of thoracic outlet compression syndrome. The relationship of major surrounding anatomic structures is depicted. IJV, internal jugular vein; SCM, sternocleidomastoid muscle. (From Machleder HI, Moll FL: In Trout HH 3rd, DePalma RG [eds]: Reoperative Vascular Surgery. New York, Marcel Dekker, 1987.)

rib removal (when present) results in significant relief of symptoms (Fig. 33–9).[25]

Scalenotomy or scalenectomy, as a single operation or combined with first rib resection, has become an accepted surgical approach to this problem (Figs. 33–10 and 33–11).[26, 27] Kashyap and coworkers have recently reviewed the most common surgical approaches, to discuss the advantages and limitations.[28]

5. Venography, which is indispensable in the evaluation of the acutely swollen upper extremity when the possibility of Paget-Schroetter syndrome exists
6. Angiography, which should generally be reserved for patients who have evidence of ischemia or embolization; this identifies any arterial damage that may be associated with the compressive syndrome

The most recent test of high sensitivity and specificity for the diagnosis of neurogenic thoracic outlet compression is the electromyogram-guided selective scalene block. The method and results have been reported by Jordan and Machleder.[24A]

Although therapy for this condition undergoes periodic revisions, a number of standard surgical approaches have been successful. Cervical rib resection is the oldest documented therapy in the English literature and is still used as an isolated procedure in selected cases. More often, resection of the first thoracic rib concomitant with cervical

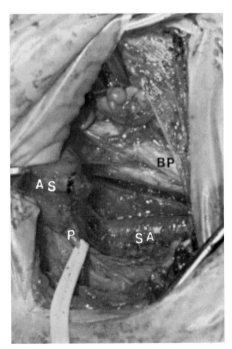

Figure 33–11. Operative view of transcervical approach after resection of anterior scalene muscle. AS, anterior scalene muscle stump; BP, brachial plexus; P, phrenic nerve; SA, subclavian artery.

References

1. Raynaud M: New researches on the nature and treatment of local asphyxia of the extremities. Arch Générales Médecin January 1874.
2. Burth DE: Digital Plethysmography. New York, Grune & Stratton, 1954.
3. Summer DS: Hemodynamics and pathophysiology of arterial venous fistulas. In Rutherford RB (ed): Vascular Surgery. Philadelphia, WB Saunders, 1977, pp 737–765.
4. Fan PT, Davis JA, Somer T, et al: A clinical approach to systemic vasculitis. Semin Arthritis Rheum 9:248–304, 1980.
5. Fauci AS, Hanes BF, Katz P: The spectrum of vasculitis: Clinical, pathologic, immunologic and therapeutic considerations. Ann Intern Med 89:660–676, 1978.
6. Bauer GM, Porter JM, Bardana EJ, et al: Rapid onset of hand ischemia of unknown etiology. Ann Surg 186:184, 1977.
7. Edwards JM, Harker CT, Taylor LM Jr, Porter JM: Small artery disease of the upper extremity. In Machleder HI (ed): Vascular Disorders of the Upper Extremity, 2nd ed. Mt. Kisco, NY, Futura Publishing, 1989.
8. Rivera R: Roentgenographic diagnosis of Buerger's disease. Cardiovasc Surg 14:40–46, 1973.
9. Kofoed H, Hansen HJ: Arterial embolism in the upper limb. Acta Chir Scand [Suppl]47:113–115, 1976.
10. Savelyev BS, Zatevakhin II, Stephanov NV: Arterial embolism of the upper limbs. Surgery 81:367–375, 1977.
11. Chaise LS, Comerota AJ, Sonlen RL, et al: Selective intraarterial streptokinase therapy in the immediate postoperative period. JAMA 247:2397–2400, 1982.
11A. Zoon KC: Important Drug Warning Center for Biologics Evaluation PHS-FDA Letter 1/25/1999. Available at http://www.fda.gov/cber/ltr/abb012599.htm
12. Davis FM, Stewart JM: Radial artery cannulation: A prospective study. Br J Anaesthesiol 52:41–47, 1980.
13. Machleder HI, Sweeney JP, Barker WF: The pulseless arm after brachial artery catheterization. Lancet I:407–409, 1972.
14. Quiñones-Baldrich WJ, Freischlag JA, Machleder HI, Busuttil RW, Moore WS: Inflow failure of grafts originating in the axillary artery. Ann Vasc Surg 2:303–308, 1988.
15. Quiñones-Baldrich WJ, Baker JD, Busuttil RW, et al: Intraoperative infusion of lytic drugs for thrombotic complications of revascularization. J Vasc Surg 10:408–417, 1989.
15A. Zoon KC: Letter posted on the Food and Drug Administration (FDA) Website, Department of Health and Human Services, Public Health Service, FDA Center for Biologics Evaluation and Research, 14 July 1999. Available at http://www.fda.gov/
15B. Gelabert HA, Machleder HI: Diagnosis and management of arterial compression at the thoracic outlet. Ann Vasc Surg 11:359–366, 1997.
16. Hughes ESR: Venous obstruction in the upper extremity (Paget-Schroetter's syndrome). Int Abstr Surg 88:89217, 1949.
17. Machleder HI: Evaluation of a new treatment strategy for Paget-Schroetter's syndrome. J Vasc Surg 17:305–317, 1993.
18. Machleder HI: Thrombolytic therapy and surgery for primary axillo-subclavian vein thrombosis: Current approach. Semin Vasc Surg 9:46–48, 1996.
19. Machleder HI: Effort thrombosis of the axillosubclavian vein: A disabling vascular disorder. Compr Ther 17:18–24, 1991.
19A. Zoon KC: Important Drug Warning Food and Drug Administration-Center for Biologics Evaluation and Research. Available at http://www.fda.gov/cber/ltr/abb012599.htm
19B. Machleder HI: Thrombolytic therapy and surgery for primary axillo-subclavian vein thrombosis: Current approach. Semin Vasc Surg 9:46–49, 1996.
20. Machleder HI: Thoracic outlet compression syndrome: New concepts from a century of discovery. Cardiovasc Surg 2:137–145, 1994.
21. Makhoul RG, Machleder HI: Developmental anomalies at the thoracic outlet: An analysis of 200 consecutive cases. J Vasc Surg 16:534–545, 1992.
22. Machleder HI, Moll F, Verity MA: The anterior scalene muscle in thoracic outlet compression syndrome: Histochemical and morphometric studies. Arch Surg 121:1141–1144, 1986.
23. Siivola J, Pokela R, Sulg I: Somatosensory evoked responses as a diagnostic aid in thoracic outlet syndrome (a postoperative study). Acta Chir Scand 149:147–150, 1983.
24. Machleder HI, Moll F, Nuwer M, Jordan S: Somatosensory evoked potentials in the assessment of thoracic outlet compression syndrome. J Vasc Surg 6:177–184, 1984.
24A. Jordan SE, Machleder HI: Diagnosis of thoracic outlet syndrome using electrophysiologically guided anterior scalene blocks. Ann Vasc Surg 12:260–264, 1998.
25. Machleder HI: Transaxillary operative management of thoracic outlet syndrome. In Ernst C, Stanley J (eds): Current Therapy in Vascular Surgery, 2nd ed. Philadelphia, BC Dekker, 1991.
26. Dale WA: Thoracic outlet compression syndrome. Critique in 1982. Arch Surg 117:1437–1445, 1982.
27. Roos DB: The place for scalenectomy and 1st rib resection in thoracic outlet syndrome. Surgery 92:1077–1085, 1982.
28. Kashyap VS, Ahn SS, Machleder HI: Thoracic outlet neurovascular compression: Approaches to anatomic decompression and their limitations. Semin Vasc Surg 11:60–264, 1998.

Review Questions

1. Allen's test is useful in evaluating
   (a) thoracic outlet compression
   (b) presence of cervical rib
   (c) integrity of palmar arch
   (d) digital blood flow
   (e) acute effort thrombosis

2. The thoracic outlet is bounded by which of the following structures? (may choose more than one)
   (a) medial border of sternum
   (b) first thoracic rib
   (c) clavicle
   (d) subclavian artery
   (e) subclavian tendon

3. The thoracic outlet is traversed by which of the following structures? (may choose more than one)
   (a) subclavian artery
   (b) brachial plexus
   (c) scalenus anticus muscle
   (d) pectoralis major tendon
   (e) scalenus medius muscle

4. Digital gangrene is frequently associated with
   (a) Raynaud's syndrome
   (b) Swan-Ganz central monitoring
   (c) Raynaud's disease
   (d) thoracic outlet compression
   (e) McLeary's syndrome

5. Digital plethysmographic tracings are most apt to be misinterpreted secondary to
   (a) cuff malfunction
   (b) transducer malfunction
   (c) segmental arterial occlusions
   (d) changes in sympathetic activity
   (e) poor light

6. A common cause of prominent right-sided supraclavicular pulsation is
   (a) common carotid aneurysm
   (b) subclavian aneurysm
   (c) subclavian tortuosity or elongation
   (d) innominate artery aneurysm
   (e) mycotic aneurysm

7. Effort thrombosis of the subclavian vein is often associated with
   (a) straining at bowel movement
   (b) hypercoagulation syndrome
   (c) thoracic outlet compression syndrome
   (d) calcinosis cutis, Raynaud's phenomenon, sclerodactyly, and telangiectasia (CRST syndrome) or scleroderma
   (e) collagen vascular disease in general

8. When peripheral pulses are absent following fracture dislocation of the humerus
   (a) arteriography should be done promptly before reduction
   (b) arterial exploration should be done at the fracture site as the first step
   (c) fracture reduction should be followed by arterial reevaluation
   (d) sympathetic block should be performed immediately

   (e) pulses should be rechecked in about 1 hour, before fracture manipulation

9. Gunshot injuries to the axillobrachial vessels have a poor prognosis owing to
   (a) particularly poor collateral circulation in these areas
   (b) associated vein injury
   (c) associated nerve injury
   (d) difficulty in maintaining patency in these arteries even after appropriate repair
   (e) forearm compartment syndrome

10. Volkmann's ischemic contracture occurs most commonly (may choose more than one)
   (a) in adults
   (b) in children
   (c) after radial artery cannulation and thrombosis
   (d) after fracture of the humeral neck
   (e) in collagen vascular diseases

Answers

1. c 2. b, c, e 3. a, b 4. a 5. d 6. c 7. c 8. c 9. c 10. b, d

34

Hemodialysis and Vascular Access

Robert S. Bennion and Samuel E. Wilson

Direct access to the vascular system for the delivery of medications and for the removal of life-threatening endogenous or exogenous chemicals from the circulation is one of the foundations of modern clinical practice. In broad terms, vascular access includes any form of cannulation of arteries or veins. This chapter briefly reviews the historical aspects; provides a practical consideration of external cannulation or shunts, autogenous fistulas, and internal bridge fistulas; and discusses the selection of prosthetic materials. The complications and outcome of each type of vascular access are analyzed.

Temporary access to the venous system for the infusion of drugs and, somewhat surprisingly, considering the outcome, for the transfusion of blood products has been in fairly common practice for well over 300 years. Sir Christopher Wren, the great 17th century English architect, is generally credited with the development of an instrument for intravenous therapy in 1656, which was used for injecting drugs (opium and crocus metallorum) into the veins of dogs.[1] It consisted of a cannula, made from a goose quill, with a pointed tip, which permitted penetration of the skin and underlying vein. In 1663, Robert Boyle described and published Wren's experiments and was the first person to extend intravenous infusions to humans, using prison inmates in London as subjects.[2]

The development of long-term cannulation of the circulatory system, however, was spurred by the introduction of a practical hemodialysis machine by Willem Kolff in the mid-1950s.[3] Initial enthusiasm for hemodialysis was blunted by the major technical problems associated with the need for repeated vascular access. Having to perform a cutdown on the artery and vein for each dialysis access, and then to ligate these vessels at the termination of each procedure, essentially limited early hemodialysis to short-term therapy for acute renal failure. In 1960, the development of the Scribner arteriovenous shunt[4] afforded long-term, relatively safe access to the circulation, and prolonged use of hemodialysis in the treatment of chronic renal failure became a reality.

As is shown in Figure 34–1, the number of individuals requiring vascular access for hemodialysis continues to rise. In the 10 years between 1988 and 1997, the number of patients on hemodialysis more than doubled.[5] In addition, the number of vascular access procedures exceeded 125,000 in 1996, with over 50,000 being revisions of existing permanent vascular access sites.[6] Figure 34–2A and B shows how the number of these procedures performed in the outpatient setting continues to rise.

SHORT-TERM HEMODIALYSIS ACCESS

The external arteriovenous shunt described by Quinton, Dillard, and Scribner[4] in 1960 consisted of a loop of silicone rubber tubing lying on the volar aspect of the forearm connecting polytetrafluoroethylene (PTFE) catheters placed in both the radial artery and nearby wrist vein (Fig. 34–3). Although quickly and widely adopted as a practical means of providing access in chronic renal failure patients, three major disadvantages to long-term use of external shunts became apparent: (1) high infectibility because of the likelihood of bacterial contamination along the silicone rubber tubing entrance sites into the skin; (2) frequent clotting due to the small diameter of the silicone rubber and PTFE conduits; and (3) restriction of patients' daily activities by the external appliance, the extra care necessary to prevent dislodgment or infection, and the additional strain the shunt placed on their already heavily burdened tolerance. Consequently, patency rates of external shunts were very low.[7]

Although acute hemodialysis in the past was carried out primarily with external shunts, these have now been replaced by percutaneously placed central venous catheter hemodialysis.[8] This technique allows important preservation of the vascular sites best suited for later construction of subcutaneous arteriovenous fistulas. The usual indications for hemodialysis by percutaneous venipuncture are (1) acute renal failure in which only a short course of

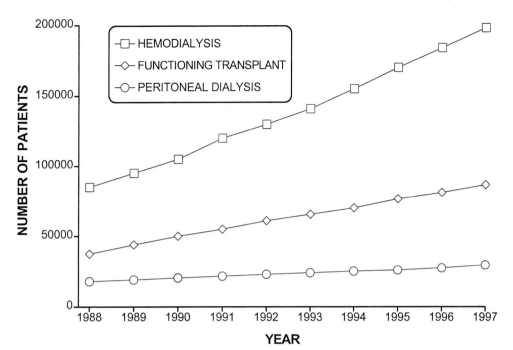

Figure 34–1. Number of treated end-stage renal disease patients in the United States by treatment modality, 1988 to 1997. (Modified from US Renal Data System USRDS 1999 Annual Data Report, Bethesda, Md, National Institutes of Health, National Institute of Diabetes and Digestive and Kidney Diseases, April 1999.)

dialysis is required; (2) during the immediate postoperative period after placement of an internal fistula in patients with chronic renal failure; (3) patients with transplantations who have thrombosed arteriovenous fistulas; (4) patients needing urgent transfer from peritoneal dialysis; and (5) treatment of poisoning.

Using this technique, short-term dialysis needs are met through the percutaneous introduction of a catheter with an external diameter of less than 2 mm (Fig. 34–4). The catheters are usually introduced by the Seldinger technique over a guidewire and may be easily left in place for a week or, with care, can last up to several months.[9] The catheters should be changed over a guidewire every 7 days, and the catheter tip cultured, with any drainage from the cutaneous entry site cultured routinely. Depending on the clinical demands, either single-catheter dialysis with pulsatile flow or double-catheter dialysis with continuous flow may be elected. The latter is usually chosen when urgent and aggressive hemodialysis is necessary, because this is 20% to 30% more efficient than single-catheter dialysis. Thrombosis is prevented by continuous low-dose heparin infusion or an intermittent injection of heparin every 12 hours. Stable patients may be given the option of going home with the catheter in place, receiving intermittent heparin injections for outpatient dialysis. Interestingly, patients with these catheters in place have a 40% incidence of moderate to severe ipsilateral subclavian vein stenosis on angiography, whereas no stenoses were found in a control group of

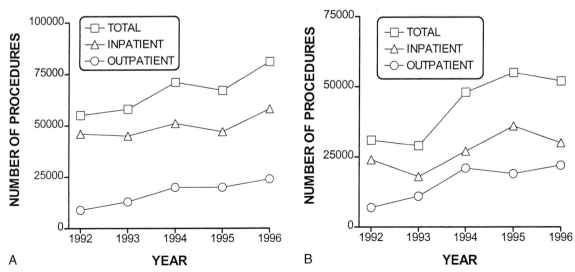

Figure 34–2. Number of primary vascular access procedures (A) and revisions (B) (excluding percutaneous procedures) for chronic hemodialysis performed in the United States, 1992 to 1996. (Modified from Orengo MF, Lawrence L: Detailed diagnoses and procedures. National Hospital Discharge Survey, 1997. National Center for Health Statistics. Vital Health Stat 13 [1–15], 1997.)

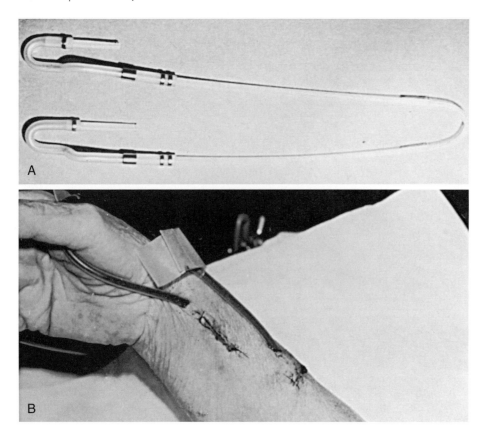

Figure 34–3. *A,* Scribner shunt apparatus. *B,* Radiocephalic Scribner shunt in place.

patients without a recent history of central venous catheters in the subclavian vein.[10] Although the effect that these stenoses may have on the function of a planned permanent vascular access is not known, avoiding placement of a percutaneous access line ipsilateral to a planned permanent access site would seem prudent.

These catheters are usually placed via the subclavian route into the superior vena cava, and are attended by the usual dangers of a percutaneous subclavian venipuncture.[11] The inferior vena cava may also be used; however, because of the danger of pelvic venous thrombosis, the catheter should not be left in place from one dialysis session to another. Although the incidence of catheter sepsis is gener-

ally low, one series reported a 28% incidence of infection in catheters left in position more than 4 weeks.[12]

Long-term use of percutaneous vascular access is becoming a more frequent alternative form of chronic hemodialysis. Using a silicone dual-lumen catheter with a Dacron cuff, a 1-year catheter survival rate of 65% and median length of catheter use of 18.5 months has been achieved.[13] Although thrombotic complications occurred in 46% of patients, the use of thrombolytic therapy was successful in restoring catheter function more than 95% of the time. Catheter exit site infection in 21% of patients (which almost always resolved with parenteral antibiotics) and bacteremia in 12% of patients were the other principal complications.

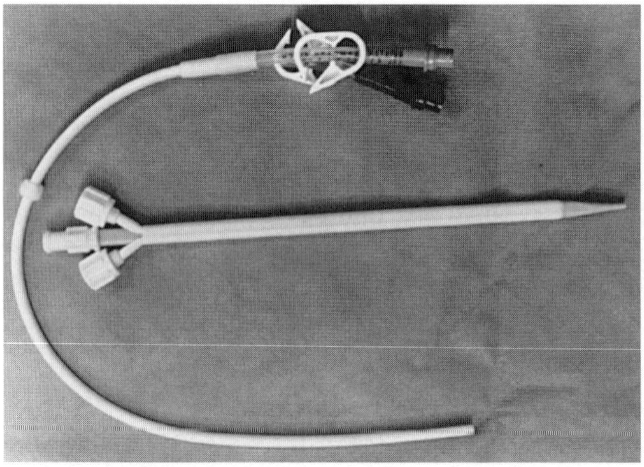

AUTOGENOUS ARTERIOVENOUS FISTULA

The autogenous arteriovenous fistula, usually constructed by joining the cephalic vein to the radial artery at the level of the wrist, remains the longest-lasting and most dependable type of long-term vascular access. One long-term prospective study demonstrated a useful patency rate for first-time fistulas of 90% at 1 year, and more than 75% at 4 years.[14] In addition, revision of a failing autogenous arteriovenous fistula can extend its longevity. An autogenous arteriovenous fistula may be unsatisfactory, however, in patients (especially those with diabetes) with advanced atherosclerotic changes extending into the radial artery, or in patients whose veins are too small, fragile, or thin-walled to mature sufficiently for repeated needle punctures.

Figure 34–4. Percutaneous hemodialysis catheter with Dacron cuff and oval dilator and sheath.

Brescia-Cimino Arteriovenous Fistula

The subcutaneous autogenous arteriovenous fistula was initially described by Brescia, Cimino, and coworkers in 1966.[15] Readily accepted by nephrologists and surgeons, the Brescia-Cimino fistula, constructed of the patient's own vessels, in great part overcomes the disadvantages of infection and early clotting found with external arteriovenous fistulas. After formation of the fistula, arterial pressure is transmitted directly into the contiguous veins, resulting in dilatation and development of a hypertrophied muscular wall (Fig. 34–5). This "arterialization" of the veins may take up to 6 weeks before sufficiently sized and thick-walled vessels have developed sufficiently to tolerate repeated venipuncture. Hemodialysis, if necessary during this postoperative period, may be accomplished using subclavian or femoral vein cannulation.

Our technique is as follows. Before operation, the veins, preferably in the nondominant arm, are distended and examined using a sphygmomanometer with the cuff applied to the upper arm and inflated to below the systolic pressure level to produce venous engorgement. All suitably sized veins are marked with an indelible pen. This is performed so that, should the fistula of choice fail just after construction, these markings can aid the surgeon in identification of other possible fistula sites. The ulnar and radial artery pulses are palpated, and if any uncertainty exists as to adequacy, the systolic pressure in each is measured with the Doppler probe. Determining beforehand by the Allen test that the ulnar artery can support the circulation of the hand is advantageous should the radial artery need to be divided or if it should subsequently clot. Digital compression, occluding both arteries at the wrist, is followed by pallor of the elevated hand. Release of compression over the ulnar artery returns a normal appearance to the hand if the blood supply is sufficient.

Local infiltration anesthesia using 0.5% to 1.0% lidocaine is usually satisfactory for construction of autogenous arteriovenous fistulas at the wrist or antecubital fossa. Although general anesthesia may be required in an extremely apprehensive or potentially uncooperative patient, a recent report of the effect of different types of anesthesia on blood flow during creation of a fistula showed that general anesthesia significantly decreased mean arterial blood pressure compared with local infiltrative anesthesia or brachial plexus block.[15, 16] In addition, brachial plexus block (supraclavicular approach) significantly increased brachial artery blood flow compared with local anesthesia. What effect these findings have on either short- or long-term patency of a fistula is not known.

The arm is prepared with povidone-iodine, abducted at a right angle from the body on an arm board, and sterilely draped. An oblique or longitudinal incision is made over the radial artery proximal to the wrist skinfold. An adjacent 4- to 5-cm length of cephalic vein is dissected free of surrounding subcutaneous tissue. Its tributaries are ligated, freeing it further so that it lies adjacent to the radial artery without kinking or twisting. A comparable length of the radial artery, found under the deep fascia of the forearm, is also isolated from surrounding structures. Adequately mobilized lengths of the two vessels are necessary so that they may rest side by side without tension. In the event that tension exists, the distal cephalic vein may be divided and its proximal segment approximated to the radial artery in an end-to-side fashion.

Four different anastomotic connections of artery and vein are in common use (Fig. 34–6), and each has its advantages and disadvantages:

1. *Side-to-side anastomosis,* with a fistula opening approximately 1 cm long. Technically, this is an easy anastomosis to construct and has the highest fistula blood flow.[17] It is also the most likely fistula to be associated with venous hypertension of the hand.[18] This complication is moderated by the presence of venous valves that prevent reversal of venous blood flow in the hand, at least in the early months.

2. *Arterial end-to-vein side anastomosis* minimizes turbulence and distal steal of blood, but results in slightly lower fistula flows and is subject to twisting of the artery during construction.

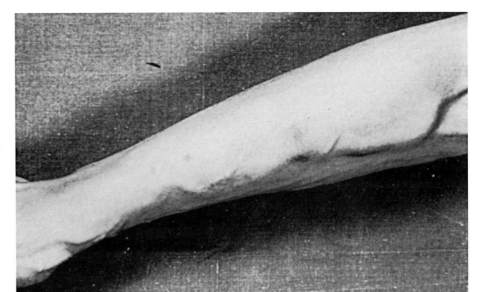

Figure 34–5. View of dilated forearm veins following construction of Brescia-Cimino radiocephalic fistula.

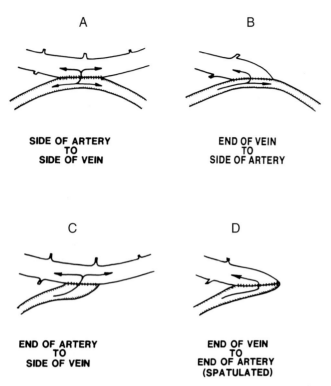

Figure 34–6. Four anastomotic options for autogenous arteriovenous fistula construction.

3. *Vein end-to-arterial side anastomosis* also decreases turbulence if constructed properly and results in the highest proximal venous flow with minimal distal venous hypertension.[19] It is technically somewhat more difficult to construct than the side-to-side fistula, and fistula flow overall is somewhat less. Most surgeons prefer this anastomosis because of the absence of vascular complications.

4. *End-to-end anastomosis* produces the least distal arterial steal and venous hypertension but has the lowest fistula flow of the four configurations.[20]

Proximal and distal control of the two vessels is gained by application of small bulldog clamps or a fine silicone rubber sling. The vessels are anastomosed in the desired configuration with 6-0 or 7-0 polypropylene suture, with knots placed outside of the lumen. One must be careful that, in approximating the artery and vein, spiral rotation of either vessel does not occur. Before the anastomosis is finally closed, a check is made by gentle passage of a coronary artery or biliary dilator to detect any stenosis. Hydrostatic dilatation with heparin-treated saline of a marginally small vein may aid in maintaining early patency.[21] Any bleeding from the anastomotic site should first be controlled by simple pressure with a gauze swab for several minutes. Too hasty a resort to suture repair is liable to produce further bleeding sites and narrowing of the anastomosis.

Upon conclusion, the artery and vein should lie beside each other without twists or kinks. A thrill should be easily felt over the fistula and propagated for a moderate distance along the contiguous venous channels. A transmitted pulse without a thrill suggests an outflow obstruction or a clotted

fistula. In this case, the proximal vein may be probed and inflated with a Fogarty catheter (avoiding intimal damage by not inflating the balloon during manipulation of the catheter) or carefully dilated with bougies. If these maneuvers do not produce a strong thrill, and the fistula is technically satisfactory, construction of the fistula at another, more proximal site should be considered. On occasion, however, the appearance of a bruit and thrill is delayed until the veins dilate and blood flow increases, especially when no outflow obstruction can be demonstrated.

After the operation, the arm is slightly elevated by the patient's side for 24 hours. Avoidance of constricting dressings, sphygmomanometer cuffs, and tight clothing is mandatory. Any swelling present usually resolves over subsequent weeks. At least 4 to 6 weeks should elapse before the fistula is used for hemodialysis. Puncturing the vessels before they are arterialized is often associated with hematoma formation, because the dilated veins are thin-walled in the first few weeks.[18] Although exercise of the forearm by squeezing a rubber ball to increase fistula flow and promote maturation of the arterialized veins has been advocated,[21] this has no reported benefit.[22]

Reverse Arteriovenous Fistula

The internal reverse arteriovenous fistula[23] (Fig. 34–7) is a method to salvage a failed or failing Brescia-Cimino fistula. This type of access procedure involves a side-to-side brachial artery-to-basilic vein anastomosis, thereby reversing blood flow into the superficial median antecubital and ulnar veins and providing an additional site for a hemodialysis fistula in patients in whom the forearm vessels have been exhausted surgically. A primary requisite for the procedure is the presence of a 4- to 5-cm segment of antecubital vein.

Three technical points are emphasized in this procedure for reversing flow in the forearm veins. First, the valves in the forearm veins just distal to the level of the anastomosis must be ruptured with a blunt probe via a basilic venotomy;

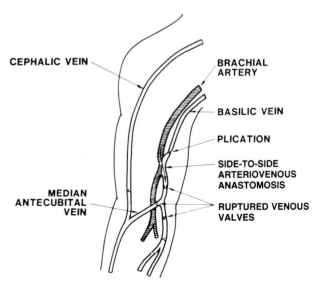

Figure 34–7. Reversed autogenous arteriovenous fistula.

however, because of the previous venous arterialization, these valves are often incompetent and require little instrumentation. Second, in carrying out rupture of the valves, care must be taken not to injure the deep brachial veins, because these eventually represent the major route of venous return in the arm, and damage to them may result in venous hypertension. Finally, the basilic vein proximal to the anastomosis is plicated to direct arterial inflow distally in the forearm. Plication rather than ligation preserves the proximal basilic vein as a future site of vascular access.

Brachiobasilic and Brachiocephalic Arteriovenous Fistulas

Brachiobasilic and brachiocephalic arteriovenous fistulas are other types of secondary upper extremity vascular access procedures that may be performed after failure of a more distal extremity arteriovenous fistula or because the forearm vessels are inadequate. Patency rates of 80% at 3 years demonstrate the usefulness of these areas of vascular access for chronic hemodialysis.[24]

The brachiobasilic fistula (Fig. 34–8C) is constructed by initially identifying the basilic vein just anterior to the medial epicondyle of the humerus and then mobilizing the vein proximal to the axilla. Care must be taken during mobilization not to injure the cutaneous nerve to the forearm, which lies adjacent to the vein. The vein is divided in the antecubital fossa and relocated in a subcutaneous tunnel running down the anterior aspect of the arm. The proximal end of the vein remains in continuity with the axillary vein. The brachial artery is isolated in the antecubital fossa, and the end of the relocated vein is anastomosed to the anterior aspect of the artery in an end-to-side fashion at this level, using a 1-cm arteriotomy. Construction of the brachiocephalic fistula (Fig. 34–8B) is similar, although technically easier. The cephalic vein already lies in a superficial position on the anterolateral aspect of the arm, so no need exists for repositioning. The vein needs only to be mobilized proximal to the antecubital fossa a sufficient distance to secure a tension-free end-to-side anastomosis.

VASCULAR GRAFTS (BRIDGE FISTULAS)

Successful long-term management of chronic renal failure frequently means that the patient outlives the usefulness of several serially constructed vascular access routes. When reconstructing an autogenous arteriovenous fistula is no longer feasible, the use of a prosthetic conduit to form a bridge arteriovenous fistula is the best alternative. Bridge fistulas can be placed between almost any suitably sized superficial artery and vein in the body. After implantation, these easily palpable conduits can be readily punctured by needle; however, if possible, this should be avoided for about 2 weeks until the prosthesis has incorporated into the patient's tissues. Premature use may result in leaking of blood from the puncture site, with formation of a perigraft hematoma.[25]

The prosthetic material used for the conduit in an arteriovenous bridge fistula is anastomosed end to side to the recipient artery and vein. If the two anastomoses are situated close by each other, the conduit takes on a U-shaped configuration; if separated by some distance, the conduit may lie straight or in a gentle curve. The conduit courses subcutaneously, allowing an adequate length for hemodialysis access.

Bridge Fistula Sites

Bridge arteriovenous fistulas may be (and have been) constructed at almost every location of the body where suitably sized arteries and veins are surgically accessible. For patient comfort, ease of handling at hemodialysis, and safety,

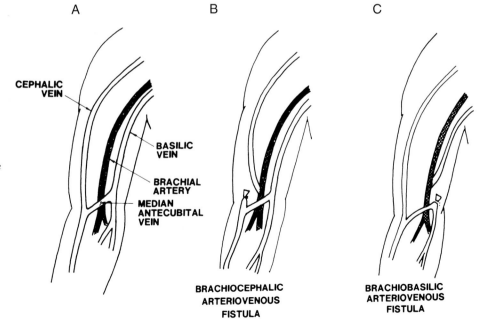

Figure 34–8. Normal anatomy (A). Brachiocephalic (B) and brachiobasilic (C) autogenous arteriovenous fistulas.

CEPHALIC VEIN

BASILIC VEIN

BRACHIAL ARTERY

MEDIAN ANTECUBITAL VEIN

BRACHIOCEPHALIC ARTERIOVENOUS FISTULA

BRACHIOBASILIC ARTERIOVENOUS FISTULA

however, the majority are constructed in either the upper extremity or thigh.

In the upper extremity, bridge arteriovenous fistulas may be satisfactorily constructed between the radial artery and an antecubital fossa vein, the brachial artery (in the antecubital fossa before its branching) and either the adjacent cephalic or basilic vein (U-configuration loop), and the brachial artery and the axillary vein (Fig. 34–9). Construction of an upper extremity bridge fistula is often more technically demanding than a thigh fistula, and its long-term patency is not as high.[26, 27] This is generally attributed to the larger vessels and greater blood flow in the thigh. The risk of infection and distal limb ischemia is less in fistulas constructed in the upper extremity,[25] however, and this is the site of preference. Patients with claudication or an ankle arterial pressure less than 80% of that at the wrist are not suitable for thigh fistulas because the proximal steal of blood through the fistula is likely to increase the ischemia in the leg.[28] Therefore, upper extremity fistulas are particularly well suited for elderly patients with significant atherosclerosis in the lower extremities. Obese patients in whom perspiration or dermatitis involving the groin skinfolds may increase the likelihood of infection should have placement of an arm fistula.

In the thigh, the arterial anastomosis should, in the first instance, be to the superficial femoral artery, immediately proximal to either the adductor canal or its more cephalad portion (Fig. 34–10A). If the superficial femoral artery is occluded, the common femoral artery may be used (Fig. 34–10B) with the understanding that if it becomes infected and ligation is subsequently necessary, leg ischemia may ensue. At times, patency of a short segment, including the origin of the superficial femoral artery, can be reestablished and used for the arterial anastomosis. The venous anastomosis is made to the proximal saphenous, common, or superficial femoral vein.

Traditionally, the site generally selected for initial placement of an arteriovenous bridge fistula was in the upper extremity from the distal radial artery to the cephalic or basilic vein in the antecubital fossa.[29] The graft should be anastomosed in an end-to-side fashion to the distal radial artery, tunneled along the lateral aspect of the forearm, and then anastomosed end to side to the largest vein in the antecubital fossa. In positioning the graft, one must ensure that the patient's arm will rest comfortably when receiving hemodialysis. Actual bridging of the elbow joint should be avoided to aid in the long-term patency of the graft.

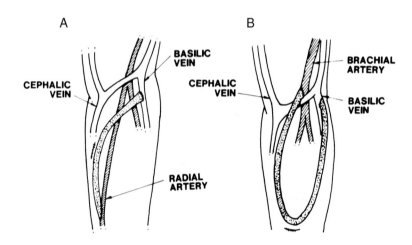

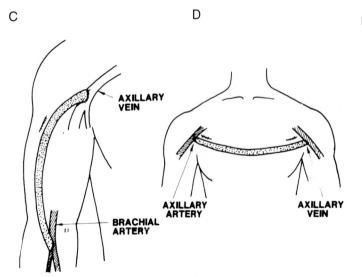

Figure 34–9. Upper extremity bridge arteriovenous fistulas.

A   B

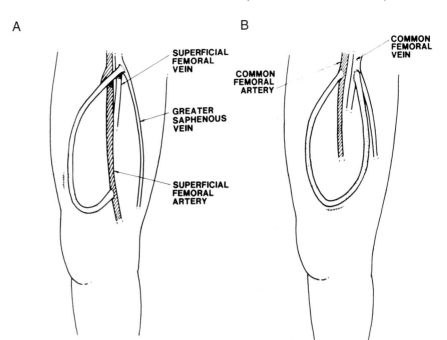

Figure 34–10. Lower extremity bridge arteriovenous fistulas.

Other vascular access sites in the upper extremity for bridge fistulas include brachiocephalic or brachiobasilic loop fistulas in the forearm and a brachioaxillary fistula in the upper arm. The loop fistulas placed in the forearm allow a large area of graft to be available for needle puncture, whereas the brachioaxillary fistula, which curves over the lateral aspect of the upper arm, allows a smaller area for needle puncture. These upper extremity loop grafts have also been found to have significantly higher patency rates at all time intervals over straight upper extremity grafts.[30] Upper extremity procedures may be easily performed using an axillary nerve block or local infiltration anesthesia.

Arteriovenous bridge fistulas in the thigh are usually constructed with the patient under a spinal or general anesthetic, although in cooperative patients a local infiltration technique can be used. Placing the arterial origin of the conduit just proximal to the adductor canal portion of the superficial femoral artery is often advisable so that, if a vascular complication should cause occlusion of the artery, adequate collateral channels would provide filling of the popliteal segment. The end-to-side arterial anastomosis should be oblique, and the graft should leave the vessel at an acute angle, to minimize turbulence. The venous anastomosis is also performed in an end-to-side fashion and as obliquely as possible. This is to counteract any purse-string effect of the suture, as well as buildup of fibrin and fibrous tissue at the venous anastomosis, which commonly causes late graft thrombosis. A vascular steal phenomenon, with reversal of flow in the distal superficial femoral artery, is more common in bridge fistulas in the lower extremity and can lead to symptoms of limb ischemia.[31] Fortunately, most patients with steal do not have symptoms, because the activity of the dialysis patient is often limited.

The femorosaphenous bridge fistula is curved subcutaneously over the lateral aspect of the thigh and is anastomosed to the proximal saphenous vein. The caudal portion of the saphenous vein may be ligated to prevent retrograde venous flow, although venous hypertension in the lower extremity is not a problem with a patent iliofemoral system. A less favorable lower extremity access configuration is the loop fistula placed in the groin from the common femoral or very proximal superficial femoral artery to the femoral vein. The high blood flow rate (greater than 700 mL/ minute) can lead to a significant increase in cardiac output. The possibility of limb loss in the event of infectious complications and the increased risk of infection could make this site less desirable.[31]

With the increased survival of chronic hemodialysis patients, the surgeon may be called to evaluate a patient who requires vascular access and may find that all extremity access sites have been expended. In this circumstance, a more central location, such as a bridge arteriovenous fistula placed between the axillary artery on one side and the axillary vein on the other side, has been used successfully.[32] The grafts are of fairly large diameter, so they are easy to cannulate, flow is reported to be excellent, and, despite the location of the access site on the anterior chest wall, patients adapt to it very promptly.[23] The major drawback of central access sites is that when complications occur, they are serious and more difficult to manage.

Bridge Fistula Materials

Both biologic and prosthetic materials have been used in the creation of arteriovenous bridge fistulas for hemodialysis since this modality came into use in 1969.[33] Although saphenous vein, bovine heterografts, human umbilical vein, and Dacron velour grafts, have all been tried during the last three decades, only expanded PTFE grafts have stood the test of time.

Expanded Polytetrafluoroethylene

Since its initial introduction as an alternative material in the creation of arteriovenous bridge fistulas in 1976,[34] expanded PTFE has become the most commonly used material. Much of its popularity stems from its ease of handling, not needing to preclot, wide availability, long shelf life, and high patency rates. PTFE bridge fistulas are consistently reported to have 24-month patency rates of over 70%,[35] and, in a large comparative clinical study comprising 187 graft placements, 36-month patency rates of PTFE grafts were significantly greater than those of bovine heterografts (62% for PTFE vs. 24% for bovine heterografts).[36] Forty-eight-month patency rates of 43% to 60% have been reported.[37, 38] However, multiple procedures for revision are usually required to maintain patency, with one study reporting an average of one operation for revision being required for every 1.1 years of graft (with a range of 1 to 16 revisions per graft).[39]

Thrombosis of the conduit appears to be a relatively common event in PTFE bridge fistulas, with figures ranging from 7% to 55%.[37, 38] Most, however, are easily dealt with by thrombectomy with good results, with some responding to simple Fogarty balloon catheter embolectomy alone.[38] Infection of PTFE fistulas is another fairly frequently encountered event, with one report of 80 fistulas monitored for 30 months showing an overall incidence of infection of 19%, with 67% of these infections occurring during the initial 4 months of use.[40] Of the infected fistulas, 73% required excision, and the remainder were treated successfully with antibiotics. Pseudoaneurysm at needle puncture sites develops in approximately 5% of fistulas.[37]

It is interesting to note that a study has demonstrated that both the primary and secondary patency rates of PTFE bridge fistulas are not significantly less than those of arteriovenous fistulas, though the arteriovenous fistulas require fewer revisions[41] (Fig. 34–11A and B).

PEDIATRIC VASCULAR ACCESS

Maintenance of chronic vascular access in children is a formidable task for vascular surgeons because small vessels are a major limiting factor. Although many of the principles and techniques are the same as for the adult, certain aspects of the placement of long-term central venous catheters for total parenteral nutrition (TPN, to be discussed later) and creation of hemodialysis access sites are sufficiently different to warrant discussion.

Dialysis (either hemodialysis or peritoneal dialysis) with subsequent renal transplantation is the preferred therapeutic regimen for end-stage renal disease in children. Transplantation is usually attempted as quickly as possible, because, in general, children tolerate dialysis poorly in that they frequently develop severe growth retardation (not reversible by transplantation), failure of maturation, renal osteodystrophy, and psychosocial problems.[42, 43] In addition, long-term hemodialysis is, at best, difficult in children younger than 10 years of age, and is extremely difficult in those younger than 5 years.

Short-term hemodialysis in children may be performed in a variety of ways with good results. Newborn or premature infants can be dialyzed via direct cannulation of the umbilical vessels using a 5- or 8-Fr catheter. Single-cannula hemodialysis may be used in older children in whom either the superior or inferior vena cava has been cannulated by either the Seldinger technique or direct venous cutdown.[43] Another method in the older child involves placement of an indwelling brachial artery catheter and a large-bore silicone rubber central venous catheter placed via the external jugular vein to separate inflow and return and provide the hemodialysis return with a large-bore egress route.[44]

The preferred method for long-term vascular access for hemodialysis in children weighing less than 20 kg is the placement of a central venous silicone rubber arteriovenous shunt inserted as described previously.[44] In addition, creation of an autogenous arteriovenous fistula between the brachial artery at the elbow and an antecubital vein using microsurgical techniques has been used in children

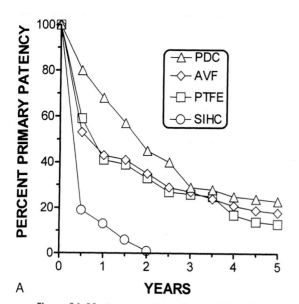

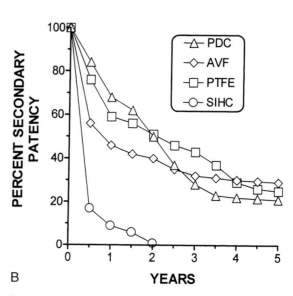

Figure 34–11. Percent primary patency (*A*) and secondary patency (*B*) of peritoneal dialysis catheters (PDC), arteriovenous fistulas (AVF), polytetrafluoroethylene grafts (PTFE), and surgically implanted dual-lumen central venous hemodialysis catheters (SIHC). (Modified from Hodges TC, Fillinger MF, Zwolek RM, et al: Longitudinal comparison of dialysis access methods: Risk factors for failure. J Vasc Surg 26:1009–1014, 1997.)

weighing between 10 kg and 23 kg, with excellent results.[45, 46]

For long-term hemodialysis access in children weighing more than 30 kg, an internal form of access, either autogenous fistula or bridge fistula, should be attempted. Children weighing between 20 and 30 kg must be individualized as regards the type of access attempted according to the size of their vessels. A Brescia-Cimino autogenous arteriovenous fistula may be created in children weighing more than 30 kg without much difficulty, and with patency rates of approximately 80% at 12 months. The use of microsurgical techniques enhances the patency rate, especially in children with small vessels to be anastomosed.[46] Bridge fistulas of PTFE have also been employed in children with good results and patency rates of more than 75% at 24 months.

The usual types of complications and their rates for both autogenous and bridge fistulas in children approximate those seen in adults. However, one of the most common complications of hemodialysis in small children is convulsions, occurring in up to 30% of patients.[47] This is probably due to two factors: (1) the use of overly efficient dialysis, and (2) the greater sensitivity of children to changes in osmolality. It can probably be avoided by tight regulation of the efficiency of the dialysis procedure based on the child's body weight.

One major disadvantage of the use of internal vascular access fistulas in children that must be specifically mentioned, however, is the physically and psychologically terrifying pain of needle puncture, which may require much time and counseling to overcome.

VASCULAR ACCESS COMPLICATIONS

Infection

Infection is a devastating complication for the chronic renal failure patient and represents the second most common cause of death among patients on chronic hemodialysis, causing 10% of all deaths in dialysis patients, exceeded only by cardiovascular disease.[48] Many of the systemic infections encountered in these patients are direct complications of an infection established at the site of hemodialysis access. In two large dialysis centers, an incidence of 0.11 septic episodes per patient-dialysis-year related specifically to the vascular access site was found.[49] This represented over 73% of the total number of septic episodes encountered.

The elevated rate of sepsis associated with hemodialysis vascular access sites is partially due to the deficient immune defense mechanisms in patients with chronic renal failure and consequent increase in infection risk.[50] The bacterial phagocytic and killing ability of polymorphonuclear leukocytes also decreases by nearly 50% in patients with chronic renal failure.[51] Lymphocytes in chronic renal failure exhibit suppressed cellular immunity, and inhibition of lymphocyte transformation, which is unaffected by dialysis, has been found.[52] In addition, the serum of uremic animals contains a nondialyzable inhibitor of the mixed lymphocyte reaction, which is probably a glycoprotein and distinct from either α-macroglobulin or immune complexes.[53] The actual ability of the animal to produce antibodies when antigen-stimu-lated, however, does not appear to be depressed in chronic renal failure.[54]

In addition to alterations in host defense mechanisms, other factors contribute to the increase in the propensity of patients on long-term hemodialysis to develop infection. Poor healing of surgical wounds is a recognized consequence of renal failure and may result in wound infections. Measurement of the bacterial colonization rate of patients receiving hemodialysis revealed that 62% of these patients carried *Staphylococcus aureus* in their oro- or nasopharynx or on the skin, and 65% of those patients with positive cultures developed infections in their hemodialysis access sites.[55] Furthermore, 30% of the dialysis staff carried *S. aureus*, whereas only 11% of normal controls had positive cultures. In the same study, more than 70% of all infections encountered were caused by *S. aureus*. The patient's own level of personal hygiene represents the best indicator for *S. aureus* colonization and vascular access site infection risk.[56]

Although infection of an autogenous arteriovenous fistula is unusual, it can occur. Repeated needling of the fistula may result in formation of a hematoma that can subsequently become infected by skin microflora. In addition, the anastomotic site of the fistula itself may become infected, resulting in an endovasculitis with subsequent septicemia and metastatic abscess formation. Treatment generally consists of therapeutic courses of appropriate antibiotic agents coupled with local measures such as drainage of a perifistula abscess from an infected hematoma. Rarely, the fistula anastomosis may have to be dismantled and the vessels ligated in the presence of an infection-induced anastomotic pseudoaneurysm.

Bridge fistulas placed for vascular access are susceptible to multiple sources of infection. Contamination from skin flora may occur during implantation and occurs more frequently when the fistula is placed on the thigh than when it is located in the upper extremity. This is owing to the greater difficulty in preparing a sterile surgical field on the medial thigh and inguinal skinfold.[57, 58] Direct inoculation of the graft by needle puncture through inadequately prepared skin also occurs, as well as inoculation of hematomas resulting in perigraft abscess formation.

The type of material in bridge fistulas also affects the infection rate, with autogenous saphenous vein fistulas demonstrating few, if any, infections, and biologic conduits (human umbilical vein graft [HUVG], bovine heterograft) being particularly susceptible to aggressive infections; synthetic conduits are also susceptible to infection by low-virulence organisms.[59] The newly implanted prosthesis is particularly susceptible to infection; however, tissue incorporation and neointima formation confer increased resistance to infection.[60] Delay in initiating hemodialysis using bridge fistulas for about 2 weeks after graft implantation allows tissue incorporation of the prosthesis and development of a neointima. Disruption of an infected bridge fistula anastomosis (Fig. 34–12) may occur at any time during the course of a prosthetic infection and does not appear to be influenced by incorporation.[59]

Treatment of an established infection of a conduit is excision of the prosthetic material. Attempts at in situ sterilization using antibiotics or povidone-iodine irrigation have not proved reliably successful. A possible exception

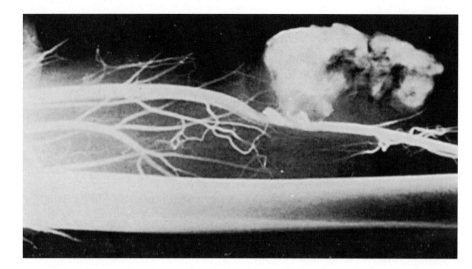

Figure 34–12. Angiogram demonstrating disruption of infected bridge fistula anastomosis.

to this would be infection surrounding an autogenous saphenous vein prosthesis, for which treatment with antibiotics has been reported.[61] After excision of the fistula, several days should be allowed to elapse before creation of a new access site for control of any associated bacteremia.

Regimens aimed at prevention of this complication should always be practiced, including the use of perioperative antibiotic administration. Randomized, prospective, double-blind studies have consistently shown the protective role of perioperative antibiotics in vascular surgery.[62, 63] This has also been confirmed in vascular access surgery, in which perioperative use of a cephalosporin in a randomized, double-blind setting resulted in a significant decrease in postoperative wound infection rates, including cellulitis.[64] Vancomycin is also very effective in the prevention of vascular access graft infections, especially in the pediatric population.[65] In addition, proper care and use of aseptic technique by the dialysis staff and the patient are required to prevent infection at the site of hemodialysis access.

Thrombosis

The most frequent complication encountered in vascular access surgery is thrombosis of the fistula or shunt. The likelihood of thrombosis depends on multiple factors, including the type of shunt or fistula constructed, the site of the arteriovenous anastomosis, the selection of prosthetic material, and the adequacy of the patient's vessels. Thrombosis at the access site may occur at any time after construction. Early thrombosis, usually defined as occurring within the first 3 months, is generally due to technical factors, whereas late thrombosis, occurring after 3 months, is usually caused by continuing trauma to the access site by needle puncture for hemodialysis or outflow stenosis.

Lack of adequate venous runoff is the primary cause of early failure of distal access sites.[66] In the operating room, this can be recognized soon after completion of the final anastomosis by the absence of pulse, bruit, or palpable thrill. Ascertaining the patency and adequate diameter of the runoff vessel by use of a Fogarty embolectomy catheter or coronary artery dilators often guards against this setback. Narrowing of the lumen of the artery or vein during con-

struction or catching the back wall of the vessel while suturing can result in immediate thrombosis. Thrombosis in the early postoperative period may also be due to compression of the fistula by a hematoma. This often results from inadequate hemostasis during the procedure or early puncture of the fistula with subsequent extravasation of blood (Fig. 34–13). Excessive pressure over the needle puncture site after a hemodialysis run may also result in fistula thrombosis. In each of these situations, early reexploration, with evacuation of any hematoma, and thrombectomy of the fistula often results in salvage of the fistula.[67]

Thrombosis of a vascular access fistula may be due to

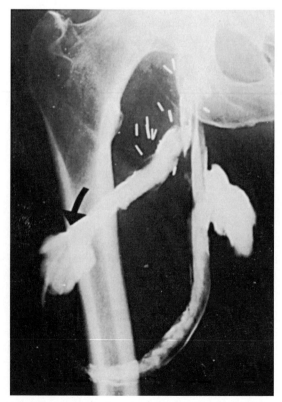

Figure 34–13. Angiogram demonstrating extravasation of blood and hematoma formation (*arrow*) following too early use of bridge fistula.

repeated trauma from needle punctures, with subsequent fibrosis and narrowing. In synthetic bridge fistulas, a needle-induced flap tear of the prosthetic wall can cause late thrombosis.

Outflow obstruction due to stenosis at the site of venous anastomosis is a relatively frequent cause of thrombosis in older bridge fistulas and may be heralded by a gradual increase in the pressure within the fistula. The combination of forceful pulsation throughout the fistula and a loud bruit at the venous end strongly suggests the development of outflow obstruction, which may be confirmed by angiography or duplex scanning (Figs. 34–14 and 34–15). True vessel aneurysmal dilatation from repeated needle punctures has also been reported as a major cause of late thrombosis in autogenous fistulas.[66] In addition, cigarette smoking significantly increases the likelihood of thrombosis and late occlusion of arteriovenous fistulas and is to be avoided if at all possible.[68]

Fistula thromboses were treated successfully by thrombectomy, restoring flow in over 80% of fistulas in one report.[69] This same study, however, indicated that approximately 70% of successfully thrombectomized fistulas reclotted within 6 months. This was thought to be due to unsuspected anatomic lesions and technical imperfections, which can be demonstrated with angiography.[70] Aggressive fistula revision, directed by angiography at the time of thrombectomy, has resulted in 6-month patency rates greater than 70%.[69]

Because elevated venous return pressure during dialysis is a very sensitive indicator of significant venous stenosis,[71, 72] we strongly recommend some type of radiologic investigation of the fistula as soon as elevation in venous return pressure is noted. Whereas fistula angiography remains the gold standard, noninvasive methods of assessing fistula flow have been described. By employing Doppler ultrasound examination of the fistula, partial or

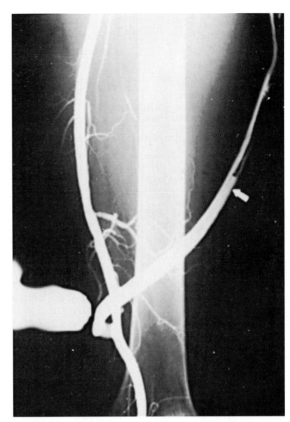

Figure 34–15. Angiogram showing partially occluding thrombus (*arrow*) in lower extremity bridge fistula.

complete thrombosis, aneurysmal dilatation, or perifistula hematoma may be diagnosed with exceptional accuracy.[73, 74] Ultrasound imaging should probably be the initial investigative technique in cases of suspected fistula malfunction. If recognized before thrombosis, many venous runoff stenoses may be corrected with percutaneous transluminal dilatation, with patency rates of 91% at 1 year and 57% at 2 years being reported.[75]

If acute thrombosis has already occurred, the use of fibrinolytic agents is successful in clearing the fistula of thrombus. In one series employing streptokinase, 52% of thrombosed fistulas were restored to function without surgical intervention, and another 21% had restoration of flow but required surgical correction of an underlying problem thereafter.[76] Another group was successful in restoring function in more than 65% of cases using urokinase.[77] The use of fibrinolytic agents in this manner appears to be most successful when the cause of failure is thrombosis secondary to hypotension, or excessive compression of fistula puncture sites after dialysis. Fistula failure associated with excessive proliferation of neointima does not respond nearly as well and usually requires surgical revision.

In an effort to improve on the thrombogenic tendency of vascular access fistulas, prophylaxis against thrombosis has been attempted with encouraging results. By using low-dose aspirin therapy (160 mg/day), one investigative group reported a highly significant reduction in fistula thrombotic episodes.[78] Another group has reported the successful establishment and maintenance of arteriovenous fistulas in nonuremic individuals by the use of aspirin and

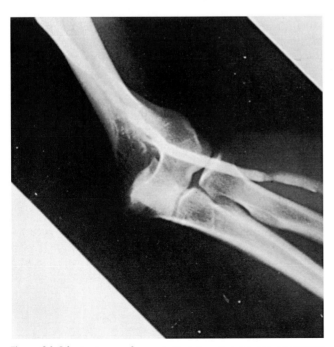

Figure 34–14. Angiogram demonstrating stenosis near venous anastomosis.

low-dose heparin therapy.[79] The use of oral pentoxifylline was found to significantly decrease access thrombosis in patients receiving long-term hemodialysis in one report, but this agent is not commonly used today.[80]

Hemodynamic Complications

The three principal hemodynamic complications of an arteriovenous fistula are congestive heart failure; peripheral vascular insufficiency, or steal phenomenon; and venous hypertension. The physiologic responses of an arteriovenous fistula for hemodialysis have been reported as a decrease in total systemic vascular resistance; an increase in cardiac output, with increases in both heart rate and, somewhat later, stroke volume; an increase in venous pressure and venous return to the heart; and reversal of flow in the artery distal to the site of the fistula when the diameter of the fistula opening exceeds the diameter of the feeding artery.[19, 20, 81] In addition, a significant decrease in subcutaneous tissue oxygen tension to levels less than 30 mm Hg occurs.[82]

Depending on the diameter of the arteriovenous communication and the size of the artery feeding it, the venous return to the heart from an arteriovenous fistula increases proportionately. This leads to a variable increase in cardiac output and work of the heart, which can be significant enough to lead to cardiomegaly and congestive heart failure. Fistula flow as low as 20% to 25% of the resting cardiac output has resulted in heart failure.[83] Because the mean blood flow rate through distal (radiocephalic) upper extremity autogenous or bridge fistulas has been measured in one report as 242 ± 89 mL/minute, high-output heart failure is unusual but does occur.[84, 85] In the same report, however, resting flow rates from more proximal upper extremity fistulas based on the brachial artery were noted to more than double, averaging as much as 641 ± 111 mL/minute. Similarly, bridge fistulas placed in the thigh arising from the superficial femoral artery had resting flow rates of 592 ± 134 mL/minute. Therefore, congestive heart failure is much more likely to result from the more proximally located fistula.

Initial blood flow through any type of arteriovenous fistula for hemodialysis is too low to cause heart failure, except in patients with underlying severely compromised cardiac function.[85] With dilatation of the venous outflow system, shunted blood flow through the fistula can increase greatly. One group of investigators, using echocardiographic evaluation of cardiac performance, has suggested that creation of any hemodialysis vascular access fistula causes a significant time-related cardiac decompensation compared with normal controls.[86] Echocardiographic assessment may also be useful preoperatively in identifying patients with poor contractility, as manifested by changes in the mean velocity of fiber shortening, ejection fraction, and left ventricular or septal wall hypertrophy.[87] Abnormal studies may warn the clinician of a propensity toward future development of heart failure and may lead to construction of the smallest, and if possible, distal, arteriovenous fistula compatible with adequate access.

When congestive heart failure arises from a high-flow arteriovenous fistula, operative correction is, fortunately, quite simple. Although revision of the fistula with narrowing of the anastomosis or construction of a completely new fistula may be used to correct the problem, the simplest procedure for correction is banding of the existing fistula by suturing a small cuff (1 cm wide) of synthetic material (Dacron, PTFE) around the prosthesis of a bridge fistula or the main venous outflow tract of an autogenous fistula. An electromagnetic flowmeter is placed around the vein proximal to the fistula and banding cuff, and continuous flow is recorded. When the fistula flow is within the range of 300 to 400 mL/minute, the banding cuff is securely sutured.

Patients who can be identified preoperatively as being at risk of access-induced congestive heart failure (e.g., elderly, existing cardiac dysfunction) and who require a bridge fistula should have either a tapered or stepped graft placed. These grafts are manufactured with the diameter of one end 2.5 to 3.0 mm smaller than the other so that when placed in the patient (with the smaller end anastomosed to the artery), flow through the graft is somewhat reduced, thereby lessening the risk of congestive heart failure.

Arterial insufficiency, or steal syndrome, in vascular access for hemodialysis was originally described as occurring in Brescia-Cimino fistulas with side-to-side anastomoses because of reversed blood flow in the distal radial artery.[88] An area of very low resistance is formed on the venous portion of the anastomosis so that the blood flow tends to course through the palmar arch from the ulnar to the radial side and steals flow from the muscles and soft tissues of the palm and fingers.[89] The syndrome is characterized by pain on exertion of the musculature of the hand, and the hand often appears cold, clammy, and pale. Severely symptomatic radial artery steal is rare, with one large study reporting only 8 of 444 (1.6%) patients who had had 516 Brescia-Cimino fistulas constructed for hemodialysis developing significant steal symptoms,[90] although up to 80% of patients with Brescia-Cimino fistulas do have mild, asymptomatic arterial steal documented by a significant decrease in thumb blood pressure.[91] Steal syndrome has also been described in 6.4% of a series of 357 patients with upper extremity bridge fistulas, one third of whom required fistula ligation to preserve function of the hand, whereas the other two thirds were successfully managed with surgical narrowing of the arterial side of the fistula.[92] Surgical correction of radial steal from a side-to-side autogenous fistula is most easily accomplished by ligation of the radial artery immediately distal to the fistula, which converts the side-to-side anastomosis to an arterial end-to-side anastomosis.[89]

Arterial insufficiency has also been noted with the use of proximally based bridge fistulas in both the upper extremity[25] and the lower extremity[28] as the result of steal from the high-flow fistulas. When steal becomes symptomatic with bridge fistulas, banding of the fistula or venous outflow tract to decrease fistula flow often causes these patients to become asymptomatic.[26] Very rarely, the entire fistula may have to be dismantled.

Arterialization of the venous system proximal to an arteriovenous fistula results in venous hypertension and, if the venous valves are incompetent, retrograde venous flow. Noted most frequently with side-to-side Brescia-Cimino fistulas and, to a lesser extent, reverse arteriovenous fistulas, retrograde venous hypertension is marked by distal extremity edema, bluish discoloration, and pigmentation of the skin (Fig. 34–16). Ulceration and neuralgias can also occur in long-standing cases.[93, 94] Surgical correction is obtained by ligation of the vein immediately distal to the fistula, converting the side-to-side anastomosis of the Brescia-Cimino fistula to a functional venous end-to-side anastomosis, and converting the bridge fistula to a functional end-to-end anastomosis.

Intimal Hyperplasia

Progressive venous stenosis occurring as a consequence of vascular access fistula placement is a recurring problem leading to thrombosis and multiple revisions or replacement fistulas of patients requiring long-term hemodialysis. Indeed, it is the main drawback associated with prosthetic conduits. Although the stenosis may be related to the technical performance of the anastomosis, in the main it can be attributed to chronic changes known to occur in the runoff veins of arteriovenous fistulas. The development of intimal fibromuscular hyperplasia may result from focal endothelial trauma caused by the shearing effect of blood flow at the site of the venous anastomosis.[95, 96] In addition, venous hypertension in the runoff vessels of an arteriovenous fistula aggravates venous atherosclerosis and intimal lipid deposition, further compounding the situation.[97] Segmental stenosis of autogenous fistulas and bridge fistulas constructed using biologic conduits has also been noted to

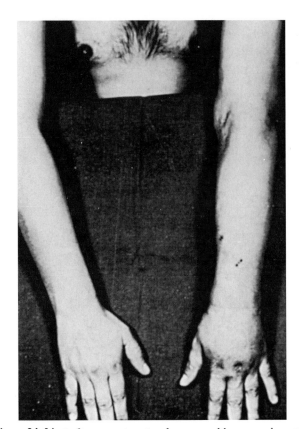

Figure 34–16. Left upper extremity edema caused by venous hypertension from Brescia-Cimino fistula.

occur from fibrosis and intimal hyperplasia secondary to the trauma of repeated needle punctures.[98]

Surgical correction of the stenotic area may be accomplished by patch angioplasty if the stenosis is extremely localized or at the site of an anastomosis by placing an extension of the graft around a larger stenotic area, by locating the venous anastomosis to a new vein, or by complete resection of the stenotic segment with placement of an interposition conduit. The use of percutaneous transluminal balloon angioplasty has been advocated for dilatation of stenotic segments in failing arteriovenous fistulas and shunts.[75] Using the Seldinger technique to gain access to the fistula, a double-lumen dilator catheter is placed at the site of the stenosis under fluoroscopic control, and the stenosis is dilated twice for 30 seconds each time. Before catheter removal, an angiogram is performed, and the dilatation repeated if a greater than 30% residual stenosis is present. Using this technique, an initial success rate of 95% has been achieved.[75]

Aneurysm Formation

Aneurysmal dilatation of bridge fistula conduits depends on the material used. True aneurysm formation occurs primarily in biologic materials (saphenous vein, bovine heterograft, HUVG) and has been attributed to degeneration over time of the graft material itself.[25] Early PTFE grafts were also prone to true aneurysm formation from nodal fracture and a gradual stretching of the PTFE fibrils[99]; however, with an increase in the wall thickness of the material, this is no longer a problem. Excessive aneurysmal enlargement of the fistula is best treated with surgical excision of the hemodialysis fistula, with placement of a new conduit of a synthetic material at another site. Pseudoaneurysm formation secondary to trauma at the site of needle punctures can occur with any of the materials used for bridge fistulas (Fig. 34–17). If no infection is apparent, treatment can be occasionally achieved by local suture repair of the defect in the graft material. Somewhat larger defects may require excision of the defect and the interposition of a new small segment of graft material. Although rare, the aneurysmal segment, once diagnosed, should be bypassed and then excluded through ligation.

VASCULAR ACCESS FOR TOTAL PARENTERAL NUTRITION OR CHEMOTHERAPY

The use of surgically created arteriovenous fistulas as a means of vascular access for reasons other than hemodialysis is increasing. Several reports have found that chronic TPN can be performed using an arteriovenous fistula with a length of patency of up to 7 years.[100, 101] The advantages are a very low incidence of infection and longevity of the access site. The primary disadvantage is that the patient must undergo a significant operation to establish vascular access. The use of an autogenous arteriovenous fistula for the delivery of chemotherapeutic agents has also been advocated.[102, 103] Bridge arteriovenous fistulas have also

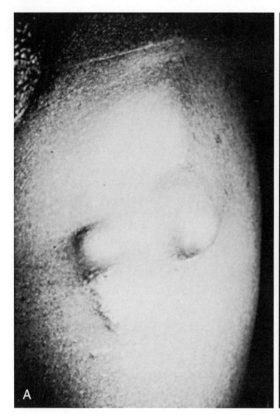
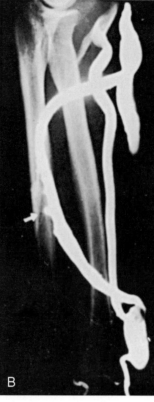

Figure 34–17. *A,* Pseudoaneurysm formation at needle puncture sites of hemodialysis fistula. *B,* Angiogram demonstrating multiple pseudoaneurysms *(arrow)* at needle puncture sites of bridge fistula.

been used; however, one series reported a significantly higher complication rate for bridge fistulas compared with Silastic right atrial catheters (48% vs. 19%, respectively) for chemotherapy use.[104]

Despite these increasing reports regarding the use of arteriovenous fistulas for chemotherapy and TPN, the more general method employed for delivering these therapeutic modalities is a chronic indwelling central venous catheter. For a number of years, the accepted method for central venous cannulation involved percutaneous catheterization with a polyethylene catheter. Recognition of the propensity of percutaneously placed polyethylene catheters toward infection and thrombosis and the inherent dangers of the technique of placing these catheters, however, has led to the development of specialized large-bore catheters that are less reactive and less thrombogenic.

The Broviac[105] and Hickman[106] central venous catheters are made of soft radiopaque rubber measuring 90 cm in length and have a small Dacron felt cuff 30 cm from the external end. The Broviac catheter has an internal diameter of 1 mm, and the Hickman modification differs only in that it has an internal diameter of 1.6 mm. Each catheter consists of a relatively thin-walled intravascular segment, and a thicker walled extravascular portion. A smaller, pediatric-sized Broviac catheter is also available, as are double-lumen catheters in various sizes. These catheters are placed via direct venous cutdown into the cephalic (Fig. 34–18), external jugular, or greater saphenous veins, and the extravascular portion of the catheter is tunneled through the subcutaneous tissue to separate the skin exit site from the venotomy site. Fibrous tissue ingrowth into the Dacron cuff located in the subcutaneous tunnel serves to anchor the catheter and presents an effective barrier to the migra-

tion of microorganisms from the skin into the venous system along the outer surface of the catheter. For further protection against infection, many of these catheters can also be ordered with an additional cuff in place that is impregnated with an antimicrobial agent. This cuff is posi-

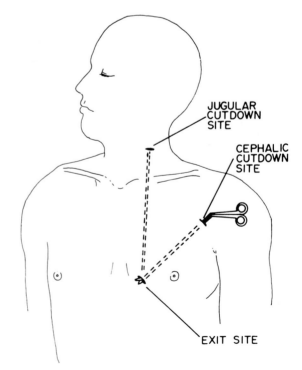

Figure 34–18. Position of subcutaneous tunnel exit site for upper body Broviac or Hickman catheter.

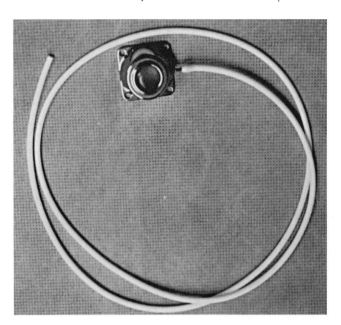

Figure 34–19. Implantable port showing reservoir with self-sealing septum and silicone catheter.

tioned in the subcutaneous tunnel between the Dacron cuff and the skin exit site. As a consequence, the sepsis rate with these catheters is relatively low.[107, 108]

Innovations in central venous access have been the introduction of the Groshong catheter and implantable ports. Unlike either the Hickman or Broviac catheters, the Groshong catheter has no clamps, comes without the hub attached, and possesses a unique two-way valve. This valve is designed to remain closed when the catheter is not in use, and opens either outward for fluid infusion or inward for blood draws. This design allows for significantly less maintenance by either the patient or the health care worker, with only a single 5-mL saline flush being recommended once a week when the catheter is not in use. One group has even suggested less frequent flushings if a heparinized saline solution is used.[109]

Implantable ports (Fig. 34–19) are central venous access devices that consist of a subcutaneously implantable reservoir containing a self-sealing septum that can withstand over 2000 needle punctures. They are connected to a silicone rubber catheter of an internal diameter ranging from 1.0 to 1.6 mm. The reservoir body, which can be constructed of plastic, stainless steel, or titanium, is placed in a subcutaneous pocket over the anterior chest or abdomen in an easily palpable location and is accessed with a Huber needle for either blood withdrawal or drug delivery. These implantable ports have the advantage of requiring little daily care and therefore interfere less with the patient's normal activities. Also, implantable ports have a catheter-related sepsis rate of 3% and show a 1% incidence of thrombosis compared with a 15% rate of catheter-related sepsis and a 22% incidence of thrombosis in external central venous catheters.[110] A prospective comparison demonstrated that external shunts have 0.13 exit site infections and 0.03 bacteremic episodes per 100 catheter-days compared with 0.06 pocket infections and 0 bacteremic episodes per 100 catheter-days for implantable ports.[111]

A newer subcutaneous port is the peripherally inserted central catheter line shown in Figure 34–20. A polyurethane catheter is placed via a cutdown in an antecubital

vein and is threaded into the superior vena cava. A small titanium port is then connected to the catheter and placed in a subcutaneous tunnel. Its primary advantage is ease of insertion; the procedure can be performed at the bedside.

The placement of any central venous catheter for TPN or chemotherapy is always considered to be an elective, sterile, operative procedure. Thus, the patient should have hypovolemia and electrolyte abnormalities corrected before catheter placement. Adequate lighting, instruments, assistance, and aseptic techniques are absolute prerequisites of safe insertion of the catheter. A thorough knowledge of the venous anatomy and adequate experience or supervision are likewise mandatory. In theory, the Broviac or Hickman catheter may be placed into any vein accessible by cutdown; but in practice, the cephalic vein in the deltopectoral groove, the external jugular vein in the neck, and the greater saphenous vein at its confluence with the common femoral vein are the preferred sites. If these are unavailable, the internal jugular, the common facial, the large pectoral radial, and the thoracoacromial veins are alternatives.[25] In patients requiring long-term central venous catheterization who have had numerous previous catheters placed, preoperative venography may be required to verify patency of the vena cava (superior or inferior), the subclavian or iliac vein, or their tributaries.

In most hospitals, Broviac or Hickman catheter insertion is performed in the controlled environment of the operating suite, where radiography or fluoroscopy is available to confirm the proper position of the catheter tip before skin closure. The cutdown site is then selected. For the cephalic vein cutdown, the skin incision is made just inferior to the coracoid process in the area of the deltopectoral groove. For the external jugular vein approach, a transverse midcervical incision is made over the vein. When the greater saphenous vein is used, a longitudinal incision over the vein and just distal to the inguinal ligament is employed.

After dissection verifies patency and adequate size of the selected vein, a subcutaneous tunnel is made from the cutdown site to a cutaneous exit either medial to the

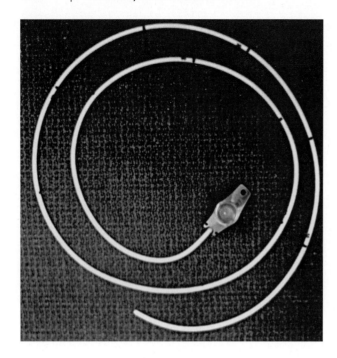

Figure 34–20. Peripherally inserted central catheter line, which is placed via cutdown in antecubital fossa.

breast (if a cephalad central vein is chosen) or the anterior abdominal wall if a caudad vein is used. A small stab wound is made at the cutaneous exit site, and the catheter is drawn through the tunnel until the Dacron cuff resides 2 to 4 cm inside the tunnel. The catheter is then shortened so that the tip just reaches the right atrium from the upper body or about the level of the renal veins from the lower body. The catheter is filled with heparin-treated saline by syringe. The vein is ligated distally, and the catheter is introduced through a small venotomy, advanced to its full length, and aspirated with the attached syringe. If dark venous blood does not return, the catheter is either kinked or misplaced, and it should be withdrawn and advanced again. A proximal ligature placed around the vein secures the catheter in place. Radiographic verification of proper

catheter tip position should always be obtained before wound closure (Fig. 34–21). The catheter is fixed to the skin at the exit site with a monofilament suture, which is removed 7 to 14 days later after fibrous ingrowth into the Dacron cuff has occurred. Povidone-iodine ointment and a sterile dressing are applied to the exit site, and the loop of redundant catheter is taped to the body wall. The catheter may either be heparin-locked or immediately connected to an intravenous infusion set.

Once properly inserted and positioned, Broviac and Hickman catheters have been left in place for more than 1 year, with an average duration reported of over 2 months.[107, 108] Because of the chronic nature of the underlying diseases often seen in patients who require long-term catheterization, multiple insertions were necessary in 13%

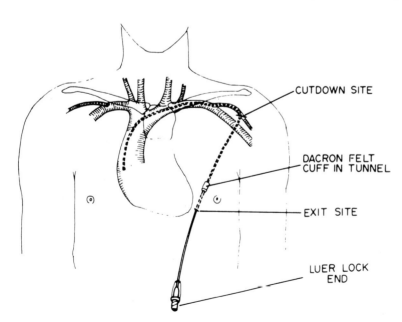

CUTDOWN SITE

DACRON FELT CUFF IN TUNNEL

EXIT SITE

LUER LOCK END

Figure 34–21. Correct position of Broviac or Hickman catheter placed via cephalic vein.

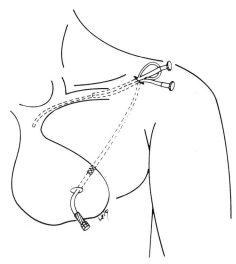

Figure 34–22. Placement of a Silastic catheter by percutaneous subclavian venipuncture.

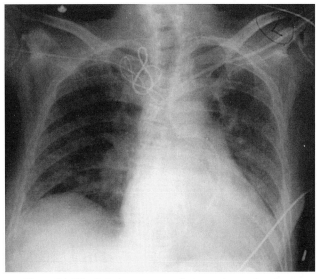

Figure 34–23. Coiled percutaneously inserted central catheter.

of patients in one study.[107] The primary complications of Broviac and Hickman catheter use are sepsis, thrombosis, and dislodgment of the catheter, which in two series comprising 199 catheter placements occurred in 12%, 5.0%, and 3.5% of cases, respectively.[107, 108] Central vein thrombosis as a result of long-term catheterization has also been noted to occur although infrequently.

An alternative technique for placement of Broviac and Hickman catheters involving direct venipuncture has been reported.[112] With this technique, two small (less than 1 cm) skin incisions are made at the proposed venous entry site and skin exit site and a subcutaneous tunnel created between them. The catheter is then brought through the tunnel until the Dacron cuff lies 2 to 4 cm within the tunnel. The chosen vein is then punctured through the vein entry incision as if for placement of a central venous pressure line. A guidewire is inserted through the needle, thus allowing the needle to be removed. A vein dilator and

peel-away sheath are then placed over the guidewire, and, once in place, the guidewire and dilator are removed. The Broviac or Hickman catheter is introduced into the vein through the peel-away sheath, and the sheath is withdrawn and peeled apart, leaving the catheter in place. Radiologic verification of catheter position is then achieved, and wound closure and catheter care are performed as with standard Broviac or Hickman catheter placement (Fig. 34–22).[23]

Although malposition of the catheter (Fig. 34–23) is the most common complication of direct venipuncture,[112] any of the complications seen with standard central venous pressure placement are possible because of the relatively blind nature of the technique. This would include pneumohemothorax, arterial laceration or perforation, arteriovenous fistula formation, brachial plexus or other nerve injury, air or catheter embolism, or lymphatic fistula formation.[11]

References

1. Garrison FH: An Introduction to the History of Medicine, 4th ed. Philadelphia, WB Saunders, 1929, p 273.
2. Wheatley HB: The Diary of Samuel Pepys, vol 2. New York, Random House, 1966, p 426.
3. Kolff WJ: The first clinical experience with the artificial kidney. Ann Intern Med 62:609–619, 1965.
4. Quinton WE, Dillard D, Scribner BH: Cannulation of blood vessels for prolonged hemodialysis. Trans Am Soc Artif Intern Organs 6:104–113, 1960.
5. US Renal Data System: USRDS 1999 Annual Data Report. Bethesda, Md, The National Institutes of Health, National Institute of Diabetes and Digestion and Kidney Diseases, April 1999.
6. Orengo MF, Lawrence L: Detailed diagnoses and procedures. National Hospital Discharge Survey, 1997. National Center for Health Statistics. Vital Health Stat 13(145), 1997.
7. Ishihara AM, Meyers CH: Longevity of arteriovenous shunts for hemodialysis. Ann Surg 168:281–286, 1968.
8. Harder F, Landmann J: Trends in access surgery for hemodialysis. Surg Annu 16:135–149, 1984.
9. Dunn J, Nylander W, Richie R: Central venous dialysis access: Experience with a dual-lumen, silicone rubber catheter. Surgery 102:784–789, 1987.
10. Surratt RS, Picus D, Hicks ME, et al: The importance of preoperative evaluation of the subclavian vein in dialysis planning. AJR 156:623–625, 1991.
11. Herbst CA: Indications, management and complications of percutaneous subclavian catheters: An audit. Arch Surg 113:1421–1425, 1978.
12. Giacchino JL, Geis WP, Wittenstein BH, Gandhi VC: Recent trends in vascular access. Am Surg 48:501–504, 1982.
13. Moss AH, Vasilakis BS, Holley JL, et al: Use of a silicone dual-lumen catheter with a Dacron cuff as a long-term vascular access for hemodialysis patients. Am J Kidney Dis 16:211–215, 1990.
14. Reilly DT, Wood RFM, Bell PRF: Prospective study of dialysis fistulas: Problem patients and their treatment. Br J Surg 69:549–553, 1982.
15. Brescia MJ, Cimino JE, Appel K, Hurwich BJ: Chronic hemodialysis using veni-puncture and a surgically created arteriovenous fistula. N Engl J Med 275:1089–1092, 1966.
16. Monquet C, Bitker MO, Bailliart O, et al: Anesthesia for creation of a forearm fistula in patients with endstage renal failure. Anesthesiology 70:909–914, 1989.
17. Johnson G: Local pathophysiology of an arteriovenous fistula. In Swam KG (ed): Venous Surgery in the Lower Extremity. St Louis, Warren H. Greene, 1975, pp 41–50.

18. Bennion RS, Williams RA: The radiocephalic fistula. Contemp Dial 3:12–16, 1982.

19. Anderson CB, Etheridge EE, Harter HR, et al: Local blood flow characteristics of arteriovenous fistulas in the forearm for dialysis. Surg Gynecol Obstet 144:531–533, 1977.

20. Johnson G, Dart CH, Peters RM, Steele F: The importance of venous circulation in arteriovenous fistula. Surg Gynecol Obstet 123:995–1000, 1966.

21. Mindich BP, Levowitz BS: Enhancement of flow through arteriovenous fistula. Arch Surg 111:195–196, 1976.

22. Moran MR, Enriquez AA, Boyero MR, et al: Hand exercise effect in maturation and blood flow of dialysis arteriovenous fistulas. Angiology 35:641–644, 1984.

23. Giacchino JL, Geis WP, Buckingham JM, et al: Vascular access: Long-term results, new techniques. Arch Surg 114:403–409, 1979.

24. Bender MHM, Bruyninckx CMA, Gerling PGG: The brachiocephalic elbow fistula: A useful alternative angioaccess for permanent hemodialysis. J Vasc Surg 20:808–813, 1994.

25. Wilson SE, Stabile BE, Williams RA, Owens ML: Current status of vascular access techniques. Surg Clin North Am 62:531–551, 1982.

26. Owens ML, Stabile BE, Gahr JE, Wilson SE: Vascular grafts for hemodialysis: An evaluation of sites and materials. Dial Transplant 8:521–525, 1979.

27. Rohr MS, Browder W, Freutz GD, McDonald JC: Arteriovenous fistulas for long-term dialysis: Factors that influence fistula survival. Arch Surg 113:153–155, 1978.

28. Fee HJ, Golding AL: Lower extremity ischemia after femoral arteriovenous bovine shunts. Ann Surg 183:42–45, 1976.

29. Humphries AL, Nesbit RP, Carnana RJ, et al: Thirty-six recommendations for vascular access operations: Lessons learned from our first thousand operations. Am Surg 47:145–151, 1981.

30. Rizzuti RP, Hale JC, Burkart TE: Extended patency of expanded polytetrafluoroethylene grafts for vascular access using optimal configuration and revisions. Surg Gynecol Obstet 166:23–27, 1988.

31. Wilson SE, Hillman M, Owens ML: Hemodynamic effects of bovine femorosaphenous fistula. Dial Transplant 6:84–89, 1977.

32. Garcia-Rinaldi R, Von Koch L: The axillary artery to axillary vein bovine graft for circulatory access. Am J Surg 135:265–268, 1978.

33. May J, Tiller D, Johnson J, et al: Saphenous-vein arteriovenous fistula in regular dialysis treatment. N Engl J Med 280:770, 1969.

34. Haimor M, Burrows L, Schanzer H, et al: Experience with arterial substitutes in the construction of vascular access for hemodialysis. J Cardiovasc Surg (Torino) 21:149–154, 1980.

35. Baker LD, Johnson JM, Goldfarb D: Expanded polytetrafluoroethylene (PTFE) subcutaneous arteriovenous conduit: An improved vascular access for chronic hemodialysis. Trans Am Soc Artif Intern Organs 22:382–387, 1976.

36. Sabanayagam P, Schwartz AB, Soricelli RR, et al: A comparative study of 402 bovine heterografts and 225 reinforced expanded PTFE grafts as AVG in the ESRD patient. Trans Am Soc Artif Intern Organs 26:88–92, 1980.

37. Munda R, First MR, Alexander JW, et al: Polytetrafluoroethylene graft survival in hemodialysis. JAMA 249:219–222, 1983.

38. Palder SB, Kirkman RL, Whittemore AD, et al: Vascular access for hemodialysis: Patency rates and results of revisions. Ann Surg 202:235–239, 1985.

39. Schuman ES, Gross GF, Hayes JF, Standage BA: Long-term patency of polytetrafluoroethylene graft fistulas. Am J Surg 155:644–646, 1988.

40. Bhat DJ, Tellis VA, Kohlberg WI, et al: Management of sepsis involving expanded polytetrafluoroethylene grafts for hemodialysis access. Surgery 87:445–450, 1980.

41. Hodges TC, Fillinger MF, Zwolak RM, et al: Longitudinal comparison of dialysis access methods: Risk factors for failure. J Vasc Surg 26:1009–1019, 1997.

42. Offner G, Aschendorff C, Hoyer PF, et al: End stage renal failure: 14 years' experience of dialysis and renal transplantation. Arch Dis Child 63:120–126, 1988.

43. Gibson TC, Dyer DP, Postlethwaite RJ, Gough DCS: Vascular access for acute hemodialysis. Arch Dis Child 62:141–145, 1987.

44. Hiatt JR, Busuttil RW: A method for vascular access in small children. Surgery 93:343–344, 1983.

45. Kinnaert P, Janssen F, Hall M: Elbow arteriovenous fistula (EAVF) for chronic hemodialysis in small children. J Pediatr Surg 18:116–119, 1983.

46. Bourquelot P, Wolfeler L, Lamy L: Microsurgery for haemodialysis distal arteriovenous fistulae in children weighing less than 10 kg. Proc Eur Dial Transplant Assoc 18:537–541, 1981.

47. Nevins TE, Kjellstrand CM: Hemodialysis for children: A review. Int J Pediatr Nephrol 4:155–169, 1983.

48. Jacobs C, Brunner SP, Chantler C, et al: Combined report on regular dialysis and transplantation in Europe. Proc Eur Dial Transplant Assoc 14:3–69, 1977.

49. Dobkin JF, Miller MH, Steigbigel NH: Septicemia in patients on chronic hemodialysis. Ann Intern Med 88:28–33, 1978.

50. Peresesuschi G, Blum M, Aviram A, Spirer ZH: Impaired neutrophil response to acute bacterial infection in dialyzed patients. Arch Intern Med 141:1301–1302, 1981.

51. Salant DJ, Glover AM, Anderson R, et al: Depressed neutrophil chemotaxis in patients with chronic renal failure on dialysis and after renal transplantation. J Lab Clin Med 88:536–545, 1976.

52. Hurst KS, Saldhana LF, Steinberg SM, et al: The effects of varying dialysis regimens on lymphocyte transformation. Trans Am Soc Artif Intern Organs 21:329–334, 1975.

53. Raskova J, Morrison AB, Shea SM, Raska K: Humoral inhibitors of the immune response in uremia, II: Further characterization of an immunosuppressive factor in uremic serum. Am J Pathol 97:277–290, 1979.

54. Nelson J, Ormrod DJ, Wilson D, Miller TE: Host immune status in uraemia, III: Humoral response to selected antigens in the rat. Clin Exp Immunol 42:234–240, 1980.

55. Kirmani N, Tuazon CU, Murry HW, et al: *Staphylococcus aureus* carriage rate of patients receiving long-term hemodialysis. Arch Intern Med 138:1657–1659, 1978.

56. Kaplowitz LG, Comstock JA, Landwehr DM, et al: Prospective study of microbial colonization of the nose and skin and infection of the vascular access site in hemodialysis patients. J Clin Microbiol 26:1257–1262, 1988.

57. Morgan AP, Knight DC, Tilney NL, Lazaris JM: Femoral triangle sepsis in dialysis patients: Frequency, management, and outcome. Ann Surg 191:460–464, 1980.

58. Wilson SE, Van Wagenen P, Passaro S: Arterial infection. Curr Probl Surg 15:1–89, 1978.

59. Bennion RS, Wilson SE, Williams RA: Vascular prosthetic infection. Infect Surg 1:45–55, 1982.

60. Moore WS, Swanson RJ, Compagna G, et al: Pseudointimal development and vascular prosthesis susceptibility to bacteremic infection. Surg Forum 25:250–251, 1974.

61. Ehrenfield WK, Wilbur BG, Olcott CN, Stoney RJ: Autogenous tissue reconstruction in the management of infected prosthetic grafts. Surgery 85:82–92, 1979.

62. Kaiser AB, Clayson DR, Mulherin JL, et al: Antibiotic prophylaxis in vascular surgery. Ann Surg 188:283–289, 1978.

63. Pitt HA, Postier RG, MacGowen WAL, et al: Prophylactic antibiotics in vascular surgery. Ann Surg 192:356–364, 1980.

64. Bennion RS, Hiatt JR, Williams RA, Wilson SE: A randomized, prospective study of perioperative antimicrobial prophylaxis for vascular access surgery. J Cardiovasc Surg (Torino) 26:270–274, 1985.

65. Fivush BA, Bock GH, Guzzetta PC, et al: Vancomycin prevents polytetrafluoroethylene graft infections in pediatric patients receiving chronic hemodialysis. Am J Kidney Dis 5:120–123, 1985.

66. Raju S: PTFE grafts for hemodialysis access. Techniques for insertion and management of complications. Ann Surg 206:666–673, 1987.

67. Bell DD, Rosental JJ: Arteriovenous graft life in chronic hemodialysis: A need for prolongation. Arch Surg 123:1169–1172, 1988.

68. Griffin PJA, Davies F, Salaman JR, Coles GA: Effects of smoking on long term patency of arteriovenous fistulas. BMJ 286:685–686, 1983.

69. Bone GE, Pomjzl MJ: Management of dialysis fistula thrombosis. Am J Surg 138:901–906, 1979.

70. Glanz S, Bashist B, Gordon DH, et al: Angiography of upper extremity access fistulas for dialysis. Radiology 143:45–52, 1982.

71. Gain JS, Fowler PR, Steinberg AW, et al: Use of the fistula assessment monitor to detect stenoses in access fistulae. Am J Kidney Dis 17:303–306, 1991.

72. Choudhury D, Lee J, Elivera HS, et al: Correlation of venography, venous pressure, and hemoaccess function. Am J Kidney Dis 25:269–275, 1995.

73. Ritgers SE, Garcia-Valdez C, McCormick JT, Posner MP: Noninvasive flow measurement in expanded polytetrafluoroethylene grafts for hemodialysis access. J Vasc Surg 3:635–642, 1986.

74. Weber M, Kuhn FP, Quintes W, et al: Sonography of arteriovenous fistulae in hemodialysis patients. Clin Nephrol 22:258–261, 1984.

75. Gmelin E, Winterhoff R, Rinast E: Insufficient hemodialysis access fistulas: Late results in treatment with percutaneous balloon angioplasty. Radiology 171:657–660, 1989.

76. Zeit RM, Cope C: Failed hemodialysis shunts: One year of experience with aggressive treatment. Radiology 154:353–356, 1985.

77. Mangiarotti G, Canavese C, Thea A, et al: Urokinase treatment for arteriovenous fistulae declotting in dialyzed patients. Nephron 36:60–64, 1984.

78. Harter HR, Burch JW, Majerus PW, et al: Prevention of thrombosis in patients on hemodialysis by low-dose aspirin. N Engl J Med 301:577–579, 1979.

79. Flye MW, Mundinger GH, Schulz SC, et al: Successful creation of arteriovenous fistulas in nonuremic patients with heparin and aspirin therapy. Am J Surg 142:759–763, 1981.

80. Radmilovic A, Boric Z, Naumovic T, et al: Shunt thrombosis prevention in hemodialysis patients—a double-blind, randomized study: Pentoxifylline vs placebo. Angiology 38:499–505, 1987.

81. Johnson G, Blythe WB: Hemodynamic effects of arteriovenous shunts used for hemodialysis. Ann Surg 171:715–721, 1970.

82. Jensen JA, Goodson WH, Omachi RS, et al: Subcutaneous tissue oxygenation falls during hemodialysis. Surgery 101:416–421, 1987.

83. Ahern DJ, Maher JF: Heart failure as a complication of hemodialysis arteriovenous fistula. Ann Intern Med 77:201–204, 1972.

84. Anderson CB, Codd JR, Graff RA, et al: Cardiac failure and upper extremity arteriovenous dialysis fistulas. Arch Intern Med 136:292–297, 1976.

85. Anderson CB, Etheridge EE, Harter HR, et al: Blood flow measurements in arteriovenous dialysis fistulas. Surgery 81:459–461, 1977.

86. Riley SM, Blackstone EH, Sterling WA, Diethelm AG: Echocardiographic assessment of cardiac performance in patients with arteriovenous fistulas. Surg Gynecol Obstet 146:203–208, 1978.

87. Von Bibra H, Castro L, Autenieth G, et al: The effects of arteriovenous shunts on cardiac function in renal dialysis patients: An echocardiographic evaluation. Clin Nephrol 9:205–209, 1978.

88. Storey BG, George CRP, Stewart JOH, et al: Embolic and ischemic complications after anastomosis of radial artery to cephalic vein. Surgery 66:325–327, 1969.

89. Bussell JA, Abbott JA, Lim RC: A radial steal syndrome with arteriovenous fistula for hemodialysis. Ann Intern Med 75:387–394, 1971.

90. Haimov M: Vascular access for hemodialysis. Surg Gynecol Obstet 141:619–625, 1975.

91. Duncan H, Ferguson L, Faris I: Incidence of the radial steal syndrome in patients with brescia fistula for hemodialysis: Its clinical significance. J Vasc Surg 4:144–147, 1986.

92. Odland MD, Kelly PH, Ney AL, et al: Management of dialysis-associated steal syndrome complicating upper extremity arteriovenous fistulas: Use of intraoperative digital photoplethysmography. Surgery 110:664–670, 1991.

93. Knezevic W, Mastaglia FL: Neuropathy associated with Brescia-Cimino arteriovenous fistulas. Arch Neurol 41:1184–1186, 1984.

94. Wood ML, Reilly GD, Smith GT: Ulceration of the hand secondary to a radial arteriovenous fistula: A model for varicose ulceration. BMJ 287:1167–1168, 1983.

95. Bond MG, Hotstetler JR, Karayannocas PE, et al: Intimal changes in arteriovenous bypass grafts: Effects of varying the angle of implantation at the proximal anastomosis and of producing stenosis in the distal runoff artery. J Thorac Cardiovasc Surg 71:907–916, 1976.

96. Telles D, Weinstein P: Intimal cellular response to microvascular anastomosis. Scanning Microsc 3:227–234, 1980.

97. Stehbens WE, Karmody AM: Venous atherosclerosis associated with arteriovenous fistulas for hemodialysis. Arch Surg 110:176–180, 1975.

98. Mennes PA, Gilula LA, Anderson CB, et al: Complications associated with arteriovenous fistulas in patients undergoing chronic hemodialysis. Arch Intern Med 138:1117–1121, 1978.

99. Owens ML, Shinaberger JH, Wilson SE, Wang SMS: Aneurysmal enlargement of e-PTFE fistulas. Dial Transplant 7:692–694, 1978.

100. Engels JGL, Skotincki SH, Buskens FGM, van Tougeren JHM: Home parenteral nutrition via arteriovenous fistulae. JPEN J Parenter Enteral Nutr 7:412–414, 1983.

101. Havill JH, Blair RD: Home parenteral nutrition using shunts. JPEN J Parenter Enteral Nutr 8:321–324, 1984.

102. Wobbes T, Slooff MJH, Lichtendahl DHE, et al: The radiocephalic fistula as vascular access for chemotherapy. World J Surg 7:532–535, 1983.

103. Wobbes T, Slooff MJH, Sleijfer DT, et al: Five years' experience in access surgery for polychemotherapy: An analysis of results in 100 consecutive patients. Cancer 52:978–982, 1983.

104. Raaf JH: Results from use of 826 vascular access devices in cancer patients. Cancer 55:1312–1321, 1985.

105. Broviac JW, Cole JJ, Scribner BH: A silicone rubber atrial catheter for prolonged parenteral alimentation. Surg Gynecol Obstet 136:602–606, 1973.

106. Hickman RO, Buckner CD, Clift RA, et al: A modified right atrial catheter for access to the venous system in bone marrow transplant recipients. Surg Gynecol Obstet 148:871–875, 1979.

107. Thomas JH, MacArthur RI, Pierce GE, Hermreck AS: Hickman-Broviac catheters: Indications and results. Am J Surg 140:791–796, 1980.

108. Weber TR, West KW, Grosfeld JL: Broviac central venous catheterization in infants and children. Am J Surg 145:791–796, 1983.

109. Bedini AV, Tavecchio L, Bonalumi MG, et al: Reliability of prolonged infusion in cancer chemotherapy with the Groshong central venous catheter. Reg Cancer Treat 3:232–234, 1990.

110. Greene FL, Moore W, Strickland G, McFarland J: Comparison of a totally implantable device for chemotherapy (Port-A-Cath) and long-term percutaneous catheterization (Broviac). South Med J 81:580–585, 1988.

111. Ross MN, Haase GM, Poole MA, et al: Comparison of totally implanted reservoirs with external catheters as venous access devices in pediatric oncologic patients. Surg Gynecol Obstet 167:141–144, 1988.

112. Stellato WE, Gauderer MW, Cohen AM: Direct central vein puncture for silicone rubber catheter insertion: An alternative technique for Broviac catheter placement. Surgery 90:896–899, 1981.

Questions

1. After creation of a radiocephalic autogenous fistula, the configuration that is associated with the lowest incidence of venous hypertension is
   (a) arterial side-to-vein side anastomosis
   (b) vein end-to-arterial side anastomosis
   (c) arterial end-to-vein side anastomosis
   (d) brachiobasilic side-to-side anastomosis
   (e) none of the above

2. The highest 3-year patency rate in vascular access procedures has been achieved with
   (a) PTFE bridge fistulas
   (b) autogenous saphenous vein bridge fistulas
   (c) Scribner shunts
   (d) autogenous radiocephalic fistulas
   (e) percutaneous double-lumen Silastic catheters

3. Postoperative hemodynamic changes that may be encountered soon after construction of a proximally located bridge fistula for hemodialysis include all the following except
   (a) increased stroke volume
   (b) reversal of flow in the distal artery when the fistula opening exceeds the diameter of the feeding artery
   (c) increased cardiac output
   (d) increased heart rate
   (e) decreased total systemic resistance

4. Which of the following is not a complication of percutaneous subclavian central venous catheterization?
   (a) hemopneumothorax
   (b) catheter embolism
   (c) brachial plexus injury
   (d) lymphatic fistula formation
   (e) all are possible complications

5. Correction of localized venous runoff stenosis can be accomplished by all of the following except
   (a) patch angioplasty of the outflow anastomosis
   (b) extension bypass graft to a more proximal vein
   (c) percutaneous transluminal dilatation
   (d) relocation of venous anastomosis to adjacent vein
   (e) replacement with new conduit

6. Characteristics of venous runoff stenosis include all of the following except
   (a) may be related to the shearing effect of blood flow at the anastomotic site
   (b) rarely develops before 2 years after fistula creation
   (c) most often seen after construction of bridge fistulas
   (d) manifests as an increase in venous return pressure during dialysis
   (e) may be due to compliance mismatch

7. The potential benefits of implantable ports over external central venous catheters for the delivery of chemotherapy include all of the following except
   (a) lower catheter-related sepsis rates
   (b) lower incidence of thrombosis
   (c) does not require constant heparinization
   (d) requires little daily care
   (e) interferes less with the patient's normal activities

8. Vascular access in children weighing less than 10 kg may be reliably accomplished by each of the following except
   (a) percutaneous central vein catheterization
   (b) forearm PTFE bridge fistula
   (c) creation of a brachial artery–antecubital vein autogenous fistula
   (d) direct cannulation of umbilical vessels if a patient is newborn
   (e) placement of an external arteriovenous shunt

9. Increased risk of infection in a prosthetic bridge fistula for hemodialysis can be related to all of the following except
   (a) poor aseptic technique during needle puncture
   (b) high colonization rate of dialysis patients and dialysis staff with *Staphylococcus aureus*
   (c) decreased chemotactic responses of polymorphonuclear leukocytes in uremia
   (d) decreased bacterial phagocytosis in uremic patients
   (e) all of the above

10. Limitations in the use of the Scribner shunt include all of the following except
   (a) long-term patency unlikely
   (b) high risk of infection
   (c) easily dislodged
   (d) cannot be used in acutely ill patients
   (e) high rate of thrombosis

Answers

1. b   2. d   3. a   4. e   5. e   6. b   7. c   8. b   9. e   10. d

35

Vascular Trauma

Malcolm O. Perry and Frederic S. Bongard

Trauma is a leading cause of death in the United States. More males younger than 18 years old die from handgun injuries than from car crashes, communicable diseases, or drugs.[1] Many victims have multiple injuries involving major vascular structures. Those who survive are frequently incapacitated due to amputation or dysfunction caused by associated soft tissue and neural injuries.

In most situations, serious injury can be ascertained with little difficulty. Multiple wounds are challenging and require careful planning, organization, and integration of resources. The basic principles of resuscitation should always assume priority.

ETIOLOGY

Major vascular wounds may occur in any environment, but the greatest incidence occurs in urban areas, where violence is endemic. Penetrating injury is more common than blunt trauma; most penetrating wounds are caused by knives and bullets. Incidental wounds may be inflicted by shards of glass or metal projections during motor vehicle accidents or industrial mishaps[2] (Table 35–1).

Among penetrating injuries, stab wounds are more common than gunshot wounds. However, because such injuries are not as deep or widespread, they are less likely to produce severe vascular wounds and often can be treated by simple débridement and ligation of superficial vessels. Deeper structures are often spared when small knives are used. These knife wounds may be meant to punish rather than kill, and the point is extended in such a fashion that only a small laceration results. Gunshot wounds usually penetrate deeply and often involve the trunk or thorax as well as the extremities; they are more likely to produce serious vascular and visceral wounds. The vessels of the extremities are most often involved, because they are longer and may be injured during attempts at self defense[2] (Table 35–2).

MECHANISMS OF INJURY

Most penetrating injuries are caused by low-velocity agents, which largely confine the damage to the wound tract. Low-velocity bullets and knives usually cause punctures, lacerations, and contusions to structures in their path. Complete vessel transection is likely with bullet wounds. The concussive effects of higher-velocity missiles produce widespread damage. The cavitation caused by a high-velocity bullet (1500 to 3000 ft/sec) may even damage a vessel remote from the wound tract. This occurs when the blast cavity collapses, causing a suction effect that draws structures into the wound. These structures may include bits of skin, clothing, or dirt particles, increasing the possibility of infection.

A high-velocity bullet or metal fragment can produce a great deal of tissue damage. The kinetic energy (KE) of a bullet is proportional to its mass (m) and the square of its velocity (v) ($KE = \frac{1}{2} mv^2$). Hence, high-velocity bullets (such as from a .458 Winchester, which also is fairly heavy) have the highest wounding potential. When the bullet strikes the tissue, it dissipates its energy rapidly. Fast-moving bullets that yaw and tumble on impact (dumdum) cause large amounts of damage because they lose virtually all of their energy as they pass through the target. Such destructive effects may not be suspected on initial inspection; only a small entrance wound may be present, yet interior damage is widespread and extensive débridement

TABLE 35–1

Relationship between Mechanism of Injury and Location*

	HEAD/NECK	THORAX	ABDOMEN	ARMS	LEGS
Gunshot wound	11	10	16	50	45
Stab wound	27	13	34	94	15
Motor vehicle accident	14	15	12	11	22
Fall	6	1	0	3	3
Other	4	0	1	3	1
Totals	62	39	63	161	86

*Data from 411 patients seen over a 9-year period in a level I trauma center.
From Bongard F, Dubrow T, Klein S: Vascular injuries in the urban battleground: Experience at a metropolitan trauma center. Ann Vasc Surg 4:415–418, 1990.

TABLE 35-2

Vascular Injuries*

Head and Neck Vessels (no. = 62)	
Carotid	13
Jugular vein	7
External jugular vein	10
Multiple arteries	5
All other	27
Thoracic Vessels (no. = 39)	
Aorta	11
Innominate/subclavian artery	9
Subclavian vein	2
Innominate/subclavian vein	2
Pulmonary vessels	2
All other	13
Abdominal Vessels (no. = 63)	
Aorta	3
Inferior vena cava/hepatic veins	23
Celiac/mesenteric arteries	19
Portal/splenic veins	3
Renal arteries	3
Iliac arteries	7
All other	5
Upper Extremity (no. = 161)	
Axillary arteries/veins	18
Brachial arteries/veins	55
Radial/ulnar arteries	64
Palmar/digital arteries	12
All other	12
Lower Extremity (no. = 86)	
Common femoral arteries	8
Superficial femoral arteries	24
Femoral veins	3
Saphenous veins	4
Popliteal arteries/veins	20
Tibial arteries/veins	5
All other	22

*Data from 411 patients seen over a 9-year period in a level I trauma center. All causes included.

From Bongard F, Dubrow T, Klein S: Vascular injuries in the urban battleground: Experience at a metropolitan trauma center. Ann Vasc Surg 4:415–418, 1990.

is required if tissue necrosis and invasive sepsis are to be avoided.

Special problems are encountered from close-range shotgun blasts. Although the muzzle velocity of a shotgun pellet is similar to that of a .22-caliber rifle bullet (approximately 1200 ft/sec), the damage inflicted by multiple pellets is usually widespread, and the shotshell wadding and bits of clothing carried into the wound greatly enhance the possibility of infection. As with high-velocity wounds, close-range shotgun blasts often cause a great deal more damage to interior structures than is apparent from inspection of the entry sites in the skin. Shotgun pellets may embolize in both the arterial and venous systems. Distal ischemia may result from the embolization of a single pellet. Plain films of the distal extremity should be obtained to exclude this possibility (Fig. 35–1).

Motor vehicle accidents continue to increase in frequency and complexity as traffic density grows and the size of the automobile decreases. These accident victims commonly have multiple injuries that often include fractures and dislocations. Direct trauma to major vessels can

occur, but in many cases the vascular injury is the result of a fracture. This is especially common with fractures near the joints, where the vessels are relatively fixed and vulnerable to shear forces. Posterior dislocations of the knee are particularly likely to injure the relatively immobile popliteal artery and vein.[3, 4]

The bending and sudden fracture of large, heavy bones such as the femur or the tibia release tremendous forces. Damage to soft tissue and neurovascular structures is frequently extensive, and the effects on these tissues are quite similar to those produced by the cavitation associated with high-velocity bullet wounds (Fig. 35–2). Remote vascular injuries can occur, but after the bones fall back into a near-normal position, the magnitude of the injury forces may not be appreciated, and the severity of damage is often underestimated. Evaluation of these patients is particularly difficult because of extensive soft tissue and bony deformity.

GENERAL PRINCIPLES

Diagnosis

Clinical Features

Physical examination is the single most important step in the evaluation of a patient with a suspected vascular injury. Complete disruption of a major vessel, regardless of mech-

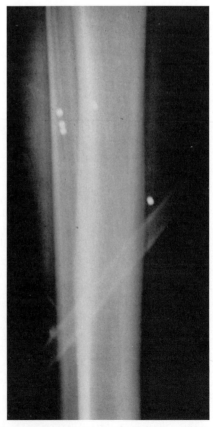

Figure 35–1. This plain radiograph shows shotgun pellet emboli to the tibial arteries. The wound is in the ipsilateral superficial femoral artery.

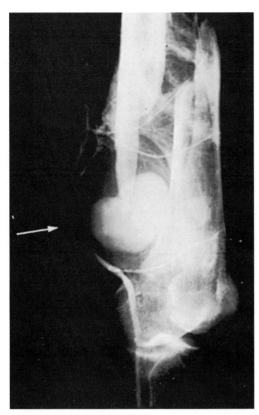

Figure 35–2. This spiral fracture of the femur caused extensive damage to the soft tissues of the thigh and punctured the superficial femoral artery.

anism, typically results in a distal pulse deficit. When the injury is due to a blunt mechanism, destruction of surrounding soft tissue may also disturb collateral pathways to the extent that distal ischemia is pronounced. When a penetrating mechanism is responsible, significant ischemia may follow injury to the common femoral or superficial femoral arteries. Severe ischemia of the upper extremity is unusual after penetrating injuries unless the brachial artery is completely transected.

The physical signs of arterial trauma are divided into two groups: hard and soft. Hard signs include severe external hemorrhage, an expanding hematoma, a palpable thrill, a continuous murmur, and any of the classic findings of acute ischemia ("six P's"), including pain, pallor, pulselessness, paresthesia, poikilothermia, and paralysis. When sufficient collateral flow is present around the injury, a pulse deficit may be present in the absence of ischemia. Recent studies suggest that the incidence of vascular injury requiring surgical repair in the absence of any sign is very small. Certain high-risk groups exist, however, and mandate further evaluation. These include patients with gunshot injuries to the calf, forearm, antecubital fossa, medial or posterior thigh, or medial or posterior arm. Extended follow-up in these patients has been limited, and the incidence of late complications such as pseudoaneurysm formation is still undefined. Physical examination alone after blunt trauma has also been advocated. Because of the frequency of associated soft tissue destruction, further evaluation of patients with abnormal pulse examinations after these injuries is mandatory.

Proximity of a penetrating injury to a major vascular structure constitutes the most common "soft sign" of injury. Other soft signs include a small nonpulsatile and nonexpanding hematoma, an ipsilateral neurologic deficit, or a history of prehospital hemorrhage or shock.

Although weak or absent pulses beyond a suspected vascular wound are fairly common, pulses may be normal in up to 20% of operatively proven arterial injuries.[5] The pulse wave is a pressure wave that reaches velocities of 7 to 13 m/second. This wave may be transmitted beyond intimal flaps, through limited areas of fresh soft clot, or via the large collateral vessels, and thus it may be detectable distal to a significant arterial injury. The flow wave of blood has a velocity of 40 to 50 cm/second and is distinct from the pulse wave. Physical examination must take these facts into account. Wounds of arteries crossing the shoulder or the pelvis, areas with rich collateral circulation, are more likely to be associated with distal pulses. Moreover, injuries of arteries such as the profunda femoris or deep brachial would not disturb distal pulses. Major venous wounds, of course, are not exposed by examination of pulses; the only finding in these patients may be hematomas or persistent bleeding. In the case of an acute traumatic arteriovenous (AV) fistula, abnormal distention of the veins is noted along with a bruit or murmur and thrill over the injury.

The detection of Doppler signals and the measurement of distal arterial systolic blood pressure by this or other techniques is helpful, but the specificity of these tests is influenced by the same hemodynamic features that govern distal pulses. Subtle abnormalities are common, but relatively normal values are also observed, compromising the reliability of these methods for the exclusion of vascular wounds. They are useful adjuncts and serve as an extension of the physical examination, but may be misleading.

Wounds of the profunda femoris or deep brachial artery do not alter distal pulses or distal limb blood pressure measurements. An injury of a single tibial artery also may not change the ankle-brachial index. In questionable cases, duplex ultrasound tests may expose the injury or may detect false aneurysms or AV fistulas. In the absence of other indications for surgical exploration, these adjunctive methods can offer helpful information regarding possible injuries to large arteries.[6, 7] Color flow duplex ultrasonography may also be helpful in screening for occult venous injuries.[8]

Injuries of the heart and great vessels present special diagnostic problems because of their inaccessibility to clinical examination. Table 35–3 lists those clinical features that suggest the presence of significant intrathoracic vascular injuries. Hemopneumothorax or mediastinal bleeding is

TABLE 35–3

Clinical Features Suggesting Injuries of the Great Vessels

Cardiac arrest
Persistent shock
Cardiac tamponade
Wide mediastinum
Recurring hemothorax

common with penetrating injuries of the chest, even without injuries of a major artery. The patient may be initially stable and thought to have only minor parenchymal lung damage until sudden hemodynamic collapse occurs. Preoperative identification of such severe injuries is important, permitting the surgeon to prepare for the possibility of major vascular reconstruction of the heart or great vessels. Many benefit from preoperative arteriography if they are sufficiently stable to permit the delay required for such studies.

A computed tomographic (CT) scan is very useful in the initial evaluation of patients with multiple injuries, especially those caused by blunt trauma. Injuries to parenchymal intraabdominal organs, hematomas, and displacement of other structures may be seen clearly by CT scanning, thus validating the need for operative exploration. Negative studies, of course, are of less value in excluding injuries, but a positive study gives compelling reasons for proceeding with surgery. The CT scan is now advocated by some as a screening technique for angiography in patients at risk of thoracic aortic disruption after blunt trauma. Because only one third of patients with this injury have any abnormal physical findings on presentation, a high index of suspicion is required. Numerous findings on chest radiographs may be suggestive of thoracic aortic disruption (see Table 35–3), although none are specific. A CT scan may be helpful in screening for angiography, because the incidence of false-negative scans is probably low when thin (5-mm) cuts are taken.[9] Recently, helical CT scanning has received attention as a diagnostic modality among victims of blunt trauma with a widened mediastinum on initial chest film. A prospective series of 112 blunt trauma patients with nine aortic ruptures found helical CT accurate in diagnosing eight.[10] The false-negative reading was in a patient who had a brachiocephalic injury. The authors suggest that all high-risk patients (high-speed deceleration) undergo helical CT scanning, irrespective of chest radiographic findings; however, the true accuracy of helical CT needs to be studied further. Magnetic resonance imaging (MRI) promises to be of more value than CT scanning; the delineation of structures is much clearer, and the detection of even minor abnormalities should be possible.

Arteriography

In the management of trauma, preoperative arteriography is used to exclude the need for surgery, to expose a suspected injury not otherwise detectable, and to plan an operation (Table 35–4). In a study of 183 patients with penetrating injuries of the extremities, the validity and usefulness of arteriography were established.[11] In those with penetrating injuries of the arms and legs, all had arteriograms and were operated on regardless of the arteriographic findings. One false-negative examination and 28 false-positive examinations were encountered. The study concluded that high-grade biplane arteriography offers reliable, but not infallible, evidence regarding the presence or absence of arterial injuries. Particular problems are encountered with preoperative arteriography in the assessment of injuries of the great vessels near the arch of the aorta, where obtaining good biplane films is difficult because of overlapping images.

Studies have shown a low yield when arteriograms are performed only because the wound is near a major artery. A study by Weaver and colleagues[12] described 157 patients with penetrating extremity injuries in whom the path of the penetrating object was judged to be in proximity to a major neurovascular bundle. None of the patients had pulse deficits, nerve deficits, hematoma, history of hemorrhage or hypotension, bruit, fracture, major soft tissue injury, or delayed capillary refill. Angiographic abnormalities were demonstrated in 17 (11%) patients; 4 abnormalities were major (3%) and 13 (8%) were minor. In a group of 216 patients with significant physical findings, the authors found 65 (30%) injuries, 22 (10%) of which were major. The majority of injuries identified by arteriography in otherwise asymptomatic patients are small intimal deficits, pseudoaneurysms, or occlusions of "noncritical" vessels. A careful physical examination usually determines the need for arteriograms.[13] Frykberg and colleagues[14] described 366 penetrating extremity wounds in 310 patients. Twenty-three patients required surgical intervention; 21 of these patients (91.3%) were initially diagnosed solely by physical examination, each producing at least one hard sign. Unfortunately, patients with no findings or "soft findings" were observed during a short hospital stay (without angiography) and were presumed to harbor no injury if signs did not manifest before discharge, making the true predictive accuracy of a negative physical examination difficult to assess. Among the patients without initial abnormal findings, two required surgery during the period of inpatient observation. For patients who are hemodynamically stable with no indications for surgical exploration, delaying arteriography is often acceptable, rather than obtaining emergency studies in the middle of the night. Careful observation is required until the tests are completed and precise treatment is initiated. Noninvasive tests may help separate these patients from those who require expedient surgery.

When firm indications for operation are present, arteriograms may be unnecessary; any untoward delay is undesirable, and in some situations dangerous. If the patient is unstable, further evaluation is best performed in the operating room, utilizing the routine commonly employed for the management of patients with leaking abdominal aortic aneurysms. The patient is taken directly to the operating room, and further assessment is performed while preparations for surgery are under way. If sudden cardiovascular collapse occurs, immediate operation can be undertaken, and control of bleeding achieved rapidly. Such a patient should not be sent to the radiology department for study

---

TABLE 35–4

Indications for Preoperative Arteriography

Blunt trauma with fractures
Penetrating injuries to the chest
Cervical injuries—base of skull and thoracic inlet (zones I and III)
Assessment of multiple pellet wounds
Injuries to forearm or leg

TABLE 35–5

Associated Injuries in Trauma Patients

	PERCENTAGE
Significant vein	34
Major nerve	18
Separate artery	7
Lung, abdominal viscera	39
Shock	36

nor admitted to an intensive care unit if unstable, because an emergency operation may be required at any time.

Priorities and Resuscitation

The management of trauma requires a rapid yet thorough evaluation. Many of these patients have associated injuries (Table 35–5), and priorities must be set. Initial attention to the airway, breathing, and control of bleeding take precedence. A dangerous situation exists when the patient has achieved cardiopulmonary stability via compensatory mechanisms, and then suddenly deteriorates. Collapse is sudden, and irreversible shock may occur. This is particularly true in older patients whose compensatory mechanisms may be unable to deal with even relatively minor injury.

Once an airway is secured and control of external bleeding has been obtained, vital signs are assessed, an overall evaluation is made, and proper priorities are set. Baseline studies are recorded and a rapid physical examination is performed to be certain that all injuries are identified and emergency measures completed. The patient must be fully undressed so that unsuspected injuries in seemingly uninvolved parts of the body can be uncovered. A carefully performed and well-documented peripheral neurologic examination (sensory and motor) of the involved extremity before surgical intervention is critical.

Fluid and blood requirements in the injured patient are often impressive, and adequate intravenous access lines are needed. Large catheters are placed into an uninjured upper extremity whenever possible. Peripheral venous cutdowns are preferable to central venous access. Hypovolemic patients have collapsed central veins, which are difficult to cannulate. Misguided and persistent attempts at subclavian venous access can result in a pneumothorax or laceration of nearby arteries. During the selection of veins for the administration of intravenous fluids, the possibility of injury to the vein proximal to the site of insertion of the line must be considered, because it may be necessary to clamp that vein to control bleeding. One line is committed to fluid replacement and another to drug administration and anesthetic manipulations. If hemorrhage is severe, large volumes of blood must be infused rapidly. Venous autografts may be needed for vascular repair; preserving the saphenous or cephalic vein in an uninjured extremity is often prudent. The treatment of shock takes priority, however, and these veins may be needed for resuscitation.

The combination of a balanced salt solution, such as lactated Ringer's solution, and blood is chosen for resuscitation. Trauma and shock cause shifts of fluid from the interstitial to the intravascular space. This fluid is best replenished with a balanced salt solution followed by blood as required. Blood should be replaced with type- and cross-matched units when possible. Type-specific and O$^-$ blood can be used until cross-matched transfusions are available. Not overtransfusing these patients is wise, especially if chest trauma or cardiac disease is present.

Often, arterial lines and Swan-Ganz catheters are helpful if the patient is hemodynamically unstable and does not respond to resuscitation as anticipated. A radial artery catheter inserted in a patient who has a normal Allen test (which demonstrates connection of the radial and ulnar artery through the palmar arch) is safe and useful. The radial artery catheter should not be irrigated with large amounts of fluid, because a thrombus in the catheter can be dislodged and can scatter multiple emboli throughout the hand. The line is kept open with a continuous infusion of minute amounts of heparinized saline (1000 units of heparin in 1 L normal saline). The brachial artery should not be chosen for continuous in-line monitoring if other sites are accessible, because brachial artery lines are associated with high complication rates related to thrombosis and embolization.

Wound Protection

During the initial treatment of patients with serious injuries, a tendency exists to overlook the problem of wound care. Because the incidence of infection and subsequent complications may be directly related to contamination of wounds at the time of resuscitation, injuries should be protected and all undamaged tissue should be conserved for future use in covering repaired vessels. When multiple wounds are present, the use of several incisions may be required, especially if fractures and other injuries are present. If incisions are poorly placed, intervening tissues may be devitalized, important collateral vessels may be divided unnecessarily, and final coverage of the vessels may be difficult to secure. Wound care is an extremely important part of initial management, especially if extensive soft tissue damage is present, as occurs with close-range shotgun wounds and motor vehicle accidents. Preservation of potentially viable soft tissue is extremely important in victims of trauma because it provides both venous and arterial collaterals around the area of injury. Remote bypass grafts to restore flow may be required because of heavy contamination of the initial wounds. Exploratory incisions should be placed to preserve areas for the use of subcutaneous grafts. Meticulous care in creating and handling these incisions is essential to avoid secondary infections.

Most trauma surgeons use "prophylactic" antibiotics in these situations. Second-generation cephalosporins are often chosen and are begun when the patient is initially examined. Customarily, they are continued while central lines are in place, or as long as specific indications exist for antibiotic therapy. The patient's tetanus immunization status should not be overlooked.

Anticoagulation

Although during the course of many vascular operations, regional or systemic anticoagulation is used while major arteries and veins are temporarily occluded during repair, administering systemic heparin to trauma patients is not generally recommended unless they have an isolated vascular injury. Distal clot propagation is a problem in such patients, especially in the face of hypotension. Thrombosis can convert an initially reasonable situation into one with risk of tissue loss. Nevertheless, systemic anticoagulation in patients with multiple injuries (especially in those with injuries of the central nervous system, eyes, and bones) carries an unacceptably high risk. Expeditious surgery rather than systemic anticoagulation is preferred.[5, 15]

OPERATIVE MANAGEMENT

Anesthesia

During preparation for surgery, the selection of anesthetic agent is important, especially in those patients who are already hypotensive. A careful assessment of the cardiodepressant action of some anesthetic agents should be kept in mind as the operation begins. Careful positioning of the neck during induction of anesthesia is necessary to avoid dislodging clots from injured vessels in the neck. Of great importance is care in positioning the patient to avoid aggravating cervical spine injuries. Most patients are placed supine in the anatomic position, thus affording access to the chest, the abdomen, and all four extremities. If the surgeon needs to enter the left chest only (for repair of a single injury of the subclavian artery), the right lateral decubitus position is preferable.

Vertical exploratory incisions are desirable because they may be extended easily and, in the extremities, parallel the neurovascular bundles. Midline abdominal incisions can be extended into the chest as a median sternal splitting incision. Vertical incisions along the anterior sternocleidomastoid muscle used to expose the carotid and jugular vessels also may be extended into a median sternal incision if injuries are present in the root of the neck.[16] Transverse incisions generally limit flexibility and are not recommended.

Control of Bleeding

External hemorrhage is best controlled with direct digital pressure. If the wound is not bleeding, not disturbing it during the early resuscitation is best, and no attempt should be made to remove foreign bodies or to evacuate clots until surgical control is possible. Penetrating objects that are still in the wound must be protected during transport and should not be removed until the patient is in the operating room and proximal and distal control of major arteries has been obtained. No attempt should be made to clamp vessels blindly before formal exploration in the appropriate environment. When fatal hemorrhage appears imminent, the wound can be extended and vascular clamps applied under direct vision.

After penetrating trauma, emergency room thoracotomy may be lifesaving. Closed chest cardiac massage for hypovolemic shock may not be effective, and open massage is often required. An aggressive approach is warranted in these infrequent situations. A team of experienced surgeons is required if these maneuvers are to be successful.[17] Resuscitative thoracotomy is generally ineffective after blunt trauma, and its use is discouraged in these situations.

Once the surgical plan has been established, the injuries are approached directly through vertical incisions. If the hematoma is large, exposing the vessels proximally and gaining control in an area in which the artery and vein can be clearly visualized is often best. In extremities with multiple distal wounds and large hematomas, exposure of the vessels can be difficult, and placing an orthopedic tourniquet around the extremity proximal to the injury may be prudent. If severe bleeding is encountered before direct control of the artery, the tourniquet can be quickly inflated, thus arresting the hemorrhage while precise identification and control are obtained. A good alternative for lower extremity injuries, especially those involving the proximal femoral vessels, is to obtain inflow control at the external iliac artery. This is accomplished by creating a flank incision and approaching the iliac artery through the retroperitoneum; the artery can then be identified easily and the bleeding controlled within several minutes. If necessary, an assistant can apply direct digital pressure over the bleeding vessel while iliac control is obtained.

Proximal control is best achieved by using soft vascular tapes, latex tubing, or vascular clamps. These measures, combined with adequate suction and direct pressure with fingers or sponge sticks, are usually satisfactory to control hemorrhage while the injuries are identified and vascular clamps are applied.

Once the injury has been exposed, clots should be evacuated carefully and the extent of the injury examined. Every effort should be made to avoid fragmenting and dislodging clots or extending the damage to the vessel. This is particularly important in patients who have atherosclerosis and fragile arteries. In some cases, using a Foley or Fogarty catheter with an attached three-way stopcock may be necessary to control hemorrhage. The catheter is inserted into the wound, inflated, and gently retracted until bleeding stops. It is left in place until precise proximal and distal control is obtained. Repairs are not begun until all hemorrhage is arrested and the extent of associated injuries is assessed. Pausing at this point to be certain that no persistent bleeding is occurring is wise. Resuscitation should be essentially complete before definitive repair of noncritical structures is begun. Organs such as the kidney and liver are more susceptible to hypoxia than others, and the repair of major vessels supplying them should be undertaken first. Such prioritization of injuries is one of the basic tenets of trauma surgery.

In the past few years, the staged laparotomy for multiply injured patients has received a great deal of attention.[18, 19] Because injuries can be extensive, it is often unwise to attempt definitive repair on initial exploration. An example is the gunshot victim with a liver injury, an iliac artery disruption, and small bowel enterotomies.[20] A reasonable approach would be repair of the iliac artery, oversewing of the small bowel injuries, and packing of the liver. A scheduled return at 24 to 48 hours accomplishes definitive repair. The advantage of such an approach is that it permits repair or control of the most significant injuries while temporizing the others. This minimizes hypothermia, reduces coagulopathy, and allows better physiologic resuscitation. Such staged laparotomy should be employed when a constellation of injuries exist that would require extensive repair and resection.

Basic Techniques

The selection of suture materials for repair of major vessels is largely the preference of the operating surgeon, but a tendency has emerged over recent years to select less-reactive plastic suture instead of the braided cardiovascular silk sutures popular in the past. Silk sutures handle well, and although they are not permanent (most of their tensile strength is gone in 6 months), this is not a major drawback in primary repairs because primarily approximated vessel ends heal to each other. Nonreactive monofilament plastic sutures are less likely to harbor bacteria than are braided sutures and may reduce the risk of postoperative infection. They are often chosen by vascular surgeons despite their relative stiffness and lack of pliability. Satisfactory results are obtained with all such materials, but polypropylene and Dacron are more popular than others.

The vessels are repaired by the usual vascular techniques. Continuous over-and-over sutures are quite effective and can be used in almost all vessels. In small vessels (less than 4 mm in diameter), using interrupted sutures may be prudent to ensure intima-to-intima coaptation, although magnification has shown that continuous sutures, even in small arteries, are equally effective when placed properly. Small vessels may be sewn end to end more easily if they are transected obliquely or spatulated to obtain a larger suture line, which also has less chance of subsequent stenosis.

Tangential lacerations of larger vessels can be successfully treated by lateral suture repair utilizing standard vascular surgical techniques. Débridement is important in the management of vascular injuries and refraining from making a firm decision as to the type of repair until the débridement has been concluded is best. Most civilian vascular wounds are inflicted by knives or low-velocity missiles, and wide débridement is generally not required. With most bullet wounds, débriding only that amount of vessel that appears to be injured is necessary. With high-velocity gunshot wounds, the injury often extends beyond that which is immediately visible to the naked eye, and approximately 5 mm of vessel beyond the apparent damage should be removed.

Smaller vessels can rarely be repaired by lateral suture techniques and require either patch-graft angioplasty or, more commonly, resection and end-to-end anastomosis. The most commonly injured vessels (femoral and brachial) can usually be mobilized to permit resection of approximately 1 cm and still allow a satisfactory end-to-end anastomosis. If the extent of the injury is such that an end-to-end anastomosis cannot be accomplished without tension, interposing a suitable autograft is better than accepting an improper repair performed under tension. The saphenous vein is usually chosen for such autografts in medium-sized and small vessels of the extremities, but the hypogastric artery, external iliac artery, and other arterial autografts may be used as necessary. When the injury involves a lower extremity, the saphenous vein should be harvested from the contralateral leg. The ipsilateral vein should be left in situ because an unexpected injury of the deep venous system leaves the saphenous vein as the only significant pathway for venous return. An arterial autograft is likely more resistant to invasive infection than are other types of prosthetic grafts.[21] When heavy bacterial contamination has occurred, arterial autografts are favored.

Studies suggest that the disruption caused by infection is not unfavorably influenced by the presence of plastic prostheses, particularly polytetrafluoroethylene (PTFE) grafts. Further, these plastic substitutes may be used even when bacterial contamination is present. This opinion is not shared by all vascular surgeons, and most use autogenous tissue if available in the appropriate size.[22] In the aortoiliac system, plastic protheses are used when extensive damage is present, because large autografts are not available. If bacterial contamination is heavy, as it may be with combined aortic and colonic injuries, oversewing the major vascular injuries and constructing remote subcutaneous prosthetic bypass grafts on a temporary basis may be best until healing is complete. Axillofemoral and femorofemoral grafts are often selected in these circumstances to avoid placing the repaired arteries in heavily contaminated areas.

Assessment of Repair in the Operating Room

In most cases, vascular repair is followed by the immediate return of pulsatile flow. In patients who are incompletely resuscitated, hypotensive, cold, and vasoconstricted, determining clinically if the repair is satisfactory can be difficult. A sterile Doppler probe is useful in documenting distal patency in such circumstances. Angiograms should be obtained in all cases to assess the adequacy of the repair and the patency of the distal runoff bed.[23]

In the postoperative period, if any question exists regarding the adequacy of flow, an arteriogram is needed. The sine qua non for viability of the extremity is continued perception of light touch and adequate intrinsic motor function. Any deterioration is a compelling reason to perform an arteriogram, regardless of skin color, temperature, presence or absence of pulses, or limb blood pressure.[5]

MANAGEMENT OF SPECIFIC PROBLEMS

Brachiocephalic Arterial Injuries

Most wounds of the cervical vessels are caused by penetrating trauma. The common carotid artery is usually involved, the left more often than the right. Associated wounds of the pharynx, esophagus, and trachea may also be present, thus increasing the likelihood of bacterial contamination. The neurologic deficit associated with some of these injuries presents a unique and often perplexing problem. The outcome in most patients appears directly related to the extent of the initial neurologic insult, unless a technical misadventure occurs.[23, 24]

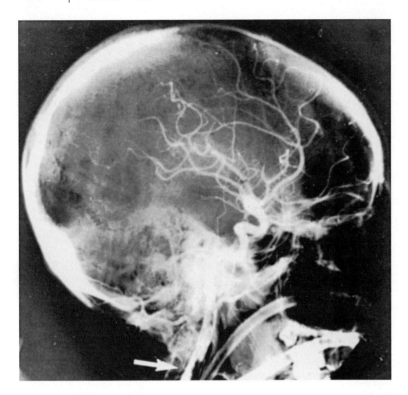

Figure 35–3. The arrow points to the area of the internal carotid artery damaged by hyperextension trauma.

Carotid Injuries

Carotid injuries are divided into three groups for evaluation and repair. The first and largest group contains those patients with common or internal carotid artery wounds but no neurologic deficit. Group 2 includes those who have a mild neurologic deficit, and group 3 includes those who have a severe neurologic deficit (coma, hemiplegia).[24]

The results of several large studies strongly support surgical repair of all carotid artery injuries in patients who have either no neurologic deficit or only a mild deficit. Thus, all of the patients in groups 1 and 2 would undergo repair of isolated carotid artery injuries. This decision is easy when the arterial injury is bleeding actively, but may be more difficult when the patient shows complete carotid artery occlusion and no neurologic symptoms.[25] In such a situation, technical problems encountered during surgery could conceivably produce brain damage, although in the reported experience this has been rare.[26] The risk does exist, however, and careful neurologic and arteriographic studies are required to assess the danger accurately before operation is undertaken in these patients. Even an artery depicted as being completely occluded by arteriography may be open at operation. MRI can be of great assistance in determining whether flow is present in a vessel. This may be helpful in patients suspected of having a hyperextension injury in which the internal carotid artery is forcibly stretched over the transverse process of C-3 and the body of C-2 (a mechanism of injury that predisposes to thromboembolic events). Until a neurologic problem appears, little evidence of carotid artery injury is usually present (Fig. 35–3).

Preoperative Evaluation

The basic management of penetrating trauma to the neck is straightforward: wounds that pierce the platysma require exploration. Dividing penetrating wounds of the neck into three zones, as suggested by Monson and colleagues,[27] is helpful. Zone III extends from the base of the skull to the angle of the mandible, zone II from the angle of the mandible to 1 cm above the head of the clavicle, and zone I from 1 cm below the head of the clavicle to include the rest of the thoracic outlet. With clinical examination, ascertaining whether injuries in zones I and III have damaged major vascular structures may be difficult. Preoperative arteriography is extremely important if these patients are hemodynamically stable. Patients with penetrating injuries in zone II who have no neurologic deficit but require surgery may undergo surgery without arteriography, although preoperative arteriography is helpful in localizing the injury.

Signs and symptoms suggesting arterial injury in the extremities apply equally to the neck, but unfortunately, these arteries may not be accessible for examination, especially after blunt trauma (Fig. 35–4). The clinical features of blunt trauma to the carotid artery are summarized in Table 35–6.[28] Few signs of injury may be present, because fewer than half of the patients will have local evidence of blunt trauma. Arteriography should be used liberally after

TABLE 35-6

Clinical Features of Blunt Trauma to Carotid Arteries

Hematoma of lateral neck
Horner's syndrome
Transient ischemic attack
Lucid interval
Limb paresis in an alert patient

From Jernigan WR, Gardner WC: Carotid artery injuries due to closed cervical trauma. Trauma 11:429, 1971.

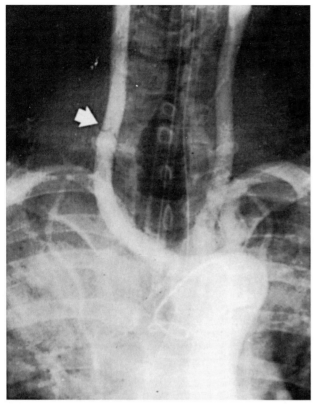

Figure 35–4. An injury inflicted by a steering wheel in an automobile accident caused pulmonary contusions and a fracture of the right common carotid artery. A graft was required to replace this section of the vessel.

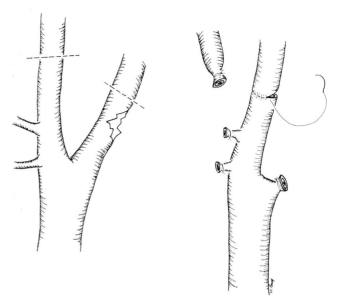

Figure 35–5. If the internal carotid artery cannot be repaired directly, the external carotid can be mobilized and used as a substitute graft.

As shown in Figure 35–5, the external carotid artery may be used to repair the internal carotid artery in certain circumstances. If lateral repair is not possible, a saphenous vein graft or an arterial autograft may be interposed, as shown in Figure 35–6. If the back-pressure from the internal carotid artery is less than 70 mm Hg, or if back-bleeding is scanty, the use of an intraluminal shunt is a satisfactory method to maintain cerebral blood flow while repairs are being completed.

blunt and penetrating trauma to the neck and thoracic outlet.

Aerodigestive injuries frequently accompany carotid artery trauma, especially after penetrating mechanisms. The surgeon must be vigilant to detect and treat these injuries, which can result in devastating complications if not addressed early. Endoscopy should include examination of the oropharynx, trachea, and esophagus. This is followed by esophagography with water-soluble media and, subsequently, barium. When aerodigestive injuries are present, the incision and repair strategy is critical to protect the vascular repair from gross contamination.

Operative Management

Patients who have carotid artery injuries and continued prograde flow are candidates for surgical repair. A patient who has complete occlusion of the internal carotid artery as a result of blunt trauma, is not bleeding, and has a severe neurologic deficit manifested by coma or hemiplegia is probably best treated nonoperatively. If operation is required for other reasons, the internal carotid artery can be ligated.[26] Complete removal of thrombus in these situations is often difficult, and residual clot may embolize and worsen the neurologic deficit.[29]

Vascular control and repair are performed as described in the preceding sections. Standard techniques are used, and every effort is made to avoid thromboembolic complications; precise suture and graft techniques are essential.

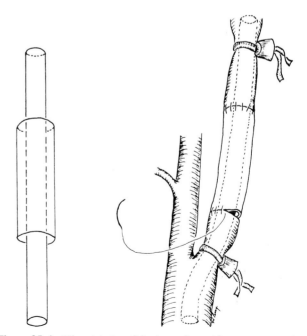

Figure 35–6. When injuries of the internal carotid artery are associated with low back-pressures (<70 mm Hg) or scanty back-bleeding, a saphenous vein graft can be placed over the temporary inlaying shunt as the repair is completed.

Postoperative Care

Although any vascular repair is susceptible to bleeding, bleeding is unusual unless multiple injuries or coagulation defects are present. Drains are not usually employed in isolated vascular wounds. However, in selected patients with cervical injuries, drains may be used for 12 to 24 hours to prevent the accumulation of blood, which may cause a compressing hematoma beneath the relatively rigid cervical fascia. Patients are carefully monitored for the appearance of neurologic deficits. Neurologic symptoms usually require arteriography or duplex ultrasonography to evaluate the status of the repair and to assess the possibility of cerebral thromboembolism. Postoperative carotid artery occlusion rarely occurs, but if it does, the patient should be returned immediately to the operating room for thrombectomy, correction of any technical errors, and reestablishment of flow. In these situations, delay for arteriography is not recommended. Thrombosis and the emergence of a stroke require immediate surgery. Expeditious restoration of flow is often successful in preventing permanent neurologic problems.

Injuries of Vessels of the Root of the Neck

Injuries of vessels in zone I (the thoracic outlet) are difficult to evaluate because the injury may be obscure. Operative exposure of the wound without proximal control can lead to fatal hemorrhage. If a penetrating wound in zone I is thought to have injured the great vessels, proximal control via a middle sternal splitting incision is recommended before exposing the wound. Similarly, if during the course of cervical exploration through an incision along the anterior sternocleidomastoid muscle border, bleeding, hematoma, or blood staining of the carotid sheath in the depths of the wound at the root of the neck are encountered, an immediate sternal splitting incision should be made to control the great vessels of the arch.[16] All the vessels of the arch, with the exception of the left subclavian artery, can be reached easily through this approach, and if necessary the incision may be extended into the second or third interspace or a separate left thoracotomy incision may be opened to control the left subclavian artery. Because of its intrapleural location, the proximal left subclavian artery is best approached through an anterolateral thoracotomy. Although this incision facilitates proximal control, the more distal extrapleural portions cannot be reached. A supraclavicular incision is added for this purpose. Although many authors speak of the "open book" created when a median sternotomy connects an anterolateral thoracotomy to a supraclavicular incision, we have found that the approach does not open easily and typically results in multiple posterior rib fractures.

Repairs of these arteries are performed in the same fashion as described in the preceding sections. In most cases, back-pressure in the innominate or left common carotid artery exceeds 70 mm Hg. Temporary shunting techniques are not required if the patient's blood pressure is maintained within a normal range. Prosthetic grafts are needed more often for repair of the great vessels of the arch, because autografts of this size are usually not available (Fig. 35–7).

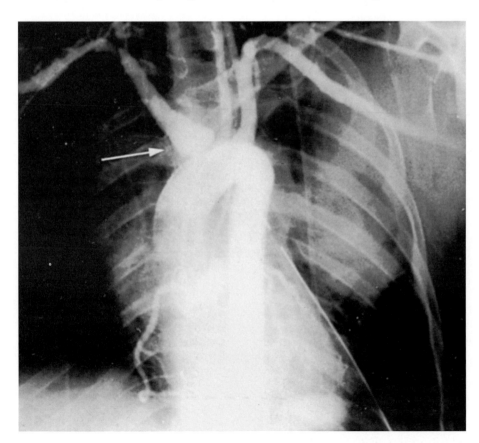

Figure 35–7. A load of lumber fell on this young man and produced lung contusions and a wide mediastinum, which prompted the arteriogram. The arrow points to the nearly avulsed innominate artery.

Injuries of the Abdominal Aorta and Its Branches

Almost all major vascular injuries in the abdomen are caused by penetrating trauma, usually gunshot wounds. Associated gastrointestinal injuries are common. This is a lethal combination, especially if multiple vascular wounds are present. Less than half of these patients survive.[17, 30]

Diagnosis

A penetrating wound of the abdomen in a hypotensive patient is a common occurrence. The usual signs and symptoms of vascular injuries can be suspected, but because the arteries are inaccessible for examination, indirect evidence of injury assumes more importance. Although abdominal distention from the accumulation of blood can occur, massive retroperitoneal bleeding can be hidden, and little blood may be present in the peritoneal cavity. This may occur with knife wounds that enter from the back, particularly if the blade passes between two of the lower ribs. Such a wound may appear benign. Moreover, pulse deficits and limb ischemia, if present, are difficult to interpret in hypotensive patients. Because of the severity of most of these injuries, little time is usually available for protracted examination and diagnostic studies. The need for surgical exploration is obvious.

Plain film radiography, CT scan, "one-shot" intravenous pyelograms, and arteriography all may be useful. Even if a vascular wound is not detected, such studies can expose other problems that require surgical correction. Abdominal paracentesis or lavage can document intraperitoneal bleeding, but false-negative results do occur, especially in the face of severe pelvic fractures.[31]

Hematuria should alert the surgeon to the possibility of a renovascular injury. If a patient shows microscopic hematuria and has not been in shock, the chance of a significant renovascular injury being present is very small, and additional evaluation is not indicated. However, if microscopic hematuria is accompanied by severe hypotension, or if gross hematuria is present, further evaluation is required, usually in the form of an intravenous contrast-enhanced CT scan. If the kidney functions normally, with no apparent parenchymal or collecting system dysfunction, hospitalization and observation are acceptable. If kidney function is impaired or absent, or if parenchymal disruption is present, renal arteriography is indicated. If the major renal vascular architecture is intact, observation is sufficient, with repeated studies. If vascular wounds are present or collecting system disruption is diagnosed, surgical correction is required.

Operative Management

Hemodynamically unstable patients are taken immediately to the operating room; preparations for surgery are completed as necessary diagnostic maneuvers are finished and interpreted. The operating team is scrubbed and ready to intervene in the event of sudden collapse.[17] This may occur upon induction of anesthesia when the tamponading effect of the tensed abdominal musculature is lost due to the use of paralytic agents.

The abdomen is opened through a long midline incision, a rapid exploration is performed, and attention is directed toward the major vessels. If a bleeding wound can be seen and exposed easily, it is controlled with vascular clamps. This is often the case with isolated wounds of the branches of the visceral arteries. Injuries of the aorta, especially the supraceliac aorta and that part containing the origins of the visceral branches (zones I and II as described by Lim and colleagues[30]), usually require a supraceliac clamp to control bleeding. This part of the aorta is approached through the gastrohepatic ligament, and the aorta is freed from the left crus of the diaphragm with finger dissection. Only the front and sides are mobilized to permit placing a long straight or slightly curved vascular clamp directly across the aorta in an anteroposterior plane. Temporary aortic occlusion at this level allows more rapid and precise exposure of wounds of the lower aorta and its branches. Control through a left thoracotomy may be required if the supraceliac approach is impractical or fails.

Infrarenal aortic wounds (Lim zone III) usually can be approached directly through the root of the mesentery using the usual methods for elective aortic operations. Wounds in the center of the mesenteric root often involve the pancreas and duodenum and can damage the major veins located there. A combination of aortic and major venous wounds is often lethal, and control of large venous injuries in this area is difficult to achieve.

When exposure of midaortic wounds is difficult because of obscuring hematomas, brisk bleeding, or multiple organ damage, mobilization of the left colon, spleen, and pancreas can allow the surgeon to reach the aorta and its branches. Reflection of the ascending colon and duodenum exposes the vena cava and aorta from the right side.

Once the vascular wounds are controlled, priorities of repair are set. Blood flow should be restored to the kidneys and liver first, because these organs are most sensitive to hypoxia. The intestine and the lower extremities can tolerate longer periods of ischemia. Repairs rarely require more than an hour to complete.

The method of vascular reconstruction is dictated by the nature of the wound. Usually, resection and end-to-end anastomosis are adequate for the aortic branches, unless tissue loss is extensive and interposition grafts are needed. Aortic wounds caused by knives and low-velocity gunshot wounds occasionally can be repaired with simple suturing; more extensive damage mandates patch angioplasty or grafting. Plastic prostheses are customarily needed to reconstruct the aortoiliac tree.

Large bowel penetration resulting in heavy bacterial soilage in association with aortic wounds presents special problems. Autogenous tissue repairs may succeed in some of these cases, but occasionally even arteries that are simply oversewn break down later because of infection. Severe contamination is an indication to restore blood flow to the lower extremities via a remote bypass rather than by aorto-iliac grafting. Axillofemoral and femorofemoral subcutaneous grafts are favored. Sewing the two common iliac arteries together may be possible, thus using one axillofemoral graft to perfuse both legs. This avoids placing a prosthetic graft into an abdominal cavity with heavy bacterial contamination. Careful closure of oversewn arterial stumps (aortic and iliac especially) is essential. The closed ends are covered and protected by pedicle flaps of the greater omentum. Antibiotics are continued until all wounds are healed and all intravenous catheters are removed. Once healing is completed, restoration of normal vascular architecture can be considered.

Injuries of the Arteries of the Extremities

Femoral arteries are among the most frequently injured vessels, constituting approximately 20% of all arterial injuries. Acute ligation of the common femoral artery results in an amputation rate of approximately 50%, only slightly less than that noted after acute occlusion of the popliteal artery. Large veins and important nerves are found within the femoral triangle, making associated injuries of these structures common.

Popliteal artery injuries are especially difficult problems, and failure to repair them results in limb loss in almost two thirds of patients.[32] Penetrating wounds are usually easily diagnosed because virtually all create pulse deficits and, frequently, ischemia of the lower extremity. Patients with blunt trauma often show more difficult problems upon evaluation. Posterior dislocations of the knee, for example, are very likely to injure the popliteal artery. As Lefrac,[4] Dart and Braitman,[3] and others have indicated, these patients should have preoperative arteriography. Lefrac reported that of 152 patients with knee dislocations, 28% sustained popliteal artery injuries; half of these eventually lost the limb.[4] Overlooking an unstable knee during the examination of a patient who has multiple injuries is very easy. Although popliteal artery injuries caused by fracture dislocations are usually easily identified because of a pulse deficit and, in most cases, ischemia, inexperienced examiners may assume that spasm is at fault. This can be a serious error that ultimately results in limb loss. Preoperative arteriography is important and may be the only way of ascertaining the extent of the injury.[23]

Preoperative Preparation

Many of these patients have suffered a great deal of blood loss by the time they are initially examined. Resuscitation should proceed in an aggressive and orderly manner prior to surgery. Stabilization of fractures should be performed early. This is easier if the patient is taken directly to the operating room, especially if hemodynamically unstable. Many surgeons favor the use of external techniques for bone stabilization to avoid introducing foreign bodies into the area of potential vascular repair. However, both internal and external fixation have been used successfully. Temporary stabilization is essential during early care to prevent further damage.

Operative Management

As with other vascular wounds, general anesthesia is usually required for operative repair. The opposite extremity is prepared so that if vascular autografts are required, the contralateral saphenous vein will be available. With concomitant femoral or popliteal vein injuries, one may wish to preserve the ipsilateral saphenous veins in case more serious venous injuries cannot be repaired. Repairing concomitant popliteal vein injuries is especially important if the saphenous vein is damaged.[32]

Rich and Spencer[33] presented compelling reasons for repair of the popliteal vein as well as the artery, pointing out that the incidence of thromboembolic events is approximately 13% after vein repair but is more than 50% after ligation. These authors and Snyder and colleagues[32] also suggested that continued popliteal artery patency is enhanced by simultaneous repair of popliteal vein injuries.

In most situations, the wounds are approached through the same medial vertical incision used for elective surgery. Proximal and distal control can be difficult to obtain when the patient is prone and the vessels are approached posteriorly through the popliteal space.

The basic techniques of repair are those used in other vascular surgery. Damaged tissue is resected and an end-to-end anastomosis with careful intimal coaptation is constructed. Popliteal arteries are especially vulnerable to injury by a vascular clamp, and soft noncrushing instruments are best for temporary occlusion. If the injury is in an atherosclerotic artery, controlling the bleeding by inserting an intraluminal catheter may be more suitable, thus avoiding wall damage that might predispose to immediate thrombosis or enhance the subsequent progress of the atheromatous disease.

For patients who have sustained blunt trauma and multiple fractures, repairing the popliteal artery and vein initially may be necessary. The vascular surgeon remains in attendance while final stabilization of the fractures is obtained by either internal or external fixation. In those situations in which ischemia is not present, such as a superficial femoral artery occlusion, completing the orthopedic repairs initially may be practical. Once the bone is stabilized, constructing an arterial repair of the proper length and tension is easier. If the foot is ischemic and extensive orthopedic repairs are required, temporary inlaying shunts can be placed in the popliteal artery and vein. These decisions should be made through consultation of the vascular surgeon and the orthopedic surgeon; both should be in attendance during bony repair to avoid disruption of the vascular suture lines.

Postoperatively, patency of the repair is usually apparent by the immediate reappearance of pedal pulses. If any question exists as to the adequacy of the repair, or if distal thromboembolism appears likely, operative arteriography is indicated. Failure to restore pulses is usually a technical problem and is seldom caused by persistent spasm.

Tibial Artery Injuries

Injuries to the tibial arteries present a difficult problem because, in most cases, they do not result in severe ischemia unless two of the three arteries are damaged. In patients who have penetrating trauma but otherwise would not require operative exploration, if only one tibial artery is occluded and no bleeding is present, such an injury can be accepted without repair. Arteriographic survey of these patients is essential to determine if a significant problem is present. In the absence of other indications, exploration of a tibial artery would be performed only if it were bleeding or if arteriography revealed an AV fistula or a false aneurysm.

False Aneurysms and Arteriovenous Fistulas

Complications of vascular injuries such as thrombosis, delayed bleeding, AV fistulas, and false aneurysms are more likely to occur, and much more difficult to manage, if the injury is not treated promptly. False aneurysms and AV fistulas can occur immediately after the injury; bleeding occurs into a cavity that is confined by surrounding tissue and a hematoma forms (sometimes false aneurysms are called pulsating hematomas). Although spontaneous regression of AV fistulas and false aneurysms can occur, the studies of Shumacker and Wayson[34] have demonstrated that this is unlikely. Fewer than 3% of AV fistulas and fewer than 6% of false aneurysms heal spontaneously.

These lesions resolve only when they thrombose, and thrombosis of major arteries is not tolerated without unacceptable ischemia. Because spontaneous regression is unlikely, and because most AV fistulas and false aneurysms increase in size and complexity with the passage of time, operative repair becomes much more difficult if surgery is delayed. Increasing edema, inflammation, and expansion of the lesion slowly encroach on and involve surrounding neurovascular structures, making repair more difficult (Fig. 35–8).

A false aneurysm is the result of an incomplete injury that permits continued bleeding from a laceration. Transection of an artery is customarily followed by retraction and clotting and, in the case of small vessels, cessation of bleeding. Contiguous tangential wounds of arteries and veins may develop into AV fistulas, even acutely.

The most apparent clinical feature of a false aneurysm is a pulsatile mass that is associated with either an acute or a chronic penetrating wound. A murmur may be heard over the mass because the tangential laceration of the artery permits the escape of blood into the surrounding tissues, ultimately forming a tamponading clot. Although the physical diagnosis is usually easy when the mass is located in the extremities, arteriography is important to ascertain the exact number and location of the involved vessels and to plan operative repair properly.

An AV fistula may be associated with a false aneurysm, or a clean endothelial channel may form in a chronic AV fistula. In some cases, very little inflammation may be present about the lesion, although the entrance of high-pressure arterial blood flow into the veins produces varicosities if the veins are thin-walled and fragile. Occasionally, false aneurysms and AV fistulas are combined.

The Nicoladoni-Branham sign can be elicited in some patients with an AV fistula. Digital occlusion of the fistula results in a slowing of the heart rate because of the reduction of flow into the right atrium. A continuous, machinery-like murmur usually occurs over the fistula, and evidence may exist of venous hypertension and adjacent varicosities.

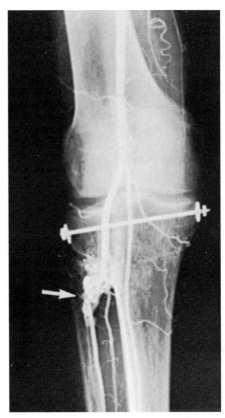

Figure 35–8. An arteriovenous fistula of the anterior tibial artery and vein is marked by the arrow. Orthopedic repairs were completed previously, without knowledge of the vascular wound.

When the shunt is large, ischemia of the distal extremity may result from shunting of large amounts of arterial blood into the low-pressure venous system. On rare occasions, large traumatic AV fistulas between the aorta and the vena cava cause florid heart failure as a result of the recirculation of enormous amounts of blood. Emergency operations may be required to treat congestive heart failure.

Large AV fistulas produce relentless enlargement of the feeding vessels and an increase in the number and complexity of the veins in the drainage system. The arteries become elongated and tortuous and their walls become thinner. Spontaneous rupture is unusual, but trauma can lead to dangerous hemorrhage.

Mural thrombosis within the system occurs occasionally. Intravascular coagulation can cause bleeding tendencies as clotting factors are depleted. Such complications should be identified and corrected before surgical repair is undertaken.

Initial surgical treatment of identified arterial injuries reduces the incidence of delayed traumatic AV fistulas and false aneurysms. Only those injuries that were missed on the initial examination and are not immediately apparent will subsequently become large enough to develop symptoms. These clearly are few in number when appropriate repair is undertaken after the initial trauma.

Preoperative arteriographic survey of AV fistulas and false aneurysms is an important step for the planning of the operation, because the lesion may be much more extensive than it appears clinically. This is especially true of

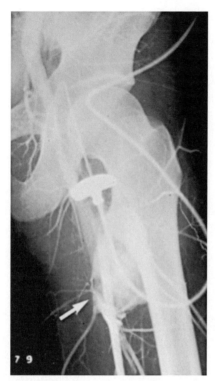

Figure 35–9. This large false aneurysm of the profunda femoral artery (*arrow*) was diagnosed only by arteriography.

deep-seated lesions involving the root of the neck, the cervical vessels, or the abdominal vessels. Even in the extremities, these lesions can be formidable. Before entering them, proximal and distal control of major arteries and veins must be achieved. In the extremities, this may be facilitated by the use of a proximal pneumatic orthopedic tourniquet. In other areas, careful dissection remote from the area of the AV fistula is required to gain control before the lesion is entered (Fig. 35–9).

For nonessential small vessels involved with a false aneurysm or AV fistula, ligation may be satisfactory. For major muscular arteries, however, repair is indicated. This is performed in the usual fashion once the vessels are controlled and identified. With large false aneurysms, the most expedient method generally involves obtaining proximal and distal control without entering the immediate area of the pseudoaneurysm. Once the vessels are clamped, the aneurysm is opened and feeding branches are controlled from within the aneurysm sac by using intraluminal occlusion catheters (such as a Fogarty catheter with an attached three-way stopcock) or special balloon occlusion catheters designed for this purpose. Repair is then completed in the usual fashion. This often requires only lateral arteriorrhaphy, because most false aneurysms result not from complete transection of the artery but from a tangential laceration that does not permit the vessel to retract and clot. If lateral repair is not possible without undue narrowing, patch-graft angioplasty may be performed. Resection and anastomosis, with appropriate graft interposition, are also used for repair.

The postoperative care of these patients is similar to that applied after repair of other arterial lesions. Not only must the pulses be monitored but neuromuscular function of the extremity must be tested to ascertain if the repair remains patent.

Intraluminal endovascular techniques are now being used to place stent-grafts across traumatic AV fistulas and pseudoaneurysms. Although most reports include only a few patients, increased expertise is being gained rapidly.[35] The presence of a fistula is suspected initially on physical examination and is confirmed with angiography or duplex sonography. Percutaneous stent placement is guided by either angiography or intravascular sonography. Duplex ultrasonography is used postoperatively to assess patency and graft position. Although deployed in a number of locations, the most practical use of these techniques appears to be in those locations where traditional operative exposure is difficult to obtain, such as the axillosubclavian system[36] (Fig. 35–10). Experience with these devices has generally been primarily limited to case reports, although some small series have been reported.[37, 38] Although initial success rates appear to be favorable, conclusions about long-term results cannot yet be reached because such series admix acute and chronic patients and those with iatrogenic and truly traumatic causes.[37] Some of the reported disadvantages of endovascular management of these injuries include fatigue of the materials, the need for a large introducer, failure of molding of the stent-graft to the arterial wall (especially in rapidly tapering or tortuous vessels), and wrinkling at its ends.[38, 39] Additional stents may be required at the end(s) of the graft. Intimal hyperplasia and the need for subsequent angioplasty have also been reported.[38] At present, the use of such endovascular techniques should be reserved for anatomically difficult lesions. Prospective trials are required before they can be recommended routinely, even for larger vessels such as the thoracic aorta.[40] Close postprocedure follow-up is required to ensure patency and maintenance of stent integrity.

Minimal (Nonocclusive) Vascular Injury

In conjunction with the trend away from routine angiography for suspected extremity injuries, some have begun to question the need to repair "minimal" vascular injuries.[41] Many of these injuries, although occurring in major or critical arteries, consist of intimal fractures, small pseudoaneurysms, mural stenoses, and small AV fistulas (Fig. 35–11). Based on the fact that arteries punctured and dilated for vascular access usually heal without incident, the need to repair all vascular injuries is being examined. The nonocclusive lesions involved vary somewhat among authors, but typical angiographic findings include (1) intimal defects (eccentric irregularities of the contrast column adjacent to the arterial wall), (2) intimal flaps (non–flow-limiting injuries that appear as a longitudinal band of decreased contrast concentration extending across the lumen), (3) pseudoaneurysms (usually smaller than 0.5 cm), (4) arterial stenoses, and (5) small AV fistulas.[41, 42]

A number of series have reported good outcomes in patients with minimal injuries treated nonoperatively. Unfortunately, in many of these studies, the duration of follow-up was limited either to inpatient observation or to a few clinic visits.[41, 42] Although some of the studies have more

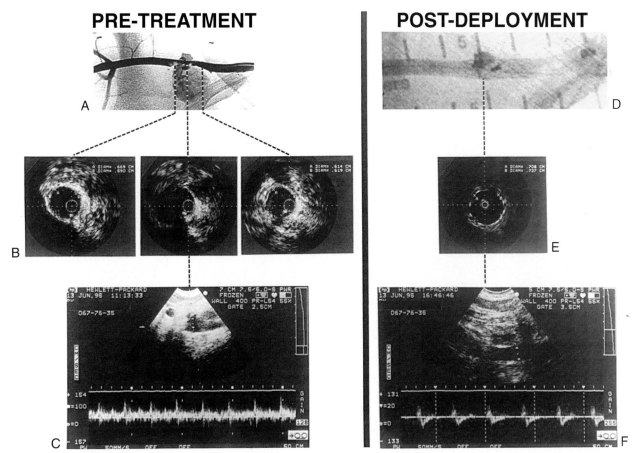

PRE-TREATMENT

POST-DEPLOYMENT

Figure 35–10. Composite photograph of the pretreatment and post-treatment images acquired during intravascular ultrasonographically guided deployment of an endoluminal graft to treat an arteriovenous (AV) fistula of the right axillary artery caused by gunshot injury. Intravascular ultrasound images acquired at the beginning of the procedure revealed dimensions of the proximal and distal artery and the length of the injury to the vessel. A corresponding duplex gray-scale surface ultrasound image of the lesion taken prior to beginning the intervention demonstrates the AV connection. The postdeployment angiogram demonstrates complete isolation and exclusion of the AV fistula, which is confirmed by the intravascular ultrasound inspection and postprocedure gray-scale surface duplex imaging of the device. (From White RA, Donayre CE, Walot I, et al: Preliminary clinical outcome and imaging criterion for endovascular prosthesis development in high risk patients with aortoiliac and traumatic arterial lesions. J Vasc Surg 24:556–571, 1996.)

longitudinal information, the natural history of these untreated lesions is not well defined. Pseudoaneurysms seem to have the greatest propensity to thrombose or expand and require the closest follow-up when treated nonoperatively. Small intimal flaps and defects probably have a better prognosis. AV fistulas that enlarge can usually be treated with endovascular techniques such as embolization. Tufaro and coworkers[43] questioned the wisdom of the nonoperative approach in their experience with seven patients treated for "minor" intimal flaps. All of the patients were monitored after their initial injury with repeat ankle-brachial index measurements for up to 48 hours before discharge. Six of the seven returned with acute onset of pain or paresthesias. Identified abnormalities included thrombosis, pseudoaneurysms, and an AV fistula, all of which required surgery. In an experimental canine model reported by Neville and colleagues[44] intimal flaps with stenosis greater than 75% were at high risk of thrombosis, even though they were not initially occlusive after formation.

The long-term outcome of minimal vascular injuries is precarious. Clearly, a difference exists between injuries caused by the low-velocity–directed punctures produced by an angiography needle and those caused by a knife or bullet. Associated soft tissue and venous trauma in the latter group clearly contributes to outcome. If nonoperative management is elected, it should be done only in those patients whose lesions are clearly nonocclusive and who will return regularly for evaluation. The duration of such follow-up is still uncertain but should last at least several years and should include duplex sonography.

Injuries of the Inferior Vena Cava

Wounds of the inferior vena cava are among the most lethal vascular injuries.[45] One in every 50 gunshot wounds and 1 in every 300 knife wounds of the abdomen injures the vena cava. Because of the serious nature of these injuries, one third of patients die before they reach the hospital, and half of the remainder die during their hospitalization. Most deaths during treatment are caused by bleeding, because of difficulties in controlling injuries of large veins, but many patients also have associated injuries. As described by Perry,[5] 79% of patients with penetrating

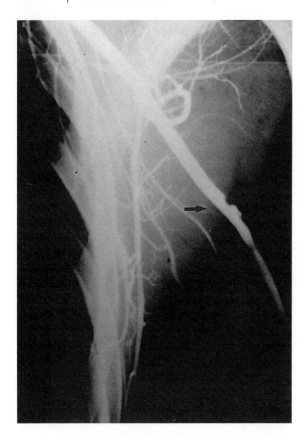

Figure 35–11. An enlargement of an angiogram obtained after a gunshot wound to the left axilla. The patient had a normal ipsilateral neurovascular examination. This is an example of a nonocclusive "minimal vascular injury" (*arrow* points to intimal defect).

trauma causing inferior vena cava wounds had injuries of other retroperitoneal structures that adversely affected survival. The renal vein, portal vein, and aorta are vulnerable to these injuries, as are the colon, liver, pancreas, and duodenum. Table 35–7 lists those injuries often associated with vena cava wounds.

The cause of the vena cava injury affects the mortality (Table 35–8). Patients who have blunt trauma and shotgun injuries are more likely to die than those who have stab wounds, especially if the injury is located in the upper part of the vena cava (Table 35–9).

Most patients, when initially examined, have an obviously serious injury: hypotension and occasional abdominal distention. Few laboratory results are of diagnostic value, except perhaps the presence of hematuria or gastrointesti-

nal bleeding, which suggests the presence of other injuries. Routine radiographic studies of the chest and abdomen are recommended if the patient is stable, but except for inferior venacavography, these tests are rarely specific. The predictors of high mortality are summarized in Table 35–10.

Operative Management

Most patients can be managed with a midline abdominal incision from the xiphoid to the pubis. In some instances, thoracotomy may be required if a suprarenal caval injury is present. The chest should be prepared in case the incision must be extended into the thorax.

A rapid abdominal exploration usually exposes major vascular injuries; this allows the surgeon to establish priorities of repair. Controlling the bleeding initially, completing the resuscitation, then assigning priorities is preferable. Control of retroperitoneal bleeding may require direct

TABLE 35–7

Injuries Associated with 110 Inferior Vena Cava Injuries

	NO.
Aorta, iliac artery	13
Major splanchnic vessel	26
Renal artery or vein	20
Liver	46
Duodenum	27
Kidney	21
Pancreas	18
Spleen	10
Colon	27
Other	21

TABLE 35–8

Etiology of Inferior Vena Cava Injuries

	NO.	DIED	MORTALITY (%)
Bullet	74	24	32
Shotgun pellets	8	6	75
Stab wound	15	2	13
Blunt trauma	13	11	85
Totals	110	43	39

TABLE 35-9

Mortality from Inferior Vena Cava Injuries by Location

	NO.	DIED	MORTALITY (%)
Above renal veins	20	11	55
At renal veins	22	13	59
Below renal veins	52	15	29
Bifurcation	16	4	25

pressure with fingers or sponge sticks while the vein is exposed and the vascular clamps are placed. Use of vascular clamps prior to adequate mobilization of the vena cava virtually guarantees additional iatrogenic injury. Sponge sticks should be used until exposure is adequate.

The suggestion has been made that some retroperitoneal injuries do not need to be explored unless they are expanding or pulsatile, but this has not been our experience. In a study of 110 patients with penetrating caval injuries, the size of the hematoma did not predict the injury.[5] Moreover, three fourths of the patients had an associated injury of some kind. In contrast, pelvic hematomas caused by fractures are not opened unless specific injuries have been identified by arteriography or other studies. Bleeding from cancellous pelvic bones is often profuse and difficult to control. Hemorrhage from pelvic fractures is best diagnosed preoperatively by CT scan, which reveals a contained retroperitoneal hematoma. When these patients undergo surgery for other indications, the hematoma should not be entered because the resulting hemorrhage is extremely difficult to control.[46] These injuries are best managed by radiographic embolization of the bleeding vessels. Lateral retroperitoneal hematomas and central hematomas should be opened when expanding or pulsatile. Inflow control should be obtained before entering the hematoma. All central hematomas after penetrating injury should be explored.

Simple lacerations or punctures are usually seen, and these can be repaired by venorrhaphy and tangential repair. If the wound is large, a partially occluding clamp may be placed about it and the lesion oversewn with a continuous suture. In patients who have anterior and posterior injuries

TABLE 35-10

Predictors of High Mortality after Vena Cava Injuries

History
    Blunt trauma
Resuscitation
    Admission blood pressure <70 mm Hg
    Failure to respond to volume resuscitation
    Preoperative cardiac arrest
    Need for emergency room thoracotomy
Operative findings
    Retrohepatic caval injury
    Associated cardiac or aortic injury
    Severe liver injury
    Multiple-organ or vascular injuries
    Severe central nervous system injury

of the vena cava, repair of the posterior wound may be effected by rotation of the cava (perhaps requiring ligation of lumbar veins) and direct suture. In some instances, the anterior caval wound can be enlarged and the posterior wall laceration repaired from the inside under direct vision.[31]

Transections of the vena cava usually can be repaired by end-to-end vascular techniques, although the vena cava does not permit loss of a long segment. If the cava is severely lacerated, if multiple wounds are present that require complicated grafts, or if repair poses a prohibitive risk in a patient with multiple injuries, ligation of the infrarenal cava is acceptable. This is rarely necessary, however.

Wounds at or above the renal veins are difficult to expose and carry a higher mortality; over half of the patients die.[45] If bleeding from behind the liver is encountered and cannot be easily identified as coming from a laceration of the anterior cava below the caudate lobe, other maneuvers may be needed. Division of the supporting ligaments permits the liver to be displaced medially a considerable distance, and, in some people, adequate exposure can be obtained for primary repair of the cava.[15, 47] Sudden interruption of the inferior vena cava blood flow returning to the heart may result in cardiac arrest. Temporary caval occlusion should be approached cautiously, with careful monitoring of blood pressure and heart rate. If extensive suprarenal caval injuries are seen after mobilization of the liver, or if two or three hepatic veins are involved in the injury, employing an intracaval shunt as described by Schrock and colleagues[48] may be necessary (Fig. 35–12). A 38-Fr Tygon shunt with appropriate openings can be inserted by the transatrial technique, although

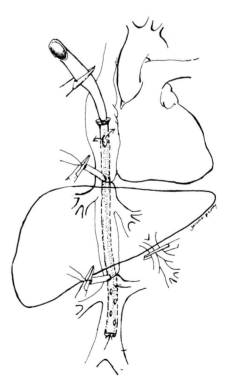

Figure 35–12. A transatrial intracaval shunt in place. (Redrawn from Schrock T, Blaisdell FW, Mathewson C Jr: Management of blunt trauma to the liver and hepatic veins. Arch Surg 96:698, 1968.)

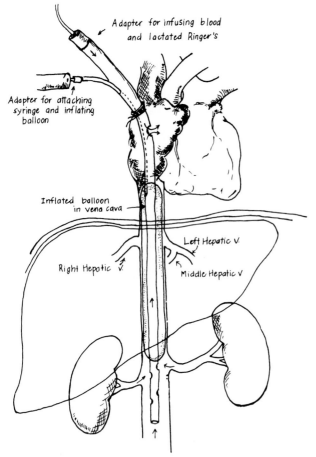

Figure 35–13. The Madding-Kennedy intracaval shunt. (Redrawn from Madding GF, Kennedy PA: Trauma to the Liver. Philadelphia, WB Saunders, 1971.)

McClelland and associates[31] have described a method using an infrarenal caval shunt. In most situations, this technique is not required, because adequate mobilization permits temporary occlusion and repair. If an intracaval shunt is used, the balloon shunt described by Madding and Kennedy[47] may be the simplest to use for these procedures (Fig. 35–13).

Concomitant repair of hepatic vein injuries is easier in

TABLE 35–11

Mortality with Bleeding Inferior Vena Cava Injuries

	NO.	DIED	MORTALITY (%)
Active bleeding	45	34	78
Tamponade	62	9	16
Not specified	3	0	0

these situations if an intracaval shunt is in place, but one of the hepatic veins may be safely ligated if repair is not possible.

These vena cava repairs usually can be completed within 30 minutes, a period of ischemia that is well tolerated by the normothermic liver. Almost inevitably, hypothermia occurs with these injuries, because of infusion of large amounts of blood and electrolyte solutions. Further regional hypothermia for liver protection may be induced by irrigating the liver directly with a saline solution at 4°C. This offers additional protection if prolonged liver ischemia occurs during caval repair (and especially if temporary hepatic artery occlusion is required).

In patients with isolated wounds of the inferior vena cava below the renal veins, direct suture is usually effective and complications are few; operative mortality is approximately 11%. However, in our experience, 67% of patients with a vena cava injury associated with one or more major vessel injuries had a fatal outcome. All of the patients with inferior vena cava wounds at or above the renal veins had associated injuries, usually to the liver or bowel and occasionally to the pancreas, stomach, or colon. Mortality is very high in this group of patients regardless of the cause of injury, but mortality is especially high if the vena cava is injured as a result of blunt trauma or a shotgun blast and is actively bleeding at the time of surgery (Table 35–11).

Late thromboembolic phenomena are uncommon, although few studies have described serial inferior venacavograms. Most patients with isolated vena cava wounds do not have recurrent thrombosis or thromboembolic phenomena. These data strongly suggest that repair of the vena cava is an effective procedure and is associated with fewer problems than is ligation.

References

1. California Wellness Foundation: Fact Sheet, Feb 12, 1995.
2. Bongard F, Dubrow T, Klein S: Vascular injuries in the urban battleground: Experience at a metropolitan trauma center. Ann Vasc Surg 4:415–418, 1990.
3. Dart CH, Braitman HE: Popliteal artery injury following fracture or dislocation at the knee. Arch Surg 112:969–973, 1977.
4. Lefrac EA: Knee dislocation. Arch Surg 111:1021, 1976.
5. Perry MO: Management of Acute Vascular Injuries. Baltimore, Williams & Wilkins, 1981.
6. Lynch J, Johansen KH: Can Doppler pressure measurement replace "exclusion" arteriography in the diagnosis of arterial trauma? Ann Surg 214:737–741, 1991.
7. Bynoe RP, Miles WS, Bell RM, et al: Noninvasive diagnosis of vascular trauma by duplex ultrasonography. J Vasc Surg 14:346–352, 1991.
8. Gagne P, Cone JB, McFarland D, et al: Proximity penetrating extremity trauma: The role of duplex ultrasound in the detection of occult venous injuries. J Trauma 39:1152–1163, 1995.
9. Morgan PW, Goodman LR, Aprahamian C, et al: Evaluation of traumatic aortic injury: Does dynamic contrast-enhanced CT play a role? Radiology 182:661–666, 1992.
10. Demetriades D, Gomez H, Velmahos G, et al: Routine helical computed tomographic evaluation of the mediastinum in high-risk blunt trauma patients. Arch Surg 133:1084–1088, 1998.
11. Snyder WH III, Thal ER, Bridges RA, et al: The validity of normal arteriography in penetrating trauma. Arch Surg 113:424–426, 1978.
12. Weaver FA, Yellin AE, Bauer M, et al: Is arterial proximity a valid indication for arteriography in penetrating extremity trauma? Arch Surg 125:1256–1260, 1990.
13. Reid JDS, Weigelt JA, Thal ER, et al: Assessment of proximity of a wound to major vascular structures as an indication for arteriography. Arch Surg 128:942–946, 1988.
14. Frykberg ER, Dennis JW, Bishop K, et al: The reliability of physical examination in the evaluation of penetrating extremity trauma for vascular injury: Results at one year. J Trauma 31:502–511, 1991.

15. Rich N, Spencer F: Vascular Trauma. Philadelphia, WB Saunders, 1978.
16. Flint LM, Snyder WH, Perry MO, Shires GT: Management of major vascular injuries in the base of the neck. Arch Surg 106:407–413, 1973.
17. Mattox KL, McCollum WB, Beall AC, et al: Management of penetrating injuries of the suprarenal aorta. J Trauma 15:808–815, 1975.
18. Moore EE, Burch JM, Francoise RJ, et al: Staged physiologic restoration and damage control surgery. World J Surg 22:1184–1190, 1998.
19. Hirshberg A, Walden R: Damage control for abdominal trauma. Surg Clin North Am 77:813–820, 1997.
20. Carillo EH, Spain DA, Wilson MA, et al: Alternatives in the management of penetrating injuries to the iliac vessels. J Trauma 44:1024–1029, 1998.
21. Ehrenfeld WK, Wilbur BG, Olcott CN, Stoney RJ: Autogenous tissue reconstruction in the management of infected prosthetic grafts. Surgery 85:82–92, 1979.
22. Bongard FS, White GH, Klein SR: Management strategy of complex extremity injuries. Am J Surg 158:151–155, 1989.
23. Bongard FS: Management strategy for combined vascular and orthopedic injuries. Perspect Vasc Surg 3:8–30, 1991.
24. Thal ER, Snyder WH, Hays RJ, Perry MO: Management of carotid artery injuries. Surgery 76:955–962, 1974.
25. Yamada S, Kindt GW, Youmans JR: Carotid artery occlusion due to nonpenetrating injury. J Trauma 7:333–342, 1967.
26. Liekweg WG, Greenfield LJ: Management of penetrating carotid injury. Ann Surg 188:587–592, 1978.
27. Monson DO, Saletta JD, Freeark RJ: Carotid-vertebral trauma. J Trauma 9:987, 1969.
28. Jernigan WR, Gardner WC: Carotid artery injuries due to closed cervical trauma. Trauma 11:429–435, 1971.
29. Perry MO, Snyder WH, Thal ER: Carotid artery injuries caused by blunt trauma. Ann Surg 192:74–77, 1980.
30. Lim RC, Trunkey DD, Blaisdell FW: Acute abdominal aortic injury. Arch Surg 109:706, 1974.
31. McClelland RN, Canizaro PC, Shires GT: Repair of hepatic venous, intrahepatic vena caval and portal venous injuries. Major Probl Clin Surg 3:146–153, 1971.
32. Snyder WH, Watkins WL, Bone GE: Civilian popliteal artery trauma: An eleven year experience with 83 injuries. Surgery 85:101, 1979.
33. Rich N, Spencer F: Venous injuries. In Vascular Trauma. Philadelphia, WB Saunders, 1978.
34. Shumacker HB, Wayson EE: Spontaneous care of aneurysms and arteriovenous fistulas with some notes on intravascular thrombosis. Am J Surg 79:532, 1950.
35. Marin ML, Veith FJ, Panetta TF, et al: Transluminally placed endovascular stented graft repair for arterial trauma. J Vasc Surg 20:466–472, 1994.
36. White RA, Donayre CE, Walot I, et al: Preliminary clinical outcome and imaging criterion for endovascular prosthesis development in high-risk patients with aortoiliac and traumatic arterial lesions. J Vasc Surg 24:556–571, 1996.
37. Parodi JC, Schonholz C, Ferreira LM, Bergan J: Endovascular stent-graft treatment of traumatic arterial lesions. Ann Vasc Surg 13:121–129, 1999.
38. Sanchez LA, Veith FJ, Ohki T, et al: Early experience with the Corvita endoluminal graft for treatment of arterial injuries. Ann Vasc Surg 13:151–157, 1999.
39. Patel AV, Marin ML, Veith FJ, et al: Endovascular graft repair of penetrating subclavian artery injuries. J Endovasc Surg 3:382–388, 1996.
40. Rousseau H, Soula P, Perreault P, et al: Delayed treatment of traumatic rupture of the thoracic aorta with endoluminal covered stent. Circulation 99:498–504, 1999.
41. Stain SC, Yellin AE, Weaver FA, et al: Selective management of nonocclusive arterial injuries. Arch Surg 124:1136–1141, 1989.
42. Frykberg ER, Crump JM, Dennis JW, et al: Nonoperative observation of clinically occult arterial injuries: A prospective evaluation. Surgery 109:85–96, 1991.
43. Tufaro A, Arnold T, Rummel M, et al: Adverse outcome of nonoperative management of intimal injuries caused by penetrating trauma. J Vasc Surg 20:656–659, 1994.
44. Neville RF, Hobson RW 2nd, Watanabe B, et al: A prospective evaluation of arterial intimal injuries in an experimental model. J Trauma 31:669–675, 1991.
45. Graham JM, Mattox KL, Beall AC, DeBakey ME: Traumatic injuries of the inferior vena cava. Arch Surg 113:413–418, 1978.
46. Klein SR, Bongard FS, Mehringer CM: Management strategy of vascular injuries associated with pelvic fractures. J Cardiovasc Surg (Torino) 33:349–357, 1992.
47. Madding GF, Kennedy PA: Trauma to the Liver. Philadelphia, WB Saunders, 1971.
48. Schrock T, Blaisdell FW, Mathewson C Jr: Management of blunt trauma to the liver and hepatic veins. Arch Surg 96:698, 1968.

Questions

1. A 20-year-old man had a stab wound of the right groin near the common femoral artery. Arterial bleeding occurred initially, but now a 2 × 2 cm hematoma overlies the vessels. Which of the following protocols is preferred?
   (a) immediate exploration in the operating room
   (b) arteriogram with runoff films
   (c) B mode sonogram
   (d) hospitalization and observation for a few days

2. Arterial injuries as a result of blunt trauma are especially likely with which of the following injuries?
   (a) shoulder dislocation
   (b) posterior knee dislocation
   (c) midfemoral shaft fracture
   (d) clavicular fracture

3. A 25-year-old man is admitted because of a bullet wound of the right flank. He is not in shock and has no hematuria or gastrointestinal bleeding. At exploration, a moderate collection of blood overlies the aorta and inferior vena cava above the bifurcation. What should be done now?
   (a) if the colon and small bowel are intact, nothing
   (b) exposure and exploration of the right kidney
   (c) arteriogram on the table
   (d) exploration of midline hematoma

4. A 22-year-old man is admitted with a gunshot wound to the right groin. His leg is pulseless and cool. At exploration he is found to have extensive soft tissue destruction and a 3-cm defect in the superficial femoral artery. He is hemodynamically stable during the exploration. The best strategy at this time is to
   (a) replace the missing segment with an appropriately sized PTFE graft
   (b) replace the missing segment with ipsilateral saphenous vein
   (c) replace the missing segment with contralateral saphenous vein
   (d) ligate the proximal and distal ends of the vessel and plan reoperation as indicated if the limb becomes ischemic

5. A 17-year-old boy experienced a penetrating wound of his left medial thigh during a motor vehicle accident. When examined, he had no ischemia, but moderate swelling surrounded the wound. A continuous murmur was heard in this area. Which of the following clinical features is least likely to be present?
   (a) Nicolodani-Branham sign
   (b) tachycardia
   (c) empty veins
   (d) decreased ankle blood pressure

6. The patient in question number 5 should
   (a) be admitted for observation awaiting resolution
   (b) have observation and measurements of the ankle-brachial index every 4 hours
   (c) be scheduled for MRI of the legs
   (d) be admitted for arteriography

7. A patient presents with a gunshot wound of the right medial thigh near the course of the superficial femoral artery. Distal pulses are normal, but a murmur is heard over the injury site. Which of the following treatment options is most appropriate?
   (a) admit to observe with serial ankle-brachial indices
   (b) obtain duplex ultrasonography as an outpatient
   (c) explore immediately with on-table angiography
   (d) admit for angiography

8. Which of the following "minimal" vascular injuries has the highest incidence of subsequent complications?
   (a) intimal flap
   (b) stenosis
   (c) intimal defect
   (d) pseudoaneurysm

9. Which of the following is true with regard to injuries of the inferior vena cava?
   (a) infrarenal injuries carry the best chance for survival
   (b) posterior injuries usually do not need to be explored
   (c) posterior injuries cannot be repaired through an anterior venotomy
   (d) pulmonary emboli occur frequently after repair

10. Concomitant tibial bone fractures causing transection of the popliteal vein and artery should be treated by
    (a) immediate external fixation and stabilization of the tibia
    (b) initial traction and internal fixation with arterial repair
    (c) repair of the vein and artery and internal fixation of bones
    (d) exploration and repair of the artery

Answers

| 1. a | 2. b | 3. d | 4. c | 5. c | 6. d | 7. d | 8. d | 9. a | 10. c |

36

Acute Arterial and Graft Occlusion

Niren Angle and William J. Quiñones-Baldrich

One of the most common clinical problems in vascular surgery is acute ischemia from a native vessel or graft occlusion. The consequences of acute limb ischemia are dependent on the speed and accuracy of diagnosis and treatment. This is made difficult by the fact that the presentation of acute limb ischemia can range from the subtle to the dramatic. Vascular specialists, and ideally every physician, must be aware of the different manifestations of acute limb ischemia so that appropriate measures can be taken and proper diagnostic and therapeutic measures instituted. A delay in diagnosis and treatment results in increased morbidity and mortality.

There are two distinct phases in the physiology of acute vascular and graft occlusion, namely ischemia and reperfusion, which can have grave and distinct consequences for the afflicted patient. The greater the period of ischemia, the more likely it is that the tissue deprived of flow will not be viable. Reperfusion of ischemic tissue can have both local and systemic effects, the latter in the form of hemodynamic instability and remote organ injury. In the last 15 to 20 years, there has been a tremendous amount of basic science research in this area, and quite fascinating insights have been gained. It behooves the vascular surgeon to be intimately aware of the pathophysiology of ischemia and reperfusion because knowledge of this phenomenon has profound consequences for management and patient outcome.

This chapter focuses on the etiology, pathophysiology, clinical manifestations, and medical and surgical management of the patient with an acutely ischemic limb. Ischemia may be secondary to native artery occlusion from thrombosis or embolism, or the patient may have thrombosis from a previous vascular reconstruction. Although both may have similar clinical presentations, the etiology and management of these two entities are different and thus are considered separately. Acute cerebral ischemia and visceral ischemia are addressed in other chapters in this book.

PATHOPHYSIOLOGY

The ultimate consequence of ischemia is the progressive depletion of high-energy substrate owing to lack of oxygen delivery to the tissue and subsequent conversion to anaerobic metabolism. The balance between supply and demand determines the magnitude and speed of the depletion of the cellular energy compounds. Different tissues have different rates of metabolism, and the consequences of interruption of blood flow or a decrease in blood flow are different for a given period of ischemia. Tissues such as heart and brain extract oxygen maximally at rest, and thus any increase in their oxygen demand can only be met by an increase in blood flow. Tissues such as kidney and skeletal muscle do not extract oxygen maximally at rest, and thus an increase in metabolic demand is compensated for by increased tissue extraction of oxygen and an increase in blood flow.

Oxygen demand is a function of metabolic activity, and, thus, one potential therapeutic intervention is reduction of tissue metabolism. Efforts at reducing ischemic myocardial infarct size concentrate on reducing metabolic demand by unloading the heart during the critical recovery phase by the use of β-blockers and afterload-reducing agents. The brain, on the other hand, is exquisitely sensitive to ischemia, because it is incapable of significantly reducing its metabolic demand. Adjunctive measures, such as the use of barbiturates, are used to reduce basal metabolism, thus reducing the consequences of ischemia after an ischemic brain injury.

In an extremity, tissues differ in their ability to tolerate ischemia, reflecting their basal metabolic demand. Skin and subcutaneous tissue appear relatively resistant to ischemia. On the other hand, peripheral nerve has been shown by Chervu and colleagues[1] to be exquisitely sensitive to ischemia and reperfusion, with prolonged functional deficit demonstrable after 3 hours of ischemia. The prior impression that peripheral nerve was relatively resistant to ischemia might have been a reflection of the lack of dramatic morphologic changes under microscopic examination.

Skeletal muscle makes up the majority of tissue mass in the extremities. It is relatively tolerant of ischemia owing to its slow resting metabolic rate, stores of glycogen, and high-energy phosphate bonds in the form of creatine phosphate, as well as its ability to function by anaerobic glycolysis.

In the clinical situation, the supply side of this equation is variable and largely depends on the location of the vascular occlusion, the rapidity with which such occlusion has developed, and the presence of collateral circulation before the occlusion. Thus, a specific ischemic interval has variable effects, depending on all of the above parameters. The concept of a safe period of ischemia beyond which the viability of the tissue is unlikely cannot be substantiated. Thus, other parameters must be used in the assessment of the ischemic extremity. In the experimental animal, measurement of contractile function is much more reliable than time as a predictor of ischemic injury.[2]

When tissues are injured by ischemia or anoxia, their ability to control the metabolism of oxygen is compromised.[3] For some time, the cell can continue cellular functions by drawing on stored adenosine triphosphate (ATP). If the rate of metabolism is slowed, the energy sources can be replenished by anaerobic glycolysis, or by use of stored energy sources such as creatine. With increasing time of ischemia, energy stores are depleted and ATP is metabolized to adenosine diphosphate (ADP), and eventually to adenosine monophosphate (AMP). The cell is unable to sustain cellular function and transmembrane gradients cannot be maintained. The cell membrane becomes compromised and there is a net cellular calcium influx.

Reperfusion or reoxygenation causes increased oxygen free radical production, associated tissue injury, and functional impairment. Injured tissues may produce superoxide radicals by various mechanisms, not necessarily involving neutrophils. Isolated organ preparations perfused with buffer, in the absence of neutrophils, still produce abundant free radicals. In tissues containing abundant xanthine dehydrogenase, ischemia results in massive catabolism of the adenine nucleotide pool owing to the low energy status of the tissue. Adenosine is broken down to inosine, and then to hypoxanthine, which accumulates.[4] Approximately 10% of a tissue's xanthine dehydrogenase exists as xanthine oxidase; ischemia induces proteolytic conversion, resulting in a marked increase in xanthine oxidase, which accumulates within the cell. This results in an abundance of the superoxide-producing xanthine oxidase and its substrate hypoxanthine. On reintroduction of the second substrate, molecular oxygen, during reperfusion, a burst of superoxide is produced.

There is a great variability in species and tissue concerning the amount of xanthine dehydrogenase or xanthine oxidase that is present.[5, 6] Reperfused organs are dramatically protected by inhibitors of xanthine oxidase or by superoxide dismutase (SOD).[7, 8] McCord and colleagues[9] have used the rabbit heart as a model of the xanthine oxidase–deficient human heart, and in that model, enzyme-inhibiting doses of allopurinol do not protect the heart, but SOD does.[9] This finding implies the existence of xanthine oxidase–independent mechanisms of free radical production, most likely resulting from ischemic changes to the mitochondria.[10] Oxygen radical injury has been demonstrated in most tissues subjected to ischemia and reperfusion.[11] Reperfusion results in lipid peroxidation and destruction of cellular membrane integrity.[12] Although reperfusion injury to ischemic muscle is mediated by super-

oxide and hydroxyl radicals, the source of these free radicals is not known; however, the xanthine oxidase pathway in skeletal muscle is of questionable clinical significance.[13]

Administration of free radical scavengers during the time of reperfusion has been advocated with the goal of retrieving injured skeletal muscle.[14] Potential sources of these radicals are present in other cellular components, and specifically in white blood cells that may be resident in the tissues during the ischemic period or introduced during the early phases of reperfusion. The ischemia may result in upregulation of the CD11b/CD18 integrin complex, which is necessary for neutrophil-endothelial cell adhesion to occur.[15, 16] Leukocyte accumulation in reperfused muscle was demonstrated by Rubin and coworkers.[17]

Acute occlusion results in a series of events, each of which potentiates the ischemic insult and amplifies the injury. The thrombus can propagate to involve and occlude collateral side branches. The ischemic tissues accumulate fluid and swell, leading to compression of the vascular channels within a fascial compartment. This results in endothelial swelling and luminal narrowing, with subsequent microvascular obstruction.

An additional feature of the reperfusion injury is the "no-reflow" phenomenon. Reperfusion injury also results in other changes—besides free radical injury directly—that cause progressive microcirculatory obstruction. There is some evidence demonstrating leukocyte-capillary plugging, causing impairment in the reflow process.[18] This leads to an increase in resistance, which has been found to correlate with the extent of tissue damage after a brief period of ischemia.[19] Leukocyte adhesion to the venules and leukocyte extravasation[20] are both mechanisms that are operative in tissue injury after ischemia-reperfusion. These two mechanisms can lead to an increased permeability of the microvascular endothelial barrier, which has been shown to be a mechanism of ischemia-reperfusion injury after prolonged ischemia.[21, 22] Additionally, ischemia-reperfusion results in endothelial swelling, which itself can lead to capillary closure, exacerbating the damage done by leukocyte plugging.[23] Thus, the no-reflow phenomenon prevents nutrient delivery, in spite of restoration of blood flow, and prolongs the ischemic injury. Another study using a model of 3 hours of ischemia and 2 hours of reperfusion demonstrated that the loss of capillary perfusion associated with the ischemia-reperfusion injury was the consequence of macromolecular leakage and resultant tissue edema and not due to leukocyte-capillary plugging.[24] Elimination of white blood cells from the initial perfusate was of no advantage in an experimental model of ischemia and reperfusion of skeletal muscle.[25] The role of the leukocyte in the no-reflow phenomenon is, therefore, uncertain. In our laboratory, we have observed that this process becomes more prevalent with increasing length of ischemia. Whereas muscles that are made ischemic from 1 to 3 hours are easily reperfused without evidence of the no-reflow phenomenon, muscles subjected to 5 hours or more of ischemia demonstrate this phenomenon in up to 40% to 50% of specimens.[26] Blood is a non-Newtonian fluid, the rheology of which takes on special significance in this phenomenon. The energy required to reestablish movement of the blood after it has stopped flowing is proportional to the third power of the red blood cell mass and the second power of the fibrinogen content.[27] Thus, the concept of "opening pressure" may be important in the early phases of reperfusion.

Thus, two major components appear responsible for reperfusion injury. Initially, the ischemic period results in the depletion of glycogen stores and stores of high-energy substrate. At some point, molecular oxygen is introduced into this milieu, and the superoxide anion and other free radicals are produced. This phase of the reperfusion has been experimentally dealt with by administration of a xanthine oxidase inhibitor, allopurinol; by administration of free radical scavengers[14, 28]; by leukocyte depletion[29]; and by controlling the rate of reperfusion[30]—all with varying degrees of success. The second major component is the no-reflow phenomenon, which prolongs the ischemic component at the cellular level.

Reperfusion, especially after prolonged ischemia, leads to changes in vasomotor tone and responsiveness, and also to an increase in microvascular permeability with resultant tissue edema. It has been hypothesized that the alteration in vasomotor tone is due to a reduction in nitric oxide (NO) levels. NO diffuses freely through the cell membrane into the surrounding smooth muscle and initiates a cascade of events culminating in smooth muscle relaxation.[31] At the same time, it diffuses into the luminal side of the endothelium where it helps to prevent platelet aggregation and adhesion to vessel walls.[32] Huk and colleagues[33] demonstrated that ischemia results in a significant depletion of tissue NO. Administration of the substrate L-arginine can significantly decrease superoxide production and increase accumulation of NO, resulting in protection from vasoconstriction.[33] In another model of ischemia-reperfusion, pentoxifylline, a xanthine-derived phosphodiesterase inhibitor, was shown to reduce reperfusion-associated membrane injury, suppress leukocyte adhesion, and improve hindlimb flow.[34]

After acute occlusion of an artery, the clinical presentation depends in large part on the presence or absence of collateral circulation. This, in turn, depends on the preexistence of occlusive arterial disease and the site of occlusion. After the initial event, ischemia may be aggravated by proximal or distal thrombus propagation or both. This impairs collateral circulation, further aggravating the process. This fragmentation, on the other hand, may produce intermittent changes of improvement and worsening depending on its severity and location. Venous thrombosis may accompany acute extremity ischemia, usually as a secondary event due to the low flow and thrombogenicity of the system. This further aggravates the ischemic process and may complicate revascularization.

Reperfusion of ischemic tissue can result in striking and sometimes lethal effects on remote organ function. The release from ischemic tissue of cytokines such as tumor necrosis factor-α, interleukin-1β, platelet-activating factor (PAF), prostaglandins such as thromboxanes and leukotrienes can cause profound perturbations in hemodynamics and organ injury such as acute lung injury. However, a more immediate systemic effect, one that can be lethal in severe cases, was described by Haimovici[35] and termed the "myonephropathic-metabolic syndrome." It is similar to the deleterious effects seen in crush injury. Upon restoration of flow, acidic blood enters the systemic circulation, capable of causing an abrupt and lethal metabolic acidosis. Some authorities recommend administration of bicarbonate during the early phase of reperfusion in anticipation of this problem. Ischemic muscle that is not salvageable can leak potassium in levels high and fast enough to produce acute hyperkalemia. This problem can be compounded by acute renal insufficiency due to myoglobinuria. Anticipation of this problem helps avoid or at least minimize its consequences. Insulin and glucose cause potassium to shift into cells and should be used to treat the hyperkalemia. Myoglobin precipitates in the renal tubules at a pH of less than 5.8, and so alkalization of the urine by the administration of bicarbonate or ammonium chloride is important to prevent acute tubular necrosis as a result of myoglobinuria. In addition, a vigorous rate of fluid administration is vital.

The pathophysiologic changes underlying acute ischemia and reperfusion are not yet completely understood, but the years have seen a blossoming of research and insights in the field of ischemia-reperfusion. Among the principles discussed in this section, our current understanding suggests that for optimal results, the quality and content of the initial perfusate represent a promising area of clinical research.

ETIOLOGY

The etiology of acute limb ischemia, whether secondary to native vessel or vascular graft occlusion, can be grouped into two distinct categories: thrombosis and embolism (Table 36–1). Although older reports suggested that embolic disease is far more common,[36, 37] more recent series suggest that thrombotic occlusions outnumber embolic occlusions by a 6:1 ratio.[38] Thrombosis in native vessels or grafts usually occurs due to an underlying lesion in the conduit itself, whereas an embolus tends to lodge in an otherwise healthy vessel, originating from another site. Bypass graft thrombosis occurs more frequently than native arterial occlusion.

Acute Arterial Occlusion

Embolism

Most emboli to the lower extremities originate in the heart, with 60% to 70% of patients having underlying myocardial disease.[39] This is most common after a myocardial infarction, because the dyskinetic portion of the heart serves as a reservoir of stagnant blood and thrombus formation. Mural thrombi can occur within hours to weeks after a myocardial infarction.[40] An embolus may, not infrequently, be the first manifestation of a silent myocardial infarction. In addition, arrhythmias may also predispose to atrial thrombus formation.

Peripheral arterial embolism is much more consequential, because there are usually few collateral vessels to the affected bed. Arterial embolism commonly lodges at vessel bifurcations, obstructing flow into two parallel channels. The upper extremities are less commonly affected than the lower extremities. Common sites of emboli are the femoral bifurcation, iliac artery bifurcation, and the tibioperoneal

Etiology of Acute Arterial Ischemia

Embolism	Trauma
Heart	Penetrating trauma
Atherosclerotic heart disease	Direct vessel injury
Coronary artery disease	Indirect injury
Acute myocardial	Missile emboli
infarction	Proximity
Arrhythmia	Blunt trauma
Valvular heart disease	Intimal flap
Rheumatic	Spasm
Degenerative	Iatrogenic
Congenital	Intimal flap
Bacterial	Dissection
Prosthetic	Presence of medical device
Artery-to-artery	Space-occupying thrombosis
Aneurysm	Clot propagation
Atherosclerotic plaque	External compression
Idiopathic	Drug abuse
Paradoxical embolus	Intraarterial administration
Thrombosis	Drug toxicity
Atherosclerosis	Contaminant
Low-flow states	Microembolization
Congestive heart failure	*Outflow Venous Occlusion*
Hypovolemia	Compartment syndrome
Hypotension	Phlegmasia
Hypercoagulable states	*Low-Flow States*
Vascular grafts	Cardiogenic shock
Progression of disease	Hypovolemic shock
Intimal hyperplasia	Drug effect
Mechanical	Mesenteric
	Digoxin
	H$_2$ blockers

trunk. Emboli to the visceral vessels account for 7% to 10% of recognized emboli. Although rheumatic disease has significantly declined in incidence, embolization from prosthetic cardiac valves now occurs more frequently, with an increasing segment of the population receiving prosthetic valves and living longer. Chronic anticoagulation is essential, because the risk of recurrent peripheral embolization is significant. Atrial myxomas can also present as a peripheral embolus of either the tumor or the clot organized around the tumor. Bacterial endocarditis remains an important consideration in the young patient appearing with a peripheral embolus without any underlying risk factors.

Patients with deep vein thrombosis and an acute arterial occlusion should be investigated for the presence of a patent foramen ovale that can produce a paradoxical embolism. Other rare causes of embolization from a central origin include tumor invasion of the intrathoracic vessels or direct arterial invasion with concomitant tumor or thrombus embolization.[41]

Proximal aneurysms frequently harbor thrombus that can embolize. The most common are abdominal and popliteal artery aneurysms. Atherosclerotic plaque can embolize and cause acute ischemia, particularly from the arch of the aorta or the descending thoracic aorta.[42] This may result in acute ischemia of the lower extremities (Fig. 36–1), the viscera, or even a stroke if the atheromatous plaque originates from the arch itself. Emboli to the lower extremities may manifest in a variety of ways. In its most dramatic

presentation, a microembolus can produce acute ischemia of a toe, leading to gangrene of the digits. This is referred to as the blue toe syndrome. Blue toes should prompt a search for a proximal source of embolization, either in the heart or the proximal vasculature.

Thrombosis

Thrombosis usually occurs in the setting of an underlying lesion in the blood vessel. It represents the final stage in the progression of atherosclerotic arterial disease. One of the most common sites of vessel occlusion is the superficial femoral artery at the adductor canal. Although atherosclerotic disease has been noted to occur equally along the entire femoral artery, the occlusion tends to occur preferentially at the adductor canal.[43] It has been hypothesized that the normal process of arterial enlargement in response to atheroma deposition is blunted at the adductor canal, thus explaining the preferential localization of the lesion at that site.

The progression from a mild atherosclerotic lesion to thrombosis begins with the deposition of lipids in the intima of the artery. A lipid-calcium core is then developed. Initially, there is a "fibrous cap" that shields the lipid-rich core from the vessel lumen. A subsequent stimulus such as macrophage infiltration, activation of matrix metalloproteinases, or the release of other proteases results in a disruption of the cap. Exposure of the underlying core is then postulated to result in accelerated thrombosis.[44] It may indeed be the case that the thickness of the cap may be more predictive of the risk of occlusion than the degree of stenosis as determined by arteriography.

The ongoing process of atherosclerosis and thrombus formation is slow, allowing gradual development of symptoms, probably due to development of collaterals. However, propagation of thrombus can also occur quite rapidly and may require immediate attention. The distinction between a thrombus and an embolus is very important because the therapy for each is very different. A low-flow state in the presence of an underlying diseased intima can induce rapid thrombosis. This is important to keep in mind in the general management of an elderly patient. Hemodynamics should be optimized and attention paid to subtle manifestations of increasing ischemia.

Thrombosis may be secondary to hypercoagulable conditions. These constitute a long list of factors that predispose to thrombosis in an otherwise unaffected arterial segment. Heparin-induced thrombosis is an important cause, usually recognized by a significant drop in the platelet count during heparin therapy and occurrence of a thrombotic event. When not recognized in a timely fashion, this may lead to limb- or life-threatening complications.[45, 46] Most other hypercoagulable states are properly treated with heparin (with concomitant administration of fresh-frozen plasma for antithrombin III deficiency), with intervention indicated by the severity of the ischemia. Malignancy may be an important underlying cause in elderly individuals with a hypercoagulable condition.[47] Chemotherapy may actually temporarily aggravate the process and lead to arterial embolism or thrombosis.[48]

Traumatic injury of an axial artery may lead to immedi-

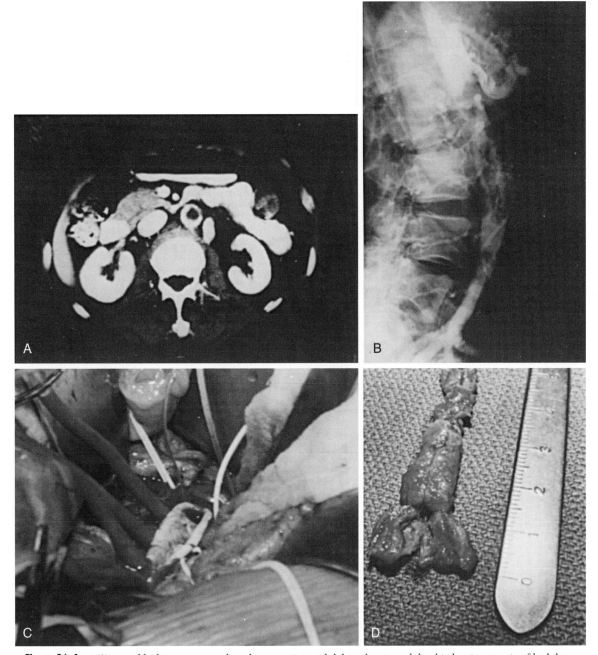

Figure 36–1. A 72-year-old white woman at clinical presentation with bilateral acute and distal ischemic rest pain of both lower extremities secondary to microembolization. *A,* Computed tomography scan with intravenous contrast shows intraluminal defect in abdominal aorta. *B,* Lateral aortogram demonstrates intraluminal defect starting at the level of the superior mesenteric artery. *C,* Operative view of infrarenal aorta with temporary control of lumbar arteries, bilateral renal artery control with vessel loops, and supraceliac aortic cross-clamping. *D,* Operative specimen after complete abdominal aortic thrombectomy. Angioscopy was helpful in assessing the completeness of the suprarenal portion of the embolectomy.

ate thrombosis, disruption, or embolization. Penetrating trauma may disrupt an artery, thus causing acute extremity ischemia. Embolization of a missile has been reported and must be kept in mind in a patient with a remote penetrating injury developing acute extremity ischemia.[49] Injuries due to proximity are usually seen with high-velocity missiles and are secondary to intimal disruption of the adjacent artery. Blunt trauma may cause acute arterial obstruction secondary to intimal disruption of the adjacent artery, intimal flap, or, on occasion, spasm due to a large expanding

hematoma. Blunt trauma to an extremity may cause fractures with associated arterial injury. This is most commonly seen with supracondylar fractures of the upper extremity, where the brachial artery is in intimate relationship with the humerus. In the lower extremity, fractures of the distal femur and posterior knee dislocations, with or without tibial plateau fractures, are most commonly associated with arterial injury. These may range from complete disruption of the artery to intimal tears and fractures, leading to secondary thrombosis (Fig. 36–2). Ascribing severe distal

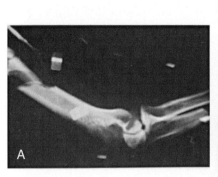
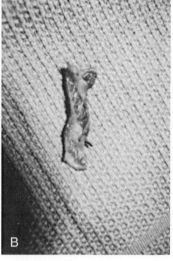
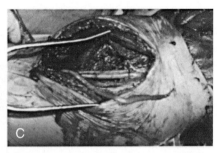

Figure 36–2. A 27-year-old patient involved in a motorcycle accident at clinical presentation with fracture of the left humerus. *A*, Arteriogram shows complete occlusion of the midbrachial artery and fracture of the distal third of the humerus. *B*, Operative specimen showing spiral disruption of the intima with thrombosis. *C*, Operative appearance of segmental vein interposition repair. Note that complete transection of the median nerve accompanied this injury and was the major cause of morbidity.

extremity ischemia to spasm without appropriate arteriographic evaluation is to be condemned and may lead to unnecessary tissue loss. Comparing distal pressures obtained by Doppler examination of the involved extremity with that of an uninvolved extremity has been suggested as an accurate means to determine which patients need arteriography. In a review of 509 consecutive patients with isolated upper or lower extremity penetrating injury, Weaver and colleagues[50] found that only pulse deficit or an ankle-brachial index less than 1.0 was a predictor of significant arterial injury.

Acute aortic dissection may occasionally appear with acute limb ischemia. Patients are usually hypertensive and complain of severe chest and back pain. Arteriography before intervention is of utmost importance to establish the diagnosis and assess visceral ischemia. On occasion, a patient taken to the operating room, misdiagnosed as having an embolic occlusion to a limb, may be suspect for aortic dissection when passage of the Fogarty catheter fails to go beyond the occlusion or does not retrieve clot or induce blood flow. The artery itself may appear friable, with easy separation of the intima through the medial plane. The inner layers of the vessel may be retrieved by the Fogarty catheter, thus compounding the problem. Failure to establish the proper diagnosis may prove fatal.

With the increased use of percutaneous endovascular techniques, iatrogenic arterial trauma is acquiring importance as a cause of acute extremity ischemia. This is usually secondary to intimal flaps, dissection, or thrombosis, and frequently requires operative therapy. Treatment may prove difficult in the patient with preexisting peripheral vascular disease. Although arteriography may be omitted in the young patient without occlusive disease, it is highly recommended in those instances in which preexisting disease may mandate an involved vascular reconstruction to reestablish circulation. The presence of a medical device, in and of itself, within the arterial system may cause significant extremity ischemia. Intraaortic balloon pumps may lead to ipsilateral or contralateral extremity ischemia sec-

ondary to clot around the device, embolization, or thrombosis. The clinical manifestations are aggravated usually because of the low-flow state requiring the device. Temporizing with heparinization is a reasonable alternative, if it is anticipated that the intraaortic balloon will be removed within the next few hours. Otherwise, construction of an extra-anatomic bypass distal to the balloon insertion site may be limb-saving.

Hand ischemia secondary to a radial artery line is usually the result of inadequate preinsertion evaluation. The performance of the Allen test before the insertion of an arterial line in the upper extremity to document the integrity of the palmar arch is an underemphasized maneuver. Failure to do this procedure inevitably results in patients experiencing hand ischemia because of interruption of radial artery flow. Removal of the radial artery cannula may result in improvement, with an occasional patient requiring operative intervention.

External compression secondary to either tourniquet or cast application to an extremity is an important preventable cause of acute extremity ischemia. Patients with peripheral vascular disease undergoing orthopedic procedures should be managed with caution, because subcutaneous collateral vessels serving to irrigate the distal extremity are most susceptible to external compression and, because of the rheology of stagnant blood, may require higher pressures to spontaneously open once they are collapsed. Emergency reconstructions in these patients may prove difficult because of the orthopedic device and preexisting peripheral vascular process. These patients are best evaluated before the orthopedic intervention so that appropriate recommendations can be made, the tourniquet avoided altogether, and intervention facilitated if a complication occurs.

Accidental intraarterial administration of illicit drugs can lead to devastating extremity ischemia secondary to toxicity of the drug itself, or contaminant microembolization. Treatment is usually supportive, and tissue loss is common with this entity.

Occlusion of venous outflow of an extremity may be

secondary to the compartment syndrome. The latter may be seen after revascularization following prolonged ischemia, trauma, or any other process that may increase compartmental pressures. As the pressure in a fascial compartment increases, venous outflow is impeded, thus producing further increase in the compartmental pressures. If this process is left unchecked, arterial inflow is restricted, leading to nerve and muscle ischemia. Early fasciotomy can be limb-saving. Outflow occlusion secondary to venous thrombosis is rare but should be recognized in the markedly swollen and painful extremity. As the venous thrombotic process progresses, arterial inflow is impeded, leading to limb-threatening ischemia (phlegmasia). Treatment alternatives include heparinization, thrombolytic therapy, and venous thrombectomy, singly or in combination.

Extreme low-flow states usually seen in patients with cardiogenic or hypovolemic shock can lead to extremity ischemia, especially in those patients with preexisting peripheral vascular disease. This process is aggravated by vasoactive drugs, which are frequently needed to support the patient. Correction of the hemodynamic derangement is the primary goal, with intervention reserved for those patients with persistent ischemia. Heparinization may be of benefit, preventing thrombosis in these poorly perfused extremities.

Vascular Graft Failure

Early and late failures of arterial reconstructions clearly can be caused by processes that have been discussed before in the section on acute arterial occlusion. In addition, processes specifically involving the graft and either the inflow or outflow vascular bed influence the performance of these reconstructions.

For the purposes of discussion, the causes of graft failure are divided into those affecting prosthetic reconstructions and those affecting autogenous reconstructions. Reconstructions involving the aortofemoral segment are discussed separately from infrainguinal reconstructions. We limit the scope of these discussions to lower extremity bypasses. The reader is referred to specific chapters dealing with other areas where failure of vascular reconstructions may be affected by similar or alternative mechanisms. Infection is an important cause of vascular graft failure and is discussed at length in Chapter 38. It suffices to say that autogenous reconstructions are more resistant to infection and, in fact, may be utilized as an alternative to a prosthetic implant in the presence of infection.[51] Acute infection of an autogenous graft usually requires graft replacement through uninvolved tissue. Chronic late-occurring infections of prosthetic grafts may be appropriately treated with autogenous reconstruction in the same bed. Exceptions to this are organisms causing necrotizing infections such as *Pseudomonas* and *Salmonella*.

Autogenous reconstruction of the lower extremities is usually seen in infrainguinal bypasses where either reversed, nonreversed, or in situ saphenous vein is used. Early failures of such reconstructions are usually secondary to technical defects that are best avoided by the liberal use of angiography, duplex scanning, or another modality at the completion of the original operation to document the technical success of the repair. Early failure may also be secondary to a defect in the graft, usually the result of previous episodes of superficial phlebitis, which may have led to sclerotic changes in a segment of the vein.[52] Additionally, injury may be caused at the time of harvest or preparation. Preservation of endothelial function should be the goal and is best accomplished by careful technique, avoiding trauma to the vein. Distention of the graft should be accomplished gently, preferably using heparinized blood. Alternatively, distention may be accomplished by the arterial pressure itself, after connecting the graft in its proximal anastomosis. One of the potential advantages of the in situ technique is that it minimizes the degree of ischemia suffered by the vein graft. Other causes of early failure include external compression or kinks, the latter avoided by assuring no twists in the vein (either in situ or reversed). Marking the proximal and distal ends of the veins before mobilization may help to accomplish this with minimal effort. Tunnels performed anatomically for autogenous grafts may produce external compression on the vein. This can be identified on completion angiography by the effacement of the contrast during injection. Subcutaneous tunnels may have an advantage in this regard, with the additional benefit of being readily accessible if revision becomes necessary.

In situ saphenous vein bypasses, in addition, may fail acutely secondary to residual arteriovenous (AV) fistulas or inadequate valve lysis. Residual AV fistulas do not lead to clinical symptoms in most instances. On occasion, however, they manifest with limb edema out of proportion to the expected swelling. They can be readily diagnosed on physical examination by the presence of a murmur over the fistula. Inadequate valve lysis can manifest as an early or late failure, due to stenosis of the segment. The use of angioscopy has been suggested by some as a means of assuring complete valve lysis in preparation of the in situ graft. Alternatively, these may be identified on continuous wave Doppler examination by a change in signal quality, implying high velocities through that segment. Completion angiography also detects these defects and avoids early failure.[53]

Intimal hyperplasia of either the proximal or distal anastomosis, or of the vein graft itself, continues to be the most frequent cause of late failure of autogenous infrainguinal reconstruction.[54] These lesions tend to occur within the first year after implantation and are rare beyond 2 years. In a series of 109 primary femoropopliteal bypasses, failures within the first 30 days resulted primarily from technical or judgmental errors. Stenotic lesions developing within the vein graft were noted to be the most common cause of failure within the first year. Progression of distal disease was the leading cause of failure after 2 years.[55] Thus, the point in time when failure occurs aids in determination of the etiologic mechanism.

Other lesions may affect autogenous vein grafts in their long-term performance. Aneurysmal dilatation is rare. When it occurs, it threatens the patency of the bypass, usually by either thrombosis or distal embolization. Stenotic lesions may develop at the inflow or outflow portion of the aneurysm, usually secondary to a kink. Rupture is rare. Repair is indicated when the lesion threatens patency of the reconstruction.

Failure of prosthetic vascular reconstructions differs from autogenous grafts in that intrinsic graft problems are extremely unusual. With the exception of the umbilical vein graft, aneurysmal dilatation is not seen. Prosthetic graft stenoses are usually the result of external compression, or twists during implantation. Externally supported grafts may avoid some of these problems. Kinking of the outflow popliteal artery in above-knee femoropopliteal bypass has been described and may account for some failures of above-knee reconstructions.[56] By far the most common cause of failure within the first 2 years after implantation of a prosthetic infrainguinal reconstruction is progression of distal disease. In a review of 111 failures of polytetrafluoroethylene (PTFE) infrainguinal bypasses over a 10-year interval, 64% of failures occurred within the first year. Fifty-six percent were due to either severity or progression of the distal disease. Progression of inflow disease occurred in 25% of instances and was most commonly seen as progression of iliac disease in patients operated on to relieve claudication and thrombosis of an inflow reconstruction in limb salvage patients. Only 8% of cases had isolated intimal hyperplasia as a cause of failure, although half of patients in whom progression of distal disease was seen had some degree of intimal hyperplasia at the distal anastomosis.[57]

Infection is a rare but important cause of failure of infrainguinal prosthetic reconstructions. When it occurs, graft excision with alternative revascularization, when indicated, is the preferred treatment.

If, after a thorough search for the cause of early failure, none is identified, a hypercoagulable condition should be suspected. A history of superficial or deep thrombophlebitis, prior bypass failure, or other thrombotic events in the past would suggest this origin. Identification of the specific abnormality is important in directing management. From a clinical standpoint, however, heparin is the treatment of choice, with the exception of heparin-induced thrombosis and the need for supplementation of antithrombin III in deficient patients. Identification of heparin-induced thrombosis is of paramount importance to avoid continued thrombotic events. Serial platelet counts during heparin therapy are most helpful, with confirmation of the diagnosis by in vitro platelet aggregation studies. Although most commonly seen in the early postoperative period, hypercoagulable conditions may play a role in early failures during the first few months after surgery. Specifically with prosthetic grafts, due to their initial thrombogenicity, some patients show acute thrombosis and no identifiable cause for failure can be determined. These patients may benefit from long-term anticoagulation.[58]

CLINICAL MANIFESTATIONS

Acute Arterial Occlusion

The clinical manifestations of acute extremity ischemia vary depending on the level and severity of the obstruction and, most important, the adequacy of collateral circulation. The latter is mostly dependent on the presence or absence of concomitant arterial occlusive disease and, to a lesser degree, location of the occlusion. In obtaining a history, one should determine the functional status of the extremity before the event. Patients with no history of claudication or previous vascular reconstruction are most likely affected by peripheral embolization.

Acute occlusion of an otherwise normal, noncollateralized artery leads to the classic manifestations of acute extremity ischemia: pulselessness, pain, pallor, paresthesia, and paralysis (the "five P's"). Certainly, the disappearance of a previously palpable pulse or the absence of a pulse in a patient with these symptoms and normal pulses in the opposite extremity is pathognomonic of an acute arterial occlusion. The presence or severity of these manifestations depends on the severity of the ischemia.

In addition to the disappearance of the pulse, an arterial occlusion may cause tenderness over the affected artery. This is usually proximal to the ischemic changes. The ischemic manifestations are usually most severe one joint distal to the level of obstruction. The classic example is the patient with foot ischemia with a relatively well-perfused calf secondary to an embolus to the level of the trifurcation of the popliteal artery.

Pain is the most common manifestation of an acute arterial occlusion. Characteristically, it is severe and progressive, with the most distal part of the extremity affected early. As the ischemia progresses, however, sensory deficits may ensue that may mask the pain, confusing the inexperienced clinician. The pain is slowly replaced by a feeling of numbness, which denotes progression of the ischemic progress and demands immediate attention.

Pallor is one of the initial manifestations of acute ischemia. The extremity rapidly develops a waxy appearance secondary to complete emptying and vasospasm of the arterial circulation. With progression, however, this is replaced by mottling, secondary vasodilatation, and stagnant circulation in the capillary bed. Blanching of these mottled areas with application of digital pressure denotes a retrievable capillary bed. Once the mottled areas become nonblanching, a manifestation of capillary sludging, early gangrene, is likely. This represents advanced ischemia. Without revascularization, this leads to blistering of the skin with further discoloration established; as water is lost, desiccation occurs with changes typical of dry gangrene.

Paralysis and sensory deficits are usually late manifestations of severe ischemia. Because of lack of nutrient flow, skeletal muscle and nerve dysfunction lead to decreasing ability of the patient to move the extremity. As the energy stores within the muscle decrease, inability to relax the muscles leads to rigor, a sign of far-advanced ischemia. Large sensory nerve fibers are responsible for pressure, deep pain, and temperature sensations that may be maintained until ischemia is advanced. Proprioception and light touch are usually lost early. Careful sensory examination may help the clinician estimate the severity of ischemia. Palpation of the muscle groups may denote tenderness initially, but, as the ischemia progresses, the muscles may become hard (rigor), a sign of skeletal muscle death. Even with prompt revascularization, functional impairment is likely, limb loss often occurs, and systemic effects of revascularization are a major risk. Revascularization at this late stage is likely to fail, with systemic manifestations of such an undertaking profound and sometimes lethal. This has led some authors to suggest that ischemia of this severity and duration is best treated with systemic anticoagulation, allowing demarcation of the extremity and early amputation.[59]

Physical examination of the patient with an acutely ischemic extremity is of utmost importance in planning appropriate management. Examination of the contralateral extremity may provide clues as to the preischemic status of the involved extremity. The exact location of the embolus or thrombosis may be determined by the level of clinical manifestations of the ischemic process. Pain and temperature changes are usually seen one joint below the level of obstruction. Tenderness over an arterial segment usually implies the presence of thrombus within its lumen. A pale, waxy extremity implies early ischemia. Mottling of the skin that blanches with elevation or digital pressure implies a retrievable capillary bed with prompt revascularization. Nonblanching represents advanced ischemia. Retrievability may require prompt revascularization and adjunctive measures, such as fibrinolytic therapy. Paralysis may occur early. If the muscle mass is hard, with marked resistance to passive motion (rigor), ischemia is far advanced. Appropriate planning for therapy may be guided by these findings.

Vascular Graft Occlusion

The clinical manifestations of vascular graft occlusion also vary widely and deserve special emphasis. The indication of the original intervention influences the presentation, with patients operated on for disabling claudication usually manifesting recurrent symptoms, and patients operated on for limb salvage presenting with limb-threatening ischemia. In the former group, however, when late occlusions occur, the patient may show limb-threatening ischemia. The cause of failure influences clinical presentation. When we analyzed the pattern and causes of primary failure of PTFE grafts in a series of patients operated on for claudication, when failure was due to progression of proximal or distal disease, most commonly patients presented with limb-threatening ischemia.[57] Of 14 patients initially operated on for severe claudication whose graft failed because of progression of distal occlusive disease, 12 manifested severe limb-threatening ischemia after failure of the reconstruction. Similarly, 50% of patients operated on for claudication whose graft failed due to progression of disease in the inflow arterial segment manifested limb-threatening ischemia, whereas the rest manifested recurrent claudication. Thus, although most patients operated on for limb salvage manifest limb-threatening ischemia upon failure of the reconstruction, patients with claudication manifest recurrent claudication unless significant progression of disease occurs in the inflow or outflow segments.

When the cause of failure is graft-related, which most commonly occurs with autogenous grafts, clinical manifestations are usually similar to the original presentation and indication for the reconstruction. This is particularly true within the first 12 to 18 months after reconstruction. Beyond that time, other factors, mainly progression of disease, influence the clinical presentation of the failed vascular graft.

After healing of their affected areas, a small number of patients whose initial indication for reconstruction was limb-threatening ischemia (specifically, those with tissue loss) may show failure of the reconstruction and perhaps symptoms of claudication without clinical symptoms of severe ischemia. This is evident in most series of infrainguinal reconstructions where limb salvage figures are almost universally higher than primary patency rates. Most of these patients do not require intervention because their symptoms may be managed conservatively with control of risk factors and exercise.

More recently, the concept of the failing vascular graft has been emphasized with several series documenting improved results when intervention is directed at the time when the graft is still patent. Clinical manifestations of failing grafts include diminished pulses, recurrent symptoms of claudication, or failure of areas of tissue loss in the foot to heal completely after an initial period of rapid healing. Most commonly, however, failing grafts have no clinical manifestations, and therefore it behooves the physician caring for the patient to identify these by noninvasive means. Serial ankle-arm indices have not been found sensitive enough to predictably detect the failing graft.[60] The most important mode of identification is with duplex scanning by insonating the entire graft, identifying areas of stenosis that lead to increased velocities in that segment. In addition, average velocity throughout the graft may decrease over time, again suggesting that the graft may be failing. Although cutoff points for velocities have been proposed, these have not been sensitive enough to be completely reliable. Although most grafts with velocities higher than 45 cm/second continue to have long-term patency, grafts below this cutoff point do not necessarily fail nor does a demonstrable lesion appear on arteriography. Additional duplex scan criteria to detect failing grafts have been proposed and include diameter reduction and peak and end-systolic velocities.[61-63] This is specifically evident in very distal reconstructions at the ankle, where the outflow bed may not allow for velocities in this range throughout the graft. Nevertheless, experience has shown excellent long-term results without the need for further interventions.

Perhaps a more sensitive way to monitor these grafts is to obtain velocity measurements early in the postoperative period using these values as baseline for that particular reconstruction. On follow-up, decreasing velocities would suggest further evaluation with arteriography. Identification of the failing graft is perhaps the most important factor in assuring excellent long-term results in patients with infrainguinal reconstructions.

MANAGEMENT

Initial Evaluation

Acute Arterial Occlusion

The morbidity and mortality of an acute arterial occlusion largely depend on the overall medical condition of the patient, the degree of ischemia of the extremity at presentation, and the promptness of management. All three of these aspects must be carefully evaluated and documented.

In general, prompt revascularization should be the goal after stabilization and control of coexistent medical conditions in patients showing an acute, ischemic extremity.

At clinical presentation, the majority of patients with acute arterial occlusion of an extremity have atherosclerotic heart disease, which must be addressed before any intervention. An acute myocardial infarction must be excluded by appropriate clinical and laboratory evaluation. Although its presence does not preclude surgical intervention, it mandates appropriate maneuvers, such as placement of a Swan-Ganz catheter or arterial line to minimize the morbidity and mortality associated with surgical intervention. Stabilization of hemodynamics is of primary importance, including correction of arrhythmias, replenishment of circulating volume, and establishment of an adequate urine output.

The history gives the clinician clues as to the status of the extremity before the acute arterial occlusion. Patients without a history of claudication or previous vascular reconstruction are more likely victims of embolization. Patients with a history of peripheral vascular disease, claudication, or previous vascular reconstruction are more likely affected by an arterial thrombosis. The importance of attempting to differentiate between these two processes is evident when one considers their management. Whereas patients with embolization are appropriately managed by thromboembolectomy, patients with preexisting vascular disease usually require a much more involved vascular reconstruction. Careful preoperative planning may make the difference in their outcome. Therefore, a patient with an identifiable source of an embolus, without claudication and with a normal contralateral extremity, is a classic presentation for an embolus. Patients without an identifiable source of emboli, with a history of claudication, and with physical findings specifically in the opposite limb suggestive of the presence of peripheral vascular disease are more likely suffering from an arterial thrombosis. A history of a previous embolic event is seen in up to one third of patients with an embolus, and a history of atrial fibrillation in up to 74% of these patients. In contrast, patients with an acute thrombotic occlusion have atrial fibrillation in their history in only 4% of instances.[64] Symptoms tend to be much more acute in patients with an embolic occlusion, with a fairly well-established area of demarcation. Patients with a thrombotic occlusion are likely to show less severe symptoms and a larger area of transition.

Heparinization of patients presenting with an acutely ischemic extremity is well established. In general, at least 10,000 units of intravenous heparin are recommended to establish immediate and complete anticoagulation. The goals of immediate anticoagulation are prevention of proximal and distal thrombus propagation, prevention of distal thrombosis, and prevention of venous thrombosis. In general, patients experience an almost immediate improvement in their symptoms, likely secondary to the nonanticoagulant effects of heparin. Clearly, patients with a history of heparin-induced thrombosis should be excluded from this recommendation. Patients with associated traumatic injuries or other systemic diseases that may present an unacceptable bleeding risk, who are not candidates for systemic heparinization, may receive local instillation of a dilute heparin solution in the vascular bed during operative therapy.

Once the patient has been stabilized and adequate anticoagulation accomplished, a decision regarding preoperative arteriography should be made. The desirability of arteriography is increased in patients with preexisting vascular disease or reconstruction. Arteriography should be avoided, however, if it is going to significantly delay revascularization. Alternatively, operative arteriograms can be obtained at the time of intervention. Nevertheless, if the patient can tolerate the ischemia, preoperative arteriography may be extremely helpful in elucidating the cause and planning the proper surgical approach. A patient whose history and physical examination are suggestive of an embolus may be properly handled without arteriography. If arteriography is undertaken, typically the outflow vascular bed is not well visualized and the increased time necessary for this study prolongs the ischemia without adding useful information. When the differentiation between an embolic and thrombotic event cannot be made, or in cases in which the cause is uncertain, arteriography is appropriate. A sharp cutoff with a crescent-shaped (meniscus sign) occlusion in an otherwise normal artery is suggestive of an embolus. Multiple filling defects are also suggestive of an embolic occlusion. The location of the occlusion may also be helpful, with emboli tending to lodge in areas of bifurcations (Fig. 36–3). Clot propagation, following either an embolic or thrombotic event, may make this distinction difficult.

Doppler examination of the extremity can be most helpful in determining patency of the distal outflow tract. In patients with an embolic occlusion, its presence is reassuring, because it implies an open distal tree and, therefore, a retrievable situation. In a patient with preexisting vascular disease, Doppler examination may help identify the most suitable distal bed for bypass reconstruction. Doppler examination of the venous system may disclose an otherwise unsuspected venous thrombosis.

Patients with concomitant injuries, such as fractures or dislocations, should have prompt restitution of blood volume and restoration of adequate blood pressure. Stabilization of the extremity is essential to prevent further injury and, on occasion, to restore distal circulation. Life-threatening injuries should take precedence over limb-threatening injuries. The use of temporary arterial shunts in these circumstances may help in preservation of the limb.

Vascular Graft Occlusion

Initial evaluation of a patient presenting with vascular graft occlusion is influenced by the clinical presentation. Patients showing recurrent claudication may be evaluated electively. Anticoagulation is not indicated in these patients. Intervention is indicated only in those patients whose claudication is disabling. Patients with limb-threatening ischemia, on the other hand, are best evaluated on an urgent basis, considering that some of the nonoperative means of management (including thrombolytic therapy) may be most effective within a short time after thrombosis. In most instances, the initial management is similar to that of patients with acute ischemia secondary to native vessel occlusion.

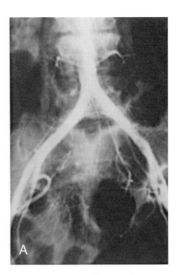

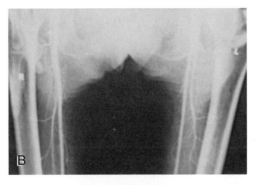

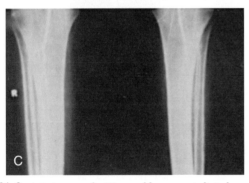

Figure 36–3. Arteriogram of a 67-year-old woman at clinical presentation with acute left lower extremity ischemia. *A,* Left iliac filling defect at the level of the bifurcation typical of an embolus. Some fragmentation has occurred, with filling defects also involving the distal external iliac and proximal common femoral. The patient had flow around this embolus to produce a normal femoral pulse. *B,* Open superficial femoral and profunda system without evidence of significant atherosclerotic disease. *C,* Evidence of distal fragmentation of the embolus with occlusion of the posterior tibial and peroneal arteries. Successful embolectomy was carried out through a combined transfemoral and infrapopliteal approach.

Patients with indications for intervention (disabling claudication or limb-threatening ischemia) due to failure of a previous vascular reconstruction are best evaluated with thorough arteriography. This study should include both inflow and outflow systems, with an attempt to establish the cause of failure. Herein lies one of the main advantages of thrombolytic therapy in the initial management of the failed infrainguinal reconstruction. Although both early and long-term results remain unclear when compared to surgi-

cal intervention, thrombolytic therapy in most instances identifies the cause of failure, allowing directed intervention.

Examination of the patient should include not only the presence or absence and quality of pulses in the involved extremity but also alternative inflow sites that may be necessary and, most important, availability of autogenous tissue for secondary reconstruction. Experience within the last 15 years suggests that patients requiring secondary bypasses after failure of an infrainguinal reconstruction are best managed with a new autogenous reconstruction. In addition to physical examination, duplex scanning of the remaining venous segments may be of benefit, if properly performed. This examination should be performed either with application of a proximal tourniquet to distend the vein, or with the patient semierect. Failure to do so usually results in an underestimate of the size and quality of available veins.

Surgical Management

In a review of 682 cases at the Massachusetts General Hospital, a trend toward increasing use of surgical management in patients with acute extremity ischemia was noted.[36] With the introduction of the Fogarty catheter in 1963, surgical intervention in patients with peripheral emboli has been greatly simplified. Nevertheless, the systemic effects of this very effective intervention must be appropriately managed to minimize mortality. In addition, the principles of embolectomy must be adhered to, avoiding common pitfalls that may lead to failure.

The surgical approach is greatly influenced by the results of the initial evaluation. Decisions regarding patients with significant peripheral vascular disease suspected of having a thrombotic occlusion are guided by the results of arteriography. In any event, wide preparation and draping are highly recommended to avoid unnecessary delays if a change in operative plan is required. The choice of anesthetics is influenced by the general condition of the patient and the planned operative procedure. By and large, femoral and brachial embolectomies can be adequately performed under local anesthesia with careful cardiac monitoring. Similarly, patients requiring femorofemoral reconstruction for a thrombotic iliac occlusion may be operated on under local anesthesia with the understanding that if a more involved procedure is required, general anesthesia may be necessary. A general anesthetic is recommended for more difficult embolectomies, such as popliteal or axillary, and in instances in which involved vascular procedures such as endarterectomy or bypass are required. Patients operated on because of a failed bypass graft frequently require a relatively involved procedure, and thus general anesthesia is preferred. If a simple thrombectomy is anticipated, local anesthesia is appropriate, provided it can be converted to general anesthesia if the need arises. Because of the general medical condition of these patients and the expected effects of reperfusion, adequate monitoring with arterial lines and Swan-Ganz catheters is recommended. These adjunctive maneuvers, however, should not delay revascularization. Regional anesthesia is usually not feasible, because these patients are most likely fully anticoagulated by the time they reach the operating room.

Embolectomy

Before 1963, an embolus to an arterial segment was usually retrieved by direct exposure, by passage of suction catheters, or with the use of rigid instruments that were very traumatic and ineffective.[65–67] With the introduction of the Fogarty catheter, the surgical technique was markedly simplified, allowing exposure remote to the level of occlusion with retrieval of the embolus by the use of the balloon catheter.

Femoral embolectomy is perhaps the most common operation done for lower extremity emboli. A vertical groin incision is made over the femoral pulse and exposure of the artery is carried out in standard fashion (Fig. 36–4). Control of the common, profunda, and superficial femoral arteries is obtained. The arteriotomy should allow visualization of the profunda and superficial femoral artery orifices. If the artery is normal to palpation, a transverse arteriotomy may be made over the profunda orifice. In diseased arteries, however, a longitudinal arteriotomy is preferable because it allows better manipulation of the catheter and, if necessary, endarterectomy or bypass. Otherwise, closure with a patch is frequently necessary to avoid narrowing of the artery (its only disadvantage).

The size of the Fogarty catheter selected should be appropriate for the artery. For the superficial femoral and popliteal arteries, a No. 4 Fogarty catheter is appropriate. For the iliac system, a No. 4 or 5 Fogarty catheter is best. For more distal insertion and for the profunda system, a No. 3 Fogarty catheter is utilized. Insertion into the profunda should not be beyond 25 cm. The catheter is gently inflated with saline as traction is maintained, avoiding overinflation, without movement of the catheter. This helps to determine when appropriate balloon inflation has been obtained, avoiding forceful traction. The catheter is handled by a single operator, because both maneuvers must be coordinated to avoid arterial injury. Inability to pass the catheter beyond the point of obstruction is usually the result of occlusive disease rather than embolus. Nevertheless, well-organized embolic material may prevent passage of the catheter, requiring more distal or direct exploration. From the femoral approach, almost 90% of distal insertions pass the catheter into the peroneal artery.[68] Several maneuvers may be helpful in orienting the catheter toward either the anterior tibial or posterior tibial artery. Bending the tip of the catheter to the appropriate side with rotation during insertion may allow cannulation of the desired artery. Use of fluoroscopy may be helpful, especially if a second small catheter is placed in the peroneal artery with the balloon gently inflated to promote passage of the catheter to the remaining vessels. More recently, endoscopy has been useful in direct visualization and cannulation of the tibial arteries. Palpation of the posterior tibial artery at the ankle or the dorsalis pedis artery in the foot during retrieval of a

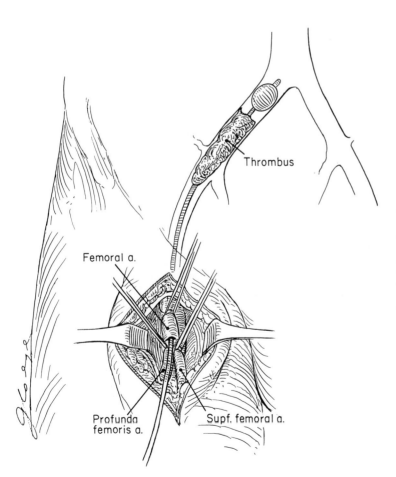

Thrombus

Femoral a.

Profunda femoris a.

Supf. femoral a.

Figure 36–4. The operative technique for femoral embolectomy. Note the control of common, superficial, and profunda femoral arteries with slings, which allow passage of the Fogarty catheter without undue blood loss from back-bleeding. The arteriotomy is placed over the profunda orifice. A transverse arteriotomy is preferred if the artery is normal and without evidence of significant atherosclerotic disease. Proximal passage of the Fogarty catheter should not be beyond the midinfrarenal aorta to avoid inadvertent cannulation of visceral vessels, overdistention of the balloon, and potential vessel injury.

distally placed catheter may help identify which vessel is being maneuvered.

The establishment of adequate inflow is usually not difficult to assess. Completeness of the distal embolectomy, however, can prove difficult to determine, because no reliable clinical guidelines are available. The presence or adequacy of back-bleeding after embolectomy is an unreliable indication of the completeness of the distal embolectomy. Operative arteriography is mandatory, unless the patient's critical condition dictates otherwise. In fact, when operative arteriograms are reviewed after embolectomy, up to 30% of cases show residual thrombi.[69] In these instances, repassage of the embolectomy catheter, more distal exploration, or infusion of intraoperative fibrinolytic agents may help in resolution of these distal thrombi.[70–77] Evaluation of the distal circulation by Doppler ultrasonography can be extremely helpful, especially in instances in which complete retrieval of all occlusive material cannot be accomplished.

Popliteal embolectomy is best carried out through an infrageniculate incision. Although a suprageniculate incision is technically easier, it offers little advantage because tibial branches are not readily accessible. Figure 36–5 illustrates the preferred approach for transpopliteal embolectomy. The goal is individual cannulation of all three tibial branches, so that distal emboli can be retrieved. Our preference is to use this approach when radiographic evidence of infrapopliteal embolism exists, or when clinical evidence exists that the embolus is distal (e.g., palpable popliteal pulse). The popliteal artery is exposed through a standard infrageniculate incision. The origin of the soleus muscle

usually requires proximal division to expose the tibial-peroneal trunk. The anterior tibial artery is exposed after careful ligation of the anterior tibial vein to allow encircling of the origin of the anterior tibial artery with vessel loops for control. Dissection beyond the tibial-peroneal trunk is rarely necessary, because digital compression of each branch allows selective cannulation of either the posterior tibial or peroneal trunks. A longitudinal arteriotomy is preferred, because it permits better visualization of the origin of the anterior tibial artery and manipulation of the catheter. In addition, if a bypass is required, extension of the arteriotomy can be performed for distal anastomosis. Otherwise, patch closure is preferred.

Evidence of persistent ischemia after popliteal embolectomy, or the presence of residual thrombus inaccessible to the thromboembolectomy catheter from this approach, is an indication for more distal exploration or, alternatively, intraoperative fibrinolytic therapy (see Chapter 41). Exploration of the tibial vessels at the ankle and foot may allow retrieval of thrombi not accessible through the transpopliteal approach.[77] A cutdown is performed over the appropriate distal vessel (posterior tibial or dorsalis pedis) and proximal and distal control is obtained with vessel loops. If the artery has no evidence of calcification or atherosclerosis, a transverse arteriotomy is preferable, because it allows easier closure with interrupted, fine monofilament vascular sutures. If the vessel is diseased, a longitudinal arteriotomy is preferred, with either patch closure or distal bypass.

Upper extremity emboli are usually approached through a cutdown in the brachial artery, just above the elbow. A

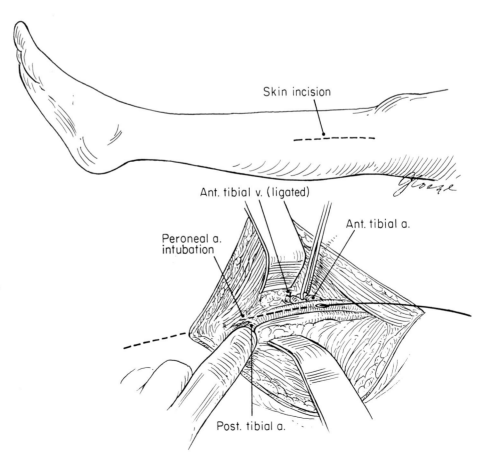

Figure 36–5. Operative technique for popliteal embolectomy. An infrageniculate incision is preferred because it allows individual cannulation of the anterior tibial, posterior tibial, and peroneal arteries. The arteriotomy is performed over the orifice of the anterior tibial artery, with selective passage into the peroneal or posterior tibial artery facilitated by digital compression of one while cannulating the other. Care must be taken during ligation of the anterior tibial vein, a critical maneuver in obtaining adequate control of the anterior tibial artery at its origin. Closure usually requires an autogenous patch to avoid narrowing.

Skin incision

Ant. tibial v. (ligated)

Ant. tibial a.

Peroneal a. intubation

Post. tibial a.

transverse arteriotomy is usually preferred, because this vessel is rarely involved with significant atherosclerotic changes. A No. 3 Fogarty catheter can be directed into the radial and ulnar artery, recognizing that reestablishing patency to one or the other is usually sufficient. Care should be taken to protect the median nerve, which runs adjacent to the artery. More proximal emboli may be approached through an infraclavicular incision similar to the one used for axillofemoral reconstructions. Preservation of branches of the axillary artery is recommended, because they serve as an important collateral pathway.

Intraoperative assessment of the adequacy of the embolectomy cannot be overemphasized. Doppler examination of the distal part of the extremity is useful but unreliable in terms of the completeness of the procedure. Intraoperative arteriography remains the best method to ensure complete removal of all embolic material. Our preference is to drape the distal extremity with a transparent sterile bag so that clinical assessment of skin perfusion can be readily made. Instillation of fluid into the bag and sterile petroleum jelly on the outside of the bag allow for Doppler examination of the various sites. The rest of the draping should reflect appropriate planning for the approach. Alternative inflow and outflow sites should be included in the operative field so that delays in revascularization are minimized.

Spasm of the runoff arteries, specifically tibial vessels in younger individuals and upper extremity vessels at all ages, is frequent after embolectomy. Intraarterial administration of papaverine or other vasodilators is recommended, although not infrequently it results in little resolution of this spastic process. This may be secondary to unrecognized residual thrombus with release of platelet vasoactive substances, specifically thromboxane. Intravenous administration of prostaglandin E_1 may be helpful, although it is of unproven value. Repeated mechanical dilatations are to be avoided because the spasm not only quickly returns but may lead to further intimal injury. If the presence of residual occlusive material can be excluded by adequate arteriography, maintaining the patient fully anticoagulated with administration of a mixture of dextran (40 mg) and papaverine (300 mg in 500 mL of saline at 50 mL/hour) is preferable to maintain patency of the circulation while the spasm spontaneously resolves. This may prove most difficult in the upper extremities in younger individuals, where very reactive distal vessels are present. Provided that no residual occlusive material is present and that flow through the vessel can be maintained with appropriate antithrombotic regimens, resolution usually occurs within the first 12 hours.

A large embolus to the aortic bifurcation (saddle embolus) can produce severe ischemia and major systemic changes upon revascularization. The transfemoral approach is still preferable, with bilateral groin incisions and simultaneous passage of No. 5 or 6 Fogarty catheters to avoid spillage of material to the contralateral side. Concomitant atherosclerotic disease may prevent reestablishment of flow to one or both sides. If adequate inflow is established to one side, a femorofemoral reconstruction may suffice to preserve both limbs. Transperitoneal exploration is indicated with failure to establish inflow on at least one side or suspicion of visceral embolization. Maintaining adequate intravascular volume is important because blood loss from

flushing is considerable and the systemic effects of reperfusion are amplified because of bilateral lower extremity involvement.

The surgeon involved in revascularization of acutely ischemic limbs must be familiar with the systemic effects of such intervention. Initiation of management of systemic effects of revascularization should be carried out in the operating room and maintained throughout the initial postoperative period. These effects are discussed in detail later in this chapter.

Bypass Graft Thrombectomy

The principles of Fogarty catheter embolectomy are applicable to thrombectomy of bypass grafts. The technique is similar, with care taken specifically in autogenous reconstructions not to overinflate the balloon, which will likely lead to intimal disruption and, occasionally, tears in a fibrotic segment of the vein graft. In this regard, vein graft thrombectomy is much more demanding than prosthetic graft thrombectomy.

Thrombectomy of the graft, with patch angioplasty of the distal anastomosis, is a well-accepted option.[78] The current trend is toward replacement of the bypass graft rather than thrombectomy.[79] Surgical thrombectomy of a prosthetic graft is a relatively simple and straightforward procedure. Proper planning, however, eliminates unnecessary delay and incisions. Our practice is to approach a failed infrainguinal prosthetic bypass at its distal anastomosis. This allows evaluation of the outflow system and identification and correction of the most common site of intimal hyperplasia. Unless a lesion away from this area has been demonstrated by preoperative evaluation, distal exploration is preferred. If a lesion limited to the first 1 or 2 cm of the distal anastomosis is identified, patch angioplasty to include the distal portion of the graft is a very reasonable alternative. If, on the other hand, the problem is distal to this site, extensions with prosthetic or autogenous graft material have had limited long-term results, with patency of 30% to 40% at 3 years.[57] In this instance, we prefer to construct an entirely new graft, preferably with autogenous tissue.

Graft thrombectomy of autogenous vein grafts is usually best for early failures or in patients in whom a hypercoagulable condition may have led to failure of the bypass. Late failures, however, are usually complicated not only by progression of the disease proximal and distal to the reconstruction but also by a fibrotic thickened graft, which is difficult to repair after graftotomy. In addition, the compliance of the graft is such that balloon embolectomy usually leads to significant intimal injury. Long-term results of saphenous vein graft thrombectomies have been notoriously poor.

Bypass Graft Revision or Replacement

Perhaps the most important element in ensuring a successful secondary reconstruction after failure of an infrainguinal bypass is identification of the cause of failure. This may allow directed intervention. Such is the case with the identification of a stenotic lesion in the midportion of a vein graft. When the lesions are short (less than 5 cm), they may be appropriately treated with balloon angioplasty. The 24-month patency rate for lesions less than 1.5 cm in vein grafts greater than 3 mm in diameter has been excellent, with a significant lower patency demonstrated in longer lesions in smaller grafts.[80] Recurrent stenosis, on the other hand, or lesions that are not suitable for balloon angioplasty are best treated with either surgical vein patch angioplasty or interposition graft replacement as the situation may dictate. If the graft is placed deep in the thigh or leg, revision requires a more extensive operative dissection. With most grafts in the subcutaneous tissue, however, surgical intervention can be both simple and effective.

Similarly, identification of residual AV fistulas may be treated with a simple incision and ligation. This may be done under local anesthesia on an outpatient basis. Presence of an incompletely lysed valve usually requires patch angioplasty with autogenous tissue. Lesions at the proximal or distal anastomosis of an otherwise good vein graft can also be treated with patch angioplasty quite effectively. As already mentioned, this is best done while the graft has maintained patency. Otherwise, when graft thrombectomy is necessary to the angioplasty, the results are significantly affected.

The surgical management of a failed infrainguinal prosthetic graft also depends on the cause of failure. Patch angioplasty may be appropriate for lesions that are limited to the first 1 to 2 cm at the proximal or distal anastomosis. Our practice is to transect the stenotic lesion and not to attempt an endarterectomy of the area, unless one is dealing with a late failure where atherosclerotic changes are present. A patch is then placed across the lesion to allow relief of the stenosis. Other alternatives include a new prosthetic bypass to a more distal site, extension of the failed bypass with prosthetic or vein graft, or a new vein graft to a more distal site. The technical aspects of these reconstructions are covered elsewhere. But it suffices to say that the results of a new bypass with autogenous saphenous vein are superior to any of the other alternatives.[57]

Fasciotomy

One of the most common manifestations of reperfusion injury after prolonged ischemia is marked swelling of skeletal muscle. Because these muscles are enveloped in fascial compartments, increased pressure within the compartment can cause poor capillary perfusion, increased venous resistance, and a vicious cycle leading to further ischemia. Normal tissue pressure within the compartment is approximately zero. As pressure within the compartment rises, tissue perfusion declines progressively and at a level of about 20 mm Hg becomes impaired. When the pressure is within 30 mm Hg of the diastolic blood pressure, flow is significantly decreased unless adequate decompression can be carried out.[81]

The decision to proceed with fasciotomy is usually based on clinical findings. Palpation of the specific compartment may reveal a very tense muscle group with tenderness. Pain on passive motion implies significant increase in tissue pressure. Numbness in the distribution of the nerves within the compartment implies nerve ischemia. The presence of

these findings indicates the need for fasciotomy. Compartmental pressure may be measured by use of a slit catheter, with commercial kits available that can be connected to pressure transducers.

Fasciotomy may be achieved in a semiclosed manner when the indication is the anticipation of increased compartmental pressures after revascularization. This is performed through a small incision in the proximal portion of the compartment, incising the fascia using either long scissors or a meniscectomy knife. For a fully established compartment syndrome, this method likely results in inadequate decompression, mainly because of difficulty in assessing the completeness of the fasciotomy. In addition, the skin may become the limiting factor, with continued elevated compartmental pressure until complete skin incision is performed. Thus, semiclosed fasciotomies should be reserved for very mild cases or as a prophylactic maneuver. Selection mainly relies on the experience of the operator.

Open fasciotomy can be limb-saving after revascularization after prolonged ischemia when muscle swelling rapidly develops. Figure 36–6 illustrates one method of achieving decompression of all four compartments through a single incision. A longitudinal incision is made over the fibula, and anterior and posterior flaps are developed. The fascia is incised to allow identification of the four specific compartments and placement of the fasciotomy incisions. The disadvantage of this approach is the creation of fairly extensive skin flaps in potentially compromised skin. In the anterior compartment, care must be taken not to injure the superficial branch of the peroneal nerve. Alternatively, medial and lateral incisions may be made that avoid the creation of skin flaps (Fig. 36–7) while achieving complete decompression. A third approach involves complete fibulectomy. Although the last achieves complete four-compartment decompression, it is fairly morbid, with injury to the peroneal artery, vein, and nerve being common complications. It also may interrupt important collateral circulation. The medial and lateral incision technique is preferred by us.

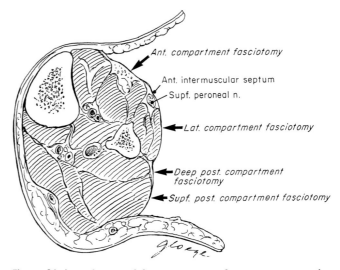

Figure 36–6. Technique of four-compartment fasciotomy via a single lateral incision. Creation of anterior and posterior flaps is necessary, which may be undesirable after revascularization for acute ischemia. Care must be taken to avoid injury to the superficial peroneal nerve, which runs just anterior to the fibula.

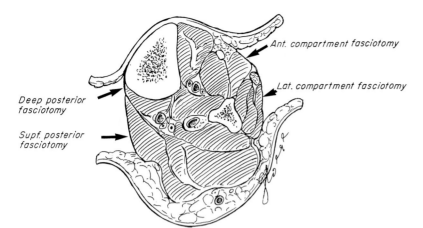

Deep posterior
fasciotomy

Supf. posterior
fasciotomy

Ant. compartment fasciotomy

Lat. compartment fasciotomy

Figure 36–7. Preferred technique for four-compartment fasciotomy of the lower extremity using a medial and a lateral incision. Note that the lateral incision is placed along the fibula to allow fasciotomy of the anterior and lateral compartments. The superficial and deep posterior compartment decompression may be facilitated by an initial transverse incision in the fascia to properly identify the compartments. Care must be taken during anterior compartment fasciotomy to avoid injury to the superficial peroneal nerve.

Most recently, foot fasciotomy has been advocated in patients with persistent foot ischemia after more proximal fasciotomy and revascularization.[82] Although it may improve foot salvage in selected cases, it is rarely necessary.

Complications after fasciotomy are usually related to wound infection. In the semiclosed method, bleeding may be a problem, mainly because these patients are thoroughly anticoagulated. Nerve injury, specifically of the superficial branch of the peroneal nerve, is a risk with this method. Maintaining the incision in the fascia close to the tibia minimizes the risk of peroneal nerve injury.

Postoperative management of open fasciotomy incisions is critical to reducing morbidity. Sterile techniques should be used for dressing changes until adequate granulation tissue has developed. As the swelling decreases, the use of Steri-Strips (3M, St. Paul, Minn.) for progressive closure of the incision usually results in almost complete closure in most cases. Skin grafting may be necessary if this cannot be accomplished. Blistering of the skin secondary to the Steri-Strip application can be minimized by alternating the site of placement.

Controversy exists as to the need for or role of fasciotomy after limb revascularization. Some authors have suggested that a significant tradeoff occurs between its usefulness and the increased risk of infection after fasciotomy.[83] The argument has been made that swelling occurring after revascularization is indicative of cell death, and thus little is gained by decompression. The majority of the reported experience, however, would support fasciotomy in selected patients. In our experience, timely fasciotomy can be limb-saving.

Delayed Embolectomy

A small but significant group of patients may experience mild to moderate symptoms after an acute arterial embolus, with gradual improvement over subsequent weeks. This is followed by either symptoms of claudication or, more important, progressive ischemia because of clot propagation. Delayed arterial embolectomy can be safely performed in these cases.[84, 85] Usually the procedure can be planned electively, with appropriate arteriographic evalua-

tion. Embolectomy is guided by arteriographic and clinical findings.

The technique is similar to acute embolectomy, recognizing that direct exposure of the occluded segment is necessary. Passage of the catheter from a remote exposure may be difficult, because the material is organized and rubbery. The surgeon must be familiar with the appearance of a thrombosed arterial segment and carefully develop a plane between the thrombus and the intima. Failure to do so may result in significant intimal injury and early rethrombosis. Heparinization in the immediate postoperative period is indicated, with chronic anticoagulation based on the clinical risk factors leading to the embolism. The thrombogenicity of the chronically embolectomized segment would dictate an aggressive use of anticoagulants. Long-term results are variable, with some patients experiencing early reocclusion due to thrombosis or marked intimal hyperplasia, or both. Intimal hyperplasia may be secondary to intimal injury from the procedure or the presence of the chronic thrombus.

Nonoperative Management

Because of the high mortality associated with revascularization of acutely ischemic limbs in most surgical series, some authors have advocated routine high-dose heparinization in patients with an acutely ischemic limb. The rationale is to select those patients with nonviable extremities, proceeding with elective planned revascularizations in those with maintained viability of the extremity after this initial treatment. Using this approach, Blaisdel and colleagues[86] found a decrease in mortality to 7.5% with limb salvage of 67% in 59 patients. Very high doses of heparin were used, with an initial bolus of 20,000 units followed by 2000 to 4000 units/hour. This report has been criticized because these results were compared with historical controls.

Controversy exists as to the appropriateness of nonoperative treatment in severely ischemic extremities. Clearly, extremities that are nonviable at the time of presentation are best treated nonoperatively. This approach is aimed at reduction in mortality. More recent series have documented an improvement in limb salvage without an increase in operative mortality with modern techniques of revascularization. Thus, considering surgical intervention in most patients is appropriate. With adequate medical support, this results in both limb and life preservation.

Thrombolytic Therapy

An attractive alternative in patients with acute limb ischemia is the use of thrombolytic therapy. This modality, however, should be reserved for patients with clearly viable extremities and should be performed in centers that are familiar with the use and complications of thrombolytic agents. In patients with prior multiple vascular reconstructions, thrombolytic therapy may facilitate recognition of the causative lesion with either percutaneous or surgical correction done in a timely fashion. When ischemia is severe, however, thrombolytic therapy, especially when carried out by inexperienced clinicians, may delay revascularization and increase tissue loss.

The technique of thrombolysis has undergone significant modifications from that described by McNamara and colleagues.[87] The thrombolytic agent is now infused through multiple side-hole catheters and allows more efficient delivery of the thrombolytic agent into a longer segment of the thrombus. The protocol that has been confirmed by multiple trials utilizes urokinase at a dose of 4000 IU/minute for 4 hours, decreasing to 2000 IU/minute until the thrombus is fully dissolved. However, urokinase has been taken off the market by the Food and Drug Administration for reasons unrelated to its efficacy, and the vascular community is attempting to learn about the efficacy and dose responses of other thrombolytics, such as tissue-type plasminogen activator (t-PA), and reteplase.

Patients Appropriate for Thrombolysis

An acute native vessel occlusion or graft occlusion can be treated initially with thrombolytic therapy. This allows restoration of flow while simultaneously providing an opportunity to discover the underlying lesion that may have precipitated the thrombosis.

There are a series of multicenter trials that have reported data that may help stratify the patients best treated with thrombolysis. The study of Surgery or Thrombolysis for the Ischemic Lower Extremity (STILE) compared two thrombolytic agents, recombinant t-PA (rt-PA) and urokinase, with primary surgery for lower extremity symptoms of less than 6 months' duration.[88] The primary end point was a composite outcome index including various factors such as, but not limited to, ongoing ischemia, death or major amputation, severe hemorrhage, or wound complications. This study was terminated prematurely by the safety committee at the first interim analysis because of poorer results in the thrombolysis groups, primarily due to a higher rate of recurrent or ongoing ischemia. Amputation or mortality was not different between groups.

The Thrombolysis or Peripheral Arterial Surgery (TOPAS) trial randomized patients with acute limb ischemia of various different etiologies to treatment with recombinant urokinase or immediate operation.[89] There were no statistically significant differences between the thrombolysis group and the surgery group with regard to the primary end point of amputation-free survival at 6 months. The authors concluded that the thrombolysis group required, on average, fewer surgical procedures than the surgical group—a conclusion that is hardly surprising given that the surgery group was randomized to an operation from entry into the trial. In an accompanying editorial, Porter[90] pointed out that the study was flawed with regard to its designated primary end points, amputation-free survival, and mortality. Thirty-two patients (12.5%) in the thrombolysis group had major bleeding, including intracranial hemorrhage in four patients, one of whom died. It must be concluded that thrombolytic therapy is not benign, does not offer any significant outcome benefits compared with surgery, and should be used selectively.

Percutaneous Thromboembolectomy

A catheter-guided system has been developed specifically for the aspiration of thrombotic material from the pulmonary vasculature.[91] Initially used for the treatment of iatrogenic emboli secondary to balloon angioplasty, this technique has now been reported in primary embolism, with a carefully selected group of patients achieving limb salvage in 40 of 42 instances. At this point, however, this procedure should be considered experimental and should be performed only by those experienced in its development.

COMPLICATIONS

Complications seen after revascularization of an acutely ischemic extremity can be divided into those related to the surgical intervention, those secondary to limb reperfusion, and those secondary to the primary cause of the event. Discussion of the last is beyond the scope of this chapter because it relates to management of the primary disease such as cardiac or peripheral vascular disease. Suffice it to say that patients with emboli originating from the heart or sources that are not surgically correctable require long-term anticoagulation to prevent further events. This particular aspect is discussed further.

Recurrent Embolization

The reported incidence of recurrent emboli after an embolic event to an extremity or viscera ranges from 6% to 45%. Prevention of recurrent emboli is of utmost importance in the management of these patients. Chronic long-term anticoagulation is indicated after an embolic event when the source of emboli cannot be surgically corrected. Anticoagulation should be started immediately after operation. In a series reported by Green and colleagues[66] only 9% of patients developed recurrent emboli when adequately anticoagulated, in contrast to 31% of those not receiving anticoagulants. This difference has been noted by others.[33, 37, 92–94] Recurrent embolization carries significantly higher morbidity and mortality than the initial event. The random distribution of emboli from the heart places these patients at risk of stroke or visceral embolization, a major cause of morbidity and mortality. Thus, chronic anticoagulation is of utmost importance in their long-term management.

Rethrombosis

After successful revascularization, recurrent limb ischemia may occur secondary to a second embolus or rethrombosis of the manipulated arterial segment. The latter is more common, because recurrent emboli to the same site are unlikely, especially when the source is the heart. Rethrombosis may occur secondary to (1) residual thrombus in the extremity not recognized at the time of the initial intervention, (2) proximal thrombus that may have been left behind, or (3) inadequate anticoagulation.

When recurrent ischemia occurs, prompt reoperation is indicated unless the patient's general condition dictates otherwise. The secondary procedure may be planned according to the clinical manifestations of the recurrent event. Reexploration of the initial operative site is indicated, with liberal use of operative arteriography or endoscopy, or both. Reoperation may be necessary in up to 21% of patients after balloon embolectomy and is usually successful in ensuring limb salvage.[95] In patients with a previously failed vascular graft, rethrombosis of the thrombectomized or revised graft usually mandates consideration for placement of a new bypass graft, preferably with autogenous tissue. The liberal use of anticoagulants (including heparin, dextran, and warfarin) in the postoperative period may benefit patients who experience this complication.

Arterial Injuries Secondary to the Balloon Catheter

Although the surgical technique for arterial embolectomy is familiar to vascular surgeons, complications of such intervention are perhaps more common than actually recognized.[96, 97] Manifestations may be delayed and appear as distal arterial occlusions secondary to intimal hyperplasia incited by aggressive embolectomy. Perforation is uncommon and usually self-limited if it occurs in a small branch of the artery. Because these patients are usually fully anticoagulated, however, they may show compartment syndromes secondary to an expanding hematoma. Alternatively, the injury may appear at a later date as a pseudoaneurysm. Perforation into an adjacent vein can occur, as illustrated in Figure 36–8. The clinical presentation can be subtle, with a decrease in palpable distal pulses or mild ischemic symptoms. Diagnosis may be established by the astute clinician with auscultation of a bruit over the fistula site. Treatment may involve direct repair, with percutaneous embolization successful in some instances.

Myonephropathic Metabolic Syndrome

One of the most dramatic and often lethal complications of revascularization of an acute severely ischemic extremity

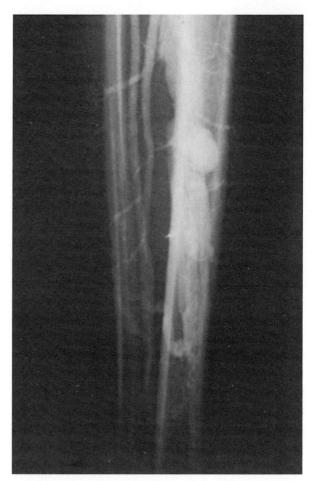

Figure 36–8. Arteriogram 6 weeks after transfemoral embolectomy showing the posterior tibial artery and vein arteriovenous fistula. The patient developed persistent swelling in the extremity with decreasing distal arterial perfusion. Careful ausculation of the calf suggested the presence of the arteriovenous fistula. The fistula was treated successfully by percutaneous embolization.

is a series of systemic processes that have been termed the "myonephropathic metabolic syndrome."[98] This is the end result of the outpouring of metabolites and cellular debris into the venous circulation after revascularization. Its severity depends on the amount of tissue involved, the degree of ischemia at revascularization, and the completeness of revascularization. Patients with clearly nonviable extremities at presentation are best treated with heparinization and early amputation to avoid this devastating syndrome. Table 36–2 summarizes drugs of potential benefit in the management of these patients.

With reestablishment of blood flow to the extremity, a general outpouring of acidic blood into the systemic circulation occurs that is capable of causing a rapid, progressive metabolic acidosis. This may lead to poor cardiac function, further acidosis, arrhythmias, and death. Judicious but aggressive use of sodium bicarbonate just before and during the initial minutes of reperfusion is advisable, with frequent evaluation of pH and arterial blood gases. If areas of the extremity remain ischemic, acidosis may persist, requiring continued monitoring and correction.

Hyperkalemia after revascularization of an acutely ischemic extremity can be dramatic and can lead to arrhythmias

TABLE 36-2

Drugs of Potential Benefit in the Medical Management of Patients with Acute Limb Ischemia

DRUG	INDICATION	CONTRAINDICATION	DOSE	EFFECT	REMARKS
Heparin	Acute limb ischemia	Heparin-induced thrombosis; contraindication to anticoagulation	5000–10,000 units IV constant infusion to maintain PTT at 1.5–2.0 × control	Potentiate antithrombin III	—
Warfarin	Reduce risk of recurrent emboli	Contraindication to anticoagulation	To maintain PTT at 1.5–2.0 × control	Decrease factors II, VII, IX, and X	—
Sodium bicarbonate	Metabolic acidosis	Lactic acidosis; metabolic alkalosis; fluid overload; hypernatremia	Guided by blood pH, ½ body weight × base deficit	Reduce H^+	Do not correct deficit with single dose; monitor pH
Mannitol	Maintenance of urine output Reperfusion	Congestive heart failure; anuria and established renal failure	12.5–25 g IV	Osmotic diuresis	Hydroxy radical scavenger
Insulin and glucose	Hyperkalemia	Diabetic ketoacidosis; hypoglycemia; hypokalemia	12.5–25 g glucose, 5–10 units insulin	Intracellular shift	—
Prostaglandin E_1	Improve renal perfusion	Severe hypotension; hypoxemia	0.005 µg/kg/min; increase q 15 min to reach 0.15–0.2 µg/kg/min	Vasodilation	Unproven value
Acetazolamide	Prevention of myoglobin precipitation in urine	Hypokalemia; severe, uncorrected acidosis	500 mg IV	Alkalization of urine; increased K^+ excretion	Not effective if $HCO_3^- <18$ mEq/L

IV, intravenous; PTT, partial thromboplastin time.

and cardiac standstill. Administration of glucose and insulin can be lifesaving by the reintroduction of potassium into cells. Hyperkalemia may be aggravated by concomitant renal failure. After this initial phase, the use of ion exchange resins, brisk diuresis, or, in some cases, hemodialysis may be necessary.

Myoglobin leakage into the venous circulation may eventually lead to renal failure by precipitation of myoglobin in the collecting tubules. This is best prevented by maintaining a brisk diuresis with the use of mannitol, adequate hydration, and general hemodynamic support. Alkalization of the urine may be achieved by the use of acetazolamide, with increased urinary excretion of potassium a secondary benefit. Myoglobinuria may continue for 24 to 48 hours after revascularization, and thus this aggressive support and maintenance of the urine output absolutely must be continued until the urine is clear. Acute renal failure may be sudden and progressive, with poor chance of recovery. Most recently, we have been impressed with the use of prostaglandin E_1 to improve renal perfusion during this acute phase. Although the experience is anecdotal, the results have been encouraging.

The effects of the venous effluent from the revascularized extremity on the pulmonary circulation can be dramatic and can lead to early respiratory failure.[86] Maintaining these patients with respiratory support, avoiding early extubation, is prudent. The chest radiograph may disclose a pattern typical of the adult respiratory distress syndrome, a sign of nonspecific pulmonary injury. The exact cause of this lung injury is not clear. Experiments carried out by Blaisdell[83] suggest a relationship between the venous effluent of the extremity and the lung injury, because experimental animals in which the venous effluent from the revascularized extremity was prevented from reaching the lungs did not show the injury. Treatment is supportive, avoiding fluid overload.

RESULTS OF THERAPY

Acute Arterial Occlusion

Since the introduction of the Fogarty catheter for the management of acute extremity ischemia, significant improvements have occurred in the morbidity and mortality of patients with this condition. Initially, improved limb salvage was noted in spite of intervention in previously untreatable ischemic limbs. In the 1960s and early 1970s, limb salvage rates averaged 50% to 60%,[6, 99–107] with further improvement noted in the decade of the 1970s, when average limb salvage rates ranged from 70% to 80%.[34, 66, 92, 108, 109] Mortality, however, remained high, averaging 20% to 30% during these two decades.

With improved recognition, surgical technique, and medical management, the decade of the 1980s saw improvement in both morbidity and mortality, with limb salvage rates routinely in the 85% to 95% range and mortality decreasing to 10% to 15%.[31–33, 93, 95, 110, 111] Clearly, aggressive and early management of recognized complications of reperfusion have had a significant impact on the overall mortality of these patients. The clinician must recognize those patients with nonviable extremities who are best treated with early amputation, leading to improved survival. The majority of patients, however, can be managed properly by timely surgical intervention, which can achieve excellent survival and limb salvage.

The presence of atherosclerotic disease negatively influences the outcome. Mortality is lower with improved limb salvage in patients with nonatherosclerotic causes of acute limb ischemia, whereas patients with atherosclerotic heart disease or severe peripheral vascular disease are at a higher risk of limb loss and death.[6, 98] The overall results are likely influenced by underlying cardiac disease and the severity of the ischemia at the time of presentation.

Advancing age in this population is likely to stall further improvement in the overall results.

Vascular Graft Occlusion

The results of treatment after occlusion of an infrainguinal reconstruction vary depending on the specific intervention carried out as secondary revascularization. By and large, the best results are obtained with a new autogenous vein graft to a more distal site. In our own series of PTFE grafts for infrainguinal bypass, comparing the alternatives for treatment of the failed reconstruction, a new bypass at the first reintervention with vein had an 88% primary patency at 30 months. This compares favorably with interventions involving extension with vein or prosthetic material, a new bypass with prosthetic material, and thrombectomy with or without patch angioplasty with patency rates at 30 months ranging from 30% to 33%. Limb salvage rates vary also with the intervention, with the best limb salvage rate obtained with a new bypass with vein at the first reoperation.

In analyzing secondary femoropopliteal reconstructions for failed autogenous infrainguinal revascularization, no correlation was found between the mode of failure and the results of secondary popliteal-tibial reconstruction. An overall 50% 5-year cumulative salvage rate was obtained, with the highest long-term patency achieved when frequent postoperative follow-up allowed recognition of graft failure before total occlusion. In the management of the failing vein graft, a simple vein patch angioplasty yielded an 85% 5-year graft patency. When thrombosis occurred, however, the highest 5-year patency rate was accomplished when reconstruction was performed using a new vein graft. When prosthetic material was used for secondary reconstruction, no graft remained patent beyond 3 years.[55]

Based on the reported experience, secondary reconstructions, even with a new autogenous vein bypass to a more distal site, clearly carry a lower patency rate than do primary reconstructions. Nevertheless, the limb salvage rate is respectable. The 5-year primary patency rate in a series reported by Edwards and colleagues[103] was 80% for primary grafts, whereas it was 57% for secondary reconstructions with autogenous tissue. Limb salvage rates for failed bypass were excellent and no different from those achieved with the initial intervention.

Prevention of recurrent graft thrombosis is the greatest challenge for vascular disease specialists managing patients after intervention. Whereas antiplatelet agents have been suggested as important in the prevention of recurrent graft thrombosis, to date no prospective randomized study has established this concept. Routinely, however, patients are maintained on aspirin after reconstructions, because some experimental evidence does suggest a decreased incidence of recurrent thrombosis. Warfarin (Coumadin) therapy with long-term anticoagulation, on the other hand, significantly reduces the incidence of graft thrombosis in patients after saphenous vein femoropopliteal bypass. This study showed a significant reduction in graft occlusions in 18% of patients treated with warfarin versus 37% among controls at a mean follow-up of 30 months.[112] The increased complication rate associated with warfarin therapy, however, suggests a selective approach in patients with infrainguinal reconstruction. Our practice has been to consider warfarin therapy in patients with no significant contraindication who have suffered a graft thrombosis and required reintervention, or in patients after prosthetic graft failure in whom no cause of thrombosis could be identified.

The overall results of secondary revascularizations after failed infrainguinal reconstructions have steadily improved. This is likely secondary to the ability to perform reconstructions to very distal arteries in the extremity, the use of thrombolytic therapy to specifically identify the cause of failure, and overall improved patient care and surgical technique.

References

1. Chervu A, Homsher E, Moore WS, et al: Differential recovery of skeletal muscle and peripheral nerve function after ischemia and reperfusion. J Surg Res 47:12, 1989.
2. Colburn MD, Quiñones-Baldrich WJ, Gelabert HA, et al: Standardization of skeletal muscle ischemic injury. J Surg Res 52:309, 1992.
3. McCord JM: Oxygen derived free radicals in post-ischemic tissue injury. N Engl J Med 312:159, 1985.
4. Saugstad OD, Schrader H, Aasen AO: Alteration of the hypoxanthine level in cerebrospinal fluid as an indicator of tissue hypoxia. Brain Res 112:118, 1976.
5. Grum CM, Ragsdale RA, Ketai LH, et al: Absence of xanthine oxidase or xanthine dehydrogenase in the rabbit myocardium. Biochem Biophys Res Commun 141:1104, 1986.
6. Eddy LJ, Stewart JR, Jones HP, et al: Free-radical producing enzyme, xanthine oxidase, is undetectable in human hearts. Am J Physiol 253:H709, 1987.
7. Granger DN, Rutuli G, McCord JM: Superoxide radicals in feline intestinal ischemia. Gastroenterology 82:9, 1982.
8. Granger DN, McCord JM, Parks DA, et al: Xanthine oxidase inhibitors attenuate ischemia-induced vascular permeability changes in the cat intestine. Gastroenterology 90:80, 1986.
9. McCord JM, Omar BA, Russell WJ: Sources of oxygen derived radicals in ischemia-reperfusion. In Hayaishi O, Niki E, Kondo M, et al (eds): Medical, Biochemical, and Chemical Aspects of Free Radicals. Amsterdam, Elsevier Science, 1989, p 1113.
10. Turrens JF, Beconi M, Barilla J, et al: Mitochondrial generation of oxygen radicals during reoxygenation of ischemic tissues. Free Radic Res 12:681, 1991.
11. McCord JM, Roy S: The pathophysiology of superoxide: Roles in inflammation and ischemia. Can J Physiol Pharmacol 60:1346, 1982.
12. Rao PS, Mueller HS: Lipid peroxidation in acute myocardial ischemia. Adv Exp Med Biol 161:347, 1983.
13. Roy S, McCord JM: Superoxide and ischemia: Conversion of xanthine dehydrogenase to xanthine oxidase. In Greenwald RG (ed): Oxy Radicals and Their Scavenger Systems. Cellular and Molecular Aspects, vol 2. New York, Elsevier Sciences, 1983, p 145.
14. Lee KR, Cronenwett JL, Shalafer M, et al: Effect of superoxide dismutase plus catalase on calcium transport in ischemic and reperfused skeletal muscle. J Surg Res 42:24, 1987.
15. Harlan JM: Neutrophil mediated vascular injury. Acta Med Scan 715(Suppl):123, 1987.
16. Simpson P, Fantone J, Mickelson J, et al: Identification of a time window for therapy to reduce experimental canine myocardial injury: Suppression of neutrophil activation during 72 hours of reperfusion. Circ Res 63:1070, 1988.
17. Rubin B, Smith A, Liauw K, et al: Skeletal muscle ischemia stimulates an immune system mediated injury. Surg Forum 40:297, 1989.
18. Del Zoppo GJ, Schmid-Schonbein GW, Mori E, et al: Polymorphonuclear leukocytes occlude capillaries following middle cerebral artery occlusion and reperfusion in baboons. Stroke 22:1276, 1986.

19. Harris AG, Skalak TC: Effects of leukocyte-capillary plugging in skeletal muscle ischemia-reperfusion injury. Am J Physiol 15:H2653, 1996.

20. Carden DL, Smith JK, Korthuis RJ: Neutrophil-mediated microvascular dysfunction in postischemic canine skeletal muscle: Role of granulocyte adherence. Circ Res 66:1436, 1990.

21. Jerome SN, Smith WC, Korthuis RJ: CD18 dependent adherence reactions play an important role in the development of the no-reflow phenomenon. Am J Physiol 264:H479, 1993.

22. Menger MD, Steiner D, Messmer K: Microvascular ischemia-reperfusion injury in striated muscle: Significance of "no reflow." Am J Physiol 263:H1892, 1992.

23. Mazzoni MC, Borgstrom P, Intaglietta M, et al: Capillary narrowing in hemorrhagic shock is rectified by hyperosmotic saline-dextran reinfusion. Circ Shock 31:407, 1990.

24. Harris AG, Steinbauer M, Leiderer R, et al: Role of leukocyte plugging and edema in skeletal muscle ischemia-reperfusion injury. Am J Physiol 273:H989, 1997.

25. Quiñones-Baldrich WJ, Chervu A, Hernandez JJ, et al: Skeletal muscle after ischemia: No reflow versus perfusion injury. J Surg Res 5:5, 1991.

26. Quiñones-Baldrich WJ: The role of fibrinolysis during reperfusion of ischemic skeletal muscle. Microcirc Endothelium Lymphatics 5:299, 1989.

27. Merril EW: Rheology of blood. Physiol Rev 49:863, 1969.

28. Perry MO, Fantini G: Ischemia: Profile of an enemy. Reperfusion injury of skeletal muscle. J Vasc Surg 6:231, 1987.

29. Belkin M, LaMorte WL, Wright JG, et al: The role of leukocytes in the pathophysiology of skeletal muscle ischemic injury. J Vasc Surg 10:14, 1989.

30. Wright JG, Fox D, Kerr JC, et al: Rate of reperfusion blood flow modulates reperfusion injury in skeletal muscle. J Surg Res 44:754, 1988.

31. Malunski T, Taha Q, Grunfeld S, et al: Diffusion of nitric oxide in the wall monitored in situ by porphyrinic microsensors. Biochem Biophys Res Commun 193:1076, 1993.

32. Malinski T, Radomski MW, Taha Z, et al: Direct electrochemical measurement of nitric oxide released from human platelets. Biochem Biophys Res Commun 194:960, 1993.

33. Huk I, Nanobashvili J, Neumayer C, et al: L-Arginine treatment alters the kinetics of nitric oxide and superoxide release and reduces ischemia/reperfusion in skeletal muscle. Circulation 96:667, 1997.

34. Kishi M, Tanaka H, Setyama A, et al: Pentoxifylline attenuates reperfusion injury in skeletal muscle after partial ischemia. Am J Physiol 274:H1435, 1998.

35. Haimovici H: Muscular, renal, and metabolic complications of acute arterial occlusions: Myonephropathic-metabolic syndrome. Surgery 85:461, 1979.

36. Abbott WM, Maloney RD, McCabe CC, et al: Arterial embolism: A 44 year perspective. Am J Surg 143:460, 1982.

37. Elliott JP Jr, Hageman JH, Szilagyi DE, et al: Arterial embolization: Problems of source, multiplicity, recurrence, and delayed treatment. Surgery 99:833, 1980.

38. Ouriel K, Veith FJ, Sasahara AA: A comparison of recombinant urokinase with vascular surgery as initial treatment for acute arterial occlusion of the legs. N Engl J Med 338:1105, 1998.

39. Sheiner NM, Zeltzer J, MacIntosh E: Arterial embolectomy in the modern era. Can J Surg 25:373, 1982.

40. Hellerstein HK, Martin JW: Incidence of thromboembolic lesions accompanying myocardial infarction. Am Heart J 33:443, 1947.

41. Harris RW, Andros G, Dulawa LB, et al: Malignant melanoma embolus as a cause of acute aortic occlusion: Report of a case. J Vasc Surg 3:550, 1986.

42. Kempzinski RF: Lower extremity arterial emboli from ulcerating atherosclerotic plaques. JAMA 241:807, 1979.

43. Zarins CK, Weisenberg E, Kolettis G, et al: Differential enlargement of artery segments in response to enlarging atherosclerotic plaques. J Vasc Surg 7:386, 1988.

44. Fernandez-Ortiz A, Badimon JJ, Falk E, et al: Characterization of the relative thrombogenicity of atherosclerotic plaque components: Implications for consequences of plaque rupture. J Am Coll Cardiol 23:1562, 1994.

45. Becker PS, Miller VT: Heparin induced thrombocytopenia. Stroke 20:1449–1459, 1989.

46. Laster J, Cikrit D, Walker N, Silver D: The heparin induced thrombocytopenia syndrome: An update. Surgery 102:763, 1987.

47. Bick RL: Alterations of hemostasis associated with malignancies. Semin Thromb Hemost 5:1, 1978.

48. Levine MN, Gent M, Hirsh J, et al: The thrombogenic effect of anti-cancer drug therapy in women with stage II breast cancer. N Engl J Med 318:404, 1988.

49. Symbas PN, Harlaftis N: Bullet emboli in the pulmonary and systemic arteries. Ann Surg 185:318, 1977.

50. Weaver FA, Schwartz MR, Yellin AE, Bauer M: Refining the indications for arteriography in penetrating extremity trauma: A prospective analysis [abstract]. Presented at the 46th Annual Meeting of the Society for Vascular Surgery, Chicago, June 8, 1992.

51. Quiñones-Baldrich WJ, Gelabert HA: Autogenous tissue reconstruction in the management of aortoiliofemoral graft infection. Ann Vasc Surg 4:223, 1990.

52. Panetta TF, Marin ML, Veith FJ, et al: Unsuspected preexisting saphenous vein disease: An unrecognized cause of vein bypass failure. J Vasc Surg 15:102, 1992.

53. Gilbertson JJ, Walsh DB, Zwolak RM, et al: A blinded comparison of angiography, angioscopy, and duplex scanning in the intraoperative evaluation of in situ saphenous vein bypass grafts. J Vasc Surg 15:121, 1992.

54. Donaldson MC, Mannick JA, Whittemore AD: Causes of primary graft failure after in situ saphenous vein bypass grafting. J Vasc Surg 15:113, 1992.

55. Barboriak JJ, Pintar K, VanHorn DL, et al: Pathologic findings in the aortocoronary vein grafts. Atherosclerosis 29:69, 1978.

56. Matsubara J, Nagasue M, Tsuchishima S, et al: Clinical results of femoropopliteal bypass using externally supported (EXS) Dacron grafts: With a comparison of above- and below-knee anastomosis. J Cardiovasc Surg (Torino) 31:731, 1990.

57. Quiñones-Baldrich WJ, Prego A, Ucelay-Gomez R, et al: Failure of PTFE infrainguinal revascularization: Patterns, management alternatives, and outcome. Ann Vasc Surg 5:163, 1991.

58. Quiñones-Baldrich WJ, Busuttil RW, Baker JD, et al: Is the preferential use of PTFE grafts for femoral-popliteal bypass justified? J Vasc Surg 8:219, 1988.

59. Blaisdell FW, Steele M, Allen RE: Management of acute lower extremity arterial ischemia due to embolism and thrombosis. Surgery 84:822, 1978.

60. Barnes RW, Thompson BW, MacDonald CM, et al: Serial noninvasive studies do not herald postoperative failure of femoropopliteal or femorotibial bypass grafts. Ann Surg 210:486, 1989.

61. Bandyk DF, Cato RF, Towne JB: A low flow velocity predicts failure of femoropopliteal and femorotibial bypass grafts. Surgery 98:799, 1985.

62. Sladen JG, Reid JDS, Cooperberg PL, et al: Color flow duplex screening of infrainguinal grafts combining low- and high-velocity criteria. Am J Surg 158:107, 1989.

63. Buth J, Disselhoff B, Sommeling C, Stam L: Color-flow duplex criteria for grading stenosis in infrainguinal vein grafts. J Vasc Surg 14:716, 1991.

64. Cambria RP, Abbott WM: Acute arterial thrombosis of the lower extremity. Arch Surg 119:784, 1984.

65. Dale WA: Endovascular suction catheters. J Thorac Cardiovasc Surg 44:557, 1962.

66. Green RM, De Weese JA, Rob CG: Arterial embolectomy before and after the Fogarty catheter. Surgery 77:24, 1975.

67. Lerman J, Miller FR, Lund CC: Arterial embolism and embolectomy. JAMA 94:1128, 1930.

68. Short D, Vaughn GD III, Jachimczyk J, et al: The anatomic basis for the occasional failure of transfemoral balloon catheter thromboembolectomy. Ann Surg 190:555, 1979.

69. Plecha FR, Pories WJ: Intraoperative angiography in the immediate assessment of arterial reconstruction. Arch Surg 105:802, 1972.

70. Cohen LH, Kaplan M, Bernhard VM: Intraoperative streptokinase: An adjunct to mechanical thrombectomy in the management of acute ischemia. Arch Surg 121:708, 1986.

71. Comerota AJ, White JV, Grosh JD: Intraoperative intraarterial thrombolytic therapy for salvage of limbs in patients with distal arterial thrombosis. Surg Gynecol Obstet 169:283, 1989.

72. Greep JM, Aleman PJ, Jarrett F, Bast TJ: A combined technique for peripheral arterial embolectomy. Arch Surg 105:869, 1972.

73. Gupta SK, Samson RH, Veith FJ: Embolectomy of the distal part of the popliteal artery. Surg Gynecol Obstet 153:254, 1981.

74. Norem RS, Short DH, Kerstein MD: Role of intraopertive fibrino-

lytic therapy in acute arterial occlusion. Surg Gynecol Obstet 167:87, 1988.

75. Parent FN III, Bernhard VM, Pabst TS III, et al: Fibrinolytic treatment of residual thrombus after catheter embolectomy for severe lower limb ischemia. J Vasc Surg 9:153, 1989.

76. Quiñones-Baldrich WJ, Baker JD, Busuttil RW, et al: Intraoperative infusion of lytic drugs for thrombotic complications of revascularization. J Vasc Surg 10:408, 1989.

77. Youkey JR, Clagett GP, Cabellon S, et al: Thromboembolectomy of arteries explored at the ankle. Ann Surg 199:367, 1984.

78. Veith FJ, Gupta S, Daly V: Management of early and late thrombosis of expanded polytetrafluoroethylene (PTFE) femoropopliteal bypass grafts: Favorable prognosis with appropriate reoperation. Surgery 87:581, 1980.

79. Edwards JE, Taylor LM Jr, Porter JM: Treatment of failed lower extremity bypass grafts with new autogenous vein bypass grafting. J Vasc Surg 11:136, 1990.

80. Sanchez LA, Gupta SK, Veith FJ, et al: A ten-year experience with one hundred fifty failing or threatened vein and polytetrafluoroethylene arterial bypass grafts. J Vasc Surg 14:729, 1991.

81. Whitesides TE, Haney TC, Harada H, et al: A simple method for tissue pressure determination. Arch Surg 110:1311, 1975.

82. Ascer E, Strauch B, Calligaro KD, et al: Ankle and foot fasciotomy: An adjunctive technique to optimize limb salvage after revascularization for acute ischemia. J Vasc Surg 9:594, 1989.

83. Blaisdell FW: Is there a reason for controversy regarding fasciotomy? J Vasc Surg 9:828, 1989.

84. Jarrett F, Dacumos GC, Crummy AB, et al: Late appearance of arterial emboli: Diagnosis and management. Surgery 86:898, 1979.

85. Levin BH, Giordano JM: Delayed arterial embolectomy. Surg Gynecol Obstet 155:549, 1982.

86. Blaisdell FW, Lim RC, Amberg JR, et al: Pulmonary microembolism: A cause of morbidity and death after major vascular surgery. Arch Surg 93:776, 1966.

87. McNamara TO, Bomberger RA, Merchant RF: Intraarterial urokinase therapy for acutely ischemic limbs. Presented at the Fourth Annual Meeting of the Western Vascular Society, Kauai, Hawaii, Jan 18, 1989.

88. Weaver FA, Comerota AJ, Youngblood M, et al: Surgical revascularization versus thrombolysis for nonembolic lower extremity native artery occlusions: Results of a prospective randomized trial. The STILE Investigators: Surgery versus Thrombolysis for Ischemia of the Lower Extremity. J Vasc Surg 24:513, 1996.

89. Oureil K, Veith FJ, Sasahara AA: A comparison of recombinant urokinase with vascular surgery as initial treatment for acute arterial occlusion of the legs. N Engl J Med 338:1105, 1998.

90. Porter JM: Thrombolysis for acute arterial occlusion of the legs [editorial]. N Engl J Med 338:1148, 1998.

91. Greenfield LJ, Kimmell GO, McCurdy WC III: Transvenous removal of pulmonary emboli by vacuum-cup catheter technique. J Surg Res 9:347, 1969.

92. Hight DW, Tilney NL, Couch NP: Changing clinical trends in patients with peripheral arterial emboli. Surgery 79:172, 1976.

93. Silvers LW, Royster TS, Mulcare RJ: Peripheral arterial emboli and factors in their recurrence rate. Ann Surg 192:232, 1980.

94. Tawes RL Jr, Beare JP, Scribner RG, Sydorak GR, Brown WH, Harris EJ: Value of postoperative heparin therapy in peripheral arterial thromboembolism. Am J Surg 146:213, 1983.

95. Tawes RL Jr, Harris EJ, Brown WH, et al: Arterial thromboembolism: A 20-year perspective. Arch Surg 120:595, 1985.

96. Dainko EA: Complications of the use of the Fogarty balloon catheter. Arch Surg 105:79, 1972.

97. Dobrin PB: Mechanisms and prevention of arterial injuries caused by balloon embolection. Surgery 106:457, 1989.

98. Haimovici H, Moss CM, Veith FJ: Arterial embolectomy revisited. Surgery 78:409, 1975.

99. Barker CF, Rosato FE, Roberts B: Peripheral arterial embolism. Surg Gynecol Obstet 123:22, 1966.

100. Billig DM, Hallman GI, Cooley DA: Arterial embolism: Surgical treatment and results. Arch Surg 95:1, 1967.

101. Buxton B, Morris P: Arterial embolism of the lower limbs: Experience with the use of the Fogarty embolectomy balloon catheter. Aust N Z J Surg 39:179, 1969.

102. Cranley JJ, Krause RJ, Strasser ES, et al: Peripheral arterial embolism: Changing concepts. Surgery 55:57,63, 1964.

103. Edwards EA, Tilney NL, Lindquist RR: Causes of peripheral embolism and their significance. JAMA 196:133, 1966.

104. Fogarty TJ, Cranley JJ: Catheter technique for arterial embolectomy. Ann Surg 161:325, 1965.

105. Karageorgis BP: Experience with the catheter technique in arterial embolectomy. J Cardiovasc Surg (Torino) 8:375, 1967.

106. McMahon JW, Sako Y: Arterial embolism and embolectomy. Geriatrics 23:132, 1968.

107. Tarnay TJ: Arterial embolism of the extremities: Experience with 62 patients. Arch Surg 99:615, 1969.

108. Satiani B, Gross WS, Evans WE: Improved limb salvage after arterial embolectomy. Ann Surg 188:153, 1978.

109. Thompson JE, Sigler L, Raut PS, et al: Arterial embolectomy: A 20-year experience. Surgery 67:212, 1970.

110. Dale WA: Differential management of acute peripheral arterial ischemia. J Vasc Surg 1:269, 1984.

111. Kendrick J, Thompson BW, Read RC, et al: Arterial embolectomy in the leg: Results in a referral hospital. Am J Surg 142:739, 1981.

112. Kretschmer G, Wenzl E, Piza F, et al: The influence of anticoagulant treatment on the probability of function in femoropopliteal vein bypass surgery: Analysis of a clinical series (1970 to 1985) and interim evaluation of a controlled clinical trial. Surgery 102:453, 1987.

37

Myointimal Hyperplasia

Wesley S. Moore and Michael M. Farooq

The development of strategies designed to suppress myointimal hyperplasia after peripheral vascular interventions has become increasingly important with the current enthusiasm for less invasive but more locally injurious percutaneous therapies. More durable prosthetic vascular reconstructive procedures also succumb to this healing response, most prominently at the points of surgical anastomosis. Autogenous vein bypass serves as the primary means of limb salvage for patients with tibial occlusive changes and limb-threatening ischemia but ultimately develops a form of myointimal hyperplasia arising in concert with the vein graft "arterialization" process. The long-term patency of vein bypass grafts is ultimately limited by progressive stenosis along the length of the graft and at anastomoses due to this inexorable process of myointimal hyperplasia.[1–3] Among the medical advances made to increase patient longevity, peripheral vascular interventions may remain temporary and palliative rather than durable and potentially curative, unless advances in the treatment of myointimal hyperplasia achieve important milestones toward its suppression.

Intimal thickening is formed by the migration of smooth muscle cells from the medial to the intimal layer of the vessel wall after an endothelial injury. Subsequent proliferation of these cells and the ensuing deposition of extracellular matrix material produce thickening of the intimal layer, luminal narrowing, and eventual thrombosis of the affected vessel. This hyperplastic intimal response is a characteristic fibromuscular cellular response of the vascular system to injury and is a normal feature of vascular healing. However, in some instances, progression of this process ultimately leads to graft failure, and it is therefore not an insignificant clinical problem. In fact, intimal hyperplasia is the most common cause of failures occurring between 2 and 3 years postoperatively. In one series, 50% of late failures identified in 5000 arterial reconstructions, including both endarterectomy and bypass operations, were due to this exuberant hyperplastic intimal process.[1]

Early graft failures related to technical errors can often be corrected and should ultimately be preventable with continued technologic improvements and appropriate training. Likewise, late graft failures are generally related to the nature of the systemic atherosclerotic process and factors external to the bypass graft. Therefore, an increasingly large portion of modern basic science vascular research has been focused on the problem of graft failure related to intimal hyperplasia. The poor long-term success rates of many vascular procedures can be accounted for, in large part, by the process of intimal hyperplasia. Appreciating how this process represents a substantial cause of morbidity in patients undergoing operations on the vascular system and why investigations into methods to prevent or reverse this process are of great importance is therefore not difficult.

Increased interest and laboratory effort have been focused on the area of pharmacologic therapy for hyperplastic intimal lesions. The ability of various agents to alter the growth and characteristics of intimal hyperplastic lesions has been studied by many investigators. Clearly, if effective therapy to suppress the growth of intimal hyperplasia and prevent the associated recurrent arterial stenoses could be developed, this would have a major impact on the durability of vascular procedures and would lower their associated morbidity, mortality, and cost. Also, in addition to suppressing the development of intimal hyperplasia, research in this area may identify agents capable of reversing established hyperplastic lesions. The development of alternative pharmacologic therapy for the patient with a failing previous vascular procedure would represent a significant advance in the management of this highly morbid and potentially lethal complication of peripheral vascular surgery.

In this chapter, we summarize the current concepts regarding the pathology, pathophysiology, clinical manifestations, and current management of hyperplastic intimal lesions. In addition, we use the molecular pathways that are important in the formation of intimal hyperplasia as a framework for rationalizing and surveying the current pharmacologic approaches to inhibiting this lesion. Finally, we speculate on possible future directions for research in this area.

PATHOLOGY

Intimal hyperplasia can be described as the abnormal continued proliferation of cells and connective tissue elements that occurs at sites of endothelial injury. During the first

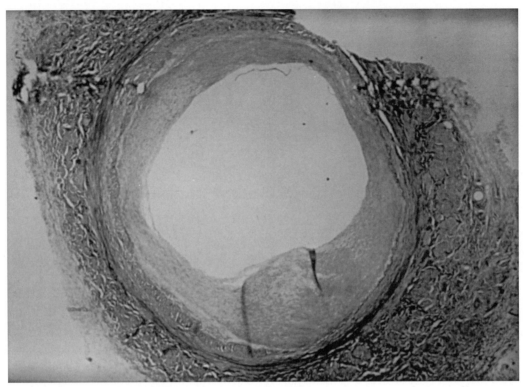

Figure 37–1. Photomicrograph of a failed infrainguinal autogenous vein bypass graft showing a large amount of hyperplastic intimal proliferation. (Verhoeff-van Gieson stain; original magnification ×20.)

decade of the 20th century, investigators noted that "within a few days after the operation, the stitches placed in making the anastomosis became covered with a glistening substance similar in appearance to the normal endothelium."[4] This early description of arterial healing probably represents the normal response of an artery to injury. Intimal hyperplasia, alternatively, is more likely to be the result of the inability to control, or the continued stimulation of, this normal regenerative process. Grossly, when operations are repeated for stenosis or graft failure, a pale, firm, homogeneous lesion is uniformly encountered. The area is smooth, shiny, and appears subendothelial. Some have suggested that, in fact, a true new intima does not form on the surface of the injured lumen. Rather, these investigators prefer the term *myointimal hyperplasia*, highlighting the origin of the proliferating tissue as the medial smooth muscle cell. Histologic examination of the lesion shows features consisting of many stellate cells surrounded by a clear fibromyxomatous-appearing stroma and connective tissue. The morphologic (external lamina, dense bodies, and myofilaments), immunocytologic (positive staining for smooth muscle cell–specific actin chains), and histochemical (positive staining for sulfated glycosaminoglycans) characteristics of these stellate cells have identified them as smooth muscle cells.[5, 6] These cells probably, but not definitely, originate in the media as differentiated smooth muscle cells. In response to injury, these smooth muscle cells undergo a series of distinct changes, the earliest of which is replication. This is followed by migration from the media across the internal elastic lamina into the intima. Once in the intima, they proliferate and, ultimately, synthesize and secrete extracellular matrix.[7] This cellular proliferation, as

well as the deposition of connective tissue elements, forms the basis of the observed intimal changes in the lumen of a traumatized vessel (Fig. 37–1).

Because the cellular component of intimal hyperplasia is derived from smooth muscle cells, an understanding of the normal physiology of these cells and their role in the healing response of a vascular wound is crucial to our understanding of intimal hyperplasia. The normal arterial wall consists primarily of three layers: intima, media, and adventitia. Normally, smooth muscle cells are located within the media along with a connective tissue mixture of collagen, elastin, and, possibly, some fibroblasts. The smooth muscle cells are responsible for maintaining the configuration and tone of the vascular wall. The intima is generally considered to consist of a single layer of endothelial cells on the luminal surface as well as a thin basal lamina. One striking characteristic of the normal, healthy vessel wall is the slow growth rate of both the intimal endothelial cells and their underlying medial smooth muscle cells. Damage to the vascular endothelium somehow triggers a complex series of events by which these cells undergo a transformation from this resting state to one of great activity. This leads to the migration of smooth muscle cells into the intima and, ultimately, to intimal hyperplasia.

PATHOPHYSIOLOGY

The precise pathophysiologic pathways leading to the development of intimal hyperplasia have not been characterized. The initiating event is thought to be damage to the vascular endothelium. Subsequent exposure of the subendothelial arterial wall elements triggers the activation of a myriad of cellular and enzymatic events that ultimately lead to the migration and proliferation of medial smooth muscle cells.[7] The response of the medial smooth muscle cell to vascular injury can be divided into four distinct stages: (1) an initial medial proliferative response, (2) migration from the media across the external elastic lamina and into the intima, (3) subsequent proliferation within the neointima, and (4) synthesis and deposition of extracellular matrix. The end result of this complex process is intraluminal thickening and reduction of the luminal diameter. Traditionally, several theories have attempted to characterize the precise mechanisms responsible for controlling each of these four stages. Among those most often cited have been hemodynamic factors such as turbulence and compliance mismatch, as well as complex interactions between endothelial and smooth muscle cells and circulating factors such as platelets and components of the inflammatory system.[8] More recently, a much more complex view has emerged that involves the synergistic action of several biologic pathways. The remainder of this section reviews, separately, the experimental basis for the hypothesized involvement of each of these systems.

Hemodynamic Factors

A wide variety of hemodynamic factors, including high- and low-flow velocities,[9] high and low wall shear stress,[10] and mechanical compliance mismatch,[11] have been implicated in the formation of intimal hyperplasia. The common pathway shared by all of these forces is likely to be the resulting damage to the endothelial cell layer.

The effects of flow velocity on the subsequent development of intimal hyperplasia have been studied in a variety of models. In a high-flow renal artery-to-vena caval anastomosis, significant intimal thickening was documented by electron microscopic examination 3 months after formation.[12] Similar intimal lesions have also been noted in arteriovenous fistulas constructed for hemodialysis access.[13] However, in a canine carotid vein interposition model, segments with low-flow velocities developed significantly thicker intimal layers.[14] Furthermore, others have found that 6 months after construction of an arteriovenous fistula in monkey iliac vessels, no increase in intimal thickening occurred on the experimental side.[15] In this study, although flow rate and velocity were increased markedly on the side of the arteriovenous fistula, the calculated wall shear stress was equal on both sides. This equality of shear stress, despite a significant difference in flow velocities, was the result of a twofold increase in diameter of the vessel lumen. This finding has been confirmed by data from other researchers. Together, these findings support the concept that flow velocity may not be a major determinant of intimal hyperplasia. Rather, tangential or wall shear stress may be the essential hemodynamic factor leading to the development of this lesion.

In an ideal tube, the flow pattern is defined as being laminar or having a parabolic wave profile. The layer of fluid adjacent to the wall is known as the boundary layer and is usually a region of low shear stress. In the human arterial tree, blood flow tends to be turbulent with sudden changes in geometric configuration. This creates areas with complex flow patterns involving the cessation or reversal of flow in the boundary layer. The flow separation that occurs in these areas leads to the generation of shear stress forces. Confusingly, some have postulated that both high and low wall shear stress may contribute, adversely, to the development of intimal hyperplasia. Probably, however, the mechanism by which each end of the shear stress spectrum stimulates this response is very different. Regions of low wall shear stress may increase intimal proliferation, possibly by increasing the time for lipid transport.[9, 14] The results of postmortem studies have shown that early atherosclerotic lesions occurred more commonly in areas of low wall shear stress.[16] Conversely, areas with extremely high shear stress cause endothelial injury, and this may lead to development of intimal lesions.[17]

A model incorporating the effects of both high and low wall shear stress has been suggested.[18] In a model of the human carotid artery bifurcation, dye injected into the central high-velocity flow lines of the common carotid segment is noted to strike the vessel wall near the bifurcation (a high shear stress region) and then, with loss of momentum, to traverse circumferentially along the carotid sinus wall to enter the adjacent boundary layer area. This is a low shear stress area and corresponds to the region across from the external carotid origin, where most atherosclerotic plaques occur. Some have hypothesized that platelet activation from intimal damage may occur in the region of high shear stress and that these same activated platelets may then enter the area of boundary layer separation and cause further intimal damage by virtue of the increased exposure time afforded by the low shear stress forces. This hypothesis is strongly supported by the spectral analysis of pulsed Doppler velocity waveforms in carotid artery bifurcations of young healthy individuals. These studies demonstrate similar zones of flow separation.[19]

Compliance mismatch is also reported as an important hemodynamic factor in the production of anastomotic intimal hyperplasia. Compliance is defined as the percentage of radial change per unit pressure and is a useful index of vessel wall distensibility to a pressure force. Although experimental and clinical studies have shown that grafts with compliance values approaching the native artery have increased patency, in none of these studies did the design control for differences in graft surfaces. An intriguing experiment was reported, which attempted to control for the vessels' flow surfaces.[20] In this study, autografts were made from one carotid artery, and after preparation, bilateral femoropopliteal grafts were constructed. The compliant graft was infused with 0.025% glutaraldehyde and externally bathed with saline solution for 30 minutes. The stiff graft was infused with a similar concentration of glutaraldehyde but was bathed in 10% glutaraldehyde for 60 minutes. At explant, only 43% of stiff grafts were patent compared with 86% of compliant grafts. Although these results did demonstrate increased patency with more compliant grafts, no effect on intimal hyperplasia was demonstrated. The authors concluded that the role of compliance mismatch in the development of intimal hyperplasia is questionable.[20] The compliance of a vein graft at the time of implantation is similar to that of a native artery, and, according to the results of one study, the compliance values remain within the normal range for a median follow-up of 33 months.[21] Textile and fabric prostheses, on the other hand, are relatively noncompliant. Furthermore, 4 months after implantation, a significant loss of compliance is noted in both polyester fabric and polytetrafluoroethylene (PTFE) grafts.[22] For this reason, some authors have suggested imposing a short cuff of autogenous vein between native artery and prosthetic grafts.[23]

When taken together, operative manipulation and hemodynamic factors may contribute, in part, to the development of intimal hyperplasia. Clinically, overaggressive dissection while harvesting vein grafts may lead to injury of the vasa vasorum and disruption of the endothelial layer.[24] Mechanical distention of a vein segment above 200 mm Hg leads to endothelial cellular damage.[25] However, these factors are probably only facilitative, and numerous other contributing elements are necessary for the development of the full hyperplastic response of a vessel wall to injury.

Alterations in Lipid Metabolism

Histologic examination of hyerplastic intimal lesions reveals an architecture that is strikingly similar to that seen in specimens of atherosclerosis. Both contain abundant lipid and connective tissue elements as well as proliferating smooth muscle cells. This observation has led to the hypothesis that intimal hyperplasia may, in fact, be a variant form of atherosclerosis. In this theory, atherosclerosis and intimal hyperplasia share a common pathophysiologic pathway but differ in the kinetics of lesion formation.

Atherosclerotic plaques are a diverse group of lesions that differ in composition depending on their age and anatomic location and the physiologic status of the individual in whom they form. The lesions consist of a matrix of connective tissue proteins in which smooth muscle cells and varying amounts of extracellular lipid are embedded. Early lesions are called fatty streaks and consist primarily of lipid-saturated cells and cholesterol deposits. Fibrous plaques are more advanced lesions characterized by a necrotic lipid core surrounded by proliferating smooth muscle cells and a connective tissue matrix. Ultimately, the variant of atherosclerosis that is expressed by each person is determined by the relative proportions of these components.

Atherosclerosis forms over decades and appears somehow connected to the slow accumulation of lipids. The association of atherogenesis and high levels of plasma low-density lipoprotein (LDL) has long been recognized. Population studies measuring the plasma concentration of LDL among Alaskan Natives have shown much lower levels in this group compared with age-matched Danes.[26] This difference may be related to the very low incidence of atherosclerotic heart disease in the Alaskan Native population. Lipids are essential components of all cells, and they are involved in a number of cellular structures (particularly membranes) and functions. Furthermore, they play an important carrier function: delivering cholesterol for cellular use. Normally, the vascular smooth muscle cell regulates the accumulation of lipid and cholesterol at the level of a surface membrane high-affinity LDL receptor.[27, 28] These receptors bind LDL and internalize the bound compounds by endocytosis. The lipids are incorporated by the cellular membranes and the cholesterol is transported to the liposomes, where it is degraded and processed for use by the cell. In atherosclerosis, many years of oversaturation with high concentrations of plasma LDL may lead to increased storage of intracellular cholesterol esters and the development of foam cells. Later, necrosis of these cells, liberation of their lipid contents, and, finally, calcification may lead to the necrotic, lipid-rich extracellular debris of mature atherosclerosis. Intimal hyperplasia, on the other hand, is characterized by a higher proportion of smooth muscle cell proliferation and less lipid-laden necrosis. This may be the result of a sudden loss of endothelial integrity, immediately exposing the underlying smooth muscle cells to large amounts of plasma-bound LDL. The smooth muscle cells respond by both upregulating production of LDL receptors and initiating cellular replication. LDL is a potent smooth muscle cell mitogen.[29] Thus, in this theory, both intimal hyperplasia and atherogenesis are related to alterations in lipid metabolism. However, the rapid kinetics of intimal hyperplasia formation leads to a predominantly cellular lesion with moderate amounts of extracellular matrix, whereas atherosclerosis develops slowly over many decades, leading to necrotic, lipid-laden lesions with a relatively sparse cellular component.

Platelets

Platelets have long been known to play a central role in the reaction of a vessel wall to injury. To date, most research in this area has focused on the activation of platelets by the injured endothelium as the major factor in the development of intimal hyperplasia. Denudation of the arterial wall exposes the subendothelial matrix, which leads to adherence of platelets. This adherence requires the interaction of subendothelial collagen, a platelet membrane glycoprotein receptor (GPIb), plasma von Willebrand's factor, and fibronectin. After adherence, platelets undergo a morphologic change, stretch to cover the exposed surface, and release a variety of stored granule products. Classically, these secreted products have been discussed and categorized according to the three types of granules in which they are stored: lysosomes, alpha granules, and dense granules. Lysosomes contain a large variety of hydrolases and other enzymes. Alpha granules contain the adhesive glycoprotein molecules, coagulation factors, and important cellular mitogens such as platelet factor 4 and platelet-derived growth factor (PDGF). Dense granules are primarily composed of adenosine triphosphate (ATP), adenosine diphosphate (ADP), serotonin, and calcium. Alternatively, when describing platelet interaction with an injured vessel wall, organizing the discussion of these activated platelet products by grouping those that act to promote platelet aggregation and those that are primarily involved in smooth muscle cell activation is helpful.

Activated platelets subsequently release ADP and activate the arachidonic acid pathway to release thromboxane A_2 (TxA_2). Both of these factors lead to platelet aggregation. Recruitment of platelets requires the rapid expression of the platelet membrane receptor complexes GPIIb and GPIIIa, both of which promote platelet aggregation through the binding of circulating fibrinogen. Platelet adhesion and granule release also lead to a parallel acceleration of the coagulation cascades. This activation of clotting pathways, combined with high local concentrations of fibrinogen mediated by binding to the GPIIb/IIIa complex, creates a fibrin protein network that further stabilizes the aggregated platelet plug. Once platelet aggregation is initiated by the pathways mentioned earlier, its further formation is actively inhibited by an intact endothelium. Thus a damaged endothelium not only initiates platelet activation but also impairs its inhibition.

With activation of platelets, secretion of PDGF occurs along with that of other granule constituents, including platelet factor 4, thromboglobulin, and thrombospondin. PDGF is a cationic protein with a molecular weight of 28,000 Da to 31,000 Da. It comprises two subunits (α and β). Physiologically, PDGF functions as both a chemoattractant and a mitogen for smooth muscle cells and fibroblasts. Because it binds with high affinity to smooth muscle cells, some have suggested that PDGF may attract the smooth muscle cells from the media into the intima, bind to them, and finally stimulate their proliferation. Interestingly, evidence has shown that the platelet may not be the only source of this protein. PDGF (α and β subunits) is produced by human umbilical vein and saphenous vein endothelial cells. In fact, a large increase in PDGF production can be measured in injured endothelial cells. Also, both α-subunit and β-subunit messenger ribonucleic acid (mRNA) have been noted in fresh endarterectomy specimens obtained during carotid surgery.[30] Lastly, smooth muscle cells themselves produce PDGF-like activity in response to arterial injury, and smooth muscle cells from human atheroma contain mRNA for the PDGF α subunit.[31] Taken together, these findings may explain how intimal proliferation continues after re-endothelialization occurs. PDGF may be released by both platelets and endothelial cells, causing activation migration of smooth muscle cells, which then secrete additional PDGF leading to proliferation.

Although platelet release of PDGF may play a role in early response to vessel injury, attempts to modify intimal hyperplasia by interfering with these activation pathways have yielded disappointing results. This work is discussed in the section on the experimental basis for pharmacologic therapy.

Inflammatory Cell Pathways

For many years, a close relationship between the biologic pathways of inflammation and cellular proliferation has been suspected. Frequently, these processes occur together during normal physiologic responses to injury. Evidence connecting these pathways is particularly strong in the case of vascular injury. At any time, a significant portion of the intravascular pool of polymorphonuclear neutrophil leukocytes (PMNs) are adherent to the vascular endothelium. Furthermore, PMN adhesion and infiltration is a common finding after arterial wall injury. Electron microscopic studies after balloon catheter intimal injury show that leukocytes attach to the de-endothelialized surface of an arterial lumen.[32] Both monocytes and lymphocytes also adhere to damaged endothelium and, in some instances, even penetrate through it. Finally, in addition to being physically present at the site of vessel wall injury, studies have demonstrated that white blood cells secrete substances capable of stimulating the growth of intimal lesions.[33]

The association between inflammation and intimal proliferation was impressively demonstrated experimentally in an in vivo model of vasculitis.[34] In this study, endotoxin-soaked thread was placed on one half of a rat femoral artery to produce an inflammatory response. This technique consistently caused a significant leukocyte infiltration that only occurred on the treated side of the vessel. Histologic examination performed 14 days later revealed nonuniform intimal lesions in which proliferating smooth muscle cells were located exclusively on the side of the lumen adjacent to the treated half of the arterial wall. Clearly, these findings suggest an association between inflammatory and proliferative biologic pathways. The mechanisms controlling this relationship are an obvious target for therapeutic intervention and have, therefore, become an intense area of ongoing investigation.

PMN adhesion to the surface of endothelial cells is controlled by several complex glycoproteins located on the surface of both endothelial and white blood cells. Together, these binding molecules constitute a sophisticated communication system. To date, two endothelial cell adhesion molecules involved in neutrophil binding have been well characterized: the endothelial leukocyte adhesion molecule-1 (ELAM-1) and the intercellular adhesion molecule-1 (ICAM-1). ELAM-1 is either unexpressed or simply remains intracellular in the nonactive endothelial cell. However, after activation by a variety of different cytokines, this adhesion complex is rapidly induced and can be seen on the membrane surface of the stimulated endothelial cell. Both the physiologic function of this molecule and the specific leukocyte receptor to which it binds remain unknown. ICAM-1 is located in small amounts on the surface of nonactive endothelial cells. After activation by either injury or a variety of stimulating agonists, the expression of this binding complex is significantly increased. ICAM-1 is the binding ligand for the CD11a/CD18 receptor on the leukocyte membrane.

Histochemically, the adhesion molecules located in the surface membranes of white blood cells that are responsible for leukocyte binding to endothelial cells can be separated into three related heterodimers. Each of these heterodimer protein complexes are composed of an α and a β subunit. The α subunit differs between the three glycoproteins complexes (either CD11a, CD11b, or CD11c) whereas the β subunit remains constant (CD18). The CD11a/CD18 complex is found on the surface of all white blood cells and mediates the attachment of unstimulated PMNs to stimulated endothelial cells. This binding probably occurs through an interaction with the ICAM-1 receptor that, as mentioned, is expressed on the luminal surface of activated or injured endothelial cells. The binding of the CD11a/CD18 complex to the ICAM-1 receptor may also play a role in cytokine-induced transendothelial migration of PMNs. The CD11b/CD18 adhesion complex is referred to as either Mac-1 or the C3b complement receptor. This glycoprotein has been implicated in the adhesion of chemotactically stimulated PMNs and controls several cellular functions such as aggregation and cytotoxicity. The third heterodimer complex, CD11c/CD18, exists both on PMNs and monocytes, but its role in binding to endothelial cells remains undetermined.

During inflammatory states, the attachment of PMNs to the involved endothelium is greatly increased due primarily to the upregulation and enhanced expression of the earlier-described binding glycoproteins. A variety of substances are capable of stimulating this enhanced PMN adherence, and together these are thought to be the primary mediators of the inflammatory response to tissue injury. Interleukin-1, tumor necrosis factor-α, lymphotoxin, and bacterial endotoxins (lipopolysaccharide [LPS]) all increase the production of both ELAM-1 and ICAM-1 on the surface of affected endothelial cells. In addition, PMN activation can be stimulated by several substances that are released secondary to inflammation. Examples include the complement factors C5a and C3b, which stimulate PMN chemotaxis and phagocytosis, respectively. Likewise PMN adhesion and chemotaxis can also be stimulated by interleukin-1, xanthine oxidase, PDGF, and the lipid mediators leukotriene B and platelet-activating factor. Finally, tumor necrosis factor is an important mediator of PMN phagocytosis and can lead to increased lysosomal enzyme release.

After activation and adhesion to the damaged vessel lumen, white blood cells migrate into the arterial wall. In one study,[35] 42 days after a denuding injury, leukocytes were shown to penetrate the arterial media and were seen deep within the hyperplastic lesions. The mechanisms triggering this leukocyte migration remain unknown. One possibility is that this process is mediated by exposure of medial smooth muscle cells, which occurs after an endothelial injury. A serum-containing medium that has been conditioned with smooth muscle cells has stimulated leukocyte migration. More important, others have shown that smooth muscle cells and macrophages elaborate potent chemotactic factors for leukocytes, implying that these cells could sustain continued white blood cell recruitment.[36] Other chemotactic agents for leukocytes include PDGF and, in some reports, factors released by fibroblasts. Smooth muscle cells removed from atherosclerotic plaques express ICAM-1, implicating a possible connection between these medial cells and leukocyte recruitment and activation.

The mechanism by which leukocytes may initiate the formation of intimal hyperplasia after penetrating the injured arterial wall remains unknown. Again, several pathways have been suggested. After a denuding endothelial injury and the deposition of inflammatory cells, a variety of inflammatory products may be elaborated. These include chemotactic factors, growth factors, complement components, and enzymes. One of the most studied substances is monocyte- and macrophage-derived growth factor (MDGF). MDGF is a well-known stimulator of smooth muscle cell and fibroblast proliferation. This growth factor is similar and, in fact, may be identical to PDGF. Thus, the stimulation of smooth muscle cell proliferation may be one mechanism by which inflammatory cells may contribute to the formation of intimal hyperplasia. A second possibility involves the production of lysosomal degradation enzymes. Activated leukocytes secrete several potent proteases capable of degrading collagen, basement membranes, and other important extracellular structural proteins. One example of a PMN-derived enzyme that has been implicated in peri-inflammatory extracellular damage

is myeloperoxidase. Liberation of these destructive enzymes into the wall of an injured vessel may weaken the extracellular matrix. This "loosening" of the vessel wall may facilitate the migration of smooth muscle cells from the medial layer toward the lumen. Lastly, leukocytes may also act directly at sites of vessel injury to worsen the degree of endothelial injury. PMNs can produce oxygen free radicals through the action of the reduced nicotinamide adenine dinucleotide phosphate (NADPH) oxidase system present on their membranes. The toxic substances elaborated by these activated PMNs, including superoxide anion, hydrogen peroxide, and hydroxyl radicals, can damage endothelial cells and alter capillary permeability. With PMN activation, marginally injured endothelial cells bordering a lesion may therefore be destroyed, increasing the magnitude of the damage to the vessel wall. This further exposure of the subendothelial layer allows more platelet cell adherence, aggregation, and activation, as well as the recruitment of more leukocyte mediators and, therefore, the stimulation of a continued cycle of inflammatory injury.

The Renin-Angiotensin System

The classic view of the regulatory function of the renin-angiotensin system is that it is primarily an endocrine-based system designed for the homeostatic control of hemodynamic and electrolyte balance. This mechanism can be simplified conceptually as follows. In response to low perfusion pressures, renin is released by renal tissue and circulates in the plasma, where it cleaves angiotensinogen, produced by the liver, into angiotensin I. Angiotensin I is converted into active angiotensin II by angiotensin-converting enzyme (ACE) located primarily in the pulmonary vasculature. Finally, angiotensin II exerts its homeostatic hemodynamic effects via specific angiotensin II receptors located in peripheral vascular arterial beds. This traditional view of the renin-angiotensin system has been revised, and a much more complex concept has emerged. In this new description, the primary site of angiotensin II production is not the pulmonary vasculature, but rather at local sites within the affected tissues themselves. This portion of the entire renin-angiotensin axis has been referred to as the "tissue renin-angiotensin system."

The concept that active angiotensin II in the vascular wall is synthesized locally, and not delivered via the systemic circulation, was originally suggested by Swales and Thurston.[37] In this report, the authors noted that the amount of angiotensin antiserum required to inhibit endogenous angiotensin effects in sodium-loaded rats could not be explained solely on the basis of systemic production. In addition, several investigators had noticed residual renin-like activity after bilateral nephrectomy in animal studies.[38] More convincing evidence for the existence of a locally active vascular renin-angiotensin system, operating independently of the classic systemic circuit, has been provided by several studies. First, angiotensinogen mRNA, the only known precursor of the angiotensin peptides, has recently been detected in several extrahepatic vascular tissues, including the aorta.[39, 40] Second, using monoclonal antirenin antibodies, immunohistochemical studies have stained positively for the presence of renin in cells located throughout the vascular wall.[41] To specifically identify the cells in the arterial wall responsible for this renin production, tissue culture techniques have been used. These studies have demonstrated that both vascular smooth muscle and endothelial cells can synthesize renin in vitro.[42, 43] Also, mRNA coding for renin has been identified in human vascular smooth muscle cells.[38, 44] Finally, ACE is primarily located on the luminal surface of vascular endothelial cells.[45] Thus, the normally functioning vascular wall possesses all of the necessary components for the independent local production of angiotensin II.

The physiologic function of locally produced angiotensin II is an area of continued controversy. Angiotensin II receptors have been identified on vascular endothelial cells,[38] smooth muscle cells,[46, 47] and circulating platelets.[48] Angiotensin II stimulation of endothelial cell–bound receptors leads to the secretion of prostacyclin (PGI_2) and possibly endothelial-derived relaxant factor (EDRF).[49, 50] Both these substances cause medial smooth muscle cell quiescence and relaxation. On the other hand, activation of the angiotensin receptors located directly on the smooth muscle cells themselves causes the opposite effect. Campbell-Boswell and Robertson[51] reported that angiotensin II stimulated the proliferation of human vascular smooth muscle cells in vitro. Also, Geisterfer and associates[52] found that the protein content of these smooth muscle cells increased by 20% when stimulated by angiotensin II for 4 days. Furthermore, this stimulation was abolished by the angiotensin II receptor antagonist saralasin. Finally, the *mas* proto-oncogene, located on the surface of medial smooth muscle cells, increases mitogenic activity when stimulated and has been identified as a functional angiotensin II receptor.[53] Therefore, one possibility for the physiologic function of a locally active renin-angiotensin system seems to be the autocrine balance of vascular wall metabolic activity and tone.

This view has led many investigators to study the effect of the local production of angiotensin II on the subsequent development of intimal hyperplasia. In this hypothesis, denudation of the arterial endothelium disrupts the balance of the local renin-angiotensin system and allows the anabolic and mitogenic effects of angiotensin II on the medial smooth muscle cells to proceed unchecked. Another possible mechanism for the promotion of hyperplastic neointimal growth by the local production of angiotensin II involves the activation of platelet metabolic pathways. As mentioned previously, human platelets possess specific binding sites for angiotensin II[48] and platelet activation and the subsequent release of PDGF may play a role in the development of intimal hyperplasia. In a 1990 study by Swartz and Moore,[54] angiotensin II enhanced both collagen-induced platelet aggregation and the production of TxA_2. Finally, the expression of PDGF by activated smooth muscle cells is upregulated in the presence of angiotensin II.[55]

Cellular Growth Factors

The stimulation of vascular smooth muscle cell growth is the final common pathway of all postulated mechanisms leading to the development of intimal hyperplasia. The view that the vascular wall is a complex integrated organ, complete with its own endogenous local autocrine system, is gaining increasing support. In this theory, intimal hyperplasia is postulated to result from an imbalance of these local hormonal systems. This could be due to either an excess of stimulatory molecules or, alternatively, smooth muscle cell proliferation may result from the absence or reduction of inhibitory hormones.

Angiotensin II, PDGF, and MDGF are all examples of cellular growth factors believed to be involved in the formation of hyperplastic intimal lesions; each has been reviewed in detail earlier. In addition to these mitogens, basic fibroblast growth factor (bFGF) is another promoter of smooth muscle cell growth that deserves comment. bFGF is a potent stimulator of angiogenesis. Interest in this protein has developed in the field of intimal hyperplasia research for several reasons. Direct smooth muscle cell damage may be an important stimulus to subsequent activation. These data come from research showing that the response of an arterial wall to injury varies depending on the method of injury. Balloon catheterization, which damages both the medial smooth muscle cells and the endothelium, causes a large proliferative response.[56] On the other hand, wire denudation, which significantly damages the endothelium but does not injure the medial cells, results in much less smooth muscle cell activation.[57] Furthermore, recent reports have shown that intimal lesions after a balloon catheter injury occur even in the absence of platelets.[58] This work implies that elaboration of PDGF in this setting may not be required for the subsequent stimulation of smooth muscle cell replication. Thus, damaged smooth muscle cells may stimulate replication of adjacent undamaged medial cells by the release of an endogenous intracellular growth factor. Because bFGF is synthesized by smooth muscle cells and the expression of bFGF mRNA in these cells is increased after injury, bFGF has been postulated to be this endogenous growth factor.

Several studies have investigated the role of bFGF in the development of hyperplastic intimal lesions. In one such study by Lindner and associates,[59] arteries were exposed to bFGF after an injury with a balloon catheter. In this experiment, smooth muscle cell replication increased from 11.5% to 54.8% after exposure to bFGF. Also, an equivalent increase was seen in vessels denuded by the wire loop technique, suggesting the ability of bFGF to upregulate undamaged medial cells. When bFGF was administered to normal nondenuded arteries, no effect on smooth muscle growth was observed. Lastly, prolonged exposure of the growth factor was found to result in a twofold increase in intimal thickness compared with control vessels. In a related study, Cuevas and colleagues[60] demonstrated that the direct local infusion of bFGF into either normal adventitia or injured media results in proliferation of both vasa vasorum and vascular smooth muscle cells.

Up until this point, all of the cellular growth factors we have discussed are peptide cellular mitogens. Nonpeptide molecules have also been shown to be important modulators of smooth muscle cell growth. Nitric oxide (NO), previously identified as EDRF, is normally secreted by endothelium, and its levels are decreased after endothelial damage. Although the exact pathways are still being determined, NO inhibits vascular smooth muscle cell proliferation and DNA synthesis in vitro.[61] Ways to manipulate NO production at sites of arterial injury may be an important new tool in the pharmacologic control of hyperplastic intimal lesions.

In summary, the balance of locally produced cellular growth factors such as bFGF and NO probably plays an important role in the regulation of smooth muscle cell activity and the subsequent development of intimal hyperplasia. Clearly, research into methods of influencing this balance will have meaningful implications for the pharmacologic management of these lesions.

Coagulation Pathways and the Locally Active Fibrinolytic System

The establishment of a mature intimal lesion after an arterial insult requires the combination of several biologic pathways. The components and pathways that make up the body's coagulation system are extremely important. The products of these pathways probably participate in complex and diverse ways in the development of intimal hyperplasia. As mentioned, the formation of a fibrin matrix in an area of endothelial damage helps to stabilize the aggregating platelet plug. Furthermore, many other substances released by the adjacent organizing thrombus may affect nearby medial smooth muscle cells independently. One important and intensely studied coagulation product is plasmin.

The establishment of a mature intimal lesion after an arterial insult requires the combination of several biologic pathways. From the perspective of the medial smooth muscle cell, many steps in the proper sequence must be coordinated for these lesions to progress. Specifically, smooth muscle cell activation within the media is followed by migration across the internal elastic lamina and finally by replication within the neointimal lining. The regulation of smooth muscle cell activation and proliferation has been extensively studied and is described thoroughly in the previous sections. Conversely, how these cells pass through the physical barrier imposed by the thick medial collagenous extracellular matrix and the mechanisms regulating this migration remain a perplexing and unresolved issue. One theory, proposed to explain this phenomenon, involves the locally active vascular fibrinolytic system.

The active end product of the tissue plasminogen-plasmin system is the proteolytic enzyme plasmin. Other important components of this system include the precursor plasminogen and its main endogenous activators: urokinase-type plasminogen activator (u-PA) and tissue-type plasminogen activator (t-PA). The catalytic action of these proteases is inhibited in vivo by the plasmin inhibitors α_2-antiplasmin, α_2-macroglobulin, and a group of related plasminogen activator inhibitory proteins (PAIs). Increased knowledge regarding the interactions of all these components at the cellular level has been accumulating.

The hypothesis that the protease plasmin is involved in smooth muscle cell migration after an arterial injury is built on several related observations. First, circulating plasminogen is a relatively large protein that is normally prevented from entering the medial layer by an intact endothelium. However, after endothelial damage, this protein can readily diffuse into this area.[62] Once present in the extracellular medial layer, conversion of plasminogen into plasmin can directly degrade several matrix proteins and activate other potent collagenases.[63] The key to this conversion depends on the local presence of specific plasminogen activators. Smooth muscle cells express plasminogen activator activity in tissue culture.[64, 65] Finally, in an in vivo model of arterial repair, Clowes and associates[66] demonstrated that vascular smooth muscle cells contain increased levels of both u-PA and t-PA. Furthermore, these two plasminogen activators appear to act synergistically, and their secretion depends on the functional state of the smooth muscle cells. During cellular proliferation u-PA is the major product, whereas during migration t-PA expression predominates. The combination of these experimental observations suggests the following hypothesis. Injury to the endothelium may allow the local penetration of plasminogen and chemotactic substances (elaborated from activated platelets and leukocytes) into the arterial wall. The conversion of extracellular plasminogen into plasmin by medial smooth muscle cells degrades the structural matrix proteins. This process may be enhanced by the presence of leukocyte-derived enzymes. Finally, activation of smooth muscle cells by the elaborated growth and chemotactic factors initiates migration of these cells through the weakened arterial wall. The direction of migration is determined automatically by the gradient of plasminogen and mitogenic activity, which is highest adjacent to the endothelial defect. Precise characterization of the role of local plasminogen-plasmin pathways in the development of intimal hyperplasia requires further research.

Vein Graft Myointimal Hyperplasia and Arterialization

Autogenous vein bypass grafting provides the primary means of long-term revascularization in patients suffering from ischemic conditions of both the heart and the peripheral circulation. Myointimal hyperplasia has been studied to a large degree in the arterial circulation but is poorly understood as it occurs in vein grafts. Vein graft myointimal hyperplasia occurs by pathobiologically distinct mechanisms relative to its counterpart in arterial injury. Prominent features in rodent models of vein grafting are referred to in this section. These features include extensive early denudation of the endothelium and smooth muscle cell layers, attachment of leukocytes and platelets to the subendothelial matrix, and elaboration of cytokine and growth factor products by these cells. This is thought to result in the activation, migration, and proliferation of vein graft adventitial myofibroblasts to form a neointima.[67–71]

The normal histology of the vein is manifestly different from that of the arterial wall. Veins possess no discernible media in the traditional sense. One or at most two layers of smooth muscle cells subtend the endothelium. Internal and external elastic laminae are not discernible, although some elastic fibers can be visualized with trichrome-elastin stain. The majority of the vessel wall consists of adventitial collagen (Fig. 37–2).

Pathologically, the trauma resulting from exposure of the vein graft to arterial pressure and flow results in complete denudation of the endothelial and smooth muscle cell layers within the first 24 hours (Fig. 37–3). The vein re-

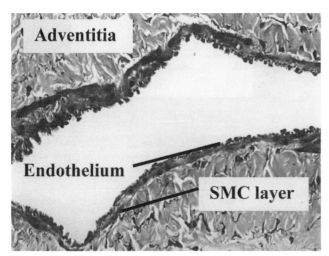

Figure 37–2. Trichrome/elastin stain of normal rat external jugular vein. Note the single layer of endothelium (granular due to preparation) and subjacent single layer of smooth muscle cells (dark nuclei and surrounding cytoplasm). The gray whorls and intercalated black streaks represent adventitial collagen and elastic fibers, respectively. SMC, Smooth muscle cells.

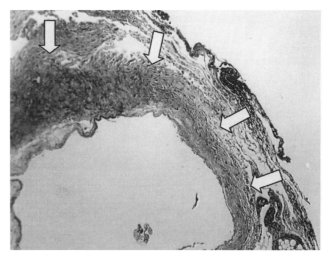

Figure 37–4. Trichrome/elastin stain of 2-week vein graft. Arrows denote the region of the external elastic lamina, within which resides the neointima. Many of the nuclei visualized in the neointima prove to be macrophages when stained with ED-2 macrophage stain (not depicted due to black-and-white limitations).

endothelializes by 1 week, but controversy remains regarding the source of actin-positive cell constituents in the ensuing myointimal lesion. Hoch and coworkers[67] have hypothesized that unlike models of arterial injury, resident smooth muscle cells are denuded and therefore not the source of actin-positive cells constituting the developing myointimal lesion. Rather, adventitial progenitor fibroblasts have been implicated, providing a pool of undifferentiated cells from which "myofibroblast" cell types are thought to proliferate and migrate into the vein graft neointima.

A prominent component of vein graft remodeling is the attachment of leukocytes and platelets early after denudation of the endothelium and smooth muscle cell layers. Macrophage infiltration dominates the early inflammatory changes observed with vein graft pathobiology. This promi-

nent inflammatory response peaks during the first 2 weeks of vein graft adaptation, which exceeds the response observed in models of arterial injury (Fig. 37–4). Hoch and coworkers have elegantly demonstrated that by inhibiting macrophage activity early in this inflammatory process, a significant reduction in myointimal hyperplasia was achieved.[69, 70]

Vein graft myointimal changes persist and can progress despite re-endothelialization, in contrast to arterial myointimal proliferation, which tends to halt its progression upon restitution of the endothelial cell layer. It is believed that the ongoing myointimal thickening associated with vein graft myointimal hyperplasia is an adaptive response to arterial blood flow physiology. It has been suggested that vein grafts respond to vessel wall shear stress, which is thought to modulate wall thickness more so than restoration of the endothelial surface.[72] Vein grafts may also experience a form of continuous injury owing to their chronic exposure to arterial pressure. In an attempt to adapt to these altered hemodynamic forces, the vessel responds by developing an exuberant thickening comprised of myointimal hyperplastic changes. The hyperplastic changes occurring in response to these multifactorial processes have been referred to as vein graft "arterialization." This process can progress throughout the life of the graft, resulting in hemodynamically significant lesions, which ultimately threaten long-term patency. We use a rat model of vein graft arterialization in which the graft maintains its myointimal-thickened characteristics at 12 weeks, including the development of focal degenerative areas comprised of calcific lesions (Fig. 37–5).

CLINICAL MANIFESTATIONS AND CURRENT MANAGEMENT

The number of procedures performed annually for occlusive vascular disease continues to increase. Currently, ap-

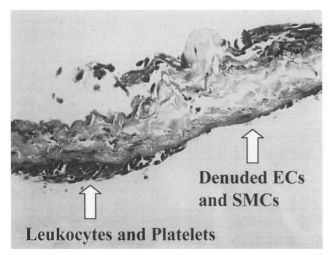

Figure 37–3. Trichrome/elastin stain of 72-hour vein graft. The luminal side is depicted on the bottom edge of this tissue section. There is evidence of endothelial and smooth muscle cell denudation with adherence of leukocytes and platelets. EC, endothelial cells; SMC, smooth muscle cells.

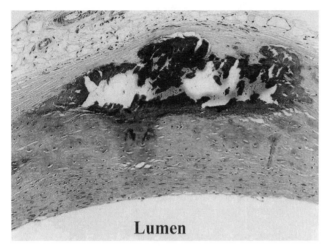

Figure 37–5. Hematoxylin/eosin stain of 12-week vein graft. Note the prominent calcification within the neointima.

proximately 500,000 patients undergo reconstructive vascular surgery each year; half of these are coronary bypass procedures and the remainder include various operations on the peripheral vascular tree. These peripheral interventions encompass a wide assortment of procedures, including autogenous and prosthetic bypass grafts, endarterectomies, and a variety of new endovascular procedures.

Most established vascular procedures, as well as the new technologies and applications, have proved both technically feasible and safe. The value of any surgical procedure, however, must be measured not only by the success by which it can be initially performed but also in terms of the durability of the results. Although the in-hospital success rates are excellent, the long-term durability of most of these procedures has been disappointing. Furthermore, the common culprit accounting for much of the poor long-term success rate of these procedures is intimal hyperplasia. Clearly, this process is a significant cause of morbidity in patients undergoing procedures on the vascular system, and investigations into methods to prevent or reverse this process are of great importance.

Restenosis after Peripheral Bypass

The 3-year primary patency rates for infrainguinal bypass grafts range from 40% to 60% with prosthetic conduits to 60% to 80% when an autogenous graft is used.[73] Of those grafts that fail between 6 months and 2 years, most fail because of intimal hyperplasia.[1, 74] In prosthetic grafts, the area most affected by hyperplastic change is the distal anastomosis. Although this location is also the likely point of obstruction in autogenous tissue grafts, focal lesions throughout the entire length of the graft are also common.

Treatment options for a failed or failing peripheral bypass graft due to intimal hyperplasia are limited. Chronically thrombosed vein grafts can rarely be salvaged and invariably need to be replaced. Often, when this is not technically possible and when the patient is suffering from severe ischemia, an amputation is required. Thrombosed grafts that are recognized early can frequently be reopened with use of thrombolytic therapy. After flow through the graft is reestablished, the lesion responsible for the occlusion is sometimes visualized. Even though some of these hyperplastic lesions may be treated percutaneously with balloon dilatation or atherectomy devices, results of these techniques are usually less than satisfactory. Immediate patency is usually excellent; however, because of the fibrous character and progressive growth of these lesions, recurrence rates are unacceptably high. Therefore, reoperation for distal anastomotic graft stenoses is generally recommended. Reconstruction usually requires implantation of a new graft, construction of a jump graft, or patch angioplasty of the existing bypass.

Restenosis after Carotid Endarterectomy

The mean incidence of asymptomatic carotid restenoses ranges from 7% to 15%, and between 1% and 5% of patients develop restenoses associated with recurrent symptoms.[75–85] In those rare instances in which a recurrent lesion becomes symptomatic, the management algorithm is straightforward. Most surgeons consider this an indication for intervention. Unfortunately, as with primary carotid lesions, little information exists regarding the natural history of recurrent carotid stenoses in asymptomatic patients; therefore, the appropriate management of these individuals remains unclear. The risk of subsequent stroke or ischemic events in these patients is clearly different from that of patients with primary atherosclerotic lesions. Smooth, fibrous, intimal hyperplastic lesions, even those of the same or greater degree of stenosis than the original atherosclerotic plaque, are well tolerated by most patients. This is probably because of the low risk of embolic events related to these lesions relative to the soft necrotic atherosclerotic plaques originally found in these patients. The majority of patients who become symptomatic due to a recurrent carotid stenosis do so on the basis of a hemodynamic flow-related mechanism or because of recurrence of a mixed plaque with a significant atherosclerotic component. This may explain the observation that patients with symptomatic recurrences often have tight stenoses or occlusions of the contralateral carotid artery.[76, 78] In general, the decision to operate on an asymptomatic patient with a recurrent carotid stenosis should be individualized and based on several factors, including the degree and rate of progression of the stenosis, the histologic character of the lesion, the condition of the remainder of the cerebral circulation, and the age and overall general medical condition of the patient.

The incision and principles of exposure when managing a recurrent carotid lesion are the same as for a standard endarterectomy. The dissection is invariably more difficult because of scarring from the previous procedure, and extra care must be taken to avoid injury to the cranial nerves. The hypoglossal nerve is particularly vulnerable because it can be draped over the bifurcation by the scar tissue. Once completely dissected, the common, external, and internal carotid vessels are clamped, and the bifurcation is opened via a longitudinal arteriotomy. The histologic property of carotid bifurcation atherosclerotic lesions that allows for the performance of a standard endarterectomy is the ease in developing a plane of dissection between the plaque and the circular medial fibers of the arterial wall. Unfortunately, recurrent carotid lesions composed of hyperplastic intimal tissue do not share this property. Thus, forming a precise plane of dissection that allows for removal of the lumen-narrowing plaque without dangerously thinning the remaining arterial wall is not possible. The surgical approach to recurrent carotid lesions, therefore, is patch angioplasty rather than endarterectomy. On the other hand, when the recurrent lesion is composed of ordinary atheroma, a standard endarterectomy can be performed.

The choice of patch material varies among surgeons treating this disease. Some use prosthetic material as their first choice, whereas others prefer the use of autogenous vein. A theoretical argument exists that prosthetic material may contribute to the hyperplastic intimal process, but this has not been proved experimentally. In fact, autogenous vein, with its intact endothelium that elaborates humoral growth factors, may be a greater stimulus to a continued hyperplastic reaction in the patched arterial segment. When vein is chosen, saphenous vein is most frequently used. Experience has shown that vein segments taken from the neck ordinarily are too thin and should be avoided. Regardless of the material chosen, the patch should always be constructed in such a way as to reapproximate the native size of the carotid bulb. Large patulous repairs increase the luminal diameter of the reconstructed carotid bulb and, by application of the law of Laplace, lead to abnormally increased tangential wall tension. This could result in a blowout of the patch suture line. Alternatively, saccular patch repairs may lead to the accumulation of laminar thrombus and result in distal embolization. Occasionally, the recurrent disease is so advanced that patch angioplasty is not feasible. In these rare cases, reconstruction can be accomplished by the use of an interposition graft.

Restenosis after Endovascular Surgery

Endovascular surgery is a relatively new field that originated with the development of percutaneous transluminal balloon angioplasty (PTA) and evolved to include angioscopy, laser and mechanical atherectomy, and intravascular stents and endovascular grafts. Together, these techniques have managed to achieve impressive initial success rates. However, with the test of time, complications such as dissections, perforations, and especially restenosis have limited their application. Advances such as "over" catheter systems and "smart" laser technology have reduced the incidence of early technical complications. Unfortunately, the problem of restenosis remains the Achilles heel of endovascular interventions and threatens to limit their ultimate usefulness.

Results after PTA in the lower extremity have been published by several authors. The combined failure rate after 1 year of follow-up ranges from 2% to 40%.[86] Some of these recurrences are no doubt due to either a progression of atherosclerosis or other mechanisms such as intraplaque hemorrhage. However, the majority are the result of intimal hyperplasia. Likewise, long-term results after laser-assisted angioplasty have not been encouraging. In one representative study, White and colleagues[87] reported their results of laser-assisted balloon angioplasty for advanced lesions of the lower extremity. In this study, several different technologies were used, including argon, neodymium:yttrium-aluminum-garnet (Nd:YAG), and metal hot-tipped systems. Although the initial recanalization rate was 67%, only 11% patency was present after 1 year. Results from other investigators have been similar. The results of peripheral atherectomy differ depending on the device used and the anatomic location of the lesion. At the University of California, Los Angeles (UCLA), we have had experience treating arterial occlusions with the Auth Rotablator (Heart Technology, Inc., Bellevue, Wash.).[88] Initial success was achieved in 92% of cases and primary patency was 67% at 6 months. However, follow-up at 24 months noted only a 9.5% patency rate. Unfortunately, the long-term outcomes of other devices have not shown any significant improvement over these results. Again, the majority of these failures can be attributed to intimal hyperplasia.

The treatment for restenotic lesions after endovascular surgery depends on the site affected, the degree of symptoms, and the overall condition of the patient. In general, redo endovascular procedures are possible, but they uniformly suffer a fate similar to the original intervention. Most frequently in this setting, conventional vascular surgical techniques have been used, including formal bypass grafts or limited endarterectomies. Of course, as described earlier, these methods also possess a small but definite risk of failure due to intimal hyperplasia and therefore do not guarantee long-term success.

EXPERIMENTAL BASIS FOR PHARMACOLOGIC CONTROL

The ability of various pharmacologic agents to suppress the development of intimal hyperplasia has been well documented. Particularly striking is the large variety of medications that have been effective in limiting this response. At least five different classes of drugs have been studied and are at least partially successful in this regard (Table 37–1). These classes of drugs are lipid metabolites,[89–91] antiplatelet agents,[92–94] anti-inflammatory agents,[95, 96] antihypertensive agents,[97–100] and anticoagulants.[101] In addition, many other substances that interfere with normal cellular growth have also shown some promise.[59, 102–106] This clearly attests to the complexity of the pathways leading to the development of this lesion and implies that no one agent will likely be totally effective in its elimination. Unfortunately, the nonuniformity of the models of intimal hyperplasia studied and the doses and duration of the agents investigated make comparison of the results of these trials unreliable. Therefore, the clinical usefulness of pharmacologic therapy in this setting remains undetermined. Nevertheless, if effective pharmacologic therapy to suppress the growth of intimal hyperplasia and prevent the associated recurrent arterial stenoses could be developed, this would have a major impact on the durability of vascular procedures and would lower their associated morbidity, mortality, and cost. Also, in addition to suppressing the development of intimal hyperplasia, one or more of these medications may prove effective in reducing established hyperplastic lesions. This would be an alternative therapy for the patient with a

TABLE 37-1

Pharmacologic Agents Effective in Suppressing the Formation of Intimal Hyperplasia

Lipid metabolites
  ω-3 polyunsaturated fatty acids (eicosapentaenoic
    acid)
Antiplatelet agents
  Aspirin
  Dipyridamole
  Thromboxane synthetase inhibitors
Anti-inflammatory agents
  Dehydroepiandrosterone
  Dexamethasone
  Cyclosporin
Antihypertensive agents
  ACE inhibitors
    Cilazapril, captopril, enalaprilat
  Calcium channel blockers
    Verapamil, nimodipine
  α$_1$-Adrenergic inhibitors
    Prazosin
Growth factor inhibitors
  Angiopeptin
  bFGF-saporin
  Ornithine decarboxylase inhibitors
Anticoagulant agents
  Heparins and heparinoids
Insulin-sensitizing agents
  Thiazolidinediones
    Troglitazone
    Rosiglitazone
    Pioglitazone

ACE, angiotensin-converting enzyme; bFGF, basic fibroblast growth factor.

failing previous vascular procedure and would represent a significant advance in the management of this highly morbid and potentially lethal complication of peripheral vascular surgery.

Experimental Models

Several models have been used in an attempt to elucidate the pathophysiologic mechanisms leading to the development of intimal hyperplasia. These include both in vitro and animal replicas of this lesion. Smooth muscle and endothelial cells have been grown in tissue culture. Although these studies have been helpful in determining the isolated effects of various mitogens, growth factors, and hormones on the growth patterns of these vascular cells, the investigations suffer greatly from the abnormal cellular relationships inherent to their preparation. Conventional anatomic descriptions of the vascular wall depict the endothelial cell as being separated from the underlying smooth muscle cells by a continuous elastic lamina. This concept of two independently functioning and autonomous cell layers has more recently been replaced by a more complex description portraying mechanisms of mutual regulation between the two cell systems.

The possibility of endothelial–smooth muscle cell interaction was first suggested by electron microscopic evidence of smooth muscle cell cytoplasmic extensions traversing holes in the elastic lamina and projecting into the overlying endothelial cell cytoplasm.[107] The subsequent description

of several endothelial cell–derived substances that either promote or inhibit the growth and activation of the medial smooth muscle cell lends further support to the concept of the vascular walls functioning as an interrelated organ system. In addition, contact of the endothelial cell layer with the cellular and serum components of flowing blood further complicates the normal functioning environment of these vascular elements. Making useful conclusions based on data collected from in vitro systems in which the processes being studied clearly exist in an artificial environment is very difficult. In an attempt to study the pathophysiology of this lesion in a setting in which the normal regulatory interrelationships have not been disturbed, most investigators have turned to animal models of intimal hyperplasia.

The classic animal model of smooth muscle cell intimal hyperplasia is a balloon catheter arterial injury model. The induction of smooth muscle cell growth after a balloon catheter–denuding injury was first described by Baumgartner[108] in 1963. Since that time, this procedure has undergone several modifications; however, the basic concepts of the model remain the same. A segment of artery to be studied is isolated, and a balloon catheter is introduced into the lumen. By inflating the balloon and withdrawing the catheter, complete denudation of the endothelial layer can be achieved. After this injury, a lesion is formed that is histologically identical to that observed clinically. The advantages of this model are its ease and reproducibility. In addition, the anatomic injury produced mimics the cleavage plane that occurs clinically in the endarterectomized vessel. Criticisms of this model include the vessel distention that occurs at the time of injury and its failure to address the intimal hyperplasia that occurs at graft anastomotic sites. A second type of injury model involves hydrostatic stretching of the vessel without deliberate denuding of the endothelial surface.[109] This model attempts to isolate and define the role of vascular distention as a contributing factor in the development of these lesions. This mode of injury does produce an increase in medial smooth muscle cell activity and lends support to the mechanical theories of hyperplasia. A third type of arterial injury model is the denudation of the intimal layer by a loop of fine nylon wire.[7] This model differs from balloon injury in that the wire removes the endothelium without the complicating effects of distention. This model suffers, however, from difficulty in standardizing the degree of vessel injury and its lack of a true anatomic correlate in clinical situations. Finally, to study the development of intimal hyperplasia at anastomotic sites, several animal models using bypass grafts of both autogenous and prosthetic material have been successful in reproducing the lesions seen clinically in humans.[10, 96]

Agents Studied

Lipid Metabolites

As mentioned, Alaskan Natives have extremely low plasma levels of LDL and this may explain their low incidence of atherosclerotic heart disease.[26] Further characterization of Alaskan Native plasma lipid composition has demonstrated low levels of circulating arachidonic acid and unusually high concentrations of eicosapentaenoic acid (EPA).[110] EPA is an ω-3 polyunsaturated fatty acid that is present in large amounts in fish but cannot be synthesized de novo by humans. After ingestion, EPA enters the prostaglandin synthesis pathway and competes directly with arachidonic acid. In contrast to arachidonic acid metabolism, which leads to the formation of TxA_2 (a potent stimulator of platelet aggregation), EPA is converted into TxA_3, which has no effect on platelet function.

Several studies have tested the hypothesis that high levels of EPA present at the time of an endothelial injury may inhibit the production of intimal hyperplasia. Both Cahill and colleagues[89] and Landymore and colleagues[90] have reported the ability of small doses of marine oils to reduce intimal thickening in vein graft models. O'Hara and colleagues[91] reported a marked suppression of intimal hyperplasia after treatment with EPA in a rabbit PTFE graft model.

Further investigation is needed to establish both the precise mechanism by which EPA prevents intimal hyperplasia and the dose and duration of exposure at which this effect is optimal.

Antiplatelet Agents

Excitement about the possibility of limiting intimal hyperplasia by inhibiting platelet pathways began with the work of Friedman and colleagues,[111] who reported reduced hyperplasia after an aortic balloon catheter injury in thrombocytopenic rabbits. Unfortunately, inhibition of intimal hyperplasia using a number of different antiplatelet drugs has yielded mixed results. Antiplatelet drugs inhibit the synthesis of prostaglandins by blocking arachidonic acid metabolic pathways. Aspirin irreversibly acetylates platelet cell cyclooxygenase. Dipyridamole increases platelet cyclic adenosine monophosphate and inhibits the precursors TxA_1 and TxB_2. Thus, both aspirin and dipyridamole inhibit platelet adherence and aggregation by interfering with the production of prostaglandin metabolites.

Clinically and in experimental models, aspirin decreases platelet adherence to prosthetic vascular grafts.[112–114] The addition of dipyridamole may or may not enhance this effect. Findings from other studies, however, have demonstrated that although antiplatelet agents may decrease subsequent platelet aggregation and thrombus formation, they have no effect on initial platelet deposition.[115] The effect of these agents on patency and the development of intimal hyperplasia has also been inconsistent. In one study, bilateral vein bypass grafts were placed to ligated iliac arteries in rhesus monkeys.[116] These monkeys were given aspirin (165 mg administered twice daily) and dipyridamole (25 mg administered twice daily) beginning 3 weeks before the surgical procedure. Sixteen weeks after the procedure, at sacrifice, the intimal areas were compared and were significantly reduced in the experimental group. On the other hand, in a follow-up study using a balloon catheter injury model in rabbits, no significant difference between the two groups in tritiated thymidine incorporation, nuclear proliferation, or progression of intimal hyperplasia was established.[94] In a similar study performed in rabbits, aspirin significantly increased the patency of an end-to-side iliac

anastomosis but had no effect on the development of intimal hyperplasia.[92]

Thromboxane synthetase converts cyclic endoperoxide precursors from the arachidonic acid pathways into TxA_2. TxA_2 is synthesized and stored in the developing platelet. It is a powerful mediator of both platelet aggregation and vascular constriction. Inhibitors of thromboxane synthetase block this conversion of intermediate endoperoxide precursors into TxA_2. Furthermore, in doing so the intracellular prostaglandin metabolic pathways are shifted toward the production of PGI_2. Thus, theoretically, thromboxane synthetase inhibitors can block platelet-derived TxA_2 while actually enhancing the production of endothelial cell–derived PGI_2. These agents may therefore be more specific inhibitors of platelet function. The efficacy of thromboxane synthetase inhibition in the prevention of distal anastomotic intimal hyperplasia was investigated and compared with aspirin.[117] A bilateral aortoiliac bypass graft model was used and two different types of grafts were evaluated: thin-walled PTFE and PTFE seeded with autogenous endothelial cells. Treatment groups consisted of antiplatelet therapy with either aspirin or the thromboxane synthetase inhibitor U-63,577A. Interestingly, in both types of grafts, aspirin was significantly more effective in maintaining patency and inhibiting intimal hyperplasia. Within the thromboxane synthetase inhibitor group, however, the agent was more effective when the bypass grafts were seeded. Also, the success of both types of grafts were improved compared with the graft accompanied by no therapy at all. In conclusion, in combination with other antiplatelet drugs, these agents could prove to be potent inhibitors of platelet function. However, no clinical trials are yet available.

At present, antiplatelet drugs appear to increase the patency of vein and prosthetic bypass grafts, but probably do not significantly alter the development of intimal hyperplasia. New approaches and agents, however, are continually being studied. Platelet aggregation in response to collagen and ADP has been reduced by blocking GPIIb and GPIIIa with a murine monoclonal antibody (LJ-CP8).[118] Unfortunately, in an arteriovenous shunt model, this antibody failed to decrease deposition of platelets on Dacron or PTFE grafts.[119] More work is necessary to determine the role of newer agents in complementing or enhancing these effects.

Anti-inflammatory Agents

Several investigators have postulated that leukocyte pathways may play a role in the development of intimal hyperplasia. This theory is supported by the fact that leukocyte infiltration is observed in hyperplastic intimal lesions. Also, these accumulated white blood cells possess sufficient enzymatic and mitogenic activity to stimulate medial smooth muscle cells. Although many approaches designed to modulate the inflammatory contribution to the formation of intimal hyperplasia have been described, most work in this area has focused on the immunosuppressive glucocorticoids and cyclosporin.

In 1979, Hoepp and colleagues[96] did not find any significant differences in patency or intimal response between steroid-treated and control groups in a canine femoropop-

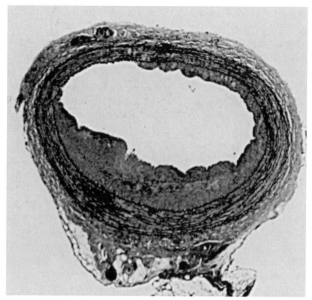

Figure 37–6. Photomicrograph of a control rabbit carotid artery, 12 weeks following a balloon catheter endothelial injury, demonstrating a large amount of intimal hyperplasia. (Verhoeff-van Gieson stain; original magnification ×20.) (From Colburn MD, Moore WS, Gelabert HA, Quiñones-Baldrich WJ: Dose responsive suppression of myointimal hyperplasia by dexamethasone. J Vasc Surg 15:510–518, 1992.)

liteal polyester fabric bypass graft model. However, the animals in this experiment were given a relatively low dose of a short-acting steroid (methylprednisolone), and the agent was administered after the procedure and not given preoperatively. A report by Gordon and associates[120] in 1988 was among the earliest to suggest that glucocorticoids could inhibit smooth muscle cell proliferation after an endothelial injury. These investigators found that the administration of the endogenous steroid dehydroepiandrosterone led to a decrease in the production of atheroscle-

rotic plaques in hypercholesterolemic rabbits. More recently, clinical trials have been attempted. The Multi-Hospital Eastern Atlantic Restenosis Trial (M-HEART) project, a large, randomized, double-blind clinical study, investigated whether steroids could decrease the rate of restenosis after balloon angioplasty.[121] In this study, a single large dose of methylprednisolone (1 g) was given intravenously before the procedure. No significant difference was found between steroid- and placebo-treated groups. Perhaps significantly, the period of maximal intimal proliferation after arterial injury is 2 to 4 weeks.[56] Furthermore, many studies have demonstrated that beginning steroid treatment before the arterial injury may be important. This may explain the negative results found in the M-HEART project study in which a relatively short-acting steroid was given as a single one-time dose. With these principles in mind, our laboratory investigated the use of steroids in a balloon catheter injury model performed in rabbits. Dexamethasone (0.10 mg/kg given intramuscularly) was administered 2 days before the endothelial injury and was continued for a period of 8 weeks. This treatment was found to result in a dramatic reduction of intimal growth.[95] Furthermore, in a follow-up study, this response to dexamethasone therapy was found to be dose-dependent[122] (Figs. 37–6 and 37–7).

How glucocorticoids prevent or suppress the development of intimal hyperplasia remains unclear. One theory involves the well-known actions these agents have on fibroblast growth and wound healing. Glucocorticoids can slow the growth of cultured fibroblast cell lines,[123] and in vitro studies clearly demonstrate decreased leukocyte aggregation to several chemotactic factors in the presence of steroids.[124] In addition, steroids decrease adhesion between leukocytes and endothelial cells.[125] Although the mechanism of this inhibition remains unknown, in some neoplastic cell lines dexamethasone has been related to ICAM-1 inhibition.[126] Lastly, steroids alter white blood cell cytotoxic function. In this setting, steroids decrease the

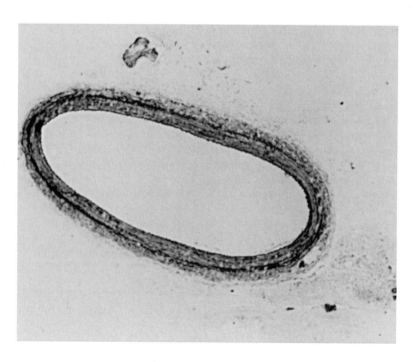

Figure 37–7. Photomicrograph of a carotid artery, 12 weeks after a balloon catheter endothelial injury, demonstrating an absence of significant intimal hyperplasia after treatment for 8 weeks with dexamethasone 0.125 mg/kg. (Verhoeff-van Gieson stain; original magnification ×20.) (From Colburn MD, Moore WS, Gelabert HA, Quiñones-Baldrich WJ: Dose responsive suppression of myointimal hyperplasia by dexamethasone. J Vasc Surg 15:510–518, 1992.)

production of superoxide anions and inhibit the release of zymogen granules.[127]

More recently, our laboratory determined that dexamethasone inhibits smooth muscle cell proliferation in cell culture by means of cell cycle arrest in the late G_1 phase.[128] At present, this effect has been localized to the inhibition of phosphorylation of the retinoblastoma protein.[129] This phosphorylation event is a final common pathway toward cell cycle progression from G_1 into S phase. Efforts continue regarding the potential effects that steroid compounds may have on the migratory activity of the activated smooth muscle cell.

In addition to these experimental data, in vivo studies have suggested a mechanism by which steroids may prevent intimal hyperplasia. In one such study, high-dose methylprednisolone was found to prevent endothelial sloughing in vein grafts.[130] This effect on endothelial sloughing may decrease one of the main stimuli leading to smooth muscle cell activation: an absent endothelium. Finally, dexamethasone has an inhibitory effect on t-PA activity.[131] Therefore, inhibition of medial smooth muscle cell migration may represent another mechanism by which steroids prevent the formation of intimal lesions.

The effect of cyclosporin treatment on the subsequent development of intimal hyperplasia was studied in a rat common iliac artery injury model.[132] Before the arterial injury, animals were given parenteral cyclosporin at a dose of 5 mg/kg/day. The drug was continued for 2 and 6 weeks. Results demonstrated that arteries treated with cyclosporin formed significantly less medial thickening at each time interval. As with steroids, the mechanism of cyclosporin's efficacy in this model has not been characterized. Atherosclerotic plaques contain activated lymphocytes and smooth muscle cells, and these cells do express class II major histocompatibility antigens. Interaction of these antigens and immune cells may propagate an immune response that results in release of other inflammatory mediators and cytokines. Determination of the exact role of the immune system in the evolution of intimal hyperplasia and whether modulation of these pathways will lead to a clinically useful strategy for preventing these lesions requires further investigation.

Antihypertensive Agents

ACE inhibitors, calcium channel blockers, and α_1-adrenergic antagonists are all agents used clinically in the treatment of systemic hypertension. Each of these categories of antihypertensive drugs is also effective in suppressing intimal hyperplasia.

The first study to report the ability of an ACE inhibitor to reduce myointimal proliferation after a vascular injury was reported in a paper by Powell and associates[98] in 1989. In this study, rats were subjected to an endothelial denudation injury using a balloon catheter. Experimental animals received 10 mg/kg of cilazapril mixed with their normal chow beginning 6 days before the endothelial injury. Therapy was continued daily for 14 days. The results showed a significant inhibition of intimal hyperplasia in the treated group, and this effect was independent of any changes in blood pressure. In another study, Clowes and

Reidy observed a reversal of this effect after the intravenous infusion of angiotensin II.[133] In 1991, O'Donohoe and associates[134] reported the inhibition of intimal hyperplasia in experimental vein grafts by the long-term administration of an ACE inhibitor. For this study, a carotid interposition vein graft model was utilized. Experimental animals received oral doses of captopril, 10 mg/kg/day. The drug was started 1 week before grafting and continued until sacrifice at 28 days. Results documented a 40% reduction in intimal thickness compared with that of control animals. Lastly, captopril also causes a significant decrease in aortic atherosclerosis in a heritable hyperlipidemic rabbit model.[135]

Unfortunately, all of these previous in vivo studies relied on oral consumption of the pharmacologic agent. This route of drug administration in any animal model makes the interpretation of the observed results difficult and unreliable. Both captopril and enalapril are available in an injectable form, whereas cilazapril is not. Enalaprilat is an active free metabolite of enalapril and it is the form of the drug that is administered parenterally. Enalaprilat is more potent and much longer acting then the injectable form of captopril, and it is therefore better suited for animal studies in which once-a-day dosing is better tolerated and more practical.[136] Also, the in vivo mechanism of action of captopril is complicated by the fact that, unlike other ACE inhibitors, it contains a sulfhydryl (—SH) group. The (—SH) group can act as a free radical scavenger,[137] and one postulated mechanism for the development of intimal hyperplasia at sites of endothelial injury is the production of free radicals by activated PMNs.[138] At least one study investigating the ability of parenterally administered enalaprilat to inhibit intimal hyperplasia has been completed. The report suggests that this agent is effective in this regard.[139]

Calcium channel antagonists are effective agents used in a variety of cardiovascular disorders. In general, the common mechanism of action of all these agents is interruption of memberane calcium channels, thereby reducing the availability of this cation for a variety of intercellular processes. Calcium has been implicated in several events involved in the development of intimal hyperplasia, including platelet activation, release of PDGF, medial smooth muscle cell proliferation, and formation of extracellular matrix. Treatment with calcium antagonists significantly reduces the development of intimal hyperplasia after mechanical arterial injury.[140] In addition, both verapamil and nimodipine have been effective in reducing intimal hyperplasia in vein bypass graft models.[100, 101]

Another important mediator of vascular tone is the α_1-adrenergic receptor. These receptors are found on vascular smooth muscle cells and, when stimulated, result in profound contraction. Experimental studies have demonstrated that endothelial denudation is accompanied by a selective increase in the sensitivity of the α_1-adrenergic receptor.[141] Also, the cytoplasmic secondary messenger system for this receptor response involves an increase in the turnover of the intracellular phosphatidylinositol cycle.[142] PDGF function has also been linked to an upregulation of the intracellular phosphatidylinositol cycle. Intermediates of this cycle stimulate protein kinase C to initiate a series of phosphorylating reactions that ultimately lead to cellular mitosis.[143] Therefore, the intracellular mechanisms of smooth muscle cell proliferation and contraction are connected through a common cytoplasmic pathway: the phosphatidylinositol cycle. Prazosin is a selective α_1-adrenergic receptor blocker that has been studied for its ability to prevent intimal hyperplasia. In a balloon catheter injury model in the rabbit aorta, prazosin produced a statistically significant reduction in the development of intimal hyperplastic lesions.[97] No clinical trials using this agent have been reported.

Growth Factor Inhibitors

Somatostatin is a widely occurring peptide hormone that acts as a modulator of a diverse class of endogenous growth promoters. If intimal hyperplasia is the result of an imbalance in local vascular autocrine systems after endothelial injury, somatostatin may be effective in limiting this response. Unfortunately, because of storage instability and a very short half-life, somatostatin is unsuitable for use in in vivo models. Angiopeptin is a stable octapeptide somatostatin analog that is an effective long-acting somatostatin receptor agonist. This analog has been extensively studied as a potential inhibitor of intimal hyperplasia.

Several authors have reported the success of angiopeptin in suppressing the development of intimal hyperplasia in animal models.[102–104] In one publication, angiopeptin significantly reduced the degree of post-transplant coronary artery intimal hyperplasia in rabbits.[105] This study was complicated, however, by the fact that these rabbits also received cyclosporin immunosuppression, which, as discussed earlier, also affects the development of hyperplastic lesions. Whether angiopeptin is actually antagonizing the trophic effects of growth promoters in this setting is not clear. In vitro work has also demonstrated the ability of angiopeptin to directly inhibit the proliferation of smooth muscle cells.[144] This suggests that the action of angiopeptin may not be related to an inhibition of the somatostatin receptor. This is further supported by the fact that some somatostatin analogues have not been successful in limiting the intimal hyperplastic response.[104] Nonetheless, the concept of the vascular tree functioning as a complex local hormonal system and the possibility of altering and controlling this balance with pharmacologic therapy remain exciting areas of investigation.

Another approach to inhibiting the effects of peptide mitogens involves use of conjugated toxins. This concept relies on the competitive inhibition of a mitogenic receptor by a "mitotoxin" comprising a specific growth factor that has been bound to a cytotoxin. A potent cellular growth inhibitor has recently been described that competes for the bFGF receptor.[145] This compound is formed by conjugating bFGF to the ribosome-inactivating protein saporin. In one in vivo study, bFGF-saporin caused a marked reduction in the number of replicating smooth muscle cells found in an arterial wall after a denuding injury.[59] Whether this or other conjugated mitotoxins are effective in reducing the degree of intimal hyperplasia after arterial injury requires further investigation.

Finally, rather than inhibiting the effects of peptide growth factors at the level of their membrane-bound receptors, attempts have been made to inhibit cellular growth by interfering with cellular proliferative pathways at the cytoplasmic level. Polyamines are important compounds in the regulation of cell growth and differentiation.[146] Because polyamines are synthesized from ornithine by the action of ornithine decarboxylase (ODC), and because this enzyme constitutes the rate-limiting step in this reaction, ODC inhibition has been postulated as a possible method of preventing cellular proliferation. This concept is supported by the fact that ODC activity increases in tissues undergoing active cell division.[147] The ability of ODC inhibition to reduce the amount of intimal hyperplasia after an arterial injury has been studied in an animal model.[106] In this study, animals treated with the ODC inhibitor α-difluoromethylornithine developed significantly less intimal hyperplasia than did similarly injured controls.

Anticoagulants

Heparin is a naturally occurring polymer containing chains of sulfonated mucopolysaccharides. In vivo, it is concentrated in mast cells and is found in several different tissues, including the endothelium. The length and thus the molecular weight of heparin polymers is highly variable. Furthermore, different-sized polymers have different anticoagulant potency.[148] Because of this variability, heparin has unpredictable biologic activity and is therefore quantified in international units rather than by weight.

Heparin works through its inhibition of the plasmabound proteolytic clotting cascades. Antithrombin III is a potent naturally occurring anticoagulant that inhibits several of the activated coagulant proteins. Heparin polymers of a certain size combine with antithrombin III. This binding greatly enhances the enzymatic action of antithrombin III. Also, because these bound cofactors are not consumed by the inhibition reaction, only a small amount of heparin is required when the plasma load of activated coagulant proteins is moderate. This forms the basis of low-dose heparin therapy for prophylaxis.

Clinically, heparin has been used most frequently in the prophylaxis and treatment of venous thrombosis and pulmonary emboli. A few studies have concluded that perioperative high-dose heparin can prevent early thrombosis in peripheral bypass grafts.[149] This action is presumably due to the drug's ability to shift the balance of the coagulation cascades and counteract the thrombotic forces of low-flow states and thrombogenic surfaces. Heparin also prevents smooth muscle cell migration and proliferation both in vitro and in vivo.[101, 150–154] The mechanism of this action has not yet been established. One theory is that heparin inhibits bFGF, which is released by damaged medial smooth muscle cells.[133] Alternatively, Clowes and Reidy[133] have postulated that heparin inhibits smooth muscle cell migration by interfering with the degradation of the surrounding extracellular matrix. Evidence supporting this view comes from the demonstration that heparin decreases the expression of both t-PA and collagenase in the arterial media.[133] Finally, available data indicate that both anticoagulant and nonanticoagulant fractions of heparin possess this antiproliferative activity.[101] Low-molecular-weight (LMW) heparin is a combination of short-chain heparin polymers with significantly lower anticoagulant activity than standard heparin preparations. Interest in this heparin derivative stems from its potential in modulating intimal hyperplasia without affecting the coagulation system. At least one study has shown that LMW heparin may be effective in this regard.[101]

Insulin-Sensitizing Agents

Aside from the beneficial vascular effects of reducing insulin production through increased sensitization, the thiazolidinediones have proved to have direct inhibitory effects on arterial myointimal hyperplasia. These agents bind to peroxisome proliferator-activated receptors (PPARs), members of the steroid hormone superfamily of nuclear receptors.[155] Troglitazone, a first-generation thiazolidinedione, inhibited intimal hyperplasia after balloon injury in the rat aorta.[156] The mechanism of action relates to the inhibition of mitogen-activated protein (MAP) kinase–dependent nuclear events that in turn block vascular smooth muscle cell migration and proliferation. The ramifications of this effect are not fully appreciated to date, as it is known that PPARs are present on macrophages as well. The influence of thiazolidinediones on early inflammation in myointimal hyperplasia remains to be addressed.

FUTURE DIRECTIONS

Photodynamic Therapy

Another way to view the intimal hyperplastic response is as a process akin to that of a benign neoplastic lesion. In this scheme, the proliferating intimal smooth muscle cell is pictured as an undifferentiated pluripotent medial myofibroblast whose growth continues in the absence of normal cellular controls. The resulting lesion can be considered a form of "vascular keloid." Photodynamic therapy is safe and effective in the treatment of several rapidly growing benign neoplasms. In photodynamic therapy, a chemosensitizing agent is administered to living tissue. Differential absorption and clearance favor selective concentration of the agent in rapidly dividing cells.[157] After exposure to light of a specific wavelength, "photoactivation" results. Once photoactivated, the chemosensitizing agent injures the tissue exposed to the light.

The mechanism by which photodynamic therapy induces cellular toxicity is still being elucidated. Photoactivation of hematoporphyrin derivatives has been hypothesized to result in the formation of oxygen species and other free radicals. These in turn induce several changes, including oxidation of membrane components, alteration of surface charges, and ultimate loss of cell membrane integrity.[158] The initial site of drug accumulation appears to be the cell membrane, but other intracellular organisms such as lysosomes, mitochondria, and nuclei are also affected.[159] Boegheim and colleagues[160] reported that photodynamic therapy inactivates cytosolic, mitochondrial, and lysosomal enzymes, decreases cellular ATP, and reduces glutathione concentration in murine fibroblasts. Enzymes involved in transport across the cell membrane and related to deoxy-

nucleic acid regulation are also inactivated after exposure to light.[160]

Because intimal hyperplasia also involves cells exhibiting increased mitotic activity, photodynamic therapy has been proposed as a means to modulate this hyperplastic response. In 1988, Neave and colleagues[161] reported the destruction of fibrocellular atheromas in the aorta of rabbits treated with dihematoporphyrin ether porphyrin-II. Mackie and colleagues,[162] Hundley and coworkers,[163] and Spears and colleagues[164] have reported that atherosclerotic paque preferentially absorbs hematoporphyrin-II (photofrin) and that photodynamic therapy leads to ablation of only the fibrous portion of the atherosclerotic lesion. These investigators were discouraged that the atherosclerotic plaque could not be ablated completely due to the remaining calcified noncellular material. Nevertheless, these experiments showed that photodynamic therapy could ablate a fibrosclerotic plaque.

The potential for using photodynamic therapy for intimal hyperplasia (rather than atherosclerosis) was perhaps most convincingly suggested by Dartsch and colleagues,[165–167] who showed that human-derived intimal hyperplasia smooth muscle cells preferentially absorbed photofrin-II and that subsequent exposure to light significantly inhibited growth of the photofrin-II–bound cells. Meanwhile, cells derived from normal arteries remained uninhibited in vitro. The ability of human intimal hyperplastic lesions to selectively absorb porphyrin compounds in vivo has not been demonstrated. However, photodynamic therapy remains an intriguing area of investigation in the treatment of intimal hyperplasia.

Modulation of the Immune System

Activated T lymphocytes have already been detected in atherosclerotic plaques.[168] These lymphocytes produce interferon-γ and various interleukins that promote expression of class II major histocompatibility antigens and perpetuate the immune response. The contribution of inflammatory mediators to the pathophysiology of intimal hyperplasia has already been discussed. These same pathways might be manipulated to control these same processes. Immunotherapy for a variety of neoplastic conditions has emerged as an exciting new area of research. The basic idea of programming the body's own immune defenses against specific antigens located on the surface of offending tumor cells is likely to be applicable to other conditions.

With increased information regarding the biologic pathways controlling leukocyte activation, specifically blocking the receptors responsible for stimulating the development of intimal hyperplasia without inhibiting the systemic inflammatory response will likely soon be possible. A murine IgG monoclonal antibody, MoAb 60.3, binds the CD18 epitope on the surface of leukocytes. This antibody reduces PMN-mediated tissue injury in a variety of physiologic settings. Administration of MoAb 60.3 to rabbits has reduced PMN adherence and prevented PMN tissue migration.[169] Of concern, however, is that patients exposed to this antibody could develop a symptom complex similar to that found in leukocyte adhesion molecule deficiency. In this disorder, the CD18 subunit is lacking and affected individuals suffer from severe recurrent bacterial infections and abnormal wound healing. Monoclonal antibody therapy directed at the leukocyte-binding adhesion molecules that are expressed on the surface of vascular endothelial cells constitutes another, perhaps more promising, approach. This more specific therapy may reduce the severity of any adverse systemic effects of PMN inhibition. Several antibodies that recognize both the ELAM-1 and ICAM-1 complexes have already been developed and are potential candidates for this type of anti-intimal hyperplasia therapy. Despite the fact that these alternative approaches have not been specifically tested, they remain an exciting area of potential future research.

In Vivo Gene Transfer

The development of the technology to transfer genetic material into human vascular cells has opened up new frontiers in the treatment of vascular disorders. Gene transfer methods are yielding important information regarding the biology of several types of vascular cells, and treatment strategies for problems such as thrombosis, atherosclerosis, vasculitis, and restenosis are already being devised.

The basic technique involves the introduction of new genetic material into the genome of various vascular cells. These genetically engineered cells subsequently express specific proteins or traits for which they have been programmed that ultimately alter the local biology of the vessel wall. The endothelial cell is often proposed as the ideal recipient for human gene therapy. This is largely due to its accessibility to recombinant vectors, as well as the possibility for any produced products to be secreted directly into the blood stream. Furthermore, endothelial seeding of vascular grafts and stents is an area of research that is currently in relatively advanced stages of development. Gene transfer into vascular endothelial cells has primarily been accomplished by one of two different methods. The first method involves the introduction of genes into cultured endothelial cells in vitro. Later, these "engineered" cells are reintroduced into the vessel wall of the recipient. Alternatively, in vivo gene transfer into the vessel wall has been performed by injecting the genetic material directly into the lumen of the host vessel. This method requires either a retroviral or plasmid vector to successfully transfer the new genes.

Several in vitro experiments have documented the ability to transfer specific genes into cultured endothelial cells.[170–172] In these studies, genes coding for neomycin resistance,[170, 172] β-galactosidase,[171, 172] growth hormone,[170] PGI,[172] and t-PA[171] have all been successfully expressed. Furthermore, transduced endothelial cells grow on both vascular prostheses[170] and stainless steel stents.[171]

Recombinant gene expression by transduced endothelial cells has also been achieved in vivo. In a series of experiments, Nabel and associates[173, 174] have successfully transferred the genes responsible for β-galactosidase production into iliofemoral arterial segments of pigs. These investigators have documented detectable levels of the transduced gene in this model for as long as 5 months.[174] The ability of avascular graft lined with genetically modified endothelial cells to maintain activity of the transduced gene has also been demonstrated.[175] In this study, grafts continued to express the β-galactosidase gene for up to 5 weeks after implantation. Furthermore, this activity was documented in both the seeded cells and their progeny.

The potential of genetically engineered vascular cells to modify the vessel wall and affect the development of vascular disorders is clear, and research in this area is rapidly progressing. However, several problems with this technology must still be overcome and, as with any new area of research, perplexing questions are as frequent as are new advances. For example, the use of retroviral vectors limits the size of the gene that can be transduced. Also, transduction rates using these methods remain quite low and alternative methods to improve the efficiency of this process are needed. Areas requiring further investigation include the effect of transduced genes on the function of host cells, the duration of activity of these genes within the host cells, and the potential of foreign genetic material to induce a host immunologic response. Nonetheless, the potential exists for this technology to someday play a role in altering the complex pathways leading to the development of intimal hyperplasia.

References

1. Imparato AM, Bracco A, Kim GFE: Intimal and neointimal fibrous proliferation causing failure of arterial reconstruction. Surgery 72:1007–1017, 1972.
2. Veith FJ, Gupta SK, Ascer E: Six-year prospective multicenter randomized comparison of autologous saphenous vein and expanded polytetrafluoroethylene grafts in infrainguinal arterial reconstructions. J Vasc Surg 3:104–114, 1986.
3. Fitzgibbon GM, Leach AJ, Kafka HP, Keon WJ: Coronary bypass graft fate: Long-term angiographic study. J Am Coll Cardiol 17:1075–1080, 1991.
4. Carrel A, Guthrie CC: Anastomosis of blood vessels by the patching method and transplantation of the kidney. JAMA 47:1648–1651, 1906.
5. Spaet TH, Stemerman MB, Veith FJ, Lejnieks I: Intimal injury and regrowth in the rabbit aorta: Medial smooth muscle cells as a source of neointima. Circ Res 36:58–70, 1975.
6. Clowes AW, Schwartz SM: Significance of quiescent smooth muscle migration in the injured rat carotid artery. Circ Res 56:139–145, 1985.
7. Clowes AW, Clowes MM, Fingerle J, Reidy MA: Regulation of smooth muscle cell growth in injured artery. J Cardiovasc Pharmacol 14(Suppl 6):S12–S15, 1989.
8. Chervu A, Moore WS: An overview of intimal hyperplasia. Surg Gynecol Obstet 171:433–447, 1990.
9. Rittgers SE, Karayannacos PE, Guy JF, et al: Velocity distribution and intimal proliferation in autologous vein grafts in dogs. Circ Res 42:792–801, 1978.
10. Morinaga K, Okadome K, Kuroki M, et al: Effect of wall shear stress on intimal thickening of arterially transplanted autogenous veins in dogs. J Vasc Surg 2:430–433, 1985.
11. Sottiurai VS, Kollros P, Glagov S, et al: Morphological alteration of cultured arterial smooth muscle cells by cyclic stretching. J Surg Res 35:490–497, 1983.
12. Imparato AM, Baumann FG, Pearson J, et al: Electron microscopic studies of experimentally produced fibromuscular arterial lesions. Surg Gynecol Obstet 139:497–504, 1976.
13. Bond MG, Hostetler JR, Karayannacos PE, et al: Intimal changes in arteriovenous bypass grafts: Effects of varying the angle of implan-

tation at the proximal anastomosis and of producing stenosis in the distal runoff artery. J Thorac Cardiovasc Surg 71:907–916, 1976.

14. Berguer R, Higgins RF, Reddy DJ: Intimal hyperplasia: An experimental study. Arch Surg 115:332–335, 1980.

15. Zarins CK, Zatina MA, Giddens DP, et al: Shear stress regulation of artery lumen diameter in experimental atherogenesis. J Vasc Surg 5:413–420, 1987.

16. Caro CG, Fitz-Gerald JM, Schroter RC: Arterial wall shear: Observation, correlation and proposal of a shear dependent mass transfer mechanism for atherogenesis. Proc R Soc Lond B Biol Sci 177:109–159, 1971.

17. Fry DL: Acute vascular endothelial changes associated with increased blood velocity gradients. Circ Res 22:165–167, 1968.

18. LoGerfo FW, Nowak MD, Quist WC, et al: Flow studies in a model carotid bifurcation. Atherosclerosis 1:235–241, 1981.

19. Phillips DJ, Greene FM, Langlois Y, et al: Flow velocity patterns in the carotid bifurcations of young, presumed normal subjects. Ultrasound Med Biol 9:39–49, 1983.

20. Abbott WM, Megerman J, Hasson JE, et al: Effect of compliance mismatch on vascular graft patency. J Vasc Surg 5:376–382, 1987.

21. Lye CR, Sumner DS, Strandness DE: The transcutaneous measurement of the elastic properties of the human saphenous vein femoropopliteal bypass graft. Surg Gynecol Obstet 141:891–895, 1975.

22. Hokanson DE, Strandness DE: Stress-strain characteristics of various arterial grafts. Surg Gynecol Obstet 127:57–60, 1968.

23. Miller JH, Foreman RK, Ferguson L, Faris A: Interposition vein cuff for anastomosis of prosthesis to small artery. Aust N Z J Surg 54:283–285, 1984.

24. Corson JD, Leather RP, Balko A, et al: Relationship between vasa vasorum and blood flow to vein bypass endothelial morphology. Arch Surg 120:386–388, 1985.

25. Abbott WM, Weiland S, Austen WG: Structural changes during preparation of autogenous venous grafts. Surgery 76:1031–1040, 1974.

26. Bang HO, Dyerberg J, Nielsen A: Plasma lipid and lipoprotein pattern in greenlandic West-coast Eskimos. Lancet 1:1143–1145, 1971.

27. Brown MS, Faust JR, Goldstein JL: Role of the low density lipoprotein receptor in regulating the content of free and esterified cholesterol in human fibroblasts. J Clin Invest 55:783–793, 1975.

28. Goldstein JL, Brown MS: The low-density lipoprotein pathway and its relation to atherosclerosis. Annu Rev Biochem 46:897–930, 1977.

29. Wissler RW: Biochemistry of Artherosclerosis, vol 7. New York, Marcel Dekker, 1979, p 345.

30. Barrett T, Benditt E: Platelet-derived growth factor gene expression in human atherosclerotic plaques and in normal artery wall. Proc Natl Acad Sci U S A 85:2810–2814, 1988.

31. Libby P, Warner S, Salomon R, Birinyi L: Production of platelet-derived growth factor–like mitogen by smooth muscle cells from human atheroma. N Engl J Med 318:1493–1498, 1988.

32. Cole C, Lucas J, Mikat E, et al: Adherence of polymorphonuclear leukocytes to injured rabbit aorta. Surg Forum 35:440–442, 1984.

33. Shimokado K, Raines E, Madtes D, et al: A significant part of macrophage-derived growth factor consists of at least two forms of PDGF. Cell 43:277–286, 1988.

34. Prescott MF, McBride CK, Venturini CM, Gerhardt SC: Leukocyte stimulation of intimal lesion formation is inhibited by treatment with diclofenac sodium and dexamethasone. J Cardiovasc Pharmacol 14(Suppl 6):S76–S81, 1989.

35. Lucas J, Makhoul R, Cole C, et al: Mononuclear cells adhere to sites of vascular balloon catheter injury. Current Surgery 43:112–115, 1986.

36. Mazzone T, Jensen M, Chait A: Human arterial wall cells secrete factors that are chemotactic for monocytes. Proc Natl Acad Sci U S A 80:5094–5097, 1983.

37. Swales JD, Thurston H: Generation of angiotensin II of peripheral vascular level: Studies using angiotensin II antisera. Clin Sci 45:691–700, 1973.

38. Dzau VJ: Vascular angiotensin pathways: A new therapeutic target. J Cardiovasc Pharmacol 10(Suppl 7):S9–S16, 1987.

39. Campbell DJ, Habener JF: Angiotensinogen gene is expressed and differentially regulated in multiple tissues of the rat. J Clin Invest 78:31–39, 1986.

40. Campbell DJ: Tissue renin-angiotensin system: Sites of angiotensin formation. J Cardiovasc Pharmacol 10(Suppl 7):S1–S8, 1987.

41. Molteni A, Dzau VJ, Fallon JT, Haber E: Monoclonal antibodies as probes of renin gene expression. Circulation 70(Suppl II):II-196, 1984.

42. Re R, Fallon JT, Dzau VJ, Ouay SC, Haber E: Renin synthesis by canine aortic smooth muscle cells in culture. Life Sci 30:99–106, 1982.

43. Lilly LS, Pratt RE, Alexander RW, et al: Renin expression by vascular endothelial cells in culture. Circ Res 57:312–318, 1985.

44. Ohashi H, Matsunaga N, Pak CH, Kawai C: Serial change in renin release by the cultured human vascular smooth muscle cells. J Hypertension 4(Suppl 6):S472–S473, 1986.

45. Drouet L, Baudin B, Baumann FC, Caen JP: Serum angiotensin-converting enzyme: An endothelial cell marker. J Lab Clin Med 112:450–457, 1988.

46. Penit J, Faure M, Jard S: Vasopressin and angiotensin II receptors in rat aortic smooth muscle cells in culture. Am J Physiol 244:E72–E82, 1983.

47. Griendling K, Tsuda T, Berk BC, Alexander RW: Angiotensin II stimulation of vascular smooth muscle. J Cardiovasc Pharmacol 14(Suppl 6):S27–S33, 1989.

48. Moore T, Williams G: Angiotensin II receptors on human platelets. Circ Res 51:314–320, 1982.

49. Gimbrone M, Alexander RW: Angiotensin II stimulation of prostaglandin production in cultured human vascular endothelium. Science 189:219–220, 1975.

50. Toda N: Endothelium-dependent relaxion induced by angiotensin II and histamine in isolated arteries of dog. Br J Pharmacol 81:301–307, 1984.

51. Campbell-Boswell M, Robertson AL: Effects of angiotensin II and vasopressin on human smooth muscle cells in vitro. Exp Mol Pathol 35:265, 1981.

52. Geisterfer AA, Peach MJ, Owens JK: Angiotensin II induces hypertrophy, not hyperplasia, of cultured rat aortic smooth muscle cells. Circ Res 62:749–756, 1988.

53. Jackson TR, Blair LAC, Marshall J, et al: The mas oncogene encodes an angiotensin receptor. Nature 335:437–440, 1988.

54. Swartz S, Moore T: Effect of angiotensin II on collagen-induced platelet activation in normotensive subjects. Thromb Haemost 63:87–90, 1990.

55. Naftilan AJ, Pratt RE, Dzau VJ: Induction of platelet-derived growth factor A-chain and c-myc gene expressions by angiotensin II in cultured rat vascular smooth muscle cells. J Clin Invest 83:1419–1424, 1989.

56. Clowes AW, Reidy MA, Clowes MM: Kinetics of cellular proliferation after arterial injury, I: Smooth muscle growth in the absence of endothelium. Lab Invest 49:327–333, 1983.

57. Fingerle J, Au YPT, Clowes AW, Reidy MA: Intimal lesion formation in the rat carotid arteries after endothelial denudation in the absence of medial injury. Arteriosclerosis 10:1082–1087, 1990.

58. Fingerle J, Johnson R, Clowes AW, et al: Role of platelets in smooth muscle proliferation and migration after vascular injury in rat carotid artery. Proc Natl Acad Sci U S A 86:8412–8416, 1989.

59. Lindner V, Lappi DA, Baird A, et al: Role of basic fibroblast growth factor in vascular lesion formation. Circ Res 68:106–113, 1991.

60. Cuevas P, Gonzalez AM, Carceller F, Baird A: Vascular response to basic fibroblast growth factor when infused onto the normal adventitia or into the injured media of the rat carotid artery. Circ Res 69:360–369, 1991.

61. Garg UC, Hassid A: Nitic oxide–generating vasodilators and 8-bromo-cyclic guanosine monophosphate inhibit mitogenesis and proliferation of cultured rat vascular smooth muscle cells. J Clin Invest 83:1774–1777, 1989.

62. Clowes AW, Collazzo RE, Karnovsky MJ: A morphologic and permeability study of luminal smooth muscle cells after arterial injury in the rat. Lab Invest 39:141–150, 1978.

63. Werb Z, Mainardi C, Vater CA, Harris ED: Endogenous activation of latent collagenase by rheumatoid synovial cells: Evidence for a role of plasminogen activator. N Engl J Med 296:1017–1023, 1977.

64. Levin EG, Loskutoff DJ: Comparative studies of the fibrinolytic activity of cultured vascular cells. Thromb Res 15:869–878, 1979.

65. Goldsmith GH, Ziats NP, Robertson AL: Studies on plasminogen activator and other proteases in subcultured human vascular cells. Exp Mol Pathol 35:257–264, 1981.

66. Clowes AW, Clowes MM, Au YPT, et al: Smooth muscle cells express urokinase during mitogenesis and tissue-type plasminogen activator

during migration in injured rat carotid artery. Circ Res 67:61–67, 1990.

67. Hoch JR, Stark VK, Turnipseed WD: The temporal relationship between the development of vein graft intimal hyperplasia and growth factor gene expression. J Vasc Surg 22:51–58, 1995.

68. Stark VK, Warner TF, Hoch JR: An ultrastructural study of progressive intimal hyperplasia in rat vein grafts. J Vasc Surg 26:94–103, 1997.

69. Stark VK, Hoch JR, Warner TF, Hullett DA: Monocyte chemotactic protein-1 is associated with the development of vein graft intimal hyperplasia. Arterioscler Thromb Vasc Biol 17:1614–1621, 1997.

70. Hoch JR, Stark VK, van Rooijen N, et al: Macrophage depletion alters vein graft intimal hyperplasia. Surgery 126:428–437, 1999.

71. Faries PL, Marin ML, Veith FJ, et al: Immunolocalization and temporal distribution of cytokine expression during the development of vein graft intimal hyperplasia in an experimental model. J Vasc Surg 24:463–471, 1996.

72. Kraiss LW, Clowes AW: Response of the arterial wall to injury and intimal hyperplasia. In Sidaway AN, Sumpio BE, DePalma RG (eds): The Basic Science of Vascular Disease, Armonk, NY, Futura, 1997, pp 289–317.

73. Dalman RL, Taylor LM Jr: Basic data related to infrainguinal revascularization procedures. Ann Vasc Surg 3:309–312, 1990.

74. Szilagyi DE, Elliott JP, Hageman JH, et al: Biologic fate of autologous vein implants as arterial substitutes: Clinical, angiographic and histologic observations in femoropopliteal operations for atherosclerosis. Ann Surg 178:232–246, 1973.

75. Stoney RJ, String ST: Recurrent carotid stenosis. Surgery 80:705–710, 1976.

76. Cossman D, Callow AD, Stein A, Matsumoto G: Early restenosis after carotid endarterectomy. Arch Surg 113:275–278, 1978.

77. Kremen JE, Gee W, Kaupp HA, McDonald KM: Restenosis or occlusion after carotid endarterectomy: A survey with ocular pneumoplethysmography. Arch Surg 114:608–610, 1979.

78. Hertzer NR, Martinez BD, Benjamin SP, Beven EG: Recurrent stenosis after carotid endarterectomy. Surg Gynecol Obstet 149:360–364, 1979.

79. Cossman DV, Treiman RL, Foran RF, et al: Surgical approach to recurrent carotid stenosis. Am J Surg 140:209–211, 1980.

80. Catelmo NL, Cutler BS, Wheeler HB, et al: Noninvasive detection of carotid stenosis following endarterectomy. Arch Surg 116:1005–1008, 1981.

81. Zierler RE, Bandyk DF, Thiele BL, Strandness DE: Carotid artery stenosis following endarterectomy. Arch Surg 117:1408–1415, 1982.

82. Baker WH, Hayes AC, Mahler D, Littooy FN: Durability of carotid endarterectomy. Surgery 94:112–115, 1983.

83. Salvian A, Baker JD, Machleder HI, et al: Cause and noninvasive detection of restenosis after carotid endarterectomy. Am J Surg 146:29–34, 1983.

84. Pierce GE, Iliopoulus JI, Holcomb MA, et al: Incidence of recurrent stenosis after carotid endarterectomy determined by digital subtraction angiography. Am J Surg 148:848–854, 1984.

85. O'Donnell TF, Callow AD, Scott G, et al: Ulrasound characteristics of recurrent carotid disease: Hypothesis explaining the low incidence of symptomatic recurrence. J Vasc Surg 2:26–41, 1985.

86. Wilson SE, Sheppard B: Results of percutaneous transluminal angioplasty for peripheral vascular occlusive disease. Ann Vasc Surg 4:94–97, 1990.

87. White RA, White GH, Mehringer MC: A clinical trial of laser thermal angioplasty in patients with advanced peripheral vascular disease. Ann Surg 212:257–265, 1990.

88. Ahn SS, Eton D, Mehigan JT: Preliminary clinical results of rotary atherectomy. In Yao JST, Pearce WH (eds): Technologies in Vascular Surgery. Philadelphia, WB Saunders, 1992, pp 388–401.

89. Cahill PD, Sarris GE, Cooper AD, et al: Inhibition of vein graft intimal thickening by eicosapentaenoic acid: Reduced thromboxane production without change in lipoprotein levels or low-density lipoprotein receptor density. J Vasc Surg 7:108–117, 1988.

90. Landymore RW, Manku MS, Tan M, et al: Effects of low-dose marine oils on intimal hyperplasia in autologous vein grafts. J Thorac Cardiovasc Surg 98:788–791, 1989.

91. O'Hara M, Esato K, Harada M, et al: Eicosapentaenoic acid suppresses intimal hyperplasia after expanded polytetrafluoroethylene grafting in rabbits fed a high cholesterol diet. J Vasc Surg 13:480–486, 1991.

92. Quiñones-Baldrich W, Ziomek S, Henderson T, Moore W: Patency and intimal hyperplasia: The effect of aspirin on small arterial anastomosis. Ann Vasc Surg 2:50–56, 1988.

93. Landymore RW, Karmazyn M, MacAulay MA, et al: Correlation between the effects of aspirin and dipyridamole on platelet function and prevention of intimal hyperplasia in autologous vein grafts. Can J Cardiol 4:56–59, 1988.

94. Radic ZS, O'Malley MK, Mikat EM, et al: The role of aspirin and dipyridamole on vascular DNA synthesis and intimal hyperplasia following deendothelialization. J Surg Res 41:84–91, 1986.

95. Chervu A, Moore WS, Quiñones-Baldrich WJ, Henderson T: Efficacy of corticosteroids in suppression of intimal hyperplasia. J Vasc Surg 10:129–134, 1989.

96. Hoepp LM, Elbadawi A, Cohn M, et al: Steroids and immunosuppression: Effect on anastomotic intimal hyperplasia in femoral arterial Dacron bypass grafts. Arch Surg 114:273–276, 1979.

97. O'Malley MK, McDermott EW, Mehigan D, O'Higgins NJ: Role for prazosin in reducing the development of rabbit intimal hyperplasia after endothelial denudation. Br J Surg 76:936–938, 1989.

98. Powell JS, Clozel JP, Müller RK, et al: Inhibitors of angiotensin-converting enzyme prevent myointimal proliferation after vascular injury. Science 245:186–188, 1989.

99. El-Sanadiki MN, Cross KS, Murray JJ, et al: Reduction of intimal hyperplasia and enhanced reactivity of experimental vein bypass grafts with verapamil. Ann Surg 212:87–96, 1990.

100. Guyotat J, Pelissou-Guyotat I, Lievre M, Chignier E: Inhibition of subintimal hyperplasia of autologous vein bypass grafts by nimodipine in rats: A placebo-controlled study. Neurosurgery 29:850–855, 1991.

101. Dryjski M, Mikat E, Bjornsson TD: Inhibition of intimal hyperplasia after arterial injury by heparins and heparinoid. J Vasc Surg 8:623–633, 1988.

102. Calcagno D, Conte JV, Howell MH, Foegh ML: Peptide inhibition of neointimal hyperplasia in vein grafts. J Vasc Surg 13:475–479, 1991.

103. Conte JV, Foegh ML, Calcagno D, et al: Peptide inhibition of myointimal proliferation following angioplasty in rabbits. Transplant Proc 21:3686–3688, 1989.

104. Lundergan C, Foegh ML, Vargas R, et al: Inhibition of myointimal proliferation of the rat carotid artery by the peptides, angiopeptin and BIM 23034. Atherosclerosis 80:49–55, 1989.

105. Foegh ML, Khirabadi BS, Chambers E, et al: Inhibition of coronary artery transplant atherosclerosis in rabbits with angiopeptin, an octapeptide. Atherosclerosis 78:229–236, 1989.

106. Endean ED, Kispert JF, Martin KW, O'Connor W: Intimal hyperplasia is reduced by ornithine decarboxylase inhibition. J Surg Res 50:634–637, 1991.

107. Ryan US, Whitaker C, Hart MA, et al: Structural interaction between endothelial and smooth muscle cells [abstract]. J Cell Biol 79:207a, 1979.

108. Baumgartner HR: Eine neue Methode zur Erzeugung von Thromben durch gezielte Überdehnung der Gefässwand. Z Ges Exp Med 137:227, 1963.

109. Clowes AW, Clowes MM, Reidy MA: Role of acute distension in the induction of smooth muscle proliferation after arterial denudation [abstract]. FASEB J 46:270, 1987.

110. Dyerberg J, Bang HO, Stoffersen E, et al: Eicosapentaenoic acid and prevention of thrombosis and atherosclerosis. Lancet 2:117–119, 1978.

111. Friedman RJ, Stemerman MB, Wenz B, et al: The effect of thrombocytopenia on experimental arteriosclerotic lesion formation in rabbits: Smooth muscle cell proliferation and reendothelialization. J Clin Invest 60:1191–1201, 1977.

112. McCollum C, Crow M, Rajah S, Kester R: Anti-thrombotic therapy for vascular prosthesis: An experimental model testing platelet inhibitory drugs. Surgery 87:668–676, 1980.

113. Oblath R, Buckley F, Green R, et al: Prevention of platelet aggregation to prosthetic vascular grafts by aspirin and dipyridamole. Surgery 84:37–44, 1978.

114. Zammit M, Kaplan S, Sauvage L, et al: Aspirin therapy in small-caliber arterial prostheses: Long-term experimental observations. J Vasc Surg 1:839–851, 1984.

115. Plate G, Stanson A, Hollier L, Dewanjee M: Drug effects on platelet deposition after endothelial injury of the rabbit aorta. J Surg Res 39:258–266, 1985.

116. McCann R, Hagen P-O, Fuchs J: Aspirin and dipyridamole decrease intimal hyperplasia in experimental vein grafts. Ann Surg 191:238–243, 1980.

117. Graham LM, Brothers TE, Darvishian D, et al: Effects of thromboxane synthetase inhibition on patency and anastomotic hyperplasia of vascular grafts. J Surg Res 46:611–615, 1989.

118. Hanson S, Pareti F, Ruggeri Z, et al: Antibody-induced platelet inhibition reduces thrombus formation in vivo. Clin Res 34:658, 1986.

119. Torem S, Schneide P, Hanson S: Monoclonal antibody–induced inhibition of platelet function: Effects on hemostasis and vascular graft thrombosis in baboons. J Vasc Surg 7:172–180, 1988.

120. Gordon GB, Bush DE, Weisman HF: Reduction of atherosclerosis by administration of dehydroepiandrosterone. J Clin Invest 82:712–720, 1988.

121. Pepine CJ, Hirshfeld JW, Macdonald RG, et al: A controlled trial of corticosteroids to prevent restenosis after coronary angioplasty. Circulation 81:1753–1761, 1990.

122. Colburn MD, Moore WS, Gelabert HA, Quiñones-Baldrich WJ: Dose responsive suppression of myointimal hyperplasia by dexamethasone. J Vasc Surg 15:510–518, 1992.

123. Ruhmann AG, Berliner DL: Effect of steroids on growth of mouse fibroblasts in vitro. Endocrinology 76:916–927, 1965.

124. Majeski JA, Alexander JW: The steroid effect on the in vitro human neutrophil chemotactic response. J Surg Res 21:265–271, 1976.

125. Mishler J: The effects of corticosteroids on mobilization and function of neutrophils. Exp Hematol 5:15–32, 1977.

126. Hess AD, Esa AH, Colombani PM, et al: Mechanisms of action of cyclosporin: Effect on cells of the immune system and on subcellular events in T-cell activation. Transplant Proc 20(Suppl 2):29, 1988.

127. Goldstein I, Roos D, Weissmann G, Kaplan H: Influence of corticosteroids on human polymorphonuclear leukocyte function in vitro enzyme release and superoxide production. Inflammation 1:305–315, 1976.

128. Reil TD, Sarkar R, Kashyap VS, et al: Dexamethasone suppresses vascular smooth muscle cell proliferation. J Surg Res 85:109–114, 1999.

129. Reil TD, Kashyap VS, Sarkar R, et al: Dexamethasone inhibits the phosphorylation of retinoblastoma protein in the suppression of human vascular smooth muscle cell proliferation. J Surg Res 92:108–113, 2000.

130. Pearce J, Dujovny M, Ho K, et al: Acute inflammation and endothelial injury in vein grafts. Neurosurgery 17:626–634, 1985.

131. Cwikel BJ, Barouski-Miller PA, Coleman PL, Gelehrter TD: Dexamethasone induction of an inhibitor of plasminogen activator in HTC hepatoma cells. J Biol Chem 259:6847–6851, 1984.

132. Wengrovitz M, Selassie LG, Gifford RRM, Thiele BL: Cyclosporine inhibits the development of medial thickening after experimental arterial injury. J Vasc Surg 12:1–7, 1990.

133. Clowes AW, Reidy MA: Prevention of stenosis after vascular reconstruction: Pharmacologic control of intimal hyperplasia—a review. J Vasc Surg 13:885–891, 1991.

134. O'Donohoe MK, Schwartz LB, Radic ZS, et al: Chronic ACE inhibition reduces intimal hyperplasia in experimental vein grafts. Ann Surg 214:727–732, 1991.

135. Chobanian AV, Haudenschild CC, Nickerson C, Drago R: Antiatherogenic effect of captopril in the watanabe heritable hyperlipidemic rabbit. Hypertension 15:327–331, 1990.

136. Cushman DW, Ondetti MA, Gordon EM, et al: Rational design and biochemical utility of specific inhibitors of angiotensin-converting enzyme. J Cardiovasc Pharmacol 10(Suppl 7):S17–S30, 1987.

137. Chopra M, Scott N, McMurray J, et al: Captopril: A free radical scavenger. Br J Clin Pharmacol 27:396–399, 1989.

138. Sacks T, Moldow C, Craddock P, Bowers T: Oxygen radicals mediate endothelial cell damage by complement-stimulated granulocytes: An in vitro model of immune vascular damage. J Clin Invest 61:1161–1167, 1978.

139. Law MM, Colburn MD, Hajjar GE, et al: Suppression of intimal hyperplasia in a rabbit model of arterial balloon injury by enalaprilat but not dimethyl sulfoxide. Ann Vasc Surg 8:158–165, 1994.

140. El-Sanadiki M, Cross K, Mikat E, Hagen P-O: Verapamil therapy reduces intimal hyperplasia in balloon injured rabbit aorta. Circulation 76(Suppl):314, 1987.

141. O'Malley MK, Mikat EM, McCann RL, Hagen P-O: Increased vascular sensitivity to norepinephrine following injury. Surg Forum 35:445–447, 1984.

142. O'Malley M, Cotecchia S, Hagen P-O: Receptor mediated noradrenaline supersensitivity in rabbit aortic intimal hyperplasia. Eur Surg Res 18:43, 1986.

143. Mark J: The polyphosphoinositides revisited. Science 228:312–313, 1985.

144. Vargas R, Bormes GW, Wroblewska B, et al: Angiopeptin inhibits thymidine incorporation in rat carotid artery in vitro. Transplant Proc 21:3702–3704, 1989.

145. Lappi DA, Martineau D, Baird A: Biological and chemical characterization of basic FGF-saporin mitotoxin. Biochem Biophys Res Commun 160:917–923, 1989.

146. Pegg AE, McCann PP: Polyamine metabolism and function. Am J Physiol 243:C212–C221, 1982.

147. Heby O, Gray JW, Lindl PA, et al: Changes in L-ornithine decarboxylase activity during the cell cycle. Biochem Biophys Res Commun 71:99–105, 1976.

148. Cifonelli J: The relationship of molecular weight, and sulfate content and distribution to anticoagulant activity of heparin preparations. Carbohydr Res 37:145–154, 1974.

149. Schweiger H, Klein P, Ruf S, Meister R: Avoiding early failure of tibial prosthetic bypass grafts. Thorac Cardiovasc Surg 35:148–150, 1987.

150. Hoover RL, Rosenberg R, Haering W, Karnovsky MJ: Inhibition of rat arterial smooth muscle cell proliferation by heparin II: In vitro studies. Circ Res 47:578–583, 1980.

151. Majack RA, Clowes AW: Inhibition of vascular smooth muscle cell migration by heparin-like glycosaminoglycans. J Cell Physiol 118:253–256, 1984.

152. Clowes AW, Clowes MM: Kinetics of cellular proliferation after arterial injury, II: Inhibition of smooth muscle growth by heparin. Lab Invest 52:611–616, 1985.

153. Clowes AW, Clowes MM: Kinetics of cellular proliferation after arterial injury, IV: Heparin inhibits rat smooth muscle mitogenesis and migration. Circ Res 58:839–845, 1986.

154. Majesky MW, Schwartz SM, Clowes MM, Clowes AW: Heparin regulates smooth muscle S phase entry in the injured rat carotid artery. Circ Res 61:296–300, 1987.

155. Hsueh WA, Law RE: Diabetes is a vascular disease. J Invest Med 46:387–390, 1998.

156. Law RE, Meehan WP, Xi XP, et al: Troglitazone inhibits vascular smooth muscle cell growth and intimal hyperplasia. J Clin Invest 98:1897–1905, 1996.

157. Figge F, Wieland G, Manganiello L: Cancer detection and therapy. Affinity of neoplastic, embryonic, and traumatized tissue for porphyrins and metalloporphyrins. Proc Soc Exp Biol Med 68:640–641, 1948.

158. Weishaupt KR, Gomer CJ, Dougherty TJ: Identification of single oxygen as the cytotoxic agent in photo-inactivation of a murine tumor. Cancer Res 36:2326–2329, 1976.

159. Kessel D: Porphyrin localization: A new modality for detection and therapy of tumors. Biochem Pharmacol 33:1389–1393, 1984.

160. Boegheim JPJ, Scholte H, Dubbleman TMAR: Photodynamic effects of hematoporphyrin-derivative on enzyme activities of murine L929 fibroblasts. J Photochem Photobiol 1:61–73, 1987.

161. Neave V, Giannotta S, Hyman S, Schneider J: Hematoporphyrin uptake in atherosclerotic plaques: Therapeutic potentials. Neurosurgery 23:307–312, 1988.

162. Mackie RW, Vincent GM, Fox J, et al: In vivo canine coronary artery laser irradiation: Photodynamic therapy using dihematoporphyrin ether and 632 nm laser: A safety and dose-response relationship study. Lasers Surg Med 11:535–544, 1991.

163. Hundley RF, Weinstein R, Spears JR: Photodynamic cytolysis of rat arterial smooth muscle cells with hematoporphyrin derivative in vitro. Lasers Life Sci 2:19–27, 1988.

164. Spears JR, Serur J, Shopshire D, et al: Fluorescence of experimental atheromatous plaques with hematoporphyrin derivative. J Clin Invest 71:395–399, 1983.

165. Dartsch PC, Ischinger T, Betz E: Differential effect of photofrin II on growth of human smooth muscle cells from nonatherosclerotic arteries and atheromatous plaques in vitro. Arteriosclerosis 10:616–624, 1990.

166. Dartsch PC, Ischinger T, Betz E: Responses of cultured smooth muscle cells from human nonatherosclerotic arteries and primary stenosing lesions after photoradiation: Implications for photodynamic therapy of vascular stenoses. J Am Coll Cardiol 15:1545–1550, 1990.

167. Dartsch PC, Betz E, Ischinger T: Effect of dihematoporphyrin derivatives on cultivated human smooth muscle cells from normal and atherosclerotic vascular segments: Overview of results and implications for photodynamic therapy. Z Kardiol 80:6–14, 1991.

168. Hansson GK, Holm J, Jonasson L: Detection of activated T lymphocytes in the human atherosclerotic plaque. Am J Pathol 135:169–175, 1989.

169. Arfors KE, Lundberg C, Lindbom L, et al: A monoclonal antibody to the membrane glycoprotein complex CD18 inhibits polymorphonuclear accumulation and plasma leakage in vivo. Blood 69:338–340, 1987.

170. Zwiebel JA, Freeman SM, Kantoff PW, et al: High-level recombinant gene expression in rabbit endothelial cells transduced by retroviral vectors. Science 243:220–222, 1989.

171. Dichek DA, Neville RF, Zwiebel JA, et al: Seeding of intravascular stents with genetically engineered endothelial cells. Circulation 80:1347–1353, 1989.

172. Brothers TE, Stanley JC: Impact of genetic engineering on vascular disease and biology. In Veith FJ (ed): Current Critical Problems in Vascular Surgery. St Louis, Quality Medical, 1990, pp 42–50.

173. Nabel EG, Plautz G, Boyce FM, et al: Recombinant gene expression in vivo within endothelial cells of the arterial wall. Science 244:1342–1344, 1989.

174. Nabel EG, Plautz G, Nabel GJ: Site-specific gene expression in vivo by direct gene transfer into the arterial wall. Science 249:1285–1288, 1990.

175. Wilson JM, Birinyi LK, Salomon RN, et al: Implantation of vascular grafts lined with genetically modified endothelial cells. Science 244:1344–1346, 1989.

Questions

1. The origin of the proliferating cells found in intimal hyperplastic lesions is most likely
   (a) fibroblasts from the adventitia
   (b) circulating immune cells
   (c) neutrophils
   (d) endothelial cells
   (e) medial smooth muscle cells

2. Which hemodynamic force has been implicated as a contributing factor leading to the subsequent development of intimal hyperplasia?
   (a) vessel wall compliance
   (b) high shear stress
   (c) flow velocity
   (d) low shear stress
   (e) all of the above

3. Which surface membrane receptor regulates vascular smooth muscle cell accumulation of low-density lipoprotein (LDL)?
   (a) glycoprotein receptor GPIb
   (b) high-affinity LDL receptor
   (c) glycoprotein receptor GPIIb/IIIa
   (d) low-affinity LDL receptor
   (e) high-affinity high-density lipoprotein receptor

4. Platelet aggregation is stimulated by
   (a) adenosine triphosphate
   (b) platelet-derived growth factor
   (c) adenosine diphosphate (ADP)
   (d) LDL
   (e) prostacyclin

5. Angiotensin-converting enzyme (ACE) is primarily located on the membrane surface of
   (a) platelets
   (b) neutrophils
   (c) fibroblasts
   (d) vascular endothelial cells
   (e) macrophages

6. Which peptide has *not* been implicated in smooth muscle cell stimulation after an endothelial layer injury?
   (a) basic fibroblast growth factor
   (b) platelet-derived growth factor (PDGF)
   (c) angiotensin II
   (d) macrophage-derived growth factor
   (e) insulin

7. The incidence of restenosis after endarterectomy for carotid artery bifurcation lesions is approximately
   (a) 5%
   (b) 35%
   (c) 1%
   (d) 25%
   (e) 50%

8. Intimal hyperplasia is the most common cause of bypass graft failure when the graft fails
   (a) within 1 month
   (b) between 1 and 6 months
   (c) between 6 months and 2 years
   (d) after 5 years
   (e) after 10 years

9. Dipyridamole inhibits platelet function by
   (a) increasing thromboxane A_2
   (b) blocking the enzyme cyclooxygenase
   (c) increasing platelet ADP
   (d) increasing platelet cyclic adenosine monophosphate
   (e) decreasing prostacyclin

10. Prazosin is a selective inhibitor of which of the following receptors?
    (a) high-affinity LDL
    (b) PDGF
    (c) β_1-adrenergic receptor
    (d) α_2-adrenergic receptor
    (e) α_1-adrenergic receptor

Answers

1. e   2. e   3. b   4. c   5. d   6. e   7. a   8. c   9. d   10. e

38

Prosthetic Graft Infections

Niren Angle and Julie A. Freischlag

The development of prosthetic biomaterial devices has made possible the treatment and salvage of conditions that would otherwise, if left untreated, have resulted in significant morbidity and mortality. Examples of such clinical conditions include but are not limited to treatment of aortic aneurysms, hemodialysis access in the patient in whom autologous fistulas are not possible, and infrainguinal bypass for limb ischemia. The advent of the use of prosthetic conduits has also resulted in the attendant problem of the prosthetic graft infection. The morbidity associated with an infected prosthetic vascular graft is considerable and can be catastrophic, resulting in limb loss, sepsis, and, not infrequently, death. This chapter examines the cause, diagnosis, and management of prosthetic graft infections.

INCIDENCE

Prosthetic graft infection is relatively uncommon, with reported incidence ranging from 0.2% to 5%. There are very few prospectively obtained data analyzing the true incidence of prosthetic graft infection, but a survey of retrospective data with extended follow-up would suggest that graft infections are influenced by the implant site, indications for operation, and host defense, as manifested in the patient's comorbid disease. A prospective, multicenter Canadian study of repair of unruptured abdominal aortic aneurysms revealed a graft infection rate of 0.2%.[1] Szilagyi's analysis of 2145 patients undergoing a variety of vascular reconstructions, which included aortofemoral, aortoiliac, and femoropopliteal reconstructions, revealed an overall graft infection rate of 1.5%.[2] The insertion of a prosthetic graft in the femoropopliteal or femorotibial positions has a higher rate of infection, ranging in some reports up to 5%.

An emergency operation (e.g., ruptured abdominal aortic aneurysm) carries with it a higher rate of infection than does an elective operation. The consequences of an infected prosthesis are also different, depending on the location of the graft. The mortality rate is higher with an infected aortic prosthesis, and the risk of limb loss is highest with lower extremity graft infections. A graft infection can manifest months to years after implantation, and

this insidious presentation itself may yield some insight into the biology of graft infections.

MICROBIOLOGY

Insight into the cause of vascular graft infections can be gained by examining the microorganisms most commonly recovered from infected grafts. Although any microorganism can potentially cause a graft infection, *Staphylococcus aureus* is the most prevalent bacterium.[3] *S. aureus* is responsible for 25% to 50% of vascular graft infections, based on anatomic location. Over the last 15 to 20 years, *Staphylococcus epidermidis* has become increasingly recognized as the responsible pathogen for a significant proportion of graft infections, predominantly the late-appearing, indolent type.

Graft infections are labeled as early (occurring <4 months after implantation) or late (occurring >4 months after implantation). Early-appearing graft infections are most commonly caused by more virulent organisms, and this is most commonly *S. aureus*. Coagulase-positive strains elaborate toxins that result in a vigorous host inflammatory response. Late-appearing graft infections are caused by less virulent gram-positive bacteria such as *S. epidermidis*. This organism is indolent and normally harbored in natural skin. It has the ability to adhere to prosthetic material and to secrete a glycocalyx biofilm that insulates the bacterium. This biofilm, over time, induces an inflammatory response resulting in perigraft inflammation, which is clinically seen as perigraft fluid. This organism is fastidious in its attachment and is not easily isolated. *S. epidermidis* graft infections appear to have a sterile exudate, resulting in poor graft incorporation. Rarely do the patients have a leukocytosis. This innocuous presentation has led many to view *S. epidermidis* infections as inflammatory allergic responses rather than bacterial graft infections.[4] Bergamini and colleagues elegantly demonstrated that ultrasonication is required to physically separate *S. epidermidis* from the graft surface in order to culture it. Also, broth culture yielded a higher rate of recovery than agar plating.[5] Bacterial recovery, which was only 30% when plated on agar media, rose to 72% in broth media. The combination of ultrasonication and broth culture resulted in a positive culture in 83% in this report.

Other microorganisms such as fungi and gram-negative bacteria can also result in graft infections. Gram-negative bacteria such as *Pseudomonas, Escherichia coli, Enterobacter,* and *Proteus* are very virulent and result in quite dramatic clinical manifestations such as anastomotic disruption and frank hemorrhage.[6] These organisms are able to secrete potent proteases, which accounts for the tissue disruption that results in artery-graft disruption. Gram-negative infections also induce a substantial host inflammatory response that contributes to the disruption as well. *Pseudomonas* is most commonly associated with graft disruption and hemorrhage. Severely immunosuppressed patients are also vulnerable to fungal graft infections, an otherwise rare clinical entity in the general population.

ETIOLOGY AND PATHOPHYSIOLOGY

The fundamental question regarding the etiology of prosthetic graft infections concerns when the graft is exposed to the microorganisms that eventually result in a clinically evident infection. The three major potential mechanisms that can result in prosthetic graft colonization and subsequent infection are the following:

1. Intraoperative contamination
2. Hematogenous spread of bacteria
3. Direct contamination of graft by infection emanating from the skin, the soft tissue, or both; gastrointestinal tract; or the genitourinary tract

Although all of these factors can result in a graft infection, the last mechanism listed is the least common.

Intraoperative Contamination

The host is the most significant source of bacterial contamination resulting in surgical site infection. The resident microflora, usually referred to as the indigenous microflora, is made up of a complex mixture of microbial species ranging from nonpathogenic saprophytes to pathogens. Endogenous bacteria are a more important source of surgical site infection than exogenous bacteria.

The patient's endogenous flora—especially from a colonized site such as the skin or gut—which is close to the prosthetic bed, is a very common site of graft infection. Most of the intertriginous areas of the body, which contain large numbers of eccrine sweat glands, such as the axillae, the groin, and the interdigital spaces of the foot, harbor large bacterial populations.[7] A good example of this phenomenon is the well-characterized propensity of prosthetic grafts placed in the groin to develop *S. aureus* infection. *S. aureus* bacteria from the groin area may contaminate only the wound, or they may also contaminate the graft surface if inadvertently dragged across the skin. The lymphatics in the groin may be contaminated at the time of surgery, especially if the patient has an open infected wound in an extremity. These lymphatics can also be a source of intraoperative graft infection. It is exceedingly rare for bacterial contamination to originate from the surgical team, from the graft, or from surgical instruments. The surgeon's hands are seldom a major source of wound contamination.[8]

Bacteria can be present in diseased vessels or in the thrombus lining an aortic aneurysm.[9] Van der Vliet and colleagues cultured the contents of the aneurysms of 216 patients and then followed the patients for more than 3 years.[10] Positive cultures were found in 55 patients (23.5%). Only four graft infections occurred (1.9%). Three of these four patients had positive cultures, but only two patients had the same organism as the original cultures. The authors concluded that bacteria in aneurysm contents have no demonstrable link to subsequent graft infections. A prospective study demonstrated that in patients undergoing peripheral vascular bypass surgery, 41% had positive arterial tissue cultures, 68% of which were coagulase-negative *Staphylococcus*.[11] Subsequent graft infections were not reported, so the significance of the cultures is intriguing but unclear.

Hematogenous Spread of Bacteria

Seeding of an indwelling prosthesis by hematogenous spread of bacteria is potentially very important; the frequency with which this occurs is unknown. In experimental animals, infusion of 10^7 organisms of *S. aureus* immediately after implantation of a prosthetic aortic graft resulted in a 100% incidence of graft infection.[12, 13] Later studies demonstrated a lower incidence of graft infection with longer time after implantation, suggesting that graft incorporation and the development of a pseudointima may provide some protection.[14, 15] Vulnerability to infection from bacteremia has been documented as late as 1 year after implantation, with 30% of aortic grafts becoming infected after a single bacterial infusion at that time.[12] The anatomic difference between the infected and noninfected grafts was the presence of a complete neointimal lining. Parenteral antibiotics significantly reduced the incidence of graft infection, particularly when culture-directed therapy was applied to the treatment of a remote infection. The significance of remote infection is unclear, but it suggests that transient bacteremia associated, for example, with dental procedures or colonoscopy, may account for the very late infections.

Direct Contamination

This category is the most easily diagnosed and the least common. The development of an intraabdominal abscess from a variety of clinical conditions can directly infect a recently placed aortic graft. Similarly, the failure of the skin incision to heal after an operation places the underlying graft at a significant risk of bacterial contamination and subsequent infection. For these reasons, it is prudent to avoid any operation on the gastrointestinal tract at the time of insertion of an aortic prosthetic graft. The exception to this is the performance of a cholecystectomy, but this too is done only after the graft is inserted and the retroperitoneum is closed over the graft.

PREVENTION

The best way to avoid graft infection is to attempt to prevent it in the operating room and during the subsequent postoperative period. It has been clearly shown that patients who are hospitalized for any length of time have an alteration in their cutaneous microflora.[16] It is unclear whether this is caused by the underlying illness or by antibiotics. The preoperative stay, if any, should be as short as possible to avoid colonization with resistant bacteria. Prophylactic antibiotics have been shown to decrease the incidence of wound infections that potentially could lead to graft infections. Most authors recommend the administration of a first-generation cephalosporin approximately a half hour before incision, with a scheduled dose continued for the first 24 hours. If the operation proceeds for an extended length of time, additional doses should be administered to maintain adequate circulating levels. There is no evidence to support the use and continuation of prophylactic antibiotics until indwelling lines such as central venous or urinary bladder catheters are removed. The prolonged use of postoperative antibiotics may even be detrimental because the patient can develop antibiotic-associated colitis or other resistant organism infections.

Meticulous surgical technique is very important in preventing wound and graft infections. The graft must be handled carefully and not allowed to be indiscriminately in contact with the patient's skin. Adhesive drapes are used commonly to aid in preventing the aforementioned contact, although it must be stated that there is not a single study demonstrating a reduced incidence of wound or graft infection with the use of the adhesive drapes, with or without iodine impregnation. If the adhesive plastic drape is separated from the skin during the operation, the infection rate increases.[17, 18] Simultaneous gastrointestinal procedures should be avoided to prevent intraoperative contamination. If an unplanned enterotomy is performed, graft implantation should be postponed, if possible. Dead space in surgical wounds should be minimized with the least possible amount of suture material. Irrigation of the peritoneal cavity is routine, but it may lead to washout of macrophages and opsonins. Irrigation should be used to remove all blood from the peritoneal cavity, because blood acts as an adjuvant for bacterial proliferation. If irrigation of a wound is performed, every effort should be made to evacuate the fluid.

DIAGNOSIS

Graft infections can result in limb loss, systemic sepsis, and, sometimes, death, even in the setting of the correct diagnosis and treatment. For these reasons, prompt diagnosis is essential to avoid or minimize the complications. Accurate diagnosis requires that the surgeon be aware of the subtle manifestations of graft infection. Every attempt should be made to confirm or exclude the diagnosis, either by imaging or operative exploration. The consequences of a missed diagnosis in this setting can be catastrophic.

Clinical Presentation

The clinical presentation of graft infection can be subtle and is influenced by the anatomic location of the graft. An infection of an infrainguinal graft frequently appears as cellulitis, soft tissue infection, drainage tract, or pseudoaneurysm. The clinical presentation of an extracavitary graft is usually not subtle. An intraabdominal graft may appear as systemic sepsis, or, alternatively, as an ileus or abdominal distention, with or without tenderness. Occasionally, an aortic graft infection may result in an aortoenteric fistula, the first sign of which is a herald bleed. A patient with upper gastrointestinal bleeding and an aortic graft must be presumed to have an aortoenteric fistula until the diagnosis is proved otherwise (Fig. 38–1).

Early graft infections can manifest with fever, leukocytosis, and purulent drainage from the graft site. Splinter hemorrhages can be present. Blood cultures may be positive if taken in the distal arterial circulation downstream from the graft infection. A late graft infection, usually caused by an indolent organism such as *S. epidermidis*, appears as a healing complication such as a seroma, a pseudoaneurysm, or a late graft thrombosis without an anatomic reason. Systemic signs of illness such as fever are usually not present.

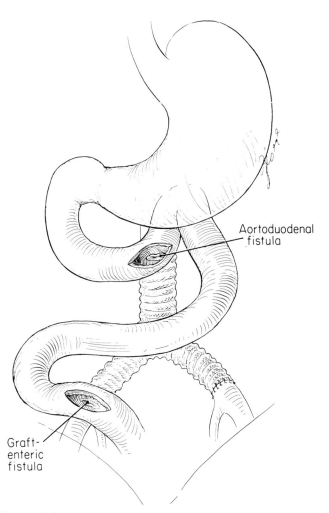

Figure 38–1. A communication may develop between the bowel lumen and the graft. Hemorrhage may be due to a direct communication between the aorta and the bowel (aortoenteric fistula) or from vessels in the bowel wall that have been eroded by the prosthetic graft (enteroparaprosthetic fistula).

Aortoduodenal fistula

Graft-enteric fistula

Laboratory Studies

A leukocytosis with a left shift and an elevated erythrocyte sedimentation rate (ESR) often accompany graft infection, but their lack of specificity limits their usefulness. Late-appearing perigraft infections with *S. epidermidis* may have none of these laboratory abnormalities.

Imaging

Imaging plays an important role in the diagnosis of prosthetic graft infection. The particular imaging modality used depends on the site being investigated and the information desired. Computed tomography (CT), angiography, ultrasonography, nuclear medicine, and magnetic resonance imaging (MRI) comprise the diagnostic armamentarium for the evaluation of potential graft infection.

Computed Tomography

CT scanning is helpful in the diagnosis of graft infections. Perigraft fluid collections, perigraft gas, anastomotic aneurysms, and distortion of tissue planes are all findings suggestive of graft infection and are all well visualized by a contrast-enhanced CT scan. Presence of gas or fluid around a graft more than 6 to 8 weeks after implantation is definitely abnormal and is presumptive evidence of graft infection. CT-guided aspiration of perigraft fluid is very reliable, offers a very good yield, and provides material for Gram stain and culture.

Ultrasonography

A duplex ultrasound scan is an excellent initial test for identification of upper and lower extremity graft infections. It is not as accurate in identifying aortic pseudoaneurysms because of difficulty in imaging owing to bowel gas. It is quick, portable, noninvasive, and very reliable in distinguishing an anastomotic pseudoaneurysm from perigraft fluid collections. The accuracy of the test depends on the technician's expertise, but in skilled hands, it is very informative and reliable.

Magnetic Resonance Imaging

MRI is a useful modality for identification of perigraft fluid, because of its ability to distinguish fluid from tissue by recognizing differences in signal intensity between T1- and T2-weighted images. The efficacy of this test was highlighted in a study by Olofsson and colleagues[19] in which 18 patients suspected of having an aortic graft infection underwent preoperative MR scanning. Twelve patients also underwent CT scanning. MRI successfully identified 14 of 16 patients who were found to have an aortic graft infection at time of operation, whereas CT was accurate in only 5 of 12 patients. It has been shown that there is only mild enhancement on the T2-weighted images in grafts undergoing normal incorporation, whereas infected perigraft tissue demonstrates increased signal intensity.[20] As MR scanning is increasingly used, its role in the diagnosis of aortic graft infections may become increasingly prominent.

Angiography

Although angiography can identify graft pseudoaneurysms (Fig. 38–2), it is not the test of choice because CT scanning and MRI are better and noninvasive. Patients with suspected graft infection should undergo preoperative arteriography to determine vessel patency and also to evaluate the proximal and distal vasculature for revascularization options.

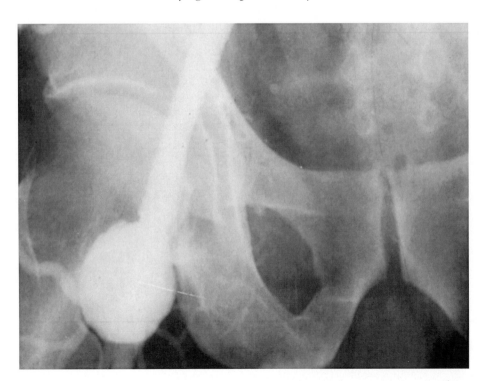

Figure 38–2. Graft infection was first manifested by the development of a false aneurysm.

White Blood Cell Scanning

Gallium 67 (^{67}Ga)- or indium 111 (^{111}In)-labeled white blood cell scanning is very sensitive for graft infection. ^{111}In-labeled leukocyte or IgG scan is quite reliable and offers an advantage over ^{67}Ga scanning because there is minimum nonspecific bowel uptake resulting in a high target-to-background ratio and better results.[21] ^{111}In-labeled leukocyte IgG scanning has been used by LaMuraglia and colleagues[22] with impressive results. In 10 patients with positive scans, graft infection was confirmed at operation at the same site. Of the 15 patients with negative scans, the only one who had a false-negative result was a patient with an aortoduodenal fistula. The advantage of IgG scanning is that preparation is easier because the patient's own blood is not required for the test and the tracer has a longer half-life.

Endoscopy

Endoscopy is a vital diagnostic tool in the evaluation of upper gastrointestinal tract bleeding.[23] A patient with an aortic prosthesis and upper gastrointestinal bleeding must be suspected of having an aortoenteric fistula until proved otherwise. The initial test for this diagnosis is upper gastrointestinal endoscopy, which should be performed expeditiously once the diagnosis of aortoenteric fistula has been considered. The examination must be performed cautiously. The finding of an adherent blood clot in the duodenum should confirm the diagnosis, and the patient should be taken immediately to the operating room. If the endoscopy does not reveal any pathology, such as bleeding varices, gastritis, or a stomach or duodenal ulcer, an aortoenteric fistula may still be present although not seen. Again, the patient should undergo exploratory surgery in the operating room.

MANAGEMENT OF GRAFT INFECTION

General Principles

Preoperative Preparation

A patient with ongoing hemorrhage, or a patient in hemorrhagic shock from an anastomotic rupture, or a patient with an aortoenteric fistula is managed according to the standard principles of resuscitation. In these categories of patients, there is not much time for preoperative planning, diagnosis, or adjuvant therapy.

Fortunately, most patients with graft infections do not appear emergently, and adequate time is available for diagnostic tests and optimization of conditions for a potentially extensive operation. The patient and family must understand that the treatment may involve a very demanding operation, both physiologically and psychologically. The patient's cardiac and pulmonary status must be evaluated and optimized. Hemodynamic volume status must be optimized. Antibiotic coverage must be initiated to contain the graft infection and to prevent progression to sepsis or septic shock. Routine total parenteral nutrition should not be used preoperatively in these patients. The only patients shown in a prospective, randomized trial to have benefited from preoperative total parenteral nutrition were those who were severely malnourished, as evaluated by the Subjective Global Assessment.[24] Glycemic control is essential, because hyperglycemia causes suppression of neutrophil function; this is, in part, one of the factors that predisposes the diabetic patient to infectious complications. Appropriate imaging studies are performed to evaluate possible options for extra-anatomic revascularization or for autogenous in situ reconstruction, which can include CT scan, MRI, IgG scanning, and angiography.

Removal of the Graft

The involvement of a suture line with the infectious process is an absolute indication for removal of the entire infected graft. Any compromise on the issue of an infected anastomosis inevitably leads to eventual rupture and hemorrhage. Many authorities have advocated conservative treatment consisting of drainage, débridement, and systemic and local antibiotic coverage for management of perigraft infection, usually limited to inguinal and infrainguinal graft infection. Calligaro and colleagues[25] have been the leading proponents of graft preservation and have realized success in more than 70% of cases. Towne and associates reported on their treatment of 20 infected grafts, 14 of which were aortofemoral grafts. In the 14 aortofemoral grafts, only the femoral limbs were excised; the proximal incorporated segment was left in situ. An interposition polytetrafluoroethylene graft was used to replace the explanted segment. Subsequent graft ultrasonication revealed that 17 out of 20 grafts grew *S. epidermidis,* one grew coagulase-positive *Staphylococcus,* and two grafts grew both. All of the surgical incisions healed, and graft patency was 100%. There was no limb loss. The authors concluded that biofilm graft infections may be safely treated with in situ replacements.[32] The requirements for selecting patients for graft preservation are that the graft anastomosis is not involved with infection and that the patient does not demonstrate systemic signs of sepsis. Tissue coverage of the débrided area can be achieved with a rotational flap or a free flap.[26] *Pseudomonas aeruginosa* infections represent a high-risk infection for which the graft salvage option is a poor choice. The risk of hemorrhage from anastomotic rupture is significantly higher. The optimal treatment for an infected graft, particularly one with involvement of the suture line, is still excision of the entire infected graft, with reconstruction through uninfected tissue planes, preferably with autogenous tissue.

Aortoenteric fistulas, particularly aortoduodenal fistulas, require complete excision of the graft and closure of the duodenal wall defect. There is no role for in situ replacement of the graft in the treatment of patients with this entity. Although lesser procedures than complete graft excision have been attempted, the data clearly show that complete graft excision (and, if necessary, placement of an extra-anatomic bypass) is clearly superior. Lesser procedures are associated with a higher rate of fistula recurrence and death. The graft must be completely excised and the defect in the duodenum oversewn. Given that the best treatment consists of graft excision, closure of the enteric defect, and extra-anatomic bypass, the sequence of these procedures becomes important. In an actively bleeding patient or one in whom the diagnosis has been made at celiotomy, graft excision must precede extra-anatomic bypass. It is often difficult to determine which patient needs a remote bypass in such a setting; therefore, the safest approach is to perform immediate revascularization in the majority of cases.

Débridement

Blowout and late hemorrhage from the proximal aortic stump occur not infrequently in some patients in whom successful excision of the graft was achieved. This is most likely due to residual infection in the bed of the graft in the perigraft and para-aortic tissues. The débridement must be generous enough to ensure eradication of all infected tissue. The aorta must then be oversewn in two layers, if possible, with polypropylene suture. If the infecting organism is of low virulence, removal of the graft is usually all that is necessary. With a more virulent organism, aggressive débridement is a must.

Antibiotic Therapy

Preoperative administration of culture-specific antibiotics is ideal. If the infecting organism is not known, broad-spectrum antibiotics, in doses adequate to reach minimal inhibitory concentration (MIC), are administered. Some authorities advocate irrigation of tissues with topical antibiotic solution, although the usefulness of this is questionable.[27] Subsequent therapy with antibiotics should be tailored to culture results. The appropriate duration of antibiotic therapy is unclear. The San Francisco group[28] has advocated at least a 2-week duration of systemic antibiotic therapy. Patients treated with at least 6 weeks of parenteral antibiotics had significantly better outcomes than those treated for 2 weeks or less.

Revascularization

Removal of an infected graft usually mandates some revascularization procedure. Reilly and colleagues[28] and Trout and associates[29] have conclusively shown that a staged operation with initial revascularization followed by graft excision in 1 to 2 days is associated with significantly less morbidity and mortality. The overall mortality rate was 53% (40/75) if graft excision preceded extra-anatomic bypass, and 17% (5/29) if bypass preceded graft excision. The physiologic stress on the patient is probably decreased with a staged approach, and performing the revascularization before graft excision obviates the need for systemic heparinization, probably enabling more radical débridement. Throughout this time period, systemic antibiotic therapy is continued.

The ideal conduit is autogenous vein or endarterectomy-treated artery. If a prosthetic conduit is chosen for the extra-anatomic bypass, polytetrafluoroethylene (PTFE) is preferable to Dacron because experimental evidence indicates that PTFE is more resistant to bacterial colonization than other prosthetic conduits.[30] This experimental information has been validated in a clinical retrospective analysis that discovered a lower infection rate for PTFE compared

with Dacron.[31] Towne and coworkers[32] suggested that aortic grafts infected with the low-virulence *S. epidermidis* may, under strict selection criteria, be safely treated with an in situ prosthetic graft composed of PTFE. Over a 9-year period, 28 patients were treated with in situ PTFE grafts for aortoiliofemoral graft infections with *S. epidermidis*. Over a mean follow-up of 4.5 years, there was no mortality and all grafts remained patent. There were two patients who had recurrent infection in the proximal limb of the old graft. These data suggest that in carefully selected patients, in situ replacement with PTFE may be safe and effective.

TREATMENT OF SPECIFIC GRAFT SITE INFECTIONS

Aortoiliac and Aortic Interposition Grafts

Aortoiliac graft infections are best treated by preliminary axillobifemoral bypass through uninfected tissue planes, followed by aortic graft excision (Fig. 38–3). This approach

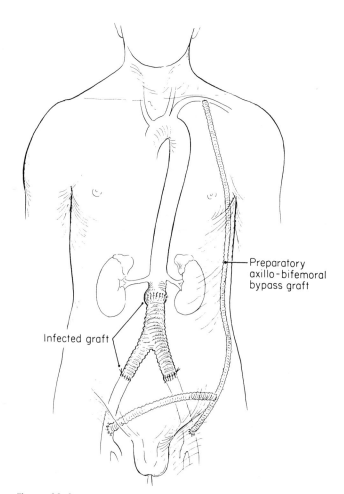

Figure 38–3. Before removing an infected intraabdominal prosthetic graft, perfusion of the lower extremities is established by an axillobifemoral bypass graft. This technique provides uninterrupted perfusion of the lower limbs and reduces the morbidity associated with ischemic changes that occur when reconstitution of flow is delayed until after the aortic graft has been removed.

(i.e., a staged approach) is associated with significantly less morbidity than the traditional mode of treatment.[28, 29] The distal anastomoses can be constructed at both common femoral arteries because the distal limbs of the aortic graft are confined to the abdomen. A European prospective, randomized trial has shown that an axillobifemoral graft with a flow splitter had a better 2-year patency rate (84%) than either an axillounifemoral bypass or a femorofemoral bypass. This operation can be immediately followed by graft excision, or, alternatively, graft excision can be performed 1 to 2 days later.

For aortic graft excision, celiotomy is performed, and the aortic graft is isolated. Although systemic heparin is indicated for the axillofemoral bypass, the advantage of the staged operation is that no anticoagulation is necessary during the aortic graft excision. If the procedures are done consecutively, the heparin should be reversed before the aortic graft is approached. Careful dissection in the abdomen is performed, and the graft is separated from adherent bowel and viscera. Once the entire graft is exposed, proximal control is obtained, probably best at the supraceliac aorta, particularly if there is a proximal anastomotic aneurysm. The iliac arteries distal to the anastomoses are also similarly isolated and control is obtained. The entire graft is then excised, and the aorta is débrided back to normal, healthy-appearing tissue. The aortic stump is then closed with locking monofilament suture. The distal aorta and iliacs are similarly closed. Perigraft tissue that may be infected is carefully but completely débrided. Closed suction drains may be placed. Care is taken to avoid injury to the ureters. If débridement is necessary above the renal arteries, it should be performed without compromise. The renal arteries are then revascularized by antegrade bypasses from one or two of the branches of the celiac axis, such as the hepatic or splenic arteries. Perfusion of the pelvic circulation is maintained by retrograde flow from the axillofemoral bypass through the external and internal iliac arteries. If the distal anastomoses are to the external iliac arteries and require excision, perfusion to at least one internal iliac artery should be maintained by means of a bypass.

Aortobifemoral Graft Infections

Although the principles regarding treatment of an aortofemoral graft infection are fundamentally the same, the issue of revascularization is more troublesome. The distal femoral anastomoses of an aortofemoral graft preclude the attachment of distal limbs of an extra-anatomic bypass to the common femoral artery. Hence, the distal anastomosis of the extra-anatomic bypass must be at the profunda femoris artery, the superficial femoral artery, or the popliteal artery.

If the graft was performed for occlusive disease in an end-to-side fashion, it may be possible to excise the graft and close the aorta, relying on flow through the native vessels to the lower extremities. Although the native vessels are undoubtedly diseased, there may be adequate flow to avoid the need for immediate revascularization. This is an issue best assessed preoperatively, because an intraoperative assessment of the adequacy of flow may result in the graft's being excised first, with subsequent extra-anatomic bypass if the flow through the native vessels is inadequate. This would be a return to the traditional method of treating infected aortic grafts, an approach that was previously documented to result in increased morbidity.[28]

If the graft infection is localized to the groin, and the proximal and distal anastomoses are not involved, an attempt at graft preservation can be made. This is done by draining the abscess, aggressively débriding the perigraft tissues, and ensuring tissue coverage.[25] The patients selected for graft preservation must meet all of the previously mentioned criteria. Contraindications to graft preservation techniques include an occluded graft, the presence of sepsis, or a virulent organism, particularly *Pseudomonas aeruginosa*. Patients treated with graft preservation should be observed in a closely monitored setting, not on a floor designed for routine nursing care.

If the femoral anastomosis is involved with the infection, that graft limb must be excised. The limb can be approached by means of an ipsilateral retroperitoneal exposure (Fig. 38–4). If the retroperitoneal portion of the graft

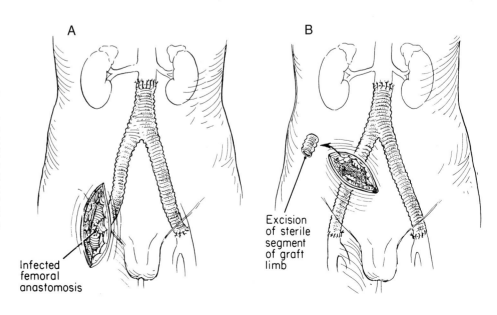

Figure 38–4. Through a retroperitoneal approach, the sterility of the proximal portion of the graft limb is determined. *A*, The sterile graft above is isolated from the area of infection at the groin by excision of a segment of graft and obliteration of the communicating tissue planes between the two areas. *B*, The distal portion of the graft limb is then removed from below after the clean procedure has been carried out in the retroperitoneal space and the wound has been closed.

A

B

Infected femoral anastomosis

Excision of sterile segment of graft limb

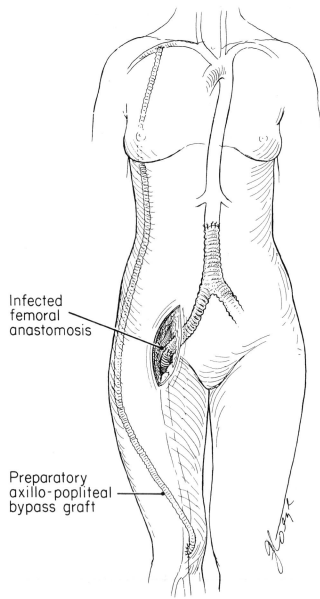

Infected
femoral
anastomosis

Preparatory
axillo-popliteal
bypass graft

Figure 38–5. Perfusion of an ischemic extremity in the presence of sepsis in the ipsilateral groin is achieved with an axillopopliteal bypass graft. Care is taken to bring the graft wide of the groin through unaffected tissue planes.

by tunneling via a retropubic route, or through the obturator canal, or by medial tunneling of a femorofemoral bypass. The choice of the vessel for distal bypass depends upon the condition of the native vasculature. The bypass conduit has to be routed through clean, uninfected territory (Fig. 38–5). If the entire graft must be excised, an extra-anatomic bypass originating from the axillary artery must be fashioned and anastomosed to the profunda artery, the superficial artery, or the popliteal artery (Fig. 38–6). It is preferable to use ring-reinforced PTFE grafts to aid in the prevention of external compression of the graft.

Femoropopliteal Bypass Graft Infection

The infected femoropopliteal bypass graft must be excised in its entirety. The same principles apply, including radical

is well incorporated, proximal control can be obtained at that level and the graft limb excised. All ligation sites should be covered with viable tissue. The graft-artery anastomosis is excised and the artery débrided. The femoral arteriotomy is then closed with patch angioplasty, preferably with autologous tissue. If a portion of the common femoral artery at that level must be débrided or excised, an attempt should be made to perform an end-to-end anastomosis of the superficial femoral artery to the profunda femoris artery to maintain retrograde perfusion of the pelvis. If the proximal anastomosis is involved, the entire graft must be excised according to the principles elucidated earlier.

An extra-anatomic bypass is then fashioned, depending on the need for revascularization of the limb. If only the unilateral limb is excised, the limb can be revascularized

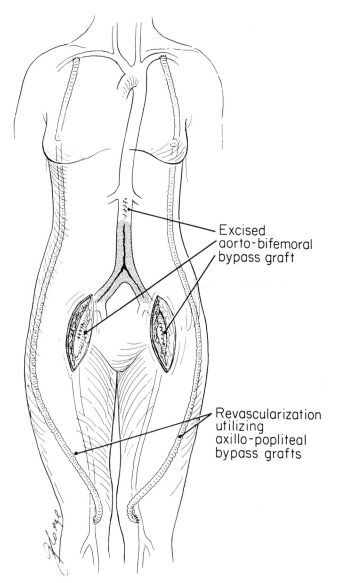

Excised
aorto-bifemoral
bypass graft

Revascularization
utilizing
axillo-popliteal
bypass grafts

Figure 38–6. Ischemia of lower extremities returned to dependence on the native circulation after removal of an infected aortic graft may be successfully managed by bilateral axillopopliteal bypass grafts.

débridement of infected tissue, débridement of the artery to healthy viable tissue, and closure of the artery with monofilament suture. The viability of the limb determines the need for immediate versus delayed revascularization. Should immediate revascularization be needed, it is ideally performed with autogenous vein, and only if the anastomosis is not done in an infected area. An alternative is to perform a semiclosed endarterectomy of the superficial femoral artery. Revascularization is performed with adherence to the same principles outlined earlier, with the route of the graft through clean, uninfected tissue.

Endovascular Stent Graft Infection

With the rapid increase in insertion of endovascular grafts, there have been a few early reports of endovascular graft infections and their management. Owing to the novelty of the experience, case series and solid guidelines are lacking. The diagnosis can also be uncertain, especially soon after graft insertion. There is a well-described postimplantation inflammatory profile of fever and leukocytosis. Velasquez and colleagues[33] described their first 12 patients' experiences after endovascular repair with Dacron-covered stent-grafts. A majority of those patients had fever (>101.4°F), leukocytosis, and CT-scan evidence of perigraft air. All patients became afebrile with resolution of their leukocytosis, and none had any evidence of graft infection on follow-up. Thus, it appears that the early postimplantation inflammatory profile does not represent evidence of graft infection.

The management of graft infections in this setting, in the absence of long-term data, should follow the same principles as the management of any prosthetic graft infection. Deiparine and associates[34] reported a case of infection of an iliac artery stent that resulted in necrosis of the common femoral artery and severe inflammation of the external iliac artery and the retroperitoneum. The patient survived after a very prolonged stay in an intensive care unit and required an above-knee amputation. The authors recommended that endovascular stent or prosthesis placement (or both) should be preceded by prophylactic antibiotics; attention to sterile technique is mandatory. Heikkinen and coworkers[35] reported on a patient with a *Listeria* infection of an endovascular bifurcated stent graft. That patient was treated with resection and débridement of the aorta and in situ replacement with a PTFE graft. Clearly, there is not enough long-term experience with endovascular grafting to yield any information about the incidence and pattern of graft infections. However, the consequences can be just as devastating. It is clear that meticulous adherence to sterile technique and, perhaps, routine antibiotic prophylaxis should not be neglected in the performance of this "less invasive procedure."

FUTURE DIRECTIONS IN THE MANAGEMENT OF GRAFT INFECTION

In the past few years, there has been a plethora of reports studying the use of a rifampin-bonded aortic prosthesis for the treatment of aortic graft infection. Colburn and colleagues[36] demonstrated the efficacy of collagen-impregnated grafts bonded to rifampin and placed in the bed of an explanted infected graft in a dog model. The use of systemic antibiotics optimized the results and outcome. Subsequent studies have confirmed these findings.[37, 38] A prospective, randomized trial in the United Kingdom[39] attempted to define the role of the rifampin-bonded prosthesis in extra-anatomic bypass grafts to see whether they resulted in a decreased risk of graft infection compared with that of controls. Two hundred fifty-seven patients were randomized at 14 vascular centers to either rifampin-bonded grafts or regular collagen-impregnated grafts. There was no significant difference in the incidence of graft infection on early follow-up (1 month). The long-term results should be interesting with regard to the primary use of an antibiotic-bonded prosthesis to prevent graft infection.

The underwhelming success of traditional modes of management of graft infections has spurred experimentation with alternative modes of management, such as selective graft preservation, antibiotic-bonded grafts, and the use of autogenous vein for reconstruction in situ. Our current understanding of graft infection and its causes and treatment is inchoate. Although evolution in the management of graft infection is ongoing and encouraging, the most fruitful endeavor may be an enhanced understanding of the pathophysiologic factors that predispose certain patients to develop graft infection. The interaction of a foreign body with the host and the subsequent response of the host determine the clinical outcome. With a better understanding of this interaction and the disparate responses of different hosts, a more successful attempt at immunomodulation may yield success in reducing the incidence of graft infection and the considerable attendant morbidity and mortality.

References

1. Johnston KW: Multicenter prospective study of nonruptured abdominal aortic aneurysm: Part II. Variables predicting morbidity and mortality. J Vasc Surg 9:437, 1989.
2. Szilagyi DE, Smith RF, Elliott JP, et al: Infection in arterial reconstruction with synthetic grafts. Ann Surg 175:321, 1972.
3. Bandyk DF: Infection in prosthetic vascular grafts. In Rutherford R (ed): Vascular Surgery. Philadelphia, WB Saunders, 1999, p 737.
4. Belletnot F, Chatenet T, Kantelip B, et al: Aseptic periprosthetic fluid collection: A late complication of Dacron arterial bypass. Ann Vasc Surg 2:220, 1988.

5. Bergamini TM, Bandyk DF, Govostis D, et al: Identification of *Staphylococcus epidermidis* vascular graft infections: A comparison of culture techniques. J Vasc Surg 9:665, 1989.
6. Geary KJ, Tomkiewicz ZM, Harrison HN, et al: Differential effects of a gram-negative and a gram-positive infection on autogenous and prosthetic grafts. J Vasc Surg 11:339, 1990.
7. Bjorson HS: Microbiology of surgical infection. In Meakins J (ed): Surgical Infections. New York, Scientific American, 1994.
8. Dougherty S: Prosthetic devices. In Meakins J (ed): Surgical Infections. New York, Scientific American, 1994.

9. Macbeth GA, Rubin JR, McIntyre KE Jr, et al: The relevance of arterial wall microbiology to the treatment of prosthetic graft infections: Graft infection vs. arterial infection. Vasc Surg 1:750, 1984.

10. Van der Vliet JA, Kouwenberg PP, Muytjens HL, et al: Relevance of bacterial cultures of abdominal aortic aneurysm contents. Surgery 119:129, 1996.

11. Lalka SG, Malone JM, Fisher DF Jr, et al: Efficacy of prophylactic antibiotics in vascular surgery: An arterial wall microbiologic and pharmacokinetic perspective. J Vasc Surg 10:501, 1989.

12. Malone JM, Moore WS, Campagna G, et al: Bacteremic infectibility of vascular grafts: The influence of pseudointimal integrity and duration of graft function. Surgery 78:211, 1975.

13. Moore WS, Rosson CT, Hall AD, et al: Transient bacteremia. A cause of infection in prosthetic vascular grafts. Am J Surg 117:342, 1969.

14. Moore WS, Malone JM, Keown K: Prosthetic arterial graft material: Influence on neointimal healing and bacterial infectibility. Arch Surg 115:1379, 1980.

15. Moore WS, Swanson RJ, Campagna G, et al: Pseudointimal development and vascular prosthesis susceptibility to bacteremic infection. Surg Forum 15:250, 1974.

16. Larson EL, McGinley KJ, Foglia AR, et al: Composition and antimicrobic resistance of skin flora in hospitalized and healthy adults. J Clin Microbiol 23:604, 1986.

17. Alexander JW, Aerni S, Plettner JP: Development of a safe and effective one-minute preoperative skin preparation. Arch Surg 120:1357, 1985.

18. Lewis DA, Leaper DJ, Speller DCE: Prevention of bacterial colonization of wounds at operation: Comparison of iodine-impregnated ("Ioban") drapes with conventional methods. J Hosp Infect 5:431, 1984.

19. Olofsson PA, Auffermann W, Higgins CB, et al: Diagnosis of prosthetic aortic graft infection by magnetic resonance imaging. J Vasc Surg 8:99, 1988.

20. Auffermann W, Olofsson PA, Rabahie GN, et al: Incorporation versus infection of retroperitoneal aortic grafts: MR imaging features. Radiology 172:359, 1989.

21. Lawrence PF, Dries DJ, Alazraki N, et al: Indium[111]-labeled leukocyte scanning for detection of prosthetic vascular graft infection. J Vasc Surg 2:165, 1985.

22. LaMuraglia GM, Fischman AJ, Strauss HW, et al: Utility of the indium 111-labeled human immunoglobulin G scan for the detection of focal vascular graft infection. J Vasc Surg 10:20, 1989.

23. Champion MC, Sullivan SN, Coles JC, et al: Aortoenteric fistula: Incidence, presentation, recognition, and management. Ann Surg 195:314, 1982.

24. Buzby GP et al: Perioperative total parenteral nutrition in surgical patients. The Veterans Affairs Total Parenteral Nutrition Cooperative Study Group. N Engl J Med 325:525, 1991.

25. Calligaro KD, Veith FJ, Gupta SK, et al: A modified method of management of prosthetic graft infections involving an anastomosis to the common femoral artery. J Vasc Surg 11:485, 1990.

26. Perler BA, Vander Kolk CA, Dufresne CR, et al: Can infected prosthetic grafts be salvaged with rotational muscle flaps? Surgery 110:30, 1991.

27. DiGiglia JD, Leonard GL, Oschner JL: Local irrigation with an antibiotic solution in the prevention of infection in vascular prosthesis. Surgery 67:836, 1970.

28. Reilly LM, Stoney RJ, Goldstone J, et al: Improved management of aortic graft infection: The influence of operation sequence and staging. J Vasc Surg 5:421, 1987.

29. Trout HH, Kozioff L, Giordano JM: Priority of revascularization in patients with graft enteric fistulas, infected arteries or infected arterial prosthesis. Ann Surg 199:669, 1984.

30. Rosenman JE, Pearce WH, Kempczinski RF: Bacterial adherence to vascular grafts after in vitro bacteremia. J Surg Res 38:648, 1985.

31. Bacourt F, Koskas F: Axillobifemoral bypass and aortic exclusion for vascular septic lesions: A multicenter retrospective study of 98 cases. Ann Vasc Surg 6:119, 1992.

32. Towne JB, Seabrook JR, Bandyk D, et al: In situ replacement of arterial prosthesis infected by bacterial biofilms: Long-term follow-up. J Vasc Surg 19:226, 1994.

33. Velasquez OC, Carpenter JP, Baum RA, et al: Perigraft air, fever, and leukocytosis after endovascular repair of abdominal aortic aneurysms. Am J Surg 178:185, 1999.

34. Deiparine MK, Ballard JL, Taylor FC, et al: Endovascular stent infection. J Vasc Surg 23:529, 1996.

35. Heikkinen L, Valtonen V, Lepantalo M, et al: Infrarenal endoluminal bifurcated stent graft infected with *Listeria monocytogenes*. J Vasc Surg 29:554, 1999.

36. Colburn MD, Moore WS, Chvapil M, et al: Use of an antibiotic-bonded graft for in situ reconstruction after prosthetic graft infections. J Vasc Surg 16:651, 1992.

37. Goeau-Brissoniere O, Mercier F, Nicolas MH, et al: Treatment of vascular graft infection by in situ replacement with a rifampin-bonded gelatin sealed Dacron graft. J Vasc Surg 19:739, 1994.

38. Lachapelle K, Graham AM, Symes JF: Antibacterial activity, antibiotic retention, and infection resistance of a rifampin-impregnated gelatin-sealed Dacron graft. J Vasc Surg 19:675, 1994.

39. Braithwaite BD, Davies B, Heather BP, Earnshaw JJ: Early results of a randomized trial of rifampicin-bonded Dacron grafts for extra-anatomic vascular reconstruction. Joint Vascular Research Group. Br J Surg 85:1378, 1998.

39

Noninfectious Complications in Vascular Surgery

Glenn C. Hunter and Alex Westerband

Complications after aortoiliac and peripheral arterial reconstruction often develop and progress rapidly to produce disastrous consequences related to life and limb and major organ failure. They may be the result of technical errors, the extent of the pathologic process, or one or more of a group of frequently associated diseases. A timeworn surgical principle applies especially to vascular surgery: "A complication not anticipated is sure to be experienced."

The primary problems reviewed in this chapter are those of operative bleeding, thrombosis, operative embolization, iatrogenic injury, major organ failure, graft deterioration, progressing atherosclerotic disease, chylous ascites, anastomotic false aneurysm, and postoperative lower extremity edema. To be concise and avoid repetition, a given problem is discussed generically in relation to its most prominent area of occurrence or severity and then reviewed briefly to highlight details and bring out differences in other circumstances.

AORTOILIAC SURGERY

Complications of aortoiliac arterial reconstruction are similar whether the procedure is for abdominal aortic aneurysmal or occlusive disease.

Operative Bleeding

Operative bleeding is most commonly due to venous injury because of venous anomalies and the close anatomic relationship of the aorta and iliac arteries to the inferior vena cava and to the inferior mesenteric, left renal, left gonadal, lumbar, and iliac veins[1] (Fig. 39–1). Careful operative dissection, a thorough understanding of the anatomy, and familiarity with the characteristics of major venous anomalies are essential to avoid this complication.[2] Anomalies of the left renal vein (retroaortic and circumaortic veins) and inferior vena cava (left-sided cava and caval duplication)

can be detected by either computed tomographic (CT) scans or venography in 2% to 7% of patients.[2–4] The most vulnerable point is the area of tight adherence of the right posterolateral surface of the aorta and common iliac artery to the adjacent wall of the vena cava and right iliac vein at the level of the aortic bifurcation. Complete separation of these structures by circumferential dissection is usually unnecessary, because temporary occlusion can usually be

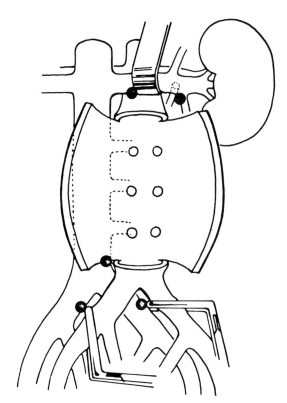

Figure 39–1. Sites of venous injury. (From Downs A: Problems in resection of aortoiliac and femoral aneurysms. In Bernhard VM, Towne JB [eds]: Complications in Vascular Surgery. New York, Grune & Stratton, 1980, p 68.)

achieved without this maneuver by clamp control or by use of intraluminal balloon catheters. If one of these veins is inadvertently lacerated, bleeding should be controlled by gentle finger tamponade and the venous laceration closed with a few stitches of fine monofilament suture. Application of clamps is hazardous and may enlarge the rent in the vein.

The left renal vein should be routinely identified early during dissection of the aorta above an aneurysm or proximal to the area of major aortic occlusive disease. The caudal border of the left renal vein should be clearly defined so that this structure can be easily retracted out of harm's way. Division of its branches enhances its mobility and improves exposure. Failure to find the left renal vein in its usual position suggests its aberrant location behind the aorta (Fig. 39–2). This anomaly occurs in approximately 2% of patients, and, when present, the vein is somewhat more caudal in position and may be readily injured during circumferential dissection of the infrarenal aorta preparatory to application of an occluding clamp.[1–4]

An arteriovenous (AV) fistula involving the aorta or iliac arteries is an uncommon complication of spontaneous aneurysm rupture into an adjacent vein (about 80%) or of retroperitoneal injury to these major vessels. The incidence of this complication is quite low, occurring in less than 1% of all aneurysms and in only 3% to 4% of ruptured aneurysms.[5–8] The presence of an AV fistula is suggested by a continuous bruit over the aneurysm associated with the sudden onset of lower extremity venous hypertension, oliguria, hematuria, and congestive heart failure. If suspected, the diagnosis of aortocaval or iliac AV fistula can be confirmed by color Doppler imaging, CT scanning, or angiography. In the series reported by Brewster and associates,[7] the presence of an AV fistula was unsuspected in 25% of the patients at the time of aortic aneurysm surgery. Occasionally, the fistula may be unsuspected intraoperatively because it is small or obscured by the laminated thrombus within the aneurysm, only to become apparent when sudden massive venous hemorrhage occurs within the lumen of the aorta during evacuation of the laminated thrombus from the aneurysmal sac.[9] In this case, direct

finger pressure over the fistula followed by proximal and distal caval compression with sponge sticks usually controls bleeding so that the venous defect can be visualized and closed with a running suture from within the aortic sac (Fig. 39–3). No attempt should be made to separate the aneurysm wall from the cava at the fistula site. In all patients undergoing aortic aneurysm repair, it is wise to palpate the inferior vena cava for the presence of a thrill, indicating an aortocaval fistula in the otherwise unsuspected case. If a fistula is suspected, the inferior vena cava should then be occluded with a sponge stick or a clamp adjacent to the neck of the aneurysm before opening the aneurysm to prevent embolism of clot or air to the lungs.[6]

Intraoperative bleeding from iliac AV fistulas is often more difficult to control because of their location deep within the pelvis, the size of the defect, and the intimate relationship between the vein and artery. Elective placement of occlusion balloon catheters above and below the aneurysm via the femoral vein before entering the aneurysm may control venous bleeding and permit closure of the defect without massive blood loss. Autotransfusion is a useful adjunct in the management of aortocaval and iliac fistulas.[5] Placement of an endoluminal stent-graft may be an alternative method of treating aortocaval and iliac fistulas when recognized preoperatively.[10, 11]

Arterial bleeding usually arises from the lumbar or the inferior mesenteric arteries during circumferential aortic dissection or after the aorta has been opened.[12] Lumbar vessel injury can be avoided in aneurysm surgery by limiting the dissection to its anterior surface and suture ligature of the lumbar orifices from within the sac after the aneurysm has been opened.[8] A tear in a fragile aortic wall may occur from suture placement during anastomosis. Additional sutures, frequently with polytetrafluoroethylene (PTFE) pledgets, may be required to control these bleeding points.[1] The aorta should be clamped briefly while additional repair sutures are being placed and tied to avoid further tears in the aortic wall.

Bleeding in the immediate postoperative period usually comes from suture lines, inadequately ligated lumbar vessels, or the inferior mesenteric vein. This is manifested by

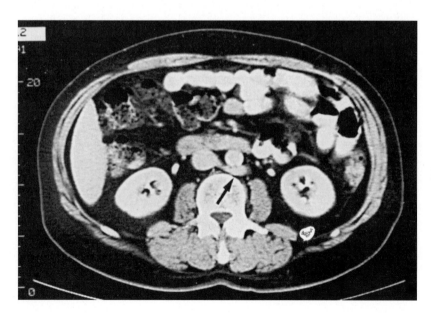

Figure 39–2. Retroaortic renal vein. Computed tomography scan demonstrating a retroaortic left renal vein (*arrow*).

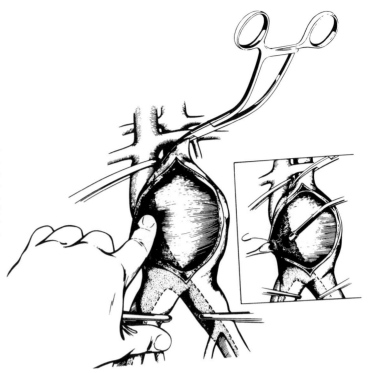

Figure 39–3. Aortocaval fistula. The fistula orifice is exposed through the aneurysm and controlled by simple digital occlusion of the hole into the inferior vena cava. The fistula is closed with a simple over-and-over suture from within the aneurysmal sac. A clear and unencumbered field is provided by rapid aspiration and autotransfusion of blood pouring into the aneurysmal sac from the cava. (From Bernhard VM: Aortocaval fistulas. In Haimovici H (ed): Vascular Emergencies. New York, Appleton-Century-Crofts, 1982, p 357.)

a continuing need for blood replacement and the development of a retroperitoneal hematoma. This can be identified by palpating the flank, usually the left, which loses its normal soft concavity and becomes distended and tense. When aortic or iliac suture line bleeding is rapid, shock is more obvious and the patient complains of severe backache similar to the pain of a ruptured aortic aneurysm.

Postoperative hemorrhage is treated by immediate return to the operating room for identification and control of the bleeding site under fully monitored general anesthesia. Prevention of this complication requires thorough inspection of the intraabdominal anastomoses and the periaortic area, with special attention to the orifices of the lumbar vessels, the inferior mesenteric artery, and the ligated or oversewn stumps of the aorta or the iliac vessels. The surgeon should search for the potential bleeding site when blood volume and pressure are at the patient's normal level before closing the retroperitoneum over the aortoiliac reconstruction.

Bleeding due to unrecognized coagulopathy usually can be prevented by careful preoperative history and evaluation of the platelet count, bleeding time, prothrombin time, and partial thromboplastin time.[13] These preliminary screening studies reliably identify the need to search for precise factor deficiencies and direct their replacement before and during surgery. Intraoperative monitoring of the activated clotting time before and after heparin administration is the most effective means of identifying variations in the individual response to intraoperatively administered heparin and to determine the adequacy of its reversal before closing the incision.[13] Transfusion reaction and disseminated intravascular coagulopathy are rare causes of operative or early postoperative bleeding; however, consumption coagulopathy secondary to massive blood loss and replacement is more common and requires the judicious use of fresh-frozen plasma and platelets. Proper management of bleeding due to congenital or acquired deficiencies requires repeated monitoring of pertinent coagulation parameters during and immediately after the operative procedure.

Thombosis

Graft thrombosis in the early postoperative period is almost invariably due to technical problems (Fig. 39–4) that usually occur at the distal anastomoses.[14–16] These include an elevated intimal flap; narrowing of the artery at the anastomotic suture line; failure to remove clot adherent to the inner wall of the graft before completion of the anastomosis; twisting or kinking in the retroperitoneal tunnel; compression of the femoral limb of the graft by the inguinal ligament; unrecognized inflow disease; or inadequate runoff secondary to unappreciated iliac, profunda, superficial femoral, or infrapopliteal disease. Rarely, thrombosis after aortofemoral bypass or aneurysm replacement is due to hypercoagulability from antithrombin III deficiency, protein C or S deficiency, a mutation in factor V Leiden or prothrombin genes, homocysteinemia, anticardiolipin antibodies or heparin-induced platelet aggregation, or stasis due to reduced cardiac output.[17–20]

The adequacy of pulsatile blood flow through the graft or endarterectomy should be evaluated in the operating room before the wounds are closed, not only by palpation of the graft itself and the arteries immediately distal to anastomoses but also by palpation of distal pulses and direct inspection of the pedal circulation beneath the drapes. If necessary, noninvasive measurements such as Doppler flow, ankle pressure, or pulse-volume recorder (PVR) tracings can be obtained intraoperatively.[14, 15, 21–23]

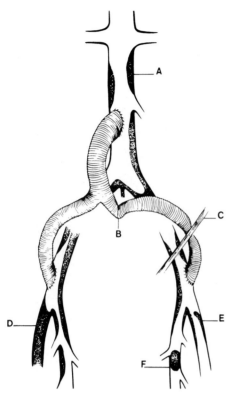

Figure 39–4. Mechanical factors that may cause early thrombosis of aortofemoral graft. *A,* Aortic anastomosis distal to obstructing atherosclerosis at subrenal level. *B,* Kinking of graft limb due to placement of the proximal anastomosis low on the aorta with too long an aortic graft segment. *C,* Compression by the inguinal ligament. *D,* Inadequate runoff due to occlusion of the superficial femoral artery and severe stenosis of the profunda. *E,* Elevation of distal intima. *F,* Peripheral embolization or thrombosis. (From Bernhard VM: The failed arterial graft: Lost pulses and gangrene. In Condon RE, DeCosse JJ [eds]: Surgical Care. Philadelphia, Lea & Febiger, 1980, p 155.)

Intraoperative completion angiograms should be obtained in all patients who have had extensive reconstructive procedures of the common femoral, superficial femoral, or profunda femoris arteries to ensure the adequacy of the repair. Noninvasive studies should be performed routinely in the recovery room when pulses cannot be felt distal to the repair or when the anticipated improvement in circulation has not occurred. Objective information obtained from these easily performed studies is particularly valuable in the immediate postoperative period when patients are frequently hypothermic and peripherally vasoconstricted. Detection of unsatisfactory graft function mandates immediate direct evaluation of involved anastomoses before wound closure or by prompt return to the operating room if graft flow deteriorates subsequently.

Treatment of immediate postreconstructive thrombosis consists of thorough inspection of the intraluminal aspect of the involved anastomosis. This is best accomplished through an incision in the distal end of the graft or by takedown of the anastomosis to directly view the intima and the runoff vessels adjacent to the arteriotomy. Effective revision may require stabilization of an elevated plaque, extension of an iliac limb to the common femoral artery, or patch angioplasty of a profunda or proximal superficial femoral stenosis. Infrequently, complementary bypass from

the femoral to the popliteal or the infrapopliteal vessels may be required when adequate runoff cannot be achieved through the profunda.[24, 25] The lie of the graft should always be inspected throughout its length to ensure that there is no kinking, twisting, or external compression within the retroperitoneal tunnel.

Prevention of early graft thrombosis depends on an accurate evaluation of the distal runoff bed by preoperative arteriography, noninvasive hemodynamic testing, and direct palpation of the iliac artery throughout its length before the selection of this vessel, rather than the femoral, as the site for distal anastomosis. The orifices of the runoff vessels should be inspected and calibrated. Special attention should be given to the profunda orifice, which often requires angioplasty when the distal anastomosis is performed at the common femoral level. Finally, technical perfection in the performance of anastomoses is mandatory to avoid narrowing of the runoff vessels. Tacking sutures may be required to prevent distal intimal dissection.

Thrombosis is the most frequent late complication of aortoiliac and aortofemoral procedures[26, 27] and usually appears as unilateral limb ischemia[28–34] (see Fig. 39–4*D*). Impaired outflow through the external iliac artery or the major branches of the common femoral is the most common etiology and is caused by progressive downstream atherosclerosis or anastomotic fibrointimal hyperplasia (Fig. 39–5*A*). Anastomotic fibrointimal hyperplasia causes stenosis, usually at distal anastomoses, by the circumferential development of fibrous tissue at the distal graft-artery interface; occlusion occurs when flow diminishes sufficiently to result in stasis thrombosis.[33] The majority of patients initially managed with aortofemoral bypass have occlusion of the superficial femoral artery at the time of the primary procedure. Therefore, an adequate lumen at the origin of the deep femoral artery is the most significant factor in ensuring long-term patency of these grafts.[22, 27, 29, 32, 34] Underestimating the severity of outflow disease at the time of primary reconstruction is an important cofactor of progressing atherosclerosis that increases susceptibility to late graft limb occlusion.[35] Despite an adequate primary procedure, progression of femoral or infrapopliteal atherosclerotic disease is more likely to occur in patients with continued exposure to atherogenic risk factors, particularly those who continue to smoke.[28, 35]

Impaired inflow is the second most common cause of late postrevascularization thrombosis. Although it is four to nine times less frequent than impaired outflow,[35] it is the most common cause of simultaneous bilateral postreconstructive lower limb ischemia after aortoiliac or femoral surgery.[27, 30] The most common mechanism is obstruction from progressive infrarenal aortic atherosclerosis proximal to the site of previous repair (see Fig. 39–4*A*). This is usually the consequence of placing the proximal anastomosis too low on the aorta (i.e., at or below the inferior mesenteric artery) (see Fig. 39–5*B*). The area between this site and the renal arteries is an active site of progressive atherosclerosis.[22] Likewise, following aortoiliac endarterectomy, late occlusion is more likely if the proximal infrarenal aorta is not included in the endarterectomy.[36] The use of an end-to-end rather than an end-to-side aortic anastomosis may be associated with fewer thrombotic failures, although this has not been clearly defined. Superior hemodynamic

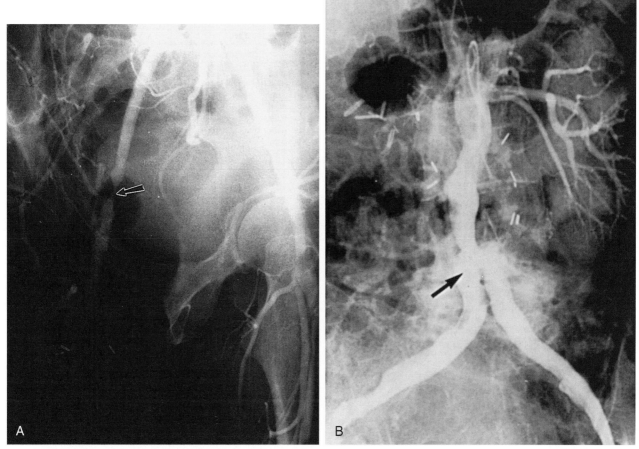

Figure 39–5. Progressive inflow and outflow obstruction. A, Outflow of obstruction due to atherosclerosis at the distal limb of an aortobifemoral graft *(arrow)*. B, An aortogram demonstrating progressive atherosclerosis proximal to an incorrectly placed bifurcation graft *(arrow)*.

flow characteristics, the absence of competitive flow, less chance of embolization from the host aorta, and less angulation of the limbs as they arise from the body graft[22, 36] have been cited as the advantages of the end-to-end aortic anastomosis.

Angulation of the graft limb at the bifurcation may produce kinking due to failure to pull the graft limb out to full length before the distal anastomoses are performed or excessive length of the graft body, resulting in too wide a bifurcation angle (see Fig. 39–4B). Inadequate retroperitoneal tunneling of the graft limbs may promote thrombosis as a consequence of extrinsic compression from the mesentery of the sigmoid colon or the recurrent portion of the inguinal ligament[35] (see Fig. 39–4C).

Less frequent causes of late thrombosis of aortoiliac and femoral reconstructions include accumulation of mural thrombus and false aneurysm. Mural thrombus develops when the graft diameter is significantly larger than the outflow artery. The flow pattern of the larger graft adjusts itself to the smaller outflow artery, leaving a peripheral layer of slowly moving blood that clots to form the mural thrombus. The normal, smooth, firmly adherent fibrous neointima becomes lined with a thick, gelatinous, loosely adherent mural thrombus that reduces the functioning lumen to the diameter of the outflow vessel. Fragmentation

with distal embolization or progressive narrowing of the graft lumen with secondary acute thrombotic occlusion may then occur.[33] Anastomotic false aneurysms, although relatively rare causes of late limb ischemia, may also produce peripheral embolization or thrombosis of the aneurysm and the adjacent vessel lumen.[35] Finally, an aortoiliac reconstruction can progress suddenly to thrombosis in the presence of cardiac embolization or decreased cardiac output secondary to myocardial infarction or congestive heart failure. Rarely, no apparent cause for late thrombosis can be identified, implicating thrombogenicity of the graft surface or degeneration and disruption of the neointima.

The diagnosis of late thrombosis is suggested by the sudden or progressive recurrence of symptoms, a decrease or loss of previously present distal pulses, and a concomitant reduction in ankle pressure, Doppler flow, or PVR waveform. The degree of ischemia after thrombosis of a reconstruction is usually more severe than before the primary revascularization procedure.[27, 30] The frequency of late thrombosis increases from 5% to 10% in the first 5 years to 20% to 30% at 10 years.[22, 34, 37–39] Therefore, routine and long-term follow-up of these patients at regular intervals is required to monitor the adequacy of graft function. If significant stenosis can be demonstrated before complete thrombosis, surgical correction is simplified. When either abrupt or gradual change is apparent, prompt aortography should be performed to determine the status of the graft, the anastomoses, the inflow, and the runoff bed.[21, 40]

The severity of recurrent ischemia, which may range from minimal to severe claudication, rest pain, or pregangrene, depends on the extent of compensating collaterals and the vigor of the patient's normal activity. Arteriography is required to determine whether further surgery is feasible and to guide the surgeon in the selection of the most appropriate reoperative procedure, considering the patient's age, state of health, and general level of activity.[28, 35]

Correction of late thrombosis requires operative determination of the underlying mechanical problem followed by appropriate corrective maneuvers.[35, 41] The occlusion of one limb of an aortoiliac bifurcation graft is usually due to overlooked or progressing disease in the external iliac and femoral arteries. Retroperitoneal exposure of the occluded limb, balloon catheter thrombectomy, and graft extension to the femoral level is a reliable solution. Femorofemoral bypass is the alternative if the donor iliofemoral inflow is satisfactory, especially in the higher risk patient. Axillofemoral bypass may be required if neither of the preceding methods is feasible.[2, 24]

The most commonly encountered situation is a thrombosed aortofemoral graft limb with impaired outflow. Inflow can usually be restored by graft thrombectomy using a balloon thromboembolectomy catheter[41] (Fig. 39–6). A thromboendarterectomy stripper or adherent clot catheter is often required to complete the extraction of adherent clot and old pseudointima. The Fogarty catheter is passed through the ring of the stripper into the patent aortic portion of the graft and its balloon fully inflated and pulled down to occlude the proximal end of the limb to control bleeding and prevent crossover embolization. The stripper is passed back and forth around the catheter within the occluded graft limb up to the distended balloon to scrape thrombus from the graft wall. Thereafter, the balloon is deflated just enough to permit its tight withdrawal through the graft limb en masse with the stripper and detached thrombus (see Fig. 39–6A and B). Use of the Fogarty adherent clot catheter obviates the need for the thromboendarterectomy stripper and may be more effective in removing adherent thrombus. The patient is systemically heparinized (100 to 125 units/kg) during all of these maneuvers.

Thrombectomy is usually combined with a profundaplasty of varying extent to provide outflow. However, femoropopliteal or femoral distal bypass may be required, depending on the extent and location of outflow disease.[24, 25, 41, 42] If an occluded graft limb cannot be reopened by thrombectomy, a femorofemoral graft can be inserted. Replacement of the graft limb is another alternative but is technically more difficult.

If an entire bifurcation graft is thrombosed, a problem at the proximal anastomosis such as low placement of the graft with proximal disease, kinking, or anastomotic aneurysm is a likely cause. A CT scan is required to identify the last-named. If no proximal problem can be demonstrated, thrombectomy with either a balloon or adherent clot catheter can be attempted but is usually not successful. The alternatives are to replace the original prosthesis or insert an axillobifemoral bypass. The latter procedure is less technically demanding and less hazardous and is the reoperation of choice in the physiologically compromised patient.[41]

When groin scarring is especially intense, bypass to the midprofunda simplifies the outflow repair of the reoperative procedure by avoiding a tedious and hazardous dissection in the area of a previous femoral anastomosis.[43] In certain circumstances, intraarterial thrombolytic therapy can be a helpful adjunct to the management of occluded aortoiliac reconstructions.[44]

An aggressive attitude toward reoperation after thrombotic failure of aortoiliac reconstruction is warranted, especially if the patient will derive sustained benefit from long-term patency and improved limb function,[41] because operative morbidity and mortality rates are low. Reoperative mortality rates of 3%, with cumulative 3-year patency rates of 68% to 75% have been reported.[27, 41] Judicious use of extraabdominal approaches has contributed significantly to reduced reoperative morbidity and mortality.[35]

Lytic Therapy for Graft Thrombosis

Whereas thrombectomy has been the treatment of choice in the management of occluded aortofemoral and femoropopliteal bypass grafts, incomplete removal of thrombotic material and the difficulties associated with reoperation have led to the evaluation of direct intraarterial infusion of thrombolytic agents, either preoperatively or intraoperatively, for the management of this problem. The potential benefits of lytic therapy include delineation of the cause of the graft thrombosis (most commonly distal occlusion due to neointimal fibrous hyperplasia or progression of disease) and, as a consequence, a shorter operation, reduced blood loss, and the ease of extraction of any residual thrombus. Potential disadvantages and complications of thrombolytic therapy include the need for monitoring in an intensive care unit, delay in surgical intervention, and the risks of bleeding or renal impairment from the contrast load requisite to frequent arteriographic evaluations.

Furthermore, mechanical thrombectomy for aortofemoral graft limb occlusion is at least as effective as clot lysis and adds little to the operative procedure required to restore outflow. Successful lysis, which does not appear to be affected by the duration and cause of the graft thrombosis, can be achieved in 50% to 90% of occluded prosthetic graft limbs, 50% to 77% of saphenous veins, and 38% to 71% of prosthetic grafts.[45–50] Gardiner and colleagues[51] reported an overall success rate of 69% of the patients with an 84% success rate when urokinase (UK) was used, compared with 48% in those receiving streptokinase. Presently, although both agents are effective in dissolving thrombus, UK appears to have some advantage over streptokinase because of its more predictable response, fewer bleeding complications, and shorter infusion time. In addition, infusion with streptokinase often cannot be repeated due to the development of antibodies. Although the cost of streptokinase is considerably less than UK, the shorter infusion time and lower complication rates negate the benefits of the initial lower cost of the former.[52]

For effective therapy, the catheter is usually embedded within the thrombus. Most radiologists initially "lace" the

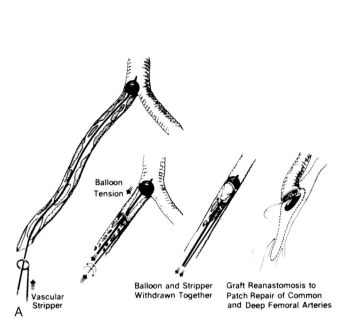

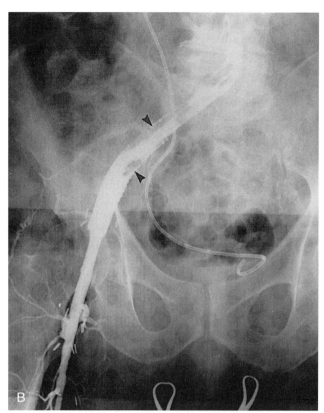

Figure 39–6. *A*, A ring endarterectomy stripper is used in conjunction with a balloon catheter to remove thrombus and pseudointima adherent to the wall of an occluded limb of an aortofemoral graft. The cleared graft limb is thereafter sutured to the common or profunda femoral outflow after patch angioplasty. *B*, An intraoperative arteriogram demonstrating residual thrombus after attempted thrombectomy. (*A*, From Bernhard VM: Late vascular graft thrombosis. In Bernhard VM, Towne JB [eds]: Complications in Vascular Surgery, 2nd ed. Orlando, FL, Grune & Stratton, 1985, p 193. *B*, From Hunter GC, Bull DA: The healing characteristics, durability, and long-term complications of vascular prostheses. In Bernhard VM, Towne TB [eds]: Complications in Vascular Surgery. St. Louis, Quality Medical Publishing, 1991, p 65.)

thrombus with a bolus dose of 250,000 units of UK distributed through the length of the graft thrombus and continue with an hourly infusion of 120,000 to 240,000 units.[47, 48] Either low-dose heparin or the lytic agent is infused into the sheath surrounding the infusion catheter to prevent pericatheter thrombosis. There are no useful laboratory tests available to evaluate the efficacy of lytic therapy, although titration of the lytic infusion to maintain a serum fibrinogen level of greater than 100 mg/dL is used by most investigators to monitor therapy. The duration of therapy ranges from 18 to 48 hours.

Bleeding, the major complication of lytic therapy, occurs after 7% to 48% of infusions.[48, 52] The most common sources of bleeding are arteriography or venous puncture sites, the interstices of prosthetic grafts, and systemic bleeding from remote sites. Central nervous system bleeding is rare with UK. Bleeding from a groin arterial puncture site may also result in femoral pseudoaneurysm or retroperitoneal hematoma, which may compress the femoral nerve within the iliac fascia or in the thigh. The resulting femoral neuralgia, reported to occur in up to 30% of patients, may persist for as long as 1 year.[53, 54] Rarely, patients develop a femoral nerve palsy, which may be debilitating, especially in patients with claudication or amputation of the contralateral limb.

The most important determinant of long-term success in the study by Gardiner and coworkers was the presence of a lesion correctable by surgical revision or balloon catheter dilatation. Such lesions responsible for the occlusion can be identified in approximately 50% of patients. Gardiner and associates reported an 84% 1-year patency in 25 grafts with underlying stenotic lesions, compared with 37% of a similar number of grafts without detectable lesions.[51]

Three prospective studies compared the efficacy of intraarterial thrombolysis and surgery in patients with lower limb ischemia.[55–57] In their initial study, Ouriel and colleagues[55] randomized 114 patients with acute lower limb ischemia of less than 7 days' duration to receive either thrombolytic therapy or surgery. The authors achieved clot dissolution in 70% of their patients and observed no difference in limb salvage rates (82%) at 1 year. However, they did observe improved patient survival (82% vs. 58%) in the patients receiving thrombolytic therapy, which they attributed to the more frequent occurrence of cardiopulmonary complications in the patients undergoing surgery. In a subsequent study,[56] Ouriel and associates randomized 213 patients with acute limb ischemia of less than 14 days' duration to either recombinant urokinase (r-UK) or surgery. Clot lysis was achieved in a similar number of patients (71%). The authors found no differences in either mortality rates (14% vs. 16%) or amputation-free survival rates (75% vs. 65%) between the two groups at 1 year. In the STILE (Surgery Versus Thrombolysis for Ischemia of the Lower Extremity) trial,[57] the efficacy of recombinant tissue-type plasminogen activator (rt-PA) and UK was compared with that of surgery in 393 patients with limb ischemia of less than 6 months' duration. Failure of catheter placement occurred in 28% of patients. Patients with ischemia of less than 14 days' duration receiving lytic therapy had lower amputation rates than surgical patients, whereas patients with ischemic symptoms of more than 14 days' duration fared better with surgery. The results of these studies suggest that in selected patients, thrombolytic therapy may be a useful adjunct or alternative to surgical therapy. However, long-term patency rates of 28% to 37% of thrombolysed grafts are clearly inferior to those obtained with surgery.[51, 58] Thrombolytic therapy may be extremely valuable in patients with limb-threatening ischemia secondary to thrombosed popliteal aneurysm. Thrombolysis may improve the chances of achieving long-term patency and limb salvage.[59]

With the recent unavailability of UK, other lytic agents are being evaluated for the treatment of occluded grafts. The three available alternatives are streptokinase, anisoylated plasminogen streptokinase activator complex (APSAC), and rt-PA. Neither streptokinase nor APSAC is currently widely used to treat acute peripheral arterial occlusions. Tissue plasminogen activator (t-PA; alteplase) and reteplase (Retavase, Roche Diagnostics, Mannheim, Germany; Centocor, Inc., Malvern, Pa.) are two of the agents currently being evaluated. Alteplase initiates local fibrinolysis by binding to fibrin in thrombus, where it converts entrapped plasminogen to plasmin. Alteplase is cleared rapidly from the plasma, primarily by the liver: more than 50% of the drug present in plasma is cleared within 5 minutes and approximately 80% within 10 minutes. Neither alteplase nor reteplase is Food and Drug Administration (FDA)–approved for intraarterial use in peripheral arterial occlusion and no optimal dosing regimen exists. An initial dose of 5 to 10 mg of t-PA into the thrombus followed by an infusion dose of 0.001–0.02 mg/kg/hour has been recommended.[60] Although there have not been any large trials evaluating alteplase in the treatment of peripheral arterial occlusion, anecdotal reports suggest an increased incidence of local and remote bleeding, predominantly intracranial hemorrhage, with its use. Whether this is due to the use of inappropriately large doses of alteplase or the concomitant administration of heparin remains to be determined.

Reteplase, a nonglycosylated deletion mutant of t-PA, offers some attraction as an alternative to UK. Reteplase catalyzes the cleavage of endogenous plasminogen to generate plasmin, which degrades the fibrin matrix of the thrombus, resulting in its dissolution. The half-life of reteplase is 13 to 16 minutes and catheter-directed infusion doses vary between 0.5 and 1.0 units/hour for a duration of 5 to 24 hours. Lacing or infiltrating the thrombus with a 2-to 5-unit bolus dose may be beneficial in some patients.[61] In approximately half the patients, low-dose heparin is infused concomitantly. Reteplase differs from alteplase both in its structure and biochemical composition and its lower affinity for thrombin.

McNamara[62] reported a 34% incidence of bleeding in a series of 40 patients treated with alteplase compared with 3% with retevase with doses of 2 to 8 mg/hour. Even reducing the dosage of alteplase to 0.5 to 1.0 mg/hour was still associated with a 25% incidence of bleeding requiring transfusion.[62]

The indications for and contraindications to the use of these two agents are similar to those of UK. The status of the use of these newer lytic agents is presently not well defined; therefore, there are few reliable data to guide the practicing clinician. It behooves us all to carefully evaluate the risks and benefits of the use of lytic therapy in the reatment of patients with graft limb occlusions.

The relatively low incidence of complications, improved technique of administration, and efficacy of thrombolytic agents have reduced the need for urgent thrombectomy in patients with noncritical limb ischemia. Successful lytic therapy readily identifies the cause of the graft limb occlusion and may allow a less extensive repair. In addition, lytic therapy may reduce the risk of wound and graft complications associated with extensive redo procedures.

Mechanical Thrombectomy

Mechanical thrombectomy (MT) devices that theoretically permit rapid revascularization of an ischemic extremity using minimally invasive techniques are gaining increasing popularity. The use of mechanical energy to cause fragmentation, dissolution, and aspiration of thrombus is appealing. These devices can be broadly classified into (a) aspiration thrombectomy catheters that remove thrombus by steady manual suction through a large-lumen aspiration catheter, (b) pull-back thrombectomy catheters that withdraw thrombus with a balloon catheter or basket into a trapping device allowing the clot to be removed, (c) recirculation thrombectomy devices that ablate thrombus by hydrodynamic vortices, which pulverize the thrombus into microscopic fragments, (d) nonrecirculation thrombectomy devices, which macerate the thrombus mechanically into fragments that are larger than those produced by recirculation catheters, and (e) energy-assisted devices, which use either ultrasound, laser, or radiofrequency to lyse thrombus or enhance the effects of pharmacologic agents.[63] None of these devices are presently FDA-approved. A number of these devices are currently being evaluated clinically, with complete angiographic success reported in approximately 50% of patients and partial success in an additional 27%.[64] Concomitant lytic therapy or balloon angioplasty is often a necessary adjunct.

Operative Embolization

Atherothrombotic debris is present to some degree in most atherosclerotic arteries and especially in the distal aorta. Protruding atheromas of the aortic arch and descending aorta have assumed increasing importance as potential sites for embolization during cardiac catheterization or bypass surgery.[65] Readily detectable by transesophageal echocardiography, lesions larger than 0.5 cm are most likely to be associated with embolic events.[66, 67] Variable amounts of this material may be dislodged and carried into the downstream arterial territory as a consequence of manipulation during arterial dissection.[21, 67, 68] Embolization may also occur on reestablishment of circulation due to the accumulation of fresh thrombus in the temporarily static blood column above or below the clamps that is not carefully evacuated before circulation is restored.

Larger emboli lodging in major vessels can usually be retrieved with a balloon thrombectomy catheter. Smaller embolic particles that cannot be retrieved will be flushed into end arteries of the foot or toes, leading to the "trash foot" syndrome.[1, 21, 67, 68] The end result is the appearance of patchy areas of painful skin gangrene at these sites (Fig. 39–7). This may be a minor and self-limited problem, or it may produce extensive gangrene of all of the digits and the forefoot.

Prevention is the key issue, because it is frequently difficult or impossible to treat this complication. A variety of technical maneuvers have been employed to prevent operative embolization.[1] Unnecessary and overly vigorous handling of vessels before the application of clamps should be avoided. Effective preclamping heparinization, preferably monitored by intraoperative measurement of the activated clotting time, reduces stasis thrombus formation above the proximal clamp and in the sluggish circulation distally. In patients with suspected or demonstrable atheromatous debris within the aorta on CT scans, the distal clamps should be applied to the common femoral or iliac arteries prior to proximal occlusion to avoid downstream displacement of debris when the aortic clamp is placed. The proximal clamp may need to be placed at the level of the diaphragm if the pararenal segment of the aorta appears to be involved. The lumen of the aortic prosthesis should be thoroughly aspirated to remove blood and debris after testing the proximal suture line, and efforts should be made to prevent the accumulation of blood within the

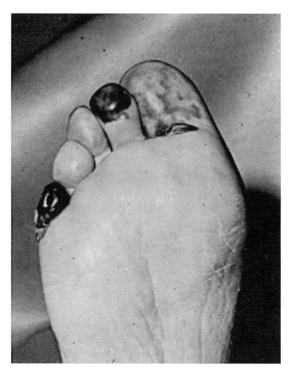

Figure 39–7. Atheroembolic ischemic lesions of the toes. (From Eastcott HHG: Complication of aortoiliac reconstruction for occlusive disease. In Bernhard VM, Towne JB [eds]: Complications in Vascular Surgery. New York, Grune & Stratton, 1980, p 59.)

prosthesis while distal iliac or femoral anastomoses are being performed. Vigorous prograde flushing of the proximal vessel and retrograde flushing from the distal arteries as the last few stitches are being placed in an anastomosis before restoration of circulation is the most reliable maneuver for ensuring that retained debris and clot are effectively removed.[68]

Treatment depends on the severity of embolization. Minor patchy areas of cyanosis or necrosis can be observed since spontaneous recovery can be anticipated. More extensive involvement with threatened viability of the distal foot requires attempted removal of embolic material with small Fogarty catheters passed into the distal vessels through the patent popliteal artery, accompanied by distal intraarterial infusion of UK. Occasionally, when there is severe ischemia of a single or multiple digits, lumbar sympathectomy or amputation may be necessary. In patients with a patent superficial femoral artery and severe forefoot ischemia, intraarterial lytic therapy may reduce the level of amputation.

Declamping Hypotension

A sudden decrease in blood pressure should be anticipated after removal of the aortic clamp to restore flow to one or both extremities after aortoiliac reconstruction.[69–72] The cause is hypovolemia due to incompletely replaced blood loss and fluid sequestration during surgery, compounded by a variable degree of preoperative dehydration that is usually present.[12] Contributing factors are peripheral vasodilatation secondary to limb ischemia during the period of aortic occlusion and a decrease in cardiac output caused by a sudden return of acidic blood and other vasoactive metabolites to the central circulation on restoration of limb perfusion. The major consequences are significant reduction in coronary perfusion, which may promote myocardial injury, especially in patients with significant coronary artery disease, and temporary renal ischemia, which may contribute to renal failure. Prevention is preferable to treatment after a hypotensive insult has occurred and depends on adequate hydration and effective restoration of intravascular volume during the procedure, and especially prior to clamp release.[71–73] Effective volume replacement requires careful monitoring of blood loss and accurate estimation of the extracellular fluid shifts due to sequestration and loss from evaporation. The extent of intravascular depletion is directly related to the duration of intraperitoneal and retroperitoneal exposure during surgery.

The most reliable guide to ensuring adequate volume replacement without circulatory overload is the use of the Swan-Ganz catheter to monitor left heart filling pressures and myocardial performance.[73] Cooperation between the surgeon and the anesthesiologist is essential during the critical moments prior to clamp release. Left atrial filling pressures should be optimized prior to release of the clamps. The arterial pressure must be continuously observed while blood flow is slowly restored to the extremities by gradual release of the clamp until full flow can be tolerated without hypotension. Finally, when a bifurcation graft is inserted, it is best to complete the anastomosis to one limb and restore its circulation immediately so that lower body perfusion can be resumed with the least amount of delay to avoid washout acidosis and reduce declamping hypotension.

Renal Failure

Acute renal failure (ARF) accompanying aortic surgery has a major impact on operative mortality. The reported incidence of ARF following elective aortic aneurysmectomy is 1% to 8%, with a mortality rate of 40%. However, if the aneurysmectomy is emergent, the reported incidence of ARF is 8% to 46%, with a mortality of 57% to 95%.[74, 75] The major cause is reduced renal perfusion due to decreased cardiac output, decreased blood volume, and dehydration. A contributing factor is renal cortical vasospasm produced by infrarenal application of the aortic clamp, which stimulates the renin angiotensin mechanism.[76, 77] Other promoting factors include suprarenal aortic cross-clamping, which totally eliminates renal perfusion; ligation of the left renal vein; and intraoperative renal arterial embolization.[78] The last may originate from debris and clot accumulating proximal to the aortic clamp or from manipulation of the juxtarenal aorta.[75, 79] Renal artery obstruction may be produced by displacement of large atherosclerotic plaques at the orifices of the renal arteries when an aortic clamp is applied. Preoperative angiography may produce a mild to moderate degree of renal dysfunction, which may be compounded by hypotension and dehydration during the operative procedure.[75] Myoglobinemia can occur after restoration of circulation to limbs that have been severely ischemic for an extended period. Finally, nephrotoxic antibiotics employed perioperatively must be considered.

Although the consequences of ischemic injury to the kidney are complex, injury to the tubules is central to the development of oliguria. Obstruction of the tubular lumen by cellular debris and casts results in reduction of the ultrafiltration pressure and sequestration of tubular fluid within obstructed tubules, in addition to back-leak of fluid into the interstitium.[80]

The critical issue is prevention, which is primarily related to the maintenance of an effective circulating blood volume and adequate hydration in the immediate perioperative period.[75, 81] It is essential that the patient be well hydrated and have a good urinary output at the commencement of surgery. Any significant extracellular fluid volume deficits should be restored the evening before surgery, especially if angiography or a mechanical bowel preparation has been recently performed. The creatinine level should be measured after angiography, and if a decrease in renal function is identified, surgery should be delayed, if possible. Central filling pressures should be monitored perioperatively to ensure that volume replacement is optimal in relation to cardiac output and myocardial performance.[73] It is appropriate to give mannitol and commence an infusion of renal-dose dopamine just before cross-clamping the aorta to promote an osmotic diuresis and reduce the effects of renal cortical vasospasm.[76] Bicarbonate is given to alkalinize the urine if there is any question of significant myoglobin washout from renewed perfusion of limbs that have undergone prolonged ischemia. Renal insufficiency is a

significant complication of surgical procedures requiring cross-clamping of the suprarenal aorta. Currently, a number of therapeutic agents, including insulin-like growth factor,[82] urodilatin (Ularitide),[83, 84] and endothelin[85] antagonists are being evaluated to determine their efficacy in reducing the incidence of ARF.

During dissection required to gain proximal control of large infrarenal or juxtarenal aneurysms, the left renal vein is vulnerable to injury. Access to this portion of the aorta is facilitated by division of the left renal vein.[86] In the past, this maneuver was viewed as one of little long-term consequence. However, Huber and coworkers[87] and Abu Rahma and associates[88] have demonstrated increased serum creatinine concentrations in patients who have had renal vein ligation. Whether the renal dysfunction following renal vein ligation is a consequence solely of the resultant increased venous pressure or develops because of a combination of venous hypertension and transient ischemia from intraoperative suprarenal clamp placement (which is required more frequently in these patients) is not yet clear. Nonetheless, it would appear prudent to repair the renal vein when possible, as advocated by Szilagyi and associates.[86]

Renal arteries should be dissected free and temporarily clamped in patients with total aortic occlusion in which thrombus extends up to the renal orifices. The quality of the renal pulses must be evaluated and blood flow assessed by Doppler scan after restoration of circulation through the aorta in any patient who has had significant juxtarenal aortic manipulation or if urine output should suddenly diminish. Immediate renal repair is required if renal artery occlusion is identified.

Postoperatively, the continued retroperitoneal and intraperitoneal sequestration of extracellular fluid requires replacement with Ringer's lactate solution, within the limits imposed by left heart filling pressures, to ensure adequate renal output.[12] Volume replacement should be reduced after the second postoperative day to prevent fluid overload from the mobilization of large volumes of sequestered extravascular fluid. The urinary output is monitored continuously and should be maintained at or above 0.5 mL/kg/hour. The specific gravity is determined frequently, and the blood urea nitrogen and creatinine measured daily for 2 or 3 days to determine the quality of renal function. Diuretics should not be given until intravascular volume has been fully restored. If ARF is diagnosed, fluid replacement should be restricted to maintain central filling pressure in the normal range. Dialysis is used aggressively to control excess volume and relieve azotemia and hyperkalemia.[75, 89] Intravenous hyperalimentation should be instituted early in the clinical course of patients with ARF to minimize protein catabolism.[90]

The liberal use of aortography before surgery is recommended to identify renal anomalies, renal artery stenoses, or suprarenal extension of an aneurysm so that appropriate alterations in operative management can be planned. These may include the use of temporary renal perfusion with cold lactated Ringer's solution containing heparin, mannitol, and methylprednisolone.[75] Postoperatively, a renal scan and aortography should be performed immediately if total renal shutdown appears, because this suggests a renal artery occlusion. This requires immediate reoperation to restore kidney circulation.

Intestinal Ischemia

Intestinal ischemia may complicate aortic bypass or endarterectomy for occlusive disease, but the majority of cases follow aneurysmectomy.[91, 92] Almost all reported instances of intestinal ischemia following aortic surgery are a result of arterial obstruction; venous ischemia is extremely rare.[93] Small bowel ischemia occurs in 0.15% of cases.[91] The clinical presentation of ischemic colitis occurs in 0.2% to 10% of aortic procedures and most commonly involves the rectosigmoid area.[94] However, if routine colonoscopy is performed, a much higher incidence of intestinal ischemia is noted because of the identification of subclinical ischemic colitis. Hagihara and associates[95] found a 6% incidence in patients undergoing elective or urgent reconstruction of the abdominal aorta for aneurysmal or occlusive disease, whereas the incidence of ischemic colitis was 60% following repair of ruptured aneurysm. The overall mortality rate for patients with colon ischemia is approximately 50% and approaches 90% for transmural colon involvement.

The cause of bowel ischemia is operative atheroembolization or interruption of the primary or collateral arteries to the bowel wall.[91, 92] There are two sets of vessels that are critical to colon perfusion: (1) the superior rectal branch of the inferior mesenteric artery that connects with the middle and inferior rectal branches of the hypogastric vessels, thus connecting the visceral with the systemic circulation; and (2) the inferior mesenteric artery and its left colic branch that connect with the superior mesenteric through the arc of Riolan and, to a lesser extent, the marginal artery of Drummond.[94] The former connection is referred to as the "meandering mesenteric artery," especially when it becomes enlarged as a collateral to compensate for superior or inferior mesenteric artery obstruction.[96] This vessel is present in about two thirds of normal people and can be seen on angiography in 27% to 35% of patients who have aneurysmal or occlusive disease.[97] Areas of deficiency in this normal anatomic relationship are at Griffith's point at the splenic flexure and in the collateral vessels of the rectosigmoid (Fig. 39–8).

Obstruction of the primary arteries supplying the viscera makes viability of the bowel dependent on this collateral circulation. Occlusion of the orifice of the inferior mesenteric artery is frequently associated with aneurysmal disease and obstructive aortic atherosclerosis, thus placing the burden of bowel circulation on collaterals from the superior mesenteric artery and the hypogastric vessels. Severe obstruction or occlusion of the superior mesenteric artery is compensated for by branches from the celiac artery and retrograde flow from the inferior mesenteric artery through the left colic and middle colic. Hypogastric obstruction requires collateral flow from branches of the inferior mesenteric artery. When this source is also impaired, colon circulation must depend on more tenuous connections between the arch of Riolan and the marginal artery and the distal branches of the hypogastric, which in turn derive their blood supply from the parietal circulation.

A critical loss of blood flow to an intestinal tract that is

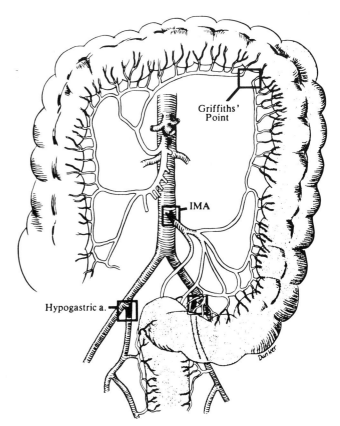

Figure 39–8. Lack of marginal artery continuity at splenic flexure (Griffiths' point) with inferior mesenteric (IMA) and hypogastric arterial occlusions predisposing to left colon ischemia. (From Ernst CB: Colon ischemia following abdominal aortic reconstruction. In Bernhard VM, Towne JB [eds]: Complications in Vascular Surgery. New York, Grune & Stratton, 1980, p 383.)

dependent on this extensive collateral network may occur if a patent inferior mesenteric artery is ligated during aortic surgery. Collateral flow may be further compromised by ligating the inferior mesenteric artery peripherally rather than flush with the aortic wall, because this may occlude the connection between the left colic and the superior rectal arteries. Failure to ensure perfusion through at least one hypogastric may promote colon ischemia if this is the primary supply in the absence of the inferior mesenteric artery or effective collateral flow from the meandering artery. Loss of the inferior mesenteric artery or the meandering artery produces right colon and small bowel ischemia when these viscera depend on retrograde flow because of superior mesenteric arterial occlusion (Fig. 39–9). The large hematoma associated with a ruptured aneurysm may compress significant collateral vessels, which may explain the high incidence of colon ischemia in this circumstance.[91] Furthermore, angiography is almost never available before repair of a ruptured aneurysm, and the surgeon does not have precise information regarding intestinal circulation to design an operative procedure that will conserve or augment colon perfusion.

Depending on the severity of ischemia and the thickness of bowel wall involved, three forms of ischemic colitis are recognized. Type I is mucosal ischemia, which is transient and mild. Type II, with mucosal and muscularis involve-

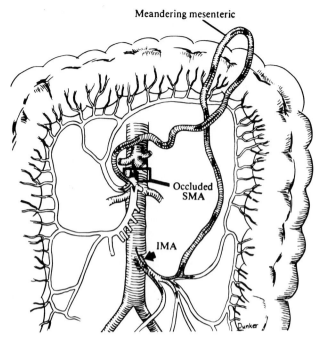

Figure 39–9. When superior mesenteric artery (SMA) is occluded, meandering mesenteric blood flow is from inferior mesenteric artery (IMA) to SMA. Meandering mesenteric sacrifice under these conditions predisposes to small bowel as well as colonic ischemia. (From Ernst CB: Colon ischemia following abdominal aortic reconstruction. In Bernhard VM, Towne JB [eds]: Complications in Vascular Surgery. New York, Grune & Stratton, 1980, p 385.)

ment, reflects more severe ischemia that may result in healing with fibrosis, scarring, and stricture. Type III is transmural ischemia, which produces irreparable damage with gangrene and bowel perforation.[98]

The clinical manifestations of intestinal ischemia immediately after aortic surgery are often masked by incisional discomfort and other problems that may explain abdominal pain, tenderness, fever, an elevated white blood cell count, and fluid sequestration. Findings that suggest the presence of intestinal ischemia and progressing infarction of the colon include progressive distention, sepsis, increasing peritoneal signs, and unexplained metabolic acidosis. The most common clinical presentation is diarrhea, either brown liquid or bloody, which occurs in 65% to 76% of patients with intestinal ischemia.[94, 99] Although the onset may occur as long as 14 days after operation, diarrhea usually appears within 24 to 48 hours after surgery.[94] Bloody diarrhea has been reported to be a more ominous prognostic sign than nonbloody diarrhea[100]; however, some investigators have noted no correlation between extent of ischemic injury and presence of bloody diarrhea.[100]

Postoperative *Clostridium difficile* colitis may mimic ischemic colitis. Therefore, in critically ill patients who develop fever, abdominal distention, diarrhea, and leukocytosis after emergency aortic procedures, stool specimens for culture and for *C. difficile* toxin should be obtained and endoscopic evaluation of the colon performed. Appropriate antibiotic therapy (metronidazole or vancomycin) should be instituted if the diagnosis of *C. difficile* is confirmed.[101, 102]

Early diagnosis of ischemia is the key to effective management of ischemic colitis. The diagnosis depends on a high index of suspicion and the prompt performance of endoscopy with the flexible sigmoidoscope or colonoscope. Sigmoid colon pH monitoring begun before surgery and continued postoperatively has been used with some success by Björk and Hedberg[103] to identify patients at risk for ischemic colitis. They found that a sigmoid colon pH below 6.86 for 9 to 12 hours had a sensitivity of 100% and specificity of 97% for predicting ischemic colitis. Furthermore, when sigmoid colon acidosis below 7.10 was reversed within 2 hours, no major complications developed, but when it was prolonged, 8 of 10 patients developed major complications. Future evaluation of sigmoid colon pH monitoring appears warranted prior to its widespread application. Occurrence of ischemic colitis without left colon involvement is rare enough that endoscopy to 40 cm is usually sufficient to establish the diagnosis.[91] Once detected, endoscopy should be terminated to avoid perforation. Mild changes of ischemic colitis consist of submucosal hemorrhage and edema that is usually circumferential. Pseudomembranes, erosions, and ulcers indicate more advanced ischemia. A yellowish-green, necrotic, noncontractile surface indicates gangrene.[94] Repeated endoscopy, every other day by the same individual, is required to document resolution or progression of the process.

Patients under observation for intestinal ischemia are managed by frequent reexamination; serial endoscopy; sigmoid colon and gastric intramucosal pH monitoring; monitoring of blood gases, urine output, and fluid requirements; institution of broad-spectrum antibiotic coverage; and bowel rest with nasogastric suction. If the colon appears distended, either clinically or radiographically, it should be decompressed by the gentle insertion of a rectal tube, because increased intraluminal pressure may further compromise colon blood flow.[94, 103]

Improvement of the patient, as evidenced by diminishing diarrhea, improvement in vital signs, clinical examination, laboratory values, and resolution of the ischemia documented by endoscopy, permits continuation of nonoperative management.[91] Reversible ischemic lesions should improve within 7 to 10 days.[98, 104] Continuing clinical evidence of ischemia beyond 2 weeks requires operative intervention because this usually reflects a walled-off perforation with local peritonitis.[94] Finally, progression of the intestinal ischemia during the period of observation, identified by deteriorating clinical signs and symptoms, requires prompt celiotomy. Surgery for transmural ischemic colitis requires resection of nonviable bowel, end-colostomy, and formation of a Hartmann's pouch or resection of the rectum, if involved.[105]

Prevention of intestinal ischemia depends on an appreciation of the potential for this complication and the institution of appropriate steps to either avoid injury to the collateral circulation of the colon or augment circulation to the bowel as part of the aortic reconstructive procedure.[106] Routine preoperative aortography identifies a patent inferior mesenteric artery with retrograde flow through a large meandering artery that is functioning as a collateral pathway for an obstructed superior mesenteric artery.[107] In this circumstance, flow through the inferior mesenteric must be preserved by sparing this orifice through construction of an end-to-side aortic anastomosis or by reimplantation of the inferior mesenteric onto the side of an aortic graft using a variation of the Carrel patch technique.[91] Spiral CT angiography is being used with increasing frequency to evaluate the abdominal aorta and its visceral branches. This technique permits multiple views of complex aortic lesions, reflects the true diameter of aortic aneurysms, and may alleviate the need for angiography.[108]

In a prospective study of 100 patients undergoing aortic reconstructive procedures, Zelenock and associates[109] observed a 3% incidence of endoscopic colonic ischemia. Adjunctive procedures were used in 12% of the patients, compared with 4% in earlier studies from their institution. Bypass to the superior mesenteric should also be considered.[106] A large meandering artery with flow from the superior mesenteric toward the sigmoid and rectum in the presence of inferior mesenteric artery occlusion is strong evidence for adequate collateral supply to the bowel.[96] Ischemic colitis is unlikely under these circumstances if this collateral is not impaired by surgery. The status of the hypogastric vessels should be identified on the aortogram so that arterial reconstruction can be designed to maintain flow through at least one of these arteries by direct revascularization or by retrograde perfusion from a femoral anastomosis, especially if a patent inferior mesenteric artery must be ligated.[104]

Measurement of the inferior mesenteric artery backpressure during aortic reconstruction may be a useful guide to the need for restoration of flow to the inferior mesenteric artery.[104] A mean pressure greater than 40 mm Hg and an inferior mesenteric artery–systemic pressure ratio of greater than 0.4 indicate satisfactory collateral circulation without the need for mesenteric arterial repair.

Thorough mechanical preparation of the bowel before aortic surgery will reduce the fecal burden to which the potentially ischemic bowel is exposed.[91] During aortic surgery, every effort should be made to prevent injury to the mesenteric vessels. Undue traction on the left colon mesentery should be avoided. When inferior mesenteric ligation is required, this should be carried out by suture ligature within the aortic lumen or immediately adjacent to the aortic wall to avoid injury to its ascending and descending branches.[91] Finally, the presence of Doppler flow signals over the base of the bowel mesentery and the serosal surface of the colon suggests that adequate collateral circulation is present.[99] Absence of a flow signal after reconstruction suggests the need to restore perfusion through the inferior mesenteric artery or through some other major collateral vessel.

Spinal Cord Ischemia

Spinal cord ischemia occurs most frequently during repair of thoracic and thoracoabdominal aneurysms but is occasionally encountered during resection of an abdominal aortic aneurysm and, rarely, following aortoiliac bypass for ischemia.[78, 110, 111] The overall incidence of this complication for abdominal aortic surgery has been reported to be 0.23% and is 10 times higher after the repair of ruptured abdominal aortic aneurysms than following elective aneurysm resection.[111, 112] The incidence of spinal cord ischemia after thoracic aortic reconstruction is in the range of 1% to 10%, depending on the extent of the lesion repaired.

The upper level of the neurologic deficit was found to be T-10 to L-2 in 39 (88.6%) of 44 patients reviewed at the Henry Ford Hospital.[112] Postoperative mortality was directly related to the severity of paraplegia. When the neurologic deficit initially was complete, involving both sensory and motor function, 76% of the patients died; there were only two complete neurologic recoveries and one partial. By contrast, when the initial loss was only partial motor or sensory loss, 24% died and some degree of recovery was noted in all but one patient.[111, 113, 114]

The major cause of spinal cord ischemia is interruption of flow through the great radicular artery of Adamkiewicz, which is the major source of supply to the anterior spinal artery at the lower end of the cord.[110, 115] The great radicular artery is a major branch of the posterior division of one of the intercostal vessels arising between T-8 and L-1. On occasion, it may originate from a lumbar branch of the infrarenal aorta. The anterior spinal artery itself is long and has rather poor collateral contributions from the posterior spinal arteries or from the radicular arteries derived from more proximal intercostal vessels. Because the spinal cord is only tenuously supplied in its lower portion by vessels other than the great radicular, any injury to this vessel during aortic reconstruction may lead to some degree of cord infarction. The effectiveness of collateral pathways may be further compromised by hypotension, especially in patients with ruptured aneurysm. The placement of a high aortic clamp for temporary control of a ruptured aneurysm, however, does not clearly correlate with the incidence or severity of cord ischemia.[111]

Williams and colleagues[116] and Kieffer and coworkers[117] reported successful angiographic visualization of the origin of the artery of Adamkiewicz in 49% and 69% of patients with thoracoabdominal aneurysms, respectively. The very low incidence of spinal cord ischemia after operations on the *infrarenal* aorta and the risks associated with preoperative or operative angiographic demonstration of the major blood supply to the lower spinal cord render visualization impractical and potentially dangerous.[88, 115–117] Moreover, the occurrence of this complication has been unpredictable and may be unpreventable in association with infrarenal aortic reconstruction. Monitoring of somatosensory evoked potentials during thoracic surgery has been shown to correlate with cord ischemia.[118] These abnormal findings have been reversed by temporary shunting and implantation of intercostal vessels into the thoracic aortic graft. Practical application of this technique to abdominal aortic surgery is undergoing continued investigation.[118–121]

Although there are no data to identify specific preventive measures, it would seem prudent to avoid high aortic clamping unless absolutely necessary, to maintain cord perfusion pressure by avoiding systemic hypotension, and to prevent stasis thrombosis in collateral vessels by effective heparinization. Suturing a patch of posterior aortic wall with its intercostal vessel orifices into a window cut out of the graft has been recommended for thoracoabdominal aneurysms.[78] Finally, it is important to ensure pelvic perfusion through one or both hypogastric arteries to maximize collateral contribution to the spinal cord.[122]

When ischemic injury to the spinal cord occurs, treatment is palliative and supportive.[111]

Ureteral Injury and Obstruction

The ureters are immediately adjacent to the operative field and may be easily injured during dissection and arterial repair.[123] This is especially important in patients with large iliac and hypogastric aneurysms or when there is increased adherence to vascular structures in the presence of an "inflammatory" aneurysm or retroperitoneal fibrosis.[124] Nachbur and associates,[125] in a study of 220 patients with asymptomatic aneurysms evaluated with CT scanning, observed 20 cases of ureteral obstruction. In eight patients, ureteral obstruction was associated with inflammatory aneurysms, and in the remaining 12, with abdominal aortic, common iliac, and hypogastric atherosclerotic aneurysms. A thorough knowledge of the anatomic relationships of the ureters at the level of the iliac bifurcation is essential. Occasionally, multiple ureters may be present, or they may be in an aberrant position owing to congenital anomalies. These variations may be defined by a preoperative intravenous pyelogram (IVP) or a pyelographic film during the preoperative aortogram or CT scan. A preoperative IVP or contrast-enhanced CT scan is especially indicated in reoperative aortoiliac surgery to identify postoperative changes in the ureteral anatomy or demonstrate possible injury incurred during the initial surgery.

Direct injury to the ureter can best be avoided by keeping the dissection close to the iliac artery at the point at which the ureter normally crosses the common iliac bifurcation in transit to the bladder. This is especially important during the blind development of the retroperitoneal tunnel for aortofemoral bypass. The ureter should be elevated away from the iliac vessels so that the graft will lie dorsal to it. Inadvertent passage of the graft ventral to the ureter may cause it to be compressed between the graft limb and the underlying iliac artery, producing hydronephrosis. The incidence of ureteral obstruction after aortic grafting in one prospective study was 2%.[126] However, the ureter may be entrapped in perigraft scar, even if it is placed in its proper position ventral to the prosthesis.[123]

Both ureters should be demonstrated before closing the retroperitoneum. The right ureter must be carefully protected during retroperitoneal closure, since this structure can easily be caught up in the suture line. Iatrogenic ureteral injuries sustained during placement or revision of a vascular graft should be repaired primarily. Although renal salvage is possible when the diagnosis is delayed, nephrectomy is often necessary if there has been extensive contamination of the graft.[127] Occasionally, an intraoperative ureteral injury is overlooked, and the diagnosis is delayed for days or weeks. Once recognized, placement of a percutaneous nephrostomy tube may be associated with a shorter hospital stay and lower infection rates than with open repair.[128]

Retroperitoneal fibrosis secondary to the surgical procedure is the most common cause of ureteral obstruction after aortic surgery. Postoperative hydronephrosis can be categorized as early (occurring within 6 months) or late (after 6 months). Temporary asymptomatic hydronephrosis can be detected on CT scans in 12% to 30% of patients and mild to moderate permanent ureteral dilatation in 2% to 14% of patients undergoing aortic surgery. The fibrosis is usually secondary to bleeding; excessive dissection, ligation, or devascularization of the ureter; or pseudoaneurysm formation. Ureteral obstruction is believed to be more common when the limb of the graft is tunneled anterior to the ureter. However, hydronephrosis secondary to anterior graft placement occurs in only 30% of cases. The majority of patients have a clinical presentation within a year of the procedure, but delayed presentation up to 14 years has been reported. Approximately 30% of patients manifest with symptoms, including pain, recurrent bouts of urinary tract infection, azotemia, or hematuria.[129-131]

Wright and associates[132] reported a 35-year experience with 58 ureteral complications in patients undergoing aortoiliac reconstructions. Two of the six patients who had ureteral obstruction treated before, or in conjunction with, repair of their aneurysms developed graft complications (one graft limb thrombosis and one graft infection). The remaining 44 patients had 46 complications, including hydronephrosis (42), ureteral leaks (3), and ureteral necrosis (1). Twenty-four patients had 36 graft complications, including anastomotic aneurysms (19), graft limb thrombosis (8), graft infections (6), and aortoenteric fistulas (3). Twenty-nine of the 44 patients underwent graft or ureteral operations, or both, with a mortality rate of 21%.

Patients in whom hydronephrosis is recognized preoperatively may benefit from ureteral stent placement to decompress the obstruction and facilitate ureteral identification during repair. Postoperative hydronephrosis detected on ultrasonography, CT scans, or IVP may initially be followed expectantly, as it often resolves. Only 12 of the 58 patients reported by Wright and coworkers[132] required surgical intervention for progressive hydronephrosis. The selective use of stents and antibiotics in conjunction with operative repair is essential if the high incidence of graft complications is to be reduced (Fig. 39–10).

Impotence

The loss of ability to achieve or maintain an erection adequate for satisfactory coitus may be due to vasculogenic, psychogenic, neurogenic, endocrinogenic, or medication-related factors.[133-137] Eighty percent of patients who have aortoiliac occlusive disease have significant erectile dysfunction.[133] Nearly 25% of patients undergoing direct aortic reconstruction will suffer iatrogenic erectile dysfunction if appropriate technical modifications are not employed. Therefore, careful evaluation of penile erectile function by history, noninvasive techniques, and angiography should be included in the preoperative evaluation before elective aortic surgery.[137, 138] This will determine whether there is normal sexual function that should be preserved or whether there is already an established pattern of impotence that may possibly be relieved by altering pelvic blood flow. This information may also provide valuable insights into the psychogenic and cultural factors contributing to an existing problem and provides the surgeon with an estimate of the importance of sexual function to the patient. Such preoperative information may alter the type of aortic operation previously planned.

Preoperative evaluation of erectile function includes nocturnal tumescence studies. The absence of tumescence during an adequate sleep study is strong evidence of or-

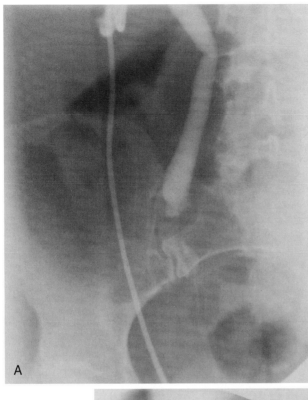

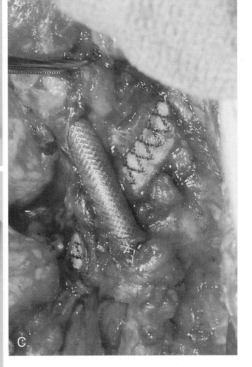

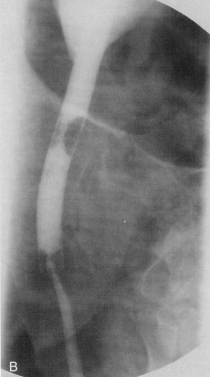

Figure 39–10. *A,* A stricture is present in the distal ureter as it crosses over the limb of an aortofemoral graft. *B,* After dilatation of the stricture, a stent was placed. *C,* Erosion of the ureter by the stent resulted in a 3-cm defect in the ureter and exposure limb of the graft.

ganic impotence. Documentation of normal erections during rapid eye movement sleep establishes the psychogenic basis of the patient's erectile dysfunction. Unfortunately, the failure of erection is often qualitative rather than complete, making tumescence studies less discriminating between organic and psychogenic impotence.[133, 138]

If organic impotence is suspected, the next step is non-invasive vascular testing. At present, the most reliable measurement is the penile systolic pressure and the penile-brachial ratio (penile-brachial index, or PBI).[133] Kempczinski and Birinyi[133] found that age had a deleterious effect on the PBI that was independent of sexual potency. Patients younger than age 40 years had a mean PBI of 0.99, compared with a PBI of 0.74 for equally potent males older than 40. This difference was statistically significant. By contrast, impotent males older than 40 had a mean PBI of 0.58, also a statistically significant difference. Despite the significant differences in PBI measurements in these three groups, there is a failure of correlation between PBI and the degree of erectile dysfunction.[138, 139] Although a low PBI is not sufficient to establish the diagnosis of vasculogenic impotence, the finding of a PBI greater than 0.8 confirms the adequacy of penile blood flow and suggests that a vasculogenic etiology is extremely unlikely.[133]

Neurogenic impotence is commonly a result of neuropathy secondary to diabetes mellitus or may follow autonomic nerve injury from genitourinary or abdominopelvic surgery. This diagnosis is often one of exclusion, but abnormal pudendal nerve velocity studies (sacral latency testing) and abnormal cystometrography (the anatomic pathways in micturition and erection being similar) can implicate this etiology.[133, 140]

The diagnosis of endocrinologic impotence requires measurement of thyroid function and serum levels of testosterone and other associated hormones. Finally, a thorough medication history is required.[140]

Preoperative angiography is useful in identifying the patency of the hypogastric vessels and their contribution to pelvic perfusion. Unfortunately, angiographic findings correlate poorly with the patient's erectile function.[133] Selective injections to identify the flow through the pudendal vessels into the penis may be required to more accurately assess patients being evaluated primarily for vasculogenic impotence.[133]

Although the findings on preoperative angiograms correlate poorly with erectile function, preservation of adequate perfusion into at least one hypogastric artery appears to be a vital component in minimizing iatrogenic impotence.[133] When possible, direct antegrade perfusion of the internal iliac artery should be ensured. This may require thromboendarterectomy of the hypogastric orifice. If both external iliac arteries are occluded or stenotic, and bypass into the common femoral arteries is anticipated, precluding retrograde iliac flow, the proximal aortic anastomosis should be constructed end to side, when feasible, to preserve pelvic blood flow. When proximal aortic disease is extensive, requiring an end-to-end proximal anastomosis, and impaired penile perfusion has been diagnosed by preoperative noninvasive testing, it may be necessary to reimplant the hypogastric artery into one limb of an aortobifemoral graft or add a jump graft to one hypogastric artery to improve pelvic inflow.[133, 140] Finally, careful flushing of the graft in both directions before completion of the final suture line is important to prevent embolization of small particles into the pelvic arteries. DePalma and colleagues[141] reported spontaneous erectile function in 58% of patients with impotence undergoing aortoiliac reconstruction, compared with 27% after microvascular procedures.

Retrograde Ejaculation

Ejaculatory dysfunction is not an uncommon occurrence after aortic surgery. Earlier series have reported an incidence of 30% to 75%, but in more contemporary series the incidence was found to be only 3%.[142] This lower incidence is clearly the result of an increased awareness of the anatomy controlling ejaculation and improved surgical technique. Emission and closure of the bladder neck to ensure antegrade ejaculation is dependent on innervation by postganglionic fibers of the lumbar sympathetic nerves arising from T-11 to L-3. The loss of one or both functions as a result of dissection in the region of the aortic bifurcation results in dry ejaculation.[143, 144]

Careful preservation of the sympathetic-parasympathetic plexus overlying the aorta and its bifurcation and maintenance of blood flow through the hypogastric and pudendal arteries are the important factors to be considered in preventing impotence in men undergoing elective aortic surgery.[135, 137, 145] Dissection should be carried down to the aortic wall on its right anterolateral surface and the para-aortic structures gently retracted to the left to avoid trauma to the nerves contained within these tissues (Fig. 39–11A and B). During aneurysm resection, the inferior mesenteric artery should not be dissected free but should be controlled by suture ligature from inside the aorta after the aneurysm has been opened to avoid disruption of nerve fibers at the junction of the inferior mesenteric artery with the aorta (see Fig. 39–11B and C). There should be minimal division of the longitudinal periaortic tissues to the left of the infrarenal aorta, and the nerve plexuses that cross

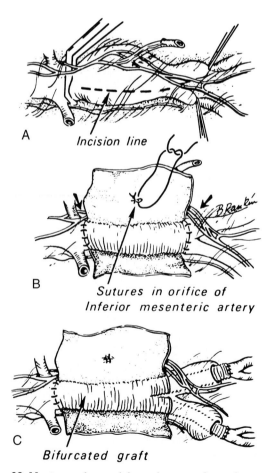

Figure 39–11. Approaches to abdominal aortic and aortoiliac aneurysm. Sac is left intact and sutured over inlay graft. (From DePalma RG: Impotence as a complication of aortic reconstruction. In Bernhard VM, Towne JB [eds]: Complications in Vascular Surgery. New York, Grune & Stratton, 1980, p 437.)

the left common iliac artery should be spared.[133, 145] The limbs of bifurcation grafts should be placed within the lumina of common iliac aneurysms to avoid external dissection and minimize injury to perivascular nerve fibers.

Anastomotic False Aneurysm

False aneurysms can develop at any anastomotic site. They are almost invariably associated with prosthetic rather than autogenous tissue suture lines.[146–152] The most common sites of occurrence are femoral anastomoses following placement of aortofemoral bypass grafts.[147, 149, 152] Pathologically, there is a partial separation of the graft from the arterial wall.[146, 149, 151] The perianastomotic fibrous tissue prevents immediate hemorrhage and forms a capsule around the hematoma that gradually expands owing to the pressure transmitted from the arterial lumen. The fibrous capsule may rupture, with rapid painful enlargement of the mass, or erode the overlying skin to produce infection and external hemorrhage. In the abdomen, false aneurysms are prone to erode into adjacent bowel, forming aortoenteric fistulas.[152–154] Because blood flow within the pseudoaneurysm is static, its lumen becomes partially filled with thrombus, which may embolize.[146, 152] The luminal distortion produced by the pseudoaneurysm and its thrombus may also cause occlusion of a graft.[152]

In the immediate postoperative period, all vascular anastomoses are entirely dependent on suture material alone. With time, a prosthetic-artery junction is maintained by the integrity of the suture material and also by external fibrous bonding caused by scarring.[155] The important factors involved in the development of an anastomotic false aneurysm include arterial wall weakness,[151] endarterectomy at the anastomotic site,[156] compliance mismatch between the graft and host artery,[157, 158] dilatation of the graft material,[154, 159] prosthetic deterioration or an actual flaw in the graft material,[160] increased tension at the anastomotic site due to insufficient length of the prosthesis,[160] deterioration of suture material,[161] and uneven tension on the anastomosis as a result of beveling of the end of the graft.[155]

Pseudoaneurysm is occasionally due to underlying infection, although this is infrequently identified.[149, 152] When infection is the causative factor, a purulent perigraft exudate is usually, but not necessarily, present. Therefore, during repair of any pseudoaneurysm, its wall and contents should be routinely cultured by aerobic and anaerobic techniques.

The incidence of false aneurysm formation ranges between 1.4% and 4.0%.[150] Recognition is usually quite simple at groin anastomoses, where a large, pulsatile, and sometimes tender mass becomes apparent to both the patient and the examining physician. False aneurysms developing in the retroperitoneum at an aortic or iliac anastomosis rarely become palpable and go unnoticed until rupture produces pain and shock or erosion occurs in an adjacent loop of bowel, with gastrointestinal hemorrhage.[162] Occasionally, false aneurysms are identified during routine arteriography for some other vascular problem. Ultrasonography and CT are reliable methods for evaluating grafts and anastomoses for dilatation and pseudoaneurysm formation.[163] Diagnosis of a pseudoaneurysm is usually confirmed by arteriography, which demonstrates widening at the anastomosis and an extraluminal accumulation of dye at the point of anastomotic disruption. Because the false aneurysm is partially filled with thrombus, the extent of extraluminal dye accumulation only partially outlines the full extent of the process. A more accurate measure of the true size of the defect can be obtained by ultrasonography or CT scanning.[162]

Retroperitoneal false aneurysms should be repaired as soon as they are identified to avoid rupture or bowel erosion.[150, 153, 162] Unfortunately, this complication is frequently the first indication that a false aneurysm is present. When there is no evidence of infection, the suture line defect can be dissected free and repaired either directly or by the interposition of fresh graft material. When infection or visceral erosion has taken place, the graft must be removed entirely and the aorta and iliac vessels closed. Management of this problem is discussed in detail elsewhere in this text.

Generally, peripheral false aneurysms should be repaired as soon as they are identified. However, false aneurysms that are small, stable, and asymptomatic may be observed, especially if the patient is at increased risk for reoperation.[149, 151, 152] If surgery is delayed, reexamination at frequent intervals is mandatory so that repair can be carried out when expansion is evident but before complications develop.

Surgical repair of a false aneurysm is usually carried out through the site of the original incision. Dissection is carried down to the graft wall proximally so that it can be controlled with a circumferential tape. Further dissection is then carried distally along the graft to define the anastomosis, the aneurysmal bulge, and the branches of the common femoral artery. It is usually difficult and tedious to dissect out the major branches of the artery at the anastomotic site. When extensive scarring is encountered, further dissection may be abandoned, and the patient is given intravenous heparin. The graft is then clamped and disconnected from the aneurysm, and branch control is achieved by the insertion of balloon occlusion catheters into the lumina of the major branches.[150] The anastomotic site is carefully surveyed to identify the cause of the pseudoaneurysm. The distal frayed end of the graft at the anastomosis is resected, and the edges of the artery are trimmed back to healthy tissue. To avoid tension at the new anastomosis, a short piece of new graft material is usually required to connect the proximal end of the old prosthesis with the freshened arterial orifice. The diameter of the interposed graft segment should usually not exceed 8 mm to more closely approximate the size of the outflow tract rather than the larger inflow prosthetic limb.[159] Unless retrograde flow up the external iliac must be preserved, it is best to convert the femoral anastomosis from end to side to end to end.[150] Before repairing the anastomosis, the orifices of the superficial femoral and profunda should be inspected so that significant stenoses can be repaired by endarterectomy or patch angioplasty to ensure adequate runoff.

Overall mortality for repair of anastomotic femoral false aneurysms was 3.5%, and the amputation rate was 2.8% in a 1985 review.[155] Results are distinctly better if this lesion is repaired electively rather than as an emergency.[151, 152]

The recurrence rate of anastomotic femoral false aneurysms after initial repair has been reported to be 5.7%; these are amenable to secondary repair.[155, 159]

Recurrent Anastomotic Aneurysm

Femoral anastomotic aneurysms (FAAs) develop in approximately 3% of all femoral anastomoses and in 6% of patients undergoing aortofemoral bypass. Repair of FAAs remains durable in approximately 80% of patients; however, a small percentage of patients develop recurrent FAAs (RFAAs). In a series of 43 FAAs, Ernst and colleagues[164] reported a 19% incidence of this complication.

Factors predisposing to RFAA include graft dilatation, local wound complications, and previous repair of an FAA in a woman.[159, 164] Although there appears to be an inverse relationship between atherosclerotic heart disease and RFAA, the significance of this observation is difficult to explain. Furthermore, factors that have been implicated in the development of FAA (e.g., hypertension, smoking, diabetes, suture material, type of graft, and performance of an endarterectomy) have not been related to the development of RFAAs.

RFAAs are subject to the same complications as primary FAAs, including rupture, thrombus, and peripheral embolization.

Repair is indicated in good-risk patients with RFAAs larger than 2 cm. Management includes careful follow-up for anastomotic aneurysms smaller than 2 cm, especially if coexisting medical problems make surgical intervention risky. The principles of repair are similar to those for primary FAAs and include careful dissection of the distal outflow vessels, use of graft material approximately the size of the outflow vessel, and conversion from end-to-side to end-to-end anastomosis.[159, 164]

Chylous Ascites

Chylous ascites, issuing from a damaged cisterna chyli and its tributaries at the root of the mesentery, is a rare complication of aortic reconstruction.[165] In a review of the literature, Pabst and coauthors[166] found that 75% of cases occurred following abdominal aortic aneurysm resection, 19% after aortic reconstruction for occlusive disease, and the remaining 7% after resection of infected aortic grafts. Interruption of the lymphatics and chylous ascites are not invariably related, since the lymphatics are often interrupted during aortic operations without apparent sequelae.[165]

Patients with chylous ascites present usually within 2 or 3 weeks of aortic repair with anorexia and progressive abdominal distention. Ascites is usually evident on physical examination and can be confirmed by abdominal radiographs, ultrasound, or CT scans. The fluid obtained by abdominal paracentesis is milky, with a high lymphocyte count and lipid content, and is bacteriologically sterile. An additional complication is leakage of ascites to the outside through a defect in the incision; this increases the fluid and protein loss and heightens the risk of infection. Such a leak should be repaired under sterile conditions and prophylactic antibiotic coverage.

The management of chylous ascites includes abdominal paracentesis, a low-fat diet rich in medium-chain triglycerides, and total parenteral nutrition (TPN). However, repeated paracentesis may result in the loss of large amounts of protein and lipid that cannot readily be replaced. An additional risk is that of line-related sepsis. In patients who do not respond to repeated paracentesis, a peritoneal venous shunt, in addition to diet control or TPN, may relieve the ascites. Operative ligation may be necessary in resistant cases.[165, 166]

Ventral Hernias

Midline, oblique, and transverse incisions are commonly used to expose the abdominal aorta.[167–170] Although transverse incisions are associated with the lowest complication rate, their use is often limited to patients with pulmonary insufficiency. Despite the reported benefits of oblique incisions, a significant number of late wound complications, including wound bulging in 11% to 23% and incisional hernias in 7% of patients, have been reported.[170, 171] Presumably, the diffuse bulging is due to muscle atrophy as a result of division of the intercostal nerves. Gardner and colleagues[172] were able to decrease the incidence of bulging from 11% to 0.03% by preserving the 11th intercostal nerve.

The incidence of ventral hernias ranges from 10% to 37%.[171, 173] Two distinct types of defects can be identified. Focal periumbilical defects are almost invariably the result of poor technique. The diffuse defects associated with lateral retraction of the recti is by far the more common of the two defects for incisional hernias in patients undergoing aortic aneurysmal resection. A number of studies have found no differences in the incidence of the usual risk factors—age, chronic obstructive pulmonary disease, diabetes, smoking, wound infection, length of intensive care unit stay, and amount of blood transfused—between patients who developed incisional hernias and those who did not.

Mass suturing of the musculoaponeurotic layers of the abdominal wall using monofilament or braided suture is the most frequently used technique to close midline incisions. It cannot be overemphasized that careful suture technique with placement of bites 2 cm from the edge and 1 cm apart is essential if this complication is to be prevented. Whether using an interrupted closure with braided or monofilament nonabsorbable sutures decreases the incidence of this complication is unknown.

Primary repair using monofilament nonabsorbable suture is appropriate for closure of small periumbilical defects. Prosthetic mesh is usually necessary to repair the large defects in the upper abdomen.

INFRAINGUINAL ARTERIAL RECONSTRUCTION

Femoropopliteal and femoroinfrapopliteal bypasses are the most commonly performed procedures for revascularization of the lower extremity below the inguinal ligament.

Specific problems related to endarterectomy of the superficial femoral, popliteal, or profunda femoris arteries are reviewed in the discussion of these procedures. The basic principles of infrainguinal bypass are similar to those for aortoiliac reconstruction, with the following significant differences: the vessels involved are smaller, and the length of the bypass conduit is greater, with a consequent increase in the incidence of early and late thrombosis; vein grafts rather than prostheses are used for the majority of procedures; and there is a tendency for less severe systemic complications owing to the more peripheral and less traumatic nature of the operative procedure.

Bleeding

Major blood loss or hemorrhage is not a frequent complication during this surgery but may become a problem in the immediate postoperative period. The most common sources are the anastomoses, insecure ligatures on branches of a vein graft, laceration of the vein wall by instruments in the in situ technique, blind disruption of small vessels encountered during blunt dissection of thigh and leg tunnels, inadequate hemostasis during the dissection of the major vessels, incomplete reversal of heparin anticoagulation, and oozing from antiplatelet medication.[174] In the immediate postoperative period, bleeding usually appears as wound swelling of the extremity, and the severity of hypotension, if present, mirrors the extent and rapidity of hemorrhage. Prompt return to the operating room is required to control the source of bleeding and to evacuate the hematoma, which may interfere with healing and promote infection. Long-term graft patency has been shown to be significantly reduced in patients who develop wound hemorrhage in the immediate postoperative period.[174] Wound hemorrhage that occurs after 48 to 72 hours is frequently due to infection involving the graft at an anastomosis and is less likely to be caused by mechanical factors.[174] However, hemorrhage may occur later in the immediate postoperative period in patients who have been maintained on anticoagulants or in whom fibrinolytic agents have been infused for graft thrombosis within 10 days to 2 weeks of surgery.[175]

Thrombosis

The most common significant complication of infrainguinal bypass or endarterectomy is thrombosis of the reconstruction. In the early postoperative period (less than 30 days), thrombosis is usually related to technical factors[21, 40, 176, 177] (Fig. 39–12). The most common of these is imprecise construction of the suture line, resulting in stenosis or elevation of a distal intimal flap that obstructs flow; this is especially important at a distal anastomosis to a small-caliber tibial or peroneal vessel. A prosthetic or reversed saphenous vein graft may become twisted when drawn through the thigh tunnel. Kinking or entrapment may occur owing to compression by nerve trunks or other tissues crossing the tunnel or by tracking the graft inappropriately in relation to the adductor muscles of the thigh or the medial head of the gastrocnemius. Vein graft stenosis may

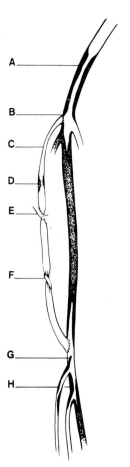

Figure 39–12. Mechanical factors underlying early thrombosis of femoropopliteal and femorotibial grafts. *A,* Stenosis of iliac inflow. *B,* Stenosis of proximal anastomosis produced by suturing a small vein to a thick-walled femoral artery. *C,* Proximal vein graft less than 4 mm in diameter. *D,* Recanalized saphenous phlebitis. *E,* External compression tissue bands in tunnel. *F,* Graft twist. *G,* Elevation of distal intima. *H,* Inadequate runoff. (From Bernhard VM: The failed arterial graft: Lost pulses and gangrene. In Condon RE, DeCosse JJ [eds]: Surgical Care. Philadelphia, Lea & Febiger, 1980, p 156.)

be produced by a branch ligature placed too close to the main saphenous trunk. For reversed saphenous vein grafts, factors leading to early thrombosis are vein diameter less than 3.5 to 4.0 mm, thick-walled vein, marked varicosities, and evidence of previous phlebitis.[178, 179] In the in situ saphenous vein bypass, technical factors causing early thrombosis are platelet deposition at sites of endothelial damage from improper intraluminal instrumentation; missed valves or incomplete cusp lysis; diversion of the flow by significant fistulas; venospasm; and torsion or kinking of the proximal or distal-free segments of the vein. Atherosclerotic disease in the inflow or outflow arteries inadequately evaluated prior to surgery is another significant cause of graft thrombosis. Other technical errors include inadequate heparinization, improper flushing of the arterial system before restoration of graft flow, and clamp injury to the inflow or outflow vessels or the bypass conduit.[40, 180] Nonmechanical causes of early thrombosis are decreased cardiac output, arterial vasospasm, and hypercoagulability.[40, 181]

Thrombosis that occurs after 1 month and up to 1 year

is most frequently due to degenerative changes in the graft itself or at an anastomosis.[176, 177, 182, 183] In reversed saphenous vein bypass, thrombosis is usually caused by fibrosis of a valve or fibrotic changes in the vein graft wall due to injury during harvest and preparation before insertion.[40, 177, 184] These intrinsic vein graft defects are more common in the narrow proximal portion of reversed vein grafts.[177] In in situ saphenous vein bypass grafts, stenoses of the conduit have been reported at the mobilized upper or lower ends of the graft due to fibrous dysplastic lesions and in the midportion as the result of thickening around a valve cusp.[185] For all types of arterial bypasses, intimal fibroplasia at or just beyond the distal anastomosis may be produced by turbulent flow secondary to alteration of the arterial stream at the junction of graft and artery,[33, 186–188] a compliance mismatch,[157, 189] and the interplay of platelets and other blood factors at anastomoses.[190] Fibrointimal hyperplasia may also be a consequence of clamp injury to the graft or artery incurred at the time of surgery.[177]

Thrombosis occurring after 1 to 2 years is most frequently due to progressive atherosclerosis in the arteries proximal or distal to the arterial repair.[177, 178, 182, 191, 192] Arterialized venous conduits in the atherosclerotic patient also tend to become atherosclerotic themselves[192]; this appears to apply only to reversed, but not in situ, vein bypass grafts.[179, 185]

There is a higher incidence of thrombosis when prosthetic conduits are employed, especially when they are carried below the knee to the distal popliteal or infrapopliteal vessels.[193–198] Thrombosis after vein grafting appears to level off between 1 and 2 years, whereas it is progressive in prosthetic grafts.[177, 196] The specific causes of prosthetic thromboses are the absence of a true intima with its antithrombotic characteristics; the tendency to develop progressive fibrointimal hyperplasia, usually at the distal anastomosis due to the complex interactions between the more rigid prosthetic graft and the arterial wall; and the greater likelihood of kinking of prosthetic materials as they cross the knee joint. Thrombosis may also occur as a consequence of false aneurysm formation, which is more frequent with prostheses than with vein grafts.

Thrombosis in a bypass graft may involve only the graft itself without loss of flow in the segments of the vessel proximal and distal to the points of anastomosis. Under these circumstances, the leg will return to its previous degree of ischemia, assuming that there has been no significant change in the inflow or outflow vessels and collateral pathways. If thrombosis extends beyond the anastomosis into the popliteal and infrapopliteal arteries, however, ischemia will invariably be more severe and the limb may become acutely nonviable unless circulation can be restored.[21]

When a reversed vein graft becomes thrombosed in the immediate postoperative period, the intima and muscularis suffer prolonged anoxic injury due to loss of nutritive blood flow from the lumen in addition to the absence of normal graft wall perfusion through the vasa vasorum that was disrupted during vein graft harvest.[182] The vein thus becomes a less satisfactory conduit, even though flow can be restored within a few hours. This is reflected in the reduced long-term patency of those vein grafts that have undergone thrombosis and initially successful thrombectomy.[177, 186]

In the case of late or neglected thrombosis of a vein conduit, either reversed or in situ, the vein tends to undergo changes that make retrieval irreversible. The vein wall becomes thick and edematous, and the lumen becomes stringlike. Thrombus usually cannot be removed by any means, and dilatation of the vein by a balloon catheter may result in splitting of the wall.[185]

In the immediate postoperative period, peripheral vasospasm may make clinical evaluation unreliable. However, noninvasive tests will permit identification of thrombosis at the earliest possible moment.[23, 199, 200] Therefore, quality of graft flow and overall limb circulation should be evaluated by noninvasive hemodynamic techniques, as well as clinical observation intraoperatively, immediately after completion of the reconstruction, and at frequent intervals in the early postoperative period.[39, 201] Doppler waveform analysis, ankle pressures, and PVRs provide reliable objective information. Surgical reintervention should be carried out immediately in the event of obstructed graft flow to limit propagation of thrombus into distal vessels and minimize the period of ischemia to the limb and the wall of a vein graft.

Beyond the immediate postoperative period, patients with infrainguinal arterial reconstruction, especially with vein grafts, should continue to be examined at regular intervals at least every 3 to 4 months for 12 to 18 months and every 6 months thereafter. A history of increasing claudication, the recognition of reduced distal pulses, and the development of new bruits over the graft or its anastomoses are important findings that should be documented at each visit. In addition, noninvasive hemodynamic tests, including duplex scanning, which provide quantitative and objective information, should be carried out, since they identify impending thrombosis in the absence of symptoms or clinical findings.[200–203] Any evidence of decreasing graft function signals the need for prompt angiography to identify the problem before thrombosis occurs.

Correction of abnormalities within the graft or in the vessels adjacent to a failing graft should be carried out as soon as reduced perfusion has been identified.[200] When possible, intervention should occur before thrombosis has taken place or in the early post-thrombotic period when mechanical disobliteration or lytic therapy is most effective. Delay of an aggressive surgical approach may be required in patients who are poor operative risks. Anticoagulants may prevent thrombosis in the presence of progressing stenosis if surgery must be delayed. However, once occlusion has occurred, the longer the thrombus has been present, the less effective recanalization attempts will be.

Areas of isolated stenosis within the graft, at an anastomosis or in the inflow or outflow arteries, may be successfully managed by percutaneous balloon angioplasty.[175] If this technique cannot be satisfactorily employed, a direct surgical approach at the site of the stenosis is indicated.[21, 177] Vein patch angioplasty can usually be accomplished with relative ease to relieve stenosis of the graft itself or at an anastomosis (Fig. 39–13). If the proximal segment of a reversed saphenous vein graft is too narrow, it can be widened (Fig. 39–14). Progressive disease in the inflow vessels will require a jump graft from the lower end of the original graft to a patent distal popliteal or infrapopliteal artery to bypass the obstruction.[177]

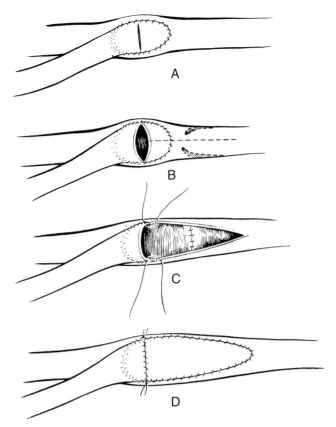

Figure 39–13. Technical sequence for inspection and repair of distal anastomosis of femoropopliteal or femorotibial graft. *A,* Transverse incision in wide "cobra head" overlying the distal anastomosis facilitates thrombus extraction, visualization of internal aspect of suture line, and closure without stenosis. *B* and *C,* When distal intima is elevated, arteriotomy is extended beyond area of injury, redundant intima is removed, and cut edge secured with tacking sutures. *D,* Closure of defect with vein patch. (From Bernhard VM: The failed arterial graft: Lost pulses and gangrene. In Condon RE, DeCosse JJ [eds]: Surgical Care. Philadelphia, Lea & Febiger, 1980, p 160.)

When thrombosis has already occurred and is recent, the graft lumen may be restored by mechanical extraction of thrombus with a balloon thromboembolectomy catheter; prosthetic grafts are more amenable to this procedure than are vein grafts.[21, 177, 204] Thrombectomy of a fresh reversed saphenous vein graft usually requires exposure of both anastomoses. A transverse incision is made at the distal wider end of the graft so that thrombus at that level can be removed and the internal aspect of the distal anastomosis viewed directly (see Fig. 39–13). A second incision over the proximal anastomotic vein hood or partial takedown of the proximal suture line is required for passage of balloon thromboembolectomy catheters and for vigorous forward flushing, since retrograde manipulations will be impeded by valves (Fig. 39–15). Prosthetic graft declotting can sometimes be accomplished through a single distal graft opening if thrombosis has been recent. The thoroughness of thrombus removal is determined by the vigor of flow through the graft from the proximal to the distal end, which also suggests that there is no inflow obstruction. Operative arteriography or angioscopy is required after declotting of either venous or prosthetic grafts to confirm that thrombus has been completely extracted, to view both

anastomoses, to evaluate the entire length of the intervening graft to identify areas of stenosis that need to be repaired, and to reevaluate the inflow and the runoff bed.[205]

The direct intraarterial infusion of thrombolytic agents is an alternative to balloon catheter thrombectomy in the patient who does not have sensory or motor deficits or signs of impending muscle necrosis.[48, 175, 185, 206, 207] Thrombolytic therapy has been successfully applied to vein grafts, prostheses, and endarterectomized segments at all levels of the lower extremity arterial system. The endothelial lining of vein grafts and of small runoff vessels is spared the trauma of mechanical thrombectomy, which may be an important factor in restored vein graft function over the long term. Although effective lysis can be accomplished several weeks after an occlusion has occurred,[44, 208] best results with this form of therapy are usually achieved within hours or days of thrombosis.[209] The technique of percutaneous intraarterial thrombolytic therapy is discussed elsewhere in this book.

As soon as the clot has been effectively cleared from the graft by lytic therapy, angiographic investigation of the entire length of the graft, both anastomoses, the inflow, and the runoff bed is required to identify the cause of graft failure that must be corrected to avoid reocclusion. In the

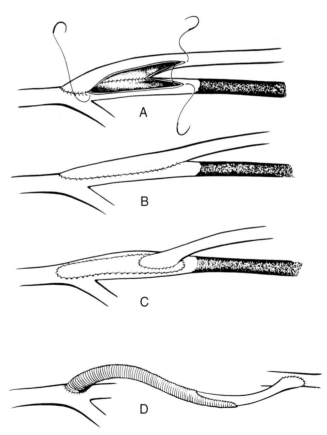

Figure 39–14. Techniques for revision of the femoral anastomosis to avoid stenosis caused by narrow vein and thick intima of artery. *A,* Proximal superficial femoral artery is incised to match long incision in vein graft; the vein graft incision is carried distally until vein diameter is at least 4 mm. *B,* Completion of anastomosis. *C,* Alternate technique using vein patch to increase diameter of artery; vein graft is then anastomosed to the patch. *D,* Composite vein-Dacron graft is another alternative solution when available saphenous vein is too short. (From Bernhard VM: The failed arterial graft: Lost pulses and gangrene. In Condon RE, DeCosse JJ [eds]: Surgical Care. Philadelphia, Lea & Febiger, 1980, p 165.)

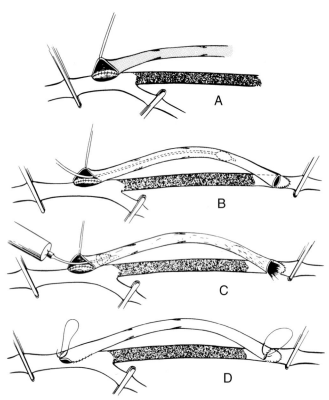

Figure 39–15. Partial detachment of the proximal anastomosis and graft thrombectomy. *A*, Partial takedown of proximal suture line. *B*, Passage of Fogarty catheter to distal end of graft and retrograde extraction of clot. *C*, Vigorous flushing of thrombectomized graft with heparinized Ringer's lactate solution. *D*, Resuture of proximal anastomosis and distal transverse venotomy. (From Bernhard VM: The failed arterial graft: Lost pulses and gangrene. In Condon RE, DeCosse JJ [eds]: Surgical Care. Philadelphia, Lea & Febiger, 1980, p 161.)

interim between lytic recanalization and correction of the causes of graft thrombosis, patients must be effectively anticoagulated to forestall rethrombosis.[44] It is important to recognize that although lytic recanalization of occluded grafts can be achieved, thrombolytic therapy alone suffices in only the minority of patients. Graft stenoses or deterioration of inflow or runoff vessels must be identified and corrected to achieve long-term patency and limb salvage.[48, 200, 208, 210]

A number of reports[211–213] indicate that intraoperative fibrinolytic therapy is an effective adjunct to catheter thrombectomy in select cases when residual clot remaining in the distal artery threatens the success of thrombectomy. The use of intraoperative fibrinolytic agents has not been associated with significant bleeding complications.[211, 212]

Graft thrombosis that is old or that cannot be reopened by mechanical or lytic therapy will require a secondary bypass procedure if the limb is in jeopardy or claudication is truly incapacitating. Autogenous vein is preferable to prosthetic material, especially for bypasses to the infrapopliteal arteries. When the saphenous vein is not available for reoperation, arm veins and lesser saphenous veins, when available, are preferable to prosthetic conduits. The long-term results with prosthetic material are poor when employed for secondary bypass, whereas arm veins have been

shown to have long-term patency rates that may be nearly equal to those of the saphenous vein.[214]

It is important to emphasize the need to search for nonmechanical reasons for decreased graft flow, such as diminished cardiac output or hypercoagulability, especially when no other causes of thrombosis can be identified. Failure to identify and correct the reason for graft occlusion usually suggests a poor prognosis, because the underlying cause has not been removed.[42] However, thrombosis in PTFE grafts may occur for no apparent reason other than presumed platelet adherence to a relatively thrombogenic surface. For this reason, antiplatelet therapy in the immediate postoperative period is indicated.[190, 215] Long-term anticoagulation with warfarin sodium should be considered in patients who have recurrent thrombosis for no apparent reason.

Reoperation to maintain extremity circulation is worthwhile, since prolonged limb salvage can be achieved in 40% to 60% of patients undergoing as many as four or more reoperative procedures.[177] The best results after reoperation for failure of an infrainguinal reconstruction are achieved in patients who only require a vein patch to relieve a stenosis that is repaired before thrombosis takes place.[177, 201] For example, Whittemore and associates[177] achieved a 19% 5-year patency after thrombectomy and patch angioplasty of thrombosed femoropopliteal vein grafts, a 36% patency at 5 years after secondary autogenous vein bypass, and an overall 50% long-term limb salvage. However, vein patch angioplasty of a stenotic graft or anastomotic lesion prior to thrombosis yielded an 86% 5-year patency. For 72 early and late occlusions of PTFE femoropopliteal grafts that placed the limb in jeopardy, Veith and colleagues[216] reported a 5-year graft patency rate of 37% and a 5-year limb salvage rate of 56% in patients undergoing reoperation. PTFE femoropopliteal bypasses appear to be unusual in that thrombectomy alone, even when delayed up to 30 days after thrombosis, can sometimes restore long-term patency. The success rate for reoperation for thrombosis of PTFE grafts to infrapopliteal arteries is considerably lower than that for femoropopliteal bypasses.

Whether the long-term use of anticoagulants can prevent thrombosis of autogenous and prosthetic infrainguinal grafts as suggested by the studies of Kretschmer and coworkers needs further evaluation.[217, 218]

Wound Complications

Major wound complications following lower extremity bypass grafting to the tibial or pedal vessels are not often reported but may jeopardize the success of these procedures.

The reported incidence of significant wound complications following autogenous infrainguinal bypass grafting ranges from 7.5% to 11%.[219–221] In a prospective study of 77 inguinal incisions, Kent and coworkers[222] reported a 10% incidence of wound complications; however, complications occurred in 44% of 79 distal (popliteal or tibial) incisions. Predisposing factors are said to include age, obesity, diabetes mellitus, renal failure, anemia, steroid therapy, ipsilateral limb ulceration or infection, and the severity of ischemia. Technical factors, including the length and placement of the incision, location of the distal anastomosis, and the technique of wound closure, may all influence the ultimate healing of these incisions.[219–222]

The use of a continuous incision increases the risk of wound hematoma or seroma and, if not positioned directly over the saphenous vein, may necessitate a large posterior flap. The two parallel incisions required to mobilize the artery and vein for in situ grafting to the dorsalis pedis artery risk necrosis of the intervening skin bridge. Wound complications range from erythema and superficial necrosis of the margins to infection of the deeper layers with exposure of the graft. Gram-positive cocci and mixed bacterial flora are frequently cultured from these wounds.[219–222]

Several steps help prevent wound complications following infrainguinal bypass procedures. Preoperative mapping of the course of the saphenous vein with duplex scanning minimizes the likelihood of creating a large posterior flap. Isolation of necrotic or ulcerative skin lesions of the foot prior to preparation of the skin limits contamination of the operative field. In patients undergoing in situ vein bypasses, valve incision under angioscopic guidance with ligation of side branches using small incisions may obviate the need for long continuous incisions and, as a consequence, reduce the incidence of wound complications.[223–225] If a continuous incision is used, careful placement of the incision, meticulous hemostasis, and careful skin closure also reduce the incidence of wound complications. Once a wound complication has occurred, however, the treatment should be tailored to the severity of infection. Wound erythema with minimal necrosis of the wound margins usually responds to appropriate antibiotics and local wound care. More extensive wound infection and necrosis require extensive débridement and often skin grafting, muscle transfers, or myocutaneous free flaps.

Rarely, an exposed vein graft ruptures, requiring removal of the graft and placement of a new conduit routed through uninvolved sites. If this is not feasible, amputation may be necessary.

GRAFT SURVEILLANCE

Vein Grafts

The increase in frequency of autogenous vein bypass procedures has increased the number of grafts at risk for late changes, including fibrosis, valvular stenosis, dilatation, aneurysm formation, and atherosclerosis, as described by Szilagyi and associates.[192]

When implanted in the arterial system, vein grafts undergo a series of morphologic changes that include thickening of the wall, fibrosis, and myointimal cellular proliferation as an adaptive response to arterial blood pressure. There is also experimental evidence to suggest that vein grafts produce more prostacyclin than normal veins, although the amount produced is still considerably less than that produced by normal arteries.[226] The introduction of better valvulotomes and the use of angioscopically assisted side branch occlusion has increased the utility of the in situ saphenous vein bypass grafts. Whether the vein should be left in situ or reversed remains a topic of considerable

debate. Proponents of the in situ technique emphasize the theoretical benefits of better endothelial preservation and compliance characteristics, but there is limited objective evidence to support this assumption. Actually, the in situ technique may entail more manipulation and damage to the intima from the use of valvulotomes.

Graft failure within the first 30 days is usually due to fibrin platelet thrombus, retained valves, twists, unrecognized AV fistulas, or technical problems with the anastomoses, and occurs in up to 3% to 10% of grafts.[227, 228] Careful intraoperative assessment of the entire length of the graft with Doppler spectral analysis, angiography, or angioscopy is essential if these early complications are to be avoided.[224, 225] Woelfle and colleagues,[229] in a series of 120 infragenicular bypass grafts evaluated by both angiography and angioscopy, found defects in 7 of 90 grafts with normal completion angiograms. Bush and coworkers[230] reported a 10% incidence of competent valves in the presence of "normal" operative arteriograms. Bandyk and associates[231] performed intraoperative arteriography and pulse Doppler evaluation on 50 in situ vein grafts. Severe flow disturbances were present in 14% of the distal anastomoses, 5% of valve incision sites, and 2% of proximal anastomoses.

Platelet thrombi occur at the sites of valve incision or splits in the intima along the length of the vein. Exploration of these sites, with careful removal of any thrombotic material and repair by patch angioplasty or replacement of the damaged vein segment, is often necessary.

Beyond the initial postoperative period, approximately one third of infrainguinal vein grafts develop stenoses that may predispose to thrombosis. Reoperation to correct such defects prior to graft occlusion permits salvage of the grafts and prevention of recurrent ischemia. Unfortunately, between 20% and 40% of grafts occlude without prior warning or with recently recorded normal ankle pressure indices.[232] Because of the propensity of these grafts to fail, every attempt should be made to detect obstructive changes within the graft, at anastomoses, or in the inflow or runoff vessels before occlusion.

A hemodynamically significant graft stenosis can be detected during carefully executed duplex scanning of the graft. Few of these patients have recurrent symptoms despite the presence of a flow-limiting lesion. The value of a vein graft duplex surveillance program allowing early detection, close follow-up, and timely revision of these lesions meeting duplex criteria for high-grade stenosis has been well established.[233–236] However, controversy remains regarding the exact criteria mandating graft revision to prevent graft thrombosis. Our personal observations have suggested that when the peak systolic velocity progresses to 350 cm/second or greater or the velocity ratio to 3.5 or greater, the graft is at significant risk of failure.[237] These threshold criteria may seem to be high compared with other published criteria, and larger surveillance studies are necessary to resolve this remaining controversy. Other important parameters are a decreased graft velocity of less than 45 cm/second and a fall in the ankle-brachial index of more than 0.15[237] (Fig. 39–16). The former is particularly suggestive of a more proximal lesion, whereas the latter, if isolated, may be indicative of an outflow lesion or a missed graft stenosis on duplex scan. Nonetheless, these abnormal values warrant our immediate attention with closer follow-

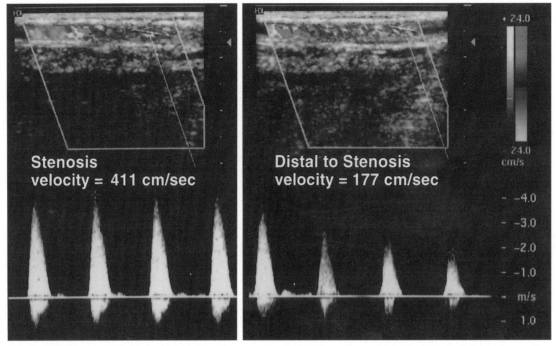

Figure 39–16. Duplex scan of a vein graft stenosis demonstrating a velocity of 441 cm/sec at the site of the stenosis and 117 cm/sec distally.

up, further evaluation, or immediate intervention, as dictated by the information obtained. After revision or the initial bypass procedure, the patient is seen every month for 1 year and every 6 months thereafter.[232, 238]

Although some of the focal lesions observed angiographically during late follow-up appear suitable for balloon catheter dilatation, the recurrence rate is high; patch angioplasty or replacement of a segment of vein offers superior long-term results.

An interesting complication of infrainguinal bypass grafts is functional failure despite continued graft patency and is manifest by extension of necrosis or failure to control the infective processes in the foot.[239] The incidence of this complication ranges from 2% to 4% for reversed vein grafts, up to 7.5% for in situ vein grafts, and 8.1% to 9.5% for PTFE grafts.[240, 241] Amputation may be required unless graft extension to an additional tibial or pedal vessel is possible. An alternative may be microvascular free flap transfer of healthy muscle to cover a persistent defect that usually involves exposed tendons, bones, or joints.

Prosthetic Graft Dilatation

With the continued increase in life expectancy of patients undergoing aortofemoral and femoropopliteal bypass grafting, the need for continued surveillance to detect deterioration in the graft material or complications resulting from implantation of prosthetic devices is becoming increasingly apparent.

Although florid rupture of Dacron grafts and dilatation of PTFE grafts have almost been eliminated by improvement in graft manufacture of the former and by increasing wall thickness or the application of an external wrap around the latter, deterioration in prosthetic grafts continues to occur.

Dacron Grafts

The true incidence of dilatation is unknown, since patients with apparently well-functioning grafts as evidenced by palpable distal pulses or normal ankle pressure indices on follow-up examinations are seldom evaluated unless some problem, such as an anastomotic aneurysm or acute occlusion of a graft limb, supervenes.

Textile grafts initially dilate approximately 15% to 20% after implantation. This is believed to be due to yarn slippage and is accompanied by a small decrease in tensile strength, which then stabilizes but may continue throughout the life span of the graft. Three factors are believed to contribute to dilatation of Dacron grafts: (1) a flattening of the crimp when the graft is subjected to arterial pressure, (2) an increase in diameter and decrease in length due to rearrangement of textile structure (i.e., the lighter the graft fiber, the greater the porosity and the more likely it is to dilate), and (3) an increase in diameter and length due to deformation of the graft material.[154, 242–245]

Dilatation is most likely to occur in knitted rather than woven grafts, as documented in a study by Nunn and associates,[244] who evaluated 95 Dacron grafts implanted for a mean of 33 months using Doppler ultrasound. The mean dilatation was 17.6% and was somewhat more severe in hypertensive patients (21%) than in their normotensive counterparts (15%). However, some grafts enlarged by more than 100%. In a CT study of 178 aortic grafts, Berman and coworkers[245] reported mean dilatation of 49.2% ± 4.0% for knitted Dacron prostheses, 28.5% ±

3.0% for woven Dacron grafts, and 20.6% ± 1.9% for PTFE grafts from their preimplantation diameter (Fig. 39–17). Complications, including supragraft aneurysms (seven), distal anastomotic aneurysms (five), proximal anastomotic aneurysms (three), graft infections (two), perigraft fluid collections (two), graft aneurysms with thrombus and distal embolization (two), and nonvascular complications (three), occurred in 13.5% of the patients.

Prosthetic rupture and anastomotic aneurysm formation have been reported in patients with dilated grafts; however, the natural history of such grafts left in place is presently unknown.[154, 159, 246, 247] Nevertheless, removal of a grossly dilated graft may be prudent in an asymptomatic patient without significant cardiorespiratory problems that increase operative risk. In practice, dilated segments of grafts associated with anastomotic aneurysms are replaced. Care should be taken to use a graft corresponding to the diameter of the outflow vessel, and no attempt should be made to match the diameter of the interposition graft to that of the dilated implanted graft.

Umbilical Veins

Umbilical veins have been used as a substitute for saphenous veins, with a 5-year patency of approximately 45%.[248] Dardik and colleagues,[249, 250] in a series of 756 glutaraldehyde-stabilized umbilical vein grafts (UVGs) implanted over a 7-year period, identified aneurysmal change in seven (1%) in the entire series. The incidence of such aneurysms has increased over time from 1.2% at 4 to 6 years to 7.7% at 6 to 8 years. It should be noted that this incidence may be underestimated, as follow-up arteriography was performed only in one third of the patients at risk. The mechanisms for UVG dilatation include mechanical fatigue, reversal of cross-linking, and immunologic factors. Julien and coworkers,[251] in a study of 80 UVG segments removed from 70 patients studied by light and electron microscopy, found aneurysmal dilatation in 4 of 80 specimens, bacterial

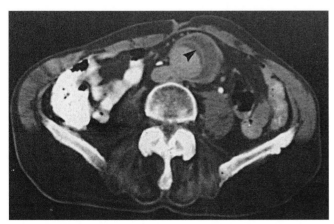

Figure 39–17. Abdominal computed tomography scan demonstrating a dilated graft *(arrow)* and the surrounding thrombus from an aortic anastomotic aneurysm. (From Hunter GC, Bull DA: The healing characteristics, durability, and long-term complications of vascular prostheses. (From Bernhard VM, Towne TB [eds]: Complications in Vascular Surgery. St. Louis, Quality Medical Publishing, 1991, p 65.)

colonization in the absence of overt infection in 26%, and irregular wall thickness with folds on the intraluminal surface in one third of the grafts. Anastomotic thrombus is often associated with this problem.

Because of the small but definite risk of continued deterioration of these grafts, Dardik and colleagues[249, 250] have recommended that an arteriogram be performed 3 to 4 years after implantation in addition to noninvasive surveillance.

Polytetrafluoroethylene

When first introduced, PTFE grafts were manufactured without an external wrap. This was associated with aneurysmal dilatation of the grafts. No further aneurysms have been reported since the application of the wrap (Gore-Tex, W. L. Gore and Associates, Inc., Flagstaff, Ariz.) or by increasing the thickness of the graft wall (Impra, C. R. Bard Inc., Tempe, Ariz.). Furthermore, PTFE does not dilate significantly over time, which makes it the material of choice for repair of anastomotic aneurysms and possibly for aortofemoral bypass.[252, 253]

Edema

Some degree of lower extremity edema accompanies the majority of successful infrainguinal arterial reconstructions. The reported incidence is as high as 70% to 100%.[42] The most important factor in the development of this edema appears to be lymphatic interruption, probably at the inguinal, thigh, and popliteal areas during the lower extremity arterial reconstruction. Microcirculatory derangements that exist in the ischemic limb, such as loss of arteriolar autoregulation, loss of the orthostatic vasoconstrictor reflex, capillary recruitment, and focal capillary endothelial injury, all apparently contribute to this lymph-related edema by increasing the net flux of interstitial fluid into the lymphatic system[254-256] (Fig. 39–18). Venous thrombosis has been shown to be a very infrequent cause of postreconstructive edema.[256, 257]

The severity of the edema increases in relation to the severity of prebypass ischemia. Furthermore, it is less frequent after aortoiliofemoral reconstruction, presumably because there is less limb lymphatic disruption.[224]

Technical modifications to minimize inguinal and popliteal lymphatic injury during infrainguinal arterial reconstruction may reduce the incidence of postoperative edema.[258] We have observed much less edema in patients undergoing in situ femorotibial bypass grafting when the branches are identified angioscopically and occluded using small interrupted incisions than in patients with continuous incisions. Once this complication occurs, bed rest, elevation, the use of elastic support stockings, and diuretics will control edema by shifting capillary dynamics in favor of fluid reabsorption.[255] Fortunately, in most instances, postreconstructive edema is self-limited and improves or disappears during the first few postoperative months.[42]

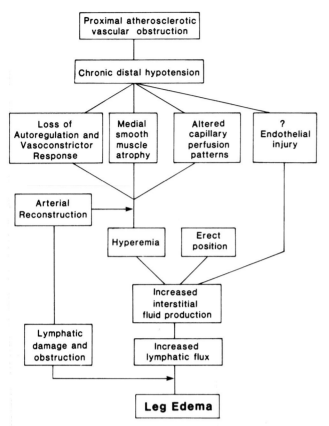

Figure 39–18. Schematic overview of the factors involved in postoperative lower extremity edema after femorodistal reconstruction. (From Schubart PJ, Porter JM: Leg edema after femorodistal bypass. In Bergan JJ, Yao JST [eds]: Reoperative Arterial Surgery. Orlando, Fla., Grune & Stratton, 1986, p 328.)

Lymphoceles and Lymph Leaks

The accumulation of lymph after groin surgery usually appears as an asymptomatic mass without evidence of overlying inflammation. If the lymphocele is small and located some distance from the incision, it may be followed expectantly. Should the lymphocele increase in size, communicate with the incision, or begin to leak, it should be explored and treated as in patients with lymph leaks.

Drainage of lymphatic fluid from the groin incision is a relatively infrequent complication of arterial reconstruction. In the series reported by Kent and associates,[222] a seroma lymph leak was present in 4% of the patients with groin incisions prospectively evaluated. The leak appears as a persistent, clear, watery drainage through the wound after the first few postoperative days or as an onset of drainage as the patient resumes ambulation.[42] The frequent presence of bacteria in the lymphatic channels draining ulcerative or gangrenous lesions of the extremity may lead to graft infection and anastomotic disruption.

Lymphatic leakage results from transected and unligated lymphatic channels and lymph nodes in the groin incision. Possible contributing factors include poor wound edge and tissue layer approximation and subcutaneous fat necrosis.[42]

Nonoperative treatment of lymphorrhea includes bed rest and leg elevation to reduce lymph flow while allowing the lymphatics to heal. Wound care must be meticulous, and systemic prophylactic antibiotics should be administered to reduce the risk of secondary infection.[42]

If the wound continues to drain for more than 2 to 3 days, the patient should be returned to the operating room and the wound explored. The divided lymphatic channels are suture-ligated and the wound closed in layers over suction drainage, care being taken to separate the drain from the prosthesis. This technique controls wound drainage and decreases the risk of secondary infection of the lymphatic cavity.[259, 260] This reported experience with early wound reexploration suggests shortened hospitalization and reduction in the incidence of graft infection. Because the site of lymphatic disruption may not be recognized on reexploration of the wound, manual massage of the thigh or staining of the lymphatic system by injection of a vital dye in the foot several hours before surgery is recommended to aid in identifying the leak site.

References

1. Downs AR: Complications of abdominal aortic surgery. In Bernhard VM, Towne JB (eds): Complications in Vascular Surgery. Orlando, Fla, Grune & Stratton, 1985, pp 25–36.
2. Brener BJ, Darling RC, Frederick PL, et al: Major venous anomalies complicating abdominal aortic surgery. Arch Surg 108:159–169, 1974.
3. Reed MD, Friedman AC, Nealey P: Anomalies of the left renal vein: Analysis of 433 CT scans. J Comput Assist Tomogr 6:1124–1126, 1982.
4. Bartle EJ, Pearce WH, Sun JH, Rutherford RB: Infrarenal venous anomalies and aortic surgery: Avoiding vascular injury. J Vasc Surg 6:590–593, 1987.
5. Bernhard VM: Aortocaval fistulas. In Haimovici H (ed): Vascular Emergencies. New York, Appleton-Century-Crofts, 1982, pp 353–363.
6. Duppler DW, Herbert WE, Dillihunt RC, et al: Primary arteriovenous fistulas of the abdomen. Arch Surg 120:786–790, 1985.
7. Brewster DC, Cambria RP, Moncure AC, et al: Aortocaval and iliac arteriovenous fistulas: Recognition and treatment. J Vasc Surg 13:253–265, 1991.
8. Calligaro KD, Savarese RP, DeLaurentis DA: Unusual aspects of aortovenous fistulas associated with ruptured abdominal aortic aneurysms. J Vasc Surg 12:586–590, 1990.
9. Dardik H, Dardik I, Strom MG: Intravenous rupture of arteriosclerotic aneurysms of the abdominal aorta. Surgery 80:647–653, 1976.
10. Zajko AB, Little AF, Steed DL, Curtiss EI: Endovascular stent-graft repair of common iliac artery to inferior vena cava fistula. J Vasc Interv Radiol 6:803–806, 1995.
11. Parodi JC, Criado FJ, Barone HD, et al: Endoluminal aortic aneurysm repair using a balloon-expandable stent-graft device: A progress report. Ann Vasc Surg 8:523–529, 1994.
12. Thompson JE, Hollier LH, Patman RD, et al: Surgical management of abdominal aortic aneurysms: Factors influencing mortality and morbidity. A 20 year experience. Ann Surg 181:654–688, 1975.
13. Effeney DJ, Goldstone J, Chin D, et al: Intraoperative anticoagulation in cardiovascular surgery. Surgery 90:1068–1074, 1981.
14. Crawford ES, Manning LG, Kelly FT: "Redo" surgery after operations for aneurysm and occlusion of the abdominal aorta. Surgery 81:41–52, 1977.
15. O'Hara PJ, Brewster DC, Darling RC, et al: The value of intraoperative monitoring using the pulse volume recorder during peripheral vascular reconstructive operations. Surg Gynecol Obstet 152:275–281, 1981.
16. Strom JA, Bernhard VM, Towne JB: Acute limb ischemia following aortic reconstruction: A preventable cause of increased mortality. Arch Surg 119:470–473, 1984.

17. Kapsch DN, Adelstein EH, Rhodes GR, et al: Heparin-induced thrombocytopenia, thrombosis, and hemorrhage. Surgery 86:148–154, 1979.
18. Towne JB: Hypercoagulable states and unexplained vascular thrombosis. In Bernhard VM, Towne JB (eds): Complications in Vascular Surgery. Orlando, Fla, Grune & Stratton, 1985, pp 381–404.
19. Towne JB, Bernhard VM, Hussey C, et al: Antithrombin III deficiency: A cause of unexplained thrombosis in vascular surgery. Surgery 89:735–747, 1981.
20. Towne JB, Bernhard VM, Hussey C, et al: White clot syndrome: Peripheral vascular complications of heparin therapy. Arch Surg 114:373–379, 1979.
21. Bernhard VM: The failed arterial graft: Lost pulses and gangrene. In Condon RE, DeCosse J (eds): Surgical Care: A Physiologic Approach to Clinical Management. Philadelphia, Lea & Febiger, 1980, pp 153–167.
22. Brewster DC, Darling RC: Optimal methods of aorto-iliac reconstruction. Surgery 84:739–748, 1978.
23. O'Mara CS, Flinn WR, Johnson ND, et al: Recognition and surgical management of patent but hemodynamically failed arterial grafts. Ann Surg 193:467–476, 1981.
24. Baird RJ, Feldman P, Miles JT, et al: Subsequent downstream repair with aortoiliac and aortofemoral bypass operations. Surgery 82:785, 1977.
25. Baird RJ: Downstream revascularization after aortofemoral bypass grafting. In Bergan JJ, Yao JST (eds): Reoperative Arterial Surgery. Orlando, Fla, Grune & Stratton, 1986, pp 223–230.
26. Mulcare RJ, Royster TS, Lynn RA, et al: Long-term results of operative therapy for aortoiliac disease. Arch Surg 113:601–604, 1978.
27. Nevelsteen A, Suy R, Daenen W, et al: Aorto-femoral grafting: Factors influencing late results. Surgery 88:642–653, 1980.
28. Charlesworth D: The occluded aortic and aorto-femoral graft. In Bergan JJ, Yao JST (eds): Reoperative Arterial Surgery. Orlando, Fla, Grune & Stratton, 1986, pp 271–278.
29. Fulenwider JT, Smith RB III, Johnson RW, et al: Reoperative abdominal arterial surgery. A ten year experience. Surgery 93:20–27, 1983.
30. Robbs JV, Wylie EJ: Factors contributing to recurrent lower limb ischemia following bypass surgery for aorto-iliac occlusive disease and their management. Ann Surg 193:346–352, 1981.
31. Frisch N, Bour P, Berg P, Fieve G, Frisch R: Long term results of thrombectomy for late occlusions of aortofemoral bypass. Ann Vasc Surg 5:16–20, 1991.
32. Nevelsteen A, Suy R: Graft occlusion following aortofemoral Dacron bypass. Ann Vasc Surg 5:32–37, 1991.
33. LoGerfo FW, Quist WC, Nowak MD, et al: Downstream anastomotic hyperplasia. Ann Surg 197:479–483, 1983.
34. Malone JM, Moore WS, Goldstone J: The natural history of bilateral aortofemoral grafts for ischemia of the lower extremities. Arch Surg 110:1300–1306, 1975.
35. Rhodes RS, Hutton MC, Lalka SG: Reoperation for intra-abdominal vascular disease. In Fry DE (ed): Reoperative Surgery of the Abdomen. New York, Marcel Dekker, 1986, pp 153–174.
36. Wylie EJ, Olcott C: Aortoiliac thromboendarterectomy. In Varco RL, Delaney JP (eds): Controversy in Surgery. Philadelphia, WB Saunders, 1976, pp 437–450.
37. Crawford ES, Bomberger RA, Glaeser DH, et al: Aorto-iliac occlusive disease: Factors influencing survival and function following reconstructive operation over a twenty-five year period. Surgery 90:1055–1067, 1981.
38. Satiani B, Liapis CD, Evans WE: Aortofemoral bypass for severe limb ischemia: Long-term survival and limb salvage. Am J Surg 141:252–256, 1981.
39. Yao JST, McCarthy WJ: Surgical correction of hemodynamic failure of bypass grafts. In Bergan JJ, Yao JST (eds): Reoperative Arterial Surgery. Orlando, Fla, Grune & Stratton, 1986, pp 257–270.
40. Bernhard VM: Late vascular graft thrombosis. In Bernhard VM, Towne JB (eds): Complications in Vascular Surgery. Orlando, Fla, Grune & Stratton, 1985, pp 187–204.
41. Bernhard VM, Ray LI, Towne JB: The reoperation of choice for aorto-femoral graft occlusion. Surgery 82:867–876, 1977.
42. Brewster DC: Early complications of vascular repair below the inguinal ligament. In Bernhard VM, Towne JB (eds): Complications in Vascular Surgery. Orlando, Fla, Grune & Stratton, 1985, pp 37–53.
43. DePalma RG, Malgieri JJ, Rhodes RS, et al: Profunda femoris bypass for secondary revascularization. Surg Gynecol Obstet 151:387–390, 1980.
44. Van Breda A, Robison JC, Feldman L, et al: Local thrombolysis in the treatment of arterial graft occlusions. J Vasc Surg 1:103–110, 1984.
45. Battey PM, Fulenwider JT, Smith RB, et al: Intraarterial thrombolysis for acute limb ischemia: A three-year experience. South Med J 80:479–482, 1987.
46. Katzen BT, Edwards KC, Albert AS, et al: Low dose direct fibrinolysis in peripheral vascular disease. J Vasc Surg 1:718–722, 1984.
47. McNamara TO, Bomberger RA: Factors affecting initial and 6 month patency rates after intra-arterial thrombolysis with high dose urokinase. Am J Surg 152:709–712, 1986.
48. McNamara TO, Fischer JR: Thrombolysis of peripheral arterial and graft occlusions: Improved results using high-dose urokinase. AJR 144:769–775, 1985.
49. Sicard GA, Schier JJ, Totty WG, et al: Thrombolytic therapy for acute arterial occlusion. J Vasc Surg 2:65–78, 1985.
50. Van Breda A, Katzen BT, Deutsch AS: Urokinase versus streptokinase in local thrombolysis. Radiology 165:109–111, 1987.
51. Gardiner GA, Harrington DP, Kolun W, et al: Salvage of occluded arterial bypass grafts by means of thrombolysis. J Vasc Surg 9:426–431, 1989.
52. Belkin M, Belkin B, Bucknam CA, et al: Intra-arterial fibrinolytic therapy. Arch Surg 121:769–773, 1986.
53. Hallett JW, Wolk SW, Cherry KJ, et al: The femoral neuralgia syndrome after arterial catheter trauma. J Vasc Surg 11:702–706, 1990.
54. Gaglani RD, Turk AA, Mehra MR, et al: Contralateral femoral neuropathy: An unusual complication of anticoagulation following PTCA. Cathet Cardiovasc Diagn 24:176–178, 1991.
55. Ouriel K, Shortell CK, DeWeese JA, et al: A comparison of thrombolytic therapy with operative revascularization in the initial treatment of acute peripheral arterial ischemia. J Vasc Surg 19:1021–1030, 1994.
56. Ouriel K, Veith FJ, Sasahara AA: Thrombolysis or peripheral arterial surgery: Phase I results. J Vasc Surg 23:64–75, 1996.
57. STILE Investigators: Results of a prospective randomized trial evaluating surgery versus thrombolysis for ischemia of the lower extremity. Ann Surg 220:251–268, 1994.
58. Hye RJ, Turner C, Valji K, et al: Is thrombolysis of occluded popliteal and tibial bypass grafts worthwhile? J Vasc Surg 20:588–597, 1994.
59. Garramone RR, Gallager JJ, Drezner AD: Intra-arterial thrombolytic therapy in the initial management of thrombosed popliteal artery aneurysms. Ann Vasc Surg 8:363–366, 1994.
60. Cina CS, Goh RH, Chan J, et al: Intraarterial catheter-directed thrombolysis: Urokinase versus tissue plasminogen activator. Ann Vasc Surg 13:571–575, 1999.
61. Laird JR, Dangas G, Jaff M, et al: Intra-arterial reteplase for the treatment of acute limb ischemia. J Invasive Cardiol 11:757–762, 1999.
62. McNamara TO: New pharmacologic therapies in the treatment of peripheral vascular disease. Presented at 11th Annual Symposium on Transcatheter Cardiovascular Therapeutics (TCT-11), Sept 22–26, 1999, Washington, DC.
63. Sharafuddin MJA, Hicks ME: Current status of percutaneous mechanical thrombectomy. Part II. Devices and mechanisms of action. Vasc Interv Radiol 9:15–31, 1998.
64. Ouriel K: Percutaneous recirculation mechanical thrombectomy catheter (Angiojet) in the management of limb threatening ischemia [abstract]. In 26th Annual Critical Problems and New Horizons and Techniques in Vascular and Endovascular Surgery, November 18–21, 1999, JP 2.1–2.3.
65. Demopoulos LA, Tunick PA, Bernstein NE, et al: Protruding atheromas of the aortic arch in symptomatic patients with carotid artery disease. Am Heart J 129:40–44, 1995.
66. Lagattolla NRF, Burnand KG, Stewart A: Role of transoesophageal echocardiography in determining the source of peripheral arterial embolism. Br J Surg 82:1651, 1995.
67. Kazmier PJ, Sheps SG, Bernatz PE, et al: Livedo reticularis and digital infarcts: A syndrome due to cholesterol infarcts arising from abdominal aortic aneurysms. Vasc Dis 3:12–22, 1966.
68. Starr DS, Lawrie GM, Morris GC: Prevention of distal embolism during arterial reconstruction. Am J Surg 138:764–771, 1979.

69. Attia RR, Murphy JD, Snider M, et al: Myocardial ischemia due to infrarenal aortic cross-clamping during aortic surgery in patients with severe coronary artery disease. Circulation 53:961–965, 1976.

70. Bush HL, LoGerfo FW, Weisel RD, et al: Assessment of myocardial performance and optimal volume loading during elective abdominal aortic aneurysm resection. Arch Surg 112:1301–1306, 1977.

71. Dauchot PJ, DePalma R, Grum D, et al: Detection and prevention of cardiac dysfunction during aortic surgery. J Surg Res 26:574–580, 1979.

72. Silverstein PR, Caldera DL, Cullen DJ, et al: Avoiding the hemodynamic consequences of aortic cross-clamping and unclamping. Anesthesiology 50:462–466, 1979.

73. Whittemore AD, Clowes AW, Hechtman HB, et al: Aortic aneurysm repair: Reduced operative mortality associated with maintenance of optimal cardiac performance. Ann Surg 192:414–421, 1980.

74. Abbott WM, Abel RM, Beck CH, et al: Renal failure after ruptured aneurysm. Arch Surg 110:1110, 1975.

75. Castonuovo JJ, Flanigan DP: Renal failure complicating vascular surgery. In Bernhard VM, Towne JB (eds): Complications in Vascular Surgery. Orlando, Fla, Grune & Stratton, 1985, pp 258–274.

76. Abbott WM, Austen WG: The reversal of renal cortical ischemia during aortic occlusion by mannitol. J Surg Res 16:482–486, 1974.

77. Berkowitz HD, Shetty S: Renin release and renal cortical ischemia following aortic cross clamping. Arch Surg 109:612–618, 1974.

78. Crawford ES, Synder DM, Cho GC, et al: Progress in treatment of thoraco-abdominal and abdominal aortic aneurysms involving the celiac, superior mesenteric and renal arteries. Ann Surg 188:404–422, 1978.

79. Iliopoulos JI, Zdon MJ, Crawford BG, et al: Renal microembolization syndrome. Am J Surg 146:779–783, 1983.

80. Myers BD, Moran SM: Hemodynamically mediated acute renal failure. N Engl J Med 314:97–105, 1986.

81. Bush HL, Huse JB, Johnson WC, et al: Prevention of renal insufficiency after abdominal aortic aneurysm reaction by optimal volume loading. Arch Surg 116:1517–1522, 1981.

82. Franklin SC, Moulton M, Sicard GA, et al: Insulin-like growth factor I preserves renal function postoperatively. Am J Physiol 272:F257–F259, 1997.

83. Meyer M, Wiebe K, Wahlers T, et al: Urodilatin (INN:ularitide) as a new drug for the therapy of acute renal failure following cardiac surgery. Clin Exp Pharmacol Physiol 24:374–376, 1997.

84. Wiebe K, Meyer M, Wahlers T, et al: Acute renal failure following cardiac surgery is reverted by administration of Urodilatin (INN: ularitide). Eur J Med Res 22:259–265, 1996.

85. Krause SM, Walsh TF, Greenlee WJ, et al: Renal protection by a dual ETA/ETB endothelin antagonist, L-754,142, after aortic cross-clamping in the dog. J Am Soc Nephrol 8:1061–1071, 1997.

86. Szilagyi DE, Smith RF, Elliot JP: Temporary transection of the left renal vein: A technical aid to aortic surgery. Surgery 65:32–40, 1969.

87. Huber D, Harris JP, Walker PJ, et al: Does division of the left renal vein during aortic surgery adversely affect renal function? Ann Vasc Surg 5:74–79, 1991.

88. Abu Rahma AF, Robinson PA, Boland JP, Lucente FC: The risk of ligation of the left renal vein in resection of the abdominal aortic aneurysm. Surg Gynecol Obstet 173:33–36, 1991.

89. Olsen PS, Schroeder T, Perko M, et al: Renal failure after operation for abdominal aortic aneurysm. Ann Vasc Surg 4:580–583, 1990.

90. Mandal AK, Visweswaran RK, Kaldas NR: Treatment considerations in acute renal failure. Drugs 44:567–577, 1992.

91. Ernst CB: Postoperative intestinal ischemia. In Haimovici H (ed): Vascular Emergencies. New York, Appleton-Century-Crofts, 1982, pp 493–513.

92. Johnson WC, Nasbeth DC: Visceral infarction following aortic surgery. Ann Surg 180:312–321, 1974.

93. Ottinger LW, Darling RC, Nathan MJ, et al: Left colon ischemia complicating aorto-iliac reconstruction. Arch Surg 105:481, 1972.

94. Ernst CB: Intestinal ischemia following abdominal aortic reconstruction. In Bernhard VM, Towne JB (eds): Complications in Vascular Surgery. Orlando, Fla, Grune & Stratton, 1985, pp 325–350.

95. Hagihara PF, Ernst CB, Griffen WO: Incidence of ischemic colitis following abdominal aortic reconstruction. Surg Gynecol Obstet 149:571–573, 1979.

96. Moskowitz M, Zimmerman H, Felson B: The meandering mesenteric artery of the colon. AJR 92:1088, 1964.

97. Ernst CB, Hagihara PF, Daugherty ME, et al: Ischemis colitis incidence following abdominal aortic reconstruction: A prospective study. Surgery 80:417–423, 1976.

98. Boley SJ, Brandt LF, Veith FJ: Ischemic disorders of the intestines. Curr Probl Surg 15:1–85, 1978.

99. Hobson RW, Wright CB, O'Donnell JA, et al: Determination of intestinal viability by Doppler ultrasound. Arch Surg 114:165–168, 1979.

100. Bicks RO, Bale GF, Howard H, et al: Acute and delayed colon ischemia after aortic aneurysm surgery. Arch Intern Med 122:249, 1968.

101. Yee J, Dixon CM, McLean APH, Meakins JL: Clostridium difficile disease in a department of surgery: The significance of prophylactic antibiotics. Arch Surg 126:241–246, 1991.

102. Teasley DG, Gerding DN, Olson MM, et al: Prospective randomized trial of metronidazole versus vancomycin for Clostridium difficile–associated diarrhoea and colitis. Lancet 2:1043–1046, 1983.

103. Björk M, Hedberg B: Early detection of major complications after abdominal aortic surgery: Predictive value of sigmoid colon and gastric intramucosal pH monitoring. Br J Surg 81:25–30, 1994.

104. Ernst CB, Hagihara PF, Daugherty ME, et al: Inferior mesenteric artery stump pressure: A reliable index for safe IMA ligation during abdominal aortic aneurysmectomy. Arch Surg 187:641–649, 1978.

105. Welling RE, Roedersheimer R, Arbaugh JJ, et al: Ischemic colitis following repair of ruptured abdominal aortic aneurysms. Arch Surg 120:1368–1370, 1985.

106. Connolly JE, Kwann JHM: Prophylactic revascularization of the gut. Ann Surg 190:514–522, 1985.

107. Brewster DC, Retana A, Waltman AC, et al: Angiography in the management of aneurysms of the abdominal aorta. N Engl J Med 292:822–825, 1975.

108. Rubin GD, Dake MD, Semba CP: Current status of three-dimensional spiral CT scanning for imaging the vasculature. Vasc Imaging 33:51–70, 1995.

109. Zelenock GB, Strodel WE, Knol JA, et al: A prospective study of clinically and endoscopically documented colonic ischemia in 100 patients undergoing aortic reconstructive surgery with aggressive colonic and direct pelvic revascularization, compared with historic controls. Surgery 106:771–780, 1989.

110. DiChiro G, Doppman JL: Paraplegia after resection of aneurysm. N Engl J Med 281:799–803, 1969.

111. Elliot JP, Szilagyi DE, Hageman JH, et al: Spinal cord ischemia: Secondary to surgery of the abdominal aorta. In Bernhard VM, Towne JB (eds): Complications in Vascular Surgery. Orlando, Fla, Grune & Stratton, 1985, pp 291–310.

112. Szilagyi ED, Hageman JH, Smith RF, et al: Spinal cord damage in surgery of the abdominal aorta. Surgery 83:38, 1978.

113. Ferguson LRJ, Bergan JJ, Conn J Jr, et al: Spinal ischemia following abdominal aortic surgery. Ann Surg 181:267, 1975.

114. Grace RR, Mattox KL: Anterior spinal artery syndrome following abdominal aortic aneurysmectomy. Arch Surg 112:813, 1977.

115. DiChiro G, Wener L: Angioplasty of the spinal cord. J Neurosurg 39:1–11, 1973.

116. Williams GM, Perler BA, Burdick JF, et al: Angiographic localization of spinal cord blood and its relationship to postoperative paraplegia. J Vasc Surg 13:23–35, 1991.

117. Kieffer E, Richard T, Chiras J, et al: Preoperative spinal cord arteriography in aneurysmal disease of the descending thoracic and thoracoabdominal aorta: Preliminary results in 45 patients. Ann Vasc Surg 3:34–46, 1989.

118. Cunningham NJ Jr, Laschinger JC, Merkin HA, et al: Measurement of spinal cord ischemia during operations upon the thoracic aorta. Initial experience. Ann Surg 196:285–296, 1982.

119. Coles JG, Wilson GJ, Sima AF, et al: Intraoperative detection of spinal cord ischemia using somotosensory cortical evoked potentials during thoracic aortic occlusion. Ann Thorac Surg 34:299, 1982.

120. Laschinger JC, Cunningham JN, Nathan IM, et al: Detection and prevention of intraoperative spinal cord ischemia after cross-clamping the thoracic aorta: Use of somatosensory evoked potentials. Surgery 92:1109, 1982.

121. Laschinger JC, Cunningham JN, Nathan IM, et al: Experimental and clinical assessment of the adequacy of partial bypass in the maintenance of spinal cord flow during operations on the thoracic aorta. Ann Thorac Surg 36:417, 1983.

122. Picone AL, Green RM, Ricotta JR, et al: Spinal cord ischemia following operations on the abdominal aorta. J Vasc Surg 3:94–103, 1986.

123. Lambardini MM, Ratliff RK: The abdominal aortic aneurysm and the ureter. J Urol 98:590–601, 1967.

124. Goldstone J, Malone JM, Moore WS: Inflammatory aneurysm of the abdominal aorta. Surgery 83:425–435, 1978.

125. Nachbur B, Marincek B, Jakob R, Ackerman D: The impact of computed tomography in the diagnosis and postoperative followup of ureteric obstruction in aorto-iliac aneurysmal disease. Eur J Vasc Surg 3:475–492, 1989.

126. Egeblad K, Brochner-Mortensen J, Krarup T, et al: Incidence of ureteral obstruction after aortic grafting: A prospective analysis. Surgery 103:411–414, 1988.

127. Spirnak JP, Nehemia H, Resnick MI: Ureteral injuries complicating vascular surgery: Is repair indicated? J Urol 141:13–14, 1989.

128. Lask D, Abarbanel J, Luttwak Z, et al: Changing trends in the management of iatrogenic ureteral injuries. J Urol 154:1693–1695, 1995.

129. Cangiano TG: Urologic complications of vascular surgery. In Ball TP Jr (ed): AUA Update Series Lesson 39, vol 17. Houston, Tex, American Urological Association, 1998.

130. Sant GR, Heaney JA, Parkhurst EC, Blaivas JG: Obstructive uropathy—a potentially serious complication of reconstructive vascular surgery. J Urol 129:16–22, 1983.

131. Goldenberg SL, Gordon PB, Cooperberg PL, McLoughlin MG: Early hydronephrosis following aortic bifurcation graft surgery: A prospective study. J Urol 140:1367–1369, 1988.

132. Wright DJ, Ernst CB, Evans JR, et al: Ureteral complications and aortoiliac reconstruction. J Vasc Surg 11:29–37, 1990.

133. Kempczinski RF, Birinyi LK: Impotence following aortic surgery. In Bernhard VM, Towne JB (eds): Complications in Vascular Surgery. Orlando, Fla, Grune & Stratton, 1985, pp 311–324.

134. Merchant RF, DePalma RG: Effects of femoro-femoral grafts on postoperative sexual function: Correlation with penile pulse volume recordings. Surgery 90:962–970, 1981.

135. Ohshiro T, Kosaki G: Sexual function after aorto-iliac vascular reconstruction: Which is more important, the internal iliac artery or hypogastric nerve? J Cardiovasc Surg 25:47–50, 1984.

136. Queral LA, Flinn WR, Bergan JJ, et al: Sexual function and aortic surgery. In Bergan JJ, Yao JST (eds): Surgery of the Aorta and Its Body Branches. Orlando, Fla, Grune & Stratton, 1979, pp 263–276.

137. Queral LA, Whitehouse WM, Flinn WR, et al: Pelvic hemodynamics after aortoiliac reconstruction. Surgery 86:799–809, 1979.

138. Kempczinski RF: Role of the vascular diagnostic laboratory in the evaluation of male impotence. Am J Surg 138:278, 1979.

139. Nath RL, Menzoian JO, Kaplan KH, et al: The multidisciplinary approach to vasculogenic impotence. Surgery 89:124, 1981.

140. Flanigan DP, Sobinsky KR, Schuler JJ, et al: Internal iliac artery revascularization in the treatment of vasculogenic impotence. Arch Surg 120:271–274, 1985.

141. DePalma RG, Olding M, Yu GW, et al: Vascular interventions for impotence: Lessons learned. J Vasc Surg 21:576–585, 1995.

142. Flanigan DP, Schuler JJ: Sexual function in aortic surgery. In Bergan JJ, Yao JST (eds): Aortic Surgery. Philadelphia, WB Saunders, 1989, pp 547–660.

143. Donohue JP, Thornhill JA, Foster RS, et al: Retroperitoneal lymphadenectomy for clinical stage A testis cancer (1965 to 1989): Modifications of technique and impact on ejaculation. J Urol 149:237–243, 1993.

144. Colleselli K, Poisel S, Schachtner W, Bartsch G: Nerve-preserving bilateral retroperitoneal lymphadenectomy: Anatomical study and operative approach. J Urol 144:293–298, 1990.

145. DePalma RG: Impotence in vascular disease: Relationship to vascular surgery. Br J Surg 69:514, 1982.

146. Chavez CM: False aneurysm of the femoral artery: A challenge in management. Ann Surg 183:694–700, 1976.

147. Gardner TJ, Brawley RK, Gott VL: Anastomotic false aneurysms. Surgery 72:474–483, 1972.

148. Knox WG: Peripheral vascular anastomotic aneurysm: A fifteen year experience. Ann Surg 183:694–703, 1976.

149. Read RC, Thompson BW: Uninfected anastomotic false aneurysms following arterial reconstruction with prosthetic grafts. J Cardiovasc Surg 16:558–567, 1975.

150. Satiani B, Kazmers M, Evans WE: Anastomotic arterial aneurysms: A continuing challenge. Ann Surg 192:674–682, 1980.

151. Szilagyi DE, Smith FR, Elliot JP, et al: Anastomotic aneurysms after vascular reconstruction: Problems of incidence, etiology and treatment. Surgery 178:800–816, 1975.

152. Satiani B: False aneurysms following arterial reconstruction. Surg Gynecol Obstet 152:357–363, 1981.

153. Bernhard VM: Aortoduodenal and other aortoenteric fistulas. In Veith FJ (ed): Critical Problems in Vascular Surgery. New York, Appleton-Century-Crofts, 1982, pp 399–410.

154. Kim GE, Imparato AM, Nathan I, et al: Dilatation of synthetic grafts and junctional aneurysms. Arch Surg 114:1296–1303, 1979.

155. Evans WE, Hayes JP, Vermilion B: Anastomotic femoral false aneurysms. In Bernhard VM, Towne JB (eds): Complications in Vascular Surgery. Orlando, Fla, Grune & Stratton, 1985, pp 205–212.

156. Moore WS: Anastomotic aneurysms. In Rutherford RB (ed): Vascular Surgery. Philadelphia, WB Saunders, 1984, pp 821–827.

157. Clark RE, Apostolou S, Kardos JL: Mismatch of mechanical properties as a cause of arterial prosthesis thrombosis. Surg Forum 27:208–210, 1978.

158. Mehigan DG, Fitzpatrick B, Browne JL, et al: Is compliance mismatch the major cause of anastomotic arterial aneurysms? J Cardiovasc Surg 26:147–150, 1985.

159. Carson SN, Hunter GC, Palmaz J, Guernsey JM: Recurrence of femoral anastomotic aneurysms. Am J Surg 146:774–778, 1983.

160. Courbier R, Larranaga J: Natural history and management of anastomotic aneurysms. In Bergan JJ, Yao JST (eds): Aneurysms: Diagnosis and Treatment. Orlando, Fla, Grune & Stratton, 1982, pp 567–580.

161. Starr DS, Weatherford SC, Lawrie GM, et al: Suture material as a factor in occurrence of anastomotic aneurysms: An analysis of 26 cases. Arch Surg 114:412–415, 1979.

162. Perdue GD, Smith RB, Anoley JD, et al: Impending aortoenteric hemorrhage: The effects of early recognition on improved outcomes. Ann Surg 192:237–243, 1980.

163. Gooding GAW, Effeney DJ, Goldstone J: The aortofemoral graft: Detection and identification of healing complications by ultrasonography. Surgery 89:94–101, 1981.

164. Ernst CB, Elliot JP, Ryan CJ, et al: Recurrent femoral anastomotic aneurysms. Ann Surg 208:401–409, 1988.

165. Williams RA, Vetto J, Quiñones-Baldrich W, et al: Chylous ascites following abdominal aortic surgery. Ann Vasc Surg 5:247–252, 1991.

166. Pabst TS, McIntyre KE, Schilling JD, et al: Management of chyloperitoneum after abdominal aortic surgery. Am J Surg 166:194–199, 1993.

167. Cambria RP, Brewster DC, Abbolt WM, et al: Transperitoneal versus retroperitoneal approach for aortic reconstruction. J Vasc Surg 11:314–329, 1990.

168. Stevick CA, Long JB, Jamasbi B, Nash M: Ventral hernia following abdominal aortic reconstruction. Am Surg 54:287–289, 1988.

169. Hall KA, Peters B, Smyth SH, et al: Abdominal wall hernias in patients with abdominal aortic aneurysmal versus aortoiliac occlusive disease. Am J Surg 170:572–576, 1995.

170. Honig MP, Mason RA, Giron F: Wound complications of the retroperitoneal approach to the aorta and iliac vessels. J Vasc Surg 15:28–34, 1992.

171. Sicard GA, Freeman MB, VanderWoude JC, Anderson CB: Comparison between the transabdominal and retroperitoneal approach for reconstruction of the infrarenal abdominal aorta. J Vasc Surg 5:19–27, 1987.

172. Gardner GP, Josephs LG, Rosca M, et al: The retroperitoneal incision. Arch Surg 129:753–756, 1994.

173. Lord RSA, Crozier JA, Snell J, Meek AC: Transverse abdominal incisions compared with midline incisions for elective infrarenal aortic reconstruction: Predisposition to incisional hernia in patients with increased intraoperative blood loss. J Vasc Surg 20:27–33, 1994.

174. Craver JM, Ottinger LW, Darling RC, et al: Hemorrhage and thrombosis as early complications of femoral popliteal bypass grafts: Causes, treatment and prognostic implications. Surgery 74:839–846, 1973.

175. Hargrove WC, Barker CF, Berkowitz HD, et al: Treatment of acute peripheral arterial and graft thromboses with low-dose streptokinase. Surgery 92:981–993, 1982.

176. LiCalzi LK, Stansel HC: Failure of autogenous reversed saphenous vein femoro-popliteal grafting: Pathophysiology and prevention. Surgery 91:352–358, 1982.

177. Whittemore AD, Clowes AW, Couch NP, et al: Secondary femoropopliteal reconstruction. Ann Surg 193:35–42, 1981.

178. Buxton B, Lambert RP, Pitt TTE: The significance of vein wall thickness and diameter in relation to the patency of femoropopliteal saphenous vein bypass grafts. Surgery 87:425–431, 1980.

179. Corson JD, Shah DM, Leather RP, et al: Reversed autogenous saphenous vein bypass grafts: Complications of their use in the lower extremity. In Bernhard VM, Towne JB (eds): Complications in Vascular Surgery. Orlando, Fla, Grune & Stratton, 1985, pp 589–610.

180. Bunt TJ, Manship L, Moore W: Iatrogenic vascular injury during peripheral revascularization. J Vasc Surg 2:491–498, 1985.

181. Samson RH, Gupta SK, Scher LA, et al: Arterial spasm complicating distal vascular bypass procedures. Arch Surg 117:973–975, 1982.

182. Fuchs CA, Mitchener JS III, Hagen PO: Postoperative changes in autologous vein grafts. Ann Surg 188:1–11, 1978.

183. LiCalzi LK, Stansel HC: The closure index: Prediction of long term patency of femoro-popliteal vein grafts. Surgery 91:413–418, 1982.

184. Gundry SR, Jones M, Ishihara T, et al: Optimal preparation techniques for human saphenous vein grafts. Surgery 88:785–794, 1980.

185. Karmody AM, Leather RP, Shah DM, et al: The in situ saphenous vein arterial bypass: Current problems and solutions. In Bernhard VM, Towne JB (eds): Complications in Vascular Surgery. Orlando, Fla, Grune & Stratton, 1985, pp 561–588.

186. Brewster DC, LaSalle AJ, Robison JG, et al: Factors affecting patency of femoropopliteal bypass grafts. Surg Gynecol Obstet 157:437–442, 1983.

187. DeWeese JA: Anastomotic neointimal fibrous hyperplasia. In Bernhard VM, Towne JB (eds): Complications in Vascular Surgery. Orlando, Fla, Grune & Stratton, 1985, pp 157–170.

188. Green RM, Thomas M, Luka N, et al: A comparison of rapid healing prosthetic arterial grafts and autogenous veins. Arch Surg 114:944–947, 1979.

189. Echave V, Kovenick AR, Haimov M, et al: Intimal hyperplasia as a complication of the use of polytetrafluoroethylene graft for femoral-popliteal bypass. Surgery 86:791–800, 1979.

190. Harker LA: Platelet mechanisms in the genesis and prevention of graft related vascular injury reactions and thromboembolism. Nature of the vascular interface. In Sawyer PN, Kaplitt HJ (eds): Vascular Grafts. New York, Appleton-Century-Crofts, 1978, pp 153–159.

191. Schuler JJ, Flanigan DP: Alternate inflow for repeated failure of femorodistal grafts. In Bergan JJ, Yao JST (eds): Reoperative Arterial Surgery. Orlando, Fla, Grune & Stratton, 1986, pp 393–406.

192. Szilagyi DE, Elliot JP, Hageman JG, et al: Biologic fate of autogenous vein implants as arterial substitute. Ann Surg 178:232–251, 1973.

193. Bergan JJ, Veith FJ, Bernhard VM, et al: Randomization of autogenous vein and polytetrafluoroethylene grafts in femoral-distal reconstruction. Surgery 92:921–930, 1982.

194. Corson JD, Johnson WC, LoGerfo FW, et al: Doppler ankle systolic pressure: Prognostic value in vein bypass grafts of the lower extremity. Arch Surg 113:932–935, 1977.

195. Kempczinski RF: Infrainguinal arterial bypass using prosthetic grafts. In Kempczinski RF (ed): The Ischemic Leg. St Louis, Mosby–Year Book, 1985, pp 437–454.

196. O'Donnell TF, Farber SP, Richmind DM, et al: Above-knee polytetrafluoroethylene femoro-popliteal bypass graft: Is it a reasonable alternative to the below-knee reversed autogenous vein graft? Surgery 94:26, 1983.

197. Robison JG, Brewster DC, Abbott WM, et al: Femoro-popliteal and tibioperoneal artery reconstruction using human umbilical vein. Arch Surg 118:1039, 1983.

198. Rosenthal D, Levine K, Stanton PE, et al: Femoropopliteal bypass: The preferred site for distal anastomosis. Surgery 93:1, 1983.

199. Marinelli MR, Beach KW, Glass MJ, et al: Non-invasive testing versus clinical evaluation of arterial disease: A prospective study. JAMA 241:2031–2034, 1979.

200. Yao JST: Postoperative evaluation of graft failure. In Bernhard VM, Towne JB (eds): Complications in Vascular Surgery. Orlando, Fla, Grune & Stratton, 1985, pp 1–24.

201. Painton JF, Avellone JC, Plecha FR: Effectiveness of reoperation after late failure of femoro-popliteal reconstruction. Am J Surg 135:235–241, 1978.

202. Berkowitz HD, Hobbs CL, Roberts B, et al: Value of routine vascular laboratory studies to identify vein graft stenosis. Surgery 90:971–979, 1981.

203. Bandyk DF: Postoperative surveillance of femoro-distal grafts: The application of echo-Doppler (duplex) ultrasonic scanning. In Bergan JJ, Yao JST (eds): Reoperative Arterial Surgery. Orlando, Fla, Grune & Stratton, 1986, pp 59–80.

204. Baker WH, Hadcock MM, Littooy FN: Management of polytetrafluoroethylene graft occlusion. Arch Surg 115:508–513, 1980.

205. White GH, White RA, Kopchok GE, et al: Endoscopic intravascular surgery intraluminal flaps, dissections, and thrombus. J Vasc Surg 11:280–288, 1190.

206. Goldberg L, Ricci MT, Sauvage LR, et al: Thrombolytic therapy for delayed occlusion of knitted Dacron bypass grafts in the axillofemoral, femoropopliteal and femorotibial positions. Surg Gynecol Obstet 160:491–498, 1985.

207. Graor RA, Risius B, Denny KM, et al: Local thrombolysis in the treatment of thrombosed arteries, bypass grafts, and arteriovenous fistulas. J Vasc Surg 2:406–414, 1985.

208. Hargrove WC, Berkowitz HD, Freiman DB, et al: Recanalization of totally occluded femoropopliteal vein grafts with low-dose streptokinase infusion. Surgery 92:890–895, 1982.

209. Dardik H, Sussman BC, Kahn M, et al: Lysis of arterial clot by intravenous or intraarterial administration of streptokinase. Surg Gynecol Obstet 158:137–140, 1984.

210. Husson JM, Fiessinger JN, Aiach M, et al: Streptokinase after late failure reconstructive surgery for peripheral arteriosclerosis. J Cardiovasc Surg 22:145–152, 1981.

211. Quiñones-Baldrich WJ, Zierlar RE, Hiatt JC: Intraoperative fibrinolytic therapy: An adjunct to catheter thromboembolectomy. J Vasc Surg 2:319–326, 1985.

212. Parent FN 3rd, Bernhard VM, Pabst TS, et al: Fibrinolytic treatment of residual thrombus after catheter embolectomy for severe limb ischemia. J Vasc Surg 9:153–160, 1989.

213. Cohen L, Kaplan M, Bernhard VM: Intraoperative streptokinase: An adjunct to mechanical thrombectomy in the management of acute ischemia. Arch Surg 121:708–716, 1986.

214. Andros G, Harris RW, Salles-Cunha SX, et al: Arm veins for arterial revascularization of the leg: Arteriographic and clinical observations. J Vasc Surg 4:416–427, 1986.

215. Harker LA, Slichter SJ, Sauvage LR: Platelet consumption by arterial prostheses: The effects of endothelialization and pharmacologic inhibition of platelet function. Ann Surg 186:594–601, 1977.

216. Veith FJ, Gupta SK, Ascer E, et al: Reoperations and other reinterventions for thrombosed and failing polytetrafluoroethylene grafts. In Bergan JJ, Yao JST (eds): Reoperative Arterial Surgery. Orlando, Fla, Grune & Stratton, 1986, pp 377–392.

217. Kretschmer G, Wenzl E, Piza F, et al: The influence of anticoagulant treatment on the probability of function in femoropopliteal vein bypass surgery: Analysis of a clinical series (1970 to 1985) and interim evaluation of a controlled clinical trial. Surgery 102:453–459, 1987.

218. Kretschmer G, Wenzl E, Schemper M, et al: Influence of postoperative anticoagulant treatment on patient survival after femoro-popliteal vein bypass surgery. Lancet 1:797–798, 1988.

219. Wengrovitz M, Atnip RG, Gifford RRM, et al: Wound complications of autogenous subcutaneous infrainguinal arterial bypass surgery: Predisposing factors and management. J Vasc Surg 11:156–163, 1990.

220. Johnson JA, Cogbill TH, Strutt PJ, Gundersen AL: Wound complications after infrainguinal bypass: Classification, predisposing factors, and management. Arch Surg 123:859–862, 1988.

221. Schwartz ME, Harrington EB, Schanzer H: Wound complications after in situ bypass. J Vasc Surg 7:802–807, 1988.

222. Kent KC, Bartek S, Kuntz KM, et al: Prospective study of wound complications in continuous infrainguinal incisions after lower limb arterial reconstruction: Incidence, risk factors, and cost. Surgery 119:378–383, 1996.

223. Mehigan JT, Olcott C: Video angioscopy as an alternative to intraoperative arteriography. Am J Surg 52:139–145, 1986.

224. La Muraglia GM, Cambria RP, Brewster DC, Abbott WM: Angioscopy guided semiclosed technique for in situ bypass. J Vasc Surg 12:601–604, 1990.

225. Stierli P, Banz M, Wigger P, Aeberhard P: Angioscopy guided in situ bypass versus angioscopy guided nonreversed bypass for infrainguinal arterial reconstructions: A comparison of outcome. J Cardiovasc Surg 36:211–217, 1995.

226. Henderson VJ, Mitchell RS, Kosek JC, et al: Biochemical (functional) adaptation of "arterialized" vein graft. Ann Surg 203:339–345, 1986.

227. Bandyk DF, Kaebnick HW, Stewart GW, Towne JB: Durability of the in situ saphenous vein arterial bypass: A comparison of primary and secondary patency. J Vasc Surg 5:256–268, 1987.

228. Levine AW, Bandyk DF, Bonier PH, Towne JB: Lessons learned in adopting the in situ saphenous vein bypass. J Vasc Surg 2:145–153, 1985.

229. Woelfle KD, Kugelmann U, Bruijnen H, et al: Intraoperative imaging techniques in infrainguinal arterial bypass grafting: Completion angiography versus vascular endoscopy. Eur J Vasc Surg 8:556–561, 1994.

230. Bush HL, Corey CA, Nasbeth DC: Distal in situ saphenous vein grafts for limb salvage. Increased operative blood flow and postoperative patency. Am J Surg 145:542–548, 1983.

231. Bandyk DF, Jorgensen RA, Towne JB: Intraoperative assessment of in situ saphenous vein arterial grafts using pulsed Doppler spectral analysis. Arch Surg 121:292–299, 1986.

232. Bandyk DF, Cato RF, Towne JB: A low flow velocity predicts failure of femoropopliteal and femorotibial bypass grafts. Surgery 98:799–809, 1985.

233. Mills JL, Fujitani RM, Taylor SM: The characteristics and anatomic distribution of lesions that cause reverse vein graft failure: A five-year prospective study. J Vasc Surg 17:195–206, 1993.

234. Mills JL, Bandyk DF, Gahtan V, Esses GE: The origin of infrainguinal vein graft stenosis. A prospective study based on duplex surveillance. J Vasc Surg 21:16–25, 1995.

235. Caps MT, Cantwell-Gab K, Bergelin RO, Strandness DE: Vein graft lesions: Time of onset and rate of progression. J Vasc Surg 22:466–475, 1995.

236. Passman MA, Moneta GL, Nehler MR, et al: Do normal early color-flow duplex surveillance examination results of infrainguinal vein grafts preclude the need for late graft revision? J Vasc Surg 22:476–484, 1995.

237. Westerband A, Mills JL, Kistler S, et al: Prospective validation of duplex criteria for intervention in infrainguinal vein grafts undergoing duplex surveillance. Ann Vasc Surg 11:44–48, 1997.

238. Mills JL, Harris EJ, Taylor LM, et al: The importance of routine surveillance of distal bypass grafts with duplex scanning: A study of 379 reversed vein grafts. J Vasc Surg 12:379–389, 1990.

239. Fowl RJ, Patterson RB, Bodenham RJ, Kempczinski RF: Functional failure of patent femorodistal in situ grafts. Ann Vasc Surg 3:200–204, 1989.

240. Taylor LM, Phinney ES, Porter JM: Present status of reversed vein bypass for lower extremity revascularization. J Vasc Surg 3:288–297, 1986.

241. Veith FJ, Gupta SK, Daly VD: Femoropopliteal bypass to the isolated popliteal segment: Is a polytetrafluoroethylene graft acceptable? Surgery 89:296–303, 1981.

242. Berger K, Sauvage LR: Late fiber deterioration in Dacron arterial grafts. Ann Surg 193:477–491, 1980.

243. Clagett GP, Salander JM, Eddleman WL, et al: Dilatation of knitted Dacron aortic prostheses and anastomotic false aneurysms: Etiologic considerations. Surgery 93:9–16, 1983.

244. Nunn DB, Freeman MH, Hudgins PC: Postoperative alterations in the size of Dacron grafts. Ann Surg 189:741–744, 1979.

245. Berman SS, Hunter GC, Smyth SH, et al: Application of computed tomography for surveillance of aortic grafts. Surgery 118:8–15, 1995.

246. Pourdeyhimi B, Wagner D: On the correlation between the failure of vascular grafts and their structural and material properties: A critical analysis. J Biomed Mater Res 20:375–409, 1986.

247. Cooke PA, Nobis PA, Stoney RJ: Dacron aortic graft failure. Arch Surg 108:101–103, 1974.

248. Cranley JJ, Karkow WS, Hafner CO, Flanagan LD: Aneurysmal dilatation in umbilical vein grafts. In Bergan JJ, Yao JST (eds): Reoperative Arterial Surgery. Orlando, Fla, Grune & Stratton, 1986, pp 343–358.

249. Dardik H, Ibrahim IM, Sussman B, et al: Biodegradation and aneurysm formation in umbilical vein graft. Ann Surg 199:61–68, 1984.

250. Dardik H: Reoperative surgery for complications following femorodistal bypass with umbilical vein grafts. In Bergan JJ, Yao JST (eds): Reoperative Arterial Surgery. Orlando, Fla, Grune & Stratton, 1986, pp 331–342.

251. Julien S, Gill F, Guidoin R, et al: Biologic and structural evaluation of 80 surgically excised human umbilical vein grafts. Can Soc Vasc Surg 32:101–107, 1989.

252. Roberts AK, Johnson N: Aneurysm formation in an expanded microporous polytetrafluoroethylene graft. Arch Surg 113:211–213, 1978.

253. Selman SH, Rhodes RS, Anderson JM, et al: Atheromatous changes in expanded polytetrafluoroethylene grafts. Surgery 87:630–637, 1980.

254. Eickhoff JF, Engell HC: Local regulation of blood flow and the occurrence of edema after arterial reconstruction of the lower limbs. Ann Surg 195:474–478, 1982.

255. Schubart PJ, Porter JM: Leg edema following femorodistal bypass. In Bergan JJ, Yao JST (eds): Reoperative Arterial Surgery. Orlando, Fla, Grune & Stratton, 1986, pp 311–330.

256. Husni EA: The edema of arterial reconstruction. Circulation 35(Suppl 1):I-169–I-173, 1967.

257. Storen EJ, Myhre HO, Stiris G: Lymphangiographic findings in patients with leg edema after arterial reconstruction. Acta Clin Scand 140:385–387, 1974.

258. Porter JM, Lindell TD, Lakin PC: Leg edema following femoropopliteal autogenous vein bypass. Arch Surg 105:883–888, 1972.

259. McShannic JR, O'Hara PJ: Management of femoral lymphatic complications following synthetic lower extremity revascularization: Early and late results. Vasc Surg 31:703–711, 1997.

260. Reifsnyder T, Bandyk D, Seabrook G, et al: Wound complications of the in situ saphenous vein bypass technique. J Vasc Surg 15:843–850, 1992.

Questions

1. Venous injury is the most common source of intraoperative bleeding because
   (a) venous pressure is lower than arterial pressure
   (b) veins are often adherent to adjacent arteries
   (c) circumferential mobilization is always necessary to gain control
   (d) anomalies occur in 2% to 7% of patients

2. Aortocaval fistulas
   (a) most commonly result from retroperitoneal trauma
   (b) occur in 1% of ruptured aneurysms
   (c) are often associated with a bruit over the aneurysm
   (d) may precipitate congestive heart failure
   (e) may be treated with a stented graft

3. The commonest cause of aortic graft limb occlusion is
   (a) hypercoagulable state
   (b) improved inflow
   (c) fibrointimal hyperplasia or atherosclerosis at the distal anastomosis
   (d) angulation of the graft
   (e) extrinsic compression by the inguinal ligament

4. Acute renal failure associated with aortic surgery
   (a) occurs more often after emergency surgery
   (b) has a mortality rate between 57% and 95%
   (c) has etiologic factors including vasospasm, suprarenal clamping, ligation of the left renal vein, and operative embolization
   (d) may benefit from the administration of fluid and mannitol intraoperatively

5. In intestinal ischemia,
   (a) incidence is 60% after rupture of aneurysms
   (b) the arc of Riolan and marginal artery of Drummond are important collaterals
   (c) preservation of hypogastric flow is important
   (d) ligation of the inferior mesenteric artery may be a precipitating factor
   (e) measurement of inferior mesenteric artery back-pressure may be helpful

6. Spinal cord ischemia
   (a) occurs in 0.23% of patients undergoing aortic surgery

(b) has a higher incidence after repair of thoracic and ruptured abdominal aneurysms
(c) is characterized by deficits between T-10 and L-2
(d) has increased mortality if patients are paraplegic at the
outset

7. Anastomotic false aneurysms
(a) occur most frequently at femoral anastomoses
(b) have partial disruption of the anastomosis as a characteristic feature
(c) are most commonly due to infection
(d) have endarterectomy as a possible contributing factor
(e) are seldom due to suture failure

8. Chylous ascites
(a) occurs most often with aortic reconstruction for aneurysmal disease

(b) is associated with progressive abdominal distention
(c) has a diagnosis confirmed by paracentesis
(d) usually requires surgical correction

9. Lower extremity edema following femoropopliteal bypass
(a) occurs in 70% to 100% of patients
(b) is related to the severity of ischemia
(c) has multifactional etiology

10. Lymphatic drainage from an incision
(a) may be prevented by careful ligation of tissue during
groin dissection
(b) occurs in 4% of groin incisions
(c) is treated with bed rest
(d) rarely requires surgical correction

Answers

1. b, d   2. b, c, d, e   3. c   4. a, b, c, d   5. a, b, c, d, e   6. a, b, c, d   7. a, b, d, e   8. a, b, c   9. a, b, c   10. a, b, c, d

40

Portal Hypertension

Hugh A. Gelabert

Portal hypertension and variceal hemorrhage remain an important clinical problem and one in which vascular surgeons have a significant interest and concern. New developments have altered the once-familiar face of this disease. At the same time, they have created confusion as to the best approach to these patients.

The role of the vascular surgeon in treating these patients remains vital. It is of paramount importance to have a clear understanding of the impact of underlying liver disease, of the pathophysiology of portal hypertension, and of the management of these problems. The goal of this chapter is to serve as an introduction to portal hypertension. The material presented should provide a solid basis for determining the cause of hepatic disease, understanding the presentation, and managing portal hypertension.

DEFINITION

Portal hypertension is a condition in which the circulation of blood in the portal venous system is impeded, resulting in an increase in portal venous pressure. Elevation of the portal venous blood pressure results in a series of physiologic alterations, including ascites, hypersplenism, and variceal hemorrhage. Normal portal venous pressures are between 5 and 10 mm Hg. Portal hypertension is said to be present when portal pressures are elevated above 15 mm Hg. Clinically significant portal hypertension exists when the portal pressure is elevated beyond 10 mm Hg above systemic pressure as measured at the inferior vena cava (IVC) (corrected portal pressure).

The natural history of patients with portal hypertension differs, depending on the cause of the condition and the stage of presentation. The patient's ability to withstand the stress of hemorrhage or surgery largely depends on the functional hepatic reserve.

PATHOGENESIS

Physiologically, portal hypertension results from either an increase in the portal blood flow (rare), or an obstruction to the outflow of blood from the portal circulation (most common). Obstructions to the portal circulation have been classified anatomically by referring to their location with regard to the hepatic sinusoids. Accordingly, the obstruction may be presinusoidal, sinusoidal, or postsinusoidal. The presinusoidal and postsinusoidal obstructions have been further subclassified as intra- or extrahepatic (Table 40–1).

Extrahepatic Presinusoidal Obstruction

Presinusoidal extrahepatic obstruction is most commonly due to thrombosis of the portal vein. Although less common than other forms of obstructive portal hypertension, portal vein thrombosis occurs in a significant number of children. It may occur in adults, but the causes are remarkably different between children and adults.

Portal vein thrombosis in children occurs as a complication of an infectious process such as omphalitis and appendicitis (most common causes). In adults, the most common cause of portal vein thrombosis is a gradual and relentless decrease in the portal blood flow secondary to the high resistance in the hepatic circulation caused by cirrhosis. Other causes in adults include pancreatitis, hypercoagulable states or tumor thrombus, and mechanical obstruction of portal venous flow. The last may be the result of malignant invasion, lymphadenopathy, or caudate lobe compression. Hypercoagulable conditions may result from polycythemia, cancer, or hypovolemia. Sepsis may lead to portal vein thrombosis by several mechanisms: low-flow states, hypovolemia, and, perhaps, activation of the coagulation system.

Intrahepatic Presinusoidal Obstruction

Most causes of intrahepatic presinusoidal obstructive portal hypertension relate to fibrosis and compression of the portal venules with subsequent restriction of portal flow. Included among these diseases are congenital hepatic fibrosis, sarcoidosis, chronic arsenic exposure, Wilson's disease, hep-

TABLE 40-1

Etiology of Portal Hypertension

Presinusoidal

Extrahepatic: portal vein thrombosis
    Omphalitis
    Pancreatitis
    Trauma
    Malignancy
    Polycythemia
    Periportal lymphadenopathy
Intrahepatic
    Biliary atresia
    Schistosomiasis
    Sarcoidosis
    Arsenic toxicity
    Congenital hepatic fibrosis
    Myeloproliferative disorders
    Primary biliary cirrhosis
    Hepatoportal sclerosis

Sinusoidal

Cirrhosis
Toxic hepatitis
Fatty metamorphosis

Postsinusoidal

Intrahepatic
    Cirrhosis
        Postnecrotic
        Portal
        Hemochromatosis
    Veno-occlusive disease
    Extrahepatic
        Budd-Chiari syndrome
        Hepatic vein webs
        Malignant obstruction
        Oral contraceptives
        Pregnancy
        Plant alkaloids
    Cardiac causes
        Congestive heart failure
        Constructive pericarditis

Increased Blood Flow: Arteriovenous Fistulas

Splenic artery to splenic vein
Hepatic artery to portal vein

atoportal sclerosis, primary biliary cirrhosis, schistosomiasis, and myeloproliferative disorders.

Schistosomiasis is the most common cause of portal hypertension in Third World countries. Deposition of ova in the portal vein walls results in a granulomatous inflammatory reaction, which in turn results in fibrosis and portal flow restriction. Hepatic function is preserved in the early stages, but later stages of this disease are characterized by advanced cirrhosis and loss of hepatic function.[1] Myeloproliferative disorders such as myelosclerosis and myeloid leukemia occasionally lead to presinusoidal hypertension by virtue of the deposition of primitive cellular material infiltrating the portal zones.[2] Sarcoidosis causes portal hypertension by two mechanisms: (1) sarcoid granulomas within the portal vein leading to obstruction and (2) increased portal blood flow.

Hepatic function is usually preserved in the early stages of these diseases. In later stages, significant hepatic impairment may result from progressive cirrhosis. Hemodynamic characteristics are similar to those of extrahepatic portal

vein obstruction: low hepatic wedge pressure and elevated portal venous pressure.

Intrahepatic Sinusoidal and Postsinusoidal Obstruction

Sinusoidal portal hypertension may be the sequela of alcoholic hepatitis or toxic hepatitis. Pure sinusoidal obstruction is a rare cause of portal hypertension. It occurs most frequently as a sequela of acute alcoholic hepatitis, viral hepatitis, or toxic hepatitis. As such, it is the most common cause of portal hypertension in the United States.

Although pure sinusoidal obstruction is relatively rare, it frequently is present as part of a combined sinusoidal and postsinusoidal obstructive picture. Postsinusoidal obstruction is seen most commonly in cases of alcoholic liver disease, postnecrotic cirrhosis, or hemochromatosis. As would be expected in these diseases, hepatic function is usually significantly impaired.

In the United States, this is estimated to be the 10th leading cause of death. Two mechanisms account for the portal hypertension in these patients. First is the mechanical obstruction of the portal blood flow by the regenerating hepatic nodules and cirrhotic bands within the damaged liver. These changes may extend beyond the confines of the hepatic sinusoids, accounting for the presence of presinusoidal, sinusoidal, and postsinusoidal distortion of the hepatic architecture. The second element is an increase in the splanchnic perfusion, in part attributed to the genesis of multiple arteriovenous (AV) shunts and collateral channels. One third of portal blood flow may bypass functional hepatocytes through these channels.[3] The clinical correlate of this increased blood flow is the hyperdynamic state that typifies cirrhosis: elevated cardiac output and a diminished systemic resistance.[4]

The portal hemodynamic characteristics of these diseases are usually those of elevated hepatic wedge pressure along with elevated portal vein pressure. Because most of these diseases directly affect hepatocytes, hepatic function is frequently impaired, even in the early stages of disease. These patients frequently have poor hepatic reserve and decompensate with each bleeding episode. Selection and timing of interventions become important steps in their management.

Extrahepatic Postsinusoidal Obstruction

Postsinusoidal hepatic vein obstruction is usually the result of thrombosis in the hepatic veins. Although the cause of most cases is unknown, a series of associated diseases have been identified. Membranous webs of the hepatic veins, malignancies (hepatomas, renal carcinomas, adrenal carcinomas), trauma, pregnancy, contraceptives, acute alcoholic hepatitis, veno-occlusive disease, or *Senecio* toxicity may all result in hepatic vein thrombosis.[5] Constrictive pericarditis and chronic congestive heart failure may also cause postsinusoidal obstruction.

Budd-Chiari syndrome is the result of hepatic venous

occlusive disease and is characterized by massive ascites, esophageal varices, variceal hemorrhage, hepatic failure, and death. Chiari's disease is due to primary hepatic vein ostial occlusion. The clinical progression after hepatic vein occlusion may be fulminant or gradual. Hepatic failure is the result of chronic congestion and ischemia from impaired hepatic blood flow. The factors that determine the rate of progression are not well understood. Angiography is essential in establishing the diagnosis; it identifies the presence of thrombus and its location.[6, 7]

The fulminant course is marked by rapid development of ascites, fatigue, and jaundice. Additionally, elevations of liver enzymes and prothrombin time indicate hepatocellular damage. Patients who do not improve with anticoagulation should be considered for either shunting or liver transplantation.

The more gradual presentation may have many similar features, such as ascites and chronic fatigue, but hepatic function is preserved to a greater degree. Hypersplenism and variceal hemorrhage may be more prominent features in these patients.

An initial trial of anticoagulation may allow endogenous fibrinolysis to resolve the venous thrombosis. Patients whose course is gradually progressive and have intact hepatocellular function should be considered for portal decompression by either a portacaval, mesocaval, or mesoatrial shunt. The selection of shunt is dependent on the patient's anatomy as defined by angiography. When the Budd-Chiari syndrome leads to deterioration of hepatic function, as demonstrated by abnormalities of liver function tests, hepatic transplantation is the procedure of choice.[8]

Arteriovenous Fistulas

As a cause of portal hypertension, AV fistulas are relatively rare. Most fistulas are either traumatic or splenic. Traumatic AV fistulas may occur as a consequence of transhepatic biliary manipulations or as a result of penetrating trauma. Splenic fistulas may be associated with splenic artery aneurysms, sarcoidosis, Gaucher's disease, myeloid metaplasia, or tropical splenomegaly. Women of childbearing age are at greatest risk. The portal hypertension results initially from increased flow in the portal circulation. At later stages, fibrosis, along with secondary obstruction of the presinusoidal spaces, exacerbates the portal hypertension.

DIAGNOSIS

The diagnosis of portal hypertension rests upon demonstrating the increased portal venous pressure or the anatomic evidence of this increased pressure. In practical terms, the diagnosis of portal hypertension is made by identifying signs of elevation of portal venous pressure and a history that would support these findings.

The signs of elevated portal venous pressure include the presence of esophageal varices, splenomegaly, ascites, or abdominal wall collaterals. Of these, ascites, splenomegaly, and abdominal wall collateralization may be apparent on physical examination. Esophagogastric endoscopy is currently considered the most reliable means of identifying gastroesophageal varices.

Signs of underlying hepatic disease include spider angiomas, palmar erythema, gynecomastia, muscle wasting, loss of pubertal hair growth, and testicular atrophy. Encephalopathy, asterixis, fetor hepatis, and fatigue may also be noted in chronic hepatic insufficiency. The presence of liver disease does not conclusively signify that the patient has significant portal hypertension.

Historical support for the diagnosis of portal hypertension includes identification of any of the diseases that are known to lead to portal hypertension (alcohol ingestion, hepatitis, hepatotoxins, and so forth). Not only the presence but also the duration of these problems are important in substantiating the diagnosis of portal hypertension. Both alcoholic toxicity and viral hepatitis lead to cirrhosis and usually portal hypertension, but the time course between the onset of these insults and the development of the hypertension may be as long as 10 or more years.

Adjunctive means of demonstrating portal hypertension include angiography and hemodynamic measurements. Neither is essential to making the diagnosis; both are supportive. Angiography may reveal both splenomegaly and collateralization in the portal region and the gastroesophageal axis. Additionally, angiography may provide information regarding the direction of portal blood flow (hepatopetal or hepatofugal).

Hemodynamic measurement of the portal circulation is most commonly accomplished by transjugular venous catheterization and measurement of the wedged hepatic vein pressure (WHVP).[9] This technique is able to record the pressure in the hepatic veins and the hepatic sinusoids. Elevations of the wedge pressure reflect elevations in the portal venous pressure. False-negative results may be encountered in patients with presinusoidal obstruction and in instances of catheter malfunction. Normal hepatic venous pressure is essentially the same as the right atrial pressure (0 to 5 mm Hg); portal venous pressure is about 2 to 6 mm Hg higher than the hepatic venous pressure. A gradient greater than 10 mm Hg is considered abnormal.

Other methods of measuring portal venous pressure have been developed but have largely been abandoned because of the increased risk associated with them. This group of tests includes direct cannulation of the portal vein (requires surgical exposure), percutaneous transhepatic portal venous catheterization, transjugular portal vein catheterization, and percutaneous splenic pulp pressure measurement.[10]

The most recent development in assessing the portal circulation is the application of noninvasive ultrasonography. Duplex scanning has been used to establish patency and measure the direction and velocity of portal blood flow. Information gathered from this technique detects portal vein thrombosis, hepatopetal and hepatofugal flow, and portal hypertension.[9–12] Bolondi and associates[13] have documented high sensitivity and specificity with these techniques.

DIAGNOSTIC EVALUATION
Laboratory Testing

The initial point of departure in evaluating most patients is to assess their serum chemistries. Specific attention should be placed on the values of the liver enzymes (serum glutamic-oxaloacetic transaminase [SGOT], serum glutamate pyruvate transaminase [SGPT], lactate dehydrogenase [LDH], alkaline phosphatase), and tests of hepatic synthetic function (prothrombin time and serum albumin). Information from these two sets of tests identifies patients who are suffering acute hepatocellular damage and those who have had sufficient damage to reduce the liver's ability to synthesize essential proteins. This represents two distinct gradations of hepatic dysfunction. The first is indicative of an acute insult; the second represents the degree of hepatic dysfunction. The presence and degree of abnormalities in liver function tests correlate with the outcome of patients: the more abnormal the tests, the worse the prognosis.[14, 15]

Abnormalities of liver function tests combined with physical findings and historical data form the basis of the Child classification of portal hypertension patients. The Child classification, or, more recently, the combined Child-Pugh classification, serves as a prognosticator of survival in cirrhotic patients who undergo both emergent and elective surgery[16] (Table 40–2).

Additional laboratory investigations should include a determination of serum ammonia and complete blood count (white blood cells [WBCs], red blood cells [RBCs], and platelets). Serum ammonia may be elevated in instances of severe hepatic dysfunction and coma. It correlates loosely with mentation but may serve as an indicator of a treatable cause of encephalopathy: hyperammonemia.[17]

The complete blood count (CBC) serves to detect the presence of anemia and hypersplenism. Anemia in cirrhotic patients may result from a number of causes other than hemorrhage. Chronic malnutrition is a particularly important cause of anemia in these patients. Although splenomegaly is present in virtually all portal hypertensive pa-

tients, hypersplenism may not develop until later in the course of their disease. The size of the spleen does not correlate directly with either the degree of portal hypertension or the severity of hypersplenism, but an enlarged spleen is found in virtually all patients with portal hypertension and hypersplenism.[18] Hypersplenism is defined principally in terms of splenic sequestration and destruction of platelets and WBCs. This leads to significant depressions in the platelet and WBC counts. Platelet counts below $50,000/mm^3$ and WBC counts below $2000/mm^3$ support this diagnosis.

Upper Gastrointestinal Endoscopy

Endoscopy plays a pivotal role in the management of portal hypertensive patients. For both diagnostic and therapeutic reasons, endoscopy should be one of the first tests performed. Endoscopy defines not only the presence of varices but also identifies the source of bleeding in patients who have hemorrhage.

The diagnosis of portal hypertension may be established by noting the presence of varices. The size, appearance, and location of the varices may significantly alter the management of the patient. Endoscopy also serves to note the presence of other sources of bleeding in portal hypertensive patients, such as hypertensive gastropathy, gastritis, gastric ulceration, duodenal ulceration, gastric mucosal lacerations (Mallory-Weiss tears), or esophageal ulcerations. Because of the variety of possible bleeding lesions and significant differences in the management of these lesions, patients admitted for hemorrhage must undergo upper gastrointestinal endoscopy on each admission. As many as 40% to 60% of patients with documented varices have

TABLE 40-2

Classifications of Portal Hypertension Patients as Prognosticators of Survival

	CHILD CLASSIFICATION		
	Risk		
Criteria	*Good*	*Moderate*	*Poor*
Bilirubin (mg/dL)	<2.0	2.0–3.0	>3.0
Albumin (mg/dL)	>3.5	3.0–3.5	<3.0
Ascites	Absent	Easily controlled	Poorly controlled
Encephalopathy	Absent	Minimal	Advanced
Nutrition	Excellent	Good	Poor
	PUGH CLASSIFICATION		
	Points Scored for Increasing Abnormality		
Criteria	*1*	*2*	*3*
Albumin (mg/dL)	>3.5	2.8–3.5	<2.8
Bilirubin (mg/dL)	1.0–2.0	2.0–3.0	>3.0
Ascites	Absent	Slight	Significant
Encephalopathy	Normal	1 or 2	3 or 4
Prothrombin time (seconds prolonged)	1–4	4–6	>6
Grade A is 5 or 6 points			
Grade B is 7–9 points			
Grade C is 10–15 points			

associated gastritis or peptic ulcer disease.[19] In patients with esophageal and gastric varices, the gastric varices have been documented as the site of bleeding in up to 18%.[20]

Liver Biopsy

The role of liver biopsy in the preoperative evaluation of portal hypertensive patients has been a focus of controversy. The goal of liver biopsy in this setting is to identify those patients who have active hepatitis. In alcoholic patients, this is most commonly denoted by the presence of Mallory bodies, which signifies acute hyaline necrosis. Mallory bodies may also be seen in patients with Wilson's disease, cholestasis, and primary biliary cirrhosis. The reason for identifying patients with acute hepatic necrosis is that these patients are thought to be at increased risk of dying in the course of shunt surgery.

Mikkelsen and others noted an operative mortality of 69% in elective shunt cases and 83% in emergent cases in the presence of acute hyaline necrosis.[20, 21] Other authors have contested the point of whether acute alcoholic hepatitis alters survival.[14, 22] Finally, it should be noted that Mallory bodies disappear when patients abstain from alcohol and the liver recovers from its insult.[23]

The current recommendation is that patients suspected of having acute hepatitis and who are candidates for elective shunt surgery should undergo percutaneous liver biopsy. If Mallory bodies are identified, consideration should be given to postponing the elective operation for a period of time to allow the liver to recover. This must be carefully balanced against the risk of recurrent hemorrhage and the likelihood of the patient's compliance.

Duplex Scanning

Duplex scanning is finding increased application in the evaluation of portal hypertensive patients. In patients who are to be considered for portacaval shunting or for hepatic transplantation, the duplex scan is frequently sufficient to document portal vein patency. Duplex scanning determines both the patency of the portal vein and the direction of portal venous blood flow. This is the minimal anatomic information required to proceed with the operations mentioned earlier. The combination of color flow imaging with duplex scanning has resulted in improved accuracy and extended the range of diagnostic abilities of the duplex scanners.[11]

Angiography

Preoperative anatomic definition is essential for optimal surgical management, particularly when peripheral shunts are being considered. If possible, angiography should be performed on all patients who are to undergo elective shunting procedures. Techniques primarily of historical interest include splenoportography[24] (introduction of radiopaque material into the spleen), umbilical vein catheterization, and transhepatic percutaneous portal venography.[21–30]

Currently, the vast majority of portal angiography is performed by selective cannulation of the celiac and superior mesenteric arteries, as well as observation of the venous phase of these angiograms. Additional studies that should be obtained include an injection of the renal veins and a hepatic wedge angiogram and pressure recording. The combination of these studies is commonly referred to as a "liver package."

The goal of these studies is to delineate the major portal tributaries: the splenic vein, the superior mesenteric vein (SMV), the portal vein itself, and their relation to the renal vein. An additional goal of the liver package study is to measure the hepatic wedge pressure and visualize the hepatic sinusoidal circulation. These last two elements are helpful in confirming the presence of portal hypertension, estimating the severity of the hypertension, and determining the etiology of the elevated pressure. Low hepatic wedge pressure (less than 10 to 12 mm Hg) in a patient with variceal hemorrhage should prompt a careful search for evidence of portal vein thrombosis.[31] The wedged hepatic vein catheter allows determination of the morphology of the sinusoids, as well as the direction of blood flow (Fig. 40–1). The wedge hepatic venogram in cirrhotic patients demonstrates irregular sinusoids with multiple scattered filling defects. Retrograde portal vein filling indicates hepatofugal flow.[24]

The delineation of the portal tributary anatomy is essential in planning an elective portal decompressive procedure because the choice of procedure is limited by the patient's anatomy. The angiographic findings correlate with the degree of cirrhosis. In early cirrhosis, no definite angiographic abnormalities are present. As cirrhosis becomes more severe, one sees the development of collateral pathways, dilatation of the hepatic artery, and pruning of intrahepatic portal vein branches (Fig. 40–2). In advanced cirrhosis, reversal of flow in the portal vein may be detected.

COMPLICATIONS

Esophageal Varices

Esophageal varices develop in about 30% of cirrhotic patients. Of those who at presentation have upper gastrointestinal bleeding, about 30% bleed from their varices. The other 70% bleed from chemical gastritis, hypertensive gastritis, ulceration, erosions, mucosal tears, and neoplastic growth. Of the cirrhotic patients who bleed from esophageal varices, about 5% to 15% have massive hemorrhage that is difficult to control. The mortality of these patients—bleeding to death from esophageal varices—is about 30% to 50%.

The pathogenesis of esophageal varices centers around the development of collateral circulatory pathways for blood exiting the portal circulation. The impetus for the development of these collaterals is the difference in pressure between the portal system and the systemic venous circulation. Several major collateral networks have been described in cirrhotic patients: the coronary-esophageal veins, the umbilical vein, the hemorrhoidal veins, and the retroperitoneal veins (veins of Retzius). Each of these ve-

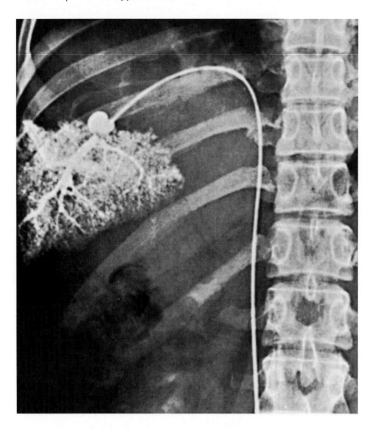

Figure 40–1. Abnormal wedged hepatic venogram demonstrating a coarse, mottled parenchymal pattern consistent with cirrhosis.

nous systems may develop into significant collateral networks.

Any blood vessel that is attenuated and distended under supranormal pressures is at risk of disruption and bleeding. The addition of mechanical trauma or chemical irritation may further serve to induce bleeding. Consequently, any of the collaterals that develop because of portal hypertension may bleed. Hemorrhoidal vessels, intestinal varices, and stomal varices have all been documented as bleeding sites in cirrhotic patients. The mechanical and chemical irritants that bathe the gastroesophageal region result in esophagitis, attenuation of the mucosal layers, and disrup-

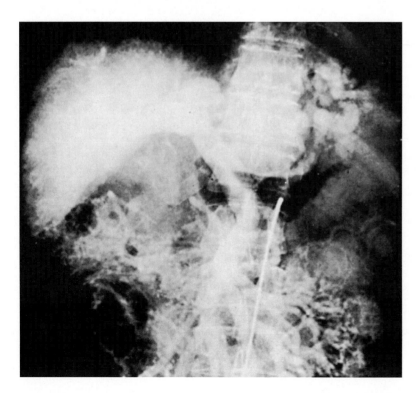

Figure 40–2. Venous phase superior mesenteric angiogram demonstrating superior mesenteric, portal, and dilated coronary vein.

tion of the varices. In combination with the increased blood pressure within the varices, and periodic exacerbations of this pressure by activities that increase the intraabdominal and intrathoracic pressure (such as coughing or retching), the risk of bleeding from esophageal varices is significantly increased. The elevation of portal pressures results in dilatation of all these collateral pathways (Fig. 40–3).

Several attempts have been made to predict the risk of hemorrhage from esophageal varices. Characterization of the severity of portal hypertension on the basis of corrected sinusoidal pressure has not correlated with subsequent hemorrhage. Factors that do predict the risk of bleeding include the size of the varices, the Child class of the patient, and the presence of erosions on the varices (red-dot signs).[32–36]

Encephalopathy

Although not usually considered a life-threatening complication of hepatic failure, encephalopathy may have a pro-foundly disabling effect on patients. The clinical manifestations of encephalopathy are varied, and cover a spectrum from mild inattention to frank coma. The most commonly used system of staging encephalopathy classifies patients on a scale from stage I through stage IV. The progression begins with mild personality alterations, occasionally with asterixis or clonus in stage I. Stage II may be characterized by drowsiness, sometimes with mild confusion. Stage III is typified by stupor and obtundation. Coma is the hallmark of stage IV. Electroencephalography is not specifically diagnostic, characteristically showing only slow wave activity, primarily in the frontal regions.[37]

The mechanism by which liver failure leads to coma is not clearly understood. Several agents have been postulated as encephalopathic, especially in the presence of a diseased liver. Ammonia, nitrogenous amines, increased false neurotransmitters, decreased true neurotransmitters, and an increased ratio of aromatic to branched chain amino acids are the most likely candidates.

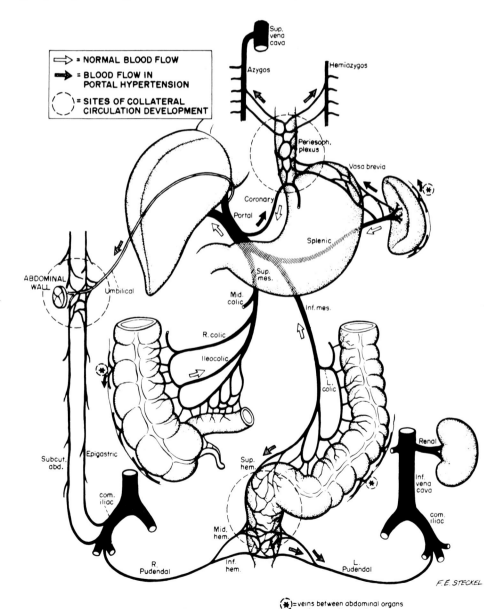

Figure 40–3. Schematic diagram of collateral venous pathways. (From Sedgwick CE, et al: Portal Hypertension. Boston, Little, Brown, 1967.)

Elevated ammonia levels have several significant repercussions. First, they elevate glucagon levels. This in turn stimulates gluconeogenesis, which produces more ammonia. Additionally, the gluconeogenesis leads to elevated insulin levels. The elevated insulin promotes catabolism of branched chain amino acids. This ultimately leads to increased levels of straight chain amino acids such as phenylalanine, tyrosine, and methionine. An elevated ratio of straight chain to branched chain amino acids drives neutral amino acids past the blood-brain barrier. The cerebral uptake of these neutral amino acids is possible because ammonia stimulates brain glutamine synthesis, allowing rapid equilibration of brain glutamine for straight chain neutral amino acids. These same neutral amino acids may act as false neurotransmitters and are thought to produce encephalopathy.[38]

The treatment of encephalopathy is based on reduction of the ammonia levels, and supplementation of branched chain amino acids. Lactulose and neomycin reduce ammonia uptake from the gut by altering the intestinal pH, reducing the number of intestinal bacteria, and reducing intestinal transit of protein. Other agents such as levodopa have been used with mixed results in improving encephalopathy.[39]

Ascites

Ascites is a common symptom of portal hypertensive patients. Up to 80% of these patients may have some degree of ascites. The mechanism by which ascites develops is a combination of hemodynamic, physiologic, and metabolic factors. The hemodynamics of the portal circulatory system in the face of cirrhosis is primarily driven by the increased portal venous pressure. In such a state, the Starling forces tend to drive fluids out of the vessels and into the interstitial space. Compounding this problem is the low oncotic pressure that characterizes many cirrhotic patients by virtue of their hypoalbuminemia. Finally, many of these patients chronically register relatively low effective intravascular volume, which in turn triggers the renal aldosterone, renin-angiotensin system, and, perhaps, an additional natriuretic hormone. These then produce a state in which the patients retain free water and salt, both of which aggravate the ascites. The net effect is the translocation of fluid from the intravascular space to the interstitial space and the abdominal cavity.

The compensatory mechanism that normally counteracts the accumulation of interstitial and peritoneal fluid is primarily the lymphatic system. In the cirrhotic patient, the lymph flow is frequently increased. Ascites accumulates when the ability of the lymphatics to reabsorb this fluid is overwhelmed.

The cornerstone of the management of ascites is restriction of salt intake and judicious use of diuretics. These measures control the vast majority of ascitic patients. In only 5% of cases can ascites be considered to be intractable, and other means of addressing the ascites are required.

MEDICAL THERAPY
General Medical Care

Medical care is based on evaluating and defining the cause of the liver disease. First is addressing any factors related to the cause of the liver disease that are amenable to change (e.g., stopping alcohol consumption). The second element is establishing the patient's current state of health and hepatic function: defining the presence of portal hypertension, splenomegaly, ascites, or varices. An assessment of the hepatic disease and the degree of hepatic deterioration helps in predicting the eventual course of the patient. The next step involves maintenance of nutrition, supplementation of vitamins and minerals, and avoidance of salt (especially in ascitic patients).

Management of Acute Complications

The management of acute complications is a very specialized area in the care of these patients. The most common problem, which requires urgent care, is hemorrhage. The significance of hemorrhage in these patients is difficult to understate. Up to 70% mortality may be associated with hemorrhage, depending on the cause and severity of the liver disease and the degree of decompensation of the patient at the time of presentation. Further, the risk of a second hemorrhage within 1 year may be as high as 60%.[16]

The essential steps in caring for a cirrhotic patient with an upper gastrointestinal hemorrhage include establishing peripheral venous access, volume-resuscitating the patient, and determining the source of bleeding. This is best accomplished by upper gastrointestinal endoscopy. As mentioned previously, between 40% and 60% of cirrhotic patients with known varices who have an upper gastrointestinal hemorrhage are not bleeding from their varices.[40]

Should the patient be bleeding from an esophageal varix or hypertensive gastritis, several specific steps are to be promptly taken. First, an assessment must be made of the rate of bleeding. Second, the patient must be adequately resuscitated. Third, the patient must be prepared for a possible therapeutic intervention.

Assessing the rate of bleeding is essential. The assessment is largely based on the progressive change in the patient's vital signs, mentation, and perfusion in the course of resuscitation. A nasogastric tube also provides information as to continued bleeding. Emergency endoscopy may provide insight into whether the patient is suffering a massive hemorrhage or is bleeding at a moderate rate. The change in the patient's hematocrit is not necessarily the best indicator of bleeding because there may be a significant lag between the bleeding episode and the subsquent drop in hematocrit.

Patients with relatively minor bleeding episodes frequently stop bleeding spontaneously. The few patients who are actively bleeding at the time of admission almost always respond to an infusion of octreotide. The key to managing these patients is to avoid overloading them with fluid and salts because this may precipitate a rebleed with further decompensation.

Patients with moderate bleeding rates stand a reasonable chance of having their bleeding stopped without surgical intervention. These patients frequently respond to infusions of octreotide, emergency sclerotherapy, or balloon tamponade.

Patients who bleed massively often require some form of more advanced intervention. This is often in addition to the octreotide and balloon tamponade. Emergent endoscopy is frequently impaired by the massive bleeding. Subsequent steps include angiographic embolization, percutaneous attempts at creating an intrahepatic shunt (transjugular intrahepatic portasystemic shunt, TIPS), or emergency surgical shunting.

The fluids used in resuscitation vary with the severity of the hemorrhage. In minor bleeds, the patients may be resuscitated with intravenous crystalloid solutions. In patients with more severe hemorrhages, it may be necessary to supplement this with infusions of albumin. In severe hemorrhages, it is necessary to infuse both packed red blood cells (PRBCs), and fresh-frozen plasma. Occasionally, infusions of other blood components are required such as platelets or cryoprecipitate, yet these instances are relatively rare. The goals of resuscitation are to maintain the patient at a level where he or she is able to perfuse vital organs while the bleeding source is addressed. The indicators of a successful resuscitation include the ability of the patient to mentate, to produce urine, and to maintain acid-base balance.

The preparation of these patients for possible therapeutic interventions include cleansing of the gastrointestinal tract, stabilization of the blood volume, identification of the bleeding source, and administration of blood components as needed to allow the proposed interventions.

SPECIFIC MEASURES FOR THE CONTROL OF ACUTE HEMORRHAGE

Protein and Gut Lavage

Hemorrhage into the gastrointestinal tract poses a significant risk of encephalopathy, particularly in patients with bleeding varices. The combination of a large protein load in the intestinal tract along with poor hepatic function frequently results in encephalopathy. The intestinal tract must be cleansed of the blood and any other nitrogenous substances by a combination of enemas and oral cathartics or gastric lavage.

The upper gastrointestinal tract should be laved with the aid of a large-bore tube (e.g., Ewald tube) to remove the clotted blood from the stomach. The rest of the tract is cleansed at the appropriate time by the administration of lactulose and neomycin by mouth.

Neomycin and lactulose are given to alter the intestinal absorption of ammonia. Neomycin is a relatively nonabsorbable antibiotic; it destroys urease-producing bacteria and thereby decreases ammonia production. Lactulose is converted by lactase-containing intestinal bacteria into lactic acid and acetic acid, thus decreasing the intraluminal intestinal pH. The lower pH ionizes ammonia into ammonium (NH_4^+), which is less able to diffuse through the colonic mucosa. Lactulose also promotes diarrhea, cleansing the intestine of its contents.[17, 41, 42]

Vasopressin

Vasopressin (Pitressin) should no longer be considered first-line therapy in the management of active bleeding varices. Still, information from its use has provided significant insight into early management of variceal bleeding. Its use is specifically directed at slowing and stopping variceal hemorrhage. It has been recognized since 1917 for its vasoconstrictive effects and its ability to decrease portal pressure.[43] Vasopressin is a naturally occurring nonapeptide that demonstrates general vasoconstrictive effects, with particular efficacy in the splanchnic bed. This splanchnic vasoconstriction leads to decreasing portal flow. Vasopressin is also known to diminish cardiac output by an average of 14% and heart rate by 11%. This in turn reduces hepatic blood flow by approximately 44% and WHVP is decreased by 11%. As much as a 23% reduction in the gradient between the hepatic venous and WHVP has been documented.[44]

A consequence of the vasoconstrictive effects of vasopressin is the potential exacerbation of cardiac ischemia. In order to counter these ischemic effects, a number of pharmacologic agents have been used in conjunction with vasopressin.[44–46] These include isoproterenol and nitroglycerin. Isoproterenol, when administered with intravenous vasopressin, resulted in equivalent reduction of portal vein pressure but maintenance of cardiac output.[45] Sublingual nitroglycerin plus vasopressin has been shown to reduce the deleterious effects of vasopressin alone while preserving the decrease in portal vein pressure.[44, 47] In the course of a controlled trial, Gimson and associates[48] noted that nitroglycerin may reverse some of the cardiac suppressive effects of vasopressin, as well as enhance the portal hypotensive effects.

Intravenous vasopressin should be used before balloon tamponade. It stops variceal bleeding in at least 80% of cases. The initial dosage is 0.2 to 0.4 units/minute. If bleeding does not cease with the initial dose, the dosage may be increased up to 1.0 unit/minute.

Somatostatin and Octreotide

Because of reduced side effects and efficacy equal to that of vasopressin, octreotide has become the agent of choice in managing acute variceal hemorrhage. Somatostatin is a tetradecapeptide derived from the hypothalamus, which has demonstrated an ability to decrease splanchnic blood. Octreotide is a synthetic octopeptide analogue of somatostatin. It has a longer half-life than somatostatin (100 minutes vs. 2 to 3 minutes). Both have been demonstrated to be as effective as vasopressin for control of acute bleeding, yet with fewer complications.[49] Hemodynamic studies have indicated that somatostatin does decrease the portal venous pressure gradient.[42, 50] Randomized studies have shown equal efficacy and meta-analysis has demonstrated no survival benefit. Somatostatin has been repeatedly shown to have fewer side effects than vasopressin.[49, 51]

Octreotide is effective in reducing and halting variceal hemorrhage in 80% of cases. Intravenous octreotide should be used before, and along with, balloon tamponade. It should be started before endoscopy. The initial dose of octreotide is a bolus infusion of 50 µg. This is followed by an infusion of 50 µg/hour. As with vasopressin infusions, the octreotide infusion should be continued over a 3-day period. After this period, the drug should be gradually discontinued.[46]

Propranolol

Propranolol, a β-blocking drug, is an agent that has been found to be useful in chronically controlling portal hypertension and reducing the risk of recurrent bleeding from esophageal varices. Its action is thought to be mediated on the basis of reduced cardiac output, reduced systemic pressure, and the subsequent reduction in portal venous pressure.

Evidence of its efficacy in the reduction of recurrent bleeding has been mixed. Burroughs and colleagues[52] compared propranolol with placebo and found no significant difference in rebleeding or survival. Fleig and colleagues[53] randomized 70 patients to sclerotherapy or propranolol and found no difference in the rebleeding rate or survival. The propranolol did decrease the size of the varices significantly after 3 months of treatment. In a prospective, controlled, randomized study of 79 patients, Lebrec and associates[54, 55] noted that after 3 months 2.6% of patients maintained on propranolol had recurrent gastrointestinal tract bleeding compared with 66% maintained on a placebo drug. Similar findings have been reported by others.[56] Poynard and coauthors[57] analyzed 127 patients treated with propranolol and found five factors that were associated with rebleeding: (1) hepatocellular carcinoma, (2) lack of persistent decrease in heart rate, (3) lack of abstinence from alcohol, (4) lack of compliance, and (5) prior history of rebleeding.

Propranolol has been specifically used as maintenance therapy to decrease the risk of recurrent esophageal variceal bleeding in patients with portal hypertension. Its use in acute bleeding episodes has not been studied.

Balloon Tamponade

Balloon tamponade is a technique that employs compression by an intragastric balloon to stem the bleeding of esophageal and gastroesophageal varices. The technique dates to the early 1950s, when Linton, Nachlas, Sengstaken, and Blakemore developed the tubes that came to bear their respective names.

All of these tubes work on the same principle: tamponade of varices. The design variations include the presence of one or two balloons for compression of the stomach alone or of the esophagus and stomach (Linton-Nachlas vs. Sengstaken tube); and the presence of adjunctive ports for aspiration of the stomach and the esophageal secretions (Sengstaken-Blakemore vs. Edlich modification or Minnesota tube).[58, 59] The Sengstaken-Blakemore tube is probably more commonly used because it is able to compress both esophageal and gastric varices, whereas the Linton-Nachlas tube is able to compress only the gastric varices.

The Sengstaken-Blakemore Tube

The Sengstaken-Blakemore tube may be passed through either the mouth or nose. Passage of this tube must be

performed carefully and precisely to prevent associated complications. The manufacturers recommend that the gastric balloon be inflated with a low volume of air (250 mL), and that an abdominal radiograph be taken to ensure that the gastric balloon is on the stomach before full inflation (with 750 mL of air). This should avoid the problem of fully inflating the gastric balloon in the esophagus, where it could tear open the esophageal wall.

Once the gastric balloon is inflated, it is taped to the facemask of a football helmet with approximately 1 kg of pressure. The gastric and esophageal ports are connected to intermittent low Gompco suction. The position of the gastric balloon is checked periodically to ensure that migration into the esophagus has not occurred. If bleeding does not cease with gastric balloon inflation and tension, the esophageal balloon is inflated to 24 to 45 mm Hg pressure. If bleeding ceases with the Sengstaken-Blakemore tube insertion, it is left inflated for 24 hours. After this period, the esophageal balloon should be deflated. Twenty-four hours later, the gastric balloon is deflated. If bleeding does not recur, the tube is deflated and left in place. It should be removed after an additional day.[60] Esophageal variceal tamponade results in cessation of hemorrhage in 45% to 92% of cases.[60-63] Bleeding recurs shortly after the Sengstaken-Blakemore tube is deflated in 24% to 42% of cases, however, and cannot be controlled in 33% to 37% of cases.[60-62] The incidence of recurrent bleeding after a second period of balloon control is 40%.[62]

This tube has been associated with significant complications: gastroesophageal tears, ulceration, and perforation. Pulmonary complications include aspiration pneumonia and asphyxia from tracheal intubation. Conn and Simpson[64] reported a complication rate of 41% and a mortality rate of 20%. The more commonly encountered incidence of major complications is in the range of 4% to 9%.[60-62]

SURGICAL CORRECTION

Shunt Nomenclature

The nomenclature of shunts changed as different operations were devised at various periods. Many of these terms remain in use, and an understanding of them is necessary. Two basic sets of nomenclature prevail: the anatomy-based descriptive names, and the taxonomic names. A final set of shunt names are the eponyms, which are presented for completeness.

The anatomic naming of shunts is based on the elements of the shunt. Thus, the principal shunts are portacaval, mesocaval, and splenorenal. The first portion of the name denotes the donor vessel, and the second portion of the name denotes the recipient vessel. Because of some ambiguity associated with these names, modifiers are applied. A portacaval shunt may be either a side-to-side portacaval shunt or an end-to-side portacaval shunt. Similarly, a splenorenal shunt may be either a proximal or a distal splenorenal shunt (DSRS). The principal advantage of this system is that it allows a clear, descriptive means of labeling an operation. This is probably the most widely used shunt nomenclature.

The taxonomic nomenclature is derived from both physiologic and anatomic considerations. These names are ingrained in the lexicon of surgery and should be understood. The two principal sets of names are central and remote and selective and nonselective. A central shunt is one constructed in the region of the porta hepatis, or at the center of the portal confluence. Included among these are the various portacaval shunts. The term is used to distinguish shunts that involve the portal vein itself from those that are remote from the portal vein, such as the splenorenal and mesocaval shunts. The distinction has regained some usefulness in the context of distinguishing shunts that are recommended for patients who are considered potential liver transplant candidates.

Selective and nonselective shunts are the second set of taxonomic names. Selectivity of a shunt refers to the effect of the shunt on the portal venous blood flow. Selective shunts preserve the flow of mesenteric blood through the portal vein to the liver while decompressing the esophageal varices. Nonselective shunts drain all portal blood flow into the vena cava. The selective shunts include the DSRS (Warren) and the coronary-caval (Inokuchi) shunts. Nonselective shunts include the end-to-side portacaval shunt, side-to-side portacaval shunt, mesocaval shunt, and proximal splenorenal shunt. Currently, the term "selective" is used almost as a synonym for a DSRS.

The last set of shunt names is the eponyms. Many shunts have been associated with the name of a proponent. These names are still frequently used. Included among these are the following: the Warren shunt (DSRS), the Linton shunt (proximal splenorenal), the Clatworthy shunt (mesocaval shunt using the IVC), the Drapanas shunt (mesocaval shunt using a Dacron interposition graft), the Inokuchi shunt (coronary-caval), and the Sarfeh shunt (portacaval polytetrafluoroethylene [PTFE] interposition graft).

Development of Shunting

Eck,[65] in 1877, performed in a dog the first portal systemic shunt. He demonstrated that not only could the portal vein be anastomosed to the IVC but that the animal could survive with total diversion of the portal vein blood flow. Pavlov, in 1893, was the first to recognize the development of a severe neuropsychiatric disorder when a widely patent portacaval shunt was present and that protein ingestion exacerbated the syndrome. Furthermore, he described the portaprival syndrome, consisting of gross liver atrophy with fatty infiltration following shunts.[66] It was not until 1945, however, that Whipple,[67] as well as Blakemore and Lord,[68] presented their results on the systematic application of portasystemic bypasses for complications of portal hypertension. The end-to-side portacaval shunt was the first to be used clinically for the control of variceal hemorrhage, and the initial results with this procedure formed the basis for the enthusiasm for shunting patients with variceal bleeding.[18] With the initial reports demonstrating overall recurrence of variceal hemorrhage of only 2.8%, little attention was directed toward the quality or length of life.[69]

Prophylactic Shunting

Proponents of prophylactic shunting argued that variceal hemorrhage could be prevented by creating a shunt in patients with varices before they had opportunity to bleed. Four prospective controlled studies addressed this question.[19, 21, 70, 71] These four early studies were similar in design. The patients were divided between medical and surgical treatment and were followed for recurrent bleeding, development of encephalopathy, and survival.

The Boston Interhospital Liver Group (BILG) allocated 45 patients to the medical group and 48 to the surgical group. At 1-, 3-, and 5-year intervals, there was no difference in survival; at 5 years the survival rate was 50%. Encephalopathy was likewise equal (21%).[72] The Veterans Administration (VA) study demonstrated an incidence of encephalopathy of 45% after shunting, almost twice that of medical therapies. Most disconcerting was that the 5-year survival after shunting (51%) was less than for medical therapy (64%).[19] Similarly, the experience of the Yale group demonstrated again decreased survival after shunting, with an increased incidence of encephalopathy.[70, 71]

Finally, indications for prophylactic variceal decompression have been studied by the Cooperative Study Group of Portal Hypertension in Japan. By comparing only nondecompressive transection procedures and selective shunts, this group found no difference in survival rates at 2 years, and suggested that in certain patients, prophylactic procedures may be indicated.[21] It should, however, be noted that these patients were primarily nonalcoholic, and the applicability of these results has been widely debated in the United States.

These studies have demonstrated that prophylactic shunts do not benefit patients with asymptomatic varices. Although the incidence of variceal hemorrhage is virtually eliminated, these patients tend to suffer from hepatic encephalopathy and die of hepatic failure. Encephalopathy is increased following portacaval shunting, and long-term survival may in fact be decreased by a shunt procedure. These results are not surprising, in that only 30% of patients who have varices bleed and that the decreased incidence of death from bleeding may be offset by the operative mortality of a shunt procedure, as well as by the effects of subsequent hepatic encephalopathy.

Therapeutic Shunting

The efficacy of portasystemic shunting has been studied with prospective randomized clinical trials. Four prospective randomized clinical trials were performed in the United States and France to evaluate the fundamental question of whether therapeutic shunts prolong survival and maintain the quality of life compared with conventional medical therapy.[73–76]

The VA study, begun in 1961, followed the survival of 155 selected patients over a 5.5-year period. Although 78 patients were randomized into the surgical group, in only 67 were shunts actually performed. Operative mortality following therapeutic portacaval shunts was 8%. Recurrence of variceal bleeding was 7% in the surgical group and 65% in the medical group. Encephalopathy occurred with approximately equal frequency in both groups, but was more severe in the shunted group. The long-term survival rate at 5 years was 57% in the shunt group and

36% in the medical group. The increase in long-term survival was not, however, statistically significant.[73]

In the BILG study,[74] patients underwent end-to-side portacaval shunt, side-to-side portacaval shunt, or medical therapy. The long-term survival was better in the shunt group than in the medically treated group, but this difference was not statistically significant. On the basis of both the VA and BILG studies, Conn[77] concluded, despite lack of statistical significance, that therapeutic portacaval shunts prolong the mean duration of life of cirrhotic patients who have suffered from variceal hemorrhage.

Researchers at the University of Southern California (USC) published a 12-year follow-up of a prospective randomized study comparing end-to-side portacaval shunts with medical therapy. One hundred ninety episodes of bleeding occurred with medical therapy compared with 11 in the surgical group. Encephalopathy of a moderate to severe degree occurred in 35% of shunt patients. A 5-year life-table analysis of survival revealed a 44% shunt survival and 24% medical therapy survival. This difference is not, however, statistically significant.[21]

Rueff and associates,[76] in a study at the Hôpital Beaujon in Clichy, France, compared therapeutic end-to-side portacaval shunts with medical therapy. The long-term survival was 47% in the shunt group and 56% in the medical group. The diminished long-term survival in the shunt group is unique to this study and may be due to their high operative mortality (19%, compared with 13% for the BILG study and 8% for the VA study). Encephalopathy was equally common in both medical and surgical groups, with an incidence of 40%. As in the other studies, it tended to be more severe and chronic in the shunt groups. Recurrent bleeding occurred in 8% of the shunt group and in 72% of the medical group.

The most compelling conclusions drawn from these studies is that they failed to demonstrate a survival advantage. Portacaval shunts were clearly superior in preventing recurrent variceal bleeding. Encephalopathy is no more common in patients undergoing a portacaval shunt, but tends to be more severe and chronic in medically treated patients.

Emergency Portacaval Shunting

Portacaval shunting on an emergency basis is no longer widely used because of the reported high mortality. Despite this, it has proved highly efficacious in its ability to stop bleeding and prevent further recurrent bleeding.[78] Orloff and colleagues[79] have continued to advocate the portacaval shunt in the acute setting, and they have achieved a 4-year actuarial survival of 69%. Villeneuve and coworkers[80] have also supported the use of this shunt in acutely bleeding patients if the patients have mild to moderate liver disease and other forms of treatment have failed. In general, emergency surgical intervention is being performed less frequently as nonsurgical options have become more effective.

Most Common Portasystemic Shunts

Nonselective Shunts

Portacaval Shunts

Both end-to-side and side-to-side portacaval shunts are nonselective and cause diversion of portal flow into the systemic circulation. The only specific indication for the portacaval shunt is esophageal variceal hemorrhage. Whereas previously intractable ascites was often treated with a side-to-side portacaval shunt, this technique has now been discarded in favor of peritoneovenous shunting and TIPS.[81, 82]

The question of whether an end-to-side or side-to-side portacaval shunt is a more effective procedure is still debated. An end-to-side portacaval shunt is certainly not indicated in the presence of Budd-Chiari syndrome because the portal vein serves as a decompressive outflow tract for intrahepatic portal blood. Uncontrolled studies comparing end-to-side with side-to-side shunts indicate that the side-to-side shunt is associated with a lower surgical mortality in patients with poor hepatic function.[83] Others find the side-to-side portacaval shunt to be more technically demanding. Encephalopathy has been shown to be somewhat more common in side-to-side than in end-to-side portacaval shunts.[84] Investigators have previously found that in addition to allowing total diversion of portal venous flow, the side-to-side shunt may also create a siphon effect permitting egress of hepatic arterial blood through the portal vein rather than the hepatic vein. This may be an explanation for the increased incidence of encephalopathy with side-to-side portacaval shunts.

Certain technical considerations preclude a portacaval shunt. First, the portal vein must be patent and free of thrombus. The portal vein diameter should also be at least 1.0 to 1.5 cm (in adults) and should not have previously undergone thrombosis with recanalization. Thrombectomy of a recanalized portal vein is contraindicated because it does not result in long-term shunt patency. Previous surgery in the right upper quadrant is a relative contraindication to a portacaval shunt procedure because of the numerous well-vascularized adhesions, which always result in excessive bleeding.

END-TO-SIDE PORTACAVAL SHUNT. Two approaches have been described: the midline incision and the right subcostal incision. After the abdomen has been entered, the duodenum is mobilized medially to expose the IVC. The dissection is carried up along the IVC to the level of the first hepatic vein under the liver. The portal vein should be exposed by rotating the bile duct and hepatic artery using a vein retractor or peanut sponges. The division of the portal vein should be done after it has been securely clamped (proximally and distally) and the hepatic portion of the vein suture ligated.

A Satinsky clamp is placed at the appropriate point on the vena cava, and an ellipse of cava is removed to allow anastomosis. Pressure in the portal vein should be measured to document the adequacy of the decompression and detect any unobserved technical problems. A 50% reduction in portal venous pressures should be expected after the shunt is completed.[85, 86]

ARTERIALIZATION OF END-TO-SIDE PORTACAVAL SHUNTS. In an attempt to reduce the morbidity of end-to-side portacaval shunts, a variety of measures have been employed to maintain portal perfusion of the liver. Portal vein arterialization refers to the anastomosis of an arterialized conduit to the hepatic end of the portal vein. Various arteries have been used for this purpose, including the right gastroepiploic artery, splenic artery, and saphenous vein grafts from the hypogastric artery or aorta.

Although a number of studies have indicated that there is no increase in morbidity or mortality, and encephalopathy may be reduced, the procedure has not been universally adopted. Maillard's group[87] divided the splenic artery close to the spleen and anastomosed it to the hepatic stump of the portal vein. They found that total hepatic blood flow with arterialization is equal to—or slightly greater than—that before the shunt. Immediate postoperative complications were fewer, and the incidence of encephalopathy was less than with the portacaval shunt alone as well. As this group pointed out, however, the fistula is not likely to remain open after 1 year.[87] Otte and associates[89] reported a retrospective study in which the 5-year survival was 48% in arterialized patients compared with 44% in other series. Encephalopathy occurred in 27% of the arterialized patients compared with 40% not arterialized.[88] No definitive conclusions may be drawn as to the benefit of arterialization of a portacaval shunt in prolonging life or decreasing encephalopathy. Because of the added time and technical difficulty in performing arterialization, it is unlikely that this technique will gain widespread use.

SIDE-TO-SIDE PORTACAVAL SHUNT. The side-to-side portacaval shunt is technically more difficult than the end-to-side shunt. The initial approach is similar to the end-to-side shunt; a longer segment of the vena cava is exposed and circumferentially dissected so as to lift it out of its bed. The portal vein must also be exposed for a greater length because a 4-cm segment is necessary for the anastomosis. Portal pressures are measured before the shunt is performed. After applying the vascular clamps, an elliptic segment measuring approximately 2 cm is then excised from the IVC and portal vein directly opposite each other. Again, mesenteric venous pressure measurements should reflect a 50% reduction in portal vein pressure.[85]

PORTACAVAL H GRAFT. An alternative to the side-to-side portacaval shunt is the portacaval H graft. Technically easier than the side-to-side shunt, the large-diameter H grafts (16 to 20 mm) effectively prevent variceal rebleeding, but encephalopathy occurs frequently. Building on this experience, Sarfeh and colleagues[89] systematically reduced portacaval H graft diameters, and found that an 8-mm PTFE graft combined with portal collateral ablation effectively prevented rebleeding, maintained hepatic perfusion, and reduced encephalopathy. The 5-year cumulative late patency rate was 97%.[89]

Mesocaval Shunts

In 1955, Clatworthy and associates[90] devised a new portasystemic shunt procedure involving division of the IVC above its bifurcation and anastomosis of the proximal cava to the side of the SMV.

The portasystemic shunt procedure has been particularly successful in children with extrahepatic portal vein thrombosis. In adults, massive lower extremity edema has limited its usefulness. Because of the extensive dissection necessary to expose the vena cava, a number of alternative graft materials have been used, including cadaveric IVC, iliac vein, PTFE, and Dacron, which is currently favored.[90–95]

There has been considerable debate as to whether portal perfusion (hepatopetal flow) is maintained by mesocaval shunts. Drapanas and colleagues[96] documented continued hepatopetal flow in 44% of their patients. Others have noted, however, that portal perfusion can persist only if there is partial or total H graft occlusion.[97] Misinterpretation of angiographic studies may also be attributable to the phenomenon of portal pseudoperfusion, as explained by Fulenwider and coauthors.[98] Overall, H graft mesocaval shunts are considered nonselective shunts.

CLINICAL ROLE OF MESOCAVAL SHUNTS. The primary use of the interposition H graft mesocaval shunt has been for the urgent control of massive variceal hemorrhage. This graft is technically easier to perform than a portacaval or a selective shunt and is frequently indicated in the emergency management of variceal hemorrhage.[99] In the case of previous surgery in the right upper quadrant, a portacaval shunt of any type is especially challenging and is usually contraindicated. If a selective shunt is contraindicated, a mesocaval shunt may be a good alternative. This is true in patients with significant ascites. Other factors that favor mesocaval shunting include extensive periportal fibrosis, a large overriding caudate lobe, an obliterated portal vein, extreme obesity, and Budd-Chiari syndrome.[100]

INTERPOSITION MESOCAVAL H GRAFT. The operation as described by Drapanas and coauthors in 1975 remains essentially unchanged to this day.[96] The transverse mesocolon is elevated superiorly and the small intestine retracted inferiorly. At the root of the small intestine mesentery, the peritoneum is opened transversely to expose the superior mesenteric vessels. Anatomically, the superior mesenteric vein lies anterior and to the right of the superior mesenteric artery. During isolation of the vein, only one or two small tributaries need to be divided. An important goal is to preserve as many branches of the SMV as needed to preserve intestinal venous flow. After the SMV is isolated, the anterior surface of the vena cava is exposed through the right transverse mesocolon. Only sufficient dissection to permit use of a Satinsky clamp on the vena cava is required. Once the vena cava is partially isolated, the third and fourth portions of the duodenum must usually be mobilized to allow the duodenum to ride above the graft. Failure to do this may cause obstruction of the occasional low-lying duodenum or occlusion of the interposed graft.

The vena cava anastomosis is performed first because it lies in the depth of the field and is potentially more hazardous. A partially occluding vascular clamp is placed on the IVC, a small ellipse of vein is excised, and an 14- to 18-mm knitted Dacron graft is anastomosed. Construction of the SMV anastomosis is particularly demanding. The SMV lies anteriorly and courses at a 20- to 30-degree angle counterclockwise to the vena cava. Because of this angulation, it is advisable to rotate the graft 20 to 30 degrees clockwise before constructing the SMV anastomosis. The graft length should be only 3 to 6 cm to minimize kinking of the prosthesis. Anastomosis is performed in the posterior surface of the vein with a continuous suture of 5-0 polypropylene (Prolene). With the clamps removed, the graft should distend quickly. In most instances, a palpable thrill should be present. Postshunt pressures are then measured in the SMV; if the shunt is functioning properly, there should be at least a 50% reduction of pressure with the shunt open.

A notable variation on this shunt is the C loop graft as reported by Cameron and coworkers.[101, 102] In their procedure, a longer graft was used, and this had the configuration of the letter C. To accomplish this, the SMV anastomosis is placed at the point where the SMV disappears under the neck of the pancreas. The proposed advantage of this variation is that the SMV diameter is greater at a more proximal anastomosis, and this allows for improved shunt flow. Despite this theoretical advantage, there is the distinct disadvantage of a more difficult dissection, particularly in patients who have had pancreatitis. The obvious drawback is a longer length of prosthetic material.

CLINICAL RESULTS. Sarr and colleagues[103] published a series of 33 patients who underwent the mesocaval C shunt procedure. There was a 24% operative mortality (all Child class C nonelective cases), 8% rebleed rate, and 46% incidence of encephalopathy. However, there were no graft thromboses.

The average incidence of encephalopathy after a mesocaval graft is about 25%.[100, 104] The reported incidence of encephalopathy ranges from 9% to 45%[97, 101] (Table 40–3). Late graft occlusion is caused by excessive layering of thrombus, possibly aggravated by perigraft scarring, leading to kinking and constriction.[97] The incidence of shunt occlusions ranges from 4% to 24%.[96, 97, 102, 105–107] Rebleeding occurs in approximately 14% of mesocaval shunts (range, 12% to 16%). One third of these may be related to occlusion of the graft.[99] Overall, the mortality is approximately 15%. The cumulative long-term mortality ranges from 28% to 57%. The long-term mortality is probably dependent on the state of liver function rather than the type of shunt.

Mortality related to H mesocaval shunts is not significantly different from that for other types of shunts and is dependent on the Child classification of the patient. Initial hospital mortality is related to the urgency of surgery, significant elevation of SGOT or bilirubin, or the presence of encephalopathy.[97]

Proximal Splenorenal Shunts

Currently of historical interest only, the nonselective splenorenal shunt, or Linton shunt, was first developed by Blakemore and Lord in 1945 utilizing a Vitallium tube.[68] Linton and coworkers[108] advocated this shunt in the years that followed and considered it the operative procedure of choice for correction of portal hypertension. Early reports of noncontrolled studies suggested a decreased incidence of encephalopathy with this shunt compared with the portacaval shunt.[109] This finding, however, has not been substantiated. Other investigators have failed to demonstrate significant differences between central splenorenal and portacaval shunts in regard to encephalopathy or long-term survival. In fact, some reports have noted an increased incidence of thrombosis associated with the central splenorenal shunt.[1, 110] The group at Massachusetts General Hospital reported a 10% incidence of recurrent variceal hemorrhage, 19% hepatic encephalopathy, and 18% terminal hepatic failure. Overall operative mortality was 12%.[111] Unlike the DSRS, the central splenorenal shunt functions hemodynamically as a side-to-side portasystemic shunt. Hepatic blood flow, as well as portal vein pressures, is markedly diminished, and angiography does not demonstrate persistent hepatopetal flow in the presence of a patent shunt.[108] Thus, it is generally accepted that a central splenorenal shunt has no distinct advantage over portacaval or mesocaval shunts, except possibly in the instance of severely symptomatic hypersplenism. In this event, the central splenorenal shunt may be combined with splenectomy.

Selective Shunts

Splenorenal Shunts

Portacaval shunts suffer two significant problems: progressive hepatic failure and progressive, occasionally disabling, encephalopathy. These are thought to be due to the diversion of portal blood away from the liver. In an attempt to avoid the complications of total diversion of portal flow, the DSRS, or Warren shunt, was developed in the late 1960s.[66, 112]

This operation is based on the principle of compartmentalization, as discussed by Malt[1]: the portal-azygous system and the portal-splanchnic system may be surgically separated into parallel and independent hemodynamic units. Decompression of the portal-azygous system may thus be accomplished without reducing the portal-splanchnic system perfusion pressure or blood flow.[1, 100] Hence, one should be able to decompress esophageal varices and prevent hemorrhage without diverting the hepatopetal flow of

TABLE 40–3

Results of Mesocaval Shunt Series

STUDY	PATIENTS (n)	OPERATIVE MORTALITY (%)	HEPATIC ENCEPHALOPATHY (%)	SHUNT OCCLUSION (%)	OVERALL MORTALITY (%)
Cameron et al.[101]	44	23	9	9	57
Reichle et al.[105]	28	18		7	36
Thompson et al.[106]	54	11	10	7	36
Drapanas et al.[91]	80	9	11	4	28
Smith et al.[97]	79	13	45	24	48
Busuttil et al.[119] (collected review)	409	12	25	10	

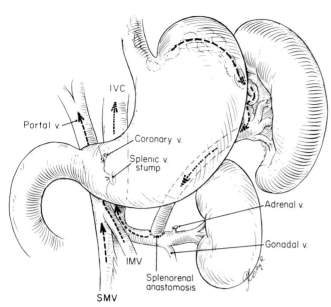

Figure 40–4. Diagrammatic illustration of the selective distal splenorenal shunt. IMV, inferior mesenteric vein; IVC, inferior vena cava; SMV, superior mesenteric vein.

the portal-splanchnic blood. In principle, this is accomplished in two steps. First, by disrupting the coronary vein and right gastroepiploic vein, blood flow into the esophageal variceal system is reduced. Second, by anastomosing the distal splenic to the left renal vein, without performing a splenectomy, blood is able to freely drain from the esophageal varices through the short gastrics into the lower pressure systemic circulation (Fig. 40–4).

The promised benefits of the DSRS shunt include preservation of hepatic perfusion and function with consequent prolongation of survival and lower risk of disabling encephalopathy. The search for evidence of this promise has led to the creation of several randomized trials. Five trials compared the DSRS against portacaval shunts. Three trials compared the DSRS with best nonsurgical management and sclerotherapy.

THE DISTAL SPLENORENAL SHUNT COMPARED WITH OTHER SHUNTS. The DSRS was compared with the end-to-side portacaval shunt in three randomized studies: by Langer and colleagues in Toronto,[113] by Resnick and coworkers in the Boston–New Haven trial,[114] and by Harley and associates at the USC Medical Center (Fig. 40–5).[115] Langer's group reported an incidence of postshunt encephalopathy

of only 14% in the selectively shunted patients but 50% in the end-to-side portacaval group. There was no difference in the long-term survival.[113] Preliminary data from Resnick's group did not indicate any substantial difference between the two operations with regard to either encephalopathy or long-term survival. It should, however, be noted that their follow-up period was relatively short.[114] Harley and associates randomized 54 patients between the two shunts and failed to demonstrate any superiority of one shunt over the other with respect to encephalopathy or survival. They did experience an unusually high rate of rebleeding with the DSRS (27%).[115]

A study in Atlanta compared the DSRS with nonselective shunts, most commonly interposition mesorenal shunts.[116, 117] The operative mortality was similar for the two groups: 12% for the DSRS and 10% for nonselective shunts. Early postoperative angiography demonstrated persistent hepatopetal flow in 88% of the DSRS patients but in only 5% of the nonselective shunt patients. Corresponding to this were quantitative measurements of hepatic function, maximal rate of urea synthesis, and the Child score, which were similar to the preoperative values in the DSRS group but greatly decreased in the nonselective group. The incidence of encephalopathy correlated with preservation of hepatopetal blood flow. Patients with hepatopetal flow suffered no encephalopathy; patients with hepatofugal flow experienced a 45% incidence of encephalopathy. Overall, encephalopathy occurred in 27% in the DSRS group and 52% in the nonselective group ($P < .001$). Recurrent variceal hemorrhage occurred in 4% of selective and 8% of nonselective shunts. Although survival was similar for the two groups, it appears that the quality of survival was improved in the DSRS group.

These results were reproduced by others in Philadelphia[105] and Toronto.[113] The Philadelphia study compared the DSRS with the H mesocaval shunt. Again, for elective shunts, the operative mortality was similar: 7%. Encephalopathy was significantly much less common with the DSRS, consistent with continued hepatopetal flow in 86% of selective but in no nonselective shunts. Hemorrhage did not recur in either group undergoing elective surgery. The long-term survival rate of 62% was comparable with that in the Atlanta study. Rebleeding in emergency cases was 2%.

Nonrandomized Studies. Two nonrandomized comparative studies also indicated excellent results with the DSRS.[118, 119] In a matched controlled study comparing the DSRS with the portacaval shunt, Busuttil and associates[119] demonstrated an incidence of significant encephalopathy of 85% in

Figure 40–5. Combined experience of the distal splenorenal shunt versus the portacaval shunt (Data from randomized trials by Rikkers et al,[116] Langer et al,[113] Reichle et al,[105] and Harley et al.[115]). PCS, portacaval shunt; PSE, portasystemic encephalopathy.

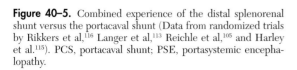
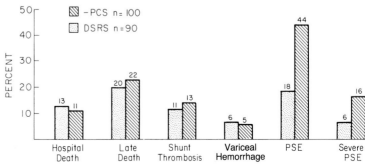

the portacaval group and only 7.6% in the DSRS group.[120, 121] Furthermore, this group demonstrated a statistically significant increase in the number of late deaths.[122] There were no recurrent variceal hemorrhages in either group.[119]

Zeppa's group[118] demonstrated that the 5-year survival of patients with nonalcoholic cirrhosis after DSRS was 89% compared with 39% in the alcoholic cirrhotic group. It should be noted that improved survival in nonalcoholic cirrhotic patients was also suggested by Warren,[117] but other investigators have contested this point.[19] In addition, a number of other unmatched studies have demonstrated excellent results with the DSRS.[122–130] A combined review of the literature comparing H mesocaval grafts to DSRSs unequivocally demonstrated the latter to be superior in decreasing the incidence of both encephalopathy and recurrent hemorrhage.[99]

THE DISTAL SPLENORENAL SHUNT AND SCLEROTHERAPY.
Warren and colleagues[131] presented the results of their randomized study of esophageal variceal bleeders who were randomized between DSRS and sclerotherapy (with salvage DSRS). A total of 71 patients were entered over a 4-year period. There was a significant difference between the two groups with regard to the preservation of portal perfusion, the maintenance of hepatic function, the rate of rebleeding, and survival. Although the sclerotherapy patients had a significantly higher rate of rebleeding (53% vs. 3%), only one of these patients died of uncontrollable hemorrhage. The 2-year survival of the group treated with sclerotherapy (and salvage surgery) was 84% (vs. 59% for those undergoing surgery alone).[131] The study clearly demonstrated that the optimal management of these patients involved the use of sclerotherapy as the initial means of controlling their bleeding. Surgery appears to work best when used to manage those patients who are not controllable with sclerotherapy. This study is important because it set the basis for the current method of managing portal hypertensive patients with esophageal variceal hemorrhage.

SPLENOPANCREATIC DISCONNECTION.
Because of the results of trials indicating that, with the passage of time, the DSRS gradually became a nonselective shunt, Warren modified the operation. In 1986,[131a] he proposed that the DSRS include complete dissection of the splenic vein and division of the splenocolic ligament (splenopancreatic disconnection). In theory, this should reduce the pancreatic sump or siphon effect: the tendency of pancreatic branches of the splenic vein to progressively enlarge and serve as an outflow collateral for the portal mesenteric circulatory system. This modification is intended to prolong and preserve the selective quality of the DSRS. Clinically, Warren's group found that this modification did preserve postoperative portal perfusion in alcoholic cirrhotic patients better than the DSRS alone. It also considerably extended the magnitude of the operation.[126]

INDICATIONS FOR THE DISTAL SPLENORENAL SHUNT.
The principal indication for a DSRS is to prevent recurrent variceal hemorrhage that is not controllable with sclerotherapy. The specific strengths of the DSRS include its lower incidence of encephalopathy and its anatomic remoteness from the porta hepatis. For these reasons it is considered the shunt of choice in elective patients who require shunting and do not present a specific contraindication to the DSRS. The most important specific contraindication to DSRS is the presence of significant ascites. In practice, this means ascites that is difficult to control by the administration of diuretics. Additionally, patients should have an adequately sized patent splenic vein. Some authors consider the presence of hepatofugal portal blood flow to be a contraindication to the DSRS. In cases of portal hypertension due to extrahepatic portal vein thrombosis, the DSRS has been demonstrated to be effective in preventing recurrent hemorrhage.[131] Finally, although the DSRS has been performed as an emergency procedure, it is not widely considered the shunt of choice in these circumstances because of the relative difficulty of the operation.

SURGICAL TECHNIQUE: DISTAL SPLENORENAL SHUNT.
The technique used for the DSRS is essentially the method described by Warren and Millikan.[132] The first goal of this operation is to anastomose the distal splenic vein to the left renal vein. The second goal is to disconnect the portal-azygous system from the splanchnic-venous system. A bilateral subcostal incision provides optimal exposure. The splenic vein may be approached either through the lesser sac or from below the transverse mesocolon. Most surgeons use the lesser sac approach. As part of this approach, the right gastroepiploic vein is divided, but the short gastric veins are carefully preserved. The pancreas is identified, and the peritoneum covering its inferior border is incised. Careful blunt dissection of the retroperitoneal tissue allows the pancreas to be rotated anteriorly and exposes the splenic vein. The splenic vein dissection is the most delicate portion of this operation. It should be carried out to the point of confluence with the SMV. The left renal vein is located by incising the posterior parietal peritoneum in the lesser sac just superior to the fourth position of the duodenum. Often, the ligament of Treitz must be incised and the duodenum reflected inferiorly to locate the vein. Dividing the adrenal vein may allow better mobilization of the renal vein. To prepare the anastomosis, the splenic vein is occluded with vascular clamps and transected close to its junction with the SMV. The stump is ligated with a suture ligature to decrease the incidence of portal vein thrombosis secondary to traumatic manipulation of the splenic vein stump.[92, 119] A partial occluding clamp is placed on the left renal vein, and the anastomosis is performed.

After completing the devascularization and the splenorenal anastomosis, measurements are made of the superior mesenteric, renal, and splenic veins. Superior mesenteric (portal) pressures should not be altered if a total portal-azygous disconnection has been performed. Splenic vein pressure will be decreased by 60% to 70%. If this pressure fails to fall, intraoperative angiography should be employed to demonstrate a technically sound anastomosis.[33]

Graft Interposition. In instances in which complete mobilization of the splenic vein cannot be accomplished because of pancreatic encasement of fibrosis, shunting may be accomplished by the interposition of a 14- to 16-mm Dacron graft between the side of the splenic vein and the side of the renal vein. After this anastomosis, the portal end of the splenic vein must be ligated if the selective nature of the shunt is to be maintained.

Portal-Azygous Disconnection. Once the anastomosis is completed and the clamps are removed, attention is focused on completing the portal-azygous disconnection. This requires interrupting all collaterals between the portal-mesenteric and portal-azygous systems. Dividing the umbilical vein and the falciform ligament completes the first step of the portal-azygous disconnection. Division of the right gastroepiploic vein constitutes the second portion of the portal-azygous disconnection. Finally, division of the coronary vein completes the portal-azygous disconnection.

Results: Patency and Portal Perfusion. The maintenance of portal perfusion in the early postoperative period has been documented in more than 90% of patients.[99, 105, 116, 130] The principal question regarding this operation, however, is one of durability: How long does the benefit of the DSRS last? It has been shown that the incidence of early partial portal vein thrombosis may be as high as 22%, and that of complete portal vein occlusion, 6%. When followed over a 6-month period, most nonocclusive portal vein thromboses resolve spontaneously.[133] A 10-year follow-up by Warren and coworkers of the DSRS group revealed that 75% had persistent portal perfusion at 10 years. Patients who were demonstrated to have portal perfusion at 3 years maintained this until the conclusion of the study at 7 years.[66, 117, 124]

The DSRS has several advantages over other nonselective shunts: it preserves portal flow to the liver; it maintains hepatotrophic perfusion; it permits the metabolism of toxic metabolites; and it maintains a high portal perfusion pressure in the intestinal venous bed, decreasing the absorption of toxic substances.[66] It is the best procedure to perform under elective conditions in a patient with hepatopetal flow. Child class A and B patients under emergent conditions also benefit from selective shunts. It should be noted that the DSRS has not been clearly demonstrated to improve survival by itself, but, when used in conjunction with judicious sclerotherapy, it appears to provide the best survival to these patients.

NONSHUNT SURGICAL PROCEDURES

Emergency portasystemic shunting results in an operative mortality of approximately 47%.[15] Furthermore, in the presence of certain clinical laboratory tests, including an SGOT greater than 300 units/L, as well as the presence of ascites or other determinants of a Child C− classification (i.e., bilirubin > 6 mg/dL, hyaline necrosis, and severe muscle wasting), a portasystemic shunt is almost sure to result in death. Because of this, numerous nonshunting surgical procedures have been developed.

Splenectomy

Based on Banti's theory, that the diseased spleen caused portal hypertension and ascites, splenectomy was one of the first operations proposed for the treatment of Banti's syndrome (splenomegaly, hypersplenism, and ascites, often accompanied by esophageal varices).

The use of splenectomy in this setting was in great part due to its advocacy by Osler, a great admirer of Banti's work. It was not until 1936, when Rousselot reviewed the experience at Columbia University in New York, that the failings of this operation were noted: a significant incidence of recurrent hemorrhage after splenectomy and the consequent loss of the splenic and portal veins, which would preclude possible shunt surgery.[134] In 1940, Thompson[135] was able to demonstrate statistically that splenectomy was of value only to those patients with isolated splenic vein thrombosis. Finally, in 1945, Pemberton and Kieman[136] reported a 54% incidence of recurrent variceal hemorrhage with splenectomy alone.

Collateralization

Development of collateral pathways between the portal circulation and the systemic circulation was the goal of several procedures. Omentopexy, introduced by Talma in 1898, produces collateral pathways by suturing the omentum to the peritoneum.[137] It was thought to be particularly beneficial in the resolution of ascites. It was sometimes used in conjunction with splenectomy for the relief of ascites associated with splenomegaly and decreased WBC counts.

Another collateral-promoting operation was the transposition of the spleen into the thorax.[138, 139] Like omentopexy, its goal was to allow the development of large venous collateral pathways between the portal venous system and the systemic venous circulation. Unfortunately, these collateral pathways were never able to adequately decompress esophageal varices. Thus, the patients were doomed to repeated hemorrhage.

Ablation

Ablative procedures to remove the source of bleeding were first advocated in 1947 by Phemister and Humphreys,[20] who recommended total gastrectomy. Peters and Womack[140] later encouraged splenectomy with obliteration of both the intra- and extraluminal vasculature of the distal varices-bearing esophagus and proximal stomach. Keagy and colleagues[141] reviewed the long-term results of the so-called Womack procedure and found the risk to be prohibitively high—a 54% incidence of rebleeding and a 35% operative mortality. They concluded that this procedure should be used only in highly selected patients who do not have suitable anatomy for a shunt.[141]

A variation of the Womack procedure was the transthoracic ligation of the esophageal varices without the splenectomy. This operation was introduced in 1949 by Boerema[142] and in 1950 by Crile.[143] Wirthlin and associates[144] reported on 55 patients who underwent transeophageal ligation of varices, with a 29% operative mortality and a 33% incidence of recurrent hemorrhage resulting in an additional 23% mortality.

Despite these results, the procedure was not abandoned. Technologic innovation in the form of the EEA (end-to-end anastomosis) stapler allowed transection and reanastomosis of the distal esophagus with greater facility. The innovation resulted in reduced operative mortality and improved reduction of postoperative hemorrhage. Wexler[145] reported that of six Child class C patients undergoing this procedure, none had recurrent bleeding. Cooperman and associates[146] reported five patients with severe hepatic dysfunction and massive variceal bleeding who underwent transabdominal EEA variceal stapling, none of whom developed recurrent bleeding up to 2 years postoperatively.

In a logical extension of these devascularization procedures, other surgeons proposed more extensive operations. Delaney[147] promulgated a devascularization procedure performed through a left thoracotomy, which involves devascularization of the upper half of the stomach and proximally to the level of the left inferior pulmonary vein, as well as splenectomy, staple interruption of intramural gastroesophageal collateral vessels, truncal vagotomy with pyloroplasty, and fundoplication. The major disadvantage of this procedure is that the splenectomy precludes performance of selective shunts at a later time. Delaney reported, however, that none of his four patients had recurrent variceal bleeding.[147]

Perhaps the most successful devascularization procedure was that developed by Suguira in Japan.[137, 148, 149] Because of the significant risk of encephalopathy, shunt procedures were abandoned in favor of an extensive periesophagogastric devascularization accompanied by esophageal transection. The procedure is performed via separate thoracic and abdominal incisions; in poor-risk patients, a two-stage procedure is indicated. The esophagus is devascularized from the gastroesophageal junction to the left inferior pulmonary vein. The vagus nerve is carefully preserved. At the level of the diaphragm, the esophagus is partially transected, leaving only the posterior muscular layer intact. Esophageal varices are occluded, not ligated, by oversewing each with interrupted sutures. The esophageal muscle is closed, but the mucosa is not sutured. The abdominal operation is performed through a separate midline incision and includes splenectomy, devascularization of the abdominal esophagus and proximal stomach, and a pyloroplasty and fundoplication.

The early results of this operation, as reported by Suguira and Futagawa,[137] were excellent. The authors reported an overall operative mortality of 4.6%. Their emergency operative mortality was 20%. Varices were eradicated in 97% of patients, and recurrent bleeding occurred in only 2.5%. Their long-term survival was 84%.[137] A follow-up report by the authors on 276 patients indicated equally good survival rates with excellent control of variceal bleeding and no encephalopathy.[148] In a later report, they analyzed their results according to the patients' Child classification. They found that in class C patients both operative mortality and long-term survival were discouraging. For class A and B patients, the results were very good, with combined (A, B, and C) 15-year survival as high as 72%.[150]

Reports by Suguira's group have been confirmed by others in Japan, as well as by selected investigators in the United States.[151, 152] A number of other reports have suggested esophageal transection procedures in the management of selected patients with poor hepatic reserves (Child class C patients). The EEA stapler has made this a relatively simple procedure, but the possibility of esophageal perforation and leakage still make the procedure one of considerable risk.[153] Overall, these studies demonstrate

that esophageal transection should be considered a reasonable option in the management of acute hemorrhage in the debilitated patient with both gastric and esophageal varices.[154–156]

POSTOPERATIVE CARE

The most common problem in the postoperative period is the development of significant ascites. Fluid management is the key to minimizing this problem. Postoperative fluids should be restricted to free water and salt-poor albumin or fresh-frozen plasma. These should be given to maintain adequate intravascular volume yet avoid overexpansion of the patient's intravascular space. A diuretic should be started as soon as the patient is begun on oral fluids. Spironolactone is frequently used because of its potassium-sparing characteristics. Caution is advised in its use because of the potential complication of metabolic alkalosis. Sodium intake should be restricted to less than 90 mg/day. Prophylactic antibiotics, which should be started 12 hours before surgery, are continued for only 1 to 2 days. Chylous ascites may develop in the immediate postoperative period as a result of interruption of retroperitoneal lymphatics, and a 30-g/day fat restriction should be maintained for 4 weeks to minimize the risk of this problem.[132]

Recurrent Bleeding

If variceal hemorrhage occurs within the immediate postoperative period, angiography should immediately be performed to accurately define the anatomy and patency of the shunt. If a patent collateral such as the coronary vein is identified, one should consider percutaneous transhepatic embolization. If other collateral pathways are present, reexploration may be indicated in order to ligate them. If the shunt is occluded and the patient is bleeding, then reexploration should be undertaken to repair the shunt or to perform another shunt.

THE TRANSJUGULAR INTRAHEPATIC PORTASYSTEMIC SHUNT

A most impressive development in the management of portal hypertensive patients with variceal hemorrhage was the introduction of the TIPS. This shunt is a combination of several procedures and techniques that were developed in parallel. The TIPS shunt has borrowed conceptually from the small-diameter Sarfeh portacaval interposition shunt, balloon angioplasty techniques, and the Palmaz balloon-expandable stent.

The essence of the TIPS is the creation of a fistula between a hepatic vein and a branch of the portal vein. This fistula is created by passing a needle-directing guidewire through the jugular vein into a hepatic vein and then into a branch of the portal vein. Once this connection has been established, balloon dilatation is used to enlarge the tract to a size adequate for the decompression of the portal hypertension. Because of the fibrotic nature of the end-stage liver, the tract must be stented open to ensure its patency. This is accomplished by placing a Palmaz-type stent at the time of balloon dilatation.

The attraction of the TIPS is that it may be a minimally invasive procedure that may effectively reduce portal hypertension. In optimal circumstances, the TIPS may be placed in a relatively short period of time, using only local anesthetic techniques. It thus avoids a major surgical procedure and a general anesthetic in a debilitated patient. An additional advantage is the preservation of the patient's normal intraabdominal anatomy. The last is of particular importance to patients who are considered potential candidates for hepatic transplantation because it avoids the scarring, neovascularization, and alteration of portal perfusion associated with shunt operations.

A final advantage is that the successful TIPS would be expected to maintain patency of the portal vein as long as the shunt itself is patent. This is of particular importance in patients who may be at risk of portal vein thrombosis, such as those with sluggish hepatopetal or hepatofugal portal flow. The sequelae of portal vein thrombosis range from asymptomatic to massive ascites to hepatic failure and death. The surgical consequence of portal vein thrombosis is that it may preclude further surgery for the patient. In patients who are to be considered for transplantation, portal vein thrombosis may affect both operability and survival.

The principal disadvantage of the TIPS is that it is a new and untested procedure. Only a few centers have any experience with this technique. A clinical trial begun in 1993 should answer the questions of initial success, complications, and early patency. The long-term track record of these procedures will require several years to establish. Accordingly, the final analysis of the role of the TIPS remains to be established.

Three reports comprising 11 patients have recorded the very early experience with the procedure.[157–159] Of these, three died in the early postshunt period, one from uncontrolled hemorrhage associated with a percutaneous embolization attempt. One shunt became occluded at 3 months after creation but was successfully reopened; another required redilatation. This initial experience served to establish the feasibility of the procedure and has generated considerable enthusiasm.

The most recent report is from Ring and associates in San Francisco.[160] They described their initial experience with 25 patients who underwent the TIPS procedure for active bleeding (12), recurrent bleeding (12), and ascites secondary to Budd-Chiari syndrome (1). They were able to place the shunts in all patients. Their 30-day mortality was 20%. Eight of their patients eventually underwent liver transplantation. Of the 12 patients who were available for prolonged follow-up (average of 5.5 months), three suffered shunt occlusion. All three shunts were reopened. Notable complications included encephalopathy and the development of intimal hyperplasia in the shunt. They concluded that the TIPS procedure provides good reduction of portal hypertension and control of bleeding but that long-term efficacy is far from established.[160]

In a review of these and other results of the TIPS, Conn[161] suggested that the long-term results of the TIPS should not be considered comparable with those of surgical shunts. He noted an incidence of restenosis approaching 15%, and occlusion occurring in 5% to 10%. In aggregate, almost one fourth of these shunts fail within the first year after implantation. The incidence of postshunt encephalopathy is about 24%. Conn noted that this is commensurate with several series of surgical shunts. Recurrent bleeding after placement of the TIPS occurs in about 10% of cases. This, however, does not include significant hemorrhagic complications that may attend the creation of these shunts. Conn further stated that these procedures should be considered experimental until adequate prospective study has been completed.[161]

Grace,[162] in a similar review, noted that the principal benefit of the TIPS procedure is that it appears to control acute bleeding in patients who do not respond to sclerotherapy and are awaiting transplantation. Given the high rates of stenosis, occlusion, recurrent hemorrhage, and encephalopathy, these shunts are best reserved for patients who are in need of transplantation and whose bleeding cannot be controlled with sclerotherapy (Table 40–4).

The role of the TIPS in management of portal hypertension was reviewed at a conference sponsored by the National Digestive Diseases Advisory Board.[163] Shiffman and associates noted that the lack of long-term follow-up data, as well as the absence of a controlled study comparing

TABLE 40-4

Results of Largest Reported Series of Transjugular Intrahepatic Portasystemic Shunt Procedures

AUTHORS	YEAR	PATIENTS (n)	Stenosis/ Occlusion (%)	Bleed (%)	PSE (%)	Died (%)
Richter et al.[159]	1990	9	11			22
LaBerge et al.[160]	1992	25	12		4	20
Noldge et al.[207]	1992	24	5	15	5	27
LaBerge et al.[208]	1993	100	15	10	7	27
Helton et al.[209]	1993	59	32	20		25
Simpson et al.[210]	1993	22	22	33	11	11
Rossle et al.[211]	1994	100	33	16	25	10
Jalan et al.[212]	1994	44	23	23	17	39

PSE, postshunt encephalopathy.

TIPS with surgical shunts, represents a significant deficit in our understanding of this technology. The authors also noted that the reported incidence of encephalopathy (15% to 30%) and restenosis (33% to 66%) is a problem that requires further improvement. Currently, they recommend the TIPS for patients who fail sclerotherapy and for those with uncontrolled variceal bleeding who are about to undergo transplantation. Specific recommendations were reviewed and classified as accepted, unproven but promising, unproven, and contraindicated. Acceptable indications include the control of hemorrhage not controlled by sclerotherapy or pharmacotherapy. Unproven but promising indications include control of refractory ascites and Budd-Chiari syndrome. Unproven indications include initial therapy for variceal hemorrhage, prophylaxis of esophageal varices, adjunct therapy to liver transplantation. Absolute contraindications include polycystic liver disease, severe hepatic failure (TIPS in place of transplantation), and severe right-sided heart failure. Relative contraindications include encephalopathy, portal vein thrombosis, and active systemic or hepatic bacterial infections.

Patients with good hepatic function and a prolonged expected survival should still be considered candidates for surgical shunts such as the DSRS. The long-term patency, low rate of recurrent hemorrhage, and low incidence of postshunt encephalopathy make this procedure superior to the TIPS in these patients.

ORTHOTOPIC LIVER TRANSPLANTATION

With the advent of liver transplantation as an established modality for the care of patients with end-stage liver failure, the role of nontransplant procedures (shunt surgery in particular) has been the subject of considerable debate. Current best transplant survival rates are generally more favorable than most of the reported survival of Child class C patients after the best care with a combination of sclerotherapy and shunting. This issue has been the subject of two reports from Iwatsuki and colleagues at the University of Pittsburgh Liver Transplant Unit.[164, 165] These reports described the survival of 302 patients who had bleeding esophageal varices. According to the authors, these patients were all ranked as Child class C with regard to hepatic function. The survival of these patients was reported in a life table format as 79% at 1 year, 74% at 2 years, and 71% at 5 years. The authors then compared these results with shunt survival as reported in the medical literature and concluded that in Child class C patients who present with bleeding varices, liver transplantation should be considered as the treatment of choice—assuming that the patients are reasonable transplant candidates.

Our experience at the University of California, Los Angeles (UCLA), has revealed that superior survival is afforded to Child class C patients by transplantation (Table 40–5). In a series of 761 patients operated on between January 1986 and December 1991, 77 underwent portasystemic shunting as their initial procedure, and 684 underwent hepatic transplantation. Of those receiving transplants, 86% were Child class C patients, whereas only 16% of the shunt patients were Child class C patients. Despite

TABLE 40 – 5

Results of Portasystemic Shunting and Liver Transplantation from January 1986 to December 1991*

	n	CHILD CLASS C (%)	5-YEAR SURVIVAL
Portasystemic shunt	77	16	64
Liver transplantation	684	87	73
Total	761		

*University of California, Los Angeles, experience. Distal splenorenal shunts constituted 50% of shunt operations; 15% of shunt patients eventually underwent liver transplantation because of deterioration of hepatic function.

this, 15% of shunt patients eventually required liver transplantation for progressive hepatic deterioration. Furthermore, the 5-year survival of the shunt group was 64% in contrast to a 73% 5-year survival of the transplant patients. These data support the impression that portasystemic shunting is an appropriate form of therapy for Child class A and B patients, but that the Child class C patients who are transplant candidates are best managed by liver transplantation.

Further complicating the issue is the effect of a prior shunt operation on a subsequent transplant operation. It has been reported that patients who must undergo a liver transplant after a prior portacaval shunt have a considerably increased blood loss, longer operative procedure, increased morbidity, and higher mortality.[166] The portacaval shunt is a particularly troublesome procedure to overcome because the technique of performing a successful liver transplant in this situation requires dissection through the scarred tissues about the portal structures, disconnection of the shunt, and reconstitution of the normal caval anatomy; only then may the liver transplant operation may begin. This is in contrast to peripheral shunt operations such as the mesocaval shunt or the DSRS. Although these shunts have an impact on the transplant procedure, they are not as difficult to manage as the central shunts. In the case of a mesocaval shunt, the shunt must be disconnected or occluded before the transplant operation is completed, or the new liver may be deprived of portal nutrient blood flow. A similar problem may arise even with the DSRS, although by the nature of this shunt, the siphon effect (drainage of portal blood through peripancreatic collaterals into the shunt) is usually relatively minor and the shunt frequently does not require dismantling.

The essential features of any consideration of the role of shunting versus liver transplantation are the underlying cause of the hepatic disease, the current stage of hepatic dysfunction, and the expected progression (the natural and treated history) of the hepatic disease. Assuming that the patient is a reasonable transplantation candidate and that the liver disease is approaching the end stage (Child class C), transplantation should be strongly considered. If the patient requires an emergent procedure for control of bleeding before being able to undergo transplantation, all efforts should be made to provide a peripheral shunt. If the patient is not a transplant candidate, treatment should consist of the best therapy available: sclerotherapy sup-

TABLE 40–6

Sclerotherapy versus Medical Management

STUDY	Follow-up (mo)	SCLEROTHERAPY			CONTROL		
		n	Rebleed (%)	Survival (yr)	*n*	Rebleed (%)	Survival (yr)
Terblanche et al.[178]	60	37	43	45% (5)	38	73	45% (5)
Paquet & Feussner[173]	9–52	93	48	36% (2)	97	54	25% (2)
Westaby et al.[177]	3–60	56	55	60% (4)	60	80	31% (4)
Korula et al.[180]	3–35	63	44	60% (2)	57	70	56% (2)
Soderlund & Ihre[179]	12–48	57	†	49% (2)	50	†	34% (2)

*There was a significant decrease in transfusion requirements in the sclerotherapy group as well as fewer rebleeding episodes per patient-month if followed up.
†Overall recurrent hemorrhage was 3.6 times more frequent in the control group.

ported by either esophageal transection with devascularization or shunting.

VARICEAL SCLEROTHERAPY

Esophageal variceal sclerotherapy was introduced by Craafoord and Frenckner in 1939.[167] These authors demonstrated a single patient who underwent rigid endoscopic sclerotherapy to prevent further variceal bleeding. With the upsurge in the variety of surgical procedures for variceal hemorrhage in the 1940s, however, sclerotherapy was soon forgotten. Once it was recognized that therapeutic portacaval shunts, with their inherent operative mortality and risk of encephalopathy, were not the ultimate surgical procedure, attention was redirected toward less invasive, more direct methods of treatment, and there was renewed interest in sclerotherapy after the results of several controlled trials.

The first major review of sclerotherapy was by Johnston and Rodgers in 1973.[168] In 117 patients, bleeding was initially controlled in 92%, and the hospital mortality per admission was 18%. The average time to recurrence of variceal hemorrhage was 10 months. This group, however, made no attempt to perform sequential variceal sclerotherapy and recommended a shunt for long-term variceal control. Similar mortality and variceal hemorrhage control rates were reported by Terblanche from South Africa.[169–172]

Endoscopy is necessary to confirm the presence of varices and differentiate those who are actively bleeding from those who have ceased to bleed. The use of sclerotherapy to stop acute bleeding at the time of initial endoscopy has been advocated as the treatment of choice.[169, 170] Urgent or emergent sclerotherapy is used in many institutions after stabilization with balloon tamponade or after failure of conservative supportive therapy and somatostatin. Several controlled trials have compared sclerotherapy with medical management with the Sengstaken-Blakemore tube in the acute setting.[173–177] Three studies demonstrated a significantly lower early rebleeding rate,[173–175] and all the studies supported the use of sclerotherapy for acute bleeding. Only Paquet and Feussner demonstrated significantly improved overall survival with sclerotherapy.[173]

The ability of sclerotherapy to prevent recurrent variceal hemorrhage and improve long-term survival with extended treatment has been examined in numerous controlled trials[176–180] (Table 40–6). When sclerotherapy was performed to eradicate all varices and compared with conservative medical management, sclerotherapy patients had fewer recurrent bleeds[178, 180] and improved long-term survival.[177] Terblanche and colleagues[178] were able to demonstrate complete eradication of varices in 95% of sclerotherapy patients; however, they could not demonstrate a significant difference in survival, and varices recurred in more than 60% of the sclerotherapy patients.

Only since 1984 has sclerotherapy been systematically compared with portasystemic shunts in the management of variceal hemorrhage. Cello and associates[181, 182] compared the portacaval shunt to sclerotherapy in Child class C patients, showing greater rebleeding, increased rehospitalization, and higher blood transfusion requirements in the sclerotherapy group, with 40% of sclerotherapy patients ultimately requiring surgical therapy. However, they were unable to demonstrate any significant difference in survival (Table 40–7). The authors concluded that in high-risk patients, sclerotherapy and portacaval shunting are equal in the acute setting, but one must consider shunt surgery if varices are not totally obliterated.[181, 182]

With the resurgence of endoscopic sclerotherapy, the DSRS has been compared with this form of treatment for the long-term management of variceal bleeding in three controlled trials (Table 40–8). Warren and coworkers[183] showed that although early mortality was the same, there was a higher rebleeding rate with sclerotherapy and one third of the patients failed treatment and required surgery.

TABLE 40–7

Sclerotherapy versus Portacaval Shunt in Management of Variceal Hemorrhage

	SCLEROTHERAPY (*n* = 32)	SHUNT (*n* = 32)	*P*-VALUE
Rebleed rate	50%	19%	< .009
Encephalopathy	13%	13%	NS
Surgery not required	7 (22%)		
Long-term cost	$23,000	$28,000	NS
18-month survival	28%	13%	NS

NS, not significant.
Data from Cello J, Grendell J, Crass R, et al: Endoscopic sclerotherapy versus portacaval shunt in patients with severe cirrhosis and variceal hemorrhage. N Engl J Med 311:1589–1594, 1984.

TABLE 40-8

Sclerotherapy versus Distal Splenorenal Shunt (DSRS) in Long-Term Management of Variceal Hemorrhage*

	SCLEROTHERAPY	DSRS	*P*-VALUE
Warren et al.[183]			
No. of patients	36	35	
Rebleed rate	53%	3%	< .05
Portal perfusion	95%	53%	< .05
Patients requiring surgery	10 (28%)		
2-yr survival	84%	59%	< .01
Rikkers et al.[185]			
No. of patients	30	27	
Rebleed rate	57%	19%	.003
Encephalopathy	7%	16%	
2-yr survival	61%	65%	NS
Teres et al.[187]			
No. of patients	55	57	
Rebleed rate	37.5%	14.3%	< .02
Encephalopathy	8%	24%	< .05
2-yr survival	68%	71%	NS

*All controlled trials.
NS, not significant.

Treatment with sclerotherapy allowed significant improvement in liver function when successful, with less encephalopathy and improved survival when backed up by surgical therapy for patients with uncontrolled bleeding. Therefore, the improved survival in the sclerotherapy group actually represents a combination of sclerotherapy and surgical therapy. Teres and colleagues[184] found no difference in early and long-term mortality, nor did Rikkers and coworkers.[185] However, the rebleeding rate was greater in those patients who had sclerotherapy, and encephalopathy rates were higher in shunt patients in the study of Teres and colleagues.[184]

Burroughs and associates,[186] in 1989, concluded a prospective randomized study comparing staple transection with sclerotherapy for emergency control of variceal bleeding. They found no difference in overall mortality and improved control of bleeding with esophageal transection compared with a single injection, but a similar incidence of hemorrhage after three injection treatments. Teres and colleagues[187] randomized cirrhotic patients with uncontrolled bleeding to portacaval shunt or staple transection in low-risk patients and staple transection or sclerotherapy in high-risk patients. Survival was similar in both groups. In the low-risk patients, portacaval shunt had a greater hemostatic effect, but a greater incidence of encephalopathy. In high-risk patients, sclerotherapy and staple transection had similar rebleeding rates and survival, but fewer complications were observed in the sclerotherapy group. The authors therefore recommended staple transection for low-risk patients and sclerotherapy for the initial management of high-risk patients. Although a consensus on sclerotherapy has not yet been reached, sclerotherapy may well represent an appropriate alternative ablative procedure in selected patients with hepatic dysfunction.[155, 173, 187-195]

A number of complications of varying degrees of severity result from esophageal variceal sclerotherapy. Frequently, the patients complain of odynophagia lasting from hours to days. This may also be associated with retrosternal chest pain, lasting for several days. Not infrequently, as a result of pyrogens within the sclerosing solution, a fever of greater than 101°F develops that abates within 2 to 3 days and is not associated with a leukocytosis. Bacteremias have been documented in as many as 50% of procedures.[196] Pleural effusion sometimes occurs but does not necessarily indicate esophageal perforation.[197] Variceal ulceration of varying degrees, depending on the amount of sclerosant injected, is not uncommon and usually resolves spontaneously.[198] Rare serious complications, including esophageal perforation, spinal cord paralysis, and bradyarrhythmias, have also been described.[25, 27, 28, 30, 172, 192, 195]

More recently, interest has increased in an alternative endoscopic technique: variceal banding. This has the advantage of avoiding the caustic agents required for sclerotherapy. In comparison studies, the rates of efficacy in halting bleeding are similar between the two techniques. There is debate as to whether the incidence of complications with banding is reduced compared with sclerotherapy. Clearly, the same major complications attend both techniques: recurrent bleeding as well as esophageal ulceration and perforation.[199]

Endoscopic variceal sclerotherapy and variceal banding have the distinct advantages of no risk of portal vein thrombosis, good control of variceal hemorrhage, and easy accessibility for repeat sclerotherapy. There is no question that in patients with acute variceal bleeding who have had a prior splenectomy or portasystemic shunt that has failed, endoscopic therapy is indicated. Because of the high mortality associated with emergency shunting procedures, variceal sclerotherapy in conjunction with octreotide is indicated in the acute management of variceal hemorrhage. Recurrent variceal hemorrhage is likely if follow-up routine sclerotherapy is not performed. Hence, sclerotherapy should be considered as an adjunctive therapeutic management tool for the acute control of variceal bleeding rather than its definitive treatment.

TREATMENT PLAN FOR VARICEAL HEMORRHAGE

When a patient has an upper gastrointestinal tract hemorrhage, and the history and physical examination suggest esophageal varices in association with hepatic disease, a preset treatment plan should rapidly be followed. It is important to consider that in these patients time is of the essence, and that delays to consider, define, and formulate a new plan of action frequently jeopardize the patient's life. The initial care of the bleeding portal hypertensive patient should be as routine as the initial care of a trauma patient. The A, B, and C steps should be routinely followed. Special variations are implemented because of the underlying hepatic disease and the associated risks that this presents.

Initial laboratory studies should include a CBC, electrolytes, blood typing, and cross-matching. Additionally, determinants of liver function, to include bilirubin, SGOT, LDH, SGPT, prothrombin time, partial thromboplastin time, albumin, total protein, and alkaline phosphatase should also be obtained. Nasogastric tubes must be placed in all of these patients; if blood is present in the stomach, gastric lavage and emergency endoscopy are indicated. This allows verification of the source of the hemorrhage and emergent sclerotherapy, if required.

Initial fluid management is crucial. Treatment with fluids and blood products should be directed at maintaining adequate tissue perfusion. Resuscitation should include PRBCs and fresh-frozen plasma as needed. Cryoprecipitates and calcium may be required in massive bleeding. It is generally preferable to resuscitate with a combination of crystalloid and blood components (albumin and PRBCs) rather than saline only. Thiamine should be administered to prevent Wernicke's encephalopathy. Propranolol or diazepam (Valium) may be required for the symptoms of alcohol withdrawal.

If bleeding does not stop during the resuscitation and transfusion, octreotide should be administered intravenously and repeat sclerotherapy performed. Balloon tamponade may be especially helpful at this juncture. If the patient fails to stop bleeding after injections and balloon tamponade, emergent intervention is indicated. Depending on the institution's resources, the patient should be considered for either a TIPS, a portasystemic shunt, or an esophageal transection with devascularization. The choice of portasystemic shunt is largely dependent on the abilities of the surgeons involved. If the patient is a potential liver transplant candidate, a peripheral shunt (DSRS or mesocaval) should be performed. The choice of TIPS or surgical shunt should probably be based on the local expertise and ability of the managing physicians.

Once bleeding is controlled, patients with relatively good hepatic function (Child class A or B) should undergo long-term sclerotherapy until varices are obliterated. If this is successful, the patient should continue to be observed and no further interventions planned. If the patient has breakthrough bleeding from noncompliance, gastric varices, or hypertensive gastritis and is an appropriate candidate for elective shunt, a preoperative evaluation should be done (angiography, duplex scan) and a shunt performed.

Patients with poor hepatic function should be considered for transplantation if they fulfill the appropriate criteria. While the patient is awaiting orthotopic liver transplant, a peripheral shunt may be necessary as a bridge to transplantation. Child class C− patients with marked muscle wasting and obvious hyaline necrosis have a prohibitively high operative mortality rate and should undergo endoscopic sclerotherapy followed by transplantation. If this technique is not available, esophageal transection with or without the EEA stapler and ligation of portal-azygous collateral pathways is indicated, although the mortality can be expected to be greater than 60% (Fig. 40–6).

MANAGEMENT OF ASCITES

Ascites predisposes portal hypertensive patients to potentially lethal complications, including renal failure, peritonitis, variceal hemorrhage, pleural effusions with respiratory insufficiency, abdominal wall hernias, anorexia, and generalized malaise. Most patients with ascites may be controlled with a restricted salt diet and diuretic regimen. Only 5% of ascitic patients can be considered to have truly intractable

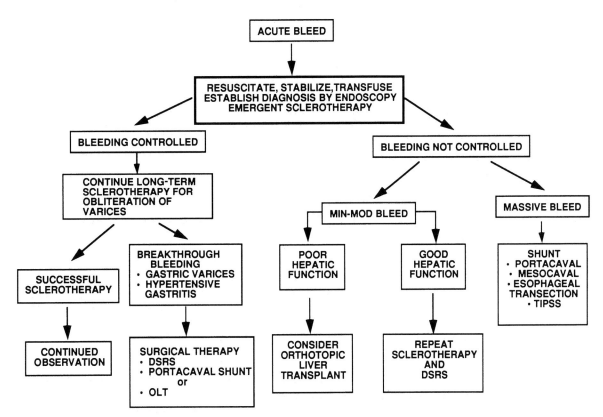

Figure 40–6. Schematic of protocol for management of variceal hemorrhage. DSRS, distal splenorenal shunt; OLT, orthotopic liver transplant; TIPS, transjugular intrahepatic portosystemic stent shunt.

ascites, and it is these patients who may require surgical intervention.[200]

Patients who have ascites related to liver disease should be admitted to the hospital for complete evaluation and therapy. The admission workup should include a careful neurologic status examination as well as measurements of electrolytes and renal and liver function tests. These patients should be placed at strict bed rest, because this will increase the amount of diuresis. Encephalopathy should be monitored by checking for asterixis at least once or twice a day.

A fluid restriction of no more than 1 L/day should be ordered in addition to a 20 mEq/day sodium diet. With this regimen one would expect a diuresis of 500 mL to 1 L/day. If such a diuresis does not occur, progressive diuretic therapy is indicated. This usually involves a gradual increase in the dosages and varieties of diuretics. Frequently, the first diuretic used is spironolactone, a potassium-sparing diuretic. It should be started at a dosage of 100 mg/day and doubled at 2-day intervals until a maximum dosage is obtained. If further diuresis is required, other agents, such as metolazone, hydrochlorothiazide, and furosemide (Lasix) may be used.

At the first sign of encephalopathy or elevation of blood urea nitrogen by 10 mg/dL or creatinine by 0.5 mg/dL, all diuretics must be discontinued to avoid development of the hepatorenal syndrome. If, after such a trial of intensive nonsurgical therapy no significant response occurs, surgery is indicated.[201]

In 1974, LeVeen introduced the peritoneovenous shunt. This device consists of a Silastic tube that runs from the peritoneum to the superior vena cava. It is controlled by a one-way valve so that a pressure gradient of 5 cm H_2O suffices to transfer the ascitic fluid from the abdomen to the intravascular space.[202]

The Denver shunt, a variation of the LeVeene shunt, incorporates a pump in line with the shunt and is implanted in the subcutaneous tissues on the chest wall. Its proposed benefit is its ability to clear the shunt of debris by using the pump mechanism.[125]

Although promising innovations, both of these shunts are dogged by complications. Early complications include congestive heart failure (from the infusion of ascitic fluid) and disseminated intravascular coagulation (DIC). In 39% to 100% of patients, changes consistent with DIC may be detected by laboratory studies. Clinically apparent DIC is much less common.[69, 203] Coagulation values tend to improve after the first postoperative week, possibly related to diminished ascitic flow into the venous system.[204] If clinically apparent DIC develops, the only definitive treatment possible is shunt ligation.[203] Some authors have been concerned that the increased intravascular volume may result in increased variceal hemorrhage. Finally, high perioperative mortality rates (20%) have been reported by a number of institutions.[205]

Late complications include shunt infection, shunt occlusion, and death. Infection may occur in up to 26% of patients. Shunt occlusion is thought to result from the precipitation of the ascitic protein in the shunt tubing. Death related to inherent liver dysfunction is not uncommon.

Usually, the infusion of ascitic fluids results in a brisk diuresis. The exact mechanism for this is not clear. Proposed mechanisms include volume expansion, increased renin levels from the ascitic fluid, and relief of intraabdominal pressure.[6] The hepatorenal syndrome is the name given to the concomitant loss of renal function in patients with hepatic failure and no intrinsic renal disease. Although the cause is unknown, it may be related to a redistribution of blood within the cortex of the kidney. The mortality from untreated hepatorenal syndrome is usually 100%. The peritoneovenous shunt is considered a potential treatment of these patients. Successful resolution of the syndrome by placement of such a shunt has been reported.[206]

Contraindications to the placement of peritoneovenous shunts include the presence of infected ascitic fluid, recurrent sepsis, or encephalopathy. Another absolute contraindication includes a bilirubin greater than 6 mg/dL or prolongation of prothrombin time longer than 4 seconds. These have been shown to be associated with a prohibitively high incidence of postoperative coagulopathy, resulting in death. DIC resulting from an intravenous test infusion of ascitic fluid is another relative contraindication to peritoneovenous shunting. Finally, a large pleural effusion associated with an elevated intrathoracic pressure may preclude use of these shunts.[200]

In general, peritoneovenous shunting is an effective method to treat ascites. It should be kept in mind as an adjunct to the care of these patients and may not be as simple in practice as it is in concept. It should not be expected to result in prolongation of survival or alteration of the natural course of the hepatic disease.

SUMMARY

The management of portal hypertension and its sequelae of ascites, encephalopathy, and recurrent variceal hemorrhage continues to be a significant challenge to the clinician. Its etiology and pathogenesis have been well described. Alcoholic cirrhosis resulting in intrahepatic sinusoidal and postsinusoidal obstruction continues to be the most common cause.

Long-term survival depends on rapid control of hemorrhage and institution of the most appropriate care for the patient according to the nature and severity of the hepatic disease. A patient who has variceal hemorrhage should be quickly resuscitated. Endoscopy should then be performed to establish the source of gastrointestinal tract bleeding and then sclerotherapy should be given. Initial management should include intravenous vasopressin followed by balloon tamponade. Angiography or duplex Doppler studies should be performed in patients considered for shunting. Emergent shunt surgery should be avoided if at all possible because the mortality is excessive.

Selective shunt procedures (DSRS), although they do not extend long-term survival, produce less encephalopathy and stop bleeding. Patients should be considered for elective shunting if they cannot be controlled with sclerotherapy and have relatively good hepatic function (Child class A or B). Child class C patients and "unshuntable" patients are best initially treated with nonshunt procedures or transplantation. Esophageal variceal sclerotherapy provides effective control of acute variceal hemorrhage, but, if it is unsuccessful after several attempts, a portal-azygous devascularization procedure should be attempted. Ultimately, the survival of these patients depends upon their degree of hepatic function. Patients with end-stage liver disease should be considered for liver transplantation.

Encephalopathy is a consequence of hepatic failure. It may be ameliorated by a medical regimen of neomycin, lactulose, and a low-protein diet. Ascites usually can be managed with salt restriction and diuretics. In a patient with intractable ascites, a peritoneovenous shunt provides effective control.

The best treatment for patients with portal hypertension relies on the recognition that the hepatic disease dictates the progression of liver failure. Depending on the stage of hepatic dysfunction, different options are available for each patient. In deciding how best to manage a patient, it is necessary to keep in mind that the goal is not merely survival but also quality of life.

References

1. Malt R: Portasystemic venous shunts. N Engl J Med 295:24–29, 1976.
2. Shaldon S, Sherlock S: Portal hypertension in the myeloproliferative syndrome and the reticuloses. Am J Surg 32:758, 1962.
3. Shaldon S, Chiandussi L, Guevara L: The measurement of hepatic blood flow and intrahepatic shunted blood flow by colloid, heat denatured serum albumin labeled with I131. J Clin Invest 40:1038, 1969.
4. Gordon M, DelGuerco L: Late effects of portal systemic shunting procedures on cardiorespiratory dynamics in man. Ann Surg 176:672–679, 1972.
5. Langer B, Stone R, Colapinto R: Clinical spectrum of the Budd-Chiari syndrome and its surgical management. Am J Surg 129:137–145.
6. Ludwick J, Markel S, Child L: Chiari's disease. Arch Surg 91:697–704, 1965.
7. Sherlock S: Classification and functional aspects of portal hypertension. Am J Surg 127:121–128, 1974.
8. Ahn S, Yellin A, Sheng F, et al: Selective surgical therapy of the Budd-Chiari syndrome provides superior survival rates than conservative medical management. J Vasc Surg 5:28–37, 1987.
9. Bosch J, Navasa M, Garcia-Pagan J, et al: Portal hypertension. Med Clin North Am 73:931–953, 1989.
10. Bosch J, Mastai R, Kravetz D, et al: Hemodynamic evaluation of the patients with portal hypertension. Semin Liver Dis 6:309–317, 1986.
11. Koslin D, Berland L: Duplex Doppler examination of the liver and portal system. Clin Ultrasound 15:675–686, 1987.
12. Ohnishi K, Saito M, Koen H, et al: Pulsed Doppler flow as a criterion of portal venous velocity: Comparison with cineangiographic measurements. Radiology 154:495–498, 1985.
13. Bolondi L, Gandolfi L, Arienti V, et al: Ultrasonography in the diagnosis of portal hypertension: Diminished response of portal vessels to respiration. Radiology 142:167–172, 1982.
14. Cello J, Deveney K, Trunkey D: Factors influencing survival after therapeutic shunts. Am J Surg 141:257–265, 1981.
15. Orloff M, Duguay L, Kosta L: Criteria for selection of patients for emergency portacaval shunt. Am J Surg 134:146–152, 1977.
16. Schwartz S: Liver. In Schwartz S (ed): Principles of Surgery. New York, McGraw-Hill, 1984, pp 1257–1305.
17. Rueff B, Benhamou J: Management of gastrointestinal bleeding in cirrhotic patients. Clin Gastroenterol 4:426–438, 1975.
18. Rikkers L: Operations for management of esophageal variceal hemorrhage. West J Med 136:107–121, 1982.
19. Resnick R: Portal hypertension. Med Clin North Am 59:945–953, 1975.
20. Phemister D, Humphreys E: Gastroesophageal resection and total gastrectomy in the treatment of bleeding varicose veins in Banti's syndrome. Ann Surg 125:397, 1947.
21. Mikkelsen W: Therapeutic portacaval shunt. Arch Surg 108:302–305, 1974.
22. Bell R, Miyai K, Orloff M: Outcome in cirrhotic patients with acute alcoholic hepatitis after emergency portacaval shunt for bleeding esophageal varices. Am J Surg 147:78–84, 1984.
23. Eckhauser F, Appelman H, O'Leary T: Hepatic pathology as a determinant of prognosis after portal decompression. Am J Surg 139:105–112, 1980.
24. Viamonte M, Warren W, Famon J: Angiographic investigations in portal hypertension. Surg Gynecol Obstet 130:37–53, 1970.
25. Huizinga W, Keenan J, Marszaley A: Sclerotherapy for bleeding esophageal varices. A case report. S Afr Med J 65:436–438, 1984.
26. Mikkelsen W, Turrill F, Kern W: Acute hyaline necrosis of the liver. A surgical trap. Am J Surg 116:266–272, 1968.
27. Seidman E, Neber A, Morin C: Spinal cord paralysis following sclerotherapy for esophageal varices. Hepatology 4:950–954, 1981.
28. Perakos P, Cirbus J, Camara D: Persistent bradyarrhythmia after sclerotherapy for esophageal varices. South Med J 77:531–532, 1984.
29. Lunderquist A, Vang J: Transhepatic catheterization and obliteration of the coronary vein in patients with portal hypertension and esophageal varices. N Engl J Med 291:646–649, 1974.
30. Abecossis M, Makowka L, Lanser B: Sclerotherapy for esophageal varices. Can J Surg 27:561–566, 1984.
31. Reynolds T: The role of hemodynamic measurements in portasystemic shunt surgery. Arch Surg 108:276–281, 1974.
32. Lebrec D, DeFleury P, Rueff B, et al: Portal hypertension, size of esophageal varices and risk of gastrointestinal bleeding in alcoholic cirrhosis. Gastroenterology 79:1139–1144, 1980.
33. Paquet K: Prophylactic endoscopic sclerosing treatment of the esophageal wall in varices—a prospective controlled randomized trial. Endoscopy 14:4–5, 1982.
34. Witzel L, Wolbergs E, Merki H: Prophylactic endoscopic sclerotherapy of esophageal varices. A prospective controlled study. Lancet 1:773–775, 1985.
35. The North Italian Endoscopic Club for the Study and Treatment of Esophageal Varices: Prediction of the first variceal hemorrhage in patients with cirrhosis of the liver and esophageal varices: A prospective multicenter trial. N Engl J Med 319:983–989, 1988.
36. Dagradi ZA: The natural history of esophageal varices in patients with alcoholic cirrhosis. Am J Gastroenterol 57:520–540, 1972.
37. Schenker S, Breen K, Hoyumpa A: Hepatic encephalopathy: Current status. Gastroenterology 66:121–151, 1974.
38. Fischer J, James J, Jeppsson B: Hyperammonemia, plasma amino acid imbalance and blood-brain amino acid transport. Lancet 2:772–778, 1979.
39. Fischer J, Furovics J, Folcao H: L-Dopa in hepatic coma. Ann Surg 183:386–391, 1976.
40. Waldram R, Davis M, Nunnerly H: Emergency endoscopy after gastrointestinal hemorrhage in 50 patients with portal hypertension. BMJ 4:94–96, 1974.
41. Maddrey W, Weber F: Chronic hepatic encephalopathy. Med Clin North Am 59:937–944, 1975.
42. Elkington S: Lactulose. Gut 11:1043–1048, 1970.
43. Bainbridge F, Trevan J: Some actions of adrenaline upon liver. J Physiol 51:460–468, 1917.
44. Graszmann R, Kravetz D, Bosch J: Nitroglycerin improves the hemodynamic response to vasopressin in portal hypertension. Hepatology 2:757–762, 1982.
45. Sirinek K, Thomford N: Isoproterenol in offsetting adverse effect of vasopressin in cirrhotic patients. Am J Surg 129:130–136, 1975.
46. Chandler J: Vasopressin and splanchnic shunting. Ann Surg 195:543–553, 1982.
47. Mols P, Hallemans R, Van Kuyk M: Hemodynamic effects of vasopressin alone and in combination with nitroprusside in patients with liver cirrhosis and portal hypertension. Ann Surg 199:176–181, 1984.
48. Gimson A, Westaby D, Hegarty J: A randomized trial of vasopressin and vasopressin plus nitroglycerin in the control of acute variceal hemorrhage. Hepatology 6:410–413, 1986.
49. Kravetz D, Bosch J, Teres J, et al: Comparison of intravenous somatostatin and vasopressin infusions in treatment of acute variceal hemorrhage. Hepatology 4:442–446, 1984.

50. Bosch J, Kravetz D, Rodes J: Effects of somatostatin on hepatic and systemic hemodynamics in patients with cirrhosis of the liver. Comparison with vasopressin. Gastroenterology 80:518–525, 1985.

51. Chan LY, Sung JJY: Review article: The role of pharmacotherapy for acute variceal hemorrhage in the era of endoscopic hemostasis. Aliment Pharmacol Ther 11:45–50, 1997.

52. Burroughs A, Jenkins W, Sherlock S: Controlled trial of propranolol for the prevention of recurrent variceal hemorrhage in patients with cirrhosis. N Engl J Med 309:1539–1542, 1983.

53. Fleig W, Stange E, Hunecke R, et al: Prevention of recurrent bleeding in cirrhotics with recent variceal hemorrhage: Prospective randomized comparison of propranolol and sclerotherapy. Hepatology 7:355–361, 1987.

54. Lebrec D, Poynard T, Hillani P: Propranolol for prevention of recurrent gastrointestinal bleeding in patients with cirrhosis. N Engl J Med 805:1371–1374, 1981.

55. Lebrec D, Bernjau J, Rueff B: Gastrointestinal bleeding after abrupt cessation of propranolol administration in cirrhosis. N Engl J Med 807:560, 1982.

56. Maringhini A, Simonetti R, Marceno M: Propranolol for gastrointestinal bleeding in cirrhosis. N Engl J Med 307:1710, 1982.

57. Poynard T, Lebrec D, Hillon P, et al: Propranolol for prevention of recurrent gastrointestinal bleeding in patients with cirrhosis: A prospective study of factors associated with rebleeding. Hepatology 7:447–451, 1987.

58. Edlich R, Lande A, Goodale R: Prevention of aspiration pneumonia by continuous esophageal aspiration during esophagogastric tamponade and gastric cooling. Surgery 67:405–408, 1968.

59. Burcharth F, Malmstrom J: Experience with the Linton-Nachlas and the Sengstaken-Blakemore tubes for bleeding esophageal varices. Surg Gynecol Obstet 142:529–531, 1976.

60. Bauer J, Kreel I, Kark A: The use of the Sengstaken-Blakemore tube for the control of bleeding esophageal varices. Ann Surg 179:273–277, 1974.

61. Hermann R, Traul D: Experience with the Sengstake-Blakemore tube for bleeding esophageal varices. Surg Gynecol Obstet 130:879–885, 1970.

62. Pitcher J: Safety and effectiveness of the modified Sengstaken-Blakemore tube: A prospective study. Gastroenterology 61:291–298, 1971.

63. Johnson W, Nabseth D, Widrich W: Bleeding esophageal varices. Ann Surg 195:893–400, 1982.

64. Conn H, Simpson J: Excessive mortality associated with balloon tamponade or bleeding varices. JAMA 202:135, 1967.

65. Eck N: On the question of ligature of the portal vein. Voyenno Med 130:1–2, 1877.

66. Warren W: Control of variceal bleeding. Reassessment of rationale. Am J Surg 145:8–16, 1983.

67. Whipple A: The problem of portal hypertension in relation to the hepatosplenopathies. Ann Surg 122:449–475, 1945.

68. Blakemore A, Lord JJ: The technique of using Vitallium tubes in establishing portacaval shunts for portal hypertension. Ann Surg 122:476–488, 1945.

69. Greig P, Langer B, Blendis L, et al: Complications of the peritoneovenous shunting for ascites. Am J Surg 139:125–131, 1980.

70. Conn H, Lindemuth: Prophylactic portacaval anastomosis in cirrhotic patients with esophageal varices: A progress report of a continuing study. N Engl J Med 272:1255–1263, 1965.

71. Conn H, Lindemuth W, May L, et al: Prophylactic portacaval anastomosis: A tale of two studies. Medicine (Baltimore) 51:27–40, 1972.

72. Resnick R, Chalmers T, Ishihara A: The Boston Interhospital Liver Group: A controlled study of the prophylactic portacaval shunt. A final report. Ann Intern Med 70:675–688, 1969.

73. Jackson F, Perrin E, Felix W, et al: A clinical investigation of the portacaval shunt. Ann Surg 174:672–701, 1971.

74. Resnick R, Iber F, Ishihara A, et al: A controlled study of the therapeutic portacaval shunt. Gastroenterology 67:843–857, 1974.

75. Reynolds T, Donovan A, Mikkelsen W, et al: Results of a 12-year randomized trial of portacaval shunt in patients with alcoholic liver disease and bleeding varices. Gastroenterology 80:1005–1011, 1981.

76. Rueff B, Prandi D, Degos F, et al: A controlled study of portacaval shunt in alcoholic cirrhosis. Lancet 1:655–659, 1976.

77. Conn H: Therapeutic portacaval anastomosis: To shunt or not to shunt. Gastroenterology 67:1065–1071, 1974.

78. Sarfeh I, Carter J, Welch H: Analysis of operative mortality after portal decompressive procedures in cirrhotic patients. Am J Surg 140:306–311, 1980.

79. Orloff M, Bell R, Hyde P, Skivolocki W: Long-term results of emergency portacaval shunt for bleeding esophageal varices in unselected patients with alcoholic cirrhosis. Ann Surg 192:325–340, 1980.

80. Villeneuve J, Pomier-Layrargues G, Duguay L, et al: Emergency portacaval shunt for variceal hemorrhage. A prospective study. Ann Surg 206:48–52, 1987.

81. LeVeen H, Wapnick S, Grosberg S, et al: Further experience with peritoneovenous shunt for ascites. Ann Surg 184:574–581, 1976.

82. Burchell A, Rousselot L, Panke W: A seven-year experience with side-to-side portacaval shunts for cirrhotic ascites. Ann Surg 168:655–670, 1968.

83. Turcotte J, Wallin V, Child C: End-to-side versus side-to-side portacaval shunts in patients with hepatic cirrhosis. Am J Surg 117:108–116, 1979.

84. Iwatsuki S, Mikkelsen W, Redeker A, et al: Clinical comparison of the end-to-side and side-to-side portacaval shunt. Ann Surg 178:65–69, 1973.

85. Blakemore W: The technique of portal systemic shunt surgery. Surgery 57:778–786, 1965.

86. Hermann R: Shunt operations for portal hypertension. Surg Clin North Am 55:1073–1087, 1975.

87. Maillard J, Rueff B, Prandi D: Hepatic arterialization and portacaval shunt in hepatic cirrhosis. Arch Surg 108:315–320, 1979.

88. Otte J, Reynaent M, Hemptinne B, et al: Arterialization of the portal vein in conjunction with a therapeutic portacaval shunt. Ann Surg 196:656–663, 1982.

89. Sarfeh I, Rypins E, Mason G: A systematic appraisal of portacaval H-graft diameters. Clinical and hemodynamic perspectives. Ann Surg 204:356–363, 1986.

90. Clatworthy H, Wall T, Watman R: A new trial of portal-to-systemic venous shunt for portal hypertension. Arch Surg 71:588, 1955.

91. Drapanas T, LoCicero J, Dowling J: Interposition meso-caval shunt for treatment of portal hypertension. Ann Surg 176:435, 1972.

92. Lord J, Rossi G, Daliana M, et al: Mesocaval shunt modified by the use of a Teflon prosthesis. Surg Gynecol Obstet 130:525–526, 1970.

93. Nay H, Fitzpatrick H: Mesocaval "H" graft using autogenous vein graft. Am Surg 183:114–119, 1976.

94. Read R, Thompson B, Wise W, et al: Mesocaval H venous homografts. Arch Surg 101:785, 1970.

95. Thompson B, Reed B, Casall R: Interposition grafting for portal hypertension. Am J Surg 130:733–739, 1975.

96. Drapanas T, LoCiciero J, Dowling J: Hemodynamics of the interposition mesocaval shunt. Ann Surg 181:523–532, 1975.

97. Smith R, Warren W, Salam A, et al: Dacron interposition shunts for portal hypertension. Ann Surg 92:9–17, 1980.

98. Fulenwider J, Nordlinger B, Millikan W: Portal pseudoperfusion: An angiographic illusion. Ann Surg 189:257, 1979.

99. Cargenas A, Busuttil R: A comparative analysis of the mesocaval H graft versus the distal splenorenal shunt. Curr Surg 39:151–157, 1982.

100. Malt R: Portasystemic venous shunts. N Engl J Med 295:80–86, 1976.

101. Cameron J, Zuidema G, Smith G, et al: Mesocaval shunts for the control of bleeding esophageal varices. Surgery 85:257–262, 1979.

102. Cameron J, Harrington D, Maddrey W: The mesocasval C shunt. Surg Gynecol Obstet 150:401, 1980.

103. Sarr M, Herlong H, Cameron J: Long-term patency of the mesocaval C shunt. Am J Surg 151:98–103, 1986.

104. Resnick R, Langer B, Taylor B, et al: Results and hemodynamic changes after interposition mesocaval shunt. Surgery 95:275–280, 1984.

105. Reichle F, Fahmy W, Golsorkhi M: Prospective comparative clinical trial with distal splenorenal and mesocaval shunts. Am J Surg 137:13–21, 1979.

106. Thompson B, Casall R, Reed R, et al: Results of interposition "H" grafts for portal hypertension. Ann Surg 187:515–522, 1978.

107. Mulcare R, Halleran D, Gardine R: Experience with 49 consecutive Dacron interposition mesocaval shunts. A unified approach to portasystemic decompression procedures. Am J Surg 147:393–399, 1984.

108. Linton R, Ellis D, Geary J: Critical comparative analysis of early and late results of splenorenal and direct portacaval shunts performed in 169 patients with portal cirrhosis. Ann Surg 154:446–449, 1961.

109. Pliam M, Adson M, Foulk W: Conventional splenorenal shunts. Arch Surg 110:588–599, 1975.

110. Bismuth H, Franco D, Hepp J: Portal-systemic shunt in hepatic cirrhosis: Does the type of shunt decisively influence the clinical result? Ann Surg 179:209–218, 1974.

111. Ottinger L: The Linton splenorenal shunt in the management of the bleeding complications of portal hypertension. Ann Surg 196:664–668, 1982.

112. Warren W, Zeppa R, Fomon J: Selective transsplenic decompression of gastroesophageal varices by distal splenorenal shunt. Ann Surg 166:431, 1967.

113. Langer B, Rotstein L, Stone R: A prospective randomized trial of the selective distal splenorenal shunt. Surg Gynecol Obstet 150:45–48, 1980.

114. Resnick R, Atterbury L, Grace N, et al: Distal splenorenal shunt versus portal systemic shunt: Current status of a controlled trial. Gastroenterology 77:433, 1979.

115. Harley H, Morgan T, Redeker A, et al: Results of a randomized trial of end-to-side portacaval shunt and distal splenorenal shunt in alcoholic liver disease and variceal bleeding. Gastroenterology 91:802–809, 1986.

116. Rikkers L, Rudman D, Galambos J: A randomized controlled trial of distal splenorenal shunt. Ann Surg 188:271–282, 1978.

117. Millikan W, Warren W, Henderson J, et al: The Emory prospective randomized trial: Selective versus nonselective shunt to control variceal bleeding. Ten year follow-up. Ann Surg 201:712–722, 1985.

118. Zeppa R, Hensley G, Levi J: The comparative survivals of alcoholics versus nonalcoholics with the distal splenorenal shunts. Ann Surg 187:510–514, 1978.

119. Busuttil R, Brin B, Tompkins R: Matched control study of distal splenorenal and portacaval shunts in the treatment of bleeding esophageal varices. Am J Surg 138:62–67, 1979.

120. Busuttil R: Selective and nonselective shunts for variceal bleeding. A prospective study of 103 patients. Am J Surg 148:27–35, 1984.

121. Hen R, Halbfass H, Rossle M, et al: Mesocaval and distal splenorenal shunts: Effect on hepatic function, hepatic hemodynamics, and portal systemic encephalopathy. Klin Wochenschr 63:409–413, 1985.

122. Adson M, Van Heerden J, Illstrup D: The distal splenorenal shunt. Arch Surg 119:609–614, 1984.

123. Busuttil R, Maywood B, Tompkins R: The Warren shunt in treating bleeding esophageal varices. West J Med 130:304–308, 1979.

124. Fulenwider J, Smith R, Millikan W, et al: Variceal hemorrhage in the veteran population. To shunt or not to shunt? Am Surg 50:264–269, 1984.

125. Lund R, Newkirk J: Peritoneovenous shunting system for surgical management of ascites. Contemp Surg 14:31–45, 1979.

126. Maksoud J, Mies S: Distal splenorenal shunt in children. Ann Surg 195:401–405, 1982.

127. Martin E, Molnar J, Cooperman M, et al: Observations on fifty distal splenorenal shunts. Surgery 84:379–383, 1978.

128. Mosimman R, Loup P: Efficacy and risks of the distal splenorenal shunt in the treatment of bleeding esophageal varices. Am J Surg 133:163–168, 1977.

129. Silver D, Puckett C, McNeer J: Evaluation of selective transsplenic decompression of gastroesophageal varices. Am J Surg 127:30–34, 1974.

130. Warren W, Millikan W, Henderson J: Ten years of portal hypertension surgery at Emory. Ann Surg 195:530–542, 1982.

131. Warren W, Henderson J, Millikan W, et al: Management of variceal bleeding in patients with non-cirrhotic portal vein thrombosis. Ann Surg 207:623–634, 1988.

131a. Warren W, Henderson J, Millikan W, et al: Splenopancreatic disconnection. Improved selectivity of distal splenorenal shunt. Ann Surg 204:346–355, 1986.

132. Warren W, Millikan W: Selective transsplenic decompression procedure: Changes in technique after 300 cases. Contemp Surg 18:11–29, 1981.

133. Henderson J, Millikan W, Chippani J: The incidence and natural history of thrombus in the portal vein following distal splenorenal shunt. Ann Surg 196:1–7, 1982.

134. Rousselot L: The role of congestion (portal hypertension) in so-called Banti's syndrome: A clinical and pathological study of thirty-one cases with late results following splenectomy. JAMA 107:1788–1793, 1936.

135. Thompson W: The pathogenesis of Banti's disease. Ann Intern Med 14:255–262, 1940.

136. Pemberton J, Kiernan P: Surgery of the spleen. Surg Clin North Am 25:880–890, 1945.

137. Suguira M, Futagawa S: A new technique for treating esophageal varices. J Thorac Cardiovasc Surg 66:677–685, 1973.

138. Strauch G: Supradiaphragmatic splenic transposition. Am J Surg 119:379–384, 1970.

139. McClelland R, Bashour F: Supradiaphragmatic transposition of the spleen in portal hypertension. Arch Surg 98:175–179, 1969.

140. Peters R, Womack N: Surgery of vascular distortions in cirrhosis of the liver. Ann Surg 154:432, 1961.

141. Keagy B, Schwartz J, Johnson G: Should ablative operations be used for bleeding esophageal varices? Ann Surg 203:463–469, 1986.

142. Boerema I: Surgical therapy of bleeding varices of esophagus during hepatic cirrhosis and Banti's disease. Ned Tijdschr Geneeskd 93:4174–4182, 1949.

143. Crile GJ: Transesophageal ligation of bleeding esophageal varices. Arch Surg 61:654–660, 1950.

144. Wirthlin L, Linton R, Ellis D: Transthoracoesophageal ligation of bleeding esophageal varices. Arch Surg 109:688–692, 1974.

145. Wexler M: Treatment of bleeding esophageal varices by transabdominal esophageal transection with the EEA stapling instrument. Surgery 88:406–416, 1980.

146. Cooperman M, Fabri P, Martin E, et al: EEA esophageal stapling for control of bleeding varices. Am J Surg 140:821–824, 1980.

147. Delaney J: A method for esophagogastric devascularization. Surg Gynecol Obstet 150:899–900, 1980.

148. Suguira M, Futagawa S: Further evaluation of the Suguira procedure in the treatment of esophageal varices. Arch Surg 112:1317–1321, 1977.

149. Koyarna K, Takagi Y, Ouchi K, et al: Results of esophageal transection for esophageal varices. Am J Surg 139:204–209, 1980.

150. Suguira M, Futagawa S: Results of six hundred thirty-six esophageal transections with paraesophagogastric devascularization in the treatment of esophageal varices. J Vasc Surg 1:254–260, 1984.

151. Superina R, Weber J, Shandling B: A modified Suguira operation for bleeding varices in children. J Pediatr Surg 18:794–799, 1983.

152. Weese J, Starling J, Yale C: Control of bleeding esophageal varices by transabdominal esophageal transection, gastric devascularization and splenectomy. Surg Gastroenterol 3:31–36, 1984.

153. Wanamaker S, Cooperman M, Carey L: Use of the EEA stapling instrument for control of bleeding esophageal varices. Surgery 94:620–626, 1983.

154. Wexler M: Esophageal procedures to control bleeding from varices. Surg Clin North Am 63:905–914, 1983.

155. Spence R, Anderson J, Johnston G: Twenty-five years of injection sclerotherapy for bleeding varices. Br J Surg 72:195–198, 1985.

156. Huizinga W, Angorn I, Baker L: Esophageal transection versus injection sclerotherapy in the management of bleeding esophageal varices in patients of high risk. Surg Gynecol Obstet 160:539–546, 1985.

157. Colapinto R, Stronell R, Birch S, et al: Creation of an intrahepatic portosystemic shunt with a Gruntzig balloon catheter. Can Med Assoc J 126:267–268, 1982.

158. Roberts J, Ring E, Lake J, et al: Intrahepatic portacaval shunt for variceal hemorrhage prior to liver transplantation. Transplantation 1;52:160–162, 1991.

159. Richter G, Noeledge G, Palmaz J, Roessle M: The transjugular intrahepatic portosystemic stent-shunt (TIPSS): Results of a pilot study. Cardiovasc Int Radiol 13:200–207, 1990.

160. LaBerge JM, Ring E, Lake J, et al: Transjugular intrahepatic portosystemic shunts: Preliminary results in 25 patients. J Vasc Surg 16:258–267, 1992.

161. Conn H: Transjugular intrahepatic portal-systemic shunts: The state of the art. Hepatology 17:148–158, 1993.

162. Grace N: The side-to-side portacaval shunt revisited. N Engl J Med 330:208–209, 1994.

163. Shiffman M, Jeffers L, Hoofnagle J, Tralka T: The role of transjugular intrahepatic shunt (TIPS) for treatment of portal hypertension and its complications. Hepatology 22:1591–1597, 1995.

164. Iwatsuki S, Starzl T, Todo S, et al: Liver transplantation in the treatment of bleeding esophageal varices. Surgery 104:697–705, 1988.

165. Reyes J, Iwatsuki S: Current management of portal hypertension with liver transplantation. Adv Surg 25:189–208, 1992.

166. Brems J, Hiatt J, Klein A, et al: Effect of a prior portasystemic shunt on subsequent liver transplantation. Ann Surg 209:51–56, 1989.

167. Crafoord C, Frenckner P: New surgical treatment of varicose veins of the esophagus. Acta Otolaryngol 27:422, 1939.

168. Johnston G, Rodgers H: A review of 15 years experience in the use of sclerotherapy in the control acute hemorrhage for esophageal varices. Br J Surg 60:797–799, 1973.

169. Paquet K, Kalk J, Koussouris P: Immediate endoscopic sclerosis of bleeding esophageal varices: A prospective evaluation over 5 years. Surg Endosc 2:18–23, 1988.

170. Schubert T, Smith O, Kirkpatrick S, et al: Improved survival in variceal hemorrhage with emergent sclerotherapy. Am J Gastroenterol 82:1134–1137, 1987.

171. Terblanche J, Northover J, Bornman P, et al: A prospective evaluation of injection sclerotherapy in the treatment of acute bleeding esophageal varices. Surgery 85:239–245, 1979.

172. Terblanche J, Yakoob H, Bornman P, et al: Acute bleeding varices: A five-year prospective evaluation of tamponade and sclerotherapy. Ann Surg 194:521–529, 1981.

173. Paquet K, Feussner H: Endoscopic sclerosis and esophageal balloon tamponade in acute hemorrhage from esophagogastric varices: A prospective controlled randomized trial. Hepatology 5:580–583, 1985.

174. Larson A, Cohen H, Zweiban B, et al: Acute esophageal variceal sclerotherapy: Results of a prospective randomized controlled trial. JAMA 255:497–500, 1986.

175. Barsoum M, Bolous F, El-Rooby A, et al: Tamponade and injection sclerotherapy in the management of bleeding oesophageal varices. Br J Surg 69:76–78, 1982.

176. Project CEVS: Sclerotherapy after first variceal hemorrhage in cirrhosis. A randomized multicenter trial. N Engl J Med 311:1594–1600, 1984.

177. Westaby D, MacDougall B, Williams R: Improved survival following injection sclerotherapy for esophageal varices: Final analysis of a controlled trial. Hepatology 5:827–830, 1985.

178. Terblanche J, Bornman P, Kahn D, et al: Failure of repeated injection sclerotherapy to improve long term survival after esophageal variceal bleeding. A five year prospective controlled clinical trial. Lancet 2:1328–1332, 1983.

179. Soderlund C, Ihre T: Endoscopic sclerotherapy v. conservative management of bleeding oesophageal varices. Acta Chir Scand 151:449–156, 1985.

180. Korula J, Balart L, Radvan G, et al: A prospective randomized controlled trial of chronic esophageal variceal sclerotherapy. Hepatology 5:584–589, 1985.

181. Cello J, Grendell J, Crass R, et al: Endoscopic sclerotherapy versus portacaval shunt in patients with severe cirrhosis and variceal hemorrhage. N Engl J Med 311:1589–1594, 1984.

182. Cello J, Grendell J, Crass R, et al: Endoscopic sclerotherapy versus portacaval shunt in patients with severe cirrhosis and acute variceal hemorrhage. Long-term follow-up. N Engl J Med 316:11–15, 1987.

183. Warren W, Henderson J, Millikan W, et al: Distal splenorenal shunt versus endoscopic sclerotherapy for long-term management of variceal bleeding. Preliminary report of a prospective, randomized trial. Ann Surg 203:454–462, 1986.

184. Teres J, Bordas J, Bravo D, et al: Sclerotherapy vs. distal splenorenal shunt in the elective treatment of variceal hemorrhage: A randomized controlled trial. Hepatology 7:430–436, 1987.

185. Rikkers L, Burnett D, Volentine G, et al: Shunt surgery versus endoscopic sclerotherapy for long-term treatment of variceal bleeding. Early results of a randomized trial. Ann Surg 206:261–271, 1987.

186. Burroughs A, Hamilton G, Phillips A, et al: A comparison of sclerotherapy with staple transection of the esophagus for the emergency control of bleeding from esophageal varices. N Engl J Med 321:857–862, 1989.

187. Teres J, Baroni R, Bordas M, et al: Randomized trial of portacaval shunt, stapling transection and endoscopic sclerotherapy in uncontrolled variceal bleeding. J Hepatol 4:159–167, 1987.

188. Terblanche J, Bornman P, Kirsch R: Sclerotherapy for bleeding esophageal varices. Annu Rev Med 35:83–94, 1984.

189. Yassin Y, Sherif S: Randomized controlled trial of injection sclerotherapy for bleeding esophageal varices. Br J Surg 70:20–22, 1983.

190. Reilly J, Schade R, Roh M, et al: Esophageal variceal sclerosis. Surg Gynecol Obstet 155:497–502, 1982.

191. Palani L, Abvabara S, Kraft A, et al: Endoscopic sclerotherapy in acute variceal hemorrhage. Am J Surg 141:164–168, 1981.

192. Lewis J, Chung R, Allison J: Sclerotherapy of esophageal varices. Arch Surg 115:476–480, 1980.

193. Johnston G: Bleeding esophageal varices: The management of shunt rejects. Ann R Coll Surg Engl 63:3–8, 1981.

194. Goodale R, Silvis S, O'Leary J, et al: Early survival for bleeding esophageal varices. Surg Gynecol Obstet 155:523–528, 1982.

195. Lewis J, Chung R, Allison J: Injection sclerotherapy for control of acute variceal hemorrhage. Am J Surg 142:592–595, 1981.

196. Cohen L, Rorsten M, Scherl E, et al: Bacteremia after endoscopic injection sclerosis. Gastrointest Endosc 29:198–200, 1983.

197. Bacon A, Bauley-Newton R, Connors A: Pleural effusions after endoscopic variceal sclerotherapy. Gastroenterology 88:1910–1914, 1985.

198. Tripodis S, Buenskin A, Wenser J: Gastric ulcers after endoscopic sclerosis of esophageal varices. J Clin Gastroenterol 7:77–79, 1985.

199. Laine L, Cook D: Endoscopic ligation compared with sclerotherapy for treatment of esophageal varicela bleeding. A meta-analysis. Ann Intern Med 123:280–287, 1995.

200. Stanley M: Treatment of intractable ascites in patients with alcoholic cirrhosis by peritoneovenous (LeVeen) shunting. Med Clin North Am 63:523–536, 1979.

201. Frakes J: Physiologic considerations in the medical management of ascites. Arch Intern Med 140:620–623, 1980.

202. LeVeen H, Christovadias G, Ip M, et al: Peritoneovenous shunting for ascites. Ann Surg 180:580, 1974.

203. Harman D, Demirjian Z, Ellman L, et al: Disseminated intravascular coagulation with the peritoneovenous shunt. Ann Intern Med 90:774–776, 1979.

204. Reinhardt G, Stanley M: Peritoneovenous shunting for ascites. Surg Gynecol Obstet 145:419–424, 1977.

205. Epstein M: Peritoneovenous shunt in the management of ascites and the hepatorenal syndrome. Gastroenterology 82:790–799, 1982.

206. Fullen W: Hepatorenal syndrome: Reversal by peritoneovenous shunt. Surgery 83:337–341, 1977.

207. Noldge G, Richter G, Rossle M, et al: Morphologic and clinical results of the transjugular intrahepatic portosystemic stent-shunt (TIPSS). Cardiovasc Intervent Radiol 15:342–348, 1992.

208. LaBerge JM, Ring E, Gordon R, et al: Creation of transjugular intrahepatic portosystemic shunts with the Wallstent endoprosthesis: Results in 100 patients. Radiology 187:413–420, 1993.

209. Helton W, Belshaw A, Althaus S, et al: Critical appraisal of the angiographic portacaval shunt (TIPS). Am J Surg 165:566–571, 1993.

210. Simpson K, Chalmers N, Redhead D, et al: Transjugular intrahepatic portasystemic stent shunting for control of acute and recurrent upper gastrointestinal hemorrhage related to portal hypertension. Gut 34:968–973, 1993.

211. Rossle M, Haag K, Ochs A, et al: The transjugular intrahepatic portosystemic stent shunt procedure for variceal bleeding. N Engl J Med 330:165–171, 1994.

212. Jalan R, Redhead D, Simpson K, et al: Transjugular intrahepatic portosystemic stent shunt (TIPSS): Long-term follow-up. Q J Med 87:565–573, 1994.

Questions

1. A 35-year-old woman with a history of viral hepatitis and cirrhosis, status postcholecystectomy, has a clinical presentation of variceal hemorrhage unresponsive to medical therapy. Which surgical procedure is indicated if sclerotherapy fails?
   (a) end-to-side portacaval shunt
   (b) side-to-side portacaval shunt
   (c) H-graft mesocaval shunt
   (d) EEA abdominal esophageal transection
   (e) distal splenorenal shunt

2. A 10-year-old boy with a history of omphalitis experiences his first episode of variceal hemorrhage. Which is the most appropriate therapy?
   (a) distal splenorenal shunt
   (b) medical regimen

(c) variceal sclerotherapy
(d) end-to-side portacaval shunt
(e) H-graft mesocaval shunt

3. Specific contraindications to peritoneovenous shunts include all of the following except
   (a) hepatic necrosis
   (b) bilirubin greater than 6
   (c) hepatorenal syndrome
   (d) infected ascitic fluid
   (e) prothrombin time more than 4 seconds prolonged

4. Prophylactic portacaval shunts have been shown to
   (a) prolong longevity
   (b) decrease encephalopathy
   (c) have a greater than 50% recurrent hemorrhage rate
   (d) be associated with a prohibitively high operative mortality
   (e) not be indicated

5. The Budd-Chiari syndrome may be treated by all of the following except
   (a) anticoagulants
   (b) side-to-side portacaval shunt
   (c) end-to-side portacaval shunt
   (d) mesoatrial shunt
   (e) mesocaval shunt

6. Technical considerations in favor of performing a distal splenorenal shunt include
   (a) cavernomatous transformation of the splenic vein
   (b) acute hyaline necrosis
   (c) splenic vein greater than 4 mm in diameter
   (d) intractable ascites
   (e) hepatopetal flow

7. False statements regarding sclerotherapy include
   (a) percutaneous transhepatic coronary vein occlusion is associated with a 20% portal vein thrombosis rate
   (b) sclerotherapy should not be used in the acute setting because of a higher mortality

(c) sodium morrhuate and ethanolamine oleate are appropriate sclerosing agents
(d) repeated sclerotherapy is necessary for control of hemorrhage
(e) esophageal ulcerations usually resolve spontaneously without sequelae

8. Advantages of selective shunts are
   (a) continued portal perfusion
   (b) gastric and esophageal varix decompression
   (c) no greater incidence of shunt thrombosis than with portacaval shunts
   (d) decreased incidence of encephalopathy
   (e) all of the above

9. A 40-year-old man has hematemesis and hypotension. Initial diagnostic measures to be performed after stabilization include
   (a) superior mesenteric arteriography
   (b) splenoportography
   (c) esophagogastroscopy
   (d) celiac angiogram with venous phase
   (e) upper gastrointestinal series

10. The most common site(s) of obstruction causing portal hypertension in the Western world is/are
    (a) portal vein thrombosis
    (b) extrahepatic postsinusoidal
    (c) intrahepatic presinusoidal
    (d) intrahepatic sinusoidal and postsinusoidal
    (e) extrahepatic presinusoidal

11. A 40-year-old man with cirrhosis is a Child's A candidate; his bleeding has been controlled with sclerotherapy and vasopressin. The most appropriate treatment plan would be
    (a) emergency shunt surgery
    (b) a Warren shunt
    (c) a mesocaval shunt
    (d) a TIPS shunt procedure
    (e) periodic sclerotherapy

Answers _____

1. c   2. b   3. c   4. e   5. c   6. e   7. b   8. e   9. c   10. d   11. e

41

Venous Thromboembolic Disease

Lazar J. Greenfield

The critical connection between venous thrombosis and pulmonary thromboembolism was made by Virchow in 1856. He not only proved by experimental studies that venous thrombi would embolize to the lungs but also defined the triad of mechanisms by which intravascular thrombosis could occur. This triad remains the basis of our understanding of the disorder and consists of stasis, vessel wall injury, and hypercoagulability of the blood. The importance of the disorder is reflected in the estimates of the development of deep venous thrombosis (DVT) in more than 500,000 hospital patients in the United States each year and a mortality rate of more than 50,000 deaths per year from pulmonary thromboembolism. Hull and Pineo[1] have shown that the cost of hospitalization alone is more than $207,000 per 100 patients treated for DVT. Of the patients who survive DVT, more than half develop chronic venous insufficiency with disabling edema and potential stasis ulcerations, representing a costly outcome in terms of lost productivity and demands on health care services. In the older patient with "idiopathic" DVT, the likelihood is increased that this presentation represents the first manifestation of a hidden malignancy as originally described by Trousseau.[2–5] In some tumors this prothrombotic state is due to the elaboration of tissue factor, which may either activate procoagulant proteins or stimulate the release of a protease from circulating blood cells, thus activating the coagulation cascade.[6, 7]

In postoperative and post-trauma patients, stasis is probably the most important and most treatable of the etiologic factors. When venous contrast medium is injected into the feet of supine immobilized patients, it may remain in soleal vein valvular sinuses for as long as an hour. This is the favored location for the formation of a nidus of thrombus. The original thrombus may become attached to the opposite wall, causing interruption of flow, retrograde thrombosis, and signs of venous stasis in the extremity. Subsequent edema formation within the confines of the deep muscular fascia produces pain. However, the thrombus may propagate without interrupting flow and develop a long floating "tail" that is highly susceptible to breaking loose from its tenuous anchor within the valvular sinus. This sequence of events is the most dangerous aspect of the disorder because major pulmonary embolism can occur without premonitory signs or symptoms at its point of origin.

The site of venous obstruction determines the level at which swelling is observed clinically. Swelling at the thigh level always implies obstruction at the level of the iliofemoral system, whereas swelling of the calf or foot suggests obstruction at the femoropopliteal level. Thrombi more commonly originate in the soleal veins and then propagate proximally in 20% to 30% of cases.[8, 9] Evidence also exists of primary thrombosis of femoral and iliac venous tributaries.

In addition to stasis, hypercoagulability must be considered a causative factor. Earlier efforts to find differences in coagulation factors among patients with or without DVT were unrewarding, but a naturally occurring inhibitor of activated factor X exists, called antithrombin III. Congenital deficiency in antithrombin III levels predisposes patients to venous thrombosis and pulmonary embolism, and similar susceptibility occurs with deficiencies of protein C, protein S, or heparin cofactor II. Factor V Leiden has also been recognized among the prothrombotic factors predisposing to venous thromboembolism, being found in 40% of patients undergoing a hypercoagulability evaluation after an episode of DVT.[10] Other unexplained hypercoagulable states seem to be associated with recent trauma, major surgical procedures, and sepsis. When stasis develops, the substances that promote platelet aggregation, including activated factor X, thrombin, fibrin, and catecholamines, remain at a high concentration in a particular area. This leads to platelet aggregation, which initiates coagulation and thrombin generation with release of adenosine diphosphate (ADP), which further aggregates platelets as the fibrin complex propagates. Opposing this process is the fibrinolytic system of the blood and vein walls. The endothelium of the vein wall contains an activator that converts plasminogen to plasmin, which lyses fibrin. As might be expected, however, the fibrinolytic system is inhibited after surgery and trauma, and less activity occurs in the veins of the lower extremity than in the upper extremity. Inadequate fibrinolytic activity has been associated with both adequate levels of nonfunctioning plasminogen and low levels of adequately functioning plasminogen.[11] The third major causative factor of Virchow's triad, vessel wall damage, usually is not demonstrable in areas of thrombosis. Obesity, aging, and malignancy also increase the risk of developing DVT by mechanisms that are not well understood.

DIAGNOSIS

Major venous thrombosis involving the deep venous system of the thigh and pelvis produces a characteristic but nonspecific clinical picture of pain, extensive pitting edema, and blanching that has been termed "phlegmasia alba dolens." Association with pregnancy may derive from hormonal effects on blood, relaxation of vessel walls, or mechanical compression of the left iliac vein at the pelvic brim, giving rise to the term "milk leg of pregnancy." Investigators originally believed that the blanching was due to spasm and compromise of arterial flow, but the subcutaneous edema is responsible for the blanching. In addition to pregnancy, mechanical factors that can affect the left iliac vein include compression from the right iliac artery or an overdistended bladder and congenital webs within the vein. These factors are responsible for the observed 4:1 preponderance of left versus right iliac vein involvement.

With further progression of venous thrombosis to impede most of the venous return from the extremity, danger of limb loss occurs from cessation of arterial flow. The clinical picture is characteristic, with sufficient congestion to produce phlegmasia cerulea dolens, or a painful blue leg. With the loss of sensory or motor function, venous gangrene is likely unless blood flow is restored. A variant of this disorder occurs peripherally in the leg and is associated with concurrent malignant disease and a high mortality rate.

As indicated earlier, these major complications affect less than 10% of patients with venous thrombosis. In fact, only 40% of patients with venous thrombosis have any clinical signs of the disorder. False-positive clinical signs occur in up to 50% of patients studied. Because of this, a great deal of interest exists in the development of better diagnostic tests. Of course, contrast venography provides direct evidence of both occlusive and nonocclusive thrombi, but it is invasive, may result in an allergic reaction to the contrast material, and requires movement of the patient to a radiographic suite. In addition, interobserver disagreement occurs regarding interpretation of the study in 10% of cases, and in an additional 5%, the study is not technically possible or the result is not diagnostic.[12]

Duplex Examination

The Doppler probe can be used at the bedside to detect major venous thrombi with a high degree of accuracy, but it is a subjective form of testing dependent on the examiner's

experience. The principle is straightforward and is based on the impairment of an accelerated flow signal produced by intraluminal thrombi. The examination begins at the ankle with identification of the posterior tibial vein signal adjacent to the artery. The flow signal should be altered by distal and proximal compression producing, respectively, augmentation and interruption of flow. The same maneuvers are repeated over the superficial and deep femoral veins and can be done over the popliteal vein. Failure to augment flow on compression below or release of interruption of flow above the probe suggests venous thrombi. The sensitivity of the test exceeds 90%, but the specificity is 5% to 10% lower owing to the interference with venous flow by other mechanical problems (e.g., Baker's cyst, hematoma). A negative Doppler ultrasound examination is reassuring, but a positive or equivocal test should be confirmed by B mode ultrasound imaging. A negative test is not reassuring when thromboembolism is suspected, because the thrombus may have embolized from the extremity.

Real-time B mode ultrasonography to visualize extremity veins has gained wide acceptance and offers a more direct technique to visualize intraluminal thrombus noninvasively.[13] Valvular movement and accelerated blood flow can be visualized in the presence of a partially obstructing thrombus. When pressure is applied by the probe, normal vein walls are easily compressed, but resistance to compression is noted when a thrombus is present, increasing with increased age of the thrombus. Chronic thrombi are characterized by greater echogenicity, heterogeneity, and an irregular surface. The addition of color to the duplex scan has increased the sensitivity and specificity of the study in symptomatic patients with proximal DVT to 96% and 100%, respectively, with a negative predictive value of 98% and accuracy of 99%.[14–16] Color-flow Doppler scanning has also improved the sensitivity and specificity of ultrasound scanning when used as a screening test in asymptomatic patients, even when used for distal veins. Acceptance of this technique has reduced the need for venography.

Plethysmography

Impedance plethysmography measures the volume response of the extremity to temporary occlusion of the venous system. The diagnosis of venous thrombosis depends on the changes in venous capacitance and rate of emptying after release of the occlusion. A proximal thigh cuff is inflated until maximum filling has occurred by plateau of the electrical signal and then deflated, allowing rapid outflow and reduction of volume. Prolongation of the outflow wave suggests major venous thrombosis with 95% accuracy. The deficiency with this technique, as with all of the noninvasive methods, is in its detection of calf vein thrombosis or the definition of new abnormalities in patients with old post-thrombotic sequelae. This test is limited to patients who can cooperate with the requirements and bear weight on the extremity. The strain gauge plethysmograph can also be used to make therapeutic decisions in the absence of clinical conditions that can produce false-positive results, such as cardiac failure, constrictive pericarditis, hypotension, arterial insufficiency, or external compression of veins.

Air plethysmography is a noninvasive technique that measures absolute limb blood volume change. It provides quantification of venous reflux, muscle pump action, venous capacitance, and noninvasive ambulatory venous pressure, thus providing a useful index of the severity of venous disease. It is used primarily to quantitate chronic venous insufficiency.

Venography

The injection of contrast material for direct visualization of the venous system is the most accurate method of confirming the diagnosis of venous thrombosis and the extent of the involvement. Injection is usually made into the foot while the superficial veins are occluded by a tourniquet. A supplementary injection into the femoral veins may be required to visualize the iliofemoral system. Both filling defects and nonvisualization can be found and provide an assessment of the threat of a thrombus, such as one seen to be floating free and extending into the iliofemoral system. This finding has been associated with a greatly increased risk of thromboembolism despite anticoagulation.[17] Potential false-positive examinations may result from external compression of a vein or washout of the contrast material from collateral veins.

Assay of Fibrin and Fibrinogen Products

The degradation of intravascular fibrin can be detected by measuring the plasma products of the lysis of fibrin or fibrinogen. Both fibrinopeptide A and fibrin fragment E can be detected by radioimmunoassay, but these are not specific for acute venous thrombosis. A negative test result could conceivably have some value in ruling out the diagnosis, but the tests are difficult and require more investigation and simplification. D-dimers or cross-linked degradation products serve as markers for the action of plasmin on fibrin. When used in conjunction with clinical assessment, proximal and distal sensitivities are 98.4% and 90.5%, respectively, and negative predictive values are 99.3% and 98.6%.[18] Thrombin-antithrombin III (TAT) complexes in plasma are correlated with activation of coagulation. These factors lack specificity as indicators of thromboembolic disease but, if sensitive enough, may be useful in ruling out DVT in certain subgroups.[19, 20]

PROPHYLAXIS

In theory, the formation of venous thrombi should be prevented either by eliminating or reducing venous stasis or by altering blood coagulability. The belief that early ambulation prevents stasis and reduces the formation of thrombi has been controversial and is not supported by studies using tagged fibrinogen. However, in patients younger than 40 years old with no additional risk factors,

it is adequate.[21] The benefit may be lost if patients sit with the legs dependent, resulting in greater stasis.

Considerable interest has developed in the prophylactic use of anticoagulant drugs and antiplatelet drugs such as aspirin. Strong data support the use of preoperative oral anticoagulation therapy with coumarin derivatives in high-risk patients. Unfortunately, this increases the risk of hemorrhage, and with the added difficulties of laboratory control of prothrombin time, the approach has not been widely accepted except by some orthopedic surgeons doing elective arthroplasty. Fixed "minidose" warfarin is both safe and efficacious in various surgical and medical patients, especially women with breast cancer receiving chemotherapy via central venous lines. This regimen offers protection against thromboembolism without the risks of hemorrhage or the cost of laboratory monitoring.[22–25] Dextran is rarely used due to the associated risks of allergic reaction, hemorrhage, or congestive failure.

In an effort to minimize the problems associated with anticoagulant prophylaxis, the current recommendation is to use heparin before and after surgery in doses that do not alter the laboratory clotting profile. Generally, a 5000-unit dose is given subcutaneously 2 hours preoperatively and then every 12 hours postoperatively for 5 days. This treatment provides protection for most high-risk patients, with the exception of trauma victims or those undergoing orthopedic or urologic procedures. The beneficial effect may be due to the enhancement of heparin cofactor (antithrombin III) as a natural inhibitor of activated factor X. Kakkar and colleagues[26] showed protection against fatal pulmonary embolism in a randomized series of 4121 patients, as well as against DVT. Low-molecular-weight heparins are Food and Drug Administration (FDA) approved for several prophylactic indications, including elective orthopedic procedures and abdominal surgery in patients with malignancy. Indications are currently being sought for trauma and medical admissions. Doses differ for each compound and are based on anti-Xa units.[27]

Three factors need to be considered when choosing a method of prophylaxis: the age of the patient, the number of inherent risk factors, and the length of the surgical procedure. For the general population of surgical patients younger than 40 years, the risk of DVT is low, and prophylaxis can be limited to early ambulation with or without graduated compression stockings. For patients older than 40 years who are undergoing major surgical procedures, the risk is moderate, and prophylaxis, such as intermittent pneumatic compression or low-dose heparin administered subcutaneously twice daily, should be considered. The patients at highest risk (age older than 40 years and obese, with malignant disease, history of DVT, or major trauma) need more protection, which might include low-dose heparin, sequential intermittent pneumatic compression, oral anticoagulants, dextran, or a combination of methods. Low-dose heparin should not be used in neurosurgical patients because of the consequences of intracranial bleeding. For these patients, external pneumatic compression is the prophylaxis of choice. Specific and detailed recommendations based on the best available evidence are summarized by Guyatt and coauthors.[21]

As experience with use of the Greenfield vena caval filter has grown and percutaneous insertion has been facilitated by a 12-French carrier system, interest has increased in the prophylactic use of this device in high-risk patients who have additional risks from anticoagulants.[28–32]

TREATMENT

Management of the patient with DVT must attempt to minimize the risk of pulmonary embolism, limit further thrombosis, and facilitate resolution of existing thrombi to avoid the post-thrombotic syndrome. The patient may initially be placed on bed rest, with the foot of the bed elevated 8 to 10 inches. Pain, swelling, and tenderness generally resolve over a 5- to 7-day period with anticoagulation. Ambulation with continued elastic stocking support can be permitted. Standing still and sitting should be prohibited to avoid increased venous pressure and stasis.

Anticoagulation

The foundation of therapy for DVT is adequate anticoagulation, initially with heparin and then with coumarin derivatives for prolonged protection against recurrent thrombosis. Unless specific contraindications exist, heparin should be administered in an initial dose of 100 to 150 units/kg intravenously. The patient should reach the therapeutic range within the first 24 hours, with an activated partial thromboplastin time of 1.5 to 2.0 times the laboratory control. At these levels, bleeding complications are minimized. Heparin is an acid mucopolysaccharide that neutralizes thrombin, inhibits thromboplastin, and reduces the platelet release reaction. It may be administered by continuous or intermittent intravenous doses regulated by activated partial thromboplastin clotting time. Continuous intravenous infusion regulated by an infusion pump seems to minimize the total dose required for control and is associated with a lower incidence of complications.

The low-molecular-weight heparins (LMWHs) have also been used to treat thromboembolic disease. Early animal studies indicated that the LMWH fractions that are derived from standard heparin retained their ability to inhibit factor Xa while producing less bleeding. They also have a longer biologic half-life, making them an attractive alternative to unfractionated heparin. Because LMWH has a predictably high bioavailability, these agents can be administered by once- or twice-daily subcutaneous injections. Dosing differs among agents but is weight adjusted. Patients who are ambulatory at the time of diagnosis have been successfully managed in an outpatient setting, which is extremely cost-effective.[33–38]

The side effects associated with heparin treatment include bleeding, thrombocytopenia, hypersensitivity, arterial thromboembolism, and osteoporosis. Bleeding is more likely to occur in elderly women, in patients treated with aspirin, or in patients after recent surgery or trauma. Bleeding can occur when the results of laboratory monitoring tests are within the therapeutic range, which may be due to the effect of heparin on platelets.

Arterial thromboembolism can complicate heparin administration by any route and is more common in the elderly. It tends to occur after 7 to 10 days of therapy and is associated with thrombocytopenia. This complication carries high morbidity and mortality rates and requires immediate cessation of heparin treatment. Thrombocytopenia is due to an immunoreaction and is rapidly reversed when heparin is stopped, usually within 2 days. Hypersensitivity to heparin may take the form of a skin rash or, rarely, may produce anaphylaxis. Subcutaneous injections that show urticaria may become necrotic as an unusual form of sensitivity. Osteoporosis has been noted in patients on long-term heparin therapy in excess of 6 months. It is probably due to a direct effect on bone resorption and can be avoided by shorter periods of treatment and dosage less than 15,000 units/day.

Oral administration of anticoagulants is begun shortly after initiation of heparin therapy, because several days usually are required to bring the prothrombin time to an international normalized ratio (INR) of 2.0 to 3.0. Using a maintenance dose rather than a larger loading dose when initiating therapy is also preferable to avoid suppression of the natural anticoagulant, protein C. The coumarin derivatives block the synthesis of several clotting factors, and prolongation of the prothrombin time beyond the range suggested is associated with a high incidence of bleeding complications. Nonhemorrhagic side effects are uncommon but include skin necrosis, dermatitis, and a syndrome of painful erythema in areas of large amounts of subcutaneous fat. Most changes are reversible if the drug is stopped. Also, the administration of fresh-frozen plasma usually restores the prothrombin time. After an episode of acute DVT, anticoagulation should be maintained for a minimum of 3 months; some investigators favor 6 months for thrombi in the larger veins or after a second thromboembolic event. Many drugs alter the pharmacodynamics of warfarin (Coumadin), as do some foods that have high levels of vitamin K, by altering its metabolic clearance, rate of absorption, or inhibition of vitamin K–dependent coagulation factor synthesis or altering other hemostatic factors. Phenylbutazone, sulfinpyrazone, disulfiram, metronidazole, and trimethoprim-sulfamethoxazole all potentiate warfarin's action.[29] Therefore, a routine for regular monitoring of prothrombin time is essential after the patient leaves the hospital. In addition, levels of concurrent medications ought to be monitored, because warfarin may compete for binding sites, thus altering plasma levels of these drugs. Oral anticoagulants are teratogenic and should not be used during established or planned pregnancy. In the pregnant patient, heparin is the drug of choice, and for long-term management subcutaneous self-administration should be taught. This regimen allows a normal delivery and can be continued postpartum.

Fibrinolysis

Great interest has been shown in the use of fibrinolytic agents to activate the intrinsic plasmin system. Tissue-type plasminogen activator, streptokinase, and urokinase have been found effective although associated with a high incidence of hemorrhagic complications. Ten percent of patients treated with streptokinase suffer allergic reactions, which vary from urticaria to anaphylaxis. In addition, streptokinase offers no advantage over heparin in the treatment

TABLE 41-1

Indications for Insertion of a Vena Caval Filter

Recurrent thromboembolism in spite of adequate anticoagulation
Deep venous thrombosis or documented thromboembolism in a patient who has a contraindication to anticoagulation
Complication of anticoagulation forcing therapy to be discontinued
Chronic pulmonary embolism with associated pulmonary hypertension and cor pulmonale
Immediately after pulmonary embolectomy
Relative indications
   Patient who has more than 50% of the pulmonary vascular bed occluded and who would not tolerate any additional embolism
   Patient with a propagating iliofemoral thrombus despite anticoagulation
   High-risk patient with a large free-floating iliofemoral thrombus on venogram

of recurrent venous thrombosis or thrombosis that has existed for over 72 hours. Lytic agents are contraindicated in the postoperative or post-traumatic patient and may be associated with an increased risk of pulmonary embolism.

Regional lysing with specialized catheters may be used to deliver recombinant tissue-type plasminogen activator directly to the thrombus. This technique may result in early thrombus resolution with long-term valve preservation and a reduced incidence of post-thrombotic syndrome.[39–43] Mewissen and colleagues[44] have reported outcomes from a registry of DVT patients treated with lytic therapy. Acute thrombosis completely lysed in 34% of cases but at the expense of major bleeding in 11%. One-year primary patency was 60%. Venous stents were used adjunctively in 104 of 473 patients.[44]

Surgical Approaches

Operative Thrombectomy

Thrombectomy directly removes thrombi from the deep veins of the leg. Despite early efficacy, venographic follow-up most often shows rethrombosis. However, when creation of an arteriovenous fistula is added to the procedure, patency is improved. Long-term follow-up is necessary to determine the incidence of post-thrombotic syndrome. The procedure is now usually reserved for limb salvage in the presence of phlegmasia cerulea dolens and impending venous gangrene.

Vena Cava Interruption

Adequate anticoagulation usually is effective in managing DVT, but if recurrent pulmonary embolism occurs during anticoagulant therapy or if a contraindication to anticoagulation exists, a mechanical approach is necessary. Mechanical protection is also indicated as prophylaxis against recurrence of embolism for the patient who has required pulmonary embolectomy and for some high-risk patients who could not tolerate recurrence. Because of the ease of insertion, the low incidence of adverse events, and the proven efficacy, interest exists in extending prophylactic indications (Table 41–1).

The cone-shaped Greenfield filter was developed to prevent pulmonary embolism while maintaining caval patency, preventing lower extremity venous stasis, and facilitating lysis of the embolus (Fig. 41–1). Before implementation of percutaneous placement techniques, the filter was commonly placed via the jugular vein; however, the femoral vein was used when the jugular vein was inadequate or an open neck wound was present. A 20-year review of our data revealed a 4% rate of recurrent embolism and a caval patency rate of 95%.[45, 46] The high caval patency rate makes it possible to position the filter above the renal vein when thrombus extends into the inferior vena cava or in young women with childbearing potential. A long-term follow-up study of patients with suprarenal filters demonstrated the safety and efficacy of such placements.[47]

The complications of filter insertion range in severity from minor wound hematoma resulting from early resumption of anticoagulation to potentially lethal migration of the device into the pulmonary artery, as documented with the bird's nest filter. The most common complication with the

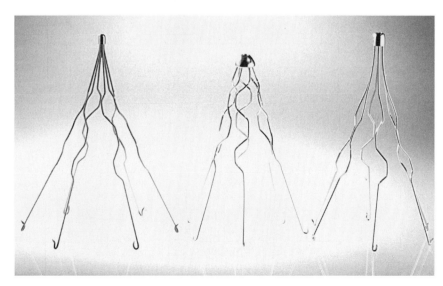

Figure 41–1. The original Greenfield filter (*center*) is made from stainless steel and inserted via a no. 24-French carrier. The titanium model of the filter (*left*) is inserted via a no. 12-French carrier system. The newer percutaneous stainless steel filter (*right*) allows placement over a guidewire. (From Greenfield LJ, Proctor MC, James EA, et al: Staging of fixation and retrievability of Greenfield filters. J Vasc Surg 20:745, 1994.)

original stainless steel Greenfield filter (SGF) was misplacement, which occurred in 7% of cases. This rate fell to 4% when the use of a guidewire became standard. When the filter is misplaced, the patient has inadequate protection, but the location (renal or iliac vein) poses no regional problem. A second filter can be placed in the appropriate location. Follow-up has shown that filters misplaced in the right ventricle or pulmonary artery need not be retrieved unless an arrhythmia or tricuspid insufficiency develops. When obesity precludes fluoroscopy, intravascular ultrasonography may be used to identify the renal veins and guide filter placement.

Recurrent embolism after filter placement has occurred in 2% to 4% of cases may be caused by a source of thrombus outside of the filtered flow, such as the upper body veins or the right atrium. In one case, a tilted filter allowed proximal thrombus formation, but this responded to treatment with urokinase and oral anticoagulation.[48] Recurrent embolism is an indication for inferior venacavography to evaluate the filter for possible proximal thrombus. This is a rare finding and can be managed either by thrombolytic therapy if the amount of thrombus is small or by placement of a second filter in the suprarenal vena cava.

Secondary infection of a captured thrombus within a Greenfield filter has been produced in the laboratory, but it was possible to sterilize the stainless steel filter and thrombus with a 2-week course of antibiotic therapy.[49] Sepsis is not a contraindication to filter insertion. The capture of a very large embolus within a filter may suddenly occlude the vena cava, with a precipitous fall in blood pressure. In a patient with known prior pulmonary embolism, this event can be mistaken for recurrent pulmonary embolism with disastrous results from vasopressor therapy. The basic distinction between functional hypovolemia of caval occlusion and right ventricular overload from recurrent pulmonary embolism can be made at the bedside by the measurement of central venous pressure and arterial oxygen tension. The response to volume resuscitation for the patient with sudden vena caval occlusion should be dramatic.

Failure to adequately flush the filter delivery system may result in thrombus formation, which may tether the limbs, prevent expansion, and allow migration on delivery. The improved technique of percutaneous insertion over a guidewire should minimize this complication.[50]

PERCUTANEOUS FILTER INSERTION

Favorable experience with the Seldinger technique for percutaneous introduction of catheters and devices has led to considerable enthusiasm on the part of radiologists for using this approach to insert a variety of innovative vena caval filter devices (Fig. 41–2). As early as 1977, a device was described made from nitinol, which is a nickel-titanium alloy that exists as a pliable wire when cool but rapidly transforms into a previously imprinted rigid shape when warmed.[51] The nitinol filter has a cone shape with an overlying dome. Clinical experience with follow-up in 102 of 224 patients revealed a 4% incidence of recurrent pulmonary embolism. The caval occlusion rate was 19%. Insertion site thrombosis was observed in 11% (Table 41–2). In

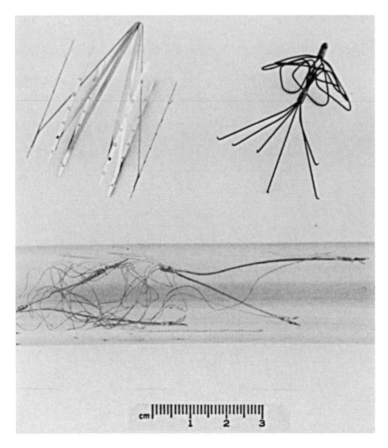

Figure 41–2. Alternative vena caval filters that have been developed for percutaneous introduction: Vena Tech filter (*top left*), Simon Nitinol filter (*top right*), and bird's nest filter (*bottom*).

TABLE 41-2

Summary of the Most Recent Published Outcome Studies of the Marketed Vena Caval Filters

SOURCE	GREENFIELD SGF 24F (GREENFIELD & PROCTOR, 1995[46])	GREENFIELD TGF-MH (GREENFIELD ET AL, 1994[45])	VENA TECH (CROCHET ET AL, 1993[56])	BIRD'S NEST (LORD AND BENN, 1994[64])	SIMON NITINOL (McCOWAN ET AL, 1992[52])
No. placed	642	173	142	61	20
No. monitored	246	113	137	37	16
Recurrent PE (%)	4	4	4	5	0
Caval patency	96	99	70	97 (85% in Mohan et al[65])	75
Filter patency (%)	96	99	NR	95	NR
Insertion site DVT (%)	1	2	8	NR	NR
Migration (%)	NR	7	18	0	6
Penetration (%)	NR	< 1	0	NR	31
Follow-up period (yr)	20	4	6	3.5	2
Follow-up tests	AP and lateral radiographs	AP and lateral radiographs	AP radiograph	AP radiograph	AP radiograph
	Duplex ultrasonography Venacavography	Duplex ultrasonography Venacavography	Duplex ultrasonography Venacavography	Duplex ultrasonography	Duplex ultrasonography Venacavography

AP, anteroposterior; CT, computed tomography; DVT, deep vein thrombosis; NR, not reported; PE, pulmonary embolism; SGF, stainless steel Greenfield filter; TGF-MH, titanium Greenfield filter with modified hook.
From Greenfield LJ, Proctor MC: Indications and techniques of inferior vena cava interruption. In Gloviczki P, Yao JST (eds): Handbook of Venous Disorders: Guidelines of the American Venous Forum. London, Chapman & Hall, p. 314.

a review of 20 patients, a 25% incidence of penetration, a 20% incidence of occlusion, and a 10% incidence of filter leg fracture occurred.[52]

Another device, the bird's nest filter,[53] has also become popular because of its ease of insertion. It consists of four stainless steel wires, each of which is 25 cm long and 0.18 mm in diameter. The wires are intended to be packed into a 7-cm length of the vena cava to trap thromboemboli. In the largest series of patients, only 37 of the 481 patients in whom the filter had been in place for 6 months or more had objective evaluation at follow-up by means of venacavography or ultrasonography. Seven (19%) had caval occlusion. A more significant problem with this device has been proximal migration after what appeared to be secure placement. This has been seen both experimentally and clinically, with published reports in five patients, including one death. Subsequent to this, a change in hook design was done in an effort to provide better fixation. Despite its small introducer system, the deployment of the device is more operator dependent than other vena caval filters. In addition, it requires 6 to 7 cm for adequate deployment, which is not always possible when the infrarenal caval segment is short, thus requiring placement extension into the iliac veins.[54]

Another of the newer cone-shaped devices, known as the Vena Tech filter, has added hooked stabilizers with sharp ends intended to center and fix the device. The initial experience was from France and consisted of 100 attempted insertions resulting in 98 filters discharged, 82 of which were positioned correctly.[55] Eight filters had a 15-degree tilt or more, five opened incompletely, and an additional three were both incompletely opened and tilted. Nine of the filters migrated distally and four in a cephalad direction, for a 13% migration rate. At follow-up at 1 year, seven occlusions (8%) had occurred, and recurrent pulmonary embolism occurred in two patients with incompletely opened filters. At later follow-up, 13 filters had

migrated, nine to the iliac vein and four to the renal veins. Studies indicate a 2% rate of recurrent pulmonary embolism, an 8% vena caval occlusion rate, insertion site thrombosis in 23%, migration greater than 10 mm in 14%, and a 6% incidence of incomplete opening (see Table 41-2). Although the initial follow-up reports were acceptable, further study up to 6 years after placement indicated an unacceptable (30%) rate of filter obstruction.[56]

The advantages of the percutaneous technique have prompted the development of a titanium Greenfield filter (TGF) that can be inserted through a 14-French sheath or operatively (Fig. 41-3). A titanium filter with an 80-degree angled hook was developed, which could be compressed into a 12-French delivery system. A multicenter study was completed in 186 patients, with a 3% rate of recurrent pulmonary embolism. Initially incomplete opening was noted in 2% of the cases and asymmetry of the legs in 5%. Apparent movement of the filter greater than 9 mm occurred in 11% of the patients, and increased filter base diameter occurred in 14%. Insertion site thrombosis was noted by duplex scanning in 9%. The use of a sheath during insertion reduced the incidence of premature discharge, and the modification of the hook reduced the migration and penetration noted with the initial titanium design.[57] The TGF is placed through a sheath, not over a wire. To regain this feature, a percutaneous stainless steel filter was developed (PSGF).

In clinical trials, the PSGF functioned in a manner comparable to the SGF and TGF with respect to the incidence of recurrent pulmonary embolism and caval patency but was superior with respect to ease of placement. Long-term evaluation of this device continues to show a high level of safety and efficacy, with a recurrent pulmonary embolism rate of 3.5% and caval patency of 99%.[58] This modified percutaneous device of stainless steel that allows placement over a guidewire was approved by the FDA in 1996. It demonstrates the same long-term protection from

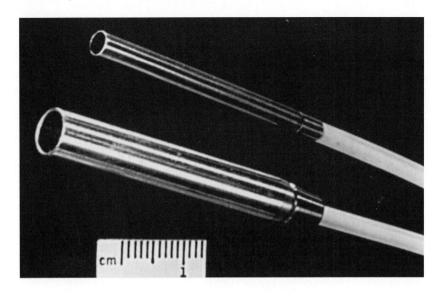

Figure 41–3. Comparison of the carrier systems used for the titanium Greenfield filter (*top*) and the standard stainless steel filter (*bottom*).

pulmonary embolism and maintenance of vena caval patency.[50] Current review after 4 years of use reveals rates of 2% and 99%, respectively.

PULMONARY THROMBOEMBOLISM

The most serious complication of DVT is pulmonary thromboembolism. Knowing the exact incidence of the disorder is difficult, because the clinical diagnosis is inherently inaccurate and is often confused with myocardial infarction, pneumothorax, sepsis, or pneumonia. Management of acute, massive pulmonary thromboembolism depends on an accurate diagnosis that documents the presence and location of an intravascular thrombus. This usually requires angiography, which has the added advantage of allowing pressure measurement in the pulmonary circulation. Because of its inherent nonspecificity, the perfusion lung scan is most useful as a screening test to exclude the diagnosis in patients with minor degrees of embolism. Spiral computed tomography and magnetic resonance angiography are effective alternative diagnostic methods. In suspected massive embolism, the patient should receive heparin sodium (150 to 200 units/kg) and be taken directly to the angiographic suite for selective pulmonary angiography. In addition to insertion of the angiographic catheter, usually through the femoral vein, a radial artery cannula is inserted for monitoring arterial blood gases, and anesthesia standby is requested should the patient require intubation and ventilatory control. If the patient's condition is too unstable for angiography and other objective signs of venous thrombosis or embolism are present, such as a prior scan showing large or multiple defects, it is reasonable to proceed to diagnosis under fluoroscopy by injection of contrast material through an embolectomy catheter.

Pulmonary Embolectomy

Open pulmonary embolectomy is most appropriate for patients with chronic pulmonary embolism and elevated pulmonary pressure, those who require closed cardiac massage to maintain blood pressure, or those in whom the catheter embolectomy procedure fails to remove thrombi.

Transvenous Catheter Embolectomy

Catheter embolectomy offers a safe, effective alternative to remove emboli that does *not* require general anesthesia or a sternotomy or risk hemorrhagic complications of lytic agents.

Access for insertion of the catheter is obtained by isolation of either the jugular or the common femoral vein (Fig. 41–4). Using the jugular vein is technically easier and quicker, although in some patients the straighter route from the femoral vein and the opportunity to perform local thrombectomy may be advantageous. The absence of projecting thrombi in the pelvis above the level of insertion is confirmed by injection of contrast medium before advancement of the catheter. If thrombi are encountered, they can be extracted readily with a Fogarty catheter. The embolectomy catheter is filled with heparinized saline through an intravenous extension tube attached to the handle, and a guidewire may be used during introduction to facilitate positioning in the pulmonary artery, although it is rarely necessary. The cup-catheter is inserted through a transverse venotomy, and the radiopaque cup is readily visualized under fluoroscopy as it is guided into the vena cava with the left hand while the right hand holds the control unit to provide tip deflection. Passage into the right ventricle is aided by medial angulation and anterior deflection, which then allow the cup to enter the pulmonary artery. Electrocardiographic monitoring should be maintained to detect premature ventricular contractions and other rhythm disturbances. The arrhythmias that occur during passage almost always respond to withdrawal or change in position of the catheter. The left main pulmonary artery is entered the most easily, and the cup may then be positioned according to the angiographic location of the major embolus on that side (usually the left lower lobe). Entry into the right main pulmonary artery requires deflection of the cup in that direction as it reaches the

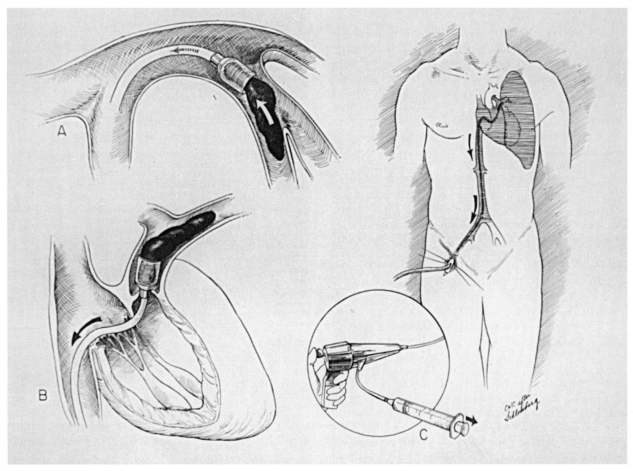

Figure 41–4. Technique of catheter embolectomy based on positioning the steerable cup catheter (*A*) adjacent to the embolus and using syringe suction to aspirate a portion of the embolus into the cup. The catheter is then withdrawn (*B*), maintaining syringe vacuum (*C*) as the embolus is removed. Repeated insertions are usually necessary to clear the pulmonary circuit and improve cardiac output.

superior edge of the heart shadow. Rotation of the tip also aids in advancement of the catheter. Juxtaposition of the cup and the embolus is confirmed by injection of 5 to 10 mL of contrast medium through the catheter. Limiting the volume of contrast is important.

A large syringe is attached to the control handle via the intravenous extension tubing, and the barrel is pulled back sharply by the assistant. A sustained jet of blood in the syringe can result if the cup is not in apposition to the thrombus, and a vacuum is produced if the embolus is

suctioned into the cup. Sustained vacuum is used to hold the embolus in the cup as the entire catheter and attached embolus are withdrawn through the right ventricle, down the inferior vena cava, or up the superior vena cava and out of the venotomy (see Fig. 41–4). Multiple retrievals are usually necessary to remove additional emboli or fragments if the embolus cannot be withdrawn intact (Fig. 41–5). Any blood that is aspirated in the syringe can be returned to the patient. The cup should be cleansed for free passage of fluid and effective suctioning before each

Figure 41–5. Specimens obtained during suction pulmonary embolectomy.

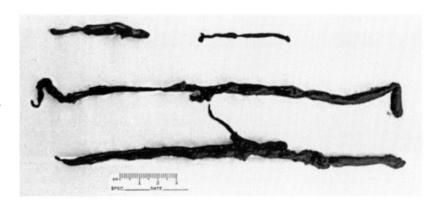

attempted retrieval. Although access and extraction from the jugular vein are easier technically in most patients, severe dyspnea in some patients may preclude this approach.

Emboli that are refractory to extraction are usually found in patients with a history of embolism of more than 72 hours and consequent fixation of the embolus to the pulmonary arterial wall. In these patients, however, subsequent embolism usually is responsible for acute decompensation, and the unfixed emboli can often be retrieved to allow hemodynamic stabilization. If the patient remains in shock and no emboli have been extracted after 30 to 40 minutes, an inferior vena cava filter should be inserted and the patient taken to the operating room for open embolectomy on cardiopulmonary bypass.

Our recent clinical experience with the technique in 35 patients showed that emboli could be extracted in 32 (91%), with overall survival of 77%, which is similar to our earlier report.[59] In this series, open embolectomy during bypass also was performed for acute thromboembolism in nine patients, five of whom survived (55%). The most common complication after catheter embolectomy is wound hematoma, due usually to resumption of heparin sodium administration within 12 hours of operation. Pulmonary infarctions occurred in two patients but not in areas where perfusion had been restored. Preventable deaths occurred in three patients, one from Swan-Ganz balloon rupture of the pulmonary artery and two from large-bolus contrast medium injection in the main pulmonary artery at the time of angiography. No myocardial damage has been seen with the steerable catheter. The procedure is always completed by insertion of a Greenfield filter to prevent recurrent embolism. Some have proposed a percutaneous approach with a large sheath; however, the sheath may not accommodate a large thrombus and may either displace it or shear it off, causing reembolization. It also may be associated with a higher incidence of air embolism.[60]

OTHER TYPES OF VENOUS THROMBOSIS

The term "thrombophlebitis" is usually applied to the disorder of the superficial veins characterized by a local inflammatory process that is usually aseptic. The cause in the upper limb is usually acidic fluid infusion or prolonged cannulation. In the lower extremities, it is usually associated with varicose veins and may coexist with DVT. The association with the injection of contrast material can be minimized by washout of the contrast material with heparinized saline.

Thrombophlebitis Migrans

Thrombophlebitis migrans, a condition of recurrent episodes of superficial thrombophlebitis, has been associated with visceral malignancy, systemic collagen-vascular disease, and blood dyscrasias. Involvement of the deep veins and the visceral veins has also been described.

Subclavian Vein Thrombosis

Subclavian vein thrombosis is most likely to be secondary to an indwelling catheter and can occur in children. It may also occur as a primary event in a young, athletic person ("effort thrombosis"), presumably as a result of chronic compressive injury at the thoracic outlet. If the patient is seen late, usually a satisfactory response to elevation and anticoagulation occurs, although some venous insufficiency and discomfort with exercise may persist. Pulmonary thromboembolism can occur from these thrombi, with an incidence of 12% reported in two series. Although it is rarely necessary, we have inserted a Greenfield filter in the superior vena cava in an inverted position in more than 20 patients.

Increased use of the axillary and subclavian veins for diagnostic and therapeutic procedures has resulted in a higher incidence of traumatic and foreign body thrombosis. Often these thrombi are asymptomatic because of gradual onset, short-segment involvement, or only partial occlusion. Thrombolytic therapy may be of value and should be considered with any acute subclavian vein thrombus occurring within 3 to 4 days of onset.[61] If the thrombus lyses, a contrast venogram should be obtained to outline any anatomic site of compression that could be treated surgically. Direct venolysis with first rib or medial clavicular excision can be used and should be considered for younger patients and manual laborers. Thrombectomy should always be performed in conjunction with creation of an ipsilateral arteriovenous fistula for angioaccess if proximal venous thrombosis is present. If the fistula is made without recognizing the proximal occlusion, the extremity may be endangered by massive edema. Operative correction is still possible without loss of the fistula, however, even if a jugular venous bypass is necessary, because the fistula assists in maintaining patency of the repair or bypass.

Abdominal Vein Thrombosis

Thrombosis of the inferior vena cava can result from tumor invasion or a propagating thrombus from the iliac veins. Most often, however, it results from ligation, plication, or insertion of occluding caval devices. Thrombosis of the renal vein is most likely to be associated with the nephrotic syndrome. It can be a source of thromboembolism and has been treated successfully by suprarenal placement of the Greenfield filter.[62]

Portal vein thrombosis may occur in the neonate, usually secondary to propagating septic thrombophlebitis of the umbilical vein. Collateral development leads to the occurrence of esophageal varices. Thrombosis of the portal, hepatic, splenic, or superior mesenteric vein in an adult can occur spontaneously, but usually it is associated with hepatic cirrhosis. Thrombosis of mesenteric or omental veins can simulate an acute abdomen but usually results in prolonged ileus rather than intestinal infarction.

Hepatic vein thrombosis (Budd-Chiari syndrome) usually produces massive hepatomegaly, ascites, and liver failure. It can be associated with a congenital web, endophlebitis, or polycythemia vera. Although some success has been reported using a direct approach to the congenital webs, the usual treatment is a side-to-side portacaval shunt to allow decompression of the liver or liver transplantation. The development of pelvic sepsis after abortion, tubal infection, or puerperal sepsis can lead to septic thrombophlebitis of the pelvic veins and septic thromboembolism. Ovarian vein and caval ligation has been the traditional treatment, but emphasis should be on drainage or excision

of the abscesses and appropriate antibiotic therapy. We have also used the Greenfield filter for septic thrombosis because the filter is inert stainless steel or titanium and does not lead to the development of an intraluminal abscess, which could occur after the traditional approach of ligation of the vena cava.[63] Long-term follow-up of patients with suprarenal filters has shown no obstruction and consequently no interference with renal function.

References

1. Hull RD, Pineo GF: Low molecular weight heparin treatment of venous thromboembolism. Prog Cardiovasc Dis 37:71–78, 1994.
2. Trousseau A: Phlegmasia Alba Dolens. Clinique Medicale de l'Hotel-Dieu de Paris, vol 3. Paris, JB Balliere et Fils, 1865, pp 654–712.
3. Prins MH, Lensing AW, Hirsh J: Idiopathic deep venous thrombosis: Is a search for malignant disease justified? Arch Intern Med 154:1310–1312, 1994.
4. Tisdale JF, Snowden TR, Johnson DR: Case report: Poorly differentiated carcinoma of unknown primary presenting as Trousseau's syndrome. Am J Med Sci 309:183–187, 1995.
5. Burgers JA, Wagenaar J: Screening for malignancies in patients with recurrent venous thrombosis. Br J Urol 74:669–670, 1994.
6. Glassman AB, Jones E: Thrombosis and coagulation abnormalities associated with cancer. Ann Clin Lab Sci 24:1–5, 1994.
7. Donati MB: Cancer and thrombosis. Haemostasis 24:128–131, 1994.
8. Lohr JM, Kerr TM, Lutter KS, et al: Lower extremity calf thrombosis—to treat or not to treat. J Vasc Surg 14:618–623, 1991.
9. White R, McGahan J, Daschbach M, Hartling R: Diagnosis of deep-vein thrombosis using duplex ultrasound. Ann Intern Med 111:297–304, 1989.
10. Solomon O, Steinberg DM, Zivelin A, et al: Single and combined prothrombotic factors in patients with idiopathic venous thromboembolism. Prevalence and risk assessment. Arterioscler Thromb Vasc Biol 19:511–518, 1999.
11. Perler B: Review of hypercoagulability syndromes: What the interventionalist needs to know. J Vasc Intervent Radiol 2:183–193, 1991.
12. Naidich J, Feinberg A, Karp-Harman H, et al: Contrast venography: Reassessment of its role. Radiology 168:97–100, 1988.
13. Flanagan LD, Sullivan ED, Cranley JJ: Venous imaging of the extremities using real-time B-mode ultrasound. In Bergan JJ, Yao JST (eds): Surgery of the Veins. Orlando, Fla, Grune & Stratton, 1985, p 89.
14. Leibovitch I, Foster RS, Wass JL, et al: Color Doppler flow imaging for deep venous thrombosis screening in patients undergoing pelvic lymphadenectomy and radical retropubic prostatectomy for prostatic carcinoma. J Urol 153:1866–1869, 1995.
15. Leutz DW, Stauffer ES: Color duplex Doppler ultrasound scanning for detection of deep venous thrombosis in total knee and hip arthroplasty patients: Incidence, location, and diagnostic accuracy compared with ascending venography. J Arthroplasty 9:543–548, 1994.
16. Mattos M, Londrey G, Leutz DW, et al: Color-flow duplex scanning for the surveillance and diagnosis of acute deep venous thrombosis. J Vasc Surg 15:366–375, 1992.
17. Norris CS, Greenfield LJ, Barnes RW: Free-floating iliofemoral thrombosis: A risk of pulmonary embolism. Arch Surg 120:806–808, 1985.
18. Aschwanden M, Labs KH, Jeanneret C, et al: The value of rapid D-dimer testing combined with structured clinical evaluation for the diagnosis of deep vein thrombosis. J Vasc Surg 30:929–935, 1999.
19. Sie P: The value of laboratory tests in the diagnosis of venous thromboembolism. Haematologica 80:57–60, 1995.
20. Tengborn L, Palmblad S, Wojciechowski J, et al: D-dimer and thrombin/antithrombin III complex—diagnostic tools in deep venous thrombosis? Haemostasis 24:344–350, 1994.
21. Guyatt GH, Cook DJ, Sackett DL, et al: Grades of recommendation for antithrombotic agents. Chest 114:441S–444S, 1998.
22. Poller L, McKernan A, Thomson J, et al: Fixed minidose warfarin: A new approach to prophylaxis against venous thrombosis after major surgery. BMJ 295:1309–1312, 1987.
23. Bern M, Lokich J, Wallach S, et al: Very low doses of warfarin can prevent thrombosis in central venous catheters. Ann Intern Med 112:423–428, 1990.
24. Turpie AGG, Hirsh J, Gunstensen J, et al: Randomized comparison of two intensities of oral anticoagulant therapy after tissue heart valve replacement. Lancet 1(8597):1242–1245, 1988.
25. MacCallum P, Thomson J, Poller L: Effects of fixed minidose warfarin on coagulation and fibrinolysis following major gynaecological surgery. Thromb Haemost 64:511–515, 1990.
26. Kakkar VV, Carrigan TP, Spindler JR, et al: Efficacy of low doses of heparin in prevention of deep vein thrombosis after major surgery: A double-blind, randomized trial. Lancet 2:101, 1972.
27. Bara L, Planes A, Samama MM: Occurrence of thrombosis and haemorrhage, relationship with anti-Xa, anti-IIa activities, and D-dimer plasma levels in patients receiving a low molecular weight heparin, enoxaparin or tinzaparin, to prevent deep vein thrombosis after hip surgery. Br J Haematol 104:230–240, 1999.
28. Walker H, Pennington D: Inferior vena caval filters in heart transplant recipients with perioperative deep vein thrombosis. J Heart Transplant 9:579–580, 1990.
29. Fink J, Jones B: The Greenfield filter as the primary means of therapy in venous thromboembolic disease. Surg Gynecol Obstet 172:253–256, 1991.
30. Alexander JJ, Yuhas JP, Piotrowski JJ: Is the increasing use of prophylactic percutaneous IVC filters justified? Am J Surg 168:102–106, 1994.
31. Rodriguez JG, Lopez JM, Proctor MC, et al: Early placement of prophylactic vena caval filters in injured patients at high risk for a pulmonary embolism. J Trauma 40:797–804, 1994.
32. Rogers FB, Shackford SR, Ricci MA, et al: Routine prophylactic vena cava filter insertion in severely injured trauma patients decreases the incidence of pulmonary embolism. J Am Coll Surg 180:641–647, 1995.
33. Bounameaux H: Unfractionated versus low-molecular-weight heparin in the treatment of venous thromboembolism. Vasc Med 3:41–46, 1998.
34. Buller HR, Kraaijenhagen RA, Koopman MMW: Early discharge strategies following venous thrombosis. Vasc Med 3:47–50, 1998.
35. Albada J, Nieuwenhuis H, Sixma J: Treatment of acute venous thromboembolism with low molecular weight heparin (Fragmin). Circulation 80:935–940, 1989.
36. Ten Cate JW, Koopman MMW, Prins MH, Buller HR: Treatment of venous thromboembolism. Thromb Haemost 74:197–203, 1995.
37. Agnelli G, Iorio A, Renga C, et al: Prolonged antithrombin activity of low-molecular-weight heparins: Clinical implications for treatment of thromboembolic diseases. Circulation 92:2819–2824, 1995.
38. Tapson VF, Hull RD: Management of venous thromboembolic disease: The impact of low-molecular-weight heparin. Clin Chest Med 16:281–294, 1995.
39. Hirsh J: Oral anticoagulant drugs. N Engl J Med 324:1865–1875, 1991.
40. Comerota AJ, Aldridge SC: Thrombolytic therapy for deep venous thrombosis: A clinical review. Can J Surg 36:359–364, 1993.
41. Robinson DL, Teitelbaum G: Phlegmasia cerulea dolens: Treatment by pulse-spray and infusion thrombolysis. AJR Am J Roentgenol 160:1288–1290, 1993.
42. Levine M, Weitz J, Turpie A, et al: Recombinant tissue plasminogen activator in patients with venous thromboembolic disease. Chest 97:168–171, 1990.
43. Bookstein J, Fellmeth B, Roberts A, et al: Pulsed-spray pharmacomechanical thrombolysis: Preliminary clinical results. AJR Am J Roentgenol 152:1097–1100, 1989.
44. Mewissen MW, Seabrook GR, Meissner MH, et al: Catheter-directed thrombolysis for lower extremity deep venous thrombosis: Report of a national multicenter registry. Radiology 211:39–49, 1999.

45. Greenfield LJ, Proctor MC, Cho KJ, et al: Extended evaluation of the titanium Greenfield vena caval filter. J Vasc Surg 20:458–465, 1994.

46. Greenfield LJ, Proctor MC: Twenty-year clinical experience with the Greenfield filter. Cardiovasc Surg 3:199–205, 1995.

47. Greenfield LJ, Proctor MC: Suprarenal filter placement. J Vasc Surg 28:432–438, 1998.

48. Greenfield LJ, Crute SL: Retrieval of Kimray-Greenfield vena caval filter. Surgery 88:719, 1980.

49. Peyton JWR, Hylemon MB, Greenfield LJ, et al: Comparison of Greenfield filter and vena caval ligation for experimental septic thromboembolism. Surgery 93:533–537, 1983.

50. Cho KJ, Greenfield LJ, Proctor MC, et al: Evaluation of a new percutaneous stainless steel Greenfield filter. J Vasc Intervent Radiol 8:181–187, 1997.

51. Simm M, Athanasoulis CA, Kim D, et al: Simon Nitinol inferior vena cava filter: Initial clinical experience. Radiology 172:99–103, 1989.

52. McCowan T, Ferris E, Carver D, Molphus M: Complications of the Nitinol vena caval filter. J Vasc Intervent Radiol 3:401–408, 1992.

53. Roehm JOF Jr, Johnsrude IS, Barth MH, Gianturco C: The bird's nest inferior vena cava filter progress report. Radiology 168:745–749, 1988.

54. Vesely T, Darcy M, Picus D, Hicks M: Technical problems associated with placement of the bird's nest inferior vena cava filter. AJR Am J Roentgenol 158:875–880, 1992.

55. Ricco JB, Crochet D, Sebilotte P, et al: Percutaneous transvenous caval interruption with the "LGM" filter: Early results of a multicenter trial. Ann Vasc Surg 3:142–147, 1988.

56. Crochet DP, Stora O, Ferry D, et al: Vena Tech-LGM filter: Long-term results of a prospective study. Radiology 188:857–860, 1993.

57. Greenfield L, Cho KJ, Proctor M, et al: Results of a multicenter study of the modified hook titanium Greenfield filter. J Vasc Surg 14:253–257, 1991.

58. Greenfield LJ, Proctor MC, Cho KJ, et al: Extended evaluation of the titanium Greenfield vena caval filter. J Vasc Surg 20:458–465, 1994.

59. Greenfield LJ: Complications of venous thrombosis and pulmonary embolism. In Greenfield LJ (ed): Complications in Surgery and Trauma, 2nd ed. Philadelphia, JB Lippincott, 1989, pp 430–438.

60. Greenfield LJ, Proctor MC, Williams D, Wakefield T: Long-term experience with transvenous catheter pulmonary embolectomy. J Vasc Surg 18:450–458, 1993.

61. Mealy K, Shanik DG: Axillary vein thrombosis—local treatment with streptokinase. Ir Med J 78:289, 1985.

62. Greenfield LJ, Peyton R, Crute SL: Hemodynamics and renal function following experimental suprarenal vena caval occlusion. Surg Gynecol Obstet 155:37, 1982.

63. Greenfield LJ, Michna BA: Twelve-year experience with the Greenfield vena caval filter. Surgery 104:706–712, 1988.

64. Lord R, Benn I: Early and late results after bird's nest filter placement in the interior vena cava: Clinical and duplex ultrasound followup. Aust N Z J Surg 64:106–114, 1994.

65. Mohan CR, Hoballah JJ, Sharp WJ, et al: Comparative efficacy and complications of vena caval filters. J Vasc Surg 21:235–246, 1995.

Questions

1. The following statement(s) is(are) true concerning venous thrombosis
   (a) the type of operation rather than its length increases the risk of deep vein thrombosis (DVT)
   (b) contrast medium can be seen to pool in soleal veins during any type of anesthesia
   (c) the presence of a thrombus in a vein produces typical pain and swelling
   (d) appropriate coagulation tests can identify the postoperative acquired thrombotic state

2. A young man with recurrent venous thrombosis after minor soft tissue injury has a family history in which other members have suffered pulmonary embolism. The following statement(s) is(are) true
   (a) the most likely underlying disorder is antithrombin III deficiency
   (b) diagnostic workup for inherited thrombotic disorder should be delayed until the patient is not receiving anticoagulants
   (c) the presence of a family history mandates the need for investigation of an inherited disorder
   (d) diagnosis of an inherited coagulation disorder indicates a need for lifelong oral anticoagulation

3. A 31-year-old woman in her third trimester of pregnancy has a painful, swollen, and pale left leg. The following statement(s) is(are) true
   (a) the optimal initial diagnostic study is a venous duplex ultrasound examination
   (b) venography is indicated because of discoloration of the leg
   (c) if venous thrombosis is found, the appropriate treatment is warfarin anticoagulation
   (d) if the thrombus progresses, the pregnancy should be terminated

4. The patient from the previous question develops progressive swelling of the entire extremity, with dusky discoloration and paresthesia. The following statement(s) is(are) true
   (a) the proximal extent of the thrombus involves the entire femoral system
   (b) the change is most likely due to hemorrhage into the extremity
   (c) venography is indicated
   (d) the changes reflect ischemia

5. A 55-year-old man has a 2-day history of calf pain without antecedent trauma. The following statement(s) is(are) true
   (a) a positive Homans sign justifies anticoagulation
   (b) absence of swelling makes DVT unlikely
   (c) venography is indicated
   (d) color-flow duplex examination of the venous system can diagnose infrapopliteal DVT

6. When using venous duplex examination, the following statement(s) is(are) true
   (a) venous thrombi are identified by their echogenicity
   (b) probe compression helps to identify veins as opposed to arteries
   (c) comparison of vein size between extremities can assist in the diagnosis of DVT
   (d) thrombus echogenicity is related to thrombus age

7. The following statement(s) is(are) true regarding a 62-year-old woman with unilateral leg swelling
   (a) impedance plethysmography (IPG) measures the rate of emptying of the congested lower extremity
   (b) a positive IPG is specific for venous thrombosis
   (c) radiolabeled antifibrin monoclonal antibodies are preferred over radiolabeled fibrinogen
   (d) a negative D-dimer test is of more value clinically in the diagnosis of pulmonary embolism than is a positive test

8. A 57-year-old obese white man with a history of prostate cancer is being considered for hip arthroplasty. The patient experienced DVT after prostatectomy 1 year ago. The following statement(s) is(are) true
   (a) prophylactic subcutaneous heparin should be used because of its ability to inhibit factor IX
   (b) low-molecular-weight heparin is preferred because of its greater anti-Xa effect
   (c) to avoid bleeding complications, dextran should be used prophylactically

(d) prophylactic warfarin derivatives are effective but are associated with increased hemorrhage

9. A 47-year-old woman with documented metastatic breast cancer has an iliofemoral DVT confirmed by duplex ultrasound examination. The following statement(s) is(are) true
   (a) the patient should be kept at bed rest for a minimum of 10 days
   (b) heparin should be administered by intravenous infusion
   (c) warfarin should be administered at the same time that heparin is started to decrease the hospital stay

(d) platelet counts should be monitored during heparin administration

10. A 72-year-old man underwent radical prostatectomy 4 days ago and is now experiencing an iliofemoral DVT. He shows massive swelling and pain in the left leg. The following statement(s) is(are) true
    (a) if sensation and motor function are lost, an indication for venous thrombectomy exists
    (b) the patient has an indication for fibrinolytic therapy
    (c) the patient has an indication for a vena caval filter
    (d) the patient should be heparinized

Answers

1. b   2. b, c, d   3. a   4. d   5. d   6. c, d   7. a, c, d   8. b, d   9. b, d   10. a, c

42

Varicose Veins: Chronic Venous Insufficiency

Niren Angle and John J. Bergan

Vascular surgery, more than most disciplines, lends itself to a systematic approach to diagnosis and treatment of disease. When examining a patient with a vascular problem, categorizing the problem as arterial or venous is useful. Venous disorders may be divided into acute thromboembolic problems or chronic venous stasis. This chapter deals with the latter subject. Disorders of chronic venostasis include primary varicose veins, superficial venous incompetence, and deep venous incompetence. Primary varicose veins can be treated for cure, whereas chronic venous insufficiency due to deep vein abnormality is treatable but not curable. More important, varicose veins should be approached as symptomatic manifestations of venous disease rather than as a mere cosmetic problem.

Varicose veins are a disease of Western civilization. More than half of adult men and two thirds of adult women have physically identifiable varicosities. Severe chronic venous insufficiency (CVI) is found in nearly 20% of working men and women. Varicose veins range in severity from the undesirable appearance of venectasia or telangiectasia to protuberant, tortuous varicosities with or without associated dermatitis, cutaneous ulcerations, or severe pigmentation. CVI produces findings identical to those of primary venostasis.

The cause of varicose veins is linked to genetics, and the problem is exacerbated by changes in the hormonal milieu. The precise origin of varicose veins is probably multifactorial and is addressed later. The appearance of varicose veins in childhood is rare, although examination of adolescents with a strong family history of varicosities reveals that some have venous valves that are incompetent. Primary varicose veins in the young adult are common. The precise cause is difficult to pinpoint, and our present understanding of this disease does not allow selection of treatment on the basis of cause.

SYMPTOMS

Primary varicosities consist of elongated, tortuous, superficial veins that are protuberant and contain incompetent valves. These produce the symptoms of mild swelling, heaviness, and easy fatigability. In this situation, the skin and subcutaneous tissue are normal, and edema, when present, is mild.

Primary varicose veins merge imperceptibly into more severe, CVI. Swelling is moderate to severe, an increased sensation of heaviness occurs with larger varicosities, and early skin changes of mild pigmentation and subcutaneous induration appear. The induration is termed "liposclerosis" by the English. Here, edema is regularly present.

When CVI becomes severe, marked swelling and calf pain occur after standing, sitting, or ambulation. Multiple dilated veins are seen associated with varicose clusters and heavy medial and lateral supramalleolar pigmentation. Marked liposclerosis and scars from previously healed ulcerations or current ulceration are also noted.

In the genesis of varicosities, female hormones in general, and progesterone in particular, have profound effects. For example, progesterone, the hormone of the second phase of the menstrual cycle and the principal hormone of pregnancy, causes passive dilatation of varicosities under the influence of venous hypertension. This fact is of importance in explaining clinical symptoms. Observant women know that the aching, heaviness, and tiredness caused by venous insufficiency is worse in the second 14 days of a menstrual cycle and that symptoms peak just before the menstrual period or during the first 2 days of the period. Furthermore, the multiparous woman who is a good observer notes the appearance or exacerbation of symptoms of varicosities when she becomes pregnant, sometimes even before the first menstrual period is missed.

PATHOGENESIS

Cutaneous venectasias develop under the same influences and may become symptomatic similarly. Textbooks of venous disease in the past and recent present have referred to venectasias as cosmetic and not symptomatic, yet ample documentation exists to the contrary. Effective treatment of venectasias can relieve symptoms of venostasis.

Fundamental defects in the strength and characteristics of the venous wall enter into the pathogenesis of varicose veins. These defects may be generalized or localized and consist of deficiencies in elastin and collagen. Gandhi and colleagues[1] compared the collagen and elastin content of varicose veins with those of normal greater saphenous veins and discovered a significant increase in the collagen content and a significant reduction in the elastin content of varicose veins. No difference in proteolytic activity was demonstrated, thereby diminishing the likelihood that enzymatic degradation is an essential component of varicose vein formation.

Anatomic differences in the location of the superficial veins of the lower extremities may contribute to the pathogenesis. For example, the main saphenous trunk is not always involved in varicose disease. Perhaps this is because it contains a well-developed medial fibromuscular layer and is supported by fibrous connective tissue that binds it to the deep fascia. In contrast, tributaries to the long saphenous vein are less supported in the subcutaneous fat and are superficial to the membranous layer of superficial fascia. These tributaries also contain less muscle mass in their walls. Thus these, and not the main trunk, may become selectively varicose.[2]

When these fundamental anatomic peculiarities are recognized, the intrinsic competence or incompetence of the valve system becomes important. For example, failure of a valve protecting a tributary vein from the pressures of the long saphenous vein allows a cluster of varicosities to develop. This is not an uncommon history for pregnant women who describe a sudden development of a cluster of varicosities of unknown cause. Failure of the protective valve is the mechanism for such development.

Our group has been interested in finding the fundamental cause of valve failure. It was our hypothesis that acquired valve damage was responsible for axial reflux, and this could explain perforating vein outflow or failure of check valve function of perforating vein valves. It was possible for us to identify monocytic infiltration into venous valves in patients with venous insufficiency.[3] This led to an animal model of modest venous hypertension in which microvenous pressure was raised to approximately 31 mm Hg. This allowed monitoring of parenchymal cell death in the mesentery by propidium iodide. With videomicroscopy we could identify a number of rolling, adherent, and migrating leukocytes.[4] All of the changes indicating leukocyte activation and parenchymal cell death were modified by a purified flavonoid fraction in a dose-dependent fashion.

The Middlesex Hospital (London, England) group has carried those observations into the clinical situation, where the micronized purified flavonoids were given as treatment for 60 days to patients with chronic venous disease.[5] Monitoring soluble endothelial adhesion molecules revealed that there was a reduction in the level of intercellular adhesion molecule 1 (ICAM-1), vascular cell adhesion molecules (VCAMs), and plasma lactoferrin, suggesting that pharmacologic intervention in CVI may be possible in the foreseeable future.

Furthermore, communicating veins connecting the deep with the superficial compartment may have valve failure.

Pressure studies show that two sources of venous hypertension exist. The first is gravitational and is a result of venous blood coursing in a distal direction down linear axial venous segments.[6] This is referred to as hydrostatic pressure and is the weight of the blood column from the right atrium. The highest pressure generated by this mechanism is evident at the ankle and foot, where measurements are expressed in centimeters of water or millimeters of mercury. The second source of venous hypertension is dynamic. It is the force of muscular contraction, usually contained within the compartments of the leg. If a perforating vein fails, high pressures (ranging from 150 to 200 mm Hg) developed within the muscular compartments during exercise are transmitted directly to the superficial venous system. Here, the sudden pressure transmitted causes dilatation and lengthening of the superficial veins. Progressive distal valvular incompetence may occur. If proximal valves such as the saphenofemoral valve become incompetent, systolic muscular contraction pressure is supplemented by the weight of the static column of blood from the heart. Furthermore, this static column becomes a barrier. Blood flowing proximally through the femoral vein spills into the saphenous vein and flows distally. As it refluxes distally through progressively incompetent valves, it is returned through perforating veins to the deep veins. Here, it is conveyed once again to the femoral veins, only to be recycled distally.

Changes also occur at the cellular level. In the distal liposclerotic area, capillary proliferation is seen and extensive capillary permeability occurs as a result of the widening of interendothelial cell pores. Transcapillary leakage of osmotically active particles, the principal one being fibrinogen, occurs. In CVI, venous fibrinolytic capacity is diminished and the extravascular fibrin remains to prevent the normal exchange of oxygen and nutrients in the surrounding cells.[7, 8] However, little proof exists for an actual abnormality in the delivery of oxygen to the tissues.[9] Instead, research suggests that many pathologic processes are involved, and at present difficulty exists in identifying which are active and which are bystanders. Fundamental investigations into this problem in the future should improve the care of patients with severe venous stasis disease.[10] An understanding of the source of venous hypertension and its differentiation into hydrostatic and hydrodynamic reflux is important. The presence of hydrostatic reflux implies the need for surgical correction of this abnormality, and the presence of hydrodynamic reflux implies the need for ablation of the perforating vein mechanism, allowing exposure of the subcutaneous circulation to compartment pressures.

Hormonal Influence

Venous function is undoubtedly influenced by hormonal changes. In particular, progesterone liberated by the corpus luteum stabilizes the uterus by causing relaxation of smooth muscle fibers. This effect directly influences venous function. The result is passive venous dilatation, which, in many instances, causes valvular dysfunction. Although progesterone is implicated in the first appearance of varicosities in pregnancy, estrogen also has profound effects. It produces the relaxation of smooth muscle and a softening of collagen fibers.[11, 12] Further, the estrogen-progesterone ratio influences venous distensibility. This ratio may explain the predominance of venous insufficiency symptoms on the first day of a menstrual period when a profound shift occurs from the progesterone phase of the menstrual cycle to the estrogen phase.[13, 14]

SYMPTOMS

Many causes of leg pain are possible, and most may coexist. Therefore, defining the precise symptoms of venostasis is necessary. These symptoms may be of gradual onset or may be initiated by a lancinating pain, and they may precede the clinical appearance of the varicosity. Discomfort usually occurs during warm temperatures and after prolonged standing.[15] Varicose vein symptoms are often disproportionate to the degree of pathologic change. Patients with small, early varices may complain more than those with large, chronic varicosities.[16] The initial symptoms may vary from a pulsating pressure or burning sensation to a feeling of heaviness. The pain is characteristically dull, does not occur during recumbency or early in the morning, and is exacerbated in the afternoon, especially after long standing. The discomforts of aching, heaviness, fatigue, or burning pain are relieved by recumbency, leg elevation, or elastic support.

Cutaneous itching is also a sign of venostasis and is often the hallmark of inadequate external support. It is a manifestation of local congestion and may precede the onset of dermatitis. This, and nearly all the symptoms of stasis disease, can be explained by the irritation of superficial nerve fibers by local pressure or accumulation of metabolic end products with a consequent pH shift. External hemorrhage may occur as superficial veins press on overlying skin within this protective envelope.

DIAGNOSTIC EVALUATION IN VENOUS DYSFUNCTION

The most important of all noninvasive tests available to study the venous system are the physical examination and a careful history that elucidates the symptoms mentioned earlier. Clinical examination of the patient in good light provides nearly all the information necessary. It determines the nature of the venostasis disease and ascertains the presence of intercutaneous venous blemishes and subcutaneous protuberant varicosities, the location of principal points of control or perforating veins that feed clusters of varicosities, the presence and location of ankle pigmentation and its extent, and the presence and severity of subcutaneous induration. After these facts have been obtained, the physician may turn to noninvasive techniques to corroborate the clinical impression. Visual examination can be supplemented by noting a downward-going impulse on coughing. Tapping the venous column of blood also demonstrates pressure transmission through the static column to incompetent distal veins.

The Perthes test for deep venous occlusion and the Brodie-Trendelenburg test of axial reflux have been re-

placed by in-office use of the continuous wave, handheld Doppler instrument supplemented by duplex evaluation.[17] The handheld Doppler instrument can confirm an impression of saphenous reflux, and this, in turn, dictates the operative procedure to be performed in a given patient. A common misconception is belief that the Doppler instrument is used to locate perforating veins. Instead, it is used in specific locations to determine incompetent valves (e.g., the handheld, continuous wave, 8-MHz flow detector placed over the greater and lesser saphenous veins near their terminations). With distal augmentation of flow and release, with normal deep breathing, and with performance of a Valsalva maneuver, accurate identification of valve reflux is ascertained.[18] Formerly, the Doppler examination was supplemented by other objective studies. These included the photoplethysmograph, the mercury strain-gauge plethysmograph, and the photorheograph. These are no longer in common use.

Another instrument reintroduced to assess physiologic function of the muscle pump and the venous valves is the air displacement plethysmograph.[19, 20] This instrument was discarded after its use in the 1960s because of its cumbersome nature. Computer technology has allowed its reintroduction as championed by Nicolaides and his coworkers.[21] It consists of an air chamber that surrounds the leg from knee to ankle. During calibration, leg veins are emptied by leg elevation and the patient is then asked to stand so that leg venous volume can be quantitated and the time for filling recorded. The filling rate is then expressed in milliliters per second, thus giving readings similar to those obtained with the mercury strain-gauge technique.

Duplex technology more precisely defines which veins are refluxing by imaging the superficial and deep veins. The duplex examination is commonly done with the patient supine, but this gives an erroneous evaluation of reflux. In the supine position, even when no flow is present, the valves remain open. Valve closure requires a reversal of flow with a pressure gradient that is higher proximally than distally.[22] Thus, the duplex examination should be done with the patient standing or in the markedly trunk-elevated position.[23, 24]

Imaging is obtained with a 10- or 7.5-MHz probe, and the pulsed Doppler consists of a 3.0-MHz probe. The patient stands with the probe placed longitudinally on the groin. After imaging, sample volumes can be obtained from the femoral or saphenous vein. This flow can be observed during quiet respiration or by distal augmentation. Sudden release of augmentation allows assessment of valvular competence. The short saphenous vein and popliteal veins are similarly examined. Imaging improves the accuracy of the Doppler examination. For example, short saphenous venous incompetence can be differentiated from gastrocnemius venous valvular incompetence by the imaging and flow detection of the duplex or triplex scans.

Widespread use of duplex scanning has allowed a comparison of findings between standard clinical examination with duplex Doppler studies.[25] In a study in which each patient was examined by three surgeons using different techniques, one using clinical examination, a second using the handheld Doppler instrument, and a third using a color duplex scanner, it was found that clinical examination failed in assessing main axial reflux at the saphenofemoral junction and saphenopopliteal junction. Whenever a Doppler instrument was added to the examination, the evaluation became more accurate. Based on preoperative assessments using clinical examination alone, inappropriate surgery would have been performed in 20% of the limbs. Clinical examination plus Doppler study would have produced a 13% incidence of inappropriate surgery.

Phlebography

In general, phlebography is unnecessary in diagnosis and treatment of primary venostasis disease and varicose veins.[26] In the complex problems of severe CVI, phlebography has specific utility.[27, 28] Ascending phlebography defines obstruction. Descending phlebography identifies specific valvular incompetence suspected on B mode scanning and clinical examination.

TREATMENT

Indications for treatment are pain, easy fatigability, heaviness, recurrent superficial thrombophlebitis, external bleeding, and appearance.[29] Treatment of venous insufficiency is similar to surgical treatment elsewhere; that is, it may be ablative or restorative. Most of the restorative venous surgical techniques remain experimental, and only a few can be considered standard therapy. On the other hand, ablative treatment has not been employed sufficiently for such a long time that the operations have undergone marked improvement and modernization[30–33] (Fig. 42–1).

Venous Ablation

Cutaneous venectasias with vessels smaller than 1 mm in diameter do not lend themselves to surgical treatment. If their cause is saphenous or tributary venous incompetence,

these conditions can be treated surgically. The venectasias themselves can be ablated successfully using modern sclerotherapy technique. Dilute solutions of sclerosant (e.g., 0.2% sodium tetradecyl) can be injected directly into the vessels of the blemish.[34] Care should be taken to ensure that no single injection dose exceeds 0.1 mL but that multiple injections completely fill all vessels contributing to the blemish. When all of the ramifications of the blemish have been filled with sclerosant, and before the subsequent inflammatory reaction has progressed, a pressure dressing can be applied to keep vessels free of return blood for 24 to 72 hours. At 14 to 21 days post injection, incision and drainage of entrapped blood are performed and a second pressure dressing is applied for 12 to 18 hours. This liberation of entrapped blood is as important to success as the primary injection. Such therapy is remarkably successful in achieving an excellent cosmetic result and relief of stasis symptoms.

In allergic patients, a solution of hypertonic saline can be used for sclerotherapy.[35] On the other hand, the use of newer technologies such as the laser in treatment of telangiectasias has proved disappointing.[36]

Venules larger than 1 mm and less than 3 mm in size can also be injected with sclerosant of slightly greater concentration (e.g., 0.5% sodium tetradecyl) but limiting the amount injected to less than 0.5 mL. Pressure dressings for these venules must be in place for 72 hours or more. Evacuation of entrapped blood is of paramount importance to prevent recanalization of these vessels after treatment.

Surgical treatment may be used to remove clusters with varicosities greater than 4 mm in diameter (Fig. 42–2). Ambulatory phlebectomy may be performed using the stab avulsion technique with preservation of the greater and lesser saphenous veins, if they are unaffected by valvular incompetence.[37] When greater or lesser saphenous incompetence is present, the removal of clusters is preceded by limited removal of the saphenous vein (stripping). Stripping techniques are best done from above downward to avoid lymphatic and cutaneous nerve damage. A number of tech-

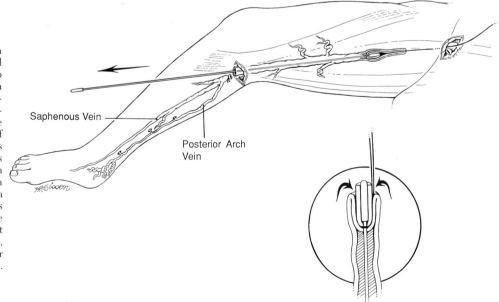

Figure 42–1. The modern variation of vein stripping consists of removal of the saphenous vein from groin to knee. The stripper is introduced in a retrograde fashion because preoperative duplex testing has shown reflux throughout the length of the saphenous vein. The objective of this removal is to detach tributaries to the saphenous vein as well as perforating veins. The inversion technique illustrated in the *inset* can be used to minimize tissue trauma in the removal of the saphenous vein from groin to knee. Note the posterior arch vein in the leg. It receives the Cockett perforators, and these perforators do not enter the saphenous vein below the knee.

Saphenous Vein

Posterior Arch Vein

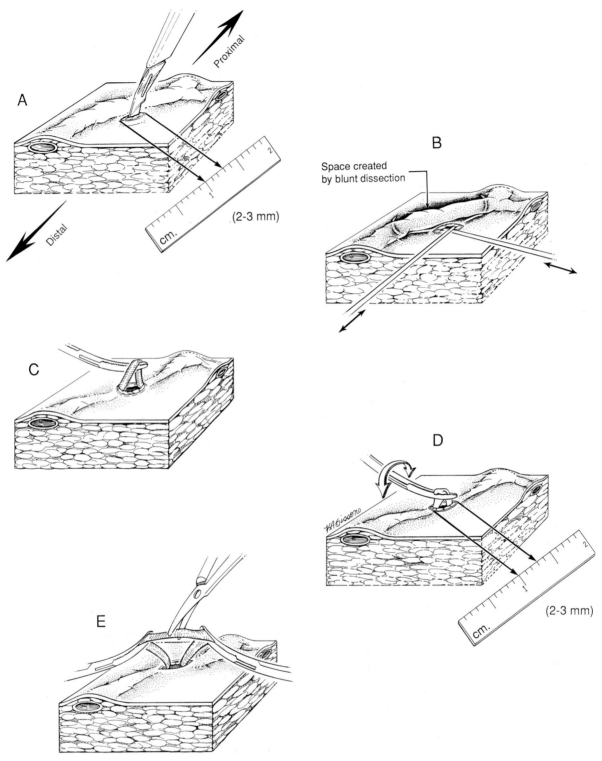

Figure 42–2. Mini-phlebectomy or stab avulsion may be performed in conjunction with saphenous vein stripping or as an isolated procedure. As an isolated procedure, this is termed ambulatory phlebectomy, and dilute solutions of local anesthesia are utilized. *A,* The incisions are placed vertically except at joint creases and where skin lines are clearly transverse. These should be no more than 2 to 3 mm in length. *B,* Mobilization of the subcutaneous space is done with blunt instruments, such as a hemostat or specially designed hooks. *C,* The instrument catches the adventitia of the vein and lifts it to the surface, where it can be clamped. *D,* The loop of vein is exteriorized and drawn into the field so that the loop can be doubly clamped. *E,* After the vein is divided, each end can be removed by stab avulsion. A minimum number of incisions are utilized, and they are kept short enough to be closed by tape strips without sutures.

niques have been described that adapt new instruments to minimally invasive removal of the saphenous vein.[38–40]

At the present time, when the greater saphenous vein is used for coronary artery bypass and peripheral arterial reconstruction, there has been an interest in preserving the saphenous vein while relieving the symptoms of venous insufficiency. However, a number of studies have shown the advantage of stripping in prevention of varicose vein recurrence. Methodologic flaws in these studies failed to convince interested surgeons.[41–46]

The question of preservation or stripping of the saphenous vein is an important one and therefore a 5-year clinical and duplex scan follow-up examination of a group of patients has been welcomed.[47] Patients were randomized to stripping of the long saphenous vein during varicose vein surgery versus saphenofemoral ligation with stab avulsion of varices. It was found that reoperation, either done or awaited, was necessary for only 3 of 52 legs that underwent stripping as compared with 12 of 58 limbs in which proximal ligation had been done. Neovascularization at the saphenofemoral junction was responsible for 10 of 12 recurrent varicose veins that underwent reoperation, and it was the cause of recurrence of saphenofemoral incompetence in 12 of the 52 limbs that were stripped versus 30 of the 58 limbs in which ligation was done. Clearly, the problem of neovascularization and recurrent varicose veins was not solved by the stripping operation, but stripping reduced the risk of reoperation by two thirds after 5 years of observation. It was the conclusion of the authors of the study that stripping "should be routine for primary long saphenous varicose veins."[47]

Surgery for Severe Chronic Venous Insufficiency

What is new in the treatment of venous stasis is a rearranging of, and modifications to, older methods.[48] What has not changed is that conservative treatment of CVI always precedes consideration of intervention. Such conservative treatment relies on limb compression to counteract the effects of venous hypertension.

While conservative therapy is being pursued or ulcer healing achieved, appropriate diagnostic studies should reveal patterns of venous reflux or segments of venous occlusion so that specific therapy can be prescribed for the individual limb being examined. Imaging by duplex Doppler suffices for detection of reflux if the examination is carried out in the standing individual. Such noninvasive imaging may prove the only testing necessary beyond the handheld, continuous wave Doppler instrument if superficial venous ablation is contemplated. If direct venous reconstruction by bypass or valvuloplasty techniques is planned, ascending and descending phlebography is required.

Surprisingly, superficial reflux may be the only abnormality present in advanced chronic venous stasis. Correction goes a long way toward permanent relief of the chronic venous dysfunction and its cutaneous effects. Using duplex technology, Menzoian and colleagues found that in 95 extremities with current venous ulceration, 16.8% had only superficial incompetence, and another 19% showed super-

ficial incompetence combined with perforator incompetence.[49] Similarly, the Middlesex group, in a study of 118 limbs, found that "in just over half of the patients with venous ulceration, the disease was confined to the superficial venous system."[50]

We studied 58 limbs with class 3 venous insufficiency. Ten limbs (17%) exhibited only superficial reflux, and superficial reflux was a major contributor to chronic venous dysfunction in another 17 limbs. Of some importance is the fact that primary, nonthrombotic deep (superficial femoral vein and popliteal vein) incompetence may accompany superficial reflux. This is explained by reflux proceeding distally down the greater saphenous vein and overloading the deep venous system.[51] One would presume this causes dilatation and elongation of the deep vessels so that their valves become incompetent. Our own study of limbs following greater saphenous vein stripping in which superficial femoral and popliteal venous incompetence was present has revealed correction of the deep reflux by superficial venous stripping in a vast majority of limbs.[52] Clearly, a significant proportion of patients with venous ulceration have normal function in the deep veins, and surgical treatment is a useful option that can definitively address the hemodynamic derangements. Maintaining that all venous ulcers are surgically incurable is not reasonable when these data suggest that superficial vein surgery holds the potential for ameliorating the venous hypertension.

In the early 1940s, Cockett and Linton[53] emphasized the importance of perforating veins, and direct surgical interruption of these was advocated. This has fallen into disfavor because of a high incidence of postoperative wound healing complications. However, video techniques that allow direct visualization through small-diameter scopes have made endoscopic subfascial exploration and perforator vein interruption the desirable alternative to the Linton technique (Fig. 42–3), minimizing morbidity and wound complications.[54, 55] The connective tissue between the fascia cruris and the underlying flexor muscles is so loose that this room can be easily opened up and dissected with the endoscope.[48] This operation, done with a vertical proximal incision, accomplishes the objective of perforator vein interruption on an outpatient basis.

The availability of subfascial endoscopic perforator vein surgery had a dramatic impact on the care of venous ulcers in Western countries.[56, 57] As patient limbs with severe CVI were studied accurately, the term "post-thrombotic syndrome" had to give way to the term "chronic venous insufficiency,"[58] and a link to platelet and monocyte aggregates in the circulation reflected the leukocytic infiltrate of the ankle skin with its lipodermatosclerosis and healed and open ulcerations.[59]

Data regarding leukocytes in CVI accumulated and were consistent, showing that the activation of leukocytes sequestered in the cutaneous microcirculation during venous stasis was important to the development of the skin changes of CVI. This is reflected in the finding of adhesion markers between leukocytes and endothelial cells and an increased production of leukocyte degranulation enzymes and oxygen free radicals. Nevertheless, experimental evidence was still required for decisive proof of the leukocyte hypothesis.[60]

In America, several groups have performed perforating vein division using laparoscopic instrumentation. Perforator

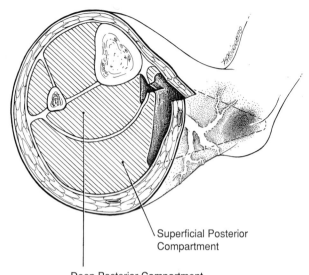

Superficial Posterior Compartment

Deep Posterior Compartment

Figure 42–3. The space created by the subfascial dissection. The scope is introduced into the leg and into the subfascial portion of the superficial posterior compartment. This allows the medial perforating veins to be interrupted from the posterior midline of the leg to the ankle. A further incision into the deep posterior compartment is necessary to ablate paratibial perforating veins, among which is the important Cockett III perforator. Clinical examination will determine the need for exploration of the deep posterior compartment.

interruption produced rapid ulcer healing and a very low rate of recurrence.[61] The North American Registry,[62] which voluntarily recorded the results of perforating vein surgery, confirmed a low 2-year recurrence rate of ulcers and a more rapid ulcer healing. Our group pursued the development of an open-scope dedicated instrument for subfascial perforator vein surgery and achieved modest success in treating patients with CVI using nondisposable instrumentation.[63]

A comparison of the three methods of perforator vein interruption, including the classic Linton procedure, the laparoscopic instrumentation procedure, and the single open-scope procedure revealed that the endoscopic techniques produced results comparable with those of the open Linton operation, with much less scarring and much greater tendency toward a fast recovery. More perforating veins were identified with the open technique. However, the mean hospital stay and the period of convalescence were more favorable with the scope procedures.[64]

In general, the registry reports and individual institution clinical experience showed that patients with true postthrombotic limbs were disadvantaged by the procedure, enough so that at Leicester (England), the students of the procedure said, "We conclude that perforating vein surgery is not indicated for the treatment of venous ulceration in limbs with primary deep venous incompetence."[65] Nevertheless, studies were reported in which previous superficial reflux was corrected with failures of such treatment. Rescue of such limbs with perforating vein division produced very satisfactory results and verified the fact that perforating veins are important in the genesis of venous ulceration and that their division accelerates healing and may reduce recurrence of ulceration.[66]

Part of the difficulty in understanding the need for

perforating vein division is the disparity between venous hemodynamics and the severity of cutaneous changes. This should not be surprising because the cutaneous changes of CVI are dependent upon leukocyte endothelial interactions and these may not be directly related to venous hemodynamics. Yet, endoscopic perforator vein division has improved venous hemodynamics in some limbs, as would be expected, by removing superficial reflux and perforating vein outflow.[67]

Direct Venous Reconstruction

Historically, the first successful procedures done to reconstruct major veins were the femorofemoral crossover graft of Eduardo Palma and the saphenopopliteal bypass described by him and used also by Richard Warren of Boston.[68, 69] These operations were elegant in their simplicity, use of autogenous tissue, and reconstruction by a single venovenous anastomosis.[70, 71]

With regard to femorofemoral crossover grafts, the only group to provide long-term physiologic study of a large number of patients is Halliday and colleagues[72] from Sydney, Australia. Although phlebography was used in selecting patients for surgery, no other details of preoperative indications are given. They were able to document that 34 of 50 grafts remained patent in the long term as assessed by postoperative phlebography. They believed the best clinical results were achieved in relief of postexercise calf pain, but they had the impression that a patent graft also slowed the progression of distal liposclerosis and controlled recurrent ulceration. No proof of this was given in their report.

The history of application of bypass procedures for venous obstruction is a fascinating one. Nevertheless, the advent of endovascular techniques has made those operations nearly obsolete.[73, 74]

Perforator interruption combined with superficial venous ablation has been effective in controlling venous ulceration in 75% to 85% of patients. However, emphasis on failures of this technique led to Kistner's significant breakthrough in direct venous reconstruction with valvuloplasty in 1968 and the general recognition of this procedure after 1975.[75] Late evaluation of direct valve reconstruction indicates good to excellent long-term results in over 80% of the patients.[76]

One cannot overestimate the contributions of Kistner. The technique of directing the incompetent venous stream through a competent proximal valve via venous segment transfer was his next achievement. After Kistner's contributions, surgeons were provided with an armamentarium that included Palma's venous bypass,[77] direct valvuloplasty (of Kistner), and venous segment transfer (of Kistner). Moreover, external valvular reconstruction as performed by various techniques, including monitoring by endoscopy, holds the promise of a renewed interest in this form of treatment of venous insufficiency.

Axillary-to-popliteal autotransplantation of valve-containing venous segments has been considered since the early observations of Taheri.[78] Verification in the long term of some preliminary excellent results has not been accomplished.

The advent of perforator vein surgery and the fine

results achieved with it have displaced direct valvuloplasty into a position of less importance and even less interest than the procedure had called for during the 1980s.

CONCLUSIONS

The door has been opened to a better understanding of the pathophysiology of venous disease, and the exploitation of that knowledge is the promise of the future. Not only are the hemodynamic derangements better understood but the cellular mechanisms of injury in chronic venous dysfunction are being discovered. More direct surgical approaches will be applied with increasing success. Importantly, the wider application of the principle of correcting deep venous incompetence by superficial venous ablation holds the promise of definitive therapy for a group of patients who, in the past, would have been relegated to "conservative" treatment founded on resignation to a chronic, unyielding disease.

References

1. Gandhi RH, Irizarry E, Nackman GB, et al: Analysis of the connective tissue matrix and proteolytic activity of primary varicose veins. J Vasc Surg 18:814–820, 1993.
2. Mashiah A, Rose SS, Hod I: The scanning electron microscope in the pathology of varicose veins. Isr J Med Sci 27:202–206, 1991.
3. Ono T, Bergan JJ, Schmid-Schönbein GW, Takase S: Monocyte infiltration into venous valves. J Vasc Surg 27:158–166, 1998.
4. Takase S, Delano F, Lerond L, et al: Inflammation in chronic venous insufficiency: Is the problem insurmountable? J Vasc Res 38(Suppl 1):3–10, 1999.
5. Shoab SS, Porter J, Scurr JH, Coleridge Smith PD: Endothelial activation response to oral micronized flavonoid therapy in patients with chronic venous disease: A prospective study. Eur J Vasc Endovasc Surg 17:313–318, 1999.
6. Bjordal RI: Hemodynamic studies of varicose veins and the postthrombotic syndrome. In Hobbs JT (ed): The Treatment of Venous Disorders. London, MTP Press, 1977, pp 37–56.
7. Burnand KG, O'Donnell TF, Thomas ML, et al: The relative importance of incompetent communicating veins in the production of varicose veins and venous ulcers. Surgery 82:9–14, 1997.
8. Burnand KG, Whimster IW, Clemenson G, et al: The relationship between the number of capillaries in the skin of the venous ulcer-bearing area of the lower leg and the fall in foot vein pressure during exercise. Br J Surg 68:297–300, 1981.
9. Scurr JH, Coleridge Smith PD: Pathogenesis of venous ulceration. Phlebologie 1(Suppl):1:13–16, 1992.
10. Scott HJ, McMullin GW, Coleridge Smith PD, Scurr JH: Histological study of white blood cells and their association with lipodermatosclerosis and venous ulceration. Br J Surg 78:210–211, 1991.
11. Wahl LM: Hormonal regulation of macrophage collagenase activity. Biochem Biophys Res Commun 74:838, 1977.
12. Woolley DE: On the sequential changes in levels of oestradiol and progesterone during pregnancy and parturition and collagenolytic activity. In Pez KA, Eddi AH (eds): Extracellular Matrix Biochemistry. New York, Elsevier Science, 1984.
13. McCausland AM, Holmes F, Trotter AD: Venous distensibility during the menstrual cycle. Am J Obstet Gynecol 86:640, 1963.
14. Marazita AJD: The action of hormones on varicose veins in pregnancy. Med Rec 159:422, 1946.
15. Conrad P: Painful legs: The GP's dilemma. Aust Fam Physician 9:691–694, 1980.
16. Lofgren KA: Varicose veins: Their symptoms, complications, and management. Postgrad Med 65:131–139, 1979.
17. Hoare MC, Royle JP: Doppler ultrasound detection of saphenofemoral and saphenopopliteal incompetence and operative venography to ensure precise saphenopopliteal ligation. Aust N Z J Surg 54:49, 1984.
18. Nicolaides A, Christopoulos DG, Vasdekis S: Progress in investigation of chronic venous insufficiency. Ann Vasc Surg 3:278–292, 1989.
19. Christopoulos DG, Nicolaides AN: Noninvasive diagnosis and quantitation of popliteal reflux in the swollen and ulcerated leg. J Cardiovasc Surg 29:535–539, 1988.
20. Christopoulos DG, Nicolaides AN, Szendro G, et al: Air plethysmography and the effect of elastic compression on the venous hemodynamics of the leg. J Vasc Surg 5:148–157, 1987.
21. Christopoulos DG, Nicolaides AN, Szendro G: Venous reflux: Quantification and correlation with the clinical severity of chronic venous disease. Br J Surg 75:352–356, 1988.
22. van Bemmelen PS, Beach K, Bedford G, et al: The mechanisms of venous valve closure. Arch Surg 125:617, 1990.
23. van Bemmelen PS, Beach K, Bedford G, et al: Quantitative segmental evaluation of venous valvular reflux with ultrasound scanning. J Vasc Surg 10:425, 1989.
24. Vasdekis SN, Clarke GH, Nicolaides AN: Quantification of venous reflux by means of duplex scanning. J Vasc Surg 10:670, 1989.
25. Singh S, Lees TA, Donlon M, et al: Improving the preoperative assessment of varicose veins. Br J Surg 84:801–802, 1997.
26. Wesolawski SA, Greenfield H, Sawyer PN, et al: Diagnostic value of phlebography in venous disorders of the lower extremity. J Cardiovasc Surg (Torino) 8(Suppl):8:133–135, 1965.
27. Darke SG, Andress MR: The value of venography in the management of chronic venous disorders of the lower limb. In Greenhalgh RM (ed): Diagnostic Techniques and Assessment Procedures in Vascular Surgery. London, Grune & Stratton, 1985.
28. Lea Thomas M, McDonald LM: Complications of phlebography of the leg. BMJ 2:307–315, 1978.
29. Bergan JJ: Surgical treatment of the veins. In Nora PJ (ed): Operative Surgery. Philadelphia, Lea & Febiger, 1991.
30. Doran FSA, White M: A clinical trial designed to discover if the primary treatment of varicose veins should be Fegan's method or by an operation. Br J Surg 62:72–76, 1975.
31. The treatment of varicose veins [editorial]: Lancet 1:311–312, 1975.
32. Fegan WG: Continuous compression technique of injecting varicose veins. Lancet 1:109–112, 1963.
33. Marston A: Treatment of varicose veins. Lancet 1:453, 1975.
34. Goldman MP: A comparison of sclerosing agents: Clinical and histologic effects of intravascular sodium morrhuate, ethanolamine oleate, hypertonic saline (11.7%), and sclerodex in the dorsal rabbit ear vein. J Dermatol Surg Oncol 17:354–362, 1991.
35. Sadick NS: Sclerotherapy of varicose and telengiectatic leg veins. Minimal sclerosant concentration of hypertonic saline and its relationship to vessel diameter. J Dermatol Surg Oncol 65:65–70, 1991.
36. Goldman MP, Martin DE, Fitzpatrick DE, et al: Pulsed dye laser treatment of telangiectasias with and without subtherapeutic sclerotherapy. J Am Acad Dermatol 23:23–30, 1991.
37. Bishop CCR, Jarrett PEM: Outpatient varicose vein surgery under local anesthesia. Br J Surg 73:821–822, 1986.
38. Conrad P: Groin-to-knee downward stripping of the long saphenous vein. Phlebology 7:20–22, 1992.
39. Fischer R: Das invaginierende Strippen in der Varicenchirurgie. Chirurg 65:736–738, 1994.
40. Goren G, Yellin A: Minimally invasive surgery for primary varicose veins. Ann Vasc Surg 9:401–414, 1995.
41. Munn SR, Morton JB, MacBeth WAAG, McLeish AR: To strip or not to strip the long saphenous vein? A varicose veins trial. Br J Surg 68:426–428, 1981.
42. Woodyer AB, Reddy PJ, Dormandy JA: Should we strip the long saphenous vein? Phlebology 1:221–224, 1986.
43. Hammarsten J, Pedersen P, Cederlund C-G, Campanello M: Long saphenous vein–saving surgery for varicose veins: A long-term follow-up. Eur J Vasc Surg 4:361–364, 1990.
44. Neglen P, Einarsson E, Eklof B: The functional long-term value of different types of treatment for saphenous vein incompetence. J Cardiovasc Surg (Torino) 34:295–301, 1993.
45. Rutgers PH, Kitslaar PJEHM: Randomized trial of stripping versus

high ligation combined with sclerotherapy in the treatment of incompetent greater saphenous vein. Am J Surg 168:311–315, 1994.

46. Sarin S, Scurr JH, Coleridge Smith PD: Stripping of the long saphenous vein in the treatment of primary varicose veins. Br J Surg 81:1455–1458, 1994.

47. Dwerryhouse S, Davies B, Harradine K, Earnshaw JJ: Stripping the long saphenous vein reduces the rate of reoperation for recurrent varicose veins: Five-year results of a randomized trial. J Vasc Surg 29:589–592, 1999.

48. Bergan JJ: New developments in surgery of the venous system. J Cardiovasc Surg 1:624, 1993.

49. Hanrahan LM, Araki CT, Rodriguez AA, et al: Distribution of valvular incompetence in patients with venous stasis ulceration. J Vasc Surg 13:805, 1991.

50. Shami SK, Sarin S, Cheatle TR, et al: Venous ulcers and the superficial venous system. J Vasc Surg 17:487, 1993.

51. Hach W: Sekundare popliteal und femoral Veneninsuffizienz, die Cockettschen Vv. perforantes und die paratibiale Fasziotomie. Med Welt 32:619–622, 1989.

52. Walsh JC, Bergan JJ, Beeman S, Comer TP: Femoral venous reflux is abolished by greater saphenous vein stripping. Ann Vasc Surg 8:56, 1994.

53. Linton RR: The communicating veins of the lower leg and the operative technique for their ligation. Ann Surg 107:582, 1938.

54. Jugenheimer M, Junginger TH: Endoscopic subfascial sectioning of incompetent perforating veins in the treatment of primary varicosis. World J Surg 16:971, 1992.

55. Fischer R: Erfahrungen mit der endoskopischen perforanten Sanierung. Phlebologie 21:224, 1992.

56. Perrin M: Venous leg perforating veins [in French]. J Mal Vasc 24:19–24, 1999.

57. Bergan JJ: Venous insufficiency and perforating veins [editorial]. Br J Surg 85:721–722, 1998.

58. Haenen JH, Janssen MCH, van Langen H, et al: The postthrombotic syndrome in relation to venous hemodynamics as measured by means of duplex scanning and strain-gauge plethysmography. J Vasc Surg 29:1071–1076, 1999.

59. Powell CC, Rohrer MJ, Barnard MR, et al: Chronic venous insufficiency is associated with increased platelet and monocyte activation and aggregation. J Vasc Surg 30:844–853, 1999.

60. Carpentier PH: Leukocytes in chronic venous insufficiency [in French]. J Mal Vasc 23:274–276, 1998.

61. Gloviczki P: Subfascial endoscopic perforator vein surgery: Indications and results. Vasc Med 4:173–180, 1999.

62. Gloviczki P, Bergan JJ, Rhodes JM, et al, and the North American Study Group: Mid-term results of endoscopic perforator vein interruption for chronic venous insufficiency: Lessons learned from the North American Subfascial Endoscopic Perforator Surgery (NASEPS) Registry. J Vasc Surg 29:489–502, 1999.

63. Murray JA, Bergan JJ, Riffenburgh RH: Development of open-scope SEPS: Lessons learned from the first 67 cases. Ann Vasc Surg 13:372–377, 1999.

64. Lacroix H, Smeets A, Nevelsteen A, Suy R: Classic versus endoscopic perforating vein surgery: A retrospective study. Acta Chir Belg 98:71–75, 1998.

65. Scriven JM, Bianchi V, Hartshorne T, et al: A clinical and hemodynamic investigation into the role of calf perforating vein surgery in patients with venous ulceration and deep venous incompetence. Eur J Vasc Endovasc Surg 16:148–152, 1998.

66. Proebstle TM, Weisel G, Paepcke U, et al: Light reflection rheography and clinical course of patients with advanced venous disease before and after endoscopic subfascial division of perforating veins. Dermatol Surg 24:771–776, 1998.

67. Rhodes JM, Gloviczki P, Canton L, et al: Endoscopic perforator vein division with ablation of superficial reflux improves venous hemodynamics. J Vasc Surg 28:839–847, 1998.

68. Palma EC, Riss F, Del Campo F, et al: Tratamiento de los trastornos postflebiticos mediante anastomosis venosa safenofemoral contralateral. Bull Soc Surg Uruguay 29:135–145, 1958.

69. Palma EC, Esperon R: Vein transplants and grafts in the surgical treatment of the post-phlebitic syndrome. J Cardiovasc Surg (Torino) 1:94–107, 1960.

70. Dale WA: Crossover vein grafts for iliac and femoral venous occlusion. Resident Staff Physician June 1983, 58–64.

71. Danza R, Navarro T, Baldizan J, Olivera D: Injerto veno-venoso libre: Indicaciones, tecnica y resultados (11 anos de experiencia). Cir Uruguay 50:485–494, 1980.

72. Halliday P, Harris J, May J: Femorofemoral crossover grafts (Palma operation): A long term follow-up study. In Bergan JJ, Yao JST (eds): Surgery of the Veins. Orlando, Fla, Grune & Stratton, 1985, pp 255–265.

73. Heniford BT, Senler SO, Olsofka JM, et al: May-Thurner syndrome: Management by endovascular surgical techniques. Ann Vasc Surg 12:482–486, 1998.

74. Molina JE, Hunter DW, Yedlicka JW: Thrombolytic therapy for iliofemoral thrombosis. Vasc Surg 39:630–637, 1992.

75. Kistner RL: Surgical repair of the incompetent femoral vein valve. Arch Surg 110:1336, 1975.

76. Kistner RL: Late results of venous valve repair. In Yao JST, Pearce WL (eds): Long-Term Results of Vascular Surgery. Philadelphia, WB Saunders, 1993, pp 451–466.

77. Palma EC, Esperon R: Vein transplants and grafts in the surgical treatment of the postphlebitic syndrome. J Cardiovasc Surg (Torino) 1:94, 1960.

78. Taheri SA, Lazar L, Elias S, et al: Surgical treatment of postphlebitic syndrome with vein valve transplant. Am J Surg 144:221, 1982.

Questions

1. Symptoms of varicose veins include aching pain and fatigue. These are greatest in which of the following?
   (a) telangiectasias
   (b) reticular varicosities
   (c) large subcutaneous varicosities
   (d) symptoms unrelated to size
   (e) symptoms may be equal in all of the above

2. In a patient with symptomatic varicose veins, after the complete history and physical examination are done, which of the following needs to be added to the evaluation?
   (a) duplex reflux examination
   (b) phlebography
   (c) handheld continuous wave Doppler evaluation
   (d) photoplethysmography

3. Treatment of telangiectasias and reticular, flat, blue-green varicosities is done to
   (a) improve the cosmetic appearance of the legs
   (b) ameliorate symptoms of aching, heaviness, and pain
   (c) neither of the above
   (d) both (a) and (b)

4. Nocturnal leg cramps are chiefly associated with
   (a) arteriosclerotic occlusive disease
   (b) lymphedema
   (c) telangiectasias
   (d) telangiectasias and varicose veins

5. Venous leg ulcer may be due to
   (a) saphenous reflux and varicose veins
   (b) deep venous reflux without superficial reflux
   (c) incompetent ankle perforating veins
   (d) all of the above

6. Severe venous dysfunction is characterized by ankle hyperpigmentation, induration, and open leg ulcers. The correct term for this condition is
   (a) stasis ulcer
   (b) postphlebitic state
   (c) chronic venous insufficiency
   (d) Marjoin's ulcer

7. The anatomic cause of venous leg ulcer is
   (a) superficial reflux
   (b) deep venous reflux
   (c) perforator reflux
   (d) all of the above, singly or in combination

8. The Linton and Cockett perforator vein operations were disappointing because of
   (a) recurrent ulceration
   (b) delayed healing of skin grafts
   (c) systemic infection
   (d) general morbidity

9. Conservative treatment of severe venous dysfunction includes
   (a) induced hyperthermia
   (b) intermittent pneumatic compression
   (c) fitted support
   (d) all of the above

10. The fundamental objective of perforator vein interruption is
    (a) improved calf muscle pump function
    (b) decreased ambulatory venous hypertension
    (c) diminished leukocyte trapping and activation
    (d) all of the above

Answers

1. d   2. c   3. d   4. d   5. d   6. c   7. a   8. d   9. c   10. d

43

Physiology and Imaging of the Peripheral Lymphatic System

Charles L. Witte and Marlys H. Witte

> The living organism does not really exist in the millieu extérieur . . . but in the liquid millieu intérieur formed by the circulating organic liquid which surrounds and bathes all the tissue elements; this is the lymph or plasma, the liquid part of the blood which . . . is diffused through the tissues.
>
> —CLAUDE BERNARD

GENERAL PRINCIPLES

Blood-Lymph Loop

From an evolutionary standpoint, a tissue fluid "circulation" long antedates a blood vascular system. Whether as a single giant coelom or an intricate network of thin-walled channels, a distinct process of tissue fluid exchange, or turnover, can be consistently identified in all vertebrate and invertebrate life. Although the term *vascular system* usually refers specifically to arteries and veins, the true extracellular fluid circulation is liquid flowing rapidly in the blood stream as a suspension of red blood cells in plasma and slowly in body tissues and lymphatics as a suspension of immunocytes in tissue fluid and lymph.

This blood-lymph loop and the partition of extracellular fluid compartments is regulated at the microvascular interface and depends primarily on the balance of the transcapillary hydrostatic and protein osmotic pressure gradients as modified by the permeability and surface area of filtering blood capillaries.[1] Normally, a small excess of tissue fluid forms, enters lymphatics, and then returns to the blood stream. In healthy individuals, net capillary filtration (i.e., lymph formation) and lymph drainage are exactly balanced, and tissues and body cavities are free of edema. When lymphatic pathways are congenitally absent or become blocked or obliterated, plasma normally escaping from the blood stream gradually accumulates as protein-rich edema or effusion. This phenomenon of static insufficiency or low-output failure of lymph flow is generally referred to as *lymphedema*. On the other hand, when microvascular fil-

tration increases to the point of overwhelming a rapidly draining but nonetheless inadequate lymphatic system (e.g., nephrosis, phlegmasia cerulea dolens, "cirrhotic" ascites), tissues also swell. This other form of edema or effusion represents dynamic insufficiency or high-output failure of lymph flow. In some circumstances, both features exist together either at the outset or during progression of disease. This phenomenon is usually referred to as the "law" of edema and is commonly expressed as

$$\Delta IFV = \int K_f[(P_c - P_t) - \sigma(\pi_p - \pi_t)] - \int L_v$$

where ΔIFV = change in interstitial fluid volume; K_f = blood capillary filtration coefficient; P_c = capillary hydrostatic pressure; P_t = tissue hydrostatic pressure; σ = solute reflection coefficient; π_p = plasma protein osmotic pressure; π_t = tissue protein osmotic pressure; and L_v = lymph flow.

Proteins in lymph and edema fluids originate primarily from corresponding tissue fluids, which, in turn, derive almost entirely from circulating plasma. Compared with plasma, lymph and tissue fluid generally contain each protein fraction but in a lower concentration and with a slightly higher proportion of albumin (molecular weight, 69 kD) and lower proportions of higher-molecular-weight globulins such as immunoglobulin M (IgM) (molecular weight, 1200 kD), a phenomenon termed *restrictive diffusion* or *molecular sieving*.[2]

Lymphatic System

The mammalian lymphatic system arises either from veins[3] or independently from mesenchymal tissue closely linked to tissue spaces[4] as a complex network of capillaries that join to form progressively larger channels and collecting ducts. In its entirety, it is composed not only of vessel conduits but also of lymph nodes, spleen, Peyer's patches, thymus, nasopharyngeal tonsils, and circulating cellular elements such as lymphocytes and macrophages. These migrating cells cross the blood-capillary barrier along with a multitude of immunoglobulins, polypeptides, plasma protein complexes, and cytokines to circulate in lymph through lymph nodes back to the blood stream (see Blood-Lymph Loop). As a specialized subcompartment of the extracellular space, therefore, the lymphatic system completes a continuous closed loop for the circulation by returning liquid, macromolecules, and other blood elements that "escape" or "leak" from blood capillaries.

Except for the central nervous system and cortical bony skeleton, lymphatics are ubiquitous and closely parallel venous tributaries. In general, lymph from the lower torso and viscera enters the blood stream via the thoracic duct at the left subclavian–jugular venous junction. Lymphatics from the head and neck and those draining the arms enter central veins either independently or via a common supraclavicular cistern. Numerous interconnections exist within this rich lymphatic vascular network, and alternative anatomic pathways are plentiful. Whereas topographic variants only indirectly influence the development and progression of peripheral lymphedema, they are nonetheless pivotal to an in-depth understanding of swelling syndromes, accompanied by visceral lymphatic abnormalities, celomic effusions, and chylous reflux.

Interstitial Dynamics

As an afferent (unidirectional) vascular network, the lymphatics originate within the interstitium as specialized capillaries, although in certain organs such as the liver, they seem to emanate from nonendothelialized precapillary channels (e.g., the space of Disse).[5] Lymphatic capillaries are extremely porous and permit the entry of even large macromolecules (e.g., IgM). In this respect, they resemble the "leaky" fenestrated sinusoids of the liver but are in distinct contrast to most other blood capillaries, which are relatively impermeable to large molecules, even those the size of albumin.[2]

Under light microscopy without pre–paraffin-embedded tracer or intravascular latex injection, it is difficult to distinguish blood from lymph microvessels, although the latter are usually thin-walled and tortuous, have a wider, more irregular lumen, and are generally devoid of erythrocytes. Many staining features have been advocated to differentiate the blood and lymph microvasculature, including the endothelial marker factor VIII:von Willebrand's factor (F8:vWf). Staining features, however, vary both in pathologic and normal states as well as at different sites related to endothelial cell proliferation and dedifferentiation. Overall, lymphatic endothelial staining resembles, but is generally less intense than, that of arteries or veins. In brief, the staining differences, if any, are more quantitative than qualitative.[6–8]

Ultrastructurally, lymph capillaries display "open" and "closed" or so-called tight endothelial junctions, often with prominent convolutions.[9] Depending on fluid filtration rate at the blood capillary, lymph microvessels can drastically alter their state and lumen size to accommodate surplus tissue fluid (i.e., edema). In contrast to blood capillaries, a basal lamina or basement membrane is tenuous or absent altogether in lymph capillaries.[9, 10] Moreover, complex elastic fibrils termed "anchoring filaments" tether the abluminal surface of the endothelium to a fibrous-gel matrix in the interstitium[11, 12] (Fig. 43–1). These unique filaments allow the initial lymphatics to open widely and to accommodate an increased tissue fluid–macromolecular load associated with increased interstitial pressure while adjacent blood capillaries collapse,[11, 12] thereby restricting plasma filtration. In contrast to more proximal and larger lymphatics, initial and terminal lymph vessels are devoid of smooth muscle, although the endothelia contain F-actin, a contractile protein.[6] Intraluminal bicuspid valves are also prominent features of lymphatic collectors and serve to partition lymph vessels into discrete contractile segments termed "lymphangions"[13–15] (Fig. 43–2). These special features of the lymphatic network facilitate the performance of this delicate apparatus in absorbing and transporting lymph nodal cellular elements and large protein moieties, other cells, and foreign particles (viruses, bacteria) that have gained access to the interstitial space.

Microvascular Forces

Although body water makes up 60% to 70% of total body weight, and more than two thirds of this volume resides within cells, it is the remaining one third of liquid outside cells that continuously circulates. Whereas the compartmentalization of extracellular fluid between plasma and interstitium depends on the "Starling forces" (transcapillary hydrostatic and protein osmotic pressure gradients), the magnitude of these hydrodynamic forces and the nature of the capillary barrier vary widely.[1] For example, hepatic sinusoids have a very low hydrostatic pressure (5 mm Hg) and are lined by a discontinuous endothelium with high permeability to plasma proteins.[16, 17] Unrestrained by an "effective" protein osmotic pressure gradient, intrahepatic transcapillary fluid flux is extremely sensitive to changes in perfusion pressure.[16, 17] Accordingly, hepatic lymph flow increases sharply in response to small increments in sinusoidal pressure. In contrast, peripheral blood microvessels are far less permeable to transcapillary protein movement and thereby maintain a relatively steep protein osmotic pressure gradient between plasma and interstitium. Whereas a rise in peripheral capillary pressure also increases outward fluid flux from plasma, adjustments (autoregulation) in extremity arterial inflow and dilution of tissue protein content oppose further blood capillary filtration ("edematogenic safety factors").[18] Nonetheless, persistent elevation in blood microvascular hydrostatic pressure increases regional lymph flow, and when the capacity of the lymphatic system is overwhelmed, edema or effusion (ascites, hydrothorax) supervenes.

Lymph Propulsion

Although blood flows in a circular pattern at 5 to 6 L/minute, lymph flow is entirely in one direction and at rest totals only 1.5 to 2.5 L/day.[19] This limited volume represents a small tissue fluid excess arising from a slight imbalance in the Starling hydrodynamic forces that favor move-

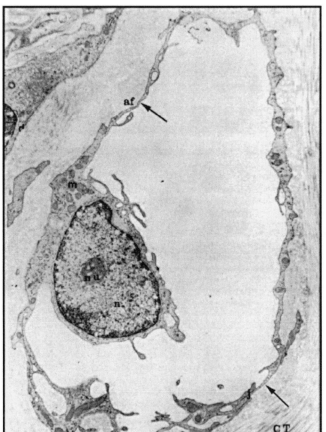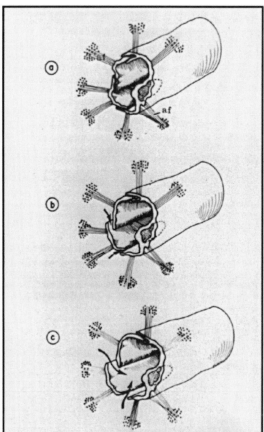

Figure 43–1. *Left panel,* Ultrastructure of a lymphatic capillary in cross-section. The close association of the adjoining connective tissue components (CT) with the lymphatic wall is maintained by numerous anchoring filaments (af), which join the abluminal surface to the adjacent interstitium as a meshwork. The endothelium is extremely attenuated at various points *(arrows),* and the nucleus (n) with its nucleolus (nu) protrudes into the lumen. Several intercellular junctions (j) are visible. Mitochondria (m) appear in the juxtanuclear region as well as in the thin cytoplasmic rims. (× 11,000.) *Right panel,* Response of lymphatic capillaries to an increase in interstitial fluid volume. As the matrix expands, the tension of the anchoring filaments (af) rises, and the lymphatic capillaries gradually open widely (a–c) to allow more rapid entry of liquid and solute. (*Left panel* from Leak LV: Electron microscopic observations on lymphatic capillaries and the structural components of the connective tissue–lymph interface. Microvasc Res 2:361–391, 1970; *right panel* from Leak LV: The fine structure and function of the lymphatic vascular system. In Meesen H [ed]: Handbüch der Allgemeinen Pathologie. Berlin and New York, Springer-Verlag, 1972, pp 149–196.)

ment of salt, water, and plasma proteins into tissues. Unlike the blood circulation, however, which is propelled by a powerful, highly specialized muscular pump (the heart), lymph flow derives from rhythmic contractions of large and probably also smaller lymph trunks[20–22] and, to a limited extent, from breathing, sighing, yawning, bowel peristalsis, and transmitted arterial pulsations.[23] Indeed, the contractions of lymphatic segments between intraluminal valves (lymphangions) are unusually responsive to lymph volume. Thus, an increase in formation of tissue fluid and lymph promotes a greater amplitude and frequency in lymphangion contraction.[13, 14, 24] This lymph dynamic response resembles Starling's other well-known physiologic principle, "the law of the heart." Furthermore, like blood vessel vasomotion, lymphatic contractility is also upregulated by α-adrenergic agonists, prostaglandins, and neural mediators but downregulated by β-adrenergic stimulators, thromboxanes, extravasated hemoglobin, and oxygen metabolites[25–32] (Fig. 43–3).

Lymph nodes, which play a central role in mammalian immunity, are potentially an anatomic site of restriction to the free flow of lymph. Unlike frogs, which lack lymph nodes but possess several strategically placed lymph hearts (cor lymphaticum) that propel large volumes of lymph back to the blood stream,[33] mammals have widely dispersed lymph nodes, which when diseased (swollen, fibrotic, or atrophic) may initiate or aggravate lymph stasis.[34] Perhaps the intrinsic contraction of mammalian lymphatic trunks represents a phylogenetic vestige of amphibian lymph hearts.

Although lymphatics, like veins, are thin-walled, flexible conduits that return liquid to the heart, the pressure-flow dynamics in the two systems are considerably different. The energy to propel both arterial and venous blood derives primarily from the thrust of the heart *(vis a tergo).* The cardiac propulsive boost maintains a pressure head throughout the blood stream that is sufficient to overcome blood vascular resistance. Skeletal muscle contraction, as in running and walking, in conjunction with intact venous valves, supplements cardiac performance in facilitating venous return. At their origin in tissues, however, lymphatics are not contiguous with the blood stream, and the chief source of energy for lymph propulsion emanates from intrinsic lymphatic wall contraction.[35] Compared with the low

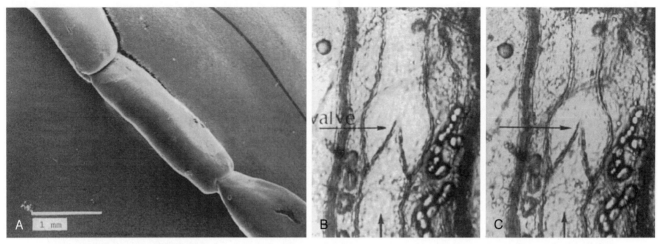

Figure 43–2. *A,* Cast preparation of a lymphatic collector—the valves produce deep fissures in the hardened resin, and the orientation of the valve slit axis changes from one segment to the next. *B* and *C,* Arrangement of bileaflet valves in a 75-μm collecting lymphatic in the mesentery of the rat. In *B,* the upper portion of the vessel is in the dilator phase of its spontaneous vasomotor activity, whereas the lower section below the valve is narrowed. In *C,* with narrowing of the distal portion of the vessel, the bulbous nature of the valve region is further exaggerated as the valves are forced shut. The propulsion is clearly peristaltic in nature. (Original magnification × 160.) (*A,* From Olszewski WL: Lymph Stasis; Pathophysiology, Diagnosis and Treatment. Boca Raton, FL, CRC Press, 1991. *B* and *C,* from Zweifach BW, Prather JW: Micromanipulation of pressure in terminal lymphatics in the mesentery. Am J Physiol 228:1326–1345, 1975.)

vascular resistance to venous flow, resistance to lymph flow is comparatively high,[36] but the contractile capability of lymphatics can overcome this impedance by generating luminal pressures of 30 to 55 mm Hg and even higher[20, 36, 37] (Figs. 43–4 and 43–5). This formidable lymphatic ejection force, as previously noted, is affected by sympathomimetics, temperature, oxygen radicals, and locally released paracrine and autocrine cytokine secretions.[25–31]

In contrast to the liquid in veins, the column of liquid (lymph) in peripheral lymphatics is incomplete. Therefore, with normal intralymphatic pressure and in the absence of edema, skeletal muscle compression has no effect on lymph propulsion, although by local agitation it moves some tissue

fluid into initial lymphatics and transiently raises the force and rate of lymphatic contraction[37] (see Fig. 43–5). Studies on the effects of gravity on hindlimb lymphatic and venous pressure conform to these findings. The assumption of the erect position dramatically raises distal venous pressure, but distal intralymphatic pressure hardly changes (see Fig. 43–4), although again, lymphatic propulsion may increase both in frequency and in amplitude.[38] On the other hand, with chronic lymphatic obstruction and persistent lymph stasis, hydrostatic pressure in the draining tissue watersheds and lymphatics rises because lymphatic contraction is unable to expel lymph completely. Now, the fluid column in the lymphatics becomes continuous (i.e., "fully primed"),

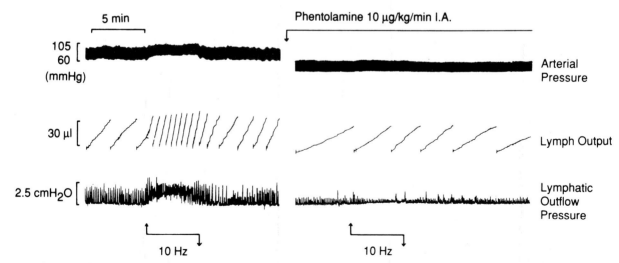

Figure 43–3. The effect of stimulating the sympathetic chain at 10 Hz on arterial pressure, popliteal efferent lymph flow, and lymphatic contraction frequency *(bottom record)* before and after an infusion of phentolamine into the femoral artery. (From McGeown JG, McHale NG, Thornbury KD: The effect of electrical stimulation of the sympathetic chain on peripheral lymph flow in the anaesthetized sheep. J Physiol (Lond) 393:127, 1987.)

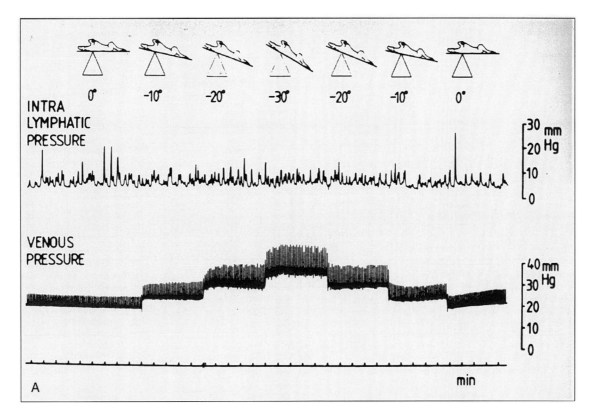

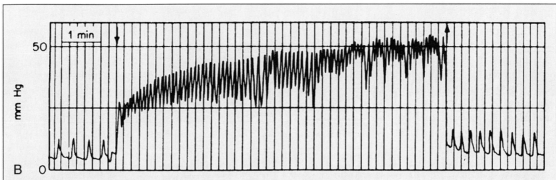

Figure 43–4. *A,* The effect of tilting the sheep on pressure in an adjacent lymphatic and vein in the metatarsal region. Note: Whereas venous pressure rises dramatically with dependency, lymphatic pressure is unaltered, although rate and amplitude of lymphatic contractions often increase. *B,* The effects of occlusion of the flow from a lymphatic vessel on the lymphatic pressure and the frequency of the intrinsic contractions of the lymph vessel wall. (*Panel A* from Pippard C, Roddie IC: Comparison of fluid transport systems in lymphatics and veins. Lymphology 20:224–229, 1987; *panel B* from Hall JG, Morris B, Woolley G: Intrinsic rhythmic propulsion of lymph in the unanesthetized sheep. J Physiol (Lond) 180:336–349, 1965.) (Compare with Figure 43–5.)

and skeletal muscle contraction or forceful external compression (e.g., massage, pneumatic) helps to move lymph onward.[37, 38]

The flow-pressure dynamic differences between veins and lymphatics can now be summarized. Veins operate with a pressure gradient that is higher distally and gradually diminishes as venous blood approaches the right atrium. The venous system is characterized by the transport of high fluid volume under low pressure and against low vascular resistance. Lymphatics, in contrast, operate with a pressure gradient that is atmospheric (or slightly subatmospheric) distally and gradually rises as central lymph approaches the great veins. The lymphatic system is charac-

terized by the transport of low fluid volume under low pressure and against high vascular resistance. Whereas venous flow is generated primarily by the thrust of the heart and muscle contraction, lymphatic flow is generated primarily by intrinsic lymph vessel contraction. Only when low-output failure of lymph flow supervenes (lymphedema) do muscle contraction and external compression augment lymph propulsion.

Lymphangiogenesis

Although an explosion of interest in angiogenesis has focused primarily on the regulation of blood vessel growth,

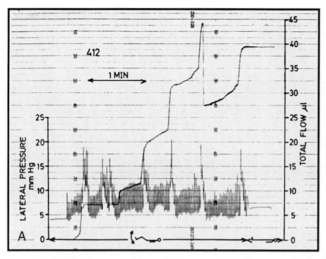 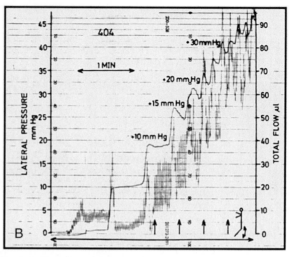

Figure 43–5. *A,* Pressure and flow record in a human superficial leg lymphatic in a horizontal position during foot exercise (dorsal and plantar flexion—40 per min). Two to three spontaneous pressure peaks (12 mm Hg) with simultaneous "bursts" of lymph flow are seen. Calf muscle contractions generate pressures of 5 mm Hg amplitude with only minimal promotion of lymph flow. *B,* A human leg lymphatic was cannulated in a retrograde fashion, and the external tip of the cannula was raised stepwise to increase hydrostatic pressure above the level of the cannulated lymphangion. With the subject in the upright position, raising outflow pressures by tiptoeing produced more frequent pulsations. Whereas contraction of the lymphatic propelled lymph flow, pressures generated by skeletal muscle contraction did not. Note that at higher lymphatic pressures, a slight retrograde flow occurred, probably from valve incompetence in the overly distended lymphatic vessel. (From Olszewski WL: Lymph Stasis; Pathophysiology, Diagnosis and Treatment. Boca Raton, FL, CRC Press, 1991.)

similar physiochemical signals and mediators are likely involved in lymphangiogenesis and lymphangiodysgenesis. Lymphatic regeneration is ordinarily a rapid and vigorous phenomenon.[39, 40] After experimental circumferential skeletonization of the neurovascular bundle of the hindlimb, new lymphatics bridge the incision site as early as the fourth day postoperatively, and by the eighth day, lymphatic reconnection is restored.[41] Bellman and Odén[42, 43] meticulously documented the time course and extensiveness of newly formed lymph vessels in wounds. As the lymphatics increased in caliber, intraluminal valves and sinuous dilatations appeared. In 1932, Clark and Clark[44] demonstrated the outgrowth of capillaries from preexisting lymph vessels, without a tendency for anastomosis with adjacent blood microvessels. Pullinger and Florey,[45] after examining lymphatic proliferation during inflammation, emphasized that despite the similar appearance of vascular endothelium, lymphatics were connected to lymphatics, veins to veins, and arteries to arteries without crossover.

More recent studies provide quantitative and qualitative information on the proliferation rate of lymphatic endothelium in vivo. Although blood vascular endothelium is considered dormant,[46, 47] lymphatic endothelial turnover is almost nonexistent. On the other hand, with injury or inflammation, increased endothelial radiolabeling with tritiated thymidine occurs with fetal lymphatic growth, demonstrating lymphatic proliferation greater than that in the neonate, which, in turn, is greater than lymphatic regrowth in the adult. Mesenteric lymphatic endothelium also shows greater proliferative potential than peripheral lymphatic endothelium.[48]

In 1984, pure cultures of lymphatic endothelium were isolated from bovine mesenteric lymphatics for the first time.[49] Our group obtained pure cultures of lymphatic

endothelium from a human patient with a cervical-mediastinal lymphangioma.[50] Like blood vascular endothelium, lymphatic endothelium has now been grown in culture from a wide variety of hosts in monolayers of "cobblestone" sheets and on microcarrier beads. Lymphangiogenesis has also been demonstrated spontaneously in lymphatic endothelial cultures from lymphangiomas by sprouting and cyst-like formation, and after treatment with collagen type I, migration, sprouting, and increase in dimension and length of lymphatic endothelial tubules have also been observed.[51]

Growing evidence implicates the genetic control of lymphangiogenesis.[52] It has been proposed that a gene or genes expressed from nonactivated portions of the inactive X chromosome or from the Y chromosome are involved in the development of lymphatics and that a deficiency of gene products is responsible for phenotypic changes in Turner's syndrome. Moreover, other chromosomal aneuploid disorders, including the common trisomy 21 (Down syndrome), also occasionally present with strangulating fetal cystic hygroma, lymphedema, and intestinal lymphangiectasia along with cardiac anomalies.

A variety of hereditary lymphedema-angiodysplasia syndromes (generally with autosomal dominant inheritance) also point to an array of "lymphangiogenesis genes." Thus, Milroy's disease, a familial disorder of lymphedema from birth or early childhood, is characterized by severe lymphatic hypoplasia and occasional intestinal lymphangiectasia. Vascular endothelial growth factors (specifically VEGF-C) have now been implicated in lymphatic new growth[53] with a "lymphedema" or more accurately a lymphangiodysplasia gene linked to the distal arm of chromosome 5 (q34–35) in some but not all families with possible associated VEGF receptor (*flt*-4) mutations in this coding region.[54–56] Nonetheless, with varied phenotypic expression and more than 30 distinct familial lymphedema syndromes, gene heterogeneity is likely, given the broad clinical manifestations of angiodysplastic and associated anomalies.

DISORDERED LYMPH FLOW

Definition

Lymphatic insufficiency or *failure* is a generic term for the pathologic buildup of liquid and solute in the extracellular matrix from an impaired or overburdened lymphatic drainage system. *Lymphedema,* on the other hand, is the specific clinical term when the outward manifestations are rooted in stagnant or decreased lymph return (low-output failure) either from lymphatic hypoplasia or aplasia (primary lymphedema) or after radical ablation or obliteration of lymph nodes and trunks (secondary lymphedema). Whereas the expression *lymphedema* usually conjures up a brawny swollen extremity or an elephantine skin disorder caused by parasites in a far-off land, it should be recognized that the physiologic principles governing the distribution of extracellular fluid, including interstitial fluid flux and lymph flow, properly apply to all tissues and organ systems.[57]

Peripheral Lymphedema

In chronic lymphedema of the extremities, the prototype disorder for lymph stasis, there is commonly a long latent period before evolution of unremitting edema, interspersed with periodic episodes of inflammation or infection and often culminating in brawny induration with tissue fibrosis. In the extreme, as with filariasis (*Wuchereria bancrofti, Brugia malayi*), deformities are grotesque and come to resemble the skin and soft tissue pedestals of a pachyderm (elephantiasis). For many years, the relation between impaired lymphatic drainage and the gross manifestations was obscure because of variable swelling and often long delay between lymphatic ablation and onset of edema, cellulitis, and the seemingly infinite capacity for lymphatic regeneration. Although complete understanding is still elusive, it is now clear that the bulk of these extremity changes can satisfactorily be explained by lymph stagnation alone and the buildup of cells and protein in the extracellular matrix. First recognized by Danese and associates[58] and later further clarified by Olszewski[59] and Clodius and Altorfer,[60] the natural history of experimental interruption of peripheral lymphatics is transient swelling (acute lymphedema) and disappearance of edema for several months or years (latent lymphedema), followed by gradual reappearance and persistence (chronic lymphedema). During the latent period when edema is not overt, oil-contrast lymphography displays diffuse lymphatic disruption and obliteration, which, over time, gradually worsens[59, 60] (Fig. 43–6). Thus, lymphatic tortuosity, dilatation, and pools of contrast progress to massive lymphangiectasia, valvular incompetence, and retrograde lymph flow. Histopathologically, round cell infiltration, destruction of lymphatic truncal musculature, and replacement of the tissue matrix with bundles of collagen become prominent.

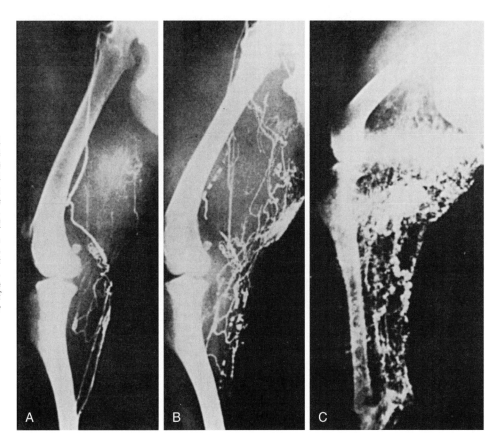

Figure 43–6. Sequential conventional lymphograms of dog hindlimb 9 *(A),* 14 *(B),* and 48 *(C)* months after operative manipulation to reproduce peripheral lymphedema. During the first year, gross edema was absent, but lymphatic channels displayed progressive dilatation and collateralization with dermal backflow (latent phase). At 48 months, when clinical edema was intractable, lymphography reveals similar albeit more extensive lymphatic dysplasia. (Modified from Olszewski WL: On the pathomechanism of development of postsurgical lymphedema. Lymphology 6:35–52, 1973.)

Lymphedema Sequelae

Fibrosis

Although the precise relationship between excessive tissue protein accumulation and matrix fibrosis with long-standing lymphedema is unclear, it seems plausible that fibrin or other cell agglutinins such as fibronectin (surface-binding α_2-macroglobulin) released into the interstitium provide the scaffolding for fibroblast proliferation and deposition of collagen.[61, 62] Another contributing factor may be insufficient removal of newly sequestered protein and deranged matrix by macrophages[63] or neutrophil proteases.[64] Finally, lymph stasis with trapped protein in the interstitium attracts mononuclear cells, which, through chemotaxis and induced release of local growth factors (e.g., cytokines), ultimately stimulates fibroblast replication and deposition of collagen.[65] The key observation or clinical implication is the common occurrence of a long interval between obliteration of lymph trunks and the development of refractory edema. This occurrence helps to explain the inconsistency and unpredictability of limb swelling after radical operations for treatment of cancer and other disorders of defective lymphatic drainage. As with deep vein occlusive disease, which is accompanied by venous stasis, gradual valve destruction, and, eventually, frank edema (postphlebitic syndrome) with trophic skin changes (brownish pigmentation and distal ulceration), lymphatic blockage is associated with intraluminal valve incompetence, lymph stagnation, and, eventually, intractable edema (postlymphangitic syndrome) with trophic skin changes (thickened digital skin folds, warty overgrowth, and brawny induration) (Fig. 43–7).

Cellulitis

Recurrent infection is potentially a devastating complication of peripheral lymphedema. Erysipelas resulting from β-hemolytic streptococci is probably the most common example, but fulminant infection occurs with a variety of microorganisms. Why there is the extraordinary susceptibility of a lymphedematous limb to secondary bacterial infection remains perplexing. Studies in canine and human filarial lymphedema suggest defective complement activation and immunodysregulation.[66] Alternative theories implicate cellular depopulation of regional lymph nodes, their replacement by fat and scar tissue,[34] and deficient proteolysis by "wandering" macrophages.[67] It remains problematic, however, whether these immune dysregulations are systemic, local, or even unique to lymphedema.

Neoplasia

A rare complication of long-standing peripheral lymphedema is development of a (lymph)angiosarcoma. This aggressive vascular neoplasm was originally thought to arise exclusively as a consequence of radical mastectomy and irradiation for treatment of breast cancer (Stewart-Treves syndrome).[68, 69] But lymphangiosarcoma has now been described in other secondary lymphedemas and even in congenital (primary) lymphedema.[70] Because brawny limb swelling has typically existed for many years and occurs in either congenital or acquired lymphedema, with or without prior radiation therapy, the lymphedema process itself is thought to be the primary causative factor (see Fig. 43–7).

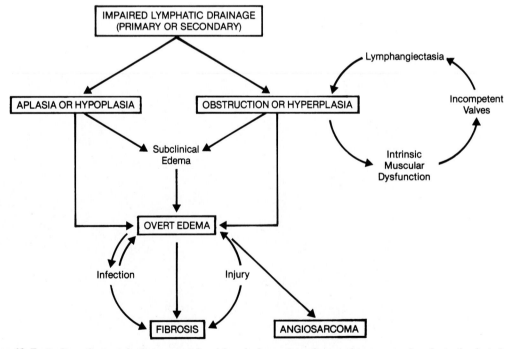

Figure 43–7. Outline of events leading to peripheral lymphedema. According to this concept, lymphatic dysplasia leads to gradual destruction of lymphatic valves and intrinsic contractile elements (lymphangioparalysis), which ultimately culminate in overt edema. Superimposed infection and injury with recurring lymphangitis aggravate underlying lymphedema and contribute to fibrosis. On rare occasions, lymphatic regeneration (lymphangiogenesis) degenerates into malignant endothelial overgrowth (angiosarcoma).

Of interest, Kaposi's sarcoma, an angiosarcoma akin to Stewart-Treves syndrome and at present associated with acquired immunodeficiency syndrome (AIDS) often complicated by lymphedema, has also been linked to an origin from lymphatic endothelium.[71–73]

Lymphangiodysgenesis

Vigorous lymphangiogenesis and lymphatic dysplasia is characteristic of long-standing experimental lymph stasis and lymphedema from surgically induced lymphatic obstruction or filarial infection and is often accompanied by concomitant hemangiogenesis.[74–76] Clinically, hemangiogenesis in lymphedema is displayed in the dermal hyperemia of the swollen limb. Thus, in both primary and secondary lymph stasis, proliferation of the blood vasculature and the heightened surface area for microvascular filtration of liquids and macromolecules into the interstitium further burdens the already compromised lymphatic network. Indiscriminate vascular hyperplasia may take on bizarre angiomatoid distortion and may even progress to highly aggressive malignant vascular tumors (e.g., Stewart-Treves angiosarcoma) in long-standing congenital or acquired lymphedema of the limbs, irradiated breast, or other sites.

The following sequence of events probably takes place in chronic lymphedema. Anatomic or functional lymph stasis generates intralymphatic hypertension, which is transmitted to the endothelial lining cells as mechanical stress. This shear-strain effect in turn signals the lymphatic endothelium to release vasoactive angiogenic chemical mediators the same or similar to those described for blood vascular endothelium. These signaling agents initiate mitogenesis and cell migration in lymphatics and perhaps indiscriminately also in nearby blood microvessels. Continued accumulation of macromolecules and trapped immune cells in the interstitium further disrupt attachments and adhesions in various cell types, thereby promoting lymphatic remodeling and collateralization. This angiogenic process involves release of growth factors not only from endothelial and other neighboring cell types but also from ground substance proteoglycans. Exacerbated by inadequate lymphatic drainage and extracellular matrix alteration, an array of different cell types is stimulated to proliferate, culminating in dysplastic soft tissue overgrowth of the limb or body part (Fig. 43–8) and, occasionally, (lymph)angiosarcoma (Fig. 43–9).

Chylous Reflux

Because cholesterol and long-chain triglycerides in the form of chylomicrons are absorbed exclusively by intestinal lymphatics from the digestive tract, malfunction (disruption, compression, obstruction, fistulization) of mesenteric lacteals, the cisterna chyli, or the thoracic duct, singly or in combination, may be accompanied by chylothorax, chylous ascites, and chyluria. In some patients with high-grade dysfunction of intestinal lymph flow, retroperitoneal lymph trunks gradually dilate, intraluminal lymphatic valves become incompetent, and lactescent lymph flows retrograde (chylous reflux) into the soft tissues of the pelvis, genitalia, and lower extremities, with prominence of chylous skin vesicles or dermal lymphatic varices (see later).

LYMPHATIC IMAGING

In patients suspected of arterial or venous disease the diagnosis is usually verified before definitive treatment is undertaken, but the diagnosis and treatment of peripheral lymphatic circulatory disorders often rest entirely on clinical impression. For example, patients who undergo axillary treatment of breast cancer and later develop arm edema

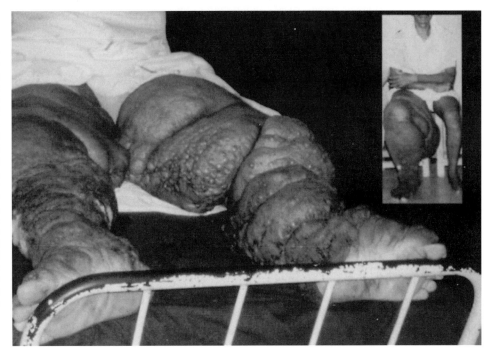

Figure 43–8. Middle-aged man from Chennai, India, with bilateral elephantine changes in both legs secondary to filariasis *(Wuchereria bancrofti).* A photograph 14 years earlier (inset) shows advanced filarial lymphedema only of the right leg and scrotum. In the interim, he underwent debulking of the right thigh and scrotum in conjunction with an inguinal nodal-venous shunt (Dr. S. Jamal). Of interest, the left leg, which now also displays advanced elephantiasis, was still grossly normal as recently as 3 years before the later, larger photograph was taken. Thus, in a relatively short time span, massive edema, acanthosis, fibrosis, and likely lipid deposition developed in the left leg, suggesting the importance of locally generated growth factors and cytokines from trapped trafficking of immune cells in addition to tissue fluid sequestration from secondary lymphedema.

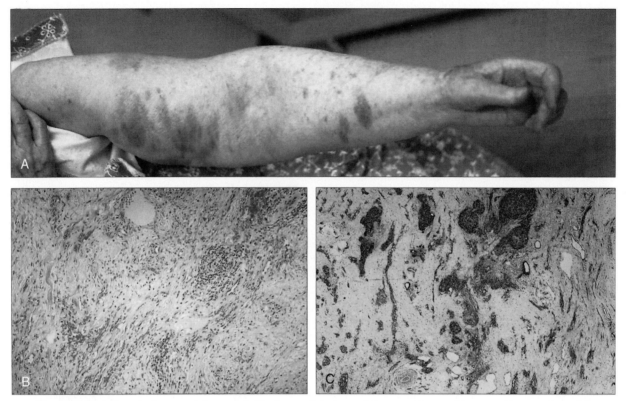

Figure 43–9. *A,* Lymphedematous left arm with blotchy purplish skin nodules in an 81-year-old woman 20 years after a left modified radical mastectomy and regional irradiation for the treatment of breast cancer. *B,* Histology of the forearm nodule after incisional biopsy showing the characteristic malignant endothelial neoplastic changes of (lymph) angiosarcoma corroborated by factor VIII–von Willebrand factor tumor positivity *(C)* of endothelial cells (Stewart-Treves syndrome).

are usually and reasonably assumed to have lymphedema. Similarly, in certain endemic areas of the world, peripheral edema may logically be assumed to be linked to filariasis, as adult filarial nematodes are known to inhabit the peripheral lymphatic system. Nonetheless, even in these seemingly straightforward conditions, it is preferable to pinpoint the anatomic and physiologic derangement before embarking on a treatment program, which may be useless or even harmful if the diagnosis of lymphedema is incomplete or incorrect.

Conventional Lymphography

Traditionally, documentation of the nature and extent of lymphatic dysfunction has required the cumbersome, inconvenient, and typically one-time procedure of conventional or direct lymphography.[77] This radiologic procedure involves visualization of skin lymphatics with coloring matter after intradermal instillation of a vital dye (e.g., pontamine blue) into the hand or foot. After a small incision, the exposed lymphatic with coloring matter is directly cannulated, and an oily medium is slowly injected over many hours under graded pressure to depict both lymphatic trunks and draining lymph nodes using plain radiographs.[77] Although conventional lymphography is still the gold standard for definitive delineation of the lymphatic system, its drawbacks (operative exposure, pulmonary oil embolism, wound infection, tediousness)[78] have led most physicians to

rely on physical appearance for diagnosis and initiation of therapy.

Isotope Lymphography (Lymphangioscintigraphy)

During the past several years, technical innovations in nuclear diagnostics and computer imaging have rekindled enthusiasm for visualizing the lymphatic system in peripheral lymphedema. In lymphangioscintigraphy (LAS), a large molecule such as sulfacolloid, dextran, hetastarch, or preferably human serum albumin is linked to a radiotracer (technetium 99m) and then instilled, preferably intradermally, as a wheal between the web spaces of the fingers or toes. Except for several seconds of a burning sensation, there are no untoward sequelae. Migration of the radiotracer within the skin and subcutaneous tissue is readily monitored with a parallel collimator in a whole-body gamma camera to provide scintiscans of truncal lymphatic drainage.[79] After several hours, the tracer has largely been cleared from the extremity, with residual radiopharmaceutical remaining at the injection site or in regional nodes ("hot spots") that decay over the next 24 hours. The advantages of this technique are that it is simple, safe, rapid, and easily repeated, and the amount of exposure to radioactivity is small (5 mCi or 18.5 MBq) (Fig. 43–10).

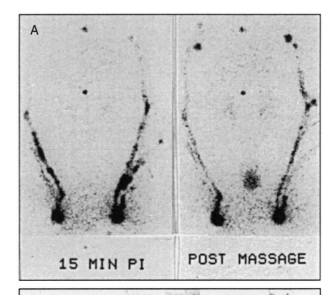

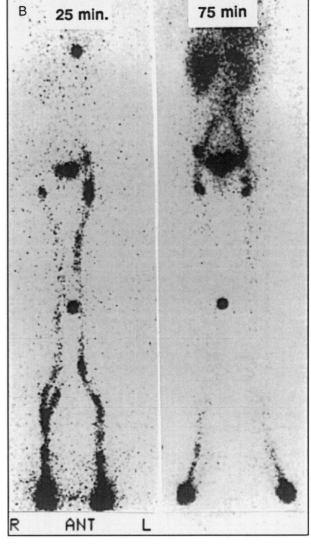

Figure 43–10. Normal appearance of lymphangioscintigram of the arms and legs *(A)* and *(B)*. In the legs, intact trunks are displayed as radioactive "bands," with rapid uptake in regional nodes. With time, the retroperitoneal or parailiac trunks are seen as the tracer (technetium 99m [^{99m}Tc]–human albumin) has cleared from both legs. Similarly in the arms, tracer transport is rapid to the axillary nodes. Rounded central densities are markers at the sternal notch, pubis, and knee.

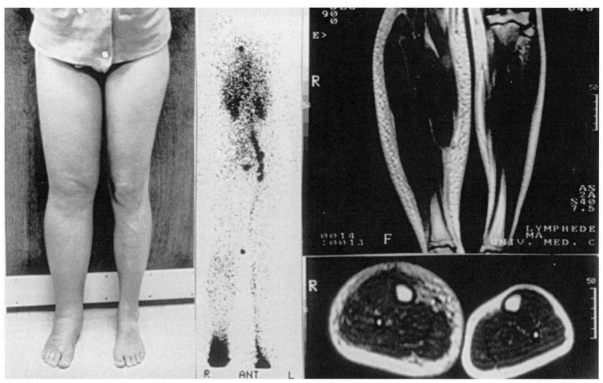

Figure 43–11. Teenage girl with lymphedema praecox. Whereas the left leg shows normal tracer transport, on the right edematous leg, no movement of the radiopharmaceutical is seen, even after several hours. Transaxial magnetic resonance views of the lower leg show subcutaneous thickening with superficial dermal lymphatics and edema. Note that the subfascial compartment (skeletal muscle) is without edema, although muscle enlargement is evident, probably from increased work hypertrophy in moving the swollen leg. (Modified from Case TC, Witte CL, Witte MH, et al: Magnetic resonance imaging in human lymphedema: Comparison with lymphangioscintigraphy. Magn Res Imag 10:549–558, 1992.)

Primary Lymphatic Dysplasia

With a wide spectrum of clinical manifestations of primary lymphedema in an age range that varies from soon after birth (congenital lymphedema or Milroy's disease) to 25 years (lymphedema praecox), it is not surprising that LAS images vary. Nonetheless, certain features are prominent, and many of these are distinctive from secondary lymphedema (see later). Typically, there is either lack of radiotracer transport altogether (Fig. 43–11) or prompt migration of tracer into the interstitium (dermal dispersion or "backflow") without evidence of intact truncal flow (i.e., lymphatic hypoplasia) (Fig. 43–12). In this context, it is imperative that a definite wheal be raised at the interdigital site of tracer injection to ensure intradermal instillation. Factitious failure of forward tracer movement may occur when the radiopharmaceutical has been introduced subcutaneously. Most patients with congenital lymphedema (i.e., onset before 8 years of age) demonstrate complete or near-complete lymphatic aplasia; however, other patients with primary lymphedema, including those with lymphedema praecox, display some tracer transport but typically in superficial dermal lymphatics (or in tissue spaces) and not in mainline lymphatic collectors. Characteristically, lymph transport is therefore retarded, and regional nodal visualization is faint, absent, or markedly delayed. In some patients with primary lymphedema, lymphatic dysplasia of the viscera is a major component of the lower extremity edema syndrome. These disorders are highlighted by re-

gurgitation of opalescent lacteal lymph into chylous vesicles or external leakage of milky lymph (Fig. 43–13) and often can be well depicted on LAS, especially after injection into the intact (nonedematous) contralateral leg (Fig. 43–14).

In summary, LAS in patients with primary lymphedema displays absent or delayed tracer transport after intradermal injection, absence of mainline lymphatic collectors, dermal backflow, poorly visualized regional nodes (without preexistent chemotherapy, extirpation, or irradiation), and, if leg edema is compounded by visceral reflux, evidence of retrograde tracer transport (Table 43–1).

TABLE 43–1

Lymphangioscintigraphy (LAS) Compared with Magnetic Resonance (MR) Imaging

LAS	MR IMAGING
Discrete or poorly defined trunks	Soft tissue (dermal and subcutis) edema and increased fat
Dermal diffusion ("backflow")	Deep (extremity) compartment unremarkable; occasional muscle ("work") hypertrophy
Delayed or nonvisualized regional nodes	Regional nodes atrophic, absent, enlarged, or unremarkable
Delayed tracer transport	Dermal lymphatic collaterals, "lakes," or "cisterns"
Crossover with retrograde tracer flow ('reflux')	Retroperitoneal or other visceral soft tissue abnormality

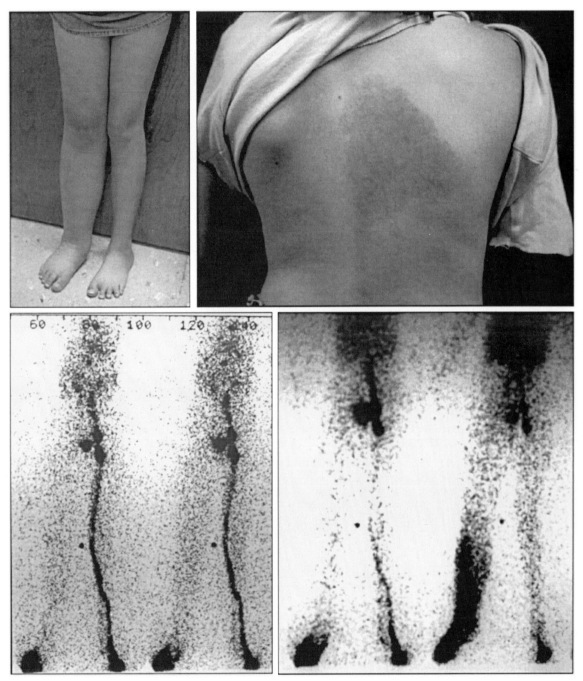

Figure 43–12. A 13-year-old girl with congenital lymphedema. Intradermal injection of technetium 99m (^{99m}Tc)–human albumin initially shows no tracer transport, but after several hours, there is diffuse dispersion of the radiopharmaceutical into the interstitium (dermal backflow). As commonly seen with lymphatic dysplasia syndromes, a prominent birthmark (blood vessel capillary angioma) is present between the scapulae.

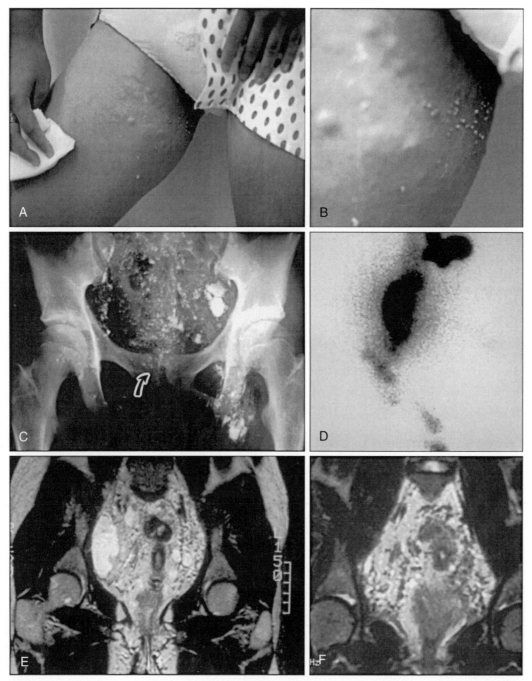

Figure 43–13. A 15-year-old girl with chylous reflux syndrome. *A* and *B*, Note milky lymph, associated with chylous vesicles, leaking from the inner thigh. *C*, Conventional lymphography displays massive "lakes" in the pelvis, with contrasting leaking from the vagina *(arrow)* (chylometrorrhagia). *D*, After instillation of a radioactive tracer into these ectatic and incompetent retroperitoneal lymphatics, the radiopharmaceutical can be seen to drain toward the pelvis and escape from the vagina. *E* and *F*, After percutaneous catheter obliteration of these dysplastic lymphatics under computer tomographic guidance (doxycycline), magnetic resonance imaging (T2-weighted) shows marked involution of the lymphangiectasia. After several treatments, chylous leakage from both the vagina and leg were nearly eliminated.

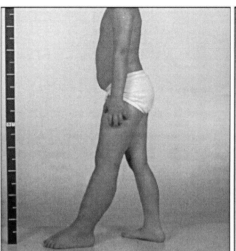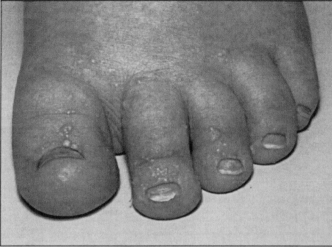

Figure 43–14. A 10-year-old boy with congenital lymphedema of the left leg. Close examination of the left foot displays chylous skin vesicles of the toes, and after instillation of a radioactive tracer in the right foot only, tracer reflux into the left leg all the way to the foot is highlighted. This lymphangioscintigraphic appearance is consistent with reflux of intestinal lymph into the left leg and foot. Separate isotope lymphographic study of the left leg (not shown) depicted severe lymphatic truncal hyperplasia as well.

Secondary Lymphatic Dysplasia

Although in many respects, LAS images in secondary lymphedema resemble those of primary lymphedema, there are nonetheless characteristic differences. With lymphatic obstruction, mainline lymphatic trunks are often well seen (Figs. 43–15, 43–16, and 43–17) in contradistinction to their attenuation or absence in congenital or hypoplastic syndromes. Although continued or long-standing lymphatic obstruction often culminates in diffuse obliteration of main lymphatic trunks (so-called die-back) because of lymph stagnation with intraluminal coagulum-gel formation and reactive inflammation, some lymphatic truncal activity usually persists, particularly in the first few minutes after intradermal injection. Regardless of the etiology, how-

ever, secondary, like primary, lymphedema is almost always associated with diffuse dermal backflow. Dermal diffusion is intense and seen early after injection in primary lymphedema but more variably in secondary lymphedema, depending on its severity and chronicity. In this regard, it is essential in performing LAS that early scintiscans (1–5 minutes) be obtained to corroborate truncal activity and that late scintiscans (approximately 3–4 hours) be obtained to detect delayed dermal backflow before an LAS study can be deemed complete (Fig. 43–18). The whole-body technique not only provides an accurate overall topographic view but also allows a global image so that subtle dermal backflow is not overlooked. In some patients, local lymph transport may initially be accelerated (perhaps related to increased amplitude and rate of truncal contraction) (see Lymph Propulsion and Fig. 43–3), but most commonly, as

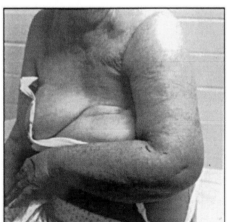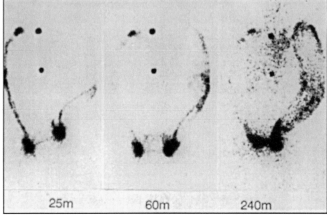

Figure 43–15. A 75-year-old woman with left arm lymphedema after modified radical mastectomy for treatment of breast carcinoma. On lymphangioscintigraphy, tracer transport in the right arm is unremarkable with prompt visualization of paraaxillary nodes and rapid clearance. In the left arm, however, initially intact lymphatic collectors are seen, but thereafter, there is progressive dermal backflow (tracer dispersion) and, after several hours, considerable retention of the radiopharmaceutical. Left-sided paraaxillary lymph nodes are not seen. (Modified from Case TC, Witte CL, Witte MH, et al: Magnetic resonance imaging in human lymphedema: Comparison with lymphangioscintigraphy. Magn Res Imag 10:549–558, 1992.)

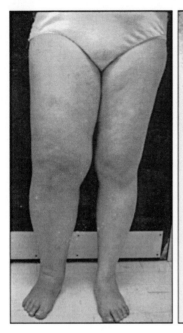
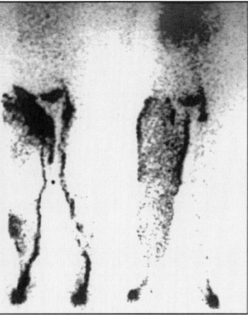

Figure 43–16. A 50-year-old woman with severe right-sided leg edema 8 months after radical hysterectomy and irradiation for treatment of carcinoma of the endometrium. Note the rapid migration of the tracer through intact lymphatics to the groin with subsequent extravasation (dermal backflow) and minimal clearance on the right after several hours. Despite the apparent symmetry of lymph node extirpation and irradiation, lymphatic transport in the left leg is apparently unaffected.

in primary lymphedema, tracer transport and regional nodal visualization are delayed and dermal backflow intensifies. Occasionally, as in early filariasis[80] or AIDS-associated Kaposi's sarcoma,[81] mild lymphedema is accompanied only by ectatic lymphatics and sluggish lymph transport. Functionally, sluggish lymph transport may also be seen in "disuse" (e.g., patients in wheelchairs), but clearance of the tracer, although slow, is complete. In some patients with morbid obesity, moreover, whose limbs resemble lymphedematous ones (e.g., "lipedema"), the diagnosis can be corroborated by a normal LAS (Fig. 43–19).

Similar LAS patterns are seen in filariasis (*W. bancrofti* and *B. malayi*). Thus, lymphangiectasia, dermal backflow, poor nodal visualization, hydrocele "filling," perirenal ex-

travasation (in chyluria), and even chylous reflux or total absence of transport are prominent features.[80]

Magnetic Resonance Imaging

Among the more vivid imaging tools for soft tissue detail is magnetic resonance (MR) imaging. In experimental animals[82] and patients with lymphedema,[83] MR has provided spectacular images of dermal edema, collateral lymph vessels, lymph nodal architecture, and the edema-free deep (subfascial) skeletal muscle compartment. The last finding explains how patients with advanced arm and leg swelling caused by lymphatic disorders typically display intact limb

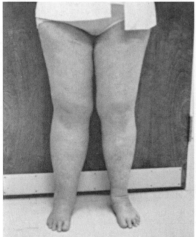
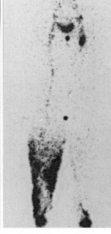
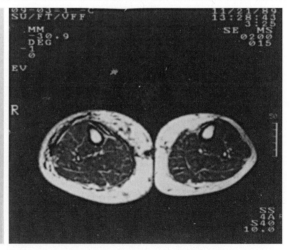

Figure 43–17. A 50-year-old woman with right leg edema after multiple stripping and ligation procedures for varicose veins. On lymphangioscintigraphy, there is tracer dispersion in the right lower leg (dermal backflow), but lymphatic collectors superiorly in the thigh and retroperitoneum are intact. Magnetic resonance imaging confirms lymphedema (liquid and collateral lymphatics) in the skin and subcutis (epifascial compartment). The subfascial (skeletal muscle) compartment is unremarkable except for slight muscle or "work" hypertrophy. Note that a duplex-Doppler study demonstrated an intact deep venous system. (Modified from Case TC, Witte CL, Witte MH, et al: Magnetic resonance imaging in human lymphedema: Comparison with lymphangioscintigraphy. Magn Res Imag 10:549–558, 1992.)

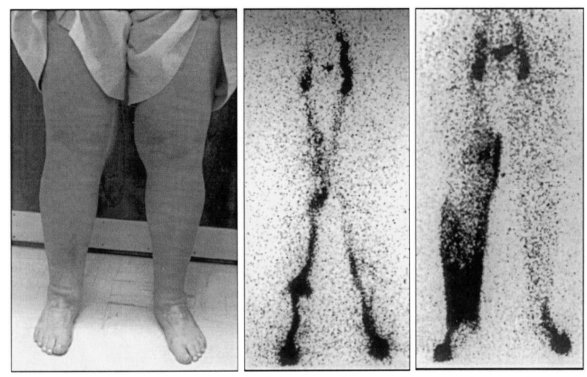

Figure 43–18. A 73-year-old woman with right leg lymphedema 7 years after excision of the greater saphenous vein for coronary artery bypass grafting complicated by severe thigh infection and regional lymphadenitis. Note on lymphangioscintigraphy early in the study, lymphatic collectors are well seen, tracer transport is rapid, and except for two small areas of dermal backflow (dispersion), the appearance is otherwise normal. At 3.5 hours (*far right panel*), however, a large amount of tracer has persisted and accumulated in the superficial lymphatics of the right leg, consistent with secondary lymphedema.

function limited only by the heaviness or unwieldy nature of the swollen extremity. Parenthetically, the apparent restriction of muscle swelling by natural myofascial binding also lends credence to the popular clinical usage of outer circumferential compression bandages or elastic stockinettes to restrict soft tissue (epifascial) swelling. In contrast to LAS, MR images characteristically show diffuse dermal and subcutaneous edema, a nonedematous, occasionally work-hypertrophied skeletal muscle compartment, serpiginous channels or "lakes" consistent with dermal collateral lymphangiectasia and sequestered lymph, and increased subcutaneous fat (see Figs. 43–11 and 43–17). Of equal

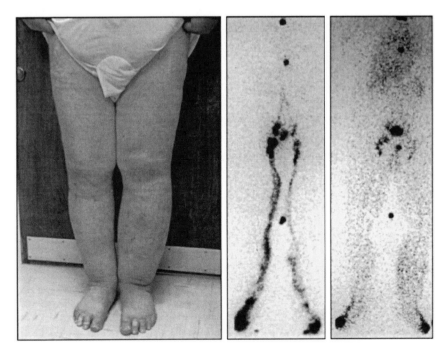

Figure 43–19. A 35-year-old man with "swollen" legs that resemble lymphedema. Lymphangioscintigraphy, however, reveals the lymphatic system to be intact. This condition is known as lipedema or simply obesity. This patient had gained more than 75 pounds in the year before presentation in the outpatient clinic.

importance, the status of proximal lymph nodes and other more central structures that may contribute to lymphatic obstruction but are not detectable after distal injection of standard contrast or radioisotopic imaging agents[83] can be assessed (see Table 43–1). Although the use of MR for depicting lymphatic abnormalities is costly and still in its infancy, newer superparamagnetic agents (e.g., iron oxide) injected interstitially dramatically reduce the signal intensity (i.e., enhance the visibility) of regional lymph nodes and adjacent lymphatics (lymphangiomagnetograms).[84] Finally, transaxial imaging (both MR and computed tomography [CT]) has even allowed percutaneous guidance to access ectatic retroperitoneal lymph trunks in chylous reflux syndromes and instill sclerosing agents (e.g., absolute alcohol or doxycycline) for obliteration of these collectors (Fig. 43–20) and control of external lymph leakage[85] (see Fig. 43–13).

Ultrasonography

Although ultrasonography usage in most patients with lymphedema is limited to verification of accumulation of subcutaneous edema fluid, recent findings indicate a

unique role in the evaluation of filariasis in endemic areas. Using a standard 7.5-MHz transducer, Amaral and colleagues[86] have detected indwelling adult nematode worms (the causative parasite) in the groin lymphatics of patients in Recife, Brazil, an endemic region for *W. bancrofti*. Using real-time Doppler-duplex studies, these workers have corroborated the nonstop, twisting motion ("Bahia dance") of these intralymphatic adult worms, a phenomenon first described in ferrets infected with *B. malayi*.[87]

Miscellaneous Techniques

A variety of other imaging methods also show promise in depicting the lymphatic system. For example, intravital fluorescence microangiography using fluorescein isothiocyanate dextran displays the superficial peripheral microvasculature, including the contractility, permeability, and diffusion characteristics of local blood and lymph capillaries[88] (Fig. 43–21). The diameters of lymph capillaries can even be determined from sequential video-recorded images of the intradermally injected field.[89] Preliminary findings suggest that patients who have had lymphedema since infancy have complete aplasia of lymphatic microvessels, whereas

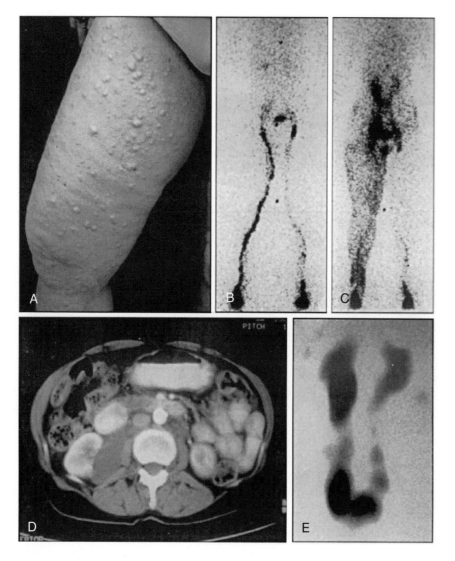

Figure 43–20. *A*, A 65-year-old woman with right leg lymphedema and prominent lymphatic varices (chylous vesicles) of the right thigh. These vesicles were filled with chylous lymph from which "milky" fluid occasionally drained. *B*, Lymphangioscintigraphy initially shows intact lymphatic collectors in the legs with rapid upward tracer transport. Thereafter, "pooling" of the tracer in the retroperitoneum is depicted (*C*) especially well on single photon emission tomography on the coronal view (*E*). In the later scintiscan (*C*), the tracer is seen to flow retrograde into the right leg with massive dermal backflow. In conjunction with computed tomographic (CT) scans demonstrating huge retroperitoneal ectatic lymphatics ("lymphangioma"), (*D*) this condition represents cavernous transformation of the thoracic duct (obstruction of the cisterna chyli). Treatment entailed CT-guided percutaneous obliteration of the ectatic incompetent retroperitoneal lymphatics using a sclerosing solution (doxycycline) in conjunction with combined physical therapy of the right leg.

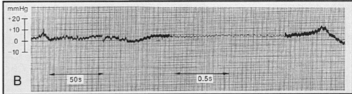

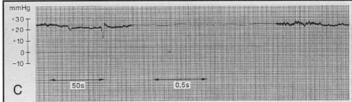

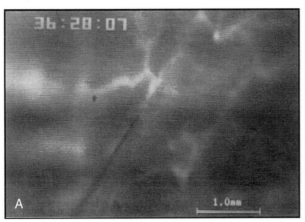

Figure 43–21. *A,* Fluorescence microlymphangiopathy demonstrating a network of superficial peripheral lymphatics punctured with a fine needle *(black)* in a human subject. After a single lymphatic has been micropunctured, normal lymphatic capillary pressure has been recorded in a healthy person *(B)* compared with high lymphatic pressure in one with primary lymphedema *(C).* (From Zaugg-Vesti B, Dorffler-Melly J, Spiegel M, et al: Lymphatic capillary pressure in patients with primary lymphedema. Microvasc Res 46:128–134, 1993.)

those whose onset of lymphedema was in puberty (e.g., lymphedema praecox) have ectatic lymphatic capillaries (initial lymphatics) in conjunction with more proximal hypoplastic lymph trunks.[90]

Direct interstitial injection of water-soluble contrast media (indirect lymphography) has also been used to depict dermal lymphatics,[91] but ready diffusibility of the contrast agent usually precludes consistent filling and accurate assessment of more proximal trunks and nodes.

Perflubron (Alliance Pharmaceutical Corp., San Diego) is a versatile, brominated fluorocarbon (perfluorooctylbromide) that shows promise for highlighting lymph nodes using CT scanning. Studies in ferrets with filariasis (*B. malayi*) demonstrate that after interstitial injection into the paw, perflubron is rapidly absorbed into peripheral lymphatics and is concentrated within macrophages in regional lymph nodes, producing vivid nodal and early lymphatic images on CT scan that are visible even on plain radiographs.[92]

SUMMARY

Physiology

Disturbances in microcirculatory perfusion and exchange of liquid, macromolecules, and cells across intact and abnormal microvessels and deranged lymph kinetics are, individually and together, associated with disorders of tissue swelling. Peripheral lymphedema manifesting as low-output failure of the lymph circulation is characteristically indolent for many years before lymphatic insufficiency and tissue swelling accelerate and become persistent. Nonetheless, impedance to lymph flow by itself is sufficient to explain at least mild to moderate forms of lymphedema. Chronic lymphedema is characterized by trapping in the skin and subcutaneous tissues of fluid, extravasated plasma proteins, and other macromolecules. It is typical to find impaired trafficking of immune cells (lymphocytes, Langerhans cells, monocytes), abnormal transport of autologous and foreign antigens, intact hydrodynamic (Starling) trans-

capillary forces, and an increased propensity to superimposed infection. Additional characteristics include progressive obliteration of lymphatics (lymphangiopathy "die-back" or lymphangitis), defective lymphangion contractility, mononuclear cell infiltrate, epidermal cell-fibroblast proliferation, collagen and fat deposition, altered immunoreactivity, and vasoactive mediator imbalance with increased production of local cytokines and growth factors, including autocrine and paracrine hormones.

In contrast to the blood circulation, in which flow depends primarily on the propulsive force of the myocardium, lymph propulsion depends predominantly on intrinsic truncal contraction. Venous plasma flows rapidly (2.5 to 3.0 L/minute) against low vascular resistance, whereas lymph "plasma" flows slowly (1 to 2 mL/minute) against high vascular resistance. On occasion, impaired transport of intestinal lymph may be associated with reflux and accumulation or leakage of intestinal chyle into swollen legs. In extreme circumstances, these factors operating together may be responsible for the hideous deformities seen in elephantiasis.

Transdifferentiation and transformation of endothelium and other vascular accessory cells associated with lymph stasis may also be pivotal factors in a wide range of dysplastic and neoplastic vascular disorders, including Stewart-Treves syndrome, AIDS-associated Kaposi's sarcoma, and lymphangitic metastatic carcinomatosis. These phenomena likely have their origin in uncontrolled or disordered lymphangiogenesis and are probably regulated at specific sites in the genome, the manipulation of which holds great promise for future therapy for patients with primary or secondary lymphedema and related angiodysplasia syndromes.

Imaging

Direct oil-contrast (conventional) lymphography has been the mainstay for depicting lymphatics for more than 40 years, but its notable shortcomings have severely curtailed usage. Improvements and refinements in isotope lymphography, however, are now providing vivid images of peripheral lymphatics and insight into lymph flow dynamics. Moreover, the procedure is essentially noninvasive, easy to perform repeatedly, and harmless to the lymphatic vascular endothelium. Besides the obvious advantage of providing a positive image of lymph vessels, LAS, equally importantly, establishes in patients with limbs that resemble those with lymphedema (e.g., in obesity) intact lymphatic truncal anatomy and tracer transport.

Although costly, MR also shows promise as an imaging tool of the lymphatic system. T_2-weighted images in particular depict pathologic dermal lymphatics without added contrast, as well as more proximal lymph flow and obstructing masses. This modality has established that the subfascial compartment in peripheral lymphedema is intact and that lymphedema is primarily a disorder of the skin and subcutaneous tissue (the epifascial compartment). Moreover, MR has readily permitted visualization of retroperitoneal ectatic lymphatic trunks (e.g., chylous reflux syndromes) and provided access for lymphatic truncal obliteration in management of lymphangiectasia syndromes characterized by lymph fistulization often in conjunction with intestinal (lacteal) lymph retrograde flow.

Although of limited value, ultrasonography has proved to be of great benefit in screening for filariasis in endemic areas. Adult nematode worms can be seen thrashing and undulating violently within scrotal lymphatics, providing new insights into the incidence of occult filariasis in the absence of peripheral edema or microfilaremia, as well as illuminating the pathomechanism of lymphatic drainage in filarial lymphedema (physical destruction of intraluminal valves and lymphatic contractility by living worms and lymphatic thrombosis after host immune responsiveness to dying or dead worms).

Peripheral lymphatics can now be visualized as easily as arteries and veins have been for several decades. Because LAS can readily be applied before and after treatment, it should become an integral adjunct to physical examination and a useful outcome measure to evaluate drugs, operations, and physical methods designed to facilitate lymph flow. Indeed, any patient who carries the provisional diagnosis of peripheral lymphatic dysfunction or idiopathic edema should undergo diagnostic LAS to verify the accuracy of diagnosis and provide a blueprint for subsequent therapy.

References

1. Mayerson HS: Physiologic importance of lymph. In Hamilton WF, Dow P (eds): Handbook of Physiology, vol. 2. Washington, DC, American Physiological Society, 1962, pp 1035–1073.
2. Leak LV: Physiology of the lymphatic system. In Abramson DI, Dobrin PB (eds): Blood Vessels and Lymphatics in Organ Systems. Orlando, Fla, Academic Press, 1984, pp 134–164.
3. Sabin FR: Further evidence of the origin of the lymphatic endothelium from the endothelium of the blood vascular system. Anat Rec 2:46, 1908.
4. Rusznyak I, Földi M, Szabo G: Lymphatics and Lymph Circulation. New York, Pergamon Press, 1967, p 33.
5. Casley-Smith JR: Lymph and lymphatics. In Kaley G, Altura BM (eds): Microcirculation. Baltimore, University Park Press, 1977, p 423.
6. Way D, Hendrix M, Witte MH, et al: Lymphatic endothelial cell line (CH3) from a recurrent retroperitoneal lymphangioma. In Vitro Cell Dev Biol Anim 23:647, 1987.
7. Gnepp DR, Chandler W: Tissue culture of human and thoracic duct endothelium. In Vitro Cell Dev Biol Anim 21:200, 1985.
8. Johnston MG, Walker MA: Lymphatic endothelial and smooth-muscle cells in tissue culture. In Vitro Cell Dev Biol Anim 20:566, 1984.
9. Casley-Smith JR: The lymphatic system. In Földi M, Casley-Smith JR (eds): Lymphangiology. Stuttgart, Germany, Schattauer-Verlag, 1983, p 89.
10. Leak LV, Burke JF: Fine structure of the lymphatic capillary and the adjoining connective tissue area. Am J Anat 118:785, 1966.
11. Leak LV: The fine structure and function of the lymphatic vascular system. In Meesen H (ed): Handbuch der allgemeinen Pathologie. Berlin, Springer-Verlag, 1972, pp 149–196.
12. Leak LV: Electron microscopic observations on lymphatic capillaries and the structural components of the connective tissue-lymph interface. Microvasc Res 2:361, 1970.
13. Mislin H: The lymphangion. In Földi M, Casley-Smith JR (eds): Lymphangiology. Stuttgart, Germany, Schattauer-Verlag, 1983, p 165.
14. Olszewski WL: Lymph Stasis: Pathophysiology, Diagnosis and Treatment. Boca Raton, Fla, CRC Press, 1991, p 377.
15. Zweifach BW, Prather JW: Micromanipulation of pressure in terminal lymphatics in the mesentery. Am J Physiol 228:1326, 1975.
16. Laine GA, Hall JF, Laine SH, Granger HJ: Transsinusoidal fluid dynamics in canine liver during venous hypertension. Circ Res 45:317, 1979.
17. Granger DN, Miller T, Allen R, et al: Permselectivity of cat liver sinusoids to endogenous macromolecules. Gastroenterology 77:103, 1977.
18. Taylor AE: The lymphatic edema safety factor: The role of edema dependent lymphatic factors (EDLF). Lymphology 23:111, 1990.
19. Yoffey JM, Courtice FC: Lymphatics, Lymph, and the Lymphomyeloid Complex. London, Academic Press, 1970, p 206.
20. Hall JG, Morris B, Wooley G: Intrinsic rhythmic propulsion of lymph in the unanesthetized sheep. J Physiol (Lond) 180:336, 1965.
21. Harens AR, Zweifach BW: Contractile stimuli in collecting lymph vessels. Am J Physiol 233:H57, 1979.
22. Olszewski WL, Engeset A: Intrinsic contractility of prenodal lymph vessels and lymph flow in the human leg. Am J Physiol 239:H775, 1980.
23. Gnepp DR: Lymphatics. In Staub NC, Taylor AE (eds): Edema. New York, Raven Press, 1984, p 263.
24. McHale NG, Roddie IC: The effect of transmural pressure on pumping activity in isolated bovine lymphatic vessels. J Physiol (Lond) 261:255, 1976.
25. McHale NG, Roddie IC: The effect of intravenous adrenaline and noradrenaline infusion on peripheral lymph flow in the sheep. J Physiol (Lond) 341:517, 1983.
26. Zawieja DC, Davis KL: Inhibition of the active lymph pump in rat mesenteric lymphatics by hydrogen peroxide. Lymphology 26:135, 1993.
27. Zawieja DC, Greiner ST, Davis KL, et al: Reactive oxygen metabolites inhibit spontaneous lymphatic contractions. Am J Physiol 260:H1935, 1991.
28. Johnston MG, Kanalec A, Gordon JL: Effects of arachidonic acid and its cyclooxygenase and lipooxygenase products on lymph vessel contractility in vitro. Prostaglandins 25:85, 1983.
29. Ohhashi T, Kawai Y, Azuma T: The response of lymphatic smooth muscles to vasoactive substances. Pflugers Arch 375:183, 1978.
30. McHale NG, Roddie IC, Thornbury K: Nervous modulation of spontaneous contractions in bovine mesenteric lymphatics. J Physiol (Lond) 309:461, 1980.
31. Sjöberg T, Steen S: Contractile properties of lymphatics from the human lower leg. Lymphology 24:16, 1991.
32. McGeown JG, McHale NC, Thornbury KD: The effect of electrical stimulation of the sympathetic chain on peripheral lymph flow in the anaesthetized sheep. J Physiol (Lond) 393:123, 1987.
33. Kampmeier OF: Lymphatic system of the amphibians. In Evolution and Comparative Morphology of the Lymphatic System. Springfield, Ill, Charles C Thomas, 1969, p 266.
34. Kinmonth JB, Wolf JH: Fibrosis in the lymph nodes in primary lymphedema. Ann R Coll Surg 62:344, 1980.

35. Johnston MG: The intrinsic lymph pump: Progress and problems. Lymphology 22:116, 1989.
36. Pippard C, Roddie IC: Resistance in the sheep's lymphatic system. Lymphology 20:230, 1987.
37. Olszewski WL: Lymph Stasis: Pathophysiology, Diagnosis and Treatment. Boca Raton, Fla, CRC Press, 1991, p 109.
38. Pippard C, Roddie IC: Comparison of fluid transport systems in lymphatics and veins. Lymphology 20:224, 1987.
39. Yoffey JM, Courtice FC (eds): Lymphatics, Lymph and the Lymphomyeloid Complex. London, Academic Press, 1970, pp 363–369.
40. Casley-Smith JR: The regenerative capacity of the lymphovascular system. In: Földi M, Casley-Smith JR (eds): Lymphangiology. Stuttgart, Schattauer-Verlag, 1983, pp 276–278.
41. Reichert FL: The regeneration of the lymphatics. Arch Surg 14:871, 1926.
42. Bellman S, Odén B: Regeneration of surgically divided lymph vessels. An experimental study on the rabbit's ear. Acta Chir Scand 116:99, 1958–59.
43. Odén B: A micro-lymphangiographic study of experimental wounds healing by secondary intention. Acta Chir Scand 120:100, 1960.
44. Clark ER, Clark EL: Observations on the new growth of lymphatic vessels as seen in transparent chambers introduced into the rabbit's ear. Am J Anat 51:49, 1932.
45. Pullinger DB, Florey HW: Proliferation of lymphatics in inflammation. J Pathol 45:157, 1937.
46. Jaffe EA: Cell biology of endothelial cells. Hum Pathol 8:234, 1987.
47. Denekamp J: Angiogenesis, neovascular proliferation and vascular pathophysiology as targets for cancer therapy. Br J Radiol 66:181, 1993.
48. Trevella W, Dugan MC: Endothelial interactions. In Nishi M, Uchino S, Yabuki S (eds): Progress in Lymphology—XII. Amsterdam, Elsevier Science, 1990, p 269.
49. Johnston M, Walker M: Lymphatic endothelial and smooth muscle cells in tissue culture. In Vitro Cell Dev Biol Anim 20:566, 1989.
50. Bowman C, Witte MH, Witte CL, et al: Cystic hygroma reconsidered: Hamartoma or neoplasm? Primary culture of an endothelial cell line from a massive cervicomediastinal cystic hygroma with bony lymphangiomatosis. Lymphology 17:15, 1984.
51. Leak LV, Jones M: Lymphangiogenesis in vitro: Formation of lymphatic capillary-like channels from confluent monolayers of lymphatic endothelial cells. In Vitro Cell Dev Biol Anim 30:512, 1994.
52. Greenlee R, Hoyme H, Witte M, et al: Developmental disorders of the lymphatic system. Lymphology 26:156–168, 1993.
53. Joukov V, Pajusola K, Kaipanen A, et al: A novel vascular endothelial growth factor is a ligand for the lflt4 (VEGFR-3) and kDR (VEGFR-2) receptor tyrosine kinases. EMBO J 15:290, 1996.
54. Ferrell RE, Levinson KL, Esman JH, et al: Hereditary lymphedema: Evidence for linkage and genetic heterogeneity. Hum Mol Genet 7:2073, 1998.
55. Witte M, Erickson R, Bernas M, et al: Phenotypic and genotypic heterogeneity in familial Milroy lymphedema. Lymphology 31:145, 1998.
56. Evans AL, Brice G, Sotirova V, et al: Mapping of primary congenital lymphedema to the 5q35.3 region. Am J Hum Genet 64:547, 1999.
57. Witte CL, Witte MH, Dumont AE: Pathophysiology of chronic edema, lymphedema, and fibrosis. In Staub NC, Taylor AE (eds): Edema. New York, Raven Press, 1984, p 521.
58. Danese CA, Georgalas-Bertakis M, Morales LE: A model of chronic postsurgical lymphedema in dogs' limbs. Surgery 64:814, 1968.
59. Olszewski W: On the pathomechanism of development of postsurgical lymphedema. Lymphology 6:35, 1973.
60. Clodius L, Altorfer J: Experimental chronic lymphostasis of extremities. Folia Angiologia 25:137, 1977.
61. Postlethwaite AE, Keski-Oja J, Balian G, Kang AH: Induction of fibroblast chemotaxis by fibronectin. J Exp Med 153:494, 1981.
62. Bitterman PB, Rennard SI, Adelberg S, Crystal RG: Role of fibronectin as a growth factor for fibroblasts. J Cell Biol 97:1925, 1983.
63. Casley-Smith JR, Piller NB, Morgan RG: Treatment of lymphedema of the arms and legs with 5,6-benzo-α-pyrone. N Engl J Med 329:1158, 1993.
64. McDonald JA, Baum S, Rosenberg D, et al: Destruction of a major

65. extracellular adhesive glycoprotein (fibronectin) of human fibroblasts by neutral proteases from polymorphonuclear leukocyte granules. Lab Invest 40:350, 1979.
65. Földi M: Insufficiency of lymph flow. In Földi M, Casley-Smith JR (eds): Lymphangiology. Stuttgart, Germany, Schattauer-Verlag, p 195.
66. Olszewski WL: Peripheral Lymph: Formation and Immune Function. Boca Raton, Fla, CRC Press, 1985, p 39.
67. Casley-Smith JR: High Protein Oedemas and the Benzopyrones. Sydney, Australia, JB Lippincott, 1986, pp 126.
68. Stewart FW, Treves N: Lymphangiosarcoma in post mastectomy lymphedema. A report of six cases in elephantiasis chirurgica. Cancer 1:64, 1948.
69. Unruh H, Robertson DI, Karasewich E: Post mastectomy lymphangiosarcoma. Can J Surg 22:586, 1979.
70. Woodward AH, Ivins JC, Sorle EH: Lymphangiosarcoma arising in chronic lymphedematous extremities. Cancer 30:562, 1972.
71. Dorfman RF: Kaposi's sarcoma. Evidence supporting its origin from the lymphatic system. Lymphology 21:45, 1988.
72. Witte MH, Stuntz M, Witte CL: Kaposi's sarcoma: A lymphologic perspective. Int J Dermatol 28:561, 1989.
73. Beckstead JH, Wood GS, Fletcher V: Evidence for the origin of Kaposi's sarcoma from lymphatic endothelium. Am J Pathol 119:294, 1985.
74. Casley-Smith JR: High Protein Oedemas and the Benzopyrones. Sydney, Australia, JB Lippincott, 1986.
75. Daroczy J: Pathology of lymphedema. Clin Dermatol 13:433, 1995.
76. Snowden K, Hammerberg B: Vascular patterns in the filaria-infected canine limb. Lymphology 19:77, 1986.
77. Kinmonth JB: Lymphangiography in man. A method of outlining lymphatic trunks at operation. Clin Sci 11:13, 1952.
78. Koehler PR: Complications of lymphography. Lymphology 1:117, 1968.
79. McNeill GC, Witte MH, Witte CL, et al: Whole-body lymphangioscintigraphy: Preferred method for initial assessment of the peripheral lymphatic system. Radiology 172:495, 1989.
80. Witte MH, Jamal S, Williams W, et al: Lymphatic abnormalities in human filariasis as depicted by lymphangioscintigraphy. Arch Intern Med 153:737, 1993.
81. Witte MH, Fiala M, McNeill GC, et al: Lymphangioscintigraphy in AIDS-associated Kaposi's sarcoma. AJR Am J Roentgenol 155:311, 1990.
82. Case TC, Unger E, Bernas MJ, et al: Lymphatic imaging in experimental filariasis using magnetic resonance. Invest Radiol 27:293, 1992.
83. Case TC, Witte CL, Witte MH, et al: Magnetic resonance imaging in human lymphedema: Comparison with lymphangioscintigraphy. Magn Res Imaging 10:549, 1992.
84. Tanoura T, Bernas M, Darkazanli A, et al: MR lymphography with iron oxide compound AMI-227. Studies in ferrets with filariasis. AJR Am J Roentgenol 159:875, 1992.
85. Molitch HI, Unger EC, Witte CL, van Sonnenberg E: Percutaneous sclerotherapy of lymphangiomas. Radiology 194:343, 1995.
86. Amaral F, Dreyer G, Figueredo-Silva J, et al: Live adult worms detected by ultrasonography in human bancroftian filariasis. Am J Trop Med 50:753, 1994.
87. Case TC, Witte MH, Way DL, Witte CL: Videomicroscopy of intra-lymphatic-dwelling *Brugia malayi*. Ann Trop Med Parasitol 86:435, 1992.
88. Bollinger A, Jaeger K, Sgier F, Seglias J: Fluorescence microlymphography. Circulation 64:1191, 1981.
89. Zaugg-Vesti B, Dorffler-Melly J, Spiegel M, et al: Lymphatic capillary pressure in patients with primary lymphedema. Microvasc Res 46:128, 1993.
90. Pfister G, Saesseli B, Hoffmann U, et al: Diameters of lymphatic capillaries in patients with different forms of primary lymphedema. Lymphology 23:140, 1990.
91. Partsch H, Urbanek A, Wenzel-Hora B: The dermal lymphatics in lymphedema visualized by indirect lymphography. Br J Dermatol 110:431, 1984.
92. Bernas M, Witte C, Pond G, et al: Enhanced lymphatic imaging using Imagent LN in filariasis infected ferrets. Lymphology 27(Suppl):265, 1994.

Questions

1. Which of the following statements is most accurate?
   (a) lymph formation derives from lymphatic endothelial secretion, as governed by cytokine stimulants released by circulating lymphocytes into the interstitium
   (b) lymph formation is a byproduct of excess intercellular water generated by catabolism of substrates in high metabolic organs such as the liver
   (c) lymph formation derives primarily from net blood capillary filtration, as governed by the hydrostatic and plasma protein osmotic pressure gradients operating across the blood microvasculature
   (d) lymph formation is directly proportional to the plasma volume and percentage of erythrocytes circulating in the blood stream
   (e) lymph formation derives from a complex formula involving renal perfusion, plasma atrial natriuretic hormone, and plasma aldosterone levels

2. The protein composition of lymph
   (a) derives mainly from plasma proteins escaping from the blood vasculature into the interstitium by diffusion and convection
   (b) derives mainly from catabolism of interstitial lymphocytes and adjacent parenchymal cells
   (c) derives mainly from synthesis of albumin and other proteins by the liver, pancreas, and skeletal muscle
   (d) is identical to the protein content ingested in the diet or the amount of amino acids administered by parenteral nutrition, or both
   (e) derives mainly from breakdown of muscle mass

3. Which of the following statements is most accurate?
   (a) lymphatics usually parallel veins except in the brain, where they empty via the arachnoid villi into large venous sinuses
   (b) lymphatics normally represent an alternative circulating route for red blood cells and platelets
   (c) lymphatics represent a compensatory efferent route to nourish parenchymal cells, especially during ischemia (i.e., reduced blood flow)
   (d) lymphatics represent an alternative source of glomerular filtration when kidney function fails
   (e) lymphatics usually parallel veins except in the gut, where mesenteric lymph in contrast to mesenteric blood returns directly to the systemic blood circulation without traversing the liver

4. In contrast to the adult human blood flow rate of 5 to 6 L/minute, total lymph flow is
   (a) 1 L/minute
   (b) 2.5 L/hour
   (c) 2.5 L/day
   (d) 2.5 L/week
   (e) 1/10 blood flow per hour

5. Lymph propulsion in humans is primarily governed by
   (a) the sucking action of the heart and deep breathing
   (b) the extent of tissue edema
   (c) strategically placed lymph hearts (cor lymphaticum) located in the groin and para-axillary regions
   (d) intrinsic lymphatic contraction modified by "haphazard" forces such as peristalsis, sighing, and adjacent arterial pulsations
   (e) skeletal muscle contraction and blood flow rate

6. Although veins and lymphatics are both conduits that return liquid back to the heart, which of the following is most accurate?
   (a) the lymphatic system, unlike the venous system, has a higher distal and lower proximal intraluminal hydrostatic pressure
   (b) lymphatics transport a small liquid volume under low pressure against relatively high vascular resistance, whereas veins transport a large liquid volume under low pressure against low vascular resistance
   (c) lymphatics transport a small liquid volume under low pressure against low vascular resistance, whereas veins transport a large liquid volume under high pressure against low vascular resistance
   (d) lymphatics transport a small liquid volume under high pressure against low vascular resistance, whereas veins transport a large liquid volume under low pressure against low vascular resistance
   (e) except for minor differences in the capillary ultrastructure of the two systems, liquid propulsion in both lymph and blood is governed by cardiac action and skeletal muscle "squeezing"

7. With an increase in interstitial volume
   (a) both lymph capillaries and blood capillaries collapse, thereby restricting further accumulation of tissue fluid and protein
   (b) lymph capillaries dilate and blood capillaries collapse, thereby facilitating fluid and protein resorption into the blood stream via lymphatics while minimizing further plasma filtration
   (c) lymph capillaries collapse while blood capillaries open, favoring rapid resorption of protein and liquid into the blood stream
   (d) both lymph capillaries and blood capillaries dilate, favoring rapid absorption of tissue fluid and protein into the blood stream
   (e) lymph capillaries collapse, thereby autoregulating a decrease in endothelin and nitric oxide release with cessation of regional blood flow

8. The pathophysiology of lymphedema is characterized by
   (a) progressive loss of lymphatic truncal contractility, intraluminal valve incompetence, and lymphangiectasis; often several months or years pass with no symptoms before edema becomes apparent, with progressive deposition of fat, fluid, and collagen in the skin and subcutaneous tissue
   (b) rapid onset of limb swelling, accumulation of protein-poor edema fluid, and progressive insufficiency of the greater and lesser saphenous venous systems, with dermal hyperpigmentation and paramalleolar skin ulceration
   (c) acute, unremitting extremity swelling, prompt response of diuretic drugs, and gradual remission of edema over many years
   (d) low protein edema fluid, progressive improvement with diuretic drugs, and dietary salt restriction, often in conjunction with limb-threatening ischemic foot ulcers
   (e) progressive limb swelling, hyperpigmentation, subcutaneous fibrosis, and development of painful skin ulceration

9. The current preferred imaging method to initially evaluate patients with peripheral lymphedema is
   (a) conventional (direct) oil-contrast lymphography
   (b) fluorescence microlymphangiography
   (c) lymphangioscintigraphy (isotope lymphography)
   (d) Computed tomography
   (e) Magnetic resonance imaging

10. Chylous reflux syndrome
    (a) refers to pancreatic dysfunction with malabsorption of ingested fats
    (b) is a synonym for serum lactescence with high serum triglyceride level
    (c) is a synonym for protein-losing enteropathy
    (d) refers to regurgitation of intestinal lymph into the pelvis, retroperitoneum, kidneys, or lower extremities
    (e) refers to incompetence of hepatic lymphatic valves with improper processing of chylomicrons by the liver

11. From MR imaging of the limbs in patients with lymphedema
    (a) both the subcutaneous (epifascial) and skeletal muscle compartments (subfascial) are edematous
    (b) fat deposition is seldom seen
    (c) metabolic changes in the cortical bone are dramatic
    (d) dermal backflow is especially prominent
    (e) only the skin and subcutaneous (prefascial) tissues are edematous; the skeletal (subfascial) compartment either is unremarkable or shows mild hypertrophy

Answers

1. c   2. a   3. e   4. c   5. d   6. b   7. b   8. a   9. c   10. d
11. e

44

Lymphedema and Tumors of the Lymphatics

Lance E. Wyatt and Timothy A. Miller

Lymphedema is the accumulation of protein-rich interstitial fluid within the skin and subcutaneous tissues, which occurs as a result of lymphatic dysfunction. It has been estimated that there are approximately 140 million cases worldwide. Those cases in which the etiology is congenital or unknown are known as *primary lymphedema*. All forms of lymphedema that occur as a result of a known cause, including infection, surgery, or radiation therapy, are termed *secondary lymphedema*.

Lymphatic malformations and a significant portion of lymphedema are probably caused by embryologic aberrations in the lymphatic system. The numerous different approaches to the treatment of lymphedema document our frustration in finding an effective way to deal with these problems.

ANATOMY

Although lymphatic vessels were first observed over 2200 years ago, recognition of the lymphatics as a discrete system did not occur until the 17th century. It is now generally agreed that lymphatics and lymph nodes arise from endothelial sprouting of the primordial venous system.[1, 2] This development begins in four areas: the paired jugular and iliac systems, the cisterna chyli, and the retroperitoneal system. Between the third and eighth weeks of gestation, these sprouting endothelial sacs develop peripherally and invade almost all tissues of the body, with the exception of the epidermis, central nervous system, bone marrow, muscle, cartilage, tendon, coats of the eye, internal ear, and intralobar portions of the liver. The thoracic duct arises from fusion of the cisterna chyli and left jugular buds. The lymphatic channels and regional nodes of each extremity are eventually formed by this peripheral growth and drain into either the cisterna chyli (lower extremities) or directly into the thoracic duct (upper extremities), thereby returning lymph to the venous system. Variations in the communications between the major lymphatic trunks and the subclavian veins are relatively common.[3]

The lymphatic system is composed of three major elements: initial lymphatics (also referred to as terminal lymphatics), collecting ducts, and lymph nodes. The initial lymphatic vessels are similar to capillaries, except that their basement membrane is absent or poorly defined, facilitating the absorption of lymph fluid from the interstitial space. The lymphatic capillaries progress in size, becoming collecting lymphatics. A valved system of collecting lymphatics normally ascends alongside the primary blood vessels of an extremity and transports lymph to regional lymph nodes. Collecting lymphatics have intimal, medial, and adventitial layers. The elastic fibers and smooth muscle in the media vary in direct proportion to lymphatic size.

Lower Extremity Lymphatics

The lower extremity lymphatics consist of separate *superficial* and *deep* systems. In the *superficial lymphatic system*, medial and lateral pathways of lymphatic vessels exist that closely correspond to the venous drainage of the leg. The *medial superficial pathway* consists of three or four vessels that follow the course of the lesser saphenous vein and then drain into the popliteal lymph nodes or join the medial pathway in the thigh. The superficial lymphatics normally drain the subcutaneous compartment, the site of fluid accumulation in lymphedema.

The *deep lymphatic system* of the lower extremities consists of several vessels that run parallel to the anterior and posterior tibial veins and the peroneal vein. Normally, the four vessels drain into the popliteal lymph nodes, while four to six vessels ascend the thigh medially, following the course of the superficial femoral vein and subsequently draining into the inguinal nodes.

The inguinal nodes are divided into a superficial group (around the fossa ovalis) and a deep group (within the fatty tissues of the femoral sheath). These nodes (approximately 15) drain into the iliac lymph nodes. Although virtually all lymph flow from the lower extremities passes through the inguinal nodes, studies have shown that lymph drainage can bypass these nodes and drain directly into the iliac area.[4] Lymph from these nodes is subsequently returned to the venous circulation via the cisterna chyli.

Upper Extremity Lymphatics

The anatomy of the upper extremity lymphatics is similar to that of the lower extremities. The *superficial lymphatic system* consists of medial and lateral groups of vessels. The medial group of lymphatics parallels the basilic vein and then drains into the axillary lymph nodes. The lateral group of vessels follows the course of the cephalic and median veins and drains primarily into the supraclavicular lymph nodes. (This lateral group of lymphatics may serve as a collateral path of lymph drainage in patients who have undergone axillary lymph node dissection.) The *deep lymphatic system* of the arms parallels the brachial vessels and also drains into axillary lymph nodes.

Regional Lymphatic Drainage

Lymphatic drainage of the extremities is generally a regional process. Normally, the superficial and deep lymphatic systems do not communicate until the vessels drain into common lymph nodes. Only under abnormal conditions, such as with proximal obstruction, do the two systems communicate.[5, 6] There are no significant direct lymphovenous communications in the extremities.[7] There is also little communication between the medial and lateral superficial pathways distal to the knee.[8] Some evidence exists that lymphatic channels draining the lower leg do not receive tributaries from the thigh. Lymphangiographic studies have shown that the thigh drains into the superior inguinal lymph nodes, whereas the lower leg drains into the more inferior inguinal lymph nodes.[9] Because of this, in some patients with acquired lymphedema, the swelling may be limited to the lower leg.

PHYSIOLOGY

The lymphatic system transports interstitial fluid and macromolecular protein lost from the capillary system, as well as infectious agents and other foreign material, back into the circulation. Edema results when the formation of protein-rich interstitial fluid exceeds the lymphatic transport capacity. Several factors influence the rate of lymph formation and the lymphatic transport capacity.

Formation of Interstitial Fluid and Lymph

Interstitial fluid is essentially an ultrafiltrate of plasma, formed by capillary filtration. According to Starling's hypothesis, the rate of capillary filtration is determined by the difference in hydrostatic and colloid osmotic pressures between the intravascular/capillary space and the interstitial space. Under normal physiologic conditions, the larger hydrostatic pressure in the capillaries is opposed by a comparably large capillary osmotic pressure. This allows relatively small net amounts of fluid and protein to enter the interstitial space. An abnormally elevated venous pressure can increase capillary hydrostatic pressure and subsequently increase fluid shift into the interstitial space.[10] However, the lymphatic system compensates by increasing lymph flow to return this interstitial fluid to the systemic circulation.[8, 11, 12]

Lymph is formed primarily by absorption of interstitial fluid by the initial lymphatic vessels. The concentration of protein within the interstitial fluid depends on the permeability of capillaries and the ability of the lymphatics to clear excessive interstitial protein. Over a 24-hour period, the capillaries normally allow 40% to 80% of intravascular protein to enter the interstitial space, where it is then transported via the lymphatics back to the circulation.[13]

Lymphatic Function and Transport Capacity

The propulsion of lymph proximally results from a combination of several factors. Muscular contractions adjacent to lymphatic vessels increase the surrounding interstitial tissue pressure, which propels lymph proximally. Lymphatic valves prevent the regress of lymph on subsequent muscle relaxation and generally encourage the unidirectional flow of lymph by lowering lymphatic pressure relative to interstitial pressure. Proximal lymph flow has also been shown to be promoted by adjacent arterial pulsations.[14] Additionally, the alternating negative, then positive intrathoracic and intraabdominal pressures associated with respiration and Valsalva's maneuvers act to pump lymph through the thoracic and abdominal cavities.[13]

In addition to the extrinsic factors promoting lymph flow, considerable evidence supports an intrinsic contractile mechanism that promotes the flow of lymph. All lymphatics, except for terminal lymphatics, have smooth muscle fibers and nerve endings in their walls and have been shown to contract spontaneously and rhythmically.[15, 16]

Lymph flow can be impeded by abnormalities in lymphatic anatomy that increase resistance, by gravity, and by an elevated central venous pressure, which impedes the return of lymph to the left innominate vein by increasing the thoracic duct pressure.[17]

Pathophysiology of Lymphedema

Lymphedema is confined to the subcutaneous compartment; the deep muscle compartments remain uninvolved. The accumulation of protein-rich lymphatic fluid results when fluid formation exceeds lymphatic transport capacity. Normal lymphatics have a substantial reserve capacity and may increase their flow rate by a factor of 10.[18] An increase in the rate of interstitial fluid formation by itself does *not* produce lymphedema.[19] Lymphatic dysfunction is a prerequisite of the accumulation of protein-rich fluid.

Early in the course of lymphedema, the accumulation of protein-rich interstitial fluid results only in a soft, pitting edema. In time, low oxygen tension, decreased macrophage function, and the presence of increasing amounts of protein-rich fluid give rise to a chronic inflammatory state and consequent fibrosis.[20] Moreover, this protein-rich fluid combined with lymphatic stasis provides an ideal environment for bacterial proliferation. Recurrent episodes of lymphangitis are a common complication, involving approximately 25% of lymphedema patients.[21] Lymphangitis and cellulitis further accelerate the rate of subcutaneous fibrosis and subsequent lymphatic obstruction.

PRIMARY LYMPHEDEMA

All forms of primary lymphedema result from some congenital abnormality in the anatomy or function, or a combination of both, of the lymphatic system. Primary lymphedema has generally been classified on the basis of age of onset but can also be classified by lymphangiographic findings.

Classification by Age of Onset

Primary lymphedema is classically subdivided into three groups on the basis of age of disease onset.[22, 23]

Congenital lymphedema presents at birth and accounts for approximately 10% to 15% of patients with primary lymphedema. Milroy's disease is a specific congenital form of lymphedema characterized by aplasia of the lymphatic trunks and a familial, sex-linked incidence. A family history is present in fewer than 5% of patients with congenital lymphedema.[24, 25] This congenital form can be associated with other diseases of the lymphatic system, such as cystic hygroma and lymphangiectasia.

Lymphedema praecox presents during adolescence and accounts for approximately 80% of patients with primary lymphedema. This represents another form of congenital lymphatic system disease but with a later onset of symptoms.

Lymphedema tarda generally presents after age 35 and accounts for approximately 10% to 15% of patients. It is unclear why normal middle-aged adults would suddenly develop lymphedema without any known precipitating event. Nor can we adequately explain (1) why women are afflicted at least three times more frequently than men and often develop edema around the time of menarche, (2) why the left leg is affected significantly more often than the right, or (3) why the upper extremities are seldom involved. The general category designated as "primary lymphedema" encompasses several conditions with varying and incompletely understood etiologies.

Classification by Lymphangiographic Findings

Lymphedema may be classified by lymphangiography into hypoplastic and hyperplastic forms.

Hypoplastic Lymphedema

Ninety-two percent of all cases of primary lymphedema show a hypoplastic pattern on lymphangiogram.[26] The hypoplasia can be further classified as distal, proximal, or both distal and proximal. In distal hypoplasia, usually fewer than five vessels are visualized at the thigh. If any lymphatics are seen, they are narrow and few. A *distal hypoplastic pattern* is most often seen in female adolescents with lymphedema praecox, which may be related to puberty or pregnancy. The associated lymphedema is mild and nonprogressive and generally affects both lower legs. *Aplasia* is an extreme form of distal hypoplastic lymphedema that is usually seen in congenital lymphedema and accounts for 15% of all cases of primary lymphedema. In these patients, lymphangiography reveals no lymphatic trunks.

A *proximal hypoplastic pattern* is seen in patients with pelvic obstruction. This is a less common but more severe form of primary hypoplastic lymphedema. Its incidence is equal in males and females, and it is seen in 17% to 34% of patients with primary lymphedema.[27–29] In these patients, lymphangiography reveals only a few small lymph nodes and vessels in the groin and pelvis, with numerous distended lymphatics distal to the site of hypoplasia. The edema is generally unilateral but most often affects the entire lower extremity.[30]

In *combined proximal and distal hypoplasia* the lymphangiographic findings and clinical characteristics are a combination of those of the two categories just described.

Hyperplastic Lymphedema

Lymphangiography reveals a hyperplastic pattern in approximately 8% of primary lymphedema patients.[26] Hyperplastic lymphedema can be further categorized as *bilateral hyperplasia* or *megalymphatics*.[31] Bilateral hyperplasia is presumed to be secondary to obstruction caused by an abnormal thoracic duct or cisterna chyli. The lymphangiogram demonstrates numerous, slightly dilated lymphatics distal to the obstruction. Large edematous pelvic lymph nodes are seen bilaterally. Mediastinal and intercostal lymph nodes may also be visualized, but the thoracic duct is seldom seen.

In patients with a megalymphatic pattern, the lymphangiogram demonstrates large, tortuous, varicose-like lymphatics. Edema of the extremity is often mild or absent. More important, the incompetent lymphatic valves allow the reflux of chyle into the pelvis. This pattern may be associated with angioma of the lower extremity or trunk or bowel lymphangiectasia.

SECONDARY (ACQUIRED) LYMPHEDEMA

The most common worldwide cause of secondary lymphedema is direct infestation of lymph nodes by the parasite *Wuchereria bancrofti* (filariasis).[32, 33] Damage or removal of regional lymph nodes by surgery, trauma, radiation, tumor invasion, or as a result of infection (e.g., filariasis, tuberculosis, lymphogranuloma, actinomycosis, or cat-scratch fever) or inflammation (e.g., chronic lymphangitis, snake bite, or insect bite) is the most common cause of secondary lymphedema in Western countries.

Approximately 10% to 15% of patients undergoing radical mastectomy will develop significant postoperative arm swelling.[34, 35] A study of 200 operable breast cancer patients found that radiation to the axilla after radical node dissection significantly increased the risk of postmastectomy lymphedema in the ipsilateral extremity.[36] In addition to patients undergoing radiation therapy, obese patients and patients with postmastectomy wound healing problems exhibit a higher incidence of lymphedema. In these patients, the swelling may not become clinically evident for as long as 1 year. This delay is a result of ongoing soft tissue fibrosis, which compresses the remaining lymphatics and possibly acts as a barrier to the regeneration of new lymphatic vessels. Factors that increase the formation of fibrous tissue, such as irradiation and infection, increase the chances that lymphedema will develop.

Lymphedema due to malignant disease occurs late in the disease process after there is extensive spread of tumor.

Lymphedema may also develop following lower extremity arterial reconstruction and appears to be more frequent after using an autologous vein graft.[37] During dissection of arterial segments or during harvest of the greater saphenous vein, lymphatic vessels may be damaged. To reduce lymphatic injury, some surgeons have proposed careful dissection with the aid of a diffusible dye to directly visualize the lymphatics.[38] In patients with secondary lymphedema, lymphangiography reveals a varicose-type pattern with dilatation of the distal lymphatics and obstruction at the operative site.

DIAGNOSIS

Patient Presentation and History

In the vast majority of patients, the diagnosis of lymphedema can and should be made by the history and physical examination alone. The gradual ascent of a soft pitting edema beginning at the ankle and proceeding proximally over a period of several months, unassociated with other symptoms, is characteristic. An increase in limb diameter produces an even greater increase in limb weight, causing lymphedema patients to often complain of fatigue in the involved extremity. As the subcutaneous fibrosis progresses, the limb becomes indurated and develops a nonpitting, spongy edema. Eventually, the skin becomes thick and hyperkeratotic.

The patient with lymphedema may present at any age. Patients with primary lymphedema classically present at birth, puberty, or middle age. Patients with secondary lymphedema present sometime after the inciting event, such as surgery, irradiation, infection, trauma, or tumor growth. The time interval between the occurrence of the inciting event and the onset of disease is variable and may range from weeks to years.

Laboratory Studies

Initial laboratory studies should include a differential white blood cell count to detect the eosinophilia often seen with filariasis and a peripheral blood smear to search for *W. bancrofti* microfilariae. Serum albumin, total protein, and electrolyte levels should be obtained, and renal function tests, liver function tests, and urinalysis should be performed to rule out other causes of limb edema.

Lymphangiography and Lymphoscintigraphy

Lymphedema can usually be diagnosed on the basis of history and physical examination alone. Laboratory tests can help exclude other causes of extremity edema. If the diagnosis is still in doubt, then lymphoscintigraphy is indicated. Lymphangiography should be avoided, as it can lead to further lymphatic damage.

Lymphangiography is an anatomic study that provides some functional information. In contrast, lymphoscintigraphy is a functional study that can provide some anatomic information. In the lower extremities, lymphangiography is performed by injecting a blue dye into the first intradigital web space bilaterally. The web spaces are massaged, and the extremity moved to promote dye dispersion. Dye uptake and proximal movement through the subcutaneous lymphatics can be easily visualized through intact skin of the normal extremity. In the lymphedematous extremity, dye diffusion may be limited to the dermal lymphatic plexus giving the foot a diffuse bluish tinge ("dermal backflow"). If any subcutaneous lymphatic channels are identified by dye uptake, they are canalized directly, and a radiopaque dye is injected. Dye progression is followed radiographically. While informative, lymphangiography may damage the remaining lymphatics and exacerbate existing lymphedema. Other potential complications include wound infection, skin staining, allergic reaction, and pulmonary or cerebral embolization. Because lymphangiography seldom influences the medical or surgical management of the lymphedematous patient, it should not be routinely performed.

Lymphoscintigraphy assesses lymphatic function by quantitating the rate of lymphatic isotope clearance. The study has emerged as the diagnostic study of choice for lymphedema and has been used by some to select patients for microsurgical lymphatic reconstruction.[39] Several radioisotopes (such as radioiodinated [^{131}I] human serum albumin [RIHSA], gold [^{198}Au] colloid, and technetium 99m [^{99m}Tc]–labeled colloid) have been used to study lymphatic function. RIHSA is now rarely used, since approximately 10% of the isotope will enter the vascular system after subdermal injection. This reduces the study's ability to differentiate between lymphatic and other causes of edema. Lymphoscintigraphy with radiolabeled colloidal suspensions can more accurately quantitate lymphatic function. The beta emitter ^{198}Au was used initially but then abandoned in favor of ^{99m}Tc-labeled sulfide colloid. Lymphoscintigraphy is performed by measuring the amount of radioactivity at the inguinal nodes at 30 minutes and at 1 hour after bipedal isotope injection. The normal range of inguinal node uptake is 0.6% to 1.6%. Uptake values below 0.3% are considered abnormal, and most patients with distal hypoplasia lymphedema exhibit uptake values less than 0.1%.[40, 41] Parameters, such as time of first isotope appearance, lymph speed, change in the rate and isotope uptake before and after exercise, and condensed image and factorial analysis techniques have been developed to derive even more information from lymphoscintigraphy. Variables such as the actual tissue depth of radioisotope injection, the volume injected, the patient's activity during the test, and the position of the extremity must be controlled. Fortunately, variation in the interstitial fluid content (degree of swelling) does not significantly change the rate of isotope clearance.

Differential Diagnosis

Lymphedema can usually be differentiated from other causes of limb edema on a clinical basis (Table 44–1). The most common causes of bilateral edema are systemic (e.g., cardiac, renal, or hepatic insufficiency). These are easily differentiated from lymphedema by history and physical findings or, occasionally, with the aid of laboratory tests. Venous disease is the most common cause of unilateral limb edema. The characteristic atrophic skin and brawny pigmentation make long-standing venous stasis easy to differentiate from lymphedema. Additionally, edema secondary to venous disease demonstrates decreased capillary perfusion, characteristic dark brawny edema, and ulceration of the skin secondary to impaired perfusion and tissue anoxia. In lymphedema, ulceration is extremely rare, and the deep-brown discoloration of venous disease is unusual. Although limb elevation rapidly improves venous edema, usually within hours, lymphedema resolves more slowly, often requiring days of limb elevation.

Left leg swelling (which is seen in 60% of lymphedema patients) has also been attributed to obstruction of the left iliac vein produced by crossing the right iliac artery. This has been termed the "iliac compression syndrome" and is proposed as an explanation of the lymphedema.[42] However, few of these patients demonstrate any classic evidence of peripheral venous disease, and it is difficult to see how venous hypertension can be reflected as lymphedema without a high incidence of chronic skin changes and ulceration.

Venography in such cases is useful but not always easily interpreted.[43] Doppler findings are valuable in differentiating *acute venous thrombosis* from lymphedema.[32]

Two additional uncommon conditions are *lipedema* and the *yellow nail syndrome* (YNS). Lipedema is a relatively rare condition generally affecting women. This lipodystrophy is characterized by diffuse, symmetric, nonpitting enlargement of the subcutaneous tissue of the extremity.[44] A weight-reduction regimen often has limited effectiveness, and surgery can be helpful in selected cases. YNS was first described in patients with lymphedema and yellow nails.[45] The triad of yellow dystrophic nails, primary lymphedema, and bilateral effusions is also associated with an increased incidence of maxillary sinusitis. One report of YNS included a refractory pericardial effusion.[46] The etiology of YNS remains obscure.[47, 48]

TREATMENT

Lymphatic insufficiency leads to the interstitial accumulation of protein-rich fluid, with subsequent stagnation, inflammation, and eventual fibrosis of the subcutaneous tissue. Elevation, compression, and other means that remove the interstitial fluid without removing a significant fraction of the accumulated interstitial proteins only provides transient relief and must be maintained indefinitely. To effect a cure, lymphatic drainage must be restored to effectively remove the protein-rich fluid prior to the onset of significant subcutaneous fibrosis. Unfortunately, this objective is largely unattainable. The patient must understand that lymphedema is a chronic condition and that none of the available medical or surgical treatment options completely restores the affected limb.

Medical Management

Medical therapy is the initial form of treatment for all lymphedema patients. Many patients can be adequately managed without subsequent surgical intervention. The medical management of the lymphedematous limb is accomplished through (1) the prevention of skin infection and the prompt treatment of all cutaneous complications, (2) the mechanical reduction of the interstitial fluid con-

TABLE 44–1

Differential Diagnosis of Chronic Leg Edema

	LYMPHATIC INSUFFICIENCY	**VENOSTASIS**	**CARDIAC, RENAL, OR HEPATIC INSUFFICIENCY**	**LIPEDEMA (NOT TRUE EDEMA)**
Consistency of edema	Initially soft and pitting Eventually spongy and firm	Brawny and pitting	Pitting	Nonpitting
Distribution of edema	Diffuse, greatest distally Usually unilateral	Greatest at ankles and legs, feet spared Usually unilateral	Diffuse, greatest distally Always bilateral	Greatest at ankles and legs; feet spared Always bilateral
Resolution with elevation	Mild, over several days	Complete, within hours	Complete, within hours	Minimal
Skin changes	Initially none Eventually hypertrophic, hyperkeratotic, and thick Ulceration is rare	Atrophic with brawny pigmentation Possible ulceration	Shiny, no trophic changes	None

tent, and (3) the pharmacologic reduction of interstitial proteins. Of course, identifiable conditions such as filariasis or tuberculosis, which can damage the remaining lymphatics, must be appropriately treated.

Cutaneous infection leads to increased fibrosis and must be avoided. All patients must be taught meticulous hygiene and skin care. Fungal infection of the web space can precipitate skin breakdown and must be avoided. Careful drying of the toes and web space after washing and use of an antifungal powder are important preventive measures. Some physicians advocate the use of a low-pH, lanolin-based skin lotion to prevent skin cracking and subsequent infection.[49] However, lotions with additives should be avoided, since they can sensitize the skin and trigger an inflammatory reaction.[31]

When infections occur, they must be treated immediately and aggressively. The patient should receive a systemic antistaphylococcal and antistreptococcal agent and be restricted to bed rest with the extremity elevated until the infection subsides. Urgent care is necessary because the infection can be fulminant, and each inflammatory episode leads to more subcutaneous fibrosis. In patients with recurrent infectious episodes of unknown origin, a prophylactic penicillin is the drug of choice; *Streptococcus* species represent the most common etiologic agent.

Reduction of interstitial fluid is the mainstay of medical therapy. Several treatment modalities are available to mechanically reduce the accumulation of interstitial fluid in the lymphedematous limb. In the United States, compression garments and pneumatic compression pumps are the most common treatments. In Europe, a special massage technique, manual lymph drainage (MLD), and compressive bandaging therapy (CBT) are popular.

Pneumatic compression pump therapy has proved to be an effective method of reducing the volume of interstitial fluid in the lymphedematous limb. An inflatable sleeve or stocking is placed over the edematous limb and intermittently inflated, thus forcing edema fluid proximally. These pneumatic devices vary from the single-chamber, single-pressure type to the segmental, sequential, adjustable pressure gradient pump (Lympha-Press, Biocompression Pump, Camp International, Inc., Jackson, Mich.).[50] These more sophisticated pumps use multiple chambers to sequentially compress the extremity. The pump pressure decreases as the "wave" advances proximally, thus "milking" the edema fluid out of the limb. Studies have shown that pump compression therapy is effective in reducing limb volume by 30% to 47%.[51–53] Compression pump therapy must be continued or else the limb edema rapidly reaccumulates. To maintain the newly reduced limb volume, elastic support garments should be worn continuously between treatment sessions. Ideally, the garments should be custom-fitted with a 30- to 60-mm Hg gradient pressure at the ankle.[31, 54]

Compressive garments (e.g., support stockings, sleeves, gloves, pantyhose) should not be prescribed as the sole treatment for nonpitting lymphedema. In the nondecompressed lymphedematous limb, the constant compression delivered by these garments may collapse and occlude the few existing lymphatic vessels and restrict lymphatic return. Support garments are best used to maintain a normal or near-normal limb volume.[31, 49, 55] Pump therapy and com-

pression garments are most effective in the early stages of lymphedema before the onset of significant subcutaneous fibrosis.

Manual lymph drainage and CBT have been popular treatment modalities in Europe for several years.[55] They have been introduced in the United States and are gaining in popularity. MLD is a superficial massage technique of lymphatic vessels developed in 1936 by Vodder to promote lymph drainage.[56, 57] Generally, normal functioning lymphatic vessels immediately adjacent to the lymphedematous limb are first massaged to promote lymph flow. The edematous limb is massaged repeatedly in a distal-to-proximal direction beginning with the proximal part of the limb and finishing with the distal end. This reportedly increases the function of existing lymphatics and directs lymph past the diseased or obstructed lymphatic vessels to the functional vessels that were previously "cleared" by massage. Subsequent European studies have reported that MLD increases lymph flow in collecting channels, increases local blood flow, increases the rate of contraction of lymphatic vessels, and promotes protein reabsorption.[58–60]

Compressive bandaging therapy was first described by Winiwater in 1892 for the treatment of elephantiasis.[61] It entails wrapping the lymphedematous limb with several layers of a minimal-stretch (nonelastic) bandage, such that distal pressure is greater than proximal pressure. This reportedly reestablishes the tissue pressure and subcutaneous mechanism support, which is compromised as a result of the destruction of subcutaneous elastic fibers. Moreover, this bandaging reportedly prevents the reaccumulation of lymph fluid and increases lymph flow. During normal activities or while performing prescribed exercises, the patient contracts the muscles of the bandaged limb within an almost nonyielding space. This reportedly increases tissue pressure and also promotes lymph flow. Most practitioners who use CBT apply the bandages after MLD. In one study, MLD combined with CBT over a 3-week period resulted in a 20% reduction of arm volume in postmastectomy lymphedema patients.[62] In 1989, Földi and colleagues described their experience treating 399 patients with benign, postmastectomy lymphedema.[20a] Ninety-five percent of their patients had a significant reduction in limb volume, and 56% of their patients had a greater than 50% reduction. At 3-year follow-up, 54% had fully maintained their therapeutic results.[20a]

Although diuretics have been used widely in the past, they are of little value in the treatment of lymphedema. In fact, some physicians believe they may be harmful. By decreasing limb water content, diuretics may increase the interstitial protein concentration, accelerating the rate of subcutaneous fibrosis.[20, 31, 49]

Reduction of interstitial protein can be accomplished pharmacologically. The benzopyrones are a family of diverse compounds that increase the number of macrophages in the interstitium of lymphedematous tissue as well as the rate of protein breakdown by macrophages.[63, 64] In clinical trials, benzopyrones given orally for 6 months produced a 15% to 20% decrease in excess limb volume, a decrease in perceived limb heaviness and discomfort, and an increase in skin softness.[65] Multiple clinical trials in both Europe and Australia have documented moderate improvement in lymphedema patients.[65–69]

Benzopyrones are inexpensive oral agents with little demonstrable toxicity. They do not offer rapid relief but can slowly improve clinical high-protein lymphedema.[65-66] Although they are not currently available in the United States, they have been used as adjuvant therapy in other affluent countries.[70] They may be most useful, however, in impoverished nations where filariasis is widespread and where patient access to more effective treatment modalities is limited.

Limb hyperthermia has been reported as a treatment for lymphedema.[71] An electric oven is used to heat the leg to approximately 40°C (1 hour/day for 20 days). Following treatment, the leg is tightly wrapped in elastic bandage. In a series of 1000 patients, good results have been reported, with the improvement attributed to lymphatic regeneration.*

Surgical Management

If optimal medical therapy is ineffective in controlling lymphedema, surgical intervention may be considered. The aim of surgical therapy is to drain or excise the lymphedematous skin and subcutaneous tissue and thereby improve function and appearance as well as decrease the frequency of recurrent infection. All patients must understand that surgery is palliative and that a cosmetically perfect result is unattainable. Functional impairment caused by inability to control the size of the extremity is the best indication for surgery. The patient with restricted movement secondary to gross extremity enlargement is most likely to benefit from surgical intervention. Those with primary hypoplastic lymphedema of moderate severity who seek surgical correction for cosmetic reasons are less likely to be satisfied.

The frustration encountered in the surgical management of lymphedema is reflected in the numerous procedures described over the past 80 years. In general, these operations can be divided into physiologic procedures and excisional procedures (Table 44–2). The physiologic operations attempt to reconstruct lymphatic drainage by either (1) establishing communication between a lymphatic-rich flap and the edematous limb or (2) bypassing a segmental lymphatic obstruction by introducing a lympholymphatic or lymphovenous shunt. The excisional operations remove varying amounts of subcutaneous tissue and skin. Most pedicle flap procedures also include a significant amount of excision. Thompson's buried dermis flap is intended to be both an excisional and a physiologic operation.

Physiologic Operations

Lymphangioplasty was first proposed by Handley[72] in 1908. He implanted silk threads in the subcutaneous tissues in lymphedematous limbs (lymphangioplasty). He argued that fibrous channels would form around the foreign body and transport lymph by capillary action. While some patients

---

*Lin WY: Heating and bandage treatment for treating chronic lymphedema of the extremity. Unpublished report from the Department of Plastic and Reconstructive Surgery, The Ninth People's Hospital, Shanghai's Second Medical College, 1982.

TABLE 44–2

Operations for Lymphedema

Physiologic Operations

Alloplastic implants (lymphangioplasty)
Pedicle flap operations
  Skin pedicle flap
  Omental pedicle flap
  Enteromesenteric pedicle flap (small bowel flap)
Microsurgical reconstruction
  Lymphonodal-venous or lymphovenous anastomoses
  Lympholymphatic anastomoses

Excisional Operations

Total subcutaneous excision (Charles' procedure)
Buried dermis flap (Thompson's procedure)*
Subcutaneous excision underneath flaps (modified Homans' procedure)

---

*This operation is intended to be both excisional and physiologic.

---

who underwent lymphangioplasty had early postoperative improvement, no patient demonstrated long-term benefit.[73] Clearly, any channel that forms around an alloplastic implant will fibrose with time.

As new and less immunogenic implant materials become available, interest in this operation is periodically renewed.[74-76] In the most recent report, 16 patients underwent multifilament. Teflon-wick lymphangioplasty, and their cases were followed for 10 years.[74] In this report, several patients experienced an initial reduction in limb circumference lasting as long as 13 months, but all patients had returned to their baseline or a worse state by the fifth postoperative year.

Lymphangioplasty is a very simple but ineffective operation. This procedure should play no role in the long-term management of either primary or secondary lymphedema.

Microsurgical Lymphatic Reconstruction

Microsurgical procedures designed to reestablish lymphatic drainage to an affected extremity can be divided into two operative categories: (1) lymphonodal-venous shunts or lymphovenous shunts and (2) lympholymphatic shunts. The aim of each procedure is to reroute lymphatic flow around the diseased lymphatic vessels or nodes. As with arterial reconstruction, a limited segmental obstruction with good distal vessel function provides the optimal setting in which to perform a bypass procedure.

Lymphonodal-venous and lymphovenous shunts were first reported in the early 1960s.[77, 78] In the lower extremity, a lymphonodal-venous shunt is created by identification and transection of a lymph node (usually femoral), removal of the lymphoid pulp, and anastomosis of the transected node onto the anterior surface of a neighboring vein (usually femoral or saphenous). Care is taken to avoid injuring the afferent lymphatic vessels entering the node. Alternatively, a lymphovenous shunt is established by identification of patent functional lymphatic vessels in the proximal medial thigh and creation of an end-to-end anastomosis with a branch of the saphenous vein immediately distal to the saphenofemoral junction. (A complete description of these operations is provided by Olszewski[79] and by Gloviczki.[39])

By the late 1960s, Nielubowicz and Olszewski[80] had performed these operations in patients with lymphedema. Their operative results were described as "fair" to "very good" in 74% of patients with secondary lymphedema and in 55% of patients with primary hyperplastic lymphedema. However, the reduction in limb circumference was modest. Furthermore, in patients with primary hypoplastic lymphedema, these procedures were ineffective. Only 24% of these patients who underwent surgery improved, whereas 28% improved with conservative therapy alone. More recent studies have reported even better results.[81–83]

After more than 25 years of clinical experience, the question of long-term anastomotic patency remains unsettled. Sequential limb volume determination continues to be one of the predominant methods of perioperative patient assessment, and it only provides indirect evidence of anastomotic function. While lymphangiography is capable of visualizing the anastomosis directly, this method has been shown to damage residual lymphatics and should not be used in postoperative patient evaluation. Lymphoscintigraphy can estimate the rate of lymphatic flow and document perioperative changes in the flow rate. It cannot directly demonstrate flow across a lymphonodal-venous or lymphovenous shunt, since any radiolabeled colloid that enters the vein is rapidly diluted. Lymphoscintigraphy, however, can demonstrate flow across a lympholymphatic anastomosis, since rapid colloid washout does not occur.

Lympholymphatic shunts are promising procedures that were developed in the late 1970s. These procedures use functional, autologous lymphatic vessels harvested from a nondiseased extremity to bypass a segmental lymphatic obstruction.[84–87] Baumeister and Siuda have the most experience with this operation and have recently published their experience with 55 patients.[88] A segmental lymphatic obstruction is the principal indication for surgery; patients with primary hypoplastic lymphedema are not operative candidates. Of the 55 patients studied, only 4 had primary lymphedema (unilateral pelvic lymphatic atresia with functional distal lymphatics). Eighty percent of study patients had achieved significant postoperative volume reduction of the affected extremity when their cases were followed for more than 3 years. Anastomotic patency was demonstrated in several patients using lymphoscintigraphy, although the patency rate was not cited. Overall, the lymphatic transport index was improved by 30% in the recipient limb, while none of the donor extremities developed lymphedema.

In summary, shunt procedures in general are most likely to benefit patients with a limited segmental lymphatic obstruction and good distal lymphatic vessel function. Secondary lymphedema of short duration (less than 5 years) provides the best indication for microsurgical reconstruction. Clearly, however, it is the functional state of the distal lymphatic vessels and not the duration of disease that best predicts the probability of shunt success. Primary lymphedema patients with distal hypoplasia (most common form) are unlikely to benefit significantly from microsurgical reconstruction.[89]

Pedicle flap operations juxtapose lymphatic-rich pedicle flaps and lymphedematous tissue in hopes of inducing lymphatic communication and providing drainage for the lymphedematous tissue. To date, skin, omentum, and small bowel have been used as pedicle flaps.

Gillies and Fraser[90] were the first to use skin pedicle flap to drain lymphedematous tissue. Significant volume reduction was achieved in a patient with secondary lymphedema in whom a tubed skin flap presumably functioned as a lymphatic bridge across a segmental obstruction. However, subsequent attempts to drain the affected limbs of patients with primary lymphedema met with predictable failure. Other surgeons have tried to provide drainage by rotating an inguinal skin flap from an uninvolved extremity to the contralateral lymphedematous limb.[91] This approach is usually not effective and may threaten the lymphatic function of the uninvolved limb. Other skin flap procedures have been devised, but they are usually unsuccessful.

Use of the omental pedicle flap was popularized by Goldsmith and others in the 1960s.[71, 92] Although initial reports were encouraging, the omental pedicle flap provides little long-term benefit.[93] The omentum is rich in lymphatics, but the vessels are small and the lymphatic flow rate is low. Experimental studies have failed to demonstrate any postoperative lymphatic connections between the omental flap and the lymphedematous tissue.[94, 95] In addition, at reoperation a bursa-like sac is often found to have formed around the flap that may act as a physical barrier against lymphatic anastomoses. Because this operation is largely ineffective and may result in serious complications (e.g., abdominal wall hernia, intestinal obstruction, or gangrene), it has been abandoned.

A small bowel pedicle flap has been developed and successfully used in the laboratory.[96] The operation is performed by raising an ileal flap on its mesenteric pedicle and stripping the mucosa to expose the submucosal lymphatics. The iliac or inguinal lymph nodes are transected (depending on the obstruction site) and sutured onto the denuded submucosa.[97] Early clinical results have been encouraging.[98] However, the mesenteric pedicle is of limited length, and the operation must be limited to patients with a very proximal segmental obstruction.

Excisional Operations

Total subcutaneous excision was originally described by Charles[99] in 1912 and is the most extensive of the excisional procedures. In the lower extremity, all of the skin and subcutaneous tissues are excised from the tibial tuberosity to the malleoli (except for tissue overlying the tendo calcaneus). While some surgeons remove the deep fascia in its entirety, others resect only heavily fibrosed segments. Tapering of tissue at the proximal and distal margins is performed to prevent a step deformity. The defect is closed using a split-thickness or full-thickness skin graft from the resected specimen or a split-thickness skin graft from an uninvolved donor site (the operative procedure is described in detail by Hoopes[100]). Coverage with a split-thickness skin graft is technically easier and gives a satisfactory initial appearance. However, these grafts are easily injured, ulcerate frequently, scar extensively, become hyperpigmented, and may develop a severe hyperkeratotic, weeping chronic dermatitis. The end result is almost always far worse than the original problem. We strongly oppose the use of split-thickness graft resurfacing after subcutaneous excision.[101] Coverage with a full-thickness skin graft is technically more demanding but produces a more durable graft site. Nevertheless, regions of graft breakdown and substantial scar formation can also occur with full-thickness grafts.

The long-term efficacy of the Charles procedure has been evaluated in very few studies. Preliminary results of patients who had undergone the operation at the Johns Hopkins Hospital were reported in 1959,[102] with a long-term follow-up study of the same patients in 1977.[103] Some degree of hyperpigmentation and hyperkeratosis of the grafted skin was reported in all 10 patients in the follow-up study. However, both conditions were more frequently observed in areas covered with split-thickness skin grafts than with full-thickness grafts. Two of the 10 patients had recurrent cellulitis that required hospitalization. Two had notable swelling of the extremity distal to the graft, and two required a subsequent procedure to revise scars or release contractures, but none of the patients required a second operation for recurrent lymphedema. All patients had mild to moderate swelling after prolonged standing that was well controlled by compression stockings. Overall, all patients were "pleased" with the improved appearance and function.[103]

In 1965, Taylor[104] reported a series of 34 patients who had undergone total subcutaneous excision followed by a split-thickness skin graft. Twelve patients (35%) had a "good" result, 12 had a "satisfactory" result, and 10 (29%) had an "unsatisfactory" result. Despite its obvious limitations, this procedure is sometimes the only surgical option for patients with very extensive swelling and extreme skin changes.

Suction curettage has been reported as a useful adjunct to the surgical management of primary and secondary lymphedema.[105, 106] This method is useful for debulking lymphedematous limbs but cannot be used to treat extremity lymphedema of any significant magnitude without a concomitant resection of the expanded skin envelope. Excisional procedures continue to be the mainstay of surgical treatment for chronic, whole-limb edema with poor distal lymphatic function.

Thompson's buried dermis flap is an operation in which a portion of the lymphedematous subcutaneous tissue is resected beneath flaps, a flap edge is de-epithelialized, and the resulting dermis flap is buried into the underlying muscle compartment. Thompson's operation has three theoretical advantages: (1) the buried dermis permits the formation of lymphatic connections between the subdermal lymphatic plexus of the flap and the deep lymphatics of the muscle compartment, (2) muscle contraction will increase the lymphatic flow rate through the subdermal plexus, and (3) the buried flap provides a physical barrier to deep fascia regeneration.[107] The operation is intended to be both excisional and physiologic in approach.

In the thigh, a medial incision is made approximately 3 cm posterior to the course of the femoral vessels and carried distally about 1 cm behind the posterior border of the tibia. The posterior flap is elevated, and a 4- to 5-cm-wide split-thickness skin graft is harvested from the flap edge. The subcutaneous tissue and the underlying fascia are excised, and the shaved flap edge is buried beneath the anterior flap. The buried segment lies next to the femoral

vessels in the thigh and next to the tibial vessels in the leg. If required, a lateral operation is performed at a later date. (The operation is presented in more detail by Thompson.[107])

In 1980, Thompson and Wee[108] published their long-term results using this procedure. One hundred fifty-one operations were performed on 140 patients (11 were bilateral). Of these, 88 operations were performed for primary lymphedema of the leg, 14 for secondary lymphedema of the leg, and 49 for secondary lymphedema of the arm. One third of the cases were followed for 5 years, one third for 5 to 10 years, and the remainder for 10 to 20 years. Operative results were reported as "good," "satisfactory," or "unimproved." A good result indicated reduction of excess swelling by more than 75%, a return to normal activity, and relief from the main complaints. A satisfactory outcome indicated a significant but less than 70% reduction of swelling, a return to moderate activity, and alleviation of most complaints.

In patients with primary lymphedema, 51% of the limbs had a good surgical result, and another 32% had a satisfactory outcome. Comparable results were reported for patients with secondary lymphedema of the lower extremity. In the upper extremity, 61% had a good result, and 14% were satisfactory. Flap necrosis was the most common complication and occurred in 47% of all operative patients. While most areas of tissue loss were small, 12% of patients had significant tissue necrosis (exceeding 10 sq cm) and required excision and skin grafting under anesthesia. An additional 14% of patients developed a draining sinus at the surgical incision. Two patients had inadvertent nerve injury during dissection.

Although operative success is attributed to the formation of lymphatic connections between the flap and the muscle compartment, postoperative lymphangiography has failed to demonstrate any lymphatic anastomosis. RIHSA clearance studies have demonstrated postoperative improvement in the rate of lymphatic isotope clearance. However, comparable improvement in RIHSA clearance was noted after skin and subcutaneous excision alone, suggesting that the tissue excision may account for postoperative improvement.[109]

Staged subcutaneous excision underneath flaps was first described by Sistrunk in 1918[110] and later popularized by Homans.[111] In our opinion, this approach provides the most reasonable surgical compromise of the excisional procedures. It offers reliable improvement and a minimum of unfavorable postoperative complications. It produces results comparable to those of Thompson's operation but has a lower complication rate. (The third excisional operation, the Charles procedure, should be reserved for patients with severe skin changes.)

Improvement is directly related to the amount of skin and subcutaneous tissue removed and the postoperative care. The surgical procedure is offered to patients as a means of managing their lymphedema and not as a cure.[112] During the operation, the surgeon removes as much subcutaneous tissue and skin as possible while attempting to maintain a viable skin flap and achieve primary skin closure.[112–114] An experience with 652 cases over 40 years demonstrated the safety and efficacy of this approach.[115]

The following section describes our preferred surgical approach.

The Authors' Preferred Surgical Approach

Preoperative Care

All patients are given bed rest, and the extremity is elevated. Although this step can be started at home, the patient is usually admitted to the hospital 1 to 3 days preoperatively, and the lower extremity is elevated using a modified Thomas orthopedic splint suspended from an overhead frame. The rate of edema resolution depends on the chronicity of the condition and the amount of subcutaneous fibrosis. While the patient is in the hospital, the extremity is washed daily. Other than a single preoperative dose, antibiotics are not routinely used.

Operative Technique

The procedure is done in two stages. The medial side is usually done first and involves the largest amount of tissue resection. A pneumatic tourniquet is placed as proximally as possible.

LOWER EXTREMITY. A medial incision is made in the leg approximately 1 cm posterior to the tibial border and extended proximally into the thigh. Flaps about 1.5 cm thick are elevated anteriorly and posteriorly to the midsagittal plane of the calf (Fig. 44–1). The dissection is less extensive in the thigh and ankle. All subcutaneous tissue underneath the flap is removed. After excising the subcutaneous fat from the periosteum of the tibia, the deep fascia is incised, permitting an easy plane of dissection to develop. The sural nerve is identified and preserved. All of the attached subcutaneous fat and deep fascia along the medial aspect of the calf are removed (Fig. 44–2). The dissection is kept superficial to the deep fascia at the knee and ankle. Flaps in the ankle are rarely longer than 6 cm. The redundant skin is excised after removal of the subcutaneous fat (Fig. 44–3). A suction catheter is placed in the dependent portion of the posterior flap and is left in place for 5 days. Interrupted and continuous 4–0 nylon is employed for skin closure. No subcutaneous or dermal sutures are placed. The extremity is immobilized with a posterior splint and gauze dressing and kept elevated. Sutures are usually removed on the eighth day. The patient is measured for an elastic stocking, and dependency of the leg is begun on the ninth day. Ambulation is started on the 11th postoperative day, but only with the leg tightly wrapped.

The second stage is performed on the lateral aspect of the limb 3 months later. The operation is essentially identical, except that the deep fascia is not removed. Great care is taken to avoid damaging the peroneal nerve.

UPPER EXTREMITY. A medial incision is made from the distal ulna across the medial epicondyle of the humerus to the posterior medial upper arm. Flaps approximately 1 cm thick are elevated to the midsagittal aspect of the forearm, and the dissection is tapered distally and proximally. The edematous subcutaneous tissue is removed, but the deep

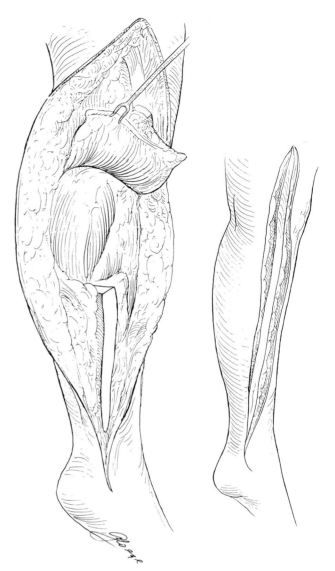

Figure 44–1. The incision is made along the midmedial aspect of the leg extending from the midthigh to the area posterior to the medial malleolus. Flaps are elevated anteriorly and posteriorly. All of the underlying fatty tissue beneath the flaps, including the deep muscle fascia investing the gastrocnemius and soleus muscles, is removed.

fascia is not spared. The ulnar nerve is identified in the region of the medial epicondyle and preserved. The redundant skin is excised. If necessary, the tourniquet can be removed, the area prepared, and the operation continued into the axilla. A suction catheter is placed, and the skin is closed with 4–0 nylon suture. No subcutaneous or dermal sutures are used. The arm is immobilized and elevated for 5 days. The suction catheter can often be removed after the third day. Otherwise, postoperative management is similar to that described for the leg.

Operative Results

We performed 82 lower extremity operations on 49 patients. Thirty-two (65%) patients had a significant reduction in extremity size. Of the remaining patients, 10% have had some improvement that has lasted through 2 years of fol-low-up. The remainder have returned to postoperative levels of swelling or continued to progress. Men have a worse prognosis than women, although the explanation for this is unclear. Only three postoperative complications related to ischemic necrosis of the flap have occurred. All have healed by second intention, and none have required further surgery. Although many patients experience decreased sensation at the incision site, this has not been a source of complaint. None of these patients had inadvertent nerve injury, nor has any alteration in hand or foot sensation been observed. All patients have some recurrence of swelling and must continue to wear support stockings.

The operative results for postmastectomy lymphedema have been more varied. In patients with massive swelling, the postoperative improvement is usually significant, and function can often be restored. In 10 patients, the postoperative arm volume was reduced by 250 to 1200 mL; the reduced volume was maintained through 6 years of follow-up. In the remaining four patients, arm swelling continued to progress despite the initial surgical reduction. Three of these patients had a progressive increase in hand edema following surgery. Whether this was the result of surgery or merely a continued progression of the underlying disease is unclear. The mechanism of improvement with staged subcutaneous excision underneath flaps is unclear. Extensive surgical dissection may establish lymphatic venous

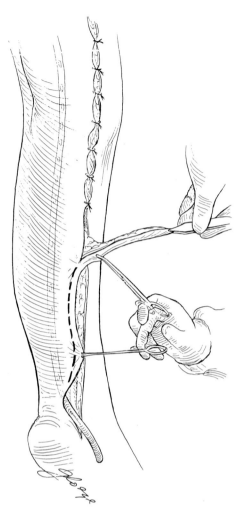

Figure 44–3. Upon closure, additional amounts of skin can be removed. As shown in Figure 44–1, some of the skin can be excised at the time of initial incision. The closure should leave no redundant skin. Large drains, inserted in the most dependent position, are left in place to drain blood and lymph for at least a 5-day period. During this time, the leg is immobilized in a posterior, well-padded plaster splint and elevated. The patient walks on the ninth postoperative day, at which time the leg is wrapped securely with elastic bandage.

anastomoses during the process of healing, and the procedure may favorably alter the balance of lymph flow by reducing the amount of lymph-forming tissue. The excision of substantial tissue and skin may result in external compression effecting an increase in interstitial pressure much like an elastic stocking, thus improving lymph flow.

The discouraging fact remains that no procedure cures lymphedema. A degree of edema inevitably follows any operative procedure. In our opinion, compared with all available methods of surgical management, skin and subcutaneous excision is the most reliable, consistently beneficial, and uncomplicated means of surgically managing the symptoms of lymphedema.

TUMORS OF LYMPHATICS

Lymphatic Malformations

Lymphatic malformations (LMs) are frequently observed at birth and are most apparent before 2 years of age. LMs

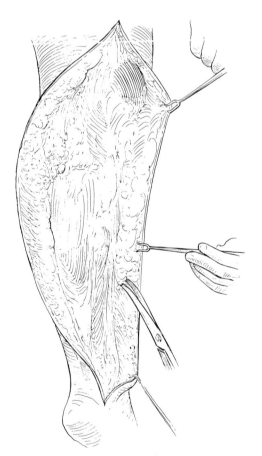

Figure 44–2. Additional amounts of subcutaneous tissue are removed from the skin flaps with scissors, thinning them to approximately 1.75 cm in thickness. The flaps are thinner around the ankle but are undermined only 4 to 8 cm. Hemostasis is accomplished after release of the pneumatic tourniquet.

can appear suddenly in an older child and on occasion in adolescence or adulthood. LMs are characterized as microcystic, macrocystic, or combined. Previously used terms are "lymphangioma" for microcystic LM and "cystic hygroma" for macrocystic LM. They are thought to have their origin in the embryologic development of the lymphatic system. Sabin[116] and, later, Goetsch[117] postulated that during the development of the lymphatic system, cell buds of lymphatic primordium occasionally fail to establish communication with veins, resulting in isolated lymphatic spaces. Portions of the lymphatic system can become sequestered and retain the ability to produce lymph and form endothelial cysts. These lymphatic cysts slowly enlarge and infiltrate the surrounding tissues by pushing other structures aside.

These tumors are all benign. The majority are present at birth, and 90% can be identified by the end of the first year of life.[91, 118] They grow in proportion to the growth of the child and can greatly enlarge at times of infection.

LMs appear as soft, cystic, discrete, nontender masses that transilluminate. They vary in size from a few millimeters to several centimeters. They can be located on any portion of the body; however, the majority are found in the head and neck region. LMs of the neck, tongue, and intraoral regions can present significant respiratory problems in the newborn and on occasion require emergent excision. These lesions must be distinguished from hemangiomas, branchial cleft cysts, lipomas, and, occasionally, neoplasms such as rhabdomyosarcoma.[119]

Treatment

Spontaneous remission of LMs is extremely rare. Percutaneous aspiration is intralesional and usually followed by prompt recurrence and, occasionally, hemorrhage or the development of infection. Introduction of sclerosing agents has been proposed, and this therapy is more effective for macrocytic LMs. Excision subsequent to sclerosis is

technically difficult.[119] Radiation therapy has no place in the treatment of LMs.

Treatment of LMs should be surgical excision, taking care to preserve all normal structures in the area. At times, a stage excision is appropriate. These lesions are nonmalignant, and care should be taken to preserve all normal anatomy. Excision is usually deferred until the age of 6 months if there is no compression of the trachea or respiratory difficulty.[118, 120]

Lymphangiosarcoma

Stewart and Treves,[121] in 1948, described the association between postmastectomy lymphedema and lymphangiosarcoma. The incidence varies between 0.07% and 0.45%.[122] This malignant lesion of the lymphatics is nearly always associated with lymphedema, most commonly with postmastectomy lymphedema, but also with filariasis.[32, 123–125] The lesion generally appears 10 years after the onset of lymphedema and pursues an aggressive malignant course. Average survival is 19 months following initiation of treatment. The lesion is described as a reddish-purple discoloration or nodule and has been confused with Kaposi's sarcoma. Satellite lesions are occasionally found, but the tumor spreads primarily by a hematogenous route.

Treatment

The mainstay of therapy has traditionally been early radical amputation.[125–127] Because of the very small number of these tumors, it has been impossible to study the effects of various forms of therapy in a randomized fashion.

Successful treatment of other soft tissue sarcomas with preoperative radiation therapy and chemotherapy, surgical excision, and postoperative adjunct chemotherapy makes a similar approach to lymphangiosarcoma justified.[128] However, insufficient evidence exists to strongly recommend any one form of therapy for this highly malignant tumor, and the prognosis remains poor.

References

1. Crockett DJ: Lymphatic anatomy and lymphoedema. Br J Plast Surg 18:12, 1965.
2. Sabin FR: The development of the lymphatic system. In Kelbel F, Mall FP (eds): Manual of Human Embryology, vol 2. Philadelphia, JB Lippincott, 1992.
3. Anson BJ (ed): Atlas of Human Anatomy. Philadelphia, WB Saunders, 1950.
4. Selkurt E (ed): Physiology. Boston, Little, Brown, 1966.
5. Melak P, Belan A, Kocandrie VL: The superficial and deep lymphatic system of the lower extremities and their mutual relationship under physiological and pathological conditions. J Cardiovasc Surg 5:686, 1964.
6. Thompson N: The surgical treatment of chronic lymphedema of the extremities. Surg Clin North Am 47:445, 1967.
7. Futrell JW, Pories W: Physiologic and immunologic considerations of the lymphatic system in tumours and transplants. Surg Gynecol Obstet 140:273, 1975.
8. Pflug JJ, Calnan JS: The normal anatomy of the lymphatic system in the human leg. Br J Surg 58:925–930, 1971.
9. Rodbard S, Feldman P: Functional anatomy of the lymphatic fluids and pathways. Lymphology 8:49, 1975.
10. Baylis W, Starling EH: Observations on venous pressure and their relationship to capillary pressures. J Physiol (Lond) 16:159, 1894.
11. Field M, Drinker C: The rapidity of interchanges between the blood and the lymph in the dog. Am J Physiol 98:378, 1931.
12. Jacobsson S: Studies of the blood circulation in lymphedematous limbs. Scand J Plast Reconstr Surg 3(Suppl):1, 1967.
13. Yoffey JM, Courtice FC: [Chapter 2]. Lymphatics, Lymph and the Lymphomyeloid Complex. London, Academic Press, 1970.
14. Parsons R, McMaster P: The effect of pulse upon the formation and flow of lymph. J Exp Med 68:353, 1938.
15. Kinmonth JB, Taylor GW: Spontaneous rhythmic contractility in human lymphatics. J Physiol (Lond) 133:3, 1956.
16. Olszewski WL, Engaset A: Intrinsic contractility of prenodal lymphatic vessels and lymph flow in human leg. Am J Physiol 239:H775, 1980.
17. Wegria R, Zekert H, Walter K, et al: Effect of systemic venous pressure on drainage of lymph from the thoracic duct. Am J Physiol 204:284, 1963.
18. Olszewski WL: Peripheral Lymph: Formation and Immune Function. Boca Raton, Fla, CRC Press, 1985.
19. Kirk RM: Capillary filtration rates in normal and lymphedematous legs. Clin Sci 27:363, 1964.
20. Casley-Smith JR, Casley-Smith JR: High-Protein Oedemas and the Benzopyrones. Sydney, Australia, JB Lippincott, 1986.

20a. Földi E, Földi M, Clodius L: The lymphedema chaos: A lancet. Ann Plast Surg 6:505, 1989.

21. Schirger A, Harrison E, Janes J: Idiopathic lymphedema: Review of 131 cases. JAMA 182:14, 1962.

22. Allen E: Lymphedema of the extremities. Classification, etiology, and differential diagnosis: Study of 300 cases. Arch Intern Med 54:606, 1934.

23. Kinmonth JB, Taylor GW, Tracey GD, et al: Primary lymphedema: Clinical and lymphangiographic studies of a series of 107 patients in which the lower limbs were affected. Br J Surg 45:1, 1957.

24. Milroy WF: An undescribed variety of hereditary oedema. N Y Med J 56:505, 1957.

25. Ersek RA, Danese CA, Howard J: Hereditary congenital lymphedema (Milroy's disease). Surgery 50:1098, 1966.

26. Kinmonth JB: Primary lymphedema: Classification and other studies based on oleolymphography and clinical features. J Cardiovasc Surg (Torino) Special Edition for 27th Congress of European Society of Cardiovascular Surgery 65:1969.

27. Olszewski W, Mackowshki J, Sawicki Z, Nielubowicz J: Clinical studies in primary lymphedema. Pol Med J 11:1560, 1972.

28. Thompson N: Buried dermal flap operation for chronic lymphedema of the extremities. Ten year survey of results in 79 cases. Plast Reconstr Surg 45:541, 1970.

29. Wolfe JHN, Kinmonth JB: The outcome of primary lymphedema of the leg. Arch Surg 116:1157, 1981.

30. Kinmonth JB, Wolfe JHN: Fibrosis in the lymph nodes in primary lymphedema. Ann R Coll Surg Engl 62:344, 1980.

31. Wolfe JHN: The management of lymphedema. In Rutherford RB (ed): Vascular Surgery, 3rd ed. Philadelphia, WB Saunders, 1989, pp 1648–1679.

32. Dale A: The swollen leg. Curr Probl Surg 140:1, 1973.

33. Stone E, Hugo N: Lymphedema. Surg Gynecol Obstet 135:635, 1972.

34. Pitts WT, Keuhnelian JG, Ravdin IS, Schor S: Swelling of the arm after radical mastectomy. Surgery 35:460, 1954.

35. Treves N: An evaluation of the etiological factors of lymphedema following radical mastectomy. Cancer 10:444, 1957.

36. Kissin MW, della Rovere GQ, Easton D, et al: Risk of lymphoedema following the treatment of breast cancer. Br J Surg 73:580, 1986.

37. Person NH, Takolander R, Bergovist D: Edema after lower limb arterial reconstruction: Influence of background factors, surgical technique and potentially prophylactic methods. Vasa 20(1):57–62, 1991.

38. Leaper D, Evans M, Pollock A: Colour lymphography in clinical surgery. Br J Surg 66:51, 1979.

39. Gloviczki P: Microsurgical treatment for chronic lymphedema: An unfilled promise? In Bergan JJ, Yao JST (eds): Venous Disorders. Philadelphia, WB Saunders, 1991, pp 344–360.

40. Baulieu F, Vaillant L, Baulieu JL, et al: The current role of lymphoscintigraphy in the study of lymphedema of the limbs. J Mal Vasc 15:152–156, 1990.

41. Browse NL: The diagnosis and management of primary lymphedema. J Vasc Surg 3:181, 1986.

42. Crockett F: The iliac compression syndrome. Br J Surg 52:391, 1967.

43. Yoffey JM, Courtice FC: Lymphatics, Lymph and Lymphoid Tissue. Cambridge, Mass, Harvard University Press, 1956.

44. Rudkin GH, Miller TA: Lipedema: A clinical entity distinct from lymphedema. Plast Reconstr Surg 94:841, 1994.

45. Samman PD, White WF: The "yellow nail" syndrome. Br J Dermatol 76:153, 1964.

46. Wakasa M, Imaizumi T, Suyama A, et al: Yellow nail syndrome associated with chronic pericardial effusion. Chest 92:366–367, 1987.

47. David I, Crawford FA Jr, Hendrix GH, et al: Thoracic surgical implications of the yellow nail syndrome. Thorac Cardiovasc Surg 91:788, 1986.

48. Gupta AK, Davies GM, Haberman HF: Yellow nail syndrome. Cutis 37:371, 1986.

49. Lerner R: Complete decongestive physiotherapy (CDP): The ideal treatment for lymphedema. Massage Ther J, winter 1992, 37.

50. Zelikovski A, Manoach M, Giler S, Urca I: Lympha-Press, a new pneumatic device for the treatment of lymphedema of the limbs. Lymphology 13:68, 1980.

51. Baulieu F, Baulieu JL, Vaillant L, et al: Factorial analysis in radionuclide lymphography: Assessment of the effects of sequential pneumatic compression. Lymphology 22:178, 1989.

52. Raines JK, O'Donell TR, Kalisher L, et al: Selection of patients with lymphedema for compression therapy. Am J Surg 133:430–437, 1977.

53. Richman DM, O'Donnell TF, Zelikovski A: Sequential pneumatic compression for lymphedema. Arch Surg 120:1116, 1985.

54. Van der Molen HR: Compression in lymphedema. Plebologie 41:391–396, 1988.

55. Földi M: Lymphedema. In Földi M, Casley-Smith JR (eds): Lymphangiology. Stuttgart, Germany, Schattauer, 1983, pp 667–668.

56. Vodder E: Le drainage lymphatique, une nouvelle méthode thérapeutique. Santé pour tous. Paris, 1936.

57. Vodder E: Foreword. In Wittlinger H, Wittlinger G (eds): Textbook of Dr. Vodder's Manual Lymph Drainage. Vol 1. Basic Course, 3rd rev ed. Translated by Harris RH. Heidelberg, Germany, Haug 1990.

58. Hutzschenreuter P, Bruemmer H, Epperfeld K: Experimentelle und klinische Untersuchungen zur Wirkungsweise der manuellen Lymphdrainage-Therapie. Lymphology 14:62–64, 1989.

59. Hutzschenreuter P, Bruemmer H: Influence of complex physical decongesting therapy on positive interstitial pressure and on lymphangiomotor activity. In Partsch H (ed): Progress in Lymphology. Amsterdam, vol 2. Amsterdam, Excerpta Medica, 1988, pp 557–560.

60. Leduc O, Bourgeois P, Leduc A: Manual lymphatic drainage: Scintigraphic demonstration of its efficacy on colloidal protein reabsorption. In Partsch H (ed): Progress in Lymphology, vol 2. Amsterdam; Excerpta Medica, 1988, p 551.

61. Winiwater A: Die Elephantiasis. In Deutsche Chirugie. Stuttgart, Germany, Enke, 1892.

62. Hutzschenreuter P, Wittlinger H, Wittlinger G, Kurz I: Postmastectomy arm lymphedema: Treated by manual lymph drainage and compression bandage therapy. Eur J Phys Med Rehabil 1:161–170, 1991.

63. Piller NB, Morgan G, Casley-Smith JR: A double-blind trial of 5,6 benzo-α-pyrone in human lymphoedema. In Casley-Smith JR, Piller NB (eds): Progress in Lymphology X. Adelaide, Australia, University of Adelaide Press, 1985, p 37.

64. Piller NB: Macrophage and tissue changes in the developmental phases of secondary lymphoedema and during conservative therapy with benzopyrone. Arch Histol Cytol 53(Suppl):209, 1990.

65. Piller NB, Morgan RG, Casley-Smith JR: A double-blind, crossover trial of O-(β-hydroxyethyl)-rutosides (benzopyrones) in the treatment of lymphoedema of the arms and legs. Br J Plast Surg 41:20, 1988.

66. Casley-Smith JR, Casley-Smith JR: The pathophysiology of lymphedema and the action of benzopyrones in reducing it. Lymphology 21:190, 1988.

67. Jamal S, Casley-Smith JR, Casley-Smith JR: The effects of 5,6 benzo-α-pyrone (coumarin) and DEC on filaritic lymphoedema and elephantiasis in India: Preliminary results. Trop Med Parasitol 83:287, 1989.

68. Clodius L, Piller NB: The conservative treatment of postmastectomy lymphoedema in patients with coumarin results in a marked continuous reduction in swelling. In Bartos V, Davidson JW (eds): Advance in Lymphology. Prague, Avicenum, 1982, p 267.

69. Knight KR, Khazanchi RK, Pederson WC, et al: Coumarin and 7-hydroxycoumarin treatment of canine obstructive lymphoedema. Clin Sci 77:69, 1989.

70. Pecking A: Medical treatment of lymphedema with benzopyrones. Experimental basis and application. J Mal Vasc 15:157, 1990.

71. Goldsmith HS, de los Santos R: Omental transposition in primary lymphedema. Surg Gynecol Obstet 125:607, 1967.

72. Handley WS: Lymphangioplasty: A new method for the relief of the brawny edema of breast cancer and for similar conditions of lymphatic oedema: Preliminary note. Lancet 1:783, 1908.

73. Handley WS: Hunterian lectures on the surgery of the lymphatic system. BMJ 1:853, 1910.

74. Silver D, Puckett CL: Lymphangioplasty: A ten year evaluation. Surgery 80:748, 1976.

75. O'Reilly K: Treatment by nylon setons of lymphoedema of the arm following radical mastectomy. Med J Aust 59:1269, 1972.

76. Degni M: New technique of drainage of the subcutaneous tissue of the limbs with nylon net for the treatment of lymphedema. Vasa 3:329, 1974.

77. Laine JB, Howard JM: Surg Forum 14:111, 1963.

78. Nielubowicz J, Olszewski W: Experimental lymphovenous anastomosis. Br J Surg 55:440, 1968.

79. Olszewski WL: The treatment of lymphedema of the extremities with microsurgical lymphovenous anastomosis. Int Angiol 7:312, 1988.

80. Nielubowicz J, Olszewski WL, et al: Late results of lymphovenous anastomosis. J Cardiovasc Surg (Torino) 14(special issue):113, 1973.

81. Nieuborg L: The Role of Lymphatico-Venous Anastomoses in the Treatment of Postmastectomy Oedema. Alblasserdam, Holland, Offsetdrukkenji Kanters BV, 1982.

82. O'Brien BMcC, Mellow CG, Khazanchi RK, et al: Long-term results after microlymphaticovenous anastomoses for the treatment of obstructive lymphedema. Plast Reconstr Surg 85:562, 1990.

83. Gong-Kang H, Ru-Qi H, Zong-Zhao L, et al: Microlymphaticovenous anastomosis in the treatment of lower limb obstructive lymphedema: Analysis of 91 cases. Plast Reconstr Surg 76:671, 1985.

84. Acland RD, Smith P: Experimental lymphatico-lymphatic anastomoses. In Abstract Book of the Seventh International Congress of Lymphology, Florence, 1979.

85. Baumeister RG, Seifert J, Wiebecke B: Homologous and autologous experimental lymph vessel transplantation: Initial experience. Int J Microsurg 3:19, 1981.

86. Baumeister RG, Seifert J, Wiebecke B: Experimental basis and first application of clinical lymph vessel transplantation of secondary lymphedema. World J Surg 5:401, 1981.

87. Baumeister RG, Seifert J, Wiebecke B: Transplantation of lymph vessels on rats as well as a first therapeutic application on the experimental lymphedema of the dog. Eur Surg Res 12(Suppl 2):7, 1980.

88. Baumeister RG, Siuda S: Treatment of lymphedemas by microsurgical lymphatic grafting: What is proved? Plast Reconstr Surg 85:64, 1990.

89. Gloviczki P, Fisher J, Hollier LH, et al: Microsurgical lymphovenous anastomosis for treatment of lymphedema: A critical review. J Vasc Surg 7:647, 1988.

90. Gillies H, Fraser FR: The treatment of lymphoedema by plastic operation: A preliminary report. BMJ 1:96, 1935.

91. Clodius L, Piller NB: Conservative therapy for postmastectomy lymphedema. Chir Plast 4:193, 1978.

92. Goldsmith HS, de los Santos R, Beattie EJ: Relief of chronic lymphedema by omental transposition. Ann Surg 166:572, 1967.

93. Goldsmith HS: Long term evaluation of omental transposition for chronic lymphedema. Ann Surg 180:847, 1974.

94. Kinmonth JB: The Lymphatics: Disease, Lymphograph and Surgery. Baltimore, Williams & Wilkins, 1972.

95. Danese CA, Papioannou AN, Morales LE, et al: Surgical approaches to lymphatic blocks. Surgery 56:821, 1968.

96. Hurst PA, Kinmonth JB, Rutt DL: A gut and mesentery pedicle for bridging lymphatic obstruction. J Cardiovasc Surg 19:589, 1978.

97. Kinmonth JB, Hurst PAE, Edwards JM, Rutt DL: Relief of lymph obstruction by use of a bridge of mesentery and ileum. Br J Surg 65:829, 1979.

98. Hurst PA, Stewart G, Kinmonth J, Browse NL: Long term results of the enteromesenteric bridge operation in treatment of primary lymphoedema. Br J Surg 72:272, 1985.

99. Charles RH: Elephantiasis scroti. In Latham A (ed): A System of Treatment, vol 3. London, Churchill, 1912.

100. Hoopes JE: Lymphedema of the extremity. In Cameron JL (ed): Current Surgical Therapy, 3rd ed. Philadelphia, BC Decker, 1989.

101. Miller TA: Charles procedure for lymphedema: A warning. Am J Surg 139:290, 1980.

102. McKee DM, Edgerton MT: The surgical treatment of lymphedema of the lower extremities. Plast Reconstr Surg 23:480, 1959.

103. Dellon AL, Hoopes JB: The Charles procedure for primary lymphedema. Plast Reconstr Surg 60:589, 1977.

104. Taylor GW: Surgical management of primary lymphedema. Proc R Soc Med 58:1024, 1965.

105. Louton RB, Terranova WA: The use of suction curettage as adjunct to the management of lymphedema. Ann Plast Surg 22:354, 1989.

106. Nava VM, Lawrence WT: Liposuction on a lymphedematous arm. Ann Plast Surg 21:366, 1988.

107. Thompson N: Surgical treatment of chronic lymphedema of the lower limb. With preliminary report of new operation. BMJ 11:1566, 1962.

108. Thompson N, Wee JTK: Twenty years' experience of the buried dermis flap operation in the treatment of chronic lymphedema of the extremities. Chir Plast 5:147, 1980.

109. Kondoleon E: Die operative Behandlung der elephantiastichen Oedeme. Zentralbl Chir 39:1022, 1912.

110. Sistrunk WE: Further experiences with the Kondoleon operation for elephantiasis. JAMA 71:800, 1918.

111. Homans J: The treatment of elephantiasis of the legs: A preliminary report. N Engl J Med 215:1099, 1936.

112. Miller TA: Surgical management of lymphedema of the extremity. Plast Reconstr Surg 56:633, 1975.

113. Fonkalsrud EW, Coulson WF: Management of congenital lymphedema in infants and children. Ann Surg 177:280, 1973.

114. Miller TA: Surgical approach to lymphedema of the arm after mastectomy. Am J Surg 148:152, 1984.

115. Servelle M: Surgical treatment of lymphedema. A report on 652 cases. Surgery 101:484, 1987.

116. Sabin FR: Direct growth of veins by sprouting. In Contributions to Embryology, Washington, DC, Carnegie Institution of Washington. vol 14. 1933, p 1.

117. Goetsch E: Hygroma colli cysticum and hygroma axillare. Pathologic and clinical study and report of twelve cases. Arch Surg 36:394, 1938.

118. Fonkalsrud EW: Surgical management of congenital malformations of the lymphatic system. Am J Surg 128:152, 1974.

119. Fonkalsrud EW: Malformation of the lymphatic system and hemangiomas. In Holder TH, Ashcraft KW (eds): Pediatric Surgery. Philadelphia, WB Saunders, 1980.

120. Bill AH Jr, Summer DS: A united concept of lymphangioma and cystic hygroma. Surg Gynecol Obstet 120:79, 1965.

121. Stewart FW, Treves N: Lymphangiosarcoma in postmastectomy lymphedema: A report of six cases in elephantiasis chirurgica. Cancer 1:64, 1948.

122. Janse AJ, van Coevorden F, Peterse H, et al: Lymphedema-induced lymphangiosarcoma. Eur J Surg Oncol 21:155, 1995.

123. Unruh H, Robertson DI, Karasewich E: Postmastectomy lymphangiosarcoma. Can J Surg 22:586, 1979.

124. Shafiroff BB, Nightingale G, Baxter JJ, O'Brien B: Lymphaticolymphatic anastomosis. Ann Plast Surg 3:199, 1979.

125. Woodward AH, Ivins JC, Soule EH: Lymph angiosarcoma arising in chronic lymphedematous extremities. Cancer 30:562, 1972.

126. Sordillo PP, Chapman R, Haidu SI, et al: Lymphangiosarcoma. Cancer 48:1674, 1981.

127. Tomita K, Yokogawa A, Oda Y, et al: Lymphangiosarcoma in postmastectomy lymphedema (Stewart-Treves syndrome): Ultra-structural and immunohistologic characteristics. J Surg Oncol 38:275, 1988.

128. Rosenberg SA, Suit HD, Baker LH, Rosen E: Sarcomas of the soft tissues and bone. In Devita VT Jr, Hellman S, Rosenberg SA (eds): Cancer: Principles and Practice of Oncology. Philadelphia, JB Lippincott, 1982.

Questions

1. All of the following lymphatic structures have valves except
   (a) interdermal lymphatics
   (b) dermal level lymphatics
   (c) collecting channels
   (d) main lymphatic trunks

2. Lower leg lymphatics drain principally into
   (a) superior inguinal nodes
   (b) iliac nodes
   (c) inferior inguinal nodes
   (d) periaortic nodes

3. There is communication between superficial and deep vein lymphatics
   (a) in normal extremities
   (b) in 50% of normal extremities
   (c) only under abnormal conditions
   (d) only after trauma

4. Complications of lymphangiography include all except
   (a) lymphangitis
   (b) pulmonary embolus
   (c) fever
   (d) pancytopenia

5. Normal lymph contains what concentration of protein?
   (a) 0.01 to 0.05 g/dL
   (b) 0.1 to 0.5 g/dL
   (c) 1.0 to 5.0 g/dL
   (d) 5.0 to 10 g/dL

6. Lymphedema is characterized by all of the following except
   (a) nonpitting edema
   (b) reduction of edema with elevation over days
   (c) skin ulceration
   (d) normal skin color

7. What percentage of patients with primary lymphedema present during adolescence (lymphedema praecox)?
   (a) 10%
   (b) 40%
   (c) 60%
   (d) 80%

8. "Stage subcutaneous excision" of lymphedematous tissue
   (a) decreases postoperative lymphangitis and cellulitis
   (b) does not change radioactive iodine–tagged human serum albumin clearance
   (c) involves extensive skin grafting
   (d) cures lymphedema in the affected extremity

9. Therapy for congenital lymphatic malformations causing respiratory obstruction in the neonatal period is
   (a) sclerosis
   (b) radiation therapy
   (c) simple surgical excision
   (d) radical surgical excision

10. Lymphangiosarcoma
   (a) arises only after radical mastectomy
   (b) occurs within 2 to 3 years of onset of lymphedema
   (c) has 80% 5-year survival
   (d) responds poorly to currently available therapy

Answers

1. a   2. c   3. c   4. d   5. b   6. c   7. d   8. a   9. c   10. d

45

Lower Extremity Amputation

James M. Malone

OVERVIEW AND HISTORICAL PERSPECTIVE

Amputation surgery is thought to be one of the oldest surgical procedures.[1] The earliest artificial limb dates from the Samnite Wars of 300 BC. Until the time of Ambroise Paré (1510–1590), the techniques for amputation surgery and amputation level selection were extremely crude. Paré not only improved the surgical technique of amputation through the use of vascular ligatures but also developed many guidelines for the selection of appropriate levels of amputation. Because many of his original drawings and descriptions are not greatly different from our surgical and prosthetic practices of today, he is considered to be the originator of the modern principles of amputation surgery. Paré's work was expanded by Dominique Jean Larrey (1776–1842) during the Napoleonic Wars. Larrey advocated early amputation for traumatic limb injuries and was instrumental in the acceptance of both complete stump débridement and modern surgical techniques, whereby bone was buried deep in the amputation stump, rather than the previous method of suturing skin tightly over the bone. Larrey was also involved in developing methods of early mobilization of war amputees.[2]

The idea of immediate or rapid fitting of an artificial leg after lower extremity amputation is relatively recent. Credit for the concept of rapid fit is generally given to Berlemont based on his work with patients with delayed healing after lower extremity amputation,[3] while the concept of immediate postsurgical prosthetic fitting was developed by Weiss.[4] In the late 1960s, Burgess and colleagues[5] and Burgess and Romano (1968) noted accelerated rehabilitation, increased acceptance of a prosthesis, and less psychological trauma associated with loss of a limb when a prosthesis was applied immediately after lower extremity amputation. In the past, advances in lower extremity amputation have included the development of new techniques for amputation level selection, the extension of the frontiers for limb salvage, and the fabrication of prosthetic limbs that have incorporated new designs and materials as well as energy storage.

Despite the long and colorful history attached to amputation surgery, amputation has been considered by most surgeons as a surgical defeat and an uninteresting and unrewarding surgical procedure. In many surgical institutions, amputation surgery was traditionally passed down to the youngest and least experienced member of the surgical team, who often operated without senior supervision. A report from the European surgical literature suggests that amputation failure is statistically linked to the amputation experience of the surgeon.[6]

There has been a resurgence of interest in amputation surgery and rehabilitation. It is my view that amputation surgery is not a failure; it is clearly a reconstructive surgical technique. In addition, the surgeon who performs the amputation *owes the patient the debit of rehabilitation* following surgery.

Historically, amputations were performed by orthopedic rather than general surgeons. However, since two thirds of all lower extremity amputations are now performed as a result of complications of peripheral vascular disease or diabetes mellitus, or both, it is not surprising that the majority of lower extremity amputations are now performed by general and vascular surgeons. Unfortunately, most general surgical training programs fail to provide education in prosthetics, prosthetic design, biomechanics, and rehabilitation. The qualifications of the surgeon performing the amputation are not nearly as important as the interest of the surgeon in providing postoperative rehabilitation for the newly amputated patient.

This chapter reviews important features of lower extremity amputation surgery and amputation rehabilitation and includes detailed subsections on patient evaluation and preparation for amputation; techniques of amputation level selection; the indications, surgical techniques, and prosthetic requirements for each level of amputation; a review of surgical morbidity and mortality; an overview of common principles of lower extremity prosthetics; a discussion on techniques of postsurgical rehabilitation; and finally, some thoughts on future trends.

PATIENT EVALUATION AND PREPARATION FOR AMPUTATION

A review of the literature suggests that the mortality rates for below-knee and above-knee amputation are 4% to 16%

and 12% to 40%, respectively.[7–12] It has been estimated that two thirds of patients undergoing lower extremity amputation have diabetes mellitus and that one half to two thirds have symptoms of cardiorespiratory diseases.[7, 9, 13] A review of the causes of late mortality following successful amputation surgery discloses that two thirds of the patients die of cardiovascular diseases, approximately one half of whom die from myocardial infarction.[7, 14]

There are between 30,000 and 50,000 new lower extremity amputations performed in the United States each year.[7, 9] At the present time, the data are unclear with respect to whether the increase in distal revascularization has decreased the number of amputations. It is clear that diabetes-related amputation rates exhibit high regional variation, even after age, sex, and race adjustment (Wrobel et al, 2001). The indications for lower extremity amputation are listed in Table 45–1. For those patients with diabetes mellitus, it has been estimated that the risk of losing their second leg in the ensuing 5 years after amputation of the first leg ranges from 15% to 33% (3% to 7% per year);[16–18] however, one third to one half of amputees with diabetes mellitus die of complications of diabetes or cardiorespiratory diseases prior to undergoing an amputation of their second extremity.[16, 18, 19]

In view of the mean age of patients undergoing lower extremity amputation (62 years),[7, 8, 13–15] the incidence of associated diseases, and the morbid and nonmorbid complications associated with surgery, the importance of a careful preoperative physical examination cannot be overly stressed. The physical examination should include a search for physical signs and symptoms suggestive of cardiorespiratory diseases. Documentation of all pulses, as well as careful assessment of the presence or absence of physical findings suggestive of extremity ischemia (pain, paresthesias, elevation pallor, rubor, alteration of sensory or motor function), should be clearly documented. The extent and depth of infection or gangrene should be noted. The presence of malnutrition or systemic diseases, such as diabetes mellitus, collagen-vascular diseases, and immunodeficiency syndromes, or the systemic administration of anti-inflammatory drugs such as steroids should be noted, because their presence may have a major influence on the preoperative preparation and timing of lower extremity amputation, as well as postsurgical recovery. All diabetic patients should be carefully screened for silent but significant coronary artery disease. A paper by Pinzur and colleagues[20] reinforced the concept that multidisciplinary presurgical evaluation helps correct amputation level selection, correct prosthetic limb fitting, and improves patient rehabilitation.

The presence of lower extremity infection in a diabetic patient requires special mention. Historically, most studies have suggested that the primary organisms were *Staphylococcus aureus* and enteric gram-negative bacilli. More recent information, however, suggests that 60% of lower extremity infections in patients with diabetes mellitus involve both obligate and facultative anaerobic organisms.[21] Fierer and associates[21] also pointed out that patients with mixed infections required more operations than those with simple staphylococcal infections and that their surgical wounds tended to heal more slowly. We therefore recommend that appropriate antibiotic coverage for diabetics with lower extremity infections should include drugs that provide broad-spectrum bactericidal aerobic and anaerobic coverage. A note of caution: there were increasing reports of MRSA (methicillin-resistant *Staphylococcus aureus*) infections, especially in patients with wound complications after vascular surgery (Naylor and coworkers, 2001).

In the absence of acute arterial embolization, diabetes mellitus, immunodeficiency syndromes, collagen-vascular diseases, or drugs that inhibit the immune system, it is unusual to see tissue loss with or without infection in patients without multilevel vascular occlusive disease. Chronic single-level arterial obstruction is not usually associated with limb loss. As a general guideline, chronic occlusion of the superficial femoral artery does not cause limb loss without outflow (tibial trifurcation) or inflow (iliofemoral or profunda) occlusive disease.

The aims of the surgeon when recommending amputation are to remove gangrenous tissues, relieve pain, obtain primary healing of the most distal amputation possible, and obtain maximal rehabilitation after amputation. For purposes of further discussion, indications and management of patients undergoing amputation are divided into three general categories: (1) acute ischemia; (2) progressive chronic ischemia; and (3) ischemia complicated by infection.

Acute Ischemia

The choice of amputation for the management of acute ischemia in a patient whose arterial tree is considered unreconstructable or in a patient who presents late in the course of acute ischemia, such that arterial reconstruction may be contraindicated, is a decision that will tax the judgment of even the most experienced surgeon (Malone, 2000). In addition, urgent or emergent amputation following acute arterial occlusion is generally associated with the greatest risk of morbidity and mortality in the entire field of amputation surgery. The degree of urgency for amputation in the face of acute arterial ischemia is governed by multiple factors that include, but are not limited to, the extent of extremity ischemia, especially the muscle mass; the pain that the patient is experiencing from the ischemic tissues; and the presence of signs of systemic toxicity resulting from products of necrotic muscle or bacteria reaching the general circulatory system. If the affected ischemic area is small, such as the toes or forefoot, the pain is relatively moderate, and there are no signs of supervening

TABLE 45–1

Indications for Lower Extremity Amputation

	PERCENTAGE (RANGE)
Complications of diabetes mellitus	60–80
Nondiabetic infection with ischemia	15–25
Ischemia without infection	5–10
Chronic osteomyelitis	3–5
Trauma	2–5
Miscellaneous (neuroma, frostbite, tumor, pain, nonhealing)	5–10

Data from references 7, 9, 13–15.

infection or systemic toxicity, then amputation can and should be postponed as long as possible to allow maximum development of collateral circulation. Delay of amputation in such a case improves the likelihood that a more distal limited amputation will heal. Mild to moderate pain can be controlled with narcotics. Adjunctive therapy, including systemic heparin, low-molecular-weight dextran, or the use of fibrinolytic agents (in the absence of urokinase, t-PA [tissue plasminogen activator or TNKase] or Retavase [reteplase recombinant] may be used), may be valuable in preventing progression of thrombus within capillary beds during the period of reduced blood flow, thus maintaining the viability of marginally ischemic tissues during the time the collateral channels are beginning to enlarge. The presence of severe pain, extensive muscle necrosis, or systemic toxicity may require more emergent amputation with less patient preparation preoperatively. If muscle necrosis is extensive, the need for urgent or emergent amputation is critical because of the risk of renal damage that may occur secondary to circulating myoglobin. In addition to renal dysfunction, necrotic muscle tissue may cause cardiovascular or respiratory compromise and further push the need for emergent amputation. The presence of systemic toxicity, especially a necrotizing infection, often necessitates emergent amputation. For those patients with significant medical comorbidities or systemic toxicity, cryologic or physiologic amputation allows extended time for patient preparation for surgery and decreases mortality.[22]

Several features of patient evaluation and clinical progression are helpful in this decision-making process. The first consideration is the extent of nonviable skin. Although discoloration or gangrene is readily apparent, hyposensitive areas due to severe skin ischemia do not allow adequate healing and may not be so easily identified. Excluding patients with diabetic neuropathy, sensation to pinprick and light touch is a useful discriminant. If there is diminished sensation below the knee, for example, the chances of being able to perform a successful below-knee amputation are small, and morbidity may be avoided by proceeding expeditiously to an above-knee amputation. The presence of significant calf muscle swelling or muscle rigidity is an ominous sign suggestive of myonecrosis. Careful monitoring of calf circumference, skin sensation, urine color and output, and signs of systemic toxicity such as lethargy, confusion, or hallucinations must be employed on an hourly basis. The presence of systemic toxicity or significant changes in physical examination represent indications for proceeding with immediate amputation or physiologic amputation.[22] Similarly, the presence of myoglobinuria or cardiovascular instability represents an indication for immediate amputation. It is generally impossible to obtain rapid myoglobin determinations in serum or urine, but the presence of a urinary heme (blood)-positive dipstick in the absence of red blood cells under microscopic examination or pink serum (hemoglobin) is consistent with a diagnosis of myoglobinuria. In addition, the presence of markedly elevated creatine phosphokinase or lactate dehydrogenase isoenzymes in the serum is suggestive of myonecrosis in the absence of trauma, myocardial infarction, or recent surgery. If continued observation is elected, prophylaxis against renal damage from myoglobin pigment is recommended and includes maintenance of a diuresis in the

range of 75 to 100 mL/hour by the administration of osmotic diuretics such as mannitol and fluids. In addition, the urine should be maintained at an alkaline pH, since myoglobin precipitates in the renal tubules at a pH less than 7. Usually a mixture of mannitol and sodium bicarbonate in a balanced salt solution can be used to titrate urine output and pH. Finally, the presence of infection in the ischemic extremity is an ominous complication requiring very careful consideration. The presence of such an infection in a diabetic is even more ominous because of the sometimes rapid progression of seemingly innocuous infections. Any evidence of systemic toxicity or progressive infection is an indication for immediate surgical débridement, which may be in the form of a débriding amputation or a physiologic amputation followed later by a formal surgical amputation.

As long as there is continued improvement in collateral blood supply to an acutely ischemic extremity and there is no sign of systemic or renal toxicity, observation may be continued. As soon as circulatory improvement ceases or signs of toxicity develop, amputation should be performed promptly. An alternative to amputation in an unstable or high-risk patient is physiologic amputation, as previously discussed.

Evaluation for potential vascular reconstruction in a patient with clear-cut demarcation of a nonviable area of a lower extremity after a period of observation for acute ischemia is not likely to be beneficial; however, if there is a question of marginal viability of tissue above an area that is believed to be nonviable and the questionably viable tissue might permit a lower amputation level, then evaluation for vascular reconstruction may be beneficial.[23] For example, the presence of a nonviable forefoot and a marginal lower extremity between the knee and ankle may be an indication for evaluation for vascular reconstruction in an attempt to salvage a below-knee rather than an above-knee amputation.

Progressive Chronic Ischemia

The patient with progressive chronic ischemia who ultimately presents for amputation has experienced one or more of the following problems: rest pain, nonhealing skin lesion or ulceration, gangrene, or gangrene with superimposed infection. Gangrene complicated by infection is a special problem and is discussed in a separate section.

From the patient's point of view, ischemic rest pain is one of the most compelling indications for amputation. Characteristically, the patient will seek relief by sitting up and allowing his or her leg(s) to hang over the side of the bed or by ambulation. The dependent position provides relief of ischemic rest pain because gravity favors improved collateral blood flow, which augments arterial perfusion pressure. In its more severe forms, ischemic rest pain forms part of a vicious circle. As the patient more frequently uses dependency to achieve pain relief, the extremity becomes edematous and lymphatic return decreases, which eventually results in more ischemia. The end result of this vicious circle is a massively swollen, very painful ischemic extremity. Mild to moderate rest pain may often be successfully managed with narcotics. There have been reports that early mild rest pain may be relieved by sympathectomy. As long as there are no signs of systemic toxicity or supervening infection and if mild ischemic rest pain can be controlled with medication, a patient can be followed and amputation postponed.

Another manifestation of chronic ischemia is the presence of ischemic skin ulceration or nonhealing skin lesions on the lower extremity. Unfortunately, many of these skin ulcers occur in hospitalized patients as a result of abrasion of the foot or pressure necrosis (due to poor foot protection in the hospital bed). In the diabetic patient, ulceration usually occurs at pressure points, and the patient will often be unaware of the problem because of diabetic neuropathy. Patients without peripheral neuropathy will be very much aware of these ischemic ulcers because they are typically extremely painful. Besides obvious areas of pressure necrosis such as the heel and the lateral and medial malleoli, other common points of ulceration include the bony prominences over the metatarsal heads and midphalangeal joints or between the toes.

Fortunately, most patients with chronic progressive ischemia come to medical attention before the presence of frank tissue loss. Even patients with tissue loss usually present early with involvement of one or more toes, or under more severe circumstances, the entire forefoot. Under these circumstances, there is usually ample opportunity to fully prepare and evaluate the patient for lower extremity amputation or arterial reconstruction if possible. Preoperative evaluation and management should include proper medical attention to all associated diseases and a careful evaluation for potential critical organ dysfunction, especially the heart, lungs, and kidneys.

All patients with chronic ischemia should undergo consideration for vascular reconstruction for limb salvage. Angiographic evaluation from the infrarenal abdominal aorta down to and including the pedal arches is mandatory. In general, the surgeon should ensure good inflow to the level of the profunda femoris artery. Reconstruction distal to the level of the profunda femoris artery should be done only if chances for success are reasonably high and if a successful procedure would obviate the need for a major amputation. There is continuing controversy over the effect of prior revascularization on amputation level.[24–32] In my opinion, revascularization should always be attempted unless contraindicated by the patient's medical condition. If vascular reconstruction is brought below the knee, the incision required for approaching the distal popliteal artery and tibial trifurcation vessels should be planned along the lines of the posterior skin flap that might be required for a subsequent below-knee amputation. Techniques for evaluating amputation level selection are discussed in a subsequent section. However, one of the interesting spinoffs from studies of amputation level selection is the identification of patients who are not able to heal a low-level amputation and in whom the chance for rehabilitation at a high level of amputation is unlikely. When such objective information is available, attempts at proximal or extended distal extremity bypass to salvage a knee joint, for example, may be indicated to keep a patient ambulatory.[23, 25, 26]

Gangrene Complicated by Infection

The presence of dry gangrene is not an emergent surgical problem or necessarily the hallmark of an ominous clinical situation. Dry gangrene, limited to the toes, for example, may be treated conservatively and requires little, if any, surgical or ancillary medical support; however, infection complicating dry gangrene (i.e., wet gangrene), especially in a diabetic patient, is a limb- and life-threatening emergency. Control of sepsis may sometimes be achieved with antibiotic therapy plus limited débridement and drainage, or it may require radical excision and débridement; however, antibiotic therapy alone is seldom adequate treatment for gangrene complicated by infection. Failure to institute prompt therapy, especially in diabetic patients, will result in rapid ascension of the infectious process, the loss of potentially salvageable tissue, and a large increase in patient mortality. As noted earlier, in patients with systemic toxicity, cryoamputation prior to definitive surgical amputation will help decrease mortality.

The first step in the management of infected or wet gangrene is identification of the infecting organisms. Usually the urgency of the clinical situation does not allow the time required for identification of specific organisms by culture, although culture should be obtained and submitted for both anaerobic and aerobic organisms. It has been our practice to assume that gangrene complicated by infection of necessity includes a mixture of aerobic and anaerobic organisms, and therefore, broad-spectrum bactericidal antibiotic coverage is used.[21]

Once antibiotic therapy has been started, the patient must be very carefully monitored. The indicators usually followed include pulse rate, white blood cell count, blood pressure, temperature, extent of infection, severity of pain, and diffuse signs of systemic toxicity such as lethargy, hallucinations, and general mental status. In a diabetic patient, serum glucose and insulin requirements are additional useful monitoring parameters. If a prompt response to antibiotic therapy is noted, therapy should be continued for maximum effect and a definitive amputation then performed. If the patient does not respond promptly to antibiotic management or if undrained purulent material was initially evident, débridement of gangrenous tissue and establishment of drainage should be employed as an early adjunct to antibiotic therapy.

If the gangrenous infection extensively involves the foot and contaminates tendon and tissue spaces, especially in a diabetic patient, then radical débridement should be performed. One of the better methods to obtain radical débridement and establish open drainage is a guillotine amputation of the foot carried out at the level of the malleoli (Fig. 45–1). Guillotine amputation will eliminate the septic focus and allow drainage of contaminated lymphatics and tissue spaces in the lower leg. The presence of cellulitis and lymphangitis at the level of ankle guillotine is not a contraindication to this type of débridement technique. After performance of a guillotine-type amputation for débridement, systemic antibiotics are continued until the definitive amputation is performed usually 3 to 5 days after ankle Guillotine amputation). Definitive amputation is performed after ascertaining that the infection has been controlled and the patient's preoperative status has been optimized.

The incidence of stump infection in patients who present with a septic foot is decreased if a preparatory ankle guillotine amputation is performed before definitive ampu-

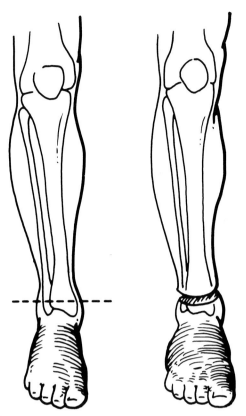

Figure 45–1. Schematic representation of an open ankle guillotine, or preparatory amputation, in a patient with a septic foot.

tation. In our experience, such a two-stage surgical approach decreased the stump infection rate from 22% to 3% ($P \leq .01$).[33] This approach was reaffirmed in a prospective randomized study by Fischer and colleagues,[34] in which the incidence of stump infection was decreased from 21% (one stage) to 0% (two stage) ($P \leq .05$).

Amputation for Trauma

In general, patients undergoing traumatic lower extremity amputation tend to be young and in good medical health, so patient evaluation and preparation for amputation are easier than those described for the geriatric patient with peripheral vascular disease and diabetes. As a general principle, formal traumatic amputation is performed to achieve healing at the lowest amputation level possible, and amputation level selection is usually predetermined by the injury. Adequate débridement of dead tissue is mandatory. The presence of a large amount of marginally viable tissue or potentially infected tissue may be an indication for débridement and open amputation followed at a later date by formal amputation with skin closure. A special effort should be made to rule out proximal bony or ligamentous injuries. Careful attention must be paid to looking for other potentially life- or limb-threatening injuries, and management of such injuries must be handled in a sequence that is appropriate for the best overall salvage of the patient. The use of a proximal extremity tourniquet for control of bleeding is optional but to be discouraged in a dysvascular

patient. The use of drains after traumatic amputation is controversial, although there is some evidence to suggest that drainage after traumatic amputation results in a more rapid resolution of postamputation stump edema. If drains are used they should be of the closed-system type (and not open Penrose drains).

AMPUTATION LEVEL DETERMINATION

The objective of preoperative amputation level selection is to determine the most distal amputation site that will heal. The general requirements are that (1) the amputation must remove all necrotic, painful, or infected tissue; (2) the amputation stump must be able to be fitted with a functional and easily applied prosthesis; and (3) the blood supply at the level of the proposed amputation must be sufficient to allow primary skin healing. Appropriate amputation level selection is of critical importance. If the surgeon elects too proximal an amputation, such as a midthigh amputation, the patient may be deprived of the opportunity for subsequent ambulation and rehabilitation, although the amputation might heal without difficulty. If a distal amputation site is selected and the blood supply is inadequate for amputation healing, further surgery will be required to achieve healing of an amputation at a higher level. This latter approach may result in increased morbidity and mortality and, in addition, may ultimately result in rehabilitation failure.

The inherent advantages of a below-knee amputation as opposed to an above-knee amputation should be obvious. It is easier to ambulate on a below-knee prosthesis, a fact that is extremely important, especially in geriatric patients. In general, a unilateral below-knee amputee requires a 10% to 40% increase in energy expenditure for ambulation compared with the energy required for walking with an intact extremity. In contrast, a unilateral above-knee amputee (using a prosthesis with a locked or unlocked knee) requires approximately a 50% to 70% increase in energy expenditure. Crutch walking without a lower extremity prosthesis utilizes approximately a 60% increase in energy expenditure, whereas wheelchair use necessitates only a small increase in energy expenditure (9%). Patients with severe coronary artery disease or severe chronic obstructive pulmonary disease may be physically unable to provide the additional energy expenditure required for ambulation on an above-knee compared with a below-knee prosthesis.

It is usually possible for the surgeon to decide on an amputation level that will remove necrotic, painful, or infected tissue as well as to plan an amputation stump that can be fitted with a prosthesis. However, the decision regarding the adequacy of blood supply at the proposed amputation level is one of the most difficult problems facing the amputation surgeon.

The earliest attempts at amputation level selection utilized presence of pulses in the affected extremity, skin temperature, correlation of arteriographic findings, and "clinical judgment." It has been well documented that none of these selection techniques has a consistent enough correlation with amputation healing to provide a sound basis for clinical decision making. In a study by Robbs and Ray,[35] the morbidity, mortality, and rates of healing of lower limb amputations in 214 patients, wherein the amputation level was determined by nonobjective criteria, were retrospectively analyzed. Six of 67 (8.9%) primary above-knee amputations and 37 of 147 (25%) primary below-knee amputations had to be revised to a higher level. The authors concluded "that flap viability could not be predicted by the extent of ischemic lesion in relation to the ankle joint, the popliteal pulse status, or lower limb angiography."[35] In a 1992 study comparing clinical parameters and skin perfusion pressure for amputation level selection, Dwars and coworkers[36] noted that the presence of palpable pulses immediately above the selected level correlated well with primary healing. However, the absence of palpable pulses and angiographic patency scores were of no clinical value in amputation level selection. However, Golbranson and colleagues[37] presented promising data on improved methods of skin temperature measurement that had a high degree of accuracy (90%) for selecting below- versus above-knee amputation levels. In addition, Spence and Walker[38] demonstrated a clear correlation between three different temperature isotherms (1.8°C separation) and isotopically derived skin blood flow ($P < .001$). Stoner and associates[39] reported that when the ratio of temperatures at the posterior and anterior incision sites (Burgess posterior flap below-knee amputation) was greater than 0.98, healing was improved. In a study comparing several modalities for amputation level selection, Wagner and colleagues[40] noted (for above- and below-knee amputations) that the average skin temperature at the amputation site was higher (34.3°C) in patients who healed primarily compared with those that required operative stump revision (33.3°C) ($P \leq .001$). One physical finding that has some value in differentiating proposed amputation levels is the presence of dependent rubor. Skin that develops dependent rubor is clearly ischemic, and hence skin with dependent rubor, like gangrenous tissue, is an absolute contraindication to amputation at that level; however, the absence of dependent rubor does not necessarily ensure healing ability. Early workers in the field of amputation surgery solved the problem of level selection by performing above-knee amputations on almost all patients. In the 1960s, Lim and coworkers[41] demonstrated that 83% of all patients requiring a lower extremity amputation would heal following a below-knee amputation. However, using empirical below-knee amputation selection potentially deprives some patients who might have healed following a more distal amputation, such as a transmetatarsal or Syme's amputation. In addition, identifying the 20% to 30% of patients in whom a below-knee amputation is doomed to failure would be advantageous so that either a knee disarticulation or above-knee amputation could be performed primarily, saving the patient additional surgical procedures.

The need for more sensitive and objective methods for preoperative amputation level selection has led to the development of numerous noninvasive techniques, including Doppler ankle and calf systolic blood pressure determinations, with or without pulse volume recordings[42–49]; xenon 133 skin blood flow studies[50–56]; digital or transmetatarsal photoplethysmographic pressures[47]; transcutaneous oxygen determination (Misuri et al, 2000)[11, 56–64]; skin fluorescence after intravenous fluorescein dye[65–68]; laser Doppler skin blood flow measurements[52, 69] (F. A. Matsen, personal communication, 1978); pertechnetate skin blood pressure studies[70, 71]; and photoelectrically measured skin color changes.[72]

An overview of the various selection criteria for prediction of healing of digit and forefoot amputations is shown in Table 45–2. Totals from Table 45–2 suggest that preoperative amputation level selection techniques correctly predicted primary healing in 174 of 180 toe and forefoot amputations (97%). Similar data for preoperative below-knee amputation level selection are summarized in Table 45–3. Excluding empirical below-knee selection, the tests shown in Table 45–3 were able to correctly predict primary healing of below-knee amputations in 522 of 554 elective amputations (94%). Clearly, objective amputation level selection is able not only to predict potential healing of a more distal level of amputation (see Table 45–2) but also to accurately assess the likelihood of healing of a below-knee compared with an above-knee amputation (see Table 45–3). It is my opinion that elective lower extremity amputation should not be performed without some type of preoperative testing to ensure primary healing of the most distal amputation possible.

The techniques for the use of ankle, calf, and popliteal Doppler systolic blood pressure determinations have been well described[42–46, 48, 49] and are not covered in this chapter. Similarly, use of the photoplethysmograph for determina-

TABLE 45–2

Toe and Forefoot Amputation Selection Criteria

SELECTION CRITERIA	REFERENCE	AMPUTATION LEVEL	HEALING PATIENTS (*n* [%])
Doppler ankle systolic pressure			
70 mm Hg	42	Forefoot	38/44 (86)
	47	Digit/forefoot	25/27 (93)
35 mm Hg	48	Digit	44/46 (96)
Fiberoptic fluorometry DFI > 44	68	Foot/forefoot	18/20 (90)
Photoplethysmographic digit or TMA pressure 20 mm Hg	47	Digit	20/20 (100)
Xenon skin clearance > 2.6 mL/100 g tissue/min	54	Digit/forefoot	25/28 (89)
Transcutaneous P_{O_2} > 20 mm Hg	62	Forefoot	4/4 (100)
		Total	174/180 (97)

DFI, dye fluorescence index; TMA, transmetatarsal-ankle.

T A B L E   4 5 – 3

Below-Knee Amputation Selection Criteria

SELECTION CRITERIA	REFERENCE	HEALING PATIENTS (n [%])
Doppler systolic ankle pressure 30 mm Hg + calf pressure 65 mm Hg + pulsatile PVR	46	27/27 (100)
Doppler systolic calf pressure 70 mm Hg	43	32/32 (100)
Doppler systolic thigh pressure 80 mm Hg or calf pressure 50 mm Hg	49	36/36 (100)
Empirical below-knee	41	38/46 (83)
Fiberoptic fluorometry DFI > 44	68	12/12 (100)
Fluorescein dye	66	24/30 (80)
^{99}Tc pertechnetate skin blood pressure	82	24/26 92
Laser-Doppler velocimetry > 20 mV	74	25/26 96
Photoelectric skin pressure 20–100 mm Hg	72, 83	60/71 85
Transcutaneous Po_2		
> 10 mm Hg or > 10 mm Hg increase on 100% O_2	59, 76	76/80 95
> 35 mm Hg	57, 61, 64	51/51 100
> 20 mm Hg	62	16/16 (100)
> 0 < 40 mm Hg	57	17/19 89
0 mm Hg	57	0/3 0°
Index > 0.59	61	17/17 100
Index > 0.20	73	33/34 97
Xenon skin clearance		
= 3.1 mL blood flow/100 g tissue/min	51	23/26 88
> 2.6 mL blood flow/100 g tissue/min	54	35/36 97
Epicutaneous > 0.9 mL/100 g tissue/min	50, 53	14/15 93
	Total	522/554 94

° Excluded from total.

DFI, dye fluorescence index; PVR, pulse volume recording.

tion of digital and transmetatarsal blood pressures has been well described by Schwartz and coworkers[47] and is not presented here. The potential advantages of both the Doppler and the photoplethysmograph are that they are relatively simple, inexpensive, and totally noninvasive. The problem with the use of these instruments is that the presence of a blood pressure of less than a predetermined level does not necessarily guarantee failure of amputation healing at that level (negative predictive value). This problem was nicely summarized by Verta and colleagues,[48] who noted that "for forefoot amputation a high Doppler ankle pressure did not guarantee successful healing and a low ankle pressure did not contraindicate primary healing." In an effort to increase the accuracy of Doppler ankle pressures, both Gibbons and coworkers[45] and Raines and associates[46] have suggested the ancillary use of pulse volume recordings. Although Raines and associates[46] reported 100% successful healing in 27 below-knee amputations where the Doppler systolic ankle pressure was greater than 30 mm Hg, calf pressure was greater than 65 mm Hg, and there was a pulsatile pulse volume recording in the foot, Gibbons and colleagues[45] were unable to duplicate those results, and concluded that "we find no consistent criteria which are more accurate and reliable than clinical judgment and no ankle pressure above which primary healing was guaranteed." Gibbons and coworkers also noted decreased accuracy in amputation level prediction using pulse volume recording and Doppler ankle systolic pressures in

patients with diabetes mellitus. Most probably, the problem with diabetic patients (falsely high systolic pressure measurements) is due to medical calcinosis of their vessels. Wagner and colleagues[40] reported that Doppler pressures at the thigh, popliteal, midcalf, or ankle levels were unreliable in predicting healing of a below-knee amputation.

Theoretically, the measurement of skin fluorescence with a Wood's ultraviolet lamp after intravenous injection of fluorescein dye (Funduscein) should form the basis for a reliable test for amputation level selection. Although this technique is somewhat more invasive than Doppler ankle systolic pressure measurements or pulse volume recordings, it is less complicated and noninvasive than ^{133}Xe skin blood flow or pertechnetate skin perfusion measurements. The commercial availability of two new types of fluorometers (Fiberoptic Perfusion Fluorometer, Diversatronics, Broomall, Pa., and Fluoroscan, V. Elings, PhD, University of California, Santa Barbara, CA), which are able to provide objective numeric readings quickly and in the absence of a Wood's lamp, may further enhance the use of this technique.[65, 67, 68] Development of a computerized video camera system to analyze skin perfusion after oral ingestion of fluorescein obviates the risk of intravenous injection and allows easy data manipulation for limb mapping. Such a system has been under study at Maricopa Medical Center in Phoenix. McFarland and Lawrence[66] reported an accuracy rate of 80% for skin fluorescence compared with 47% for Doppler popliteal systolic blood pressure (50 mm Hg) for prediction of healing of below-knee amputation (see Table 45–3). In addition, when skin fluorescence and Doppler pressure did not agree on the level of amputation, fluorescein always predicted a more distal level. Silverman and associates,[68] in 1985, reported their data on fiberoptic fluorometry for amputation level selection at the below-knee, below-ankle, and above-knee levels in dysvascular limbs. The overall success rate was 92% (36 of 39), and individual rates were 18 of 20 below-ankle (90%), 12 of 12 below-knee (100%), and 6 of 7 above-knee (86%) amputations. Discriminate analysis demonstrated an optimal reference point between healing and nonhealing amputations, and a dye fluorescence index of greater than 44 had 93% accuracy. Two later studies, however, did not demonstrate such promising results.[73, 74] In a blinded prospective review of 56 patients undergoing below-knee amputation, objective measurement of fluorescein perfusion did not correlate with amputation healing.[75] In a study comparing multiple methods of amputation level selection, Wagner and colleagues[40] found that qualitative skin fluorescence was not as successful as cutaneous oxygen measurement.

Promising work with a modified Clark-type oxygen electrode (with a heating element and thermostat for temperature control; Transoxode, Hellige-Orager, FRG; U.S. manufacturer, Litton Industries) for amputation level selection has been reported by several groups.[57, 59, 61, 62, 64, 76] Franzeck and colleagues[59] reported that the mean transcutaneous partial pressure of oxygen (PO_2) values of patients who primarily healed a lower extremity amputation compared with those that failed to heal were 36.5 ± 17.5 and less than 0.3 mm Hg, respectively. However, in those patients with a transcutaneous PO_2 less than 10 mm Hg, six of nine failed to heal while three of nine healed primarily. In a study on below-knee amputations, Burgess and coworkers[57] found that 15 of 15 amputations healed primarily if the transcutaneous PO_2 was greater than 40 mm Hg, 17 of 19 healed if the transcutaneous PO_2 was greater than 0 mm Hg but less than 40 mm Hg, and none of the three amputations with a PO_2 of 0 mm Hg healed. Katsamouris and coworkers[61] reported that 17 of 17 lower extremity amputations healed if the PO_2 was greater than 38 mm Hg or if the PO_2 index (chest wall control site) was greater than 0.59. Ratliff and colleagues[64] noted that 18 below-knee amputations healed if the PO_2 was greater than 35 mm Hg, while 10 of 15 failed if the PO_2 was less than 35 mm Hg. Kram and associates[73] noted success in 33 of 34 (97%) below-knee amputations with multisensor transcutaneous oxygen mapping when the critical PO_2 index was greater than 0.20. In addition, none of the six patients healed with an index of less than 0.20. All investigators have reported that some amputations healed in patients with low PO_2 values. A partial explanation for this observation might be the nonlinear relationship between PO_2 and cutaneous blood flow. In a very careful study, Matsen and coworkers[63] reported that PO_2 measurements are most dependent on arteriovenous gradients and cutaneous vascular resistance. Techniques to improve the accuracy of transcutaneous PO_2 probes include local heating (44°C; minimizes local vascular resistance and makes PO_2 more linear with respect to cutaneous blood flow), measurements before and after oxygen administration, oxygen isobar extremity

mapping, and transcutaneous oxygen recovery half-time (TORT).[77] Oishi and associates[78] noted—in a study comparing skin temperature, Doppler pressure, and transcutaneous oxygen—that after the inhalation of oxygen, if the PO_2 increased 10 mm Hg or more, the PO_2 predicted amputation healing with a sensitivity of 98%. In another study, the authors prospectively compared the following tests for their accuracy in amputation level selection: transcutaneous oxygen, transcutaneous carbon dioxide, transcutaneous oxygen-to-transcutaneous carbon dioxide, foot-to-chest transcutaneous oxygen, intradermal ^{133}Xe, ankle-brachial index, and absolute popliteal artery pressure.[62] All metabolic parameters had a high degree of statistical accuracy in predicting amputation healing, whereas none of the other tests had statistical reliability. All amputations, transmetatarsal, below-knee, and above-knee, healed primarily if the transcutaneous PO_2 level was greater than 20 mm Hg, and there was a 0% incidence of false-positive and false-negative studies. Most authors of transcutaneous oxygen testing studies for amputation level selection suggest using a cutoff point of 35–40 mm Hg. The author has used 20 mm Hg with excellent results. Recent data reconfirm the accuracy of a threshold of 20 mm Hg, especially in distal limb amputations (Miguri et al, 2000). Also of importance was the observation that amputation site healing was not affected by the presence of diabetes mellitus, nor were the test results for any of the metabolic parameters. Similar data have been reported by Bacharach and colleagues,[79] who stated that 51 of 52 limbs healed (primary and delayed) (98%) with a PO_2 greater than or equal to 40 mm Hg, and a PO_2 of less than 20 mm Hg was associated with universal failure. In that study, PO_2 measurements during limb elevation improved predictability of outcome for patients with supine PO_2 values greater than 20 mm Hg but less than 40 mm Hg.

Theoretically, laser-Doppler velocimetry should be an ideal tool for skin blood flow determination, since it is noninvasive and "measures" capillary blood flow (good correlation between laser-Doppler blood flow measurements using microspheres and electromagnetic flow probes and ^{133}Xe clearance[80]); however, data by Holloway and Burgess,[51] Holloway and Watkins,[52] Holloway,[80] and Matsen (personal communication, 1978) suggest that although there is a linear relationship among techniques, there is a fair amount of variance. These groups, however, have noted that the use of local skin heating may enhance the accuracy of the laser-Doppler and make it a more valuable adjunct for amputation level selection.[80] Holloway and Burgess[69] reported their experience with laser-Doppler velocimetry in 20 lower extremity amputations at the foot, forefoot, below- and above-knee levels, and the accuracy rates were as follows: foot and forefoot, two of six (33%); below-knee, eight of eight (100%); and above-knee, six of six (100%).

Malone and coworkers'[54] and Moore's[55] greatest postsurgical experience was with the use of ^{133}Xe skin clearance for amputation level selection. The techniques for utilization of ^{133}Xe skin blood flow have been well described by Moore,[55] Daly and Henry,[81] and subsequently, Malone and associates.[54] One of the major difficulties with the application of ^{133}Xe skin clearance for amputation level selection is its reproducibility by other investigators. In an earlier publication, Holloway and Burgess[51] were not able to document a clear-cut end point above which all amputations healed. On the other hand, Silberstein and others[56] reported that 38 of 39 patients (11 above-knee and 18 below-knee or transmetatarsal amputations, and 9 no amputation) healed when ^{133}Xe skin blood flow was greater than 2.4 mL/100 g tissue per minute, and that when flow was less than 2.4 mL/100 g tissue per minute, only four of seven patients healed. One significant advantage of ^{133}Xe clearance techniques that may offset both of these problems, if its ultimate reliability is demonstrated in other centers, is its potential ability to successfully predict healing at all levels of lower extremity amputation.[54]

A final problem with the intradermal use of ^{133}Xe for skin blood flow measurements is that the manufacturer no longer supplies ^{133}Xe. The product must be made by nuclear medicine departments. This limitation may further preclude widespread use of the intradermal ^{133}Xe technique. Finally, despite past publications[54, 55, 81] and previously published excellent results, I no longer use ^{133}Xe skin clearance for amputation level selection. In part this change was made because of the enumerated difficulties; however, for the most part this change was made as a result of a study[62] wherein ^{133}Xe was not found to be statistically reliable as a selection method for amputation level determination. (As noted previously, transcutaneous oxygen was very reliable.)

Using the disappearance of intradermal technetium 99m pertechnetate, Na[^{131}I], ^{131}I antipyrine, or ^{133}Xe in the presence of external pressure, Holstein[70] and Holstein and Lassen[82] have reported amputation level selection data comparable to data reported by Moore, Daly, Henry, Malone, and others. Because ^{133}Xe is trapped in subcutaneous fat, there are solid theoretical issues that support the use of an isotope other than ^{133}Xe. Holstein and associates[71] found no significant difference among Na[^{131}I], ^{131}I antipyrine, and ^{99m}Tc pertechnetate for the measurement of skin perfusion pressure.

Stockel and coworkers[72] and Ovesen and Stockel[83] have reported preliminary data that correlate well with the ^{133}Xe skin perfusion pressure techniques of Holstein[70] and Holstein and colleagues[71] on the use of a photodetector and plethysmography (Medimatic, Copenhagen, Denmark) for amputation level selection. This technique uses a blood pressure cuff placed over a photoelectric detector, which is connected to a plethysmograph, to measure the minimal external pressure required to prevent skin reddening after blanching. To date, 66 of 71 (85%) below-knee amputations healed with skin pressures between 20 and 100 mm Hg. In 1992, Dwars and associates[36] reported that skin perfusion pressure measurements were of excellent predictive value for the healing of lower extremity amputations (positive predictive value, 89%; negative predictive value, 99%).

In summary, it is my opinion that elective lower extremity amputation should not be performed in the absence of objective testing to determine the most distal amputation that will primarily heal yet allow removal of infected, painful, or ischemic tissue. A variety of techniques are available, and which of the various techniques is chosen depends on available equipment, the amputation level under consideration, and the current accuracy rates for the reported techniques. However, in the opinion of the author, the most reliable, easiest to use, and best overall technique for prospective amputation level selection is transcutaneous oxygen testing.

LOWER EXTREMITY AMPUTATION LEVELS: INDICATIONS, CONTRAINDICATIONS, TECHNIQUE, ADVANTAGES, DISADVANTAGES, PROSTHETIC REQUIREMENTS, AND REHABILITATION POTENTIAL

This section discusses only those amputation levels that are relevant to patients with peripheral vascular disease or diabetes mellitus. Amputation levels that are less desirable from the standpoint of healing or rehabilitation or those that present specific prosthetic fitting problems are omitted. In my experience and that of others, Chopart, Lisfrank, and Boyd forefoot amputations have been fraught with controversy because of healing problems, prosthetic fitting problems, and equinus deformities.[84] Since these amputation levels are occasionally used by vascular surgeons, they are reviewed here only briefly.

Toe Amputation

Toe amputation is the most frequently performed peripheral amputation. It is especially common in patients with diabetes mellitus, since these patients are prone to lesions that necessitate amputation (ulceration, osteomyelitis, and gangrene).

Patients who present with dry gangrene allow the surgeon a choice between direct surgical intervention and autoamputation. In the absence of supervening infection or pain, expectant management permits epithelialization to take place under the dry gangrenous eschar. As soon as epithelialization is complete, the toe will drop off, leaving a cleanly healed stump. Autoamputation is preferable to direct surgical intervention because it removes the necessity for healing after amputation and probably results in a more distal site of healing than would be achieved with surgical intervention. However, this process often requires months before it is complete.

Indications

The gangrene, infection, neuropathic ulceration, or osteomyelitis should be confined to the midphalanx or distal phalanx. There must be no dependent rubor, and venous filling time should be less than 20 to 25 seconds. Sizer and Wheelock[85] demonstrated that the presence of pedal pulses, even in patients with diabetes, is associated with a very high rate of healing after toe amputation (98%).

Contraindications

Cellulitis proximal to the area of proposed toe excision, the presence of dependent rubor, forefoot infection, and involvement of the metatarsophalangeal joint or (distal) metatarsal head all represent specific contraindications to toe amputation.

Surgical Technique

A single toe should never be amputated by disarticulation but should be transected through the proximal phalanx, leaving a small button of bone to protect the metatarsal head. Skin flaps can be of any design, so long as they obey basic surgical principles and have adequate base for length of flap. The flaps can be fish-mouth, plantar base, dorsal base, side to side, or any variation or combination; however, they must be long enough to close without tension. The most commonly used incision is circular (Fig. 45–2). Amputation through the metatarsophalangeal joint or an interphalangeal joint should be avoided because of the avascular nature of cartilage and the likelihood of supervening infection or failure to heal.

Careful atraumatic edge-to-edge skin closure without the use of forceps will maximize the chances of primary healing. Suture material that produces minimal reaction when left in place for long periods of time should be employed, such as monofilament wire or plastic. A soft postoperative dressing that provides gentle wound compression should be applied.

Chronic osteomyelitis of the great toe without gangrene in a diabetic patient presents a difficult surgical problem. Since complete healing is not common and total resection of the great toe results in some imbalance in walking (which can be accommodated with proper shoe orthotics), débridement and resection of the infected phalanges through a medial or lateral incision, leaving a soft tissue toe remnant in place, is probably the best surgical procedure from a functional standpoint.

Advantages and Disadvantages

The primary advantage of toe amputation is the lack of requirement for prosthetic rehabilitation and the fact that minimal tissue is excised.

Except for the risk of nonhealing or secondary infection and stump breakdown, requiring a higher level of amputation, there are no disadvantages to this level of amputation.

Rehabilitation Potential

Rehabilitation potential is 100%. However, the performance of a toe amputation in a patient with peripheral vascular disease, especially with concomitant diabetes, is an ominous sign with respect to long-term prognosis. Little and coworkers[56] found that by 3.5 years after toe amputation, almost three fourths of their patients required a more proximal major amputation.

Ray Amputation

Indications

If the gangrenous skin or infectious process approaches the metatarsophalanged crease or includes the (distal) metatarsal head, this precludes a toe amputation. A conservative partial distal forefoot amputation can still be performed by extending the toe amputation to include the distal metatarsal shaft and head.

Contraindications

Gangrene, infection, cellulitis, and dependent rubor involving skin proximal to the metatarsophalangeal crease are contraindications to the ray amputation. In addition, involvement of multiple toes is a relative contraindication, since a transmetatarsal amputation would be a more suitable surgical procedure. Ray amputation for gangrene or infection of the great toe also is a relative contraindication, since removal of the first metatarsal head leads to unstable weight bearing and difficulties with ambulation; however, with proper shoe orthotics, ray amputation of the first or great toe results in an excellent foot salvage and provides patients with a stable gait pattern.

Surgical Technique

The incision begins vertically on the dorsum of the foot, bifurcates laterally and medially to encircle the toe, meets on the plantar aspect of the foot, and extends for a variable distance on the plantar aspect of the foot. The plantar incision is extended proximally as needed to allow removal

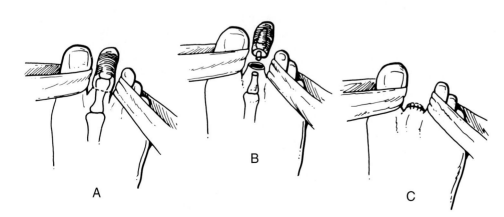

A

B

C

Figure 45–2. A single-toe amputation using a circular incision and transverse wound closure.

of the toe and distal metatarsal head. Care should be taken not to injure the digital arteries or nerves adjacent to the metatarsal bone and not to enter into the deep tension or joint spaces of the medial and lateral toes. The distal metatarsal shaft is divided at its neck, and soft tissues are removed by sharp dissection. The surgical specimen consists of the toe, metatarsophalangeal joint, and distal portion of the metatarsal shaft and head. If possible, the surgical specimen should be removed in continuity. The metatarsal shaft must be transected in an area of normal bone. "Soft bone" suggests osteomyelitis, especially in diabetic patients, and mandates higher (i.e., more proximal) bone division.

We recommend that the surgical wound be generously irrigated with an antibiotic solution (the content of which is based on preoperative cultures, if available). Once again, attention is paid to meticulous hemostasis and an atraumatic deep tissue and skin closure. Interrupted monofilament sutures that achieve edge-to-edge skin coaptation (without the use of forceps) should be placed (Fig. 45–3). The postoperative dressing can either be a soft dressing with an outer elastic wrap (which allows compression of the forefoot and removes tension from the suture line) or a combination of a soft dressing with foot and lower leg plaster cast that provides maximum skin and wound protection. In the event that adequate hemostasis cannot be obtained, the use of a drain is suggested. In the presence of infection in either the metatarsophalangeal joint or skin flaps, consideration should be given to leaving the wound open and doing a delayed primary closure or allowing secondary healing.

Advantages and Disadvantages

This relatively conservative amputation results in minimal cosmetic deformity and maximum (100%) rehabilitation potential. There are no prosthetics required; however, ray resection of the first metatarsal head will cause some walking imbalance, and the foot should be fitted with a specially constructed shoe to minimize foot trauma and improve ambulatory balance.

There are no disadvantages except for the risk of hematoma formation, nonhealing, secondary infection, or chronic osteomyelitis of the remaining metatarsal shaft.

Transmetatarsal Amputation

Indications

The indication for transmetatarsal amputation is gangrene or infection involving several toes or the great toe (on the same foot). This amputation may also be used if the gangrenous or infectious process extends a small distance on the dorsal skin past the metatarsophalangeal crease (but not up to the distal third or midthird junction of the forefoot), provided that the plantar skin is uncompromised.

Contraindications

Deep forefoot infection, cellulitis, lymphangitis, or dependent rubor involving the dorsal forefoot proximal to the metatarsophalangeal crease all represent contraindications to amputation at this level. In addition, gangrenous changes on the plantar skin of the foot, even those extending only a small distance past the metatarsophalangeal crease, is a specific contraindication to amputation at this level. Foot pulses are not necessary for healing, and venous refill should probably be less than 25 seconds.

Surgical Technique

An excellent description of the technique for transmetatarsal amputation was presented by McKittrick and associates in 1949.[87] A skin incision is designed that uses a total plantar flap. A slightly curved dorsal incision is carried from side to side of the foot at the level of the midmetatarsal shafts. The incision extends to the base of the toes medially and laterally in the midplane axis of the foot and then across the plantar surface at the metatarsophalangeal crease. It is important to place the dorsal skin incision slightly distal to the anticipated line of bone division. The dorsal skin incision is carried down to the metatarsal bones, and each metatarsal shaft is transected with an air-driven oscillating saw approximately 4 mm to 1 cm proximal to the skin incision (Fig. 45–4).

The plantar tissues in the distal forefoot are separated from the metatarsal shafts with a scalpel. The tissues of the plantar flap are thinned sharply, excising exposed tendons

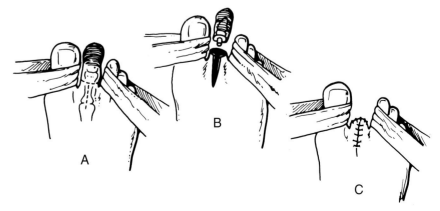

Figure 45–3. A single-digit ray amputation of the foot. The dorsal and plantar incisions are closed in their original direction; the toe incision can be closed either vertically or transversely.

A

B

C

A well-padded short leg plaster cast is the best postoperative dressing, since it will control edema and prevent stump trauma. I do not prefer early ambulation after transmetatarsal amputation because of problems with flap necrosis and stump healing. If wound healing is satisfactory at the first cast change (7 to 10 days after surgery) and if the surgeon chooses, then a rubber heel may be incorporated into the second cast for ambulation. Subsequent casts are changed when they become loose, generally once every 7 to 14 days, and a rigid dressing is used until the transmetatarsal flap is well healed, usually 3 to 4 weeks after surgery.

Advantages and Disadvantages

Transmetatarsal amputation provides an excellent result compared with more proximal foot or lower extremity amputations. Disability is minimal, and the prosthetic requirements are relatively simple.

The primary disadvantages of a transmetatarsal amputation are the risks of nonhealing, infection, hematoma formation, and the resultant necessity for a secondary higher level amputation.

Prosthetic Requirements and Rehabilitation Potential

To achieve maximum ambulation potential, some minor prosthetic requirements should be considered. Shoe modification that incorporates a steel shank in the sole of the shoe will allow normal toe-off during ambulation. The spring steel shank reproduces the action of the longitudinal arch of the foot during ambulation. A custom-molded foam pad or lamb's wool can be used to fill the toe portion of the shoe. An alternative approach is the use of a custom-molded shoe that uses a roller-shaped sole to provide toe-off motion during walking.

There are relatively few, if any, limitations in rehabilitation for a transmetatarsal amputation. With proper shoe modification, there should be no discernible physical disability for a transmetatarsal amputee during ambulation. It is important, however, that a shoe or other prosthetic device be properly constructed to avoid stump ulceration and breakdown. There are increased numbers of anecdotal reports combining guillotine forefoot amputation with secondary distal split-thickness skin graft(s) to achieve successful healing at this amputation level. Although this latter technique will allow salvage of more proximal transmetatarsal amputations, it is not a technique that I favor because of frequent problems with distal stump (skin graft) breakdown in active patients.

Lisfranc and Chopart Amputations

Indications

Recent publications have called attention to foot-sparing amputations when a transmetatarsal amputation is pre-

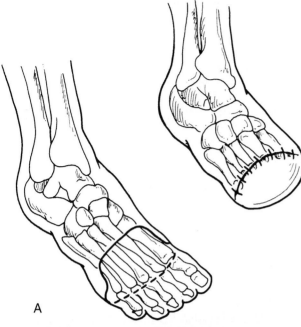

A

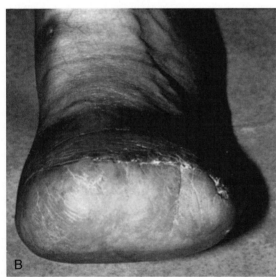

B

Figure 45–4. *A*, The planned transmetatarsal plantar-based skin flap and appearance of the completed closure. *B*, A healed right transmetatarsal amputation treated with immediate postsurgical prosthetic fitting, 1 month after amputation.

and leaving the underlying musculature attached to the skin flap. The plantar flap is then rotated dorsally for closure. Further tailoring or thinning of the plantar flap may be necessary to achieve good skin coaptation.

Attention to absolute hemostasis cannot be overemphasized. A simple closure with a deep layer of absorbable interrupted sutures and a skin closure with a monofilament suture utilizing a vertical mattress technique is used. Once again, careful approximation of skin edges is important, and I recommend that forceps not be used on the skin.

If adequate hemostasis cannot be readily achieved, use of a closed drainage system is suggested. Bone wax should not be used to control bleeding from the metatarsal shafts; the use of electrocautery to achieve hemostasis is preferable.

cluded because of the extent of ischemia and/or infection (Early, 1999; Reyzelman et al, 1999; Sanders 1997; Chang et al, 1994). The Lisfranc amputation is a tarsometatarsal joint amputation, and the Chopart amputation is a midtarsal joint amputation. The author would agree with Chang et al (1994) that both of these midforefoot amputations are easier to perform than a Syme amputation and may improve long-term ambulation (Hirsch et al, 1996).

Contraindications

Both the Lisfranc and Chopart amputations result in the development of equinovarus deformity and require lengthening the Achilles tendon to achieve maximum rehabilitation potential (Reyzelman et al, 1999; Sanders, 1997). In addition, Hirsch et al (1996) documented force plate data showing that an abnormal pattern characterized by reduced stance duration and deficient forward propulsion on the amputated side was greater in a Chopart prosthesis than in a transmetatarsal prosthesis. That study also documented stump problems as the principal difficulty with Chopart amputations over time.

Surgical Technique

Both the Lisfranc (tarsometatarsal joint amputation) and the Chopart (midtarsal joint amputation) amputations are well described in articles by Sanders (1997) and Chang and coworkers (1994), to which the interested reader is referred.

Prosthetic Requirements and Rehabilitation Potential

The author would agree with a modified version of the conclusion reached by Chang and associates (1994) that ischemic foot necrosis extending beyond the limits of conventional transmetatarsal amputation *does not necessarily have to be treated with a major limb amputation*. With improvements in patient selection and surgical technique, the Lisfranc and Chopart amputations are viable options to *consider when attempting salvage of mid- to hindfoot structures*. From a prosthetic standpoint, fitting of these more distal and conservative amputation levels should emphasize unloading the distal part of the stump and smoothing out the impulsive force peak on the stump in late stance to minimize pain, decrease stump breakdown, and enhance ambulation capacity (Hirsch et al, 1996).

Syme's Amputation

James Syme first described this amputation in 1843.[88] Then, as now, there have been arguments as to its merit. Harris (Toronto) has championed Syme's amputation and has written several excellent articles concerning its development and the surgical technique necessary for successful results.[89, 90] We believe the Syme's amputation level to be

the most technically demanding lower extremity amputation, and attention to surgical detail is crucial for its success.

Indications

If the gangrenous or infectious process precludes transmetatarsal amputation, then the next level to be considered is an ankle disarticulation or Syme's amputation.

Contraindications

If the gangrenous or infectious process involves the heel, if there are open lesions on the heel or about the ankle, if there is cellulitis or lymphangitis ascending up the distal leg, or if dependent rubor is present at the heel, then the Syme's amputation is contraindicated. The presence of a neuropathic foot in a diabetic patient, where there is absence of heel sensation, is also a relative contraindication to a Syme's amputation. A high rate of primary healing for a Syme's amputation demands the use of preoperative objective noninvasive amputation level selection techniques and preservation of the posterior tibial artery (if patent).

Surgical Technique

The skin incision is placed to construct a posterior flap using the heel pad. The dorsal incision extends across the ankle from the tip of the medial malleolus to the tip of the lateral malleolus. The plantar incision begins at a 90-degree angle from the dorsal incision and progresses around the plantar aspect of the foot distal to the heel pad (Fig. 45–5). The dorsal incision is deepened through subcutaneous tissues and carried down to bone without dissection in the tissue planes. The anterior tendons (tibialis anterior, extensor hallucis longus, and extensor digitorum longus) are pulled down into the wound, transected, and allowed to retract. The anterior tibial artery is identified, clamped, divided, and suture-ligated. The incision is then deepened and the capsule of the tibial-talar joint is opened. The tibialis posterior tendon is divided, and the foot is forced into plantar flexion to provide increased visualization of the tibial-talar joint. Great care should be taken during medial dissection to preserve the posterior tibial artery. The joint is further dislocated by incising the posterior capsule. The peroneus brevis and tertius tendons are transected. The plantar aspect of the incision is deepened through all layers of the sole of the foot down to the neck of the calcaneus. The calcaneus is then carefully and sharply dissected from the heel pad. Dissection of the calcaneus is the most difficult part of the operation, and great care is taken to maintain the dissection on the bony surface of the calcaneus to avoid damaging the soft tissues of the heel, prevent injury to the posterior tibial artery, and prevent buttonholing of the posterior skin as the Achilles' tendon is transected. Performance of the Syme's amputation by the one-stage and two-stage techniques is identical to this point.

If the surgeon chooses the one-stage technique, then the lateral and medial malleoli are transected flush with

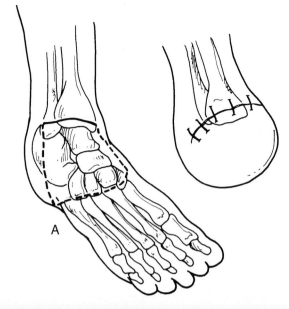

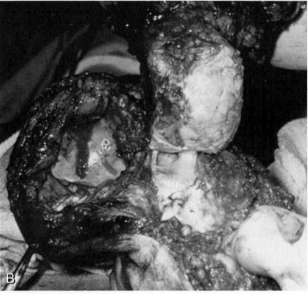

Figure 45–5. *A,* The Syme's level amputation with the posterior heel-based skin flap performed with the one-stage surgical technique. *B,* Intraoperative photograph of a Syme's amputation showing the Achilles' attachment of the calcaneus *(midsuperior portion of picture),* the tibial plateau, and the heel flap *(lower left corner).*

the articular surface of the tibial-talar joint with an air-driven reciprocating saw. Once again, the importance of hemostasis cannot be overemphasized. If adequate hemostasis cannot be achieved, then a closed drainage system should be incorporated. Even in dry surgical wounds, the use of a drain is advocated by some authors.[84, 89, 90] I prefer to irrigate the surgical wound with copious amounts of antibiotic solution before closure. The heel pad is rotated anteriorly and sutured to the proximal dorsal skin edge with a single layer of interrupted vertical mattress sutures. Once again, atraumatic placement of skin sutures is mandatory, and forceps should not be used on the skin edges.

If the two-stage technique is selected,[84] the lateral and medial malleoli are not transected. A drain is placed, and

the wound is closed as previously described. Approximately 6 weeks after performance of the first stage, the patient is returned to surgery for the second stage (which can be done under local anesthesia). Medial and lateral incisions are made over the dog ears on the amputation stump and the incisions carried down to bone with sharp dissection. The malleoli are removed flush with the ankle joint. The tibial articular cartilage is not disturbed. The distal tibia and fibula are exposed subperiosteally approximately 6 cm above the ankle joint, and the tibial and fibular flares are removed with an osteotome and a smooth rongeur. This last procedure produces a relatively square stump that simplifies postoperative prosthetic fitting and improves cosmesis. If the heel pad is loose after removal of the malleoli, it can be secured to the tibia and fibula through drill holes in the bones.

The postoperative dressing for a Syme's amputation stump for both the one- and two-stage surgical procedures is extremely important because it is critical to maintain correct alignment of the heel pad over the end of the tibia and fibula during healing. Either a soft compression dressing or a rigid plaster cast can be used as a postoperative dressing; however, most authors prefer the application of a short-leg plaster cast. If a cast is used, great care must be taken to avoid injury to the medial and lateral skin flaps (dog ears). Weight bearing should not occur during the early phases of healing of a Syme's amputation because of the risks of nonhealing and flap necrosis. When the first cast is removed, usually 7 to 10 days after surgery, a second cast that incorporates a walking heel can be applied if healing is satisfactory. I prefer to keep the Syme's amputation patients nonambulatory for 3 weeks after amputation to allow good heel pad fixation and healing. After ambulation begins, the patients are kept in a short leg walking cast for an additional 3 to 4 weeks prior to construction of a temporary removable prosthesis.

Advantages and Disadvantages

The Syme's amputation stump is extremely durable because it is end–weight bearing. It provides minimal disability from the standpoint of walking. Performance of a one-stage Syme's amputation procedure results in a somewhat bulbous distal stump compared with a two-stage Syme's amputation. For cosmetic reasons, a two-stage procedure is probably preferable in female patients, although I generally will not perform a Syme's amputation in young female patients because of concerns about cosmesis. Clinical evaluation by patients, prosthetists, and surgeons has consistently shown the Syme's amputation to be superior to levels above the ankle. Oxygen uptake, gait velocity, cadence, and stride length are significantly better in patients with the Syme's amputation than in patients with higher-level amputations.[91]

Delayed healing or healing complications due to hematoma formation or infection are not uncommon. Careful preoperative amputation level selection helps to ensure primary healing of the Syme's amputation. Failure to heal a Syme's amputation almost always results in performance of a more proximal amputation. Long-term follow-up of our diabetic patients, in whom a Syme's level was chosen with normal or "almost normal" sensation, has demonstrated a high incidence of revision to the below-knee level because of problems resulting from a progressive insensate Syme's stump (i.e., progressive neuropathy). Other authors have not reported similar problems.

Prosthetic Requirements and Rehabilitation Potential

Ambulation in the home can be achieved without the application of a prosthetic appliance; however, ambulation outside the home requires some type of prosthetic device. The usual cosmetic prosthesis consists of a foot and a plastic shell that incorporates the lower leg. A typical prosthesis for a patient with a one-stage Syme's amputation is shown in Figure 45–6. Ambulation in the home or for limited distances can be achieved with the application of a simple strap on a cup slipper with a built-up heel.

A patient with a successful Syme's amputation and an appropriately fitted prosthesis can expect a minimal degree of disability. Energy consumption compared with that of a nonamputee is, at most, 10% above normal. Many patients with Syme's amputations continue to be employed, including some who perform heavy manual labor. The salvage of a Syme's amputation, especially in those patients who are likely to become bilateral amputees, may be the ultimate difference for continued ambulation and nonambulation.

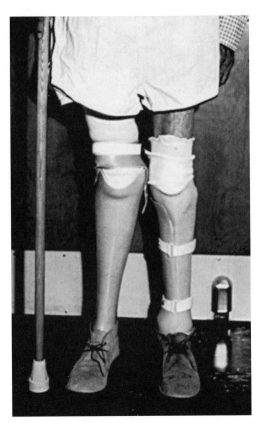

Figure 45–6. A bilateral lower extremity amputee with a right below-knee and left Syme's amputation. The Syme's prosthesis is a standard medial window design for a one-stage Syme's amputation. Notice the bulbous distal ankle on the Syme's *(left)* compared with the cosmetic ankle on the below-knee prosthesis *(right).*

Below-Knee Amputation

Indications

Below-knee amputation is the most common amputation level selected for management of lower extremity gangrene, infection, or ischemia with nonhealing lesions that preclude more distal amputations. When the blood supply is inadequate for healing at more distal levels, amputation at the below-knee level can be expected to have adequate blood supply for healing in the majority of cases. In fact, as previously noted, 83% of all patients undergoing lower extremity amputation can expect healing of a below-knee amputation[41] (see Table 45–3). Through the use of objective amputation level selection, primary healing of below-knee amputation in excess of 94% can be expected.

Contraindications

A below-knee amputation is contraindicated if the gangrenous or infectious process extends to involve skin on the anterior portion of the lower extremity within 4 to 5 cm of the tibial tuberosity or skin to be used to construct the posterior flap. A flexion contracture of the knee greater than 20 degrees also represents a contraindication to below-knee amputation. Great caution should be used in attempting below-knee amputation in patients with an occluded profunda femoris artery (the superficial femoral is almost always occluded) in the absence of objective amputation level selection data that suggest that the amputation will heal. Finally, a patient with stroke or neurologic dysfunction on the side of proposed amputation, in whom muscle spasticity or rigidity is marked, should not have a below-knee amputation because following amputation, spastic muscles force the knee into flexion and result ultimately in amputation failure.

Surgical Technique

There have been two significant advances in amputation technique that have contributed to better results after below-knee amputation: use of a long posterior flap and the application of a rigid dressing in the immediate postoperative period. There is considerable clinical and theoretical information available to support the use of a long posterior flap. The gastrocnemius and soleus muscles and the overlying posterior calf skin derive their major blood supply through the sural arteries, which originate proximal to the knee joint. Blood flow is maintained to this area in many patients, particularly diabetic patients, in whom flow through the popliteal artery and its major branches is restricted. Blood supply via the anterior tibial artery and geniculate collaterals to the skin and soft tissues of the anterior lower leg is so poor that even if equal anterior and posterior below-knee skin flaps are utilized, there is a high incidence of rehabilitation failure due to wound necrosis of the anterior skin flap.

The operation can be performed under general or spinal anesthesia, with the patient in the supine position on the operating table. If there are open infected lesions on the foot, a plastic bag or plastic adherent drape can be placed over the open infected portion of the extremity to isolate it. As mentioned previously, in patients with a septic foot, a preparatory ankle guillotine amputation followed by a delayed primary below-knee amputation will result in a higher rate of healing and fewer stump infections than the performance of a one-stage primary below-knee amputation.[33, 34] An alternative to the two-stage approach (one-stage technique with delayed primary closure) that works well for all diabetic patients except those with Wagner grade 5 foot infection was reported by Kernek and Rozzi.[92]

We prefer to use a long posterior flap and no anterior flap for reasons previously stated; however, there is at least one prospective randomized study comparing sagittal technique and long posterior musculocutaneous flaps that shows no significant difference with respect to healing, limb fitting, ambulation, and ultimate rehabilitation.[93] Another report of sagittal incisions for below-knee amputation by Persson[94] pointed out the utility of this type of incision in patients in whom a long posterior flap may be contraindicated because of infection or skin necrosis. A report by Ruckley and coworkers[95] noted that, for below-knee amputations in patients with end-stage peripheral vascular disease, the skew flap is an excellent alternative to the long posterior flap. The techniques for construction of a long posterior flap in below-knee amputation have been well documented in many previous publications;[10, 96-98] however, the salient features of the amputation are outlined here.

For a standard below-knee amputation, I select a point of bone division approximately a handbreadth, including the thumb, below the tibial tuberosity. In those patients in whom there is concern that the posterior flap may impinge on distal infection or ischemia, a palmbreadth (minus the thumb) can be used for a point of division below the tibial tuberosity. The absolute minimum length for a below-knee amputation is three fingerbreadths (7 to 8 cm) below the tibial tuberosity. The skin incision should be approximately 1 cm distal to the intended point of bone division. The transverse diameter of the midshaft calf at the level of the anterior incision, plus 1 inch, represents the approximate length of the posterior skin flap. It is usually my preference to outline the flap with a marking pencil prior to making a skin incision. The anterior skin incision represents the anterior half of the circumference of the extremity. The skin incision then abruptly turns distally with gentle curves and proceeds down the medial and lateral aspects of the extremity, in the midplane axis of the leg, to the point of distal extent of the posterior skin flap. The two lateral incisions are then connected posteriorly. My preference is to then incise the flap through skin and fascia in all areas before muscle transection. Use of a proximal tourniquet for hemostatic control is optional in patients undergoing traumatic below-knee amputation but is relatively contraindicated in patients undergoing elective below-knee amputation for ischemia. Use of electrocautery is preferred for division of all muscles. The anterior tibial muscle is divided at the level of bone division, and the anterior tibial neurovascular bundle is identified, clamped, divided, and suture-ligated. Electrocautery is used to incise the tibial periosteum circumferentially, and a periosteal elevator is used to mobilize the periosteum of the tibia proximal to the point

of proposed bone division. The tibia is then divided with an air-driven reciprocating saw. Using electrocautery, the fibula is isolated at the level of the transected tibia and divided approximately 0.25 inch proximal to the tibia, using the saw. Following division of fibula and tibia, proximal traction is placed on the transected tibia (use of a bone hook is easiest) and the lower extremity is bent at 90 degrees and retracted distally. The posterior tibial artery and vein and the common peroneal artery and vein are identified, clamped, transected, and individually suture-ligated. The posterior tibial nerve is identified, pulled into the wound, ligated, transected, and allowed to retract out of the area of surgical incision. The posterior calf muscle musculature is transected, leaving the gastrocnemius muscle as part of the posterior skin flap. The surgical specimen is then divided at the same point as the posterior flap skin incision, which permits removal of the surgical specimen. Care should be taken not to thin the posterior flap so much as to provide inadequate coverage for the tibia when the flap is closed. The saw is used to bevel the tibia at a 45- to 60-degree angle, and bony edges are filed smooth. Care is also taken to make sure that the distal ends of the fibula are smooth (Fig. 45–7).

The wound is copiously irrigated with an antibiotic solution. Once again, the importance of meticulous hemostasis cannot be stressed enough. Generally, drains are not necessary on below-knee amputations for peripheral vascular disease; however, drains are frequently used in below-knee amputations performed for trauma or reasons other than peripheral vascular insufficiency. If a drain is required, I prefer a closed suction drain, which is brought through a separate stab wound in the lateral aspect of the lower leg. The sural nerve (posterior flap) is identified, pulled down, ligated, transected, and allowed to retract back from the edge of the flap. The flap is rotated anteriorly, and the muscle fascia of the posterior flap is approximated to anterior fascia with interrupted absorbable sutures. The skin is carefully approximated with interrupted vertical mattress sutures using a monofilament plastic or metal suture. I avoid the use of tissue forceps and believe that the closure of the below-knee stump, especially in patients with peripheral vascular disease, should be performed with the care of a plastic surgical procedure. Tailoring the corner of the skin flap may be required to prevent excessive dog ears.

The use of a rigid plaster of Paris dressing incorporating the knee is ideal, regardless of whether an immediate postoperative prosthesis is to be used. A rigid dressing will control edema, promote healing, and protect the stump during the postoperative period. In addition, a rigid dressing will prevent a flexion contracture. Application of an immediate postoperative prosthesis as part of the rigid dressing is described in detail in a subsequent section.

Advantages and Disadvantages

The below-knee amputation has been shown to be an extremely durable amputation. The likelihood of primary healing is very good, and the ability to rehabilitate a patient on a below-knee prosthesis is excellent. In a report by Kim and coworkers[99] in 1976, 90% of their patients with unilateral below-knee amputations were able to ambulate.

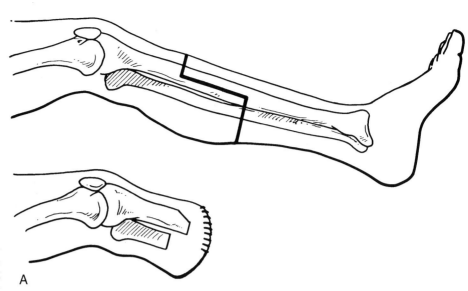

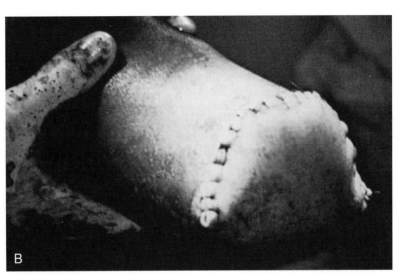

Figure 45–7. *A*, The standard posterior flap below-knee amputation. Notice the beveled tibia and the proximal shortening of the fibula compared to the tibia. *B*, An intraoperative photograph showing a below-knee amputation. Notice the skin coaptation with interrupted sutures and the minimal dog-ears.

Roon and colleagues[14] achieved a 100% ambulation rate with unilateral below-knee amputations and a 93% ambulation rate in patients with bilateral below-knee amputations. In addition, 91% of the patients reported by Roon and colleagues[14] were still ambulatory an average of 44 months following amputation.

In the absence of the ability to perform a more distal amputation, there are no specific disadvantages of a below-knee amputation.

Prosthetic Requirements and Rehabilitation Potential

A below-knee prosthesis is required for ambulation at this level of amputation. A variety of prostheses are available but in general involve total stump contact (with or without a prosthesis liner) with weight bearing on the patellar tendon and tibial-fibular condyles. Newer types of below-knee prostheses incorporate total contact and total weight-bearing designs. The prosthesis can be suspended with a variety of techniques, including a thigh lacer with external

joints, Silastic sleeve suspension, standard patellar tendon-bearing (PTB) strap, supracondylar medial clip, suction, and self-suspension secondary to muscle control. These prostheses can incorporate a variety of feet, some of which have flexion and extension motion or "ankle rotation" (with weight loading) or energy storage (Seattle Foot; Flex-Foot). The energy requirement for a unilateral below-knee amputee is increased approximately 40% to 60% compared with normal (energy consumption with an energy-storing leg has not yet been reported).

It has been our experience, as well as that of others, that any patient, irrespective of age, who was ambulatory prior to below-knee amputation and who undergoes amputation within 30 days of hospital entrance can ambulate successfully on a below-knee prosthesis. In fact, most patients who require bilateral below-knee amputations can ambulate successfully, as shown by Roon and associates.[14] The importance of aggressive rehabilitation after unilateral below-knee amputation in patients who are at high risk for bilateral lower extremity amputation was stressed in a report by Inderbitzi and coworkers.[100] Delay in rehabilitation resulted in a high rate of nonambulatory patients after their second amputation. The time required for gait training for a unilateral below-knee amputee approximates 2 to 3 weeks, and the gait pattern most patients develop is very good. There are some physical limitations for a geriatric below-knee amputee; however, young below-knee amputees are able to negotiate ladders, stairs, and other obstacles with minimal difficulty.

Knee Disarticulation

Indications

The indications for knee disarticulation amputation are limited, and it is primarily performed on young, active males for whom the advantages of strength and serviceability outweigh prosthetic cosmesis. Disarticulation amputation of the knee is the second most technically difficult lower extremity amputation procedure following the Syme's amputation. Successful performance of a knee disarticulation amputation with a high degree of primary healing usually requires some type of objective preoperative amputation level selection technique. The primary indication for knee disarticulation is when the gangrenous process, infection, trauma, tumor, or orthopedic disability encroaches too close to the anterior and posterior (or sagittal) limits of a below-knee amputation flap or has resulted in a nonsalvageable knee joint. Another potential indication for knee disarticulation is a patient who has had either acute or chronic failure of a below-knee amputation in whom skin flaps at the knee are viable enough to consider knee disarticulation. In general, British surgeons have been more enamored with knee disarticulation than their American colleagues. Interest in this level of amputation has arisen as a result of advances in cosmetic prosthetic components and prosthetic fitting techniques. Moreover, in a study of 169 unilateral lower extremity amputees, Houghton and coworkers[101] found that rehabilitation results were better for through-knee amputation (62%) than for above-knee (33%) ($P <.02$) or Gritti-Stokes amputations (44%).

Contraindications

Contraindications to knee disarticulation are primarily inadequate blood flow of the skin in the region or ulceration, gangrene, or infection involving tissues about the knee joint or the joint space.

Surgical Technique

There are two excellent reviews that describe the advantages and disadvantages and surgical techniques of disarticulation of the knee;[102, 103] therefore, the techniques are only briefly described in the following paragraphs. We prefer the knee disarticulation technique described by Burgess,[102] having reached this conclusion after failures with other types of knee disarticulation amputation and success using the modified Burgess technique.

Anesthetic management of knee disarticulation is best handled with either spinal or general anesthesia with the patient in the prone position. The operation can be performed, but is more difficult, with the patient in the supine position. At the discretion of the surgeon, a gown or pack can be placed beneath the thigh to hyperextend the hip joint and provide an easier working surface on the anterior portion of the knee and lower leg. The leg is held in a flexed position. Depending on the availability of suitable skin, either a classic long anterior, equal flap, or sagittal flap-type incision can be used (Fig. 45–8). A marking pencil should be used to outline the skin flaps prior to making the skin incision. Construction of the knee disarticulation skin flaps is crucial to avoid tension on the skin suture line when the amputation stump is closed. Dissection is first carried anteriorly down to the insertion of the patellar tendon on the tibia. The tendon is severed at its insertion and sharply dissected proximally. Deep dissection on the medial side of the knee results in exposure of the hamstring muscles. The tendons are sectioned and allowed to retract. The deep fascia is reflected with the overlying tendon and skin flap. On the lateral side of the knee, the tendon of the biceps femoris muscle and iliotibial band are sectioned low.

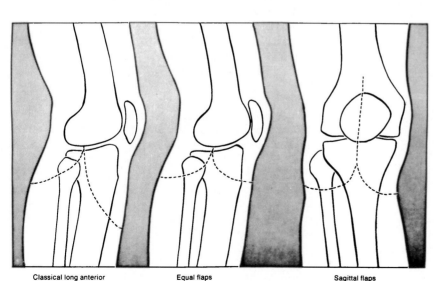

Classical long anterior   Equal flaps   Sagittal flaps

Figure 45–8. The three types of skin incisions commonly used for knee disarticulation amputation. (From Burgess EM: Disarticulation of the knee. A modified technique. Arch Surg 117:1251, 1977.)

The knee joint is entered anteriorly, the knee is flexed, and the cruciate ligaments are transected at their tibial insertion. The posterior knee capsule structures are divided, and the individual members of the popliteal vascular sheath are clamped, transected, and suture-ligated. The tibial and peroneal nerves are identified, retracted under moderate tension, ligated, sectioned with a sharp knife, and allowed to retract into the proximal amputation stump. The patella is removed subperiosteally, and the fascial defect in the patellar tendon is closed with interrupted sutures.

The femoral condyles are now transected transversely, approximately 1.5 cm above the level of the knee joint (Fig. 45–9). Sharp distal femoral margins are carefully contoured. The patellar tendon is pulled down into the intracondylar notch under moderate tension and sewn to the stump of the crus ligaments. The semitendinosus and biceps tendons are likewise pulled into the notch, tailored, and sewn to the stump of the patellar tendon and cruciate ligaments. This approximation of the tendons and ligaments allows muscle stability. The superficial skin fascia is approximated with interrupted absorbable sutures, and once again the skin is meticulously closed using a vertical mattress technique with monofilament metal or plastic sutures but without the use of forceps. Alternatively, skin staples may be used. The use of a through-and-through or a suction drain is optional and left to the discretion of the surgeon. A rigid dressing, with or without the incorporation of an immediate postoperative prosthesis, should be applied.

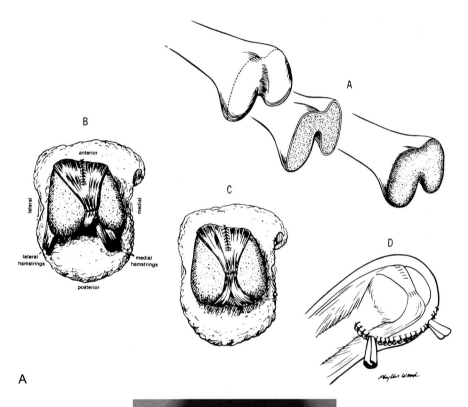

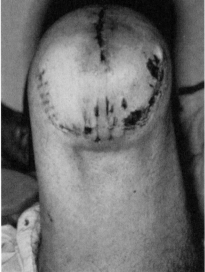

Figure 45–9. *A,* The femur is transected 1.5 cm above the condylar ends (A), the patellar tendon is sewn to the cruciate ligaments (B), hamstring tendons are sutured to the cruciate/patellar ligaments (C), and the wound is closed over a drain (D). *B,* An anterior flap knee disarticulation amputation at the first immediate postoperative cast change (7–10 days) with the patient in the supine position (in this case, the patella was removed transcutaneously). (From Burgess EM: Disarticulation of the knee. A modified technique. Arch Surg 117:1253, 1977.)

Advantages and Disadvantages

The advantages of a knee disarticulation amputation include excellent durability and end–weight-bearing capacity; retention of a long and powerful, muscle-stabilized femoral lever arm; improved proprioception; and a limb-socket interface with improved prosthetic suspension and rotational control (compared with an above-knee amputation). This amputation level is almost as good as a below-knee amputation and therefore is a tremendous benefit to the patient in comparison to the next higher level, the above-knee amputation.

The absence of a knee joint and increased energy expenditure make this amputation level less advantageous than a below-knee amputation.

Prosthetic Requirements and Rehabilitation Potential

Historically, knee disarticulation amputations were not well liked in the prosthetic community because of cosmetic and knee-thigh length problems resulting from existing prosthetic components (nonequal knee centers); however, the availability of lightweight polycentric hydraulic knee joints and endoskeletal systems has helped to solve these problems. The usual knee disarticulation socket incorporates some type of medial window to allow the bulbous stump to pass through the smaller lower thigh portion of the socket.

Knee disarticulation level amputation probably has its greatest usefulness in a young, active, nonperipheral vascular amputee. However, this amputation is also an excellent choice for a geriatric patient. Patient performance is better than that of a patient with a mid- to high above-knee amputation although not nearly as good as that of a patient with a standard below-knee amputation. There are some limitations of physical activities resulting from the absence of a knee joint, specifically involving those tasks such as climbing stairs and ladders and physical tasks that require rotational or flexion-extension knee motions.

Above-Knee Amputation

Indications

The indications for an amputation at the above-knee level are inadequate blood flow for healing at a more distal level, a disabled patient who is not expected to walk again, profound life-threatening infection with questionable viability of the lower extremity, and extensive infection or gangrene that would preclude a knee disarticulation or below-knee amputation. Historically, above-knee amputation has been the operation of choice for many surgeons because greater than 90% primary healing can be anticipated, regardless of the vascular status of the patient.

Contraindications

Extension of the infectious or gangrenous process to the level of the proposed above-knee amputation is the most common contraindication. Severe necrotizing lower extremity infection is a relative contraindication unless a high above-knee amputation is performed.

Surgical Technique

There are three basic levels for the above-knee amputation (Fig. 45–10). In general, the longer the above-knee amputation stump, the more likely the patient is to ambulate, so the stump should be as long as possible. If an amputation is being performed to control sepsis or toxicity, a midthigh or high-thigh amputation will provide greater assurance of healing and control of systemic toxicity, although the chances of rehabilitation are lessened.

Either a circular or sagittal-type incision can be used. I prefer the use of a circular (or fish-mouth) incision appropriate for the level of anticipated bone division. A circumferential line of incision is drawn with a marking pen 2 to 3 cm below the level of the proposed bone transection. The incision is then carried down through skin and fascia. The skin and fascia are retracted superiorly to allow more proximal muscle division. I prefer the use of electrocautery for muscle division. The femoral artery and vein are identified, clamped, divided, and suture-ligated in the subsartorial canal. All the muscles of the anterior, medial, and lateral thigh are transected. The muscle mass is then retracted proximally, the proposed line of bone transection is exposed, and the periosteum is cut using electrocautery. An air-driven reciprocating saw is then used to transect the femur. The posterior muscles are transected using electrocautery. The sciatic nerve is identified, pulled down into the wound, ligated, transected, and allowed to retract into

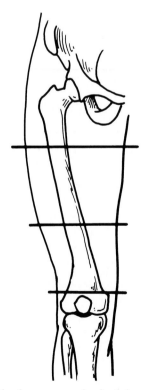

Figure 45–10. The three common levels of above-knee amputation.

the proximal amputation stump. The rough edges of the femur are filed smooth. Again, the amputation stump should be irrigated with an antibiotic solution, especially if the amputation is being performed for infection. The soft tissues and skin are drawn distally to ensure adequacy of soft tissue coverage for the femur. If soft tissue coverage is adequate, the wound is closed in two layers. The fascia is closed with an interrupted absorbable suture, and the skin is closed with interrupted vertical mattress sutures of plastic or metal monofilament. Again, good skin coaptation is important, and the use of forceps on the skin is to be avoided. If the soft tissue coverage for the bone is inadequate, then the femur is shortened as required, so as to allow adequate soft tissue coverage without tension on the skin suture line (Fig. 45–11). If the amputation is being performed for infection, especially a necrotizing infection, then the wound should be left open. If a fishmouth incision is used, then the apex of the "angle of the mouth" approximates the point of bony division. Closure, although spatially different, encompasses the careful atraumatic technique described previously.

A rigid dressing can be applied and is advantageous for control of stump edema, but it is much more cumbersome and less valuable than a rigid dressing used at lower amputation levels. I prefer to use a soft dressing suspended with a silesia type of elastic bandage or a modified waist suspension belt.[104] After the wound has healed satisfactorily (1 to 2 weeks after surgery), a temporary removable prosthesis can be provided if appropriate.

Advantages and Disadvantages

The primary advantage of an above-knee amputation is the very high likelihood of primary healing. Prosthetic rehabilitation is very difficult at this level of amputation. Whereas 80% to 90% of all patients with unilateral or bilateral below-knee amputations can be expected to ambulate, only 40% to 50% of unilateral above-knee amputees can be expected to ambulate. It has been my experience that fewer than 10% of bilateral lower extremity amputees, where one side is an above-knee amputation, will successfully ambulate.

Prosthetic Requirements and Rehabilitation Potential

A variety of prostheses are available for the above-knee amputee. Newer prosthetic devices incorporate contoured axially aligned sockets, ultralightweight materials, endoskeletal design, hydraulic-assisted knee joints, the use of ankle rotators and motion feet, and energy storage. There is a direct correlation between successful ambulation at this level of amputation and the weight of the prosthesis because of the energy expenditure required for walking. Compared with normal, the energy expenditure of an above-knee amputee is increased 80% to 120%.

As noted, the rehabilitation potential for a unilateral above-knee amputee is only fair and averages 10% to 50%.

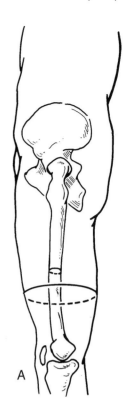

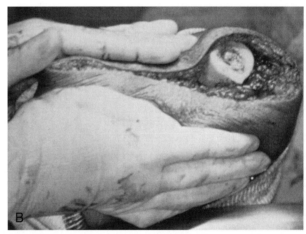

Figure 45–11. *A*, The standard circular incision technique for above-knee amputation. Sagittal flaps can be used if appropriate. The key to closure is adequate femur shortening to avoid later bone protrusion through the distal end of the stump. *B*, This intraoperative photograph of an above-knee amputation stump demonstrates why skin/soft tissue length for bone coverage should be checked prior to closure. Proximal femur shortening was required to decrease wound tension.

Hip Disarticulation Amputation

In general, hip disarticulation amputation is not an amputation that the usual general or vascular surgeon performs, because almost all patients will heal after a high above-knee amputation.

Indications

The indications for hip disarticulation are inadequate blood flow (usually in patients with occlusion of both the profunda femoris and superficial femoral arteries) for healing of a more distal amputation, a life-threatening infection or extensive gangrene that precludes amputation at a lower level, trauma, tumor, and failed hip reconstruction.[105] Wound complications occur frequently, and their incidence is increased for urgent or emergent operations and prior above-knee amputations.[106] In addition, both limb ischemia and infection increase the mortality rate.

Contraindications

In our experience, infection that precludes hip disarticulation amputation is almost uniformly a fatal event. There are no contraindications to this level of amputation, except infection and gangrene (or tumor) that extends above the level of the proposed amputation.

Surgical Technique

Since this procedure is performed only occasionally by the general and vascular surgeon and since there are excellent articles published describing this operation,[105–109] the surgical technique for performance of this level of amputation is not presented here. Based on a limited experience, I favor a posterior flap technique (Fig. 45–12A).

Advantages and Disadvantages

In the absence of healing at an above-knee level, there is a higher likelihood of primary healing.

Prosthetic rehabilitation at this level of lower extremity amputation is uncommon (less than 10%), even with unilateral amputation in geriatric patients.

Prosthetic Requirements

Various types of prostheses have been described and created for the hip disarticulation amputation. Most of them entail a pelvic bucket (Canadian-type) prosthesis (Fig. 45–12B). Most prostheses are endoskeletal in construction (to save weight), and very few involve the use of sophisticated knee joints, ankle joints, or motion feet. A full discussion of prosthetic requirements for this level of amputation is beyond the scope of most general and vascular surgeons, and the interested reader is referred to appropriate references.[105–108] Compared with normal, the energy expenditure of a hip disarticulation amputee is increased 1.5 to 2.5 times.

COMPLICATIONS OF LOWER EXTREMITY AMPUTATION

Historically, postoperative morbidity and mortality following major lower extremity amputation were common, and the incidence of fatal complications was high enough that there was considerable debate as to the optimal preoperative, operative, and postoperative management. In general, however, the morbidity and mortality following a major lower extremity amputation have decreased with time.[110–112]

The major postoperative complications following lower extremity amputation with ranges of frequency of occur-

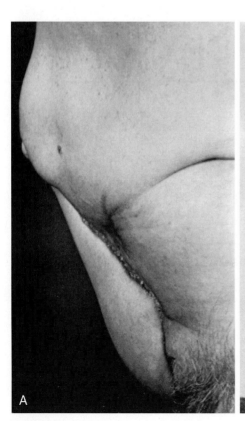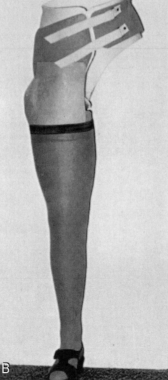

Figure 45–12. *A,* Photograph of a left hip disarticulation stump 6 months after amputation. The operation was performed with a posterior/gluteal flap technique. *B,* An ultralightweight (4.5 lb) left hip disarticulation prosthesis based on an Aqualite plastic endoskeletal system with cosmetic cover (US Manufacturing Co, Pasadena, CA) and Scotchcast Canadian-type socket (bucket).

TABLE 45-4

Postoperative Complications

	INCIDENCE (%)	REFERENCES
Stump pain/phantom pain	5–80	9, 14, 15, 113–120
Death	0–35	7, 9, 15, 91, 110, 111, 121, 122
Pulmonary complications	8	14
Stump infection	12–28	111, 122
Nonhealing stump	3–28	9, 14, 15, 110, 111, 121
Pulmonary embolus	4–38	7, 14
Deep venous thrombosis	1–3	9, 14, 15
Flexion contracture	1–3	9, 14, 15, 54
Renal insufficiency	1–3	9, 14, 15

rence are listed in Table 45–4. Each of these complications is addressed separately in the following paragraphs.

Early Postoperative Complications

Pain

The literature suggests that the incidence of disabling stump pain and phantom limb pain following major lower extremity amputation ranges from 5% to 30%.[113–118] In a retrospective random survey of 5000 Veterans Administration (VA) amputees, Sherman and coworkers[119, 120] noted that 85% of the amputees responding to their survey noted significant phantom limb pain. Their explanation for the high incidence of pain problems was, in part, based on the fact that most reports, especially those citing pain treatment modalities, do not have adequate post-treatment follow-up. In addition, Sherman and associates suggested that most amputees quickly learn that physicians are not interested in pain problems and therefore fail to give accurate responses when questioned, often to protect their credibility and relationship with their physician (thereby guaranteeing long-term care). Of more concern was the fact that statistical analysis of 42 of the most common treatment modalities for phantom limb pain, including drug therapy, local injections, and surgery, failed to show that any treatment gave satisfactory results.[119, 120] At most, 8.4% of survey respondents could be said to have been helped to any real extent. In my experience, based on an amputation program that uses immediate postsurgical prosthetic fitting and aggressive postamputation rehabilitation, the incidence of disabling pain problems following major lower extremity amputations is less than 5%. I have no objective explanation for the difference between reports in the surgical literature and our personal experience, but I believe that the rapidity and success of rehabilitation, as well as postoperative rigid dressings, with or without a pylon, have a positive impact in decreasing postamputation pain problems.

In the author's personal experience, the perioperative administration of gabapentin (Neurontin) in dogs, ranging from 100 to 300 mg orally twice a day, seems to be associated with less postoperative pain and phantom pain.

Death

The incidence of death following major lower extremity amputation ranges from 0% to 35%.[7, 9, 15, 17, 110, 111, 121, 122] Although the postoperative death rate has decreased each decade since the 1950s, an overall death rate of 6% to 10% is still the average for centers treating large numbers of amputees.[9, 14, 15] As might be expected, the postoperative death rate for above-knee amputation (20% to 40%) exceeds that for below-knee amputation (3% to 10%).[9, 14, 15, 91, 110, 111, 122] Two thirds of all postoperative deaths are due to cardiovascular complications, including myocardial infarction, stroke, congestive heart failure, and visceral ischemia, with approximately one third to one half of these deaths due to myocardial infarction alone. Death after lower extremity amputation is related to patient age. In my experience and that of others, the mortality increases for patients over the age of 75.[123]

Nonhealing

Nonhealing of an amputation stump represents a major complication, since it almost always results in an amputation at a higher level. Nonhealing represents failure due to inadequate blood supply at the level selected for amputation, to rough or traumatic intraoperative handling of marginally vascularized tissue, or to a stump hematoma with or without secondary infection. The incidence of nonhealing after major lower extremity amputation ranges from 3% to 28%.[9, 14, 15, 110, 111, 121, 124] In other words, the primary healing rate after major lower extremity amputation ranges from 63% to 97%. Because, in previous sections, we have shown that the literature suggests an overall healing rate of 97% for digit and forefoot amputations (see Table 45–2) and 94% for below-knee amputations (see Table 45–3) when objective amputation level selection techniques were used, it can be anticipated that the failure of an amputation stump to heal is probably directly related to the methods used for amputation level selection. In a modern amputation program using objective preoperative amputation level selection techniques, the rate of nonhealing should not be greater than 4% to 8%. In my last 250 consecutive lower extremity amputations there has been one failure (0.8%) due to nonhealing from ischemia (if the TcPo$_2$ was > 20 mm Hg).

The literature is somewhat controversial on healing differences between patients with and without diabetes mellitus. However, it has been my experience, as well as that of others, that there is no significant difference in the healing rates of major lower extremity amputation between diabetic and nondiabetic patients.[9, 15, 51, 54, 57, 62, 72, 125] The rate of infectious stump complications might be slightly higher in diabetics; however, this has not been my experience.

In a review of 59 consecutive lower extremity amputations in diabetics, Bailey and associates[126] noted that the preoperative hemoglobin level was statistically significantly lower in patients whose amputations healed primarily. Eighteen amputations done in patients with a preoperative hemoglobin value of less than 12 g/dL healed primarily, whereas all 30 amputations in patients with a hemoglobin level greater than 13 g/dL failed to heal.

It seems reasonable to consider isovolemic hemodilution in patients with marginally viable skin or borderline values by amputation level selection techniques. In a study on skin flap survival, Gatti and colleagues[127] suggested that isovolemic hemodilution might be a valuable technique for the salvage of marginally ischemic tissues.

Stump Infection

The incidence of infection in an amputation stump following major lower extremity amputation ranges from 12% to 28%.[9, 15, 18, 54, 111] As might be expected, the incidence of postoperative stump infection is directly related to the reason for performing the amputation. The incidence of this complication can be reduced by appropriate management of preexisting infections, including the use of perioperative antibiotic therapy, as well as wide débridement or drainage of infection before definitive amputation. Reviews by McIntyre and coworkers[33] and Fischer and colleagues[34] noted a statistically significant decrease in the rate of stump infection in patients undergoing definitive below-knee amputation for a septic foot in whom prior ankle guillotine amputation was performed to control infection. The incidence of below-knee stump infection in patients managed with a one-stage surgical procedure was 22% and 21%, respectively, whereas the incidence in those patients who had undergone preparatory guillotine ankle amputation was 3% and 0%, respectively ($P < .05$).[33, 34] My most recent incidence of stump infection is 3% (4 of 134), and most of these infections represent aggressive closure of contaminated wounds or amputations in limbs with distal ipsilateral septic foci.

I would recommend the use of prophylactic antibiotics in all patients undergoing lower extremity amputation, even in the absence of established limb infection. It has been my practice to treat patients with preoperative infections with broad-spectrum antibiotics that provide bactericidal aerobic and anaerobic coverage. The necessity for aerobic and anaerobic coverage is especially important in diabetic patients, in whom the incidence of mixed facultative and obligate anaerobic infections may be as high as 60%.[21]

Once an infection is established in an amputation stump, the wound must be opened widely to provide adequate drainage. In general, this means that amputation will have to be revised to a higher level, so that, for example, a stump infection in a below-knee amputation usually results in an above-knee amputation. The importance of this complication is emphasized by the fact that for a geriatric patient, conversion from a below-knee to an above-knee amputation is often the difference between successful ambulation and lack of ability to walk.

Stump hematoma after lower extremity amputation is a catastrophic complication, especially when the amputation has been performed for distal extremity infection. Although the correlation between stump hematoma and stump infection is not 1:1, it is high enough to make the avoidance of a postamputation stump hematoma highly desirable. The importance of meticulous hemostasis after amputation cannot be emphasized enough. If an amputation is not dry, then the wound should be closed with drains (closed drainage system, not Penrose drains), although several studies have suggested that the use of drains increases the risk of infection.[128]

Pulmonary Embolism and Deep Venous Thrombosis

The incidence of pulmonary embolism and deep venous thrombosis following major lower extremity amputation is 1% to 3%[7, 14] and 4% to 38%,[9, 14] respectively. The postoperative lower extremity amputee is at high risk for venous thromboembolic complications. Usually these patients have had a prolonged period of hospitalization and bed rest prior to amputation. In addition, many have undergone attempts at prior vascular surgical reconstruction that may cause injury to the deep veins in the leg and prolong preamputation immobilization. The amputation itself involves division of veins, which may result in stagnation and thrombosis in these vein segments postoperatively. When an active rehabilitation program is not begun on the first day after surgery, an additional period of inactivity or immobilization may follow the amputation and further predispose the patient to venous thromboembolic complications. The morbidity and mortality from venous thromboembolic complications may be significant, and in addition, impairment of blood oxygenation may further compromise the healing of ischemic tissues.

For those patients undergoing elective major lower extremity amputation in whom major risk factors for venous thromboembolic complications exist, appropriate prophylaxis for pulmonary embolism should be instituted. Since there is a slight increase in stump hematoma formation, the use of a closed suction drainage system in those patients is advisable. Probably the most important factor in preventing thromboembolic complications is not to allow patients undergoing major lower extremity amputation to become bedridden either preoperatively or postoperatively. The patient being prepared for lower extremity amputation should be undergoing preoperative physical therapy for range of motion and strengthening of the contralateral leg and upper extremities. The postoperative amputee, even if an immediate postoperative prosthesis is not used, should be going to physical therapy for similar body conditioning. Attention should be paid to the nonamputated extremity, and the use of thromboembolic elastic stockings is recommended during the perioperative period. A final factor that must be considered is the state of hydration of the amputee patient, both preoperatively and postoperatively. This is especially true in those patients who have undergone prior attempts at vascular reconstruction or angiography.

Pulmonary Complications

The incidence of pulmonary complications, including pneumonia, atelectasis, and sepsis, has been estimated to approximate 8% in patients undergoing a major lower extremity amputation.[14] These complications are significantly higher in patients undergoing above-knee amputation, as noted by Huston and colleagues,[7] in whom the incidence of pneumonia and sepsis ranged from 8% to 60%. The same conditions of bed rest, inactivity, dehabilitation, and dehydration that predispose to thromboembolic complications also predispose a patient to atelectasis and pneumonia. Next to myocardial infarction, pulmonary complications are probably the biggest problem with geriatric patients undergoing lower extremity amputation. Attention to good pulmonary toilet, increased muscular activity, and active exercise (physical therapy) are all valuable adjuncts to preoperative and perioperative care.

Flexion Contractures

Flexion contractures of the knee or hip joint can occur quite rapidly following major lower extremity amputation, especially in geriatric patients. In my experience, the incidence of such postoperative flexion contractures has been 1% to 3%.[9, 14, 15, 54]

Irreversible flexion contracture will prohibit successful fitting of a prosthesis and, subsequently, successful patient ambulation. Such a problem may also necessitate amputation at a higher level. The use of a rigid postoperative dressing, with or without an immediate postoperative pylon, will help decrease the incidence of this complication. In those patients not receiving immediate postoperative prosthetic treatment, physical therapy directed toward range of motion and muscle strengthening should be instituted preoperatively if possible and as rapidly as possible after amputation.

Renal Insufficiency

Renal insufficiency represents a low-frequency complication following major lower extremity amputation, with an incidence of 1% to 3%.[9, 54] This complication is, for the most part, avoidable if proper attention is paid to adequate preoperative and postoperative hydration. In addition, in patients requiring prolonged antibiotic therapy for perioperative infections, attention must be paid to antibiotic dosage to avoid renal insufficiency as a complication of antibiotic therapy.

Long-Term Complications

Stump Revision

There is little information available in the literature regarding the frequency of stump revision in those patients who have been successfully discharged from the hospital following lower extremity amputation. A previous report by Malone and associates,[15] in which there was a 97% rate of primary healing after lower extremity amputation, noted that 88% of their lower extremity amputees were followed without stump revision for up to 18 months after surgery. The incidence of prosthesis use in those patients was 100%. Similar information was reported by Roon and others,[14] who noted that 91% of their patients were ambulatory on their prostheses 44 months following amputation. I believe that the frequency of stump revision is probably related to methods of amputation level selection, the quality of prosthesis fit, and careful postoperative follow-up. My current incidence of late stump revision is 2.3% (10 of 450).

Death

Approximately one third of all lower extremity amputees will die within 5 years of their amputation, and two thirds of these deaths will be due to cardiovascular causes.[111] Roon and coworkers[14] reported a 45% overall 5-year survival following lower extremity amputation, compared with an expected 85% 5-year survival for the age-adjusted normal population. More striking, however, was the analysis of Roon and associates of the projected 5-year survival following lower extremity amputation for diabetic and nondiabetic amputees. They reported a 5-year survival for nondiabetics of 75% and only a 39% 5-year survival for patients with diabetes mellitus (Fig. 45–13). Analysis of the cause

Figure 45–13. Life-table representation of survival after lower extremity amputation for both diabetic and nondiabetic amputees compared with the age-adjusted normal population. (From Roon AJ, Moore WS, Goldstone J: Below knee amputation: A modern approach. Am J Surg 134:153–158, 1977.)

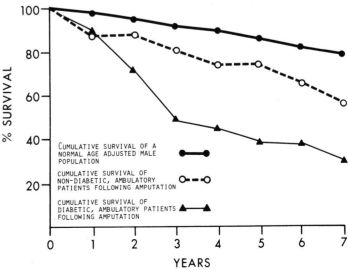

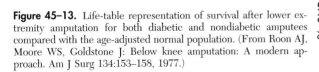

of death of patients in the series reported by Roon and colleagues disclosed that 35% were due to myocardial infarction, and two thirds were due to cardiovascular causes.[14]

There are good multivariate data to show that in dialyzed diabetic patients, Apo-A-I, fibrinogen, age, and stroke were independent predictors of both cardiac and noncardiac deaths (Koch et al, 1997). In addition, in type 1 diabetic patients, in spite of intensified insulin therapy, nephropathy is the strongest predictor of mortality and end-stage complications, including amputation. (Muhlhauser et al, 2000).

Contralateral Limb Loss

It can be estimated that the rate of contralateral limb loss ranges from 15% to 33% in 5 years following major lower extremity amputation.[16–18] In all probability, however, the diabetic amputee is likely to die before contralateral limb loss.[14, 111] Because of the risk of contralateral limb loss, significant care and attention should be paid to examination of the contralateral limb as well as education of the patient in prophylactic skin and foot care. Patient instructions for the care of diabetic feet that are used at the Tucson VA Medical Center and Maricopa Medical Center (Phoenix) are shown in Figure 45–14.

Data from a randomized prospective educational study at the Tucson VA Medical Center of diabetics who present with foot ulcers, infection, prior amputation, or high-risk lesions suggest that an audiovisual education program decreased the incidence of subsequent amputation significantly (at 1 year).[16] Two hundred three patients were randomized into two groups: education and no education. There were no significant differences in medical management or clinical risk factors between the two groups. There was no significant difference in the incidence of infection; however, the rate of ulceration and amputation was three times higher in the no-education subgroup (26 of 177 vs. 8 of 177 ulceration, $P \leq .005$; 21 of 177 vs. 7 of 177 amputation, $P \leq .025$). That study demonstrated that a simple education program significantly reduced the incidence of ulcer or foot and limb amputation in diabetic patients.[16] Other studies have documented the importance of diabetes education, protective footwear, and preventive footcare (Rivera, 1998; Lehto et al, 1996).[129, 130]

Lehto et al (1996) have clearly demonstrated that there is a dose-response relationship between plasma glucose or HbA1 and the risk of amputation. Similar data have been published by Muhlhauser and colleagues (2000) showing that the end-stage complications of blindness, amputation, and dialysis were statistically linked to a level of glycosylated hemoglobin. Flores Rivera (1998) has documented an increased risk for amputation in diabetic patients with cholesterol greater than 450 mg. Muhlhauser and coworkers (2000) linked serum cholesterol levels to the combined end points of blindness or amputation or dialysis. Clearly, good blood glucose control should decrease the incidence of amputation in diabetics. However, the benefit, if any, of cholesterol-lowering drugs in decreasing the risk of amputation in both diabetic and nondiabetic patients is not known.

Patient Instructions for Care of the Diabetic Foot

1. Inspect your feet daily for blisters, cuts, scratches, and areas of possible infection. Do not miss looking between your toes. A mirror can help you see the bottom of your feet or between the toes. If it is not possible for you to inspect your feet yourself, seek the help of a family member or friend.

2. Wash your feet and toes daily, and dry very carefully, especially between the toes. It is also important to dry carefully after showering or swimming.

3. Avoid extreme temperatures for your feet. Test bath water with your hand to ensure that it is not too hot, and be extremely careful of hot pavement or concrete during the summer.

4. If your feet feel cold at night, wear socks. Do not apply hot water bottles or heating pads.

5. Do not use chemical agents to remove corns or calluses.

6. Inspect your shoes daily for foreign objects, nail points, torn linings, or other problems that might damage your feet.

7. Wear properly fitting stockings, and try to avoid stockings with seams and stockings that are mended. It is important to change stockings daily.

8. All shoes should be comfortable and loose fitting at the time of purchase. Do not depend on shoes to stretch or break in. Try to avoid shoes that are pointed or apply pressure on the toes.

9. Do not wear shoes without stockings.

10. Do not wear sandals with thongs between the toes. Never walk barefoot, especially on hot surfaces. Be extremely careful of walking barefoot at home owing to danger from pins, tacks, or other items dropped on the floor.

11. Toenails should be cut straight across, and if there is a question, please consult your physician or podiatrist.

12. Do not cut corns or calluses yourself; seek counseling from your physician or podiatrist. See your physician or podiatrist regularly, and be sure that your feet are examined on each visit.

13. If your vision is impaired or you have other difficulties with examining your feet, have a family member or friend inspect your feet, trim nails, and otherwise ensure adequate foot care.

14. Be sure to tell your podiatrist or physician that you are diabetic.

15. Do not smoke.

16. Remember that even minor infections can cause significant problems in diabetics, and a physician or podiatrist should be consulted when infection occurs.

Figure 45–14. Patient instruction sheet for care of the diabetic foot.

PROSTHETIC CONSIDERATIONS FOLLOWING MAJOR LOWER EXTREMITY AMPUTATION

In general, as the level of amputation moves proximally up the lower extremity and the age of the patient increases, the success rates for rehabilitation decline and the length of time required to achieve ambulation increases.[17, 131–137] Before discussions on prosthetic considerations after major lower extremity amputation, a review of some of the problems with rehabilitation of geriatric amputees is worthwhile.

TABLE 45–5

Overview of Postsurgical and Rehabilitation Outcome for Several Series*

AUTHORS	AMPUTATIONS (n)	PRIMARY HEALING (%)	EVENTUAL HEALING (%)	MORTALITY RATE (%)	REHABILITATION WITH PROSTHESIS (%)	AVERAGE TIME OPERATION TO REHABILITATION (DAYS)
Warren & Kihn	121	48.8	66.9	4.1	69.4	180–270
Chilvers et al.	53	50.0	67.9	7.5	60.4	—
Robinson	47	77.0	—	17.0	83.0	—
Bradham & Smoak	84	85.7	88.0	—	—‡	—
Block & Whitehouse	43	88.0	95.0	0.0†	53.5	120–180
Cranley et al.	101	76.0	86.0	7.0	73.3	—
Lim et al.	55	53.0	83.0	16.0	51.0	70
Ecker & Jacobs	69	77.0	85.0	8.7	52.2	201
Wray et al.	174	92.0	—	3.5	70.0	49–77
Nagrendran et al.	174	80.5	91.4	—	—	—
Berardi & Keonin	44	—	61.4	4.5	29.5	111
Averaged totals	965	74.9	82.0	6.7	63.8	133

*Series reporting their results with conventional techniques of rehabilitation after below-knee amputation. Note that the overall rehabilitation rate was 64% and the average time to achieve ambulation was 133 days.

†Two patients died before discharge, and were not included as postoperative deaths.

‡Authors commented that very few patients attained ambulation; however, no numbers were given.

From Malone JM, Moore WS, Goldstone J, Malone SJ: Therapeutic and economic impact of a modern amputation program. Ann Surg 189:801, 1979.

Rehabilitation of Elderly Amputees

In the mid- to late 1960s, the literature was replete with reports on problems with rehabilitation of geriatric amputees. Many of these reports have been forgotten; however, the information they presented is still valid. Among the most important surveys of that period was that of Mazet and associates[17] involving a 10-year follow-up of 1770 geriatric patients from the VA and county hospitals in Los Angeles. Among the findings from that study was the fact that 60% of patients who were given limbs discarded them within 6 months. Thirteen years later, Jamieson and Hill[138] reported, in their review of amputation for peripheral vascular disease, that over half the patients fitted with an artificial leg never used it effectively. In addition, they reported that if the rehabilitation process was not started for 2 or more months after amputation, the likelihood of ultimate ambulation was very poor. In a more recent review on delays in rehabilitation following lower extremity amputation, Kerstein and colleagues[139] noted that it required an

average of 27 weeks (189 days) to achieve the maximum benefits of rehabilitation, and it was approximately 6 months before the successfully rehabilitated amputee was returned to society. In an earlier article analyzing the influence of age on rehabilitation, Kerstein and coauthors[133] found that many patients over age 65 required a year to achieve maximum benefit from the rehabilitation process. Malone and coworkers[9] analyzed contemporary series on below-knee amputation in patients treated with conventional rehabilitation techniques and found that the average rate of rehabilitation was 64% and the average time from operation to rehabilitation (ambulation) was 133 days (Table 45–5). In a later review, Malone and coworkers[15] noted that the rehabilitation times for patients treated with conventional techniques versus accelerated rehabilitation techniques (including amputation level selection and immediate postoperative prosthesis) were 128 and 31 days, respectively (Table 45–6). The same review pointed out that the success rate for ambulation after amputation with conventional rehabilitation techniques was 70%, whereas it was

TABLE 45–6

Comparison of Rehabilitation Time with Conventional and Accelerated Techniques*

LEVEL OF AMPUTATION	GROUP 1 (DAYS)		GROUP 2 (DAYS)		P VALUE
	Range	Mean	Range	Mean	
Transmetatarsal	20–60	47.0	10–24	18.4	NS
Syme's	—	—	15–17	23.0	—
Below-knee	60–330	132.0	18–140	32.5	.0001
Knee disarticulation	—	—	15–140	60.7	—
Above-knee	360	—	27–30	28.5	NS
Hip disarticulation	—	—	35	—	—
Overall	20–360	128.4	10–140	30.8	.0001

*Rehabilitation time following lower extremity amputation for patients treated with conventional surgical and prosthetic techniques (group 1: 128 days) and accelerated techniques incorporating immediate postoperative prostheses (group 2: 31 days) (P<.001).

NS, not significant.

From Malone SM, Moore WS, Leal JM, Childers SJ: Rehabilitation for lower extremity amputation. Arch Surg 116:97, 1981.

100% for amputees treated with accelerated rehabilitation techniques. In addition, it has been my experience with geriatric amputees that if a patient is nonambulatory for either a month before amputation or a month after amputation (rehabilitation is delayed), the likelihood for rehabilitation is significantly less than if the patient is maintained in an ambulatory status in the perioperative period.

Part of the problem with rehabilitation of geriatric amputees is their decreased cardiorespiratory reserve and the increased energy expenditures required after lower extremity amputation, especially at more proximal amputation levels. These problems are complicated by the fact that individual surgeons probably see too few amputees to treat them with maximum efficiency, and the few patients they see create a large burden on beds, resources, and physician time.

In a review on the energy cost of walking for amputees, Waters and colleagues[136] found that in both unilateral traumatic and vascular amputees, performance was directly related to the level of amputation. Walking velocity, cadence, and stride length were all decreased in amputation patients compared with control groups. In a detailed analysis of velocity of ambulation, rate of oxygen uptake, respiratory quotient, and heart rate, these authors concluded that amputees adjust their gait velocity to keep their rate of energy expenditure within normal limits. The approximate energy expenditures (compared with those of controls) after lower extremity amputation are shown in Table 45–7.[136, 140–142] Note that the energy expenditures for both unilateral and bilateral below-knee amputees are less than those of unilateral above-knee amputees. This clearly demonstrates the importance of the knee joint in terms of energy used for ambulation. The additional effort of walking with an above-knee prosthesis is accomplished by the use of small muscles, which are poorly designed for locomotion.[142]

Decreased physical strength due to increasing age, decreased cardiorespiratory reserve due to the ravages of cardiovascular or pulmonary disease, and increased energy expenditures for ambulation after lower extremity amputation can all be seen to have an additive effect that complicates the rehabilitation of geriatric amputees. It is in this setting that the salvage of the most distal amputation that will heal may establish the difference between ambulation and independence and nonambulation and dependence for the elderly amputee. These factors also explain the higher

likelihood of ambulation for a young high-level amputee compared with an elderly high-level or bilateral amputee. In their evaluation of 113 amputations in 103 patients, most of whom underwent amputation for peripheral vascular disease or diabetes or both (mean age of 61 years), Roon and coworkers[14] found the following rates of success for rehabilitation for below-knee, above-knee, and combination bilateral amputations: 100% for unilateral below-knee amputation; 93% for bilateral below-knee amputation; 17% for a combination of above-knee and below-knee amputations; and no success for patients with bilateral above-knee amputations.

Postoperative Prosthetic Techniques

After major lower extremity amputation, the surgeon has three choices for prosthetic management: soft dressings or conventional technique; constant environmental treatment (CET) (which at this point is probably only of historical interest); and rigid dressings with or without a postoperative prosthesis. In addition, the surgeon may choose delayed (conventional), rapid, or immediate postoperative rehabilitation.

Conventional Stump Wrap (Soft Dressing)

The historical standard, and a technique that is still used in many institutions, is the application of a soft postoperative dressing. Cotton gauze or fluffs are used to pad the amputation stump, and the stump is wrapped with elastic bandages (Fig. 45–15). The advantage of this technique is that it does not require a prosthetist to be present in the operating room or at the time of dressing changes. The disadvantages are that it does not readily control stump edema, the dressings are difficult to maintain in place (especially for high-level amputees), there is minimal stump protection from postoperative trauma, the dressing will not prevent knee flexion contracture, and ambulation may be delayed as a result of the prolonged time period required for stump maturity (6 months).

Except for the above-knee and hip disarticulation amputation levels, where it is technically difficult to maintain a rigid dressing in good stump contact, we do not believe that there are valid reasons to continue the use of this postoperative dressing technique.

Constant Environmental Treatment Unit

Developed and used almost exclusively in Great Britain, the CET unit consists of a control console containing a multistage centrifugal air compressor. The air passes through pressure control valves, a pressure cycle timing device, a bacteriologic filter, and a thermostatically controlled heating element that controls heat and relative humidity. The dressing on the patient consists of a transparent flexible polyvinyl bag. The bag is not in direct contact with the residual limb except on the resting surface. A pleated air seal is incorporated into the proximal end of the bag to maintain a pressure seal. A sterile CET bag is

---

TABLE 45-7

Energy Expenditure (Compared with Controls) after Lower Extremity Amputation*

	INCREASE IN ENERGY EXPENDITURE (%)
Unilateral below-knee	9–25
Bilateral below-knee	41
Unilateral above-knee	25–100
Bilateral above-knee	280

*As measured by oxygen utilization per minute[136, 140, 142] or indirect calorimetry.[141] Measured at comfortable walking speeds that averaged 22% of normal.

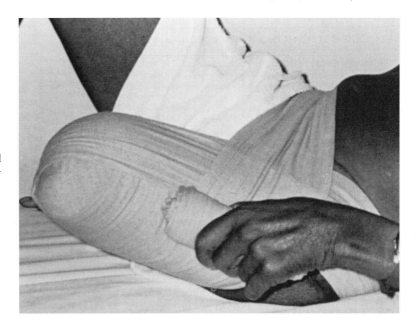

Figure 45–15. The standard conventional soft dressing and stump wrap being applied by a patient on his right above-knee amputation.

placed over the amputation stump in the operating room. The amputation stump is in essence "enclosed" in a sterile environment with cyclic pressure (which controls stump edema) and airflow set to the desired temperature and humidity (Fig. 45–16).

The CET unit was designed for use in a setting in which a prosthetist was not immediately available to the surgeon or one in which the surgeon wishes to be able to control stump edema and yet have easy ability to examine the surgical wound. The system incorporates a long flexible hose so that the patient can undergo rehabilitation training at the bedside. The use for the CET unit is relatively limited, and it is probably best used on those patients in whom there is some risk of stump infection, and the ability to have continuous observation of the wound without dressing changes is desirable. Because of its limited application, high cost, and poor patient acceptance due to noise, the CET unit, although successful, has seen limited use in the United States.[143]

Rapid and Immediate Postoperative Prostheses

The application of an immediate postoperative prosthesis has received considerable attention, support, credit, and discredit in the recent past. Proponents of the technique have waxed eloquently on the benefit to the patient, while opponents of the technique have cautioned about the potential complications to the amputation stump from the casting technique.

Berlemont is generally credited with the early work that led to establishment of the technique based on his application of temporary prostheses in patients with delayed (secondary) amputation stump healing.[3] Professor Marion Weiss of Poland is credited with adapting this technique for stumps undergoing primary healing (i.e., immediate postoperative prosthesis). The latter technique proved highly successful, and Weiss reported his initial results at the Sixth International Prosthetic Course in Copenhagen in July 1963. This early presentation and a subse-

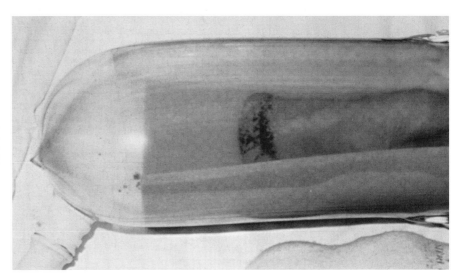

Figure 45–16. The clear polyvinyl controlled environment treatment bag, which has been placed over a left below-knee amputation. Notice the air supply hose at the distal end of the bag.

quent publication in 1966[4] came to the attention of surgeons worldwide. The Prosthetic and Sensory Aids Service of the VA was especially interested in the application of this technique for the management of veteran amputees and was instrumental in bringing this procedure to the American surgical theatre. Working with the VA, Ernest Burgess, an orthopedic surgeon in Seattle, Washington, refined and developed the application of the immediate postoperative prosthetic technique for the American surgical field.[5, 125, 144-146] Burgess and his team performed most of the early work in the United States on the use of immediate postoperative prosthetic techniques, and he was instrumental in training other investigators in its use. In the late 1960s and early 1970s, there were multiple reports extolling the virtues and possible pitfalls of the immediate postoperative prosthetic (IPOP) technique (also called IPPF, immediate postoperative prosthetic fitting).

Initially, there was general agreement that the IPOP technique was ideally suited for the nondiabetic, nondysvascular amputee. Subsequent reports in the literature, however, have shown that if properly used, the technique works perhaps ideally in the geriatric dysvascular amputee because of its ability to shorten hospitalization time and increase rates of rehabilitation.[9, 14, 15]

In general, proponents of the technique note that its benefits include an increased rate of healing, decreased hospital time, decreased rehabilitation time, decreased psychological trauma to the patient, control of stump edema, protection from trauma to the stump in the early postoperative period, and perhaps an increased rate of rehabilitation.[9, 14, 15, 84, 147-150] The paper most commonly cited against the use of the IPOP technique is that by Cohen and colleagues.[151] Using conventional surgical and prosthetic techniques, Cohen and colleagues were able to achieve 97% amputation stump healing, whereas only two of nine amputation stumps treated with immediate postoperative prostheses healed. They noted no rehabilitation advantage to the IPOP technique and recommended caution in its application. The experience reported by Cohen and coworkers is not matched by other similar reports in the literature. There are reports that note no change in the rate of wound healing,[147] but in general most papers find no deleterious effect to the stump from the use of a rigid postoperative dressing (with or without a prosthesis), decreased hospitalization time, and decreased rehabilitative time.[9, 14, 15, 147, 149, 150] Importantly, Cohen and colleagues suggested that their problems with the IPOP technique might be with the plaster technique itself or in the application of the technique. A review of their paper shows that four patients sustained what are described as second-degree blisters, which almost certainly indicate problems with plaster fabrication and application rather than problems with the IPOP technique itself. In my own experience with 600 consecutive major lower extremity amputations during the past 12 years, there has been only one stump problem related to the use of an immediate postoperative prosthesis, and that problem was directly caused by improper application of an immediate postoperative cast.

An overview of data on use of the IPOP technique reported from the San Francisco VA Hospital, the Tucson VA Hospital, and Maricopa Medical Center by Roon and colleagues[14] and Malone and associates[9, 15] is given in Table 45–8. A 1992 paper by Folsum and coworkers[152] documented the overall rate of rehabilitation at 80% and the interval from amputation to ambulation at 15.2 days and 9.3 days for below-knee and above-knee amputees, respectively. Information not tabulated in Table 45–8 suggests that the ambulatory status of the patient prior to surgery was one of the most important predeterminants of postoperative ambulation. Essentially, 100% of patients undergoing unilateral major lower extremity amputation who ambulated prior to surgery were successfully rehabilitated after amputation, whereas fewer than 15% of the patients who were nonambulatory prior to amputation surgery were successfully rehabilitated.[9, 14, 15]

The advantages of immediate or early postoperative prostheses can be divided into two categories: those derived from the rigid dressing and those derived from early weight bearing and ambulation. The advantages of the rigid dressing include edema control, stump immobilization, perhaps improved healing, prevention of joint flexion contracture, and protection of the amputation stump from external trauma. There may not be a difference between soft and rigid dressings with respect to the time required to reach eventual stump maturity (6 months), although postoperative stump edema resolves much more quickly with a rigid dressing. The advantages of immediate or early ambulation include decreased hospital time, shortened time from surgery to ambulation, increased rates of rehabilitation compared with those of patients managed in a more conventional manner, a reduction in morbid and nonmorbid complications of amputation, and an improvement in the psychological outlook of the patient after amputation.[9, 14, 15, 114]

In summary, then, there is general agreement on both the benefits and pitfalls of the IPOP technique. We agree with Friedmann's conclusions: "immediate postoperative prosthetic fitting should be confined to large centers with medical and prosthetic facilities available on short notice."[76] In other circumstances, he believed that the use of conventional amputation rehabilitation was indicated but specified that conventional amputation management should include modern postoperative techniques, specifically including the early use of temporary prostheses for evaluation and training. The best solution to the problem of choosing a postoperative prosthetic technique would be the routine use of a rigid dressing and the application or use of a temporary prosthesis when the surgeon thinks that adequate wound healing has occurred (usually 1 to 2 weeks after amputa-

TABLE 45-8

Overview: San Francisco and Tucson VA Hospitals and Maricopa Medical Center Immediate Prosthesis Data

Stump healing	138/153 (90%)
Rehabilitation time	15–32 days
Rate of rehabilitation	155/175 (88%)
Unilateral below-knee	128/129 (99%)
Bilateral below-knee	17/19 (89%)
Bilateral (above/below-knee or above/above-knee)	6/23 (26%)
Unilateral above-knee	4/4 (100%)

Data from references 9, 14, 15.

tion), thereby avoiding some of the potential hazards of immediate ambulation.[153–155]

Another variant of a postoperative rigid dressing that allows early postsurgical ambulation is the air splint.[132, 156] This device may be a practical alternative for a surgeon who wants to achieve early postoperative amputation but does not have access to a prosthetist skilled in the application of immediate postoperative prostheses or temporary removable prostheses.

Techniques of Immediate Postoperative Prosthetic Application

Immediate postoperative prosthetic use has been described for all levels of major lower extremity amputation—from the transmetatarsal through the high above-knee amputation; however, it is best suited to below-knee amputation. Specific technical details regarding application of immediate postoperative prostheses have been well described and therefore are only briefly outlined here.[98]

Transmetatarsal and the Syme's Amputation

A rigid cast with felt padding for bony prominence relief is used as the first dressing for these distal levels of lower extremity amputation; however, ambulation is not allowed until adequate primary healing has been obtained (3 weeks). Early ambulation for transmetatarsal and Syme's amputation patients results in a higher incidence of wound complications. It is extremely important for the Syme's amputation that the posterior heel flap be held in good approximation and alignment by the cast and that great care be taken to pad the distal stump and dog ears as well as the bony prominences. If a two-stage surgical approach for Syme's amputation is used,[84] it is probably best to avoid weight bearing until completion of the second stage of the

surgical procedure (6 to 8 weeks). Both transmetatarsal and Syme's amputees will ultimately ambulate well, and a short delay in the ambulation process has essentially no impact on their overall rehabilitation. Avoidance of stump trauma to ensure primary wound healing during the early postoperative period is of paramount importance, and rehabilitation efforts can be confined to range of motion and strengthening of the opposite leg and upper extremities during the early postoperative period.

Below-Knee Amputation Level

Following completion of the amputation, a thin sheet of fine mesh material (Owen's silk) is moistened in antibiotic solution or saline and applied over the suture line with care taken to avoid wrinkling (Fig. 45–17). Next, lamb's wool or polyurethane foam is placed over the end of the stump to provide stump compression and padding (Fig. 45–18). A Spandex stump sock is then carefully rolled over the stump, with care taken to avoid displacement of the distal stump padding (Fig. 45–19). Relief pads made from nonporous foam are fashioned and glued to the stump sock with Dow-Corning medical adhesive. These pads can be obtained precut or can be hand-fashioned in the operating room. They are placed so as to pad the bony prominences, specifically including the fibular head, the tibial condyles, and the patella. Care is taken to leave a relief area between the medial and lateral tibial pads (Fig. 45–20). Next, elastic plaster is used to form the inner layer of the immediate postoperative prosthesis. It is important that an assistant maintain traction on the stump sock during plaster application. Care is taken to maintain compression from posterior to anterior (direction of the posterior skin flap) and to grade compression from the distal end of the stump to the more proximal thigh (Fig. 45–21). The suspension assembly of the immediate postoperative pylon is then contoured to the inner cast after the cast has dried (Fig. 45–22). The

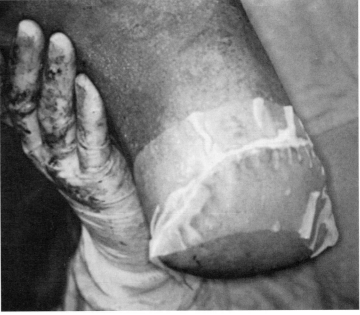

Figure 45–17. A single sheet of moistened Owen's silk is placed over the suture line on the below-knee amputation stump. Care is taken to avoid wrinkling of the silk material.

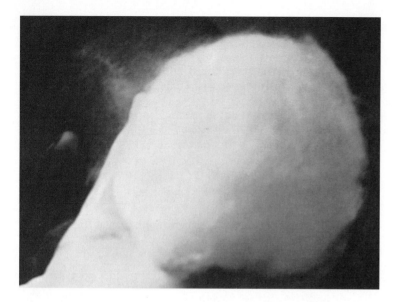

Figure 45–18. Lamb's wool, Dacron waste, or prefabricated polyurethane foam, can be placed over Owen's silk to provide distal stump padding. Care is taken to place padding material both above and below skin dog-ears, if they exist.

pylon can then be attached and static alignment achieved before incorporating the suspension assembly into the cast. The pylon is removed and the suspension assembly is secured to the inner cast using fiberglass casting tape. The use of lightweight casting tape decreases the weight of the immediate postoperative prosthesis and significantly increases its durability.[154] A completed immediate postoperative prosthesis, waist suspension belt, pylon, and foot are shown in Figure 45–23. If a drain is employed, the drain should be brought out proximally (and laterally) through a separate hole made in the cast during the fabrication process. The drain should not be secured to the skin, so that it can be pulled out through the cast when appropriate.

Most surgical pain is gone within 36 to 48 hours after surgery. Significant pain more than 48 hours after surgery is an indication that the cast is too tight or that there is a wound complication, and the cast should be removed, the wound inspected, and the cast reapplied if appropriate. Almost all patients comment that their postoperative stump pain diminishes if the heel of the prosthesis is weight-loaded (when they are in the supine position), and this test can be used as a further check for stump swelling and

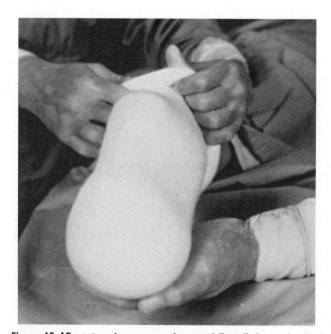

Figure 45–19. A Spandex stump sock is carefully pulled over the distal end of the below-knee stump and rolled proximally up the leg. Care is taken to not displace distal end stump padding during application of the sock. Until the postoperative cast is dry, it is necessary for an assistant to maintain traction on the stump sock.

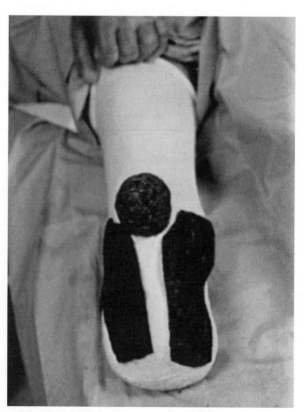

Figure 45–20. Felt relief pads are measured, trimmed, and glued to the Spandex stump sock over the bony prominences of the knee and lower leg. Care is taken to leave a relief area between the medial and lateral tibial pads.

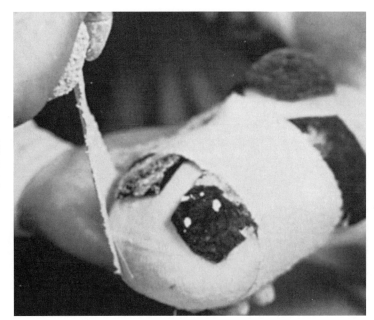

Figure 45–21. The inner layer of the postoperative rigid cast is made using elastic plaster. Elastic plaster provides good control of stump compression. Compression should be from posterior to anterior, in the direction of the posterior flap, and distal to proximal so that the compression decreases as the cast moves higher on the upper leg.

prosthesis fit. One of the most important principles in the postoperative management of these patients is that if there is any question about prosthesis fit or healing of the surgical wound, the prosthesis should be removed, the wound inspected by the surgeon and the prosthetist, and the cast reapplied at the discretion of the surgeon.

On the first postoperative morning, the patient is helped into a standing position at the bedside and instructed in techniques of touchdown weight bearing. At this time, the prosthetist will complete the initial static alignment. On the second postoperative morning, the patient will go to the physical therapy department, where he or she is taught touchdown weight bearing using the bathroom scale technique (Fig. 45–24). An alternative to the scale technique is the load cell, which is a pressure-sensing device built into

the prosthetic pylon.[157] During the first 7 to 10 days after surgery, the patient will ambulate with parallel bars with a maximum of 10 to 15 pounds touchdown weight bearing (10% of body weight). After application of the second postoperative prosthesis, the patient will increase weight bearing to approximately 50% of total body weight. At the end of 14 to 21 days, on removal of the second postoperative prosthesis, a decision is made to place the patient either in a third postoperative prosthesis (if there is a question of wound healing) or in a removable temporary prosthesis (if the wound appears to be healing satisfactorily).[154, 155] At this time the patient begins full weight bearing. By approximately 30 to 35 days after amputation surgery, most patients have achieved either independent ambulation or ambulation with some type of ancillary

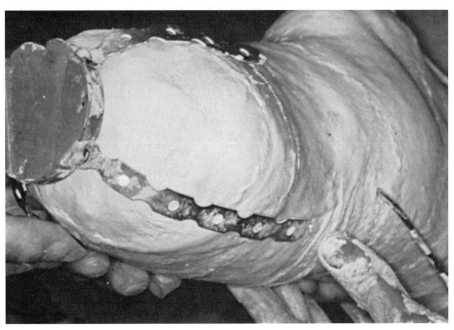

Figure 45–22. The metal arms of the immediate postoperative prosthetic bucket are molded to the contours of the inner plaster shell after the cast has dried.

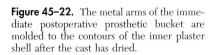

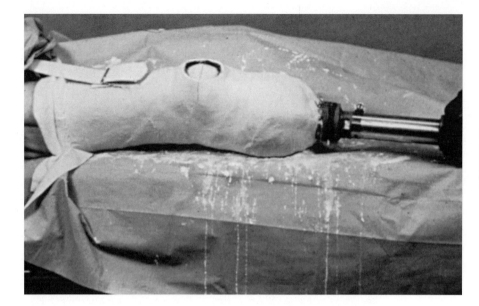

Figure 45–23. Intraoperative photograph of a completed immediate postoperative below-knee prosthesis with pylon, foot, and waist suspension belt. Note that a relief window has been placed over the area of the patella.

walking aid (cane, walker). If a patient lives close to the hospital and is able to come to daily physical therapy training as an outpatient, he or she may be discharged from the hospital shortly after receiving the second postoperative prosthesis (5 to 10 days); however, if the patient lives a great distance from the hospital, then discharge is usually delayed until surgeon, prosthetist, and therapist are happy with the rehabilitation process (4 to 5 weeks). This approach may, however, have to be modified under the economic restraints that surround current medical care. Reasonable alternatives include transfer to a rehabilitation unit or service or early discharge with outpatient care. In either case, careful follow-up by the surgeon, prosthetist, and therapist is mandatory, especially in patients undergoing early ambulation and rehabilitation.

It can be anticipated that between discharge from the hospital and construction of the first permanent prosthesis (on average, 6 months after amputation), approximately three to six changes in the socket on the temporary prosthesis will be required as a result of progressive stump shrinking. A typical lightweight removable temporary below-knee prosthesis is shown in Figure 45–25. The same pylon and foot can be used throughout all intermediate (temporary) cast changes, so that the only new prosthetic requirement is the prosthetic socket and realignment of the prosthesis. Prosthetic fit is maintained with stump socks and the primary indication for change of the temporary prosthesis is when the patient has reached a total of 15-ply stockings to maintain a good prosthetic fit. Obviously, great care is taken to educate the patient about the use of the prosthesis and stump care to avoid any stump problems due to poor prosthetic fit.

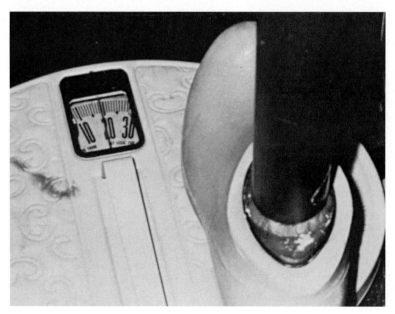

Figure 45–24. To control the amount of postoperative weight bearing by patients, a bathroom scale is used to teach them distribution of body weight. During the first week after surgery, weight bearing is limited to 10 to 15 pounds. After the second cast change, weight bearing is limited to 50% of total body weight.

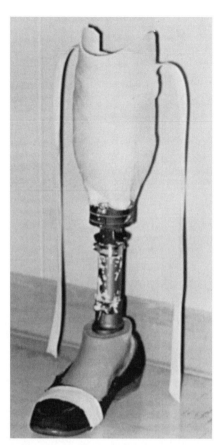

Figure 45–25. Standard removable lightweight below-knee temporary/intermediate prosthesis. This prosthesis is prescribed after removal of the last immediate postoperative prosthesis. The particular prosthesis in the photograph is constructed with 3M Scotchcast (3M, St. Paul, MN). Fabrication with Scotchcast allows construction of a lightweight, cool yet durable prosthesis.

Knee Disarticulation Amputation

The techniques for the application of an immediate postoperative prosthesis for the knee disarticulation amputation are essentially the same as those for the below-knee amputation. Because of the bulbous distal end of the knee disarticulation stump, the immediate postoperative prosthesis for this amputation level is self-suspending. Great care should be taken during cast fabrication to carefully contour the femoral flares and to bring the proximal end of the cast to at least the upper third of the thigh to minimize distal end–weight bearing. Our preference is to incorporate a polypropylene quadrilateral above-knee brim into the knee disarticulation cast so as to provide ischial weight bearing. The stump should be well-padded, since there is more stump weight bearing with this level of amputation than with a below-knee amputation. At the choice of the surgeon and prosthetist, polycentric hydraulic knee units can be incorporated with the initial immediate postoperative prosthesis or be incorporated any time during postoperative follow-up. The times for cast change, rehabilitation techniques, and use of a temporary prosthesis are approximately the same as those for a below-knee amputation.

Above-Knee Amputation

Immediate postoperative prosthetic techniques for above-knee amputation require more prosthetic attention to detail to maintain adequate suspension and socket fit. Although techniques using a modified silesia suspension (contralateral hip sling) or waist suspension belt are described and are simple to use,[104] we believe that the difficulties encountered when using immediate postoperative prostheses at the above-knee level are not offset by significant improvements in the overall rehabilitation process as to make the effort worthwhile. Our use of immediate postoperative prostheses at this amputation level is reserved for young amputees. For the dysvascular amputee, a temporary above-knee prosthesis is prescribed when primary wound healing has been achieved (2 to 3 weeks). During the postoperative period, the above-knee amputee goes to rehabilitation daily to achieve upper extremity strengthening and balance and to practice ambulation with parallel bars or other walking aids. Once a temporary prosthesis has been constructed, the times for prosthesis modification and rehabilitation techniques are similar to those for below-knee or knee disarticulation amputation postsurgical management.

Overview of Prostheses and Prosthetic Techniques

There is not one type of standard prosthetic prescription for any level of lower extremity amputation, and knowledge of available components is crucial in developing the proper prescription for each amputee based on his or her activities and lifestyle. A more complete discussion of prosthetic components is beyond the scope of this chapter; however, interested surgeons are referred to the local prosthetist or prosthetic facility with whom they should be working.

Immediate postoperative prosthetic techniques will not work in all clinical settings. The success of the technique is based on the experience and dedication of the team, and there is no question that if the immediate postoperative prosthesis is improperly applied, significant damage to the amputation stump can and will occur. In the absence of the availability of an experienced prosthetist and therapist to help the surgeon, we suggest that a rigid postoperative dressing be applied, and when primary stump healing has occurred, an appropriate temporary prosthesis can be prescribed and the rehabilitation process initiated. A delay of 1 to 2 weeks in the rehabilitation process is meaningless in the overall context of amputee rehabilitation; however, it has been my experience that if the rehabilitation process is delayed for a month or more, the ultimate success of rehabilitation, especially for high-level amputations in geriatric patients, is severely compromised. It is therefore logical and reasonable to provide a temporary prosthesis sometime between wound healing (7 to 10 days after surgery) and 1 month after surgery. Using this "between" type of approach (i.e., a rigid dressing with early prosthetic application), maximum rehabilitation results can be achieved even in the absence of a formalized rehabilitation team.

Prosthetic Components

For the occasional amputation surgeon, the number and types of prostheses and prosthetic components for lower extremity amputees can be bewildering and probably of little interest. Therefore, a general overview of prosthetic components and specific combinations of components for certain levels of lower extremity amputation may be of value.

Transmetatarsal Amputation

In general, there is minimal, if any, prosthetic requirement for a transmetatarsal amputation. A steel shank placed in the sole of the shoe will allow near-normal toe-off, and the void spot in the shoe can be filled with cotton, lamb's wool, or a soft foam material. The other available option is construction of a specially designed shoe molded to the patient's foot in which toe-off is built into the shoe during construction.

The Syme's Amputation

Depending on whether the Syme's amputation has been performed with a one- or two-stage surgical procedure, the cosmetic quality of the prosthesis will be different (two-stage is more cosmetic). In general, this is an end–weight-bearing stump, and a prosthetic foot is attached to the leg shaft portion of the prosthesis. Because of the bulbous nature of the stump, a medial window has to be cut into the prosthesis to allow the stump to pass through the narrow midportion of the prosthesis. These prostheses are usually built with a nonmotion solid ankle–cushion heel (SACH) foot. The presence of a particularly bulbous distal end will preclude a very cosmetic prosthesis and this type of amputation may be contraindicated for cosmetic reasons alone.

Below-Knee Amputation

In general, the below-knee prosthesis consists of a prosthetic socket that is attached to a pylon or ankle block (endoskeletal system) and a foot. The prosthetic shell can be composed of plastic laminate, wood, or some of the newer lightweight rolled fiberglass materials such as 3M Scotchcast (3M, St. Paul, Minn.). The socket may use no liner (skin-socket interface) or may use a liner composed of lightweight plastic such as pelite, silicone gel bonded between two sheets of soft leather, or stump socks. The prosthesis can be suspended in a variety of manners, the most common of which include a standard PTB strap, a supracondylar clip, Silastic sleeve suspension, suction, or a thigh lacer with external hinges (Fig. 45–26). Self-suspending prostheses or physiologic suspension (the prosthesis is held in place by changes in muscle shape and contour with contraction) may be used in young, active amputees. In a young, highly active amputee, an ankle-rotating unit may be placed between the prosthesis and the foot. The

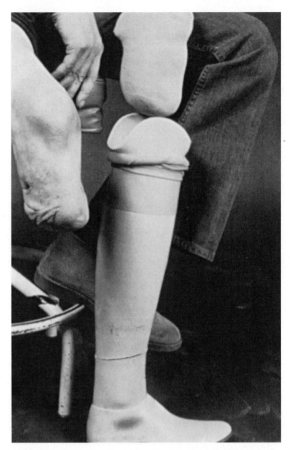

Figure 45–26. The below-knee prosthesis shown in this photograph is an ultralightweight patellar tendon weight-bearing-type prosthesis using a Silastic sleeve for suspension, a Silastic gel insert, and a SAFE motion-type foot. This is an ideal prosthetic prescription for a young, active amputee.

feet currently in use include the SACH foot, which is a nonmotion foot, the stationary attachment flexible endoskeletal (SAFE) foot, or the Griesinger 5-Way foot. The last two feet incorporate flexion, extension, and internal and external rotation when the foot is stressed under weight. The drawback to both of these motion feet is increased weight and perhaps decreased life expectancy compared with the SACH foot. The most popular motion foot, the Seattle foot, overcomes the drawbacks of the previously mentioned motion feet, and has a cosmetic design that incorporates toes. A hydraulic ankle unit has recently been developed, but the unit is quite heavy, and there are still problems with oil leakage. New energy-storing feet (energy is "stored" by deformation of carbon-plastic composites and "released" on toe-off), such as the Seattle-Boeing-Burgess Foot and the Flex-Foot, offer significant improvements in gait and activity levels (such as running), especially for the young, active amputee. The combination of a motion foot and a lightweight prosthesis provides a very high degree of function for an active amputee.

Knee Disarticulation

Historically, knee disarticulation amputations were a prosthetic nightmare because the knee centers (thigh-knee length) could not be matched; however, the availability of polycentric knee joints has allowed construction of a cosmetic knee disarticulation prosthesis. In general, this prosthesis is similar to the Syme's-type prosthesis, in that the distal bony end of the stump is passed through the proximal portion of the prosthesis via a window cut in the medial portion of the prosthesis. The prosthetic shell can again be constructed of plastic or wood. In general, the prosthetic shell extends from the end of the stump up to the ischium to provide both distal end– and ischial weight bearing. Most knee disarticulation prostheses incorporate some type of hydraulic knee unit for both cosmetic and functional reasons. The lower part of the leg can be constructed of solid wood, plastic laminate, or a metal or plastic endoskeletal system for connection to the ankle block and foot. Again, ankle rotators and energy-storing motion or nonmotion feet can be used at the discretion of the prosthetist and surgeon.

Above-Knee Amputation

The above-knee prosthesis can be constructed of plastic or wood. Suspension techniques include an external hip joint with belt, shoulder suspension, or suction socket suspension. The prosthesis is not an end–weight bearing prosthesis, and all the weight is borne by the proximal socket quadrilateral brim design (the soft tissues of the thigh and ischium). Newer prosthetic designs for above-knee sockets include the contoured adducted trochanteric-controlled alignment method (CAT-CAM) design (which holds the stump laterally and medially, providing rigid support for the femur, in contrast to the quadrilateral socket, which holds the stump anteriorly and posteriorly with poor femur support) and a variety of new flexible socket and strut designs (outer rigid strut attached to the knee joint with a soft flexible inner socket). These new designs significantly enhance function for above-knee amputees. A hydraulic, passive, or manual lock knee joint can be incorporated as required by the needs of the individual patient. The lower part of the prosthesis is constructed as outlined in the section on knee disarticulation prostheses.

Hip Disarticulation Prostheses

In general, the hip disarticulation prostheses are built along the lines of the Canadian system, which incorporates a pelvic bucket, an endoskeletal upper and lower leg, simple spring-assisted hip and knee joints, and a nonmotion foot.

AMPUTATION REHABILITATION TEAM

It is exceedingly difficult to achieve consistently reliable rehabilitation results in the absence of a formal centralized, dedicated rehabilitation team that includes active participation by a prosthetist and members of the physical medicine and therapy departments. Just as some surgical procedures are confined to regional centers because of the cost and necessity of skilled labor, it is our belief that under the best of circumstances, amputation rehabilitation should be

a centralized resource in a community or group of communities to achieve the best results. Our concept of the structure of the amputation rehabilitation team is shown in Figure 45–27. Note that the center of the rehabilitation team is the patient and that other members of the team interface with the patient through or with an amputation coordinator. This coordinator could be a physical therapist, occupational therapist, nurse, or layperson. In my opinion, this person is key to maintaining coordination and especially long-term follow-up among members of the team. It has been our experience that one break in this rehabilitation circle results in at least a 50% failure in amputee rehabilitation. This fact (i.e., a break in the rehabilitation circle) may explain why the average rate of rehabilitation after lower extremity amputation is 60% or less.

There are five primary areas of concern in successful amputee rehabilitation: (1) coordination of care, (2) education of patient and family, (3) directed access to community resources, (4) discharge planning, and (5) centralized follow-up. In essence, the coordination of health care and mobilization of resources is under the direct control of the physician; however, in actual fact, once surgery is completed, this task is best organized by the amputation program coordinator. Discharge planning for the patient should start, if possible, before amputation. Education of the patient and family and evaluation of financial and social resources available to the patient should also begin prior to amputation or as soon as possible after amputation. Centralized follow-up probably is only important if the team is interested in evaluating specific treatment techniques or prosthetic components. However, long-term follow-up is mandatory if reliable information on rehabilitation and postoperative complications is to be obtained.

The role of the physician is that of team director and provider of health care. The enthusiasm and interest of the

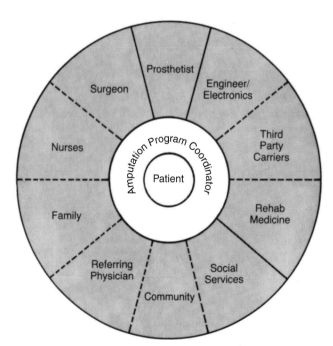

Figure 45–27. The rehabilitation team or circle of resources required for successful amputation rehabilitation. Notice that the patient is at the center, and the surgeon is only one of many coequal team members.

physician will be reflected by all other members of the health care team. In the absence of an interested physician, it can be expected that rehabilitation failures will be common.

It is my personal belief that the prosthetist should be seen as coequal to the physician in the amputation rehabilitation process. From a practical standpoint, most patients rely more on their prosthetist than their physician (in the absence of medical problems) once the acute phase of rehabilitation is completed.

The therapist is in the unique position of being able to make or break all of the efforts of the surgeon and prosthetist. Only if the rehabilitation process runs smoothly and if attention is paid to small details during the rehabilitation process will the patient successfully regain ambulation. The greatest surgery in the world or the best limb in the world can meet defeat at the hands of an unskilled therapist. The therapist is the third coequal in the rehabilitation team with the physician and prosthetist.

Finally, the patient is the most important member of the rehabilitation team. The team can provide the patient with tools and techniques for rehabilitation, but it cannot provide the patient with motivation. It is of the utmost importance that the patient be taught to take primary control of the rehabilitation process. Included in this learning process are care of the amputation stump, care of the nonamputated contralateral leg, and care of the prosthesis. Failure of the patient to take an active role in the rehabilitation process will necessarily doom it to failure.[158]

One of the areas in which we as physicians and rehabilitation team members fail our patients is in the area of posthospital discharge follow-up and home care. An excellent review article on this topic appeared in the February 1979 issue of the *Orthopedic Nurses Association Journal*. All interested rehabilitation physicians and team members are advised to review this information and pass it on to their patients.[112]

The author is now in a solo private practice without a dedicated amputation team. Although three experienced prosthetists, all of whom have significant experience with immediate postoperative prosthetic fitting, are nearby, the lack of trained therapists and capitated-directed patient care contracts makes acclerated rehabilitation difficult if not impossible. Objective amputation level selection (transcutaneous oxygen testing), early if not immediate postoperative prosthetic filling, utilization of rehabilitation facilities after discharge, education of therapists, and persistence usually lead to a successful outcome. However, the rehabilitation results, especially in elderly or frail patients, are not as good as those documented in this chapter using a dedicated amputation team or center of care model.

WHAT'S NEW IN AMPUTATION SURGERY

Instrumentation

As noted earlier, many new instruments are currently undergoing evaluation for amputation level selection. In addition to amputation level selection, many of these instruments are now being evaluated for their discriminate role

in arterial insufficiency. Once again, early information is available, but the definitive place for these instruments is undecided. Perhaps more promising than any of the specific instruments for amputation level selection will be the availability of computer software and microprocessors to integrate results from several different types of noninvasive amputation level selection techniques, resulting, in essence, in the era of the "limb viability laboratory." It can be anticipated that multi-instrument testing will have greater accuracy than single-instrument evaluation. In addition, many of these instruments will find use in the evaluation of limb ischemia, especially in the perioperative period.

Prosthetics

Three current areas of prosthetic development that are showing promising results are the emergence of ultralightweight and throwaway or temporary or intermediate prostheses (Fig. 45–28); the design and development of energy-absorbing and energy-returning prosthetic components (designed to return energy on toe-off), as exemplified by the Burgess-Seattle-Boeing foot and the Flex-Foot; and new fabrication techniques such as flexible sockets (ISNY socket), flexible suction sockets (OCERPSS and ICEPOSS sockets), and nonquadrilateral or medial-lateral–contoured above-knee sockets. The use of new plastics, fiberglass casting tapes, and carbon fiber polymers is allowing the construction of ultralightweight yet rugged, durable prostheses. These prostheses have obvious value for the geriat-

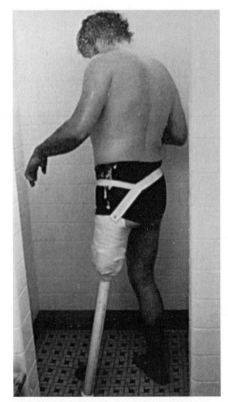

Figure 45–28. Patients with lower extremity amputations usually sit on a stool when taking a shower. The left above-knee amputee shown here is wearing an Aqualite above-knee shower prosthesis (US Manufacturing Co, Pasadena, CA).

ric amputee in terms of energy-saving characteristics, especially for the high-level amputee, but they also have value for the young, active amputee for sports or water-related activities. Lightweight prostheses constructed with these new materials are often easier to fabricate than standard plastic laminate prostheses. Artificial limbs constructed with fiberglass casting tapes, such as 3M Scotchcast, allow a decrease in skin temperature at the socket-skin interface because of the porous nature of the casting material. Preliminary work by our group demonstrated a 5°C to 7°C drop in skin temperature with 3M Scotchcast PTB below-knee prostheses, compared with standard plastic laminate PTB below-knee prostheses. The importance of decreased skin temperature is unknown with respect to stump durability, but there is no question these prostheses result in improved patient comfort in hot, humid climates.

Increasing numbers of studies are now being done with young, active amputees to improve their performance abilities in activities such as running, jumping, and other sports functions.[159] Projects such as this point not only toward directions for improvements in existing prosthetic devices but also toward directions for future research efforts, perhaps improving the efficiency with which amputees conduct their physical activities.

Surgery

There are increasing numbers of articles in the surgical literature describing arterial reconstruction with free tissue transfer to save limb length (Vermassen and van Landuyt, 2000; Lutz et al, 2000), myofasciocutaneous flaps to improve stump healing and prosthesis utilization (Bowker et al, 2000), and foot salvage and avoidance of major lower limb amputations in diabetic patients (Moore and Jolly, 2000). In 45 patients with gangrenous lesions of the foot or lower leg due to severe diabetic arterial disease resulting in extensive soft-tissue defects with exposed bones or tendons, Vermassen and van Landuyt reported excellent clinical results with arterial reconstruction and combined free-tissue transfer. Combined survival and limb salvage rate was 84% after 1 year, 77% after 2 years, and 65% after 3 years (2000). The articles quoted are only a small fraction of the published literature, and the interested reader can find many more publications using PubMed and doing Internet searches on amputation and skin flaps. The combination of distal vascular reconstruction and free flap utilization, rotational flaps, and other techniques for closure of soft-tissue defects of the extremities all offer exciting opportunities for extended limb salvage and avoidance of major limb amputation, especially in patients with diabetes.

References

1. Wangensteen OH, Wangensteen SD: The Rise of Surgery from Empiric Craft to Scientific Discipline. Minneapolis, University of Minnesota Press, 1978, p 18.
2. Boedner CW: Baron Dominique Jean Larrey, Napoleon's surgeon. ACS Bull, July 1982, 18–21.
3. Berlemont M: Notre expérience de l'appareillage précoce des amputés des membres inférieurs aux establishments helio Marins de Berk. Ann Med Phys Med 5(4): 1961.
4. Weiss M: The prosthesis on the operating table from a neurophysical point of view. Report of a workshop panel on lower extremity prosthetic fitting. Committee on Prosthetics Research Development. Presented to the National Academy of Sciences, February 1966.
5. Burgess EM, Tramb JE, Wilson AB Jr: Immediate Postsurgical Prosthetics in the Management of Lower Extremity Amputees. TR 10–5, Washington, DC, Veterans Administration, 1967.
6. Falstie-Jensen N, Christensen KB: A model for prediction of failure in amputation of the lower limb. Dan Med Bull 37:283–286, 1990.
7. Huston CC, Bivins BA, Ernst CB, Griffen WO Jr: Morbid implications of above-knee amputations. Report of a series and review of the literature. Arch Surg 115:165–167, 1980.
8. Kerstein MD, Zimmer H, Dugdale FE, Lerner E: Associated diagnoses complicating rehabilitation after major lower extremity amputation. Angiology 25:536–547, 1974.
9. Malone JM, Moore WS, Goldstone J, Malone SJ: Therapeutic and economic impact of a modern amputation program. Ann Surg 189:798–802, 1979.
10. Moore WS, Hall AD, Lim RC: Below the knee amputation for ischemic gangrene. Comparative results of conventional operation and immediate postoperative fitting technic. Am J Surg 124:127–134, 1972.
11. Porter JM, Baur GM, Taylor LM Jr: Lower-extremity amputation for ischemia. Arch Surg 116:89–92, 1981.
12. Towne JB, Condon RE: Lower extremity amputation for ischemic disease. Adv Surg 13:199–227, 1979.
13. Otteman MG, Stahlgren LH: Evaluation of factors which influence mortality and morbidity following major lower extremity amputation for arteriosclerosis. Surg Gynecol Obstet 120:1217–1220, 1965.
14. Roon AJ, Moore WS, Goldstone J: Below-knee amputation: A modern approach. Am J Surg 134:153–158, 1977.
15. Malone JM, Moore WS, Leal JM, Childers SJ: Rehabilitation for lower extremity amputation. Arch Surg 116:93–98, 1981.
16. Malone JM, Synder M, Anderson GG, et al: Prevention of amputation by diabetic education. Am J Surg 158:520–524, 1989.
17. Mazet R Jr, Schiller FJ, Dunn OJ, Alonzo NJ: The influence of prosthesis wearing on the health of the geriatric patient. Project 431. Dept HEW, Washington, DC, Office of Vocational Rehabilitation, Department of Health, Education and Welfare, March 1963.
18. Whitehouse FW, Jurgensen C, Block MA: The later life of the diabetic amputee. Another look at fate of the second leg. Diabetes 17:520–521, 1968.
19. Malone JM, Moore WS, Goldstone J: Life expectancy following aortofemoral arterial grafting. Surgery 81:551–555, 1977.
20. Pinzur MS, Littooy F, Daniels J, et al: Multidisciplinary preoperative assessment and late function in dysvascular amputees. Clin Orthop 281:239–243, 1992.
21. Fierer J, Daniel D, Davis C: The fetid foot: Lower-extremity infections in patients with diabetes mellitus. Rev Infect Dis 1:210–217, 1979.
22. Brinker MR, Timberlake GA, Goff JM, et al: Below knee physiologic cryoanesthesia in the critically ill patient. J Vasc Surg 7:433–438, 1988.
23. Johansen K, Burgess EM, Zorn R, et al: Improvement of amputation level by lower extremity revascularization. Surg Gynecol Obstet 153:707–709, 1981.
24. Kazmers M, Satiani B, Evans WE: Amputation level following unsuccessful distal limb salvage operations. Surgery 87:683–687, 1980.
25. Samson RH, Gupta SK, Scher LA, Veith FJ: Treatment of limb threatening ischemia despite a palpable popliteal pulse. J Surg Res 32:535–539, 1982.
26. Samson RH, Gupta SK, Scher LA, Veith FJ: Level of amputation after failed limb salvage procedures. Surg Gynecol Obstet 154:56–58, 1982.
27. Stoney RJ: Ultimate salvage for the patient with limb threatening ischemia: Realistic goals and surgical considerations. In Bergan JJ, Yao JST (eds): Gangrene and Severe Ischemia of the Lower Extremities. New York, Grune & Stratton, 1978, pp 383–392.
28. Stirneman P, Walpoth B, Wiursten VH, et al: Influence of failed arterial reconstruction on the outcome of major limb amputation. Surgery 111:363–368, 1992.
29. Tsang GM, Crowson MC, Hickey NC, Simms MH: Failed femorocrural reconstruction does not prejudice amputation level. Br J Surg 78:1479–1481, 1991.

30. Evans WE, Hayes JP, Vermilion BD: Effect of a failed distal reconstruction on the level of amputation. Am J Surg 160:217–220, 1990.

31. Epstein SB, Worth MH Jr, Ferzli G: Level of amputation following failed vascular reconstruction for lower limb ischemia. Curr Probl Surg 46:185–192, 1989.

32. Bloom RJ, Stevick CA: Amputation level and distal salvage of the limb. Surg Gynecol Obstet 166:1–5, 1988.

33. McIntyre KE Jr, Bailey SA, Malone JM, Goldstone J: The nonsalvageable infected lower extremity: A new look at guillotine amputation. Am J Surg 117:58–64, 1985.

34. Fischer DF, Clagett GP, Fry RE, et al: One-stage versus two-stage amputation for wet gangrene of the lower extremity: A randomized study. J Vasc Surg 8:428–433, 1988.

35. Robbs JV, Ray R: Clinical predictors of below knee stump healing following amputation for ischemia. S Afr J Surg 20:305–310, 1982.

36. Dwars BJ, Van Den Broek TA, Rauwerda JA, Bakker FC: Criteria for reliable selection of the lowest level of amputation in peripheral vascular disease. J Vasc Surg 15:536–542, 1992.

37. Golbranson FL, Yu EC, Gelberman RH: The use of skin temperature determinations in lower extremity amputation level selection. Foot Ankle 3:170–172, 1982.

38. Spence VA, Walker WF: The relationship between temperature isotherms and skin blood flow in the ischemic limb. J Surg Res 36:278–281, 1984.

39. Stoner HB, Taylor L, Marcuson RW: The value of skin temperature measurements in forecasting the healing of below-knee amputation for end stage ischemia of the leg in peripheral vascular disease. Eur J Vasc Surg 3:355–361, 1989.

40. Wagner WH, Keagy BA, Kotb MN, et al: Noninvasive determination of healing of major lower extremity amputation: The continued role of clinical judgment. J Vasc Surg 8:703–710, 1988.

41. Lim RC Sr, Blaisdell FW, Hall AD, et al: Below knee amputation for ischemic gangrene. Surg Gynecol Obstet 125:493–501, 1967.

42. Baker WH, Barnes RW: Minor forefoot amputation in patients with low ankle pressure. Am J Surg 133:331–332, 1977.

43. Barnes RW, Shanik GO, Slaymaker EE: An index of healing in below-knee amputation: Leg blood pressure by Doppler ultrasound. Surgery 79:13–20, 1976.

44. Bernstein EF: The noninvasive vascular diagnostic laboratory. In Najarian JS, Oelaney JP (eds): Vascular Surgery. Miami, Symposia Specialists. New York, Stratton Intercontinental, 1978, pp 33–46.

45. Gibbons GW, Wheelock FC Jr, Siembieda C, et al: Noninvasive prediction of amputation level in diabetic patients. Arch Surg 114:1253–1257, 1979.

46. Raines JK, Darling RC, Buth J, et al: Vascular laboratory criteria for the management of peripheral vascular disease of the lower extremities. Surgery 79:21–29, 1976.

47. Schwartz JA, Schuler JJ, O'Connor RJA, Flanigan DP: Predictive value of distal perfusion pressure in the healing of amputation of the digits and the forefoot. Surg Gynecol Obstet 154:865–869, 1982.

48. Verta MJ, Gross WS, Van Bellan B, et al: Forefoot perfusion pressure and minor amputation surgery. Surgery 80:729–734, 1976.

49. Yao JST, Bergan JJ: Application of ultrasound to arterial and venous diagnosis. Surg Clin North Am 54:23–38, 1974.

50. Cheng EY: Lower extremity amputation level: Selection using noninvasive hemodynamic methods of evaluation. Arch Phys Med Rehabil 63:475–479, 1982.

51. Holloway GA Jr, Burgess EM: Cutaneous blood flow and its relation to healing of below knee amputation. Surg Gynecol Obstet 146:750–756, 1978.

52. Holloway GA Jr, Watkins BW: Laser Doppler measurement of cutaneous blood flow. J Invest Dermatol 69:300–309, 1977.

53. Kostuik JP, Wood D, Hornby R, et al: Measurement of skin blood flow in peripheral vascular disease by the epicutaneous application of xenon-133. J Bone Joint Surg Am 58:833–837, 1964.

54. Malone JM, Leal JM, Moore WS, et al: The "gold standard" for amputation level selection: Xenon-133 clearance. J Surg Res 30:449–455, 1981.

55. Moore WS: Determination of amputation level. Measurement of skin blood flow with xenon-133. Arch Surg 107:798–802, 1973.

56. Silberstein EB, Thomas S, Cline J, et al: Predictive value of intracutaneous xenon clearance for healing of amputation and cutaneous ulcer sites. Radiology 147:227–229, 1983.

57. Burgess EM, Matsen FA, Wyss CR, Simmons CW: Segmental transcutaneous measurements of Po₂ in patients requiring below the knee amputation for peripheral vascular insufficiency. J Bone Joint Surg Am 64:378–382, 1982.

58. Clyne CAC, Ryan J, Webster JHH, Chant AOB: Oxygen tension on the skin of ischemic legs. Am J Surg 143:315–318, 1982.

59. Franzeck UK, Talke P, Berstein EF, et al: Transcutaneous Po₂ measurement in health on peripheral arterial occlusive disease. Surgery 91:156–163, 1982.

60. Harward TRS, Volny J, Golbranson F, et al: Oxygen-inhalation induced transcutaneous Po₂ changes as a predictor of amputation level. J Vasc Surg 2:220–227, 1985.

61. Katsamouris A, Brewster DC, Megerman J, et al: Transcutaneous oxygen tension in selection of amputation level. Am J Surg 147:510–516, 1984.

62. Malone JM, Anderson GG, Halka SC, et al: Prospective comparison of noninvasive techniques for amputation level selection. Am J Surg 154:179–184, 1987.

63. Matsen FA, Wyss CR, Robertson CL, et al: The relationship of transcutaneous Po₂ and laser Doppler measurements in a human model of local arterial insufficiency. Surg Gynecol Obstet 159:418–422, 1984.

64. Ratliff DA, Clune CAC, Chant ADB, Webster JHH: Prediction of amputation healing: The role of transcutaneous Po₂ assessment. Br J Surg 71:219–222, 1984.

65. Graham BH, Walton RL, Elings VB, Lewis F: Surface quantification of injected fluorescein as a predictor of flap viability. Plast Reconstr Surg 71:826–833, 1983.

66. McFarland DC, Lawrence PF: Skin fluorescence. A method to predict amputation site healing. J Surg Res 32:410–415, 1982.

67. Silverman DG, Hurford WE, Cooper HS, et al: Quantification of fluorescein distribution to strangulated reticulum. J Surg Res 34:179–186, 1983.

68. Silverman DG, Rubin JM, Reilly CA, et al: Fluorometric prediction of successful amputation levels in the ischemic limb. J Rehabil Res Dev 22:29–34, 1985.

69. Holloway GA Jr, Burgess EM: Preliminary experiences with laser Doppler velocimetry for the determination of amputation levels. Prosthet Orthot Int 7:63–66, 1983.

70. Holstein P: Level selection in leg amputation for arterial occlusive disease: A comparison of clinical evaluation and skin perfusion pressure. Acta Orthop Scand 53:821–831, 1982.

71. Holstein P, Trap-Jensen J, Bagger H, Larsen B: Skin perfusion pressure measured by isotope washout in legs with arterial occlusive disease. Clin Physiol 3:313–324, 1983.

72. Stockel M, Ovesen J, Brochner-Morstensen J, Emneus H: Standardized photoelectric technique as routine method for selection of amputation level. Acta Orthop Scand 53:875–878, 1982.

73. Kram HB, Appel PL, Shoemaker WC: Multisensor transcutaneous oximetric mapping to predict below-knee amputation wound healing: Use of critical Po₂. J Vasc Surg 9:796–800, 1989.

74. Kram HB, Appel PL, Shoemaker WC: Prediction of below-knee amputation wound healing using noninvasive laser Doppler velocimetry. Am J Surg 158:29–31, 1989.

75. Burnham ST, Wagner WH, Keagy BH, Johnson G Jr: Objective measurement of limb perfusion by dermal fluorometry. A criterion for healing of below knee amputation. Arch Surg 125:104–106, 1990.

76. Friedmann LW: The prosthesis—immediate or delayed fitting? Angiology 23:513–524, 1972.

77. Durham JR, Anderson GG, Malone JM: Methods of preoperative selection of amputation level. In Flanigan P (ed): Modern Methods of Perioperative Assessment in Peripheral Vascular Surgery. New York, Marcel Dekker, 1986.

78. Oishi CS, Fronek A, Golbranson FL: The role of noninvasive vascular studies in determining levels of amputation. J Bone Joint Surg Am 70:1520–1530, 1988.

79. Bacharach JM, Rooke TW, Osmundson PJ, Gloviczki P: Predictive value of transcutaneous oxygen pressure and amputation success by use of supine and elevation measurement. J Vasc Surg 15:558–563, 1992.

80. Holloway GA Jr: Cutaneous blood flow responses to infection trauma measured by laser Doppler velocimetry. J Invest Dermatol 74:1–4, 1980.

81. Daly MJ, Henry RE: Quantitative measurement of skin perfusion with xenon-133. J Nucl Med 21:156–160, 1980.

82. Holstein P, Lassen NA: Assessment of safe level of amputation by measurement of skin blood pressure. In Rutherford R, et al (eds): Vascular Surgery. Philadelphia, WB Saunders, 1977, pp 105–111.

83. Ovesen J, Stockel M: Measurement of skin perfusion pressure by photoelectric technique: Aid to amputation level selection in arteriosclerotic disease. Prosthet Orthot Int 8:39–42, 1984.

84. Wagner FW Jr: Amputation of the foot and ankle. Current Status. Clin Orthop 122:62–69, 1977.

85. Sizer JS, Wheelock FC: Digital amputations in diabetic patients. Surgery 72:980–989, 1972.

86. Little JM, Stephen MS, Zylstra PL: Amputation of the toes for vascular disease: Fate of the affected leg. Lancet 2:1318–1319, 1976.

87. McKittrick LS, McKittrick MB, Risby TS: Transmetatarsal amputation for infection of gangrene in patients with diabetes mellitus. Ann Surg 130:825–842, 1949.

88. Syme J: On amputation at the ankle joint. London and Edinburgh Monthly J Med Sci 3(26):93, 1843.

89. Harris RI: Syme's amputation, the technical details essential for success. J Bone Joint Surg Br 38:614–632, 1956.

90. Harris RI: The history and development of Syme's amputations. Artif Limbs 6:4–43, 1961.

91. Warren R, Kihn RB: A survey of lower extremity amputations for ischemia. Surgery 63:107–120, 1968.

92. Kernek CB, Rozzi WB: Simplified two stage below-knee amputation for unsalvageable diabetic foot infections. Clin Orthop 261:251–256, 1990.

93. Termansen NB: Below-knee amputation for ischaemic gangrene. Prospective, randomized comparison of a transverse and a sagittal operative technique. Acta Orthop Scand 48:311–316, 1977.

94. Persson BM: Sagittal incision for below-knee amputation in ischaemic gangrene. J Bone Joint Surg Br 56:110–114, 1974.

95. Ruckley CV, Stonebridge PA, Prescott RJ: Skewflap versus long posterior flap in below-knee amputations: Multicenter trial. J Vasc Surg 13:423–427, 1991.

96. Block MA, Whitehouse FW: Below-knee amputation in patients with diabetes mellitus. Arch Surg 87:682–689, 1963.

97. Dellon AL, Morgan RF: Myodermal flap closure of below the knee amputation. Surg Gynecol Obstet 153:383–386, 1981.

98. Moore WS: Immediate postoperative prosthesis. In Rutherford R, Bernhard V, et al (eds): Vascular Surgery. Philadelphia, WB Saunders, 1977, pp 1333–1343.

99. Kim GE, Imparato AM, Chu DS, Davis SW: Lower limb amputation for occlusive vascular disease. Am Surg 42:589–601, 1976.

100. Inderbitzi R, Biuttiker M, Pfluger D, Nachbur B: The fate of bilateral lower limb amputees in end stage disease. Eur J Vasc Surg 6:321–326, 1992.

101. Houghton A, Allen A, Luff R, McColl I: Rehabilitation after lower extremity amputation: A comparative study of above-knee, through knee and Gritti-Stokes amputations. Br J Surg 76:622–624, 1989.

102. Burgess EM: Disarticulation of the knee. A modified technique. Arch Surg 112:1250–1255, 1977.

103. Doran J, Hopkinson BR, Making GS: The Gritti-Stokes amputation in ischaemia: A review of 134 cases. Br J Surg 65:135–137, 1978.

104. Puddifoot PC, Weaver PC, Marshall SA: A method of supportive bandaging for amputation stumps. Br J Surg 60:729–731, 1973.

105. Ford LT, Holder BR: Disarticulation for failed surgical procedures about the hip. South Med J 70:1293–1296, 1977.

106. Endean ED, Schwarz TH, Barker DE, et al: Hip disarticulation: Factors affecting outcome. J Vasc Surg 14:398–404, 1991.

107. Boyd HB: Anatomic disarticulation of the hip. Surg Gynecol Obstet 84:346–349, 1947.

108. Hogshead HP: Experience with hip disarticulation and hemipelvectomy procedure. J Bone Joint Surg Am 53:1031, 1971.

109. Wu KK, Guise ER, Frost HM, Mitchell CL: The surgical technique for hindquarter amputation. Report of 19 cases. Acta Orthop Scand 48:479–486, 1977.

110. Baur GM, Porter JM, Axthelm S, et al: Lower extremity amputation for ischemia. Am Surg 44:472–477, 1978.

111. Berardi RS, Keonin Y: Amputations in peripheral vascular occlusive disease. Am J Surg 135:231–234, 1978.

112. Home instructions: Amputee with prosthesis. Orthop Nurses Assoc J 6:73–77, 1979.

113. Abramson AS, Feibel A: The phantom phenomenon: Its use and disuse. Bull N Y Acad Med 57:99–112, 1981.

114. Bradway JR, Racy J, Malone JM: Psychological adaptation to amputation. Orthot Prosthet 38:46–50, 1984.

115. Parkes CM: Factors determining persistence of phantom pain in the amputee. J Psychosom Res 17:97–108, 1973.

116. Sherman RA: Published treatment of phantom pain. Am J Phys Med 59:232–244, 1980.

117. Sherman RA, Tippens JK: Suggested guidelines for treatment of phantom limb pain. Orthopedics 5:1595–1600, 1982.

118. Solomon GF, Schmidt KM: A burning issue. Phantom limb pain and psychological preparation of the patient for amputation. Arch Surg 113:185–186, 1978.

119. Sherman RA, Sherman CJ, Gall NG: A survey of current phantom limb pain treatment in the United States. Pain 8:85–99, 1980.

120. Sherman RA, Sherman CJ, Parker L: Chronic phantom and stump pain among American veterans: Results of a survey. Pain 18:83–95, 1984.

121. Nagendran T, Johnson G Jr, McDaniel WJ, et al: Amputation of the leg: An improved outlook. Ann Surg 175:994–999, 1972.

122. Wray CH, Still JM Jr, Moretz WH: Present management of amputations for peripheral vascular disease. Am Surg 38:87–92, 1972.

123. Bertin VJ, Plechia FR, et al: The early results of vascular surgery in patients 75 years of age or older: An analysis of 3,259 cases. J Vasc Surg 2:769–774, 1985.

124. Gregg RO: Bypass or amputation? Concomitant review of bypass arterial grafting and major amputation. Am J Surg 149:397–401, 1985.

125. Burgess EM, Romano RL, Aettl JH, Schrock RD Jr: Amputation of the leg for peripheral vascular ischemia. J Bone Joint Surg Am 53:874–890, 1971.

126. Bailey MJ, Johnston CLW, Yates CJP, et al: Preoperative haemoglobin as predictor of outcome of diabetic amputations. Lancet 2:168–170, 1979.

127. Gatti JE, LaRossa D, Neff SR, Silverman DG: Altered skin flap survival and fluorescein kinetics with hemodilution. Surgery 92:200–205, 1982.

128. Malone JM: Complications of lower extremity amputation. In Bernhard VM, Towne J (eds): Complications in Vascular Surgery. Orlando, Fla, Grune & Stratton, 1985, pp 445–470.

129. Reiber GE, Pecoraro RE, Koepsell TD: Risk factors for amputation in patients with diabetes mellitus. A case control study. Ann Intern Med 117:97–105, 1992.

130. Ebskou LB: Epidemiology of lower limb amputations in Denmark. (1980 to 1989). Int Orthop 15:285–288, 1991.

131. Harris PL, Read F, Eardley A, et al: The fate of elderly amputees. Br J Surg 61:665–668, 1974.

132. Kerstein MD: Utilization of an air splint after below knee amputation. Am J Phys Med 53:119–126, 1974.

133. Kerstein MD, Zimmer H, Dugdale FE, Lerner E: The delays in the rehabilitation in lower extremity amputees. Conn Med 41:549–551, 1977.

134. Kihn RB, Warren R, Beebe GW: The "geriatric" amputee. Ann Surg 176:305–314, 1972.

135. Reyes RL, Leahey EB, Leahey EB Jr: Elderly patients with lower extremity amputations: Three year study in a rehabilitation setting. Arch Phys Med Rehabil 58:116–123, 1977.

136. Waters RL, Perry J, Antonelli D, Hislop H: Energy cost of walking of amputees: The influence of level of amputation. J Bone Joint Surg Am 58:42–46, 1976.

137. Weaver PC, Marshall SA: A functional and social review of lower-limb amputees. Br J Surg 60:732–737, 1973.

138. Jamieson CW, Hill D: Amputation for vascular disease. Br J Surg 63:693–690, 1976.

139. Kerstein MD, Zimmer H, Dugdale FE, Lerner E: What influence does age have on rehabilitation of amputees? Geriatrics 30:67–71, 1975.

140. Gonzalez EG, Corcoran PH, Reyes RL: Energy expenditure in below-knee amputees: Correlation with stump length. Arch Phys Med Rehabil 55:111–119, 1974.

141. Huang CT, Jackson JR, Moore NB, et al: Amputation: Energy cost of ambulation. Arch Phys Med Rehabil 60:18–24, 1979.

142. Kavanagh T, Shephard RJ: The application of exercise testing to the elderly amputee. J Can Med Assoc 108:314–317, 1973.

143. Kegel B: Controlled environment treatment (CET) for patients with below-knee amputations. Phys Ther 56:1366–1371, 1976.

144. Burgess EM, Romano RL: The management of lower extremity amputees using immediate postsurgical prosthesis. Clin Orthop 57:137–146, 1968.

145. Burgess EM, Romano RL, Zettl JH: The Management of Lower Extremity Amputation Surgery. Immediate Postsurgical Prosthetic

Fitting. Patient Care, Washington, DC, US Government Printing Office, 1969.

146. Burgess EM, Zettl JH: Amputations below the knee. Artif Limbs 13:1–12, 1969.

147. Baker WH, Barnes RW, Shurr OG: The healing of below-knee amputations. A comparison of soft and plaster dressings. Am J Surg 133:716–718, 1977.

148. Kraeger RR: Amputation with immediate fitting prostheses. Am J Surg 120:634–636, 1970.

149. Ruoff AC, Smith AG, Thoroughman JC, et al: The immediate postoperative prosthesis in lower extremity amputations. Arch Surg 101:40–44, 1970.

150. Thorpe W, Gerber LH, Lampert M, et al: A prospective study of the rehabilitation of the above-knee amputee with rigid dressings. Comparison of immediate and delayed ambulation and the role of physical therapists and prosthetists. Clin Orthop 143:133–137, 1979.

151. Cohen SI, Goldman LO, Salzman EW, Glotzer OJ: The deleterious effect of immediate postoperative prosthesis in below-knee amputation for ischemic disease. Surgery 761:992–1001, 1974.

152. Folsum D, King T, Rubin J: Lower extremity amputation with

153. Leal JM, Malone JM, Moore WS, Malone SJ: For accelerated postamputation rehabilitation: Zoroc intermediate prostheses. Orthot Prosthet 34:3–12, 1980.

154. Seery J, Leal JM, Malone JM: Impact of new casting tapes on prosthetic fabrication. Presented to the International Society for Prosthetics and Orthotics Fourth World Congress, London, September 1983.

155. Wu Y, Brncick MD, Krick HJ, et al: Scotchcast P.V.C. interim prosthesis for below-knee amputees. Bull Prosthet Res Fall:40–45, 1981.

156. Sher MH: The air splint. An alternative to the immediate postoperative prosthesis. Arch Surg 108:746–747, 1974.

157. Kegel B, Moore AJ: Load cell. A device to monitor weight bearing for lower extremity amputees. Phys Ther 57:652–654, 1977.

158. Lipp MR, Malone SJ: Group rehabilitation of vascular surgery patients. Arch Phys Med Rehabil 57:180–183, 1976.

159. Enoka RM, Miller DI, Burgess EM: Below-knee amputee running gait. Am J Phys Med 61:66–84, 1982.

immediate postoperative prosthetic placement. Am J Surg 164:370–322, 1992.

Supplemental Bibliography

Bowker JH, San Giovanni TP, Pinzur MS: North American experience with knee disarticulation with use of a posterior myofasciocutaneous flap. Healing rate and functional results in seventy-seven patients. J Bone Joint Surg Am 82-A:1571–1574, 2000.

Burgess EM, Romano RL: The management of lower extremity amputees using immediate postsurgical prostheses. Clin Orthop 57:137–156, 1968.

Chang BB, Bock, DE, Jacobs RL, et al: Increased limb salvage by the use of unconventional foot amputations. J Vasc Surg 19:341–348, 1994.

Early JS: Transmetatarsal and midfoot amputations. Clin Orthop 361:85–90, 1999.

Flores Rivera AR: Risk factors for amputation in diabetic patients: A case-control study. Arch Med Res 29:179–184, 1998.

Hirsch G, McBride ME, Murray DD, et al: Chopart prosthesis and semirigid orthosis in traumatic forefoot amputations. Comparative gait analysis. Am J Phys Med Rehabil 75:283–291, 1996.

Koch M, Kutkuhn B, Grabensee B, et al: Apolipoprotein A, fibrinogen, age, and history of stroke are predictors of death in dialysed diabetic patients: A prospective study in 412 subjects. Nephrol Dial Transplant 12:2603–2611, 1997.

Lehto S, Ronnemaa T, Pyorala K, et al: Risk factors predicting lower extremity amputations in patients with NIDDM. Diabetes Care 19:607–612, 1996.

Lutz BS, Siemers F, Shen ZL, et al: Free flap to the arteria peronea magna for lower limb salvage. Plast Reconstr Surg 105:684–687, 2000.

Malone JM: Revascularization versus amputation. In Rutherford R (ed):

Vascular Surgery, 5th ed. Philadelphia, WB Saunders, 2000, pp 2255–2266.

Misuri A, Lucertini G, Nanni A, et al: Predictive value of transcutaneous oximetry for selection of amputation level. J Cardiovasc Surg 41:83–87, 2000.

Moore JC, Jolly GP: Soft tissue considerations in partial foot amputations. Clin Podiatr Med Surg 17:631–648, 2000.

Muhlhauser I, Overmann H, Bender R, et al: Predictors of mortality and end-stage diabetic complications in patients with type 1 diabetes mellitus on intensified insulin therapy. Diabet Med 17:727–734, 2000.

Naylor AR, Hayes PD, Darke S: A prospective audit of complex wound and graft infections in Great Britain and Ireland: The emergence of MRSA. Eur J Vasc Surg 21:289–294, 2001.

Reyzelman AM, Hadi S, Armstrong DG: Limb salvage with Chopart's amputation and tendon balancing. J Am Podiatr Med Assoc 89:100–103, 1999.

Sanders LJ: Transmetatarsal and midfoot amputations. Clin Podiatr Med Surg 14:741–762, 1997.

Tepel M, van der Giet M, Schwarzfeld C, et al: Prevention of radiographic-contrast-agent-induced reductions in renal function by acetylcysteine. N Engl J Med 343:210–212, 2000.

Vermassen FE, van Landuyt K: Combined vascular reconstruction and free flap transfer in diabetic arterial disease. Diabetes Metab Res Rev 16(Suppl 1):S33–S36, 2000.

Wrobel JS, Mayfield JA, Reiber GE: Geographic variation of lower-extremity major amputation in individuals with and without diabetes in the Medicare population. Diabetes Care 24:860–864, 2001.

Questions

1. The best overall approach to postamputation prosthetic care and rehabilitation is
   (a) conventional soft dressings
   (b) rigid dressings
   (c) immediate postoperative prosthetics
   (d) rigid dressings with early ambulation
   (e) soft dressings with early ambulation

2. The advantages of a rigid dressing (without an attached prosthesis) after major lower extremity amputation include all of the following except
   (a) control of stump edema
   (b) protection of the wound from trauma
   (c) stump immobilization
   (d) prevention of joint flexion contracture
   (e) accelerated stump maturity

3. Which of the following statements about amputees or amputation rehabilitation is false?
   (a) the risk of contralateral limb loss in the 5 years following major lower extremity amputation is greater than 25%
   (b) the 5-year life expectancy for patients with diabetes after major lower extremity amputation is less than 50%
   (c) above-knee amputations should be performed in all geriatric patients because of their poor prognosis for successful rehabilitation
   (d) using noninvasive amputation level selection techniques,

primary healing can be expected in greater than 90% of all below-knee amputations
(e) none of the above

4. Which of the following statements about amputation surgery or amputees is true?
   (a) clinical judgment is the best technique for amputation level selection
   (b) there is no benefit to the patient in performing a knee disarticulation amputation
   (c) amputees reduce their walking speed to control energy expenditure
   (d) the successful rehabilitation of bilateral above-knee amputees is common
   (e) none of the above

5. The following therapeutic maneuvers are often successful for the treatment of phantom pain
   (a) surgical stump revision
   (b) psychotherapy
   (c) narcotics
   (d) physical therapy
   (e) none of the above

6. Amputation level selection techniques such as transcutaneous oxygen measurement can also be used
   (a) intraoperatively
   (b) postoperatively
   (c) to evaluate or quantitate the degree of ischemia
   (d) all of the above

7. Which statement about major lower extremity amputation is false?
   (a) 80% of all patients will heal a below-knee amputation
   (b) two thirds of patients undergoing amputation surgery have other cardiovascular diseases
   (c) the best amputation level selection technique is a combination of clinical judgment and preoperative arteriography

(d) it takes at least twice as much energy for an above-knee amputee to walk as for a below-knee amputee
(e) any patient ambulating before amputation can ambulate after amputation, irrespective of age

8. The most common cause of major lower extremity amputation is
   (a) a failed vascular reconstruction
   (b) trauma
   (c) ischemia
   (d) tumor
   (e) complications of diabetes mellitus

9. Which of the following statements about major lower extremity amputation is false?
   (a) most amputations are caused by complications of peripheral vascular disease or diabetes mellitus
   (b) the average rate of ambulation after major lower extremity amputation is 60%
   (c) occlusion of the superficial femoral artery is the most common arterial lesion that leads to below-knee amputation
   (d) patients, especially those with diabetes mellitus, who have undergone successful amputation have a decreased life expectancy
   (e) there is no difference in healing between patients with diabetes mellitus and those without diabetes

10. Which of the following statements is true?
    (a) amputation surgery is reconstructive surgery
    (b) amputation surgery may be the preferred procedure compared to extended distal bypass or multiple revisions of below-knee distal bypass if good amputee rehabilitation treatment is available
    (c) patient education and foot care of the contralateral non-amputated extremity is important
    (d) optimal results after lower extremity amputation require amputation level selection techniques and early or rapid postamputation rehabilitation
    (e) all of the above

Answers

1. d   2. e   3. c   4. c   5. e   6. d   7. c   8. e   9. c   10. e

Index

Note: Page numbers followed by f indicate figures; page numbers followed by t indicate tables.

ISBN 0-7216-9313-X

90038